Conversions between measurement systems

You may need to convert from one measurement system to another, particularly when a drug is ordered in one system but only available in another. To perform conversion calculations, you need to know the equivalent measurements for the different systems. One of the most commonly used methods for converting drug measurements is the fraction method.

Fraction method

The fraction method for converting between measurement systems involves an equation consisting of two fractions. Set up the first fraction by placing the ordered dosage over an unknown number of units of the available dosage.

For example, say a prescriber orders 7.5 ml of acetaminophen elixir to be given by mouth. To find the equivalent in teaspoons, first set up a fraction in which the top of the fraction (numerator) represents the ordered dosage in milliliters and the bottom of the fraction (denominator) represents the unknown (x) number of teaspoons:

$$\frac{7.5 \text{ ml}}{x \text{ tsp}}$$

Then, set up the second fraction, which appears on the right side of the equation. This fraction consists of the standard equivalents between the ordered (ml) and the available (tsp) measures. Because milliliters must be converted to teaspoons, the right side of the equation appears as follows:

$$\frac{5 \text{ ml}}{1 \text{ tsp}}$$

The same unit of measure should appear in the numerator of both fractions. Likewise, the same unit of measure should appear in both denominators. The entire equation should appear as:

$$\frac{7.5 \text{ ml}}{x \text{ tsp}} = \frac{5 \text{ ml}}{1 \text{ tsp}}$$

To solve for x, cross multiply:

$$x \text{ tsp} \times 5 \text{ ml} = 7.5 \text{ ml} \times 1 \text{ tsp}$$

$$x \text{ tsp} = \frac{7.5 \text{ ml} \times 1 \text{ tsp}}{5 \text{ ml}}$$

$$x \text{ tsp} = \frac{7.5 \times 1 \text{ tsp}}{5}$$

$$x \text{ tsp} = 1.5 \text{ tsp}$$

The patient should receive 1.5 teaspoons of acetaminophen elixir.

Computing drug dosages

Computing drug dosages is a two-step process that you complete after verifying the drug order. Determine whether the ordered drug is available in units in the same system of measurement in which the order was written. If not, convert the measurement for the ordered drug to the system used for the available drug.

If the ordered units of measurement are available, calculate how much of the available dosage form should be given. For example, if the prescribed dose is 250 mg, determine the quantity of tablets, powder, or liquid that would equal 250 mg. To determine that quantity, use one of the methods described below.

Fraction method

When using the fraction method to compute a drug dosage, write an equation consisting of two fractions. First, set up a fraction showing the number of units to be given over x, which represents the quantity of the dosage form you are trying to find. In this case, this dosage form is tablets (tab).

For example, if the number of units to be administered equals 250 mg, the first fraction in the equation would appear as:

$$\frac{250 \text{ mg}}{x \text{ tab}}$$

On the other side of the equation, set up a fraction showing the number of units of the drug in its dosage form over the quantity of dosage forms that supply that number of units. The number of units and the quantity of dosage forms are specific for each drug. In most cases, the stated quantity equals 1. You can find all of the information for the second fraction on the drug label.

The drug label states that each tablet contains 125 mg, so the second fraction would appear as:

$$\frac{125 \text{ mg}}{1 \text{ tab}}$$

Note that in the two equations, the numerator units are the same (mg) and the denominator units are the same (tab).

The entire equation would appear as:

$$\frac{250 \text{ mg}}{x \text{ tab}} = \frac{125 \text{ mg}}{1 \text{ tab}}$$

Solving for x by cross-multiplying determines the quantity of the dosage form—two tablets, in this example.

Ratio method

To use the ratio method, write the amount of the drug to be given and the x quantity of the dosage form as a ratio. Using the example above, you would write:

$$250 \text{ mg} : x \text{ tab}$$

Next, complete the equation by forming a second ratio from the number of units in each tablet. The drug label provides this information. The entire equation is:

$$250 \text{ mg} : x \text{ tab} :: 125 \text{ mg} : 1 \text{ tab}$$

Solve for x by multiplying the inner portions (means) and outer portions (extremes) of the equation. The patient should receive two tablets.

Desired-available method

You can also use the desired-available method, also known as the dose-over-on hand (D/H) method. This method converts ordered units into available units and computes the drug dosage all in one step. The desired-available equation appears as:

$$\begin{array}{l} x \\ \text{quantity} \\ \text{to give} \end{array} = \frac{\text{ordered}}{1} \times \begin{array}{c} \text{conversion} \\ \text{fraction} \end{array} \times \frac{\text{quantity of dosage form}}{\begin{array}{c}\text{stated quantity of drug within each dosage form}\end{array}}$$

For example, say you receive an order for grains (gr) X of a drug. The drug is available only in 300-mg tablets. To determine what number of tablets to give the patient, substitute gr X (the ordered number of units) for the first element of the equation. Then use the conversion fraction as the second portion of the formula. The conversion factor is:

$$\frac{60 \text{ mg}}{\text{gr I}}$$

The measure in the denominator must be the same as the measure in the ordered units. In this case, the order specified gr X. As a result, grains will appear in the denominator of the conversion fraction.

The third element of the equation shows the dosage form over the stated drug quantity for that dosage form. Because the drug is available in 300-mg tablets, the fraction appears as:

$$\frac{1 \text{ tab}}{300 \text{ mg}}$$

The dosage form should always appear in the numerator, and the quantity of drug in each dosage form should always appear in the denominator. The completed equation is:

$$x \text{ tab} = \text{gr X} \times \frac{60 \text{ mg}}{\text{gr I}} \times \frac{1 \text{ tab}}{300 \text{ mg}}$$

Solving for x shows that the patient should receive two tablets.

The desired-available method has the advantage of using only one equation. However, you need to memorize an equation more elaborate than the one used in the fraction method or the ratio method. Relying on your memorization of a more complicated equation may increase the chance of error.

Dimensional analysis

A variation of the ratio method, dimensional analysis (also known as factor analysis or factor labeling) eliminates the need to memorize formulas and requires only one equation. To compare the two methods at a glance, read the following problem and solutions, and then read the paragraphs that follow for a detailed explanation.

Say the prescriber orders 0.25 g of streptomycin sulfate I.M. The vial reads 2 ml = 1 g. How many milliliters should you give?

Dimensional analysis

$$\frac{0.25 \text{ g}}{1} \times \frac{2 \text{ ml}}{1 \text{ g}} = 0.5 \text{ ml}$$

Ratio method

$$1 \text{ g} : 2 \text{ ml} :: 0.25 \text{ g} : x \text{ ml}$$
$$x = 2 \times 0.25$$
$$x = 0.5 \text{ ml}$$

Explanation

When using dimensional analysis you arrange a series of ratios, called factors, in a single (although sometimes lengthy) fractional equation. Each factor, written as a fraction, consists of two quantities and their related units of measurement. For instance, if 1,000 ml of a drug should be given over 8 hours, the relationship between the dose and time is expressed by the fraction:

$$\frac{1,000 \text{ ml}}{8 \text{ hr}}$$

When a problem includes a quantity or a unit of measurement that doesn't have an equivalent in the problem, these numbers appear in the numerator of the fraction, and 1 becomes the denominator. In the problem and solutions above, 0.25 g is such a number.

Some mathematical problems contain all the information you need to identify the factors, set up the equation, and find the solution. Other problems require you to use a conversion factor. Conversion factors are equivalents (for example, 1 g = 1,000 mg) that you can memorize or get from a conversion chart. Because the two quantities and units of measurement are equivalent, they can serve as the numerator or the denominator; thus, the conversion factor 1 g = 1,000 mg can be written in fraction form as:

$$\frac{1,000 \text{ mg}}{1 \text{ g}} \text{ or } \frac{1 \text{ g}}{1,000 \text{ mg}}$$

The factors given in the problem, plus any conversion factors needed to solve the problem, are called *knowns*. The quantity of the answer, of course, is the *unknown*. When setting up an equation in dimensional analysis, work backward, beginning with the unit of measurement of the answer. After plotting all the knowns, find the solution by following this sequence:
• Cancel similar quantities and units of measurement.
• Multiply the numerators.
• Multiply the denominators.
• Divide the numerator by the denominator.

Mastering dimensional analysis can take practice, but it will be well worth it. To understand more fully how dimensional analysis works, review the following problem and the steps taken to solve it.

A prescriber orders grains X of a drug. The pharmacy supplies the drug in 300-mg

tablets (tab). How many tablets should you administer?
• Write down the unit of measurement of the answer, followed by an "equal to" symbol:

$$\text{tab} =$$

• Search the problem for the quantity with the same unit of measurement (if one doesn't exist, use a conversion factor); place this in the numerator and its related quantity and unit of measurement in the denominator:

$$\text{tab} = \frac{1 \text{ tab}}{300 \text{ mg}}$$

• Separate the first factor from the next with a multiplication symbol:

$$\text{tab} = \frac{1 \text{ tab}}{300 \text{ mg}} \times$$

• Place the unit of measurement of the first factor's denominator in the second factor's numerator. Then search the problem for the quantity with the same unit of measurement (if one doesn't exist, as in this example, use a conversion factor); place this in the numerator and its related quantity and unit of measurement in the denominator, and follow the fraction with a multiplication symbol. Repeat this step until all known factors are included in the equation:

$$\text{tab} = \frac{1 \text{ tab}}{300 \text{ mg}} \times \frac{60 \text{ mg}}{\text{gr I}} \times \frac{\text{gr X}}{1}$$

• Treat the equation as a large fraction. First, cancel similar units of measurement in the numerator and the denominator. What remains should be what you began with: the unit of measurement of the answer. If not, check your equation to find and correct the error. Next, multiply the numerators and then the denominators. Finally, divide the numerator by the denominator:

$$\text{tab} = \frac{1 \text{ tab}}{300 \text{ mg}} \times \frac{60 \text{ mg}}{\text{gr I}} \times \frac{\text{gr X}}{1}$$

$$= \frac{60 \times 10 \text{ tab}}{300}$$

$$= \frac{600 \text{ tab}}{300}$$

$$= 2 \text{ tab}$$

For more practice, study the following examples, which use dimensional analysis to solve

various mathematical problems common to dosage calculations and drug administration.

1. A patient weighs 140 lb. What is his weight in kilograms (kg)?

$$1\text{st factor (conversion factor): } \frac{1 \text{ kg}}{2.2 \text{ lb}}$$

$$2\text{nd factor: } \frac{140 \text{ lb}}{1}$$

$$kg = \frac{1 \text{ kg}}{2.2 \text{ lb}} \times 140 \text{ lb}$$

$$= \frac{140}{2.2}$$

$$= 63.6 \text{ kg}$$

2. A physician prescribes 75 mg of a drug. The pharmacy stocks a multidose vial containing 100 mg/ml. How many milliliters should you give?

$$1\text{st factor: } \frac{1 \text{ ml}}{100 \text{ mg}}$$

$$2\text{nd factor: } \frac{75 \text{ mg}}{1}$$

$$ml = \frac{1 \text{ ml}}{100 \text{ mg}} \times \frac{75 \text{ mg}}{1}$$

$$= 0.75 \text{ ml}$$

3. A nurse practitioner prescribes 1 tsp of a cough elixir. The pharmacist sends up a bottle whose label reads 1 ml = 50 mg. How many milligrams should you give?

$$1\text{st factor: } \frac{50 \text{ mg}}{1 \text{ ml}}$$

$$2\text{nd factor (conversion factor): } \frac{5 \text{ ml}}{1 \text{ tsp}}$$

$$3\text{rd factor: } \frac{1 \text{ tsp}}{1}$$

$$mg = \frac{50 \text{ mg}}{1 \text{ ml}} \times \frac{5 \text{ ml}}{1 \text{ tsp}} \times \frac{1 \text{ tsp}}{1}$$

$$= 50 \text{ mg} \times 5$$

$$= 250 \text{ mg}$$

4. A physician prescribes 1,000 ml of an I.V. solution to be given over 8 hours. The I.V. tub-ing delivers 15 drops (gtt)/ml/minute. What is the infusion rate in gtt/minute?

$$1\text{st factor: } \frac{15 \text{ gtt}}{1 \text{ ml}}$$

$$2\text{nd factor: } \frac{1,000 \text{ ml}}{8 \text{ hr}}$$

$$3\text{rd factor (conversion factor): } \frac{1 \text{ hr}}{60 \text{ min}}$$

$$gtt/min = \frac{15 \text{ gtt}}{1 \text{ ml}} \times \frac{1,000 \text{ ml}}{8 \text{ hr}} \times \frac{1 \text{ hr}}{60 \text{ min}}$$

$$= \frac{15 \text{ gtt} \times 1,000 \times 1}{8 \times 60 \text{ min}}$$

$$= \frac{15,000 \text{ gtt}}{480 \text{ min}}$$

$$= 31.3 \text{ or } 31 \text{ gtt/min}$$

5. A physician prescribes 10,000 units of heparin added to 500 ml of 5% dextrose and water at 1,200 units/hour. How many drops per minute should you give if the I.V. tubing delivers 10 gtt/ml?

$$1\text{st factor: } \frac{10 \text{ gtt}}{1 \text{ ml}}$$

$$2\text{nd factor: } \frac{500 \text{ ml}}{10,000 \text{ units}}$$

$$3\text{rd factor: } \frac{1,200 \text{ units}}{1 \text{ hr}}$$

$$4\text{th factor (conversion factor): } \frac{1 \text{ hr}}{60 \text{ min}}$$

$$gtt/min = \frac{10 \text{ gtt}}{1 \text{ ml}} \times \frac{500 \text{ ml}}{10,000 \text{ units}} \times \frac{1,200 \text{ units}}{1 \text{ hr}} \times \frac{1 \text{ hr}}{60 \text{ min}}$$

$$= \frac{10 \times 500 \times 1,200 \text{ gtt}}{10,000 \times 60 \text{ min}}$$

$$= \frac{6,000,000 \text{ gtt}}{600,000 \text{ min}}$$

$$= 10 \text{ gtt/min}$$

Special computations

The fraction, ratio, and desired-available methods, as well as dimensional analysis, can be used to compute drug dosages when the or-

dered drug and the available form of the drug occur in the same units of measure. These methods can also be used when the availability of a particular dosage form differs from the units in which the dosage form is given.

For example, if a patient is to receive 1,000 mg of a drug available in liquid form and measured in milligrams, with 100 mg contained in 6 ml, how many milliliters should the patient receive? Because the ordered and the available dosages are in milligrams, no initial conversions are needed. The fraction method would be used to determine the number of milliliters the patient should receive, in this case, 60 ml.

Because the drug will be given in ounces (oz), the number of ounces should be determined using a conversion method. For the fraction method of conversion, the equation would appear as:

$$\frac{60 \text{ ml}}{x \text{ oz}} = \frac{30 \text{ ml}}{1 \text{ oz}}$$

Solving for x shows that the patient should receive 2 oz of the drug.

To use the desired-available method, change the order of the elements in the equation to correspond with the situation. The revised equation should appear as:

$$\begin{array}{c} x \\ \text{quantity} \\ \text{to give} \end{array} = \frac{\begin{array}{c}\text{ordered}\\\text{units}\end{array}}{1} \times \frac{\begin{array}{c}\text{quantity}\\\text{of dosage}\\\text{form}\\\hline\text{stated}\\\text{quantity of}\\\text{drug within}\\\text{each dosage}\\\text{form}\end{array}}{} \times \begin{array}{c}\text{conversion}\\\text{fraction}\end{array}$$

Placing the given information into the equation results in:

$$x \text{ oz} = \frac{1,000 \text{ mg}}{1} \times \frac{6 \text{ ml}}{100 \text{ mg}} \times \frac{1 \text{ oz}}{30 \text{ ml}}$$

Solving for x shows that the patient should receive 2 oz of the drug.

Imprecision of dosage computations

Converting drug measurements from one system to another and then determining the amount of a dosage to give can easily produce inexact dosages. A rounding error made during computation or discrepancies in the dosage may occur, depending on the conversion standard used in calculation. Or, you may determine a precise amount to be given, only to find that

giving that amount is impossible. For example, precise computations may indicate that a patient should receive 0.97 tablets. Giving such an amount is impossible.

The following rule helps avoid calculation errors and discrepancies between theoretical and real dosages: No more than a 10% variation should exist between the dosage ordered and the dosage to be given. For example, if you determine that a patient should receive 0.97 of a tablet, you can safely give 1 tablet. If your calculations don't give you a clear answer, notify the prescriber and request an equivalent dosage in the form you have available.

Computing parenteral dosages

The methods for computing drug dosages can be used not just for oral but also for parenteral routes. The following example shows how to determine a parenteral drug dosage. Say a prescriber orders 75 mg of Demerol. The package label reads: meperidine (Demerol), 100 mg/ml. By using the fraction method to determine the number of milliliters the patient should receive, your equation should look like this:

$$\frac{75 \text{ mg}}{x \text{ ml}} = \frac{100 \text{ mg}}{1 \text{ ml}}$$

To solve for x, cross multiply:

$$x \text{ ml} \times 100 \text{ mg} = 75 \text{ mg} \times 1 \text{ ml}$$

$$x \text{ ml} = \frac{75 \text{ mg} \times 1 \text{ ml}}{100 \text{ mg}}$$

$$x \text{ ml} = \frac{75 \text{ ml}}{100}$$

$$x \text{ ml} = 0.75 \text{ ml}$$

The patient should receive 0.75 ml.

Reconstituting powders for injection

Although a pharmacist usually reconstitutes powders for parenteral use, nurses sometimes perform this function by following the directions on the drug label. The label gives the total quantity of drug in the vial or ampule, the amount and type of diluent to be added to the powder, and the strength and expiration date of the resulting solution.

When you add diluent to a powder, the powder increases the fluid volume. That's why the label calls for less diluent than the total volume of the prepared solution. For example, a label may tell you to add 1.7 ml of diluent to a vial of

powdered drug to obtain a 2-ml total volume of prepared solution.

To determine the amount of solution to give, use the manufacturer's information about the concentration of the solution. For example, if you want to give 500 mg of a drug and the concentration of the prepared solution is 1 g (1,000 mg)/10 ml, use the following equation:

$$\frac{500 \text{ mg}}{x \text{ ml}} = \frac{1,000 \text{ mg}}{10 \text{ ml}}$$

The patient would receive 5 ml of the prepared solution.

Intravenous drip rates and flow rates

Make sure you know the difference between I.V. drip and flow rates and also how to calculate each rate. I.V. drip rate refers to the number of drops of solution to be infused per minute. Flow rate refers to the number of milliliters of fluid to be infused over 1 hour.

To calculate an I.V. drip rate, first set up a fraction showing the volume of solution to be delivered over the number of minutes in which that volume should be infused. For example, if a patient should receive 100 ml of solution in 1 hour, the fraction would be written as:

$$\frac{100 \text{ ml}}{60 \text{ min}}$$

Multiply the fraction by the drip factor (the number of drops contained in 1 ml) to determine the number of drops per minute to be infused, or the drip rate. The drip factor varies among different I.V. sets and should appear on the package that contains the I.V. tubing administration set.

Following the manufacturer's directions for drip factor is a crucial step. Standard administration sets have drip factors of 10, 15, or 20 gtt/ml. A microdrip, or minidrip, set has a drip factor of 60 gtt/ml.

Use the following equation to determine the drip rate of an I.V. solution:

$$\text{gtt/min} = \frac{\text{total no. of ml}}{\text{total no. of min}} \times \frac{\text{drip}}{\text{factor}}$$

The equation applies to I.V. solutions that infuse over many hours or to small-volume infusions such as those used for antibiotics usually given in less than an hour. For example, if an order requires 1,000 ml of 5% dextrose in nor-

mal saline solution to infuse over 12 hours and the administration set delivers 15 gtt/ml, what should the drip rate be?

$$x \text{ gtt/min} = \frac{1,000 \text{ ml}}{720 \text{ min}} \times 15 \text{ gtt/ml}$$

$$x \text{ gtt/min} = 20.83 \text{ gtt/min}$$

The drip rate would be rounded to 21 gtt per minute.

You'll use flow-rate calculations when working with I.V. infusion pumps to set the number of milliliters to be delivered in an hour. To perform this calculation, you should know the total volume in milliliters to be infused and the amount of time for the infusion. Use the following equation:

$$\text{flow rate} = \frac{\text{total volume ordered}}{\text{number of hours}}$$

Quick methods for calculating drip rates

To give an I.V. solution through a microdrip set, adjust the flow rate (number of milliliters per hour) to equal the drip rate (gtt per minute).

Using this method, the flow rate is divided by 60 minutes and then multiplied by the drip factor, also 60. Because the flow rate and the drip factor are equal, the two arithmetic operations cancel each other out. For example, if 125 ml/hour represented the ordered flow rate, the equation is:

$$\text{drip rate (125)} = \frac{125 \text{ ml}}{60 \text{ min}} \times 60$$

Rather than spending time calculating the equation, you can use the number assigned to the flow rate as the drip rate.

For I.V. administration sets that deliver 15 gtt/ml, the flow rate divided by 4 equals the drip rate. For sets with a drip factor of 10, the flow rate divided by 6 equals the drip rate.

Critical care calculations

Many drugs given on the critical care unit are used to treat life-threatening disorders. You must be able to perform calculations swiftly and accurately, prepare the drug for infusion, give the drug, and then observe the patient closely to evaluate the drug's effectiveness.

Three calculations must be performed before giving critical care drugs:
• Calculate the concentration of the drug in the I.V. solution.

• Figure the flow rate needed to deliver the desired dose.
• Determine the needed dosage.

Calculating concentration

To calculate the drug's concentration, use the following formula:

concentration in mg/ml = mg of drug/ml of fluid

To express the concentration in mcg/ml, multiply the answer by 1,000.

Figuring flow rate

To determine the I.V. flow rate per minute, use the following formula:

$$\frac{dose/min}{x\ ml/min} = \frac{concentration\ of\ solution}{1\ ml\ of\ fluid}$$

To calculate the hourly flow rate, first multiply the ordered dose, given in milligrams or micrograms per minute, by 60 minutes to determine the hourly dose. Then use the following equation to compute the hourly flow rate:

$$\frac{hourly\ dose}{x\ ml/hr} = \frac{concentration\ of\ solution}{1\ ml\ of\ fluid}$$

Determining dosage

To determine the dosage in mg/kg of body weight/minute, first determine the concentration of the solution in milligrams per milliliter. (If a drug is ordered in micrograms, convert milligrams to micrograms by multiplying by 1,000.) To determine the dose in milligrams per hour, multiply the hourly flow rate by the concentration using the following formula:

$$\frac{dose\ in}{mg/hr} = \frac{hourly}{flow\ rate} \times concentration$$

Then calculate the dose in milligrams per minute. Divide the hourly dose by 60 minutes.

$$dose\ in\ mg/min = \frac{dose\ in\ mg/hr}{60\ min}$$

Divide the dose per minute by the patient's weight, using the following formula:

$$mg/kg/min = \frac{mg/min}{patient's\ weight\ in\ kg}$$

Finally, make sure that the drug is being given within a safe and therapeutic range. Compare the amount in milligrams per kilogram per minute to the safe range shown in this book.

The following examples show how to calculate an I.V. flow rate using the different formulas.

Example 1

A patient has frequent runs of ventricular tachycardia that subside after 10 to 12 beats. The prescriber orders 2 g (2,000 mg) of lidocaine in 500 ml of D_5W to infuse at 2 mg/minute. What's the rate in milliliters per minute? What's the rate in milliliters per hour?

First, find the concentration of the solution by setting up a proportion with the unknown concentration in one fraction and the ordered dose in the other fraction:

$$\frac{x\ mg}{1\ ml} = \frac{2,000\ mg}{500\ ml}$$

Cross multiply the fractions:

$$x\ mg \times 500\ ml = 2,000\ mg \times 1\ ml$$

Solve for x by dividing each side of the equation by 500 ml and canceling units that appear in both the numerator and denominator:

$$\frac{x\ mg \times 500\ ml}{500\ ml} = \frac{2,000\ mg \times 1\ ml}{500\ ml}$$

$$x = \frac{2,000\ mg}{500}$$

$$x = 4\ mg$$

The concentration of the solution is 4 mg/ml. Next, calculate the flow rate per minute needed to deliver the ordered dose of 2 mg/minute. To do this, set up a proportion with the unknown flow rate per minute in one fraction and the concentration of the solution in the other fraction:

$$\frac{2\ mg}{x\ ml} = \frac{4\ mg}{1\ ml}$$

Cross multiply the fractions:

$$x\ ml \times 4\ mg = 1\ ml \times 2\ mg$$

Solve for x by dividing each side of the equation by 4 mg and canceling units that appear in both the numerator and denominator:

$$\frac{x\ ml \times 4\ mg}{4\ mg} = \frac{1\ ml \times 2\ mg}{4\ mg}$$

$$x = \frac{2\ ml}{4}$$

$$x = 0.5\ ml$$

The patient should receive 0.5 ml/minute of lidocaine. Because lidocaine must be given with an infusion pump, compute the hourly flow rate. Set up a proportion with the unknown flow rate per hour in one fraction and the drip rate per minute in the other fraction:

$$\frac{x \text{ ml}}{60 \text{ min}} = \frac{0.5 \text{ ml}}{1 \text{ min}}$$

Cross multiply the fractions:

$$x \text{ ml} \times 1 \text{ min} = 0.5 \text{ ml} \times 60 \text{ min}$$

Solve for x by dividing each side of the equation by 1 minute and canceling units that appear in both the numerator and denominator:

$$\frac{x \text{ ml} \times 1 \text{ min}}{1 \text{ min}} = \frac{0.5 \text{ ml} \times 60 \text{ min}}{1 \text{ min}}$$

$$x = 30 \text{ ml}$$

Set the infusion pump to deliver 30 ml/hour.

Example 2

A 200-lb patient is scheduled to receive an I.V. infusion of dobutamine at 10 mcg/kg/minute. The package insert says to dilute 250 mg of the drug in 50 ml of D_5W. Because the drug vial contains 20 ml of solution, the total to be infused is 70 ml (50 ml of D_5W plus 20 ml of solution). How many micrograms of the drug should the patient receive each minute? How many each hour?

First, compute the patient's weight in kilograms. To do this, set up a proportion with the weight in pounds and the unknown weight in kilograms in one fraction and the number of pounds per kilogram in the other fraction:

$$\frac{200 \text{ lb}}{x \text{ kg}} = \frac{2.2 \text{ lb}}{1 \text{ kg}}$$

Cross multiply the fractions:

$$x \text{ kg} \times 2.2 \text{ lb} = 1 \text{ kg} \times 200 \text{ lb}$$

Solve for x by dividing each side of the equation by 2.2 lb and canceling units that appear in both the numerator and denominator:

$$\frac{x \text{ kg} \times 2.2 \text{ lb}}{2.2 \text{ lb}} = \frac{1 \text{ kg} \times 200 \text{ lb}}{2.2 \text{ lb}}$$

$$x = \frac{200 \text{ kg}}{2.2}$$

$$x = 90.9 \text{ kg}$$

The patient weighs 90.9 kg. Next, determine the dose in micrograms per minute by setting up a proportion with the patient's weight in kilograms and the unknown dose in micrograms per minute in one fraction and the known dose in micrograms per kilogram per minute in the other fraction:

$$\frac{90.9 \text{ kg}}{x \text{ mcg/min}} = \frac{1 \text{ kg}}{10 \text{ mcg/min}}$$

Cross multiply the fractions:

$$x \text{ mcg/min} \times 1 \text{ kg} = 10 \text{ mcg/min} \times 90.9 \text{ kg}$$

Solve for x by dividing each side of the equation by 1 kg and canceling units that appear in both the numerator and denominator:

$$\frac{x \text{ mcg/min} \times 1 \text{ kg}}{1 \text{ kg}} = \frac{10 \text{ mcg/min} \times 90.9 \text{ kg}}{1 \text{ kg}}$$

$$x = 909 \text{ mcg/min}$$

The patient should receive 909 mcg of dobutamine every minute. Finally, determine the hourly dose by multiplying the dose per minute by 60:

$$909 \text{ mcg/min} \times 60 \text{ min/hr} = 54,540 \text{ mcg/hr}$$

The patient should receive 54,540 mcg of dobutamine every hour.

Pediatric dosages

To determine the correct pediatric dosage of a drug, prescribers, pharmacists, and nurses use one of two computational methods. One is based on a child's weight in kilograms; the other is based on the child's body surface area. Other methods are less accurate and not recommended.

Dosage range per kilogram of body weight

Many drug companies provide information on the safe dosage ranges for drugs given to children. The companies usually provide the dosage ranges in milligrams per kilogram of body weight and, in many cases, give similar information for adult dosage ranges. The following example and explanation show how to calculate the safe pediatric dosage range for a drug, using the company's suggested safe

dosage range provided in milligrams per kilogram.

For a child, a prescriber orders a drug with a suggested dosage range of 10 to 12 mg/kg of body weight/day. The child weighs 12 kg. What is the safe daily dosage range for the child?

You must calculate the lower and upper limits of the dosage range provided by the manufacturer. First, calculate the dosage based on 10 mg/kg of body weight. Then, calculate the dosage based on 12 mg/kg of body weight. The answers represent the lower and upper limits of the daily dosage range, expressed in mg/kg of the child's weight.

Body surface area

A second method for calculating safe pediatric dosages uses the child's body surface area. This method may provide a more accurate calculation because the child's body surface area is thought to parallel the child's organ growth and maturation and metabolic rate.

You can determine the body surface area of a child by using a three-column chart called a nomogram. Mark the child's height in the first column and weight in the third column. Then draw a line between the two marks. The point at which the line intersects the vertical scale in the second column is the child's estimated body surface area in square meters. To calculate the child's approximate dose, use the body surface area measurement in the following equation:

$$\frac{\text{body surface area of child}}{\text{average adult body surface area } (1.73 \text{ m}^2)} \times \text{average adult dose} = \text{child's dose}$$

The following example illustrates the use of the equation. The nomogram shows that a 25-lb (11.3-kg) child who is 33 inches (84 cm) tall has a body surface area of 0.52 m². To determine the child's dose of a drug with an average adult dose of 100 mg, the equation would appear as:

$$\frac{0.52 \text{ m}^2}{1.73 \text{ m}^2} \times 100 \text{ mg} = \frac{30.06 \text{ mg}}{\text{(child's dose)}}$$

The child should receive 30 mg of the drug. Many facilities have guidelines that determine acceptable calculation methods for pediatric doses. If you work with children, familiarize yourself with your facility's policies about pediatric doses.

Drug administration routes

You will give drugs by many routes, including oral (P.O.), intravenous (I.V.), intramuscular (I.M.), subcutaneous, topical, ophthalmic, rectal (P.R.), buccal and sublingual (S.L.), inhalation, nasogastric (NG), otic, and vaginal. No matter which route you use, you need to follow the established procedure to make sure you give the right drug, in the right dose, to the right patient, at the right time, and by the right route. Immediately after giving the drug, you need to provide the right documentation. This procedure includes:

• checking the order, medication record, and label
• confirming the patient's identity
• following standard drug safety procedures
• addressing all of the patient's questions
• correctly documenting the drug administration in the patient's medical record.

Check the order

Make sure you have a written order for every drug given. Use verbal orders only in emergencies; write them out and get the prescriber to sign them within the time period specified by your facility.

If your facility has a computerized order system, it may allow prescribers to order drugs electronically from the pharmacy. The computer may indicate whether the pharmacy has the drug and trigger the pharmacy staff to fill the prescription. A computerized order also may generate a patient record, either paper or electronic, on which you can document medication administration.

Computer systems offer several advantages over paper systems. Drugs often arrive in the patient care area more quickly. Documentation is quicker and easier. Prescribers can see at a glance which drugs have been given. Errors can't result from poor handwriting (although typing mistakes may occur). Finally, computerized records are easier to store than paper records.

Check the medication record

Check the order on the patient's medication record against the prescriber's order.

Check the label

Before giving a drug, check its label three times to make sure you're giving the prescribed drug and the prescribed dose. First, check the label when you take the container from the shelf or drawer. Next, check the label right before pouring the drug into the medication cup or drawing it into the syringe. Finally, check the label again before returning the container to the shelf or drawer. If you're giving a unit-dose drug, open the container at the patient's bedside. Check the label for the third time immediately after pouring the drug and again before discarding the wrapper.

Don't give a drug from a poorly labeled or unlabeled container. Also, don't attempt to label a drug or to reinforce a label that is falling off or improperly placed. Instead, return the drug to the pharmacist for verification and proper relabeling.

Confirm the patient's identity

Before giving the drug, ask the patient his full name and confirm his identity by comparing two patient identifiers, such as the medical record number and the patient's birth date, against the medication administration record. Don't rely on information that can vary during a hospital stay, such as a room or bed number. In nonacute settings, identify the patient by picture or other specific information.

Check again that you have the correct drug, and make sure the patient isn't allergic to it. If the patient has any drug allergies, check to make sure the chart and medication administration record are labeled accordingly and that the patient is wearing an allergy wristband that identifies the allergen.

Follow safety procedures

Whenever you give a drug, follow these safety procedures:
• Never give a drug poured or prepared by someone else.

• Never allow the medication cart or tray out of your sight once you've prepared a dose.
• Never leave a drug at a patient's bedside.
• Always observe the patient during drug administration; make sure he swallows oral drugs or uses an inhaler appropriately. If the patient is giving the drug to himself, make sure his technique is correct.
• Always use safety syringes or needleless devices.
• Never return unwrapped or prepared drugs to stock containers; instead, dispose of them and notify the pharmacy.
• Keep the medication cart locked at all times.
• Follow your facility's standard precautions.

Respond to questions

If the patient questions you about his drug or dosage, check the order and his medication record again. If the drug you're giving is correct, reassure the patient and explain the reason for the drug. Explain any changes to his drug regimen or drug dosage. Instruct him, as appropriate, about possible adverse reactions, and ask him to report anything that he feels may be an adverse reaction.

Oral administration

Because oral drug administration is usually the safest, most convenient, and least expensive method, most drugs are given this way. Drugs for oral administration are available in many forms: tablets, enteric-coated tablets, capsules, syrups, elixirs, oils, liquids, suspensions, powders, and granules. Some require special preparation before administration, such as mixing with juice to make them more palatable.

Oral drugs are sometimes prescribed in higher dosages than their parenteral equivalents because after the drugs are absorbed through the gastrointestinal (GI) system, the liver breaks them down before they reach the systemic circulation.

Equipment and preparation

• Check the chart and the medication administration record.
• Make sure the patient isn't allergic to the drug or any of its components.
• Check the drug's expiration date.
• Gather the drug and medication cup.

• If the patient is a child or an elderly person, you may need to gather a mortar and pestle for crushing pills and an appropriate buffer, such as jelly or applesauce for crushed pills or juice, water, or milk for liquid drugs.

Implementation
• Wash your hands.
• Confirm the patient's identity using two patient identifiers.
• Explain the procedure to the patient.
• Assess the patient's condition, including level of consciousness and vital signs. Changes in the patient's condition may call for withholding the drug.
• Give the patient the drug. If needed and verified safe, crush the drug to facilitate swallowing or mix it with a soft food or liquid to aid swallowing, minimize adverse effects, or promote absorption.
• Stay with the patient until he has swallowed the drug. If he seems confused or disoriented, check his mouth to make sure he has indeed swallowed the drug. Return and reassess the patient's response within 1 hour of giving the drug.

Nursing considerations
• To avoid damaging or staining the patient's teeth, give acid or iron preparations through a straw. An unpleasant-tasting liquid usually can be made more palatable if taken through a straw because the liquid contacts fewer taste buds.
• If the patient can't swallow a whole tablet or capsule, ask the pharmacist if the drug is available in liquid form or if it can be given by another route. If not, ask the pharmacist if the tablet can be crushed or if capsules can be opened and mixed with food.
• Don't crush sustained-action, buccal, S.L., or enteric-coated drugs because this may counteract the safety or effectiveness of these drugs.

Intravenous bolus administration

In this method, rapid I.V. administration allows the drug level to quickly peak in the bloodstream. This method also may be used for drugs that can't be given I.M. because they're toxic or because the patient can't absorb them well. It

may also be used for drugs that can't be diluted. Bolus doses may be injected directly into a vein or through an existing I.V. line.

Equipment and preparation

• Check the chart and the medication administration record.
• Make sure the patient isn't allergic to the drug or any of its components.
• Gather the prescribed drug, 20G needle and syringe, diluent (if needed), tourniquet, alcohol sponge, sterile 2″ × 2″ gauze pad, gloves, adhesive bandage, and tape. Other materials may include a winged device primed with normal saline solution and a second syringe (and needle) filled with normal saline solution.
• Draw the drug into the syringe and dilute, if needed.
• Label the syringe with the drug name.

Implementation

• Confirm the patient's identity using two patient identifiers.
• Explain the procedure to the patient.

To give a direct injection

• Wash your hands and put on gloves.
• Select the largest vein suitable to dilute the drug and minimize irritation.
• Apply a tourniquet above the site to distend the vein, and clean the site with an alcohol sponge, working outward in a circle.
• If you're using the needle of the drug syringe, insert it at a 30-degree angle with the bevel up. The bevel should reach ¼″ (0.6 cm) into the vein. Insert a winged device bevel-up at a 10- to 25-degree angle. Lower the angle once you enter the vein. Advance the needle into the vein. Tape the wings in place when you see blood return, and attach the syringe containing the drug.
• Check for blood backflow.
• Remove the tourniquet, and inject the drug at the ordered rate.
• To ensure that the needle remained in place and the entire amount of injected drug entered the vein, check again for blood backflow.
• For a winged device, flush the line with normal saline solution from the second syringe to ensure complete delivery.
• Withdraw the needle and discard it in a biohazard container. To prevent hematoma, apply pressure to the site with the sterile gauze pad for at least 3 minutes.

• Apply an adhesive bandage when the bleeding stops.
• Remove your gloves and discard them in a designated biohazard container. Wash your hands.

To inject through an existing line

• Wash your hands and put on gloves.
• Check the drug's compatibility with the I.V. solution.
• If the drug isn't compatible with the I.V. solution, flush the line with normal saline solution before and after the injection.
• Close the flow clamp, wipe the injection port with an alcohol sponge, and inject the drug as you would a direct injection.
• Open the flow clamp and readjust the flow rate.
• Remove and discard your gloves in a designated biohazard container. Wash your hands.

Nursing considerations

• If the existing I.V. line is capped, making it an intermittent infusion device, verify patency and placement of the device before injecting the drug. Then flush the device with normal saline solution, give the drug, and follow with the appropriate flush.
• Immediately report signs of acute allergic reaction or anaphylaxis. If extravasation occurs, stop the injection, estimate the amount of infiltration, and notify the prescriber.
• When giving diazepam or chlordiazepoxide hydrochloride through a steel needle winged device or an I.V. line, flush device with bacteriostatic water before and after use to prevent precipitation.

Intravenous administration through a secondary line

A secondary I.V. line is a complete I.V. set connected to the lower Y-port (secondary port) of a primary line instead of to the I.V. catheter or needle. It features an I.V. container, long tubing, and either a microdrip or a macrodrip system, and this line can be used for continuous or intermittent drug infusion. When used continuously, it permits drug infusion and titration while the primary line maintains a constant total infusion rate.

A secondary I.V. line used only for intermittent drug administration is called a piggyback set. In this case, the primary line maintains venous access between drug doses. A piggyback set includes a small I.V. container, short tubing, and usually a macrodrip system, and it connects to the primary line's upper Y-port (piggyback port).

Equipment and preparation

- Check the chart and the medication administration record.
- Make sure the patient isn't allergic to the drug or any of its components.
- Gather the prescribed I.V. drug, diluent (if needed), prescribed I.V. solution, administration set with secondary injection port, 22G 1" needle or a needleless system, gloves, alcohol sponges, 1" (2.5 cm) adhesive tape, time tape, labels, infusion pump, extension hook, and solution for intermittent piggyback infusion.
- Wash your hands and put on gloves.
- Inspect the I.V. container for cracks, leaks, or contamination.
- Check the expiration date.
- Check compatibility with the primary solution.
- Determine whether the primary line has a secondary injection port.
- If needed, add the drug to the secondary I.V. solution (usually 50- to 100-ml of normal saline solution or D_5W). To do so, remove the seals from the secondary container and wipe the main port with an alcohol sponge.
- Inject the prescribed drug and agitate the solution to mix the drug.
- Label the I.V. mixture.
- Insert the administration set spike, and attach the needle or needleless system.
- Open the flow clamp and prime the line. Then close the flow clamp.
- Some drugs come in vials that can hang directly on the I.V. pole. In this case, inject diluent directly into the drug vial. Then spike the vial, prime the tubing, and hang the set.

Implementation

- If the drug is incompatible with the primary I.V. solution, replace the primary solution with a fluid that's compatible with both solutions, and flush the line before starting the drug infusion.
- Confirm the patient's identity using two patient identifiers.
- Explain the procedure to the patient.

- Hang the container of the secondary set and wipe the injection port of the primary line with an alcohol sponge.
- Insert the needle or needleless system from the secondary line into the injection port, and tape it securely to the primary line.
- To run the container of the secondary set by itself, lower the primary set's container with an extension hook. To run both containers simultaneously, place them at the same height.
- Open the clamp and adjust the drip rate.
- For continuous infusion, set the secondary solution to the desired drip rate; then adjust the primary solution to the desired total infusion rate.
- For intermittent infusion, wait until the secondary solution has completely infused; then adjust the primary drip rate, as needed.
- If the secondary solution tubing is being reused, close the clamp on the tubing and follow your facility's policy: Remove the needle or needleless system and replace it with a new one, or leave it taped to the injection port, and label it with the time it was first used.
- Leave the empty container in place until you replace it with a new dose of drug at the prescribed time. If the tubing won't be reused, discard it appropriately with the I.V. container.

Nursing considerations

- If institutional policy allows, use a pump for drug infusion. Place a time tape on the secondary container to help prevent an inaccurate administration rate.
- When reusing secondary tubing, change it when your facility's policy requires, usually every 2 or 3 days. Inspect the injection port for leakage with each use; change it more often, if needed.
- Except for lipids, don't piggyback a secondary I.V. line to a total parenteral nutrition line because this risks contamination.

Intramuscular administration

You'll use intramuscular (I.M.) injections to deposit up to 5 ml of drug deep into well-vascularized muscle for rapid systemic action and absorption.

Equipment and preparation

- Check the chart and the medication administration record.

- Make sure the patient isn't allergic to the drug or any of its components.
- Gather the prescribed drug, diluent, or filter needle (if needed), 1 to 5-ml safety syringe, 20G to 25G 1″ to 3″ needle, gloves, alcohol sponges, and a nonsterile cotton ball or 2″ × 2″ gauze pad.
- The prescribed drug must be sterile. The needle may be packaged separately or already attached to the syringe. Needles used for I.M. injections are longer than those used for subcutaneous injections because they must reach deep into the muscle. Needle length also depends on the injection site, the patient's size, and the amount of subcutaneous fat covering the muscle. A larger needle gauge can accommodate viscous solutions and suspensions.
- Check the drug for abnormal changes in color and clarity. If in doubt, ask the pharmacist.
- Wipe the stopper that tops the drug vial with alcohol, and draw up the prescribed amount of drug.
- Provide privacy and explain the procedure to the patient.
- Position the patient and drape him appropriately, making sure that the site is well lit and exposed.

Implementation

- Wash your hands.
- Confirm the patient's identity using two patient identifiers.
- Explain the procedure to the patient and provide privacy.
- Select an appropriate injection site. Avoid any site that looks inflamed, edematous, or irritated. Also, avoid using injection sites that contain moles, birthmarks, scar tissue, or other lesions.
- The dorsogluteal and ventrogluteal muscles are used most commonly for I.M. injections.

Dorsogluteal muscle

- Posterior superior iliac spine
- Greater trochanter of femur
- Sciatic nerve

Ventrogluteal muscle

- Iliac crest
- Anterior superior iliac spine
- Greater trochanter of femur

- The deltoid muscle may be used for injections of 2 ml or less.

Deltoid muscle

- Acromial process
- Deep brachial artery
- Radial nerve
- Humerus

- The vastus lateralis muscle is used most often in children; the rectus femoris may be used in infants.

Vastus lateralis and rectus femoris muscles

- Greater trochanter of femur
- Rectus femoris
- Vastus lateralis

- Loosen, but don't remove, the needle sheath.
- Gently tap the site to stimulate nerve endings and minimize pain.

• Clean the site with an alcohol sponge, starting at the site and moving outward in expanding circles to about 2″ (5 cm). Allow the skin to dry because wet alcohol stings in the puncture.
• Put on gloves.
• With the syringe in your dominant hand, remove the needle cap with your other hand.
• With the thumb and index finger of your non-dominant hand, gently stretch the skin.
• Position the syringe perpendicular to the skin surface and a couple of inches from the skin. Tell the patient that he'll feel a prick. Then quickly and firmly thrust the needle into the muscle.
• Pull back slightly on the plunger to aspirate for blood. If blood appears, the needle is in a blood vessel. Withdraw the needle, prepare a fresh syringe, and inject another site. If no blood appears, inject the drug slowly and steadily to let the muscle distend gradually. You should feel little or no resistance. Gently but quickly remove the needle at a 90-degree angle.
• Using a gloved hand, apply gentle pressure to the site with the cotton ball or 2″ × 2″ gauze. Massage the relaxed muscle, unless contraindicated, to distribute the drug and promote absorption.
• Inspect the site for bleeding or bruising. Apply pressure, as needed.
• Discard all equipment properly. Don't recap needles; put them in an appropriate biohazard container to avoid needle-stick injuries.
• Remove your gloves and discard them in a biohazard container. Wash your hands.

Nursing considerations

• To slow absorption, some drugs are dissolved in oil. Mix them well before use.
⚠ **ALERT:** If you must inject more than 5 ml, divide the solution and inject it at two different sites.
• Rotate injection sites for patients who need repeated injections.
• Urge the patient to relax the muscle to reduce pain and bleeding.
• To prevent leakage of irritating and discoloring medications (such as iron dextran) into the subcutaneous tissue, use the Z-track injection method of pulling the skin and subcutaneous layers out of alignment with the underlying muscle before inserting the needle.
⚠ **ALERT:** Never inject into the gluteal muscles of a child who has been walking for less than 1 year.

• Keep in mind that I.M. injections can damage local muscle cells and elevate CK levels, which can be confused with elevated levels caused by MI. Diagnostic tests can be used to differentiate between them.

Subcutaneous administration

A subcutaneous injection allows slower, more sustained administration than an I.M. injection. Drugs and solutions delivered subcutaneously are injected through a relatively short needle using sterile technique.

Equipment and preparation

• Check the chart and the medication administration record.
• Make sure the patient isn't allergic to the drug or any of its components.
• Gather drug, needle of appropriate gauge and length, 1- to 3-ml syringe, gloves, alcohol sponges, and nonsterile cotton ball or 2″ × 2″ gauze pad. Other materials may include antiseptic cleanser, filter needle, insulin syringe, and insulin pump.
• Inspect the drug to make sure it's the right color and consistency and is free of precipitates.
• Wash your hands.

For single-dose ampules

• Wrap the neck of the ampule in an alcohol sponge and snap off the top, directing it away from you.
• Attach a filter needle to the needle, slightly tip the ampule, and withdraw the desired amount of the drug.
• Tap the syringe to disperse air bubbles.
• Cover the needle with the attached safety sheath by placing the needle sheath on the counter or medication cart and sliding the needle into the sheath.
• Before discarding the ampule, check the label against the patient's medication record.
• Discard the filter needle and the ampule in a biohazard container.
• Attach the appropriate-sized needle to the syringe.

For single-dose and multidose vials

• Reconstitute powdered drugs according to the instructions on the label.

• Clean the rubber stopper on the vial with an alcohol sponge for at least 15 seconds.

• Pull the syringe plunger back until the volume of air in the syringe equals the volume of drug to be withdrawn from the vial.

• Insert the needle into the vial.

• Inject the air, invert the vial, and keep the bevel tip of the needle below the level of the solution as you withdraw the prescribed amount of drug.

• Tap the syringe to disperse air bubbles.

• Cover the needle with the attached safety sheath by placing the needle sheath on the counter or medication cart and sliding the needle into the sheath.

• Check the drug label against the patient's medication record before returning the multidose vial to the shelf or drawer or before discarding the single-dose vial.

• Attach the appropriate-sized needle to the syringe.

Implementation

• Confirm the patient's identity using two patient identifiers.

• Explain the procedure to the patient and provide privacy.

• Select the injection site from those shown below, and tell the patient where you'll be giving the injection.

• Wash your hands and put on gloves. Position and drape the patient.

• Clean the injection site with an alcohol sponge. Loosen the protective needle sheath.

• With your nondominant hand, pinch the skin around the injection site firmly to elevate the subcutaneous tissue, forming a 1″ (2.5 cm) fat fold, as shown below.

• Holding the syringe in your dominant hand, grip the needle sheath between the fourth and fifth fingers of your nondominant hand while continuing to pinch the skin around the injection site with the index finger and thumb of your nondominant hand. Pull the sheath back to uncover the needle. Don't touch the needle.

• Position the needle with its bevel up.

• Tell the patient he'll feel a prick as you insert the needle. Do so quickly, in one motion, at a 45-degree or 90-degree angle, as shown below. The needle length and the angle you use depend on the amount of subcutaneous tissue at the site. Some drugs, such as heparin, should always be injected at a 90-degree angle.

• Release the skin to avoid injecting the drug into compressed tissue and irritating the nerves. Except for insulin and heparin, pull the plunger back slightly to check for blood return. If blood appears, withdraw the needle, prepare another syringe, and repeat the procedure. If no blood appears, slowly inject the drug.

• After injection, remove the needle at the same angle you used to insert it. Using a gloved hand, apply gentle pressure to the site with the cotton ball or 2″ × 2″ gauze pad. Massage the site gently, unless contraindicated, to distribute the drug and promote absorption.

• Inspect the injection site for bleeding or bruising.

• Discard all equipment properly. Don't recap needles; put them in a biohazard container to avoid needle-stick injuries.

• Remove and discard your gloves in a biohazard container. Wash your hands.

Nursing considerations

⑤ ALERT: Don't aspirate for blood return when giving insulin or heparin. It isn't necessary with insulin and may cause a hematoma with heparin.

• Don't massage the site after giving heparin.

⑤ ALERT: Repeated injections in the same site can cause lipodystrophy, a natural immune response. Rotating injection sites can minimize this complication.

Topical administration

Topical drugs, such as patches, lotions, and ointments, are applied directly to the skin. They're commonly used for local rather than systemic effects. Certain types of topical drugs—known as transdermal drugs—are meant to enter the patient's bloodstream and to have a systemic effect after you apply them.

Equipment and preparation

• Check the chart and the drug administration record.

• Make sure the patient isn't allergic to the drug or any of its components.

• Gather the prescribed drug, sterile tongue blades, gloves, sterile gloves for open lesions, sterile 4″ × 4″ gauze pads, transparent semipermeable dressing, adhesive tape, normal saline solution, cotton-tipped applicators, gloves, and linen savers, if needed.

Implementation

• Confirm the patient's identity using two patient identifiers.

• Explain the procedure to the patient because, after discharge, he may have to apply the drug himself.

• If the procedure is uncomfortable, premedicate the patient with an analgesic. Give it time to take effect.

• Wash your hands to reduce the risk of cross-contamination, and glove your dominant hand.

• Help the patient to a comfortable position, and expose the area to be treated. Make sure the skin or mucous membrane is intact (unless the drug is for a skin lesion). Applying the drug to broken or abraded skin may cause unwanted systemic absorption and further irritation.

• If needed, clean debris from the skin. You may have to change your gloves if they become soiled.

To apply paste, cream, or ointment

• Open the container. Place the cap upside down to avoid contaminating its inner surface.

• Remove a tongue blade from its sterile wrapper, and cover one end of the blade with drug from the tube or jar. Then transfer the drug from the blade to your gloved hand.

• Apply the drug to the affected area with long, smooth strokes that follow the direction of hair growth. This technique avoids forcing the drug into hair follicles, which can cause irritation and folliculitis. Don't press too hard because it could abrade the skin and cause discomfort.

• When applying a drug to the patient's face, use cotton-tipped applicators for small areas, such as under the eyes. For larger areas, use a sterile gauze pad.

• To avoid contaminating the drug, use a new sterile tongue blade each time you remove the drug from its container.

• Remove and discard your gloves and wash your hands.

To apply transdermal ointment

• Choose the application site—usually a dry, hairless spot on the patient's chest or upper arm.

• To help absorption, wash the site with soap and warm water and dry thoroughly.

• Wash your hands and put on gloves.

• If the patient has a previously applied medication strip at another site, remove it and swab or wash this area to clear away the drug residue.

• If the area you choose is hairy, clip excess hair rather than shaving it. Shaving causes irritation, which the drug may worsen.

• Squeeze the prescribed amount of ointment onto the application strip or measuring paper. Don't get the ointment on your skin.

• Apply the strip, drug side down, directly to the patient's skin.
• Maneuver the strip slightly to spread a thin layer of the ointment over a 3″ (8-cm) area, but don't rub the ointment into the skin.
• Secure the application strip to the patient's skin by covering it with a semipermeable dressing or plastic wrap.
• Tape the covering securely in place.
• Label the strip with the date, time, and your initials, if required by your facility.
• Remove your gloves and wash your hands.

To apply a transdermal patch
• Remove the old patch and swab or wash the site to remove any residual drug or adhesive.
• Choose a dry, hairless application site.
• Clip (don't shave) hair from the chosen site. Wash the area with warm water and soap, and dry it thoroughly.
• Wash your hands and put on gloves.
• Without touching the adhesive surface, remove the clear plastic backing.
• Apply the patch to the site without touching the adhesive.
• If required by your facility's policy, label the patch with the date, time, and your initials.
• Remove your gloves and wash your hands.

To remove ointment
• Wash your hands and put on gloves.
• Gently swab ointment from the patient's skin using a sterile 4″ × 4″ gauze pad saturated with normal saline solution.
• Don't wipe too hard because you could irritate the skin.
• Remove and discard your gloves and wash your hands.

Nursing considerations
• To prevent skin irritation, always remove previous drug applications by swabbing or washing; then select a new site.
• Always wear gloves to protect your skin.
• Never apply ointment to the eyelids or ear canal. The ointment may congeal and occlude the tear duct or ear canal.
• Inspect the treated area frequently for allergic or other adverse reactions.
• Don't apply a topical drug to scarred or callused skin because this may slow absorption.
• Don't place a defibrillator paddle on a transdermal patch. The aluminum on the patch can cause electrical arcing during defibrillation, re-

sulting in smoke and thermal burns. If a patient has a patch on a standard paddle site, remove the patch and swab the skin quickly before applying the paddle, or use another site, if possible.

Ophthalmic administration
Ophthalmic drugs—drops or ointments—serve both diagnostic and therapeutic purposes. During an ophthalmic examination, drugs can be used to anesthetize the eye, dilate the pupil, and stain the cornea to identify anomalies. Therapeutic uses include eye lubrication and treatment of glaucoma and infections.

Equipment and preparation
• Check the chart and the medication administration record.
• Make sure the patient isn't allergic to the drug or any of its components.
• Gather the prescribed ophthalmic drug, sterile cotton balls, gloves, warm water or normal saline solution, sterile gauze pads, and facial tissue. An ocular dressing also may be used.
• Make sure the drug is labeled for ophthalmic use. Check the expiration date. Remember to date the container after first use. If in doubt, consult the pharmacist.
• Inspect ocular solutions for cloudiness, discoloration, and precipitation, keeping in mind that some drugs are suspensions that normally appear cloudy.

Implementation
• Make sure you know which eye you are treating because different drugs or doses may be ordered for each eye.
• Confirm the patient's identity using two patient identifiers.
• Explain the procedure to the patient.
• Wash your hands and put on gloves.
• If the patient has an eye dressing, remove it by pulling it down and away from his forehead, being careful not to contaminate your hands. (If you do, remove the contaminated gloves, wash your hands, and put on new gloves.) Don't apply pressure to the area around the eyes.
• To remove exudates or meibomian gland secretions, clean around the eye with sterile cotton balls or sterile gauze pads that have been moistened with warm water or normal saline solution. Have the patient close his eyes; then

gently wipe the eyelids from the inner to the outer canthus. Use a fresh cotton ball or gauze pad for each stroke, and use a different cotton ball or pad for each eye.

• Have the patient sit or lie on his back. Tell him to tilt his head back and toward his affected eye so that any excess drug can flow away from the tear duct, minimizing systemic absorption through the nasal mucosa.

• Remove the dropper cap from the drug container, and draw the drug into the dropper. Or, if the bottle has a dropper tip, remove the cap and hold or place it upside down to prevent contamination.

• Before instilling eyedrops, tell the patient to look up and away. This moves the cornea away from the lower lid and minimizes the risk of touching the lid with the dropper.

To instill eyedrops

• Steady the hand that's holding the dropper by resting it gently against the patient's forehead. With your other hand, gently pull down the lower lid of the affected eye, and instill the drops in the conjunctival sac. Never instill eyedrops directly onto the eyeball.

• After instilling the eyedrops, tell the patient to close his eyes gently without squeezing the lids shut and not to blink.

• Instruct the patient to place a finger in the corner of the eye between the bridge of the nose and the eyelid and to apply gentle pressure for 2 to 3 minutes to prevent systemic absorption of drops through the lacrimal sac. Then have the patient wipe away any excess drops or tears with a clean tissue before opening the eyes. Use a fresh tissue for each eye.

• Remove and discard your gloves and wash your hands.

• An elderly patient may have difficulty feeling the drops in his eye. When teaching an elderly patient how to instill drops himself, suggest that he chill the drug slightly in the refrigerator because cold drops are easier to feel.

• Have him try it himself while you observe.

To apply eye ointment

• Squeeze a small ribbon of drug on the edge of the conjunctival sac from the inner to the outer canthus, as shown below. Cut off the ribbon by turning the tube. Don't touch the eye with the tip of the tube.

• After applying ointment, tell the patient to close his eye gently without squeezing the lid shut and to roll his eye behind a closed lid to help distribute the drug over the eyeball. Have the patient sit with the eye closed for 2 to 3 minutes to facilitate absorption and avoid "clouding" of the vision from the ointment.

• Use a tissue to remove any excess drug that leaks from the eye. Use a fresh tissue for each eye to prevent cross-contamination.

• Apply a new eye dressing, if needed.

• Remove and discard your gloves and wash your hands.

Nursing considerations

• Urge the patient not to rub his eye or blink immediately after eyedrops.

• To maintain the drug container's sterility, don't put the cap down after opening the container, and never touch the eye area with the tip of the dropper or bottle. Discard any solution remaining in the dropper before returning it to the bottle. If the dropper or bottle tip is contaminated, discard it and use another sterile dropper. Never share eyedrops between patients.

Rectal administration

A rectal suppository is a small, solid drug mass, usually cone shaped, with a cocoa butter or glycerin base. It may be inserted to stimulate peristalsis and defecation or to relieve pain, vomiting, and local irritation. An ointment is a semisolid drug used to produce local effects. It may be applied externally to the anus or internally to the rectum.

Equipment and preparation
• Check the chart and the medication administration record.
• Make sure the patient isn't allergic to the drug or any of its components.
• Gather the rectal suppository or tube of ointment and applicator, 4″ × 4″ gauze pads, gloves, and a water-soluble lubricant. A bedpan also may be needed.
• To prevent softening of the drug and decreased effectiveness, store rectal suppositories in the refrigerator until needed. A soft suppository is also harder to handle and insert than a hard one. To harden a softened suppository, hold it (in its wrapper) under cold running water.

Implementation
• Confirm the patient's identity using two patient identifiers.
• Explain the procedure to the patient.
• Wash your hands.

To insert a rectal suppository
• Place the patient on his left side in Sims' position. Drape him with the bedcovers, exposing only his buttocks.
• Put on gloves. Unwrap the suppository and lubricate it with water-soluble lubricant.
• Lift the patient's right buttock with your nondominant hand to expose the anus.
• Instruct the patient to take several deep breaths through his mouth to relax the anal sphincter and to reduce anxiety and discomfort during drug insertion.
• Using the index finger of your dominant hand, insert the suppository—tapered end first—about 3″ (8 cm) until you feel it pass the internal anal sphincter, as shown below.

• Direct the tapered end of the suppository toward the side of the rectum so the drug contacts the membranes.
• Encourage the patient to lie quietly and, if possible, to contract his anal sphincter and buttocks together to retain the suppository for the correct length of time. Press on the patient's anus with a gauze pad, if needed, until the urge to defecate passes.
• Discard the used equipment and gloves. Wash your hands thoroughly.

To apply an ointment
• For external application, put on gloves and use a gauze pad to spread the drug over the anal area. For internal application, attach the end of the applicator to the tube of ointment, and coat the applicator with water-soluble lubricant.
• Use about 1″ (2.5 cm) of ointment. To gauge how much pressure to use during application, try squeezing a small amount from the tube before you attach the applicator.
• Place the patient on his left side in Sims' position. Drape him with the bedcovers, exposing only his buttocks.
• Lift the patient's right buttock with your nondominant hand to expose the anus.
• Tell the patient to take several deep breaths through his mouth to relax the anal sphincter and reduce anxiety and discomfort during insertion. Gently insert the applicator, directing it toward the umbilicus.
• Squeeze the tube to eject drug.
• Remove the applicator and place a folded 4″ × 4″ gauze pad between the patient's buttocks to absorb excess ointment.
• Disassemble the tube and applicator and recap the tube. Clean the applicator with soap and warm water and store or discard it. Remove and discard your gloves, and wash your hands thoroughly.

Nursing considerations
• Because eating and drinking stimulates peristalsis, a suppository for relieving constipation should be inserted about 30 minutes before mealtime to help soften the stool and facilitate defecation. A medicated retention suppository should be inserted between meals.
• Tell the patient to try to retain the suppository. If this is difficult, place the patient on a bedpan.

• Make sure that the patient's call button is handy, and watch for his signal because he may be unable to suppress the urge to defecate.
• Inform the patient that the suppository may discolor his next bowel movement.

Buccal and sublingual administration

Certain drugs are given buccally (between the cheek and teeth) or S.L. (under the tongue) to bypass the digestive tract and speed absorption into the bloodstream. When using either method, observe the patient carefully to make sure he doesn't swallow the drug or develop mucosal irritation.

Equipment and preparation

• Check the chart and the medication administration record.
• Make sure the patient isn't allergic to the drug or any of its components.
• Gather the prescribed drug, medication cup, and gloves.

Implementation

• Wash your hands. If you'll be placing the drug into the patient's mouth, put on gloves.
• Confirm the patient's identity using two patient identifiers.
• Explain the procedure to the patient.
• For buccal administration, place the tablet in the patient's buccal pouch, between the cheek and teeth, as shown below.

• For S.L. administration, place the tablet under the patient's tongue, as shown above right.

• Remove and discard gloves and wash your hands.

• Instruct the patient to keep the drug in place until it dissolves completely to ensure absorption. Caution the patient against chewing the tablet or touching it with his tongue to prevent accidental swallowing.
• Tell the patient not to smoke before the drug has dissolved because nicotine constricts blood vessels and slows drug absorption.

Nursing considerations

• Don't give liquids until a buccal tablet is absorbed; in some cases, this may take up to an hour.
• If the patient has angina, tell him to wet the nitroglycerin tablet with saliva and keep it under his tongue until it's fully absorbed.
• Make sure a patient with angina knows how to take nitroglycerin, how many doses to take, and when to call for emergency help.

Inhalation administration

Hand-held oropharyngeal inhalers include the metered-dose inhaler, dry-powder multidose inhaler, nasal inhaler, and turbo-inhaler. These devices deliver topical drugs to the respiratory tract, producing local and systemic effects. The mucosal lining of the respiratory tract absorbs the inhalant almost immediately. Examples of oral inhalants are bronchodilators, which improve airway patency and facilitate mucous drainage, and mucolytics, which liquefy tenacious bronchial secretions. Examples of nasal inhalants include corticosteroids, which reduce allergic symptoms.

Equipment and preparation

- Check the chart and the medication administration record.
- Gather the metered-dose inhaler, diskus, or turbo-inhaler, prescribed drug, and normal saline solution.

Implementation

- Confirm the patient's identity using two patient identifiers.
- Make sure the patient isn't allergic to the drug or any of its components.
- Wash your hands. Apply gloves if there is a risk of aerosol or secretion exposure.
- Explain the procedure to the patient.

To use a metered-dose inhaler

- Shake the inhaler bottle. Remove the cap and insert the stem into the small hole on the flattened portion of the mouthpiece, as shown.
- Place the inhaler about 1″ (2.5 cm) in front of the patient's open mouth.
- Tell the patient to exhale.
- If using a spacer, which can make the inhaler more effective, tell the patient to place the spacer mouthpiece in his mouth and to press his lips firmly around the mouthpiece.
- As you push the bottle down against the mouthpiece, tell the patient to inhale slowly through his mouth and to continue inhaling until his lungs feel full. Compress the bottle against the mouthpiece only once.
- Remove the inhaler and tell the patient to hold his breath for several seconds. Then instruct him to exhale slowly through pursed lips to keep distal bronchioles open and allow increased absorption and diffusion of the drug.
- Repeat if additional puff is ordered.
- Have the patient gargle with normal saline solution or water to remove the drug from his mouth and the back of his throat and to help prevent oral fungal infections. Warn the patient not to swallow after gargling, but rather to spit out the liquid.

To use a dry-powder multidose inhaler

- Hold the dry-powder multidose inhaler in one hand and put the thumb of your other hand on the thumbgrip. Push your thumb away from you as far as it will go, until the mouthpiece appears and snaps into position.
- Hold the dry-powder multidose inhaler level horizontally with the mouthpiece toward the patient. Slide the lever away from the patient as far as it will go until it clicks.
- Instruct the patient to exhale fully (not into the mouthpiece of the dry-powder multidose inhaler).
- Instruct the patient to breathe in quickly and deeply through the dry-powder multidose inhaler's mouthpiece, then hold the breath for 10 or more seconds. Then have the patient breathe out slowly.
- Wipe off the mouthpiece with a clean tissue, if needed, and close. (It will automatically reset for the next dose.)
- Tell the patient to rinse his mouth with water, without swallowing, after each dose.
- Never take a dry-powder multidose inhaler apart or wash any part of it. Check counter on top of dry-powder multidose inhaler to be sure dose is available and reorder five inhalations from end.

To use a turbo-inhaler

- Hold the mouthpiece in one hand. With the other hand, slide the sleeve away from the mouthpiece as far as possible, as shown.
- Unscrew the tip of the mouthpiece by turning it counter-clockwise.
- Press the colored portion of the drug capsule into the propeller stem of the mouthpiece.
- Screw the inhaler together again.
- Holding the inhaler with the mouthpiece at the bottom, slide the sleeve all the way down and then up again to puncture the capsule and release the drug. Do this only once.
- Have the patient exhale completely and tilt his head back. Instruct him to place the mouthpiece in his mouth, close his lips around it, and inhale once. Tell him to hold his breath for several seconds.

• Remove the inhaler from the patient's mouth, and tell him to exhale as much air as possible.
• Repeat the procedure until the entire amount of drug in the device is inhaled.
• Have the patient gargle and spit with normal saline solution or water, if desired, to remove the drug from his mouth and the back of his throat.

To use a nasal inhaler
• Instruct patient to clear his nasal passages before administration.
• Shake the container to ensure even distribution of contents.
• Wipe the tip of the container with a clean tissue, if needed.
• Tell patient to place a finger against the nostril not being treated to block air entrance. Instruct the patient to exhale fully through the mouth.
• Place tip of nasal container into appropriate nostril without directing it onto nasal mucosa. Instruct patient to inhale quickly and deeply through this nostril, with mouth closed, while squeezing the nasal inhaler to release spray along with inhalation.
• Remove the inhaler and have the patient gently press closed the medicated nostril, breathing through his mouth for several seconds. Treat the opposite nostril, if indicated, or give two inhalations to each nostril, if indicated, spaced 3 to 5 seconds apart.

Nursing considerations
• Teach the patient how to use the inhaler so he can continue treatments after discharge, if needed. Explain that overdose can cause the drug to lose its effectiveness. Tell him to record the date and time of each inhalation and his response.
• Some inhalants may cause restlessness, palpitations, nervousness, and other systemic effects. They also may cause hypersensitivity reactions, such as a rash, urticaria, rhinitis, nasal bleeding, or bronchospasms.
• Give oral inhalants cautiously to patients with heart disease because these drugs may lead to coronary insufficiency, cardiac arrhythmias, or hypertension. If paradoxical bronchospasm occurs, stop the drug and use a different drug.
• If the patient is prescribed a bronchodilator and a corticosteroid, give the bronchodilator

first so the air passages can open fully before the patient uses the corticosteroid.
• Instruct the patient to keep an extra inhaler handy.
• Instruct the patient to discard the inhaler after taking the prescribed number of doses and to start a new inhaler.
• Urge the patient to notify his prescriber if he notices an increased use of or need for an inhaler, or if symptoms are not relieved with the prescribed regimen.

Nasogastric administration
Besides providing another way to feed patients who can't eat normally, an NG tube allows for the instillation of drugs directly into the GI system.

Equipment and preparation
• Check the chart and the medication administration record.
• Make sure the patient isn't allergic to the drug or any of its components.
• Gather equipment for use at the bedside, including prescribed drug, towel or linen-saver pad, 50- or 60-ml piston-type catheter-tip syringe, feeding tubing, two 4″ × 4″ gauze pads, stethoscope, gloves, diluent (juice, water, or a nutritional supplement), cup for mixing drug and fluid, spoon, 50-ml cup of water, and rubber band. You may also need pill-crushing equipment and a clamp, if it's not already attached to the tube.
• Make sure that liquids are at room temperature to avoid abdominal cramping and that the cup, syringe, spoon, and gauze are clean.

Implementation
• Wash your hands and put on gloves.
• Confirm the patient's identity using two patient identifiers.
• Explain the procedure to the patient.
• Unpin the tube from the patient's gown. To avoid soiling the sheets during the procedure, fold back the bed linens and drape the patient's chest with a towel or linen-saver pad.
• Help the patient into Fowler position, if possible.
• After unclamping the tube, attach a catheter-tie or bulb syringe to the tube and try to aspirate stomach contents. Examine the aspirate and

place a small amount on a pH test strip. Probability of gastric placement is increased if the aspirate has a typical gastric fluid appearance and the pH is less than or equal to 5.

- If no gastric contents appear or if you meet resistance, the tube may be lying against the gastric mucosa. Withdraw the tube slightly or turn the patient to free it.
- Clamp the tube, detach the syringe, and lay the end of the tube on the 4″ × 4″ gauze pad.
- If the drug is a tablet, crush it before mixing it with the diluent. Make sure the particles are small enough to pass through the eyes at the distal end of the tube. Some drugs (extended release, enteric-coated, or S.L. drugs, for example) shouldn't be crushed. If you aren't sure, ask the pharmacist. Also, check to see if the drug comes as a liquid form or if a capsule may be opened and the contents poured into a diluent. Pour liquid drugs into the diluent and stir well.
- Reattach the syringe, without the piston, to the end of the tube. Holding the tube upright at a level slightly above the patient's nose, open the clamp and pour the drug in slowly and steadily, as shown below.

- To keep air from entering the patient's stomach, hold the tube at a slight angle and add more drug before the syringe empties. If the drug flows smoothly, slowly give the entire dose. If it doesn't flow, it may be too thick. If so, dilute it with water. If you suspect that tube placement is inhibiting flow, stop the procedure and reevaluate the placement.
- Watch the patient's reaction. If you see signs of discomfort, stop immediately.

- As the last of the drug flows out of the syringe, start to irrigate the tube by adding 30 to 50 ml of water (15 to 30 ml for a child). Irrigating clears drug from the tube and reduces the risk of clogging.
- When the water stops flowing, clamp the tube. Detach the syringe, and discard it properly.
- Fasten the tube to the patient's gown, and make the patient comfortable.
- Leave the patient in Fowler position or on his right side with his head partially elevated for at least 30 minutes to ease flow and prevent esophageal reflux.
- Remove and discard your gloves and wash your hands.

Nursing considerations

- If you must give a tube feeding and a drug, give the drug first to make sure the patient receives the entire drug.
- Certain drugs—such as phenytoin (Dilantin)—bind with tube feedings, decreasing the availability of the drug. Stop the tube feeding for 2 hours before and after the dose, according to your facility's policy.
- If residual stomach contents exceed 150 ml, withhold the drug and feeding, and notify the prescriber. Excessive stomach contents may indicate intestinal obstruction or paralytic ileus.
- Never crush enteric-coated, buccal, S.L., or sustained-release drugs.
- If suction is on, turn it off for 20 to 30 minutes after giving a drug.

Otic administration

Eardrops may be instilled to treat infection and inflammation, to soften cerumen for removal, to produce local anesthesia, or to remove an insect trapped in the ear.

Equipment and preparation

- Check the chart and the medication administration record.
- Make sure the patient isn't allergic to the drug or any of its components.
- Gather the eardrops, gloves, a light, and facial tissue or cotton-tipped applicators. Cotton balls and a bowl of warm water may be needed.
- First, warm the drug to body temperature in the bowl of warm water, or carry the drug in

your pocket for 30 minutes before giving. Test the temperature of the drug by placing a drop on your wrist. If the drug is too hot, it may burn the patient's eardrum.

● To avoid injuring the ear canal, check the dropper before use to make sure it's not chipped or cracked.

Implementation

● Wash your hands and put on gloves.
● Confirm the patient's identity using two patient identifiers.
● Explain the procedure to the patient.
● Have the patient lie on the side opposite the affected ear.

● Straighten the patient's ear canal. For an adult, pull the auricle up and back, as shown above. For a child younger than age 3, pull the auricle down and back, as shown below, because the ear canal is straighter at this age.

● Using a light, examine the ear canal for drainage. If you see drainage, gently clean the canal with the tissue or cotton-tipped applica-

tors because drainage can reduce the effectiveness of the drug. Never insert an applicator past the point where you can see it.

● Straighten the patient's ear canal once again, and instill the proper number of drops. For the patient's comfort, aim the dropper so that the drops fall against the sides of the ear canal, not on the eardrum. Hold the ear canal in position until you see the drug disappear down the canal. Then release the ear.

● To avoid damaging the ear canal with the dropper, especially with a struggling child, it may be necessary to gently rest the hand that is holding the dropper against the patient's head to secure a safe position before giving the drug.

● Instruct the patient to remain on his side for 5 to 10 minutes to allow the drug to run down into the ear canal.

● Tuck a cotton ball with a small amount of petroleum jelly on it loosely into the opening of the ear canal to prevent the drug from leaking out. Don't insert the cotton too deeply into the canal because this may prevent secretions from draining and may increase pressure on the eardrum.

● Clean and dry the outer ear.
● If needed, repeat the procedure in the other ear after 5 to 10 minutes.
● Help the patient into a comfortable position.
● Remove your gloves and wash your hands.

Nursing considerations

● Some conditions make the normally tender ear canal even more sensitive, so be especially gentle.

● To prevent injury to the eardrum, never insert a cotton-tipped applicator into the ear canal past the point where you can see the tip.

● After instilling eardrops to soften cerumen, irrigate the ear to remove.

● If the patient has vertigo, keep the side rails of his bed up and assist him as needed during the procedure. Also, move slowly to avoid worsening his vertigo.

● Teach the patient to instill the eardrops himself so that he can continue treatment at home. Have him try it himself while you observe.

Vaginal administration

Vaginal drugs can be inserted as topical treatment for infection, particularly *Trichomonas vaginalis* and vaginal candidiasis or inflammation. Suppositories melt when they contact the vaginal mucosa, and the drug diffuses topically.

Vaginal drugs usually come with a disposable applicator that enables placement of drug in the anterior and posterior fornices. Vaginal administration is most effective when the patient can remain lying down afterward to retain the drug.

Equipment and preparation

- Check the chart and the medication administration record.
- Make sure the patient isn't allergic to the drug or any of its components.
- Gather the prescribed drug and applicator, gloves, water-soluble lubricant, and a small sanitary pad.

Implementation

- If possible, give vaginal drugs at bedtime when the patient is lying down.
- Confirm the patient's identity using two patient identifiers.
- Wash your hands, explain the procedure to the patient, and provide privacy.
- Ask the patient to void.
- Ask the patient if she would prefer to insert the drug herself and give instruction.
- Help the patient into the lithotomy position. Drape her, exposing only the perineum.
- Remove the suppository from the wrapper and lubricate it with water-soluble lubricant.
- Put on gloves and expose the vagina by spreading the labia. If you see discharge, wash the area with several cotton balls soaked in warm, soapy water. Clean each side of the perineum and then the center, using a fresh cotton ball for each stroke. Rinse well with clean, warm water. While the labia are still separated, insert the suppository or vaginal applicator about 3″ to 4″ (7.6 to 10 cm) into the vagina, as shown below.
- After insertion, wash the applicator with soap and warm water, and store or discard it. Label it so it will be used only for this patient.
- Remove and discard gloves.

- To keep the drug from soiling the patient's clothing and bedding, provide a sanitary pad.
- Help the patient return to a comfortable position, and tell her to stay in bed for the next several hours.
- Wash your hands thoroughly.

Nursing considerations

- Refrigerate vaginal suppositories that melt at room temperature.
- Teach the patient how to insert the vaginal drug because she may have to insert it herself after she is discharged. Give her instructions in writing, if possible.
- Instruct the patient not to insert a tampon after inserting a vaginal drug because the tampon will absorb the drug and decrease its effectiveness.

4

Drug administration safety

Nurses carry a great deal of responsibility for administering drugs safely and correctly, for making sure the right patient gets the right drug, in the right dose, at the right time, and by the right route. By staying aware of potential trouble areas, you can minimize your risk of making medication errors and maximize the therapeutic effects of your patients' drug regimens.

Name game

Drugs with similar-sounding names can be easily confused. Even different-sounding names can look similar when written rapidly by hand on a prescription form. An example is Soriatane and Loxitane, which are both capsules. If the patient's drug order doesn't seem right for his diagnosis, call the prescriber to clarify the order.

Allergy alert

Once you've verified your patient's full name, check to see if he's wearing an allergy bracelet. If he is, the allergy bracelet should conspicuously display the name of the allergen. The allergy information also should be labeled on the front of the patient's chart and on his medication record. Whether the patient is wearing an allergy bracelet or not, take the time to double-check and ask the patient whether he has any allergies—even if he's in distress.

A patient who's severely allergic to peanuts could have an anaphylactic reaction to ipratropium bromide (Atrovent) aerosol given by metered-dose inhaler. Ask your patient or his parents whether he's allergic to peanuts before you give this drug. If you find that he's allergic, you'll need to use the nasal spray and inhalation solution form of the drug. Because it doesn't contain soy lecithin, it's safe for patients allergic to peanuts.

Compound errors

Many medication errors occur because of a compound problem—a mistake or group of mistakes that could have been caught at any of several steps along the way. For a drug to be

given correctly, each member of the health care team must fill the appropriate role:
● The prescriber must write the order correctly and legibly, or enter the correct order electronically.
● The pharmacist must evaluate whether the order is appropriate and fill it correctly.
● The nurse must evaluate whether the order is appropriate and give it correctly.

A breakdown anywhere along this chain of events can lead to a medication error. That's why it's so important for members of the health care team to act as a real team so that they can check each other and catch any problems that might arise before those problems affect the patient's health. Encourage an environment in which professionals double-check each other.

Route trouble

Many drug errors happen, at least in part, from problems related to the route of administration. The risk of error increases when a patient has several I.V. lines running for different purposes.

Risky abbreviations

Abbreviating drug names is risky. Abbreviations may not be commonly known and, in some cases, the same abbreviation may be used for different drugs or compounds. For example, epoetin alfa is commonly abbreviated EPO; however, some use the abbreviation EPO to stand for "evening primrose oil." Ask all prescribers to spell out drug names.

Unclear orders

A patient was supposed to receive one dose of the antineoplastic lomustine to treat brain cancer. (Lomustine typically is given as a single oral dose once every 6 weeks.) The doctor's order read, "Administer h.s." Because a nurse misinterpreted the order to mean every night, the patient received nine daily doses, developed severe thrombocytopenia and leukopenia, and died.

If you're unfamiliar with a drug, check a drug book before giving it. If a prescriber uses "h.s." and doesn't specify the frequency of ad-

31

ministration, ask him to clarify the order. When documenting orders, note "at bedtime nightly" or "at bedtime one dose today."

Color changes

If a familiar drug seems to have an unfamiliar appearance, investigate the cause. If the pharmacist cites a manufacturing change, ask him to double-check whether he has received verification from the manufacturer. Always document the appearance discrepancy, your actions, and the pharmacist's response in the patient record.

Stress levels

Committing a serious error can cause enormous stress and cloud your judgment. If you're involved in a drug error, ask another professional to give the antidote.

Drug
Classifications

Alkylating drugs

altretamine
busulfan
carboplatin
carmustine
chlorambucil
cisplatin
cyclophosphamide
dacarbazine
ifosfamide
lomustine
mechlorethamine hydrochloride
melphalan
procarbazine hydrochloride
thiotepa

Indications

▶ Various tumors, especially those with large volume and slow cell-turnover rate.

Contraindications and cautions

• Contraindicated in patients hypersensitive to these drugs.
• Use cautiously in patients receiving other cell-destroying drugs or radiation therapy.
☀ Lifespan: In pregnant women, use only when potential benefits to the mother outweigh known risks to the fetus. Breast-feeding women should stop breast-feeding during therapy because drugs are found in breast milk. In children, safety and effectiveness of many alkylating drugs haven't been established. Elderly patients have an increased risk of adverse reactions; monitor these patients closely.

Adverse reactions

The most common adverse reactions are bone marrow depression, chills, diarrhea, fever, flank pain, hair loss, leukopenia, nausea, redness or pain at the injection site, sore throat, swelling of the feet or lower legs, thrombocytopenia, secondary leukemia, infertility, and vomiting.

Action

Alkylating drugs appear to act independently of a specific cell-cycle phase. They're polyfunctional compounds that can be divided chemically into five groups: nitrogen mustards, ethylene imines, alkyl sulfonates, triazines, and nitro-

soureas. These drugs are highly reactive; they primarily target nucleic acids and form links with the nuclei of different molecules. This allows the drugs to cross-link double-stranded DNA and to prevent strands from separating for replication, which may contribute to these drugs' ability to destroy cells.

NURSING PROCESS

📑 Assessment
• Perform a complete assessment before therapy begins.
• Monitor patient for adverse reactions throughout therapy.
• Monitor platelet and total and differential leukocyte counts, hematocrit, and BUN, ALT, AST, LDH, bilirubin, creatinine, uric acid, and other levels as needed.
• Monitor vital signs and patency of catheter or I.V. line throughout administration.

🔵 Key nursing diagnoses
• Ineffective protection related to thrombocytopenia
• Risk for infection related to immunosuppression
• Risk for deficient fluid volume related to adverse GI effects

▶ Planning and implementation
• Give under the supervision of a physician experienced in the use of antineoplastics.
• Follow established procedures for safe and proper handling, administration, and disposal of chemotherapeutic drugs.
• Treat extravasation promptly.
• Give ifosfamide with mesna to prevent hemorrhagic cystitis.
• Give lomustine 2 to 4 hours after meals. Nausea and vomiting usually last less than 24 hours, although loss of appetite may last for several days.
• Maintain adequate hydration before and for 24 hours after cisplatin treatment.
• Allopurinol may be prescribed to prevent drug-induced hyperuricemia.
• Discuss reproductive effects with patient before starting therapy.
Patient teaching
• Tell patient to avoid people with bacterial or viral infections because chemotherapy can in-

crease susceptibility. Urge him to report fever and signs of infection promptly.
• Review proper oral hygiene, including cautious use of toothbrush, dental floss, and toothpicks.
• Advise patient to complete dental work before therapy begins or to delay it until blood counts are normal.
• Warn patient that he may bruise easily because of drug's effect on platelets.

✓ Evaluation
• Patient develops no serious bleeding complications.
• Patient remains free from infection.
• Patient maintains adequate hydration.

Alpha blockers (peripherally acting)
alfuzosin hydrochloride (selective)
doxazosin mesylate (nonselective)
prazosin hydrochloride (nonselective)
tamsulosin hydrochloride (selective)
terazosin hydrochloride (nonselective)

Indications
▶ Hypertension, or mild to moderate urinary obstruction in men with BPH.

Contraindications and cautions
• Contraindicated in patients with MI, coronary insufficiency, or angina or with hypersensitivity to these drugs or any of their components. Also contraindicated in combination therapy with phosphodiesterase type 5 inhibitors (sildenafil, tadalafil, vardenafil), although tadalafil may be taken with tamsulosin 0.4 mg daily.
⚖ Lifespan: In pregnant or breast-feeding women, use cautiously. In children, the safety and effectiveness of many alpha blockers haven't been established; use cautiously. In elderly patients, hypotensive effects may be more pronounced.

Adverse reactions
Alpha blockers may cause severe orthostatic hypotension and syncope, especially with the first few doses, an effect commonly called the "first-dose effect." The most common adverse

effects of alpha$_1$ blockade are dizziness, headache, drowsiness, somnolence, and malaise. These drugs also may cause tachycardia, palpitations, fluid retention (from excess renin secretion), nasal and ocular congestion, and aggravation of respiratory tract infection.

Action
Selective alpha blockers decrease vascular resistance and increase vein capacity, thereby lowering blood pressure and causing nasal and scleroconjunctival congestion, ptosis, orthostatic and exercise hypotension, mild to moderate miosis, interference with ejaculation, and pink, warm skin. They also relax nonvascular smooth muscle, especially in the prostate capsule, which reduces urinary problems in men with BPH. Because alpha$_1$ blockers don't block alpha$_2$ receptors, they don't cause transmitter overflow.

Nonselective alpha blockers antagonize both alpha$_1$ and alpha$_2$ receptors. Generally, alpha blockade results in tachycardia, palpitations, and increased renin secretion because of abnormally large amounts of norepinephrine (from transmitter overflow) released from adrenergic nerve endings as a result of the blockade of alpha$_1$ and alpha$_2$ receptors. Norepinephrine's effects are counterproductive to the major uses of nonselective alpha blockers.

NURSING PROCESS

⚖ Assessment
• Monitor vital signs, especially blood pressure.
• Monitor patient closely for adverse reactions.

⊕ Key nursing diagnoses
• Decreased cardiac output related to hypotension
• Acute pain related to headache
• Excessive fluid volume related to fluid retention

▶ Planning and implementation
• Give at bedtime to minimize dizziness or lightheadedness.
• Begin therapy with a small dose to avoid first-dose syncope.
Patient teaching
• Warn patient not to rise suddenly from a lying or sitting position.

• Urge patient to avoid hazardous tasks that require mental alertness until the drug's full effects are known.
• Advise patient that alcohol, excessive exercise, prolonged standing, and heat exposure will intensify adverse effects.
• Tell patient to promptly report dizziness or irregular heartbeat.
• Caution patient to speak to his prescriber before taking a drug for erectile dysfunction.

☑ Evaluation
• Patient maintains adequate cardiac output.
• Patient's headache is relieved.
• Patient has no edema.

Aminoglycosides

amikacin sulfate
gentamicin sulfate
neomycin sulfate
streptomycin sulfate
tobramycin sulfate

Indications

▶ Septicemia; postoperative, pulmonary, intra-abdominal, and urinary tract infections; skin, soft tissue, bone, and joint infections; aerobic gram-negative bacillary meningitis not susceptible to other antibiotics; serious staphylococcal, *Pseudomonas aeruginosa,* and *Klebsiella* infections; enterococcal infections; nosocomial pneumonia; anaerobic infections involving *Bacteroides fragilis;* tuberculosis; initial empiric therapy in febrile, leukopenic patients.

Contraindications and cautions

• Contraindicated in patients hypersensitive to these drugs.
• Use cautiously in patients with a neuromuscular disorder and in those taking neuromuscular blockades.
• Use at lower dosages in patients with renal impairment.
⚖ Lifespan: In pregnant women, use cautiously. In breast-feeding women, safety hasn't been established. In neonates and premature infants, the half-life of aminoglycosides is prolonged because of immature renal systems. In infants and children, dosage adjustment may be need-

ed. Elderly patients have an increased risk of nephrotoxicity and commonly need a lower dose and longer intervals; they're also susceptible to ototoxicity and superinfection.

Adverse reactions

Ototoxicity and nephrotoxicity are the most serious complications. Neuromuscular blockade also may occur. Oral forms most commonly cause diarrhea, nausea, and vomiting. Parenteral drugs may cause vein irritation, phlebitis, and sterile abscess.

Action

Aminoglycosides are bactericidal. They bind directly and irreversibly to 30S ribosomal subunits, inhibiting bacterial protein synthesis. They're active against many aerobic gram-negative and some aerobic gram-positive organisms.

NURSING PROCESS

📋 Assessment
• Obtain patient's history of allergies.
• Monitor patient for adverse reactions.
• Obtain results of culture and sensitivity tests before first dose, and check tests periodically to assess drug effectiveness.
• Monitor vital signs and electrolyte levels. Conduct hearing ability and renal function studies before and during therapy.
• Check serum blood levels to assess for efficacy and toxicity. Peak levels assess efficacy; trough levels assess toxicity.
• Draw blood for peak level 1 hour after I.M. injection and 30 minutes to 1 hour after I.V. infusion; for trough level, draw sample just before next dose. Time and date all blood samples. Don't use heparinized tube to collect blood samples because it interferes with results.

✛ Key nursing diagnoses
• Risk for injury related to nephrotoxicity and ototoxicity
• Risk for infection related to drug-induced superinfection
• Risk for deficient fluid volume related to adverse GI reactions

▶ Planning and implementation
• Keep patient hydrated to minimize chemical irritation of renal tubules.

• Don't add or mix other drugs with I.V. infusions, particularly penicillins, which inactivate aminoglycosides. If other drugs must be given I.V., temporarily stop infusion of primary drug.
• Follow manufacturer's instructions for reconstitution, dilution, and storage of drugs; check expiration dates.
• Shake oral suspension well before giving it.
• Give I.M. dose deep into the gluteal muscle mass or midlateral thigh; rotate injection sites to minimize tissue injury. Apply ice to injection site to relieve pain.
• Giving I.V. dose too rapidly may cause neuromuscular blockade. Infuse I.V. dose continuously or intermittently over 30 to 60 minutes for adults, 1 to 2 hours for infants; dilution volume for children is determined individually.

Patient teaching
• Teach signs and symptoms of hypersensitivity and other adverse reactions. Urge patient to report unusual effects promptly.
• Emphasize importance of adequate fluid intake.

✓ Evaluation
• Patient maintains pretreatment renal and hearing functions.
• Patient is free from infection.
• Patient maintains adequate hydration.

Angiotensin-converting enzyme inhibitors

benazepril hydrochloride
captopril
enalapril maleate
enalaprilat
fosinopril sodium
lisinopril
moexipril hydrochloride
perindopril erbumine
quinapril hydrochloride
ramipril
trandolapril

Indications

▶ Hypertension, heart failure, left ventricular dysfunction (LVD), MI (with ramipril and lisinopril), and diabetic nephropathy (with captopril).

Contraindications and cautions

• Contraindicated in patients hypersensitive to these drugs.
• Use cautiously in patients with impaired renal function or serious autoimmune disease and in those taking other drugs known to decrease WBC count or immune response.
⚖ **Lifespan:** Women of childbearing age taking ACE inhibitors should report suspected pregnancy immediately to prescriber. High risks of fetal morbidity and mortality are linked to ACE inhibitors, especially in the second and third trimesters. Some ACE inhibitors appear in breast milk. To avoid adverse effects in infants, instruct patient to stop breast-feeding during therapy. In children, safety and effectiveness haven't been established; give drug only if potential benefits outweigh risks. Elderly patients may need lower doses because of impaired drug clearance.

Adverse reactions

The most common adverse effects of therapeutic doses are angioedema of the face and limbs, dry cough, dysgeusia, fatigue, headache, hyperkalemia, hypotension, proteinuria, rash, and tachycardia. Severe hypotension may occur at toxic drug levels.

Action

ACE inhibitors prevent conversion of angiotensin I to angiotensin II, a potent vasoconstrictor. Besides decreasing vasoconstriction and thus reducing peripheral arterial resistance, inhibiting angiotensin II decreases adrenocortical secretion of aldosterone. This reduces sodium and water retention and extracellular fluid volume. ACE inhibition also causes increased levels of bradykinin, which results in vasodilation. This decreases heart rate and systemic vascular resistance.

NURSING PROCESS

⚱ Assessment
• Observe patient for adverse reactions.
• Monitor vital signs regularly, and monitor WBC count and electrolyte level periodically.

⊞ Key nursing diagnoses
• Risk for falls related to orthostatic hypotension

- Ineffective protection related to hyperkalemia
- Acute pain related to headache

▶ Planning and implementation
- To reduce risk of hypotension, stop diuretic 2 to 3 days before starting ACE inhibitor. If drug doesn't adequately control blood pressure, diuretics may be restarted.
- If patient has impaired renal function, give a reduced dosage.
- Give potassium supplements and potassium-sparing diuretics cautiously because ACE inhibitors may cause potassium retention.
- If patient becomes pregnant, stop ACE inhibitors. These drugs can cause birth defects or fetal death in the second and third trimesters.
- Give captopril and moexipril 1 hour before meals.

Patient teaching
- Tell patient that drugs may cause a dry, persistent, tickling cough that stops when therapy stops.
- Urge patient to report lightheadedness, especially in the first few days of therapy so that the dosage can be adjusted. Tell him to report signs of infection, such as sore throat and fever, because these drugs may decrease WBC count. Advise him to immediately report facial swelling or difficulty breathing.
- Advise patient to avoid sudden position changes to minimize orthostatic hypotension.
- Warn patient to seek medical approval before taking self-prescribed cold preparations.
- Tell women to report pregnancy at once.
- Warn patient to use potassium-containing salt substitutes cautiously because ACE inhibitors may cause potassium retention.

☑ Evaluation
- Patient sustains no injury from orthostatic hypotension.
- Patient's WBC count remains normal throughout therapy.
- Patient's headache is relieved by mild analgesic.

Antacids
aluminum hydroxide
calcium carbonate
magaldrate
magnesium hydroxide
magnesium oxide
sodium bicarbonate

Indications

▶ Hyperacidity; hyperphosphatemia (aluminum hydroxide); hypomagnesemia (magnesium oxide); postmenopausal hypocalcemia (calcium carbonate).

Contraindications and cautions

- Calcium carbonate, magaldrate, and magnesium oxide are contraindicated in patients with severe renal disease. Sodium bicarbonate is contraindicated in patients with hypertension, renal disease, or edema; patients who are vomiting; patients receiving diuretics or continuous GI suction; and patients on sodium-restricted diets.
- In patients with mild renal impairment, give magnesium oxide cautiously.
- Give aluminum preparations, calcium carbonate, and magaldrate cautiously in elderly patients; in those receiving antidiarrheals, antispasmodics, or anticholinergics; and in those with dehydration, fluid restriction, chronic renal disease, or suspected intestinal absorption problems.
- Lifespan: Pregnant women should consult their prescriber before using antacids. Breast-feeding women may take antacids. In infants, serious adverse effects are more likely from changes in fluid and electrolyte balance; monitor them closely. Elderly patients have an increased risk of adverse reactions; monitor them closely; also, give these patients aluminum preparations, calcium carbonate, magaldrate, and magnesium oxide cautiously.

Adverse reactions

Antacids containing aluminum may cause aluminum intoxication, constipation, hypophosphatemia, intestinal obstruction, and osteomalacia. Antacids containing magnesium may cause diarrhea or hypermagnesemia (in renal failure). Calcium carbonate, magaldrate, magnesium ox-

ide, and sodium bicarbonate may cause constipation, milk-alkali syndrome, or rebound hyperacidity.

Action

Antacids reduce the total acid load in the GI tract and elevate gastric pH to reduce pepsin activity. They also strengthen the gastric mucosal barrier and increase esophageal sphincter tone.

NURSING PROCESS

Assessment
• Assess patient's condition before therapy and regularly thereafter.
• Record number and consistency of stools.
• Observe patient for adverse reactions.
• Monitor patient receiving long-term, high-dose aluminum carbonate and hydroxide for fluid and electrolyte imbalance, especially if patient is on a sodium-restricted diet.
• Monitor phosphate level in a patient taking aluminum carbonate or hydroxide.
• Watch for signs of hypercalcemia in a patient taking calcium carbonate.
• Monitor magnesium level in a patient with mild renal impairment who takes magaldrate.

Key nursing diagnoses
• Constipation related to adverse effects of aluminum-containing antacid
• Diarrhea related to adverse effects of magnesium-containing antacid
• Ineffective protection related to drug-induced electrolyte imbalance

Planning and implementation
• Manage constipation with laxatives or stool softeners, or switch patient to a magnesium preparation.
• If patient suffers from diarrhea, give an antidiarrheal, and switch patient to an antacid containing aluminum.
• Shake container well, and give with small amount of water or juice to facilitate passage. When giving through an NG tube, make sure the tube is patent and placed correctly. After instilling the drug, flush the tube with water to ensure passage to the stomach and to clear the tube.

Patient teaching
• Warn patient not to take antacids randomly or to switch antacids without prescriber's consent.

• Tell patient not to take calcium carbonate with milk or other foods high in vitamin D.

Evaluation
• Patient regains normal bowel pattern.
• Patient states that diarrhea is relieved.
• Patient maintains normal electrolyte balance.

Antianginals
Beta blockers
acebutolol
atenolol
bisoprolol fumarate
esmolol hydrochloride
metoprolol
nadolol
propranolol hydrochloride
Calcium channel blockers
amlodipine besylate
diltiazem hydrochloride
nicardipine hydrochloride
nifedipine
verapamil hydrochloride
Nitrates
isosorbide dinitrate
isosorbide mononitrate
nitroglycerin

Indications

▶ Moderate to severe angina (beta blockers); classic, effort-induced angina and Prinzmetal angina (calcium channel blockers); recurrent angina (long-acting nitrates and topical, transdermal, transmucosal, and oral extended-release nitroglycerin); acute angina (S.L. nitroglycerin and S.L. or chewable isosorbide dinitrate); unstable angina (I.V. nitroglycerin).

Contraindications and cautions

• Beta blockers are contraindicated in patients hypersensitive to them and in patients with cardiogenic shock, sinus bradycardia, heart block greater than first degree, or bronchial asthma. Calcium channel blockers are contraindicated in patients with severe hypotension or heart block greater than first degree (except with functioning pacemaker). Nitrates are contraindicated in patients with severe anemia, cerebral hemorrhage, head trauma, glaucoma, or hyper-

thyroidism or in patients using phosphodiesterase type 5 inhibitors (sildenafil, tadalafil,
vardenafil).

• Use beta blockers cautiously in patients with
nonallergic bronchospastic disorders, diabetes
mellitus, or impaired hepatic or renal function.
Use calcium channel blockers cautiously in patients with hepatic or renal impairment, bradycardia, heart failure, or cardiogenic shock. Use
nitrates cautiously in patients with hypotension
or recent MI.

⚜ **Lifespan:** In pregnant women, use beta
blockers cautiously. Recommendations for
breast-feeding vary by drug; use beta blockers
and calcium channel blockers cautiously. In
children, safety and effectiveness haven't been
established. Check with prescriber before giving these drugs to children. Elderly patients
have an increased risk of adverse reactions; use
cautiously.

Adverse reactions

Beta blockers may cause bradycardia, cough,
diarrhea, disturbing dreams, dizziness, dyspnea,
fatigue, fever, heart failure, hypotension, lethargy, nausea, peripheral edema, and wheezing.
Calcium channel blockers may cause bradycardia, confusion, constipation, depression, diarrhea, dizziness, dyspepsia, edema, elevated liver enzyme levels (transient), fatigue, flushing,
headache, hypotension, insomnia, nervousness,
and rash. Nitrates may cause alcohol intoxication (from I.V. preparations containing alcohol),
flushing, headache, orthostatic hypotension, reflex tachycardia, rash, syncope, and vomiting.

Action

Beta blockers decrease catecholamine-induced
increases in heart rate, blood pressure, and myocardial contraction. Calcium channel blockers
inhibit the flow of calcium through muscle
cells, which dilates coronary arteries and decreases systemic vascular resistance, known as
afterload. Nitrates decrease afterload and left
ventricular end-diastolic pressure, or preload,
and increase blood flow through collateral coronary vessels.

NURSING PROCESS

📇 Assessment
• Monitor vital signs. With I.V. nitroglycerin,
monitor blood pressure and pulse rate every

5 to 15 minutes while adjusting dosage, and
every hour thereafter.
• Monitor the drug's effectiveness.
• Observe patient for adverse reactions.

⊕ Key nursing diagnoses
• Risk for injury related to adverse reactions
• Excessive fluid volume related to adverse CV
effects of beta blockers or calcium channel
blockers
• Acute pain related to headache

▷ Planning and implementation
• Have patient sit or lie down when receiving
the first nitrate dose; take his pulse and blood
pressure before giving dose and when drug action starts.
• Don't give a beta blocker or calcium channel
blocker to relieve acute angina.
• Withhold the dose and notify prescriber if patient's heart rate is slower than 60 beats/minute
or systolic blood pressure is lower than
90 mm Hg.

Patient teaching
• Warn patient not to stop drug abruptly without prescriber's approval.
• Teach patient to take his pulse before taking a
beta blocker or calcium channel blocker. Tell
him to withhold the dose and alert the prescriber if his pulse rate is slower than 60 beats/
minute.
• Instruct patient taking nitroglycerin S.L. to go
to the emergency department if 3 tablets taken
5 minutes apart don't relieve angina.
• Caution patient about the dangers of using nitrates with certain erectile dysfunction drugs.
• Tell patient to report serious or persistent adverse reactions.

☑ Evaluation
• Patient sustains no injury from adverse reac-
tions.
• Patient maintains normal fluid balance.
• Patient's headache is relieved with mild anal-
gesic.

Antiarrhythmics

adenosine
Class IA
disopyramide
procainamide hydrochloride
quinidine bisulfate
quinidine gluconate
quinidine sulfate
Class IB
lidocaine hydrochloride
mexiletine hydrochloride
phenytoin sodium
Class IC
flecainide acetate
propafenone hydrochloride
Class II (beta blockers)
acebutolol hydrochloride
esmolol hydrochloride
propranolol hydrochloride
Class III
amiodarone hydrochloride
bretylium tosylate
dofetilide
ibutilide fumarate
sotalol hydrochloride
Class IV (calcium channel blocker)
verapamil hydrochloride

Indications

▶ Atrial and ventricular arrhythmias.

Contraindications and cautions

• Contraindicated in patients hypersensitive to these drugs.
• Many antiarrhythmics are contraindicated or require cautious use in patients with cardiogenic shock, digitalis toxicity, and second- or third-degree heart block (unless patient has a pacemaker or implantable cardioverter defibrillator).
⚞ Lifespan: In pregnant women, use only if potential benefits to the mother outweigh risks to the fetus. In breast-feeding women, use cautiously; many antiarrhythmics appear in breast milk. In children, monitor closely because they have an increased risk of adverse reactions. In elderly patients, use these drugs cautiously because these patients may exhibit physiologic alterations in CV system.

Adverse reactions

Most antiarrhythmics can aggravate existing arrhythmias or cause new ones. They also may produce CNS disturbances, such as dizziness or fatigue, GI problems, such as nausea, vomiting, or altered bowel elimination; hypersensitivity reactions; and hypotension. Some antiarrhythmics may worsen heart failure. Class II drugs may cause bronchoconstriction.

Action

Class I drugs reduce the inward current carried by sodium ions, which stabilizes neuronal cardiac membranes. Class IA drugs depress phase 0, prolong the action potential, and stabilize cardiac membranes. Class IB drugs depress phase 0, shorten the action potential, and stabilize cardiac membranes. Class IC drugs block the transport of sodium ions, which decreases conduction velocity but not repolarization rate. Class II drugs decrease the heart rate, myocardial contractility, blood pressure, and AV node conduction. Class III drugs prolong the action potential and refractory period. Class IV drugs decrease myocardial contractility and oxygen demand by inhibiting calcium ion influx; they also dilate coronary arteries and arterioles.

NURSING PROCESS

⚕ Assessment
• Monitor ECG continuously when therapy starts and when dosage is adjusted.
• Monitor patient's vital signs frequently, and assess for signs of toxicity and adverse reactions.
• Measure apical pulse rate before giving drug.
• Monitor drug level as indicated.

⚕ Key nursing diagnoses
• Decreased cardiac output related to arrhythmias or myocardial depression
• Ineffective protection related to adverse reactions
• Noncompliance related to long-term therapy

⚕ Planning and implementation
• Don't crush sustained-release tablets.
• Take safety precautions if adverse CNS reactions occur.
• Notify prescriber about adverse reactions.

Prototype drug

Patient teaching

- Stress the importance of taking drug exactly as prescribed.
- Teach patient to take his pulse before each dose. Tell him to notify prescriber if his pulse is irregular or slower than 60 beats/minute.
- Instruct patient to avoid hazardous activities that require mental alertness if adverse CNS reactions occur.
- Tell patient to limit fluid and salt intake if his prescribed drug causes fluid retention.

✓ Evaluation

- Patient maintains adequate cardiac output, as shown by normal vital signs and adequate tissue perfusion.
- Patient has no serious adverse reactions.
- Patient states importance of compliance with therapy.

Antibiotic antineoplastics

bleomycin sulfate
daunorubicin hydrochloride
doxorubicin hydrochloride
epirubicin hydrochloride
idarubicin hydrochloride
mitomycin
mitoxantrone hydrochloride

Indications

▶ Various tumors.

Contraindications and cautions

- Contraindicated in patients hypersensitive to these drugs.
- �△ **Lifespan:** In pregnant women, avoid antineoplastics. Breast-feeding during therapy isn't recommended. In children, safety and effectiveness of some drugs haven't been established; use cautiously. In elderly patients, use cautiously because of their increased risk of adverse reactions.

Adverse reactions

The most common adverse reactions include anxiety, bone marrow depression, chills, confusion, diarrhea, fever, flank or joint pain, hair loss, nausea, redness or pain at the injection site, sore throat, swelling of the feet or lower legs, vomiting, and cardiomyopathy.

Action

Although classified as antibiotics, these drugs destroy cells, thus ruling out their use as antimicrobials alone. They interfere with proliferation of malignant cells in several ways. Their action may be specific to cell-cycle phase, not specific to cell-cycle phase, or both. Some of these drugs act like alkylating drugs or antimetabolites. By binding to or creating complexes with DNA, antibiotic antineoplastics directly or indirectly inhibit DNA, RNA, and protein synthesis.

NURSING PROCESS

▲ Assessment

- Perform a complete assessment before therapy begins.
- Monitor patient for adverse reactions.
- Monitor vital signs and patency of catheter or I.V. line.
- Monitor platelet and total and differential leukocyte counts, and monitor ALT, AST, LDH, bilirubin, creatinine, uric acid, BUN, and hemoglobin levels and hematocrit.
- Monitor pulmonary function tests in a patient receiving bleomycin. Assess lung function regularly.
- Check baseline cardiac function with a multiple-gated acquisition scan (MUGA) or echocardiogram to assess ejection fraction. Monitor cardiac function periodically throughout course of therapy.

⊕ Key nursing diagnoses

- Ineffective protection related to thrombocytopenia
- Risk for infection related to immunosuppression
- Risk for deficient fluid volume related to adverse GI effects

▷ Planning and implementation

- Follow established procedures for safe and proper handling, administration, and disposal of chemotherapeutic drugs.
- Try to ease anxiety in patient and family before treatment.

• Keep epinephrine, corticosteroids, and anti-histamines available during bleomycin therapy. Anaphylactoid reaction may occur.
• Daunorubicin, doxorubicin, epirubicin, idarubicin, mitomycin are vesicants; treat extravasation promptly with cold compresses.
• Ensure adequate hydration during idarubicin therapy.

Patient teaching
• Advise patient to avoid exposure to people with bacterial or viral infections because chemotherapy increases susceptibility. Urge him to report signs of infection immediately.
• Review proper oral hygiene, including cautious use of toothbrush, dental floss, and tooth-picks. Chemotherapy can increase the risk of microbial infection, delayed healing, and bleeding gums.
• Urge patient to complete dental work before therapy begins or to delay it until blood counts are normal.
• Warn patient that he may bruise easily.
• Tell patient to report redness, pain, or swelling at injection site immediately. Local tissue injury and scarring may result if I.V. infiltration occurs.
• Advise patient taking daunorubicin, doxorubicin, or idarubicin that his urine may turn orange or red for 1 to 2 days after therapy begins.
• Mitoxantrone may temporarily turn urine blue.

☑ **Evaluation**
• No serious bleeding complications develop.
• Patient remains free from infection.
• Patient maintains adequate hydration.

Anticholinergics

atropine sulfate
benztropine mesylate
dicyclomine hydrochloride
scopolamine
scopolamine hydrobromide

Indications

▶ Prevention of motion sickness, preoperative reduction of secretions and blockage of cardiac reflexes, adjunct treatment of peptic ulcers and other GI disorders, blockage of cholinomimetic

effects of cholinesterase inhibitors or other drugs, and (for benztropine) various spastic conditions, including acute dystonic reactions, muscle rigidity, parkinsonism, and extrapyramidal disorders.

Contraindications and cautions

• Contraindicated in patients hypersensitive to these drugs and in those with angle-closure glaucoma, renal or GI obstructive disease, reflux esophagitis, or myasthenia gravis.
• Use cautiously in patients with heart disease, GI infection, open-angle glaucoma, prostatic hypertrophy, hypertension, hyperthyroidism, ulcerative colitis, autonomic neuropathy, or hiatal hernia with reflux esophagitis.
⚖ Lifespan: In pregnant women, safe use hasn't been established. In breast-feeding women, avoid anticholinergics because they may decrease milk production; some may appear in breast milk and cause infant toxicity. In children, safety and effectiveness haven't been established. Patients older than age 40 may be more sensitive to these drugs. In elderly patients, use cautiously and give a reduced dosage, as indicated.

Adverse reactions

Therapeutic doses commonly cause blurred vision, constipation, cycloplegia, decreased sweating or anhidrosis, dry mouth, headache, mydriasis, palpitations, tachycardia, and urinary hesitancy and retention. These reactions usually disappear when therapy stops. Toxicity can cause signs and symptoms resembling psychosis (disorientation, confusion, hallucinations, delusions, anxiety, agitation, and restlessness); dilated, nonreactive pupils; blurred vision; hot, dry, flushed skin; dry mucous membranes; dysphagia; decreased or absent bowel sounds; urine retention; hyperthermia; tachycardia; hypertension; and increased respirations.

Action

Anticholinergics competitively antagonize the actions of acetylcholine and other cholinergic agonists at muscarinic receptors.

Assessment
• Monitor patient regularly for adverse reactions.
• Check vital signs at least every 4 hours.
• Measure urine output; check for urine retention.
• Assess patient for changes in vision and for signs of impending toxicity.

Key nursing diagnoses
• Urinary retention related to adverse effect on bladder
• Constipation related to adverse effect on GI tract
• Acute pain related to headache

Planning and implementation
• Provide ice chips, cool drinks, or hard candy to relieve dry mouth.
• Relieve constipation with stool softeners or bulk laxatives.
• Give a mild analgesic for headache.
• Notify prescriber about urine retention, and be prepared to catheterize patient, if needed.
Patient teaching
• Teach patient how and when to take the drug and caution him not to take other drugs unless prescribed.
• Warn patient to avoid hazardous tasks if he experiences dizziness, drowsiness, or blurred vision. Inform him that the drug may increase his sensitivity to or intolerance of high temperatures, resulting in dizziness.
• Advise patient to avoid alcohol because it may cause additive CNS effects.
• Urge patient to drink plenty of fluids and to eat a high-fiber diet to prevent constipation.
• Tell patient to notify prescriber promptly if he experiences confusion, rapid or pounding heartbeat, dry mouth, blurred vision, rash, eye pain, significant change in urine volume, or pain or difficulty on urination.
• Advise women to report planned or known pregnancy.

Evaluation
• Patient maintains normal voiding pattern.
• Patient regains normal bowel patterns.
• Patient is free from pain.

Anticoagulants
Coumarin derivative
warfarin sodium
Heparin derivative
heparin sodium
Low–molecular-weight heparins
dalteparin sodium
enoxaparin sodium
tinzaparin sodium
Selective factor Xa inhibitor
fondaparinux sodium
Thrombin inhibitors
argatroban
bivalirudin

Indications
▶ Pulmonary emboli, deep vein thrombosis, thrombus, blood clotting, DIC, unstable angina, MI, atrial fibrillation.

Contraindications and cautions
• Contraindicated in patients hypersensitive to these drugs or any of their components; in patients with aneurysm, active bleeding, CV hemorrhage, hemorrhagic blood dyscrasias, hemophilia, severe hypertension, pericardial effusions, or pericarditis; and in patients undergoing major surgery, neurosurgery, or ophthalmic surgery.
• Use cautiously in patients with severe diabetes, renal impairment, severe trauma, ulcerations, or vasculitis.
Lifespan: Most anticoagulants (except warfarin) may be used in pregnancy only if clearly necessary. In pregnant women and those who have just had a threatened or complete spontaneous abortion, warfarin is contraindicated. Women should avoid breast-feeding during therapy. Infants, especially neonates, may be more susceptible to anticoagulants because of vitamin K deficiency. Elderly patients are at greater risk for hemorrhage because of altered hemostatic mechanisms or age-related deterioration of hepatic and renal functions.

Adverse reactions
Anticoagulants commonly cause bleeding and may cause hypersensitivity reactions. Warfarin may cause agranulocytosis, alopecia (long-term use), anorexia, dermatitis, fever, nausea, tissue

necrosis or gangrene, urticaria, and vomiting. Heparin derivatives may cause thrombocytopenia and may increase liver enzyme levels. Nonhemorrhagic adverse reactions associated with thrombin inhibitors may include back pain, bradycardia, and hypotension.

Action

Heparin derivatives accelerate formation of an antithrombin III-thrombin complex. It inactivates thrombin and prevents conversion of fibrinogen to fibrin. The coumarin derivative warfarin inhibits vitamin K–dependent activation of clotting factors II, VII, IX, and X, which are formed in the liver. Thrombin inhibitors directly bind to thrombin and inhibit its action. Selective factor Xa inhibitors bind to antithrombin III which, in turn, initiates the neutralization of factor Xa.

NURSING PROCESS

Assessment
• Monitor patient closely for bleeding and other adverse reactions.
• Check PT, INR, or PTT.
• Monitor vital signs, hemoglobin, and hematocrit.
• Assess patient's urine, stools, and emesis for blood.
• Monitor for signs of clotting, such as deep vein thrombosis (pain and swelling in legs) or pulmonary embolism (chest pain, shortness of breath).

Key nursing diagnoses
• Ineffective protection related to drug's effects on body's normal clotting and bleeding mechanisms
• Risk for deficient fluid volume related to bleeding
• Noncompliance related to long-term warfarin therapy

Planning and implementation
• Don't give heparin I.M.; avoid I.M. injections of any anticoagulant if possible.
• Keep protamine sulfate available to treat severe bleeding caused by heparin. Keep vitamin K available to treat frank bleeding caused by warfarin.
• Notify prescriber about serious or persistent adverse reactions.

• Maintain bleeding precautions throughout therapy.
Patient teaching
• Urge patient to take drug exactly as prescribed. If he's taking warfarin, tell him to take the drug as prescribed at the same time each day.
• Advise patient to consult his prescriber before taking any other drug, including OTC medications and herbal remedies.
• Advise the patient on bleeding-prevention precautions to take in everyday activities. Urge patient to remove safety hazards and make home repairs to reduce risk of injury.
• Advise patient to eat green, leafy vegetables consistently; variation of these in the diet can affect INR.
• Instruct patient to report bleeding or other adverse reactions promptly.
• Encourage patient to keep appointments for blood tests and follow-up examinations.
• Advise a woman to report planned or known pregnancy.

Evaluation
• Patient has no adverse change in health status.
• Patient has no evidence of bleeding or hemorrhaging.
• Patient demonstrates compliance with therapy, as shown by bleeding and clotting values within therapeutic range.

Anticonvulsants
carbamazepine
clonazepam
clorazepate dipotassium
diazepam
divalproex sodium
fosphenytoin sodium
gabapentin
lamotrigine
levetiracetam
magnesium sulfate
oxcarbazepine
phenobarbital
phenobarbital sodium
phenytoin sodium
phenytoin sodium (extended)
primidone

tiagabine hydrochloride
topiramate
valproate sodium
valproic acid
zonisamide

Indications

▶ Seizure disorders; acute, isolated seizures not caused by seizure disorders; status epilepticus; prevention of seizures after trauma or craniotomy; neuropathic pain.

Contraindications and cautions

• Contraindicated in patients hypersensitive to these drugs.
• Carbamazepine is contraindicated within 14 days of MAO inhibitor use.
• Use cautiously in patients with blood dyscrasias. Also, use barbiturates cautiously in patients with suicidal ideation.
⚘ Lifespan: In pregnant women, therapy usually continues despite the fetal risks caused by some anticonvulsants (barbiturates, phenytoin). In breast-feeding women, the safety of many anticonvulsants hasn't been established. Children, especially young ones, are sensitive to the CNS depression of some anticonvulsants; use cautiously. Elderly patients are sensitive to CNS effects and may require lower doses. Also, some anticonvulsants may take longer to be eliminated because of decreased renal function, and parenteral use is more likely to cause apnea, hypotension, bradycardia, and cardiac arrest.

Adverse reactions

Anticonvulsants can cause adverse CNS effects, such as ataxia, confusion, somnolence, and tremor. Many anticonvulsants also cause CV disorders, such as arrhythmias and hypotension; GI effects, such as vomiting; and hematologic disorders, such as agranulocytosis, bone marrow depression, leukopenia, and thrombocytopenia. Stevens-Johnson syndrome, other severe rashes, and abnormal liver function test results may occur with certain anticonvulsants.

Action

Anticonvulsants include six classes of drugs: selected hydantoin derivatives, barbiturates, benzodiazepines, succinimides, iminostilbene derivatives (carbamazepine), and carboxylic acid derivatives. Magnesium sulfate is a miscellaneous anticonvulsant. Some hydantoin derivatives and carbamazepine inhibit the spread of seizure activity in the motor cortex. Some barbiturates and succinimides limit seizure activity by increasing the threshold for motor cortex stimuli. Selected benzodiazepines and carboxylic acid derivatives may increase inhibition of GABA in brain neurons. Magnesium sulfate interferes with the release of acetylcholine at the myoneural junction.

NURSING PROCESS

❧ Assessment
• Monitor drug level and patient's response as indicated.
• Monitor patient for adverse reactions.
• Assess patient's compliance with therapy at each follow-up visit.

⊕ Key nursing diagnoses
• Risk for trauma related to adverse reactions
• Impaired physical mobility related to sedation
• Noncompliance related to long-term therapy

▶ Planning and implementation
• Give oral forms with food to reduce GI irritation.
• Phenytoin binds with tube feedings, thus decreasing absorption of drug. Turn off tube feedings for 2 hours before and after giving phenytoin, according to your facility's policy.
• Adjust dosage according to patient's response.
• Take safety precautions if patient has adverse CNS reactions.
Patient teaching
• Instruct patient to take drug exactly as prescribed and not to stop drug without medical supervision.
• Urge patient to avoid hazardous activities that require mental alertness if adverse CNS reactions occur.
• Advise patient to wear or carry medical identification at all times.

☑ Evaluation
• Patient sustains no trauma from adverse reactions.
• Patient maintains physical mobility.
• Patient complies with therapy and has no seizures.

Antidepressants, tricyclic

amitriptyline hydrochloride
amoxapine
clomipramine hydrochloride
desipramine hydrochloride
doxepin hydrochloride
imipramine hydrochloride
imipramine pamoate
nortriptyline hydrochloride

Indications

▶ Depression, anxiety (doxepin hydrochloride), obsessive-compulsive disorder (clomipramine), enuresis in children older than age 6 (imipramine), neuropathic pain.

Contraindications and cautions

• Contraindicated in patients hypersensitive to these drugs and in patients with urine retention or angle-closure glaucoma.
• Tricyclic antidepressants are contraindicated within 2 weeks of MAO inhibitor therapy.
• Use cautiously in patients with suicidal tendencies, schizophrenia, paranoia, seizure disorders, CV disease, or impaired hepatic function.
⚖ Lifespan: In pregnant and breast-feeding women, safety hasn't been established; use cautiously. In children younger than age 12, tricyclic antidepressants aren't recommended. Elderly patients are more sensitive to therapeutic and adverse effects; they need lower dosages.

Adverse reactions

Adverse reactions include anticholinergic effects, orthostatic hypotension, and sedation. The tertiary amines (amitriptyline, doxepin, and imipramine) exert the strongest sedative effects; tolerance usually develops in a few weeks. Amoxapine is most likely to cause seizures, especially with overdose. Tricyclic antidepressants may cause cardiovascular effects such as T-wave abnormalities, conduction disturbances, and arrhythmias.

Action

Tricyclic antidepressants may inhibit reuptake of norepinephrine and serotonin in CNS nerve terminals (presynaptic neurons), thus enhancing the concentration and activity of neurotransmitters in the synaptic cleft. Tricyclic antidepressants also exert antihistaminic, sedative, anticholinergic, vasodilatory, and quinidine-like effects.

NURSING PROCESS

⚗ Assessment
• Observe patient for mood changes to monitor drug effectiveness; benefits may not appear for 3 to 6 weeks. For treatment of neuropathic pain, benefit may be noted within 1 week.
• Check vital signs regularly for tachycardia or decreased blood pressure; observe patient carefully for other adverse reactions and report changes. Check ECG in patients older than age 40 before starting therapy.
• Monitor patient for anticholinergic adverse reactions, such as urine retention or constipation, which may require dosage reduction.

⊕ Key nursing diagnoses
• Disturbed thought processes related to adverse effects
• Risk for injury related to sedation and orthostatic hypotension
• Noncompliance related to long-term therapy

▷ Planning and implementation
• Make sure patient swallows each dose; a depressed patient may hoard pills for suicide attempt, especially when symptoms begin to improve.
• Don't withdraw drug abruptly; instead, gradually reduce dosage over several weeks to avoid rebound effect or other adverse reactions.
Patient teaching
• When appropriate, advise patient on use of antidepressant as treatment for neuropathic pain.
• Explain to patient the rationale for therapy and its anticipated risks and benefits. Inform patient that full therapeutic effect may not occur for several weeks.
• Teach patient how and when to take the drug. Warn him not to increase dosage, stop taking the drug, or take any other drug, including OTC medicines and herbal remedies, without approval from prescriber.
• Because overdose with tricyclic antidepressants is commonly fatal, entrust a reliable family member with the drug, and warn him to store drug safely away from children.
• Advise patient not to take drug with milk or food to minimize GI distress. Suggest taking full dose at bedtime if daytime sedation is a problem.

- Tell patient to avoid alcohol.
- Advise patient to avoid hazardous tasks that require mental alertness until full effects of drug are known.
- Warn patient that excessive exposure to sunlight, heat lamps, or tanning beds may cause burns and abnormal hyperpigmentation.
- Urge diabetic patient to monitor his glucose level carefully because drug may alter it.
- Recommend sugarless gum or hard candy, artificial saliva, or ice chips to relieve dry mouth.
- Advise patient to report adverse reactions promptly.

☑ Evaluation

- Patient regains normal thought processes.
- Patient sustains no injury from adverse reactions.
- Patient complies with therapy, and his depression is alleviated.

Antidiabetics

acarbose
glimepiride
glipizide
glyburide
metformin hydrochloride
miglitol
nateglinide
pioglitazone hydrochloride
repaglinide
rosiglitazone maleate

Indications

▶ Mild to moderately severe, stable, nonketotic, type 2 diabetes mellitus that can't be controlled by diet alone.

Contraindications and cautions

- Contraindicated in patients hypersensitive to these drugs and in patients with diabetic ketoacidosis with or without coma. Metformin is also contraindicated in patients with renal disease or metabolic acidosis and generally should be avoided in patients with hepatic disease.
- Use sulfonylureas cautiously in patients with renal or hepatic disease. Use metformin cautiously in patients with adrenal or pituitary insufficiency and in debilitated and malnourished patients. Alpha-glucosidase inhibitors should be used cautiously in patients with mild to moderate renal insufficiency. Thiazolidinediones aren't recommended in patients with edema, heart failure, or liver disease.

⚕ **Lifespan:** In pregnant or breast-feeding women, use is contraindicated. Oral antidiabetics appear in small amounts in breast milk and may cause hypoglycemia in the infant. In children, oral antidiabetics aren't effective in type 1 diabetes mellitus. Elderly patients may be more sensitive to these drugs, usually need lower dosages, and are more likely to develop neurologic symptoms of hypoglycemia; monitor these patients closely. In elderly patients, avoid chlorpropamide use because of its long duration of action.

Adverse reactions

Sulfonylureas cause dose-related reactions that usually respond to decreased dosage: anorexia, headache, heartburn, nausea, paresthesia, vomiting, and weakness. Hypoglycemia may follow excessive dosage, increased exercise, decreased food intake, or alcohol use.

The most serious adverse reaction linked to metformin is lactic acidosis. It's a rare effect and most likely to occur in patients with renal dysfunction. Other reactions to metformin include dermatitis, GI upset, megaloblastic anemia, rash, and unpleasant or metallic taste.

Thiazolidinediones may cause fluid retention leading to or exacerbating heart failure. Alpha-glucosidase inhibitors can cause abdominal pain, diarrhea, and flatulence.

Action

Oral antidiabetics come in several types. Sulfonylureas are sulfonamide derivatives that aren't antibacterial. They lower glucose levels by stimulating insulin release from the pancreas. These drugs work only in the presence of functioning beta cells in the islet tissue of the pancreas. After prolonged administration, they produce hypoglycemia by acting outside of the pancreas, including reduced glucose production by the liver and enhanced peripheral sensitivity to insulin. The latter may result from an increased number of insulin receptors or from changes after insulin binding. Sulfonylureas are divided into first-generation drugs, such as chlorpropamide, and second-generation drugs, such as glyburide, glimepiride, and glipizide.

Although their mechanisms of action are similar, the second-generation drugs carry a more lipophilic side chain, are more potent, and cause fewer adverse reactions. Their most important difference is their duration of action.

Meglitinides, such as nateglinide and repaglinide, are nonsulfonylurea antidiabetics that stimulate the release of insulin from the pancreas.

Metformin decreases hepatic glucose production, reduces intestinal glucose absorption, and improves insulin sensitivity by increasing peripheral glucose uptake and utilization. With metformin therapy, insulin secretion remains unchanged, and fasting insulin levels and all-day insulin response may decrease.

Alpha-glucosidase inhibitors, such as acarbose and miglitol, delay digestion of carbohydrates, resulting in a smaller rise in glucose levels.

Rosiglitazone and pioglitazone are thiazolidinediones, which lower glucose levels by improving insulin sensitivity. These drugs are potent and highly selective agonists for receptors found in insulin-sensitive tissues, such as adipose, skeletal muscle, and liver.

NURSING PROCESS

Assessment
• Monitor patient's glucose level regularly. Increase monitoring during periods of increased stress, such as infection, fever, surgery, or trauma.
• Monitor patient for adverse reactions.
• Assess patient's compliance with drug therapy and other aspects of diabetic treatment.

Key nursing diagnoses
• Risk for injury related to hypoglycemia
• Risk for deficient fluid volume related to adverse GI effects
• Noncompliance related to long-term therapy

Planning and implementation
• Give sulfonylurea 30 minutes before morning meal for once-daily regimen or 30 minutes before morning and evening meals for twice-daily regimen. Give metformin with morning and evening meals. Alpha-glucosidase inhibitors should be taken with the first bite of each main meal three times daily.

• Patients who take a thiazolidinedione should have liver enzyme levels measured at the start of therapy, every 2 months for the first year of therapy, and periodically thereafter.
• Keep in mind that a patient transferring from one oral antidiabetic to another (except chlorpropamide) usually needs no transition period.
• Anticipate patient's need for insulin during periods of increased stress.

Patient teaching
• Emphasize importance of following the prescribed regimen. Urge patient to adhere to diet, weight reduction, exercise, and personal hygiene recommendations.
• Explain that therapy relieves symptoms but doesn't cure the disease.
• Teach patient how to recognize and treat hypoglycemia.

Evaluation
• Patient sustains no injury.
• Patient maintains adequate hydration.
• Patient complies with therapy, as shown by normal or near-normal glucose level.

Antidiarrheals

bismuth subgallate
bismuth subsalicylate
calcium polycarbophil
diphenoxylate hydrochloride and atropine sulfate
kaolin and pectin mixtures
loperamide hydrochloride
octreotide acetate
opium tincture
opium tincture, camphorated

Indications

▶ Mild, acute, or chronic diarrhea. Octreotide acetate is indicated for certain cancers that cause diarrhea.

Contraindications and cautions

• Contraindicated in patients hypersensitive to these drugs.
• Lifespan: Some antidiarrheals may appear in breast milk; check individual drugs for specific recommendations. For infants younger than age 2, don't give kaolin and pectin mix-

tures. For children or teenagers recovering from flu or chickenpox, consult prescriber before giving bismuth subsalicylate. For elderly patients, use caution when giving antidiarrheal drugs, especially opium preparations.

Adverse reactions

Bismuth preparations may cause salicylism (with high doses) or temporary darkening of tongue and stools. Kaolin and pectin mixtures may cause constipation and fecal impaction or ulceration. Opium preparations may cause dizziness, lightheadedness, nausea, physical dependence (with long-term use), and vomiting.

Action

Bismuth preparations may have a mild water-binding capacity, may absorb toxins, and provide a protective coating for the intestinal mucosa. Kaolin and pectin mixtures decrease fluid in the stool by absorbing bacteria and toxins that cause diarrhea. Opium preparations increase smooth muscle tone in the GI tract, inhibit motility and propulsion, and decrease digestive secretions.

NURSING PROCESS

Assessment
• Assess patient's condition before therapy and regularly thereafter.
• Monitor fluid and electrolyte balance.
• Observe patient for adverse reactions.

Key nursing diagnoses
• Constipation related to adverse effect of bismuth preparations on GI tract
• Risk for injury related to adverse CNS reactions
• Risk for deficient fluid volume related to GI upset

Planning and implementation
• Take safety precautions if patient has adverse CNS reactions.
• Don't substitute opium tincture for paregoric.
• Notify prescriber about serious or persistent adverse reactions.
Patient teaching
• Instruct patient to take drug exactly as prescribed; warn that excessive use of opium preparations can lead to dependence.

• Instruct patient to notify prescriber if diarrhea lasts longer than 2 days and to report adverse reactions.
• Warn patient to avoid hazardous activities that require alertness if CNS depression occurs.

Evaluation
• Patient doesn't develop constipation.
• Patient maintains adequate hydration.

Antihistamines
azelastine hydrochloride
brompheniramine maleate
cyproheptadine hydrochloride
desloratadine
diphenhydramine hydrochloride
fexofenadine hydrochloride
hydroxyzine embonate
hydroxyzine hydrochloride
hydroxyzine pamoate
loratadine
meclizine hydrochloride
promethazine hydrochloride

Indications

▶ Allergic rhinitis, urticaria, pruritus, vertigo, motion sickness, nausea and vomiting, sedation, dyskinesia, parkinsonism.

Contraindications and cautions

• Contraindicated in patients hypersensitive to these drugs and in those with angle-closure glaucoma, stenosing peptic ulcer, pyloroduodenal obstruction, or bladder neck obstruction. Also contraindicated in those taking MAO inhibitors.
Lifespan: In pregnant women, safe use hasn't been established. During breast-feeding, antihistamines shouldn't be used because many of these drugs appear in breast milk and may cause unusual excitability in the infant. Neonates, especially premature infants, may experience seizures. Children, especially those younger than age 6, may experience paradoxical hyperexcitability with restlessness, insomnia, nervousness, euphoria, tremors, and seizures; give cautiously. Elderly patients usually are more sensitive to the adverse effects of antihistamines, especially dizziness, sedation, hy-

potension, and urine retention; use cautiously and monitor these patients closely.

Adverse reactions

Most antihistamines cause drowsiness and impaired motor function early in therapy. They also can cause blurred vision, constipation, and dry mouth and throat. Some antihistamines, such as promethazine, may cause cholestatic jaundice, which may be a hypersensitivity reaction, and may predispose patients to photosensitivity. Promethazine may also cause extrapyramidal reactions with high doses.

Action

Antihistamines are structurally related chemicals that compete with histamine for histamine H_1-receptor sites on smooth muscle of bronchi, GI tract, and large blood vessels, binding to cellular receptors and preventing access to and subsequent activity of histamine. They don't directly alter histamine or prevent its release.

NURSING PROCESS

Assessment
• Monitor patient for adverse reactions.
• Monitor blood counts during long-term therapy; watch for signs of blood dyscrasia.

Key nursing diagnoses
• Risk for injury related to sedation
• Impaired oral mucous membrane related to dry mouth
• Constipation related to anticholinergic effect of antihistamines

Planning and implementation
• Reduce GI distress by giving antihistamines with food.
• Provide sugarless gum, hard candy, or ice chips to relieve dry mouth.
• Increase fluid intake or humidify air to decrease adverse effect of thickened secretions.
Patient teaching
• Advise patient to take drug with meals or snacks to prevent GI upset.
• Suggest that patient use warm water rinses, artificial saliva, ice chips, or sugarless gum or candy to relieve dry mouth. Tell him to avoid overusing mouthwash, which may worsen dryness and destroy normal flora.

• Warn patient to avoid hazardous activities until full CNS effects of drug are known.
• Tell patient to seek medical approval before using alcohol, tranquilizers, sedatives, pain relievers, or sleeping medications.
• For accurate diagnostic skin test results, advise patient to stop taking antihistamines 4 days before test.

Evaluation
• Patient sustains no injury from sedation.
• Patient maintains normal mucous membranes by using preventive measures throughout therapy.
• Patient maintains normal bowel function.

Antihypertensives
Angiotensin-converting enzyme inhibitors
benazepril hydrochloride
captopril
enalapril maleate
enalaprilat
fosinopril sodium
lisinopril
moexipril hydrochloride
perindopril erbumine
quinapril hydrochloride
ramipril
trandolapril
Angiotensin II receptor blockers
candesartan cilexetil
eprosartan mesylate
irbesartan
losartan potassium
olmesartan medoxomil
telmisartan
valsartan
Beta blockers
acebutolol hydrochloride
atenolol
bisoprolol fumarate
carvedilol
labetalol hydrochloride
metoprolol tartrate
nadolol
pindolol
propranolol hydrochloride
timolol maleate

Calcium channel blockers
amlodipine besylate
diltiazem hydrochloride
felodipine
nicardipine hydrochloride
nifedipine
nisoldipine
verapamil hydrochloride

Centrally acting alpha blockers (sympatholytics)
clonidine hydrochloride
guanfacine hydrochloride
methyldopa

Peripherally acting alpha blockers
doxazosin mesylate
prazosin hydrochloride
terazosin hydrochloride

Vasodilators
diazoxide
hydralazine hydrochloride
minoxidil
nitroprusside sodium

Indications

▶ Essential and secondary hypertension.

Contraindications and cautions

• Contraindicated in patients hypersensitive to these drugs and in those with hypotension.
• Use cautiously in patients with hepatic or renal dysfunction.
⚵ Lifespan: In pregnant women, use cautiously when potential benefits to the mother outweigh risks to the fetus. Check each drug because some are safe only in the first trimester. In breast-feeding women, use cautiously; some antihypertensives appear in breast milk. In children, safety and effectiveness of many antihypertensives haven't been established; give these drugs cautiously and monitor children closely. Elderly patients are more susceptible to adverse reactions and may need lower maintenance doses; monitor these patients closely.

Adverse reactions

Antihypertensives commonly cause orthostatic changes in heart rate, headache, hypotension, nausea, and vomiting. Other reactions vary greatly among different drug types. Centrally acting sympatholytics may cause constipation, depression, dizziness, drowsiness, dry mouth, headache, palpitations, severe rebound hyper-

tension, and sexual dysfunction; methyldopa also may cause aplastic anemia and thrombocytopenia. Rauwolfia alkaloids may cause anxiety, depression, drowsiness, dry mouth, hyperacidity, impotence, nasal stuffiness, and weight gain. Vasodilators may cause ECG changes, diarrhea, dizziness, heart failure, palpitations, pruritus, and rash.

Action

For information on the action of ACE inhibitors, alpha blockers, angiotensin II receptor blockers, beta blockers, calcium channel blockers, and diuretics, see their individual drug class entries. Centrally acting sympatholytics stimulate central alpha-adrenergic receptors, reducing cerebral sympathetic outflow, thereby decreasing peripheral vascular resistance and blood pressure. Rauwolfia alkaloids bind to and gradually destroy the norepinephrine-containing storage vesicles in central and peripheral adrenergic neurons. Vasodilators act directly on smooth muscle to reduce blood pressure.

NURSING PROCESS

⚕ Assessment
• Obtain baseline blood pressure and pulse rate and rhythm; recheck regularly.
• Monitor patient for adverse reactions.
• Monitor patient's weight and fluid and electrolyte status.
• Monitor patient's compliance with treatment.

⊞ Key nursing diagnoses
• Risk for trauma related to orthostatic hypotension
• Risk for deficient fluid volume related to GI upset
• Noncompliance related to long-term therapy or adverse reactions

▶ Planning and implementation
• Give drug with food or at bedtime, as indicated.
• When mixing and giving parenteral drugs, follow manufacturer's guidelines.
• Take steps to prevent or minimize orthostatic hypotension.
• Maintain patient's nondrug therapy, such as sodium restriction, calorie reduction, stress management, and exercise program.

Patient teaching
• Instruct patient to take drug exactly as prescribed. Warn against stopping drug abruptly.
• Review adverse reactions caused by drug, and urge patient to notify prescriber of serious or persistent reactions.
• To prevent dizziness, lightheadedness, or fainting, advise patient to avoid sudden changes in position.
• Warn patient to avoid hazardous activities until full effects of drug are known. Also, warn patient to avoid physical exertion, especially in hot weather.
• Advise patient to consult prescriber before taking any OTC medications or herbal remedies; serious drug interactions can occur.
• Encourage patient to comply with therapy.

☑ Evaluation
• Patient doesn't experience trauma from orthostatic hypotension.
• Patient maintains adequate hydration.
• Patient complies with therapy, as shown by normal blood pressure.

Antilipemics

atorvastatin calcium
cholestyramine
colesevelam hydrochloride
ezetimibe
fenofibrate
fluvastatin sodium
gemfibrozil
lovastatin
pravastatin sodium
rosuvastatin calcium
simvastatin

Indications

▶ Hyperlipidemia, hypercholesterolemia.

Contraindications and cautions

• Contraindicated in patients hypersensitive to these drugs. Also, bile-sequestering drugs are contraindicated in patients with complete biliary obstruction. Fibric acid derivatives are contraindicated in patients with primary biliary cirrhosis or significant hepatic or renal dysfunction. HMG-CoA reductase inhibitors and cho-

lesterol absorption inhibitors are contraindicated in patients with active liver disease or persistently elevated transaminase levels.
• Use bile-sequestering drugs cautiously in constipated patients. Use fibric acid derivatives cautiously in patients with peptic ulcer. Use HMG-CoA inhibitors cautiously in patients who consume large amounts of alcohol or who have a history of liver or renal disease.
⚖ Lifespan: In pregnant women, use bile-sequestering drugs and fibric acid derivatives cautiously and avoid using HMG-CoA inhibitors. In breast-feeding women, avoid using fibric acid derivatives and HMG-CoA inhibitors; give bile-sequestering drugs cautiously. In children ages 10 to 17, certain antilipemics have been approved to treat heterozygous familial hypercholesterolemia. Elderly patients have an increased risk of severe constipation; use bile-sequestering drugs cautiously and monitor patients closely.

Adverse reactions

Antilipemics commonly cause GI upset. Bile-sequestering drugs may cause bloating, cholelithiasis, constipation, and steatorrhea. Fibric acid derivatives may cause cholelithiasis and have other GI or CNS effects. Use of gemfibrozil with lovastatin may cause myopathy. HMG-CoA reductase inhibitors may affect liver function or cause rash, pruritus, increased CK levels, rhabdomyolysis, and myopathy.

Action

Antilipemics lower elevated lipid levels. Bile-sequestering drugs (cholestyramine and colesevelam) lower LDL level by forming insoluble complexes with bile salts, thus triggering cholesterol to leave the bloodstream and other storage areas to make new bile acids. Fibric acid derivatives (gemfibrozil) reduce cholesterol formation, increase sterol excretion, and decrease lipoprotein and triglyceride synthesis. HMG-CoA reductase inhibitors (atorvastatin, fluvastatin, lovastatin, pravastatin, rosuvastatin, simvastatin) interfere with the activity of enzymes that generate cholesterol in the liver. Selective cholesterol absorption inhibitors (ezetimibe) inhibit cholesterol absorption by the small intestine, reducing hepatic cholesterol stores and increasing cholesterol clearance from the blood.

⚕ Assessment
- Monitor fasting lipid profile, CK, and liver enzymes before and periodically during therapy.
- Check CK level in a patient who complains of muscle pain or muscle weakness.
- Monitor patient for adverse reactions.
- Watch for potential interactions with other drugs.

⊕ Key nursing diagnoses
- Risk for deficient fluid volume related to adverse GI reactions
- Constipation related to adverse effect on bowel
- Noncompliance related to long-term therapy

➤ Planning and implementation
- Mix powder form of bile-sequestering drugs with 120 to 180 ml of liquid. Never give dry powder alone because patient may inhale it accidentally.
- Give lovastatin with evening meal, simvastatin in the evening, and fluvastatin and pravastatin at bedtime.

Patient teaching
- Instruct patient to take drug exactly as prescribed. If he takes a bile-sequestering drug, warn him never to take the dry form.
- Stress importance of diet in controlling lipid levels.
- Advise patient to maintain adequate fluid intake and to report persistent or severe constipation.

☑ Evaluation
- Patient maintains adequate fluid volume.
- Patient doesn't experience severe or persistent constipation.
- Patient complies with therapy, as shown by normal lipid and cholesterol levels.

Antimetabolite antineoplastics
capecitabine
cytarabine
cytarabine liposomal
fludarabine phosphate
fluorouracil
hydroxyurea
mercaptopurine

methotrexate
pentostatin
thioguanine

Indications
▶ Various tumors and hematologic conditions.

Contraindications and cautions
- Contraindicated in patients hypersensitive to these drugs.
- **⚘ Lifespan:** Pregnant women should be informed of the risks to the fetus. Breast-feeding isn't recommended for women taking these drugs. In children, safety and effectiveness of some drugs haven't been established; use cautiously. Elderly patients have an increased risk of adverse reactions; monitor them closely.

Adverse reactions
The most common adverse effects include anxiety, bone marrow depression (anemia, leukopenia, thrombocytopenia), chills, diarrhea, fever, flank or joint pain, hair loss, nausea, redness or pain at injection site, stomatitis, swelling of the feet or lower legs, and vomiting.

Action
Antimetabolites are structurally similar to naturally occurring metabolites and can be divided into three subcategories: purine, pyrimidine, and folinic acid analogues. Most of these drugs interrupt cell reproduction at a specific phase of the cell cycle. Purine analogues are incorporated into DNA and RNA, interfering with nucleic acid synthesis (by miscoding) and replication. They also may inhibit synthesis of purine bases through pseudofeedback mechanisms. Pyrimidine analogues inhibit enzymes in metabolic pathways that interfere with biosynthesis of uridine and thymine. Folic acid antagonists prevent conversion of folic acid to tetrahydrofolate by inhibiting the enzyme dihydrofolic acid reductase.

⚕ Assessment
- Perform a complete assessment before therapy begins.
- Monitor patient for adverse reactions.
- Monitor vital signs and patency of catheter or I.V. line throughout administration.

• Monitor platelet and total and differential leukocyte counts, hematocrit, and ALT, AST, LDH, bilirubin, creatinine, uric acid, and BUN levels.

Key nursing diagnoses
• Ineffective protection related to thrombocytopenia
• Risk for infection related to immunosuppression
• Risk for deficient fluid volume related to adverse GI effects

Planning and implementation
• Follow established procedures for safe and proper handling, administration, and disposal of drugs.
• Try to ease patient's and family's anxiety before treatment.
• Give an antiemetic to reduce nausea before giving drug.
• Anticipate tumor lysis syndrome in treatment-sensitive, bulky disease with allopurinol and urine alkalinization. Encourage patient to drink plenty of fluids.
• Provide diligent mouth care to prevent stomatitis with cytarabine, fluorouracil, capecitabine, or methotrexate therapy.
• Anticipate the need for leucovorin rescue with high-dose methotrexate therapy.
• Treat extravasation promptly.
• Anticipate diarrhea, possibly severe, with prolonged fluorouracil and capecitabine therapy.
Patient teaching
• Teach patient proper oral hygiene, including cautious use of toothbrush, dental floss, and toothpicks. Chemotherapy can increase the incidence of microbial infection, delayed healing, and bleeding gums.
• Advise patient to complete dental work before therapy begins or to delay it until blood counts are normal.
• Tell patient to defer immunizations, if possible, until hematologic stability is confirmed.
• Warn patient that he may bruise easily because of drug's effect on platelets.
• Advise patient to avoid close contact with people who have taken oral poliovirus vaccine or who have been exposed to people with bacterial or viral infection because chemotherapy may increase susceptibility. Urge patient to notify prescriber promptly if he develops signs or symptoms of infection.

• Instruct patient to report redness, pain, or swelling at injection site. Local tissue injury and scarring may result from tissue infiltration at infusion site.
• Educate patient on potential toxicities of capecitabine and when to hold doses.
• Tell patient to contact prescriber if he becomes febrile.

Evaluation
• Patient doesn't have serious bleeding complications.
• Patient doesn't have an infection.
• Patient maintains adequate hydration.

Antiparkinsonians
amantadine hydrochloride
apomorphine hydrochloride
benztropine mesylate
bromocriptine mesylate
diphenhydramine hydrochloride
entacapone
levodopa
levodopa and carbidopa
levodopa, carbidopa, and entacapone
pergolide mesylate
pramipexole dihydrochloride
ropinirole hydrochloride
selegiline hydrochloride
tolcapone
trihexyphenidyl hydrochloride

Indications

▶ Signs and symptoms of Parkinson disease and drug-induced extrapyramidal reactions.

Contraindications and cautions

• Contraindicated in patients hypersensitive to these drugs.
• Use cautiously in patients with prostatic hyperplasia or tardive dyskinesia and in debilitated patients.
• Neuroleptic malignant–like syndrome involving muscle rigidity, increased body temperature, and mental status changes may occur with abrupt withdrawal of antiparkinsonians.
⚠ Lifespan: In pregnant women, safe use hasn't been established. Antiparkinsonians may appear in breast milk; a decision should be

made to stop the drug or stop breast-feeding, taking into account the importance of the drug to the mother. In children, safety and effectiveness haven't been established. Elderly patients have an increased risk for adverse reactions; monitor them closely.

Adverse reactions

Anticholinergics may cause blurred vision, cycloplegia, constipation, decreased sweating or anhidrosis, dry mouth, headache, mydriasis, palpitations, tachycardia, and urinary hesitancy and urine retention. Dopaminergics may cause arrhythmias, confusion, disturbing dreams, dystonias, hallucinations, headache, muscle cramps, nausea, orthostatic hypotension, and vomiting. Amantadine also causes irritability, insomnia, and livedo reticularis (with prolonged use).

Action

Antiparkinsonians include synthetic anticholinergics, dopaminergics, and the antiviral amantadine. Anticholinergics probably prolong the action of dopamine by blocking its reuptake into presynaptic neurons and by suppressing central cholinergic activity. Dopaminergics act in the brain by increasing dopamine availability, thus improving motor function. Entacapone is a reversible inhibitor of peripheral catechol-*O*-methyltransferase (commonly known as COMT), which is responsible for elimination of various catecholamines, including dopamine. Blocking this pathway when giving levodopa and carbidopa should result in higher levels of levodopa, thereby allowing greater dopaminergic stimulation in the CNS and leading to a greater effect in treating parkinsonian symptoms. Amantadine is thought to increase dopamine release in the substantia nigra.

NURSING PROCESS

Assessment
• Obtain baseline assessment of patient's impairment, and reassess regularly to monitor the drug's effectiveness.
• Monitor patient for adverse reactions.
• Monitor vital signs, especially during dosage adjustments.

Key nursing diagnoses
• Risk for injury related to adverse CNS effects

• Urinary retention related to anticholinergic effect on bladder
• Sleep disturbance related to amantadine-induced insomnia

Planning and implementation
• Give drug with food to prevent GI irritation.
• Adjust dosage according to patient's response and tolerance.
• Never withdraw drug abruptly.
• Institute safety precautions.
• Provide ice chips, drinks, or sugarless hard candy or gum to relieve dry mouth. Increase fluid and fiber intake to prevent constipation, as appropriate.
• Notify prescriber about urine retention, and be prepared to catheterize patient, if needed.

Patient teaching
• Instruct patient to take drug exactly as prescribed, and warn him not to suddenly stop taking the drug.
• Advise patient to take drug with food to prevent GI upset.
• Teach patient how to manage anticholinergic effects.
• Instruct patient to avoid hazardous tasks if adverse CNS effects occur. Tell him to avoid alcohol during therapy.
• Encourage patient to report severe or persistent adverse reactions.

Evaluation
• Patient remains free from injury.
• Patient's voiding pattern doesn't change.
• Patient's sleep pattern isn't altered by amantadine.

Barbiturates

amobarbital sodium
pentobarbital sodium
phenobarbital
phenobarbital sodium
primidone
secobarbital sodium

Indications

▶ Sedation, preanesthetic, short-term treatment of insomnia, seizure disorders.

Contraindications and cautions

• Contraindicated in patients hypersensitive to these drugs and in those with bronchopneumonia, other severe pulmonary insufficiency, or liver dysfunction.

• Use cautiously in patients with blood pressure alterations, pulmonary disease, and CV dysfunction. Use cautiously, if at all, in patients who are depressed or have suicidal tendencies.

⚖ **Lifespan:** Barbiturates can cause fetal abnormalities; avoid use in pregnant women. Barbiturates appear in breast milk and may result in infant CNS depression; use cautiously. Premature infants are more susceptible to depressant effects of barbiturates because of their immature hepatic metabolism. Children may experience hyperactivity, excitement, or hyperalgesia; use cautiously and monitor closely. Elderly patients may experience hyperactivity, excitement, or hyperalgesia; use cautiously.

Adverse reactions

CNS depression, drowsiness, headache, lethargy, and vertigo are common with barbiturates. After hypnotic doses, a hangover effect, subtle distortion of mood, and impaired judgment and motor skills may continue for many hours. After dosage reduction or discontinuation, rebound insomnia or increased dreaming or nightmares may occur. Barbiturates cause hyperalgesia in subhypnotic doses. They can also cause paradoxical excitement at low doses, confusion in elderly patients, and hyperactivity in children. High fever, severe headache, stomatitis, conjunctivitis, or rhinitis may precede potentially fatal skin eruptions. Withdrawal symptoms may occur after as little as 2 weeks of uninterrupted therapy.

Action

Barbiturates act throughout the CNS, especially in the mesencephalic reticular activating system, which controls the CNS arousal mechanism. The main anticonvulsant actions are reduced nerve transmission and decreased excitability of the nerve cell. Barbiturates decrease presynaptic and postsynaptic membrane excitability by promoting the actions of GABA. They also depress respiration and GI motility and raise the seizure threshold.

NURSING PROCESS

🕭 Assessment

• To evaluate the drug's effectiveness, assess patient's level of consciousness and sleeping patterns before and during therapy. Monitor neurologic status for alteration or deterioration.

• Assess vital signs often, especially during I.V. use.

• Monitor seizure character, frequency, and duration for changes.

• Observe patient to prevent hoarding and taking extra doses, especially if patient is depressed, suicidal, or drug dependent.

🕭 Key nursing diagnoses

• Risk for injury related to sedation

• Disturbed thought processes related to confusion

• Risk-prone health behavior related to drug dependence

▷ Planning and implementation

• When giving parenteral drug, inject I.V. or deep I.M., to avoid extravasation, which may cause local tissue damage and tissue necrosis. To avoid tissue damage, don't exceed 5 ml for any I.M. injection site.

• Keep resuscitative measures available. Giving I.V. drug too rapidly may cause respiratory depression, apnea, laryngospasm, or hypotension.

• Take seizure precautions as needed.

• Take precautions to prevent falls and injury. Raise side rails, help patient out of bed, and keep call light within easy reach.

• Stop drug slowly. Stopping drug abruptly may cause withdrawal symptoms.

Patient teaching

• Explain that barbiturates can cause physical or psychological dependence.

• Instruct patient to take drug exactly as prescribed. Warn him not to change the dosage or take other drugs, including OTC medications or herbal remedies, without prescriber's approval.

• Reassure patient that a morning hangover is common after therapeutic use of barbiturates.

• Advise patient to avoid hazardous tasks, driving a motor vehicle, or operating machinery while taking the drug, and to review other safety measures to prevent injury.

• Instruct patient to report skin eruptions or other significant adverse effects.

☑ Evaluation
- Patient sustains no injury from sedation.
- Patient maintains normal thought processes.
- Patient doesn't develop physical or psychological dependence.

Benzodiazepines

alprazolam
chlordiazepoxide hydrochloride
clonazepam
clorazepate dipotassium
diazepam
estazolam
flurazepam hydrochloride
lorazepam
midazolam hydrochloride
oxazepam
quazepam
temazepam
triazolam

Indications

▶ Seizure disorders (clonazepam, clorazepate, diazepam, midazolam, parenteral lorazepam); anxiety, tension, and insomnia (chlordiazepoxide, clorazepate, diazepam, estazolam, flurazepam, lorazepam, oxazepam, quazepam, temazepam, triazolam); conscious sedation or amnesia in surgery (diazepam, lorazepam, midazolam); skeletal muscle spasm and tremor (oral forms of chlordiazepoxide and diazepam); delirium.

Contraindications and cautions

- Contraindicated in patients hypersensitive to these drugs, in those with acute angle-closure glaucoma, and in those with depressive neuroses or psychotic reactions in which anxiety isn't prominent.
- Avoid use in patients with suicidal tendencies and patients with a history of drug abuse.
- Use cautiously in patients with chronic pulmonary insufficiency or sleep apnea and in those with hepatic or renal insufficiency.
- ⚖ Lifespan: In pregnant patients, benzodiazepines increase the risk of congenital malformation if taken in the first trimester. Use during labor may cause neonatal flaccidity. A neonate whose mother took a benzodiazepine during

pregnancy may have withdrawal symptoms. In breast-feeding mothers, benzodiazepines may cause sedation, feeding difficulties, and weight loss in the infant. In children, use caution; they're especially sensitive to CNS depressant effects. In elderly patients, benzodiazepine elimination may be prolonged; consider a lower dosage.

Adverse reactions

Therapeutic dose may cause drowsiness, impaired motor function, constipation, diarrhea, vomiting, altered appetite, urinary changes, visual disturbances, and CV irregularities. Toxic dose may cause continuing problems with short-term memory, confusion, severe depression, shakiness, vertigo, slurred speech, staggering, bradycardia, shortness of breath, difficulty breathing, or severe weakness. Prolonged or frequent use of benzodiazepines can cause physical dependency and withdrawal syndrome when drug is stopped.

Action

Benzodiazepines act selectively on polysynaptic neuronal pathways throughout the CNS. Precise sites and mechanisms of action aren't fully known. However, benzodiazepines enhance or facilitate the action of GABA, an inhibitory neurotransmitter in the CNS. These drugs appear to act at the limbic, thalamic, and hypothalamic levels of the CNS to produce anxiolytic, sedative, hypnotic, skeletal muscle relaxant, and anticonvulsant effects.

NURSING PROCESS

🕮 Assessment
- Assess level of consciousness and neurologic status before therapy and often during therapy. Monitor patient for paradoxical reactions, especially early in therapy.
- Observe sleep patterns and quality, and watch for changes in seizure character, frequency, or duration.
- Assess vital signs often during therapy. Significant changes in blood pressure and heart rate may indicate impending toxicity.

🔅 Key nursing diagnoses
- Anxiety related to underlying condition
- Risk for injury related to drug-induced CNS effects

• Decreased cardiac output related to hypotension

▶ Planning and implementation
• Don't use benzodiazepines in patients with chronic pulmonary insufficiency, sleep apnea, depressive neuroses or psychotic reactions without predominant anxiety, or acute alcohol intoxication.
• Give dose with milk or just after a meal to prevent GI upset. Give antacid, if needed, at least 1 hour before or after dose to prevent interaction and ensure maximum drug absorption and effectiveness.
• Periodically monitor renal and hepatic function to ensure adequate drug removal and prevent cumulative effects.
• Institute safety measures—raised side rails and ambulatory assistance—to prevent injury. Anticipate possible rebound excitement.
• After prolonged use, stopping drug abruptly may cause withdrawal symptoms; instead, taper gradually.
Patient teaching
• To prevent additive depressant effects, caution patient to avoid use of alcohol or other CNS depressants, such as antihistamines, analgesics, MAO inhibitors, antidepressants, and barbiturates.
• Caution patient to take drug as prescribed and not to give drug to others. Tell him not to change the dose or frequency and to call before taking OTC cold or allergy medicines because they may worsen CNS depressant effects.
• Warn patient to avoid activities requiring alertness and good psychomotor coordination until the CNS response to the drug is determined. Instruct him in safety measures to prevent injury.
• Tell patient to avoid using antacids, which may delay drug absorption, unless prescribed.
• Make sure patient understands that benzodiazepines may cause physical and psychological dependence with prolonged use.
• Warn patient not to stop taking the drug abruptly to prevent withdrawal symptoms after prolonged therapy.
• Tell patient that smoking decreases drug effectiveness. Encourage patient to stop smoking during therapy.
• Tell patient to report adverse reactions. These are often dose-related and can be relieved by dosage adjustments.

• Inform a woman of childbearing age to contact prescriber if she suspects pregnancy or intends to become pregnant during therapy.

☑ Evaluation
• Patient is less anxious.
• Patient sustains no injury from drug-induced CNS reactions.
• Patient's blood pressure stays within normal limits.

Beta blockers
Beta₁ blockers
acebutolol hydrochloride
atenolol
betaxolol
bisoprolol fumarate
esmolol hydrochloride
metoprolol tartrate
Beta₁ and beta₂ blockers
carvedilol
labetalol hydrochloride
nadolol
pindolol
propranolol hydrochloride
sotalol hydrochloride
timolol maleate

Indications

▶ Hypertension (most drugs), angina pectoris (atenolol, metoprolol, nadolol, and propranolol), arrhythmias (acebutolol hydrochloride, esmolol, propranolol, and sotalol), glaucoma (betaxolol and timolol), prevention of MI (atenolol, metoprolol, propranolol, and timolol), prevention of recurrent migraine and other vascular headaches (propranolol and timolol), pheochromocytomas or essential tremors (selected drugs), heart failure (atenolol, bisoprolol, carvedilol, metoprolol).

Contraindications and cautions

• Contraindicated in patients hypersensitive to these drugs and in patients with cardiogenic shock, sinus bradycardia, heart block greater than first degree, and bronchial asthma.
• Use cautiously in patients with nonallergic bronchospastic disorders, diabetes mellitus, im-

paired hepatic or renal function, and congestive heart failure.

☀ Lifespan: In pregnant women, use cautiously. Drugs appear in breast milk. In children, safety and effectiveness haven't been established; use only if the benefits outweigh the risks. In elderly patients, use cautiously; these patients may need reduced maintenance doses because of increased bioavailability, delayed metabolism, and increased adverse effects.

Adverse reactions

Therapeutic dose may cause bradycardia, dizziness, and fatigue; some may cause other CNS disturbances, such as depression, hallucinations, memory loss, and nightmares. Toxic dose can produce severe hypotension, bradycardia, heart failure, or bronchospasm.

Action

Beta blockers compete with beta agonists for available beta receptors; individual drugs differ in their ability to affect beta receptors. Some drugs are nonselective: they block beta$_1$ receptors in cardiac muscle and beta$_2$ receptors in bronchial and vascular smooth muscle. Several drugs are cardioselective and, in lower doses, inhibit mainly beta$_1$ receptors. Some beta blockers have intrinsic sympathomimetic activity and stimulate and block beta receptors. Others stabilize cardiac membranes, which affects cardiac action potential.

NURSING PROCESS

℞ Assessment
• Check apical pulse rate daily; alert prescriber about extremes, such as a pulse rate lower than 60 beats/minute.
• Monitor blood pressure, ECG, and heart rate and rhythm frequently; be alert for progression of AV block or bradycardia.
• If patient has heart failure, weigh him regularly; watch for weight gain of more than 2.25 kg (5 lb) per week.
• Observe diabetic patients for sweating, fatigue, and hunger. Signs of hypoglycemic shock may be masked.

Key nursing diagnoses
• Risk for injury related to adverse CNS effects
• Excessive fluid volume related to edema

• Decreased cardiac output related to bradycardia or hypotension

▷ Planning and implementation
• Stop beta blockers before surgery for pheochromocytoma. Before any surgical procedure, notify anesthesiologist that patient is taking a beta blocker.

Patient teaching
• Teach patient to take drug exactly as prescribed, even when he feels better.
• Warn patient not to stop taking the drug suddenly. Stopping suddenly can worsen angina or precipitate MI.
• Tell patient not to take OTC medications or herbal remedies without prescriber's approval.
• Explain potential adverse reactions, and stress importance of reporting unusual effects.

✓ Evaluation
• Patient remains free from injury.
• Patient has no signs of edema.
• Patient maintains normal blood pressure and heart rate.

Calcium channel blockers

amlodipine besylate
diltiazem hydrochloride
felodipine
nicardipine hydrochloride
nifedipine
nisoldipine
verapamil hydrochloride

Indications

▶ Prinzmetal variant angina, chronic stable angina, unstable angina, mild-to-moderate hypertension, arrhythmias.

Contraindications and cautions

• Contraindicated in patients hypersensitive to these drugs and in those with second- or third-degree heart block (except those with a pacemaker) and cardiogenic shock. Use diltiazem and verapamil cautiously in patients with heart failure.

☀ Lifespan: In pregnant women, use cautiously. Calcium channel blockers may appear in breast milk; instruct patient to stop breast-

feeding during therapy. In neonates and infants, adverse hemodynamic effects of parenteral verapamil are possible, but safety and effectiveness of other calcium channel blockers haven't been established; avoid use, if possible. In elderly patients, the half-life of calcium channel blockers may be increased as a result of decreased clearance; use cautiously.

Adverse reactions

Verapamil may cause bradycardia, hypotension, various degrees of heart block, and worsening of heart failure after rapid I.V. delivery. Prolonged oral verapamil therapy may cause constipation. Nifedipine may cause flushing, headache, heartburn, hypotension, lightheadedness, and peripheral edema. The most common adverse reactions with diltiazem are anorexia and nausea; it also may induce bradycardia, heart failure, peripheral edema, and various degrees of heart block.

Action

The main physiologic action of calcium channel blockers is to inhibit calcium influx across the slow channels of myocardial and vascular smooth muscle cells. By inhibiting calcium flow into these cells, calcium channel blockers reduce intracellular calcium levels. This, in turn, dilates coronary arteries, peripheral arteries, and arterioles and slows cardiac conduction.

When used to treat Prinzmetal variant angina, calcium channel blockers inhibit coronary spasm, which then increases oxygen delivery to the heart. Peripheral artery dilation reduces afterload, which decreases myocardial oxygen use. Inhibiting calcium flow into specialized cardiac conduction cells in the SA and AV nodes slows conduction through the heart. Verapamil and diltiazem have the greatest effect on the AV node, which slows the ventricular rate in atrial fibrillation or flutter and converts supraventricular tachycardia to a normal sinus rhythm.

NURSING PROCESS

Assessment
• Monitor cardiac rate and rhythm and blood pressure carefully when therapy starts or dosage increases.
• Monitor fluids and electrolytes.
• Monitor patient for adverse reactions.

Key nursing diagnoses
• Decreased cardiac output related to adverse CV reactions
• Constipation related to oral verapamil therapy
• Noncompliance related to long-term therapy

Planning and implementation
• Don't give calcium supplements while patient is taking a calcium channel blocker; they may decrease the drug's effectiveness.
• Expect to decrease dosage gradually; don't stop calcium channel blockers abruptly.
Patient teaching
• Teach patient to take drug exactly as prescribed, even if he feels better.
• Instruct patient to take a missed dose as soon as possible, unless it's almost time for his next dose. Warn him never to take a double dose.
• Warn patient not to stop drug suddenly; abrupt discontinuation can produce serious adverse effects.
• Urge patient to report irregular heartbeat, shortness of breath, swelling of hands and feet, pronounced dizziness, constipation, nausea, or hypotension.

Evaluation
• Patient maintains adequate cardiac output throughout therapy, as shown by normal blood pressure and pulse rate.
• Patient regains normal bowel pattern.
• Patient complies with therapy, as shown by absence of symptoms related to disorder.

Cephalosporins
First generation
cefadroxil monohydrate
cefazolin sodium
cephalexin monohydrate
Second generation
cefaclor
cefoxitin sodium
cefprozil
cefuroxime axetil
cefuroxime sodium
Third generation
cefdinir
cefditoren pivoxil
cefixime

cefoperazone sodium
cefotaxime sodium
cefpodoxime proxetil
ceftazidime
ceftibuten
ceftizoxime sodium
ceftriaxone sodium

Indications

▶ Infections of the lungs, skin, soft tissue, bones, joints, urinary and respiratory tracts, blood, abdomen, and heart; CNS infections caused by susceptible strains of *Neisseria meningitidis, Haemophilus influenzae,* and *Streptococcus pneumoniae;* meningitis caused by *Escherichia coli* or *Klebsiella;* infections that develop after surgical procedures classified as contaminated or potentially contaminated; penicillinase-producing *Neisseria gonorrhoeae;* otitis media and ampicillin-resistant middle ear infection caused by *H. influenzae.*

Contraindications and cautions

• Contraindicated in patients hypersensitive to these drugs.
• Use cautiously in patients with renal or hepatic impairment, history of GI disease, or allergy to penicillins.
⚖ Lifespan: In pregnant women, use cautiously; safety hasn't been definitively established. In breast-feeding women, use cautiously because drugs appear in breast milk. In neonates and infants, half-life is prolonged; use cautiously. Elderly patients are susceptible to superinfection and coagulopathies, commonly have renal impairment, and may need a lower dosage; use cautiously.

Adverse reactions

Many cephalosporins have similar adverse effects. Hypersensitivity reactions range from mild rashes, fever, and eosinophilia to fatal anaphylaxis and are more common in patients with penicillin allergy. Adverse GI reactions include abdominal pain, diarrhea, dyspepsia, glossitis, nausea, tenesmus, and vomiting. Hematologic reactions include positive direct and indirect antiglobulin in Coombs' test, thrombocytopenia or thrombocythemia, transient neutropenia, and reversible leukopenia. Minimal elevation of liver function test results occurs occasionally. Adverse renal effects may occur with any cephalo-

sporin; they are most common in older patients, those with decreased renal function, and those taking other nephrotoxic drugs.
Local venous pain and irritation are common after I.M. injection; these reactions occur more often with higher doses and long-term therapy. Bacterial and fungal superinfections may result from suppression of normal flora.

Action

Cephalosporins are chemically and pharmacologically similar to penicillin; they act by inhibiting bacterial cell wall synthesis, causing rapid cell destruction. Their sites of action are enzymes known as penicillin-binding proteins. The affinity of certain cephalosporins for these proteins in various microorganisms helps explain the differing actions of these drugs. They are bactericidal: they act against many aerobic gram-positive and gram-negative bacteria and some anaerobic bacteria but don't kill fungi or viruses.
First-generation cephalosporins act against many gram-positive cocci, including penicillinase-producing *Staphylococcus aureus* and *Staphylococcus epidermidis, S. pneumoniae,* group B streptococci, and group A beta-hemolytic streptococci. Susceptible gram-negative organisms include *Klebsiella pneumoniae, E. coli, Proteus mirabilis,* and *Shigella.*
Second-generation cephalosporins are effective against all organisms attacked by first-generation drugs and have additional activity against *Moraxella catarrhalis, H. influenzae, Enterobacter, Citrobacter, Providencia, Acinetobacter, Serratia,* and *Neisseria. Bacteroides fragilis* are susceptible to cefoxitin.
Third-generation cephalosporins are less active than first- and second-generation drugs against gram-positive bacteria but are more active against gram-negative organisms, including those resistant to first- and second-generation drugs. They have the greatest stability against beta-lactamases produced by gram-negative bacteria. Susceptible gram-negative organisms include *E. coli, Klebsiella, Enterobacter, Providencia, Acinetobacter, Serratia, Proteus, Morganella,* and *Neisseria.* Some third-generation drugs are active against *B. fragilis* and *Pseudomonas.*

NURSING PROCESS

Assessment

• Review patient's history of allergies. Try to determine whether any previous reactions were true hypersensitivity reactions or adverse effects (such as GI distress) that patient interpreted as allergy.

• Monitor patient continuously for possible hypersensitivity reactions or other adverse effects.

• Obtain culture and sensitivity specimen before giving first dose; check test results periodically to assess drug's effectiveness.

• Monitor renal function study; dosage of certain cephalosporins must be lowered in a patient with severe renal impairment. In patient with decreased renal function, monitor BUN and creatinine levels and urine output for significant changes.

• Monitor PT and platelet count, and assess patient for signs of hypoprothrombinemia, which may occur, with or without bleeding, during therapy with cefoperazone or ceftriaxone. It usually occurs in elderly, debilitated, malnourished, or immunocompromised patients and in patients with renal impairment or impaired vitamin K synthesis.

• Monitor patient receiving long-term therapy for possible bacterial and fungal superinfection; this is especially problematic in elderly or debilitated patients and in those receiving immunosuppressants or radiation therapy.

• Monitor at-risk patients for fluid retention while they are taking sodium salts of cephalosporins.

Key nursing diagnoses

• Ineffective protection related to hypersensitivity

• Risk for infection related to superinfection

• Risk for deficient fluid volume related to adverse GI reactions

Planning and implementation

• Give these drugs at least 1 hour before bacteriostatic antibiotics, such as tetracyclines, erythromycin, and chloramphenicol; the antibiotics keep bacteria from growing by decreasing cephalosporin uptake by bacterial cell walls.

• Refrigerate oral suspensions, which are stable for 14 days; to ensure correct dosage, shake well before giving.

• Give I.M. dose deep into gluteal muscle mass or midlateral thigh; rotate injection sites to minimize tissue injury.

• Don't add or mix other drugs with I.V. infusions, particularly aminoglycosides, which will be inactivated if mixed with cephalosporins. If other drugs must be given I.V., temporarily stop infusion of primary drug.

• Ensure adequate dilution of I.V. infusion and rotate site every 48 hours to help minimize local vein irritation; using a small-gauge needle in a larger available vein may be helpful.

Patient teaching

• Make sure patient understands how and when to take drug. Urge him to comply with instructions for around-the-clock dosage and to complete the prescribed regimen.

• Advise patient to take oral drug with food if GI irritation occurs.

• Review proper storage and disposal of drug, and remind him to check expiration date.

• Teach signs and symptoms of hypersensitivity and other adverse reactions, and emphasize importance of reporting unusual effects.

• Teach signs and symptoms of bacterial and fungal superinfection, especially if patient is elderly or debilitated or has low resistance from immunosuppressants or irradiation. Emphasize importance of promptly reporting signs or symptoms.

• Warn patient not to ingest alcohol in any form within 3 days of treatment with cefoperazone.

• Advise patient to add yogurt or buttermilk to diet to prevent intestinal superinfection resulting from suppression of normal intestinal flora.

• Advise diabetic patient to monitor glucose level with Diastix, not Clinitest.

• Urge patient to keep follow-up appointments.

Evaluation

• Patient has no evidence of hypersensitivity.

• Patient is free from infection.

• Patient maintains adequate hydration.

Corticosteroids

betamethasone
betamethasone sodium phosphate
cortisone acetate
dexamethasone
dexamethasone acetate

dexamethasone sodium phosphate
fludrocortisone acetate
hydrocortisone
hydrocortisone acetate
hydrocortisone cypionate
hydrocortisone sodium phosphate
hydrocortisone sodium succinate
methylprednisolone
methylprednisolone acetate
methylprednisolone sodium succinate
prednisolone
prednisolone acetate
prednisolone sodium phosphate
prednisolone tebutate
prednisone
triamcinolone

Indications

▶ Hypersensitivity; inflammation, particularly of eye, nose, and respiratory tract; to initiate immunosuppression; replacement therapy in adrenocortical insufficiency, dermatologic diseases, respiratory disorders, rheumatic disorders.

Contraindications and cautions

• Contraindicated in patients hypersensitive to these drugs or any of their components and in those with systemic fungal infection.
• Use cautiously in patients with GI ulceration, renal disease, hypertension, osteoporosis, varicella, vaccinia, exanthema, diabetes mellitus, hypothyroidism, thromboembolic disorder, seizures, myasthenia gravis, heart failure, tuberculosis, ocular herpes simplex, hypoalbuminemia, emotional instability, or psychosis.
≋ Lifespan: In pregnant women, avoid use, if possible, because of risk to the fetus. Women should stop breast-feeding because these drugs appear in breast milk and could cause serious adverse effects in infants. In children, long-term use should be avoided whenever possible because stunted growth may result. Elderly patients may have an increased risk of adverse reactions; monitor them closely.

Adverse reactions

Systemic corticosteroid therapy may suppress the hypothalamic-pituitary-adrenal (HPA) axis. Excessive use may cause cushingoid symptoms and various systemic disorders, such as diabetes and osteoporosis. Other effects may include

dermatologic disorders, edema, euphoria, fluid and electrolyte imbalances, gastritis or GI irritation, hypertension, immunosuppression, increased appetite, insomnia, psychosis, and weight gain.

Action

Corticosteroids suppress cell-mediated and humoral immunity by reducing levels of leukocytes, monocytes, and eosinophils; by decreasing immunoglobulin binding to cell-surface receptors; and by inhibiting interleukin synthesis. They reduce inflammation by preventing hydrolytic enzyme release into the cells, preventing plasma exudation, suppressing polymorphonuclear leukocyte migration, and disrupting other inflammatory processes.

NURSING PROCESS

▨ **Assessment**
• Establish baseline blood pressure, fluid and electrolyte status, and weight; reassess regularly.
• Monitor patient closely for adverse reactions.
• Evaluate drug effectiveness at regular intervals.

▨ **Key nursing diagnoses**
• Ineffective protection related to suppression of HPA axis with long-term therapy
• Risk for injury related to severe adverse reactions
• Risk for infection related to immunosuppression

▨ **Planning and implementation**
• Give drug early in the day to mimic circadian rhythm.
• Give drug with food to prevent GI irritation.
• Take precautions to avoid exposing patient to infection.
• Don't stop drug abruptly.
• Notify prescriber of severe or persistent adverse reactions.
• Avoid prolonged use of corticosteroids, especially in children.
Patient teaching
• Teach patient to take drug exactly as prescribed, and warn him never to stop it abruptly.
• Tell patient to notify prescriber if stress level increases; dosage may need to be temporarily increased.
• Instruct patient to take oral drug with food.

• Urge patient to report black tarry stools, bleeding, bruising, blurred vision, emotional changes, or other concerns.
• Encourage patient to wear or carry medical identification at all times.
• Tell patient to take dose early in the day.

✔ Evaluation
• Patient has no evidence of adrenal insufficiency.
• Patient remains free from injury.
• Patient is free from infection.

Diuretics, loop

bumetanide
ethacrynate sodium
ethacrynic acid
furosemide
torsemide

Indications

▶ Edema from heart failure, hepatic cirrhosis, or nephrotic syndrome; mild-to-moderate hypertension; adjunct treatment in acute pulmonary edema or hypertensive crisis.

Contraindications and cautions

• Contraindicated in patients hypersensitive to these drugs and in patients with anuria, hepatic coma, or severe electrolyte depletion.
• Use cautiously in patients with severe renal disease. Also use cautiously in patients with severe hypersensitivity to sulfonamides because allergic reaction may occur.
※ Lifespan: In pregnant women, use cautiously. In breast-feeding women, don't use. In neonates, use cautiously; the usual pediatric dose can be used, but dosage intervals should be extended. In elderly patients, use a lower dose, if needed, and monitor patient closely; these patients are more susceptible to drug-induced diuresis.

Adverse reactions

Therapeutic dose commonly causes metabolic and electrolyte disturbances, particularly potassium depletion. It also may cause hyperglycemia, hyperuricemia, hypochloremic alkalosis, and hypomagnesemia. Rapid parenteral administration may cause hearing loss (including deafness) and tinnitus. High doses can produce profound diuresis, leading to hypovolemia and CV collapse. Photosensitivity also may occur.

Action

Loop diuretics inhibit sodium and chloride reabsorption in the ascending loop of Henle, thus increasing excretion of sodium, chloride, and water. Like thiazide diuretics, loop diuretics increase excretion of potassium. Loop diuretics produce more diuresis and electrolyte loss than thiazide diuretics.

NURSING PROCESS

⚗ Assessment
• Monitor blood pressure and pulse rate, especially during rapid diuresis. Establish baseline values before therapy begins and watch for significant changes.
• Establish baseline CBC (including WBC count), liver function test results, and electrolyte levels including sodium, potassium, chloride, carbon dioxide, magnesium, BUN, and creatinine levels. Review periodically.
• Assess patient for evidence of excessive diuresis: hypotension, tachycardia, poor skin turgor, excessive thirst, or dry and cracked mucous membranes.
• Monitor patient for edema and ascites. Observe the legs of ambulatory patients and the sacral area of patients on bed rest.
• Weigh patient each morning immediately after he voids and before breakfast, in the same type of clothing, and on the same scale. Weight provides a reliable indicator of patient's response to diuretic therapy.
• Monitor and record patient's intake and output daily.

⊞ Key nursing diagnoses
• Risk for deficient fluid volume related to excessive diuresis
• Impaired urinary elimination related to change in diuresis pattern
• Ineffective protection related to electrolyte imbalance

▷ Planning and implementation
• Give diuretics in morning to ensure that major diuresis occurs before bedtime. To prevent nocturia, give diuretics before 6 p.m.

• Reduce dosage for patient with hepatic dysfunction, and increase dosage for patient with renal impairment, oliguria, or decreased diuresis. Inadequate urine output may result in circulatory overload, which causes water intoxication, pulmonary edema, and heart failure.

• May need to increase dosage of insulin or oral antidiabetic in diabetic patient, and reduce dosage of other antihypertensives.

• Take safety measures for all ambulatory patients until response to diuretic is known.

• Consult dietitian about need for potassium supplements.

• Keep urinal or commode readily available to patient.

Patient teaching

• Explain rationale for therapy and importance of following prescribed regimen.

• Review adverse effects, and urge patient to report symptoms promptly, especially chest, back, or leg pain; shortness of breath; dyspnea; increased edema or weight; lightheadedness or palpitations; and excess diuresis shown by weight loss of more than 0.9 kg (2 lb) daily.

• Advise patient to eat potassium-rich foods and to avoid high-sodium foods, such as lunch meat, smoked meats, and processed cheeses. Instruct him not to add table salt when cooking and eating foods.

• Encourage patient to keep follow-up appointments to monitor effectiveness of therapy.

☑ Evaluation

• Patient maintains adequate hydration.

• Patient states importance of taking diuretic early in the day to prevent nocturia.

• Patient complies with therapy, as shown by improvement in underlying condition.

Diuretics, potassium-sparing

amiloride hydrochloride
spironolactone
triamterene

Indications

▶ Edema from hepatic cirrhosis, nephrotic syndrome, and heart failure; mild or moderate hypertension; diagnosis of primary hyperaldosteronism; metabolic alkalosis produced by thiazide and other kaliuretic diuretics; recurrent calcium nephrolithiasis; lithium-induced polyuria secondary to lithium-induced nephrogenic diabetes insipidus; aid in the treatment of hypokalemia; prophylaxis of hypokalemia in patients taking cardiac glycosides; precocious puberty and female hirsutism; adjunct to treatment of myasthenia gravis and familial periodic paralysis.

Contraindications and cautions

• Contraindicated in patients hypersensitive to drug, those with a potassium level above 5.5 mEq/L, those taking other potassium-sparing diuretics or potassium supplements, and those with anuria, acute or chronic renal insufficiency, or diabetic nephropathy.

• Use cautiously in patients with severe hepatic insufficiency, because electrolyte imbalance may lead to hepatic encephalopathy, and in patients with diabetes, who are at increased risk for hyperkalemia.

⚖ **Lifespan:** In pregnant women, no controlled studies exist. Women who wish to breast-feed should consult prescriber because drug may appear in breast milk. In children, use cautiously; they're more susceptible to hyperkalemia. In elderly and debilitated patients, observe closely and reduce dosage, if needed; they're more susceptible to drug-induced diuresis and hyperkalemia.

Adverse reactions

Hyperkalemia is a serious adverse reaction; it may occur with all drugs in this class and could lead to arrhythmias. Other adverse reactions include nausea, vomiting, headache, weakness, fatigue, bowel disturbances, cough, and dyspnea.

Action

Amiloride and triamterene act directly on the distal renal tubules, inhibiting sodium reabsorption and potassium excretion, thereby reducing potassium loss. Spironolactone competitively inhibits aldosterone at the distal renal tubules, also promoting sodium excretion and potassium retention.

NURSING PROCESS

⚖ Assessment

• Monitor vital signs, intake and output, weight, and blood pressure daily; also, check patient for edema, oliguria, or lack of diuresis, which may indicate drug tolerance.

• Monitor patient with hepatic disease, for whom mild drug-induced acidosis may be hazardous; watch for mental confusion, lethargy, or stupor. Patients with hepatic disease are especially susceptible to diuretic-induced electrolyte imbalance; in extreme cases, coma and death can result.

• Watch for other signs of toxicity.

⊕ Key nursing diagnoses

• Risk for deficient fluid volume related to excessive diuresis

• Impaired urinary elimination related to change in diuresis pattern

• Ineffective protection related to electrolyte imbalance

▶ Planning and implementation

• Establish safety measures for ambulatory patients until response is known; diuretics may cause orthostatic hypotension, weakness, ataxia, and confusion.

• Give diuretics in the morning to ensure that major diuresis occurs before bedtime. To reduce the likelihood of nocturia, advise patient not to take diuretics after 6 p.m.

• Patients taking other antihypertensives and patients with renal impairment may need decreased dosages. Monitor diabetic patients; insulin dosages may need to be changed.

• Measure potassium and other electrolyte levels often to avoid imbalances that could cause arrhythmias. At baseline and periodically, monitor CBC with WBC count; carbon dioxide, BUN, and creatinine levels; and especially liver function test values.

Patient teaching

• Explain possible adverse effects and the importance of reporting unusual changes.

• Tell patient to weigh himself each morning after voiding and before dressing and eating, using the same scale. Urge him to report weight gain or loss of more than 0.9 kg (2 lb) per day.

• Teach patient how to minimize dizziness from orthostatic hypotension by avoiding sudden position changes.

• Advise patient to avoid potassium-rich food and potassium-containing salt substitutes or supplements, which increase the hazard of hyperkalemia.

• Tell patient to take drug at same time each morning to avoid interrupted sleep from nighttime diuresis.

• Advise patient to take drug with or after meals to minimize GI distress.

• Caution patient to avoid hazardous activities, such as driving or operating machinery, until response to drug is known.

• Tell patient to seek medical approval before taking OTC drugs; many contain sodium and potassium and can cause electrolyte imbalance.

☑ Evaluation

• Patient maintains adequate hydration.

• Patient states importance of taking diuretic early in the day to prevent nocturia.

• Patient complies with therapy, as shown by improvement in underlying condition.

Diuretics, thiazide and thiazide-like

Thiazide
chlorothiazide
hydrochlorothiazide
Thiazide-like
indapamide
metolazone

Indications

▶ Edema from right-sided heart failure, mild-to-moderate left-sided heart failure, or nephrotic syndrome; edema and ascites caused by hepatic cirrhosis; hypertension; diabetes insipidus, particularly nephrogenic diabetes insipidus.

Contraindications and cautions

• Contraindicated in patients hypersensitive to these drugs and in those with anuria.

• Use cautiously in patients with severe renal disease, impaired hepatic function, or progressive liver disease.

⚜ Lifespan: In pregnant women, use cautiously. In breast-feeding women, thiazides are contraindicated because they appear in breast milk.

In children, safety and effectiveness haven't been established. In elderly patients, reduce dosage, if needed, and monitor patient closely; these patients are more susceptible to drug-induced diuresis.

Adverse reactions

Therapeutic dose causes electrolyte and metabolic disturbances, most commonly potassium depletion. Other abnormalities include elevated cholesterol levels, hypercalcemia, hyperglycemia, hyperuricemia, hypochloremic alkalosis, hypomagnesemia, and hyponatremia. Photosensitivity also may occur.

Action

Thiazide and thiazide-like diuretics interfere with sodium transport across the tubules of the cortical diluting segment in the nephron, thereby increasing renal excretion of sodium, chloride, water, potassium, and calcium.

Thiazide diuretics also exert an antihypertensive effect. Although the exact mechanism is unknown, direct arteriolar dilation may be partially responsible. In diabetes insipidus, thiazides cause a paradoxical decrease in urine volume and an increase in renal concentration of urine, possibly because of sodium depletion and decreased plasma volume. This increases water and sodium reabsorption in the kidneys.

NURSING PROCESS

⚚ Assessment
● Monitor patient's intake, output, and electrolyte level regularly.
● Weigh patient each morning immediately after he voids and before breakfast, in the same type of clothing, and on the same scale. Weight provides a reliable indicator of patient's response to diuretic therapy.
● Monitor diabetic patient's glucose level. Diuretics may cause hyperglycemia.
● Monitor creatinine and BUN levels regularly. Drug isn't as effective if these levels are more than twice normal. Also, monitor uric acid level.

⊕ Key nursing diagnoses
● Risk for deficient fluid volume related to excessive diuresis
● Impaired urinary elimination related to change in diuresis pattern
● Ineffective protection related to electrolyte imbalance

▷ Planning and implementation
● Give drug in the morning to prevent nocturia.
● Provide a high-potassium diet.
● Give potassium supplements to maintain acceptable potassium level.
● Keep urinal or commode readily available to patient.
Patient teaching
● Explain the rationale for therapy and the importance of following the prescribed regimen.
● Tell patient to take drug at the same time each day to prevent nocturia. Suggest taking drug with food to minimize GI irritation.
● Urge patient to seek prescriber's approval before taking any other drug, including OTC medications and herbal remedies.
● Advise patient to record his weight each morning after voiding and before breakfast, in the same type of clothing, and on the same scale.
● Review adverse effects, and urge the patient to promptly report symptoms, especially chest, back, or leg pain; shortness of breath; dyspnea; lightheadedness; palpitations; increased edema or weight; or excess diuresis shown by weight loss of more than 0.9 kg (2 lb) daily. Warn him about photosensitivity reactions that usually occur 10 to 14 days after initial sun exposure.
● Advise patient to eat potassium-rich foods and to avoid high-sodium foods, such as lunch meat, smoked meats, processed cheeses. Instruct him not to cook with salt or add table salt to foods.
● Encourage patient to keep follow-up appointments to monitor effectiveness of therapy.

☑ Evaluation
● Patient maintains adequate hydration.
● Patient states importance of taking diuretic early in the day to prevent nocturia.
● Patient complies with therapy, as shown by improvement in underlying condition.

Estrogens

esterified estrogens
estradiol
estradiol cypionate
estradiol valerate
estrogenic substances, conjugated
estrone
estropipate

Indications

▶ Prevention of moderate to severe vasomotor symptoms linked to menopause, such as hot flushes and dizziness; stimulation of vaginal tissue development, cornification, and secretory activity; inhibition of hormone-sensitive cancer growth; female hypogonadism; female castration; primary ovulation failure; ovulation control; prevention of conception.

Contraindications and cautions

● Contraindicated in women with thrombophlebitis or thromboembolic disorders, unexplained abnormal genital bleeding, or estrogen-dependent neoplasia.
● Use cautiously in patients with hypertension; metabolic bone disease; migraines; seizures; asthma; cardiac, renal, or hepatic impairment; blood dyscrasia; diabetes; family history of breast cancer; or fibrocystic disease.
⚕ Lifespan: In pregnant or breast-feeding women, use is contraindicated. In adolescents whose bone growth isn't complete, use cautiously because of effects on epiphyseal closure. Postmenopausal women with a history of long-term estrogen use have an increased risk of endometrial cancer and stroke. Postmenopausal women also have increased risk for breast cancer, MI, stroke, and blood clots with long-term use of estrogen plus progestin.

Adverse reactions

Acute adverse reactions include abdominal cramps; bloating caused by fluid and electrolyte retention; breast swelling and tenderness; changes in menstrual bleeding patterns, such as spotting and prolongation or absence of bleeding; headache; loss of appetite; loss of libido; nausea; photosensitivity; swollen feet or ankles; and weight gain.

Long-term effects include benign hepatomas, cholestatic jaundice, elevated blood pressure (sometimes into the hypertensive range), endometrial carcinoma (rare), and thromboembolic disease (risk increases greatly with cigarette smoking, especially in women older than age 35).

Action

Estrogens promote the development and maintenance of the female reproductive system and secondary sexual characteristics. They inhibit the release of pituitary gonadotropins and have various metabolic effects, including retention of fluid and electrolytes, retention and deposition in bone of calcium and phosphorus, and mild anabolic activity. Of the six naturally occurring estrogens in humans, estradiol, estrone, and estriol are present in significant quantities.

Estrogens and estrogenic substances given as drugs have effects related to endogenous estrogen's mechanism of action. They can mimic the action of endogenous estrogen when used as replacement therapy and can inhibit ovulation or the growth of certain hormone-sensitive cancers. Conjugated estrogens and estrogenic substances are normally obtained from the urine of pregnant mares. Other estrogens are manufactured synthetically.

NURSING PROCESS

🔍 Assessment
● Monitor patient regularly to detect improvement or worsening of symptoms; observe patient for adverse reactions.
● If patient has diabetes mellitus, watch closely for loss of diabetes control.

⊕ Key nursing diagnoses
● Excessive fluid volume related to drug-induced fluid retention
● Risk of injury related to adverse effects
● Noncompliance related to long-term therapy

▶ Planning and implementation
● Notify pathologist of patient's estrogen therapy when sending specimens for evaluation.
Patient teaching
● Urge patient to read the package insert describing adverse reactions. Follow this with a

verbal explanation. Tell patient to keep the package insert for later reference.

• Advise patient to take drug with meals or at bedtime to relieve nausea. Reassure patient that nausea usually disappears with continued therapy.

• Teach patient how to apply estrogen ointments or transdermal estrogen. Review symptoms that accompany a systemic reaction to ointments.

• Teach patient how to insert intravaginal estrogen suppository. Advise her to use sanitary pads instead of tampons when using suppository.

• Teach patient how to perform routine monthly breast self-examination.

• Tell patient to stop taking drug immediately if she becomes pregnant because estrogens can harm fetus.

• Remind patient not to breast-feed during estrogen therapy.

• If patient is receiving cyclic therapy for postmenopausal symptoms, explain that withdrawal bleeding may occur during the week off, but that fertility hasn't been restored and ovulation isn't expected to occur.

• Explain that medical supervision is essential during prolonged therapy.

• Explain to a man on long-term therapy about possible temporary gynecomastia and impotence, which will disappear when therapy ends.

• Instruct patient to notify prescriber immediately if patient experiences abdominal pain; pain, numbness, or stiffness in legs or buttocks; pressure or pain in chest; shortness of breath; severe headaches; visual disturbances, such as blind spots, flashing lights, or blurriness; vaginal bleeding or discharge; breast lumps; swelling of hands or feet; yellow skin and sclera; dark urine; or light-colored stools.

• Urge diabetic patient to report symptoms of hyperglycemia or glycosuria.

☑ **Evaluation**

• Patient experiences only minimal fluid retention.

• Patient doesn't develop serious complications of estrogen therapy.

• Patient complies with therapy, as shown by improvement in condition or absence of pregnancy.

Fluoroquinolones

ciprofloxacin
gemifloxacin
levofloxacin
lomefloxacin hydrochloride
moxifloxacin
norfloxacin
ofloxacin
sparfloxacin

Indications

▶ Bone and joint infection, bacterial bronchitis, endocervical and urethral chlamydial infection, bacterial gastroenteritis, endocervical and urethral gonorrhea, intra-abdominal infection, empiric therapy for febrile neutropenia, pelvic inflammatory disease, bacterial pneumonia, bacterial prostatitis, acute sinusitis, skin and soft tissue infection, typhoid fever, bacterial UTI (prevention and treatment), chancroid, meningococcal carriers, and bacterial septicemia caused by susceptible organisms.

Contraindications and cautions

• Contraindicated in patients hypersensitive to fluoroquinolones because serious, possibly fatal, reactions can occur.

• Use cautiously in patients with known or suspected CNS disorders that predispose them to seizures or lower seizure threshold, cerebral ischemia, severe hepatic dysfunction, or renal insufficiency.

☀ Lifespan: In pregnant women, these drugs cross the placental barrier and may cause arthropathies. Breast-feeding isn't recommended because these drugs may cause arthropathies in newborns and infants, although it isn't known if all fluoroquinolones appear in breast milk. In children, fluoroquinolones aren't recommended because they can cause joint problems. In elderly patients, reduce dosage, if needed, because these patients are more likely to have reduced renal function.

Adverse reactions

Adverse reactions that are rare but need medical attention include CNS stimulation (acute psychosis, agitation, hallucinations, tremors), hepatotoxicity, hypersensitivity reactions, inter-

stitial nephritis, phlebitis, pseudomembranous colitis, and tendinitis or tendon rupture. Adverse reactions that need no medical attention unless they persist or become intolerable include CNS effects (dizziness, headache, nervousness, drowsiness, insomnia), GI reactions, and photosensitivity.

Action

Fluoroquinolones produce a bactericidal effect by inhibiting intracellular DNA topoisomerase II (DNA gyrase), which prevents DNA replication. These enzymes are essential catalysts in the duplication, transcription, and repair of bacterial DNA.

Fluoroquinolones are broad-spectrum, systemic antibacterial drugs active against a wide range of aerobic gram-positive and gram-negative organisms. Gram-positive aerobic bacteria include *Staphylococcus aureus, Staphylococcus epidermis, Staphylococcus hemolyticus, Staphylococcus saprophyticus;* penicillinase- and non–penicillinase-producing staphylococci and some methicillin-resistant strains; *Streptococcus pneumoniae;* group A (beta) hemolytic streptococci *(S. pyogenes);* group B streptococci *(S. agalactiae);* viridans streptococci; groups C, F, and G streptococci and nonenterococcal group D streptococci; *Enterococcus faecalis.* These drugs are active against gram-positive aerobic bacilli including *Corynebacterium* species, *Listeria monocytogenes,* and *Nocardia asteroides.*

Fluoroquinolones are also effective against gram-negative aerobic bacteria including, but not limited to, *Neisseria meningitidis* and most strains of penicillinase- and non–penicillinase-producing *Haemophilus ducreyi, Haemophilus influenzae, Haemophilus parainfluenzae, Moraxella catarrhalis, Neisseria gonorrhoeae,* and most clinically important Enterobacteriaceae, *Vibrio cholerae,* and *Vibrio parahaemolyticus.* Certain fluoroquinolones are active against *Chlamydia trachomatis, Legionella pneumophila, Mycobacterium avium-intracellulare, Mycoplasma hominis, Mycoplasma pneumoniae,* and *Pseudomonas aeruginosa.*

NURSING PROCESS

⌨ Assessment
● Obtain specimen for culture and sensitivity tests before starting therapy and, as needed, to detect bacterial resistance. Therapy may begin pending results.
● Obtain history of seizure disorders or other CNS diseases, such as cerebral arteriosclerosis, before starting therapy.
● Monitor renal and liver function test values in patients with impaired renal or hepatic function.
● Achilles and other tendon ruptures have occurred with fluoroquinolone use. Stop drug if patient experiences pain, inflammation, or rupture of a tendon.

⊞ Key nursing diagnoses
● Ineffective protection related to presence of bacteria
● Risk for deficient fluid volume related to drug-induced adverse GI reactions
● Risk for unstable blood glucose

▷ Planning and implementation
● Treat acute hypersensitivity reactions with epinephrine, oxygen, I.V. fluids, antihistamines, corticosteroids, pressor amines, and airway management.
● Notify prescriber if patient has symptoms of excessive CNS stimulation (restlessness, tremor, confusion, hallucination). Take seizure precautions.
● If patient develops severe diarrhea or diarrhea unresponsive to treatment suspect pseudomembranous colitis and notify prescriber.
Patient teaching
● Instruct patient to take drug as prescribed and to finish the full course of therapy.
● Tell patient to take drug with an 8-oz (240-ml) glass of water.
● Caution patient that norfloxacin should be taken on an empty stomach with water 1 hour before or 2 hours after meals.
● Instruct patient that, if a dose is missed, the next dose should be taken as soon as possible; advise patient not to double the dose.
● Advise patient to avoid use with antacids and multivitamins containing iron, zinc, aluminum, magnesium, or sucralfate. If coadministration can't be avoided, tell patient to separate doses by at least 2 hours.
● Tell patient fluoroquinolones may cause dizziness; advise patient to avoid engaging in activities that require mental alertness until CNS effects on him are known.

• Caution patient not to take other drugs without medical approval.

☑ Evaluation
• Patient is free from infection.
• Patient maintains adequate hydration throughout drug therapy.
• Patient's blood sugar level remains within normal limits.

Histamine$_2$-receptor antagonists
cimetidine
famotidine
nizatidine
ranitidine hydrochloride

Indications
▶ Acute duodenal or gastric ulcer, Zollinger-Ellison syndrome, gastroesophageal reflux.

Contraindications and cautions
• Contraindicated in patients hypersensitive to these drugs.
• Use cautiously in patients with impaired renal or hepatic function.
⚖ Lifespan: In pregnant women, use cautiously. In breast-feeding women, histamine$_2$ (H$_2$)-receptor antagonists are contraindicated because they may appear in breast milk. In children, safety and effectiveness haven't been established. Elderly patients have increased risk of adverse reactions, particularly those affecting the CNS; use cautiously.

Adverse reactions
H$_2$-receptor antagonists rarely cause adverse reactions. Cardiac arrhythmias, dizziness, fatigue, gynecomastia, headache, mild and transient diarrhea, and thrombocytopenia are possible.

Action
All H$_2$-receptor antagonists inhibit the action of H$_2$-receptors in gastric parietal cells, reducing gastric acid output and concentration, regardless of stimulants, such as histamine, food, insulin, and caffeine, or basal conditions.

NURSING PROCESS

🔍 Assessment
• Monitor patient for adverse reactions, especially hypotension and arrhythmias.
• Periodically monitor laboratory tests, such as CBC and renal and hepatic studies.

🔑 Key nursing diagnoses
• Risk for trauma related to drug-induced thrombocytopenia
• Decreased cardiac output related to adverse CV effects (cimetidine)
• Fatigue related to drug's CNS effects

▷ Planning and implementation
• Give once-daily dose at bedtime, twice-daily doses in morning and evening, and multiple doses with meals and at bedtime. A once-daily dose at bedtime promotes compliance.
• Don't exceed recommended infusion rates when giving drugs I.V.; doing so increases risk of adverse CV effects. Continuous I.V. infusion may suppress acid secretion more effectively.
• Give antacids at least 1 hour before or after H$_2$-receptor antagonists. Antacids can decrease drug absorption.
• Adjust dosage for patient with renal disease.
• Don't abruptly stop the drug.
Patient teaching
• Teach patient how and when to take drug, and warn him not to abruptly stop taking it.
• Review possible adverse reactions, and urge patient to report unusual effects.
• Caution patient to avoid smoking during therapy; smoking stimulates gastric acid secretion and worsens the disease.

☑ Evaluation
• Patient is free from trauma.
• Patient maintains a normal heart rhythm.
• Patient states appropriate management plan for combating fatigue.

Laxatives

Bulk-forming
calcium polycarbophil
methylcellulose
psyllium
Emollient
docusate calcium
docusate potassium
docusate sodium
Hyperosmolar
glycerin
lactulose
lubiprostone
magnesium citrate
magnesium hydroxide
magnesium sulfate
sodium phosphates
Stimulant
bisacodyl
senna

Indications

▶ Constipation, irritable bowel syndrome, diverticulosis.

Contraindications and cautions

- Contraindicated in patients with GI obstruction or perforation, toxic colitis, megacolon, nausea and vomiting, or acute surgical abdomen.
- Use cautiously in patients with rectal or anal conditions such as rectal bleeding or large hemorrhoids.
- **Lifespan:** For pregnant women and breastfeeding women, recommendations vary for individual drugs. Infants and children have an increased risk of fluid and electrolyte disturbances; use cautiously. In elderly patients, dependence is more likely to develop because of age-related changes in GI function. Monitor these patients closely.

Adverse reactions

All laxatives may cause flatulence, diarrhea, abdominal discomfort, weakness, and dependence. Bulk-forming laxatives may cause intestinal obstruction, impaction, or (rarely) esophageal obstruction. Emollient laxatives may cause a bitter taste or throat irritation. Hyperosmolar laxatives may cause fluid and electrolyte imbalances. Stimulant laxatives may cause urine discoloration, malabsorption, and weight loss.

Action

Laxatives promote movement of intestinal contents through the colon and rectum in several ways: bulk-forming, emollient, hyperosmolar, and stimulant.

NURSING PROCESS

Assessment
- Obtain baseline assessment of patient's bowel patterns and GI history before giving.
- Monitor patient for adverse reactions.
- Monitor bowel pattern throughout therapy. Assess bowel sounds and color and consistency of stools.
- Monitor patient's fluid and electrolyte status during administration.

Key nursing diagnoses
- Diarrhea related to adverse GI effects
- Acute pain related to abdominal discomfort
- Ineffective health maintenance related to laxative dependence

Planning and implementation
- Don't crush enteric-coated tablets.
- Anticipate when constipation is likely to occur (such as with opiate therapy) and add a preventative bowel regimen.
- Time administration so that bowel evacuation doesn't interfere with sleep.
- Make sure patient has easy access to bedpan or bathroom.
- Take precautions to prevent constipation.

Patient teaching
- Advise patient that therapy should be short-term. Point out that abuse or prolonged use can cause nutritional imbalances.
- Tell patient that stool softeners and bulk-forming laxatives may take several days to achieve results.
- Encourage patient to remain active and to drink plenty of fluids if he takes a bulk-forming laxative.
- Explain that stimulant laxatives may cause harmless urine discoloration.
- Teach patient about including foods high in fiber into diet.

☑ **Evaluation**
• Patient regains normal bowel pattern.
• Patient states that pain is relieved with stool evacuation.
• Patient discusses dangers of laxative abuse and importance of limiting laxative use.

Nonsteroidal anti-inflammatory drugs

celecoxib
diclofenac potassium
diclofenac sodium
diflunisal
etodolac
ibuprofen
indomethacin
indomethacin sodium trihydrate
ketoprofen
ketorolac tromethamine
meloxicam
nabumetone
naproxen
naproxen sodium
oxaprozin
piroxicam
sulindac

Indications

▶ Mild to moderate pain, inflammation, stiffness, swelling, or tenderness caused by headache, arthralgia, myalgia, neuralgia, dysmenorrhea, rheumatoid arthritis, juvenile arthritis, osteoarthritis, or dental or surgical procedures.

Contraindications and cautions

• Contraindicated in patients with GI lesions or GI bleeding and in patients hypersensitive to these drugs.
• Use cautiously in patients with heart failure, hypertension, risk of MI, fluid retention, renal insufficiency, or coagulation defects.
⚠ Lifespan: In pregnant women, use cautiously in the first and second trimesters; don't use in the third trimester. For breast-feeding women, NSAIDs aren't recommended. In children younger than age 14, safety of long-term therapy hasn't been established. Patients older than age 60 may be more susceptible to toxic effects

of NSAIDs because of decreased renal function.

Adverse reactions

Adverse reactions chiefly involve the GI tract, particularly erosion of the gastric mucosa. The most common symptoms are abdominal pain, dyspepsia, epigastric distress, heartburn, and nausea. CNS and skin reactions also may occur. Flank pain with other evidence of nephrotoxicity occurs occasionally. Fluid retention may aggravate hypertension or heart failure.

Action

The analgesic effect of NSAIDs may result from interference with the prostaglandins involved in pain. Prostaglandins appear to sensitize pain receptors to mechanical stimulation or to other chemical mediators. NSAIDs inhibit synthesis of prostaglandins peripherally and possibly centrally.

Like salicylates, NSAIDs exert an antiinflammatory effect that may result in part from inhibition of prostaglandin synthesis and release during inflammation. The exact mechanism isn't clear.

NURSING PROCESS

✎ **Assessment**
• Assess patient's level of pain and inflammation before therapy begins, and evaluate drug effectiveness.
• Monitor patient for evidence of bleeding. If patient needs surgery, hold drug a sufficient amount of time before the procedure, as advised by prescriber.
• Monitor ophthalmic and auditory function before and periodically during therapy to detect toxicity.
• Monitor CBC, platelet count, and hepatic and renal function studies periodically to detect abnormalities.
• Watch for bronchospasm in patients with aspirin hypersensitivity, rhinitis or nasal polyps, and asthma.
• Assess for potential drug interactions and establish management strategies.

🔅 **Key nursing diagnoses**
• Risk for injury related to adverse reactions
• Excessive fluid volume related to fluid retention

• Disturbed sensory perception (visual and auditory) related to toxicity

▶ Planning and implementation
• Give oral NSAIDs with 8 oz (240 ml) of water to ensure adequate passage into the stomach. Have patient sit up for 15 to 30 minutes after taking drug to prevent it from lodging in esophagus.
• Crush tablets or mix with food or fluid to aid swallowing. Give with antacids to minimize GI upset.
Patient teaching
• Encourage patient to take drug as directed to achieve desired effect.
• Review methods to prevent or minimize GI upset.
• Work with patient on long-term therapy to arrange for monitoring of laboratory values, especially BUN and creatinine levels, liver function test results, and CBC.
• Instruct patient to notify prescriber about severe or persistent adverse reactions.
• Inform patient of potential drug interactions and how to manage them.

☑ Evaluation
• Patient remains free from injury.
• Patient shows no signs of edema.
• Patient maintains normal visual and auditory function.

Nucleoside reverse transcriptase inhibitors
abacavir sulfate
didanosine
emtricitabine
lamivudine
stavudine
tenofovir disoproxil fumarate
zidovudine

Indications

▶ HIV infection, AIDS, prevention of maternal-fetal HIV transmission, prevention of HIV infection after occupational exposure (as by needle stick) or nonoccupational exposure to blood, genital secretions, or other potentially infectious body fluids of an HIV-infected person when there's substantial risk of transmission.

Contraindications and cautions

• Contraindicated in patients hypersensitive to these drugs and in patients with moderate to severe hepatic impairment (abacavir) or pancreatitis (didanosine).
• Use cautiously in patients with mild hepatic impairment or risk factors for liver impairment, risk for pancreatitis (didanosine), or compromised bone marrow function (zidovudine).
☀ Lifespan: In pregnant women, use drug only if benefits outweigh risks. To reduce the risk of transmitting the virus, HIV-infected mothers shouldn't breast-feed. It isn't known if NRTIs appear in breast milk. The pharmacokinetic and safety profile of NRTIs is similar in children and adults. NRTIs may be used in children age 3 months and older, but the half-life may be prolonged in neonates. In elderly patients, elimination half-life may be prolonged.

Adverse reactions

Because of the complexity of HIV infection, it's often difficult to distinguish between disease-related symptoms and adverse drug reactions. The most frequently reported adverse effects of NRTIs are anemia, leukopenia, and neutropenia. Thrombocytopenia is less common. Rare adverse effects of NRTIs are hepatotoxicity, myopathy, and neurotoxicity. Any of these adverse effects requires prompt medical attention.

Adverse effects that don't need medical attention unless they persist or are bothersome include headache, severe insomnia, myalgias, nausea, or hyperpigmentation of nails.

Action

NRTIs suppress HIV replication by inhibiting HIV DNA polymerase. Competitive inhibition of nucleoside reverse transcriptase inhibits DNA viral replication by chain termination, competitive inhibition of reverse transcriptase, or both.

NURSING PROCESS
☑ Assessment
• Obtain baseline assessment of patient's infection, and reassess regularly to monitor drug effectiveness.
• Monitor hepatic function, CBC, and platelet count regularly.

- Assess patient for risk factors for liver disease.
- Lactic acidosis and severe hepatomegaly with steatosis may occur, especially in women or patients who are obese or have prolonged exposure to nucleosides. If patient has symptoms of lactic acidosis or pronounced hepatotoxicity, stop treatment. Symptoms may include hepatomegaly and steatosis, even without elevated transaminase levels.

🔲 **Key nursing diagnoses**
- Disturbed body image related to redistribution of body fat from antiretroviral therapy
- Diarrhea related to drug-induced adverse effect on bowel
- Ineffective coping related to HIV infection

▶ **Planning and implementation**
- Combination therapy should include three or more antiretrovirals, usually two NRTIs and a protease inhibitor or nonnucleoside reverse transcriptase inhibitor.
- Give didanosine on an empty stomach, at least 30 minutes before or 2 hours after meals.
- Redistribution or accumulation of body fat, including central obesity, dorsocervical fat enlargement (buffalo hump), peripheral wasting, facial wasting, breast enlargement, and cushingoid appearance, may occur.
- Patients with renal impairment may need dosage adjustment.
- Notify prescriber about persistent GI adverse effects.

Patient teaching
- Tell patient to take drug as prescribed, no more and no less, and to finish the full course of therapy.
- Instruct patient not to miss a dose but, if a dose is missed, to take the next dose as soon as possible; caution against doubling the dose.
- Advise patient to keep scheduled appointments because important blood tests are needed to evaluate the response to this drug.
- Tell patient not to take other drugs without medical approval.
- Tell patient to practice safe sex.

✓ **Evaluation**
- Patient doesn't experience altered body image.
- Patient regains normal bowel pattern.
- Patient demonstrates adequate coping mechanisms.

Opioids

alfentanil hydrochloride
codeine phosphate
codeine sulfate
difenoxin hydrochloride
diphenoxylate hydrochloride
fentanyl citrate
hydrocodone bitartrate
hydromorphone hydrochloride
meperidine hydrochloride
methadone hydrochloride
morphine sulfate
oxycodone hydrochloride
oxymorphone hydrochloride
propoxyphene hydrochloride
propoxyphene napsylate
sufentanil citrate

Indications

▶ Moderate to severe pain from acute and some chronic disorders; diarrhea; dry, nonproductive cough; management of opioid dependence; anesthesia support; sedation.

Contraindications and cautions

- Contraindicated in patients hypersensitive to these drugs and in those who have recently taken an MAO inhibitor. Also contraindicated in those with acute or severe bronchial asthma or respiratory depression.
- Use cautiously in patients with head injury, increased intracranial or intraocular pressure, hepatic or renal dysfunction, mental illness, emotional disturbances, or drug-seeking behaviors.
⚖ Lifespan: In pregnant or breast-feeding women, use cautiously; codeine, meperidine, methadone, morphine, and propoxyphene appear in breast milk. Breast-feeding infants of women taking methadone may develop physical dependence. In children, safety and effectiveness of some opioids haven't been established; use cautiously. Elderly patients may be more sensitive to opioids, and lower doses are usually given.

Adverse reactions

Respiratory and circulatory depression (including orthostatic hypotension) are the major hazards of opioids. Other adverse CNS effects in-

clude agitation, coma, depression, dizziness, dysphoria, euphoria, faintness, mental clouding, nervousness, restlessness, sedation, seizures, visual disturbances, and weakness. Adverse GI effects include biliary colic, constipation, nausea, and vomiting. Urine retention or hypersensitivity also may occur. Tolerance to the drug and psychological or physical dependence may follow prolonged therapy.

Action

Opioids act as agonists at specific opiate-receptor binding sites in the CNS and other tissues, altering the patient's perception of pain.

NURSING PROCESS

Assessment
• Obtain baseline assessment of patient's pain, and reassess frequently to determine the drug's effectiveness.
• Evaluate patient's respiratory status before each dose; watch for respiratory rate below patient's baseline level and for restlessness, which may be compensatory signs of hypoxia. Respiratory depression may last longer than the analgesic effect.
• Monitor patient for other adverse reactions.
• Monitor patient for tolerance and dependence. The first sign of tolerance to opioids is usually a shortened duration of effect.

Key nursing diagnoses
• Ineffective breathing pattern related to respiratory depression
• Risk for injury related to orthostatic hypotension
• Ineffective coping related to drug dependence

Planning and implementation
• Keep resuscitative equipment and an opioid antagonist, such as naloxone, available.
• Give I.V. drug by slow injection, preferably in diluted solution. Rapid I.V. injection increases the risk of adverse effects.
• Give drug I.M. or subcutaneously, cautiously, to a patient with decreased platelet count and to a patient who is chilled, hypovolemic, or in shock; decreased perfusion may lead to drug accumulation and toxicity. Rotate injection sites to avoid induration.
• Chronic use may cause constipation; consider a preventive bowel regimen.

• Carefully note the strength of solution when measuring a dose. Oral solutions of varying concentrations are available.
• For maximum effectiveness, give on a regular dosage schedule rather than as needed.
• Institute safety precautions.
• Encourage postoperative patient to turn, cough, and breathe deeply every 2 hours to avoid atelectasis.
• If GI irritation occurs, give oral forms with food.
• Withdrawal symptoms—including tremors, agitation, nausea, and vomiting—may occur if drug is stopped abruptly. Monitor patient with these symptoms carefully and provide supportive therapy.

Patient teaching
• Teach patient to take drug exactly as prescribed. Urge him to call prescriber if he isn't experiencing desired effect or if he is experiencing significant adverse reactions.
• Warn patient to avoid hazardous activities until drug's effects are known.
• Advise patient to avoid alcohol while taking opioid; alcohol will cause additive CNS depression.
• Suggest measures to prevent constipation, such as increasing fiber in diet and using a stool softener.
• Instruct patient to breathe deeply, cough, and change position every 2 hours to avoid respiratory complications.

Evaluation
• Patient maintains adequate ventilation, as shown by normal respiratory rate and rhythm and pink color.
• Patient remains free from injury.
• Patient doesn't become tolerant to drug.
• Patient reports that pain is adequately controlled.

Penicillins

Natural penicillins
penicillin G benzathine
penicillin G potassium
penicillin G procaine
penicillin G sodium
penicillin V potassium

Aminopenicillins
amoxicillin and clavulanate potassium
amoxicillin trihydrate
ampicillin
ampicillin sodium and sulbactam sodium
ampicillin trihydrate
Extended-spectrum penicillins
carbenicillin indanyl sodium
piperacillin sodium and tazobactam sodium
ticarcillin disodium
ticarcillin disodium and clavulanate
   potassium
Penicillinase-resistant penicillins
dicloxacillin sodium
nafcillin sodium
oxacillin sodium

Indications

▶ Streptococcal pneumonia; enterococcal and nonenterococcal group D endocarditis; diphtheria; anthrax; meningitis; tetanus; botulism; actinomycosis; syphilis; relapsing fever; Lyme disease; pneumococcal infections; rheumatic fever; bacterial endocarditis; neonatal group B streptococcal disease; septicemia; gynecologic infections; infections of urinary, respiratory, and GI tracts; infections of skin, soft tissue, bones, and joints.

Contraindications and cautions

• Contraindicated in patients hypersensitive to these drugs.
• Use cautiously in patients with history of asthma or drug allergy, mononucleosis, renal impairment, CV diseases, hemorrhagic condition, or electrolyte imbalance.
⚘ Lifespan: In pregnant women, use cautiously. For breast-feeding patients, recommendations vary depending on the drug. For children, dosage recommendations have been established for most penicillins. Elderly patients are susceptible to superinfection and renal impairment, which decreases excretion of penicillins; use cautiously and at a lower dosage.

Adverse reactions

With all penicillins, hypersensitivity reactions range from mild rash, fever, and eosinophilia to fatal anaphylaxis. Hematologic reactions include hemolytic anemia, leukopenia, thrombocytopenia, and transient neutropenia.

Certain adverse reactions are more common with specific classes. For example, bleeding episodes are usually seen with high doses of extended-spectrum penicillins, whereas GI adverse effects are most common with ampicillin. In patients with renal disease, high doses, especially of penicillin G, irritate the CNS by causing confusion, twitching, lethargy, dysphagia, seizures, and coma. Hepatotoxicity may occur with penicillinase-resistant penicillins, and hyperkalemia and hypernatremia have been reported with extended-spectrum penicillins.

Local irritation from parenteral therapy may be severe enough to warrant administration by subclavian or centrally placed catheter or stopping therapy.

Action

Penicillins are generally bactericidal. They inhibit synthesis of the bacterial cell wall, causing rapid cell destruction. They're most effective against fast-growing susceptible bacteria. Their sites of action are enzymes known as penicillin-binding proteins (PBPs). The affinity of certain penicillins for PBPs in various microorganisms helps explain the different activities of these drugs.

Susceptible aerobic gram-positive cocci include *Staphylococcus aureus;* nonenterococcal group D streptococci; groups A, B, D, G, H, K, L, and M streptococci; *Streptococcus viridans;* and *Enterococcus* (usually with an aminoglycoside). Susceptible aerobic gram-negative cocci include *Neisseria meningitidis* and non–penicillinase-producing *N. gonorrhoeae.*

Susceptible aerobic gram-positive bacilli include *Corynebacterium, Listeria,* and *Bacillus anthracis.* Susceptible anaerobes include *Peptococcus, Peptostreptococcus, Actinomyces, Clostridium, Fusobacterium, Veillonella,* and non–beta-lactamase–producing strains of *Streptococcus pneumoniae.* Susceptible spirochetes include *Treponema pallidum, T. pertenue, Leptospira, Borrelia recurrentis*, and, possibly, *B. burgdorferi.*

Aminopenicillins have uses against more organisms, including many gram-negative organisms. Like natural penicillins, aminopenicillins are vulnerable to inactivation by penicillinase. Susceptible organisms include *Escherichia coli, Proteus mirabilis, Shigella, Salmonella, S. pneumoniae, N. gonorrhoeae, Haemophilus influenzae, S. aureus, S. epidermidis* (non–

penicillinase-producing *Staphylococcus*), and *Listeria monocytogenes*.

Penicillinase-resistant penicillins are semisynthetic penicillins designed to remain stable against hydrolysis by most staphylococcal penicillinases and thus are the drugs of choice against susceptible penicillinase-producing staphylococci. They also act against most organisms susceptible to natural penicillins.

Extended-spectrum penicillins offer a wider range of bactericidal action than the other three classes and usually are given in combination with aminoglycosides. Susceptible strains include *Enterobacter, Klebsiella, Citrobacter, Serratia, Bacteroides fragilis, Pseudomonas aeruginosa, Proteus vulgaris, Providencia rettgeri,* and *Morganella morganii.* These penicillins are also vulnerable to beta-lactamase and penicillinases.

NURSING PROCESS

Assessment
- Assess patient's history of allergies. Try to find out whether any previous reactions were true hypersensitivity reactions or adverse reactions (such as GI distress) that patient interpreted as allergy.
- Keep in mind that a patient who has never had a penicillin hypersensitivity reaction may still have future allergic reactions; monitor patient continuously for possible allergic reactions or other adverse effects.
- Obtain culture and sensitivity tests before giving first dose; repeat tests periodically to assess drug's effectiveness.
- Monitor vital signs, electrolytes, and renal function studies.
- Assess patient's consciousness and neurologic status when giving high doses; CNS toxicity can occur.
- Coagulation abnormalities, even frank bleeding, can follow high doses, especially of extended-spectrum penicillins. Monitor PT, INR, and platelet counts. Assess patient for signs of occult or frank bleeding.
- Monitor patients, especially elderly patients, debilitated patients, and patients receiving immunosuppressants or radiation, receiving long-term therapy for possible superinfection.

Key nursing diagnoses
- Ineffective protection related to hypersensitivity
- Risk for infection related to superinfection
- Risk for deficient fluid volume related to adverse GI reactions

Planning and implementation
- Give penicillin at least 1 hour before bacteriostatic antibiotics, such as tetracyclines, erythromycin, and chloramphenicol; these drugs inhibit bacterial cell growth and decrease rate of penicillin uptake by bacterial cell walls.
- To enhance GI absorption, give oral penicillin at least 1 hour before or 2 hours after meals.
- Refrigerate oral suspensions, which will be stable for 14 days; to ensure correct dosage, shake suspension well before giving it.
- To minimize tissue injury, give I.M. dose deep into gluteal muscle mass or midlateral thigh, and rotate injection sites. To relieve pain, apply ice to injection site. Don't inject more than 2 g of drug per injection site.
- With I.V. infusions, don't add or mix another drug, especially an aminoglycoside, which will become inactive if mixed with penicillin. If other drugs must be given I.V., temporarily stop infusion of primary drug.
- Infuse I.V. drug continuously or intermittently over 30 minutes. Rotate infusion site every 48 hours. Intermittent I.V. infusion may be diluted in 50 to 100 ml sterile water, normal saline solution, D_5W, D_5W and half-normal saline solution, or lactated Ringer's solution.

Patient teaching
- Make sure patient understands how and when to take drug. Urge him to complete the prescribed regimen, comply with instructions for around-the-clock scheduling, and keep follow-up appointments.
- Teach patient signs and symptoms of hypersensitivity and other adverse reactions. Urge him to report unusual reactions.
- Tell patient to check drug's expiration date and to discard unused drug. Warn him not to share drug with family or friends.

Evaluation
- Patient shows no signs of hypersensitivity.
- Patient is free from infection.
- Patient maintains adequate hydration.

Phenothiazines

chlorpromazine hydrochloride
fluphenazine
mesoridazine besylate
perphenazine
prochlorperazine
promazine hydrochloride
promethazine
thioridazine hydrochloride
thiothixene
trifluoperazine hydrochloride

Indications

▶ Agitated psychotic states, hallucinations, manic-depressive illness, excessive motor and autonomic activity, nausea and vomiting, moderate anxiety, behavioral problems caused by chronic organic mental syndrome, tetanus, acute intermittent porphyria, intractable hiccups, itching, symptomatic rhinitis.

Contraindications and cautions

• Contraindicated in patients with CNS depression, bone marrow suppression, heart failure, circulatory collapse, coronary artery or cerebrovascular disorders, subcortical damage, or coma. Also contraindicated in patients receiving spinal and epidural anesthetics and adrenergic blockers.
• Use cautiously in debilitated patients and in those with hepatic, renal, or CV disease; respiratory disorders; hypocalcemia; seizure disorders; suspected brain tumor or intestinal obstruction; glaucoma; and prostatic hyperplasia.
⚘ Lifespan: In pregnant women, use only if clearly necessary; safety hasn't been established. Women shouldn't breast-feed during therapy because most phenothiazines appear in breast milk and directly affect prolactin levels. For children younger than age 12, phenothiazines aren't recommended unless otherwise specified; use cautiously for nausea and vomiting. Acutely ill children, such as those with chickenpox, measles, CNS infections, or dehydration have a greatly increased risk of dystonic reactions. Elderly patients are more sensitive to therapeutic and adverse effects, especially cardiac toxicity, tardive dyskinesia, and other extrapyramidal effects; use cautiously and give reduced doses, adjusting dosage to patient response.

Adverse reactions

Phenothiazines may produce extrapyramidal symptoms, such as dystonic movements, torticollis, oculogyric crises, and parkinsonian symptoms ranging from akathisia during early treatment to tardive dyskinesia after long-term use. A neuroleptic malignant syndrome resembling severe parkinsonism may occur, most often in young men taking fluphenazine.

Other adverse reactions include abdominal pain, agitation, anorexia, arrhythmias, confusion, constipation, dizziness, dry mouth, endocrine effects, fainting, hallucinations, hematologic disorders, local gastric irritation, nausea, orthostatic hypotension with reflex tachycardia, photosensitivity, seizures, skin eruptions, urine retention, visual disturbances, and vomiting.

Action

Phenothiazines are believed to function as dopamine antagonists by blocking postsynaptic dopamine receptors in various parts of the CNS. Their antiemetic effects result from blockage of the chemoreceptor trigger zone. They also produce varying degrees of anticholinergic effects and alpha-adrenergic–receptor blocking.

NURSING PROCESS

Assessment
• Check vital signs regularly for decreased blood pressure, especially before and after parenteral therapy, or tachycardia; observe patient carefully for other adverse reactions.
• Check intake and output for urine retention or constipation, which may require dosage reduction.
• Establish baseline CBC, ECG (for quinidine-like effects), liver and renal function test results, electrolyte level (especially potassium), and eye examination findings. Monitor these findings periodically thereafter, especially in patients receiving long-term therapy.
• Observe patient for mood changes and monitor progress.
• Monitor patient for involuntary movements. Check patient receiving prolonged treatment at least once every 6 months.

⊕ Key nursing diagnoses
• Risk for injury related to adverse reactions
• Impaired physical mobility related to extrapyramidal symptoms
• Noncompliance related to long-term therapy

▷ Planning and implementation
• Don't stop drug abruptly. Although physical dependence doesn't occur with antipsychotic drugs, rebound worsening of psychotic symptoms may occur, and many drug effects may persist.
• Follow manufacturer's guidelines for reconstitution, dilution, administration, and storage of drugs. Slightly discolored liquids may or may not be acceptable for use. Check with pharmacist.

Patient teaching
• Teach patient how and when to take drug. Tell him not to increase the dosage or stop taking the drug without prescriber's approval. Suggest taking the full dose at bedtime if daytime sedation occurs.
• Teach signs and symptoms of adverse reactions, and urge patient to report unusual effects, especially involuntary movements.
• Instruct patient to avoid beverages and drugs containing alcohol, and warn him not to take other drugs, including OTC or herbal products, without prescriber's approval.
• Advise patient to avoid hazardous tasks until full effects of drug are established. Explain that sedative effects will lessen after several weeks.
• Inform patient that excessive exposure to sunlight, heat lamps, or tanning beds may cause photosensitivity reactions. Advise him to avoid exposure to extreme heat or cold.
• Explain that phenothiazines may cause pink or brown discoloration of urine.

☑ Evaluation
• Patient remains free from injury.
• Patient doesn't develop extrapyramidal symptoms.
• Patient complies with therapy, as shown by improved thought processes.

Protease inhibitors
atazanavir sulfate
fosamprenavir calcium
indinavir sulfate
lopinavir
nelfinavir mesylate
ritonavir
saquinavir
saquinavir mesylate
tipranavir

Indications
▶ HIV infection and AIDS.

Contraindications and cautions
• Contraindicated in patients hypersensitive to drug or its components, and in patients taking a drug highly dependent on CYP3A4 for metabolism.
• Use cautiously in patients with impaired hepatic or renal function and those with diabetes mellitus or hemophilia.
※ **Lifespan:** In pregnant women, use drug only if benefits outweigh risks. Contact the pregnancy registry at 1-800-258-4263 or www.apregistry.com to report pregnant women on therapy. To reduce the risk of transmitting HIV to the infant, HIV-infected mothers shouldn't breast-feed.

Adverse reactions
The most common adverse effects, which require immediate medical attention, include kidney stones, pancreatitis, diabetes or hyperglycemia, ketoacidosis, and paresthesia.

Common adverse effects that don't need medical attention unless they persist or are bothersome include generalized weakness, GI disturbances, headache, insomnia, and taste disturbance. Less common adverse effects include dizziness and somnolence.

Action
Protease inhibitors bind to the protease active site and inhibit HIV protease activity. This enzyme is required for the proteolysis of viral polyprotein precursors into individual functional proteins found in infectious HIV. The net effect is formation of noninfectious, immature viral particles.

NURSING PROCESS

⏏ Assessment
• If patient has hepatic dysfunction, consider the risks and potential benefits of therapy with protease inhibitors.
• Monitor patient for opportunistic infections and drug resistance.
• Observe patients with hemophilia closely for spontaneous bleeding.

⊕ Key nursing diagnoses
• Risk for disturbed body image related to redistribution of body fat from antiretroviral therapy
• Diarrhea related to drug-induced adverse effect on bowel
• Ineffective individual coping related to HIV infection

▷ Planning and implementation
• Protease inhibitors are used with other antiretrovirals. Combination therapy should include three or more antiretrovirals, including a protease inhibitor.
• Protease inhibitors have many interactions. Be aware of what drugs you shouldn't give with a protease inhibitor.
• Check blood glucose levels in patients with diabetes. Drug may cause hyperglycemia, new-onset diabetes, or worsened existing diabetes.
• Indinavir may cause nephrolithiasis. Advise increasing fluid intake.
• Redistribution or accumulation of body fat, including central obesity, dorsocervical fat enlargement (buffalo hump), peripheral wasting, facial wasting, breast enlargement, and cushingoid appearance, may occur.
Patient teaching
• Instruct patient to take drug as prescribed and to finish the full course of therapy.
• Tell patient to take the next dose as soon as possible after a missed dose but not to double the dose.
• Advise patient that drug should be taken with plenty of water 1 or 2 hours before meals and that he should drink about 48 oz (1,440 ml) of water daily.
• Instruct patient not to take other drugs without medical approval.

☑ Evaluation
• Patient doesn't experience altered body image.
• Patient regains normal bowel pattern.
• Patient demonstrates adequate coping mechanisms.

Selective serotonin reuptake inhibitors
citalopram hydrobromide
escitalopram oxalate
fluoxetine hydrochloride
fluvoxamine maleate
paroxetine hydrochloride
sertraline hydrochloride

Indications

▶ Major depression, obsessive-compulsive disorder, bulimia nervosa, premenstrual dysphoric disorders, panic disorders, post-traumatic stress disorder (sertraline).

Contraindications and cautions

• Contraindicated in patients hypersensitive to drug or its components.
• Use cautiously in patients with hepatic, renal, or cardiac insufficiency.
⚘ Lifespan: In pregnant women, use drug only if benefits outweigh risks; use of certain SSRIs in the first trimester may cause birth defects. Neonates born to women who took an SSRI during the third trimester may develop complications that warrant prolonged hospitalization, respiratory support, and tube feeding. In breast-feeding women, use isn't recommended. SSRIs appear in breast milk and may cause diarrhea and sleep disturbance in neonates. However, risks and benefits to both the woman and infant must be considered. Children and adolescents may be more susceptible to increased suicidal tendencies when taking SSRIs or other antidepressants. Elderly patients may be more sensitive to the insomniac effects of SSRIs.

Adverse reactions

Common adverse effects include headache, tremor, dizziness, sleep disturbances, GI disturbances, and sexual dysfunction. Less common

adverse effects include bleeding (ecchymoses, epistaxis), akathisia, breast tenderness or enlargement, extrapyramidal effects, dystonia, fever, hyponatremia, mania or hypomania, palpitations, serotonin syndrome, weight gain or loss, rash, urticaria, or pruritus.

Action

SSRIs selectively inhibit the reuptake of serotonin with little or no effects on other neurotransmitters such as norepinephrine or dopamine, in the CNS.

NURSING PROCESS

Assessment
• Obtain a detailed mental health history, including a family history of suicide, bipolar disorder, or depression, before therapy starts.
• Monitor patient closely for increased suicidal tendencies.
• Hyponatremia usually results from inappropriate secretion of antidiuretic hormone. This problem is most often seen in elderly patients and those treated with diuretics.
• Monitor for serotonin syndrome; signs and symptoms include diarrhea, fever, palpitations, mood swings, behavior changes, restlessness, shaking, and shivering. Hypertension and seizures may occur as well. Risk of this syndrome is highest within days after dosage increases and if patient takes another serotonergic drug.

Key nursing diagnoses
• Disturbed thought processes related to presence of depression
• Risk for injury related to drug-induced adverse CNS reaction
• Deficient knowledge related to drug therapy

Planning and implementation
• Evaluate potential for interactions with other drugs.
• Don't use an SSRI within 14 days of an MAO inhibitor.
• Don't stop therapy abruptly. Taper gradually over several weeks, and monitor the patient carefully for serotonin syndrome.
• Notify prescriber immediately if patient's depression worsens or if he's having thoughts of suicide.

Patient teaching
• Tell patient that drug may take 4 to 5 weeks to produce its full benefit. Advise patient to take drug as prescribed and not to double the next dose if a dose is missed.
• Instruct patient to stop drug and call as soon as possible if a rash or hives develops.
• Caution family members or caregivers to monitor closely for suicidal behaviors or increased agitation.
• Caution patient to avoid alcohol, drugs, or substances that have serotonergic activity.
• Tell patient to use caution when driving or performing tasks requiring alertness because these drugs may cause drowsiness or impair judgment or motor skills.

Evaluation
• Patient's thought process remains clear.
• Patient's safety is maintained.
• Patient and family state understanding of drug therapy.

Skeletal muscle relaxants
baclofen
carisoprodol
chlorzoxazone
cyclobenzaprine hydrochloride
methocarbamol

Indications

▶ Painful musculoskeletal disorders, spasticity caused by multiple sclerosis.

Contraindications and cautions

• Contraindicated in patients hypersensitive to these drugs.
• Use cautiously in patients with impaired renal or hepatic function.
⚕ Lifespan: In pregnant women and breastfeeding women, use only when potential benefits to the patient outweigh risks to the fetus or infant. In children, recommendations vary. Elderly patients have an increased risk of adverse reactions; monitor them carefully.

Adverse reactions

Skeletal muscle relaxants may cause ataxia, confusion, depressed mood, dizziness, drowsi-

ness, dry mouth, hallucinations, headache, hypotension, nervousness, tachycardia, tremor, and vertigo. Baclofen also may cause seizures.

Action

All skeletal muscle relaxants, except baclofen, reduce impulse transmission from the spinal cord to skeletal muscle. Baclofen's mechanism of action is unclear.

NURSING PROCESS

☑ Assessment
- Monitor patient for hypersensitivity reactions.
- Assess degree of relief obtained to determine when dosage can be reduced.
- Watch for increased seizures in epileptic patient receiving baclofen.
- Monitor CBC results closely.
- In patient receiving cyclobenzaprine, monitor platelet counts.
- In patient receiving methocarbamol, watch for orthostatic hypotension.
- In patient receiving long-term baclofen or chlorzoxazone therapy, monitor hepatic function.
- In patient receiving long-term therapy, assess compliance.

☺ Key nursing diagnoses
- Risk for trauma related to baclofen-induced seizures
- Disturbed thought processes related to confusion
- Noncompliance related to long-term therapy

▶ Planning and implementation
- Avoid withdrawal symptoms, such as insomnia, headache, nausea, and abdominal pain, by not abruptly stopping baclofen or carisoprodol after long-term therapy, unless patient has severe adverse reactions.
- Institute safety precautions as needed.
- Prevent GI distress by giving oral forms of drug with meals or milk.

Patient teaching
- Tell patient to take drug exactly as prescribed. Teach him to avoid withdrawal symptoms by not stopping baclofen or carisoprodol abruptly after long-term therapy.
- Instruct patient to avoid hazardous activities that require mental alertness until CNS effects of drug are known.

- Advise patient to avoid alcohol use during therapy.
- Advise patient to follow prescriber's advice regarding rest and physical therapy.
- Instruct patient receiving cyclobenzaprine or baclofen to report urinary hesitancy.
- Inform patient taking methocarbamol or chlorzoxazone that urine may be discolored.

☑ Evaluation
- Patient remains free from seizures.
- Patient exhibits normal thought processes.
- Patient complies with therapy, as shown by pain relief or improvement of spasticity.

Sulfonamides
co-trimoxazole (trimethoprim and
    sulfamethoxazole)
sulfasalazine

Indications

▶ Bacterial infections, nocardiosis, toxoplasmosis, chloroquine-resistant *Plasmodium falciparum* malaria.

Contraindications and cautions

- Contraindicated in patients hypersensitive to these drugs.
- Use cautiously in patients with renal or hepatic impairment, bronchial asthma, severe allergy, or G6PD deficiency.
- ☀ Lifespan: In pregnant women at term and in breast-feeding women, use is contraindicated; sulfonamides appear in breast milk. In infants younger than age 2 months, sulfonamides are contraindicated unless there's no therapeutic alternative. In children with fragile X chromosome and mental retardation, use cautiously. Elderly patients are susceptible to bacterial and fungal superinfection and have an increased risk of folate deficiency anemia and adverse renal and hematologic effects.

Adverse reactions

Many adverse reactions stem from hypersensitivity, including bronchospasm, conjunctivitis, erythema multiforme, erythema nodosum, exfoliative dermatitis, fever, joint pain, pruritus, leukopenia, Lyell syndrome, photosensitivity, rash,

Stevens-Johnson syndrome, and toxic epidermal necrolysis. GI reactions include anorexia, diarrhea, folic acid malabsorption, nausea, pancreatitis, stomatitis, and vomiting. Hematologic reactions include agranulocytosis, granulocytopenia, hypoprothrombinemia, thrombocytopenia, and, in G6PD deficiency, hemolytic anemia. Renal effects usually result from crystalluria caused by precipitation of sulfonamide in renal system.

Action

Sulfonamides are bacteriostatic. They inhibit biosynthesis of tetrahydrofolic acid, which is needed for bacterial cell growth. They're active against some strains of staphylococci, streptococci, *Nocardia asteroides* and *brasiliensis, Clostridium tetani* and *perfringens, Bacillus anthracis, Escherichia coli,* and *Neisseria gonorrhoeae* and *meningitidis.* Sulfonamides are also active against organisms that cause UTIs, such as *E. coli, Proteus mirabilis* and *vulgaris, Klebsiella, Enterobacter,* and *Staphylococcus aureus,* and genital lesions caused by *Haemophilus ducreyi* (chancroid).

NURSING PROCESS

▓ Assessment
• Assess patient's history of allergies, especially to sulfonamides or to any drug containing sulfur, such as thiazides, furosemide, and oral sulfonylureas.
• Monitor patient for adverse reactions.
• Obtain culture and sensitivity tests before first dose; check test results periodically to assess the drug's effectiveness.
• Monitor urine cultures, CBC, and urinalysis before and during therapy.
• During long-term therapy, monitor patient for possible superinfection.

▓ Key nursing diagnoses
• Ineffective protection related to hypersensitivity
• Risk for infection related to superinfection
• Risk for deficient fluid volume related to adverse GI reactions

▓ Planning and implementation
• Give oral dose with 8 oz (240 ml) of water. Give 3 to 4 L of fluids daily, depending on

drug; patient's urine output should be at least 1,500 ml daily.
• Follow manufacturer's directions for reconstituting, diluting, and storing drugs; check expiration dates.
• Shake oral suspensions well before giving to ensure correct dosage.

Patient teaching
• Urge patient to take drug exactly as prescribed, to complete the prescribed regimen, and to keep follow-up appointments.
• Advise patient to take oral drug with full glass of water and to drink plenty of fluids; explain that tablet may be crushed and swallowed with water to ensure maximum absorption.
• Teach signs and symptoms of hypersensitivity and other adverse reactions. Urge patient to report bloody urine, difficulty breathing, rash, fever, chills, or severe fatigue.
• Advise patient to avoid direct sun exposure and to use a sunscreen to help prevent photosensitivity reactions.
• Tell diabetic patient that sulfonamides may increase effects of oral antidiabetics.
• Inform patient taking sulfasalazine that it may cause an orange-yellow discoloration of urine or skin and may permanently stain soft contact lenses yellow.

▓ Evaluation
• Patient exhibits no signs of hypersensitivity.
• Patient is free from infection.
• Patient maintains adequate hydration.

Tetracyclines

doxycycline
doxycycline hyclate
minocycline hydrochloride
oxytetracycline hydrochloride
tetracycline hydrochloride

Indications

▶ Bacterial, protozoal, rickettsial, and fungal infections.

Contraindications and cautions

• Contraindicated in patients hypersensitive to these drugs.

• Use cautiously in patients with renal or hepatic impairment.

⚘ **Lifespan:** In pregnant or breast-feeding women, use is contraindicated; tetracyclines appear in breast milk. Children younger than age 8 shouldn't take tetracyclines; these drugs can cause permanent tooth discoloration, enamel hypoplasia, and a reversible decrease in bone calcification. Elderly patients may have decreased esophageal motility; use these drugs cautiously, and monitor patients for local irritation from slow passage of oral forms. Elderly patients also are more susceptible to superinfection.

Adverse reactions

The most common adverse effects involve the GI tract and are dose related; they include abdominal discomfort; anorexia; bulky, loose stools; epigastric burning; flatulence; nausea; and vomiting. Superinfections also are common. Photosensitivity reactions may be severe. Renal failure may be caused by Fanconi syndrome after use of outdated tetracycline. Permanent discoloration of teeth occurs if drug is given during tooth formation in children younger than age 8.

Action

Tetracyclines are bacteriostatic but may be bactericidal against certain organisms. They bind reversibly to 30S and 50S ribosomal subunits, which inhibits bacterial protein synthesis.

Susceptible gram-positive organisms include *Bacillus anthracis, Actinomyces israelii, Clostridium perfringens* and *tetani, Listeria monocytogenes,* and *Nocardia.*

Susceptible gram-negative organisms include *Neisseria meningitidis, Pasteurella multocida, Legionella pneumophila, Brucella, Vibrio cholerae, Yersinia enterocolitica, Yersinia pestis, Bordetella pertussis, Haemophilus influenzae, Haemophilus ducreyi, Campylobacter fetus, Shigella,* and many other common pathogens.

Other susceptible organisms include *Rickettsia akari, typhi, prowazekii,* and *tsutsugamushi; Coxiella burnetii; Chlamydia trachomatis* and *psittaci; Mycoplasma pneumoniae* and *hominis; Leptospira; Treponema pallidum* and *pertenue;* and *Borrelia recurrentis.*

🝫 Assessment
• Assess patient's allergic history.
• Monitor patient for adverse reactions.
• Obtain culture and sensitivity tests before first dose; check cultures periodically to assess drug effectiveness.
• Check expiration dates before giving. Outdated tetracyclines may cause nephrotoxicity.
• Monitor patient for bacterial and fungal superinfection, especially if patient is elderly, debilitated, or receiving immunosuppressants or radiation therapy; watch especially for oral candidiasis.

🟦 Key nursing diagnoses
• Ineffective protection related to hypersensitivity
• Risk for infection related to superinfection
• Risk for deficient fluid volume related to adverse GI reactions

❯ Planning and implementation
• For maximum absorption, give all oral tetracyclines except doxycycline and minocycline 1 hour before or 2 hours after meals. Don't give drug with food, milk or other dairy products, sodium bicarbonate, iron compounds, or antacids, which may impair absorption.
• Give water with and after oral drug to help it pass to the stomach because incomplete swallowing can cause severe esophageal irritation. To prevent esophageal reflux, don't give drug within 1 hour of bedtime.
• Monitor I.V. injection sites and rotate routinely to minimize local irritation. I.V. administration may cause severe phlebitis.
Patient teaching
• Urge patient to take drug exactly as prescribed, to complete the prescribed regimen, and to keep follow-up appointments.
• Warn patient not to take drug with food, milk or other dairy products, sodium bicarbonate, or iron compounds because they may interfere with absorption. Advise him to wait 3 hours after taking tetracycline before taking an antacid.
• Instruct patient to check expiration dates and to discard any expired drug.
• Teach signs and symptoms of adverse reactions, and urge patient to report them promptly.

• Advise patient to avoid direct exposure to sunlight and to use a sunscreen to help prevent photosensitivity reactions.

✔ Evaluation
• Patient shows no signs of hypersensitivity.
• Patient is free from infection.
• Patient maintains adequate hydration.

Xanthine derivatives
aminophylline
theophylline

Indications
▶ Asthma and bronchospasm from emphysema and chronic bronchitis.

Contraindications and cautions
• Contraindicated in patients hypersensitive to these drugs.
• Use cautiously in patients with arrhythmias, cardiac or circulatory impairment, cor pulmonale, hepatic or renal disease, active peptic ulcers, hyperthyroidism, or diabetes mellitus.
⚖ Lifespan: In pregnant women, use cautiously. In breast-feeding women, avoid these drugs because they appear in breast milk, and infants may have serious adverse reactions. Small children may have excessive CNS stimulation; monitor them closely. In elderly patients, use cautiously.

Adverse reactions
Adverse effects, except for hypersensitivity, are dose related and can be controlled by dosage adjustment. Common reactions include arrhythmias, headache, hypotension, irritability, nausea, palpitations, restlessness, urine retention, and vomiting.

Action
Xanthine derivatives are structurally related; they directly relax smooth muscle, stimulate the CNS, induce diuresis, increase gastric acid secretion, inhibit uterine contractions, and exert weak inotropic and chronotropic effects on the heart. Of these drugs, theophylline exerts the greatest effect on smooth muscle.

The action of xanthine derivatives isn't completely caused by inhibition of phosphodiesterase. Current data suggest that inhibition of adenosine receptors or unidentified mechanisms may be responsible for therapeutic effects. By relaxing smooth muscle of the respiratory tract, they increase airflow and vital capacity. They also slow onset of diaphragmatic fatigue and stimulate the respiratory center in the CNS.

NURSING PROCESS

⚗ Assessment
• Monitor theophylline level closely because therapeutic level ranges from 10 to 20 mcg/ml.
• Monitor patient closely for adverse reactions, especially toxicity.
• Monitor vital signs.

⊕ Key nursing diagnoses
• Insomnia related to CNS effects
• Urinary retention related to adverse effects on bladder
• Noncompliance related to long-term therapy

▷ Planning and implementation
• Don't crush or allow patient to chew timed-release forms.
• Calculate dosage from lean body weight because theophylline doesn't distribute into fatty tissue.
• Adjust daily dosage in elderly patients and in those with heart failure or hepatic disease.
• Provide patient with nondrug sleep aids, such as a back rub or milk-based beverage.
Patient teaching
• Tell patient to take drug exactly as prescribed.
• Advise patient to check with prescriber before using any other drug, including OTC medications or herbal remedies, and before switching brands.
• If patient smokes, tell him that doing so may decrease theophylline level. Urge him to notify prescriber if he quits smoking because the dosage will need adjustment to avoid toxicity.

✔ Evaluation
• Patient sleeps usual number of hours without interruption.
• Patient's voiding pattern doesn't change.
• Patient complies with therapy, as shown by maintenance of therapeutic level.

⊗ **Incompatibilities**
Don't infuse in the same line with other I.V. drugs.

Route	Onset	Peak	Duration
I.V.	Unknown	Unknown	Unknown

Contraindications and cautions

• Contraindicated in patients hypersensitive to abatacept or any component of the drug. Don't use in patients taking a TNF antagonist or anakinra.
• Use cautiously in patients with active infection, history of chronic infections, scheduled elective surgery, or COPD. Patients who test positive for tuberculosis should be treated before receiving abatacept.
⚹ **Lifespan:** In pregnant women, use drug only if clearly needed. It isn't known if drug appears in breast milk; drug could cause serious adverse reactions in a breast-fed infant and may affect the developing immune system. In elderly patients, use drug cautiously because older adults may have a higher risk of infection and malignancy.

Adverse reactions

CNS: dizziness, *headache.*
CV: hypertension.
EENT: *nasopharyngitis,* rhinitis, sinusitis.
GI: diverticulitis, dyspepsia, *nausea.*
GU: acute pyelonephritis, UTI.
Musculoskeletal: back pain, limb pain.
Respiratory: bronchitis, cough, pneumonia, *upper respiratory tract infection.*
Skin: cellulitis, rash.
Other: herpes simplex, *infections,* influenza, infusion reactions, ***malignancies.***

Interactions

Drug-drug. *Anakinra, TNF antagonists:* May increase risk of infection. Avoid use together.
Live-virus vaccines: May decrease effectiveness of vaccine. Avoid giving vaccines during abatacept treatment or within 3 months after stopping.

Effects on lab test results

None reported.

Pharmacokinetics

Absorption: Given I.V.
Distribution: Not reported.
Metabolism: Not reported.
Excretion: Not reported. *Half-life:* 13 days.

Action

Chemical effect: Inhibits T-cell activation, decreases T-cell proliferation, and inhibits production of TNF-alpha, interferon-gamma, and interleukin-2.
Therapeutic effect: Reduces pain and inflammation and improves physical function in patients with rheumatoid arthritis.

Available forms

Lyophilized powder for injection: 250 mg/15-ml single-use vial

NURSING PROCESS

▨ **Assessment**
• Screen patient for tuberculosis before giving abatacept.
• Assess patient's condition before starting therapy and regularly thereafter to monitor drug's effectiveness.
• Monitor patient carefully for infections and malignancies.
• Assess patient's and family's knowledge of drug therapy.

⊕ **Nursing diagnoses**
• Ineffective health maintenance related to underlying disease
• Risk for infection related to abatacept therapy
• Deficient knowledge related to drug therapy

▷ **Planning and implementation**
• Don't give abatacept with TNF antagonists (Enbrel, Remicade, Humira) or anakinra.
• Notify prescriber if patient develops a severe infection; therapy may need to be stopped.
• If patient has COPD, monitor patient for worsening of symptoms during drug therapy.
Patient teaching
• Urge patient to have tuberculosis screening before starting abatacept treatment.
• Tell patient to continue taking prescribed arthritis drugs. Caution against taking TNF antagonists (Enbrel, Remicade, Humira) or anakinra.
• Tell patient to avoid exposure to infections during treatment.

• Tell patient to immediately report signs and symptoms of infection, swollen face or tongue, and difficulty breathing.
• Tell patient with COPD to report worsening signs and symptoms.
• Advise patient to avoid live-virus vaccines during abatacept treatment and for up to 3 months after it's stopped.
• Advise patient to consult prescriber if she becomes pregnant or plans to breast-feed.
• Advise patient to contact prescriber before taking any other drugs or herbal supplements.
• Remind patient to contact prescriber before being scheduled for surgery.

✓ Evaluation
• Patient's rheumatoid arthritis symptoms and level of physical function improve.
• Patient is free from infection during drug therapy.
• Patient and family state understanding of drug therapy.

abciximab
(ab-SICKS-ih-mahb)
ReoPro

Pharmacologic class: glycoprotein IIb/IIIa receptor blocker
Therapeutic class: platelet-aggregation inhibitor
Pregnancy risk category: C

Indications and dosages

▶ **Adjunct for percutaneous coronary intervention (PCI) to prevent acute cardiac ischemic complications in patients at high risk for abrupt closure of treated coronary vessel.**
Adults: 0.25 mg/kg as I.V. bolus 10 to 60 minutes before PCI, followed by continuous I.V. infusion of 0.125 mcg/kg/minute (maximum, 10 mcg/minute) for 12 hours.
▶ **Patients with unstable angina not responding to conventional medical therapy who will undergo PCI within 24 hours.**
Adults: 0.25 mg/kg as I.V. bolus; then an 18- to 24-hour infusion of 10 mcg/minute, concluding 1 hour after PCI.

▽ I.V. administration
• Intended for use with heparin and aspirin.
• Anticipate hypersensitivity reactions. Have epinephrine, dopamine, theophylline, antihistamine, and corticosteroid available for immediate use.
• If solution contains opaque particles, discard it and obtain a new vial.
• For I.V. bolus, withdraw needed amount of drug into syringe; then inject through a sterile 0.2- to 5-micron syringe filter.
• For I.V. infusion, withdraw needed amount of drug through a 0.2- to 5-micron syringe filter; then inject drug into normal saline solution or D_5W, and infuse via continuous infusion pump equipped with 0.2- or 0.22-micron in-line filter.
• Discard any unused portion of vials or mixed drug.
⊗ **Incompatibilities**
• Give drug in a separate I.V. line; don't add another drug to infusion solution.

Contraindications and cautions

• Contraindicated in patients hypersensitive to a drug component or to murine proteins and in patients with active internal bleeding; bleeding diathesis; platelet count less than 100,000/mm³; intracranial neoplasm, arteriovenous malformation, or aneurysm; severe uncontrolled hypertension; a history of stroke within 2 years or with significant residual neurologic deficit; or a history of vasculitis. Also contraindicated within 6 weeks of major surgery, trauma, or GI or GU bleeding; when oral anticoagulants have been given within 7 days unless PT is 1.2 times control or less; and when I.V. dextran is used before or during PCI.
• Use cautiously in patients who weigh less than 75 kg (165 lb), have a history of GI disease, or are receiving thrombolytics because these patients are at increased risk for bleeding. Conditions that increase risk of bleeding include PCI within 12 hours of onset of symptoms of acute MI, PCI lasting longer than 70 minutes, failed PCI, and use of heparin.
※ **Lifespan:** In pregnant or breast-feeding women, use cautiously. In children, safety and effectiveness of drug haven't been established. In patients older than age 65, use cautiously.

Adverse reactions

CNS: hypoesthesia, confusion, headache, pain.

CV: hypotension, chest pain, *bradycardia,* peripheral edema.
EENT: abnormal vision.
GI: nausea, vomiting, abdominal pain.
Hematologic: *bleeding, thrombocytopenia,* anemia, leukocytosis.
Musculoskeletal: *back pain.*
Respiratory: pleural effusion, pleurisy, pneumonia.

Interactions

Drug-drug. *Antiplatelets, heparin, NSAIDs, other anticoagulants, thrombolytics:* May increase risk of bleeding. Monitor patient closely.

Effects on lab test results

• May decrease hemoglobin level and hematocrit.
• May decrease platelet counts. May increase WBC count.

Pharmacokinetics

Absorption: Given I.V.
Distribution: Rapidly binds to platelet receptors.
Metabolism: Unknown.
Excretion: Unknown. *Half-life:* Initially, less than 10 minutes; second phase, about 30 minutes.

Route	Onset	Peak	Duration
I.V.	Immediate	Immediate	24 hr

Action

Chemical effect: Prevents binding of fibrinogen, von Willebrand factor, and other adhesive molecules to receptor sites on activated platelets.
Therapeutic effect: Inhibits platelet aggregation.

Available forms

Injection: 2 mg/ml

NURSING PROCESS

℞ Assessment
• PCI patients at risk for abrupt closure include those with unstable angina, non–ST segment elevation MI (NSTEMI), ST segment elevation MI (STEMI) within 12 hours of symptom onset, two type B lesions in the artery to be dilated,

one type B lesion in the artery to be dilated in a patient with diabetes or a woman older than age 65, one type C lesion in the artery to be dilated, or angioplasty of an infarct-related lesion within 7 days of MI.
• Assess vital signs and evaluate bleeding studies before therapy.
• Monitor patient closely for bleeding, particularly bleeding at the arterial access site for cardiac catheterization and internal bleeding involving the GI or GU tract or retroperitoneal sites.
• Look for adverse reactions and drug interactions.
• Assess patient's and family's knowledge of drug therapy.

⊞ Nursing diagnoses
• Ineffective cerebral or cardiopulmonary tissue perfusion related to patient's underlying condition
• Risk for deficient fluid volume related to drug-induced bleeding
• Deficient knowledge related to drug therapy

▷ Planning and implementation
• Institute bleeding precautions. Keep patient on bed rest for 6 to 8 hours after removing sheath or stopping infusion, whichever is later.
• Drug is intended for use with aspirin, heparin, and Plavix.
⚠ **ALERT:** Keep epinephrine, dopamine, theophylline, antihistamines, and corticosteroids available in case of anaphylaxis.
Patient teaching
• Teach patient about his disease and therapy.
• Stress the importance of reporting adverse reactions.

✓ Evaluation
• Patient maintains adequate tissue perfusion.
• Patient maintains adequate hydration.
• Patient and family state understanding of drug therapy.

acamprosate calcium

(ay-CAM-proh-sate KAL-see-um)
Campral⊘

Pharmacologic class: GABA and glutamate agonist
Therapeutic class: alcohol deterrent
Pregnancy risk category: C

Indications and dosages

▶ **Maintenance of alcohol abstinence as part of a comprehensive treatment program.**
Adults: 666 mg P.O. t.i.d.
◪ **Adjust-a-dose:** If patient's creatinine clearance is 30 to 50 ml/minute, give 333 mg t.i.d.

Contraindications and cautions

• Contraindicated in patients allergic to drug or its components and in those whose creatinine clearance is 30 ml/minute or less.
• Use cautiously in patients with moderate renal impairment or a history of depression with suicidal thoughts or attempts.
✷ **Lifespan:** Use cautiously in women who are pregnant or breast-feeding and in elderly patients. Safety and effectiveness haven't been evaluated in children. In elderly patients, drug levels are likely to be increased because these patients commonly have reduced renal function; consider a reduced dosage, and monitor renal function.

Adverse reactions

CNS: abnormal thinking, amnesia, anxiety, asthenia, depression, dizziness, headache, insomnia, paresthesia, somnolence, *suicidal ideation,* syncope, tremor.
CV: hypertension, palpitations, peripheral edema, vasodilation.
EENT: abnormal vision, pharyngitis, rhinitis.
GI: abdominal pain, anorexia, constipation, *diarrhea,* dry mouth, dyspepsia, flatulence, increased appetite, nausea, taste disturbance, vomiting.
GU: impotence.
Metabolic: weight gain.
Musculoskeletal: arthralgia, back pain, chest pain, myalgia.
Respiratory: bronchitis, dyspnea, increased cough.
Skin: increased sweating, pruritus, rash.

Other: accidental injury, chills, flulike symptoms, infection, pain.

Interactions

None significant.

Effects on lab test results

• May increase ALT, AST, and bilirubin levels. May decrease hemoglobin level and hematocrit.
• May decrease platelet count.

Pharmacokinetics

Absorption: Absolute bioavailability is about 11%.
Distribution: Into plasma. Negligibly protein-bound.
Metabolism: Not metabolized.
Excretion: By the kidneys as unchanged drug. *Half-life:* 20 to 33 hours.

Route	Onset	Peak	Duration
P.O.	Unknown	3–8 hr	Unknown

Action

Chemical effect: Restores the balance of neuronal excitation and inhibition, probably by interacting with glutamate and gamma aminobutyric acid neurotransmitter systems, thus reducing alcohol dependence.
Therapeutic effect: Aids maintenance of alcohol abstinence.

Available forms

Tablets (delayed-release): 333 mg

NURSING PROCESS

⬛ Assessment
• Obtain a history of the patient's alcohol use before therapy.
• Assess the patient's support system and his involvement in a comprehensive treatment program.
• Monitor the patient for adverse reactions to drug therapy.
• Monitor the patient for development of depression or suicidal thoughts.
• Assess the patient's and family's knowledge of drug therapy.

⊕ Nursing diagnoses
• Ineffective health maintenance related to alcoholism

Reactions may be *common,* uncommon, *life-threatening*, or COMMON AND LIFE-THREATENING.

• Risk for injury related to alcoholism and drug-induced adverse CNS effects
• Deficient knowledge related to drug therapy

> **Planning and implementation**
• Use drug only after the patient has successfully achieved abstinence.
• Drug doesn't eliminate or reduce withdrawal symptoms.
• Drug doesn't cause alcohol aversion or a disulfiram-like reaction if used with alcohol.
Patient teaching
• Tell patient to continue the alcohol abstinence program, including counseling and support.
• Advise patient to notify his prescriber if he develops depression, anxiety, thoughts of suicide, or severe diarrhea.
• Caution patient's family or caregiver to watch for signs of depression or suicidal ideation.
• Tell patient that drug may be taken without regard to meals, but that taking it with meals may help him remember to take it.
• Tell patient not to crush, break, or chew the tablets but to swallow them whole.
• Advise women to use effective contraception while taking this drug. Tell the patient to contact her prescriber if she becomes pregnant or plans to become pregnant.
• Explain that this drug may impair judgment, thinking, or motor skills. Urge patient to use caution when driving or performing hazardous activities until drug's effects are known.
• Tell patient to continue taking acamprosate and to contact his prescriber if he resumes drinking.

☑ Evaluation
• Patient abstains from alcohol consumption.
• Patient abstains from alcohol and doesn't experience injury.
• Patient and family state understanding of drug therapy.

HIGH ALERT!

acarbose
(ay-KAR-bohs)
Precose

Pharmacologic class: alpha-glucosidase inhibitor
Therapeutic class: antidiabetic
Pregnancy risk category: B

Indications and dosages

▶ **To lower glucose level in patients with type 2 diabetes mellitus, along with diet, exercise, and possibly a sulfonylurea, metformin, or insulin.** *Adults:* Initially, 25 mg P.O. t.i.d. with the first bite of each main meal. Adjust dosage every 4 to 8 weeks based on glucose level and tolerance 1 hour after a meal. Maximum dosage is 50 mg P.O. t.i.d. for patients weighing 60 kg (132 lb) or less and 100 mg P.O. t.i.d. for patients weighing more than 60 kg.

Contraindications and cautions

• Contraindicated in patients hypersensitive to drug and in patients with diabetic ketoacidosis, cirrhosis, inflammatory bowel disease, colonic ulceration, partial intestinal obstruction, predisposition to intestinal obstruction, chronic intestinal disease with disorder of digestion or absorption, or conditions that may deteriorate because of increased intestinal gas formation.
• Drug isn't recommended in patients with severe renal impairment.
• Use cautiously in patients receiving insulin or a sulfonylurea. Drug may increase the hypoglycemic potential of a sulfonylurea.
✹ **Lifespan:** In pregnant or breast-feeding women, drug isn't recommended. In children, safety and effectiveness haven't been established.

Adverse reactions

GI: *abdominal pain, diarrhea, flatulence.*

Interactions

Drug-drug. *Calcium channel blockers, corticosteroids, estrogens, hormonal contraceptives, isoniazid, nicotinic acid, phenothiazines, phenytoin, sympathomimetics, thiazides and other diuretics, thyroid products:* May cause hyperglycemia and loss of glucose control during use or hypoglycemia when withdrawn. Monitor glucose level.
Digestive enzyme preparations containing carbohydrate-splitting enzymes (such as amylase, Beano enzyme, pancreatin), intestinal adsorbents (such as activated charcoal): May reduce effect of acarbose. Don't give together.
Digoxin: May decrease digoxin level. Monitor digoxin level.
Drug-herb. *Aloe, bilberry leaf, bitter melon, burdock, dandelion, fenugreek, garlic, ginseng:* May improve glucose control and allow reduced

---

antidiabetic dosage. Urge patient to discuss herbal products with prescriber before use.

Effects on lab test results
• May increase ALT and AST levels. May decrease hemoglobin level and hematocrit.

Pharmacokinetics
Absorption: Minimal.
Distribution: Acts locally in GI tract.
Metabolism: Exclusively in the GI tract, mainly by intestinal bacteria and partly by digestive enzymes.
Excretion: Almost completely excreted by the kidneys. *Half-life:* 2 hours.

Route	Onset	Peak	Duration
P.O.	Unknown	1 hr	2–4 hr

Action
Chemical effect: Delays carbohydrate digestion and glucose absorption. Inhibits the metabolism of sucrose to glucose and fructose.
Therapeutic effect: Lessens postprandial hyperglycemia.

Available forms
Tablets: 25 mg, 50 mg, 100 mg

NURSING PROCESS

Assessment
• Obtain baseline creatinine level. Drug isn't recommended in patient with a creatinine level greater than 2 mg/dl.
• Monitor glucose level 1 hour after a meal to determine effectiveness and to identify appropriate dose. Report hypoglycemia or hyperglycemia to prescriber.
• Measure glycosylated hemoglobin level every 3 months.
• In a patient receiving 50 mg t.i.d. or more, monitor transaminase level every 3 months in first year of therapy and periodically thereafter. Report abnormalities to prescriber.
• Assess patient's and family's knowledge of drug therapy.

Nursing diagnoses
• Risk for imbalanced fluid volume related to adverse GI effect

• Imbalanced nutrition: less than body requirements related to patient's underlying condition
• Deficient knowledge related to drug therapy

Planning and implementation
• If dosage exceeds 50 mg t.i.d., watch for high transaminase and bilirubin levels and low calcium and vitamin B_6 levels.
• Drug may increase hypoglycemic potential of sulfonylureas. Closely monitor any patient receiving both drugs. If hypoglycemia occurs, treat with dextrose, I.V. glucose infusion, or glucagon. Report hypoglycemia to prescriber.
• Insulin may be needed during increased stress, such as during infection, fever, surgery, or trauma.

Patient teaching
• Tell patient to take drug daily with first bite of each of three main meals.
• Explain that therapy relieves symptoms but doesn't cure the disease.
• Stress the importance of adhering to specific diet, weight reduction, exercise, and hygiene programs. Show patient how to monitor glucose level and how to recognize and treat hyperglycemia.
• Teach patient to recognize hypoglycemia and to treat symptoms with a form of dextrose rather than with a product containing table sugar.
• Instruct patient to check with the prescriber before using any OTC natural or herbal products, such as Beano.
• Urge patient to wear or carry medical identification at all times.

Evaluation
• Patient maintains adequate fluid volume balance.
• Patient doesn't experience hypoglycemia.
• Patient and family state understanding of drug therapy.

acebutolol
(as-ih-BYOO-tuh-lol)
Sectral

Pharmacologic class: beta blocker
Therapeutic class: antihypertensive, antiarrhythmic
Pregnancy risk category: B

A

Indications and dosages

▶ **Hypertension.** *Adults:* 400 mg P.O. as single daily dosage or in divided doses b.i.d. Maximum, 1,200 mg daily.

▶ **Suppression of PVCs.** *Adults:* 400 mg P.O. in divided doses b.i.d. Increase dosage to attain adequate response. Usual dosage is 600 to 1,200 mg daily.

▶ **Stable angina‡.** *Adults:* Initially, 200 mg P.O. b.i.d. Increase dosage up to 800 mg daily until angina is controlled. Patients with severe stable angina may require higher doses.

§ **Adjust-a-dose:** For patients with renal impairment, if creatinine clearance is less than 50 ml/minute, decrease dosage by 50%; if creatinine clearance is less than 25 ml/minute, decrease dosage by 75%. In elderly patients, don't exceed 800 mg daily.

Contraindications and cautions

• Contraindicated in patients with persistently severe bradycardia, second- or third-degree heart block, overt heart failure, or cardiogenic shock.

• Use cautiously in patients with heart failure, peripheral vascular disease, bronchospastic disease, diabetes, or hepatic impairment. Avoid abrupt withdrawal.

⚘ **Lifespan:** In pregnant women, use cautiously and only if benefits to mother outweigh risks to fetus. In breast-feeding women, use is contraindicated. In children, safety of drug hasn't been established. In elderly patients, use cautiously and at a reduced dosage.

Adverse reactions

CNS: abnormal dreams, depression, dizziness, *fatigue,* fever, headache, insomnia.
CV: *bradycardia,* chest pain, edema, ***heart failure,*** hypotension.
EENT: abnormal vision, dry eye, eye pain, rhinitis.
GI: constipation, diarrhea, dyspepsia, flatulence, ***mesenteric arterial thrombosis,*** nausea, vomiting.
GU: impotence.
Metabolic: hyperglycemia, ***hypoglycemia, unstable diabetes mellitus.***
Musculoskeletal: arthralgia, myalgia.
Respiratory: *bronchospasm,* cough, dyspnea.
Skin: rash.

Interactions

Drug-drug. *Alpha-adrenergic stimulants:* May increase hypertensive response. Use together cautiously.
Diltiazem: May cause excessive bradycardia and increase myocardial depression. Use together cautiously.
Insulin, oral antidiabetics: May alter dosage requirements in previously stabilized diabetic patient. Observe patient carefully.
NSAIDs: May decrease antihypertensive effect. Monitor blood pressure and adjust dosage.
Prazosin: May increase the risk of orthostatic hypotension early in use together. Help patient to stand slowly until effects are known.
Reserpine: May have an additive effect. Monitor patient closely.
Verapamil: May increase the effects of both drugs. Monitor cardiac function closely, and decrease dosages as needed.

Effects on lab test results

• May cause false-positive antinuclear antibody test result. May cause false results with glucose or insulin tolerance tests.

Pharmacokinetics

Absorption: Well absorbed after oral use.
Distribution: About 25% protein-bound. Minimal quantities detected in CSF.
Metabolism: Undergoes extensive first-pass metabolism in liver.
Excretion: 30% to 40% of dose is excreted in urine, the rest in feces and bile. *Half-life:* 3 to 4 hours.

Route	Onset	Peak	Duration
P.O.	1–1½ hr	2½ hr	< 24 hr

Action

Chemical effect: May reduce cardiac output and inhibit renin release. May decrease myocardial contractility and heart rate.
Therapeutic effect: Lowers blood pressure and heart rate and restores normal sinus rhythm.

Available forms

Capsules: 200 mg, 400 mg

NURSING PROCESS

Assessment
- Assess blood pressure and heart rate and rhythm before and during therapy.
- Monitor energy level.
- Be alert for adverse reactions and drug interactions.
- Assess patient's and family's knowledge of drug therapy.

Nursing diagnoses
- Risk for injury related to patient's underlying condition
- Fatigue related to drug-induced CNS adverse reactions
- Deficient knowledge related to drug therapy

Planning and implementation
- Drug may be removed by hemodialysis.
- Check apical pulse before giving drug; if it's slower than 60 beats/minute, withhold drug and call prescriber.
- ⚠ ALERT: Don't stop drug abruptly. Doing so may worsen angina or cause an MI or rebound hypertension.
- Before surgery, notify anesthesiologist about patient's drug therapy.
- ⚠ ALERT: Don't confuse Sectral with Factrel or Septra.

Patient teaching
- Teach patient how to take his pulse; if it's lower than 60 beats/minute, instruct him to skip the dose and notify his prescriber.
- Warn patient that drug may cause dizziness. Instruct him to avoid sudden position changes and to sit down immediately if he feels dizzy.
- Explain the importance of taking the drug as prescribed, even when feeling well.
- Tell a diabetic patient to monitor glucose level closely because this drug may mask the symptoms of hypoglycemia.

Evaluation
- Patient's blood pressure and heart rate and rhythm are normal.
- Patient effectively combats fatigue.
- Patient and family state understanding of drug therapy.

acetaminophen
(APAP, paracetamol)
(as-ee-tuh-MIH-nuh-fin)

Abenol ◆ †, Acephen†, Aceta†, Aceta Elixir*†, Acetaminophen Uniserts†, Anacin†, Anacin Maximum Strength Aspirin Free†, Apacet†, Atasol Drops ◆ †, Atasol Elixir*†, Atasol Forte Caplets ◆ †, Atasol Tablets ◆ †, FeverAll Children's†, FeverAll Infant's†, FeverAll Junior Strength†, Genapap†, Genapap Children's Elixir†, Genapap Children's Tablets†, Genapap Extra Strength†, Genapap Infant's Drops†, Genebs†, Genebs Extra Strength†, Liquiprin Infant's Drops†, Mapap†, Meda-Cap†, Meda Tab†, Neopap†, Oraphen-PD†, Panadol†, Panadol Children's†, Redutemp†, Silapap Children's, Silapap Infant's Drops, St. Joseph Aspirin-Free Fever Reducer for Children†, Tapanol Extra Strength†, Tempra†, Tempra Infant's†, Tylenol†, Tylenol Arthritis Extended Relief, Tylenol Children's Chewable Tablets†, Tylenol Children's Elixir†, Tylenol Extended Relief†, Tylenol Extra Strength†, Tylenol Infant's Drops†, Tylenol Junior Strength†

Pharmacologic class: para-aminophenol derivative
Therapeutic class: nonpioid analgesic, antipyretic
Pregnancy risk category: B

Indications and dosages

▶ **Mild pain or fever.** *Adults and children older than age 12:* Give 325 to 650 mg P.O. or P.R. every 4 hours, p.r.n. Or 1 g P.O. t.i.d. or q.i.d., p.r.n. Or two extended-release caplets P.O. every 8 hours. Maximum daily dose, 4 g. Maximum dosage for chronic alcoholics is 2 g daily.
Children ages 11 to 12: Give 480 mg P.O. or P.R. every 4 to 6 hours, p.r.n.
Children ages 9 to 10: Give 400 mg P.O. or P.R. every 4 to 6 hours, p.r.n.
Children ages 6 to 8: Give 320 mg P.O. or P.R. every 4 to 6 hours, p.r.n.
Children ages 4 to 5: Give 240 mg P.O. or P.R. every 4 to 6 hours, p.r.n.
Children ages 2 to 3: Give 160 mg P.O. or P.R. every 4 to 6 hours, p.r.n.

Reactions may be *common,* uncommon, *life-threatening,* or COMMON AND LIFE-THREATENING.

Children ages 12 to 23 months: Give 120 mg P.O. every 4 to 6 hours, p.r.n.
Infants ages 4 to 11 months: Give 80 mg P.O. every 4 to 6 hours, p.r.n.
Infants age 3 months or younger: Give 40 mg P.O. every 4 to 6 hours, p.r.n.
▶ **Osteoarthritis.** *Adults:* Up to 1 g P.O. q.i.d.

Contraindications and cautions

• Contraindicated in patients hypersensitive to drug.
• Use cautiously in patients with a history of chronic alcohol abuse because hepatotoxicity may occur after therapeutic doses.
⚘ **Lifespan:** In pregnant or breast-feeding women, use cautiously.

Adverse reactions

Hematologic: hemolytic anemia, *leukopenia, neutropenia, pancytopenia, thrombocytopenia.*
Hepatic: *liver damage* (with toxic doses), jaundice.
Metabolic: *hypoglycemia.*
Skin: rash, urticaria.

Interactions

Drug-drug. *Barbiturates, carbamazepine, hydantoins, isoniazid, rifampin, sulfinpyrazone:* May reduce therapeutic effects and enhance hepatotoxic effects of acetaminophen with high doses or long-term use of these drugs. Avoid use together.
Lamotrigine: Serum lamotrigine concentrations may be reduced and may decrease therapeutic effects.
Warfarin: May increase hypoprothrombinemic effect with long-term use of high doses of acetaminophen. Monitor PT and INR closely.
Zidovudine: May increase risk of bone marrow suppression because of impaired zidovudine metabolism. Monitor patient closely.
Drug-lifestyle. *Alcohol use:* May increase risk of liver damage. Discourage use together.

Effects on lab test results

• May decrease hemoglobin level and hematocrit.
• May decrease neutrophil, WBC, RBC, and platelet counts.
• May produce false-positive results for urinary 5-hydroxyindoleacetic acid.

Pharmacokinetics

Absorption: Rapid and complete.
Distribution: 25% protein-bound. Level isn't connected strongly with analgesic effect but is with toxicity.
Metabolism: 90% to 95% metabolized in liver.
Excretion: In urine. *Half-life:* 1 to 4 hours.

Route	Onset	Peak	Duration
P.O., P.R.	Unknown	10–60 min	4–6 hr

Action

Chemical effect: Blocks pain impulses, probably by inhibiting prostaglandin or pain receptor sensitizers. May relieve fever by acting in hypothalamic heat-regulating center.
Therapeutic effect: Relieves pain and reduces fever.

Available forms

Caplets: 165 mg†, 500 mg†, 650 mg†
Caplets (extended-release): 650 mg†
Capsules: 500 mg†
Elixir: 80 mg/2.5 ml†, 80 mg/5 ml†, 120 mg/5 ml†, 160 mg/5 ml*†
Gelcaps: 500 mg†
Geltab: 500 mg†
Geltab (extended-release): 500 mg†, 650 mg†
Infant drops: 80 mg/0.8 ml†, 100 mg/ml†
Liquid: 160 mg/5 ml†, 500 mg/15 ml†
Solution: 80 mg/1.66 ml†, 100 mg/ml†
Sprinkles: 80 mg/capsule†, 160 mg/capsule†
Suppositories: 80 mg†, 120 mg†, 125 mg†, 300 mg†, 325 mg†, 650 mg†
Tablets: 160 mg†, 325 mg†, 500 mg†, 650 mg†
Tablets (chewable): 80 mg†, 160 mg†
Tablets (disintegrating): 80 mg†, 160 mg†

NURSING PROCESS

☞ Assessment

• Assess patient's pain or temperature before and during therapy.
• Assess patient's drug history, and calculate total daily dosage accordingly. Many OTC products and combination prescription pain products contain acetaminophen.
• Be alert for adverse reactions and drug interactions.
• Assess patient's and family's knowledge of drug therapy.

⊕ Nursing diagnoses
• Acute pain related to patient's underlying condition
• Risk for injury related to drug-induced liver damage with toxic doses
• Deficient knowledge related to drug therapy

▷ Planning and implementation
• Give liquid form to children and other patients who have trouble swallowing.
⊛ **ALERT:** When giving liquid form, use caution because drops and elixir have different concentrations.
• Use P.R. in young children and patients for whom oral forms aren't practical.
Patient teaching
⊛ **ALERT:** Tell patient not to use drug for fever that's higher than 103.1° F (39.5° C), lasts longer than 3 days, or recurs.
⊛ **ALERT:** Tell patient that drug is for short-term use. Explain the need to contact the prescriber if a child takes the drug for longer than 5 days or an adult takes it for longer than 10 days.
• Warn patient that high doses or unsupervised long-term use can cause liver damage. Excessive alcohol use may increase risk of hepatotoxicity.
• Tell patient to keep track of daily acetaminophen intake, including OTC and prescription medications. Warn patient not to exceed total recommended dose of acetaminophen per day because of risk of hepatotoxicity.
• Tell a breast-feeding woman that drug appears in breast milk in levels less than 1% of dose. She may use the recommended dose safely for short-term therapy.

☑ Evaluation
• Patient reports pain relief with drug.
• Patient's liver function test results remain normal.
• Patient and family state understanding of drug therapy.

---

acetazolamide
(ah-see-tuh-ZOH-luh-mighd)
Diamox, Diamox Sequels

acetazolamide sodium
Diamox

Pharmacologic class: carbonic anhydrase inhibitor
Therapeutic class: anticonvulsant, diuretic
Pregnancy risk category: C

Indications and dosages

▶ **Secondary glaucoma; preoperative management of acute angle-closure glaucoma.** *Adults:* 250 mg P.O. every 4 hours, or 250 mg P.O. or I.V. b.i.d. for short-term therapy. For some acute glaucomas, 500 mg P.O.; then 125 to 250 mg P.O. every 4 hours.
▶ **Edema in heart failure.** *Adults:* 250 to 375 mg (5 mg/kg) P.O. daily in a.m.
▶ **Chronic open-angle glaucoma.** *Adults:* 250 mg to 1 g P.O. daily in divided doses q.i.d., or 500 mg extended-release P.O. b.i.d.
▶ **Prevention or amelioration of acute mountain sickness.** *Adults:* 500 mg to 1 g P.O. daily in divided doses every 8 to 12 hours, or 500 mg extended-release P.O. every 12 hours. Start therapy 24 to 48 hours before ascent and continue for 48 hours while at high altitude.
▶ **Adjunct treatment of myoclonic, refractory generalized tonic-clonic, absence, or mixed seizures.** *Adults and children:* 8 to 30 mg/kg P.O. daily in divided doses. Optimum dosage, 375 mg to 1 g daily. When given with other anticonvulsants, the initial dosage is 250 mg daily.
▶ **Drug-induced edema.** *Adults:* 250 to 375 mg (5 mg/kg) P.O. as a single dose for 1 or 2 days alternating with one drug-free day.
▶ **Periodic paralysis‡.** *Adults:* 250 mg P.O. b.i.d. or t.i.d., not to exceed 1.5 g daily.

▽ I.V. administration

• Reconstitute 500-mg vial with at least 5 ml of sterile water for injection.
• Inject 100 to 500 mg/minute into large vein using 21G or 23G needle.
• Intermittent or continuous infusion isn't recommended.
• Use within 24 hours.

⊗ **Incompatibilities**
Multivitamins.

Contraindications and cautions

• Contraindicated in patients hypersensitive to drug, patients undergoing long-term therapy for chronic noncongestive angle-closure glaucoma, and patients with hyponatremia, hypokalemia, renal or hepatic impairment, adrenal gland failure, or hyperchloremic acidosis.
• Use cautiously in patients receiving other diuretics and in patients with respiratory acidosis, emphysema, or COPD.
♨ **Lifespan:** In pregnant women, use cautiously. In breast-feeding women, drug is contraindicated. In children, safety and effectiveness of drug haven't been established, and cases of growth retardation have been reported.

Adverse reactions

CNS: confusion, drowsiness, paresthesia.
EENT: transient myopia.
GI: altered taste, anorexia, nausea, vomiting.
GU: crystalluria, hematuria, renal calculi.
Hematologic: *aplastic anemia,* hemolytic anemia, *leukopenia.*
Metabolic: asymptomatic hyperuricemia, *hyperchloremic acidosis,* hypokalemia.
Skin: rash.
Other: *pain at injection site,* sterile abscesses.

Interactions

Drug-drug. *Amphetamines, anticholinergics, mecamylamine, procainamide, quinidine, tricyclic antidepressants:* May decrease renal clearance of these drugs, increasing toxicity. Monitor patient closely.
Cyclosporine: May increase cyclosporine level, causing toxicity. Use cautiously together.
Lithium: May increase lithium secretion. Monitor patient.
Methenamine: May reduce acetazolamide effectiveness. Avoid use together.
Phenytoin: May increase risk of osteomalacia with long-term use. Use cautiously together.
Primidone: May decrease primidone absorption, reducing anticonvulsant effect. Use cautiously together.
Salicylates: May cause acetazolamide accumulation and toxicity, including CNS depression and metabolic acidosis. Monitor patient closely.

Effects on lab test results

• May increase uric acid level. May decrease potassium and hemoglobin levels and hematocrit. May increase or decrease glucose and theophylline levels.
• May decrease WBC count and thyroid iodine uptake.
• May cause false-positive urine protein test results.

Pharmacokinetics

Absorption: Well absorbed from GI tract.
Distribution: Throughout body tissues.
Metabolism: None.
Excretion: Mainly in urine. *Half-life:* 10 to 15 hours.

Route	Onset	Peak	Duration
P.O.			
capsules	2 hr	8–12 hr	18–24 hr
tablets	1–1½ hr	2–4 hr	8–12 hr
I.V.	2 min	15 min	4–5 hr

Action

Chemical effect: Blocks action of carbonic anhydrase, promoting urine excretion of sodium, potassium, bicarbonate, and water. Decreases secretion of aqueous humor in eye. May decrease abnormal paroxysmal or excessive neuronal discharge. Produces respiratory and metabolic acidosis that may encourage ventilation, increase cerebral blood flow, and help release oxygen from hemoglobin.
Therapeutic effect: Lowers intraocular pressure (IOP), controls seizure activity, and may improve respiratory function.

Available forms

Capsules (extended-release): 500 mg
Injection: 500 mg/vial
Tablets: 125 mg, 250 mg

NURSING PROCESS

⚕ Assessment

• In patients with glaucoma, assess eye discomfort and IOP before and during therapy; in those with heart failure, assess edema; in those with seizures, assess neurologic condition.
• Closely monitor intake and output.
• Be alert for adverse reactions and drug interactions.

- Assess patient's and family's knowledge of drug therapy.

Nursing diagnoses
- Excessive fluid volume related to patient's underlying condition
- Impaired urinary elimination related to diuretic action of drug
- Deficient knowledge related to drug therapy

▶ Planning and implementation
- Give oral form early in the morning and the second dose early in the afternoon to avoid nocturia.
- If patient can't swallow oral form, ask pharmacist to make a suspension using crushed tablets in flavored syrup. Although concentrations up to 500 mg/5 ml are possible, concentrations of 250 mg/5 ml are more palatable. Refrigeration improves palatability but doesn't improve stability. Suspensions are stable for 1 week.
- Diuretic effect decreases with acidosis but is restored by stopping drug for several days and then restarting it, or by giving drug intermittently.
- **ALERT:** Don't confuse acetazolamide with acetohexamide. Also don't confuse acetazolamide sodium (Diamox) with acyclovir sodium (Zovirax); these vials may appear similar.
- If hypersensitivity or adverse reactions occur, withhold drug and notify prescriber.

Patient teaching
- Advise patient to take drug early in the day to avoid sleep interruption caused by nocturia.
- Teach patient to monitor fluid volume by measuring weight, intake, and output daily.
- Encourage patient to avoid high-sodium foods and to choose high-potassium foods.
- Teach patient to recognize and report signs and symptoms of fluid and electrolyte imbalance.

Evaluation
- Patient is free from edema.
- Patient adjusts lifestyle to accommodate altered patterns of urine elimination.
- Patient and family state understanding of drug therapy.

acetylcysteine
(as-ee-til-SIS-teen)
Acetadote, Mucomyst

Pharmacologic class: amino acid (L-cysteine) derivative
Therapeutic class: mucolytic, antidote for acetaminophen overdose
Pregnancy risk category: B

Indications and dosages

▶ **Pneumonia, bronchitis, tuberculosis, cystic fibrosis, emphysema, atelectasis (adjunct), complications of thoracic and CV surgery.**
Adults and children: 1 to 2 ml of 10% or 20% solution by direct instillation into trachea as often as hourly; or 3 to 5 ml of 20% solution or 6 to 10 ml of 10% solution by nebulization every 2 to 3 hours p.r.n.
▶ **Acetaminophen toxicity. (Acetadote only)**
Adults and children: Initially, 140 mg/kg P.O., followed by 70 mg/kg P.O. every 4 hours for 17 doses. Or give 150 mg/kg as loading dose I.V. over 60 minutes. Then begin maintenance doses of 50 mg/kg I.V. over 4 hours, followed by 100 mg/kg I.V. over 16 hours. Adjust total volume given for patients who weigh less than 40 kg or are fluid restricted.

▼ I.V. administration

Acetadote only
- If patient weighs 40 kg (88 lb) or more, dilute loading dose in 200 ml, second dose in 500 ml, and third dose in 1,000 ml of D_5W.
- If patient weighs 25 to 40 kg (55 to 88 lb), dilute loading dose in 100 ml, second dose in 250 ml, and third dose in 500 ml of D_5W.
- If patient weighs 20 to 24 kg (44 to 53 lb), dilute loading dose in 60 ml, second dose in 140 ml, and third dose in 280 ml of D_5W.
- If patient weighs 15 to 19 kg (33 to 43 lb), dilute loading dose in 45 ml, second dose in 105 ml, and third dose in 210 ml of D_5W.
- If patient weighs 10 to 14 kg (22 to 32 lb), dilute loading dose in 30 ml, second dose in 70 ml, and third dose in 140 ml of D_5W.
- Store unopened vials at controlled room temperature of 68° to 77° F (20° to 25° C). Reconstituted solution is stable for 24 hours.

• Once the stopper is punctured, drug may turn from colorless to slightly pink or purple. This change doesn't affect potency.

⊗ **Incompatibilities**

Rubber and metals, particularly iron, copper, and nickel.

Contraindications and cautions

• Contraindicated in patients hypersensitive to drug.
• Use cautiously in debilitated patients with severe respiratory insufficiency. In patients with asthma or a history of bronchospasm, use I.V. form cautiously.
☀ **Lifespan:** In pregnant and breast-feeding women and in elderly patients with severe respiratory insufficiency, use cautiously.

Adverse reactions

EENT: hemoptysis, rhinorrhea.
GI: nausea, stomatitis, vomiting.
Respiratory: BRONCHOSPASM.

Interactions

Drug-drug. *Activated charcoal:* May limit acetylcysteine's effectiveness. Avoid use together in treating drug toxicity.

Effects on lab test results

None reported.

Pharmacokinetics

Absorption: Most inhaled acetylcysteine acts directly on mucus in lungs; remainder is absorbed by pulmonary epithelium. After oral administration, drug is absorbed from GI tract.
Distribution: 50% protein-bound.
Metabolism: In liver.
Excretion: The mean elimination terminal half-life is longer in newborns (11 hours) than in adults (5½ hours). *Half-life:* 6¼ hours.

Route	Onset	Peak	Duration
P.O., I.V., inhalation	Unknown	Unknown	Unknown

Action

Chemical effect: Increases respiratory tract fluids to help liquefy tenacious secretions. Restores glutathione in liver to treat acetaminophen toxicity.

Therapeutic effect: Thins respiratory secretions and reverses toxic effects of acetaminophen.

Available forms

I.V. injection: 200 mg/ml
Oral or inhalation solution: 10%, 20%

NURSING PROCESS

📋 Assessment

• Assess patient's respiratory secretions before and during therapy.
• Be alert for adverse reactions and drug interactions.
• Assess patient's and family's knowledge of drug therapy.

🔁 Nursing diagnoses

• Ineffective airway clearance related to patient's underlying condition
• Impaired oral mucous membrane related to drug-induced stomatitis
• Deficient knowledge related to drug therapy

▷ Planning and implementation

• Dilute oral doses with cola, fruit juice, or water to treat acetaminophen overdose. Dilute 20% solution to 5% by adding 3 ml of diluent to each ml of acetylcysteine. If patient vomits within 1 hour of initial or maintenance dose, repeat dose.
⚡ **ALERT:** If the time of ingestion is unknown or the acetaminophen level isn't available or can't be interpreted within 8 hours of ingestion, immediately give drug I.V.
⚡ **ALERT:** Don't confuse acetylcysteine with acetylcholine.
• Use plastic, glass, stainless steel, or another nonreactive metal when giving by nebulization. Drug isn't compatible with rubber or metals, especially iron, copper, and nickel.
• Hand-bulb nebulizers aren't recommended because output is too small and particle size is too large.
• Before aerosol administration, have patient clear airway by coughing.
⚡ **ALERT:** Drug is incompatible with tetracyclines, erythromycin lactobionate, amphotericin B, and ampicillin sodium. If given by aerosol inhalation, these drugs should be nebulized separately. Iodized oil, trypsin, and hydrogen

peroxide are incompatible with drug. Don't add these drugs to nebulizer.
• Have suction equipment available in case patient can't effectively clear his air passages.
• Alert prescriber if patient's respiratory secretions thicken or become purulent or if bronchospasm occurs.
• After opening, store in refrigerator, and use within 4 days.
• The vial stopper contains no natural rubber latex, dry natural rubber, or blends of natural rubber.

Patient teaching
• Instruct patient to follow directions on drug label exactly. Explain importance of using drug as directed.
• If patient's condition doesn't improve within 10 days, tell him to notify prescriber. Drug shouldn't be used for prolonged period without direct medical supervision.
• Teach patient how to use and clean nebulizer.
• Inform patient that drug may have a foul taste or smell.
• Instruct patient to clear his airway by coughing before aerosol use to achieve maximum effect.
• Instruct patient to rinse mouth with water after nebulizer treatment because it may leave a sticky coating.

☑ **Evaluation**
• Patient has clear lung sounds, decreased respiratory secretions, and reduced frequency and severity of cough.
• Patient's oral mucous membranes remain unchanged.
• Patient and family state understanding of drug therapy.

activated charcoal
(AK-tih-vay-ted CHAR-kohl)
Actidose†, Actidose-Aqua†, CharcoAid†, CharcoCaps†, Insta-Char Pediatric†, Liqui-Char†, SuperChar†

Pharmacologic class: adsorbent
Therapeutic class: antidote
Pregnancy risk category: C

Indications and dosages

▶ **Poisoning.** *Adults:* Initially, 1 g/kg (30 to 100 g) P.O. or 5 to 10 times amount of poison ingested as suspension in 180 to 240 ml of water.
Children: Five to 10 times estimated weight of poison ingested, with minimum dose being 30 g P.O. in 240 ml of water to make a slurry, preferably within 30 minutes of poisoning. If patient has food in his stomach, a larger dose is needed.
▶ **Flatulence, dyspepsia.** *Adults:* 600 mg to 5 g P.O. t.i.d. after meals.

Contraindications and cautions

None reported.

Adverse reactions

GI: black stool, constipation, nausea.

Interactions

Drug-drug. *Acetylcysteine, ipecac:* May render charcoal ineffective. Don't use together, and don't perform gastric lavage until all charcoal is removed.
Drug-food. *Milk, ice cream, sherbet:* May decrease effectiveness of activated charcoal.

Effects on lab test results

None reported.

Pharmacokinetics

Absorption: None.
Distribution: None.
Metabolism: None.
Excretion: In feces.

Route	Onset	Peak	Duration
P.O.	Immediate	Unknown	Unknown

Action

Chemical effect: Adheres to many drugs and chemicals, inhibiting their absorption.
Therapeutic effect: Used as antidote for selected poisons and overdoses.

Available forms

Liquid: 208 mg/ml
Oral suspension: 15 g†, 30 g†
Powder: 15 g†, 30 g†, 40 g†, 50 g†, 120 g†, 240 g†

NURSING PROCESS

Assessment
• Find out what substance was ingested and when it was ingested. Drug isn't effective for all drugs and toxic substances.
• Be alert for adverse reactions and drug interactions.
• Assess patient's and family's knowledge of drug therapy.

Nursing diagnoses
• Risk for injury related to ingestion of toxic substance or overdose
• Risk for deficient fluid volume related to drug-induced vomiting
• Deficient knowledge related to drug therapy

Planning and implementation
• Drug is commonly used for treating poisoning or overdose of acetaminophen, aspirin, atropine, barbiturates, cardiac glycosides, oxalic acid, parathion, phenol, phenytoin, poisonous mushrooms, propantheline, propoxyphene, strychnine, or tricyclic antidepressants. Check with poison control center for use in other types of poisonings or overdoses.
• Give after emesis because drug absorbs and inactivates syrup of ipecac.
⚡ **ALERT:** Don't give to a semiconscious or unconscious patient unless airway is protected and NG tube is in place for instillation.
• Mix powder form (most effective) with tap water to form consistency of thick syrup. Add small amount of fruit juice or flavoring to make mix more palatable.
• Give by NG tube after lavage, if needed.
• Don't give in ice cream, milk, or sherbet, which may reduce absorption.
• If patient vomits shortly after administration, repeat dose.
• Keep airway, oxygen, and suction equipment nearby.
• Follow treatment with stool softener or laxative to prevent constipation.
⚡ **ALERT:** Don't confuse Actidose with Actos.
Patient teaching
• Warn patient that feces will be black.
• Instruct patient to report respiratory difficulty immediately.

Evaluation
• Patient sustains no injury from ingesting toxic substance or from overdose.
• Patient has no signs of deficient fluid volume.
• Patient and family state understanding of drug therapy.

acyclovir sodium
(ay-SIGH-kloh-veer SOH-dee-um)
Avirax ♦ , Zovirax

Pharmacologic class: synthetic purine nucleoside
Therapeutic class: antiviral
Pregnancy risk category: B

Indications and dosages

▶ **Chickenpox.** *Adults and children weighing more than 40 kg (88 lb):* 800 mg P.O. q.i.d. for 5 days.
Children age 2 and older weighing less than 40 kg: 20 mg/kg P.O. q.i.d. for 5 days.
▶ **Acute herpes zoster.** *Adults:* 800 mg P.O. every 4 hours, five times daily for 7 to 10 days. Give within 48 hours of rash onset.
▶ **Initial genital herpes.** *Adults:* 200 mg P.O. every 4 hours during waking hours (total of five capsules daily) for 10 days. If using ointment, apply sufficient amount to cover all lesions every 3 hours, 6 times daily for 7 days.
▶ **Intermittent therapy for recurrent genital herpes.** *Adults:* 200 mg P.O. every 4 hours during waking hours (total of five capsules daily) for 5 days. Start therapy at first sign of recurrence.
▶ **Long-term suppressive therapy for recurrent genital herpes.** *Adults:* 400 mg P.O. b.i.d. for up to 12 months.
Adjust-a-dose: In patients with renal impairment, if usual dosage is 800 mg five times daily and creatinine clearance is 10 to 25 ml/minute, decrease dosage to 800 mg every 8 hours. If creatinine clearance is 10 ml/minute or less, decrease the 200- to 400-mg dosage to 200 mg every 12 hours, or the 800-mg dosage to 800 mg every 12 hours.
▶ **Initial and recurrent episodes of mucocutaneous herpes simplex virus (HSV-1 and HSV-2) infections in immunocompromised patients; severe initial episodes of herpes genitalis in immunocompetent patients.** *Adults*

and children age 12 and older: 5 mg/kg I.V. at constant rate over 1 hour every 8 hours for 7 days (5 days for herpes genitalis).

Children younger than age 12: Give 10 mg/kg I.V. at constant rate over 1 hour every 8 hours for 7 days (5 days for herpes genitalis).

▶ **Herpes simplex encephalitis.** *Adults:* 10 mg/kg I.V. infused at a constant rate over 1 hour, every 8 hours for 10 days.

Children ages 3 months to 12 years: 20 mg/kg I.V. at a constant rate over at least 1 hour, every 8 hours for 10 days.

▶ **Neonatal herpes simplex virus infections.** *Children from birth to age 3 months:* 10 mg/kg I.V. at a constant rate for over 1 hour, every 8 hours for 10 days.

▶ **Varicella zoster in immunocompromised patients.** *Adults and children age 12 and older:* 10 mg/kg I.V. infused at a constant rate over 1 hour, every 8 hours for 7 days. Give obese patients 10 mg/kg (ideal body weight). Don't exceed maximum dose equivalent to 500 mg/m² every 8 hours.

Children younger than age 12: Give 20 mg/kg I.V. every 8 hours for 7 days, or 500 mg/m² at a constant rate over at least 1 hour, every 8 hours for 7 days.

🕲 **Adjust-a-dose:** In patients with renal impairment, if creatinine clearance exceeds 50 ml/minute, give 100% of the I.V. dose every 8 hours; if it's 25 to 50 ml/minute, 100% of the dose every 12 hours; if it's 10 to 25 ml/minute, 100% of the dose every 24 hours; and if it's less than 10 ml/minute, 50% of the dose every 24 hours.

▶ **Recurrent herpes labialis (cold sores).** *Adults and children age 12 and older:* Apply cream five times daily for 4 days. Start therapy as early as possible following onset of signs and symptoms.

▶ **Genital herpes in immunocompromised patients‡.** *Adults:* 400 mg P.O. three to five times daily.

▶ **Long-term suppressive or maintenance therapy for recurrent HSV infections in patients with HIV‡.** *Adults and children older than age 12:* Give 200 mg P.O. t.i.d. or 400 mg P.O. b.i.d.

Children age 12 and younger: 600 to 1,000 mg P.O. daily in three to five divided doses.

▶ **Acute herpes zoster ophthalmicus‡.** *Adults:* 600 mg P.O. every 4 hours five times

daily for 10 days, preferably within 3 days of rash onset, but no longer than 7 days.

▶ **Rectal herpes infection‡.** *Adults:* 400 mg P.O. five times daily for 10 days or until resolved. Or, give 800 mg P.O. every 8 hours for 7 to 10 days.

▶ **Disseminated herpes zoster‡.** *Adults:* 5 to 10 mg/kg I.V. every 8 hours for 7 to 10 days. Infuse over at least 1 hour.

🕲 **Adjust-a-dose:** In patients with renal impairment, if creatinine clearance exceeds 50 ml/minute, give 100% of the I.V. dose every 8 hours; if it's 25 to 50 ml/minute, 100% of the dose every 12 hours; if it's 10 to 25 ml/minute, 100% of the dose every 24 hours; and if it's less than 10 ml/minute, 50% of the dose every 24 hours.

▼ I.V. administration

- Dissolve the contents of 500-mg vial in 10 ml (or 1,000-mg vial in 20 ml) of sterile water for injection to yield 50 mg/ml. Then dilute further in appropriate I.V. solution to 7 mg/ml or less. Concentrated solutions (10 mg/ml or more) increase the risk of phlebitis.
- Don't use bacteriostatic water containing benzyl alcohol or parabens.
- Give I.V. infusion over at least 1 hour to prevent renal tubular damage. Don't give by bolus injection.
- Don't exceed a maximum dose equivalent of 20 mg/kg every 8 hours.
- Make sure I.V. infusion is accompanied by adequate hydration. Monitor intake and output closely during administration.

⊗ **Incompatibilities**
Biological or colloidal solutions, idarubicin hydrochloride, parabens.

Contraindications and cautions

- Contraindicated in patients hypersensitive to drug, its components, or valacyclovir.
- Use cautiously in patients receiving other nephrotoxic drugs and those with underlying neurologic problems, renal disease, or dehydration.

🌢 **Lifespan:** In pregnant or breast-feeding women, use cautiously. In children younger than age 2, safety and effectiveness of drug haven't been established.

Adverse reactions

CNS: *encephalopathic changes* with I.V. use (including agitation, confusion, *coma,* hallucinations, headache, lethargy, obtundation, *seizures,* tremor), ataxia, aggressive behavior, fatigue, fever, pain.
CV: hypotension, peripheral edema.
GI: abdominal pain, diarrhea, nausea, vomiting.
GU: hematuria.
Hematologic: *DIC, hemolysis, leukopenia.*
Hepatic: *hepatitis,* hyperbilirubinemia, jaundice.
Musculoskeletal: myalgia.
Skin: itching, rash, *vesicular eruptions.*
Other: *anaphylaxis, angioedema,* inflammation, phlebitis at injection site.

Interactions

Drug-drug. *Phenytoin, valproic acid:* May decrease levels of these drugs. Monitor patient closely.
Probenecid: May increase acyclovir level. Monitor patient for toxicity.
Theophylline: May increase plasma theophylline level. Monitor levels and effects.

Effects on lab test results

• May increase BUN, creatinine, liver enzyme, and bilirubin levels. May decrease hemoglobin level and hematocrit.
• May increase or decrease platelet, neutrophil, and WBC counts.

Pharmacokinetics

Absorption: Slow, and only 15% to 30% is absorbed. Not affected by food.
Distribution: Widely to organ tissues and body fluids. CSF levels equal about 50% of serum levels, and 9% to 33% binds to plasma proteins.
Metabolism: Mainly inside viral cell to its active form.
Excretion: Up to 92% of systemically absorbed acyclovir is excreted unchanged by kidneys. *Half-life:* 2 to 3½ hours with normal renal function; up to 19 hours with renal impairment.

Route	Onset	Peak	Duration
P.O.	Unknown	Unknown	Unknown
I.V.	Immediate	Immediate	Unknown

Action

Chemical effect: Becomes incorporated into viral DNA and inhibits viral multiplication.

Therapeutic effect: Kills susceptible viruses.

Available forms

Capsules: 200 mg
Injection: 500 mg/vial, 1 g/vial
Suspension: 200 mg/5 ml
Tablets: 400 mg, 800 mg
Topical: 5% cream or ointment

NURSING PROCESS

⚖ Assessment
• Assess infection before and regularly during therapy.
• Monitor patient for renal toxicity. Dehydration, renal disease, and use of other nephrotoxic drugs increase risk.
• Monitor patient's mental condition when giving I.V. drug. Encephalopathic changes are more likely in patients with neurologic disorders and in those who have had neurologic reactions to cytotoxic drugs.
• If adverse GI reactions occur with oral use, monitor hydration.
• Assess patient's and family's knowledge of drug therapy.

🔄 Nursing diagnoses
• Risk for infection related to presence of virus
• Risk for deficient fluid volume related to adverse GI reactions to oral drug
• Deficient knowledge related to drug therapy

▷ Planning and implementation
⚠ ALERT: Don't give I.M., subcutaneously, or by bolus injection.
⚠ ALERT: Don't confuse Zovirax with Zyvox. Also, don't confuse acyclovir sodium with acetazolamide sodium. The vials may look alike.
• To prevent transmission of virus, wear finger cot or examination glove to apply cream or ointment.
Patient teaching
• Explain that drug manages herpes infection but doesn't eliminate or cure it.
• Warn patient that drug won't prevent spread of infection to others.
• Help patient recognize early symptoms of herpes infection (tingling, itching, pain) so he can take drug before infection fully develops.
• Tell patient to report pain or discomfort at I.V. injection site.

☑ Evaluation

- Patient's infection is controlled.
- Patient maintains adequate hydration.
- Patient and family state understanding of drug therapy.

adalimumab

(ay-da-LIM-yoo-mab)
Humira

Pharmacologic class: tumor necrosis factor (TNF)-alpha blocker
Therapeutic class: antirheumatic
Pregnancy risk category: B

Indications and dosages

▶ **Rheumatoid arthritis; psoriatic arthritis; ankylosing spondylitis.** *Adults:* 40 mg subcutaneously every other week. Patient may continue to take methotrexate, steroids, NSAIDs, salicylates, analgesics, or other disease-modifying antirheumatic drugs during therapy. Patients with rheumatoid arthritis who aren't also taking methotrexate may have the dose increased to 40 mg weekly, if needed.

■ **NEW INDICATION:** Moderate to severe Crohn's disease when response to conventional therapy is inadequate, or when response to infliximab is lost, or patient is unable to tolerate the drug.
Adults: Initially, 160 mg subcutaneously q.i.d. on day 1 or divided b.i.d. on days 1 and 2 of week 1, then 80 mg at week 2, followed by maintenance dose of 40 mg every other week starting at week 4.

Contraindications and cautions

- Contraindicated in patients hypersensitive to drug or any of its components. Don't start drug if patient is immunosuppressed or has a chronic or localized active infection.
- Use cautiously in patients with a history of recurrent infection, those with underlying conditions that predispose them to infections, and those who have lived in areas where tuberculosis and histoplasmosis are common. Use cautiously in patients with CNS-demyelinating disorders.

🜲 **Lifespan:** In pregnant women, give only if benefits outweigh risks to the fetus. Breastfeeding women should either stop nursing or stop taking the drug because of the risk of serious adverse reactions. It's unknown whether drug appears in breast milk or would be absorbed by a breast-feeding infant. In children, safety and effectiveness of drug haven't been established. In elderly patients, use cautiously because serious infections and malignancies are more common in these patients.

Adverse reactions

CNS: headache.
CV: hypertension.
EENT: sinusitis.
GI: abdominal pain, nausea.
GU: hematuria, UTI.
Hematologic: *leukopenia, pancytopenia, thrombocytopenia.*
Metabolic: hypercholesterolemia, hyperlipidemia.
Musculoskeletal: back pain.
Respiratory: bronchitis, upper respiratory tract infection.
Skin: rash.
Other: *accidental injury,* allergic reactions, *anaphylaxis,* flulike syndrome, injection site reactions (erythema, hemorrhage, itching, pain, swelling), *malignancy, sepsis,* serious infections.

Interactions

Drug-drug. *Anakinra:* May cause serious infections. Avoid use together.
Live-virus vaccines: May cause immunosuppression and susceptibility to disease. Avoid use together.

Effects on lab test results

- May increase alkaline phosphatase and cholesterol levels.

Pharmacokinetics

Absorption: Average absolute bioavailability is 64%.
Distribution: Levels in synovial fluid are 31% to 96% of those in serum.
Metabolism: Clearance may be higher if anti-adalimumab antibodies are present and lower in patients age 40 or older.
Excretion: Unknown. *Half-life:* Ranges from 10 to 20 days.

Route	Onset	Peak	Duration
SubQ	Variable	Variable	Unknown

Action

Chemical effect: Blocks human TNF-alpha that aids normal inflammatory and immune responses and the inflammation and joint destruction of rheumatoid arthritis.
Therapeutic effect: Reduces signs and symptoms of rheumatoid arthritis.

Available forms

Injection: 40 mg/0.8 ml in prefilled syringe or prefilled pen

NURSING PROCESS

☞ Assessment
• Assess patient for immunosuppression or active infection before therapy and regularly thereafter.
• Monitor patient for hypersensitivity reaction.

⊕ Nursing diagnoses
• Impaired physical mobility related to rheumatoid arthritis
• Deficient knowledge related to signs and symptoms of immunosuppression or infection
• Deficient knowledge related to drug therapy

▷ Planning and implementation
• Drug can be given alone or with methotrexate or other disease-modifying antirheumatics.
• Give first dose under supervision of experienced health care provider.
• Evaluate patient for latent tuberculosis and, if present, start treatment before giving drug.
• Serious infections and sepsis, including tuberculosis and invasive opportunistic fungal infections, may occur. If patient develops new infection during treatment, monitor him closely.
⊛ **ALERT:** Stop drug if patient develops a severe infection, anaphylaxis, other serious allergic reaction, or evidence of a lupuslike syndrome.
⊛ **ALERT:** The needle cover contains latex and shouldn't be handled by those with latex sensitivity.
Patient teaching
• Tell patient to report evidence of tuberculosis.
• If appropriate, teach patient or caregiver how to give drug.
• Tell patient to rotate injection sites and to avoid tender, bruised, red, or hard skin.
• Teach patient to dispose of used vials, needles, and syringes safely.

• Tell patient to refrigerate drug in its original container before use.
⊛ **ALERT:** Warn patient to seek immediate medical attention for symptoms of blood dyscrasias or infection, including fever, bruising, bleeding, and pallor.

☑ Evaluation
• Patient experiences reduced signs and symptoms of rheumatoid arthritis.
• Patient remains free from infection during therapy.
• Patient and family state understanding of drug therapy.

adefovir dipivoxil
(uh-DEPH-uh-veer dih-pih-VOCKS-ul)
Hepsera

Pharmacologic class: acyclic nucleotide analogue
Therapeutic class: antiviral
Pregnancy risk category: C

Indications and dosages

▶ **Chronic hepatitis B infection.** *Adults:* 10 mg P.O. daily.
▣ **Adjust-a-dose:** In patients with renal impairment, if creatinine clearance is 20 to 49 ml/minute, give 10 mg P.O. every 2 days. If creatinine clearance is 10 to 19 ml/minute, give 10 mg P.O. every 3 days. In patients receiving hemodialysis, give 10 mg P.O. every 7 days, after dialysis session.

Contraindications and cautions

• Contraindicated in patients hypersensitive to drug or its components.
• Use cautiously and at a reduced dosage in patients with renal impairment and in those receiving nephrotoxic drugs.
🕯 **Lifespan:** In pregnant women, use drug only if benefits to mother outweigh risks to fetus. Women should avoid breast-feeding. It's unknown if drug appears in breast milk. In children, safety and effectiveness of drug haven't been established. In elderly patients, use cautiously because of increased risk of renal or CV dysfunction.

Adverse reactions

CNS: *asthenia,* headache, fever.
EENT: pharyngitis, sinusitis.
GI: abdominal pain, diarrhea, dyspepsia, flatulence, nausea, vomiting.
GU: glycosuria, hematuria, *renal failure,* renal insufficiency.
Hepatic: *hepatic failure,* hepatomegaly with steatosis.
Metabolic: *lactic acidosis.*
Respiratory: cough.
Skin: pruritus, rash.

Interactions

Drug-drug. *Nephrotoxic drugs, such as aminoglycosides, cyclosporine, NSAIDs, tacrolimus, vancomycin:* May increase risk of nephrotoxicity. Use together cautiously.

Effects on lab test results

● May increase ALT, amylase, AST, CK, creatinine, and lactic acid levels.

Pharmacokinetics

Absorption: Readily from the GI tract with a bioavailability of 59%.
Distribution: Up to 4% bound to plasma and serum proteins.
Metabolism: Rapidly converted to adefovir diphosphate, an active metabolite.
Excretion: Undergoes renal elimination. *Half-life:* Unknown.

Route	Onset	Peak	Duration
P.O.	Unknown	1–4 hr	7½ hr

Action

Chemical effect: Inhibits hepatitis B virus reverse transcriptase, which breaks the viral DNA chain.
Therapeutic effect: Reduces symptoms of hepatitis B.

Available forms

Tablets: 10 mg

NURSING PROCESS

⬛ Assessment
● Assess patient's condition before therapy and regularly thereafter.
● Watch for hypersensitivity reaction.

● Monitor renal function, especially in patients with renal dysfunction and in those taking nephrotoxic drugs.
● Monitor hepatic function.

✚ Nursing diagnoses
● Risk for injury secondary to adverse drug effects
● Deficient knowledge related to drug therapy

▶ Planning and implementation
● The ideal length of treatment hasn't been established.
● Offer HIV antibody testing because drug may promote resistance to antiretrovirals in patients with unrecognized or untreated HIV infection.
⬥ **ALERT:** Patients may develop lactic acidosis and severe hepatomegaly with steatosis during treatment. Risk is higher in women, obese patients, and those taking other antiretrovirals.
● Monitor hepatic function. If patient develops evidence of lactic acidosis and severe hepatomegaly with steatosis, notify prescriber, who will stop drug.
⬥ **ALERT:** Stopping drug may cause severe worsening of hepatitis. Monitor hepatic function closely in patients who stop taking drug.
● Overdose causes GI adverse effects. Treating overdose includes monitoring patient for evidence of toxicity and giving supportive therapy. Dialysis may be helpful.
● Enroll pregnant women in the Antiretroviral Pregnancy Registry, which monitors fetal outcomes, by calling 1-800-258-4263.

Patient teaching
● Inform patient that drug may be taken with or without food.
● Tell patient to immediately report weakness, muscle pain, trouble breathing, stomach pain with nausea and vomiting, dizziness, lightheadedness, fast or irregular heartbeat, or feeling cold in the arms and legs.
● Warn patient not to stop taking drug unless directed because hepatitis could worsen.
● Instruct women to tell their prescriber if they become pregnant or are breast-feeding. Advise breast-feeding women to either stop breast-feeding or stop taking the drug.

✅ Evaluation
● Patient remains free from injury during therapy.

• Patient and family state understanding of drug therapy.

HIGH ALERT!
---

adenosine
(uh-DEN-oh-seen)
Adenocard

Pharmacologic class: nucleoside
Therapeutic class: antiarrhythmic
Pregnancy risk category: C

Indications and dosages

▶ **To convert paroxysmal supraventricular tachycardia (PSVT) to sinus rhythm.** *Adults:* 6 mg I.V. by rapid bolus injection over 1 to 2 seconds. If PSVT isn't eliminated in 1 to 2 minutes, give 12 mg by rapid I.V. bolus and repeat, if needed.

▼ I.V. administration

• If solution is cold, check it for crystals. If they appear, gently warm solution to room temperature. Don't use cloudy solution.
• Give by rapid I.V. injection over 1 to 2 seconds, directly into vein if possible. If I.V. line is used, inject drug into the most proximal port.
• Drug has a very short half-life. Follow with rapid saline flush to ensure that drug reaches systemic circulation quickly.
• Don't give single dose that's larger than 12 mg.
• Discard unused drug. It doesn't contain preservatives.
⊗ **Incompatibilities**
Other I.V. drugs.

Contraindications and cautions

• Contraindicated in patients hypersensitive to drug and in those with second- or third-degree heart block or sick-sinus syndrome unless artificial pacemaker is present. Don't repeat dose in patients who develop significant heart block from drug.
• Use cautiously in patients with asthma because bronchoconstriction may occur.
⚘ **Lifespan:** In pregnant and breast-feeding women and in children, safety of drug hasn't been established.

Adverse reactions

CNS: apprehension, burning sensation, *dizziness, headache,* heaviness in arms, *light-headedness,* numbness, tingling in arms.
CV: *atrial fibrillation, chest pressure, chest pain, facial flushing,* hypotension, palpitations, *ventricular fibrillation, ventricular tachycardia.*
EENT: blurred vision, metallic taste, tightness in throat.
GI: nausea.
Musculoskeletal: back pain, neck pain.
Respiratory: *dyspnea,* hyperventilation.
Skin: diaphoresis.

Interactions

Drug-drug. *Carbamazepine:* May cause higher degree of heart block. Monitor patient.
Digoxin, verapamil: In rare cases, may cause ventricular fibrillation. Use together cautiously.
Dipyridamole: May potentiate adenosine's effects. A smaller dose may be needed.
Methylxanthines: May antagonize adenosine's effects. A patient taking theophylline or caffeine may need a higher dose or may not respond to therapy.
Drug-herb. *Guarana:* May decrease therapeutic response. Discourage use together.
Drug-food. *Caffeine:* May antagonize adenosine's effects. Give higher dose.

Effects on lab test results

None reported.

Pharmacokinetics

Absorption: Given I.V.
Distribution: Rapidly taken up by erythrocytes and vascular endothelial cells.
Metabolism: Within tissues to inosine and adenosine monophosphate.
Excretion: Unknown. *Half-life:* Less than 10 seconds.

Route	Onset	Peak	Duration
I.V.	Immediate	Immediate	Seconds

Action

Chemical effect: Acts on AV node to slow conduction and inhibit reentry pathways.
Therapeutic effect: Restores normal sinus rhythm.

Available forms

Injection: 3 mg/ml

NURSING PROCESS

⚡ Assessment
• Monitor patient's heart rate and rhythm before and during therapy.
• Be alert for adverse reactions and drug interactions.
• Assess patient's and family's knowledge of drug therapy.

⊕ Nursing diagnoses
• Decreased cardiac output related to arrhythmias
• Ineffective protection related to drug-induced proarrhythmias
• Deficient knowledge related to drug therapy

▷ Planning and implementation
• If a new arrhythmia occurs, withhold drug, obtain rhythm strip, and notify prescriber immediately.
• **ALERT:** Have emergency equipment and drugs on hand to treat new arrhythmias.
Patient teaching
• Teach patient and family about the disease and therapy.
• Stress importance of alerting health care provider about chest pain or dyspnea.
• Advise patient to avoid caffeine.

☑ Evaluation
• Patient's arrhythmias are corrected and his heart maintains normal sinus rhythm.
• Patient doesn't experience proarrhythmias.
• Patient and family state understanding of drug therapy.

albumin 5%
(al-BYOO-min)
Albuminar-5, Albutein 5%, Plasbumin-5

albumin 25%
Albuminar-25, Albutein 25%, Plasbumin-25

Pharmacologic class: blood derivative
Therapeutic class: plasma volume expander
Pregnancy risk category: C

Indications and dosages

▶ **Hypovolemic shock.** *Adults:* Initially, 500 ml of 5% solution by I.V. infusion; repeat, if needed. Dosage varies with patient's condition and response. Maximum, 250 g in 48 hours. *Children:* 10 to 20 ml/kg of 5% solution by I.V. infusion, repeated in 15 to 30 minutes if response isn't adequate. Or, 2.5 to 5 ml/kg of 25% solution I.V.; repeat after 10 to 30 minutes, if needed.

▶ **Hypoproteinemia.** *Adults:* 1,000 to 1,500 ml of 5% solution by I.V. infusion daily, with maximum rate of 5 to 10 ml/minute; or 200 to 300 ml 25% solution by I.V. infusion daily, with maximum rate of 3 ml/minute. Dosage varies with patient's condition and response.

▶ **Hyperbilirubinemia.** *Infants:* 1 g albumin (4 ml of 25% solution)/kg I.V. 1 to 2 hours before transfusion.

▽ I.V. administration
• Albumin can be given undiluted or diluted with normal saline solution or D_5W. Use within 4 hours of opening the vial, and discard unused solution because it has no preservatives. Don't use cloudy solutions or those containing sediment. Solution should be clear amber.
• Avoid infusing 10 ml/minute or faster. Infusion rate is individualized according to patient's age, condition, and diagnosis. Albumin 5% is infused undiluted; albumin 25% may be undiluted or diluted with normal saline or D_5W injection.
• Follow storage instructions on bottle. Freezing may cause bottle to break.
• Don't give more than 250 g in 48 hours.
⊗ **Incompatibilities**
Verapamil hydrochloride.

Contraindications and cautions

• Contraindicated in patients hypersensitive to drug. The 5% solution is contraindicated in patients who have severe anemia or cardiac failure with normal or increased intravascular volume. The 25% solution is contraindicated in patients at risk for circulatory overload.
• Use cautiously in patients with cardiac disease, severe pulmonary infection, renal insufficiency, or hypoalbuminemia with peripheral edema.
⚘ **Lifespan:** In pregnant women, use drug cautiously.

Adverse reactions

CNS: fever.
CV: altered pulse rate, hypotension, *vascular overload.*
GI: increased salivation, nausea, vomiting.
Respiratory: altered respiration, *pulmonary edema.*
Skin: rash, urticaria.
Other: chills.

Interactions

None significant.

Effects on lab test results

• May increase albumin level.

Pharmacokinetics

Absorption: Given I.V.
Distribution: Albumin accounts for about 50% of plasma proteins. It's distributed into the intravascular space and extravascular sites, including skin, muscle, and lungs.
Metabolism: Unknown.
Excretion: Unknown. *Half-life:* 15 to 20 days.

Route	Onset	Peak	Duration
I.V.	Immediate	15 min	Up to several hr

Action

Chemical effect: Albumin 5% supplies colloid to blood and increases plasma volume. Albumin 25% causes fluid to shift from interstitial spaces to circulation, slightly increasing protein level and providing hemodilution.
Therapeutic effect: Relieves shock by increasing plasma volume and corrects plasma protein deficiency.

Available forms

albumin 5% injection: 50-ml, 250-ml, 500-ml, and 1,000-ml vials
albumin 25% injection: 20-ml, 50-ml, and 100-ml vials

NURSING PROCESS

🖎 Assessment
• Assess patient's underlying condition.
• Be alert for adverse reactions.
• Monitor fluid intake and output; protein, electrolyte, and hemoglobin levels; and hematocrit.
• Monitor patient's blood pressure often during therapy.

• Assess patient's and family's knowledge of drug therapy.

⊕ Nursing diagnoses
• Deficient fluid volume related to patient's underlying condition
• Excessive fluid volume related to adverse effects of drug
• Deficient knowledge related to drug therapy

▶ Planning and implementation
• One volume of albumin 25% is equivalent to five volumes of albumin 5% in producing hemodilution and relative anemia.
• In patient with cerebral edema, check with prescriber about whether fluids should be withheld post-infusion.
• If hypotension occurs, slow or stop infusion. Use vasopressor, if needed.
Patient teaching
• Explain how and why albumin is given.
• Tell patient to report chills, fever, dyspnea, nausea, or rash immediately.

☑ Evaluation
• Patient's deficient fluid volume is resolved.
• Patient doesn't develop fluid overload.
• Patient and family state understanding of drug therapy.

albuterol sulfate (salbutamol sulfate)
(al-BYOO-ter-oll SULL-fayt)
AccuNeb, Airomir, Asmol CFC-free, Proventil, Proventil HFA, Proventil Repetabs, Ventolin, Ventolin HFA, VoSpire ER

Pharmacologic class: adrenergic
Therapeutic class: bronchodilator
Pregnancy risk category: C

Indications and dosages

▶ **To prevent exercise-induced bronchospasm.** *Adults and children age 4 and older:* Two aerosol inhalations 15 to 30 minutes before exercise.
▶ **To prevent or treat bronchospasm in patients with reversible obstructive airway disease.** *Aerosol. Adults and children age 4 and*

older: One or two inhalations every 4 to 6 hours. More frequent use and more inhalations aren't recommended. Proventil isn't indicated for use in children younger than age 12.

Solution for inhalation. *Adults and children age 12 and older:* 2.5-mg solution for inhalation by nebulizer t.i.d. or q.i.d. To prepare solution, use 0.5 ml of 0.5% solution diluted with 2.5 ml normal saline solution. Or, use 3 ml of 0.083% solution.

Children ages 2 to 11: Initially, 0.1 to 0.15 mg/kg of solution for inhalation by nebulizer, adjusted to response. Don't exceed 2.5 mg t.i.d. or q.i.d. by nebulization.

Tablets. *Adults and children older than age 12:* Give 2- to 4-mg tablets P.O. t.i.d. or q.i.d. Maximum, 8 mg q.i.d.

Children ages 6 to 12: Give 2-mg tablets P.O. t.i.d. or q.i.d. Maximum dose is 6 mg q.i.d. Or, 4- to 8-mg extended-release tablets P.O. every 12 hours. Maximum, 12 to 16 mg b.i.d.

Syrup. *Adults and children age 15 and older:* 2 to 4 mg (5 to 10 ml) syrup P.O. t.i.d. or q.i.d. Maximum, 8 mg P.O. q.i.d.

Children ages 6 to 14: Give 2 mg (5 ml) syrup P.O. t.i.d. or q.i.d. Maximum, 24 mg daily in divided doses.

Children ages 2 to 5: Initially, 0.1 mg/kg syrup P.O. t.i.d. Starting dose shouldn't exceed 2 mg (5 ml) t.i.d. Maximum, 4 mg (10 ml) t.i.d.

⊠ Adjust-a-dose: For elderly patients and patients sensitive to beta-adrenergic stimulators, 2-mg tablets P.O. t.i.d. or q.i.d. tablets or syrup. Maximum, 8 mg t.i.d. or q.i.d.

Contraindications and cautions

• Contraindicated in patients hypersensitive to drug or its components.
• Use cautiously in patients with CV disorders (including coronary insufficiency, cardiac arrhythmias, and hypertension), hyperthyroidism, or diabetes mellitus and in those unusually responsive to adrenergics.
• Use extended-release tablets cautiously in patients with GI narrowing.

⚘ **Lifespan:** In pregnant women, use cautiously. Breast-feeding women shouldn't take drug. In children, safety of drug hasn't been established in those younger than age 6 for tablets and Repetabs, younger than age 4 for aerosol, and younger than age 2 for inhalation solution and syrup. In elderly patients, use cautiously.

Adverse reactions

CNS: dizziness, headache, insomnia, *nervousness, tremor.*
CV: hypertension, palpitations, tachycardia.
EENT: drying and irritation of nose and throat.
GI: heartburn, nausea, vomiting.
Metabolic: hypokalemia, weight loss.
Musculoskeletal: muscle cramps.
Respiratory: *bronchospasm.*

Interactions

Drug-drug. *CNS stimulants:* May increase CNS stimulation. Avoid use together.
Levodopa: May increase risk of arrhythmias. Monitor patient closely.
MAO inhibitors, tricyclic antidepressants: May increase adverse CV effects. Monitor patient closely.
Propranolol, other beta blockers: May antagonize each other. Monitor patient carefully.
Drug-herb. *Herbs containing caffeine:* May have additive adverse effects. Discourage use together.
Drug-food. *Caffeine:* May increase CNS stimulation. Discourage use together.

Effects on lab test results

• May decrease potassium level.

Pharmacokinetics

Absorption: After inhalation, most of dose is swallowed and absorbed through GI tract.
Distribution: Doesn't cross blood–brain barrier.
Metabolism: Extensively in liver to inactive compounds.
Excretion: Rapidly in urine and feces. *Half-life:* About 4 hours for inhalation, 5 to 6 hours for oral form.

Route	Onset	Peak	Duration
P.O.	15–30 min	2–3 hr	4–6 hr
Inhalation	5–15 min	1–1½ hr	3–4 hr

Action

Chemical effect: Relaxes bronchial and uterine smooth muscle by acting on beta$_2$-adrenergic receptors.
Therapeutic effect: Improves ventilation.

Available forms

Aerosol inhaler: 90 mcg/metered spray, 100 mcg/metered spray

Solution for inhalation: 0.083%, 0.5%, 0.63 mg/3 ml, 1.25 mg/3 ml
Syrup: 2 mg/5 ml
Tablets: 2 mg, 4 mg
Tablets (extended-release): 4 mg, 8 mg

NURSING PROCESS

Assessment
• Obtain baseline assessment of patient's respiratory status, and assess patient often during therapy.
• Be alert for adverse reactions and drug interactions.
• Assess patient's and family's knowledge of drug therapy.

Nursing diagnoses
• Impaired gas exchange related to underlying respiratory condition
• Risk for injury related to drug-induced adverse reactions
• Deficient knowledge related to drug therapy

Planning and implementation
• Pleasant-tasting syrup may be taken by children as young as age 2. Syrup contains no alcohol or sugar.
• If more than one dose is ordered, wait at least 2 minutes between nebulized doses. If corticosteroid inhaler also is used, first have patient use bronchodilator, wait 5 minutes, and then have patient use corticosteroid inhaler. This permits bronchodilator to open air passages for maximum effectiveness.
• Aerosol form may be prescribed for use 15 minutes before exercise to prevent exercise-induced bronchospasm.
• Patients may use tablets and aerosol together.
⚠ **ALERT:** Don't confuse albuterol with atenolol or Albutein.
Patient teaching
• Warn patient to stop drug immediately if paradoxical bronchospasm occurs.
• Give these instructions for using metered-dose inhaler: Clear nasal passages and throat. Breathe out, expelling as much air from lungs as possible. Place mouthpiece well into mouth, and inhale deeply as dose is released. Hold breath for several seconds, remove mouthpiece, and exhale slowly.

• Advise patient to wait at least 2 minutes before repeating procedure if more than one inhalation is ordered.
• Warn patient to avoid accidentally spraying inhalant into eyes, which may cause temporary blurred vision.
• Tell patient to reduce intake of foods and herbs containing caffeine, such as coffee, cola, and chocolate, when using a bronchodilator.
• Show patient how to take his pulse. Instruct him to check pulse before and after using bronchodilator and to call prescriber if pulse rate increases more than 20 to 30 beats/minute.

Evaluation
• Patient's respiratory signs and symptoms improve.
• Patient has no injury from adverse drug reactions.
• Patient and family state understanding of drug therapy.

alefacept
(ALE-fuh-sept)
Amevive

Pharmacologic class: immunosuppressive
Therapeutic class: antipsoriatic
Pregnancy risk category: B

Indications and dosages
▶ **Moderate to severe chronic plaque psoriasis in candidates for systemic therapy or phototherapy.** *Adults:* 15 mg I.M. once weekly for 12 weeks. Another 12-week course may be given if CD4+ T lymphocyte count is normal and at least 12 weeks have passed since the previous treatment.
▧ **Adjust-a-dose:** If CD4+ T lymphocyte count is below 250 cells/mm³, withhold dose. Stop drug if CD4+ count remains below 250 cells/mm³ for 1 month.

Contraindications and cautions
• Contraindicated in patients hypersensitive to drug or its components, patients with a history of systemic malignancy or clinically important infection, and patients with HIV infection.
• Use cautiously in patients at high risk for malignancy and in those with chronic or recurrent infections.

⚘ **Lifespan:** In pregnant women, use only if clearly needed because effects on fetus aren't known. Breast-feeding women should either stop nursing or stop the drug because it isn't known whether drug appears in breast milk. In children, safety and effectiveness of drug haven't been established. In elderly patients, give drug cautiously because of their increased rate of infection and malignancies.

Adverse reactions

CNS: dizziness.
CV: *coronary artery disorder, MI.*
EENT: pharyngitis.
GI: nausea.
Hematologic: *lymphopenia.*
Musculoskeletal: myalgia.
Respiratory: cough.
Skin: pruritus.
Other: antibody formation; chills; hypersensitivity reaction; infection; *injection site* bleeding, edema, *inflammation,* mass, or *pain; malignancy.*

Interactions

Drug-drug. *Immunosuppressants, phototherapy:* May increase risk of excessive immunosuppression. Avoid using together.

Effects on lab test results

● May decrease CD4+ and CD8+ T lymphocyte counts.

Pharmacokinetics

Absorption: Unknown.
Distribution: 63% bioavailable after I.M. injection.
Metabolism: Unknown.
Excretion: Unknown. *Half-life:* 270 hours.

Route	Onset	Peak	Duration
I.M.	Unknown	Unknown	Unknown

Action

Chemical effect: Interferes with lymphocyte activation and reduces CD4+ and CD8+ T lymphocyte counts.
Therapeutic effect: Reduces symptoms of psoriasis.

Available forms

Powder for injection: 15-mg single-dose vial

NURSING PROCESS

Assessment
● Make sure patient has a normal CD4+ T lymphocyte count before therapy starts, and monitor it weekly for the 12-week course.
● Monitor patient carefully for evidence of infection or malignancy, and stop drug if it appears.

Nursing diagnoses
● Impaired skin integrity related to psoriasis
● Risk for infection related to immunosuppressive drug therapy
● Deficient knowledge related to drug therapy

Planning and implementation
ALERT: Rotate I.M. injection sites to give new injection at least 1" from the old site. Avoid areas that are bruised, tender, or hard.
● Overdose may cause chills, headache, arthralgia, and sinusitis. Provide supportive care, and closely monitor total lymphocyte and CD4+ T lymphocyte counts.
● Enroll pregnant women receiving drug into the Biogen Pregnancy Registry by calling 1-866-263-8483 so that drug effects can be studied.
Patient teaching
● Warn patient about potential adverse reactions.
● Urge patient to report evidence of infection immediately.
● Inform patient that blood tests will be done regularly to monitor WBC count.
● Tell patient to notify prescriber if she is or could be pregnant within 8 weeks of receiving drug.

Evaluation
● Patient's psoriasis improves.
● Patient remains free from infection.
● Patient and family state understanding of drug therapy.

alemtuzumab
(ah-lem-TOO-zeh-mab)
Campath

Pharmacologic class: monoclonal antibody
Therapeutic class: antineoplastic
Pregnancy risk category: C

Indications and dosages

▶ **B-cell chronic lymphocytic leukemia as monotherapy or combined with alkylating drugs in patients for whom fludarabine therapy has failed.** *Adults:* Initially, 3 mg I.V. infusion over 2 hours daily; if tolerated, increase to 10 mg daily; then increase to 30 mg daily. Dosage usually can be increased to 30 mg in 3 to 7 days. As maintenance, give 30 mg I.V. three times weekly on nonconsecutive days (such as Monday, Wednesday, Friday) for up to 12 weeks. Don't give a single dose greater than 30 mg or a weekly dose greater than 90 mg.

◺ Adjust-a-dose: The first time absolute neutrophil count (ANC) is 250/mm³ or less or platelet count is 25,000/mm³ or less, stop therapy; resume at same dose when ANC is 500/mm³ or more or platelet count is 50,000/mm³ or more. If interruption is 7 days or longer, start with 3 mg and increase to 10 mg and then 30 mg as tolerated. The second time ANC is 250/mm³ or less or platelet count is 25,000/mm³ or less, stop therapy; when ANC returns to 500/mm³ or more or platelet count to 50,000/mm³ or more, resume at 10 mg; if interruption is 7 days or longer, start with 3 mg and increase only to 10 mg. The third time ANC is 250/mm³ or less or platelet count is 25,000/mm³ or less, stop therapy. If ANC or platelet count decreases to 50% or less of baseline in patients starting therapy with a baseline ANC of 500/mm³ or less or a baseline platelet count 25,000/mm³ or less, stop therapy; when ANC or platelet count returns to baseline, resume therapy. If interruption is 7 days or longer, start with 3 mg and increase to 10 mg and then 30 mg, as tolerated.

▽ I.V. administration

• Don't use solution if it's discolored or contains precipitate. Don't shake ampule before use. Filter with a sterile, low–protein-binding, 5-micron filter before dilution. Add to 100 ml normal saline solution or D₅W. Gently invert bag to mix solution.
• Premedicate with 50 mg diphenhydramine and 650 mg acetaminophen 30 minutes before initial infusion and before each dose increase. If prescribed, give 200 mg hydrocortisone to decrease severe infusion-related adverse events.
• Give anti-infective prophylaxis, such as trimethoprim-sulfamethoxazole double strength b.i.d. three times weekly and 250 mg famci-

clovir (or equivalent) b.i.d. Continue prophylaxis for 2 months or until CD4+ count is 200/mm³ or more, whichever occurs later.
• Don't give as I.V. push or bolus.
• Infuse over 2 hours.
• Protect solution from light.
• Use within 8 hours of dilution.
⊗ **Incompatibilities**
Other I.V. drugs.

Contraindications and cautions

• Contraindicated in patients with active systemic infection, underlying immunodeficiency (such as HIV), or type I hypersensitivity or anaphylactic reactions to drug or any of its components.
⚖ **Lifespan:** In pregnant women, benefits of drug should be weighed against risks to the fetus. Breast-feeding women should stop breast-feeding during treatment and for at least 3 months after taking last dose of drug. In children, safety and effectiveness of drug haven't been established.

Adverse reactions

CNS: asthenia, depression, dizziness, dysthesias, fatigue, fever, headache, insomnia, malaise, somnolence, syncope, tremor.
CV: edema, hypertension, hypotension, peripheral edema, SUPRAVENTRICULAR TACHYCARDIA, tachycardia.
EENT: epistaxis, *pharyngitis,* rhinitis.
GI: abdominal pain, anorexia, constipation, diarrhea, dyspepsia, mucositis, nausea, stomatitis, ulcerative stomatitis, vomiting.
Hematologic: *anemia,* NEUTROPENIA, *pancytopenia,* purpura, THROMBOCYTOPENIA.
Musculoskeletal: back pain, myalgias, pain, skeletal pain.
Respiratory: *acute respiratory distress syndrome,* bronchitis, *bronchospasm,* cough, dyspnea, *pneumonia,* pneumonitis.
Skin: increased sweating, pruritus, rash, urticaria.
Other: candidiasis, chills, herpes simplex, infection, rigors, SEPSIS.

Interactions

None reported.

Effects on lab test results

• May decrease hemoglobin level and hematocrit.

- May decrease CD4+, lymphocyte, neutrophil, WBC, RBC, and platelet counts.
- May interfere with diagnostic tests that use antibodies.

Pharmacokinetics

Absorption: Given I.V.
Distribution: Binds to various tissues.
Metabolism: Unknown.
Excretion: Unknown. *Half-life:* 12 hours to 6 days.

Route	Onset	Peak	Duration
I.V.	Unknown	Unknown	Unknown

Action

Chemical effect: Binds to CD52 and causes antibody-dependent destruction of leukemic cells following cell-surface binding.
Therapeutic effect: Destroys leukemic cells.

Available forms

Ampules: 10 mg/ml, in 3-ml ampules

NURSING PROCESS

Assessment

- Assess patient before therapy for evidence of active infection or compromised immune function.
- Obtain baseline CBC and platelet count before starting therapy.
- Monitor blood pressure, and watch for hypotension during administration.
- ⓢ **ALERT:** Monitor hematologic studies during therapy. Even with normal doses, patients may develop hematologic toxicity, including myelosuppression, bone marrow dysplasia, and thrombocytopenia. Initial doses greater than 3 mg aren't well tolerated. Extremely high doses cause acute bronchospasm, cough, shortness of breath, and anuria and may be fatal. Stop drug and provide supportive treatment.
- Monitor CBC and platelet counts weekly during therapy and more often if anemia, neutropenia, or thrombocytopenia worsens.
- After treatment, monitor CD4+ count until it reaches 200 cells/mm^3.

Nursing diagnoses

- Risk for infection related to immunocompromised state
- Fatigue caused by drug therapy

- Deficient knowledge related to alemtuzumab therapy

Planning and implementation

- If transfusions are needed, irradiate blood to protect against graft-versus-host disease.
- Don't immunize with live-virus vaccines.
- If therapy is stopped for longer than 7 days, restart with gradual dose increase.
- ⓢ **ALERT:** Don't confuse alemtuzumab with trastuzumab.

Patient teaching

- Tell patient to immediately report infusion reaction, such as rigors, chills, fever, nausea, or vomiting.
- Advise patient to report signs or symptoms of infection immediately.
- Inform patient that blood tests will be done often during therapy to observe for adverse effects.
- Tell women of childbearing age and men to use effective contraception during therapy and for at least 6 months afterward.

Evaluation

- Patient remains free from infection.
- Patient has no harmful drug-induced adverse reactions.
- Patient and family state understanding of drug therapy.

alendronate sodium

(ah-LEN-droh-nayt SOH-dee-um)
Fosamax◆, Fosamax Plus D

Pharmacologic class: inhibitor of osteoclast-mediated bone resorption
Therapeutic class: antiosteoporotic
Pregnancy risk category: C

Indications and dosages

▶ **Osteoporosis in postmenopausal women; to increase bone mass in men with osteoporosis.** *Adults:* 10 mg P.O. daily or 70-mg tablet, one bottle of 70-mg oral solution, or one 70 mg/2,800 international units vitamin D$_3$ tablet, P.O. once weekly with water at least 30 minutes before first food, beverage, or medication of the day.
▶ **Prevention of osteoporosis in postmenopausal women.** *Women:* 5 mg P.O. daily or

35-mg tablet P.O. once weekly taken with water at least 30 minutes before first food, beverage, or medication of the day.

▶ **Corticosteroid-induced osteoporosis, given with calcium and vitamin D supplements.**
Adults: 5 mg P.O. daily.
Postmenopausal women not receiving estrogen replacement therapy: 10 mg P.O. daily.

▶ **Paget disease of bone.** *Adults:* 40 mg P.O. daily for 6 months taken with water at least 30 minutes before first food, beverage, or drug of the day.

Contraindications and cautions

• Contraindicated in patients with hypocalcemia; severe renal insufficiency; inability to stand or sit upright for at least 30 minutes; abnormalities of the esophagus that delay esophageal emptying, such as stricture or achalasia; increased risk of aspiration (oral solution); or hypersensitivity to drug or its components.
• Use cautiously in patients with dysphagia, esophageal diseases, gastritis, duodenitis, ulcers, or mild to moderate renal insufficiency.
⚠ **Lifespan:** In pregnant women, use only if benefits outweigh risks to the fetus. In breastfeeding women and in children, safety of drug hasn't been established.

Adverse reactions

CNS: headache.
GI: abdominal distention, abdominal pain, acid regurgitation, constipation, diarrhea, dyspepsia, dysphagia, esophageal ulcer, flatulence, gastritis, nausea, taste perversion, vomiting.
Musculoskeletal: musculoskeletal pain.

Interactions

Drug-drug. *Antacids, calcium supplements, and many other oral medications:* May interfere with alendronate absorption. Give 30 minutes after alendronate dose.
Aspirin, NSAIDs: May increase risk of upper GI reactions with alendronate doses greater than 10 mg daily. Monitor patient closely.
Drug-food. *Any food:* May decrease drug absorption. Don't give drug with food.

Effects on lab test results

• May mildly decrease calcium and phosphate levels.

Pharmacokinetics

Absorption: Food or beverages can significantly decrease bioavailability.
Distribution: Initially to soft tissues, but rapidly redistributed to bone or excreted in urine. About 78% protein-bound.
Metabolism: None.
Excretion: In urine. *Half-life:* More than 10 years.

Route	Onset	Peak	Duration
P.O.	1 mo	3–6 mo	3 wk after therapy

Action

Chemical effect: Suppresses osteoclast activity on newly formed resorption surfaces, reducing bone turnover.
Therapeutic effect: Increases bone mass.

Available forms

Oral solution: 70 mg/75 ml
Tablets: 5 mg, 10 mg, 35 mg, 40 mg, 70 mg, 70-mg tablet also containing 2,800 international units vitamin D_3

NURSING PROCESS

📋 **Assessment**
• Obtain history of patient's underlying disorder before therapy.
• Monitor calcium and phosphate levels throughout therapy.
• Be alert for adverse reactions and drug interactions.
• Assess patient's and family's knowledge of drug therapy.

⊕ **Nursing diagnoses**
• Risk for injury related to decreased bone mass
• Risk for deficient fluid volume related to drug-induced GI upset
• Deficient knowledge related to drug therapy

▷ **Planning and implementation**
• Correct hypocalcemia and other disturbances of mineral metabolism (such as vitamin D deficiency) before therapy begins.
• Give drug in the morning at least 30 minutes before first meal, fluid, or other oral drugs.
Ⓢ **ALERT:** Don't confuse Fosamax with Flomax.
• The recommended daily intake of vitamin D is 400 to 800 international units. Fosamax Plus

D provides 400 international units daily in the once-weekly formulation. Patients at risk for vitamin D deficiency, such as those who are chronically ill, have a GI malabsorption syndrome, or are older than age 70, may need additional amounts.

Patient teaching

• Advise patient to take tablets when he awakes with 6 to 8 oz of water; tell him to take oral solution with at least 2 oz of water.

⦿ **ALERT:** Warn patient not to lie down for at least 30 minutes after taking drug and until after the first food of the day to aid passage to stomach and reduce risk of esophageal irritation.

• Tell patient to take calcium and vitamin D supplements if daily dietary intake is inadequate.

• Show patient how to perform weight-bearing exercises, which help increase bone mass.

• Urge patient to limit or restrict smoking and alcohol use, if appropriate.

☑ **Evaluation**

• Patient remains free from bone fracture.
• Patient maintains adequate hydration.
• Patient and family state understanding of drug therapy.

alfuzosin hydrochloride
(al-FY00-zoe-sin high-droh-KLOR-ighd)
Uroxatral, Xatral ◆

Pharmacologic class: selective postsynaptic alpha$_1$-adrenergic antagonist
Therapeutic class: benign prostatic hypertrophy (BPH) drug
Pregnancy risk category: B

Indications and dosages

▶ **BPH.** *Men:* 10 mg P.O. after the same meal daily.

Contraindications and cautions

• Contraindicated in patients hypersensitive to drug or any of its components, in those with moderate or severe hepatic insufficiency (Child–Pugh categories B and C), and those being treated with potent inhibitors of CYP3A4.

• Use cautiously in patients who develop hypotension with other drugs and patients with severe renal insufficiency, congenital or acquired prolonged QT interval, or symptomatic hypotension.

⚞ **Lifespan:** In women and children, drug is contraindicated.

Adverse reactions

CNS: dizziness, fatigue, headache, pain.
CV: angina, chest pain, orthostatic hypotension, tachycardia.
EENT: pharyngitis, sinusitis.
GI: abdominal pain, constipation, dyspepsia, nausea.
GU: impotence, priapism.
Respiratory: bronchitis, upper respiratory tract infection.
Skin: rash.

Interactions

Drug-drug. *Alpha blockers:* May interact, although use not studied. Don't use together.
Antihypertensives: May cause hypotension. Monitor blood pressure, and use together cautiously.
Atenolol: May decrease blood pressure and heart rate. Monitor blood pressure and heart rate.
Cimetidine: May increase alfuzosin level. Use together cautiously.
CYP3A4 inhibitors (itraconazole, ketoconazole, and ritonavir): May increase alfuzosin level. Don't use together.
Drug-food. *Any food:* May increase absorption by 50%. Give with food.

Effects on lab test results

None significant.

Pharmacokinetics

Absorption: When taken with food, bioavailability is 49% and levels peak in 8 hours.
Distribution: 82% to 90% bound to plasma proteins.
Metabolism: Extensive, mainly by CYP3A4.
Excretion: 11% unchanged in urine. *Half-life:* 10 hours.

Route	Onset	Peak	Duration
P.O.	Unknown	8 hr	Unknown

Action

Chemical effect: Blocks alpha$_1$-adrenergic receptors in the lower urinary tract, causing smooth muscle in the bladder, neck, and prostate to relax.

Therapeutic effect: Improves urine flow and reduces symptoms of BPH.

Available forms

Tablets (extended-release): 10 mg

NURSING PROCESS

Assessment
• Assess patient's condition before therapy and regularly thereafter.
• Monitor patient for adverse reactions.
• Assess patient's and family's knowledge of drug therapy.

Nursing diagnoses
• Risk for injury related to adverse reactions from drug therapy
• Deficient knowledge related to drug therapy

Planning and implementation
• Prostate cancer and BPH may cause similar symptoms. Make sure prostate cancer is ruled out before starting therapy.
• Orthostatic hypotension may occur within a few hours after therapy. Take safety precautions.
• If angina appears or worsens, stop drug.
• Current or previous alpha blocker therapy may predispose the patient to floppy iris syndrome during cataract surgery.
ALERT: If overdose leads to hypotension, provide CV support by restoring blood pressure and heart rate. Have patient lie down, and give I.V. fluids and vasopressors, if needed.
ALERT: Don't use alfuzosin to treat hypertension.
Patient teaching
• Tell patient to take drug with food and with the same meal each day.
• Advise patient to rise slowly to prevent orthostatic hypotension.
• Warn patient that he may be dizzy, and caution him to avoid hazardous tasks until drug effects are known.
• Advise patient not to crush or chew tablets.
• If patient plans cataract surgery, urge him to tell the ophthalmologist that he takes or has taken an alpha blocker.

Evaluation
• Patient remains free from any adverse effects.
• Patient and family state understanding of drug therapy.

New Drug

A

aliskiren
(a-LIS-KYE-ren)
Tekturna

Pharmacologic class: renin inhibitor
Therapeutic class: antihypertensive
Pregnancy risk category: C (D in second and third trimesters)

Indications and dosages

▶ **Hypertension, alone or in combination with other antihypertensives.** *Adults:* 150 mg daily, may be increased to 300 mg daily.

Contraindications and cautions

• Contraindicated in patients who are hypersensitive to aliskiren or any of its components.
• Use cautiously in patients with a history of angioedema and in those with severe renal dysfunction (creatinine of 1.7 mg/dl in women and 2 mg/dl in men, or GFR less than 30 ml/minute), history of dialysis, nephrotic syndrome, or renovascular hypertension.
Lifespan: In pregnant women, drug is contraindicated because of possible fetal injury or death. Stop drug when patient becomes pregnant. In breast-feeding women, drug is contraindicated. In children, safety and effectiveness haven't been established. Elderly patients may be more sensitive to the drug's hypotensive effects.

Adverse reactions

CNS: headache, dizziness, fatigue, *seizures.*
CV: hypotension.
EENT: nasopharyngitis.
GI: diarrhea.
Metabolic: elevated creatine kinase, *hyperkalemia,* hyperuricemia.
Musculoskeletal: back pain.
Respiratory: cough, upper respiratory infection.
Skin: rash.
Other: *angioedema.*

Interactions

Drug-drug. *Atorvastatin:* May increase aliskiren levels. Use together cautiously.
Furosemide: May reduce furosemide peak levels. Monitor patient for effectiveness.
Irbesartan: May decrease aliskiren levels. Monitor patient for effectiveness.

Ketoconazole: May significantly increase aliskiren blood levels. Use together cautiously.
Drug-food. *High fat foods:* Significantly decreases plasma concentrations of aliskiren.

Effects on lab test results

• May increase potassium, creatine kinase, BUN, and serum creatinine levels.

Pharmacokinetics

Absorption: Poorly absorbed (2.5% bioavailable).
Distribution: Peak plasma concentrations reached within 1 to 3 hours.
Metabolism: It isn't known how much of drug is metabolized. CYP3A4 is a major enzyme involved in metabolism.
Excretion: 25% excreted in urine unchanged. Steady-state blood levels are reached in 7 to 8 days. *Half-life:* 24 hours.

Route	Onset	Peak	Duration
P.O.	Unknown	1–3 hr	Unknown

Action

Chemical effect: A potent renin inhibitor that decreases renin activity, inhibiting the conversion of angiotensinogen to angiotensin I. This ultimately reduces the conversion of angiotensin I to angiotensin II, which is a powerful vasoconstrictor, thus lowering blood pressure. It indirectly reduces aldosterone secretion and sodium reabsorption.
Therapeutic effect: Dilated blood vessels lowering blood pressure.

Available forms

Tablets: 150 mg, 300 mg

NURSING PROCESS

Assessment

• Obtain history of patient's blood pressure before starting therapy and reassess regularly.
• Assess patient's and family's knowledge of drug therapy.
• **ALERT:** Monitor patient for hypotension, angioedema, hyperkalemia, and worsening renal function.

Nursing diagnoses

• Risk for injury related to drug-induced adverse effects

• Deficient knowledge related to drug therapy

Planning and implementation

• Monitor blood pressure for hypotension.
• If creatinine rises or hyperkalemia occurs, notify prescriber immediately and stop drug.
• If angioedema occurs, notify prescriber immediately and stop drug. Institute appropriate supportive therapy (epinephrine, antihistamines, steroids).

Patient teaching

• Instruct patient to report history of kidney disease to their prescriber.
• Instruct patient to take the drug exactly as prescribed. Tell him to avoid taking the medication with a high-fat meal because this may decrease the drug's effectiveness.
• Warn patient to immediately report to prescriber swelling of the face, neck, tongue, lips, or difficulty breathing and to stop drug.
• Instruct patient to monitor blood pressure daily, if possible. Have him report low blood pressure, headache, or dizziness.
• Advise patient that he'll need periodic laboratory work.
• Instruct patient to tell prescriber about all drugs he's taking to avoid undesirable adverse effects and drug interactions.

Evaluation

• Patient's blood pressure becomes normal.
• Patient's creatine kinase, creatinine, uric acid, and serum potassium remain within normal limits.
• Patient and family state understanding of drug therapy.

allopurinol
(al-oh-PYOOR-ih-nol)
Novo-Purol ◆ , Zyloprim

allopurinol sodium
Aloprim

Pharmacologic class: xanthine oxidase inhibitor
Therapeutic class: antigout drug
Pregnancy risk category: C

Indications and dosages

▶ **Gout.** *Adults:* For mild gout, 200 to 300 mg P.O. daily. For severe gout with large tophi, 400 to 600 mg P.O. daily. May be given as single dose or divided; divide doses larger than 300 mg. Maximum, 800 mg daily.

▶ **To prevent acute gouty attacks.** *Adults:* 100 mg P.O. daily; increase at weekly intervals by 100 mg to a maximum recommended dose of 800 mg daily or until uric acid level falls to 6 mg/dl or less.

▶ **Hyperuricemia secondary to malignancies.** *Adults and children older than age 10:* Give 200 to 400 mg/m²/day I.V. 1 to 2 days before chemotherapy as a single infusion or in equally divided doses every 6, 8, or 12 hours. Maximum, 600 mg daily.

Children age 10 and younger: Initially, 200 mg/m²/day I.V. as a single infusion or in equally divided doses every 6, 8, or 12 hours. Then, titrate according to uric acid level. For children ages 6 to 10, 300 mg P.O. daily or divided t.i.d. For children younger than age 6, 150 mg P.O. daily.

▶ **To prevent uric acid nephropathy during chemotherapy.** *Adults:* 600 to 800 mg P.O. daily for 2 to 3 days, with high fluid intake.

▶ **Recurrent calcium oxalate calculi.** *Adults:* 200 to 300 mg P.O. daily in single or divided doses.

🔲 **Adjust-a-dose:** In patients with renal impairment, if creatinine clearance is 10 to 20 ml/minute, give 200 mg P.O. or I.V. daily; if clearance is less than 10 ml/minute, give 100 mg P.O. or I.V. daily; if it's less than 3 ml/minute, give 100 mg P.O. or I.V. at extended intervals.

▼ I.V. administration

● Dissolve contents of vial in 25 ml sterile water for injection. Dilute solution to desired concentration (no more than 6 mg/ml) with normal saline solution for injection or D₅W. Don't use solution that contains sodium bicarbonate.

● Store solution at 68° to 77° F (20° to 25° C) and use within 10 hours. Don't use if solution has particulates or is discolored.

⊗ **Incompatibilities**
Amikacin, amphotericin B, carmustine, cefotaxime, chlorpromazine, cimetidine, clindamycin phosphate, cytarabine, dacarbazine, daunorubicin, diphenhydramine, doxorubicin, doxycycline hyclate, droperidol, floxuridine, gentamicin, haloperidol lactate, hydroxyzine,

idarubicin, imipenem and cilastatin sodium, mechlorethamine, meperidine, methylprednisolone sodium succinate, metoclopramide, minocycline, nalbuphine, netilmicin, ondansetron, prochlorperazine edisylate, promethazine, sodium bicarbonate, streptozocin, tobramycin sulfate, vinorelbine.

Contraindications and cautions

● Contraindicated in patients hypersensitive to drug and in those with idiopathic hemochromatosis.

⚠ **Lifespan:** In pregnant or breast-feeding women, use cautiously.

Adverse reactions

CNS: drowsiness, headache.
EENT: cataracts, retinopathy.
GI: abdominal pain, diarrhea, nausea, vomiting.
GU: *renal failure,* uremia.
Hematologic: *agranulocytosis,* anemia, *aplastic anemia, thrombocytopenia.*
Hepatic: *hepatitis.*
Skin: *erythema multiforme; exfoliative lesions;* ichthyosis; rash, usually maculopapular; *toxic epidermal necrolysis,* urticarial and purpuric lesions.
Other: severe furunculosis of nose.

Interactions

Drug-drug. *ACE inhibitors:* May increase risk of hypersensitivity reaction. Monitor patient closely.

Amoxicillin, ampicillin, bacampicillin: May increase risk of rash. Avoid use together.

Anticoagulants, dicumarol: May potentiate anticoagulant effect. Adjust dosage, if needed.

Antineoplastics: May increase risk of bone marrow suppression. Monitor patient carefully.

Azathioprine, mercaptopurine: May increase levels of these drugs. Adjust dosage, if needed.

Chlorpropamide: May increase hypoglycemic effect. Avoid use together.

Cyclosporine: May increase cyclosporine level. Monitor and adjust cyclosporine dosage, if needed.

Diazoxide, diuretics, mecamylamine, pyrazinamide: May increase uric acid level. Adjust allopurinol dosage, if needed.

Ethacrynic acid, thiazide diuretics: May increase risk of allopurinol toxicity. Reduce allopurinol dosage, and closely monitor renal function.

Uricosurics: May have an additive effect. Use to therapeutic advantage.

Urine-acidifying drugs: May increase possibility of kidney stone formation. Monitor patient carefully.

Xanthines: May increase theophylline level. Adjust theophylline dosage.

Drug-lifestyle. *Alcohol use:* May increase uric acid level. Discourage use together.

Effects on lab test results

● May increase alkaline phosphatase, AST, ALT, BUN, and creatinine levels. May decrease hemoglobin level and hematocrit.

● May decrease granulocyte and platelet counts.

Pharmacokinetics

Absorption: 80% to 90%.

Distribution: Widely throughout body except brain, where levels are 50% of those found elsewhere.

Metabolism: To oxypurinol by xanthine oxidase.

Excretion: Mainly in urine; minute amount in feces. *Half-life:* Allopurinol, 1 to 2 hours; oxypurinol, about 15 hours.

Route	Onset	Peak	Duration
P.O.	2–3 days	½–2 hr	1–2 wk
I.V.	Unknown	½ hr	Unknown

Action

Chemical effect: Reduces uric acid production by inhibiting needed biochemical reactions.

Therapeutic effect: Relieves gout symptoms and treats hyperuricemia secondary to malignancy.

Available forms

allopurinol

Tablets (scored): 100 mg, 200 mg ♦ , 300 mg

allopurinol sodium

Injection: 500 mg/30-ml vial

NURSING PROCESS

🔖 Assessment

● Assess patient's history. Gout may be secondary to diseases such as acute or chronic leukemia, polycythemia vera, multiple myeloma, or psoriasis.

● Assess patient's uric acid level, joint stiffness, and pain before and during therapy. Optimal benefits may take 2 to 6 weeks of therapy.

● Monitor fluid intake and output. Daily urine output of at least 2 L and urine that's neutral or slightly alkaline urine are desirable.

● Monitor CBC and hepatic and renal function at the start and periodically during therapy.

● Be alert for adverse reactions and drug interactions.

● Assess patient's and family's knowledge of drug therapy.

🔷 Nursing diagnoses

● Acute pain (joint) related to patient's underlying condition

● Risk for infection related to drug-induced agranulocytosis

● Deficient knowledge related to drug therapy

▷ Planning and implementation

● Give drug with or just after meals to minimize adverse GI reactions.

● Have patient drink plenty of fluids while taking drug, unless contraindicated.

● Notify prescriber if renal insufficiency occurs during treatment; this usually warrants dosage reduction.

🔵 **ALERT:** Don't confuse Zyloprim with ZORprin.

● Give colchicine with allopurinol at the start of treatment to reduce the risk of acute gout attacks that may occur in first 6 weeks of therapy.

Patient teaching

● Advise patient not to drive or perform hazardous tasks requiring mental alertness until CNS effects of drug are known.

● Advise patient taking allopurinol for recurrent calcium oxalate stones to reduce intake of animal protein, sodium, refined sugars, oxalate-rich foods, and calcium.

● Tell patient to stop drug at first sign of rash, which may precede severe hypersensitivity or other adverse reaction. Rash is more common in patients taking diuretics and in those with renal disorders. Tell patient to report all adverse reactions immediately.

● Advise patient not to use alcohol during drug therapy.

✓ Evaluation

● Patient expresses relief from joint pain.

● Patient is free from infection.

- Patient and family state understanding of drug therapy.

almotriptan malate
(AL-moh-trip-tan MAH-layt)
Axert

Pharmacologic class: serotonin 5-HT$_1$ receptor agonist
Therapeutic class: antimigraine drug
Pregnancy risk category: C

Indications and dosages

▶ **Acute migraine with or without aura.**
Adults: 6.25-mg or 12.5-mg tablet P.O., with one additional dose after 2 hours if headache is unresolved or recurs. Maximum, two doses in 24 hours.
◺ **Adjust-a-dose:** For patients with hepatic or renal impairment, initially, 6.25 mg P.O. daily. Maximum, 12.5 mg daily.

Contraindications and cautions

- Contraindicated in patients hypersensitive to drug or its components and in those with angina pectoris, a history of MI, silent ischemia, uncontrolled hypertension, other CV disease, hemiplegic or basilar migraine, or coronary artery vasospasm, such as Prinzmetal variant angina.
- Don't give within 24 hours after other serotonin agonists or ergotamine drugs.
- Use cautiously in patients with renal or hepatic impairment and in those with cataracts because of the risk of corneal opacities.
- Also use cautiously in patients with risk factors for coronary artery disease (CAD), such as obesity, diabetes, and a family history of CAD.
☀ **Lifespan:** In pregnant women, use only if potential benefits outweigh risks to the fetus. In breast-feeding women, use cautiously because it isn't known whether drug appears in breast milk. In children, safety and effectiveness of drug haven't been established.

Adverse reactions

CNS: dizziness, headache, paresthesia, somnolence.
CV: *coronary artery vasospasm, MI, transient myocardial ischemia, ventricular fibrillation, ventricular tachycardia.*
GI: dry mouth, nausea.

Interactions

Drug-drug. *CYP3A4 inhibitors, such as ketoconazole:* May increase almotriptan level. Monitor patient for adverse reactions. Reduce dosage, if needed.
Ergot-containing drugs, serotonin 5-HT$_{1B/1D}$ agonists: May cause additive effects. Avoid using within 24 hours of almotriptan.
MAO inhibitors, verapamil: May increase almotriptan level. No dosage adjustment is needed.
SSRIs: May cause additive serotonin effects, resulting in weakness, hyperreflexia, or incoordination. If given together, monitor patient closely.

Effects on lab test results

None reported.

Pharmacokinetics

Absorption: Rapid and extensive; peaks in 1 to 3 hours. Food doesn't affect absorption.
Distribution: High. Minimally protein-bound.
Metabolism: Mainly by MAO-A, CYP3A4, and CYP2D6.
Excretion: 75% through renal excretion. *Half-life:* 3 to 4 hours.

Route	Onset	Peak	Duration
P.O.	1–3 hr	1–3 hr	3–4 hr

Action

Chemical effect: Binds selectively to various serotonin receptors, mainly serotonin 5-HT$_{1B/1D}$ receptors, resulting in cranial vessel constriction, which inhibits migraine.
Therapeutic effect: Blocks neuropeptide release to the pain pathways to prevent migraines.

Available forms

Tablets: 6.25 mg, 12.5 mg

NURSING PROCESS

◺ **Assessment**
- Assess patient's condition before and during drug therapy.
- Obtain list of patient's drug intake within 24 hours to prevent interactions. Use caution when giving drug to patient who takes an MAO inhibitor or a CYP3A4 or CYP2D6 inhibitor. Don't give drug with other serotonin agonist or ergotamine derivatives.

Rapid onset   *Liquid form contains alcohol.*   ◆ Canada   †OTC   ✐Photoguide   ‡Off-label use

- Be alert for adverse reactions.
- Monitor ECG in patients with risk factors for CAD or with symptoms similar to those of CAD, such as chest or throat tightness, pain, and heaviness.
- Assess patient's and family's knowledge of drug therapy.

✦ Nursing diagnoses
- Acute pain related to presence of acute migraine attack
- Risk for injury related to drug-induced interactions
- Deficient knowledge related to almotriptan therapy

▷ Planning and implementation
- Give dose as soon as patient complains of migraine symptoms.
- Repeat dose after 2 hours, if needed.
- Don't give more than two doses in 24 hours.
- ⊛ **ALERT:** Don't confuse Axert with Antivert.

Patient teaching
- Advise patient to take drug only when having a migraine.
- Teach patient to avoid possible migraine triggers, such as cheese, chocolate, citrus fruits, caffeine, and alcohol.
- Tell patient to repeat dose only once in 24 hours and no sooner than 2 hours after the first dose.
- Inform patient that other common migraine drugs may interact with this drug.
- Tell patient to immediately report any chest, throat, jaw, or neck tightness, pain, or heaviness, and to stop using the drug.
- Advise patient to use caution while driving or operating machinery.

✓ Evaluation
- Patient's symptoms are alleviated, and patient is free from pain.
- Serious complications from drug interactions don't develop.
- Patient and family state understanding of drug therapy.

alosetron hydrochloride
(a-LOE-se-tron high-droh-KLOR-ighd)
Lotronex

Pharmacologic class: selective 5-HT$_3$ receptor antagonist
Therapeutic class: GI drug
Pregnancy risk category: B

Indications and dosages

▶ **Irritable bowel syndrome (IBS) in women with severe diarrhea who haven't responded adequately to conventional therapy.** *Women:* 0.5 mg P.O. b.i.d. with or without food. If, after 4 weeks, the drug is well tolerated but doesn't adequately control IBS symptoms, increase to 1 mg b.i.d. If symptoms aren't controlled after 4 weeks at this dosage, stop drug.

Contraindications and cautions

- Contraindicated in women hypersensitive to the drug or its components; those with Crohn disease, ulcerative colitis, diverticulitis, or a history of chronic or severe constipation; those with sequelae from constipation, intestinal obstruction, stricture, toxic megacolon, GI perforation, GI adhesions, ischemic colitis, impaired intestinal circulation, thrombophlebitis, or hypercoagulation; and those taking fluvoxamine.
- Women shouldn't take drug if they're constipated or the chief bowel symptom is constipation.
- ☀ **Lifespan:** In pregnant women, use only if clearly needed. In breast-feeding women, use cautiously because it isn't known if drug or its metabolites appear in breast milk. In children, drug isn't recommended because it hasn't been studied. In elderly women, use cautiously because they may be at greater risk for complications of constipation.

Adverse reactions

CNS: abnormal dreams, anxiety, depressive disorders, headache, sedation, sleep disorders.
CV: *arrhythmias, hypertension.*
EENT: *allergic rhinitis; bacterial ear, nose, and throat infections; photophobia; throat and tonsil discomfort and pain.*
GI: abdominal discomfort and pain, abdominal distention, *constipation,* dyspeptic symptoms, gaseous symptoms, GI discomfort and pain,

hemorrhoids, ileus, impaction, ischemic colitis, nausea, obstruction, *perforation,* proctitis, small-bowel mesenteric ischemia, viral GI infections.

Interactions

Drug-drug. *CYP1A2 inhibitors (cimetidine, quinolones), ketoconazole:* May increase alosetron level. Avoid use together.
Fluvoxamine: May severely increase alosetron level. Use together is contraindicated.
Hydralazine, isoniazid, procainamide: May slow metabolism and increase level of these drugs because of N-acetyltransferase inhibition. Monitor patient for toxicity.

Effects on lab test results

• May increase ALT, AST, alkaline phosphatase, and bilirubin levels.

Pharmacokinetics

Absorption: Rapid. Mean absolute bioavailability is 50% to 60%. Food decreases rate by 25%.
Distribution: 82% bound to plasma proteins.
Metabolism: Extensive, by cytochrome P-450 enzymes (CYP2C9, CYP3A4, CYP1A2).
Excretion: 7% unchanged in urine. Radiolabeled dose 73% in urine and 24% in feces. *Half-life:* 1½ hour.

Route	Onset	Peak	Duration
P.O.	Unknown	1 hr	Variable

Action

Chemical effect: Selectively inhibits 5-HT$_3$ receptors on enteric neurons in the GI tract. Blocks neuronal depolarization, which decreases visceral pain, colonic transit, and GI secretions.
Therapeutic effect: Relieves pain and decreases frequency of loose stools caused by IBS.

Available forms

Tablets: 0.5 mg, 1 mg

NURSING PROCESS

Assessment
⊛ **ALERT:** Effectiveness in men hasn't been established.
• Call 1-888-825-5249 or visit www.lotronex.com to enroll or report adverse

reactions; only physicians enrolled in the prescribing program can prescribe this drug.
• Don't use in patient whose main symptom is constipation.
• Assess patient before and during drug therapy.

Nursing diagnoses
• Diarrhea related to underlying IBS condition
• Acute pain related to underlying IBS condition
• Deficient knowledge related to drug therapy

Planning and implementation
• If patient develops constipation, therapy should be stopped and laxatives and fiber should be used until the constipation resolves.
⊛ **ALERT:** Death may occur in patients who develop ischemic colitis and serious complications of constipation. If patient complains of rectal bleeding or sudden worsening of abdominal pain, stop therapy and rule out acute ischemic colitis.
• Acute symptoms of toxicity include labored breathing, ataxia, subdued behavior, tremors, and seizures. No antidote exists for overdose. Treatment for overdose includes supportive care.

Patient teaching
⊛ **ALERT:** Explain to patient that she must be enrolled in the prescribing program. Counsel patient about the drug's risks and benefits, give instructions, answer questions, and provide information about the drug. The patient must review and sign a patient–physician agreement. A special program sticker must be affixed to all written prescriptions; no telephone, facsimile, or computerized prescriptions are permitted.
• Instruct patient not to start drug if she is constipated.
⊛ **ALERT:** Tell patient to stop drug and consult prescriber immediately if she becomes constipated or has signs and symptoms of ischemic colitis, such as rectal bleeding, bloody diarrhea, or worsened abdominal pain or cramping.
• Explain that this drug doesn't cure but may alleviate some IBS symptoms. If it doesn't adequately control symptoms after twice-daily therapy, advise patient to stop taking drug and contact prescriber.
• Inform patient that most women notice symptoms improving after about 1 week, but some may take up to 4 weeks to experience relief.

Symptoms usually return within 1 week of stopping therapy.

☑ Evaluation
• Patient's symptoms related to IBS, including pain and frequency of loose stools, are relieved.
• Patient and family state understanding of drug therapy.

HIGH ALERT!

alprazolam
(al-PRAH-zoh-lam)
Apo-Alpraz ◆, Niravam, Novo-Alprazol ◆, Nu-Alpraz ◆, Xanax⌀, Xanax XR

Pharmacologic class: benzodiazepine
Therapeutic class: anxiolytic
Pregnancy risk category: D
Controlled substance schedule: IV

Indications and dosages
▶ **Anxiety.** *Adults:* Usual initial dose, 0.25 to 0.5 mg P.O. t.i.d. Maximum, 4 mg daily in divided doses.
🔋**Adjust-a-dose:** For elderly or debilitated patients or those with advanced liver disease, usual initial dose is 0.25 mg P.O. b.i.d. or t.i.d. Maximum, 4 mg daily in divided doses.
▶ **Panic disorders.** *Adults:* 0.5 mg P.O. t.i.d., increased every 3 to 4 days in increments of no more than 1 mg. Maximum, 10 mg daily in divided doses. Or initially 0.5 to 1 mg extended-release P.O. daily, increased every 3 to 4 days by no more than 1 mg daily. Usual dosage is 3 to 6 mg P.O. once daily, preferably in the morning. Individualize dosage, as needed. Maximum, 10 mg daily. If dosage reduction is needed, decrease by no more than 0.5 mg every 3 days.
▶ **Social phobias‡.** *Adults:* 2 to 8 mg P.O. daily.

Contraindications and cautions
• Contraindicated in patients hypersensitive to drug or other benzodiazepines, those with acute angle-closure glaucoma, and those taking azole antifungals.
• Use cautiously in patients with hepatic, renal, or pulmonary disease and in patients with cardiac disease because hypotension may occur.
🌿 **Lifespan:** In pregnant women, drug may cause congenital abnormalities and fetal harm.

Avoid use, especially during the first trimester. In breast-feeding women, drug isn't recommended. In children, safety of drug hasn't been established. In elderly patients, use cautiously because they may be more sensitive to sedation and ataxia.

Adverse reactions
CNS: agitation, akathisia, *anxiety,* ataxia, *confusion, depression, difficulty speaking, dizziness, drowsiness,* dyskinesia, emergence of anxiety between doses, *fatigue, headache,* hypoesthesia, *impaired coordination, insomnia, irritability,* lethargy, *light-headedness,* malaise, mania, *memory impairment,* mental impairment, nervousness, nightmares, paresthesia, restlessness, *sedation, somnolence,* **suicidal thoughts,** syncope, tremor, vertigo.
CV: chest pain, hypotension, palpitations.
EENT: allergic rhinitis, blurred vision, nasal congestion, sore throat.
GI: abdominal pain, anorexia, *constipation, diarrhea, dry mouth,* dyspepsia, increased or decreased appetite, nausea, vomiting.
GU: difficulty urinating, dysmenorrhea, premenstrual syndrome.
Metabolic: increased or decreased weight.
Musculoskeletal: arthralgia; limb and back pain; muscle rigidity, cramps, or twitching; myalgia.
Respiratory: dyspnea, hyperventilation, upper respiratory tract infection.
Skin: dermatitis, increased sweating, pruritus.
Other: decreased or increased libido, dependence, hot flushes, influenza, injury, sexual dysfunction.

Interactions
Drug-drug. *Anticonvulsants, antidepressants, antihistamines, barbiturates, benzodiazepines, general anesthetics, opioids, phenothiazines:* May increase CNS depressant effects. Avoid use together.
Carbamazepine, propoxyphene: May decrease alprazolam level. Use together cautiously.
Cimetidine, fluoxetine, fluvoxamine, hormonal contraceptives, nefazodone: May increase alprazolam level. Use together cautiously, and consider reducing alprazolam dosage.
Digoxin: May increase digoxin level. Monitor it closely.

Fluconazole, itraconazole, ketoconazole, miconazole: May increase and prolong drug levels, CNS depression, and psychomotor impairment. Use together is contraindicated.
Tricyclic antidepressants: May increase levels of these drugs. Monitor patient closely.
Drug-herb. *Calendula, hops, lemon balm, skullcap, valerian:* May increase sedative effects. Discourage use together.
Kava: May increase CNS sedation. Discourage use together.
Drug-food. *Grapefruit:* May increase alprazolam level. Use cautiously together.
Drug-lifestyle. *Alcohol use:* May cause additive CNS effects. Strongly discourage use together.
Smoking: May decrease effectiveness of drug. Help patient quit smoking.

Effects on lab test results
• May increase ALT and AST levels.

Pharmacokinetics
Absorption: Well absorbed.
Distribution: Wide. 80% of dose is bound to plasma proteins.
Metabolism: In liver by CYP3A4 pathway, equally to alpha-hydroxyalprazolam and inactive metabolites.
Excretion: In urine. *Half-life:* Immediate-release, 12 to 15 hours; extended-release, 11 to 16 hours.

Route	Onset	Peak	Duration
P.O.	Unknown	1–2 hr	Unknown
P.O. extended	Unknown	Unknown	Unknown

Action
Chemical effect: May potentiate effects of GABA, an inhibitory neurotransmitter, and depress CNS at limbic and subcortical levels of brain.
Therapeutic effect: Decreases anxiety.

Available forms
Oral solution: 1 mg/ml (concentrate)
Tablets: 0.25 mg, 0.5 mg, 1 mg, 2 mg
Tablets (extended-release): 0.5 mg, 1 mg, 2 mg, 3 mg
Tablets (orally-disintegrating): 0.25 mg, 0.5 mg, 1 mg, 2 mg

NURSING PROCESS

Assessment
• Assess patient's anxiety before and often after therapy.
• In patient receiving repeated or prolonged therapy, monitor liver, renal, and hematopoietic function test results periodically.
• Be alert for adverse reactions and drug interactions.
• Assess patient's and family's knowledge of drug therapy.

Nursing diagnoses
• Anxiety related to patient's underlying condition
• Risk for injury related to drug-induced CNS reactions
• Deficient knowledge related to drug therapy

Planning and implementation
• Drug shouldn't be given for longer than 4 months.
• Make sure patient has swallowed tablets after you give them.
ALERT: Paradoxic excitation, hostility, mania, hypomania, and insomnia may occur.
ALERT: Don't stop drug abruptly after long-term use because withdrawal symptoms may occur. Abuse or addiction is possible.
• Withdrawal symptoms include seizures, status epilepticus, impaired concentration, muscle cramps or twitch, diarrhea, blurred vision, decreased appetite, and weight loss.
ALERT: Don't confuse alprazolam with alprostadil. Don't confuse Xanax with Zantac or Tenex.
• To switch patient from immediate-release to extended-release tablets, calculate the total daily dose of immediate-release tablets and give the same dose of extended-release tablets once daily.
Patient teaching
• Warn patient to avoid hazardous activities that require alertness and psychomotor coordination until CNS effects of drug are known.
• Tell patient to avoid alcohol and smoking while taking drug.
• Advise patient to take drug as prescribed and not to stop without prescriber's approval. Explain the risk of dependence if taken longer than directed.

- Instruct patient to swallow extended-release tablets whole and not to chew or crush them.
- Tell patient taking orally disintegrating tablets to remove tablet from bottle using dry hands and immediately place on his tongue, where the tablet will dissolve and can be swallowed with saliva.
- Tell patient taking half of a scored orally disintegrating tablet to destroy the unused portion.
- Advise patient to discard any cotton from the bottle of orally disintegrating tablets and to keep it tightly sealed to prevent moisture from entering the bottle and dissolving the tablets.
- Teach patient how to manage or avoid adverse reactions, such as constipation and drowsiness.

✓ Evaluation
- Patient is less anxious.
- Patient sustains no injury from adverse CNS reactions.
- Patient and family state understanding of drug therapy.

alprostadil
(al-PROS-tuh-dil)
Prostin VR Pediatric

Pharmacologic class: prostaglandin
Therapeutic class: ductus arteriosus patency adjunct
Pregnancy risk category: NR

Indications and dosages
▶ **Temporary maintenance of patent ductus arteriosus until surgery can be performed.**
Infants: 0.05 to 0.1 mcg/kg/minute by I.V. infusion. When therapeutic response occurs, reduce rate to lowest effective dosage. Maximum, 0.4 mcg/kg/minute. Or, drug may be given through umbilical artery catheter placed at ductal opening.

▽ I.V. administration
- Keep respiratory and emergency equipment available.
- Before giving, dilute 500 mcg of drug with sodium chloride or dextrose injection. Dilute to appropriate volume for pump delivery system.
- Drug isn't recommended for direct injection or intermittent infusion. Give by continuous infusion using constant-rate pump. Infuse through

large peripheral or central vein or through umbilical artery catheter placed at level of ductus arteriosus. If flushing occurs as a result of peripheral vasodilation, reposition catheter.
- If fever or significant hypotension develops in an infant, reduce the infusion rate.
- If apnea and bradycardia develop, stop infusion immediately. This may be a sign of drug overdose.
- In prolonged infusions, infant may develop gastric outlet obstruction, morphologic changes in pulmonary arteries, and proliferation of long bones.
- Discard solution after 24 hours.
⊗ **Incompatibilities**
Diluents that contain benzyl alcohol; fatal toxic syndrome may occur.

Contraindications and cautions
None known.
♨ **Lifespan:** In neonates with bleeding tendencies, use cautiously because drug inhibits platelet aggregation. In neonates with respiratory distress syndrome or in premature infants with a patent ductus arteriosus, drug is contraindicated. Infants on long-term infusions may experience cortical growth of long bones.

Adverse reactions
CNS: fever, *seizures.*
CV: *bradycardia, cardiac arrest,* flushing, hypotension, tachycardia.
GI: diarrhea.
Hematologic: *DIC.*
Respiratory: APNEA.
Other: *sepsis.*

Interactions
None significant.

Effects on lab test results
- May decrease potassium level.

Pharmacokinetics
Absorption: Given I.V.
Distribution: Rapid.
Metabolism: About 68% of dose is metabolized in one pass through lung, mainly by oxidation; 100% is metabolized within 24 hours.
Excretion: All metabolites are excreted in urine within 24 hours. *Half-life:* About 5 to 10 minutes.

Route	Onset	Peak	Duration
I.V.	5–10 min	20 min	1–3 hr

Action

Chemical effect: Relaxes smooth muscle of ductus arteriosus.
Therapeutic effect: Improves cardiac circulation.

Available forms

Injection: 500 mcg/ml

NURSING PROCESS

Assessment

• Obtain baseline assessment of infant's cardiopulmonary status before therapy.
• Measure drug's effectiveness by monitoring blood oxygenation of infants with restricted pulmonary blood flow and by systemic blood pressure and blood pH of infants with restricted systemic blood flow.
• Be alert for adverse reactions throughout therapy.
• Evaluate parent's knowledge of drug therapy.

Nursing diagnoses

• Ineffective cardiopulmonary tissue perfusion related to underlying condition
• Risk for injury related to drug-induced adverse reactions
• Deficient knowledge related to drug therapy

Planning and implementation

• Before drug is given, a differential diagnosis should be made between respiratory distress syndrome and cyanotic heart disease. Don't use drug in neonates with respiratory distress syndrome.
⊕ ALERT: Don't confuse alprostadil with alprazolam.
Patient teaching
• Keep parents informed of infant's status.
• Explain that parents will be allowed as much time and physical contact with infant as possible.

Evaluation

• Patient is stable with a working cardiopulmonary system.
• Patient isn't injured by adverse drug reactions.
• Parents state understanding of drug therapy.

HIGH ALERT!

alteplase (tissue plasminogen activator, recombinant; tPA)
(AL-teh-plays)
Activase, Cathflo Activase

Pharmacologic class: enzyme
Therapeutic class: thrombolytic enzyme
Pregnancy risk category: C

Indications and dosages

▶ **Lysis of thrombi obstructing coronary arteries in acute MI.** *Adults:* 100 mg I.V. infusion over 3 hours as follows: 60 mg in first hour, with 6 to 10 mg given as bolus over first 1 to 2 minutes. Then, 20 mg/hour infusion for 2 hours. Adults weighing less than 65 kg (143 lb) receive 1.25 mg/kg using the same method (60% in first hour with 10% as bolus, then 20% of total dose per hour for 2 hours). Don't exceed 100-mg dose. Higher doses may increase risk of intracranial bleeding.
▶ **Acute massive pulmonary embolism.** *Adults:* 100 mg I.V. infusion over 2 hours. Begin heparin at end of infusion when PTT or PT returns to twice normal or less. Don't exceed 100-mg dose. Higher doses may increase risk of intracranial bleeding. ‡Also, may infuse 30 or 50 mg via intrapulmonary artery over 1½ or 2 hours, respectively, with heparin therapy.
▶ **Acute ischemic stroke.** *Adults:* 0.9 mg/kg (maximum 90 mg) I.V. over 60 minutes with 10% of the total dose given as initial bolus over 1 minute.
▶ **To restore function to central venous access devices as assessed by the ability to withdraw blood.** *Adults and children older than age 2:* For patients weighing 30 kg (66 lb) or more, instill 2 mg Cathflo Activase in 2 ml sterile water into catheter. For patients weighing 10 to 30 kg (22 to 66 lb), instill 110% of the internal lumen volume of the catheter, not to exceed 2 mg. After 30 minutes of dwell time, assess catheter function by aspirating blood. If function is restored, aspirate 4 to 5 ml of blood to remove Cathflo Activase and residual clot, and gently irrigate the catheter with normal saline solution. If catheter function isn't restored after 120 minutes, instill a second dose.
▶ **To prevent reocclusion after thrombolysis for acute MI‡.** *Adults:* 3.3 mcg/kg/minute by

I.V. infusion for 4 hours with heparin immediately following initial thrombolytic infusion.

▶ **Lysis of arterial occlusion in a peripheral vessel or bypass graft‡.** *Adults:* 0.05 to 0.1 mg/kg/hour infused via the intrapulmonary artery for 1 to 8 hours.

▽ I.V. administration

• Reconstitute alteplase immediately before use in sterile water for injection, without preservatives. Check label for specific information.
• Don't use vial if vacuum seal isn't present. Reconstitute with large-bore (18G) needle, directing stream of sterile water at lyophilized cake. Don't shake, but make sure that drug dissolves completely. Slight foaming is common. Solution should be clear or pale yellow.
• Drug may be given as reconstituted (1 mg/ml) or diluted with equal volume of normal saline solution or D₅W to make 0.5-mg/ml solution.
• Drug and may be stored temporarily at 35° to 86° F (2° to 30° C), but it's stable for only 8 hours at room temperature. Discard unused solution.

To restore function of a central venous catheter
• Reconstitute Cathflo Activase with 2.2 ml sterile water; dissolve completely into a colorless to pale yellow solution of 1 mg/ml. Solution is stable up to 8 hours at room temperature.
• Assess the cause of catheter dysfunction before using Cathflo Activase. Causes of occlusion may include incorrect catheter position, mechanical failure, constriction by a suture, and lipid deposits or drug precipitates in the catheter lumen. Don't try to suction because of the risk of damage to the vascular wall or collapse of soft-walled catheters.
• Don't use excessive pressure while instilling Cathflo Activase into the catheter because it could cause catheter rupture or expulsion of the clot into circulation.
⊗ **Incompatibilities**
Don't mix with other drugs.

Contraindications and cautions

• Contraindicated in patients with active internal bleeding, intracranial neoplasm, arteriovenous malformation, aneurysm, severe uncontrolled hypertension, history of stroke, known bleeding diathesis, or intraspinal or intracranial trauma or surgery within past 2 months.

• Use cautiously in patients who had major surgery within 10 days; those receiving anticoagulants; those with organ biopsy, trauma (including cardiopulmonary resuscitation), GI or GU bleeding, cerebrovascular disease, hypertension, acute pericarditis, subacute bacterial endocarditis, septic thrombophlebitis, or diabetic hemorrhagic retinopathy; and those with mitral stenosis, atrial fibrillation, or other conditions that may lead to left-sided heart thrombus.
❋ **Lifespan:** During pregnancy, the first 10 days postpartum, and lactation, use cautiously. In children, safety of drug hasn't been established. In patients age 75 and older, use cautiously.

Adverse reactions

CNS: *cerebral hemorrhage,* fever.
CV: *arrhythmias,* edema, hypotension.
GI: *bleeding,* nausea, vomiting.
GU: bleeding.
Hematologic: *severe, spontaneous bleeding.*
Musculoskeletal: arthralgia.
Skin: urticaria.
Other: *anaphylaxis, angioedema,* bleeding at puncture sites, hypersensitivity reactions.

Interactions

Drug-drug. *Abciximab, aspirin, coumarin anticoagulants, dipyridamole, heparin:* May increase risk of bleeding. Monitor patient carefully.
Nitroglycerin: May decrease tPA antigen level. Avoid use together. If unavoidable, use the lowest effective nitroglycerin dose.
Drug-herb. *Dong quai, garlic, ginkgo:* May increase risk of bleeding. Discourage use together.

Effects on lab test results

None reported.

Pharmacokinetics

Absorption: Given I.V.
Distribution: Rapidly cleared from plasma by liver (about 80% cleared within 10 minutes after infusion stops).
Metabolism: Mainly hepatic.
Excretion: Over 85% in urine, 5% in feces.
Half-life: Less than 10 minutes.

Route	Onset	Peak	Duration
I.V.	Immediate	45 min	4 hr

Action

Chemical effect: Binds to fibrin in thrombus and locally converts plasminogen to plasmin, which initiates local fibrinolysis.
Therapeutic effect: Dissolves blood clots in coronary arteries and lungs.

Available forms

Injection: 50-mg (29 million international units), 100-mg (58 million international units) vials
Solution for intracatheter clearance: 2-mg single-use vials

NURSING PROCESS

🔲 Assessment

• Assess patient's cardiopulmonary status (including ECG, vital signs, and coagulation studies) before and during therapy.
• Be alert for adverse reactions and drug interactions.
• Monitor patient for internal bleeding, and check puncture site often.
• Assess patient's and family's knowledge of drug therapy.

🔲 Nursing diagnoses

• Ineffective cardiopulmonary tissue perfusion related to patient's underlying condition
• Risk for injury related to adverse effects of drug therapy
• Deficient knowledge related to drug therapy

🔲 Planning and implementation

• Recanalization of occluded coronary arteries and improvement of heart function require starting drug as soon as possible after onset of symptoms.
• Heparin is given often after alteplase to reduce risk of rethrombosis.
• For arterial puncture, select site on arm and apply pressure for 30 minutes afterward. Also use pressure dressings, sand bags, or ice packs on recent puncture sites to prevent bleeding.
• Notify prescriber about severe bleeding that doesn't stop with intervention; alteplase and heparin infusions will need to be stopped.
🔲 **ALERT:** Have antiarrhythmics available. Coronary thrombolysis is linked to arrhythmias induced by reperfusion of ischemic myocardium.
• Avoid invasive procedures during thrombolytic therapy.

Patient teaching
• Tell patient to immediately report chest pain, dyspnea, changes in heart rate or rhythm, nausea, and bleeding.

🔲 Evaluation

• Patient's cardiopulmonary assessment findings show improved perfusion.
• Patient has no serious adverse drug reactions.
• Patient and family state understanding of drug therapy.

amantadine hydrochloride
(uh-MAN-tah-deen high-droh-KLOR-ighd)
Symmetrel

Pharmacologic class: synthetic cyclic primary amine
Therapeutic class: antiviral, antiparkinsonian
Pregnancy risk category: C

Indications and dosages

▶ **Prevention or treatment of influenza type A virus; respiratory tract illness in elderly or debilitated patients.** *Adults age 65 and older:* 100 mg P.O. once daily. Continue for 24 to 48 hours after symptoms resolve. Start prophylaxis as soon as possible after exposure, and continue for at least 10 days. When inactivated influenza A vaccine is unavailable, may continue preventive use as long as influenza A is present in community. If used with influenza vaccine, drug is continued for 2 to 4 weeks until protection develops from vaccine.
Adults age 65 and younger and children age 13 and older: 200 mg P.O. daily in single dose or divided b.i.d.
Children ages 9 to 12: Give 100 mg P.O. b.i.d.
Children ages 1 to 8: Give 4.4 to 8.8 mg/kg P.O. daily in single dose or divided b.i.d. Maximum, 150 mg daily.
▶ **Drug-induced extrapyramidal reactions.** *Adults:* 100 mg P.O. b.i.d. Occasionally, patients whose responses aren't optimal may benefit from an increase to 300 mg P.O. daily in divided doses.
▶ **Idiopathic parkinsonism, parkinsonian syndrome.** *Adults:* 100 mg P.O. b.i.d. In patients who are seriously ill or taking other antiparkinsonians, 100 mg daily for at least

1 week; then 100 mg b.i.d., p.r.n. Maximum, 400 mg daily.

⬛ **Adjust-a-dose:** For patients with creatinine clearance of 30 to 50 ml/minute, give 200 mg the first day and 100 mg daily thereafter; for clearance of 15 to 29 ml/minute, give 200 mg the first day and then 100 mg every other day; for clearance of less than 15 ml/minute, give 200 mg once weekly.

Contraindications and cautions

• Contraindicated in patients hypersensitive to drug.
• Use cautiously in patients with seizure disorders, heart failure, peripheral edema, hepatic disease, mental illness, eczematoid rash, renal impairment, orthostatic hypotension, or CV disease. Adjust dosage in patients with renal impairment.
⚖ **Lifespan:** In pregnant and breast-feeding women, use cautiously. In children younger than age 1, safety of drug hasn't been established. In elderly patients, use cautiously.

Adverse reactions

CNS: anxiety, ataxia, confusion, depression, difficulty concentrating, dizziness, fatigue, hallucinations, headache, insomnia, irritability, light-headedness, *neuroleptic malignant syndrome,* psychosis, weakness.
CV: *heart failure,* orthostatic hypotension, peripheral edema.
GI: anorexia, constipation, diarrhea, dry mouth, nausea, vomiting.
GU: urine retention.
Skin: livedo reticularis.

Interactions

Drug-drug. *Anticholinergics:* May increase adverse anticholinergic effects. Use together cautiously.
CNS stimulants: May cause additive CNS stimulation. Use together cautiously.
Hydrochlorothiazide, sulfamethoxazole, triamterene, trimethoprim: May increase amantadine level. Use together cautiously.
Quinidine, quinine: May reduce renal clearance of amantadine. Use together cautiously.
Thioridazine: May worsen tremor in elderly patients. Monitor these patients closely.
Drug-herb. *Jimsonweed:* May adversely affect CV function. Discourage use together.

Effects on lab test results

None reported.

Pharmacokinetics

Absorption: Well absorbed from the GI tract.
Distribution: Widely throughout the body; crosses the blood–brain barrier.
Metabolism: About 10% of drug is metabolized.
Excretion: About 90% unchanged in urine, mainly by tubular secretion. Some drug may appear in breast milk. Excretion rate depends on urine pH. *Half-life:* About 24 hours; with renal dysfunction, may be prolonged to 10 days.

Route	Onset	Peak	Duration
P.O.	Unknown	2–4 hr	Unknown

Action

Chemical effect: May interfere with influenza A virus penetration into susceptible cells. In parkinsonism, action is unknown.
Therapeutic effect: Protects against and reduces symptoms of influenza A viral infection and extrapyramidal symptoms.

Available forms

Capsules: 100 mg
Syrup: 50 mg/5 ml
Tablets: 100 mg

NURSING PROCESS

📋 **Assessment**
• Obtain baseline assessment of patient's exposure to influenza A virus or history of Parkinson disease.
• Watch for adverse reactions and drug interactions.
• If adverse GI reactions occur, monitor patient's hydration status.
• Assess patient's and family's knowledge of drug therapy.

✥ **Nursing diagnoses**
• Ineffective health maintenance related to patient's underlying condition
• Risk for deficient fluid volume related to adverse GI reactions
• Deficient knowledge related to drug therapy

A

▶ Planning and implementation

• Elderly patients are more susceptible to neurologic adverse effects. Giving drug in two daily doses rather than as single dose may reduce these effects.

• For best absorption, give drug after meals.

⊕ **ALERT:** Don't confuse amantadine with rimantadine.

Patient teaching

• To prevent insomnia, advise patient to take drug several hours before bedtime.

• To prevent orthostatic hypotension, advise patient not to stand or change positions too quickly.

• Instruct patient to report adverse reactions, especially dizziness, depression, anxiety, nausea, and urine retention.

• Warn patient with parkinsonism not to stop drug abruptly because doing so could cause a parkinsonian crisis.

☑ Evaluation

• Patient shows improved health.

• Patient maintains adequate hydration.

• Patient and family state understanding of drug therapy.

❋ **New Drug**

HIGH ALERT!

ambrisentan

(am-bree-SEN-tan)
Letairis

Pharmacologic class: endothelin receptor antagonist
Therapeutic class: vasodilator
Pregnancy risk category: X

Indications and dosages

▶ **Pulmonary arterial hypertension (PAH) in patients with World Health Organization (WHO) class II or III symptoms to improve exercise ability and decrease rate of clinical worsening.** *Adults:* 5 mg P.O. once daily; may increase to 10 mg P.O. once daily, if tolerated.

⊠ **Adjust-a-dose:** Don't start therapy in patients with elevated aminotransferase (ALT) levels of more than three times the upper limit of normal (ULN) at baseline. If ALT elevations are between three and five times the ULN, remeasure. If confirmed level is in the same range, reduce

dosage or stop therapy and remeasure every 2 weeks until levels are less than three times ULN. If ALT elevations are between five and eight times the ULN, stop therapy and monitor until the levels are less than three times ULN. Restart therapy with more frequent monitoring. If ALT elevations exceed eight times the ULN, stop therapy and don't restart the drug.

Contraindications and cautions

• Contraindicated in patients who are hypersensitive to the drug or its components and in those with moderate to severe hepatic impairment. Don't begin therapy in patient with ALT levels more than three times the ULN at baseline.

• Use cautiously in patients with mild hepatic or renal impairment. Drug hasn't been studied in those with severe renal impairment.

⚖ **Lifespan:** In pregnant women drug is contraindicated because it may harm the fetus. In breast-feeding women, drug is contraindicated because it isn't known if drug appears in breast milk. In children, safety and effectiveness haven't been established. Elderly patients may experience less improvement and more episodes of peripheral edema than younger patients.

Adverse reactions

CNS: *headache.*
CV: *peripheral edema,* flushing, palpitations.
EENT: nasal congestion, sinusitis, nasopharyngitis.
GI: abdominal pain, constipation.
Hematologic: anemia.
Respiratory: dyspnea.

Interactions

Drug-drug. *CYP3A4 inducers, such as aminoglutethimide, carbamazepine, nafcillin, nevirapine, phenobarbital, phenytoin, and rifampin:* May decrease the effects of ambrisentan. Use together cautiously.
CYP2C19 inducers, such as aminoglutethimide, carbamazepine, phenytoin, and rifampin: May decrease the effects of ambrisentan. Use together cautiously.
CYP3A4 inhibitors, such as azole antifungals, clarithromycin, cyclosporine, doxycycline, erythromycin, imatinib, isoniazid, nefazodone, nicardipine, propofol, protease inhibitors, and verapamil: May increase the effects of ambrisentan. Use together cautiously.

CYP2C19 inhibitors, such as omeprazole, flu-voxamine, fluconazole, and ticlopidine: May increase the effects of ambrisentan. Use to-gether cautiously.

Drug-food. *Grapefruit or grapefruit juice:* May increase the effects of ambrisentan. Avoid use together.

Effects on lab test results

• May increase AST, ALT, and bilirubin levels.
• May decrease hemoglobin and hematocrit count.

Pharmacokinetics

Absorption: Rapidly absorbed.
Distribution: 99% bound to plasma proteins.
Metabolism: Metabolized by CYP3A4, CYP2C19, and other nonrenal pathways.
Excretion: Non-renal. *Half-life:* About 9 hours.

Route	Onset	Peak	Duration
P.O.	Rapid	2 hr	Unknown

Action

Chemical effect: Blocks endothelin-1 (ET-1) receptors on vascular smooth muscle and en-dothelin, causing vasodilation. ET-1 levels are elevated in patients with PAH leading to vaso-constriction.
Therapeutic effect: Vasodilation and de-creased pulmonary artery pressures.

Available forms

Tablets: 5 mg, 10 mg

NURSING PROCESS

Assessment

• Assess patient's underlying condition before therapy, and reassess regularly thereafter.
• Make sure patient isn't pregnant. Obtain monthly pregnancy tests.
• Serious liver injury may occur. Measure ALT levels before treatment and monthly thereafter; adjust dosage as directed.
• This drug may cause hematologic changes. Monitor hemoglobin level at baseline 1 month after start of therapy and periodically thereafter.
• Monitor the patient for adverse effects.
• Assess patient's and family's knowledge of drug therapy.

Nursing diagnoses

• Risk for injury related to drug-induced liver enzyme elevations
• Ineffective tissue perfusion (cardiopulmonary) related to underlying condition
• Deficient knowledge related to drug therapy

Planning and implementation

• Because of the dangers of liver and fetal toxi-city, this drug is supplied only through the Letairis Education and Access Program (LEAP). For enrollment call 1-866-664-LEAP (5327) or visit their Web site at www.letairis.com.
• To report adverse effects, pregnancy, or liver injury call Gilead sciences at 1-800-GILEAD-5 (option 3) or contact the FDA at 1-800-FDA-1088 or www.fda.gov/medwatch.
• The tablet must be taken whole.
• Ambrisentan may be prescribed for patients who had to stop taking an endothelin-receptor antagonist such as bosentan, because of asymp-tomatic increases in ALT, after these levels have returned to normal.
Patient teaching
• Instruct a woman of childbearing age to use two reliable forms of birth control (latex con-doms, diaphragms, cervical caps). If patient has had tubal sterilization or has a Copper T 380A IUD or LNg 20 IUD inserted, no other form of contraception is required. Inform the patient that she'll need to have a pregnancy test done monthly and tell her to immediately report sus-pected pregnancy to her prescriber.
• Tell the patient that a blood sample will be drawn monthly for certain blood tests, such as liver function tests, and periodically for other tests, such as hemoglobin.
• Remind the patient that the drug may be taken without regard to food.
• Warn the patient that drug must be taken whole and not to split, crush, or chew the tablet.
• Tell the patient to report signs or symptoms of edema, such as weight gain.
• Teach the patient the signs and symptoms of liver injury, including anorexia, nausea, vomit-ing, fever, malaise, fatigue, right upper quadrant abdominal discomfort, itching, or jaundice.

Evaluation

• Patient has no adverse reactions or liver dam-age from drug therapy.

• Patient's pulmonary artery pressure decreases, and the patient reaches pulmonary hemodynamic stability.
• Patient shows improvement in exercise ability.
• Patient and family state understanding of drug therapy.

amikacin sulfate
(am-eh-KAY-sin SULL-fayt)
Amikin

Pharmacologic class: aminoglycoside
Therapeutic class: antibiotic
Pregnancy risk category: D

Indications and dosages

▶ **Serious infections caused by sensitive strains of *Pseudomonas aeruginosa, Escherichia coli, Proteus, Klebsiella, Serratia, Enterobacter, Acinetobacter, Providencia, Citrobacter, Staphylococcus;* meningitis.** *Adults and children:* 15 mg/kg daily divided every 8 to 12 hours I.M. or I.V. infusion.
Neonates: Initially, loading dose of 10 mg/kg I.V., followed by 7.5 mg/kg every 12 hours.
◪ **Adjust-a-dose:** For patients with renal impairment, initially, 7.5 mg/kg I.M. or I.V. Later doses and interval determined by drug level and renal function test results.
▶ **Uncomplicated UTI.** *Adults:* 250 mg I.M. or I.V. b.i.d.
▶ ***Mycobacterium avium* complex, with other drugs‡.** *Adults:* 15 mg/kg I.V. daily, in divided doses every 8 to 12 hours.
◪ **Adjust-a-dose:** For patients with renal impairment, initially, 7.5 mg/kg I.M or I.V. Later doses and interval determined by drug level. Keep peak level between 15 and 35 mcg/ml. Trough level shouldn't exceed 10 mcg/ml.

▽ I.V. administration

• For adults, dilute in 100 to 200 ml of D₅W or normal saline solution. Volume for children depends on dose.
• For adults, infuse over 30 to 60 minutes. Infants should receive a 1- to 2-hour infusion.
• After I.V. infusion, flush line with normal saline solution or D₅W.
⊗ **Incompatibilities**
Amphotericin B, bacitracin, cephapirin, cisplatin, heparin sodium, other I.V. drugs, phenytoin, thiopental, vancomycin, vitamin B complex with C.

Contraindications and cautions

• Contraindicated in patients hypersensitive to drug or other aminoglycosides.
• Use cautiously in patients with impaired renal function or neuromuscular disorders.
⚕ **Lifespan:** In pregnant women, use cautiously and only if benefit outweighs risk to the fetus. In breast-feeding women, don't give drug. In neonates and infants, use cautiously. In elderly patients, use cautiously because they have a higher risk of ototoxicity.

Adverse reactions

CNS: headache, lethargy, *neuromuscular blockade.*
EENT: ototoxicity.
GU: nephrotoxicity.
Hepatic: *hepatic necrosis.*
Other: *anaphylaxis,* hypersensitivity reactions.

Interactions

Drug-drug. *Acyclovir, amphotericin B, cephalothin, cisplatin, methoxyflurane, other aminoglycosides, vancomycin:* May increase nephrotoxicity. Use together cautiously.
Atracurium, pancuronium, rocuronium, vecuronium: May increase the effects of nondepolarizing neuromuscular blockade, including prolonged respiratory depression. Dose of nondepolarizing muscle relaxant may need to be reduced.
Dimenhydrinate: May mask symptoms of ototoxicity. Use cautiously.
Indomethacin: May increase trough and peak levels of amikacin. Monitor amikacin level closely.
I.V. loop diuretics (such as furosemide): May increase ototoxicity. Use together cautiously.
Parenteral penicillins (such as ticarcillin): May cause amikacin inactivation in vitro. Don't mix.

Effects on lab test results

• May increase BUN, creatinine, nonprotein nitrogen, and urine urea levels.

Pharmacokinetics

Absorption: Rapidly after I.M. use.
Distribution: Wide. Minimally protein-bound. Drug crosses the placenta.
Metabolism: None.

Excretion: Mainly in urine by glomerular filtration. *Half-life:* 2 to 3 hours (adults); 30 to 86 hours (patients with severe renal damage).

Route	Onset	Peak	Duration
I.V.	Immediate	Immediate	8–12 hr
I.M.	Unknown	1 hr	8–12 hr

Action

Chemical effect: Inhibits protein synthesis by binding directly to 30S ribosomal subunit. Generally bactericidal.
Therapeutic effect: Kills susceptible bacteria and many aerobic gram-negative organisms (including most strains of *P. aeruginosa*) and some aerobic gram-positive organisms. Ineffective against anaerobes.

Available forms

Injection: 50 mg/ml, 250 mg/ml

NURSING PROCESS

☰ Assessment

• Assess patient's infection, hearing, weight, and renal function test values before therapy and regularly thereafter.
• Watch for signs of ototoxicity, including tinnitus, vertigo, and hearing loss.
• Monitor amikacin level. Obtain blood for peak amikacin level 1 hour after I.M. injection and 30 minutes to 1 hour after infusion ends; for trough level, draw blood just before next dose. Don't collect blood in heparinized tube because heparin is incompatible with aminoglycosides. Peak level higher than 35 mcg/ml and trough level higher than 10 mcg/ml may raise the risk of toxicity.
• Be alert for signs of nephrotoxicity, including cells or casts in urine, oliguria, proteinuria, decreased creatinine clearance, and increased BUN and creatinine levels.
• Assess patient's and family's knowledge of drug therapy.

⊕ Nursing diagnoses

• Risk for infection related to bacteria
• Impaired urinary elimination related to amikacin-induced nephrotoxicity
• Deficient knowledge related to drug therapy

▷ Planning and implementation

• Obtain specimen for culture and sensitivity tests before first dose. Therapy may begin before receiving results.
• Therapy usually lasts 7 to 10 days.
• Drug potency isn't affected if solution turns light yellow.
• Patient should be well hydrated while taking drug to minimize renal tubule irritation.
• If no response occurs after 5 days, therapy may be stopped and new specimens obtained for culture and sensitivity testing.
Ⓢ **ALERT:** Don't confuse Amikin with Amicar or amikacin with anakinra.
Patient teaching
• Tell patient to immediately report changes in hearing or in urine appearance or elimination pattern. Teach patient how to measure intake and output.
• Emphasize importance of drinking 2 L of fluid daily, unless contraindicated.
• Teach patient to watch for and promptly report signs of superinfection, such as continued fever and other signs of new infections, especially of upper respiratory tract.

☑ Evaluation

• Patient's infection is eradicated.
• Patient's renal function test values remain unchanged.
• Patient and family state understanding of drug therapy.

HIGH ALERT!

amiodarone hydrochloride
(am-ee-OH-dah-rohn high-droh-KLOR-ighd)
Cordarone, Pacerone

Pharmacologic class: benzofuran derivative
Therapeutic class: ventricular antiarrhythmic
Pregnancy risk category: D

Indications and dosages

▶ **Recurrent ventricular fibrillation, unstable ventricular tachycardia, atrial fibrillation‡, angina‡, and hypertrophic cardiomyopathy‡.** *Adults:* 800 to 1,600 mg P.O. daily for 1 to 3 weeks as loading dose until initial response occurs; then 650 to 800 mg P.O. daily for 1 month; then 200 to 600 mg P.O. daily as maintenance dosage. Or, for first 24 hours, 150 mg I.V. over 10 minutes (mix in 100 ml

---

Reactions may be *common*, uncommon, *life-threatening*, or COMMON AND LIFE-THREATENING.

D_5W); then 360 mg I.V. over 6 hours (mix 900 mg in 500 ml D_5W); then maintenance dose of 540 mg I.V. over 18 hours at 0.50 mg/minute. After first 24 hours, continue a maintenance infusion of 0.5 mg/minute in a concentration of 1 to 6 mg/ml. For infusions longer than 1 hour, don't exceed 2 mg/ml unless you use a central venous catheter. Don't use for longer than 3 weeks. **Conversion from I.V. to P.O. route.** *Adults:* After daily dose of 720 mg I.V. (assuming rate of 0.5 mg/minute) for less than 1 week, start 800 to 1,600 mg P.O. daily; for 1 to 3 weeks, give 600 to 800 mg P.O. daily; and for longer than 3 weeks, give 400 mg P.O. daily.

▶ **Supraventricular arrhythmias‡.** *Adults:* 600 to 800 mg P.O. for 1 to 4 weeks or until supraventricular tachycardia is controlled. Maintenance dose is 100 to 400 mg P.O. daily.

▼ I.V. administration

• Drug may be given I.V. if close monitoring of cardiac function and resuscitation is available. Initial dose of 5 mg/kg should be mixed in 250 ml of D_5W.
• Repeat doses should be given through central venous catheter. Patient should receive maximum of 1.2 g in up to 500 ml D_5W daily.
• Maintain ECG monitoring when therapy starts and dosage changes. Notify prescriber of significant change in ECG.
• Because of significant risk of life-threatening adverse reactions, drug is used after other antiarrhythmics have been ineffective.

⊗ **Incompatibilities**
Aminophylline, cefazolin sodium, heparin sodium, sodium bicarbonate.

Contraindications and cautions

• Contraindicated in patients hypersensitive to drug and in those with severe sinus node disease, bradycardia, second- or third-degree AV block (unless artificial pacemaker is present), or bradycardia-induced syncope.
• Use cautiously in patients receiving other antiarrhythmics and in patients with pulmonary or thyroid disease because use may result in fatal toxicity.
⚖ **ALERT:** Some I.V. Cordarone preparations contain benzyl alcohol, which may cause gasping syndrome in neonates younger than age 1 month. Monitor patient for symptoms of sudden onset of gasping respiration, hypotension, bradycardia, and CV collapse.

⚖ **Lifespan:** In pregnant women, use only when benefits outweigh risks to patient and fetus. In breast-feeding women, drug is contraindicated. In children, safety of drug hasn't been established. I.V. Cordarone leaches plasticizers from administration tubing, which can adversely affect male reproductive tract development in a fetus, infant, or toddler.

Adverse reactions

CNS: abnormal gait, ataxia, dizziness, extrapyramidal symptoms, fatigue, headache, malaise, paresthesias, peripheral neuropathy, tremor.
CV: *arrhythmias, bradycardia, heart block, heart failure,* hypotension, *sinus arrest.*
EENT: *corneal microdeposits,* vision disturbances.
GI: anorexia, constipation, *nausea, vomiting.*
Hepatic: *hepatic dysfunction.*
Metabolic: hyperthyroidism, hypothyroidism.
Musculoskeletal: muscle weakness.
Respiratory: SEVERE PULMONARY TOXICITY (ALVEOLITIS, PNEUMONITIS).
Skin: blue-gray skin, *photosensitivity.*
Other: gynecomastia.

Interactions

Drug-drug. *Antiarrhythmics:* May reduce hepatic or renal clearance of certain antiarrhythmics (especially flecainide and procainamide), and may induce torsades de pointes with other antiarrhythmics (especially disopyramide, mexiletine, procainamide, and propafenone). Monitor ECG closely.
Antihypertensives: May increase hypotensive effect. Use together cautiously.
Beta blockers, calcium channel blockers: May increase cardiac depressant effects and potentiate slowing of sinus node and AV conduction. Use together cautiously.
Cholestyramine, rifampin: May decrease amiodarone level. Use together cautiously.
Cimetidine, protease inhibitors: May increase amiodarone level. Avoid use together.
Cyclosporine: May increase cyclosporine level. Monitor patient for cyclosporine toxicity.
Digoxin: May increase digoxin level by 70% to 100%. Monitor digoxin level closely.
Phenytoin: May decrease phenytoin metabolism. Monitor phenytoin level.
Quinidine: May increase quinidine level, producing potentially fatal cardiac arrhythmias. If

drugs must be used together, monitor quinidine level closely, and adjust dosage as needed.
Theophylline: May increase theophylline level and lead to toxicity. Monitor theophylline level.
Warfarin: May increase INR by 100% within 1 to 4 weeks of therapy. Decrease warfarin dosage 33% to 50% when amiodarone starts. Monitor patient closely.
Drug-herb. *Pennyroyal:* May change the rate at which toxic metabolites of pennyroyal form. Discourage use together.
St. John's wort: May decrease amiodarone levels. Discourage use together.
Drug-food. *Grapefruit juice:* May increase amiodarone levels. Discourage use together.
Drug-lifestyle. *Sun exposure:* May cause photosensitivity reaction. Advise against prolonged or unprotected sun exposure.

Effects on lab test results

• May increase ALT, AST, alkaline phosphatase, and GGT levels.
• May increase PT and INR. May alter thyroid function test results.

Pharmacokinetics

Absorption: Slow and variable.
Distribution: Wide, accumulating in adipose tissue and in organs with marked perfusion, such as lungs, liver, and spleen. Drug is 96% protein-bound.
Metabolism: Extensive in liver to active metabolite, desethyl amiodarone.
Excretion: Mainly hepatic through biliary tree.
Half-life: 25 to 110 days (usually 40 to 50 days).

Route	Onset	Peak	Duration
P.O.	2–21 days	3–7 hr	Varies
I.V.	Unknown	Unknown	Unknown

Action

Chemical effect: Unknown; thought to prolong refractory period and duration of action potential and decrease repolarization.
Therapeutic effect: Abolishes ventricular arrhythmia.

Available forms

Injection: 50 mg/ml
Tablets: 100 mg, 200 mg, 400 mg

NURSING PROCESS

🔅 Assessment

• Assess CV status before therapy.
• Review pulmonary, liver, and thyroid function test results before and regularly during therapy.
• Continuously monitor cardiac status of patient receiving I.V. amiodarone to evaluate its effectiveness.
• Watch for adverse reactions and drug interactions.
• Monitor patient carefully for pulmonary toxicity, which can be fatal. Risk increases in patients receiving more than 400 mg daily.
• Monitor electrolytes, particularly potassium and magnesium levels, and PT and INR if on warfarin.
• Assess patient's and family's knowledge of drug therapy.

🔅 Nursing diagnoses

• Decreased cardiac output related to ventricular arrhythmia
• Risk for injury related to drug-induced adverse reactions
• Deficient knowledge related to drug therapy

▶ Planning and implementation

• Adverse reactions commonly limit drug's use.
• **ALERT:** Drug may pose life-threatening risks for patients already at risk for sudden death. It may cause fatal toxicities, including hepatic and pulmonary toxicity and should be used only in patients with life-threatening, recurrent ventricular arrhythmias unresponsive to other antiarrhythmics or when other drugs can't be tolerated.
• Divide oral loading dose into three equal doses and give with meals to decrease GI intolerance. If GI intolerance occurs, maintenance dosage may be given once daily or divided into two doses taken with meals.
• **ALERT:** Don't confuse amiodarone with amiloride.
Patient teaching
• Stress importance of taking drug exactly as prescribed.
• Emphasize importance of close follow-up and regular diagnostic studies to monitor drug action and detect adverse reactions.
• Warn patient that drug may cause blue-gray skin pigmentation.

Reactions may be *common*, uncommon, *life-threatening*, or COMMON AND LIFE-THREATENING.

A

• Advise patient to use sunscreen to prevent photosensitivity reaction (burning or tingling skin followed by erythema and possible blistering).

• Inform patient that adverse effects are more prevalent at high doses but are generally reversible when therapy stops. Resolution of adverse reactions may take up to 4 months.

• Advise patient to have yearly eye examination.

☑ Evaluation
• Patient's arrhythmia is corrected.
• Patient has no injury from adverse reactions.
• Patient and family state understanding of drug therapy.

amitriptyline hydrochloride
(am-ih-TRIP-tuh-leen high-droh-KLOR-ighd)

Pharmacologic class: tricyclic antidepressant
Therapeutic class: antidepressant
Pregnancy risk category: C

Indications and dosages

▶**Depression.** *Adults:* 50 to 100 mg P.O. at bedtime, gradually increasing to 150 mg daily; maximum dosage for a hospitalized patient is 300 mg daily, if needed.
Geriatric patients and adolescents: 10 mg P.O. t.i.d. and 20 mg at bedtime daily.
▶**Anorexia or bulimia related to depression; adjunctive therapy for neurogenic pain‡.**
Adults: If outpatient, initially 75 to 100 mg P.O. in divided doses daily. If inpatient, 100 to 300 mg P.O. in divided doses daily. After maximum effect is achieved, gradually decrease to maintenance dose of 50 to 100 mg or less P.O. daily for a minimum of 3 months.

Contraindications and cautions

• Contraindicated during acute recovery phase of MI, in patients hypersensitive to drug, and within 14 days of MAO inhibitor therapy.
• Use cautiously in patients with history of seizures, urine retention, prostatic hypertrophy, angle-closure glaucoma, or increased intraocular pressure; in those with hyperthyroidism, CV disease, diabetes, or impaired liver function; and in those taking thyroid medications.

☀ **Lifespan:** In pregnant women, use cautiously. In breast-feeding women, drug is contraindicated. In children younger than age 12, don't use drug. In elderly patients, who may experience increased falls and increased anticholinergic effects while taking this drug, use cautiously.

Adverse reactions

CNS: confusion, *drowsiness,* dizziness, EEG alterations, excitation, extrapyramidal reactions, headache, nervousness, *seizures, stroke,* tremors, weakness.
CV: *arrhythmias,* ECG changes, hypertension, *MI, orthostatic hypotension,* tachycardia.
EENT: blurred vision, mydriasis, tinnitus.
GI: anorexia, *constipation, dry mouth,* nausea, paralytic ileus, vomiting.
GU: *urine retention.*
Hematologic: *agranulocytosis, thrombocytopenia.*
Skin: diaphoresis, photosensitivity reaction, rash, urticaria.
Other: hypersensitivity reactions.

Interactions

Drug-drug. *Barbiturates, CNS depressants:* May increase CNS depression. Avoid use together.
Cimetidine, methylphenidate: May increase tricyclic antidepressant level. Monitor patient for increased antidepressant effect.
Clonidine: May cause loss of blood pressure control and potentially life-threatening increase in blood pressure. Don't use together.
Epinephrine, norepinephrine: May increase hypertensive effect. Use together cautiously.
Guanethidine: May antagonize antihypertensive action of guanethidine. Monitor patient.
MAO inhibitors: May cause severe excitation, hyperpyrexia, or seizures, especially at high dosage. Avoid using within 14 days of each other.
Drug-herb. *SAMe, St. John's wort, yohimbe:* May cause serotonin level to become too high. Discourage use together.
Drug-lifestyle. *Alcohol use:* May increase CNS depression. Discourage use together.
Smoking: May lower drug level. Monitor patient for lack of effect.
Sun exposure: May increase risk of photosensitivity reactions. Advise against prolonged or unprotected sun exposure.

Effects on lab test results

- May increase or decrease glucose level.
- May increase eosinophil count and liver function test values. May decrease granulocyte, platelet, and WBC counts.

Pharmacokinetics

Absorption: Rapid.
Distribution: Widely into body, including CNS and breast milk. 96% protein-bound.
Metabolism: By liver to active metabolite nortriptyline; significant first-pass effect may account for variable levels in different patients taking same dosage.
Excretion: Mainly in urine. *Half-life:* Varies widely.

Route	Onset	Peak	Duration
P.O., I.M.	Unknown	2–12 hr	Unknown

Action

Chemical effect: Unknown, but tricyclic antidepressant increases levels of norepinephrine, serotonin, or both in CNS by blocking their reuptake by presynaptic neurons.
Therapeutic effect: Relieves depression.

Available forms

Tablets: 10 mg, 25 mg, 50 mg, 75 mg, 100 mg, 150 mg

NURSING PROCESS

Assessment
- Assess patient's depression before therapy.
- Be alert for adverse reactions and drug interactions.
- Assess patient's and family's knowledge of drug therapy.

Nursing diagnoses
- Ineffective coping related to depression
- Risk for injury related to adverse CNS reactions
- Deficient knowledge related to drug therapy

Planning and implementation
- Oral therapy should replace injection as soon as possible.
- Give full dose at bedtime when possible.
- Don't withdraw drug abruptly.
- If signs of psychosis occur or increase, reduce dosage. Give patient minimum supply of drug.

ALERT: Drug may increase the risk of suicidal thinking and behavior in young adults ages 18 to 24 during the first two months of treatment.
- Because hypertensive episodes may occur during surgery in patients receiving tricyclic antidepressants, drug should be gradually stopped several days before surgery.

ALERT: Don't confuse amitriptyline with nortriptyline or aminophylline, or Endep with Depen.

Patient teaching
- Advise patient to take full dose at bedtime, and warn of possible morning orthostatic hypotension.
- Tell patient to avoid alcohol and smoking while taking drug.
- Warn patient to avoid hazardous activities until full CNS effects of drug are known. Drowsiness and dizziness usually subside after a few weeks.
- Advise patient to consult prescriber before taking other prescription drugs, OTC medications, or herbal remedies.
- Teach patient to relieve dry mouth with sugarless hard candy or gum. Saliva substitutes may be needed.
- Advise patient to use sunblock, wear protective clothing, and avoid prolonged exposure to strong sunlight.
- Warn patient not to stop therapy abruptly. After abrupt withdrawal of long-term therapy, patient may have nausea, headache, and malaise. These symptoms don't indicate addiction.
- Tell patient to watch for urine retention and constipation. Instruct him to increase fluids, and suggest a stool softener or high-fiber diet, as needed.
- Advise patient that effects of drug may not be apparent for 2 to 3 weeks.

Evaluation
- Patient's behavior and communication indicate improvement of depression.
- Patient sustains no injury from CNS adverse reactions.
- Patient and family state understanding of drug therapy.

amlodipine besylate

(am-LOW-dih-peen BEH-sih-layt)
Norvasc✦

Pharmacologic class: calcium channel blocker
Therapeutic class: antianginal, antihypertensive
Pregnancy risk category: C

Indications and dosages

▶ **Chronic stable angina; vasospastic angina (Prinzmetal [variant] angina).** *Adults:* Initially, 10 mg P.O. daily.
🔲 **Adjust-a-dose:** For small, frail, or elderly patients or patients with hepatic insufficiency, start with 5 mg daily. Most patients need 10 mg daily for adequate results.
▶ **Hypertension.** *Adults:* Initially, 5 mg P.O. daily. Maximum, 10 mg daily.
🔲 **Adjust-a-dose:** For small, frail, or elderly patients; patients receiving other antihypertensives; and patients with hepatic insufficiency; start with 2.5 mg daily and adjust based on patient response and tolerance. Maximum, 10 mg daily.

Contraindications and cautions

• Contraindicated in patients hypersensitive to drug.
• Use cautiously in patients taking other peripheral vasodilators (especially those with severe aortic stenosis) and in those with heart failure.
• In patients with severe hepatic disease, use cautiously and in reduced dosage because drug is metabolized by liver.
🌿 **Lifespan:** In pregnant women, use cautiously. In breast-feeding women, drug is contraindicated. In children, safety of drug hasn't been established.

Adverse reactions

CNS: fatigue, headache, somnolence.
CV: dizziness, *edema,* flushing, palpitations.
GI: abdominal pain, dyspepsia, nausea.

Interactions

Drug-food. *Grapefruit juice:* May increase drug level and adverse effects. Tell patient not to take drug with grapefruit juice. However, if he has been stabilized on the drug while routinely drinking grapefruit juice, caution him not to abruptly stop doing so.

Effects on lab test results

None reported.

Pharmacokinetics

Absorption: Absolute bioavailability from 64% to 90%.
Distribution: About 93% of circulating drug is bound to plasma proteins.
Metabolism: About 90% of drug is converted to inactive metabolites in liver.
Excretion: Mainly in urine. *Half-life:* 30 to 50 hours.

Route	Onset	Peak	Duration
P.O.	Unknown	6–9 hr	24 hr

Action

Chemical effect: Inhibits calcium ion influx across cardiac and smooth-muscle cells, thus decreasing myocardial contractility and oxygen demand. Also dilates coronary arteries and arterioles.
Therapeutic effect: Reduces blood pressure and prevents angina.

Available forms

Tablets: 2.5 mg, 5 mg, 10 mg

NURSING PROCESS

Assessment
• Assess patient's blood pressure or angina before therapy and regularly thereafter.
• Monitor patient carefully for pain. In some patients, especially those with severe obstructive coronary artery disease, increased frequency, duration, or severity of angina or even acute MI has developed after starting a calcium channel blocker or increasing dosage.
• Be alert for adverse reactions.
• Assess patient's and family's knowledge of drug therapy.

Nursing diagnoses
• Acute pain related to increased oxygen demand in cardiac tissue
• Risk for injury related to hypertension
• Deficient knowledge related to drug therapy

▶ Planning and implementation

• Give S.L. nitroglycerin as needed for acute angina.

ⓘ **ALERT:** Don't confuse amlodipine with amiloride.

Patient teaching

• Tell patient that S.L. nitroglycerin may be taken as needed for acute angina. If patient continues nitrate therapy during adjustment of amlodipine dosage, urge continued compliance.

• Advise patient to continue taking drug even when feeling better.

☑ Evaluation

• Patient's blood pressure is normal.

• Patient states anginal pain occurs with less frequency and severity.

• Patient and family state understanding of drug therapy.

amoxicillin and clavulanate potassium

(uh-moks-uh-SIL-in and KLAV-yoo-lan-ayt poh-TAH-see-um)
Amoclan, Augmentin, Augmentin ES-600, Augmentin XR, Clavulin ◆

Pharmacologic class: aminopenicillin, beta-lactamase inhibitor
Therapeutic class: antibiotic
Pregnancy risk category: B

Indications and dosages

▶ **Lower respiratory tract infections, otitis media, sinusitis, skin and skin-structure infections, and UTI caused by susceptible strains of gram-positive and gram-negative organisms.** *Adults:* 250 mg (based on amoxicillin component) P.O. every 8 hours. For more severe infections, 500 mg every 8 hours or 875 mg P.O. every 12 hours.
Children: 20 to 40 mg/kg (based on amoxicillin component) P.O. daily in divided doses every 8 hours.
Neonates and infants younger than age 12 weeks: 30 mg/kg (based on amoxicillin component) P.O. daily in divided doses every 12 hours.
▶ **Recurrent or persistent acute otitis media caused by** *Streptococcus pneumoniae,*

Haemophilus influenzae, **or** *Moraxella catarrhalis. Infants and children at least 3 months old, exposed to antibiotics during the previous 3 months, who are either age 2 or younger or attend daycare:* 90 mg/kg daily Augmentin ES 600 (based on amoxicillin component) P.O. every 12 hours for 10 days. Information about this drug in patients weighing 40 kg (88 lb) or more is unavailable.
▶ **Community-acquired pneumonia or acute bacterial sinusitis from confirmed, or suspected beta-lactamase–producing pathogens (***H. influenzae, M. catarrhalis, Haemophilus parainfluenzae, Klebsiella pneumoniae,* **or methicillin-susceptible** *Staphylococcus aureus***) and** *S. pneumoniae* **with reduced susceptibility to penicillin.** *Adults and children age 16 and older:* 2,000 mg/125 mg Augmentin XR every 12 hours for 7 to 10 days for pneumonia, or 10 days for sinusitis. Taken with meals.

Contraindications and cautions

• Contraindicated in patients hypersensitive to drug or other penicillins and in those with a history of amoxicillin-related cholestatic jaundice or hepatic dysfunction.
• Augmentin XR is contraindicated in hemodialysis patients and patients with creatinine clearance less than 30 ml/minute.
• Use cautiously in patients with other drug allergies, especially to cephalosporins (possible cross-sensitivity), and those with mononucleosis (high risk of maculopapular rash) or hepatic impairment.
✦ **Lifespan:** In pregnant and breast-feeding women, use cautiously. In children younger than age 16, safety and effectiveness of Augmentin XR haven't been established.

Adverse reactions

CNS: agitation, anxiety, behavioral changes, confusion, dizziness, insomnia.
GI: abdominal pain, black "hairy" tongue, *diarrhea,* enterocolitis, gastritis, glossitis, indigestion, mucocutaneous candidiasis, nausea, *pseudomembranous colitis,* stomatitis, vomiting.
GU: vaginal candidiasis, vaginitis.
Hematologic: *agranulocytosis,* anemia, eosinophilia, *leukopenia, thrombocytopenia, thrombocytopenic purpura.*
Other: hypersensitivity reactions (*anaphylaxis, angioedema,* pruritus, rash, urticaria), over-

growth of nonsusceptible organisms, serum sickness–like reactions (urticaria or rash accompanied by arthralgia, arthritis, myalgia, and commonly fever).

Interactions

Drug-drug. *Allopurinol:* May cause rash. Monitor patient.
Probenecid: May increase level of amoxicillin and other penicillins. Probenecid may be used for this purpose.

Effects on lab test results

• May decrease hemoglobin level and hematocrit.
• May increase eosinophil count. May decrease granulocyte, platelet, and WBC counts.
• May cause false-positive urine glucose determinations with copper sulfate tests, such as Benedict solution and Clinitest.

Pharmacokinetics

Absorption: Well absorbed.
Distribution: Both drugs are distributed into pleural fluid, lungs, and peritoneal fluid, with high urine levels. Amoxicillin also appears in synovial fluid, liver, prostate, muscle, gallbladder, middle ear effusions, maxillary sinus secretions, tonsils, sputum, and bronchial secretions. Both drugs are minimally protein-bound.
Metabolism: Amoxicillin is metabolized partially; clavulanate potassium, extensively.
Excretion: Amoxicillin mainly in urine; clavulanate potassium by glomerular filtration. *Half-life:* 1 to 1½ hours (in severe renal impairment, 7½ hours for amoxicillin and 4½ hours for clavulanate).

Route	Onset	Peak	Duration
P.O.			
Augmentin	Unknown	1–2½ hr	6–8 hr
Augmentin ES-600	Unknown	1–4 hr	Unknown
Augmentin XR	Unknown	1–6 hr	Unknown

Action

Chemical effect: Prevents bacterial cell-wall synthesis during replication. Clavulanic acid increases amoxicillin's effectiveness by inactivating beta lactamases, which destroy amoxicillin.
Therapeutic effect: Kills susceptible bacteria.

Available forms

Oral suspension: 125 mg amoxicillin trihydrate and 31.25 mg clavulanic acid/5 ml (after reconstitution); 200 mg amoxicillin trihydrate and 28.5 mg clavulanic acid/5 ml (after reconstitution); 250 mg amoxicillin trihydrate and 62.5 mg clavulanic acid/5 ml (after reconstitution); 400 mg amoxicillin trihydrate and 57 mg clavulanic acid/5 ml (after reconstitution); 600 mg amoxicillin trihydrate and 42.9 mg clavulanic acid/5 ml (after reconstitution)
Tablets: 875 mg amoxicillin trihydrate, 125 mg clavulanic acid
Tablets (chewable): 125 mg amoxicillin trihydrate, 31.25 mg clavulanic acid; 200 mg amoxicillin trihydrate, 28.5 mg clavulanic acid; 250 mg amoxicillin trihydrate, 62.5 mg clavulanic acid; 400 mg amoxicillin trihydrate, 57 mg clavulanic acid
Tablets (extended-release): 1,000 mg amoxicillin trihydrate, 62.5 mg clavulanic acid
Tablets (film-coated): 250 mg amoxicillin trihydrate, 125 mg clavulanic acid; 500 mg amoxicillin trihydrate, 125 mg clavulanic acid

NURSING PROCESS

Assessment
• Before therapy begins, assess patient's infection, ask about past allergic reactions to penicillin (although negative history is no guarantee against allergic reaction), and obtain specimen for culture and sensitivity tests. Therapy may begin pending results.
• Be alert for adverse reactions and drug interactions.
• Monitor hydration status if adverse GI reactions occur.
• Assess patient's and family's knowledge of drug therapy.

Nursing diagnoses
• Ineffective protection related to presence of susceptible bacteria
• Risk for deficient fluid volume related to drug-induced adverse GI reactions
• Deficient knowledge related to drug therapy

Planning and implementation
• Give drug with food to prevent GI distress. Adverse effects for this combination drug, especially diarrhea, are more common than with amoxicillin alone.

• Give drug at least 1 hour before bacteriostatic antibiotics.

⚠ **ALERT:** Tablets and suspension contain varying amounts of clavulanic acid. Don't assume that two 250-mg (amoxicillin) tablets replace one 500-mg tablet because amount of clavulanic acid may not change in same proportion.

⚠ **ALERT:** Augmentin (250 mg or 500 mg amoxicillin) and Augmentin XR extended-release tablets aren't interchangeable because of the different amounts of clavulanic acid in each and because Augmentin XR is an extended-release formulation.

⚠ **ALERT:** Augmentin ES-600 is intended only for children.

• This drug combination is particularly useful with amoxicillin-resistant organisms.

• After reconstitution, refrigerate oral suspension and discard after 10 days.

⚠ **ALERT:** Don't confuse amoxicillin with amoxapine.

Patient teaching

• Tell patient to take entire quantity of drug exactly as prescribed, even after he feels better.

• Tell patient to call prescriber if rash develops (sign of allergic reaction).

• Instruct patient to take drug with food to prevent GI distress.

✓ **Evaluation**

• Patient is free from infection.

• Patient maintains adequate hydration.

• Patient and family state understanding of drug therapy.

---

amoxicillin trihydrate (amoxycillin trihydrate)

(uh-moks-uh-SIL-in trigh-HIGH-drayt)

Amoxil, Apo-Amoxi, DisperMox, Novamoxin ♦, Nu-Amoxi ♦, Trimox

Pharmacologic class: aminopenicillin
Therapeutic class: antibiotic
Pregnancy risk category: B

Indications and dosages

▶ **Mild to moderate infections of the ear, nose and throat, skin and skin structure, or GU tract.** *Adults and children weighing 40 kg (88 lb) or more:* 500 mg P.O. every 12 hours or 250 mg P.O. every 8 hours.

Children older than 3 months weighing less than 40 kg: 25 mg/kg/day P.O. divided every 12 hours or 20 mg/kg/day P.O. divided every 8 hours.

Neonates and infants younger than age 3 months: Up to 30 mg/kg/day P.O. divided every 12 hours.

▶ **Mild to severe infections of the lower respiratory tract and severe infections of the ear, nose and throat, skin and skin structure, or GU tract.** *Adults and children weighing 40 kg or more:* 875 mg P.O. every 12 hours or 500 mg P.O. every 8 hours.

Children older than 3 months who weigh less than 40 kg: 45 mg/kg/day P.O. divided every 12 hours or 40 mg/kg/day P.O. divided every 8 hours.

▶ ***Helicobacter pylori* eradication to reduce the risk of duodenal ulcer, given with other drugs.** *Dual therapy. Adults:* Amoxicillin 1 g P.O. and lansoprazole 30 mg P.O., each every 8 hours for 14 days.

Triple therapy. Adults: Amoxicillin 1 g P.O., clarithromycin 500 mg P.O., and lansoprazole 30 mg P.O., each every 12 hours for 14 days.

▶ **Uncomplicated gonorrhea.** *Adults:* 3 g P.O. as a single dose.

Children older than age 2: Give 50 mg/kg with 25 mg/kg probenecid as a single dose.

▶ **Chlamydial and mycoplasmal infections during pregnancy.** *Adults:* 500 mg P.O. t.i.d. for 7 to 10 days.

▣ **Adjust-a-dose:** Patients with renal failure who need repeated doses may need an increased dose interval. If creatinine clearance is 10 to 30 ml/minute, increase to every 12 hours; if it's less than 10 ml/minute, give drug every 24 hours. Supplemental doses may be needed after hemodialysis. Don't give 875-mg tablet if creatinine clearance is less than 30 ml/minute.

▶ **Oral prophylaxis of bacterial endocarditis.** Consult current American Heart Association recommendations before giving drug. *Adults:* 2 g 1 hour before procedure.

Children: 50 mg/kg (maximum, 2 g) 1 hour before procedure.

▶ **Postexposure prophylaxis for penicillin-susceptible anthrax.** *Adults and children age 9 and older:* 500 mg P.O. t.i.d. for 60 days.

Children younger than age 9: Give 80 mg/kg/day P.O., divided t.i.d. for 60 days.

▶ **Lyme disease‡.** *Adults:* 250 to 500 mg P.O. t.i.d. or q.i.d. for 10 to 30 days.
Children: 25 to 50 mg/kg daily (maximum, 1 to 2 g daily) P.O. in three divided doses for 10 to 30 days.
▶ **Acute complicated UTI in nonpregnant women‡.** *Adults:* 3 g P.O. as a single dose.

Contraindications and cautions

• Contraindicated in patients hypersensitive to drug or other penicillins.
• Use cautiously in patients with other drug allergies, especially to cephalosporins (possible cross-sensitivity), and in those with mononucleosis (high risk of maculopapular rash), or renal impairment.
⚘ **Lifespan:** In pregnant or breast-feeding women, use cautiously.

Adverse reactions

CNS: *seizures.*
GI: diarrhea, nausea, vomiting.
Hematologic: *agranulocytosis,* anemia, eosinophilia, *leukopenia, thrombocytopenia, thrombocytopenic purpura.*
Other: hypersensitivity reactions (*anaphylaxis,* erythematous maculopapular rash, urticaria), overgrowth of nonsusceptible organisms.

Interactions

Drug-drug. *Allopurinol:* May increase risk of rash. Monitor patient.
Probenecid: May increase level of amoxicillin and other penicillins. Probenecid may be used for this purpose.

Effects on lab test results

• May decrease hemoglobin level and hematocrit.
• May increase eosinophil count. May decrease granulocyte, platelet, and WBC counts.
• May cause false-positive urine glucose determinations with copper sulfate tests (such as Benedict solution and Clinitest).

Pharmacokinetics

Absorption: About 80%.
Distribution: Appears in pleural, peritoneal, and synovial fluids; lungs; prostate; muscle; liver; gallbladder; middle ear; maxillary sinus and bronchial secretions; tonsils; and sputum. Amoxicillin readily crosses placenta and is 17% to 20% protein-bound.

Metabolism: Partial.
Excretion: Mainly in urine by renal tubular secretion and glomerular filtration; also in breast milk. *Half-life:* 1 to 1½ hours (7½ hours in severe renal impairment).

Route	Onset	Peak	Duration
P.O.	Unknown	1–2 hr	6–8 hr

Action

Chemical effect: Inhibits cell-wall synthesis during bacterial multiplication.
Therapeutic effect: Kills susceptible bacteria.

Available forms

Capsules: 250 mg, 500 mg
Suspension: 50 mg/ml (pediatric drops), 125 mg/5 ml, 200 mg/5 ml, 250 mg/5 ml, 400 mg/5 ml
Tablets (chewable): 200 mg, 400 mg
Tablets (film-coated): 500 mg, 875 mg
Tablets (for oral suspension): 200 mg, 400 mg, 600 mg

NURSING PROCESS

🝆 Assessment

• Before therapy, assess patient's infection, ask about allergic reactions to drug or other forms of penicillin (although negative history doesn't guarantee against future reaction), and obtain specimen for culture and sensitivity tests. Therapy may begin pending test results.
• Be alert for adverse reactions and drug interactions.
• If adverse GI reactions occur, monitor patient's hydration status.
• Assess patient's and family's knowledge of drug therapy.

⊕ Nursing diagnoses

• Ineffective protection related to presence of susceptible bacteria
• Risk for deficient fluid volume related to drug-induced adverse GI reactions
• Deficient knowledge related to drug therapy

▶ Planning and implementation

• Give amoxicillin at least 1 hour before bacteriostatic antibiotics.
• May be taken with or without food.

• Trimox oral suspension may be stored at room temperature for up to 2 weeks. Check individual product labels for storage information.

• For DisperMox, mix 1 tablet in 10 ml of water and have patient drink mixture. Rinse container with a small amount of water to make sure the entire tablet is taken. Don't let the patient chew or swallow tablet or let it dissolve in mouth.

⑤ **ALERT:** Don't confuse amoxicillin with amoxapine.

Patient teaching
• If drug allergy develops, advise patient to wear or carry medical identification stating penicillin allergy.
• Tell patient to take entire quantity of drug exactly as prescribed, even after feeling better.
• Tell patient to call prescriber if rash (most common), fever, or chills develop.
• Tell patient to take drug with or without food.
• Warn patient never to use leftover amoxicillin for a new illness or share it with others.
• For DisperMox, give patient these instructions: Mix tablet in 10 ml of water (only water) and drink. Rinse the container with a small amount of water and drink again to get entire dose. Don't chew or swallow tablets or let them dissolve in mouth.

☑ **Evaluation**
• Patient is free from infection.
• Patient maintains adequate hydration.
• Patient and family state understanding of drug therapy.

HIGH ALERT!

amphotericin B desoxycholate
(am-foh-TER-ah-sin bee dess-ox-ee-KOH-layt)
Amphocin, Fungizone

Pharmacologic class: polyene macrolide
Therapeutic class: antifungal
Pregnancy risk category: B

Indications and dosages

▶ **Systemic, potentially fatal fungal infections caused by susceptible organisms; fungal endocarditis; fungal septicemia.** *Adults and children:* Some clinicians recommend an initial dose of 1 mg I.V. in 20 ml D_5W infused over 20 minutes. If test dose is tolerated, then give daily doses of 0.25 to 0.3 mg/kg, gradually increasing by 5 to 10 mg daily until dosage is

0.5 to 0.7 mg/kg daily, up to 1 mg/kg daily or 1.5 mg/kg every alternate day. Duration of therapy depends on the severity and nature of infection.

▶ **Sporotrichosis.** *Adults and children:* 0.4 to 0.5 mg/kg daily I.V. for up to 9 months. Total I.V. dosage of 2.5 g over 9 months.

▶ **Aspergillosis.** *Adults and children:* 0.5 to 1.5 mg/kg daily initially and a total I.V. dose of 1.5 to 4 g over 11 months.

▶ **Disseminated or invasive candidal infections.** *Adults and children:* 0.4 to 0.6 mg/kg I.V. daily. Higher doses of up to 1.5 mg/kg have been used in rapidly progressing or potentially fatal infections. Therapy may last 7 to 14 days to more than 6 weeks depending on severity.

▶ **Coccidioidomycosis.** *Adults:* 0.5 to 1 mg/kg I.V. daily. Therapy usually lasts 4 to 12 weeks.

▶ **Cryptococcosis.** *Adults:* 0.3 to 1 mg/kg I.V. daily. Therapy may last 2 weeks to several months. Drug may be given with flucytosine P.O.

▶ **Cryptococcal meningitis in HIV-infected patients.** *Adults:* 0.7 mg/kg I.V. daily for 4 weeks followed by 0.7 mg/kg I.V. every other day for another 4 weeks.

▶ **Mucocutaneous leishmaniasis.** *Adults and children:* 0.25 to 0.5 mg/kg/day I.V., increased gradually to 0.5 to 1 mg/kg/day. Then give on alternate days. Treat for 3 to 12 weeks.

▶ **Visceral leishmaniasis.** *Adults and children:* 0.5 to 1 mg/kg/day I.V. on alternate days for 14 to 20 doses.

▶ **Paracoccidioidomycosis‡.** *Adults:* 0.4 to 0.5 mg/kg I.V. daily for 4 to 12 weeks.

▶ **Empiric therapy of presumed fungal infections in febrile, neutropenic patients, including those with cancer or bone marrow transplant‡.** *Adults:* 0.1 mg/kg daily.

▽ I.V. administration

• Reconstitute only with 10 ml sterile water. To avoid precipitation, don't mix with solutions containing sodium chloride, other electrolytes, or bacteriostatic drugs (such as benzyl alcohol).
• Don't use if solution contains precipitate or foreign matter.
• Amphotericin B appears to be compatible with limited amounts of heparin sodium, hydrocortisone sodium succinate, and methylprednisolone sodium succinate.
• Give drug parenterally only in hospitalized patients, under close supervision, after diagnosis

---

Reactions may be *common*, uncommon, *life-threatening*, or COMMON AND LIFE-THREATENING.

of potentially fatal fungal infection is confirmed.

• Be prepared to give an initial test dose, for which 1 mg is added to 20 ml of D_5W and infused over 20 to 30 minutes.

• Use an infusion pump and in-line filter with a mean pore diameter larger than 1 micron. Infuse over 2 to 6 hours because rapid infusion may cause CV collapse.

• Use I.V. sites in distal veins. If thrombosis occurs, alternate sites.

• If patient has severe adverse infusion reactions to first dose, stop infusion, notify prescriber, and give antipyretics, antihistamines, antiemetics, or small doses of corticosteroids. To prevent reactions during subsequent infusions, premedicate with these drugs or give amphotericin B on an alternate-day schedule.

• Reconstituted solution is stable for 1 week in refrigerator, 24 hours at room temperature, and 8 hours in room light.

• Store dry form at 36° to 46° F (2° to 8° C). Protect from light.

⊗ **Incompatibilities**
Amikacin, calcium chloride, chlorpromazine, cimetidine, diphenhydramine, edetate calcium disodium, gentamicin, kanamycin, lactated Ringer's injection, melphalan, methyldopa, normal saline solution, paclitaxel, penicillin G potassium, penicillin G sodium, polymyxin B, potassium chloride, prochlorperazine mesylate, streptomycin, verapamil. Give antibiotics separately; don't mix or piggyback with amphotericin B.

Contraindications and cautions

• Contraindicated in patients hypersensitive to drug or its components.

• Use cautiously in patients with impaired renal function.

⚘ **Lifespan:** In pregnant women, use cautiously. Breast-feeding women must stop breast-feeding or stop the drug. In children, safety and dosage haven't been fully established, but therapy may be successful.

Adverse reactions

CNS: encephalopathy, fever, headache, malaise, paresthesia, peripheral nerve pain, peripheral neuropathy, *seizures.*
CV: *arrhythmias, asystole,* hypertension, hypotension, phlebitis, thrombophlebitis.

EENT: hearing loss, tinnitus, vertigo, visual impairment.
GI: anorexia, diarrhea, dyspepsia, epigastric cramps, *hemorrhagic gastroenteritis,* nausea, vomiting, weight loss.
GU: abnormal renal function with anuria, hyposthenuria, nephrocalcinosis, oliguria, *permanent renal impairment,* renal tubular acidosis.
Hematologic: *agranulocytosis,* eosinophilia, normochromic normocytic anemia, *thrombocytopenia.*
Hepatic: *acute liver failure, hepatitis.*
Metabolic: azotemia, hypokalemia, *hypomagnesemia.*
Musculoskeletal: arthralgia, myalgia.
Respiratory: dyspnea, hypersensitivity pneumonitis, pulmonary edema.
Skin: burning, irritation, pain at injection site, pruritus, rash, stinging, tissue damage with extravasation.
Other: *anaphylactoid reactions,* chills, generalized pain.

Interactions

Drug-drug. *Azole antifungals (fluconazole, ketoconazole):* May induce fungal resistance. Use with caution.
Corticosteroids, corticotropin: May cause potassium depletion. Monitor potassium level.
Digoxin: May increase risk of digitalis toxicity in potassium-depleted patients. Monitor patient closely.
Flucytosine: May increase flucytosine toxicity. Monitor patient closely.
Nephrotoxic drugs (such as antibiotics and antineoplastics): May increase risk of nephrotoxicity. Use together cautiously.
Skeletal muscle relaxants: May increase effects of muscle relaxants. Monitor patient for increased effects.

Effects on lab test results

• May increase urine urea, uric acid, BUN, creatinine, alkaline phosphatase, ALT, AST, GGT, LDH, and bilirubin levels. May decrease phosphate, magnesium, and hemoglobin levels and hematocrit. May increase or decrease glucose, potassium, and calcium levels.
• May decrease platelet and granulocyte counts. May increase or decrease WBC and eosinophil counts.

Pharmacokinetics

Absorption: Poor.

Distribution: Well into pleural cavities and joints; less so into aqueous humor, bronchial secretions, pancreas, bone, muscle, and parotid gland. Drug is 90% to 95% bound to plasma proteins.

Metabolism: Not well defined.

Excretion: Up to 5% unchanged in urine. *Half-life:* Adults and children older than age 9, 24 hours; children age 9 and younger, 18 hours.

Route	Onset	Peak	Duration
I.V.	Immediate	Immediate	Unknown

Action

Chemical effect: May bind to sterol in fungal cell membrane and alter cell permeability, allowing leakage of intracellular components.
Therapeutic effect: Decreases activity of or kills susceptible fungi.

Available forms

Powder for injection: 50-mg lyophilized cake

NURSING PROCESS

⚕ Assessment

• Obtain history of fungal infection and samples for culture and sensitivity tests before first dose. Reevaluate condition during therapy.
• Be alert for adverse reactions and drug interactions.
• Monitor patient's pulse, respiratory rate, temperature, and blood pressure every 30 minutes for at least 4 hours after giving drug I.V.; fever, shaking chills, anorexia, nausea, vomiting, headache, tachypnea, and hypotension may appear 1 to 3 hours after start of I.V. infusion. Symptoms are usually more severe with initial dose.
• Monitor BUN, creatinine level or clearance, electrolyte levels, CBC, and liver function test results at least weekly.
• Drug is linked to rhinocerebral phycomycosis, especially in patients with uncontrolled diabetes. Leukoencephalopathy also may occur. Monitor pulmonary function. Acute reactions are characterized by dyspnea, hypoxemia, and infiltrates.
• Assess patient's and family's knowledge of drug therapy.

⊕ Nursing diagnoses

• Ineffective protection related to presence of susceptible fungal species
• Risk for injury related to drug-induced adverse reactions
• Deficient knowledge related to drug therapy

▶ Planning and implementation

⚠ **ALERT:** Different amphotericin B preparations aren't interchangeable, and dosages vary.
• If BUN level exceeds 40 mg/dl, or if creatinine level exceeds 3 mg/dl, prescriber may reduce or stop drug until renal function improves. Drug may be stopped if alkaline phosphatase or bilirubin level increases.

Patient teaching

• Teach patient signs and symptoms of hypersensitivity, and stress importance of reporting them immediately.
• Warn patient that therapy may take several months; teach personal hygiene and other measures to prevent spread and recurrence of lesions.
• Urge patient to comply with prescribed regimen and recommended follow-up.
• Warn patient that discomfort at injection site and adverse reactions may occur during therapy, which may last several months.

✓ Evaluation

• Patient is free from fungal infection.
• Patient sustains no injury from drug-induced adverse reactions.
• Patient and family state understanding of drug therapy.

HIGH ALERT!

amphotericin B lipid complex
(am-foe-TER-ah-sin bee LIP-id KOM-pleks)
Abelcet

Pharmacologic class: polyene antibiotic
Therapeutic class: antifungal
Pregnancy risk category: B

Indications and dosages

▶ **Invasive fungal infections, including those caused by *Aspergillus fumigatus; Candida albicans, guilliermondii, stellatoidea,* and *tropicalis; Coccidioidomycosis* sp.; *Cryptococcus* sp.; *Histoplasma* sp.; and *Blastomyces* sp. in patients refractory to or intolerant of conventional amphotericin B therapy.** *Adults and*

---

children: 5 mg/kg daily as a single I.V. infusion. Give by continuous I.V. infusion at 2.5 mg/kg/hour.

▼ I.V. administration

• To prepare, shake the vial gently until you see no yellow sediment. Using aseptic technique, draw the calculated dose into one or more 20-ml syringes, using an 18G needle. You'll need more than one vial.
• Attach a 5-micron filter needle to the syringe and inject the dose into an I.V. bag of D_5W. One filter needle can be used for up to four vials of drug. The volume of D_5W should be sufficient to yield a final concentration of 1 mg/ml.
• For children and patients with CV disease, the recommended final concentration is 2 mg/ml.
• Shake the bag, and check the contents for foreign matter.
• Don't use an in-line filter.
• If infusing through an existing I.V. line, flush first with D_5W.
• Solutions are stable for up to 48 hours when refrigerated at 36° to 46° F (2° to 8° C) and for up to 6 hours at room temperature.
• Refrigerate and protect from light. Don't freeze.
• Discard unused drug; it contains no preservatives.
• Slowing the infusion rate also may decrease the risk of infusion-related reactions.
• For infusions lasting longer than 2 hours, shake the I.V. bag every 2 hours to ensure an even suspension.

⊗ **Incompatibilities**
Electrolytes, other I.V. drugs, saline solutions.

Contraindications and cautions

• Contraindicated in patients hypersensitive to amphotericin B or its components.
• Use cautiously in patients with renal impairment.
⚘ **Lifespan:** In pregnant women, safety hasn't been established. Use only if benefits outweigh risks to the fetus. Breast-feeding women must stop breast-feeding or stop drug. In infants younger than 1 month, safety and effectiveness haven't been established.

Adverse reactions

CNS: fever, headache, pain.
CV: *cardiac arrest,* chest pain, hypertension, hypotension.

GI: abdominal pain, diarrhea, *GI hemorrhage,* nausea, vomiting.
GU: *renal failure.*
Hematologic: anemia, *leukopenia, thrombocytopenia.*
Hepatic: bilirubinemia.
Metabolic: hypokalemia.
Respiratory: dyspnea, respiratory disorder, *respiratory failure.*
Skin: rash.
Other: chills, infection, MULTIPLE ORGAN FAILURE, *sepsis.*

Interactions

Drug-drug. *Antineoplastics:* May increase risk of renal toxicity, bronchospasm, and hypotension. Use cautiously.
Azole antifungals (fluconazole, ketoconazole): May induce fungal resistance. Use with caution.
Corticosteroids, corticotropin: May enhance hypokalemia, which may lead to cardiac dysfunction. Monitor electrolytes and cardiac function.
Cyclosporin A: May increase renal toxicity. Monitor patient closely.
Digoxin: May increase risk of digoxin toxicity and induce hypokalemia. Monitor potassium level closely.
Flucytosine: May increase risk of flucytosine toxicity from increased cellular uptake or impaired renal excretion. Use together cautiously.
Imidazoles (clotrimazole, fluconazole, itraconazole, ketoconazole, miconazole): May decrease effectiveness of amphotericin B because of inhibition of ergosterol synthesis. Clinical significance is unknown.
Leukocyte transfusions: May cause acute pulmonary toxicity. Avoid use together.
Nephrotoxic drugs (aminoglycosides, pentamidine): May increase risk of renal toxicity. Use together cautiously. Monitor renal function closely.
Skeletal muscle relaxants: May enhance effects of skeletal muscle relaxants because of drug-induced hypokalemia. Monitor potassium level closely.
Zidovudine: May increase myelotoxicity and nephrotoxicity. Monitor renal and hematologic function.

Effects on lab test results

• May increase BUN, creatinine, alkaline phosphatase, ALT, AST, bilirubin, GGT, and LDH

levels. May decrease potassium and hemoglobin levels and hematocrit.

• May decrease WBC and platelet counts.

Pharmacokinetics

Absorption: Given I.V.
Distribution: Well distributed. Volume increases with dose. Amphotericin B lipid complex yields measurable amphotericin B levels in spleen, lung, liver, lymph nodes, kidney, heart, and brain.
Metabolism: Unknown.
Excretion: Rapidly cleared from blood. *Terminal half-life:* About a week, probably because of slow elimination from tissues.

Route	Onset	Peak	Duration
I.V.	Unknown	Unknown	Unknown

Action

Chemical effect: Binds to sterols in fungal cell membranes, increasing cellular permeability and cell damage. It has fungistatic or fungicidal effects, depending on fungal susceptibility.
Therapeutic effect: Decreases activity of or kills susceptible fungi.

Available forms

Suspension for injection: 50 mg/10-ml vial; 100 mg/20-ml vial

NURSING PROCESS

⚗ Assessment

• Obtain history of fungal infection and samples for culture and sensitivity tests before therapy. Reevaluate condition during therapy.
• Be alert for adverse reactions and drug interactions.
• Assess renal function before therapy starts.
• Monitor liver function, creatinine and electrolyte levels (especially magnesium and potassium), and CBC during therapy.
• Assess patient's and family's knowledge of drug therapy.

🔢 Nursing diagnoses

• Risk for infection related to presence of susceptible fungal infection
• Risk for injury related to drug-induced adverse reactions
• Deficient knowledge related to drug therapy

⧉ Planning and implementation

• If severe respiratory distress develops, stop the infusion, provide supportive therapy for anaphylaxis, and notify prescriber. Don't resume the infusion.
⚠ ALERT: Different amphotericin B preparations aren't interchangeable, and dosages vary.
• Premedicate patient with acetaminophen, antihistamines, and corticosteroids to prevent or lessen the severity of infusion-related reactions, such as fever, chills, nausea, and vomiting, which occur 1 to 2 hours after the start of infusion.

Patient teaching

• Inform patient that fever, chills, nausea, and vomiting may occur during the infusion and that these reactions usually subside with later doses.
• Instruct patient to report redness or pain at the infusion site.
• Teach patient to recognize and report symptoms of acute hypersensitivity, such as respiratory distress.
• Tell patient to expect frequent laboratory testing to monitor kidney and liver function.

☑ Evaluation

• Patient is free from fungal infection.
• Patient has no injury from adverse drug reactions.
• Patient and family state understanding of drug therapy.

HIGH ALERT!

amphotericin B liposomal
(am-foh-TER-ah-sin bee lye-poh-SOW-mul)
AmBisome

Pharmacologic class: polyene antibiotic
Therapeutic class: antifungal
Pregnancy risk category: B

Indications and dosages

▶ **Empirical therapy for presumed fungal infection in febrile, neutropenic patients.** *Adults and children:* 3 mg/kg I.V. infusion daily.
▶ **Systemic fungal infections caused by *Aspergillus*, *Candida*, or *Cryptococcus* sp. refractory to amphotericin B deoxycholate or in patients with renal impairment or unacceptable toxicity that precludes the use of amphotericin B deoxycholate.** *Adults and children:* 3 to 5 mg/kg I.V. infusion daily.

▶ **Visceral leishmaniasis in immunocompetent patients.** *Adults and children:* 3 mg/kg I.V. infusion daily on days 1 to 5, 14, and 21. A repeat course may be beneficial if initial treatment fails to clear parasites.

▶ **Visceral leishmaniasis in immunocompromised patients.** *Adults and children:* 4 mg/kg I.V. infusion daily on days 1 to 5, 10, 17, 24, 31, and 38. Expert advice regarding further treatment is recommended if initial therapy fails or relapse occurs.

▶ **Cryptococcal meningitis in HIV-infected patients.** *Adults and children:* 6 mg/kg daily I.V. infusion over 2 hours. Infusion time may be decreased to 1 hour if well tolerated or increased if discomfort occurs.

▽ I.V. administration

• Reconstitute each 50-mg vial of amphotericin B liposomal with 12 ml of sterile water for injection to yield 4 mg amphotericin B per milliliter.
• After reconstitution, shake vial vigorously for 30 seconds or until particulate matter disappears. Withdraw calculated amount of reconstituted solution into a sterile syringe and inject through a 5-micron filter into the appropriate amount of D_5W to a final concentration of 1 to 2 mg/ml. Lower concentrations (0.2 to 0.5 mg/ml) may be appropriate for children to provide sufficient volume for infusion.
• Flush existing I.V. line with D_5W before infusing drug. If this isn't feasible, give drug through a separate line.
• Use a controlled infusion device and an in-line filter with a mean pore diameter larger than 1 micron. Initially, infuse drug over at least 2 hours. Infusion time may be reduced to 1 hour if the treatment is well tolerated. If the patient has discomfort, infusion time may be increased.
• Observe patient closely for adverse reactions during infusion. If anaphylaxis occurs, stop the infusion immediately, provide supportive therapy, and notify the prescriber.
• Refrigerate unopened drug at 36° to 46° F (2° to 8° C). Once reconstituted, the product may be stored for up to 24 hours at 36° to 46° F. Don't freeze.

⊗ **Incompatibilities**
Other I.V. drugs, saline solutions, bacteriostatic water for injection and bacteriostatic drugs.

Contraindications and cautions

• Contraindicated in patients hypersensitive to drug or its components.
• Use cautiously in patients with renal impairment.

⚖ **Lifespan:** In pregnant women, safety hasn't been established. Use only if benefits outweigh risks to the fetus. Breast-feeding women must stop breast-feeding or stop drug. In infants younger than 1 month, safety and effectiveness haven't been established.

Adverse reactions

CNS: anxiety, asthenia, confusion, fever, headache, insomnia, pain.
CV: *chest pain, edema,* hypertension, *hypotension,* phlebitis, *tachycardia,* vasodilation.
EENT: *epistaxis, rhinitis.*
GI: *abdominal pain,* anorexia, *diarrhea, GI hemorrhage,* nausea, vomiting.
GU: *hematuria.*
Hepatic: hepatomegaly.
Metabolic: *hyperglycemia,* hypernatremia, *hypocalcemia, hypokalemia, hypomagnesemia.*
Musculoskeletal: *back pain.*
Respiratory: *cough, dyspnea,* hyperventilation, *hypoxia, lung disorder, pleural effusion.*
Skin: *pruritus, rash,* sweating.
Other: *anaphylaxis, blood product infusion reaction,* chills, infection, *sepsis.*

Interactions

Drug-drug. *Antineoplastics:* May increase risk of renal toxicity, bronchospasm, and hypotension. Use cautiously.
Azole antifungals (fluconazole, ketoconazole): May induce fungal resistance. Use with caution.
Corticosteroids, corticotropin: May potentiate hypokalemia, which could result in cardiac dysfunction. Monitor potassium level and cardiac function.
Digoxin: May increase risk of digoxin toxicity in potassium-depleted patients. Monitor potassium level closely.
Flucytosine: May increase flucytosine toxicity by increasing cellular uptake or impairing renal excretion of flucytosine. Monitor renal function closely.
Imidazole antifungals (clotrimazole, ketoconazole, miconazole): May induce fungal resistance to amphotericin B. Use together cautiously.
Leukocyte transfusions: May increase risk of acute pulmonary toxicity. Avoid use together.

Other nephrotoxic drugs (antibiotics, antineo-plastics): May increase risk of nephrotoxicity. Use together cautiously. Monitor renal function closely.

Skeletal muscle relaxants: May increase effects of skeletal muscle relaxants because of ampho-tericin-induced hypokalemia. Monitor potassium level.

Effects on lab test results
• May increase BUN, creatinine, glucose, sodium, alkaline phosphatase, ALT, AST, bilirubin, GGT, and LDH levels. May decrease potassium, calcium, and magnesium levels.

Pharmacokinetics
Absorption: Given I.V.
Distribution: Unknown.
Metabolism: Unknown.
Excretion: Unknown. *Initial half-life:* 7 to 10 hours with 24-hour dosing. *Terminal elimination half-life:* About 4 to 6 days.

Route	Onset	Peak	Duration
I.V.	Unknown	Unknown	Unknown

Action
Chemical effect: Binds to the sterol component of a fungal cell membrane, altering cell permeability and cell death.
Therapeutic effect: Decreases activity of or kills susceptible fungi. Treats visceral protozoal infections.

Available forms
Injection: 50-mg vial

NURSING PROCESS

Assessment
• Obtain history of fungal infection and samples for culture and sensitivity tests before therapy. Reevaluate condition during therapy.
• Carefully assess patients who are also receiving chemotherapy or bone marrow transplantation because of their increased risk of additional adverse reactions, including seizures, arrhythmias, thrombocytopenia, and respiratory failure.
• Monitor CBC, liver function test results, and creatinine, BUN, and electrolyte levels, particularly magnesium and potassium.

• Monitor patient for signs of hypokalemia, such as ECG changes, muscle weakness, cramping, and drowsiness.
• Watch for adverse reactions. Patients who receive drug may have fewer chills, decreased BUN level, a lower risk of hypokalemia, and less vomiting than patients who receive regular amphotericin B.
• Assess patient's and family's knowledge of drug therapy.

Nursing diagnoses
• Risk for infection related to presence of susceptible fungal or parasite infections
• Risk for injury related to drug-induced adverse reactions
• Deficient knowledge related to drug therapy

Planning and implementation
ALERT: Amphotericin B preparations aren't interchangeable, and dosages vary.
• To lessen the risk or severity of adverse reactions, premedicate patient with antipyretics, antihistamines, antiemetics, or corticosteroids.
• Therapy may take several weeks to months.
Patient teaching
• Teach patient signs and symptoms of hypersensitivity, and stress importance of reporting them immediately.
• Warn patient that therapy may take several months; teach personal hygiene and other measures to prevent spread and recurrence of lesions.
• Instruct patient to report adverse reactions.
• Instruct patient to watch for and report signs of hypokalemia, such as muscle weakness, cramping, and drowsiness.
• Advise patient that frequent laboratory testing will be performed.

Evaluation
• Patient is free from fungal or parasitic infection.
• Patient sustains no injury from drug-induced adverse reactions.
• Patient and family state understanding of drug therapy.

A

ampicillin
(am-pih-SIL-in)
Apo-Ampi ♦ , Nu-Ampi, Principen

ampicillin sodium

ampicillin trihydrate

Pharmacologic class: aminopenicillin
Therapeutic class: antibiotic
Pregnancy risk category: B

Indications and dosages

▶ **Respiratory tract or skin and skin-structure infection.** *Adults and children weighing 40 kg (88 lb) or more:* 250 to 500 mg P.O. every 6 hours.
Children weighing less than 40 kg: 25 to 50 mg/kg/day P.O. in equally divided doses every 6 hours. Pediatric dosages shouldn't exceed recommended adult dosages.
▶ **GI infection, UTI.** *Adults and children weighing 40 kg (88 lb) or more:* 500 mg P.O. every 6 hours. For severe infections, larger doses may be needed.
Children weighing less than 40 kg: 50 to 100 mg/kg/day P.O. in equally divided doses every 6 hours.
▶ **Bacterial meningitis or septicemia.** *Adults:* 150 to 200 mg/kg/day I.V. in divided doses every 3 to 4 hours. May be given I.M. after 3 days of I.V. therapy. Maximum, 14 g daily.
Children: 100 to 200 mg/kg I.V. daily in divided doses every 3 to 4 hours. Give I.V. for 3 days; then give I.M.
▶ **Uncomplicated gonorrhea.** *Adults and children weighing more than 45 kg (99 lb):* 3.5 g P.O. with 1 g probenecid given as a single dose.
▶ **To prevent endocarditis in patients having dental procedures.** *Adults:* 2 g I.M. or I.V. within 30 minutes before procedure.
Children: 50 mg/kg I.M. or I.V. within 30 minutes before procedure.
◨ **Adjust-a-dose:** In patients with severe renal impairment, increase drug interval to 12 hours. Use same dose.

▽ I.V. administration

• Don't give I.V. unless infection is severe or patient can't take oral dose.

• For direct injection, reconstitute with bacteriostatic water for injection. Use 5 ml for 125-mg, 250-mg, or 500-mg vials; 7.4 ml for 1-g vials; and 14.8 ml for 2-g vials. Use initial dilution within 1 hour.
• Give direct I.V. injections over 3 to 5 minutes for doses of 500 mg or less; over 10 to 15 minutes for larger doses. Don't exceed 100 mg/minute.
• For an intermittent infusion, dilute in 50 to 100 ml of normal saline solution and give over 15 to 30 minutes. Follow manufacturer's directions for stability data when ampicillin is further diluted for I.V. infusion.
• Give intermittently to prevent vein irritation. Change site every 48 hours.
⊗ **Incompatibilities**
Amikacin, amino acid solutions, chlorpromazine, dextran solutions, dopamine, erythromycin lactobionate, 10% fat emulsions, fructose, gentamicin, heparin sodium, hetastarch, hydrocortisone sodium succinate, hydromorphone, kanamycin, lidocaine, lincomycin, polymyxin B, prochlorperazine edisylate, sodium bicarbonate, streptomycin, tobramycin.

Contraindications and cautions

• Contraindicated in patients hypersensitive to drug or other penicillins.
• Use cautiously in patients with other drug allergies, especially to cephalosporins (possible cross-sensitivity), and in those with mononucleosis (high risk of maculopapular rash).
⚘ **Lifespan:** In pregnant or breast-feeding women, use cautiously.

Adverse reactions

CNS: *seizures.*
CV: thrombophlebitis, vein irritation.
GI: nausea, vomiting, diarrhea, glossitis, stomatitis.
Hematologic: *agranulocytosis,* anemia, eosinophilia, *leukopenia, thrombocytopenia, thrombocytopenic purpura.*
Other: hypersensitivity reactions (*anaphylaxis,* maculopapular rash, urticaria), overgrowth of nonsusceptible organisms, pain at injection site.

Interactions

Drug-drug. *Allopurinol:* May increase risk of rash. Monitor patient.

Probenecid: May increase level of ampicillin and other penicillins. Probenecid may be used for this purpose.

Effects on lab test results

• May decrease hemoglobin level and hematocrit.
• May increase eosinophil count. May decrease platelet, WBC, and granulocyte counts.
• May cause false-positive urine glucose determinations with copper sulfate tests (Clinitest).

Pharmacokinetics

Absorption: About 42% after P.O. use; unknown after I.M. use.
Distribution: Into pleural, peritoneal, and synovial fluids; lungs; prostate; liver; gallbladder; middle ear effusions; maxillary sinus and bronchial secretions; tonsils; and sputum. Ampicillin is minimally protein-bound at 15% to 25%.
Metabolism: Only partial.
Excretion: In urine by renal tubular secretion and glomerular filtration. *Half-life:* About 1 to 1½ hours (10 to 24 hours in severe renal impairment).

Route	Onset	Peak	Duration
P.O.	Unknown	2 hr	6–8 hr
I.V.	Immediate	Immediate	Unknown
I.M.	Unknown	1 hr	Unknown

Action

Chemical effect: Inhibits cell-wall synthesis during microorganism multiplication.
Therapeutic effect: Kills susceptible bacteria, including non-penicillinase–producing gram-positive bacteria and many gram-negative organisms.

Available forms

Capsules: 250 mg, 500 mg
Infusion: 500 mg, 1 g, 2 g
Injection: 125 mg, 250 mg, 500 mg, 1 g, 2 g
Oral suspension: 125 mg/5 ml, 250 mg/5 ml (after reconstitution)

NURSING PROCESS

◢ Assessment

• Obtain history of patient's infection before therapy, and observe throughout therapy to assess improvement.

• Ask patient about previous allergic reaction to penicillin. A negative history of penicillin allergy doesn't rule out future reaction.
• Obtain specimen for culture and sensitivity tests before giving first dose.
• Be alert for adverse reactions and drug interactions.
• If adverse GI reactions occur, monitor patient's hydration status.
• Assess patient's and family's knowledge of drug therapy.

◉ Nursing diagnoses

• Risk for infection related to presence of susceptible bacterial infection
• Risk for deficient fluid volume related to drug-induced adverse GI reactions
• Deficient knowledge related to drug therapy

▶ Planning and implementation

• Give orally either 1 hour before or 2 hours after meals. Food may interfere with absorption.
• Don't give I.M. unless infection is severe or patient can't take oral dose.
• Give at least 1 hour before bacteriostatic antibiotics.
• In children with meningitis, give with parenteral chloramphenicol for 24 hours pending culture results.
• If anaphylaxis occurs, stop drug immediately. Notify prescriber, and prepare to give immediate treatment, such as epinephrine, corticosteroids, antihistamines, and other resuscitative measures.
Patient teaching
• Tell patient to take entire quantity of drug exactly as prescribed, even after feeling better.
• Tell patient to call prescriber if a rash (most common), fever, or chills develop.
• Warn patient never to use leftover ampicillin for a new illness or to share it with others.
• Advise patient to take oral ampicillin 1 hour before or 2 hours after meals for best absorption.

☑ Evaluation

• Patient is free from infection.
• Patient maintains adequate hydration.
• Patient and family state understanding of drug therapy.

Reactions may be *common*, uncommon, *life-threatening*, or COMMON AND LIFE-THREATENING.

ampicillin sodium and sulbactam sodium

(am-pih-SIL-in SOH-dee-um and
sul-BAC-tam SOH-dee-um)
Unasyn

Pharmacologic class: aminopenicillin and
beta-lactamase inhibitor
Therapeutic class: antibiotic
Pregnancy risk category: B

Indications and dosages

▶ **Intra-abdominal, gynecologic, and skin
and skin-structure infections caused by susceptible gram-positive, gram-negative, and
beta-lactamase–producing strains.** *Adults:*
Dosage expressed as total drug (each 1.5-g vial
contains 1 g ampicillin sodium and 0.5 g sulbactam sodium). 1.5 to 3 g I.M. or I.V. every
6 hours. Maximum, 4 g sulbactam (12 g of
combined drugs) daily.

▶ **Skin and skin-structure infections caused
by susceptible organisms.** *Children older than
age 1:* Give 300 mg/kg I.V. daily in equally divided doses every 6 hours. Give children a maximum of 14 days of therapy. Children weighing
40 kg (88 lb) or more may receive the usual
adult dosage shown above.

▼ I.V. administration

• When preparing injection, reconstitute powder
with any of the following diluents: normal saline solution, D_5W, lactated Ringer's solution,
1/6 M sodium lactate, dextrose 5% in half-
normal saline solution for injection, or 10%
inert sugar. Stability varies with diluent, temperature, and concentration of solution.
• After reconstitution, let vials stand for a few
minutes to let foam dissipate and to permit visual inspection of contents for particles.
• Give dose by injection over 10 to 15 minutes,
or dilute in 50 to 100 ml of a compatible diluent
and infuse over 15 to 30 minutes. If permitted,
give intermittently to prevent vein irritation.
Change site every 48 hours.

⊗ **Incompatibilities**
Amikacin, amino acid solutions, chlorpromazine, dextran solutions, dopamine, erythromycin lactobionate, 10% fat emulsions, fructose, gentamicin, heparin sodium, hetastarch,
hydrocortisone sodium succinate, kanamycin,

lidocaine, lincomycin, netilmicin, polymyxin B,
prochlorperazine edisylate, sodium bicarbonate,
streptomycin, tobramycin. Don't add or mix
with other drugs because they might be physically or chemically incompatible.

Contraindications and cautions

• Contraindicated in patients hypersensitive to
drug or other penicillins.
• Use cautiously in patients with other drug allergies, especially to cephalosporins (possible
cross-sensitivity), and in those with mononucleosis (high risk of maculopapular rash).
☤ **Lifespan:** In pregnant and breast-feeding
women, use cautiously. In children younger than
age 1, safety of drug hasn't been established. In
children age 1 and older, drug can be used I.V.
for skin and skin-structure infections. Children
shouldn't receive the drug I.M.

Adverse reactions

CV: thrombophlebitis, vein irritation.
GI: *diarrhea,* glossitis, nausea, stomatitis, vomiting.
Hematologic: *agranulocytosis,* anemia, eosinophilia, *leukopenia, thrombocytopenia, thrombocytopenic purpura.*
Other: hypersensitivity reactions (*anaphylaxis,*
erythematous maculopapular rash, urticaria),
overgrowth of nonsusceptible organisms, pain at
injection site.

Interactions

Drug-drug. *Allopurinol:* May increase risk of
rash. Monitor patient.
Hormonal contraceptives: May decrease effectiveness of hormonal contraceptives. Advise patient to use barrier contraception until therapy is
complete.
Probenecid: May increase ampicillin level.
Probenecid may be used for this purpose.

Effects on lab test results

• May increase BUN, creatinine, ALT, AST, alkaline phosphatase, bilirubin, LDH, CK, and
GGT levels. May decrease hemoglobin level
and hematocrit.
• May increase eosinophil count. May decrease
platelet, WBC, and granulocyte counts.
• May cause false-positive urine glucose determinations with copper sulfate tests (Clinitest).

Pharmacokinetics

Absorption: Given I.V.
Distribution: Both drugs into pleural, peritoneal, and synovial fluids; lungs; prostate; liver;
gallbladder; middle ear effusions; maxillary sinus and bronchial secretions; tonsils; and sputum. Ampicillin is minimally protein-bound at
15% to 25%; sulbactam is about 38% protein-
bound.
Metabolism: Both drugs only partially.
Excretion: Both drugs in urine by renal tubular
secretion and glomerular filtration. *Half-life:*
1 to 1½ hours (10 to 24 hours in severe renal
impairment).

Route	Onset	Peak	Duration
I.V.	Immediate	Immediate	Unknown
I.M.	Unknown	Unknown	Unknown

Action

Chemical effect: Ampicillin inhibits cell-wall
synthesis during microorganism multiplication;
sulbactam inactivates bacterial beta-lactamase,
the enzyme that inactivates ampicillin and provides bacterial resistance to it.
Therapeutic effect: Kills susceptible bacteria.

Available forms

Injection: Vials and piggyback vials containing
1.5 g (1 g ampicillin sodium with 0.5 g sulbactam sodium); 3 g (2 g ampicillin sodium with
1 g sulbactam sodium)

NURSING PROCESS

Assessment

• Obtain history of patient's infection before
therapy, and observe throughout therapy to determine improvement.
• Ask patient about previous allergic reaction to
penicillin. A negative history of penicillin allergy doesn't rule out future reaction.
• Obtain specimen for culture and sensitivity
tests before giving first dose.
• Be alert for adverse reactions and drug interactions.
• Monitor patient's hydration status if adverse
GI reactions occur.
• Assess patient's and family's knowledge of
drug therapy.

Nursing diagnoses

• Risk for infection related to presence of susceptible bacterial infection
• Risk for deficient fluid volume related to
drug-induced adverse GI reactions
• Deficient knowledge related to drug therapy

Planning and implementation

• When giving drug I.M., reconstitute with sterile water for injection or with 0.5% or 2% lidocaine hydrochloride. Add 3.2 ml to a 1.5-g vial
(or 6.4 ml to a 3-g vial) to yield 375 mg/ml.
Give deep into muscle.
• In patients with renal impairment, dosage
should be reduced.
• Give drug at least 1 hour before bacteriostatic
antibiotics.
• Stop drug immediately if anaphylaxis occurs.
Notify prescriber and give immediate treatment,
such as epinephrine, corticosteroids, antihistamines; and other resuscitative measures.
Patient teaching
• Tell patient to call prescriber if rash (most
common), fever, or chills develop.
• Advise women taking hormonal contracep-
tives to use a barrier form of contraception during drug therapy.

Evaluation

• Patient is free from infection.
• Patient maintains adequate hydration.
• Patient and family state understanding of drug
therapy.

anakinra
(ann-uh-KIN-ruh)
Kineret

Pharmacologic class: recombinant human in-
terleukin-1 receptor antagonist
Therapeutic class: disease-modifying antirheumatic drug (DMARD)
Pregnancy risk category: B

Indications and dosages

▶ **Reduction in signs and symptoms and
slowing of structural damage in moderate-
to-severe active rheumatoid arthritis (RA)
after one failure with DMARDs, used alone
or combined with DMARDs other than tu-**

mor necrosis factor (TNF) blockers. *Adults:* 100 mg subcutaneously daily.

Contraindications and cautions

• Contraindicated in patients hypersensitive to *Escherichia coli*–derived proteins or components of the product. Don't use in immunosuppressed patients or in those with chronic or active infection.

• Use cautiously with TNF blockers because of the increased risk of neutropenia.

⚠ **Lifespan:** In pregnant women, use only if necessary because no adequate, well-controlled studies exist. In breast-feeding women, use cautiously because it's unknown whether drug appears in breast milk. In patients with juvenile RA, safety and effectiveness of drug haven't been established. In elderly patients, use drug cautiously because they have a greater risk of infection and are more likely to have renal impairment.

Adverse reactions

CNS: headache.
EENT: sinusitis.
GI: abdominal pain, diarrhea, nausea.
Hematologic: *neutropenia.*
Respiratory: upper respiratory tract infection.
Other: infection (bone and joint, cellulitis, pneumonia), flulike symptoms, injection site reactions (ecchymosis, erythema, inflammation, pain).

Interactions

Drug-drug. *Etanercept, other TNF blockers:* May increase risk of severe infection. Use together cautiously.
Vaccines: May decrease effectiveness of vaccines or increase risk of secondary transmission of infection with live vaccines. Avoid use together.

Effects on lab test results

• May increase differential percentage of eosinophils. May decrease neutrophil, WBC, and platelet counts.

Pharmacokinetics

Absorption: Absolute bioavailability is 95% after a 70-mg subcutaneous injection.
Distribution: In plasma.
Metabolism: Unknown.

Excretion: Renal. Clearance increases with increasing creatinine clearance and body weight. Mean plasma clearance decreases 70% to 75% in patients with creatinine clearance less than 30 ml/minute. *Half-life:* 4 to 6 hours.

Route	Onset	Peak	Duration
SubQ	Unknown	3–7 hr	Unknown

Action

Chemical effect: A recombinant, nonglycosylated form of the human interleukin-1 receptor antagonist (IL-1Ra). The level of naturally occurring IL-1Ra in synovium and synovial fluid from patients with RA isn't enough to compete with the elevated level of locally produced IL-1. Drug blocks the activity of IL-1 by competitively inhibiting IL-1 from binding to the interleukin-1–type receptors.
Therapeutic effect: Decreases inflammation and cartilage degradation.

Available forms

Injection: 100 mg/ml in prefilled glass syringe

NURSING PROCESS

Assessment
• Assess patient before therapy for signs and symptoms of chronic or active infection. If patient has active infection, don't start treatment.
• Obtain neutrophil count before treatment, monthly for the first 3 months of treatment, and then quarterly for up to 1 year.
• Monitor patient for infections and injection site reactions.

Nursing diagnoses
• Risk for infection related to anakinra therapy
• Chronic pain from underlying rheumatoid arthritis
• Risk for impaired skin integrity from injection site reaction

Planning and implementation
• Inject the entire contents of the prefilled syringe subcutaneously.
• Stop drug if patient develops a serious infection.
⚠ **ALERT:** Don't confuse anakinra with amikacin.
Patient teaching
• Tell patient to store drug in refrigerator and not to freeze or expose to excessive heat. Tell

patient to allow drug to come to room temperature before injecting.
- Teach patient proper technique for administration and disposal of syringes in a puncture-resistant container. Also, warn patient not to reuse needles.
- Urge patient to rotate injection sites.
- Review with patient the signs and symptoms of allergic and other adverse reactions and the symptoms of infection. Urge patient to contact prescriber immediately if they arise. Inform patient that injection site reactions are common, are usually mild, and typically last 14 to 28 days.
- Tell patient to avoid live-virus vaccines while taking anakinra.

☑ **Evaluation**
- Patient is free from infection or adverse reactions during drug therapy.
- Patient's symptoms of RA are relieved.
- Patient and family state understanding of drug therapy and give drug properly.

HIGH ALERT!

anastrozole
(uh-NASS-truh-zohl)
Arimidex✍

Pharmacologic class: nonsteroidal aromatase inhibitor
Therapeutic class: antineoplastic
Pregnancy risk category: D

Indications and dosages

▶ **First-line therapy for hormone-receptor–positive or hormone-receptor–unknown locally advanced or metastatic breast cancer; advanced breast cancer with disease progression following tamoxifen; adjuvant therapy for hormone-receptor–positive early breast cancer.** *Postmenopausal women:* 1 mg P.O. daily.

Contraindications and cautions
- Contraindicated in patients hypersensitive to the drug or its components.
- Use cautiously in patients with hepatic impairment.
- ⚕ **Lifespan:** In pregnant women, drug isn't recommended because it may cause fetal harm. In

breast-feeding women, use cautiously. In children, safety of drug hasn't been established.

Adverse reactions
CNS: anxiety, asthenia, depression, dizziness, headache, insomnia, pain, paresthesia.
CV: chest pain, edema, hypertension, peripheral edema, *thromboembolic disease, vasodilation.*
EENT: cataracts, pharyngitis.
GI: abdominal pain, anorexia, constipation, diarrhea, dry mouth, nausea, vomiting.
GU: pelvic pain, vaginal dryness, *vaginal hemorrhage.*
Metabolic: increased appetite, weight gain.
Musculoskeletal: arthralgia, back pain, bone pain.
Respiratory: dyspnea, increased cough.
Skin: rash, sweating.
Other: *hot flushes.*

Interactions
Drug-drug. *Estrogen-containing therapies, tamoxifen:* May decrease anastrozole's effect. Avoid use together.

Effects on lab test results
- May increase liver enzyme and cholesterol levels.

Pharmacokinetics
Absorption: Food doesn't affect extent of absorption.
Distribution: 40% bound to plasma proteins.
Metabolism: In liver.
Excretion: In urine. *Half-life:* About 50 hours.

Route	Onset	Peak	Duration
P.O.	Unknown	Unknown	Unknown

Action
Chemical effect: Lowers estradiol level.
Therapeutic effect: Hinders cancer cell growth.

Available forms
Tablets: 1 mg

NURSING PROCESS

🔍 **Assessment**
- Obtain history of patient's neoplastic disease before therapy.
- Be alert for adverse reactions.

- Assess patient's and family's knowledge of drug therapy.

✛ Nursing diagnoses
- Ineffective health maintenance related to neoplastic disease
- Risk for deficient fluid volume related to drug-induced adverse GI reactions
- Deficient knowledge related to drug therapy

▶ Planning and implementation
- Rule out pregnancy before treatment begins.
- Give drug under supervision of a prescriber experienced in using antineoplastics.
- Patients with hormone-receptor–negative disease and those who didn't respond to previous tamoxifen therapy, rarely respond to anastrozole.
- Patients with advanced breast cancer should continue therapy until tumor progresses.

Patient teaching
- Instruct patient to report adverse reactions.
- Stress importance of follow-up care.

☑ Evaluation
- Patient has positive response to therapy.
- Patient maintains adequate hydration.
- Patient and family state understanding of drug therapy.

anidulafungin
(uh-nigh-doo-lah-FUN-jin)
Eraxis

Pharmacologic class: echinocandin
Therapeutic class: antifungal
Pregnancy risk category: C

Indications and dosages

▶ **Candidemia and other *Candida* infections (intra-abdominal abscess, peritonitis).** *Adults:* A single 200-mg loading dose given by I.V. infusion at no more than 1.1 mg/minute on day 1; then 100 mg daily for at least 14 days after last positive culture.

▶ **Esophageal candidiasis.** *Adults:* A single 100-mg loading dose given by I.V. infusion at no more than 1.1 mg/minute on day 1; then 50 mg daily for at least 14 days and for at least 7 more days after symptoms resolve.

▼ I.V. administration
- Reconstitute each vial with 15 ml of supplied diluent.
- Further dilute with D_5W or normal saline solution to a final concentration of 0.5 mg/ml.
- For 50-mg dose, add to 85 ml for final infusion volume of 100 ml. For 100-mg dose, add to 170 ml for final infusion volume of 200 ml. For 200-mg dose, add to 340 ml for final infusion volume of 400 ml.
- Don't infuse at more than 1.1 mg/minute.
- Store at room temperature; don't freeze. Use reconstituted solution within 24 hours of preparation.

⊗ **Incompatibilities**
Unknown. Use only supplied diluent to reconstitute and D_5W or normal saline solution to further dilute.

Contraindications and cautions
- Contraindicated in patients hypersensitive to anidulafungin, other echinocandins, or any component of the drug.
- Use cautiously in patients with liver impairment.

☀ **Lifespan:** In pregnant or breast-feeding women, use cautiously. In children, safety and effectiveness haven't been established.

Adverse reactions
CNS: headache.
CV: *deep vein thrombosis,* hypotension.
GI: abdominal pain, dyspepsia, nausea, vomiting.
Hematologic: *leukopenia, neutropenia.*
Metabolic: hypokalemia.
Skin: flushing, pruritus, rash, urticaria.

Interactions
Drug-drug. *Cyclosporin:* Use together can cause slight increase in anidulafungin levels. Monitor levels.

Effects on lab test results
- May increase AST, ALT, alkaline phosphatase, GGT, hepatic enzyme, amylase, lipase, bilirubin, CK, creatinine, urea, calcium, glucose, potassium, and sodium levels. May decrease potassium and magnesium levels.
- May increase PT. May decrease neutrophil and WBC counts. May increase or decrease platelet count.

Pharmacokinetics

Absorption: Given I.V.
Distribution: Short distribution half-life; 84% bound to plasma proteins.
Metabolism: No observable hepatic metabolism.
Excretion: About 30% in feces; less than 1% in urine.

Route	Onset	Peak	Duration
I.V.	< 24 hr	Unknown	Unknown

Action

Chemical effect: Inhibits glucan synthase, which in turn inhibits formation of 1,3-β-D-glucan, an essential component of fungal cell walls.
Therapeutic effect: Kills susceptible fungi.

Available forms

Powder for injection: 50 mg/vial with companion diluent

NURSING PROCESS

⚡ Assessment
• Obtain specimens for culture and sensitivity tests and baseline laboratory tests before therapy begins.
• Monitor patient closely for changes in liver function and blood cell counts during therapy.
• Assess patient for signs or symptoms of liver toxicity, such as dark urine, jaundice, abdominal pain, and fatigue; notify prescriber.
• Assess patient's and family's knowledge of drug therapy.

⊕ Nursing diagnoses
• Risk for infection related to presence of fungal infection and drug-induced leukopenia and neutropenia
• Risk for injury related to drug-induced liver toxicity
• Deficient knowledge related to drug therapy

▶ Planning and implementation
• Use only the supplied diluent to reconstitute powder.
• To avoid histamine-mediated symptoms, such as rash, urticaria, flushing, itching, dyspnea, and hypotension, don't infuse more than 1.1 mg/minute.

• Patients with esophageal candidiasis who are HIV-positive may need suppressive antifungal therapy after anidulafungin treatment to prevent relapse.
• In case of overdose, monitor laboratory tests, especially liver function tests; drug isn't dialyzable.

Patient teaching
• Tell patient to report a rash, itching, trouble breathing, or other adverse effects during infusion.
• Explain that blood tests will be needed to monitor the drug's effects.

✓ Evaluation
• Patient is free from infection.
• Patient does not experience symptoms of liver toxicity.
• Patient and family state understanding of drug therapy.

apomorphine hydrochloride
(ah-poe-MORE-feen high-droh-KLOR-ighd)
Apokyn

Pharmacologic class: dopamine agonist
Therapeutic class: antiparkinsonian drug
Pregnancy risk category: C

Indications and dosages

▶ **Intermittent hypomobility, "off" episodes caused by advanced Parkinson disease (with an antiemetic).** *Adults:* Initially, give a 0.2-ml test dose subcutaneously. Measure supine and standing blood pressure every 20 minutes for the first hour. If patient tolerates and responds to drug, start with 0.2 ml subcutaneously p.r.n. (outpatient). Separate doses by at least 2 hours. Increase by 0.1 ml every few days, as needed.
  If initial 0.2-ml dose is ineffective but tolerated, give 0.4 ml at next "off" period, measuring supine and standing blood pressure every 20 minutes for the first hour. If drug is tolerated, start with 0.3 ml (outpatient). If needed, increase by 0.1 ml every few days.
  If patient doesn't tolerate 0.4-ml dose, give 0.3 ml as a test dose at the next "off" period, measuring supine and standing blood pressure as before. If drug is tolerated, give 0.2 ml (outpatient). Increase by 0.1 ml every few days,

---

p.r.n., but doses higher than 0.4 ml usually aren't tolerated if 0.2 ml is the starting dose.

Maximum recommended dose is usually 0.6 ml p.r.n. Most patients take drug about three times daily. Experience is limited at more than five times daily or more than 2 ml daily.

⊠**Adjust-a-dose:** In patients with mild to moderate renal impairment, the test and starting doses should be 0.1 ml, given subcutaneously.

Contraindications and cautions

• Contraindicated in patients allergic to apomorphine or its ingredients, including sulfites, and in patients who take 5-HT$_3$ antagonists.
• Use cautiously in patients at risk for prolonged QTc interval, such as those with hypokalemia, hypomagnesemia, bradycardia, or genetic predisposition. Also use cautiously in patients with cardiovascular or cerebrovascular disease and in those with renal or hepatic impairment.
⚖ **Lifespan:** In pregnant and breast-feeding women, drug effects are unknown. Give drug only if clearly needed. In children, safety and effectiveness haven't been established.

Adverse reactions

CNS: aggravated Parkinson disease, anxiety, *confusion,* depression, *dizziness, drowsiness,* fatigue, *hallucinations,* headache, insomnia, *somnolence,* syncope, weakness.
CV: *angina,* **cardiac arrest,** *chest pain, chest pressure, edema, flushing,* **heart failure,** *hypotension, orthostatic hypotension,* **MI.**
EENT: *rhinorrhea.*
GI: constipation, diarrhea, *nausea, vomiting.*
GU: UTI.
Metabolic: dehydration.
Musculoskeletal: arthralgia, back pain, *dyskinesias,* limb pain.
Respiratory: dyspnea, pneumonia.
Skin: bruising, injection site reaction, pallor, sweating.
Other: *falls, yawning.*

Interactions

Drug-drug. *Antihypertensives, vasodilators:* May increase risk of hypotension, MI, pneumonia, falls, and joint injury. Use together cautiously.
Dopamine antagonists, metoclopramide: May reduce apomorphine effectiveness. Use together cautiously.

Drugs that prolong the QTc interval: May prolong the QTc interval. Give cautiously with other drugs that prolong QTc interval.
5-HT$_3$ antagonists (alosetron, dolasetron, granisetron, ondansetron, palonosetron): May cause serious hypotension and loss of consciousness. Use together is contraindicated.
Drug-lifestyle. *Alcohol use:* May increase risk of sedation and hypotension. Discourage use together.

Effects on lab test results

None known.

Pharmacokinetics

Absorption: Rapid. Patients with hepatic or renal impairment may have higher serum level.
Distribution: Large, but CSF penetration is poor.
Metabolism: Unknown.
Excretion: Unknown. *Elimination half-life:* About 30 to 60 minutes in patients with normal or impaired renal function.

Route	Onset	Peak	Duration
SubQ	20 min	10–60 min	2 hr

Action

Chemical effect: Improves motor function by stimulating dopamine D2 receptors in the caudate-putamen area of the brain.
Therapeutic effect: Relieves signs and symptoms of parkinsonism.

Available forms

Solution for injection: 10 mg/ml (contains benzyl alcohol)

NURSING PROCESS

🕮 **Assessment**
• Monitor supine and standing blood pressure every 20 minutes for the first hour after therapy starts or dosage changes.
Ⓢ **ALERT:** Monitor patient for drowsiness or sleepiness, which may occur well after treatment starts. Stop drug if patient develops significant daytime sleepiness that interferes with activities of daily living.
• Watch for evidence of coronary or cerebral ischemia, and stop drug if they occur.

• Assess elderly patients carefully because adverse effects are more likely in elderly patients, particularly hallucinations, falls, CV events, respiratory problems, and GI effects.
• Assess patient's and family's knowledge of drug therapy.

🔄 Nursing diagnoses
• Impaired physical mobility related to presence of parkinsonism
• Risk for deficient fluid volume related to drug-induced nausea and vomiting
• Deficient knowledge related to drug therapy

▶ Planning and implementation
🔴 **ALERT:** Drug is for subcutaneous injection only. Avoid I.V. use.
• Give with an antiemetic to avoid severe nausea and vomiting. Start with trimethobenzamide 300 mg P.O. t.i.d. 3 days before starting apomorphine, and continue antiemetic at least 2 months.
🔴 **ALERT:** The prescribed dose should always be specified in milliliters rather than milligrams to avoid confusion. The dosing pen is marked in milliliters.
• When programming the dosing pen, it's possible to select the appropriate dose even though insufficient drug remains in the pen. To avoid insufficient dosing, track the amount of drug received at each dose and change the cartridge before drug runs out.
• Give test dose in a medically supervised setting to determine tolerability and effect.
Patient teaching
• Tell patient to avoid sudden position changes, especially rising too quickly from lying down. A sudden drop in blood pressure, dizziness, or fainting can occur.
• Urge patient to keep taking the prescribed antiemetic because nausea and vomiting are likely.
• Instruct patient or caregiver to document each dose to make sure enough drug remains in the cartridge to provide a full next dose.
• Tell patient or caregiver to wait at least 2 hours between doses.
• Show patient or caregiver how to read the dosing pen, and make sure he understands that it's marked in milliliters and not milligrams.
• Tell patient or caregiver to rotate injection sites and to wash hands before each injection. Applying ice to the site before and after the injection may reduce soreness, redness, pain, itching, swelling, or bruising at the site.
• Explain that hallucinations (either visual or auditory) may occur, and urge patient or caregiver to report them immediately.
• Explain that headaches may occur, and urge patient or caregiver to notify the prescriber if they become severe or don't go away.
• Advise patient to avoid hazardous activities that require alertness until drug effects are known.
• Caution patient to avoid consuming alcohol.

✅ Evaluation
• Patient has improved physical mobility.
• Patient doesn't experience nausea and vomiting.
• Patient and family state understanding of drug therapy.

aprepitant
(uh-pre-PIH-tant)
Emend

Pharmacologic class: substance P and neurokinin-1 receptor antagonist
Therapeutic class: centrally acting antiemetic
Pregnancy risk category: B

Indications and dosages
▶ **To prevent nausea and vomiting after moderately or highly emetogenic chemotherapy (including cisplatin); given with a 5-HT$_3$ antagonist and a corticosteroid.**
Adults: 125 mg P.O. on day 1 of treatment (1 hour before chemotherapy); then 80 mg P.O. every a.m. on days 2 and 3. Single doses up to 600 mg of aprepitant have been well tolerated.
▶ **Prevention of postoperative nausea and vomiting.** *Adults:* 40 mg P.O. within 3 hours before induction of anesthesia.

Contraindications and cautions
• Contraindicated in patients hypersensitive to drug or its components and in those taking astemizole, cisapride, pimozide, or terfenadine.
• Administration beyond 3 days per cycle of chemotherapy isn't recommended because of the potential for CYP3A4- and CYP2C9-related drug interactions.

🔆 **Lifespan:** In pregnant women, use with caution; drug hasn't been well studied. In breast-feeding women, use cautiously because it's unknown whether drug appears in breast milk. In children, safety and effectiveness haven't been established.

Adverse reactions

CNS: dizziness, *fatigue,* headache, insomnia.
CV: *bradycardia,* hypertension, hypotension.
EENT: tinnitus.
GI: abdominal pain, *anorexia, constipation, diarrhea,* gastritis, *nausea,* vomiting.
GU: proteinuria, UTI.
Hematologic: anemia, *febrile neutropenia, neutropenia.*
Respiratory: *hiccups.*
Skin: drug-induced rash with urticaria, pruritus, *Stevens-Johnson syndrome.*
Other: *angioedema.*

Interactions

Drug-drug. *Benzodiazepines, such as alprazolam and midazolam:* May increase levels of these drugs. Monitor patient for increased sedation and other CNS effects. Decrease benzodiazepine dose by 50% if use together is necessary.
Chemotherapy metabolized by CYP3A4, such as etoposide, ifosfamide, irinotecan, taxanes, and vinca alkaloids: May increase levels of these drugs, leading to increased toxicity. Avoid using together if possible.
Corticosteroids: May increase levels of these drugs, leading to increased toxicity. Decrease the dose of corticosteroids by 50% if use together is necessary.
CYP3A4 inducers (carbamazepine, phenytoin, rifampin): May decrease aprepitant level and decrease antiemetic effect. Avoid use together if possible.
CYP3A4 inhibitors (azole antifungals, diltiazem, erythromycin, nelfinavir, ritonavir): May increase aprepitant level, leading to increased toxicity. Avoid use together if possible.
Diltiazem: May increase diltiazem level. Monitor heart rate and blood pressure. Avoid use together if possible.
Hormonal contraceptives: May decrease the effectiveness of these drugs. If drugs must be used together, tell woman to use an additional form of birth control.

Phenytoin: May decrease phenytoin level. Avoid use together if possible. Monitor phenytoin level carefully; increase dose if needed.
SSRIs: May decrease the effectiveness of these drugs. Avoid use together if possible.
Tolbutamide: May decrease tolbutamide effectiveness. Monitor glucose level carefully.
Warfarin: May decrease warfarin effectiveness. Monitor INR carefully in the 2 weeks after each treatment, especially days 7 to 10. Avoid use together if possible.
Drug-herb. *St. John's wort:* May decrease antiemetic effects. Discourage use together.
Drug-food. *Grapefruit juice:* May increase drug level and toxicity. Discourage use together.

Effects on lab test results

• May increase creatinine, AST, and ALT levels.
• May decrease neutrophil counts.

Pharmacokinetics

Absorption: Well absorbed, with an average bioavailability of 60% to 65%. Food doesn't appear to have an effect. Level peaks about 4 hours after a dose.
Distribution: 95% protein-bound. May cross the placenta and blood–brain barrier.
Metabolism: Extensively in the liver by CYP3A4 and to a lesser degree by CYP1A2 and CYP2C19.
Excretion: In the urine and in the feces. *Half-life:* 9 to 13 hours.

Route	Onset	Peak	Duration
P.O.	Unknown	4 hr	9–13 hr

Action

Chemical effect: Selectively antagonizes substance P and neurokinin-1 receptors in the brain.
Therapeutic effect: Inhibits emesis caused by cytotoxic chemotherapy.

Available forms

Capsules: 40 mg, 80 mg, 125 mg

NURSING PROCESS

📝 **Assessment**

• Monitor patient thoroughly for drug and herb interactions before giving.
• Assess patient's condition before therapy and regularly thereafter.
• Watch for hypersensitivity reactions.

• Monitor therapy with other drugs for potential interactions, particularly drugs metabolized by the liver.

🔲 **Nursing diagnoses**
• Imbalanced nutrition: less than body requirements related to chemotherapy-induced nausea and vomiting
• Ineffective individual coping related to effects of chemotherapy
• Deficient knowledge related to drug therapy

🔲 **Planning and implementation**
• Give the first dose of drug 1 hour before chemotherapy.
• Give drug with other antiemetics, usually a 5-HT$_3$ antagonist and a corticosteroid.
• Don't give for longer than 3 days per chemotherapy cycle.
• Don't give for established nausea and vomiting. Make sure patient has other antiemetics to treat breakthrough emesis.
• Higher doses may lead to drowsiness and headache. Provide supportive treatment for overdose; because of the drug's mechanism of action, antiemetics may not be effective. Drug isn't removed by hemodialysis.
• Monitor CBC, liver function tests, and creatinine periodically during drug therapy.
Patient teaching
• Advise patient that drug is given with other antiemetics and shouldn't be taken alone to prevent chemotherapy-induced nausea and vomiting.
• Tell patient that you will give the first dose 1 hour before each chemotherapy cycle, and that he should take the second and third doses in the morning on days 2 and 3 of the treatment cycle. It may be taken with or without food.
• Instruct patient to treat breakthrough emesis with other antiemetics.
• Advise patient to tell his oncologist if he starts or stops any other drugs or herbal supplements during therapy because of the many drug and herb interactions.
• Advise women of childbearing age who are taking hormonal contraceptives to use an additional form of birth control during therapy.

🔲 **Evaluation**
• Patient has no chemotherapy-induced nausea or vomiting.

• Patient maintains adequate nutrition and hydration during chemotherapy treatments.
• Patient and family state understanding of drug therapy.

HIGH ALERT!

argatroban
(ahr-GAH-troh-ban)

Pharmacologic class: direct thrombin inhibitor
Therapeutic class: anticoagulant
Pregnancy risk category: B

Indications and dosages

▶ **Prevention or treatment of thrombosis in patients with heparin-induced thrombocytopenia.** *Adults:* 2 mcg/kg/minute, given as a continuous I.V. infusion; adjust dosage until steady state PTT is 1½ to 3 times the initial baseline value, not to exceed 100 seconds; maximum dose is 10 mcg/kg/minute.

The standard infusion rates for 2 mcg/kg/minute are shown below.

Body weight (kg)	Infusion rate (ml/hour)
50	6
60	7
70	8
80	10
90	11
100	12
110	13
120	14
130	16
140	17

🔲 **Adjust-a-dose:** For patients with moderate hepatic impairment, reduce initial dose to 0.5 mcg/kg/minute and give as a continuous infusion. Monitor PTT closely, and adjust dosage as needed.
▶ **Anticoagulation in patients with or at risk for heparin-induced thrombocytopenia during percutaneous coronary interventions (PCI).** *Adults:* 350 mcg/kg I.V. bolus over 3 to 5 minutes. Start a continuous I.V. infusion at 25 mcg/kg/minute. Check activated clotting time (ACT) 5 to 10 minutes after giving the bolus dose and every 5 to 10 minutes during the infusion until it stabilizes at 300 seconds or longer.

☒ **Adjust-a-dose:** See table below.

Activated clotting time	Additional I.V. bolus	Continuous I.V. infusion
< 300 sec	150 mcg/kg	30 mcg/kg/min***
300–450 sec	None needed	25 mcg/kg/min
> 450 sec	None needed	15 mcg/kg/min***

***Check ACT again after 5 to 10 minutes.

In case of dissection, impending abrupt closure, thrombus formation during the procedure, or inability to achieve or maintain an ACT longer than 300 seconds, give an additional bolus of 150 mcg/kg and increase infusion rate to 40 mcg/kg/minute. Check ACT again after 5 to 10 minutes.

⊛ **ALERT:** Check ACT every 20 to 30 minutes during a prolonged PCI.

▼ I.V. administration

• Dilute in normal saline solution, D_5W, or lactated Ringer's injection to 1 mg/ml.
• Dilute each 2.5-ml vial to 1:100 by mixing it with 250 ml of diluent.
• Mix the constituted solution by repeatedly turning over the diluent bag for 1 minute.
• Prepared solutions are stable for up to 24 hours at 77° F (25° C).
⊗ **Incompatibilities**
Other I.V. drugs.

Contraindications and cautions

• Contraindicated in patients hypersensitive to drug or its components and in patients with active bleeding.
• Use cautiously in patients with hepatic disease; diseases that increase the risk of hemorrhage, such as severe hypertension; very recent lumbar puncture, spinal anesthesia, or major surgery, especially involving the brain, spinal cord, or eye; and hematologic conditions linked to increased bleeding tendencies, such as congenital or acquired bleeding disorders and GI lesions and ulcerations.
⚖ **Lifespan:** In pregnant women, use only if clearly needed. Breast-feeding women should either stop drug or stop breast-feeding based on importance of the drug to the mother. In children, safety and effectiveness haven't been established.

Adverse reactions

CNS: fever, pain.
CV: atrial fibrillation, *cardiac arrest, cerebrovascular disorder, hemorrhage,* hypotension, vasodilation, *ventricular tachycardia.*
GI: abdominal pain, diarrhea, *GI bleeding,* hemoptysis, nausea, vomiting.
GU: abnormal renal function, groin bleeding, *hematuria,* UTI.
Hematologic: anemia.
Respiratory: cough, dyspnea, pneumonia.
Skin: bullous eruptions, rash.
Other: *allergic reactions (in patients also receiving thrombolytic therapy for acute MI),* brachial bleeding, infection, *sepsis.*

Interactions

Drug-drug. *Oral anticoagulants, antiplatelet drugs:* May prolong PT and INR and increase risk of bleeding. Avoid use together.
Thrombolytics: May increase risk of intracranial bleeding. Avoid use together.

Effects on lab test results

• May decrease hemoglobin level and hematocrit.
• May increase WBC and platelet counts, PTT, ACT, and INR.

Pharmacokinetics

Absorption: Given I.V.
Distribution: Mainly in the extracellular fluid. Drug is 54% protein-bound, of which 34% is bound to alpha$_1$-acid glycoprotein and 20% to albumin.
Metabolism: Mainly in the liver by hydroxylation. Formation of four metabolites is catalyzed in the liver by CYP3A4 and CYP3A5. Primary metabolite is 20% weaker than parent drug. Other metabolites appear in low levels in urine.
Excretion: Mainly in feces, presumably through the biliary tract. *Half-life:* 39 to 51 minutes.

Route	Onset	Peak	Duration
I.V.	Rapid	1–3 hr	Until infusion stops

Action

Chemical effect: Reversibly binds to the thrombin active site and inhibits reactions catalyzed or induced by thrombin, including fibrin formation; activation of coagulation factors V, VIII,

and XIII and protein C; and platelet aggregation. Inhibits the action of both free and clot-related thrombin.
Therapeutic effect: Prevents clot formation.

Available forms

Injection: 100 mg/ml

NURSING PROCESS

Assessment
• Assess patient for increased risk of bleeding or overt bleeding before starting therapy.
• Obtain baseline coagulation tests, platelet counts, hemoglobin level, and hematocrit before therapy. Check PTT and ACT. Note abnormalities, and notify prescriber.
• Stop all parenteral anticoagulants before giving drug.
• Assess patient's and family's knowledge of drug therapy.

Nursing diagnoses
• Ineffective tissue perfusion related to presence of blood clots
• Risk for injury related to increased PTT and increased risk of bleeding from drug therapy
• Deficient knowledge related to argatroban therapy and anticoagulant safety precautions

Planning and implementation
• If patient has unexplained drop in hematocrit or blood pressure or another unexplained symptom, suspect a hemorrhage and notify prescriber.
ALERT: Excessive anticoagulation, with or without bleeding, may occur with overdose. Symptoms of acute toxicity include loss of reflex, tremors, clonic seizures, limb paralysis, and coma. No specific antidote is available. Stop drug immediately and monitor PTT and other coagulation tests. Provide symptomatic and supportive therapy.
• To convert to oral anticoagulant therapy, give warfarin with argatroban at up to 2 mcg/kg/minute until INR is higher than 4. After stopping argatroban, repeat INR in 4 to 6 hours. If the repeat INR is below the desired therapeutic range, resume argatroban. Repeat daily until the desired therapeutic range is reached on warfarin alone.

ALERT: Don't confuse argatroban with Aggrastat.
Patient teaching
• Advise patient that drug can cause bleeding, and urge him to immediately report any unusual bruising, bleeding (nosebleeds, bleeding gums, ecchymosis, or hematuria), or tarry or bloody stools.
• Advise patient to avoid activities that carry a risk of injury or cuts, and instruct him to use a soft toothbrush and electric razor while taking argatroban.
• Tell patient to notify prescriber if she's pregnant, breast-feeding, or recently gave birth.
• Tell patient to notify prescriber if he has stomach ulcers or liver disease; if he's had recent surgery, radiation treatments, falls, or other injury; or if he develops wheezing, difficulty breathing, or rash.

Evaluation
• Patient doesn't develop blood clots while on drug.
• Patient has no unnecessary bruising or bleeding.
• Patient and family state understanding of drug therapy.

aripiprazole
(air-uh-PIP-rah-zol)
Abilify◆, Abilify Discmelt

Pharmacologic class: psychotropic
Therapeutic class: atypical antipsychotic
Pregnancy risk category: C

Indications and dosages

▶ **Schizophrenia.** *Adults:* Initially, 10 to 15 mg P.O. daily, increasing to a maximum of 30 mg daily if needed, after at least 2 weeks. Maintenance doses of 15 mg P.O. daily may be effective.
Adolescents ages 13 to 17: Initially, 2 mg P.O. daily for 2 days. Then 5 mg P.O. daily for 2 days, followed by target dosage of 10 mg P.O. daily. Further increases by 5 mg increments may be made up to maximum dosage of 30 mg daily.
▶ **Manic and mixed episodes associated with bipolar disorder.** *Adults:* Initially, 30 mg P.O.

once daily. May decrease to 15 mg daily based on patient response.

⃠ Adjust-a-dose: Give half the dose when giving with CYP3A4 or CYP2D6 inhibitors, particularly ketoconazole, quinidine, fluoxetine, or paroxetine. Double the dose when giving with CYP3A4 inducers, such as carbamazepine. Give original dose once other drugs are stopped.

▶ **Agitation in schizophrenia or in mixed or manic bipolar 1 disorder.** *Adults:* 5.25 to 15 mg by deep I.M. injection. Recommended dose is 9.75 mg. If needed, may give a second dose after 2 hours. Safety of giving more often than every 2 hours or more than 30 mg daily isn't known. Switch to P.O. route as soon as possible.

Contraindications and cautions

• Contraindicated in patients hypersensitive to drug.
• Use cautiously in patients with CV disease, cerebrovascular disease, or conditions that could predispose the patient to hypotension, such as dehydration or hypovolemia. Also use cautiously in patients with a history of seizures or with conditions that lower the seizure threshold and in those at risk for aspiration pneumonia, such as those with Alzheimer disease. Use caution in patients who engage in strenuous exercise, are exposed to extreme heat, take anticholinergic drugs, or are susceptible to dehydration.

⚖ Lifespan: In pregnant women, use only if benefits outweigh risks. In breast-feeding women, use cautiously because it's unknown whether drug appears in breast milk. In children, safety and effectiveness of drug haven't been established. In elderly patients, use cautiously because they may be more sensitive to drug.

Adverse reactions

CNS: abnormal gait, *akathisia, anxiety,* asthenia, cognitive and motor impairment, cogwheel rigidity, confusion, depression, dizziness, fatigue, fever, *headache,* hostility, *insomnia, lightheadedness,* **neuroleptic malignant syndrome, seizures,** *somnolence,* **suicidal thoughts,** tardive dyskinesia, tremor.
CV: *bradycardia,* chest pain, hypertension, orthostatic hypotension, peripheral edema, tachycardia.

EENT: blurred vision, conjunctivitis, ear pain, increased salivation, rhinitis.
GI: abdominal pain, anorexia, *constipation,* diarrhea, dry mouth, dyspepsia, esophageal dysmotility, *nausea, vomiting.*
GU: urinary incontinence.
Hematologic: anemia.
Metabolic: *hyperglycemia,* weight gain, weight loss.
Musculoskeletal: muscle cramps, neck pain, neck stiffness.
Respiratory: cough, dyspnea, pneumonia.
Skin: dry skin, ecchymosis, pruritus, rash, sweating, ulcer.
Other: flulike syndrome, inability to regulate body temperature.

Interactions

Drug-drug. *Antihypertensives:* May increase antihypertensive and orthostatic hypotensive effects. Monitor blood pressure.
Carbamazepine and other CYP3A4 inducers: May decrease level and effectiveness of aripiprazole. Double the usual aripiprazole dose, and monitor patient closely.
Fluoxetine, paroxetine, quinidine, and other CYP2D6 inhibitors; ketoconazole and other CYP3A4 inhibitors: May increase level and toxicity of aripiprazole. Halve the usual aripiprazole dose, and monitor patient closely.
Drug-food. *Grapefruit juice:* May increase drug level. Advise patient to avoid grapefruit juice during treatment.
Drug-lifestyle. *Alcohol use:* May increase CNS effects and impair motor function. Discourage use together.

Effects on lab test results

• May increase glucose and CK levels.

Pharmacokinetics

Absorption: Good. Absolute bioavailability is 87% and isn't affected by food.
Distribution: Extensive. Drug and major metabolites are 99% protein-bound, mainly to albumin.
Metabolism: Extensively through the CYP3A4 and CYP2D6 systems, with one active metabolite.
Excretion: In urine and feces. *Elimination half-life:* About 75 hours in patients with normal me-

tabolism and about 146 hours in those unable to metabolize the drug through CYP2D6.

Route	Onset	Peak	Duration
P.O.	Unknown	3–5 hr	Unknown
I.M.	Unknown	1–3 hr	Unknown

Action

Chemical effect: May exert antipsychotic effects through partial agonist activity at D2 and serotonin 5-HT$_{1A}$ receptors and antagonist activity at serotonin 5-HT$_{2A}$ receptors.
Therapeutic effect: Decreases psychotic behaviors.

Available forms

Injection: 7.5 mg/ml single-dose vial
Oral solution: 1 mg/ml
Tablets: 2 mg, 5 mg, 10 mg, 15 mg, 20 mg, 30 mg
Tablets (orally-disintegrating): 10 mg, 15 mg

NURSING PROCESS

⚖ Assessment
• Assess patient's condition before and after therapy.
• Watch for possible compliance issues.
• Be alert for adverse reactions and drug interactions.
• Assess patient's and family's knowledge of drug therapy.

⊕ Nursing diagnoses
• Disturbed thought processes related to underlying disease process
• Noncompliance related to medication regimen
• Deficient knowledge related to drug therapy

▶ Planning and implementation
⚠ **ALERT:** Neuroleptic malignant syndrome may occur. Monitor patient for hyperpyrexia, muscle rigidity, altered mental status, irregular pulse or blood pressure, tachycardia, diaphoresis, and cardiac arrhythmias. If signs and symptoms of neuroleptic malignant syndrome occur, stop drug immediately.
• Monitor patient for evidence of tardive dyskinesia. Elderly patients, particularly women, are at higher risk. If it occurs, stop drug.
⚠ **ALERT:** Monitor patients with diabetes regularly, because hyperglycemia may occur. Patients with risk factors for diabetes should have fasting

blood glucose level tested at baseline and periodically. Monitor patient for symptoms of hyperglycemia, including polydipsia, polyuria, polyphagia, and weakness. If symptoms develop, obtain fasting blood glucose test. In some cases, hyperglycemia is reversible by stopping drug.
• Give the smallest effective dose for the shortest time. Periodically reassess need for treatment.
• To reduce risk of an overdose, make sure only a small quantity of tablets is available at any time.
• The oral solution can be substituted on a milligram-per-milligram basis in place of the 5-, 10-, 15-, or 20-mg tablets up to 25 mg. Patients taking 30-mg tablets should receive 25 mg of solution.
• Overdose may cause somnolence and vomiting. Give activated charcoal during the first hour of overdose because 50% of a 15-mg dose is absorbed within the first hour. Dialysis isn't helpful because drug is highly protein-bound.

Patient teaching
• Tell patient to use caution when driving or operating hazardous machinery because psychoactive drugs may impair judgment, thinking, or motor skills.
• Tell patient that drug may be taken without regard to meals.
• Advise patient to avoid taking drug with grapefruit juice.
• Inform patient that symptoms should improve gradually over several weeks rather than immediately.
• Explain to patient that periodic blood work will be needed.
• Tell patient to avoid alcohol use while taking drug.
• Advise patient to limit strenuous activity while taking drug to avoid dehydration and becoming overheated.
• Tell patient to keep orally disintegrating tablet in blister package until ready to use. Then, with dry hands, carefully peel open the foil backing and place tablet on the tongue. It will dissolve rapidly in saliva, making liquid unnecessary. Tell patient not to split tablet.
• Tell patient to store oral solution in refrigerator and that it can be used up to 6 months after opening.

Reactions may be *common*, uncommon, *life-threatening*, or COMMON AND LIFE-THREATENING.

☑ Evaluation
- Patient has reduced symptoms of underlying disease process.
- Patient is compliant with drug regimen.
- Patient and family state understanding of drug therapy.

✳ New Drug

armodafinil
(are-moe-DAFF-ih-nihl)
Nuvigil

Pharmacologic class: CNS stimulant
Therapeutic class: analeptic
Pregnancy risk category: C

Indications and dosages

▶ **To improve wakefulness in patients with excessive sleepiness in obstructive sleep apnea/hypopnea syndrome (OAHS), narcolepsy, or shift-work sleep disorder (with continuous positive airway pressure).** *Adults:* 150 to 250 mg P.O. as a single dose in the morning. For OAHS, dosages exceeding 150 mg daily may not be more effective. For shift-work sleep disorder, 150 mg P.O. daily, 1 hour before start of shift.

⬛ Adjust-a-dose: Reduce dosage in patients who have severe hepatic impairment, with or without cirrhosis.

Contraindications and cautions

- Contraindicated in patients hypersensitive to or with a history of angioedema or anaphylactoid reaction to modafinil, armodafinil, or their active ingredients.
- Contraindicated in patients with left ventricular hypertrophy and patients with mitral valve prolapse who have developed mitral valve syndrome with other CNS stimulants.
- Use cautiously in geriatric patients; those with a history of drug abuse or dependence, psychiatric illness, cardiac disease, multi-organ hypersensitivity, or rash, including Stevens-Johnson syndrome; and those with severe hepatic impairment at a reduced dose.

⚘ Lifespan: In pregnant women, use cautiously. In breast-feeding women, use cautiously because it isn't known if the drug appears in breast milk. In patients younger than age 17 years, safety and effectiveness haven't been established.

Adverse reactions

CNS: agitation, anxiety, depression, dizziness, fatigue, *headache*, insomnia, migraine, nervousness, paresthesia, pyrexia, tremor.
CV: increased blood pressure, increased pulse, palpitations.
GI: abdominal pain, anorexia, constipation, decreased appetite, diarrhea, dry mouth, dyspepsia, loose stools, nausea, vomiting.
GU: polyuria.
Respiratory: dyspnea.
Skin: contact dermatitis, hyperhydrosis, rash, *Stevens-Johnson syndrome.*
Other: allergic reactions, flulike illness, pain, thirst.

Interactions

Drug-drug. *CNS stimulants, such as amphetamine, methylphenidate:* May produce additive effects. Use together cautiously.
Drugs metabolized by CYP2C19, such as diazepam, omeprazole, phenytoin, propranolol: May increase levels of these drugs when given with armodafinil. Monitor patient, and reduce dosages as needed.
Drugs metabolized by CYP3A, such as cyclosporine, ethinyl estradiol, midazolam, triazolam: May decrease levels of these drugs when given with armodafinil. Adjust dosages as needed.
Drugs that induce CYP3A, such as carbamazepine, phenobarbital, rifampin: May decrease armodafinil level. Check drug level, and adjust dosage as needed.
Drugs that inhibit CYP3A, such as erythromycin, ketoconazole: May increase armodafinil level. Monitor patient carefully.
Drug-food. *Any food:* May delay by several hours the onset of action and time to peak level.
Drug-lifestyle. *Alcohol use:* May counteract armodafinil's effect. Advise against consuming alcohol during therapy.

Effects on lab test results

- May increase gamma-glutamyltransferase and alkaline phosphatase levels.

Pharmacokinetics

Absorption: Readily absorbed after P.O. use. Food may delay onset of action or time to peak level.
Distribution: Moderate. About 60% bound to plasma proteins.

Metabolism: Mainly hepatic, including the cytochrome P-450 pathway.
Excretion: Mainly in feces. Less than 10% of parent compound appears in urine. *Half-life:* About 15 hours.

Route	Onset	Peak	Duration
P.O.	Unknown	2 hr	Unknown

Action

Chemical effect: Unknown. May be like sympathomimetics, such as amphetamine and methylphenidate. Also may inhibit dopamine reuptake.
Therapeutic effect: Improves daytime wakefulness.

Available forms

Tablets: 50 mg, 150 mg, 250 mg

NURSING PROCESS

Assessment
• Obtain history of patient's condition before therapy, and reassess regularly thereafter to monitor drug effectiveness.
• Assess patient's hepatic function before and during therapy.
• Assess patient's cardiac status before and during therapy.
• Assess patient's and family's knowledge of drug therapy.

Nursing diagnoses
• Sleep deprivation related to drug-induced insomnia
• Risk for injury related to drug-induced CNS adverse effects
• Deficient knowledge related to drug therapy

Planning and implementation
• Food will delay onset of action and time to peak level by several hours. Patient should take consistently with or without food.
• Armodafinil is a controlled substance; use it cautiously in patients with a history of drug abuse or dependence.
• In patients with a history of psychiatric illness, armodafinil may increase the risk of mania, delusions, hallucinations, and suicidal ideation.
• If patient develops a rash, stop therapy right away and monitor patient carefully. Armodafinil

and modafinil have been implicated in serious rash requiring hospitalization, Stevens-Johnson syndrome, toxic epidermal necrolysis, drug rash with eosinophilia and systemic symptoms, and multi-organ hypersensitivity reaction.
• Ask patient about drowsiness or sleepiness during specific activities to assess abnormal sleepiness. If patient seems excessively drowsy, advise against driving and other hazardous activities.

Patient teaching
• Instruct patient to report a history of drug abuse or dependence or liver, heart, or psychiatric disease before taking armodafinil.
• Instruct patient to stop taking armodafinil and to notify the prescriber if he develops a rash, hives, mouth sores, blisters, peeling skin, trouble swallowing, trouble breathing, or other signs of allergic reaction.
• Explain to patient that his level of wakefulness may not return to normal and that he should avoid driving and other hazardous tasks if he still feels excessive sleepiness.
• To help avoid potentially dangerous drug interactions, encourage patient to tell all prescribers about all of the drugs he takes.
• Tell a woman to notify her prescriber right away if she becomes pregnant or plans to breast-feed.

Evaluation
• Patient develops and maintains normal sleep-wake patterns.
• Patient has no adverse CNS effects.
• Patient and family state understanding of drug therapy.

aspirin (acetylsalicylic acid)
(ASS-prinn)
Ancasall†, Artria S.R.†, ASA†, ASA Enseals†, Asadol ♦ †, Asaphen ♦ †, Aspergum†, Bayer Aspirin†, Easprin†, Ecotrin†, Empirin†, Entrophen ♦ †, Halfprin†, Norwich Extra Strength†, Novasen†, Rivasa ♦ †, ZORprin†

Pharmacologic class: salicylate
Therapeutic class: nonopioid analgesic, antipyretic, anti-inflammatory, antiplatelet drug
Pregnancy risk category: C (D in third trimester)

Indications and dosages

▶ **Arthritis.** *Adults:* Initially, 2.4 to 3.6 g P.O. daily in divided doses. Maintenance dosage is 3.6 to 5.4 g P.O. daily in divided doses.
Children: 60 to 130 mg/kg P.O. daily in divided doses.
▶ **Mild pain or fever.** *Adults:* 325 to 650 mg P.O. or P.R. every 4 hours, p.r.n.
Children: For mild pain only, 65 mg/kg P.O. or P.R. daily in four to six divided doses.
▶ **Prevention of thrombosis.** *Adults:* 1.3 g P.O. daily in two to four divided doses.
▶ **Reduction of MI risk in patients with previous MI or unstable angina.** *Adults:* 160 to 325 mg P.O. daily. Give dose immediately when acute coronary syndrome is suspected.
▶ **Kawasaki syndrome (mucocutaneous lymph node syndrome).** *Children:* 80 to 100 mg/kg P.O. daily in four divided doses during febrile phase. Some patients may need up to 120 mg/kg. When fever subsides, decrease dosage to 3 to 8 mg/kg once daily, adjusted according to salicylate level.
▶ **Prophylaxis for transient ischemic attack (TIA).** *Adults:* 50 to 325 mg P.O. daily.
▶ **TIA.** *Adults:* 160 to 325 mg P.O. immediately within 48 hours of onset of stroke.
▶ **Prevention of reocclusion in coronary revascularization procedures.** *Adults:* 325 mg P.O. every 6 hours after surgery and for 1 year.
▶ **Rheumatic fever‡.** *Adults:* 4.9 to 7.8 g P.O. daily in divided doses every 4 to 6 hours for 1 to 2 weeks. Decrease to 60 to 70 mg/kg daily for 1 to 6 weeks; then gradually withdraw over 1 to 2 weeks.
Children: 90 to 130 mg/kg P.O. daily in divided doses every 4 to 6 hours.
▶ **Pericarditis after acute MI‡.** *Adults:* 160 to 325 mg P.O. daily.
▶ **Stent implantation‡.** *Adults:* 80 to 325 mg P.O. 2 hours before stent placement and 160 to 325 mg P.O. daily thereafter.

Contraindications and cautions

• Contraindicated in patients hypersensitive to drug and those with bleeding disorders such as hemophilia, von Willebrand disease, and telangiectasia; or NSAID-induced sensitivity reactions.
• Use cautiously in patients with GI lesions, impaired renal function, hypoprothrombinemia, vitamin K deficiency, thrombocytopenia, throm-
botic thrombocytopenic purpura, or severe hepatic impairment.
⚖ **Lifespan:** In pregnant women, use cautiously. In breast-feeding women, safety hasn't been established.
ⓈALERT: Because of the risk of Reye syndrome, the Centers for Disease Control and Prevention recommends not giving salicylates to children or teenagers who have or are recovering from chickenpox or flulike illness or who have acute febrile illnesses. In elderly patients, use cautiously because GI and renal adverse effects may be exacerbated.

Adverse reactions

EENT: *hearing loss, tinnitus.*
GI: dyspepsia, *GI bleeding,* GI distress, *nausea, occult bleeding, vomiting.*
GU: transient renal insufficiency.
Hematologic: *prolonged bleeding time, thrombocytopenia.*
Hepatic: *hepatitis.*
Skin: bruising, *rash,* urticaria.
Other: *angioedema,* hypersensitivity reactions (*anaphylaxis,* asthma), *Reye syndrome.*

Interactions

Drug-drug. *Ammonium chloride, other urine acidifiers:* May increase levels of aspirin products. Watch for aspirin toxicity.
Antacids in high doses (and other urine alkalinizers): May decrease levels of aspirin products. Watch for decreased aspirin effect.
Beta blockers: May decrease antihypertensive effect. Avoid long-term aspirin use if patient is taking antihypertensives.
Corticosteroids: May enhance salicylate elimination. Watch for decreased salicylate effect.
Heparin: May increase risk of bleeding. Monitor patient and coagulation studies closely if used together.
Ibuprofen, other NSAIDs: May negate the antiplatelet effect of low-dose aspirin therapy. Patients using immediate-release aspirin (not enteric coated) should take ibuprofen at least 30 minutes after aspirin, or more than 8 hours before aspirin. Occasional use of ibuprofen is unlikely to have a negative impact.
Methotrexate: May increase risk of methotrexate toxicity. Monitor patient closely.
NSAIDs: May alter pharmacokinetics of these drugs, leading to lower levels and decreased effectiveness. Avoid use together. May also in-

crease risk of GI bleeding. Monitor patient closely.
Oral anticoagulants: May increase risk of bleeding. Monitor patient for signs of bleeding.
Oral antidiabetics: May increase hypoglycemic effect. Monitor patient closely.
Probenecid, sulfinpyrazone: May decrease uricosuric effect. Avoid aspirin during therapy with these drugs.
Steroids: May increase risk of GI bleeding. Monitor patient closely.
Drug-herb. *Dong quai, feverfew, garlic, ginger, horse chestnut, red clover:* May increase risk of bleeding. Monitor patient for increased effects, and discourage use together.
Drug-food. *Caffeine:* May increase the absorption of aspirin. Monitor patient for increased effects.
Drug-lifestyle. *Alcohol use:* May increase risk of GI bleeding. Discourage use together.

Effects on lab test results

• May increase liver enzyme levels, BUN, serum creatinine, serum potassium, and may prolong bleeding times.
• May decrease WBC and platelet counts.

Pharmacokinetics

Absorption: Rapid and complete.
Distribution: Wide. Protein-binding to albumin is concentration-dependent; it ranges from 75% to 90% and decreases as level increases.
Metabolism: Hydrolyzed partially in GI tract to salicylic acid, but almost completely in liver.
Excretion: In urine as salicylate and its metabolites. *Half-life:* 15 to 20 minutes.

Route	Onset	Peak	Duration
P.O.			
buffered	5–30 min	1–2 hr	1–4 hr
enteric-coated	5–30 min	4–8 hr	1–4 hr
extended-release	5–30 min	1–2 hr	4–8 hr
regular	5–30 min	25–40 min	1–4 hr
solution	5–30 min	15–60 min	1–4 hr
P.R.	5–30 min	3–4 hr	1–4 hr

Action

Chemical effect: Produces analgesia by blocking prostaglandin synthesis (peripheral action), which may prevent lowering of pain threshold that occurs when prostaglandins sensitize pain receptors to stimulation. Drug exerts anti-inflammatory effects by inhibiting prostaglandins and other mediators of inflammatory response. Relieves fever by acting on hypothalamic heat-regulating center to cause peripheral vasodilation, which increases peripheral blood supply and promotes sweating, heat loss, and cooling by evaporation. In low doses, aspirin also appears to impede clotting by blocking prostaglandin synthesis, which prevents formation of platelet-aggregating substance thromboxane A2.
Therapeutic effect: Relieves pain, reduces fever and inflammation, and decreases risk of transient ischemic attacks and MI.

Available forms

Capsules: 325 mg†, 500 mg†
Chewing gum: 227.5 mg†
Suppositories: 60 mg†, 65 mg†, 120 mg†, 125 mg†, 130 mg†, 195 mg†, 200 mg†, 300 mg†, 325 mg†, 600 mg†, 650 mg†
Tablets: 325 mg†, 500 mg†, 600 mg†, 650 mg†
Tablets (chewable): 81 mg†
Tablets (enteric-coated): 81 mg†, 165 mg†, 325 mg†, 500 mg†, 650 mg†, 975 mg
Tablets (extended-release): 800 mg
Tablets (timed-release): 650 mg†

NURSING PROCESS

🔖 Assessment

• Obtain history of patient's pain or fever before therapy, and monitor patient throughout therapy.
• Be alert for adverse reactions and drug interactions.
• During long-term therapy, monitor salicylate level. Therapeutic level in arthritis is 10 to 30 mg/dl. With long-term therapy, mild toxicity may occur at levels of 20 mg/dl. Tinnitus may occur at levels of 30 mg/dl and above but doesn't reliably indicate toxicity, especially in very young patients and those older than age 60.
• Assess patient's and family's knowledge of drug therapy.

🔖 Nursing diagnoses

• Acute pain related to underlying condition
• Risk for injury related to drug-induced adverse GI reactions
• Deficient knowledge related to drug therapy

⟩ Planning and implementation

• Give aspirin with food, milk, antacid, or large glass of water to reduce adverse GI reactions.
• If patient has trouble swallowing, crush aspirin, combine it with soft food, or dissolve it in liquid. Give immediately after mixing with liquid because drug doesn't stay in solution. Don't crush enteric-coated aspirin.
• Enteric-coated products are absorbed slowly and not suitable for acute effects. These products cause less GI bleeding and may be more suited for long-term therapy, such as for arthritis.
• Give P.R. after a bowel movement or at night to maximize absorption.
• Hold dose and notify prescriber if bleeding, salicylism (tinnitus, hearing loss), or adverse GI reactions develop.
• Stop aspirin 5 to 7 days before elective surgery.
⚠ **ALERT:** Don't confuse aspirin with Asendin or Afrin.

Patient teaching

• Encourage patient to retain suppository for as long as possible, preferably at least 10 hours to maximize absorption.
• Advise patient receiving high-dose prolonged treatment to watch for petechiae, bleeding gums, and signs of GI bleeding and to maintain adequate fluid intake. Encourage use of a soft toothbrush.
• Because of many possible drug interactions involving aspirin, warn patient who takes prescription form to check with prescriber or pharmacist before taking herbal preparations or OTC combinations containing aspirin.
• Explain that various OTC preparations contain aspirin. Warn patient to read labels carefully to avoid overdose.
• Advise patient to avoid alcohol use during drug therapy.
• Advise patient to restrict intake of caffeine during drug therapy.
• Instruct patient to take aspirin with food or milk.
• Instruct patient not to chew enteric-coated products.
• Aspirin is a leading cause of poisoning in children. Emphasize safe storage of drugs in the home. Teach patient to keep aspirin and other drugs out of children's reach. Encourage use of child-resistant containers, even if children only visit occasionally.

☑ Evaluation

• Patient states that aspirin has relieved pain.
• Patient remains free from adverse GI effects throughout drug therapy.
• Patient and family state understanding of drug therapy.

atazanavir sulfate
(att-uh-ZAH-nuh-veer SULL-fayt)
Reyataz

Pharmacologic class: protease inhibitor
Therapeutic class: antiretroviral
Pregnancy risk category: B

Indications and dosages

▶ **HIV-1 infection, with other antiretrovirals.**
Adults: In antiretroviral-experienced patients, give 300 mg (as one 300-mg capsule or two 150-mg capsules) once daily plus 100 mg ritonavir once daily with food. For antiretroviral-naive patients, 400 mg (as two 200-mg capsules) P.O. once daily with food. When giving with efavirenz in antiretroviral-naive patients, give 300 mg atazanavir and 100 mg ritonavir with 600 mg efavirenz, all as a single daily dose with food. Recommendations for efavirenz and atazanavir in treatment-experienced patients haven't been established.
⊠ **Adjust-a-dose:** For patients with Child-Pugh class B hepatic insufficiency, reduce dosage to 300 mg P.O. once daily.

Contraindications and cautions

• Contraindicated in patients hypersensitive to drug or its components and in patients taking drugs highly dependent on CYP3A4 for clearance and for which elevated levels are linked to life-threatening effects, such as cisapride, dihydroergotamine, ergonovine, ergotamine, methylergonovine, midazolam, pimozide, triazolam.
• Use cautiously in patients with conduction system disease or hepatic impairment.
⚠ **ALERT:** May cause nephrolithiasis.
☀ **Lifespan:** In pregnant women, drug should be used only if potential benefits outweigh risk. To help monitor maternal-fetal outcomes of pregnant women, register pregnant women in the Antiretroviral Pregnancy Registry by calling 1-800-258-4263. In breast-feeding women, use cautiously because it's unknown whether drug

appears in breast milk. In children, an optimal regimen hasn't been established. In children younger than age 3, drug shouldn't be used because of a risk for kernicterus. In elderly patients, use cautiously because they may retain more of the drug.

Adverse reactions

CNS: depression, dizziness, fatigue, fever, *headache,* insomnia, pain, peripheral neurology symptoms.
CV: first-degree heart block.
GI: *abdominal pain,* diarrhea, *nausea,* vomiting.
Hepatic: *hepatitis,* jaundice, scleral icterus.
Metabolic: *lactic acidosis,* lipodystrophy, lipo-hypertrophy.
Musculoskeletal: arthralgia, back pain.
Respiratory: increased cough.
Skin: *rash.*

Interactions

Drug-drug. *Amiodarone, lidocaine (systemic), quinidine:* May increase levels of these drugs. Monitor levels.
Antacids and buffered drugs: May decrease atazanavir level. Give atazanavir 2 hours before or 1 hour after these drugs.
Atorvastatin, lovastatin, simvastatin: May increase statin level and the risk of myopathy and rhabdomyolysis. Use atorvastatin cautiously; don't use lovastatin or simvastatin.
Clarithromycin: May increase clarithromycin and atazanavir levels and decrease 14-OH clarithromycin levels. Reduce clarithromycin dose by 50% when giving with atazanavir. Because levels of the active metabolite 14-OH clarithromycin are significantly reduced, consider alternative therapy for indications other than infections caused by *Mycobacterium avium* complex.
Cyclosporine, sirolimus, tacrolimus: May increase immunosuppressant levels. Monitor immunosuppressant levels.
Didanosine buffered forms: May decrease atazanavir level. Give atazanavir 2 hours before or 1 hour after didanosine buffered forms.
Dihydroergotamine, ergonovine, ergotamine, methylergonovine: May cause life-threatening reactions, such as acute ergot toxicity characterized by peripheral vasospasm and ischemia of the limbs and other tissues. Don't use together.
Diltiazem: May increase diltiazem and desacetyl-diltiazem levels. Use cautiously. Reduce dosage of diltiazem by 50%. Monitor ECG.

Efavirenz: May decrease atazanavir level. If used together, give 300 mg atazanavir with 100 mg ritonavir and 600 mg efavirenz all as a single daily dose with food. This combination provides atazanavir exposure similar to that of 400 mg of atazanavir alone. Don't give atazanavir with efavirenz unless also given with ritonavir.
Ethinyl estradiol and norethindrone: May increase ethinyl estradiol and norethindrone levels. Use cautiously at the lowest effective dosage of each contraceptive component.
Felodipine, nicardipine, nifedipine, verapamil: May increase calcium channel blocker level. Use cautiously. Adjust calcium channel blocker dosage, and monitor ECG.
Fluticasone: May significantly increase fluticasone exposure, causing decreased serum cortisol level, leading to systemic corticosteroid effects (including Cushing syndrome). Don't use together, if possible.
H_2-receptor antagonists: May decrease atazanavir level. Give 12 hours apart.
Indinavir: May increase risk of hyperbilirubinemia. Use together isn't recommended.
Irinotecan: May interfere with irinotecan metabolism, resulting in increased irinotecan toxicities. Don't use together.
Itraconazole, ketoconazole: May interact with ritonavir-boosted atazanavir. Use together cautiously.
Midazolam, triazolam: May cause life-threatening reactions, such as prolonged or increased sedation or respiratory depression. Don't use together.
Nevirapine: May decrease atazanavir level. Use together isn't recommended.
Pimozide: May cause life-threatening reactions, such as cardiac arrhythmias. Don't use together.
Proton pump inhibitors: May substantially decrease atazanavir level and therapeutic effect. Use together isn't recommended.
Rifabutin: May increase rifabutin level. Reduce rifabutin dosage by up to 75%.
Rifampin: May decrease level of most protease inhibitors, resulting in loss of therapeutic effect and development of resistance. Don't use together.
Ritonavir: May increase atazanavir level. Give 300 mg atazanavir once daily with 100 mg ritonavir once daily, with food.
Saquinavir (soft gelatin capsules): May increase saquinavir level. Appropriate dose for this combination hasn't been established.

Reactions may be *common,* uncommon, *life-threatening*, or COMMON AND LIFE-THREATENING.

Sildenafil, tadalafil, vardenafil: May increase levels of these drugs and adverse events, including hypotension, visual changes, and priapism. Tell patient to use caution and reduced dosages: sildenafil at 25 mg every 48 hours, tadalafil at 10 mg every 72 hours, and vardenafil at 2.5 mg every 72 hours. Monitor patient for adverse events.

Tenofovir: May decrease atazanavir level, causing resistance. Give both drugs with ritonavir.

Trazodone: May increase trazodone level, causing nausea, dizziness, hypotension, and syncope. Avoid use together, or use cautiously with a lower trazodone dosage.

Tricyclic antidepressants: May increase tricyclic antidepressant level. Monitor level.

Voriconazole: May interact. Monitor patient for toxicity. Avoid use with ritonavir-boosted atazanavir.

Warfarin: May increase warfarin level. Monitor INR.

Drug-herb. *St. John's wort:* May reduce atazanavir level, resulting in loss of therapeutic effect and development of resistance. Discourage use together.

Effects on lab test results

• May increase AST, ALT, total bilirubin, amylase, and lipase levels. May decrease hemoglobin level and hematocrit.

• May decrease neutrophil count.

Pharmacokinetics

Absorption: Rapid. Level peaks at about 2½ hours. Food enhances bioavailability.

Distribution: 86% protein-bound and binds to alpha₁-acid glycoprotein and albumin to a similar extent.

Metabolism: Extensively, mainly by the liver.

Excretion: In urine and feces. About 7% excreted unchanged in urine. *Elimination half-life:* About 7 hours.

Route	Onset	Peak	Duration
P.O.	Unknown	2 hr	Unknown

Action

Chemical effect: Prevents the formation of mature virions within HIV-1 infected cells.

Therapeutic effect: Treatment of HIV infection.

Available forms

Capsules: 100 mg, 150 mg, 200 mg, 300 mg

NURSING PROCESS

Assessment

• Monitor cardiac status during therapy.

• Test women for pregnancy before starting therapy.

• Monitor liver function tests periodically during therapy.

• Assess patient's and family's knowledge of drug therapy.

Nursing diagnoses

• Ineffective protection related to underlying HIV infection

• Risk for injury related to adverse reactions

• Deficient knowledge related to drug therapy

Planning and implementation

• Drug may prolong PR interval.

• Most patients develop asymptomatic increase in indirect bilirubin, which may cause yellowing of skin or sclerae. Hyperbilirubinemia is reversible when drug is stopped.

• Various degrees of cross-resistance among protease inhibitors may occur. Resistance to this drug doesn't preclude later use of other protease inhibitors. Give drug with other antiretrovirals.

• Patient should remain under the care of a physician while taking drug.

• At high doses, jaundice is caused by indirect (unconjugated) hyperbilirubinemia (without liver function test changes), or prolonged PR interval may occur.

• Treat overdose with general supportive measures, including monitoring of vital signs and ECG. Induce vomiting or use gastric lavage to eliminate unabsorbed drug. Also give activated charcoal to aid removal of unabsorbed drug. Because drug is highly metabolized by the liver and is highly protein-bound, dialysis probably won't help.

Patient teaching

• Tell patient that sustained decreases in HIV RNA have been linked to a reduced risk of progression to AIDS and death.

• Tell patient to remain in a physician's care while taking drug.

• Tell patient to take drug with food every day and to take other antiretrovirals as prescribed.

- Inform patient that drug doesn't cure HIV and that he may develop opportunistic infections and other complications of HIV disease. Also explain that drug doesn't reduce the risk of transmitting HIV to others.
- Tell patient not to alter dose or stop therapy without consulting the prescriber.
- If a dose is delayed, advise patient to take it as soon as possible and then return to the normal schedule. If a dose is skipped, tell patient not to double the next dose.
- Tell patient to consult prescriber about dizziness or light-headedness.
- Tell patient that elevations in indirect bilirubin may occur and to report yellowing of the skin or the whites of the eyes.
- Inform patient that drug may cause redistribution or accumulation of body fat.
- To prevent postnatal transmission of HIV, tell HIV-infected mothers to avoid breast-feeding.

☑ Evaluation
- Patient remains free from infection.
- Patient sustains no injury from adverse reactions.
- Patient and family state understanding of drug therapy.

HIGH ALERT!

atenolol
(uh-TEN-uh-lol)
Apo-Atenol ◆ , Novo-Atenol ◆ , Nu-Atenol ◆ , Tenormin⌀

Pharmacologic class: beta blocker
Therapeutic class: antihypertensive, antianginal
Pregnancy risk category: D

Indications and dosages

▶ **Hypertension.** *Adults:* Initially, 50 mg P.O. once daily. Increase to 100 mg once daily after 7 to 14 days. Doses higher than 100 mg aren't likely to produce further benefit.
☒ Adjust-a-dose: *Geriatric patients:* Initially, 25 mg P.O. daily, increased slowly until desired response. Also reduce dosage in patients with renal impairment. If creatinine clearance is 15 to 35 ml/minute, maximum dosage is 50 mg daily. If clearance is less than 15 ml/minute, maximum dosage is 25 mg daily.

▶ **Angina pectoris.** *Adults:* 50 mg P.O. once daily. Increase as needed to 100 mg daily after 7 days for optimal effect. Maximum dosage is 200 mg daily.
▶ **To reduce CV mortality rate and risk of reinfarction in patients with acute MI.**
Adults: 5 mg I.V. over 5 minutes, followed by another 5 mg 10 minutes later. After another 10 minutes, 50 mg P.O., followed by 50 mg P.O. in 12 hours. Thereafter, 100 mg P.O. daily (as a single dose or 50 mg b.i.d.) for at least 7 days.
▶ **To slow rapid ventricular response to atrial tachyarrhythmias after acute MI without left ventricular dysfunction and AV block‡.**
Adults: 2.5 to 5 mg I.V. over 2 to 5 minutes, p.r.n., to control rate. Maximum, 10 mg over a 10- to 15-minute period.

▼ I.V. administration
- Mix doses with D_5W, normal saline solution, or dextrose and sodium chloride solutions.
- Give by slow injection, not to exceed 1 mg/minute.
- Solution is stable for 48 hours after mixing.
⊗ **Incompatibilities**
Other I.V. drugs.

Contraindications and cautions
- Contraindicated in patients with sinus bradycardia, greater than first-degree heart block, overt cardiac failure, or cardiogenic shock, or in those hypersensitive to atenolol or its components.
- Use cautiously in patients at risk for heart failure and in those with bronchospastic disease, diabetes, and hyperthyroidism.
▲ **Lifespan:** In pregnant women, don't use unless absolutely necessary because fetal harm can occur. In breast-feeding women, use cautiously. In children, safety of drug hasn't been established.

Adverse reactions
CNS: fatigue, fever, hallucinations, headache, lethargy.
CV: BRADYCARDIA, intermittent claudication, PROFOUND HYPOTENSION, *second- or third-degree AV block.*
EENT: visual disturbances.
GI: diarrhea, dry mouth, nausea, vomiting.
GU: impotence, Peyronie disease.
Respiratory: *bronchospasm,* dyspnea.
Skin: rash, reversible alopecia.

Reactions may be *common,* uncommon, *life-threatening,* or COMMON AND LIFE-THREATENING.

Interactions

Drug-drug. *Antihypertensives:* May increase hypotensive effect. Use together cautiously.
Digoxin, diltiazem: May cause excessive brady-cardia and increase depressant effect on myo-cardium. Use together cautiously.
Insulin, oral antidiabetics: May alter dosage re-quirements in previously stabilized patient with diabetes. Observe patient carefully.
Prazosin and terazosin: May increase the risk of orthostatic hypotension early in use together. Help patient to stand slowly until effects are known.
Reserpine: May cause hypotension. Use togeth-er cautiously.
Verapamil: May increase the effects of both drugs. Monitor cardiac function closely, and de-crease dosages as needed.

Effects on lab test results

- May increase BUN, creatinine, potassium, uric acid, transaminase, alkaline phosphatase, triglyceride, and LDH levels. May increase or decrease glucose level.
- May increase platelet count.

Pharmacokinetics

Absorption: About 50% to 60%.
Distribution: Into most tissues and fluids ex-cept brain and CSF. About 5% to 15% protein-bound.
Metabolism: Minimal.
Excretion: From 40% to 50% of dose is excret-ed unchanged in urine; remainder is excreted as unchanged drug and metabolites in feces. *Half-life:* 6 to 7 hours.

Route	Onset	Peak	Duration
P.O.	1 hr	2–4 hr	24 hr
I.V.	5 min	5 min	12 hr

Action

Chemical effect: Selectively blocks beta$_1$ re-ceptors; decreases cardiac output, peripheral re-sistance, and cardiac oxygen consumption; and depresses renin secretion.
Therapeutic effect: Decreases blood pressure, relieves angina, and reduces CV mortality rate and risk of reinfarction after acute MI.

Available forms

Injection: 5 mg/10 ml
Tablets: 25 mg, 50 mg, 100 mg

NURSING PROCESS

Assessment
- Obtain history of patient's underlying condi-tion.
- If prescribed for hypertension, monitor drug's effectiveness by checking patient's blood pres-sure often. Full antihypertensive effect may not occur for 1 to 2 weeks. For angina pectoris, monitor frequency and severity of anginal pain. For reducing CV mortality rate and risk of rein-farction after acute MI, monitor signs of rein-farction.
- Be alert for adverse reactions and drug inter-actions.
- Assess patient's and family's knowledge of drug therapy.

Nursing diagnoses
- Risk for injury related to underlying condition
- Decreased cardiac output related to drug-induced adverse CV reactions
- Deficient knowledge related to drug therapy

Planning and implementation
- Adjust dosage in patients with renal insuffi-ciency and those receiving hemodialysis.
- Check patient's apical pulse before giving drug; if slower than 60 beats/minute, withhold drug and call prescriber.
- Give as a single daily dose.
- Be prepared to treat shock or hypoglycemia because this drug masks common signs of these conditions.
- Notify prescriber immediately if patient shows signs of decreased cardiac output.
- **ALERT:** Withdraw drug gradually over 1 to 2 weeks to avoid serious adverse reactions.
- **ALERT:** Don't confuse atenolol with timolol or albuterol.

Patient teaching
- Teach patient how to take his pulse. Tell him not to take the drug and to call his prescriber if pulse rate is slower than 60 beats/minute.
- Warn patient that stopping drug abruptly can worsen angina and MI. Drug should be with-drawn gradually over 2 weeks.
- Tell patient to take drug at same time every day.
- Tell patient to notify prescriber of excessive fatigue.
- Tell a woman to notify her prescriber if she be-comes pregnant because drug must be stopped.

☑ Evaluation
• Patient's underlying condition improves with drug therapy.
• Patient's cardiac output remains unchanged throughout drug therapy.
• Patient and family state understanding of drug therapy.

atomoxetine hydrochloride
(ATT-oh-mocks-uh-teen high-droh-KLOR-ighd)
Strattera✒

Pharmacologic class: selective norepinephrine reuptake inhibitor
Therapeutic class: attention deficit hyperactivity disorder (ADHD) drug
Pregnancy risk category: C

Indications and dosages

▶ **Adjunct therapy for ADHD.** *Adults and children weighing more than 70 kg (154 lb):* Initially, 40 mg P.O. daily; increase after at least 3 days to a target total daily dose of 80 mg P.O. as a single dose in the morning or two evenly divided doses in the morning and late afternoon or early evening. After 2 to 4 weeks, increase total dosage to a maximum of 100 mg, if needed. *Children weighing 70 kg or less:* Initially, 0.5 mg/kg P.O. daily; increase after at least 3 days to a target total daily dose of 1.2 mg/kg P.O. as a single dose in the morning or two evenly divided doses in the morning and late afternoon or early evening. Don't exceed 1.4 mg/kg or 100 mg daily, whichever is less.
⧈ **Adjust-a-dose:** For patients with moderate hepatic impairment, give 50% of the normal dose; in those with severe hepatic impairment, give 25% of the normal dose.

Contraindications and cautions

• Contraindicated in patients hypersensitive to drug or its components, those who took an MAO inhibitor within the past 14 days, those who have jaundice or laboratory evidence of liver injury, and those with narrow-angle glaucoma.
• Use cautiously in patients with hypertension, tachycardia, moderate to severe hepatic insufficiency, or CV or cerebrovascular disease.
⚘ **Lifespan:** In pregnant and breast-feeding women, use cautiously. In children younger than age 6, safety and effectiveness of drug haven't been established. In the elderly, safety and effectiveness haven't been established.

Adverse reactions

CNS: abnormal dreams, crying, depression, dizziness, early morning awakening, fatigue, *headache, insomnia,* irritability, mood swings, paresthesia, pyrexia, sedation, sleep disorder, somnolence, **suicidal thoughts,** tremor.
CV: hypertension, orthostatic hypotension, palpitations, tachycardia.
EENT: ear infection, nasal congestion, mydriasis, nasopharyngitis, rhinorrhea, sinus congestion, sinusitis, sore throat.
GI: abdominal pain, constipation, decreased appetite, dry mouth, dyspepsia, flatulence, gastroenteritis, nausea, vomiting.
GU: delayed menses, difficulty in micturition, dysmenorrhea, ejaculatory problems, erectile disturbance, impotence, menstrual disorder, prostatitis, urinary hesitation, urine retention.
Metabolic: weight loss.
Musculoskeletal: arthralgia, myalgia.
Respiratory: *cough,* upper respiratory tract infection.
Skin: dermatitis, increased sweating, pruritus.
Other: decreased libido, hot flashes, influenza, rigors.

Interactions

Drug-drug. *Albuterol:* May increase CV effects. Use together cautiously.
MAO inhibitors: May cause hyperthermia, rigidity, myoclonus, autonomic instability with possibly rapid fluctuations of vital signs, and mental status changes. Separate atomoxetine and MAO inhibitor doses by 14 days.
Pressor agents: May increase blood pressure. Use together cautiously.
Strong CYP2D6 inhibitors (fluoxetine, paroxetine, quinidine): May increase atomoxetine level. Monitor patient closely.

Effects on lab test results

• May increase liver enzyme levels.

Pharmacokinetics

Absorption: Rapid.
Distribution: Mainly into total body water. 98% bound to plasma proteins, mainly albumin.
Metabolism: Mainly through CYP2D6. Absolute bioavailability is about 63% in patients

A

with extensive metabolism and 94% in those with poor metabolism.
Excretion: More than 80% of the dose in urine, and less than 17% of the dose via feces. *Half-life:* 2½ hours.

Route	Onset	Peak	Duration
P.O.	Rapid	1–2 hr	Unknown

Action

Chemical effect: Unknown. May relate to selective inhibition of presynaptic norepinephrine transporter.
Therapeutic effect: Decreases symptoms of ADHD.

Available forms

Capsules: 10 mg, 18 mg, 25 mg, 40 mg, 60 mg, 80 mg, 100 mg

NURSING PROCESS

⚞ Assessment
• Assess patient's condition before therapy and regularly thereafter.
• Watch for hypersensitivity reaction and evidence of liver injury (nausea, anorexia, pruritus, jaundice, right upper quadrant pain, flulike symptoms).
• Assess patient's and family's knowledge of disease and drug therapy.

⚙ Nursing diagnoses
• Disturbed thought processes related to underlying disease
• Imbalanced nutrition: less than the body requires, related to adverse effect of medication
• Deficient knowledge related to drug therapy

▷ Planning and implementation
• Use drug as part of a total treatment program for ADHD, with psychological, educational, and social intervention.
• Periodically reevaluate patients taking drug for extended periods to determine drug's usefulness.
⑨ **ALERT:** Monitor children and adolescents closely for agitation, irritability, and suicidal thinking or behaviors.
• Monitor growth during treatment. If growth or weight gain is unsatisfactory, consider stopping therapy.

• Monitor blood pressure and pulse at baseline, after each dose increase, and periodically during treatment.
• Monitor patient for urinary hesitancy, urine retention, and sexual dysfunction.
⑨ **ALERT:** If patient becomes jaundiced or has abnormal liver function test results, stop drug.
• The patient can stop drug without tapering.
• In case of overdose, monitor patient closely and provide supportive care. Perform gastric lavage and give activated charcoal to prevent absorption.
Patient teaching
• Advise parents to call prescriber immediately if their child develops unusual behaviors or suicidal thoughts.
• Tell pregnant women, women planning to become pregnant, and breast-feeding women to consult prescriber before taking drug.
• Tell patient to use caution when operating a vehicle or machinery until drug effects are known.
• Tell patient to report itching, yellow skin, yellow sclera, nausea or decreased appetite, abdominal pain, or flulike symptoms to prescriber immediately.

✓ Evaluation
• Patient has reduced signs and symptoms of underlying disease.
• Patient maintains adequate nutritional status.
• Patient and family state understanding of drug therapy.

atorvastatin calcium
(uh-TOR-vah-stah-tin KAL-see-um)
Lipitor⌀

Pharmacologic class: HMG-CoA reductase inhibitor
Therapeutic class: antilipemic
Pregnancy risk category: X

Indications and dosages

▶ **Adjunct to diet to reduce elevated LDL, total cholesterol, apo B, and triglyceride levels and to increase HDL level in patients with primary hypercholesterolemia (heterozygous familial and nonfamilial) and mixed dyslipidemia (Fredrickson Types IIa and IIb).**
Adults: Initially, 10 or 20 mg P.O. once daily.

Start dosage at 40 mg once daily for patients who require a reduction in LDL cholesterol level of more than 45%. Increase dosage, as needed, to maximum of 80 mg daily as single dose. Base dosage on lipid levels drawn within 4 to 6 weeks after starting therapy.

▶ **Alone or as an adjunct to lipid-lowering treatments such as LDL apheresis to reduce total cholesterol and LDL levels in patients with homozygous familial hypercholesterolemia.** *Adults:* 10 to 80 mg P.O. daily.

▶ **Heterozygous familial hypercholesterolemia.** *Children ages 10 to 17:* Give 10 mg P.O. once daily. Adjust dosage after 4 weeks to 20 mg daily.

▶ **To reduce the risk of MI, stroke, angina, and revascularization procedures in patients with no evidence of CAD but with multiple risk factors.** *Adults:* 10 mg P.O. daily.

▪ **NEW INDICATION: To reduce risk of nonfatal MI, fatal and non-fatal strokes, angina, heart failure, and revascularization procedures in patients with coronary heart disease.** *Adults:* Initially, 10 to 20 mg P.O. daily. May increase based on patient response and tolerance; usual dosage, 10 to 80 mg P.O. daily.

Contraindications and cautions

• Contraindicated in patients hypersensitive to drug and in those with active liver disease or conditions linked with unexplained persistent increases in transaminase levels. Also contraindicated in patients with serious, acute conditions that suggest myopathy and in those at risk for renal failure caused by rhabdomyolysis from trauma; major surgery; severe metabolic, endocrine, and electrolyte disorders; severe acute infection; hypotension; or uncontrolled seizures.

• Adolescent girls must be at least 1 year postmenarche.

⚘ **Lifespan:** In pregnant or breast-feeding women and in women who may become pregnant, drug is contraindicated.

Adverse reactions

CNS: asthenia, fever, *headache,* malaise.
CV: chest pain.
EENT: pharyngitis, sinusitis.
GI: abdominal pain, constipation, diarrhea, dyspepsia, flatulence.
Musculoskeletal: arthralgia, back pain, myalgia, *rhabdomyolysis.*

Skin: rash, *erythema multiforme, Stevens-Johnson syndrome, toxic epidermal necrolysis.*
Other: accidental injury, *anaphylaxis, angioedema,* flulike syndrome, hypersensitivity reaction, infection.

Interactions

Drug-drug. *Antacids:* May decrease bioavailability. Give separately.
Azole antifungals, cyclosporine, erythromycin, fibric acid derivatives, niacin: May increase risk of myopathy. Avoid use together.
Bile-acid sequestrants, such as colestipol: May decrease atorvastatin level; however, these drugs may be used together for therapeutic effect. Monitor patient.
Digoxin: May increase digoxin level. Monitor digoxin level.
Erythromycin: May increase drug level. Monitor patient.
Fluconazole, itraconazole, ketoconazole: May increase level and adverse effects of atorvastatin. Avoid this combination. If they must be given together, reduce atorvastatin dosage.
Hormonal contraceptives: May increase hormone levels. Consider when selecting a hormonal contraceptive.
Warfarin: May increase anticoagulant effect. Monitor INR and patient for bleeding.
Drug-food. *Grapefruit juice:* Large quantities may increase atorvastatin level, increasing the risk of myopathy. Advise patient to avoid consuming large amounts of grapefruit juice.

Effects on lab test results

• May increase ALT and AST levels.

Pharmacokinetics

Absorption: Rapid.
Distribution: 98% bound to plasma proteins.
Metabolism: By liver.
Excretion: In bile. *Half life:* 14 hours.

Route	Onset	Peak	Duration
P.O.	Unknown	1–2 hr	20–30 hr

Action

Chemical effect: Selectively inhibits HMG-CoA reductase, which converts HMG-CoA to mevalonate, a precursor of sterols.
Therapeutic effect: Lowers cholesterol and lipoprotein levels.

Reactions may be *common*, uncommon, *life-threatening*, or COMMON AND LIFE-THREATENING.

Available forms

Tablets: 10 mg, 20 mg, 40 mg, 80 mg

NURSING PROCESS

⚡ Assessment
• Monitor patient's lipid and liver function levels at baseline and periodically thereafter.
• Monitor patient for signs of rhabdomyolysis, especially if taking more than one class of lipid-lowering drugs.
• Assess patient's and family's knowledge of drug therapy.

✤ Nursing diagnoses
• Risk for injury related to elevated cholesterol levels
• Deficient knowledge related to drug therapy

▶ Planning and implementation
• Use drug only after diet and other nondrug treatments prove ineffective. Patient should follow a low-cholesterol diet before and during therapy.
• Drug can be given as a single dose at any time of the day, with or without food.
• Obtain liver function test results and lipid levels before therapy, after 6 and 12 weeks, after a dosage increase, and periodically thereafter.
• Check CK level if patient complains of muscle pain, tenderness, or weakness.
⊛ **ALERT:** Don't confuse Lipitor with Levatol.
Patient teaching
• Teach patient about proper diet, weight control, and exercise, and explain their role in controlling elevated lipid levels.
• Tell patient to inform prescriber of adverse reactions, such as muscle pain, tenderness, or weakness, especially if accompanied by fever or malaise.
• Urge a woman to notify her prescriber immediately if pregnancy is suspected.

☑ Evaluation
• Patient's cholesterol level is within normal limits.
• Patient and family state understanding of drug therapy.

atovaquone
(uh-TOH-vuh-kwohn)
Mepron

Pharmacologic class: ubiquinone analogue
Therapeutic class: antiprotozoal
Pregnancy risk category: C

Indications and dosages

▶ **Prevention of *Pneumocystis jiroveci* (*carinii*) pneumonia in patients who can't tolerate co-trimoxazole, including those infected with HIV.** *Adults and children age 13 and older:* 1,500 mg (10 ml) P.O. daily with food.
Infants ages 1 to 3 months and children older than 24 months‡: 30 mg/kg P.O. once daily.
Infants ages 4 to 24 months‡: 45 mg/kg P.O. daily.
▶ **Mild to moderate *P. jiroveci* (*carinii*) pneumonia in patients who can't tolerate co-trimoxazole.** *Adults and children age 13 and older:* 750 mg P.O. b.i.d. for 21 days.
▶ **Prevention of toxoplasmosis in HIV-infected patients‡.** *Adults and children age 13 and older:* 1,500 mg P.O. daily.

Contraindications and cautions

• Contraindicated in patients hypersensitive to drug.
• Use cautiously with other highly protein-bound drugs because drug is almost completely protein-bound. Also use cautiously in those with liver disease.
⚘ **Lifespan:** In pregnant and breast-feeding women, use cautiously. In children, safety of drug hasn't been established. In elderly patients, use cautiously.

Adverse reactions

CNS: asthenia, depression, dizziness, dreams, fever, *headache,* insomnia.
EENT: visual difficulties.
GI: *abdominal pain,* anorexia, diarrhea, dyspepsia, gastritis, *nausea,* oral ulcers, *vomiting.*
Musculoskeletal: myalgia.
Respiratory: cough, rhinitis, sinusitis.
Skin: pruritus, rash, sweating.
Other: flulike syndrome.

Interactions

Drug-drug. *Highly protein-bound drugs:* May compete for receptor sites affecting drug levels. Use together cautiously.
Rifabutin, rifampin: May decrease atovaquone's steady-state level. Avoid use together.

Effects on lab test results

• May increase alkaline phosphatase, ALT, and AST levels. May decrease hemoglobin level and hematocrit.
• May decrease WBC count.

Pharmacokinetics

Absorption: Limited. Bioavailability is doubled when given with meals. Fat enhances absorption significantly.
Distribution: 99.9% bound to plasma proteins.
Metabolism: Not metabolized.
Excretion: Undergoes enterohepatic cycling and is excreted mainly in feces. *Half-life:* 2 to 3 days.

Route	Onset	Peak	Duration
P.O.	Unknown	1–8 hr	Unknown

Action

Chemical effect: Unknown; may interfere with electron transport in protozoal mitochondria, inhibiting enzymes needed for synthesis of nucleic acids and adenosine triphosphate.
Therapeutic effect: Kills *P. jiroveci (carinii)* protozoa.

Available forms

Suspension: 750 mg/5 ml

NURSING PROCESS

◪ Assessment

• Obtain history of patient's protozoal respiratory infection, and reassess regularly.
• Be alert for adverse reactions.
• Monitor patient's hydration if adverse GI reactions occur.
• Assess patient's and family's knowledge of drug therapy.

◫ Nursing diagnoses

• Ineffective protection related to presence of susceptible protozoal organisms

• Risk for deficient fluid volume related to drug-induced adverse GI reactions
• Deficient knowledge related to drug therapy

◪ Planning and implementation

• Give drug with food to improve bioavailability.
Patient teaching
• Instruct patient to take drug with meals because food significantly enhances absorption.
• Warn patient not to perform hazardous activities if dizziness occurs.
• Emphasize importance of taking drug as prescribed, even if patient is feeling better.
• Tell patient to notify prescriber if serious adverse reactions occur.

☑ Evaluation

• Patient's infection is eradicated.
• Patient remains adequately hydrated throughout therapy.
• Patient and family state understanding of drug therapy.

HIGH ALERT!

atracurium besylate
(at-truh-KYOO-ree-um BESS-eh-layt)
Tracrium

Pharmacologic class: nondepolarizing neuromuscular blocker
Therapeutic class: skeletal muscle relaxant
Pregnancy risk category: C

Indications and dosages

▶ **Adjunct to general anesthesia to facilitate endotracheal intubation and cause skeletal muscle relaxation during surgery or mechanical ventilation.** *Adults and children older than age 2:* Initially 0.4 to 0.5 mg/kg by I.V. bolus. During prolonged surgery, give maintenance dose of 0.08 to 0.1 mg/kg within 20 to 45 minutes of initial dose. Maintenance doses may be given every 15 to 25 minutes in patients receiving balanced anesthesia. During prolonged surgery, a constant infusion of 5 to 9 mcg/kg/minute may be used after initial bolus.
Children ages 1 month to 2 years: Initial dose, 0.3 to 0.4 mg/kg. Frequent maintenance doses may be needed.

A

▼ I.V. administration

• Drug usually is given by rapid I.V. bolus injection but may be given by intermittent or continuous infusion.
• At 0.2 to 0.5 mg/ml, drug is compatible for 24 hours in D_5W, normal saline solution injection, or dextrose 5% in normal saline solution injection.

⊗ **Incompatibilities**
Acidic and alkaline solutions, lactated Ringer's solution.

Contraindications and cautions

• Contraindicated in patients hypersensitive to drug.
• Use cautiously in debilitated patients and patients with CV disease; severe electrolyte disorders; bronchogenic carcinoma; hepatic, renal, or pulmonary impairment; neuromuscular diseases; or myasthenia gravis.
⚖ **Lifespan:** In pregnant women, breast-feeding women, and elderly patients, use cautiously.

Adverse reactions

CV: *bradycardia, flushing,* hypotension, increased heart rate.
Respiratory: increased bronchial secretions, *prolonged dose-related apnea,* wheezing.
Skin: erythema, pruritus, urticaria.
Other: *anaphylaxis.*

Interactions

Drug-drug. *Amikacin, gentamicin, neomycin, streptomycin, tobramycin:* May increase nondepolarizing muscle relaxant effects, including prolonged respiratory depression. Use together only when necessary, and reduce dose of nondepolarizing muscle relaxant.
Carbamazepine, phenytoin, theophylline: May decrease atracurium effects. Increase atracurium dose.
Clindamycin, general anesthetics (such as enflurane, halothane, isoflurane), kanamycin, polymyxin antibiotics (colistin, polymyxin B sulfate), quinidine: May potentiate neuromuscular blockade, leading to increased skeletal muscle relaxation and prolonged effect. Use cautiously during surgical and postoperative periods.
Lithium, magnesium salts, opioid analgesics: May potentiate neuromuscular blockade, which may lead to increased skeletal muscle relaxation

and, possibly, respiratory paralysis. Reduce atracurium dose.

Effects on lab test results

None reported.

Pharmacokinetics

Absorption: Given I.V.
Distribution: Into extracellular space. About 82% protein-bound.
Metabolism: Rapidly by Hofmann elimination and by nonspecific enzymatic ester hydrolysis. The liver doesn't appear to play a major role.
Excretion: Drug and metabolites are excreted in urine and feces. *Half-life:* 20 minutes.

Route	Onset	Peak	Duration
I.V.	2 min	3–5 min	35–70 min

Action

Chemical effect: Prevents acetylcholine from binding to receptors on muscle end plate, thus blocking depolarization and resulting in skeletal muscle paralysis.
Therapeutic effect: Relaxes skeletal muscles.

Available forms

Injection: 10 mg/ml

NURSING PROCESS

🔲 **Assessment**
• Obtain history of patient's neuromuscular status before therapy, and reassess regularly.
• Be alert for adverse reactions and interactions.
• Monitor respirations closely until patient fully recovers from neuromuscular blockade, as shown by tests of muscle strength (hand grip, head lift, and ability to cough).
• A nerve stimulator and train-of-four monitoring are recommended to confirm antagonism of neuromuscular blockade and recovery of muscle strength. Before attempting reversal with neostigmine, patient should show some evidence of spontaneous recovery.
• Assess patient's and family's knowledge of drug therapy.

💠 **Nursing diagnoses**
• Risk for injury related to underlying condition
• Impaired spontaneous ventilation related to drug-induced respiratory paralysis
• Deficient knowledge related to drug therapy

Planning and implementation

• Give sedatives or general anesthetics before neuromuscular blockers. Neuromuscular blockers don't decrease consciousness or alter pain threshold.

ALERT: Use this drug only under direct medical supervision by personnel skilled in use of neuromuscular blockers and techniques for maintaining a patent airway. Don't use unless facilities and equipment for mechanical ventilation, oxygen therapy, and intubation as well as an antagonist are immediately available.

• Don't give by I.M. injection.

• Prior use of succinylcholine doesn't prolong duration of action but quickens onset and may deepen neuromuscular blockade.

• Explain all events to patient because he can still hear.

• Give analgesics for pain. Patient may have pain but be unable to express it.

• Keep airway clear. Have emergency equipment and drugs available.

• After spontaneous recovery starts, reverse atracurium-induced neuromuscular blockade with an anticholinesterase (such as neostigmine or edrophonium). These drugs usually are given with an anticholinergic (such as atropine).

Patient teaching

• Instruct patient and family about drug therapy.

• Reassure patient and family that patient will be monitored at all times and that respiratory life support will be used during paralysis.

• Reassure patient that pain medication will be given as needed.

Evaluation

• Patient's underlying condition is resolved without causing injury.

• Patient sustains spontaneous ventilation after effects of atracurium besylate wear off.

• Patient and family state understanding of drug therapy.

HIGH ALERT!

atropine sulfate

(AT-truh-peen SULL-fayt)
AtroPen Auto-Injector, Sal-Tropine

Pharmacologic class: anticholinergic, belladonna alkaloid
Therapeutic class: antiarrhythmic, vagolytic
Pregnancy risk category: C

Indications and dosages

▶ **Symptomatic bradycardia, bradyarrhythmia (junctional or escape rhythm).** *Adults:* Usually 0.5 to 1 mg I.V. push; repeat every 3 to 5 minutes to maximum of 2 mg, as needed. Lower doses (less than 0.5 mg) can cause bradycardia.
Children: 0.02 mg/kg I.V. to a maximum of 1 mg; or 0.3 mg/m²; may repeat every 5 minutes.

▶ **Anticholinesterase insecticide poisoning.** *Adults and children:* 1 to 2 mg I.M. or I.V. repeated every 20 to 30 minutes until muscarinic symptoms disappear or signs of atropine toxicity appear. Patient with severe poisoning may require up to 6 mg every hour.

▶ **Preoperatively for decreasing secretions and blocking cardiac vagal reflexes.** *Adults and children weighing 20 kg (44 lb) or more:* 0.4 mg I.M. or subcutaneously 30 to 60 minutes before anesthesia.
Children weighing less than 20 kg: 0.1 mg I.M. for 3 kg, 0.2 mg I.M. for 4 to 9 kg, 0.3 mg I.M. for 10 to 20 kg, given 30 to 60 minutes before anesthesia.

▶ **Adjunct in peptic ulcer disease; functional GI disorders such as irritable bowel syndrome.** *Adults:* 0.4 to 0.6 mg P.O. every 4 to 6 hours.
Children: 0.01 mg/kg or 0.3 mg/m² (not to exceed 0.4 mg) every 4 to 6 hours.

I.V. administration

• Give by direct injection into a large vein or I.V. tubing over 1 to 2 minutes.

⊗ **Incompatibilities**
Alkalies, bromides, iodides, isoproterenol, methohexital, norepinephrine, pentobarbital sodium, sodium bicarbonate.

Contraindications and cautions

• Contraindicated in patients hypersensitive to drug and those with acute angle-closure glaucoma, obstructive uropathy, obstructive disease of GI tract, paralytic ileus, toxic megacolon, intestinal atony, unstable CV status in acute hemorrhage, asthma, or myasthenia gravis.

• Use cautiously in patients with Down syndrome.

Lifespan: In pregnant women, use cautiously. Use in breast-feeding women isn't recommended. In children and elderly patients, use cautiously because they may have increased adverse effects.

Reactions may be *common*, uncommon, *life-threatening*, or COMMON AND LIFE-THREATENING.

A

Adverse reactions

CNS: agitation, ataxia, *coma,* confusion, delirium, disorientation, *dizziness,* excitement, hallucinations, *headache, insomnia, restlessness.*
CV: *angina,* **arrhythmias,** flushing, *palpitations, tachycardia.*
EENT: *blurred vision, mydriasis,* photophobia.
GI: *constipation, dry mouth,* nausea, thirst, vomiting.
GU: urine retention.
Hematologic: leukocytosis.
Other: *anaphylaxis.*

Interactions

Drug-drug. *Antacids:* May decrease anticholinergic absorption. Give at least 1 hour apart.
Anticholinergics, drugs with anticholinergic effects (such as amantadine, antiarrhythmics, antiparkinsonians, glutethimide, meperidine, phenothiazines, tricyclic antidepressants): May cause additive anticholinergic effects. Use together cautiously.
Ketoconazole, levodopa: May decrease absorption. Avoid use together.
Methotrimeprazine: May produce extrapyramidal symptoms. Monitor patient carefully.

Effects on lab test results

• May increase WBC count.

Pharmacokinetics

Absorption: Well absorbed after P.O. and I.M. use; unknown for subcutaneous use.
Distribution: Throughout the body, including CNS. 18% bound to plasma proteins.
Metabolism: In liver to several metabolites.
Excretion: Mainly through kidneys; small amount in feces and expired air. *Half-life:* Initial, 2 hours; second phase, 12½ hours.

Route	Onset	Peak	Duration
P.O.	½ hr	2 hr	4 hr
I.V.	Immediate	2–4 min	4 hr
I.M.	30 min	1–1½ hr	4 hr
SubQ	Unknown	Unknown	4 hr

Action

Chemical effect: Inhibits acetylcholine at parasympathetic neuroeffector junction, blocking vagal effects on SA node, enhancing conduction through AV node, and speeding heart rate.
Therapeutic effect: Increases heart rate, decreases secretions, and slows GI motility. Anti-

dote for anticholinesterase insecticide poisoning.

Available forms

Injection: 0.05 mg/ml, 0.1 mg/ml, 0.3 mg/ml, 0.4 mg/ml, 0.5 mg/ml, 0.8 mg/ml, 1 mg/ml
Tablets: 0.4 mg

NURSING PROCESS

Assessment
• Obtain history of patient's underlying condition, and reassess regularly.
• Be alert for adverse reactions and drug interactions.
• Monitor patients, especially those receiving doses of 0.4 to 0.6 mg, for paradoxical initial bradycardia, which is caused by a drug effect in CNS and usually disappears within 2 minutes.
⚠ **ALERT:** Watch for tachycardia in cardiac patients because it may cause ventricular fibrillation.
• Assess patient's and family's knowledge of drug therapy.

Nursing diagnoses
• Ineffective health maintenance related to underlying condition
• Risk for injury related to drug-induced adverse reactions
• Deficient knowledge related to drug therapy

Planning and implementation
• Give with or without food.
• If ECG disturbances occur, withhold drug, obtain a rhythm strip, and notify prescriber immediately.
• Have emergency equipment and drugs on hand to treat new arrhythmias. Other anticholinergics may increase vagal blockage.
• Use physostigmine salicylate as antidote for atropine overdose.
Patient teaching
• Teach patient about atropine sulfate therapy.
• Instruct patient to ask for assistance with activities if adverse CNS reactions occur.
• Teach patient how to handle distressing anticholinergic effects.

Evaluation
• Patient's underlying condition improves.
• Patient has no injury as a result of therapy.

• Patient and family state understanding of drug therapy.

HIGH ALERT!

azacitidine
(az-uh-SIT-uh-deen)
Vidaza

Pharmacologic class: pyrimidine nucleoside analogue
Therapeutic class: antineoplastic
Pregnancy risk category: D

Indications and dosages

▶ **Myelodysplastic syndrome, including refractory anemia, refractory anemia with ringed sideroblasts (if patient has neutropenia or thrombocytopenia or needs transfusions), refractory anemia with excess blasts, refractory anemia with excess blasts in transformation, or chronic myelomonocytic leukemia.** *Adults:* Initially, 75 mg/m^2 subcutaneously or I.V. daily for 7 days, repeating cycle every 4 weeks. May increase to 100 mg/m^2 if no response after two treatment cycles and nausea and vomiting are the only toxic reactions. At least four treatment cycles are recommended.

🔲 **Adjust-a-dose:** If bicarbonate level is less than 20 mEq/L, reduce next dose by 50%. If BUN or creatinine level rises during treatment, delay the next cycle until they're normal, and then give 50% of previous dose. Make further adjustments based on hematologic and renal toxicities.

▼ I.V. administration

• Reconstitute drug with 10 ml of sterile water for injection.
• Vigorously shake or roll the vial until powder is dissolved. The resulting solution will be 10 mg/ml. Use only clear solution.
• Withdraw proper dose and mix in a total volume of 50 to 100 ml of normal saline solution or lactated Ringer's solution.
• Give the infusion over 10 to 40 minutes. Infusion must be completed within 1 hour of reconstitution.

⊗ **Incompatibilities**
Dextrose 5%, Hespan, or solutions containing bicarbonate.

Contraindications and cautions

• Contraindicated in patients hypersensitive to azacitidine or mannitol and in patients with advanced malignant hepatic tumors.
• Use cautiously in patients with hepatic and renal disease.

🕯 **Lifespan:** In pregnant and breast-feeding women, avoid use because drug may cause cancer in an unborn or breast-fed baby. In children, safety and effectiveness haven't been established. For elderly patients, choose dose carefully. The drug is substantially excreted by the kidneys and elderly patients are more likely to have decreased renal function.

Adverse reactions

CNS: *anxiety, depression, dizziness, fatigue, headache,* hypoesthesia, *insomnia,* lethargy, *malaise,* pain, syncope, *weakness.*
CV: *cardiac murmur, chest pain, edema,* hypotension, peripheral swelling, tachycardia.
EENT: *epistaxis,* nasal congestion, *nasopharyngitis, pharyngitis,* postnasal drip, *rhinorrhea,* sinusitis.
GI: abdominal distension, *abdominal pain and tenderness, anorexia, constipation, decreased appetite, diarrhea,* dyspepsia, dysphagia, gingival bleeding, hemorrhoids, loose stools, mouth hemorrhage, *nausea,* oral mucosal petechiae, stomatitis, tongue ulceration, *vomiting.*
GU: dysuria, UTI.
Hematologic: *anemia,* FEBRILE NEUTROPENIA, hematoma, LEUKOPENIA, NEUTROPENIA, postprocedural hemorrhage, THROMBOCYTOPENIA.
Metabolic: *weight loss.*
Musculoskeletal: *arthralgia, back pain, limb pain,* muscle cramps, *myalgia.*
Respiratory: *atelectasis,* cough, crackles, *dyspnea,* pleural effusion, *rales, rhonchi, pneumonia, upper respiratory tract infection,* wheezing.
Skin: *bruising,* dry skin, granuloma, *pain,* pigmentation, pruritus, or swelling at injection site; cellulitis; *contusion; ecchymosis; erythema; increased sweating; injection site reaction;* night sweats; *pallor; petechiae; pitting edema; rash; skin lesion;* skin nodules; urticaria.
Other: herpes simplex, lymphadenopathy, *pyrexia, rigors.*

Interactions

Drug-drug. *Concomitant chemotherapy:* Monitor closely for renal dysfunction.

Effects on lab test results

• May increase creatinine and BUN levels. May decrease bicarbonate, potassium, AST, ALT, and hemoglobin levels and hematocrit.
• May decrease WBC, neutrophil, and platelet counts.

Pharmacokinetics

Absorption: Rapid.
Distribution: Mean volume isn't known.
Metabolism: By the liver.
Excretion: Mainly in urine, with less than 1% in feces. *Half-life:* About 4 hours.

Route	Onset	Peak	Duration
SubQ	Unknown	30 min	Unknown

Action

Chemical effect: Causes demethylation or hypomethylation of DNA and is toxic to abnormal hematopoietic cells in bone marrow. Hypomethylation may restore normal function to genes needed for proliferation and differentiation. Drug has little effect on nonproliferating cells.
Therapeutic effect: Restores normal bone marrow function.

Available forms

Powder for injection: 100-mg vials

NURSING PROCESS

Assessment

• Assess patient's condition before therapy and regularly thereafter.
• Check liver function test results and bicarbonate and creatinine levels before therapy starts.
• Obtain CBC before each cycle or more often.
• If patient has renal impairment, monitor him closely; check metabolic panel to assess electrolytes and renal function.
• Assess patient's and family's knowledge of drug therapy.

Nursing diagnoses

• Ineffective health maintenance related to presence of underlying disease
• Ineffective protection related to both underlying disease and drug-induced adverse hematologic reactions
• Deficient knowledge related to drug therapy

Planning and implementation

• Give antiemetic before therapy.
• Dilute using aseptic and hazardous substances techniques. Reconstitute with 4 ml sterile water for injection. Invert vial two to three times and gently rotate until a uniform suspension forms. The resulting cloudy suspension will be 25 mg/ml. Draw up suspension into syringes for injection (no more than 4 ml per syringe).
• Just before giving drug, resuspend it by inverting the syringe two to three times and gently rolling between palms for 30 seconds. Divide doses larger than 4 ml into two syringes and inject into two separate sites. Give new injection at least 1″ from previous site and never into tender, bruised, red, or hardened skin.
• Store unreconstituted vials at room temperature (59° to 86° F [15° to 30° C]).
• Reconstituted drug is stable 1 hour at room temperature and 8 hours refrigerated (36° to 46° F [2° to 8° C]). After refrigeration, suspension may be allowed to equilibrate for 30 minutes at room temperature.
⚠ ALERT: Don't confuse azacitidine with gemcitabine.

Patient teaching
• Inform patient about potential decrease in blood counts with febrile neutropenia, thrombocytopenia, and anemia.
• Advise men and women to use birth control during azacitidine therapy.

Evaluation

• Patient responds well to the drug.
• Patient doesn't develop serious complications from adverse hematologic reactions.
• Patient and family state understanding of drug therapy.

azathioprine
(ay-zuh-THIGH-oh-preen)
Azasan, Imuran

Pharmacologic class: purine antagonist
Therapeutic class: immunosuppressant
Pregnancy risk category: D

Indications and dosages

▶ **Immunosuppression in kidney transplantation.** *Adults and children:* Initially, 3 to 5 mg/kg P.O. or I.V. daily, usually starting on

day of transplantation. Maintain at 1 to 3 mg/kg daily depending on patient response.

▶ **Severe, refractory rheumatoid arthritis.**
Adults: Initially, 1 mg/kg (about 50 mg to 100 mg) P.O. daily as single dose or as two doses. If patient response isn't satisfactory after 6 to 8 weeks, increase dosage by 0.5 mg/kg daily (up to maximum of 2.5 mg/kg daily) at 4-week intervals.

▼ I.V. administration

• Reconstitute 100-mg vial with 10 ml of sterile water for injection. Inspect for particles before infusing or injecting.
• Drug may be given by direct I.V. injection or further diluted in normal saline solution or D_5W and infused over 30 to 60 minutes.
• Use only for patient who can't tolerate P.O. drugs.
⊗ **Incompatibilities**
None reported.

Contraindications and cautions

• Contraindicated in patients hypersensitive to drug.
• Use cautiously in patients with hepatic or renal dysfunction.
⚠ **Lifespan:** In pregnant women, don't use for rheumatoid arthritis. Consider potential benefit to the mother versus possible risk to the unborn baby. In breast-feeding women, drug isn't recommended.

Adverse reactions

GI: anorexia, esophagitis, mouth ulceration, nausea, *pancreatitis*, steatorrhea, vomiting.
Hematologic: anemia, *bone marrow suppression*, LEUKOPENIA, *pancytopenia*, THROMBOCYTOPENIA.
Hepatic: *hepatotoxicity*, jaundice.
Musculoskeletal: arthralgia, muscle wasting.
Skin: alopecia, pruritus, rash.
Other: *immunosuppression*, infections, *neoplasia*.

Interactions

Drug-drug. *ACE inhibitors:* May cause severe leukopenia and anemia. Monitor patient closely.
Allopurinol: May impair inactivation of azathioprine. Decrease azathioprine dose to one-fourth or one-third normal dose.
Co-trimoxazole and other drugs that interfere with myelopoiesis: May cause severe leukope-

nia, especially in renal transplant patients. Use together cautiously.
Cyclosporine: May decrease cyclosporine level. Monitor level.
Methotrexate: May increase 6-MP metabolite level. Monitor patient for increased adverse effects.
Nondepolarizing neuromuscular blockers: May decrease or reverse effects of these drugs. Monitor patient for clinical effects.
Vaccines: May decrease immune response. Postpone routine immunization.
Warfarin: May inhibit anticoagulant effect of warfarin. Monitor PT and INR.

Effects on lab test results

• May increase AST, ALT, alkaline phosphatase, and bilirubin levels. May decrease uric acid and hemoglobin levels and hematocrit.
• May decrease WBC, RBC, and platelet counts.

Pharmacokinetics

Absorption: Good.
Distribution: Throughout body. I.V. and P.O. forms are 30% protein-bound.
Metabolism: Mainly to mercaptopurine; tissue levels of thiopurine nucleotide produce clinical effects.
Excretion: Small amounts of azathioprine and mercaptopurine intact in urine; most of given dose is excreted in urine as secondary metabolites. *Half-life:* About 5 hours.

Route	Onset	Peak	Duration
P.O., I.V.	Unknown	1–2 hr	Unknown

Action

Chemical effect: Unknown.
Therapeutic effect: Suppresses immune system activity.

Available forms

Injection: 100 mg
Tablets: 25 mg, 50 mg, 75 mg, 100 mg

NURSING PROCESS

✎ Assessment

• Obtain history of patient's immune status before therapy.
• Monitor effectiveness by observing patient for signs of organ rejection. Therapeutic response usually occurs within 8 weeks.

Reactions may be *common*, uncommon, *life-threatening*, or COMMON AND LIFE-THREATENING.

- Be alert for adverse reactions and drug interactions.
- Monitor hemoglobin level, hematocrit, and WBC and platelet counts at least once monthly—more often at start of treatment.
- Assess patient's and family's knowledge of drug therapy.

🔯 Nursing diagnoses
- Ineffective protection related to threat of organ rejection
- Risk for infection related to drug-induced immunosuppression
- Deficient knowledge related to drug therapy

▶ Planning and implementation
- Give in divided doses or after meals to minimize adverse GI effects.
- Benefits must be weighed against risks with systemic viral infections, such as chickenpox and herpes zoster.
- Patients with rheumatoid arthritis previously treated with alkylating drugs, such as cyclophosphamide, chlorambucil, and melphalan, may have prohibitive risk of neoplasia if treated with azathioprine.
- To prevent irreversible bone marrow suppression, stop drug immediately when WBC count is less than 3,000/mm³. Notify prescriber.
- To prevent bleeding, avoid I.M. injections when platelet count is lower than 100,000/mm³.
- ⚠ **ALERT:** Don't confuse azathioprine with azidothymidine, Azulfidine, or azatadine. Don't confuse Imuran with Inderal.

Patient teaching
- Warn patient to report even mild infections (colds, fever, sore throat, and malaise) because drug is a potent immunosuppressant.
- Instruct woman to avoid conception during therapy and for 4 months after stopping.
- Warn patient that thinning of hair is possible.
- Tell patient taking this drug for refractory rheumatoid arthritis that it may take up to 12 weeks to be effective.

☑ Evaluation
- Patient has no signs of organ rejection.
- Patient has no signs and symptoms of infection.
- Patient and family state understanding of drug therapy.

azelastine hydrochloride
(ah-zuh-LAST-een high-droh-KLOR-ighd)
Astelin, Optivar

Pharmacologic class: H_1-receptor antagonist
Therapeutic class: antihistamine
Pregnancy risk category: C

Indications and dosages

▶ **Seasonal allergic rhinitis, such as rhinorrhea, sneezing, and nasal pruritus.** *Adults and children age 12 and older:* 2 sprays (274 mcg/2 sprays) per nostril b.i.d.
Children ages 5 to 11 years: 1 spray (137 mcg/spray) per nostril b.i.d.
▶ **Vasomotor rhinitis, such as rhinorrhea, nasal congestion, and postnasal drip.** *Adults and children age 12 and older:* 2 sprays (274 mcg/2 sprays) per nostril b.i.d.
▶ **Allergic conjunctivitis.** *Adults and children older than age 3:* Give 1 drop into affected eye b.i.d.

Contraindications and cautions

- Contraindicated in patients hypersensitive to drug.
- Use cautiously in patients with pulmonary conditions because drug can cause thickened secretions.
- ☀ **Lifespan:** In pregnant women, drug should be used only if benefit justifies risk to fetus. Breast-feeding women shouldn't take drug. In children younger than age 5, safety and effectiveness haven't been established for treating seasonal allergic rhinitis. In children younger than age 12, don't use drug for vasomotor rhinitis.

Adverse reactions

CNS: dizziness, dysesthesia, fatigue, *headaches, somnolence.*
EENT: conjunctivitis, epistaxis, eye pain, nasal burning, paroxysmal sneezing, pharyngitis, rhinitis, sinusitis, stinging, transient eye burning, temporary eye blurring.
GI: *bitter taste,* dry mouth, nausea.
Metabolic: weight increase.
Respiratory: *asthma,* dyspnea.
Skin: pruritus.
Other: flulike symptoms.

Interactions

Drug-drug. *Cimetidine:* May increase azelastine level. Avoid use together.
CNS depressants: May reduce alertness and impair CNS performance. Avoid use together.
Drug-lifestyle. *Alcohol use:* May reduce alertness and cause CNS impairment if using the nasal spray. Discourage use together.

Effects on lab test results

None reported.

Pharmacokinetics

Absorption: Ophthalmic solution has low absorption.
Distribution: Systemic bioavailability is 40%.
Metabolism: After reaching steady state, level ranges from 20% to 50%.
Excretion: Oral drug is 75% excreted in feces. Less than 10% remains unchanged. *Half-life:* 22 hours.

Route	Onset	Peak	Duration
Nasal	Unknown	2–3 hr	12 hr
Ophthalmic	3 min	Unknown	8 hr

Action

Chemical effect: Exerts H$_1$-receptor antagonist activity.
Therapeutic effect: Relieves seasonal allergic rhinitis and conjunctivitis.

Available forms

Nasal solution: 137 mcg/spray
Ophthalmic solution: 0.05%

NURSING PROCESS

Assessment
• Obtain history of patient's allergy condition before therapy begins, and reassess regularly thereafter.
• Be alert for adverse reactions and drug interactions.
• Assess patient's and family's knowledge of drug therapy.

Nursing diagnoses
• Ineffective health maintenance related to underlying allergic condition
• Deficient knowledge related to drug therapy

Planning and implementation
• Don't contaminate eye dropper tip or solution.
• Make sure patient removes contact lenses before giving eyedrops. Tell patient to wait at least 10 minutes before reinserting them.
• When using nasal spray, avoid spraying into patient's eyes.

Patient teaching
• Warn patient not to drive or perform hazardous activities if somnolence occurs.
• Advise patient not to use alcohol, CNS depressants, or other antihistamines while taking drug.
• Teach patient proper use of nasal spray: Replace child-resistant screw top on bottle with pump unit. Prime delivery system with four sprays or until a fine mist appears. If 3 or more days have elapsed since last use, reprime system with 2 sprays or until a fine mist appears. Store bottle upright at room temperature with pump closed tightly. Keep unit away from children.
• Tell patient to avoid getting nasal spray in eyes.

Evaluation
• Patient's allergic symptoms are relieved with drug therapy.
• Patient and family state understanding of drug therapy.

azithromycin
(uh-zith-roh-MIGH-sin)
Zithromax◊, Zmax

Pharmacologic class: azalide macrolide
Therapeutic class: antibiotic
Pregnancy risk category: B

Indications and dosages

▶ **Acute bacterial exacerbations of chronic obstructive pulmonary disease caused by** *Haemophilus influenzae, Moraxella catarrhalis,* **or** *Streptococcus pneumoniae;* **uncomplicated skin and skin-structure infections caused by** *Staphylococcus aureus, Streptococcus pyogenes,* **or** *Streptococcus agalactiae;* **and second-line therapy for pharyngitis or tonsillitis caused by** *S. pyogenes. Adults and children age 16 and older:* Initially, 500 mg P.O. as a single dose on day 1, followed by 250 mg daily on days 2 through 5. Total cumulative dose is 1.5 g. Or for COPD exacerbations, 500 mg P.O. daily for 3 days.

▶ **Community-acquired pneumonia caused by** *Chlamydia pneumoniae, H. influenzae, Mycoplasma pneumoniae, S. pneumoniae;* **I.V. form is also used for** *Legionella pneumophila, M. catarrhalis,* **and** *S. aureus. Adults and children age 16 and older:* 500 mg P.O. as a single dose on day 1, followed by 250 mg P.O. daily on days 2 through 5. Total dosage is 1.5 g. For patients who need initial I.V. therapy, 500 mg I.V. as a single daily dose for 2 days, followed by 500 mg P.O. as a single daily dose to complete a 7- to 10-day course. Switch from I.V. to P.O. route at prescriber's discretion and based on patient's response.
Children age 6 months and older: 10 mg/kg (maximum 500 mg) P.O. as a single dose on day 1, followed by 5 mg/kg (maximum 250 mg) daily on days 2 through 5.

▶ **Single-dose treatment for mild to moderate acute bacterial sinusitis caused by** *H. influenzae, M. catarrhalis,* **or** *S. pneumoniae;* **community-acquired pneumonia caused by** *Chlamydophila pneumoniae, H. influenzae, Mycoplasma pneumoniae,* **or** *S. pneumoniae. Adults:* 2 g P.O. (Zmax) as a single dose 1 hour before or 2 hours after a meal.

▶ **Nongonococcal urethritis or cervicitis caused by** *Chlamydia trachomatis. Adults and children age 16 and older:* 1 g P.O. as a single dose.

▶ **Prevention of disseminated** *Mycobacterium avium* **complex (MAC) disease in patients with advanced HIV infection.** *Adults:* 1,200 mg P.O. once weekly, as indicated.
Infants and children‡: 20 mg/kg P.O. (maximum, 1.2 g) weekly or 5 mg/kg (maximum, 250 mg) can be given P.O. daily. Children age 6 and older may also receive rifabutin 300 mg P.O. daily.

▶ **Disseminated MAC in patients with advanced HIV infection.** *Adults:* 600 mg P.O. daily with ethambutol 15 mg/kg daily.

▶ **Urethritis and cervicitis caused by** *Neisseria gonorrhoeae. Adults:* 2 g P.O. as a single dose.

▶ **Pelvic inflammatory disease caused by** *C. trachomatis, N. gonorrhoeae,* **or** *Mycoplasma hominis* **in patients who need initial I.V. therapy.** *Adults and adolescents age 16 and older:* 500 mg I.V. as a single daily dose for 1 to 2 days, followed by 250 mg P.O. daily to complete a 7-day course. Switch from I.V. to P.O.

route at prescriber's discretion and based on patient's response.

▶ **Genital ulcer disease caused by** *Haemophilus ducreyi* **(chancroid) in men, women‡, and children‡.** *Adults:* 1 g P.O. as a single dose.
Children and infants‡: 20 mg/kg (maximum, 1 g) P.O. as a single dose.

▶ **Acute otitis media.** *Children older than age 6 months:* 30 mg/kg P.O. as a single dose. Or, 10 mg/kg P.O. once daily for 3 days. Or 10 mg/kg P.O. on day 1; then 5 mg/kg once daily on days 2 to 5.

▶ **Pharyngitis, tonsillitis caused by** *S. pyogenes. Children age 2 and older:* 12 mg/kg (maximum, 500 mg) P.O. daily for 5 days.

▶ **Prophylaxis for sexual assault victims‡.** *Adults:* 1 g P.O. as a single dose (conventional, immediate-release tablets) with metronidazole and ceftriaxone.

▶ **Prophylaxis of bacterial endocarditis in penicillin-allergic patients at moderate to high risk‡.** *Adults:* 500 mg P.O. 1 hour before the procedure.
Children: 15 mg/kg P.O. 1 hour before the procedure. Don't exceed adult dose.

▶ *Chlamydial ophthalmia* **neonatorum‡.** *Infants:* 20 mg/kg once daily P.O. for 3 days.

▼ I.V. administration

● Reconstitute drug by adding 4.8 ml sterile water for injection to 500-mg vial and shaking until all the drug is dissolved. Further dilute in 250 to 500 ml D₅W, normal saline solution, or other compatible solution.
● Infuse over 1 to 3 hours.
● Reconstituted solution is stable for 7 days if stored in refrigerator (41° F [5° C]).
● Don't give by I.V. injection or bolus.
⊗ **Incompatibilities**
Amikacin, aztreonam, cefotaxime, ceftazidime, ceftriaxone, cefuroxime, ciprofloxacin, clindamycin, famotidine, fentanyl, furosemide, gentamicin, imipenem and cilastatin, ketorolac, levofloxacin, morphine, ondansetron, piperacillin and tazobactam sodium, potassium chloride, ticarcillin disodium and clavulanate potassium, tobramycin.

Contraindications and cautions

● Contraindicated in patients hypersensitive to erythromycin or other macrolides.

• Use cautiously in patients with impaired hepatic function.

🔥 **Lifespan:** In pregnant or breast-feeding women, use cautiously.

Adverse reactions

CNS: aggressive reaction, anxiety, dizziness, fatigue, headache, *seizures,* somnolence, vertigo.
CV: chest pain, palpitations, *QT-interval prolongation, torsades de pointes.*
EENT: hearing loss, taste perversion, tinnitus.
GI: *abdominal pain,* cholestatic jaundice, *diarrhea,* dyspepsia, flatulence, melena, *nausea, pseudomembranous colitis, vomiting.*
GU: candidiasis, nephritis, vaginitis.
Hematologic: mild neutropenia, *thrombocytopenia.*
Hepatic: cholestatic jaundice, *hepatic failure, hepatic necrosis, hepatitis.*
Skin: photosensitivity, rash, *Stevens-Johnson syndrome, toxic epidermal necrolysis,* urticaria.
Other: *anaphylaxis, angioedema.*

Interactions

Drug-drug. *Antacids containing aluminum and magnesium:* May lower peak azithromycin level. Separate doses by at least 2 hours.
Digoxin: May elevate digoxin level. Monitor patient closely.
Dihydroergotamine, ergotamine: May cause acute ergot toxicity. Avoid use together.
Drugs metabolized by cytochrome P-450 system: May elevate carbamazepine, cyclosporine, hexobarbital, and phenytoin levels. Monitor patient closely.
Theophylline: May increase theophylline level with other macrolides; effect of azithromycin is unknown. Monitor theophylline level carefully.
Triazolam: May increase pharmacologic effect of triazolam. Use together cautiously.
Warfarin: May increase PT with other macrolides; effect of azithromycin is unknown. Monitor PT and INR carefully.
Drug-food. *Any food:* May decrease rate of absorption, but not effectiveness of drug.
Drug-lifestyle. *Sun exposure:* May cause photosensitivity reactions. Advise against prolonged or unprotected sun exposure.

Effects on lab test results

None reported.

Pharmacokinetics

Absorption: Rapid. Food decreases both maximum level and amount of drug absorbed.
Distribution: Rapid throughout body and readily penetrates cells; drug doesn't readily enter CNS. Drug concentrates in fibroblasts and phagocytes. Significantly higher levels are reached in tissues compared with plasma.
Metabolism: None.
Excretion: Mostly in feces after excretion into bile. Less than 10% in urine. *Terminal elimination half-life:* 68 hours.

Route	Onset	Peak	Duration
P.O.	Unknown	2½–4½ hr	Unknown
I.V.	Unknown	Unknown	Unknown

Action

Chemical effect: Binds to 50S subunit of bacterial ribosomes, blocking protein synthesis; bacteriostatic or bactericidal, depending on concentration.
Therapeutic effect: Hinders or kills susceptible bacteria, including many gram-positive and gram-negative aerobic and anaerobic bacteria.

Available forms

Injection: 500 mg
Powder for oral suspension: 100 mg/5 ml, 200 mg/5 ml; 1,000 mg/packet
Powder for oral suspension (extended-release): 2 g
Tablets: 250 mg, 500 mg, 600 mg

NURSING PROCESS

📋 **Assessment**
• Obtain history of patient's infection before therapy, and reassess the patient regularly thereafter.
• Obtain specimen for culture and sensitivity tests before first dose. Therapy may begin pending test results.
• Be alert for adverse reactions and drug interactions.
• Assess patient's and family's knowledge of drug therapy.

⊕ **Nursing diagnoses**
• Ineffective protection related to drug-induced superinfection
• Deficient knowledge related to drug therapy

Reactions may be *common,* uncommon, *life-threatening*, or **COMMON AND LIFE-THREATENING**.

▶ Planning and implementation
⊕ **ALERT:** Don't give drug I.M. or by I.V. bolus injection.
• If patient vomits within 5 minutes of drinking extended-release solution, consider additional antibiotic treatment. If patient vomits 5 to 60 minutes after drinking it, consider alternative treatment. If patient vomits more than 60 minutes after drinking, no further treatment is needed.
• Don't give with antacids.

Patient teaching
• Tell patient that tablets or oral suspension may be taken with or without food, but that taking with food may decrease risk of nausea.
• Tell patient to take all medication as prescribed, even after he feels better.
• Instruct patient to use sunblock and avoid prolonged exposure to the sun to decrease risk of photosensitivity reactions.

☑ Evaluation
• Patient doesn't experience superinfection during therapy.
• Patient and family state understanding of drug therapy.

aztreonam
(az-TREE-oh-nam)
Azactam

Pharmacologic class: monobactam
Therapeutic class: antibiotic
Pregnancy risk category: B

Indications and dosages

▶ **UTI, lower respiratory tract infection, septicemia, skin and skin-structure infections, intra-abdominal infection, surgical infection, gynecologic infection caused by various aerobic organisms; or as adjunct therapy to pelvic inflammatory disease‡ or gonorrhea‡.**
Adults: 500 mg to 2 g I.V. or I.M. every 8 to 12 hours. For severe systemic or life-threatening infection, 2 g every 6 to 8 hours. Maximum, 8 g daily.

▶ **Infections of the respiratory or GU tract, bone, skin, or soft tissues caused by susceptible organisms‡.** *Neonates ages 1 to 4 weeks weighing more than 2 kg (4.4 lb):* 30 mg/kg I.V. every 6 hours.

Neonates ages 1 to 4 weeks weighing 2 kg or less: 30 mg/kg I.V. every 8 hours.
Neonates younger than 7 days weighing more than 2 kg: 30 mg/kg I.V. every 8 hours.
Neonates younger than 7 days weighing 2 kg or less: 30 mg/kg I.V. every 12 hours.

▽ I.V. administration
• Inject bolus dose drug over 3 to 5 minutes directly into vein or I.V. tubing.
• Give infusion over 20 minutes to 1 hour.
⊗ **Incompatibilities**
Acyclovir, amphotericin B, ampicillin sodium, azithromycin, cephradine, chlorpromazine, daunorubicin, ganciclovir, lorazepam, metronidazole, mitomycin, mitoxantrone, nafcillin, other I.V. drugs, prochlorperazine, streptozocin, vancomycin.

Contraindications and cautions
• Contraindicated in patients hypersensitive to drug.
• Use cautiously in patients with impaired renal function. Dosage adjustment may be needed.
⚘ **Lifespan:** In breast-feeding women, drug isn't recommended. In children, safety of drug hasn't been established. In elderly patients, use cautiously because dosage adjustment may be needed.

Adverse reactions
CNS: confusion, headache, insomnia, *seizures.*
CV: hypotension.
EENT: altered taste, halitosis.
GI: diarrhea, nausea, vomiting.
Hematologic: anemia, *neutropenia, pancytopenia, thrombocytopenia.*
Other: discomfort or swelling at I.M. injection site, hypersensitivity reactions (*anaphylaxis,* rash), rash or thrombophlebitis at I.V. site.

Interactions
Drug-drug. *Aminoglycosides, beta-lactam antibiotics, other anti-infectives:* May have synergistic effect and increase risk of ototoxicity, nephrotoxicity. Monitor patient closely.
Cefoxitin, imipenem: May have antagonistic effect. Avoid use together.
Furosemide, probenecid: May increase aztreonam level. Avoid use together.

Effects on lab test results

• May increase BUN, creatinine, ALT, AST, and LDH levels. May decrease hemoglobin level and hematocrit.
• May increase PT, PTT, and INR. May decrease neutrophil and RBC counts. May increase or decrease WBC and platelet counts.

Pharmacokinetics

Absorption: Rapid and complete.
Distribution: Rapid and wide to all body fluids and tissues, including bile, breast milk, and CSF.
Metabolism: From 6% to 16% metabolized to inactive metabolites by nonspecific hydrolysis of beta-lactam ring; 56% to 60% protein-bound, less if renal impairment is present.
Excretion: Mainly unchanged in urine by glomerular filtration and tubular secretion; 1.5% to 3.5% unchanged in feces. *Half-life:* Average 2 hours.

Route	Onset	Peak	Duration
I.V.	Immediate	Immediate	Unknown
I.M.	Unknown	½–1½ hr	Unknown

Action

Chemical effect: Inhibits bacterial cell-wall synthesis, ultimately causing cell-wall destruction.
Therapeutic effect: Kills susceptible bacteria.

Available forms

Injection: 500-mg, 1-g, 2-g vials

NURSING PROCESS

Assessment

• Obtain history of patient's infection before therapy, and reassess regularly thereafter.
• Obtain urine specimen for culture and sensitivity tests before giving first dose. Therapy may begin pending test results.
• Be aware of adverse reactions and drug interactions.
• Patients who are allergic to penicillins or cephalosporins may not be allergic to this drug. However, closely monitor patients who have had an immediate hypersensitivity reaction to these antibiotics.
• Assess patient's and family's knowledge of drug therapy.

Nursing diagnoses

• Ineffective protection related to drug-induced superinfection
• Deficient knowledge related to drug therapy

Planning and implementation

• Give I.M. injection deep into large muscle mass, such as the upper outer quadrant of gluteus maximus or the outer thigh. Give doses larger than 1 g by I.V. route.
• Report diarrhea to the prescriber. Pseudomembranous colitis may need to be ruled out.
• Monitor renal and hepatic function.
Patient teaching
• Tell patient to report pain or discomfort at I.V. site.
• Warn patient receiving drug I.M. that pain and swelling may develop at injection site.
• Instruct patient to report signs or symptoms that suggest superinfection.

Evaluation

• Patient doesn't develop superinfection as a result of therapy.
• Patient and family state understanding of drug therapy.

baclofen

(BAH-kloh-fen)
Kemstro, Lioresal, Lioresal Intrathecal

Pharmacologic class: chlorophenyl derivative (GABA derivative)
Therapeutic class: skeletal muscle relaxant
Pregnancy risk category: C

Indications and dosages

▶ **Spasticity in multiple sclerosis, spinal cord injury.** *Adults:* Initially, 5 mg P.O. t.i.d. for 3 days. Based on response, increase dosage at 3-day intervals by 15 mg (5 mg/dose) daily to maximum of 80 mg daily (20 mg q.i.d.).
▶ **Severe spasticity in patients who don't respond to or can't tolerate oral baclofen therapy.** *Adults (screening phase):* Give test dose of 50 mcg in 1-ml dilution into intrathecal space

by barbotage over 1 minute or longer. After test dose, give drug by implantable infusion pump. Muscle tone should be reduced or muscle spasm significantly decreased in severity or frequency in 4 to 8 hours. If response is inadequate, give a second test dose of 75 mcg/1.5 ml 24 hours after the first. If response is still inadequate, give a final test dose of 100 mcg/2 ml 24 hours later. Patients unresponsive to 100-mcg dose aren't candidates for an implantable pump.

Adults (maintenance therapy): Adjust initial dose based on the screening dose that gives an adequate response. Double effective dose and give over 24 hours. If screening-dose effectiveness is maintained for 8 hours or longer, don't double dosage. After first 24 hours, increase dose slowly, as needed and tolerated, by 10% to 30% daily until desired effects occur. Decrease dose by 10% to 20% if intolerable adverse effects occur.

Children younger than age 12: Testing dose is the same as for adults (50 mcg); but for very small children, an initial dose of 25 mcg may be given.

Contraindications and cautions

• Contraindicated in patients hypersensitive to drug. Orally disintegrating tablets are contraindicated in patients hypersensitive to aspartame.
• Use cautiously in patients with impaired renal function or seizure disorder or when spasticity is used to maintain motor function.
⚠ Lifespan: In pregnant or breast-feeding women, use cautiously. In children younger than age 12, safety of oral form hasn't been established. In children younger than age 4, safety of intrathecal form hasn't been established.

Adverse reactions

CNS: *confusion,* dizziness, drowsiness, fatigue, *headache,* **high fever,** *hypotonia,* paresthesia, SEIZURES, somnolence, weakness.
CV: ankle edema, hypotension.
EENT: blurred vision, nasal congestion.
GI: constipation, nausea, vomiting.
GU: impotence, sexual dysfunction, urinary frequency, urinary incontinence.
Metabolic: hyperglycemia, weight gain.
Musculoskeletal: dysarthria, *muscle rigidity or spasticity,* **rhabdomyolysis.**
Respiratory: dyspnea.
Skin: excessive perspiration, pruritus, rash.
Other: *multiple organ-system failure.*

Interactions

Drug-drug. *CNS depressants:* May increase CNS depression. Avoid use together.
MAO inhibitors, tricyclic antidepressants: May cause CNS and respiratory depression and hypotension. Avoid use together.
Drug-lifestyle. *Alcohol use:* May increase CNS depression. Discourage use together.

Effects on lab test results

• May increase AST, alkaline phosphatase, and glucose levels.

Pharmacokinetics

Absorption: Rapid and extensive with P.O. use; may vary.
Distribution: Wide throughout body, with small amounts crossing blood–brain barrier. About 30% protein-bound.
Metabolism: About 15% in liver by deamination.
Excretion: 70% to 80% in urine unchanged or as metabolites; remainder in feces. *Half-life:* 2½ to 4 hours.

Route	Onset	Peak	Duration
P.O.	Rapid	2–3 hr	8 hr
P.O. orally disintegrating	Rapid	1½ hr	8 hr
Intrathecal	½–1 hr	4 hr	4–8 hr

Action

Chemical effect: Unknown; appears to reduce transmission of impulses from spinal cord to skeletal muscle. For intrathecal route, effects may occur from stimulation of GABA receptors.
Therapeutic effect: Relieves muscle spasms.

Available forms

Intrathecal injection: 50 mcg/ml, 500 mcg/ml, 2,000 mcg/ml
Tablets: 10 mg, 20 mg, 25 mg
Tablets (orally-disintegrating): 10 mg, 20 mg

NURSING PROCESS

🔍 Assessment

• Obtain history of patient's pain and muscle spasms from underlying condition before therapy, and reassess regularly thereafter.

- Be alert for adverse reactions and drug interactions.
- Watch for increased seizures in patients with seizure disorder. Seizures may occur during overdose and withdrawal of intrathecal form, as well as in patients maintained on therapeutic doses. Monitor patient carefully, and institute seizure precautions.
- Assess patient's and family's understanding of drug therapy.

🔆 Nursing diagnoses
- Acute pain related to spasticity
- Risk for injury related to drug-induced adverse CNS reactions
- Deficient knowledge related to drug therapy

▶ Planning and implementation
- Give with meals or milk to prevent GI distress.
- Don't give orally to treat muscle spasm caused by rheumatic disorders, cerebral palsy, Parkinson disease, or stroke because effectiveness hasn't been established.
- Treatment for oral overdose is supportive; don't induce emesis or use respiratory stimulant in an unconscious patient.
- Implantable pump or catheter failure can make intrathecal baclofen suddenly ineffective.
- ⚠ **ALERT:** Don't give intrathecal form by I.V., I.M., subcutaneous, or epidural routes.
- The amount of relief determines whether dose (and drowsiness) can be reduced.
- Don't stop intrathecal baclofen abruptly. Early symptoms of baclofen withdrawal may include return of baseline spasticity, pruritus, hypotension, and paresthesias. Symptoms may include high fever, altered mental status, exaggerated rebound spasticity, and muscle rigidity, which could lead to rhabdomyolysis, multiple organ-system failure, and death. To treat withdrawal, resume intrathecal baclofen at or near the previous dosage. If delayed, treat with P.O. or enteral baclofen or with P.O., enteral, or I.V. benzodiazepines to prevent life-threatening withdrawal. Don't rely on P.O. or enteral baclofen alone to halt withdrawal from intrathecal baclofen.
- About 10% of patients may develop tolerance to drug. In some cases, this may be treated by hospitalizing patient and by slowly withdrawing drug over a 2-week period.

Patient teaching
- Tell patient to avoid activities that require alertness until drug's CNS effects are known. Drowsiness usually is transient.
- Inform patient with phenylketonuria that orally disintegrating tablets contain phenylalanine (3.9 mg/10-mg tablet and 7.9 mg/20-mg tablet).
- Instruct patient to remove orally disintegrating tablet from blister pack, immediately place on tongue to dissolve, and swallow with or without water.
- Tell patient to avoid alcohol while taking drug.
- Advise patient to follow prescriber's orders about rest and physical therapy.
- Advise patient to take drug with food or milk to prevent GI distress.

✓ Evaluation
- Patient reports that pain and muscle spasms have ceased with drug therapy.
- Patient doesn't experience injury as a result of drug-induced drowsiness.
- Patient and family state understanding of drug therapy.

balsalazide disodium
(bal-SAL-uh-zighd digh-SOH-dee-um)
Colazal

Pharmacologic class: GI drug
Therapeutic class: anti-inflammatory
Pregnancy risk category: B

Indications and dosages
▶ **Ulcerative colitis.** *Adults:* 2.25 g (three 750-mg capsules) P.O. t.i.d. for a total of 6.75 g daily for 8 to 12 weeks.
▶ **Mild to moderately active ulcerative colitis.** *Children age 5 and older:* Three 750-mg capsules P.O. t.i.d. (6.75 g/day) for 8 weeks. Or one 750-mg capsule P.O. t.i.d. (2.25 g/day) for 8 weeks.

Contraindications and cautions
- Contraindicated in patients hypersensitive to salicylates or balsalazide metabolites.
- Use cautiously in patients with history of renal disease or renal dysfunction.
- Use cautiously in patients with pyloric stenosis because of prolonged retention of drug.

Safety and effectiveness beyond 12 weeks of treatment haven't been established.

🍼 **Lifespan:** In breast-feeding women, use cautiously because it's unknown whether drug appears in breast milk. In children, safety and effectiveness haven't been established.

Adverse reactions

CNS: dizziness, fatigue, fever, headache, insomnia.
EENT: pharyngitis, rhinitis, sinusitis.
GI: abdominal pain, anorexia, constipation, cramps, diarrhea, dry mouth, dyspepsia, flatulence, frequent stools, nausea, rectal bleeding, vomiting.
GU: UTI.
Hepatic: *hepatotoxicity.*
Musculoskeletal: arthralgia, back pain, myalgia.
Respiratory: cough, respiratory infection.
Other: flulike symptoms.

Interactions

Drug-drug. *Azathioprine, 6-mercaptopurine:* May interfere with metabolism of these drugs. Use with caution.
Oral antibiotics and anti-infectives: May interfere with release of mesalamine in the colon. Monitor patient for worsening symptoms.

Effects on lab test results

• May increase AST, ALT, LDH, alkaline phosphatase, and bilirubin levels.

Pharmacokinetics

Absorption: Very low and variable in healthy patients; 60 times greater in patients with ulcerative colitis.
Distribution: 99% or more protein-bound.
Metabolism: To mesalamine (5-aminosalicylic acid), the active component of the drug.
Excretion: By the kidneys. Less than 1% recovered in urine. *Half-life:* Unknown.

Route	Onset	Peak	Duration
P.O.	Unknown	Unknown	Unknown

Action

Chemical effect: Probably blocks colon's production of arachidonic acid metabolites, which are increased in patients with chronic inflammatory bowel disease. Balsalazide is converted in the colon to mesalamine, which is then convert-

ed to 5-aminosalicylic acid. The mechanism of action is unknown, but it appears to be local rather than systemic.
Therapeutic effect: Decreases inflammation in the colon.

Available forms

Capsules: 750 mg

NURSING PROCESS

📋 Assessment
• Assess patient's underlying condition and note frequency of bowel movements before starting therapy.
• Hepatotoxicity, including elevated liver function test results, jaundice, cirrhosis, liver necrosis, and liver failure, has occurred with other products containing or metabolized to mesalamine. Although no signs of hepatotoxicity have been reported with balsalazide disodium, monitor patient closely for evidence of hepatic dysfunction.
• Assess patient's and family's knowledge of drug therapy and ulcerative colitis.

Nursing diagnoses
• Diarrhea related to underlying disease process
• Imbalanced nutrition: less than body requirements related to frequent bowel movements from ulcerative colitis
• Deficient knowledge related to balsalazide disodium therapy

Planning and implementation
• Notify prescriber if drug has been given for 8 to 12 weeks or longer.
Patient teaching
• Advise patient not to take drug if he's allergic to aspirin or salicylate derivatives.
• Advise patient to promptly report adverse reactions to prescriber.

✓ Evaluation
• Patient states that diarrhea has improved.
• Because of decreasing symptoms of ulcerative colitis, patient can tolerate and absorb a balanced diet.
• Patient and family state understanding of balsalazide disodium therapy.

basiliximab

(ba-sihl-IHK-sih-mab)
Simulect

Pharmacologic class: recombinant chimeric human monoclonal antibody IgG_{1k}
Therapeutic class: immunosuppressant
Pregnancy risk category: B

Indications and dosages

▶ **To prevent acute organ rejection in renal-transplant patients when used as part of immunosuppressive regimen that includes cyclosporine and corticosteroids.** *Adults and children weighing 35 kg (77 lb) or more:* 20 mg I.V. 2 hours before transplant surgery and 20 mg I.V. for 4 days after transplantation.
Children weighing less than 35 kg: 10 mg I.V. 2 hours before transplant surgery and 10 mg I.V. for 4 days after transplantation.

▽ I.V. administration

● Reconstitute 10-mg vial with 2.5 ml sterile water for injection or 20-mg vial with 5 ml sterile water for injection. Shake vial gently to dissolve powder.
● Give by infusion or bolus.
● If giving by infusion, dilute reconstituted solution to volume of 25 ml normal saline solution or D_5W for 10-mg vial and 50 ml with normal saline solution or D_5W for infusion for the 20-mg vial. When mixing solution, gently invert bag to avoid foaming. Don't shake.
● Infuse over 20 to 30 minutes by a central or peripheral vein.
● Use reconstituted solution immediately; it may be refrigerated at 36° to 46° F (2° and 8° C) for up to 24 hours or kept at room temperature for 4 hours.
⊗ **Incompatibilities**
Other I.V. drugs.

Contraindications and cautions

● Contraindicated in patients hypersensitive to drug or its components.
⚘ **Lifespan:** In pregnant women, use only if potential benefits outweigh risks to the fetus. Breast-feeding women should stop nursing or stop taking the drug because of potential for adverse effects. It's unknown whether drug appears in breast milk. In elderly patients, use cautiously.

Adverse reactions

CNS: agitation, anxiety, asthenia, depression, *dizziness,* fatigue, *fever, headache,* hypoesthesia, *insomnia,* neuropathy, paresthesia, *tremor.*
CV: abnormal heart sounds, aggravated hypertension, angina pectoris, **arrhythmias,** atrial fibrillation, chest pain, general edema, **heart failure, hemorrhage,** *hypertension,* hypotension, *leg or peripheral edema,* tachycardia.
EENT: abnormal vision, cataract, conjunctivitis, *pharyngitis, rhinitis,* sinusitis.
GI: *abdominal pain, candidiasis, constipation, diarrhea, dyspepsia,* esophagitis, enlarged abdomen, flatulence, gastroenteritis, GI disorder, **GI hemorrhage,** gum hyperplasia, melena, *nausea,* ulcerative stomatitis, *vomiting.*
GU: abnormal renal function, albuminuria, bladder disorder, *dysuria,* polyuria, genital edema, hematuria, impotence, *increased nonprotein nitrogen,* oliguria, **renal tubular necrosis,** ureteral disorder, *UTI.*
Hematologic: anemia, hematoma, *polycythemia,* **purpura, thrombocytopenia, thrombosis.**
Metabolic: *acidosis,* dehydration, **diabetes mellitus,** fluid overload, hypercalcemia, *hypercholesterolemia,* hyperglycemia, HYPERKALEMIA, hyperlipemia, *hyperuricemia, hypocalcemia, hypokalemia,* **hypomagnesemia,** hypophosphatemia, hypoproteinemia, *weight gain.*
Musculoskeletal: arthralgia, arthropathy, *back pain,* bone fracture, cramps, hernia, *leg pain,* myalgia.
Respiratory: abnormal chest sounds, bronchitis, **bronchospasm,** *cough, dyspnea,* pneumonia, pulmonary disorder, **pulmonary edema,** *upper respiratory tract infection.*
Skin: *acne,* cyst, herpes simplex, herpes zoster, hypertrichosis, pruritus, rash, skin disorder or ulceration.
Other: accidental trauma, infection, **sepsis,** *surgical wound complications, viral infection.*

Interactions

None significant.

Effects on lab test results

● May increase calcium, cholesterol, glucose, lipid, and uric acid levels. May decrease magnesium, phosphorus, protein, and hemoglobin lev-

els and hematocrit. May increase or decrease potassium level.
• May increase RBC count. May decrease platelet count.

Pharmacokinetics

Absorption: Given I.V.
Distribution: Unknown.
Metabolism: Unknown.
Excretion: Unknown. *Half-life:* About 7¼ days in adults, 9½ days in children, 9 days in adolescents.

Route	Onset	Peak	Duration
I.V.	Unknown	Immediate	Unknown

Action

Chemical effect: Binds to and blocks the interleukin (IL)-2 receptor alpha chain on the surface of activated T lymphocytes, inhibiting IL-2–mediated activation of lymphocytes, a critical pathway in the cellular immune response involved in allograft rejection.
Therapeutic effect: Prevents organ rejection.

Available forms

Injection: 10-mg and 20-mg vials

NURSING PROCESS

Assessment
• Monitor patient for anaphylactoid reactions. Be sure that drugs for treating severe hypersensitivity reactions are available for immediate use.
• Check for electrolyte imbalances and acidosis.
• Monitor patient's intake and output, vital signs, hemoglobin level, and hematocrit.
• Be alert for signs and symptoms of opportunistic infections.
• Assess patient's and family's knowledge of drug therapy.

Nursing diagnoses
• Risk for injury related to potential for organ rejection
• Ineffective protection related to drug-induced immunosuppression
• Deficient knowledge related to drug therapy

Planning and implementation
• Use drug only under supervision of prescriber experienced in management of organ transplantation.
• Patients who have a severe hypersensitivity reaction shouldn't receive the drug again.
Patient teaching
• Inform patient of potential benefits and risks of therapy, including decreased risk of graft loss or acute rejection. Advise patient that therapy increases risk of lymphoproliferative disorders and opportunistic infections. Tell him to report signs and symptoms of infection immediately.
• Tell women of childbearing age to use effective contraception before, during, and for 4 months after therapy ends.
• Instruct patient to immediately report adverse effects to prescriber.
• Explain that drug is used with cyclosporine and corticosteroids.

Evaluation
• Patient doesn't have organ rejection while taking this drug.
• Patient is free from infection and serious bleeding episodes during therapy.
• Patient and family state understanding of drug therapy.

beclomethasone dipropionate
(bek-loh-METH-eh-sohn digh-proh-PIGH-uh-nayt)
QVAR

Pharmacologic class: synthetic corticosteroid
Therapeutic class: antiasthmatic
Pregnancy risk category: C

Indications and dosages

▶ **Chronic asthma.** *Adults and children age 12 and older:* Starting dose, 40 to 80 mcg b.i.d. by aerosol inhalation when used with bronchodilators alone, or 40 to 160 mcg b.i.d. when used with other inhaled corticosteroids. Maximum, 320 mcg b.i.d.
Children ages 5 to 11: Give 40 mcg b.i.d., up to 80 mcg b.i.d. by aerosol inhalation when used with bronchodilators alone or with inhaled corticosteroids.

Contraindications and cautions

• Contraindicated in patients hypersensitive to drug or its components, and in those with status asthmaticus, nonasthmatic bronchial diseases, or asthma controlled by bronchodilators or other noncorticosteroids alone.
• Use with extreme caution, if at all, in patients with tuberculosis, fungal or bacterial infections, ocular herpes simplex, or systemic viral infections.
• Use with caution in patients receiving systemic corticosteroid therapy.

⚱ Lifespan: In pregnant or breast-feeding women, use cautiously. In children younger than age 5, safety and effectiveness haven't been established.

Adverse reactions

EENT: *fungal infection of throat, hoarseness, throat irritation.*
GI: dry mouth, *fungal infection of mouth.*
Metabolic: *adrenal insufficiency, suppression of hypothalamic-pituitary-adrenal function.*
Respiratory: *bronchospasm,* cough, wheezing.
Other: *angioedema,* facial edema, hypersensitivity reactions.

Interactions

None significant.

Effects on lab test results

None reported.

Pharmacokinetics

Absorption: Rapid from lungs and GI tract.
Distribution: No evidence of tissue storage of drug or its metabolites.
Metabolism: Mostly in liver.
Excretion: Unknown, although when drug is given systemically, its metabolites are excreted mainly in feces and, to a lesser extent, in urine.
Half-life: 15 hours.

Route	Onset	Peak	Duration
Inhalation	1–4 wk	Unknown	Unknown

Action

Chemical effect: Decreases inflammation, mainly by stabilizing leukocyte lysosomal membranes.
Therapeutic effect: Helps alleviate asthma symptoms.

Available forms

Oral inhalation aerosol: 40 mcg/metered spray, 80 mcg/metered spray

NURSING PROCESS

🔲 **Assessment**
• Obtain history of patient's asthma before therapy, and reassess regularly thereafter.
• Be alert for adverse reactions.
• Monitor patient closely during times of stress (trauma, surgery, or infection) because systemic corticosteroids may be needed to prevent adrenal insufficiency in previously steroid-dependent patients.
• Periodic measurement of growth and development may be needed during high-dose or prolonged therapy in children.
• Assess patient's and family's understanding of drug therapy.

🔲 **Nursing diagnoses**
• Impaired gas exchange related to asthma
• Impaired oral mucous membranes related to drug-induced fungal infections
• Deficient knowledge related to drug therapy

▶ **Planning and implementation**
ⓢ **ALERT:** Never give drug to relieve an emergency asthma attack because onset of action is too slow.
• Give prescribed bronchodilators several minutes before beclomethasone.
• Have patient hold breath for a few seconds after each puff and rest 1 minute between puffs to enhance drug action.
• Use of a spacer device isn't needed.
ⓢ **ALERT:** Taper oral corticosteroid therapy slowly. Acute adrenal insufficiency and death have occurred in patients with asthma who changed abruptly from oral corticosteroids to beclomethasone.
• Notify prescriber if decreased response is noted after giving drug.
• Have patient gargle and rinse mouth with water after inhalations to help prevent oral fungal infections.
Patient teaching
• Tell patient to prime the inhaler before first use and after 10 days of not using it by depressing canister twice into the air.
• Inform patient that drug doesn't relieve acute asthma attacks.

Reactions may be *common*, uncommon, *life-threatening*, or COMMON AND LIFE-THREATENING.

B

• Tell patient who needs a bronchodilator to use it several minutes before beclomethasone.
• Instruct patient to carry or wear medical identification indicating his need for supplemental systemic corticosteroids during stress.
• Advise patient to allow 1 minute to elapse between inhalations of drug and to hold his breath for a few seconds to enhance drug action.
• Tell patient it may take up to 4 weeks to feel the full benefit of the drug.
• Tell patient to keep inhaler clean by wiping it weekly with a dry tissue or cloth; don't get it wet.
• Advise patient to prevent oral fungal infections by gargling or rinsing his mouth with water after each use. Caution him not to swallow the water.
• Tell patient to report evidence of corticosteroid withdrawal, including fatigue, weakness, arthralgia, orthostatic hypotension, and dyspnea.
• Instruct patient to store drug at 77° F (25° C), and advise patient to use at room temperature.

☑ Evaluation
• Patient's lungs are clear, and breathing and skin color are normal.
• Patient doesn't develop an oral fungal infection during therapy.
• Patient and family state understanding of drug therapy.

beclomethasone dipropionate monohydrate
(bek-loh-METH-eh-sohn digh-proh-PIGH-uh-nayt mon-oh-HIGH-drayt)
Beconase AQ

Pharmacologic class: corticosteroid
Therapeutic class: anti-inflammatory
Pregnancy risk category: C

Indications and dosages

▶ **Symptoms of allergic rhinitis; prevention of recurrence of nasal polyps after surgical removal.** *Adults and children age 12 and older:* 1 to 2 inhalations or sprays in each nostril b.i.d. Maximum, 336 mcg daily.
Children ages 6 to 11: Give 1 inhalation or spray in each nostril b.i.d. Patients with more

severe symptoms may need 2 inhalations in each nostril b.i.d.

Contraindications and cautions

• Contraindicated in patients hypersensitive to drug and in those experiencing status asthmaticus or other acute episodes of asthma.
• Use cautiously, if at all, in patients with active or quiescent respiratory tract tubercular infections or untreated fungal, bacterial, systemic viral, or ocular herpes simplex infections. Also use cautiously in patients who've recently had nasal septal ulcers, nasal surgery, or trauma.
⚞ **Lifespan:** In pregnant or breast-feeding women, use cautiously. In children younger than age 6, safety and effectiveness of drug haven't been established.

Adverse reactions

CNS: headache.
EENT: epistaxis; irritation of nasal mucosa; *mild, transient nasal burning* and stinging; nasal congestion; nasopharyngeal fungal infections; sneezing; watery eyes.
GI: nausea, vomiting.

Interactions

None significant.

Effects on lab test results

None reported.

Pharmacokinetics

Absorption: Mainly through nasal mucosa, with minimal systemic absorption.
Distribution: Unknown.
Metabolism: Most of drug in liver.
Excretion: Unknown. *Half-life:* 15 hours.

Route	Onset	Peak	Duration
Inhalation	5–7 days	≤ 3 wk	Unknown

Action

Chemical effect: Decreases nasal inflammation, mainly by stabilizing leukocyte lysosomal membranes.
Therapeutic effect: Helps relieve nasal allergy symptoms.

Available forms

Nasal spray: 42 mcg/metered spray

NURSING PROCESS

🔆 Assessment

• Obtain history of patient's allergy symptoms and nasal congestion before therapy, and reassess regularly thereafter.
• Be alert for adverse reactions.
• If adverse GI reactions occur, monitor patient's hydration.
• Check for irritation of nasal mucosa.
• Assess patient's and family's understanding of drug therapy.

🔆 Nursing diagnoses

• Ineffective health maintenance related to allergy-induced nasal congestion
• Risk for deficient fluid volume related to drug-induced adverse GI reactions
• Deficient knowledge related to drug therapy

▶ Planning and implementation

• Drug isn't effective for acute rhinitis. Decongestants or antihistamines may be needed.
• Shake container and invert it. Have patient clear his nasal passages and then tilt his head backward. Insert nozzle (pointed away from septum) into nostril, holding other nostril closed. Deliver spray while patient inhales. Shake container and repeat in other nostril.
• Notify prescriber if relief isn't obtained or signs of infection appear.

Patient teaching
• Teach patient how to give himself nasal spray.
• Advise patient to pump new nasal spray three or four times before first use and once or twice before first use each day thereafter. Also tell patient to clean cap and nosepiece of activator in warm water every day and to air-dry them.
• Advise patient to use drug as prescribed because its effectiveness depends on regular use.
• Explain that drug's therapeutic effects, unlike those of decongestants, aren't immediate. Most patients achieve benefit in a few days, but some may need 2 to 3 weeks.
• Warn patient not to exceed recommended doses because of risk of hypothalamic-pituitary-adrenal function suppression.
• Tell patient to notify prescriber if symptoms don't improve within 3 weeks or if nasal irritation persists.
• Teach patient good nasal and oral hygiene.

☑ Evaluation

• Patient's nasal congestion subsides with therapy.
• Patient maintains adequate hydration throughout therapy.
• Patient and family state understanding of drug therapy.

benazepril hydrochloride
(ben-AY-zuh-pril high-droh-KLOR-ighd)
Lotensin

Pharmacologic class: ACE inhibitor
Therapeutic class: antihypertensive
Pregnancy risk category: C (D in second and third trimesters)

Indications and dosages

▶ **Hypertension.** *Adults not taking diuretics:*
Initially, 10 mg P.O. daily. Adjust dosage as needed and tolerated, usually 20 to 40 mg daily, equally divided into one or two doses. Maximum, 80 mg daily.
Adults taking diuretics: Stop diuretic 2 to 3 days before starting this drug to minimize hypotension. If unable to stop diuretic, start dose at 5 mg daily.
🔲 **Adjust-a-dose:** For adults with renal impairment, if creatinine clearance is less than 30 ml/minute (or serum creatine is less than 3 mg/dl), start dose at 5 mg daily. Don't exceed 40 mg P.O. daily.
Children age 6 and older with creatinine clearance greater than 30 ml/minute: 0.2 mg/kg P.O. daily. Doses exceeding 0.6 mg/kg (or in excess of 40 mg/day) haven't been studied.

Contraindications and cautions

• Contraindicated in patients hypersensitive to ACE inhibitors.
• Use cautiously in patients with impaired hepatic or renal function.
🔹 **Lifespan:** In pregnant women, stop drug as soon as possible; it can cause injury and death to the fetus during the second and third trimesters. With breast-feeding women, use cautiously. In children younger than age 6 years and those with a glomerular filtration rate less than 30 ml/minute, safety of drug hasn't been established.

Adverse reactions

CNS: amnesia, anxiety, asthenia, depression, dizziness, headache, insomnia, lightheadedness, nervousness, neuralgia, neuropathy, paresthesia, somnolence, syncope.
CV: angina, *arrhythmias*, edema, palpitations, *symptomatic hypotension.*
GI: abdominal pain, constipation, dyspepsia, dysphagia, gastritis, increased salivation, nausea, vomiting.
GU: impotence.
Metabolic: *hyperkalemia,* weight gain.
Musculoskeletal: arthralgia, arthritis, myalgia.
Respiratory: dry, persistent, tickling, nonproductive cough; dyspnea.
Skin: dermatitis, increased diaphoresis, photosensitivity, pruritus, purpura, rash.
Other: *angioedema,* hypersensitivity reactions.

Interactions

Drug-drug. *Digoxin:* May increase digoxin level. Monitor patient for toxicity.
Diuretics, other antihypertensives: May cause excessive hypotension. Stop diuretic or lower dose of benazepril, if needed.
Indomethacin, aspirin: May reduce hypotensive effects. Monitor blood pressure.
Lithium: May increase lithium level and toxicity. Avoid use together.
Potassium-sparing diuretics, potassium supplements: May cause hyperkalemia. Monitor patient closely.
Drug-herb. *Capsicum:* May aggravate or cause ACE inhibitor–induced cough. Discourage use together.
Licorice: May cause sodium retention, thus decreasing ACE inhibitor effects. Discourage use together.
Sodium substitutes containing potassium: May cause hyperkalemia. Monitor patient closely.

Effects on lab test results

• May increase BUN, creatinine, uric acid, glucose, bilirubin, liver enzymes, and potassium levels.

Pharmacokinetics

Absorption: At least 37%.
Distribution: Extensively protein-bound.
Metabolism: Almost completely in liver to benazeprilat, which has much greater ACE inhibitory activity than benazepril.

Excretion: Mainly in urine. *Half-life:* Benazepril, about ½ hour; benazeprilat, 10 to 12 hours.

Route	Onset	Peak	Duration
P.O.	≤ 1 hr	2–6 hr	24 hr

Action

Chemical effect: Inhibits ACE, preventing conversion of angiotensin I to angiotensin II, a potent vasoconstrictor. Reduced formation of angiotensin II decreases peripheral arterial resistance, thus decreasing aldosterone secretion. This reduces sodium and water retention and lowers blood pressure. Drug also is antihypertensive in patients with low-renin hypertension.
Therapeutic effect: Lowers blood pressure.

Available forms

Tablets: 5 mg, 10 mg, 20 mg, 40 mg

NURSING PROCESS

Assessment
• Obtain history of patient's blood pressure before therapy, and reassess regularly thereafter. Measure blood pressure when drug level is at peak (2 to 6 hours after dose) and trough (just before dose) to verify adequate blood pressure control.
• Be alert for adverse reactions and drug interactions.
• Monitor patient's ECG.
• Monitor renal and hepatic function periodically. Also monitor potassium levels.
• Monitor patient's CBC with differential every 2 weeks for first 3 months of therapy and periodically thereafter. Other ACE inhibitors have been linked to agranulocytosis and neutropenia.
• Assess patient's and family's understanding of drug therapy.

Nursing diagnoses
• Risk for injury related to hypertension
• Decreased cardiac output related to drug-induced arrhythmias
• Deficient knowledge related to drug therapy

Planning and implementation
• If patient takes a diuretic, benazepril dose should be reduced; excessive hypotension can occur when given with diuretics.
• For children who can't swallow pills, an oral suspension can be made from the tablet.

• Give drug at about the same time every day to maintain consistent effect on blood pressure.
• Give drug when patient's stomach is empty.
Patient teaching
• Instruct patient to take drug on an empty stomach; meals, particularly those high in fat, can impair absorption.
• Tell patient to avoid sodium substitutes because such products may contain potassium, which can cause hyperkalemia.
• Tell patient to rise slowly to minimize risk of dizziness, which may occur during first few weeks of therapy. Advise patient to stop taking drug and to call prescriber immediately if dizziness occurs.
• Tell patient to use caution in hot weather and during exercise. Inadequate fluid intake, vomiting, diarrhea, and excessive perspiration can lead to light-headedness and syncope.
• Urge patient to report signs of infection, such as fever and sore throat. Also tell him to call prescriber if any of the following occurs: easy bruising or bleeding; swelling of tongue, lips, face, eyes, mucous membranes, or limbs; difficulty swallowing or breathing; or hoarseness.
• Tell woman to notify prescriber if pregnancy occurs. Drug will need to be stopped.

☑ Evaluation
• Patient's blood pressure is normal.
• Patient has adequate cardiac output during drug therapy.
• Patient and family state understanding of drug therapy.

benztropine mesylate
(BENZ-troh-peen MESS-ih-layt)
Cogentin

Pharmacologic class: anticholinergic
Therapeutic class: antiparkinsonian
Pregnancy risk category: C

Indications and dosages

▶ **Drug-induced extrapyramidal disorders (except tardive dyskinesia).** *Adults:* 1 to 4 mg P.O. or I.M. once or twice daily.
▶ **Acute dystonic reaction.** *Adults:* 1 to 2 mg I.V. or I.M., followed by 1 to 2 mg P.O. b.i.d. to prevent recurrence.

▶ **Parkinsonism.** *Adults:* 0.5 to 6 mg P.O. daily. Initial dose is 0.5 to 1 mg. I.M. or P.O. Because of cumulative action, start at a low dose and increase by 0.5 mg every 5 to 6 days. Adjust to meet individual requirements. Maximum, 6 mg daily.

▽ I.V. administration
• Drug is seldom used I.V. because of small difference in onset compared with I.M. route.
⊗ **Incompatibilities**
None reported.

Contraindications and cautions
• Contraindicated in patients hypersensitive to drug or its components and in those with acute angle-closure glaucoma.
• Use cautiously in patients exposed to hot weather, those with mental disorders, and those with prostatic hyperplasia, arrhythmias, seizure disorder, obstructive disease of the GI or GU tract, or a tendency toward urine retention.
⚖ **Lifespan:** In pregnant women, use cautiously. In breast-feeding women and children younger than age 3, drug is contraindicated. In children age 3 and older and adults older than age 60, use cautiously.

Adverse reactions
CNS: confusion, depression, disorientation, hallucinations, headache, incoherence, irritability, nervousness, restlessness, sedation.
CV: flushing, palpitations, *paradoxical bradycardia,* tachycardia.
EENT: blurred vision, difficulty swallowing, dilated pupils, photophobia.
GI: *constipation,* dry mouth, epigastric distress, nausea, vomiting.
GU: urinary hesitancy, urine retention.
Musculoskeletal: muscle weakness.

Interactions
Drug-drug. *Amantadine, phenothiazines, tricyclic antidepressants:* May cause additive anticholinergic adverse reactions, such as hyperthermia or heat intolerance. Notify prescriber immediately about adverse GI effects, fever, or heat intolerance.
Other anticholinergics and antiparkinsonians: May increase anticholinergic effects and may be fatal. Use cautiously.
Cholinesterase inhibitors: May decrease effectiveness of cholinesterase inhibitors.

Reactions may be *common,* uncommon, *life-threatening,* or COMMON AND LIFE-THREATENING.

Effects on lab test results

None reported.

Pharmacokinetics

Absorption: Unknown.
Distribution: Largely unknown; however, drug crosses blood–brain barrier.
Metabolism: Unknown.
Excretion: In urine as unchanged drug and metabolites. *Half-life:* Unknown.

Route	Onset	Peak	Duration
P.O.	1–2 hr	Unknown	24 hr
I.V., I.M.	≤ 15 min	Unknown	24 hr

Action

Chemical effect: Unknown; thought to block central cholinergic receptors, helping to balance cholinergic activity in basal ganglia.
Therapeutic effect: Improves capability for voluntary movement.

Available forms

Injection: 1 mg/ml in 2-ml ampules
Tablets: 0.5 mg, 1 mg, 2 mg

NURSING PROCESS

☞ Assessment
• Obtain history of patient's dyskinetic movements and underlying condition before therapy.
• Monitor effectiveness by regularly checking body movements for signs of improvement. Full effect of drug may take 2 to 3 days.
• Be alert for adverse reactions and drug interactions. Some adverse reactions may result from atropine-like toxicity and are dose related.
• Assess patient's and family's understanding of drug therapy.

🔄 Nursing diagnoses
• Impaired physical mobility related to dyskinetic movements
• Risk for injury related to drug-induced adverse CNS reactions
• Deficient knowledge related to drug therapy

➤ Planning and implementation
⏲ **ALERT:** Never stop drug abruptly. Reduce dose gradually.
• Give drug after meals to help prevent GI distress.

• The I.M. route is preferred for parenteral administration.
• If patient will receive single daily dose, give drug at bedtime.
Patient teaching
• Warn patient to avoid activities requiring alertness until CNS effects of drug are known.
• If patient will take single daily dose, tell him to take it at bedtime.
• If patient will take drug orally, tell him to take it after meals.
• Advise patient to report signs of urinary hesitancy or urine retention.
• Tell patient to relieve dry mouth with cool drinks, ice chips, sugarless gum, or hard candy.
• Advise patient to limit activities during hot weather because drug-induced anhidrosis may result in hyperthermia.

☑ Evaluation
• Patient has improved mobility with reduced muscle rigidity, akinesia, and tremors.
• Patient sustains no injury as a result of drug-induced adverse CNS reactions.
• Patient and family state understanding of drug therapy.

HIGH ALERT!

bevacizumab
(beh-vah-SIZZ-yoo-mab)
Avastin

Pharmacologic class: monoclonal antibody
Therapeutic class: antineoplastic
Pregnancy risk category: C

Indications and dosages

➤ **Metastatic colon or rectal cancer, given with fluorouracil-based chemotherapy as first- or second-line treatment.** *Adults:* If used with bolus IFL regimen (irinotecan, 5-fluorouracil, leucovorin), give 5 mg/kg I.V. every 14 days until disease progresses. If used with FOLFOX4 regimen (5-fluorouracil, oxaliplatin, leucovorin), give 10 mg/kg I.V. every 14 days until disease progresses. Don't start therapy for at least 28 days after major surgery. Make sure incision is fully healed before therapy starts.

➤ **Unresectable, locally advanced, recurrent or metastatic, nonsquamous, non–small-cell lung cancer, given with carboplatin and**

paclitaxel as first-line treatment. *Adults:* 15 mg/kg I.V. infusion once every 3 weeks.

▽ I.V. administration

• Dilute using aseptic technique. Don't freeze or shake the vials. Withdraw proper dose and mix into I.V. bag with 100 ml normal saline solution.
• Give the first infusion over 90 minutes and, if tolerated, the second infusion over 60 minutes. Later infusions can be given over 30 minutes if patient tolerated previous infusions.
• Don't give I.V. push or bolus.
• Drug is stable for 8 hours if refrigerated at 36° to 46° F (2° to 8° C) and protected from light.
⊗ **Incompatibilities**
Dextrose solutions.

Contraindications and cautions

• Contraindicated in patients with recent hemoptysis or within 28 days of major surgery.
• Use with extreme caution if patient has significant CV disease or history of arterial thromboembolism.
• Use cautiously in patients hypersensitive to drug or its components. Also use cautiously in patients who need surgery.
☀ **Lifespan:** In pregnant women, use during pregnancy only if potential benefits to the mother outweigh risks to the fetus. Breast-feeding women should stop nursing during therapy and for 60 days after it stops because of the drug's long half-life. In children, safety and effectiveness haven't been established. In patients age 65 or older, increased risk of serious to fatal arterial thromboembolic events.

Adverse reactions

CNS: abnormal gait, *asthenia,* confusion, *dizziness, headache,* pain, syncope.
CV: *deep vein thrombosis, heart failure, hypertension,* hypotension, INTRA-ABDOMINAL THROMBOSIS, *thromboembolism.*
EENT: *epistaxis,* excess lacrimation, gum bleeding, nasal septum perforation, taste disorder, voice alteration.
GI: abdominal pain, *anorexia,* colitis, *constipation, diarrhea,* dry mouth, *dyspepsia, flatulence, GI hemorrhage, GI perforation,* nausea, *stomatitis, vomiting.*
GU: proteinuria, urinary urgency, *vaginal hemorrhage.*

Hematologic: *leukopenia, neutropenia, thrombocytopenia.*
Metabolic: bilirubinemia, *hypokalemia, weight loss.*
Musculoskeletal: myalgia.
Respiratory: dyspnea, HEMOPTYSIS, PULMONARY HEMORRHAGE upper respiratory tract infection.
Skin: *alopecia, dermatitis, discoloration, dry skin, exfoliative dermatitis,* nail disorder, skin ulcer.
Other: slow wound healing, hypersensitivity.

Interactions

Drug-drug. *Irinotecan:* May increase level of irinotecan metabolite (SN-38). Monitor patient.

Effects on lab test results

• May increase bilirubin and urine protein levels. May decrease potassium level.
• May decrease WBC, neutrophil, and platelet counts.

Pharmacokinetics

Absorption: Given I.V.
Distribution: Unknown.
Metabolism: To basic peptides via phagocytosis by the reticuloendothelial system.
Excretion: Via the reticuloendothelial system. *Half-life:* 11 to 50 days.

Route	Onset	Peak	Duration
I.V.	Unknown	Unknown	Unknown

Action

Chemical effect: Inhibits actions between proteins and surface receptors that would normally allow proliferation of endothelial cells and new blood vessel growth.
Therapeutic effect: Inhibits metastatic colon or rectal tumor growth.

Available forms

Solution: 25 mg/ml in 4-ml and 16-ml vials

NURSING PROCESS

📇 **Assessment**
• Assess patient's condition before therapy and regularly thereafter.
• Monitor CBC, platelet count, and serum electrolytes before and during therapy.

Reactions may be *common,* uncommon, *life-threatening,* or COMMON AND LIFE-THREATENING.

• Monitor patient for hypersensitivity reactions, which can occur during infusions.
• Monitor urinalysis for presence or worsening of proteinuria. Patients with 2+ or greater urine dipstick test should have 24-hour urine collection.
• Monitor patient for reversible posterior leukoencephalopathy syndrome, a rare brain-capillary leak syndrome. Signs and symptoms include hypertension, fluid retention, headache, visual disturbances, altered mental state, and seizures.
• Check patient's blood pressure every 2 to 3 weeks.
• Assess patient's and family's knowledge of drug therapy.

🖳 Nursing diagnoses
• Ineffective health maintenance related to presence of neoplastic disease
• Delayed surgical recovery related to decreased wound healing effects of drug
• Deficient knowledge related to bevacizumab therapy

▷ Planning and implementation
• Monitor patient for serious adverse effects during therapy. Stop drug if patient develops nephrotic syndrome, severe hypertension, hypertensive crisis, hemoptysis, serious hemorrhage, GI perforation, or wound dehiscence that needs intervention.
• Stop drug before elective surgery, taking into account drug's half-life of about 20 days. Don't resume therapy until surgical incision is fully healed.
🜲 **ALERT:** Drug may increase the risk of serious or fatal arterial thromboembolic events, including MI, transient ischemic attack, stroke, and angina. Patients at highest risk include those age 65 or older, those with a history of arterial thromboembolism, and those previously treated with drug. If patient has an arterial thrombotic event, stop therapy.
🜲 **ALERT:** May cause fatal GI perforation. Monitor the patient closely.
• Treat symptoms and provide supportive care if overdose occurs. Large doses may cause headache, and the maximum tolerated dose is unknown.
Patient teaching
• Inform patient about potential adverse reactions.

• Tell patient to immediately report adverse reactions, especially abdominal pain, constipation, or vomiting.
• Advise patient that blood pressure and urinalysis will be monitored during treatment.
• Caution women of childbearing age to avoid pregnancy during treatment.
• Urge patient to alert other health care providers about treatment and to avoid elective surgery during treatment.

☑ Evaluation
• Patient responds to drug therapy.
• Drug is stopped before surgery. Drug therapy isn't started until surgical incision is fully healed.
• Patient and family state understanding of drug therapy.

bimatoprost
(by-MAT-oh-prohst)
Lumigan

Pharmacologic class: prostaglandin analogue
Therapeutic class: antiglaucoma drug, ocular antihypertensive
Pregnancy risk category: C

Indications and dosages
▶ **Elevated intraocular pressure (IOP), first- or second-line treatment in patients with open-angle glaucoma or ocular hypertension.**
Adults: Instill 1 drop in the conjunctival sac of each affected eye once daily in the evening.

Contraindications and cautions
• Contraindicated in patients hypersensitive to bimatoprost, benzalkonium chloride, or the drug's components. Also contraindicated in patients with angle-closure glaucoma, inflammatory glaucoma, or neovascular glaucoma.
• Use cautiously in patients with renal or hepatic impairment, active intraocular inflammation (iritis or uveitis), aphakic patients, pseudophakic patients with a torn posterior lens capsule, or patients at risk for macular edema.
🜲 **Lifespan:** In pregnant women, drug isn't recommended. In breast-feeding women, use cautiously because it's unknown whether drug appears in breast milk. In children, safety and effectiveness of drug haven't been established.

Adverse reactions

CNS: asthenia, headache.
EENT: allergic conjunctivitis, asthenopia, blepharitis, cataract, conjunctival edema, *conjunctival hyperemia,* eye discharge, eye pain, eyelash darkening, eyelid erythema, foreign body sensation, gradual change in eye color, *growth of eyelashes,* increased iris pigmentation, ocular burning, ocular dryness, ocular irritation, *ocular pruritus,* photophobia, pigmentation of the periocular skin, superficial punctate keratitis, tearing, visual disturbance.
Respiratory: *upper respiratory tract infection.*
Skin: hirsutism.
Other: *infection.*

Interactions

None significant.

Effects on lab test results

• May cause abnormal liver function test values.

Pharmacokinetics

Absorption: Through the cornea.
Distribution: Moderately into tissues. About 12% remains unbound.
Metabolism: Mainly by oxidation.
Excretion: Metabolites are 67% eliminated in urine; 25% are eliminated in feces. *Half-life:* 45 minutes.

Route	Onset	Peak	Duration
Ophthalmic	4 hr	10 min	1½ hr

Action

Chemical effect: May increase the outflow of aqueous humor through the trabecular meshwork and uveoscleral routes.
Therapeutic effect: Reduces IOP.

Available forms

Ophthalmic solution: 0.03%

NURSING PROCESS

🔲 Assessment
🟢 **ALERT:** Obtain complete medication history. If more than one ophthalmic drug is being used, give drugs at least 5 minutes apart.
• Assess patient's underlying condition and eyes before giving eye drops.
• Monitor patient for excessive ocular irritation, and evaluate the success of treatment.

• Assess patient's and family's knowledge of drug therapy and administration.

🔲 Nursing diagnoses
• Risk for injury related to improper administration of drug
• Disturbed sensory perception (visual) related to underlying condition
• Deficient knowledge related to bimatoprost therapy

▶ Planning and implementation
🟢 **ALERT:** Contact lenses must be removed before using solution. Lenses may be reinserted 15 minutes after administration.
• Don't touch the tip of the dropper to the eye. Avoid contaminating the dropper.
• Apply light pressure on lacrimal sac for 1 minute after instillation to minimize systemic absorption of the drug.
• Store drug in original container at 59° to 77° F (15° to 25° C).
• Pigmentation of the iris, eyelid, and eyelashes may increase, and eyelashes may grow.
Patient teaching
• Explain to patients receiving treatment in only one eye the possibility for increased brown pigmentation of iris, eyelid skin darkening, and increased length, thickness, pigmentation, or number of lashes in the treated eye.
• Teach patient to instill drops properly, and advise him to wash his hands before and after. Warn him not to touch the dropper tip to the eye or surrounding tissue.
• If eye trauma or infection occurs or if eye surgery is needed, tell patient to seek immediate medical advice before continuing to use multidose container.
• Urge patient to immediately report conjunctivitis or lid reactions to prescriber.

🔳 Evaluation
• Patient demonstrates proper instillation of the drug, and no injury occurs.
• Patient's underlying eye condition responds positively to drug.
• Patient and family state understanding of drug therapy.

Reactions may be *common,* uncommon, *life-threatening*, or COMMON AND LIFE-THREATENING.

bisacodyl

(bigh-suh-KOH-dil)
**Bisac-Evac†, Bisacodyl Uniserts†,
Bisacolax ◆ †, Bisa-lax†, Caroid†,
Correctol†, Dulcolax†, Ex-Lax Ultra†,
Feen-a-Mint†, Fleet Laxative†, Modane†**

Pharmacologic class: diphenylmethane derivative
Therapeutic class: stimulant laxative
Pregnancy risk category: NR

Indications and dosages

▶ **Chronic constipation; preparation for childbirth, surgery, or rectal or bowel examination.** *Adults and children age 12 and older:* 10 to 15 mg P.O. in evening or before breakfast. Maximum, 30 mg P.O. For preparation for examination or surgery, 10 mg P.R.
Children ages 6 to 12: Give 5 mg P.O. or P.R. at bedtime or before breakfast.

Contraindications and cautions

• Contraindicated in patients hypersensitive to drug and in those with rectal bleeding, gastroenteritis, intestinal obstruction, or symptoms of appendicitis or acute surgical abdomen, such as abdominal pain, nausea, or vomiting.
⚘ **Lifespan:** In pregnant women and children younger than age 10, safety hasn't been established.

Adverse reactions

GI: *abdominal cramps, burning sensation in rectum* (with suppositories), diarrhea (with high doses), laxative dependence (with long-term or excessive use), *nausea,* protein-losing enteropathy (with excessive use), *vomiting.*
Metabolic: *alkalosis,* fluid and electrolyte imbalance, hypokalemia.
Musculoskeletal: muscle weakness (with excessive use), tetany.

Interactions

Drug-drug. *Antacids:* May cause gastric irritation or dyspepsia from premature dissolution of enteric coating. Avoid use together.
Drug-food. *Milk:* May cause gastric irritation or dyspepsia from premature dissolution of enteric coating. Avoid use together.

Effects on lab test results

• May increase phosphate and sodium levels. May decrease calcium, magnesium, and potassium levels.

Pharmacokinetics

Absorption: Minimal.
Distribution: Locally.
Metabolism: Up to 15% of P.O. dose may enter enterohepatic circulation.
Excretion: Mainly in feces; some in urine.
Half-life: Unknown.

Route	Onset	Peak	Duration
P.O.	6–12 hr	Variable	Variable
P.R.	15–60 min	Variable	Variable

Action

Chemical effect: Increases peristalsis, probably by acting directly on smooth muscle of intestine. May irritate musculature, stimulate colonic intramural plexus, and promote fluid accumulation in colon and small intestine.
Therapeutic effect: Relieves constipation.

Available forms

Enema: 10 mg/30 ml†
Suppositories: 10 mg†
Tablets (delayed-release): 10 mg†
Tablets (enteric-coated): 5 mg†

NURSING PROCESS

Assessment
• Obtain history of bowel disorder, GI status, fluid intake, nutritional status, exercise habits, and normal patterns of elimination.
• Monitor effectiveness by checking frequency and characteristics of stools.
• Be alert for adverse reactions and drug interactions.
• Auscultate bowel sounds at least once per shift. Check for pain and cramping.
• Assess patient's and family's understanding of drug therapy.

Nursing diagnoses
• Constipation related to interruption of normal pattern of elimination
• Acute pain related to drug-induced abdominal cramps
• Deficient knowledge related to drug therapy

⬎ Planning and implementation

• Don't give tablets within 60 minutes of milk or antacid.

• Insert suppository as high as possible into rectum, and try to position suppository against rectal wall. Avoid embedding in fecal material because this may delay onset of action.

• Time administration of drug so as not to interfere with scheduled activities or sleep. Soft, formed stool usually is produced 15 to 60 minutes after P.R. administration.

• Tablets and suppositories are used together to clean colon before and after surgery and before barium enema.

• Store tablets and suppositories below 86° F (30° C).

Patient teaching

• Advise patient to swallow enteric-coated tablet whole to avoid GI irritation. Tell him not to take tablet within 1 hour of milk or antacid.

• Advise patient to report adverse effects to prescriber.

• Teach patient about dietary sources of fiber, including bran and other cereals, fresh fruit, and vegetables.

• Warn patient against excessive use of drug.

☑ Evaluation

• Patient reports return of normal bowel pattern of elimination.

• Patient is free from abdominal pain and cramping.

• Patient and family state understanding of drug therapy.

---

bismuth subgallate

(BIS-muth sub-GAL-ayt)
Devrom

bismuth subsalicylate

Children's Kaopectate†, Extra Strength Kaopectate†, Kaopectate (Regular)†, Maximum Strength Pepto-Bismol†, Pepto-Bismol†

Pharmacologic class: adsorbent
Therapeutic class: antidiarrheal
Pregnancy risk category: NR

Indications and dosages

▶ **To control fecal odors in colostomy, ileostomy, or incontinence.** *Adults:* 1 to 2 subgallate tablets P.O. t.i.d. with meals. Tablet can be chewed or swallowed whole.

▶ **Mild, nonspecific diarrhea.** *Adults and children age 12 and older:* 30 ml or 2 subsalicylate tablets P.O. every 30 minutes to 1 hour up to a maximum of eight doses in 24 hours and for no longer than 2 days.

Children ages 9 to 12: Give 15 ml or 1 subsalicylate tablet P.O. every 30 minutes to 1 hour up to a maximum of eight doses in 24 hours and for no longer than 2 days.

Children ages 6 to 9: Give 10 ml or ⅔ subsalicylate tablet P.O. every 30 minutes to 1 hour up to a maximum of eight doses in 24 hours and for no longer than 2 days.

Children ages 3 to 6: Give 5 ml or ½ subsalicylate tablet P.O. every 30 minutes to 1 hour up to a maximum of eight doses in 24 hours and for no longer than 2 days.

Contraindications and cautions

• Contraindicated in patients hypersensitive to salicylates.

• Use cautiously in patients already taking aspirin.

🎇 **Lifespan:** In pregnant or breast-feeding women, use cautiously.

Adverse reactions

GI: temporary darkening of tongue and stools.
Other: salicylism (with high doses).

Interactions

Drug-drug. *Aspirin, other salicylates:* May increase risk of salicylate toxicity. Monitor patient closely.

Oral anticoagulants, oral antidiabetics: May increase effects of these drugs after high doses of bismuth subsalicylate. Monitor patient closely.

Probenecid: May decrease uricosuric effects after high doses of bismuth subsalicylate. Monitor patient closely.

Tetracycline: May decrease tetracycline absorption. Give drugs at least 2 hours apart.

Effects on lab test results

• May increase lipid levels.

Pharmacokinetics

Absorption: Poor; significant salicylate absorption may occur after taking subsalicylate form.
Distribution: Local.
Metabolism: Minimal.
Excretion: Subsalicylate form: in urine. *Half-life:* Unknown.

Route	Onset	Peak	Duration
P.O.	1 hr	Unknown	Unknown

Action

Chemical effect: May adsorb toxins and provide protective coating for mucosa.
Therapeutic effect: Relieves diarrhea.

Available forms

bismuth subgallate
Tablets (chewable): 200 mg†
bismuth subsalicylate
Caplet: 262 mg
Liquid (Children's): 87 mg/5 ml
Liquid (Extra Strength): 175 mg/5 ml
Liquid (Regular): 87.3 mg/ml
Oral suspension: 130 mg/15 ml, 262 mg/15 ml†, 524 mg/15 ml†
Tablets (chewable): 262 mg†

NURSING PROCESS

⚡ Assessment
• Obtain history of patient's bowel disorder, GI status, and frequency of loose stools.
• Monitor drug's effectiveness by checking frequency and nature of stools.
• Be alert for adverse reactions and drug interactions.
• Check patient's hearing if he takes drug in large doses.
• Assess patient's and family's understanding of drug therapy.

⊕ Nursing diagnoses
• Diarrhea related to underlying GI condition
• Disturbed sensory perception (auditory) related to drug-induced salicylism
• Deficient knowledge related to drug therapy

▷ Planning and implementation
• Avoid use before GI radiologic procedures because drug is radiopaque and may interfere with X-rays.

• Read label carefully because dosage varies with form of drug.
• If tinnitus occurs, stop drug and notify prescriber.
Patient teaching
⑤ ALERT: Oral OTC drug products containing subsalicylate form or kaolin are the only ones generally recognized as safe and effective for use as antidiarrheals.
• Advise patient that drug contains large amount of salicylate. Each tablet contains 102 mg; regular-strength liquid contains 130 mg/15 ml, and extra-strength liquid contains 230 mg/15 ml.
• Instruct patient to chew tablets well or to shake liquid before measuring dose.
• Tell patient to report diarrhea that persists for longer than 2 days or is accompanied by high fever.
• Tell patient to consult with prescriber before giving bismuth subsalicylate to children or teenagers who have or are recovering from flu or chickenpox because of risk of Reye syndrome.
• Inform patient that both liquid and tablet forms are effective against traveler's diarrhea. Tablets may be more convenient to carry.
• Tell patient that any darkening of stool or the tongue is temporary.

✔ Evaluation
• Patient reports decrease or absence of loose stools.
• Patient remains free from signs and symptoms of salicylism.
• Patient and family state understanding of drug therapy.

bisoprolol fumarate
(bis-OP-roh-lol FOO-muh-rayt)
Zebeta

Pharmacologic class: beta blocker
Therapeutic class: antihypertensive
Pregnancy risk category: C

Indications and dosages
▶ **Hypertension.** *Adults:* Initially, 5 mg P.O. once daily. If response is inadequate, increase to 10 mg or 20 mg P.O. daily. Maximum, 20 mg.

◤ **Adjust-a-dose:** For patients with renal impairment, a creatinine clearance of less than 40 ml/minute, hepatic dysfunction, cirrhosis, or hepatitis, start with 2.5 mg P.O. daily. Adjust dosage cautiously.

▶ **Heart failure‡.** *Adults:* 1.25 mg P.O. daily for 2 to 4 weeks. If dose is tolerated, increase dose to 2.5 mg daily for 2 to 4 weeks. Subsequent doses can be doubled every 2 to 4 weeks, if tolerated.

Contraindications and cautions

• Contraindicated in patients hypersensitive to drug and in those with cardiogenic shock, overt cardiac failure, marked sinus bradycardia, or second- or third-degree AV block.
• Use cautiously in patients with bronchospastic disease because blockade of beta$_1$ receptors isn't absolute and blockade of pulmonary beta$_2$ receptors may worsen symptoms. When giving drug to these patients, keep a bronchodilator available.
• Use cautiously in patients with diabetes, peripheral vascular disease, thyroid disease, or a history of heart failure.
☀ **Lifespan:** In pregnant or breast-feeding women, use cautiously. In children, safety and effectiveness of drug haven't been established.

Adverse reactions

CNS: asthenia, depression, dizziness, fatigue, headache, hypoesthesia, insomnia, vivid dreams.
CV: *bradycardia,* chest pain, *heart failure,* peripheral edema.
EENT: pharyngitis, rhinitis, sinusitis.
GI: diarrhea, dry mouth, nausea, vomiting.
Musculoskeletal: arthralgia.
Respiratory: cough, dyspnea.
Skin: sweating.

Interactions

Drug-drug. *Beta blockers:* May cause extreme hypotension. Don't use together.
Calcium channel blockers: May cause myocardial depression and AV conductive inhibition. Monitor ECG closely.
Guanethidine, reserpine: Can cause hypotension. Monitor patient closely.
NSAIDs: May decrease antihypertensive effect. Monitor blood pressure, and adjust dosage.
Rifampin: May increase metabolic clearance of bisoprolol. Monitor patient.

Effects on lab test results

None reported.

Pharmacokinetics

Absorption: After 10-mg dose, about 80%.
Distribution: About 30% protein-bound.
Metabolism: After first pass, about 20%.
Excretion: Equally by renal and nonrenal pathways, with about 50% of dose appearing unchanged in urine and remainder appearing as inactive metabolites. Less than 2% in feces.
Half-life: 9 to 12 hours.

Route	Onset	Peak	Duration
P.O.	Unknown	2–4 hr	24 hr

Action

Chemical effect: May decrease myocardial contractility, heart rate, and cardiac output; lowers blood pressure; and reduces myocardial oxygen consumption.
Therapeutic effect: Decreases blood pressure.

Available forms

Tablets: 5 mg, 10 mg

NURSING PROCESS

⚏ Assessment
• Obtain history of patient's hypertension before therapy, and check blood pressure regularly throughout therapy.
• Be alert for adverse reactions and drug interactions.
• If adverse GI reactions occur, monitor the patient's hydration.
• For patient with diabetes, monitor glucose level closely. Drug may mask evidence of hypoglycemia such as tachycardia.
• Assess patient's and family's understanding of drug therapy.

⊕ Nursing diagnoses
• Risk for injury related to presence of hypertension
• Risk for deficient fluid volume related to drug-induced adverse GI reactions
• Deficient knowledge related to drug therapy

▷ Planning and implementation
• Have a beta$_2$ agonist (bronchodilator) available for patients with bronchospastic disease.

• 1.25-mg tablet isn't available in the United States. Carefully split 5-mg tablet or request assistance from pharmacy.

⚠ **ALERT:** Don't stop drug abruptly; angina may occur in patients with unrecognized coronary artery disease.

⚠ **ALERT:** Don't confuse Zebeta with Zestril, Zetia, or Zyrtec.

Patient teaching

• Tell patient to take drug as prescribed, even when he's feeling better. Warn him that stopping drug abruptly can worsen angina and precipitate MI. Explain that drug must be withdrawn gradually over 1 to 2 weeks.

• Instruct patient to call prescriber if adverse reactions occur.

• Tell patient with diabetes to closely monitor glucose levels.

• Tell patient to check with prescriber or pharmacist before taking OTC medications or herbal remedies.

☑ **Evaluation**

• Patient's blood pressure is normal.

• Patient maintains adequate fluid balance throughout therapy.

• Patient and family state understanding of drug therapy.

HIGH ALERT!

bivalirudin

(bye-VAL-ih-roo-din)
Angiomax

Pharmacologic class: direct thrombin inhibitor
Therapeutic class: anticoagulant
Pregnancy risk category: B

Indications and dosages

▶ **Anticoagulation in patients with unstable angina undergoing percutaneous transluminal coronary angioplasty (PTCA); anticoagulation in patients with unstable angina undergoing percutaneous coronary intervention (PCI), with provisional use of a glycoprotein IIb/IIIa platelet inhibitor (GPI).** *Adults:* 0.75 mg/kg I.V. bolus followed by a continuous infusion of 1.75 mg/kg/hour for the duration of the procedure. Check activated clotting time 5 minutes after bolus dose. May give additional 0.3-mg/kg bolus dose if needed. Infusion may continue for up to 4 hours after procedure. After

4-hour infusion, may give an additional infusion of 0.2 mg/kg/hour for up to 20 hours, if needed. Use with 300 to 325 mg aspirin.

◪ **Adjust-a-dose:** For patients with creatinine clearance of 30 ml/minute or less, decrease infusion rate to 1 mg/kg/hour. For patients on hemodialysis, reduce infusion rate to 0.25 mg/kg/hour. No reduction of bolus dose is needed.

▶ **Patients with or at risk for heparin-induced thrombocytopenia (HIT) or heparin-induced thrombocytopenia and thrombosis syndrome (HITTS) undergoing PCI.** *Adults:* 0.75 mg/kg I.V. bolus followed by continuous infusion of 1.75 mg/kg/hour for the duration of the procedure. The prescriber may continue the infusion after PCI.

▽ **I.V. administration**

• Reconstitute each 250-mg vial with 5 ml of sterile water for injection. Further dilute each reconstituted vial in 50 ml D_5W or normal saline solution to yield 5 mg/ml.

• To prepare low-rate infusion, further dilute each reconstituted vial in 500 ml D_5W or normal saline solution to yield 0.5 mg/ml.

• The prepared solution is stable and may be stored for up to 24 hours at 36° to 46° F (2° to 8° C).

⊗ **Incompatibilities**

Alteplase, amiodarone, amphotericin B, chlorpromazine, diazepam, prochlorperazine edisylate, reteplase, streptokinase, vancomycin, all I.V. drugs.

Contraindications and cautions

• Contraindicated in patients hypersensitive to the drug or its components and in patients with active major bleeding. Don't use drug in patients with unstable angina who aren't undergoing PTCA or PCI, in patients with other acute coronary conditions, or in patients who aren't taking aspirin.

• Use cautiously in patients with HIT or HITTS and in patients with an increased risk of bleeding.

⚘ **Lifespan:** In pregnant women, use only if clearly needed because of the risk of maternal bleeding. In breast-feeding women, use cautiously because it isn't known whether drug appears in breast milk. In children, safety and effectiveness of drug haven't been established. In elderly patients, use with caution because

they're more likely to get puncture-site hemorrhage or catheterization-site hematoma.

Adverse reactions

CNS: anxiety, *cerebral ischemia,* confusion, fever, *headache,* insomnia, nervousness, *pain.*
CV: *bradycardia,* hypertension, hypotension, syncope, vascular anomaly, *ventricular fibrillation.*
GI: abdominal pain, dyspepsia, *nausea,* vomiting.
GU: oliguria, *renal failure,* urine retention.
Hematologic: *arterial site hemorrhage; severe, spontaneous bleeding (cerebral, GI, GU, retroperitoneal).*
Musculoskeletal: *back pain,* pelvic pain, facial paralysis.
Respiratory: *pulmonary edema.*
Other: infection, pain at injection site, *sepsis.*

Interactions

Drug-drug. *GPIIb/IIIa inhibitors:* Safety and effectiveness haven't been established. Avoid use together.
Heparin, warfarin, other oral anticoagulants: May increase risk of bleeding. Use together cautiously. If using low–molecular-weight heparin, stop it at least 8 hours before giving bivalirudin.

Effects on lab test results

• May increase activated clotting time, PTT, thrombin time, and PT.

Pharmacokinetics

Absorption: Given I.V.
Distribution: Binds rapidly to thrombin and has a rapid onset of action.
Metabolism: Rapid, through a combination of renal mechanisms and proteolytic cleavage.
Excretion: Renal. Total body clearance is similar in patients with normal renal function and mild renal impairment. Reduced about 20% in patients with moderate and severe renal impairment and about 80% in dialysis-dependent patients. Hemodialyzable. *Half-life:* 25 minutes in patients with normal renal function.

Route	Onset	Peak	Duration
I.V.	Rapid	Immediate	Duration of infusion

Action

Chemical effect: Directly inhibits both clot-bound and circulating thrombin, preventing generation of fibrin and further activation of the clotting cascade. Inhibits thrombin-induced platelet activation, granule release, and aggregation.
Therapeutic effect: Prevents blood clots.

Available forms

Injection: 250-mg vial

NURSING PROCESS

Assessment
• Obtain and monitor baseline coagulation tests and hemoglobin level and hematocrit before and throughout therapy.
• Monitor effectiveness by measuring PTT, PT, and thrombin time values regularly.
• Monitor venipuncture sites for bleeding, hematoma, or inflammation.
• Be alert for adverse reactions.
ALERT: If the patient has an unexplained drop in hematocrit, blood pressure, or other unexplained symptom, consider the possibility of hemorrhage.
• Assess access site regularly for bleeding.
• Assess patient's and family's knowledge of drug therapy.

Nursing diagnoses
• Risk for injury related to potential acute ischemic event caused by impaired CV status
• Ineffective protection related to increased risk of bleeding from anticoagulant therapy
• Deficient knowledge related to drug therapy

Planning and implementation
• Patients with renal failure require reduced dosage.
• Don't give I.M.
Patient teaching
• Advise patient that drug can cause bleeding. Urge patient to report immediately any unusual bruising or bleeding (nosebleeds, bleeding gums, petechiae, and hematuria), or tarry or bloody stools.
• Warn patient to avoid other aspirin-containing drugs and drugs used to treat swelling or pain (such as Motrin, Naprosyn, Aleve).
• Advise patient to avoid activities that carry a risk of injury, and instruct patient to use a soft toothbrush and electric razor while taking drug.

☑ Evaluation

• Patient doesn't have an acute ischemic event after PTCA or PCI.
• Patient doesn't have drug-induced adverse reactions or bleeding.
• Patient and family state understanding of drug therapy.

HIGH ALERT!

bleomycin sulfate
(blee-oh-MIGH-sin SULL-fayt)
Blenoxane

Pharmacologic class: antibiotic
Therapeutic class: antineoplastic
Pregnancy risk category: D

Indications and dosages

▶ **Hodgkin lymphoma, squamous cell carcinoma, non-Hodgkin lymphoma, testicular cancer.** *Adults:* 10 to 20 units/m² (0.25 to 0.5 units/kg) I.V., I.M., or subcutaneously once or twice weekly. After 50% response in patients with Hodgkin lymphoma, maintenance dosage is 1 unit I.V. or I.M. daily or 5 units I.V. or I.M. weekly.
▶ **Malignant pleural effusion, prevention of recurrent pleural effusions or to manage pneumothorax related to AIDS or *Pneumocystis jiroveci (carinii)* pneumonia.** *Adults:* Give 60 units as a single-dose bolus in 50 to 100 ml of normal saline solution by intrapleural injection through a chest tube. Leave in for 4 hours, then drain and resume suction. Maximum dose is 1 unit/kg.
Elderly patients receiving intrapleural injection: Don't exceed 40 units/m².
▶ **AIDS-related Kaposi sarcoma‡.** *Adults:* 20 units/m² daily I.V. continuously over 72 hours every 3 weeks.

▽ I.V. administration

• Follow facility policy for giving drug to reduce risks. Preparation and administration of parenteral form of this drug carry carcinogenic, mutagenic, and teratogenic risks.
• For I.V. use, dissolve contents of 15- or 30-unit vial with 5 or 10 ml, respectively, of normal saline for injection. Give slowly over 10 minutes.

⊗ Incompatibilities

Amino acids; aminophylline; ascorbic acid injection; cefazolin; diazepam; drugs containing sulfhydryl groups; fluids containing dextrose; furosemide; hydrocortisone; methotrexate; mitomycin; nafcillin; penicillin G; riboflavin; solutions containing divalent and trivalent cations, especially calcium salts and copper; terbutaline sulfate.

Contraindications and cautions

• Contraindicated in patients hypersensitive to drug.
• Use cautiously in patients with renal or pulmonary impairment.
⚹ **Lifespan:** In pregnant or breast-feeding women and in children, safety of drug hasn't been established.

Adverse reactions

CNS: fever, headache, hyperesthesia of scalp and fingers.
GI: diarrhea, nausea, *prolonged anorexia, stomatitis,* vomiting.
Hematologic: leukocytosis.
Musculoskeletal: swelling of interphalangeal joints.
Respiratory: *dyspnea, fine crackles, nonproductive cough,* PNEUMONITIS, *pulmonary fibrosis.*
Skin: *acne;* desquamation of hands, feet, and pressure areas; *erythema; hardening and discoloration of palmar and plantar skin; hyperpigmentation; reversible alopecia; vesiculation.*
Other: *anaphylaxis, hypersensitivity reactions (fever up to 106° F [41.1° C] with chills after injection).*

Interactions

Drug-drug. *Digoxin:* May decrease digoxin level. Monitor patient closely for loss of therapeutic effect.
Oxygen: Give supplemental oxygen, if ordered after treatment, at a fraction of inspired oxygen no higher than 25% to avoid potential lung damage.
Phenytoin: May decrease phenytoin level. Monitor patient closely.

Effects on lab test results

• May increase uric acid level.
• May increase WBC count.

Pharmacokinetics

Absorption: I.M. use yields lower levels than equivalent I.V. doses.
Distribution: Wide into total body water, mainly in skin, lungs, kidneys, peritoneum, and lymphatic tissue.
Metabolism: Unknown; however, extensive tissue inactivation occurs in liver and kidneys, with much less in skin and lungs.
Excretion: Drug and its metabolites primarily in urine. *Half-life:* 2 hours.

Route	Onset	Peak	Duration
I.V., I.M., intrapleural, SubQ	Unknown	Unknown	Unknown

Action

Chemical effect: May inhibit DNA synthesis and divide single- and double-stranded DNA.
Therapeutic effect: Kills selected types of cancer cells.

Available forms

Injection: 15- and 30-unit vials (1 unit = 1 mg)

NURSING PROCESS

Assessment

• Obtain history of patient's overall physical status (especially respiratory status, CBC, and pulmonary and renal function tests) before therapy and reassess regularly thereafter.
• Be alert for adverse reactions and drug interactions. Adverse pulmonary reactions are common in patients older than age 70.
⚠ **ALERT:** Fatal pulmonary fibrosis may occur rarely, especially when cumulative dose exceeds 400 units.
• Monitor patient for drug-induced fever, which is common and usually occurs 3 to 6 hours after giving drug.
• Watch for hypersensitivity reactions, which may be delayed for several hours, especially in patients with lymphoma.
• Assess patient for fine crackles and dyspnea.
• Assess patient's and family's understanding of drug therapy.

Nursing diagnoses

• Risk for injury related to underlying neoplastic condition

• Impaired gas exchange related to drug-induced adverse pulmonary reactions
• Deficient knowledge related to drug therapy

Planning and implementation

• Follow facility policy for giving drug to reduce risks. Preparation and administration of parenteral form of this drug carry carcinogenic, mutagenic, and teratogenic risks.
• For I.M. or subcutaneous routes, reconstitute 15-unit vial with 1 to 5 ml or the 30-unit vial with 2 to 10 ml of sterile water for injection, normal saline solution for injection, or bacteriostatic water for injection.
• Follow manufacturer's guidelines for giving subcutaneously.
• For intrapleural use, dissolve 60 units of drug in 50 to 100 ml normal saline solution for injection. Give through a chest tube after excess intrapleural fluid has been drained and complete lung expansion has been confirmed.
• Refrigerate unopened vials containing dry powder.
• Reconstituted solution for injection is stable for 4 weeks refrigerated or 2 weeks at room temperature; however, manufacturer recommends use within 24 hours of preparation and disposal of unused portion.
• If pulmonary function test shows a marked decline, stop drug.
• Don't use adhesive dressings on skin. This helps prevent streaking from drug concentrating in keratin of squamous epithelium.
• Give acetaminophen before treatment and for 24 hours after treatment in patients susceptible to post-treatment fever.

Patient teaching

• Explain the risks of drug therapy, especially the danger of serious pulmonary reactions in high-risk patients.
• Explain the need for monitoring and the type of monitoring to be done.
• Tell patient that alopecia may occur, but that it's usually reversible.

Evaluation

• Patient exhibits positive response to therapy, as shown by follow-up diagnostic test results.
• Patient's gas exchange remains normal throughout therapy.
• Patient and family state understanding of drug therapy.

Reactions may be *common*, uncommon, *life-threatening*, or COMMON AND LIFE-THREATENING.

B

bortezomib
(bore-TEHZ-uh-mihb)
Velcade

Pharmacologic class: proteasome inhibitor
Therapeutic class: antineoplastic
Pregnancy risk category: D

Indications and dosages

▶ **Multiple myeloma and mantle cell lymphoma that's progressing after at least one previous therapy.** *Adults:* 1.3 mg/m^2 by I.V. bolus twice weekly for 2 weeks (days 1, 4, 8, and 11) followed by a 10-day rest period (days 12 to 21). This 3-week period is a treatment cycle. For therapy of longer than 8 weeks, may adjust dosage schedule to once weekly for 4 weeks (days 1, 8, 15, and 22) followed by a 13-day rest period (days 23 to 35). Separate consecutive doses of drug by at least 72 hours.

▧ **Adjust-a-dose:** If patient develops a grade 3 nonhematologic or a grade 4 hematologic toxicity (excluding neuropathy), withhold drug. When toxicity resolves, restart at a 25% reduced dose. If patient has neuropathic pain, peripheral neuropathy, or both, use the following table.

Severity of neuropathy	Dosage adjustment
Grade 1 (paresthesias, loss of reflexes, or both without pain or loss of function)	No change.
Grade 1 with pain or grade 2 (function altered but not activities of daily living)	Reduce to 1 mg/m^2.
Grade 2 with pain or grade 3 (interference with activities of daily living)	Hold drug until toxicity resolves; then start at 0.7 mg/m^2 once weekly.
Grade 4 (permanent sensory loss that interferes with function)	Stop drug.

▼ I.V. administration

● Reconstitute with 3.5 ml of normal saline solution. Use caution and aseptic technique when preparing and handling drug. Wear gloves and protective clothing to prevent skin contact.
● Give by I.V. bolus within 8 hours of reconstitution.
● Drug may be stored up to 8 hours in a syringe, but total storage time for reconstituted solution mustn't exceed 8 hours when exposed to normal indoor lighting.
● Store unopened vials at a controlled room temperature, in original packaging, and protect from light.

⊗ **Incompatibilities**
None reported.

Contraindications and cautions

● Contraindicated in patients hypersensitive to bortezomib, boron, or mannitol.
● Use cautiously if patient is dehydrated, is receiving other drugs known to cause hypotension, or has a history of syncope. In patients with severe neuropathy, use cautiously and only after careful assessment of risks and benefits.
⚖ **Lifespan:** In pregnant or breast-feeding women, avoid use. Women should avoid breast-feeding or becoming pregnant during drug therapy. In children, safety and effectiveness of drug haven't been established.

Adverse reactions

CNS: anxiety, *asthenia,* dizziness, dysesthesia, *fever,* headache, insomnia, paresthesia, *peripheral neuropathy,* rigors.
CV: edema, orthostatic and postural hypotension.
EENT: blurred vision.
GI: abdominal pain, *constipation, decreased appetite, diarrhea,* dysgeusia, dyspepsia, *nausea, vomiting.*
GU: dehydration.
Hematologic: *anemia,* NEUTROPENIA, THROMBOCYTOPENIA.
Musculoskeletal: arthralgia, back pain, bone pain, limb pain, muscle cramps, myalgia.
Respiratory: cough, dyspnea, pneumonia, upper respiratory tract infection.
Skin: rash, pruritus.
Other: herpes zoster.

Interactions

Drug-drug. *Antihypertensives:* May cause hypotension. Monitor patient's blood pressure closely.
Drugs linked to peripheral neuropathy, such as amiodarone, antivirals, isoniazid, nitrofurantoin, statins: May worsen neuropathy. Use together cautiously.
Inhibitors or inducers of CYP3A4: Monitor patient closely for either toxicity or reduced effects.

Oral antidiabetics: May cause hypoglycemia or hyperglycemia. Monitor glucose levels closely.

Effects on lab test results

• May decrease hemoglobin level and hematocrit.
• May decrease neutrophil and platelet counts.

Pharmacokinetics

Absorption: Given I.V.
Distribution: 83% protein-bound.
Metabolism: Mainly in the liver by cytochrome P-450 enzymes.
Excretion: Unknown. *Half-life:* 9 to 15 hours.

Route	Onset	Peak	Duration
I.V.	Unknown	Unknown	Unknown

Action

Chemical effect: Disrupts intracellular homeostatic mechanisms by inhibiting the 26S proteasome, which regulates intracellular levels of certain proteins and causes cells to die.
Therapeutic effect: Destroys cancer cells.

Available forms

Injection: 3.5 mg

NURSING PROCESS

Assessment
• Assess patient's condition before therapy and regularly thereafter.
• Assess patient's nutrition and hydration status before and during therapy.
• Assess patient's and family's knowledge of drug therapy.

Nursing diagnoses
• Risk for injury related to potential neuropathy as an adverse effect
• Deficient fluid volume related to dehydration
• Risk for imbalanced nutrition: less than body requires related to underlying disease and drug adverse effects

Planning and implementation
• Monitor patient's reaction. An antiemetic, antidiarrheal, laxative, or, enema may be needed based on response.
• Adjust antihypertensive dosage, maintain hydration, and give mineralocorticoids to manage orthostatic hypotension.

• Watch for evidence of neuropathy, such as a burning sensation, hyperesthesia, hypoesthesia, paresthesia, discomfort, or neuropathic pain.
• If patient develops new or worsening peripheral neuropathy, change dose and schedule.
Patient teaching
• Tell patient to notify prescriber about new or worsening peripheral neuropathy.
• Urge women to use effective contraception during treatment.
• Teach patient how to avoid dehydration, and stress the need to tell prescriber about dizziness, light-headedness, or fainting spells.
• Tell patient to use caution when driving or performing potentially hazardous activities because drug may cause fatigue, dizziness, faintness, light-headedness, and vision problems.

Evaluation
• Patient has no serious drug reactions.
• Patient maintains adequate hydration.
• Patient maintains adequate nutrition.
• Patient and family state understanding of drug therapy.

bosentan
(bow-SEN-tan)
Tracleer

Pharmacologic class: endothelin receptor antagonist
Therapeutic class: vasodilator
Pregnancy risk category: X

Indications and dosages

▶ **Pulmonary arterial hypertension in patients with World Health Organization class III or IV symptoms to improve exercise ability and decrease clinical worsening.** *Adults:* 62.5 mg P.O. b.i.d. for 4 weeks. Increase to maintenance dose of 125 mg P.O. b.i.d. In patients older than age 12 who weigh less than 40 kg (88 lb), the initial and maintenance dose is 62.5 mg b.i.d. Adjust dosage based on ALT and AST levels.

Contraindications and cautions

• Contraindicated in patients hypersensitive to drug. Don't use in patients with moderate-to-severe liver impairment or in those with amino-

transferase (ALT and AST) levels more than three times upper limit of normal (ULN).
• Use cautiously in patients with mild liver impairment.

🔥 **Lifespan:** In pregnant women, drug is contraindicated. In breast-feeding women, drug isn't recommended because it's unknown whether drug appears in breast milk. In children age 12 or younger, safety and effectiveness of drug haven't been established. In elderly patients, select dose cautiously because of greater likelihood of decreased organ function.

Adverse reactions

CNS: fatigue, *headache.*
CV: edema, flushing, hypotension, lower leg edema, palpitations.
EENT: *nasopharyngitis.*
GI: dyspepsia.
Hematologic: anemia.
Hepatic: *liver failure.*
Skin: pruritus.

Interactions

Drug-drug. *Cyclosporine A:* May increase bosentan level and decrease cyclosporine level. Avoid use together.
Glyburide: May increase risk of elevated liver enzyme levels and decrease levels of both drugs. Avoid use together.
Hormonal contraceptives: May cause contraceptive failure. Advise use of a barrier birth control.
Ketoconazole: May increase bosentan level. Monitor patient for increased effects of bosentan.
Simvastatin, other statins: May decrease levels of these drugs. Monitor cholesterol levels to assess need for statin dosage adjustment.

Effects on lab test results

• May increase liver aminotransferase (such as AST, ALT, and bilirubin) levels. May decrease hemoglobin level and hematocrit.

Pharmacokinetics

Absorption: 50% bioavailability.
Distribution: More than 98% protein-bound, mainly albumin.
Metabolism: Hepatically into three metabolites. Drug induces CYP2C9 and CYP3A4, and possibly CYP2C19.

Excretion: Biliary. Less than 3% in urine. *Half-life:* About 5 hours.

Route	Onset	Peak	Duration
P.O.	Unknown	3–5 hr	Unknown

Action

Chemical effect: Antagonizes endothelin-1, which is elevated in patients with pulmonary arterial hypertension.
Therapeutic effect: Increases exercise capacity and cardiac index. Decreases blood pressure, pulmonary arterial pressure, vascular resistance, and mean right arterial pressure.

Available forms

Tablets: 62.5 mg, 125 mg

NURSING PROCESS

Assessment
• Assess patient's underlying condition before therapy, and reassess regularly thereafter.
• Make sure a woman isn't pregnant. Obtain monthly pregnancy tests.
• Serious liver injury may occur. Measure aminotransferase levels before treatment and monthly thereafter, and adjust dosage accordingly.
• This drug may cause hematologic changes. Monitor hemoglobin level after 1 and 3 months of therapy and then every 3 months thereafter.
• Be alert for adverse events.
• Assess patient's and family's knowledge of drug therapy.

Nursing diagnoses
• Risk for injury related to drug-induced liver enzyme elevations
• Ineffective tissue perfusion (cardiopulmonary) related to underlying condition
• Deficient knowledge related to drug therapy

Planning and implementation
• To decrease the possibility of serious liver injury and limit the chance of fetal exposure, Tracleer may be prescribed only through the Tracleer access program at 1-866-228-3546. Adverse effects also may be reported through this number.
• For patients who develop aminotransferase abnormalities, the dosage may need to be decreased or therapy stopped until aminotrans-

ferase levels return to normal. If liver function abnormalities with symptoms of liver injury, such as nausea, vomiting, fever, abdominal pain, jaundice, or unusual lethargy or fatigue occur, or if bilirubin level is greater than or equal to two times ULN, stop treatment and don't restart.

• Overdose may cause headache, nausea and vomiting, mildly decreased blood pressure, and increased heart rate. Massive overdose may cause severe hypotension requiring CV support. Treat symptoms, and provide supportive care.

• To avoid the potential for deterioration, gradually reduce the dosage when stopping drug.

Patient teaching

• Advise patient to take drug only as prescribed.

• Warn patient to avoid becoming pregnant while taking this drug because major birth defects may result. Reliable contraception must be used and a monthly pregnancy test performed.

• Advise patient to have liver tests and blood counts performed regularly.

• Tell woman to use barrier contraception, which includes condoms and diaphragm, with her hormonal contraceptives (oral, transdermal, implantable, and injectable) because failure may occur.

☑ **Evaluation**

• Patient has no adverse reactions or liver damage from drug therapy.

• Patient's pulmonary artery pressure decreases, and patient reaches pulmonary hemodynamic stability.

• Patient and family state understanding of drug therapy.

---

bromfenac ophthalmic solution
(BROM-fehn-ack off-THAL-mick suh-LOO-shun)
Xibrom

Pharmacologic classification: NSAID
Therapeutic classification: anti-inflammatory, ophthalmic
Pregnancy risk category: C

Indications and dosages

▶ **Postoperative inflammation and pain after cataract surgery.** *Adults:* 1 drop in affected eye b.i.d. starting 24 hours after cataract surgery and continuing for 2 weeks.

Contraindications and cautions

• Contraindicated in patients hypersensitive to any ingredient in the product. Drug contains sulfite, which may cause allergic-type reactions, including anaphylaxis and life-threatening or less severe asthmatic episodes in patients sensitive to sulfites.

• Use cautiously in patients with bleeding tendencies, patients taking anticoagulants, and patients sensitive to acetylsalicylic acid, phenylacetic acid derivatives, and other NSAIDs because of the risk of cross-sensitivity reactions. Also use cautiously in patients with complicated ocular surgeries, corneal denervation, corneal epithelial defects, diabetes mellitus, ocular surface diseases (such as dry eye syndrome), rheumatoid arthritis, or recent repeat ocular surgeries because the risk of corneal adverse effects, which may be sight-threatening, is increased.

🔥 **Lifespan:** In pregnant women, use only if potential benefit justifies the risk. Avoid giving drug late in pregnancy because NSAIDs may cause premature closure of the ductus arteriosus, a necessary structure of fetal circulation. In breast-feeding women, use cautiously. In children, safety and effectiveness haven't been established.

Adverse reactions

CNS: headache.
EENT: abnormal sensation in the eye, burning, conjunctival hyperemia, eye irritation, eye pain, eye pruritus, eye redness, iritis, keratitis, stinging.
Other: *anaphylaxis,* hypersensitivity reactions.

Interactions

Drug-drug. *Drugs that affect coagulation:* May further increase bleeding tendency or prolong bleeding time. Avoid use together, if possible, or monitor bleeding closely.
Topical corticosteroids: May disrupt healing. Avoid use together, if possible, or monitor healing closely.

Effects on lab test results

None reported.

Pharmacokinetics

Absorption: Unknown.
Distribution: Intraocular.
Metabolism: Unknown.

Excretion: Unknown. *Half-life:* Unknown.

Route	Onset	Peak	Duration
Ophthalmic	Unknown	Unknown	Unknown

Action

Chemical effect: Blocks prostaglandin synthesis by inhibiting cyclooxygenase 1 and 2.
Therapeutic effect: Reduces postoperative inflammation after cataract surgery.

Available forms

Ophthalmic solution: 0.09%

NURSING PROCESS

Assessment
• Assess patient's risk for allergic reaction; ask patient before treatment if he is sensitive to sulfites, aspirin, or other NSAIDs.
• If patient takes an anticoagulant, monitor closely for increased bleeding.
• Monitor PT and INR if appropriate.
• Assess patient's and family's knowledge of drug therapy.

Nursing diagnoses
• Disturbed visual sensory perception related to cataract surgery and potential adverse effects of medication
• Risk for activity intolerance related to decreased visual acuity
• Deficient knowledge related to drug therapy

Planning and implementation
• Patients with asthma have an increased likelihood of sulfite sensitivity.
• Begin treatment at least 24 hours after surgery, and continue for 2 weeks.
• Giving drug less than 24 hours after surgery or more than 14 days after surgery increases risk of adverse ocular effects.
• If overdose or significant adverse ocular effect occurs, stop drug and monitor ocular health closely.
Patient teaching
• Advise patient not to use drops while wearing contact lenses.
• Teach patient how to instill the drops.
• Instruct patient to start using drops 24 hours after surgery and to continue for 14 days.

• Tell him not to use drops for longer than 2 weeks after surgery or to save unused drops for other conditions.
• Review the signs and symptoms of adverse effects. If bothersome or serious adverse effects occur, inform the patient to stop the drops and contact his prescriber.
• Tell patient to store drops at room temperature.

Evaluation
• Patient has no adverse effects.
• Patient's activity level improves.
• Patient and family state understanding of drug therapy.

bromocriptine mesylate
(broh-moh-KRIP-teen MESS-ih-layt)
Parlodel, Parlodel SnapTabs

Pharmacologic class: dopamine receptor agonist
Therapeutic class: antiparkinsonian, inhibitor of prolactin and growth hormone release
Pregnancy risk category: B

Indications and dosages

▶ **Parkinson disease.** *Adults:* 1.25 to 2.5 mg P.O. b.i.d. with meals. Increase dosage every 14 to 28 days, up to 100 mg daily, as needed. Usual dosage, 10 to 40 mg daily.
▶ **Acromegaly.** *Adults:* 1.25 to 2.5 mg P.O. at bedtime with snack for 3 days. An additional 1.25 to 2.5 mg may be added every 3 to 7 days until patient receives therapeutic benefit. Usual therapeutic dose is 20 to 30 mg daily. Maximum dosage, 100 mg daily.
▶ **Amenorrhea and galactorrhea related to hyperprolactinemia; infertility or hypogonadism in women.** *Adults:* 1.25 to 2.5 mg P.O. daily. Increase by 2.5 mg daily at 2- to 7-day intervals until desired effect is achieved. Maintenance dosage is usually 5 to 7.5 mg daily, but may be 2.5 to 15 mg daily.
▶ **Premenstrual syndrome‡.** *Adults:* 2.5 to 7.5 mg P.O. b.i.d. from day 10 of menstrual cycle until menstruation starts.
▶ **Cushing syndrome‡.** *Adults:* 1.25 to 2.5 mg P.O. b.i.d. to q.i.d.

▶ **Hepatic encephalopathy‡.** *Adults:* 1.25 mg P.O. daily, increase by 1.25 mg every 3 days until 15 mg is reached.
▶ **Neuroleptic malignant syndrome related to neuroleptic therapy‡.** *Adults:* 2.5 to 5 mg P.O. two to six times daily.

Contraindications and cautions

• Contraindicated in patients hypersensitive to ergot derivatives and in those with uncontrolled hypertension, severe ischemic heart disease or peripheral vascular disease, or toxemia of pregnancy.
• Use cautiously in patients with renal or hepatic impairment or history of MI with residual arrhythmias.
⚘ **Lifespan:** In pregnant women, use only if benefits outweigh risks to fetus. In breastfeeding women, avoid use because it inhibits lactation. In children younger than age 15, safety and effectiveness of drug haven't been established.

Adverse reactions

CNS: confusion, delusions, depression, *dizziness,* fatigue, hallucinations, *headache,* insomnia, mania, nervousness, *seizures, stroke, syncope,* uncontrolled body movements.
CV: *acute MI,* hypertension, *hypotension,* orthostatic hypotension.
EENT: blurred vision, nasal congestion, tinnitus.
GI: *abdominal cramps,* constipation, diarrhea, *nausea,* vomiting.
GU: urinary frequency, urine retention.
Skin: coolness and pallor of fingers and toes.

Interactions

Drug-drug. *Antihypertensives:* May increase hypotensive effects. Antihypertensive dosage may need adjustment.
Ergot alkaloids, estrogens, hormonal contraceptives, progestins: May interfere with bromocriptine effects. Don't use together.
Erythromycin: May increase bromocriptine level. Bromocriptine dosage may need adjustment.
Haloperidol, loxapine, MAO inhibitors, methyldopa, metoclopramide, phenothiazines, reserpine: May interfere with bromocriptine effects. Bromocriptine dosage may need to be increased.
Levodopa: May have additive effects. Levodopa dosage may need adjustment.

Drug-lifestyle. *Alcohol use:* May cause disulfiram-like reaction. Discourage use together.

Effects on lab test results

• May increase BUN, alkaline phosphatase, uric acid, AST, ALT, and CK levels.

Pharmacokinetics

Absorption: 28% absorbed.
Distribution: 90% to 96% bound to albumin.
Metabolism: First-pass metabolism occurs with more than 90% of absorbed dose. Drug is metabolized completely in liver.
Excretion: Major route is through bile. Only 2.5% to 5.5% of dose excreted in urine. *Half-life:* 15 hours.

Route	Onset	Peak	Duration
P.O.	½–2 hr	1–3 hr	12–24 hr

Action

Chemical effect: Inhibits secretion of prolactin and acts as a dopamine-receptor agonist by activating postsynaptic dopamine receptors.
Therapeutic effect: Reverses amenorrhea and galactorrhea caused by hyperprolactinemia, increases fertility in women, improves voluntary movement, and inhibits prolactin and growth hormone release.

Available forms

Capsules: 5 mg
Tablets: 2.5 mg

NURSING PROCESS

⚏ Assessment

• Obtain history of patient's underlying condition before therapy, and reassess regularly thereafter.
• Before treatment, assess patient for evidence of dementia. Monitor patient for mental changes during therapy.
• Perform baseline and periodic evaluations of cardiac, hepatic, renal, and hematopoietic functions during prolonged therapy.
• Be alert for adverse reactions and drug interactions. Risk of adverse reactions is high, particularly at start of therapy and with doses greater than 20 mg. Adverse reactions are more common when drug is used for Parkinson disease.

- Assess patient's and family's knowledge of drug therapy.

Nursing diagnoses
- Ineffective health maintenance related to underlying condition
- Risk for injury related to drug-induced adverse CNS or CV reactions
- Deficient knowledge related to drug therapy

Planning and implementation
- Give drug with meals.
- Gradually adjust dose to effective level to minimize adverse reactions.
- Patients with impaired renal function may need dosage adjustment.
- For Parkinson disease, drug is usually given with either levodopa or levodopa and carbidopa.
Patient teaching
- Advise patient to use a barrier contraceptive, not a hormonal contraceptive, during treatment.
- Advise patient to rise slowly to an upright position and avoid sudden position changes to avoid dizziness and fainting.
- Advise patient that resumption of menses and suppression of galactorrhea may take 6 weeks or longer.
- Warn patient to avoid hazardous activities that require alertness until CNS and CV effects of drug are known.
- Tell patient to take drug with meals to minimize GI distress.

☑ Evaluation
- Patient shows improvement in underlying condition.
- Patient sustains no injury from drug-induced adverse reactions.
- Patient and family state understanding of drug therapy.

budesonide
(byoo-DESS-oh-nighd)
Pulmicort Flexhaler, Pulmicort Respules, Pulmicort Turbuhaler (inhalation), Rhinocort Aqua (intranasal)

Pharmacologic class: glucocorticoid
Therapeutic class: anti-inflammatory
Pregnancy risk category: B

Indications and dosages

▶ **Symptoms of seasonal or perennial allergic rhinitis and nonallergic perennial rhinitis.**
Adults and children age 6 and older: 1 spray in each nostril once daily. In adults and children age 12 and older, may increase to 4 sprays in each nostril once daily; in children younger than age 12, may increase to 2 sprays in each nostril once daily. Maintenance dosage is fewest number of sprays needed to control symptoms.
▶ **Chronic asthma.** *Adults:* 200 to 400 mcg oral inhalation via Turbuhaler b.i.d. when patient previously used bronchodilators alone or inhaled corticosteroids; 400 to 800 mcg oral inhalation b.i.d. when patient previously used oral corticosteroids. Maximum dosage 800 mcg b.i.d. Or, 360 mcg oral inhalation via Flexhaler b.i.d. Maximum dosage 720 mcg b.i.d.
Children age 6 and older: Initially, 200 mcg oral inhalation via Turbuhaler b.i.d. Maximum dosage is 400 mcg b.i.d.
Children ages 1 to 8: Give 0.5 mg respules once daily or 0.25 mg b.i.d. in child not receiving systemic or inhaled corticosteroids or 1 mg daily or 0.5 mg b.i.d. if child is receiving oral corticosteroids. Or, in children unresponsive to nonsteroidal therapy, 0.25 mg respules by jet nebulizer with compressor once daily.

Contraindications and cautions

- Contraindicated in patients hypersensitive to the drug or its components and in those who have had recent septal ulcers, nasal surgery, or nasal trauma, until total healing has occurred. Pulmicort is contraindicated for primary treatment of status asthmaticus.
- Use cautiously in patients with tuberculous infections, ocular herpes simplex, or untreated fungal, bacterial, or systemic viral infections.
☖ **Lifespan:** In pregnant or breast-feeding women, use cautiously. In children younger than age 1, don't use respules via jet nebulizer. In children younger than age 6, safety of oral inhalation via Turbuhaler hasn't been established.

Adverse reactions

CNS: *headache,* nervousness.
CV: facial edema.
EENT: epistaxis, hoarseness, nasal irritation, nasal pain, pharyngitis, reduced sense of smell, sinusitis.
GI: bad taste, dry mouth, dyspepsia, nausea, vomiting.

Metabolic: weight gain.
Musculoskeletal: myalgia.
Respiratory: candidiasis, cough, dyspnea, wheezing.
Skin: contact dermatitis, pruritus, rash.
Other: hypersensitivity reactions.

Interactions

Drug-drug. *Alternate-day prednisone therapy, inhaled corticosteroids:* May increase risk of hypothalamic-pituitary-adrenal suppression. Monitor patient closely.
Ketoconazole: May increase budesonide level. Use together cautiously.

Effects on lab test results

None reported.

Pharmacokinetics

Absorption: Intranasal dose, typically about 20% in system.
Distribution: 88% protein-bound.
Metabolism: Rapid and extensive in liver.
Excretion: About 67% in urine and 33% in feces. *Half-life:* About 2 hours.

Route	Onset	Peak	Duration
Nasal inhalation	Unknown	45 min	8–10 hr
Oral inhalation	5–15 min	30 min	Unknown

Action

Chemical effect: Decreases nasal and pulmonary inflammation, mainly by inhibiting activities of specific cells and mediators involved in allergic response.
Therapeutic effect: Decreases nasal and pulmonary congestion.

Available forms

Inhalation suspension: 0.25 mg/2 ml, 0.5 mg/2 ml, 1 mg/2 ml
Nasal spray: 32 mcg/metered spray (7-g canister)
Oral inhalation powder: 90 mcg/dose, 200 mcg/dose

NURSING PROCESS

Assessment
• Obtain history of patient's condition before therapy, and reassess regularly thereafter.
• Be alert for adverse reactions.
• Assess patient's and family's knowledge of drug therapy.

Nursing diagnoses
• Ineffective health maintenance related to allergy-induced nasal congestion
• Impaired gas exchange related to drug-induced wheezing
• Deficient knowledge related to drug therapy

Planning and implementation
ALERT: Flexhaler and Turbohaler doses aren't equivalent. Dosage adjustment may be needed if patient is switched from one to the other.
• Before using nasal inhaler, shake container. Prime by pumping 8 times before first use. Reprime with one spray if not used in more than 2 days. Reprime with 2 sprays if not used in more than 14 days. Have patient clear his nasal passages. Insert nozzle (pointed away from septum) into nostril, holding other nostril closed. Have patient tilt head slightly forward so spray is directed up nasal passage. Deliver spray while patient inhales. Have patient tilt head back for a few seconds. Repeat in other nostril. Wipe off tip of inhaler before capping.
• If relief isn't obtained or signs of infection appear, notify prescriber.
• If signs of nasal infection occur, obtain specimen for culture.
Patient teaching
• Teach patient how to use nasal inhaler, as described in "Planning and implementation," above.
• Tell patient to hold the inhaler upright while orally inhaling the dose. When loading Turbuhaler, tell him not to blow or exhale into the inhaler or shake it while loaded. Have him place the mouthpiece between his lips and inhale forcefully and deeply. Have him rinse his mouth after use to decrease risk of fungal growth.
• Respules given only by jet nebulizer connected to an air compressor with minimum airflow of 5.5 L/minute. System should be equipped with a mouthpiece or face mask. Have patient rinse mouth after administration. When using face mask, teach him to wash his face after use to decrease risk of contact dermatitis or rash.
• Inform patient that use of an oral inhaler results in improvement in asthma control in 10 to 24 hours, with maximum benefit at 1 to 2 weeks, or possibly longer.

- Advise parent that antihistamines can cause paradoxical excitement in small children.
- ⚠ **ALERT:** Advise patient that Pulmicort isn't intended to relieve acute asthma attacks.
- To prevent spread of infection, tell patient that he shouldn't share any drug-delivery devices.
- Advise patient not to break or incinerate canister or store it in extreme heat. Contents are under pressure.
- Warn patient not to exceed prescribed dose or use for long periods because of risk of hypothalamic-pituitary-adrenal axis suppression.
- Tell patient to report worsened condition or symptoms that don't improve in 3 weeks.
- Teach patient good nasal and oral hygiene.

☑ Evaluation
- Patient's nasal congestion subsides.
- Patient has adequate gas exchange.
- Patient and family state understanding of drug therapy.

budesonide (oral)
(byoo-DESS-uh-nighd)
Entocort EC

Pharmacologic class: corticosteroid
Therapeutic class: anti-inflammatory
Pregnancy risk category: C

Indications and dosages

▶ **Mildly to moderately active Crohn disease involving the ileum or the ascending colon.** *Adults:* 9 mg P.O. once daily in the morning for up to 8 weeks. For recurrent episodes of active Crohn disease, a second 8-week course may be given.

▶ **To maintain remission of mild to moderate Crohn disease involving the ileum or ascending colon.** *Adults:* 6 mg P.O. daily for up to 3 months. If symptoms are controlled at 3 months, taper drug to complete stop. Maintenance treatment beyond 3 months doesn't provide additional benefit.

Contraindications and cautions

- Contraindicated in patients hypersensitive to drug.
- Use cautiously in patients with tuberculosis, hypertension, diabetes mellitus, osteoporosis, peptic ulcer disease, glaucoma, or cataracts.

Also use cautiously in patients with a family history of diabetes or glaucoma and those with any other condition in which glucocorticosteroids may have unwanted effects.

⚘ **Lifespan:** In pregnant women, use only if potential benefit justifies risks. For breastfeeding women, the decision to breast-feed should be based on importance of drug to the mother; drug may appear in breast milk, and infants may have adverse reactions. In children, safety and effectiveness of drug haven't been established. In elderly patients, give drug cautiously, starting at the lower end of the dosage range.

Adverse reactions

CNS: agitation, asthenia, confusion, dizziness, fatigue, fever, *headache,* hyperkinesia, insomnia, malaise, migraine, nervousness, pain, paresthesia, sleep disorder, somnolence, syncope, tremor, vertigo.
CV: chest pain, dependent edema, facial edema, flushing, hypertension, palpitations, tachycardia.
EENT: abnormal vision, ear infection, eye abnormality, neck pain, *pharyngitis,* sinusitis, voice alteration.
GI: abdominal pain, aggravated Crohn disease, anus disorder, *diarrhea,* dry mouth, dyspepsia, epigastric pain, fistula, flatulence, gastroenteritis, glossitis, hemorrhoids, increased appetite, intestinal obstruction, *nausea,* oral candidiasis, taste perversion, tongue edema, tooth disorder, vomiting.
GU: dysuria, intermenstrual bleeding, menstrual disorder, polyuria, nocturia.
Hematologic: anemia, leukocytosis.
Metabolic: ADRENAL INSUFFICIENCY, *hypercorticism,* hypokalemia, weight gain.
Musculoskeletal: aggravated arthritis, arthralgia, back pain, cramps, hypotonia, myalgia.
Respiratory: bronchitis, cough, dyspnea, *respiratory tract infection.*
Skin: acne, alopecia, dermatitis, ecchymosis, eczema, increased sweating, skin disorder.
Other: flulike syndrome, infection, viral infection.

Interactions

Drug-drug. *CYP3A4 inhibitors (erythromycin, indinavir, itraconazole, ketoconazole, ritonavir, saquinavir):* May increase budesonide effects. If drugs must be given together, watch for signs of

---

hypercorticism and consider reducing budesonide dosage.

Drug-food. *Grapefruit or grapefruit juice:* May increase drug effects. Discourage use together.

Effects on lab test results

• May increase alkaline phosphatase and C-reactive protein levels. May decrease hemoglobin level and hematocrit. May increase or decrease potassium level.

• May increase erythrocyte sedimentation rate and atypical neutrophil and WBC counts.

Pharmacokinetics

Absorption: Complete.
Distribution: 85% to 90% protein-bound.
Metabolism: Extensive first-pass. Rapid, extensive biotransformation by CYP3A4 to two major metabolites that have little glucocorticoid activity.
Excretion: In urine and feces as metabolites; mainly renally. *Half-life:* Unknown.

Route	Onset	Peak	Duration
P.O.	Unknown	½–10 hr	Unknown

Action

Chemical effect: Has high affinity for glucocorticoid receptors.
Therapeutic effect: Alleviates symptoms of Crohn disease.

Available forms

Capsules: 3 mg

NURSING PROCESS

Assessment

• Assess patient's underlying condition before starting therapy, and reassess regularly thereafter.

• Monitor patient's laboratory values regularly. Monitor patient for adverse effects.

• Be alert for signs and symptoms of hypercorticism.

• Assess patient's and family's knowledge of drug therapy.

Nursing diagnoses

• Diarrhea caused by underlying Crohn disease
• Imbalanced nutrition: less than body requirements related to underlying Crohn disease
• Deficient knowledge related to drug therapy

Planning and implementation

• Patients undergoing surgery or another stressful situation may need systemic glucocorticoids in addition to budesonide.

• When a patient is transferred from systemic glucocorticoids to budesonide, watch carefully for evidence of steroid withdrawal. Taper glucocorticoid when budesonide treatment starts.

• Watch for immunosuppression, especially in a patient who hasn't had diseases such as chickenpox or measles because these diseases can be fatal in a patient who is immunosuppressed, such as one receiving glucocorticoids. Monitor adrenocortical function carefully, and reduce dosage cautiously.

• Prevent exposure to chickenpox or measles. If patient is exposed to measles, consider therapy with pooled intravenous immunoglobulin. If patient develops chickenpox, antiviral treatment and varicella zoster immune globulin may be considered.

• Treat overdose with immediate gastric lavage or emesis, followed by treatment of symptoms and supportive therapy. For chronic overdose in serious disease requiring continuous steroid therapy, dosage may be reduced temporarily. Acute toxicity after overdose is rare.

• Prolonged use of drug may cause hypercorticism (symptoms include swelling of the face and neck, acne, bruising, hirsutism, buffalo hump, and skin striae) and adrenal suppression.

• Dosage may need to be reduced in patients with moderate to severe liver disease if they have increased signs or symptoms of hypercorticism.

Patient teaching

• Tell patient to swallow capsules whole and not to chew or break them.

• Advise patient not to drink grapefruit juice while taking drug.

• Tell patient to notify prescriber immediately if exposed to chickenpox or measles.

Evaluation

• Patient's symptoms of Crohn disease, including diarrhea and abdominal pain, are relieved.

• Patient's nutrition improves as symptoms improve.

• Patient and family state understanding of drug therapy.

bumetanide
(byoo-MEH-tuh-nighd)
Bumex

Pharmacologic class: loop diuretic
Therapeutic class: diuretic
Pregnancy risk category: C

Indications and dosages

▶ **Hypertension.** *Adults:* 0.5 mg P.O. daily.
Oral maintenance dosage is 1 to 4 mg daily, not
to exceed 5 mg P.O. daily.
▶ **Heart failure.** *Children:* 0.015 mg/kg every
other day to 0.1 mg/kg daily. Use with extreme
caution in neonates.
▶ **Heart failure, hepatic or renal disease,
postoperative edema‡, premenstrual syn-
drome‡, disseminated cancer‡.** *Adults:* 0.5 to
2 mg P.O. once daily. If diuretic response isn't
adequate, give second or third dose at 4- to
5-hour intervals. Maximum, 10 mg daily. Give
parenterally if P.O. use isn't feasible. Usual initial dose is 0.5 to 1 mg given I.V. over 1 to
2 minutes or I.M. If response isn't adequate,
give second or third dose at 2- to 3-hour intervals. Maximum, 10 mg daily.
Adjust-a-dose: For patients with severe
chronic renal insufficiency, a continuous infusion of 12 mg over 12 hours may be more effective and less toxic than intermittent bolus therapy.

▼ I.V. administration

• For direct injection, use 21G or 23G needle
and give drug over 1 to 2 minutes.
• For intermittent infusion, give diluted drug
through an intermittent infusion device or piggyback into an I.V. line containing free-flowing
compatible solution. Infuse at ordered rate.
• Continuous infusion not recommended.
⊗ **Incompatibilities**
Dobutamine, midazolam.

Contraindications and cautions

• Contraindicated in patients hypersensitive to
drug or sulfonamides (possible cross-sensitivity), in those with anuria or hepatic coma, and in
those with severe electrolyte depletion.
• Use cautiously in patients with depressed renal function or hepatic cirrhosis or ascites.

※ **Lifespan:** In pregnant women, use cautiously. In breast-feeding women, drug is contraindicated. In children, safety and effectiveness of
drug haven't been established.

Adverse reactions

CNS: dizziness, headache.
CV: ECG changes, orthostatic hypotension, vol-
ume depletion and dehydration.
EENT: transient deafness.
GI: nausea.
GU: azotemia, frequent urination, nocturia,
oliguria, polyuria, *renal failure.*
Hematologic: *thrombocytopenia.*
Metabolic: asymptomatic hyperuricemia; fluid
and electrolyte imbalances, including dilutional
hyponatremia, hypocalcemia, and *hypomagne-
semia;* hyperglycemia; hypochloremic alkalo-
sis; hypokalemia; impaired glucose tolerance.
Musculoskeletal: muscle pain and tenderness.
Skin: rash.

Interactions

Drug-drug. *Aminoglycoside antibiotics:* May
cause ototoxicity. Use together cautiously.
Antihypertensives: May increase risk of hypotension. Use together cautiously.
*Chlorothiazide, chlorthalidone, hydrochloro-
thiazide, indapamide, metolazone:* May cause
excessive diuretic response, resulting in serious
electrolyte abnormalities or dehydration. Adjust
dosages carefully while monitoring patient for
excessive diuretic responses.
Digoxin: May increase risk of digitalis toxicity
from drug-induced hypokalemia. Monitor potassium and digoxin levels.
Indomethacin, NSAIDs, probenecid: May inhibit diuretic response. Use together cautiously.
Lithium: May decrease lithium clearance, increasing risk of lithium toxicity. Monitor lithium level.
Other potassium-wasting drugs: May increase
risk of hypokalemia. Use together cautiously.
Drug-herb. *Licorice:* May contribute to excessive potassium loss. Discourage use together.

Effects on lab test results

• May increase creatinine, urine urea, glucose,
and cholesterol levels. May decrease potassium,
magnesium, sodium, and calcium levels.
• May decrease platelet count.

Pharmacokinetics

Absorption: After P.O. use, 85% to 95%; food delays. Complete after I.M. use.
Distribution: About 92% to 96% protein-bound. It isn't known if drug enters CSF.
Metabolism: By liver to at least five metabolites.
Excretion: In urine (80%) and feces (10% to 20%). *Half-life:* 1 to 1½ hours.

Route	Onset	Peak	Duration
P.O.	30–60 min	1–2 hr	4–6 hr
I.V.	3 min	15–30 min	½–4 hr
I.M.	40 min	Unknown	Unknown

Action

Chemical effect: Inhibits sodium and chloride reabsorption at ascending portion of loop of Henle.
Therapeutic effect: Promotes sodium and water excretion.

Available forms

Injection: 0.25 mg/ml
Tablets: 0.5 mg, 1 mg, 2 mg

NURSING PROCESS

Assessment
• Obtain history of patient's urine output, vital signs, electrolyte levels, breath sounds, peripheral edema, and weight before therapy, and reassess regularly thereafter.
• Be alert for adverse reactions and drug interactions.
• Assess patient's and family's knowledge of drug therapy.

Nursing diagnoses
• Excess fluid volume related to underlying condition
• Impaired urinary elimination related to therapeutic effect of drug therapy
• Deficient knowledge related to drug therapy

Planning and implementation
• Give P.O. dose with food to prevent GI upset.
• To prevent nocturia, give in morning. If second dose is needed, give in early afternoon.
• The safest and most effective dosage schedule for control of edema is intermittent dosage either given on alternate days or given for 3 to 4 days with 1- or 2-day rest periods.

• Drug can be used safely in patients allergic to furosemide: 1 mg of bumetanide equals 40 mg of furosemide. Bumetanide may be less ototoxic than furosemide.
• If oliguria or azotemia develops or increases, anticipate that prescriber may stop drug.
• Notify prescriber if drug-related hearing changes occur.
⚠ **ALERT:** Don't confuse bumetanide with budesonide.

Patient teaching
• Advise patient to stand up slowly to prevent dizziness; also tell him to limit alcohol intake and strenuous exercise in hot weather to avoid worsening orthostatic hypotension.
• Teach patient to monitor fluid volume by measuring weight daily.
• Advise patient to take drug early in day to avoid sleep interruption caused by nocturia.
• Tell patient with diabetes to monitor glucose levels closely.

✓ Evaluation
• Patient is free from edema.
• Patient demonstrates adjustment of lifestyle to deal with altered patterns of urinary elimination.
• Patient and family state understanding of drug therapy.

HIGH ALERT!

buprenorphine hydrochloride
(byoo-preh-NOR-feen high-droh-KLOR-ighd)
Buprenex, Subutex

buprenorphine hydrochloride and naloxone hydrochloride dihydrate
Suboxone

Pharmacologic class: opioid agonist-antagonist, opioid partial agonist
Therapeutic class: analgesic
Pregnancy risk category: C
Controlled substance schedule: III

Indications and dosages

▶ **Moderate to severe pain.** *Adults and children age 13 and older:* 0.3 mg I.M. or slow I.V. every 6 hours, p.r.n., or around-the-clock. May repeat 0.3 mg or increase to 0.6 mg, if needed, 30 to 60 minutes after initial dose.

Children ages 2 to 12: Give 2 to 6 mcg/kg I.V. or I.M. every 4 to 6 hours.

▶ **Opioid dependence.** *Adults:* 12 to 16 mg S.L. daily. Maintenance therapy with Suboxone is preferred; target dose is 16 mg/day. Increase or decrease in increments of 2 mg or 4 mg according to withdrawal effects; usual range is 4 to 24 mg.

▶ **Postoperative pain‡.** *Adults:* 25 to 250 mcg/ hour I.V. infusion over 48 hours.

▶ **Pain‡.** *Adults:* 60 mcg epidural injection, as a single dose. Maximum, 180 mcg in 48 hours.

▶ **Circumcision‡.** *Children ages 9 months to 9 years:* 3 mcg/kg I.M. with surgical anesthesia.

▼ I.V. administration

● Give by direct I.V. injection into vein or through tubing of free-flowing compatible I.V. solution over at least 2 minutes.

⊗ **Incompatibilities**
Diazepam, furosemide, lorazepam.

Contraindications and cautions

● Contraindicated in patients hypersensitive to drug.
● Use cautiously in debilitated patients and patients with head injury, intracranial lesions, increased intracranial pressure, or severe respiratory, liver, or kidney impairment. Also use cautiously in patients with CNS depression or coma, thyroid irregularities, adrenal insufficiency, prostatic hyperplasia, urethral stricture, acute alcoholism, alcohol withdrawal syndrome, or kyphoscoliosis.

⚖ **Lifespan:** In pregnant and breast-feeding women and in elderly patients, use cautiously.

Adverse reactions

CNS: confusion, depression, *dizziness,* dreaming, euphoria, fatigue, headache, ***increased intracranial pressure,*** nervousness, paresthesia, psychosis, *sedation,* slurred speech, *vertigo,* weakness.
CV: *bradycardia, cyanosis,* flushing, hypertension, *hypotension,* tachycardia, Wenckebach block.
EENT: blurred vision, conjunctivitis, diplopia, *miosis,* tinnitus, visual abnormalities.
GI: constipation, dry mouth, *nausea,* vomiting.
GU: urine retention.
Respiratory: dyspnea, hypoventilation, ***respiratory depression.***
Skin: *diaphoresis, pruritus.*

Other: chills, *injection site reactions,* withdrawal syndrome.

Interactions

Drug-drug. *CNS depressants, MAO inhibitors:* May have additive effects. Monitor patient.
Opioid analgesics: May decrease analgesic effect. Avoid use together.
Drug-lifestyle. *Alcohol use:* May have additive effects. Discourage use together.

Effects on lab test results

● May decrease alkaline phosphatase and hemoglobin levels and hematocrit.
● May decrease erythrocyte count and sedimentation rate.

Pharmacokinetics

Absorption: Rapid.
Distribution: About 96% protein-bound.
Metabolism: In liver.
Excretion: Mainly in feces. *Half-life:* 1 to 7 hours. *Combination drug half-life:* Buprenorphine, 37 hours; naloxone, 1 hour.

Route	Onset	Peak	Duration
I.V., I.M.	15 min	1 hr	6 hr
S.L.	Unknown	Unknown	2–8 hr

Action

Chemical effect: Binds with opiate receptors in CNS, altering perception of and emotional response to pain.
Therapeutic effect: Relieves pain.

Available forms

Injection: 0.324 mg (0.3 mg base/ml)
Sublingual: 2 mg, 8 mg
Sublingual (combination): 2 mg buprenorphine and 0.5 mg naloxone, 8 mg buprenorphine and 2 mg naloxone

NURSING PROCESS

🗎 Assessment

● Obtain history of patient's pain.
● Monitor respiratory status frequently for at least 1 hour after administration. Notify prescriber if respiratory depression occurs.
● In an opioid-dependent patient, cytolytic hepatitis or hepatitis with jaundice may occur. Monitor closely.

- Assess patient's and family's knowledge of drug therapy.

⊕ Nursing diagnoses
- Acute pain related to underlying condition
- Ineffective breathing pattern related to drug-induced respiratory depression
- Deficient knowledge related to drug therapy

▶ Planning and implementation
- Safety of giving single I.M. doses greater than 0.6 mg for long-term use is unknown.
- Analgesic potency of 0.3 mg buprenorphine is equal to that of 10 mg morphine and 75 mg meperidine, but buprenorphine has a longer duration of action.
- Notify prescriber if pain isn't relieved.
- If patient's respiratory rate falls below 8 breaths per minute, withhold dose, rouse patient to stimulate breathing, and notify prescriber.
- For buprenorphine overdose, naloxone won't completely reverse respiratory depression; mechanical ventilation may be needed. Doxapram or larger-than-usual doses of naloxone may also be ordered.
- Drug may precipitate withdrawal syndrome in opioid-dependent patients.
- If dependence occurs, withdrawal symptoms may appear up to 14 days after drug is stopped.

Patient teaching
- Warn ambulatory patient about getting out of bed slowly and walking cautiously because of risk of dizziness or hypotension.
- When drug is used postoperatively, encourage patient to turn, cough, and deep-breathe to prevent atelectasis.
- Teach patient to avoid activities that require full alertness until CNS effects are known.
- Instruct patient to avoid alcohol and other CNS depressants.
- For sublingual form, tell patient to take entire dose at the same time; if he can't do so comfortably, tell him to take dose two tablets at a time.

☑ Evaluation
- Patient reports pain relief.
- Patient's respiratory status is within normal limits.
- Patient and family state understanding of drug therapy.

bupropion hydrochloride
(byoo-PROH-pee-on high-droh-KLOR-ighd)
Wellbutrin, Wellbutrin SR, Wellbutrin XL, Zyban

Pharmacologic class: aminoketone
Therapeutic class: antidepressant, smoking cessation aid
Pregnancy risk category: C

Indications and dosages

▶ **Depression.** *Adults:* Initially, 100 mg immediate-release Wellbutrin P.O. b.i.d., increased after 3 days to 100 mg P.O. t.i.d. if needed. If no response occurs after several weeks of therapy, increase to 150 mg t.i.d. Don't exceed 150 mg for a single dose. Allow at least 6 hours between doses. Maximum, 450 mg daily. Or, initially, 150 mg sustained-release Wellbutrin P.O. every morning; increase to target dose of 150 mg P.O. b.i.d. as tolerated as early as day 4 of therapy. Allow at least 8 hours between doses. Maximum, 400 mg daily. Or, initially, 150 mg extended-release Wellbutrin P.O. every morning; increase to target dose of 300 mg P.O. daily as tolerated as early as day 4 of therapy. Allow at least 24 hours between doses. Maximum, 450 mg daily.

🔲 **Adjust-a-dose:** For patients with mild to moderate hepatic cirrhosis or renal impairment, reduce dosage. For patients with severe hepatic cirrhosis, don't exceed 75 mg immediate-release P.O. daily; 100 mg sustained-release P.O. daily; 150 mg sustained-release P.O. every other day; or 150 mg extended-release P.O. every other day.

▶ **Seasonal affective disorder.** *Adults:* Start therapy in autumn before symptoms of depression start. Initially, 150 mg Wellbutrin XL P.O. once daily in the morning. After 1 week, increase to 300 mg once daily if tolerated. Continue through autumn and winter; then taper to 150 mg daily for 2 weeks before stopping therapy in early spring.

▶ **Aid to smoking cessation.** *Adults:* 150 mg Zyban P.O. daily for 3 days; increase to maximum dosage of 150 mg P.O. b.i.d. at least 8 hours apart. Start therapy 1 to 2 weeks before patient stops smoking.

▶ **Attention deficit hyperactivity disorder‡.**
Adults: 150 mg Wellbutrin P.O. daily with regu-

lar-release tablets. Adjust dosage to a maximum of 450 mg P.O. daily.

Contraindications and cautions

• Contraindicated in patients hypersensitive to drug, those who have taken MAO inhibitors during the previous 14 days, and those with seizure disorders or a history of bulimia or anorexia nervosa because of a higher risk of seizures. Also contraindicated in patients abruptly stopping alcohol or sedatives (including benzodiazepines). Don't use Wellbutrin with Zyban or other drugs containing bupropion that are used for smoking cessation.
• Use cautiously in patients with renal or hepatic impairment and in patients with recent MI or unstable heart disease.
• In adults and children with major depressive disorders, depression may worsen and suicidal ideation and behavior emerge even while taking an antidepressant. Carefully monitor patients for worsening depression or suicidal ideation, especially when therapy starts or dosage changes and in young adults ages 18 to 24 during the first 2 months of treatment. These drugs haven't been approved for use in children.
☀ Lifespan: In pregnant women, use cautiously. If drug must be given to breast-feeding woman, breast-feeding should be stopped. In children, safety and effectiveness of drug haven't been established. Clinicians are encouraged to register pregnant patients at 800-336-2176 to monitor fetal outcomes.

Adverse reactions

CNS: *agitation,* akathisia, anxiety, *confusion,* delusions, euphoria, fever, *headache,* hostility, impaired sleep quality, insomnia, sedation, *seizures,* sensory disturbance, syncope, tremor.
CV: *arrhythmias,* hypertension, hypotension, palpitations, tachycardia.
EENT: auditory disturbance, blurred vision.
GI: anorexia, constipation, dry mouth, dyspepsia, increased appetite, nausea, taste disturbance, vomiting.
GU: impotence, menstrual complaints, urinary frequency.
Metabolic: hyperglycemia, weight gain or loss.
Musculoskeletal: arthritis.
Skin: cutaneous temperature disturbance, diaphoresis, pruritus, rash.
Other: chills, decreased libido.

Interactions

Drug-drug. *Amantadine, levodopa, MAO inhibitors, phenothiazines, recent and rapid withdrawal of benzodiazepines, tricyclic antidepressants:* May increase risk of adverse reactions, including seizures. Monitor patient closely.
Antipsychotics, beta blockers, SSRIs, type IC antiarrhythmics: May inhibit metabolism by CYP2D6. If used together, consider reducing dosage.
Carbamazepine: May decrease bupropion level. Monitor patient for loss of therapeutic effect.
Nicotine-replacement drugs: May cause hypertension. Monitor blood pressure.
Ritonavir: May increase bupropion level and risk of toxicity. Monitor patient closely.
Warfarin: May alter PT and INR. Monitor patient for bleeding or clotting.
Drug-lifestyle. *Alcohol use:* May alter seizure threshold. Discourage use together.
Sun exposure: Photosensitivity reactions may occur. Advise patient to wear protective clothing and sunblock and to avoid sun exposure.

Effects on lab test results

• May decrease hemoglobin level and hematocrit. May increase or decrease glucose level.
• May decrease platelet count. May increase or decrease WBC count, PT, and INR.

Pharmacokinetics

Absorption: Unknown.
Distribution: About 80% protein-bound.
Metabolism: Probably in liver; several active metabolites have been identified.
Excretion: Mainly in urine. *Half-life:* 8 to 24 hours.

Route	Onset	Peak	Duration
P.O.	1–3 wk	2 hr	Unknown
Wellbutrin SR	Unknown	3 hr	Unknown
Wellbutrin XL	Unknown	5 hr	Unknown

Action

Chemical effect: May work through noradrenergic, dopaminergic, or both mechanisms.
Therapeutic effect: Relieves depression; smoking deterrent.

Available forms

Tablets (extended-release): 150 mg, 300 mg
Tablets (immediate-release): 75 mg, 100 mg

Tablets (sustained-release): 100 mg, 150 mg, 200 mg

NURSING PROCESS

⚡ Assessment
• Obtain history of patient's condition before therapy, and reassess regularly thereafter.
• Be alert for adverse reactions and drug interactions. Closely monitor a patient with history of bipolar disorder. Drug may cause manic episodes during depressive phase.
• Assess patient's and family's knowledge of drug therapy.

🔆 Nursing diagnoses
• Ineffective coping related to underlying condition
• Risk for injury related to drug-induced adverse CNS reactions
• Deficient knowledge related to drug therapy

▶ Planning and implementation
ⓈALERT: Minimize risk of seizure by not exceeding 450 mg/day (immediate-release) and by giving drug daily in three equally divided doses. Dosage increases shouldn't exceed 100 mg/day in a 3-day period. For sustained-release form, don't exceed 400 mg/day, and give drug daily in two equally divided doses. Dosage increases shouldn't exceed 200 mg/day in a 3-day period. Patients who have seizures often have predisposing factors, including history of head trauma, prior seizures, or CNS tumors, or they may be taking a drug that lowers seizure threshold.
ⓈALERT: Don't confuse bupropion with buspirone.
• Make sure patient has swallowed dose.
• Patient may experience period of increased restlessness, agitation, insomnia, and anxiety, especially at start of therapy.
ⓈALERT: Monitor young adults for suicidal thinking and behavior.
• Reassess patient taking warfarin regularly for changes in PT and INR, risk for bleeding, and clotting.
• For smoking cessation, begin therapy while patient is still smoking because about 1 week is needed to achieve steady state levels of drug. Treatment course is usually 7 to 12 weeks.
Patient teaching
• Advise patient to take drug as scheduled and to take each day's dose in three divided doses

(immediate-release) or two divided doses (sustained-release) to minimize risk of seizures.
• Tell patient to avoid alcohol while taking drug because alcohol may contribute to development of seizures.
• Tell patient and family to report changes in mood and behavior, especially increased suicidal thinking.
• Advise patient to avoid hazardous activities that require alertness and good psychomotor coordination until CNS effects of drug are known.
ⓈALERT: Advise patient not to take Wellbutrin with Zyban and to seek medical advice before taking other prescription drugs, OTC medications, or herbal remedies.
• Tell patient not to crush, chew, or divide sustained-release tablets.

✅ Evaluation
• Patient's behavior and communication indicate improvement of depression.
• Patient sustains no injury from drug-induced adverse CNS reactions.
• Patient and family state understanding of drug therapy.

buspirone hydrochloride
(byoo-SPEER-ohn high-droh-KLOR-ighd)
BuSpar

Pharmacologic class: miscellaneous anxioselective derivative
Therapeutic class: anxiolytic
Pregnancy risk category: B

Indications and dosages

▶ **Anxiety disorders, short-term relief of anxiety.** *Adults:* Initially, 7.5 mg P.O. b.i.d. Increase by 5 mg daily at 2- to 3-day intervals. Usual maintenance dosage is 20 to 30 mg daily in divided doses. Don't exceed 60 mg daily.
◪ **Adjust-a-dose:** When given with a CYP3A4 inhibitor, lower initial dosage to 2.5 mg P.O. b.i.d. Subsequent dosage adjustment of either drug also may be needed.

Contraindications and cautions

• Contraindicated in patients hypersensitive to drug and in those who have taken an MAO inhibitor within 14 days.

Reactions may be *common*, uncommon, *life-threatening*, or COMMON AND LIFE-THREATENING.

B

• Use cautiously in patients with hepatic or renal failure.

⚖ **Lifespan:** In pregnant women, use cautiously. In breast-feeding women, don't use. In children, safety and effectiveness of drug haven't been established.

Adverse reactions

CNS: *dizziness, drowsiness,* excitement, fatigue, headache, insomnia, nervousness.
GI: diarrhea, dry mouth, nausea.

Interactions

Drug-drug. *CNS depressants:* May increase CNS depression. Avoid use together.
Erythromycin: May increase buspirone level. Consider initial dose of 2.5 mg b.i.d.
Itraconazole: May increase buspirone level. Consider initial dose of 2.5 mg once daily.
MAO inhibitors: May elevate blood pressure. Avoid use together.
Drug-food. *Grapefruit juice:* May increase buspirone level. Don't use together.
Drug-lifestyle. *Alcohol use:* May increase CNS depression. Discourage use together.

Effects on lab test results

• May increase aminotransferase level.
• May decrease WBC and platelet counts.

Pharmacokinetics

Absorption: Rapid and complete, but extensive first-pass metabolism limits absolute bioavailability to between 1% and 13% of P.O. dose. Food slows absorption but increases amount of unchanged drug in systemic circulation.
Distribution: 95% protein-bound; doesn't displace other highly protein-bound medications.
Metabolism: In liver.
Excretion: 29% to 63% in urine in 24 hours, mainly as metabolites; 18% to 38% in feces.
Half-life: 2 to 3 hours.

Route	Onset	Peak	Duration
P.O.	Unknown	40–90 min	Unknown

Action

Chemical effect: May inhibit neuronal firing and reduce serotonin turnover in cortical, amygdaloid, and septohippocampal tissue.
Therapeutic effect: Relieves anxiety.

Available forms

Tablets: 5 mg, 7.5 mg, 10 mg, 15 mg, 30 mg

NURSING PROCESS

⚗ Assessment
• Obtain history of patient's anxiety before therapy, and reassess regularly thereafter.
• Signs of improvement usually appear within 7 to 10 days; optimal results occur after 3 to 4 weeks of therapy.
• Be alert for adverse reactions and drug interactions.
• Assess patient's and family's knowledge of drug therapy.

⊕ Nursing diagnoses
• Anxiety related to underlying condition
• Fatigue related to drug-induced adverse reactions
• Deficient knowledge related to drug therapy

▶ Planning and implementation
• Although drug has shown no potential for abuse and hasn't been classified as a controlled substance, it isn't recommended for relief from everyday stress.
• Before starting therapy, make sure patient taking a benzodiazepine doesn't stop it abruptly because withdrawal reaction may occur.
• Give drug with food or milk but not grapefruit juice.
• Dosage may be increased in 2- to 4-day intervals.
Patient teaching
• Tell patient to take drug with food but avoid grapefruit juice.
• Warn patient to avoid hazardous activities that require alertness and psychomotor coordination until the drug's CNS effects are known.
• Review energy-saving measures with patient and family.
• If patient is already being treated with a benzodiazepine, warn him not to abruptly stop it because withdrawal reaction can occur. Teach him how and when benzodiazepine can be withdrawn safely.

✔ Evaluation
• Patient's anxiety is reduced.
• Patient states that energy-saving measures help combat fatigue caused by therapy.

• Patient and family state understanding of drug therapy.

HIGH ALERT!

busulfan
(byoo-SUL-fan)
Busulfex, Myleran

Pharmacologic class: alkylating drug
Therapeutic class: antineoplastic
Pregnancy risk category: D

Indications and dosages

▶ **Palliative treatment of chronic myelocytic (granulocytic) leukemia (CML).** *Adults:* For remission induction, 4 to 8 mg P.O. daily (0.06 mg/kg or 1.8 mg/m²). For maintenance therapy, 1 to 3 mg P.O. daily. Dosages may vary. *Children:* 0.06 mg/kg or 1.8 mg/m² P.O. daily. Dosages may vary.
▶ **With cyclophosphamide as a conditioning regimen before allogeneic hematopoietic progenitor cell transplantation for CML.** *Adults:* 0.8 mg/kg of ideal body weight or actual body weight (whichever is lower) I.V. by central venous catheter as a 2-hour infusion every 6 hours for 4 consecutive days for a total of 16 doses. Give phenytoin for seizure prophylaxis. Dosages may vary.
▶ **Myelofibrosis‡.** *Adults:* Initially, give 2 to 4 mg P.O. daily, then followed by the same dose two to three times weekly. Dosages may vary.

▽ I.V. administration

• Use aseptic technique when preparing and handling drug. Wear gloves and other protective clothing to prevent skin contact.
• Dilute with normal saline solution or D_5W to a final concentration of at least 0.5 mg/ml.
• Flush catheter with diluent before and after infusion.
• Give by infusion pump over 2 hours.
• If solution is kept at room temperature, use within 8 hours of preparing; if refrigerated, within 12 hours.
• Refrigerate unopened ampules.
⊗ **Incompatibilities**
Other I.V. drugs.

Contraindications and cautions

• Contraindicated in patients with drug-resistant CML.

• Use cautiously in patients recently given other myelosuppressive drugs or radiation therapy and in those with depressed neutrophil or platelet count. Because high-dose therapy has been linked to seizures, use such therapy cautiously in patients with history of head trauma or seizures and in patients receiving other drugs that lower seizure threshold.
🎋 **Lifespan:** In pregnant women, use cautiously, if at all. In breast-feeding women, drug is contraindicated.

Adverse reactions

CNS: agitation, *anxiety, asthenia,* confusion, delirium, *depression, dizziness,* **encephalopathy,** *fever,* hallucinations, *headache, insomnia,* lethargy, *pain,* **seizures,** somnolence.
CV: cardiomegaly, *chest pain,* **ECG abnormalities,** *edema,* **heart failure,** *heart rhythm abnormalities,* hypertension, hypotension, **pericardial effusion,** *tachycardia,* **thrombosis,** *vasodilation.*
EENT: cataracts, ear disorder, *epistaxis, pharyngitis, rhinitis,* sinusitis.
GI: *abdominal pain and enlargement, anorexia, cheilosis (P.O.), constipation, diarrhea, dry mouth, dyspepsia, mucositis, nausea,* **pancreatitis,** *rectal disorder, stomatitis, vomiting.*
GU: dysuria, hematuria, hemorrhagic cystitis, *oliguria.*
Hematologic: anemia, **granulocytopenia, leukopenia, thrombocytopenia.**
Hepatic: **hepatic necrosis,** hepatomegaly, *jaundice.*
Metabolic: *hyperglycemia, hypervolemia, hypocalcemia, hypokalemia,* HYPOMAGNESEMIA, hyponatremia, *hypophosphatemia, weight gain.*
Musculoskeletal: *arthralgia, back pain, myalgia.*
Respiratory: *alveolar hemorrhage, asthma,* atelectasis, *cough, dyspnea,* hemoptysis, hypoxia, *irreversible pulmonary fibrosis, lung disorder,* pleural effusion.
Skin: acne, *alopecia,* anhidrosis, erythema nodosum, exfoliative dermatitis, *hyperpigmentation, pruritus, rash,* skin discoloration.
Other: Addison-like wasting syndrome, gynecomastia, inflammation at injection site (P.O.); *allergic reaction, chills,* **graft-versus-host disease,** hiccups, **infection.**

Interactions

Drug-drug. *Acetaminophen within 72 hours:*
May decrease busulfan clearance. Use together
cautiously.
Anticoagulants, aspirin: May increase risk of
bleeding. Avoid use together.
Cyclophosphamide: May increase risk of car-
diac tamponade in patients with thalassemia.
Monitor patient.
Cytotoxic drugs that cause pulmonary injury:
May cause additive pulmonary toxicity. Avoid
use together.
Itraconazole: May decrease busulfan clearance.
Use together cautiously.
Myelosuppressives: May increase myelosup-
pression. Monitor patient.
Phenytoin: May decrease busulfan level. Moni-
tor busulfan level.
Thioguanine: May cause hepatotoxicity,
esophageal varices, or portal hypertension. Use
together cautiously.

Effects on lab test results

• May increase serum glucose, ALT, bilirubin,
alkaline phosphatase, uric acid, creatinine, and
BUN levels. May decrease magnesium, calcium, potassium, phosphorus, sodium, and hemoglobin levels and hematocrit.
• May decrease WBC, and platelet counts.

Pharmacokinetics

Absorption: Well absorbed from GI tract.
Distribution: Unknown.
Metabolism: In liver.
Excretion: Cleared rapidly and excreted in
urine. *Half-life:* About 2½ hours.

Route	Onset	Peak	Duration
P.O.	1–2 wk	Unknown	Unknown
I.V.	Unknown	Unknown	Unknown

Action

Chemical effect: Unknown; thought to cross-
link strands of cellular DNA and interfere with
RNA transcription, causing an imbalance of
growth that leads to cell death.
Therapeutic effect: Kills selected type of cancer cell.

Available forms

Injection: 6 mg/ml
Tablets: 2 mg

NURSING PROCESS

Assessment
• Obtain history of patient's underlying neoplastic disease.
• Monitor WBC and platelet counts weekly
while patient is receiving drug. WBC count falls
about 10 days after the start of therapy and continues to fall for 2 weeks after stopping drug.
• Monitor uric acid, liver and kidney function,
and glucose levels.
ALERT: Be alert for adverse reactions and drug
interactions. Pulmonary fibrosis may occur as
late as 4 to 6 months after treatment.
• Assess patient's and family's knowledge of
drug therapy.

Nursing diagnoses
• Ineffective health maintenance related to pres-
ence of neoplastic disease
• Risk for infection related to drug-induced im-
munosuppression
• Deficient knowledge related to drug therapy

Planning and implementation
• Premedicate patient with phenytoin to de-
crease risk of seizures that can occur with I.V.
infusion.
• Follow facility policy regarding preparation
and handling of drug. Label as hazardous drug.
• Give drug at same time each day.
• Make sure patient is adequately hydrated.
• Adjust dosage based on patient's weekly
WBC counts, and if severe leukocytopenia develops, temporarily stop drug therapy. Toxicity
often accompanies therapeutic effects.
• Give with allopurinol and ensure adequate hydration to prevent hyperuricemia with resulting
uric acid nephropathy.
Patient teaching
• Warn patient to watch for signs of infection,
such as fever, sore throat, and fatigue, and for
symptoms of bleeding, such as easy bruising,
nosebleeds, bleeding gums, and melena. Advise
patient to take his temperature daily.
ALERT: Instruct patient to report symptoms of
toxicity so dosage adjustments can be made.
Symptoms include persistent cough and progressive dyspnea with alveolar exudate, suggestive of pneumonia.
• Instruct patient to avoid OTC products that
contain aspirin.

• Advise woman of childbearing age to avoid becoming pregnant during therapy. Recommend that patient consult with prescriber before becoming pregnant.
• Advise breast-feeding woman to stop breast-feeding because of possible risk of toxicity in infant.

☑ Evaluation
• Patient has positive response to drug therapy.
• Patient remains free from infection.
• Patient and family state understanding of drug therapy.

HIGH ALERT!

butorphanol tartrate
(byoo-TOR-fah-nohl TAR-trayt)
Stadol, Stadol NS

Pharmacologic class: opioid agonist-antagonist
Therapeutic class: analgesic, adjunct to anesthesia
Pregnancy risk category: C

Indications and dosages

▶ **Moderate to severe pain.** *Adults:* 0.5 to 2 mg I.V. every 3 to 4 hours, p.r.n., or around-the-clock. Or 1 to 4 mg I.M. every 3 to 4 hours, p.r.n., or around-the-clock. Maximum, 4 mg per dose. Or, 1 mg by nasal spray every 3 to 4 hours (1 spray in one nostril); repeat in 60 to 90 minutes if pain relief is inadequate.
▶ **Labor for pregnant women at full term and in early labor.** *Adults:* 1 to 2 mg I.V. or I.M., repeated after 4 hours, p.r.n.
▶ **Preoperative anesthesia or preanesthesia.** *Adults:* 2 mg I.M. 60 to 90 minutes before surgery.
▶ **Adjunct to balanced anesthesia.** *Adults:* 2 mg I.V. shortly before induction or 0.5 to 1 mg I.V. in increments during anesthesia.
Adjust-a-dose: For patients with hepatic or renal impairment and elderly patients, reduce dosage to 50% of the usual parenteral adult dose at 6-hour intervals p.r.n. For nasal spray, the initial dose (1 spray in one nostril) is the same, but repeat dose is in 90 to 120 minutes, if needed. Repeat doses thereafter every 6 hours, p.r.n.

▼ I.V. administration
• Give drug by direct I.V. injection into vein or into I.V. line containing free-flowing compatible solution.
⊗ **Incompatibilities**
Dimenhydrinate, pentobarbital sodium.

Contraindications and cautions
• Contraindicated in patients with opioid addiction; may precipitate withdrawal syndrome. Also contraindicated in patients hypersensitive to drug or to preservative (benzethonium chloride).
• Use cautiously in patients with head injury, increased intracranial pressure, acute MI, ventricular dysfunction, coronary insufficiency, respiratory disease or depression, or renal or hepatic dysfunction. Also use cautiously in patients who have recently received repeated doses of an opioid analgesic.
⚠ **Lifespan:** In pregnant women, use only when benefits outweigh risks to fetus. In breast-feeding women, drug is contraindicated. In children, safety and effectiveness haven't been established. In the elderly, mean half-life of the drug is longer; use cautiously because adverse reactions may increase.

Adverse reactions
CNS: agitation, *confusion,* euphoria, *floating sensation,* flushing, hallucinations, *headache, increased intracranial pressure,* lethargy, nervousness, *sedation,* unusual dreams, *vertigo.*
CV: fluctuation in blood pressure, palpitations.
EENT: blurred vision, diplopia, *nasal congestion* (with nasal spray).
GI: constipation, *dry mouth,* nausea, vomiting.
Respiratory: *respiratory depression.*
Skin: clamminess, excessive sweating, rash, urticaria.

Interactions
Drug-drug. *CNS depressants:* May have additive effects. Use together cautiously.
Opioid analgesics: May decrease analgesic effect. Avoid use together.
Drug-lifestyle. *Alcohol use:* May have additive depressant effects. Discourage use together.

Effects on lab test results
None reported.

Pharmacokinetics

Absorption: Good after I.M. use.
Distribution: 80% protein-bound. Drug rapidly crosses placenta, and neonatal levels are 0.4 to 1.4 times maternal levels.
Metabolism: Extensive, in liver to inactive metabolites.
Excretion: In inactive form, mainly by kidneys. About 11% to 14% of parenteral dose in feces.
Half-life: About 2 to 9¼ hours.

Route	Onset	Peak	Duration
I.V.	2–3 min	½–1 hr	2–4 hr
I.M.	10–30 min	½–1 hr	3–4 hr
Intranasal	≤ 15 min	1–2 hr	4–5 hr

Action

Chemical effect: Binds with opiate receptors in CNS, altering both perception of and emotional response to pain through unknown mechanism.
Therapeutic effect: Relieves pain and enhances anesthesia.

Available forms

Injection: 1 mg/ml, 2 mg/ml
Nasal spray: 10 mg/ml

NURSING PROCESS

Assessment
• Obtain history of patient's pain before therapy, and reassess during therapy.
• Be alert for adverse reactions and drug interactions.
• Periodically monitor postoperative vital signs and bladder function. Drug decreases both rate and depth of respirations, and monitoring arterial oxygen saturation may aid in assessing respiratory depression.
• Assess patient's and family's knowledge of drug therapy.

Nursing diagnoses
• Acute pain related to underlying condition
• Risk for injury related to drug-induced adverse CNS reactions
• Deficient knowledge related to drug therapy

Planning and implementation
• For intranasal use, have patient clear nasal passages before giving drug. Shake container. Tilt patient's head slightly backward; insert nozzle into nostril, pointing away from septum.

Have patient hold other nostril closed, and spray while patient inhales gently.
• Subcutaneous route isn't recommended.
• Monitor patient for psychological and physical addiction, which may occur.
• Notify prescriber and discuss increasing dose or frequency if pain persists.
• Keep opioid antagonist (naloxone) and resuscitative equipment available.
Patient teaching
• Caution patient to get out of bed slowly and walk carefully until CNS effects are known.
• Warn outpatient to refrain from driving and performing other activities that require mental alertness until drug's CNS effects are known.
• Warn patient that drug can cause physical and psychological dependence. Tell him to use drug only as directed and that abrupt withdrawal after prolonged use produces intense withdrawal symptoms.

Evaluation
• Patient reports relief from pain.
• Patient doesn't experience injury as a result of therapy.
• Patient and family state understanding of drug therapy.

calcitonin (salmon)
(kal-sih-TOH-nin)
Calcimar, Fortical, Miacalcin

Pharmacologic class: thyroid hormone, calcium and bone metabolism regulator
Therapeutic class: hypocalcemic, bone resorption inhibitor
Pregnancy risk category: C

Indications and dosages

▶ **Osteoporosis.** *Postmenopausal women:* 100 international units I.M. or subcutaneously every other day. Or, 200 international units (one activation) daily intranasally, alternating nostrils daily.
▶ **Paget disease of bone (osteitis deformans).** *Adults:* Initially, 100 international units daily

I.M. or subcutaneously; maintenance dosage is 50 to 100 international units daily or every other day.

▶ **Hypercalcemia.** *Adults:* 4 international units/kg every 12 hours I.M. or subcutaneously. If response is inadequate after 1 or 2 days, increase dosage to 8 international units/kg I.M. every 12 hours. If response remains unsatisfactory after 2 more days, increase dosage to maximum of 8 international units/kg every 6 hours.

▶ **Osteogenesis imperfecta‡.** *Adults:* 2 international units/kg subcutaneously or I.M. three times weekly with daily calcium supplementation.

Contraindications and cautions

• Contraindicated in patients hypersensitive to drug.

⚖ **Lifespan:** In pregnant women, use cautiously. In breast-feeding women, don't use because drug may inhibit lactation. In children, safety and effectiveness haven't been established.

Adverse reactions

CNS: dizziness, headache, paresthesia, weakness.
CV: facial flushing, hypertension.
EENT: epistaxis, nasal symptoms (irritation, redness, sores) with intranasal use, *rhinitis.*
GI: anorexia, diarrhea, *nausea,* unusual taste, *vomiting.*
GU: nocturia, urinary frequency.
Metabolic: goiter, hyperglycemia, hyperthyroidism, hypocalcemia.
Musculoskeletal: arthralgia, back pain.
Skin: facial and hand flushing, rash.
Other: *anaphylaxis;* hand swelling, tingling, and tenderness; hypersensitivity reactions; *inflammation at injection site.*

Interactions

None significant.

Effects on lab test results

• May increase glucose, T_3, and T_4 levels. May decrease calcium and thyroid-stimulating hormone levels.

Pharmacokinetics

Absorption: Rapid with intranasal use.
Distribution: Unknown; however, drug doesn't cross the placenta.

Metabolism: Rapid, in kidneys; additional activity in blood and peripheral tissues.
Excretion: In urine as inactive metabolites.
Half-life: Calcitonin human, 60 minutes; calcitonin salmon, 43 to 60 minutes.

Route	Onset	Peak	Duration
I.M., SubQ	≤ 15 min	≤ 4 hr	8–24 hr
Intranasal	Rapid	30 min	1 hr

Action

Chemical effect: Decreases osteoclastic activity by inhibiting osteocytic lysis; decreases mineral release and matrix or collagen breakdown in bone.
Therapeutic effect: Prohibits bone and kidney (tubular) resorption of calcium.

Available forms

Injection: 200 international units/ml, 2-ml ampules or vials
Nasal spray: 200 international units/activation in 2-ml bottle (0.09 ml/dose)

NURSING PROCESS

⚗ Assessment

⚡ **ALERT:** Assess postmenopausal woman's history. Only give drug if patient can't take estrogen. Patient requires continued vitamin D and calcium supplements in addition to drug.
• Assess patient's calcium level before therapy and regularly thereafter.
• If using nasal spray, assess nasal passages before therapy and periodically thereafter.
• For Paget disease, monitor alkaline phosphatase and 24-hour urine hydroxyproline levels to evaluate the drug's effectiveness.
• Monitor glucose level and thyroid studies before and periodically during treatment. Repeat DEXA bone scan to assess effectiveness of therapy at least yearly.
• Examine urine sediment periodically for casts, particularly in immobilized patients.
• Look for adverse reactions.
• Assess patient's and family's knowledge of drug therapy.

⊕ Nursing diagnoses

• Risk for injury related to patient's underlying bone condition

• Ineffective protection related to potential for drug-induced anaphylaxis
• Deficient knowledge related to drug therapy

▷ Planning and implementation

• Perform skin test before therapy.
• Give drug at bedtime to minimize nausea and vomiting; remind patient that these symptoms usually resolve after 1 to 2 months of treatment.
• If dose is larger than 2 ml, give it I.M.
• When using nasal spray, alternate nostrils daily.
• Keep parenteral calcium available during first doses in case hypocalcemic tetany occurs.
• Refrigerate calcitonin salmon at 36° to 46° F (2° to 8° C). Store open nasal spray at room temperature.
• In patient who relapses after a positive initial response, evaluate for antibody response to hormone protein.
• Systemic allergic reactions may occur because hormone is a protein; keep epinephrine handy.
• If symptoms have been relieved after 6 months, stop drug until symptoms or radiologic signs recur.
⚠ ALERT: Don't confuse calcitonin with calciferol or calcitriol.

Patient teaching
• For outpatient therapy for Paget disease, teach patient how to give drug subcutaneously.
• Teach patient to activate nasal spray before first use by holding bottle upright and depressing side arms six times until a faint mist appears, signifying pump is primed and ready for use. Patient doesn't need to reprime the pump before each use.
• Instruct patient to report signs of nasal irritation from spray.
• Tell patient to handle missed doses as follows: With daily use, take as soon as possible, but don't double the dose. With alternate-day use, take missed dose as soon as possible, and then resume alternate-day schedule from that point.
• Remind patient with postmenopausal osteoporosis to take adequate calcium and vitamin D supplements.

✓ Evaluation
• Patient's calcium level is normal.
• Patient doesn't experience anaphylaxis.
• Patient and family state understanding of drug therapy.

calcitriol (1,25-dihydroxycholecalciferol)
(kal-SIH-try-ohl)
Calcijex, Rocaltrol

Pharmacologic class: vitamin D analogue
Therapeutic class: antihypocalcemic
Pregnancy risk category: C

Indications and dosages

▶ **Hypocalcemia in patients undergoing long-term dialysis.** *Adults:* Initially, 0.25 mcg P.O. daily. Increase by 0.25 mcg daily at 4- to 8-week intervals. Maintenance dosage is 0.25 mcg every other day up to 1 mcg daily or 1 to 2 mcg I.V. three times weekly. Dosages from 0.5 to 4 mcg three times weekly may be used initially. If response to initial dose is inadequate, increase by 0.5 to 1 mcg at 2- to 4-week intervals. Maintenance dosage is 0.5 to 3 mcg I.V. three times weekly.
▶ **Hypoparathyroidism and pseudohypoparathyroidism.** *Adults and children age 6 and older:* Initially, 0.25 mcg P.O. daily. Increase dosage at 2- to 4-week intervals. Maintenance dosage is 0.25 to 2 mcg daily.
▶ **Hypoparathyroidism.** *Children and infants ages 1 to 5:* Give 0.25 to 0.75 mcg P.O. daily.
▶ **To manage secondary hyperparathyroidism and resulting metabolic bone disease in predialysis patients (moderate-to-severe chronic renal impairment with creatinine clearance of 15 to 55 ml/minute).** *Adults and children age 3 and older:* Initially, 0.25 mcg P.O. daily. Increase dosage to 0.5 mcg daily, if needed.
Children younger than age 3: Initially, 0.01 to 0.015 mcg/kg P.O. daily.

▽ I.V. administration

• For hypocalcemic patients with chronic renal impairment who are undergoing hemodialysis, give I.V. dose by rapid injection via dialysis catheter after treatment.
• Discard unused portions because drug contains no preservatives.
• Store injection at room temperature; avoid excessive heat or freezing. Protect from light.
⊗ **Incompatibilities**
None reported.

Contraindications and cautions

• Contraindicated in patients with hypercalcemia or vitamin D toxicity.

⚕ **Lifespan:** In pregnant or breast-feeding women, use cautiously.

Adverse reactions

CNS: headache, somnolence.
EENT: conjunctivitis, photophobia, rhinorrhea.
GI: anorexia, constipation, dry mouth, metallic taste, nausea, vomiting.
GU: polyuria.
Musculoskeletal: bone and muscle pain, weakness.

Interactions

Drug-drug. *Antacids containing magnesium:* May induce hypermagnesemia, especially in patients with chronic renal impairment. Avoid use together.
Cholestyramine, colestipol, excessive use of mineral oil: May decrease absorption of orally given vitamin D analogues. Avoid use together.
Corticosteroids: Counteracts vitamin D analogue effects. Avoid use together.
Digoxin: May increase risk of arrhythmias. Avoid use together.
Ketoconazole: May decrease endogenous calcitriol level. Monitor patient.
Phenytoin, phenobarbital: May reduce calcitriol level. Higher doses of calcitriol may be needed.
Thiazides: May induce hypercalcemia. Monitor calcium level and patient closely.
Verapamil: May cause atrial fibrillation because of increased risk of hypercalcemia. Monitor calcium level and patient closely.

Effects on lab test results

• May increase BUN, ALT, AST, albumin, and cholesterol levels.

Pharmacokinetics

Absorption: Readily.
Distribution: Wide; protein-bound.
Metabolism: In liver and kidneys.
Excretion: Mainly in feces. *Half-life:* 3 to 6 hours.

Route	Onset	Peak	Duration
P.O.	2–6 hr	3–6 hr	3–5 days
I.V.	Immediate	Unknown	3–5 days

Action

Chemical effect: Stimulates calcium absorption from GI tract; promotes calcium secretion from bone to blood.
Therapeutic effect: Raises calcium level.

Available forms

Capsules: 0.25 mcg, 0.5 mcg
Injection: 1 mcg/ml, 2 mcg/ml
Oral solution: 1 mcg/ml

NURSING PROCESS

⚖ Assessment

• Assess patient's calcium and phosphate levels before therapy and regularly thereafter to monitor drug effectiveness; make sure calcium level times phosphate level doesn't exceed 70. During dosage adjustment, determine calcium level twice weekly.
• Monitor patient for vitamin D intoxication, which may cause anorexia, arrhythmias, bone and muscle pain, conjunctivitis, constipation, decreased libido, dry mouth, headache, hypertension, hyperthermia, irritability, metallic taste, nausea, nephrocalcinosis, nocturia, pancreatitis, photophobia, polydipsia, pruritus, rhinorrhea, somnolence, vomiting, weakness, polyuria, and weight loss.
• Look for adverse reactions and drug interactions.
• Assess patient's and family's knowledge of drug therapy.

⊕ Nursing diagnoses

• Risk for injury related to patient's underlying condition
• Ineffective protection related to potential for drug-induced vitamin D intoxication
• Deficient knowledge related to drug therapy

▶ Planning and implementation

• Keep drug away from heat, light, and moisture.
• Give drug at same time each day.
• If hypercalcemia occurs, stop drug and notify prescriber; resume drug after calcium level returns to normal. Make sure patient receives adequate daily calcium intake.
⑤ **ALERT:** Don't confuse calcitriol with calciferol or calcitonin.

Patient teaching
• Tell patient to immediately report early symptoms of vitamin D intoxication, such as weakness, nausea, vomiting, dry mouth, constipation, muscle or bone pain, or metallic taste.
• Instruct patient to adhere to diet and calcium supplements and to avoid OTC drugs and antacids containing magnesium.
• Warn patient that drug is the most potent form of vitamin D available and that severe toxicity can occur if ingested by anyone for whom it isn't prescribed.
• Tell patient to protect drug from light, moisture, and heat.

☑ Evaluation
• Patient's calcium level is normal.
• Patient sustains no injury from drug-induced vitamin D toxicity.
• Patient and family state understanding of drug therapy.

---

calcium acetate
(KAL-see-um AS-ih-tayt)
Calphron, Phos-Lo

calcium carbonate
Alka-Mints†, Amitone†, Cal-Carb Forte†, Calci-Chew†, Chooz†, Equilet†, Florical†, Maalox†, Mallamint†, Nephro-Calci†, Os-Cal†, Oyst-Cal†, Rolaids Extra Strength Softchews†, Trial Antacid†, Tums†, Tums E-X†, Tums Extra Strength†

calcium chloride

calcium citrate
Cal-C-Caps†, Cal-CEE†, Citracal†, Citracal Liquitabs

calcium glubionate
Calcionate†, Calciquid†

calcium gluconate

calcium lactate
Cal-Lac†

calcium phosphate, dibasic
calcium phosphate, tribasic
Posture†

Pharmacologic class: mineral, electrolyte
Therapeutic class: calcium supplement, antiarrhythmic
Pregnancy risk category: NR; C (PhosLo)

Indications and dosages
▶ **Hypocalcemic emergency.** *Adults:* 7 to 14 mEq calcium I.V. May be given as 10% calcium gluconate solution or 2% to 10% calcium chloride solution.
Children: 1 to 7 mEq calcium I.V.
Infants: Up to 1 mEq calcium I.V.
▶ **Hypocalcemic tetany.** *Adults:* 4.5 to 16 mEq calcium I.V. Repeat until tetany is controlled.
Children: 0.5 to 0.7 mEq/kg calcium I.V. t.i.d. or q.i.d. until tetany is controlled.
Neonates: 2.4 mEq/kg I.V. daily in divided doses.
▶ **Adjunct in cardiac arrest.** *Adults:* 500 mg to 1 g calcium chloride I.V. Don't exceed 1 ml/minute. Determine calcium level before giving further doses.
▶ **Adjunct in magnesium intoxication.**
Adults: Initially, 7 mEq I.V. Base later doses on patient's response.
▶ **During exchange transfusions.** *Adults:* 1.35 mEq I.V. with each 100 ml citrated blood.
Neonates: 0.45 mEq I.V. with each 100 ml citrated blood.
▶ **Hyperphosphatemia in end-stage renal failure.** *Adults:* 2 to 4 tablets calcium acetate P.O. with each meal.
▶ **Gastric hyperacidity, calcium supplement.** *Adults:* 0.5 to 1.5 g p.r.n.

▽ I.V. administration
• Calcium salts aren't interchangeable. Verify preparation before use.
• Give calcium chloride and calcium gluconate only I.V.
• When adding calcium chloride to parenteral solutions that contain other additives (especially phosphorus or phosphate), inspect solution closely for precipitate. Use in-line filter.
• Monitor ECG when giving calcium I.V. If patient complains of discomfort, stop and notify prescriber. After injection, make sure patient remains recumbent for 15 minutes.

• Severe necrosis and tissue sloughing can occur after extravasation. Calcium gluconate is less irritating to veins and tissues than calcium chloride.
Direct injection
• Warm solution to body temperature.
• Give direct injection slowly through small needle into large vein or through I.V. line containing free-flowing, compatible solution at no more than 1 ml/minute (1.5 mEq/minute) for calcium chloride or 0.5 to 2 ml/minute for calcium gluconate. Don't use scalp veins in children.
• Rapid injection may cause syncope, vasodilation, bradycardia, arrhythmias, or cardiac arrest.
Intermittent infusion
• When giving intermittent infusion, infuse diluted solution through I.V. line containing compatible solution. Maximum, 200 mg/minute for calcium gluconate.
• Precipitate will form if drug is given I.V. with sodium bicarbonate or other alkaline drugs. Use an in-line filter.
⊗ **Incompatibilities**
Calcium chloride: amphotericin B, chlorpheniramine, dobutamine.
Calcium gluconate: amphotericin B, cefamandole, dobutamine, fluconazole, indomethacin sodium trihydrate, methylprednisolone sodium succinate, prochlorperazine edisylate.

Contraindications and cautions

• Contraindicated in patients with ventricular fibrillation, hypercalcemia, hypophosphatemia, or renal calculi.
• Use all calcium products cautiously in patients taking digitalis and in patients with sarcoidosis and renal or cardiac disease.
• Use calcium chloride cautiously in patients with cor pulmonale, respiratory acidosis, or respiratory impairment.
⚖ **Lifespan:** In children, use I.V. drug cautiously; safety and effectiveness haven't been established.

Adverse reactions

CNS: pain, sense of oppression or heat waves, syncope, tingling.
CV: *arrhythmias, bradycardia, cardiac arrest,* mild decrease in blood pressure, vasodilation.
GI: chalky taste; constipation, *hemorrhage,* or irritation with oral use; nausea; thirst; vomiting.
GU: polyuria, renal calculi.
Metabolic: hypercalcemia.

Skin: burning, cellulitis, necrosis, soft-tissue calcification, and tissue sloughing with I.M. use; irritation with subcutaneous injection.
Other: *vein irritation with I.V. use.*

Interactions

Drug-drug. *Atenolol, fluoroquinolones, tetracyclines:* May decrease bioavailability of these drugs and calcium when oral forms are taken together. Give drugs at different times.
Calcium channel blockers: May decrease calcium effectiveness. Avoid use together.
Ciprofloxacin, levofloxacin, lomefloxacin, moxifloxacin, norfloxacin, ofloxacin: May decrease effects of quinolone. Give antacid at least 6 hours before or 2 hours after the quinolone.
Digoxin: May increase digitalis toxicity. Use together cautiously, if at all.
Enteric-coated drugs: May cause premature release of enteric-coated drug in the stomach. Don't give within 1 hour of each other.
Sodium bicarbonate: May cause milk-alkali syndrome (confusion, headache, hypercalcemia, hypercalciuria, hypophosphatemia, metabolic alkalosis, vomiting, weakness). Discourage use together.
Sodium polystyrene sulfonate: May increase risk of metabolic acidosis in patients with renal disease. Avoid use together in such patients.
Thiazide diuretics: May increase risk of hypercalcemia. Avoid use together.
Thyroid hormone: May inhibit the absorption of thyroid drugs. Give drugs at least 2 hours apart.
Drug-food. *Foods containing oxalic acid (rhubarb, spinach), phytic acid (bran, whole cereals), or phosphorus (hard cheese, nuts, dried fruits, sardines):* May interfere with calcium absorption. Tell patient to avoid these foods.

Effects on lab test results

• May increase calcium and 11-hydroxycorticosteroid levels.
• May produce false-negative values for serum and urinary magnesium as measured with Titan yellow.

Pharmacokinetics

Absorption: Pregnancy and reduced calcium intake may enhance absorption. Vitamin D in active form is required for absorption.
Distribution: Enters extracellular fluid and is incorporated rapidly into skeletal tissue. Bone contains 99% of total calcium; 1% is distributed

equally between intracellular and extracellular fluids. Level in CSF is about half that in blood.
Metabolism: Insignificant.
Excretion: Mainly in feces, minimally in urine.
Half-life: Unknown.

Route	Onset	Peak	Duration
P.O.	Unknown	Unknown	Unknown
I.V.	Immediate	Immediate	½–2 hr

Action

Chemical effect: Replaces and maintains calcium. Reduces total acid load in GI tract, elevates gastric pH to reduce pepsin activity, strengthens gastric mucosal barrier and increases esophageal sphincter tone.
Therapeutic effect: Raises calcium level and relieves mild gastric discomfort.

Available forms

calcium acetate
Contains 253 mg or 12.7 mEq of elemental calcium/g
Capsules: 333.5 mg, 667 mg
Gelcaps: 667 mg
Tablets: 667 mg
calcium carbonate
Contains 40% calcium; 20 mEq calcium/g
Chewing gum: 300 mg†, 450 mg†, 500 mg†/piece
Oral suspension: 1.25 g/5 ml†
Tablets: 500 mg†, 600 mg†, 650 mg†, 1,250 mg†, 1,500 mg†
Tablets (chewable): 350 mg†, 400 mg†, 420 mg†, 500 mg†, 750 mg†, 850 mg†, 1,000 mg†, 1,177 mg† 1,250 mg†
calcium chloride
Contains 270 mg or 13.5 mEq of elemental calcium/g
Injection: 10% solution in 10-ml ampules and syringes
calcium citrate
Contains 211 mg or 10.6 mEq of elemental calcium/g
Capsules: 180 mg†
Effervescent tablets: 500 mg†
Powder for oral suspension: 760 mg/5 ml†
Tablets: 200 mg†, 250 mg†
calcium glubionate
Contains 64 mg or 3.2 mEq of elemental calcium/g
Syrup: 1.8 g/5 ml

calcium gluconate
Contains 90 mg or 4.5 mEq of elemental calcium/g
Injection: 10% solution in 10-ml ampules and syringes, 10-ml or 50-ml vials
Tablets: 500 mg†, 650 mg†, 1 g†
calcium lactate
Contains 130 mg or 6.5 mEq of elemental calcium/g
Capsules: 96 mg†
Tablets: 84.5 mg†, 100 mg†
calcium phosphate, dibasic
Contains 230 mg or 11.5 mEq of elemental calcium/g
Tablets: 468 mg†
calcium phosphate, tribasic
Contains 400 mg or 20 mEq of elemental calcium/g
Tablets: 600 mg†

NURSING PROCESS

Assessment
• Assess patient's calcium level before therapy and frequently thereafter to monitor the drug's effectiveness. Hypercalcemia may result after large doses in patients with chronic renal impairment.
• Look for adverse reactions and drug interactions.
• Assess patient's and family's knowledge of drug therapy.

Nursing diagnoses
• Ineffective protection related to calcium deficiency
• Risk for injury related to drug-induced adverse reactions
• Deficient knowledge related to drug therapy

Planning and implementation
• If hypercalcemia occurs, stop drug and notify prescriber. Provide emergency supportive care until calcium level returns to normal.
• Signs and symptoms of severe hypercalcemia may include stupor, confusion, delirium, and coma. Signs and symptoms of mild hypercalcemia may include anorexia, nausea, and vomiting.
ALERT: Make sure prescriber specifies which calcium form to use because code carts usually contain both calcium gluconate and calcium chloride.

Patient teaching
• Tell patient to take oral calcium 1 to 1½ hours after meals if GI upset occurs.
⚠ **ALERT:** Warn patient to avoid foods containing oxalic acid, phytic acid, and phosphorus because interactions may interfere with calcium absorption.
• Teach patient to recognize and report signs and symptoms of hypercalcemia.
• Stress importance of follow-up care and regular blood samples to monitor calcium level.
• Advise patient not to take drug indiscriminately and not to switch antacids without consulting prescriber.
• Tell patient to take calcium carbonate 1 hour after meals and at bedtime, as needed.

☑ **Evaluation**
• Patient's calcium level is normal.
• Patient doesn't experience injury from calcium-induced adverse reactions.
• Patient and family state understanding of drug therapy.

calfactant
(kal-FAK-tant)
Infasurf

Pharmacologic class: surfactant
Therapeutic class: respiratory distress syndrome (RDS) drug
Pregnancy risk category: NR

Indications and dosages

▶ **Confirmed RDS in neonates younger than 72 hours old who need endotracheal intubation.** *Neonates:* 3 ml/kg birth weight, intratracheally, given in 2 aliquots of 1.5 ml/kg. Repeat doses of 3 ml/kg of birth weight, given in 2 aliquots of 1.5 ml/kg, up to a total of three doses given 12 hours apart.
▶ **Prevention of RDS in premature infants younger than 29 weeks' gestational age at high risk for RDS.** 3 ml/kg birth weight, given intratracheally within 30 minutes of birth, in 2 aliquots of 1.5 ml/kg each.

Contraindications and cautions

None reported.
🜃 **Lifespan:** Indicated for premature infants only.

Adverse reactions

CV: BRADYCARDIA, *cyanosis.*
Respiratory: AIRWAY OBSTRUCTION, APNEA, *dislodgment of endotracheal tube, hypoventilation, reflux of drug into endotracheal tube.*

Interactions

None significant.

Effects on lab test results

None reported.

Pharmacokinetics

Absorption: Unknown.
Distribution: Unknown.
Metabolism: Unknown.
Excretion: Unknown. *Half-life:* Unknown.

Route	Onset	Peak	Duration
Intratracheal	24–48 hr	Unknown	Unknown

Action

Chemical effect: Modifies alveolar surface tension, thereby stabilizing the alveoli.
Therapeutic effect: Prevents or treats RDS in premature neonates with specific characteristics.

Available forms

Intratracheal suspension: 35 mg phospholipids and 0.65 mg proteins/ml; 6-ml vial

NURSING PROCESS

🜚 **Assessment**
• Assess patient's underlying condition before therapy and regularly thereafter.
• Monitor patient for reflux of drug into endotracheal tube, cyanosis, bradycardia, or airway obstruction. If these occur, stop the drug and stabilize infant. After infant is stable, give remainder of the dose, with appropriate monitoring.
• After giving drug, carefully monitor infant so oxygen therapy and ventilation can be adjusted for improved oxygenation and lung compliance.
• Evaluate parents' knowledge of drug therapy.

⊕ **Nursing diagnoses**
• Risk for injury related to potential for RDS
• Impaired gas exchange related to presence of RDS
• Deficient knowledge related to drug therapy

C

▷ Planning and implementation

• Give drug under supervision of a prescriber experienced in acute care of neonates with respiratory impairment who need intubation.
• Drug is intended only for intratracheal use; to prevent RDS, give immediately after birth, preferably within 30 minutes.
• Suspension settles during storage. Gently swirl or agitate the vial to redisperse, but don't shake. Visible flecks in the suspension and foaming at the surface are normal.
• Withdraw dose into a syringe from single-use vial using a 20G or larger needle; avoid excessive foaming.
• Use each single-use vial only once; discard unused material.
• Give through a side-port adapter into the endotracheal tube. Two health care providers should be present. Give dose in 2 aliquots of 1.5 ml/kg each. Continue ventilation over 20 to 30 breaths for each aliquot, with small bursts timed to occur during inspiration. Between aliquots, evaluate respiration and reposition infant.
• Store drug at 36° to 46° F (2° to 8° C). Don't warm drug before use; it's not needed. Unopened, unused vials that have warmed to room temperature can be returned to refrigerated storage within 24 hours for future use. Avoid repeated warming to room temperature.

Patient teaching
• Explain to parents the reason for using drug to prevent or treat RDS.
• Notify parents that although the infant may improve rapidly after therapy, he may still need intubation and mechanical ventilation.
• Notify parents about adverse effects of the drug, including bradycardia, reflux into endotracheal tube, airway obstruction, cyanosis, dislodgment of the endotracheal tube, and hypoventilation.
• Reassure parents that infant will be carefully monitored.

☑ Evaluation
• Premature infant doesn't develop RDS.
• Patient's gas exchange improves because of oxygenation and increased lung compliance.
• Parents state understanding of drug therapy.

candesartan cilexetil
(kan-dih-SAR-ten se-LEKS-ih-til)
Atacand

Pharmacologic class: angiotensin II receptor antagonist
Therapeutic class: antihypertensive
Pregnancy risk category: C (D in second and third trimesters)

Indications and dosages

▶ **Heart failure.** *Adults:* Initially, 4 mg P.O. once daily. Double the dose about every 2 weeks as tolerated, to a target dose of 32 mg once daily.
▶ **Hypertension (alone or with other antihypertensives).** *Adults:* Initially, 16 mg P.O. once daily when used as monotherapy; usual dosage is 8 to 32 mg P.O. daily as single dose or divided b.i.d.
☒ Adjust-a-dose: In patients with volume depletion or moderate hepatic impairment, consider giving lower initial dose.

Contraindications and cautions

• Contraindicated in patients hypersensitive to drug or its components.
• Use cautiously in patients whose renal function depends on the renin-angiotensin-aldosterone system (such as patients with heart failure) because of risk of oliguria and progressive azotemia resulting in acute renal impairment. Also use cautiously in patients who are volume- or salt-depleted because of risk of symptomatic hypotension.
⚖ Lifespan: In pregnant women, don't use because drug acts directly on the renin-angiotensin system and may harm the fetus or neonate. If drug is absolutely needed, limit to first trimester. If pregnancy is suspected, stop the drug. In breast-feeding women, use cautiously because the effects on the infant are unknown.

Adverse reactions

CNS: dizziness, fatigue, headache.
CV: chest pain, peripheral edema.
EENT: pharyngitis, rhinitis, sinusitis.
GI: abdominal pain, diarrhea, nausea, vomiting.
GU: albuminuria.
Musculoskeletal: arthralgia, back pain.

Respiratory: bronchitis, cough, upper respiratory tract infection.

Interactions

Drug-drug. *Lithium:* May increase lithium level. Carefully monitor lithium level for toxicity.

Effects on lab test results

• May increase bilirubin, lithium, BUN, creatinine, potassium, and uric acid levels. May decrease hemoglobin level and hematocrit.
• May increase liver function test results.

Pharmacokinetics

Absorption: Absolute bioavailability is about 15%.
Distribution: More than 99% protein-bound; doesn't penetrate RBCs.
Metabolism: Rapid and complete.
Excretion: About 33% is in urine (26% unchanged) and 67% in feces. *Half-life:* 9 hours.

Route	Onset	Peak	Duration
P.O.	Unknown	3–4 hr	24 hr

Action

Chemical effect: Blocks the angiotensin II receptor on the surface of vascular smooth muscle and other tissue cells.
Therapeutic effect: Dilates blood vessels and decreases blood pressure.

Available forms

Tablets: 4 mg, 8 mg, 16 mg, 32 mg

NURSING PROCESS

Assessment

• Monitor patient's electrolytes, and assess patient for volume or sodium depletion (as from vigorous diuretic use) before starting therapy.
• Carefully monitor therapeutic response and adverse reactions, especially in elderly patients and patients with renal or moderate liver impairment
• Assess patient's and family's knowledge of drug therapy.

Nursing diagnoses

• Decreased cardiac output related to risk for symptomatic hypotension in volume- or sodium-depleted patients

• Risk for imbalanced fluid volume in patients with impaired renal function related to drug-induced oliguria
• Deficient knowledge related to drug therapy

Planning and implementation

• Make sure patient is adequately hydrated before starting therapy.
• Assess patient for hypotension. If it occurs after a dose, place patient in supine position and, if needed, give an I.V. infusion of normal saline solution.
• Most of antihypertensive effect occurs within 2 weeks. Maximal antihypertensive effect is obtained within 4 to 6 weeks. If blood pressure isn't controlled by drug alone, add diuretic.
• Drug can't be removed by hemodialysis.

Patient teaching
• Advise woman of childbearing age about risk of second- and third-trimester exposure to drug. If pregnancy is suspected, tell her to notify prescriber immediately.
• Tell patient to report adverse reactions promptly.
• Instruct patient to take drug exactly as directed.
• Tell patient that drug may be taken with or without food.

Evaluation

• Patient's volume or sodium depletion is corrected so that symptomatic hypotension doesn't occur.
• Patient maintains fluid balance.
• Patient and family state understanding of drug therapy.

HIGH ALERT!

capecitabine
(kayp-SIGHT-a-been)
Xeloda

Pharmacologic class: fluoropyrimidine carbamate
Therapeutic class: antineoplastic
Pregnancy risk category: D

Indications and dosages

▶ **First-line therapy for metastatic colorectal cancer; Dukes C colon cancer after complete resection of primary tumor when fluoropyrimidine monotherapy is preferred; metasta-**

---

tic breast cancer resistant to combined pacli-taxel and anthracycline therapy, or to pacli-taxel after anthracycline therapy, or with do-cetaxel after anthracycline failure. *Adults:* 1,250 mg/m² P.O. within 30 minutes after morn-ing and evening meals for 2 weeks; followed by a 1-week rest period. Continue as an every-3-week cycle; adjust for toxicity and individual needs. Adjuvant treatment in patients with Dukes C colon cancer is recommended for a to-tal of 6 months.

Adjust-a-dose: For patients with renal impair-ment, if creatinine clearance is 30 to 50 ml/minute, reduce initial dose by 75% (from 1,250 mg/m² to 950 mg/m² b.i.d.); if patient develops NC1C grade 2, 3, or 4 toxicity, see manufacturer recommendations for dose re-ductions.

Contraindications and cautions

• Contraindicated in patients hypersensitive to 5-fluorouracil (5-FU) and in patients with a cre-atinine clearance less than 30 ml/minute.

Lifespan: In pregnant women, use only in life-threatening situations or severe disease for which safer drugs can't be used or are ineffec-tive. Breast-feeding should be stopped during therapy. In children, safety and effectiveness haven't been established. In patients older than age 80, use cautiously because they may have a greater risk of GI adverse effects.

Adverse reactions

CNS: dizziness, *fatigue, fever, headache,* in-somnia, mood alteration, *pain, paresthesia, pe-ripheral neuropathy,* tremor.
CV: dysrhythmias, *edema, **venous thrombosis.***
EENT: *eye irritation, increased lacrimation,* rhinorrhea, sore throat.
GI: *abdominal pain, anorexia, constipation, di-arrhea,* dyspepsia, *nausea, stomatitis,* taste dis-turbance, *vomiting.*
Hematologic: anemia, *leukopenia, lymphope-nia, neutropenia, thrombocytopenia.*
Hepatic: *hyperbilirubinemia.*
Musculoskeletal: *back pain,* limb pain, myal-gia.
Respiratory: cough, *dyspnea,* pharyngeal dis-order.
Skin: alopecia, *dermatitis, hand-foot syndrome,* nail disorder.
Other: dehydration.

Interactions

Drug-drug. *Leucovorin:* May increase 5-FU level and toxicity. Monitor patient carefully.
Phenytoin: May increase phenytoin level. Moni-tor level carefully. Consider decreased pheny-toin dose.
Warfarin: May increase risk of bleeding and death. Avoid this combination, or monitor PT and INR often and adjust warfarin dosage, if needed.
Drug-food. *Any food:* May decrease rate and extent of absorption. Give drug 30 minutes after a meal to decrease GI adverse events, but avoid excessive drug inactivation.

Effects on lab test results

• May increase bilirubin, AST, ALT, alkaline phosphatase, and hemoglobin levels and hemat-ocrit.
• May increase PT and INR. May decrease platelet, lymphocyte, and neutrophil counts.

Pharmacokinetics

Absorption: Good.
Distribution: About 60% protein-bound.
Metabolism: Extensively in the liver and tumor cells.
Excretion: 70% in urine. *Half-life:* About 45 minutes.

Route	Onset	Peak	Duration
P.O.	Unknown	1½–2 hr	Unknown

Action

Chemical effect: Interferes with DNA synthesis to inhibit cell division and with RNA processing and protein synthesis.
Therapeutic effect: Inhibits cell growth of se-lected cancers.

Available forms

Tablets: 150 mg, 500 mg

NURSING PROCESS

Assessment
• Assess patient's underlying condition before therapy and regularly thereafter.
• Assess patient for coronary artery disease, mild to moderate hepatic impairment caused by liver metastases, hyperbilirubinemia, and renal insufficiency.
• Monitor PT and INR in patients also taking warfarin because of increased risk of bleeding.

Patients older than age 60 are also at risk for co-agulopathies, even if they aren't taking warfarin.
• Monitor patient for severe diarrhea; if it occurs, notify prescriber.
• Monitor patient for hand-foot syndrome (numbness, paresthesia, tingling, painless or painful swelling, erythema, desquamation, blistering, and severe pain of hands or feet), hyperbilirubinemia, and severe nausea. If these reactions occur, adjust therapy immediately.
• Assess patient's and family's knowledge of drug therapy.

Nursing diagnoses
• Risk for infection related to adverse effects of drug
• Risk for impaired skin integrity related to potential for hand-foot syndrome
• Deficient knowledge related to drug therapy

Planning and implementation
• If diarrhea occurs and patient becomes dehydrated, give fluid and electrolyte replacement. Stop the drug immediately until diarrhea diminishes or resolves.
• If hyperbilirubinemia occurs, stop the drug.
• Monitor patient for toxicity. To manage toxicity, treat symptoms, stop the drug temporarily, and reduce the dosage.

Patient teaching
• Inform patient and family of expected adverse drug effects, especially nausea, vomiting, diarrhea, and hand-foot syndrome. Explain that dosage will be adjusted.
ALERT: Instruct patient to stop taking the drug and to contact prescriber immediately if he develops diarrhea (more than four bowel movements daily or diarrhea at night), vomiting (two to five episodes in 24 hours), nausea, appetite loss or decrease in amount of food taken each day, stomatitis (pain, redness, swelling or sores in mouth), hand-foot syndrome, fever of 100.5° F (38° C) or more, or other evidence of infection.
• Tell patient that most adverse effects improve within 2 or 3 days after stopping drug and that if they don't, he should contact prescriber.
• Tell patient how to take drug. Dosage cycle is usually to take drug for 14 days followed by 7-day rest period. Inform him how many cycles he should take.
• Instruct patient to take drug with water within 30 minutes after breakfast and after dinner.

• If a combination of tablets is prescribed, teach patient importance of correctly identifying the tablets.
• For missed doses, instruct patient not to take the missed dose and not to double the next one. Instead, he should continue with regular schedule and check with prescriber.
• Instruct patient to inform prescriber if he's taking folic acid.

Evaluation
• Patient doesn't develop infection.
• Patient doesn't develop hand-foot syndrome.
• Patient and family state understanding of drug therapy.

captopril
(KAP-toh-pril)
Capoten✦

Pharmacologic class: ACE inhibitor
Therapeutic class: antihypertensive, adjunct treatment of heart failure and diabetic nephropathy
Pregnancy risk category: C (D in second and third trimesters)

Indications and dosages
▶ **Hypertension.** *Adults:* Initially, 25 mg P.O. b.i.d. or t.i.d. If blood pressure isn't controlled in 1 to 2 weeks, increase dosage to 50 mg b.i.d. or t.i.d. If not controlled after another 1 to 2 weeks, add thiazide diuretic. If blood pressure needs to be reduced further, raise dosage as high as 150 mg t.i.d. while continuing diuretic. Maximum daily dose, 450 mg.
▶ **Heart failure.** *Adults:* 6.25 to 12.5 mg P.O. t.i.d. initially. Gradually increase to 50 to 100 mg t.i.d. as needed. Maximum daily dose, 450 mg.
▶ **Diabetic nephropathy.** *Adults:* 25 mg P.O. t.i.d.
▶ **Left ventricular dysfunction after MI.** *Adults:* 6.25 mg P.O. as a single dose 3 days after MI; then 12.5 mg t.i.d., increasing dosage to 25 mg t.i.d. Target dosage is 50 mg t.i.d.

Contraindications and cautions
• Contraindicated in patients hypersensitive to drug or other ACE inhibitors.
• Use cautiously in patients with renal impairment or serious autoimmune disease (particular-

ly systemic lupus erythematosus), and in patients exposed to other drugs known to affect WBC counts or immune response.

⚠ **Lifespan:** In pregnant women, use cautiously. If patient becomes pregnant, drug usually is stopped. In breast-feeding women, use cautiously. In children, safety and effectiveness haven't been established.

Adverse reactions

CNS: dizziness, fainting, fever.
CV: angina pectoris, *heart failure, hypotension,* pericarditis, tachycardia.
GI: anorexia, dysgeusia.
GU: membranous glomerulopathy, nephrotic syndrome, proteinuria, *renal impairment* (in patients with renal disease or those receiving high dosages), urinary frequency.
Hematologic: *agranulocytosis, leukopenia, pancytopenia, thrombocytopenia.*
Hepatic: cholestatic jaundice, elevated liver enzyme levels.
Metabolic: *hyperkalemia.*
Respiratory: cough.
Skin: maculopapular rash, pruritus, urticaria.
Other: *angioedema.*

Interactions

Drug-drug. *Antacids:* May decrease captopril effect. Separate doses.
Digoxin: May increase digoxin level by 15% to 30%. Monitor patient for digitalis toxicity.
Diuretics, other antihypertensives: May increase risk of excessive hypotension. Stop diuretic or lower captopril dosage.
Insulin, oral antidiabetics: May increase risk of hypoglycemia when captopril therapy starts. Monitor patient closely.
Lithium: May increase lithium level and cause lithium toxicity. Monitor patient closely.
NSAIDs: May reduce antihypertensive effect. Monitor blood pressure.
Potassium supplements, potassium-sparing diuretics: May increase risk of hyperkalemia. Avoid these drugs unless hypokalemic level is confirmed.
Probenecid: May increase captopril level. Avoid use together.
Drug-food. *Any food:* May reduce absorption of drug. Give drug 1 hour before meals.
Drug-herb. *Black catechu:* May have additional hypotensive effects of catechu. Discourage use together.

Capsaicin: May worsen captopril-related cough. Discourage herb use.
Licorice: May cause sodium retention, which counteracts ACE effects. Monitor blood pressure.

Effects on lab test results

● May increase alkaline phosphatase, bilirubin, and potassium levels and may cause a transient increase in hepatic enzyme levels. May decrease hemoglobin level and hematocrit.
● May decrease WBC, granulocyte, RBC, and platelet counts.

Pharmacokinetics

Absorption: Through GI tract; food may reduce absorption by up to 40%.
Distribution: Into most body tissues except CNS. 25% to 30% protein-bound.
Metabolism: About 50% in liver.
Excretion: Mainly in urine, minimally in feces.
Half-life: Less than 2 hours.

Route	Onset	Peak	Duration
P.O.	15–60 min	30–90 min	6–12 hr

Action

Chemical effect: Thought to inhibit ACE, preventing conversion of angiotensin I to angiotensin II. Reduced formation of angiotensin II decreases peripheral arterial resistance, thus decreasing aldosterone secretion.
Therapeutic effect: Reduces sodium and water retention, lowers blood pressure, and helps improve renal function adversely affected by diabetes.

Available forms

Tablets: 12.5 mg, 25 mg, 50 mg, 100 mg

NURSING PROCESS

▨ Assessment
● Assess patient's underlying condition before therapy and regularly thereafter.
● Monitor blood pressure and pulse rate often.
● Monitor WBC and differential counts before therapy, every 2 weeks for first 3 months, and periodically thereafter.
● Monitor potassium level and renal function (BUN and creatinine clearance levels, urinalysis).
● Be alert for adverse reactions and drug interactions.

- Assess patient's and family's knowledge of drug therapy.

⊕ Nursing diagnoses
- Risk for injury related to patient's underlying condition
- Ineffective protection related to drug-induced blood disorder
- Deficient knowledge related to drug therapy

▷ Planning and implementation
- If patient has persistent dry, tickling, nonproductive cough, watch closely for adverse reaction and respiratory impairment.
- Because antacids decrease drug's effect, separate doses.
- If patient develops fever, sore throat, leukopenia, hypotension, or tachycardia, withhold dose and notify prescriber.
- Notify prescriber about abnormal laboratory studies.
- ⊛ **ALERT:** Don't confuse captopril with carvedilol.

Patient teaching
- Instruct patient to take drug 1 hour before meals because food decreases drug absorption.
- Inform patient that light-headedness may occur, especially during the first few days of therapy. Tell patient to rise slowly to minimize this effect and to report symptoms to prescriber. Tell patient with syncope to stop taking drug and call prescriber immediately.
- Tell patient to use caution in hot weather and during exercise. Inadequate fluid intake, vomiting, diarrhea, and excessive perspiration can lead to light-headedness and syncope.
- Advise patient to report signs of infection, such as fever and sore throat.
- Tell woman to notify prescriber if she becomes pregnant because drug will be stopped.
- Tell patient to notify prescriber if cough interferes with sleep or required activities so that drug can be changed.

☑ Evaluation
- Patient's underlying condition improves.
- Patient's WBC and differential counts are normal.
- Patient and family state understanding of drug therapy.

carbamazepine
(kar-buh-MAH-zuh-peen)
Carbatrol, Epitol, Equetro, Novo-Carbamaz♦, Tegretol, Tegretol CR♦, Tegretol-XR

Pharmacologic class: iminostilbene derivative
Therapeutic class: anticonvulsant, analgesic
Pregnancy risk category: D

Indications and dosages

▶ **Generalized tonic-clonic and complex partial seizures, mixed seizure patterns.**
Adults and children older than age 12: Initially, 200 mg P.O. b.i.d. for tablets or 100 mg of suspension P.O. q.i.d. Increase at weekly intervals by 200 mg P.O. daily, in divided doses at 6- to 8-hour intervals. Adjust to minimum effective level when control is achieved. Maximum daily dosage, 1 g in children ages 12 to 15, or 1.2 g in patients older than age 15.
Children ages 6 to 12: Initially, 100 mg P.O. b.i.d., or 50 mg of suspension P.O. q.i.d. Increase at weekly intervals by 100 mg P.O. daily. Maximum daily dose is 1 g.
Children younger than age 6: Initially, 10 to 20 mg/kg P.O. daily in two to three divided doses (tablets) or four divided doses (suspension). Increase weekly to achieve optimal response. Maximum, 35 mg/kg/day.
▶ **Trigeminal neuralgia.** *Adults:* Initially, 100 mg P.O. b.i.d. or 50 mg of suspension P.O. q.i.d. with meals. Increase by 100 mg every 12 hours for tablets or 50 mg of suspension q.i.d. until pain is relieved. Maintenance dosage is 200 to 1,200 mg P.O. daily. Maximum daily dosage is 1,200 mg. Decrease dose to minimum effective level, or stop drug at least once every 3 months.
▶ **Restless leg syndrome‡.** *Adults:* 100 to 300 mg P.O. at bedtime.
▶ **Chorea‡.** *Children:* 15 to 25 mg/kg P.O. daily.
▶ **Acute manic and mixed episodes in bipolar 1 disorder (Equetro).** *Adults:* Initially, 200 mg P.O. b.i.d. Increase by 200 mg daily to achieve therapeutic response. Doses higher than 1,600 mg daily haven't been studied.

Contraindications and cautions

- Contraindicated in patients hypersensitive to drug or tricyclic antidepressants, in patients

with previous bone marrow suppression, and within 14 days of MAO inhibitor therapy.
• Use cautiously in patients with mixed seizure disorders because drugs may increase risk of seizures, usually atypical absence or generalized.
⚜ **Lifespan:** In pregnant women, use cautiously. If breast-feeding woman must take drug, breast-feeding should be stopped.

Adverse reactions

CNS: ataxia, dizziness, drowsiness, fatigue, fever, vertigo, *worsening of seizures* (usually in patients with mixed seizure disorders, including atypical absence seizures).
CV: aggravation of coronary artery disease, *heart failure,* hypertension, hypotension.
EENT: blurred vision, conjunctivitis, diplopia, dry mouth and pharynx, nystagmus.
GI: abdominal pain, anorexia, diarrhea, glossitis, nausea, stomatitis, vomiting.
GU: albuminuria, glycosuria, impotence, urinary frequency, urine retention.
Hematologic: *agranulocytosis, aplastic anemia,* eosinophilia, leukocytosis, *thrombocytopenia.*
Hepatic: *hepatitis.*
Respiratory: pulmonary hypersensitivity.
Skin: *erythema multiforme,* excessive sweating, rash, *Stevens-Johnson syndrome,* urticaria.
Other: chills, *water intoxication.*

Interactions

Drug-drug. *Atracurium, cisatracurium, pancuronium, rocuronium, vecuronium:* May decrease the effects of nondepolarizing muscle relaxant, causing it to be less effective. May need to increase the dose of the nondepolarizing muscle relaxant.
Charcoal: May decrease GI absorption of carbamazepine. Use only in cases of overdose to promote drug clearance.
Cimetidine, danazol, diltiazem, isoniazid, macrolides, propoxyphene, valproic acid, verapamil: May increase carbamazepine level. Use together cautiously.
Clarithromycin, erythromycin, troleandomycin: May inhibit carbamazepine metabolism, increasing the level and risk of toxicity. Avoid use together.
Doxycycline, haloperidol, hormonal contraceptives, phenytoin, theophylline, tiagabine, topiramate, valproate, warfarin: May decrease levels of these drugs. Monitor patient for decreased effect.

Lithium: May increase risk of CNS toxicity of lithium. Avoid use together.
MAO inhibitors: May increase depressant and anticholinergic effects. Don't use together.
Phenobarbital, phenytoin, primidone: May decrease carbamazepine level. Monitor patient for decreased effect.
Drug-herb. *Plantains:* Psyllium seeds may inhibit GI absorption. Discourage use together.

Effects on lab test results

• May increase BUN level. May decrease hemoglobin level and hematocrit.
• May increase eosinophil count. May decrease granulocyte, WBC, and platelet counts and thyroid and liver function test values.

Pharmacokinetics

Absorption: Slow.
Distribution: Widely throughout body; about 75% protein-bound.
Metabolism: By liver to active metabolite; may also induce its own metabolism.
Excretion: 70% in urine and 30% in feces.
Half-life: 25 to 65 hours with single dose; 8 to 29 hours with long-term use.

Route	Onset	Peak	Duration
P.O.			
extended-release	Unknown	4–8 hr	Unknown
suspension	1 hr	1½ hr	Unknown
tablets	1 hr	4–12 hr	Unknown

Action

Chemical effect: May stabilize neuronal membranes and limit seizure activity by increasing efflux or decreasing influx of sodium ions across cell membranes in motor cortex during generation of nerve impulses.
Therapeutic effect: Prevents seizure activity, eliminates pain caused by trigeminal neuralgia, and, by an unknown mechanism, treats bipolar disorder.

Available forms

Capsules (extended-release): 100 mg, 200 mg, 300 mg
Oral suspension: 100 mg/5 ml
Tablets: 100 mg, 200 mg, 300 mg, 400 mg
Tablets (chewable): 100 mg
Tablets (extended-release): 100 mg, 200 mg, 400 mg

NURSING PROCESS

🌡 Assessment
• Assess patient's seizure disorder or trigeminal neuralgia before therapy and regularly thereafter.
• Obtain baseline determinations of urinalysis, BUN level, liver function, CBC, platelet and reticulocyte counts, and iron level. Reassess regularly.
• Monitor drug level and effects closely. Therapeutic level is 4 to 12 mcg/ml.
• Be alert for adverse reactions and drug interactions.
• Assess patient's and family's knowledge of drug therapy.

💠 Nursing diagnoses
• Risk for injury related to seizure disorder
• Acute pain related to trigeminal neuralgia
• Deficient knowledge related to drug therapy

▶ Planning and implementation
⚠ ALERT: Don't confuse Tegretol or Tegretol-XR with Topamax or Toprol-XL.
• Give drug in divided doses to maintain consistent level.
• Give drug with food to minimize GI distress.
• Shake oral suspension well before measuring dose.
• Extended-release capsules may be opened and contents sprinkled over food, such as a teaspoon of applesauce.
• When giving by NG tube, mix dose with equal volume of water, normal saline solution, or D_5W. Flush tube with 100 ml of diluent after giving dose.
⚠ ALERT: When treating seizures or status epilepticus, never abruptly stop giving the drug. If adverse reactions occur, notify prescriber immediately. Increase dosage gradually to minimize adverse reactions.
Patient teaching
• Tell patient to take drug with food to minimize GI distress.
• Tell patient to keep tablets in original container, tightly closed, and away from moisture. Some formulations may harden when exposed to excess moisture, resulting in decreased bioavailability and loss of seizure control.
• Inform patient with trigeminal neuralgia that prescriber may try to decrease dosage or withdraw drug every 3 months.

⚠ ALERT: Tell patient to notify prescriber immediately about fever, sore throat, mouth ulcers, or easy bruising or bleeding.
• Warn patient that drug may cause mild-to-moderate dizziness and drowsiness at first. Advise patient to avoid hazardous activities until effects disappear (usually within 3 to 4 days).
• Advise patient to have periodic eye examinations.
• Tell patient not to crush or chew capsules or their contents.

✓ Evaluation
• Patient remains free from seizures.
• Patient reports pain relief.
• Patient and family state understanding of drug therapy.

HIGH ALERT!

carboplatin
(KAR-boh-plat-in)
Paraplatin, Paraplatin-AQ ♦

Pharmacologic class: alkylating drug
Therapeutic class: antineoplastic
Pregnancy risk category: D

Indications and dosages
▶ **Palliative therapy for ovarian cancer.**
Adults: 360 mg/m² I.V. on day 1 of a 28-day cycle; don't repeat until platelet count exceeds 100,000/mm³ and neutrophil count exceeds 2,000/mm³. Base later doses on blood counts.
⬛ Adjust-a-dose: For patients with renal impairment, if creatinine clearance is 41 to 59 ml/minute, starting dose is 250 mg/m² I.V. If creatinine clearance is 16 to 40 ml/minute, it's 200 mg/m². Recommended dosage adjustments aren't available for patients with creatinine clearance of 15 ml/minute or less.
▶ **Initial therapy for advanced ovarian cancer, with cyclophosphamide.** *Adults:* Initial dose is 300 mg/m² I.V. on day 1 of a 28-day cycle for six cycles. Don't repeat cycles until neutrophil count is 2,000/mm³ or more and platelet count is 100,000/mm³ or more.

▽ I.V. administration
• Have epinephrine, corticosteroids, and antihistamines available when giving drug because anaphylactoid reactions may occur within minutes of administration.

Reactions may be *common*, uncommon, *life-threatening*, or COMMON AND LIFE-THREATENING.

• Preparing and giving I.V. form is linked to mutagenic, teratogenic, and carcinogenic risks. Follow facility policy to reduce risks.

• Reconstitute powder for injection with D_5W, normal saline solution, or sterile water for injection to make 10 mg/ml. Add 5 ml of diluent to 50-mg vial, 15 ml of diluent to 150-mg vial, or 45 ml of diluent to 450-mg vial. Then, further dilute reconstituted powder or aqueous solution for injection with normal saline solution or D_5W before infusion. Concentrations as low as 0.5 mg/ml can be prepared.

• Give drug by continuous or intermittent infusion over at least 15 minutes.

• Don't give carboplatin with needles or I.V. administration sets that contain aluminum because drug may precipitate or lose potency.

• Store unopened vials at room temperature. Once reconstituted and diluted, drug is stable at room temperature for 8 hours. Discard unused drug at this time.

⊗ **Incompatibilities**
Amphotericin B cholesteryl sulfate complex, fluorouracil, mesna, sodium bicarbonate.

Contraindications and cautions

• Contraindicated in patients hypersensitive to cisplatin, platinum-containing compounds, or mannitol. Also contraindicated in patients with severe bone marrow suppression or bleeding.

☀ **Lifespan:** In pregnant women, drug is contraindicated. In breast-feeding women and in children, safety and effectiveness haven't been established. In patients older than age 65, use cautiously because of greater risk for neurotoxicity.

Adverse reactions

CNS: CENTRAL NEUROTOXICITY, confusion, dizziness, *peripheral neuropathy, stroke.*
CV: *embolism, heart failure.*
EENT: *ototoxicity.*
GI: constipation, diarrhea, *nausea, vomiting.*
Hematologic: anemia, *bone marrow suppression, leukopenia, neutropenia, thrombocytopenia.*
Hepatic: *hepatotoxicity.*
Skin: alopecia.
Other: hypersensitivity reactions.

Interactions

Drug-drug. *Bone marrow depressants, including radiation therapy:* May increase hematologic toxicity. Monitor hematologic studies.

Nephrotoxic drugs: May enhance nephrotoxicity of carboplatin. Monitor renal function tests.

Effects on lab test results

• May increase BUN, creatinine, bilirubin, AST, and alkaline phosphatase levels. May decrease magnesium, calcium, potassium, sodium, and hemoglobin levels and hematocrit.

• May decrease neutrophil, WBC, RBC, and platelet counts.

Pharmacokinetics

Absorption: Given I.V.
Distribution: Volume distributed is about equal to that of total body water; no significant protein binding occurs.
Metabolism: Hydrolyzed to form hydroxylated and aquated types.
Excretion: 65% by kidneys within 12 hours, 71% within 24 hours. *Half-life:* 5 hours.

Route	Onset	Peak	Duration
I.V.	Unknown	Unknown	Unknown

Action

Chemical effect: Probably produces cross-linking of DNA strands.
Therapeutic effect: Impairs ovarian cancer cell replication.

Available forms

Powder for injection: 50-mg, 150-mg, 450-mg vials
Solution for injection: 50 mg/5 ml, 150 mg/ 15 ml, 450 mg/45 ml

NURSING PROCESS

Assessment

• Assess patient's condition before therapy and regularly thereafter.

• Determine electrolyte, creatinine, and BUN levels; creatinine clearance; CBC; and platelet count before first infusion and before each course of therapy. Lowest WBC and platelet counts usually occur by day 21. They usually return to baseline by day 28.

• Be alert for adverse reactions and drug interactions.

• Assess patient's and family's knowledge of drug therapy.

Nursing diagnoses
• Ineffective health maintenance related to ovarian cancer
• Ineffective protection related to drug-induced adverse reactions
• Deficient knowledge related to drug therapy

Planning and implementation
• Check dose carefully against laboratory test results. Only increase dose once. Don't exceed 125% of starting dose in subsequent doses.
• Bone marrow suppression may be more severe in patients with creatinine clearance below 60 ml/minute. Adjust dosage in these patients.
• **ALERT:** Don't repeat dose unless platelet count exceeds 100,000/mm³ or neutrophil count exceeds 2,000/mm³.
• Provide antiemetic therapy. Carboplatin can produce severe vomiting.
• **ALERT:** Don't confuse carboplatin with cisplatin.

Patient teaching
• Warn patient to watch for evidence of infection (fever, sore throat, fatigue) and bleeding (easy bruising, nosebleed, bleeding gums, melena). Tell patient to take his temperature daily.
• Instruct patient to avoid OTC products that contain aspirin.
• Advise woman of childbearing age to avoid pregnancy during therapy and to consult prescriber before becoming pregnant.
• Advise breast-feeding patient to stop breast-feeding because of risk of toxicity to infant.

Evaluation
• Patient has positive response to carboplatin as shown by follow-up diagnostic tests.
• Patient doesn't experience injury from drug therapy.
• Patient and family state understanding of drug therapy.

carisoprodol
(kar-ih-soh-PROH-dol)
Soma

Pharmacologic class: carbamate derivative
Therapeutic class: skeletal muscle relaxant
Pregnancy risk category: C

Indications and dosages
▶ **Adjunct in acute, painful musculoskeletal conditions.** *Adults:* 350 mg P.O. t.i.d. and at bedtime.

Contraindications and cautions
• Contraindicated in patients hypersensitive to related compounds (such as meprobamate) and in patients with intermittent porphyria.
• Use cautiously in patients with hepatic or renal impairment. Prolonged use may lead to dependence; use cautiously in addiction-prone patients.
※ **Lifespan:** In pregnant or breast-feeding women and in children younger than age 12, safety and effectiveness haven't been established.

Adverse reactions
CNS: agitation, ataxia, depressive reactions, *dizziness, drowsiness,* fever, headache, insomnia, irritability, tremor, vertigo.
CV: facial flushing, orthostatic hypotension, tachycardia.
GI: epigastric distress, increased bowel activity, nausea, vomiting.
Hematologic: eosinophilia.
Respiratory: *asthmatic episodes,* hiccups.
Skin: *erythema multiforme,* pruritus, rash.
Other: *anaphylaxis, angioedema.*

Interactions
Drug-drug. *CNS depressants:* May increase CNS depression. Avoid use together.
Drug-lifestyle. *Alcohol use:* May increase CNS depression. Discourage use together.

Effects on lab test results
• May increase eosinophil count.

Pharmacokinetics
Absorption: Unknown.
Distribution: Widely throughout body.
Metabolism: In liver.
Excretion: In urine mainly as metabolites; less than 1% excreted unchanged. *Half-life:* 8 hours.

Route	Onset	Peak	Duration
P.O.	≤ 30 min	≤ 4 hr	4–6 hr

Action
Chemical effect: Appears to modify central perception of pain without modifying pain re-

flexes. Blocks interneuronal activity in descending reticular activating system and in spinal cord.

Therapeutic effect: Relieves musculoskeletal pain.

Available forms

Tablets: 350 mg

NURSING PROCESS

🔲 Assessment

• Assess patient's pain before and after giving drug.

• Monitor the drug's effectiveness by regularly assessing severity and frequency of muscle spasms.

• Be alert for adverse reactions and drug interactions.

🛇 **ALERT:** Watch for idiosyncratic reactions after first to fourth doses (weakness, ataxia, visual and speech difficulties, fever, skin eruptions, and mental changes) and for severe reactions (bronchospasm, hypotension, and anaphylaxis).

• Assess patient for history of drug addiction. Prolonged use of drug may lead to dependence.

• Assess patient's and family's knowledge of drug therapy.

🔲 Nursing diagnoses

• Acute pain related to patient's underlying condition

• Risk for injury related to drug-induced drowsiness

• Deficient knowledge related to drug therapy

▷ Planning and implementation

• Give drug with meals or milk to prevent GI distress.

• Once pain is adequately relieved, reduce dose.

• If unusual reactions occur, stop drug and notify prescriber immediately.

• Don't stop drug abruptly because mild withdrawal effects, such as insomnia, headache, nausea, and abdominal cramps, may result.

Patient teaching

• Warn patient to avoid activities that require alertness or physical dexterity, such as operating machinery or a motor vehicle, until drug's CNS effects are known.

• Advise patient not to consume alcohol or other CNS depressants.

• Advise patient to follow prescriber's orders about rest and physical therapy.

• Tell patient to take drug with meals or milk to prevent GI distress.

☑ Evaluation

• Patient reports pain has ceased.

• Patient doesn't experience injury from drug-induced CNS adverse reactions.

• Patient and family state understanding of drug.

HIGH ALERT!

carmustine (BCNU)

(kar-MUHS-teen)
BiCNU, Gliadel

Pharmacologic class: alkylating drug
Therapeutic class: antineoplastic
Pregnancy risk category: D

Indications and dosages

▶ **Hodgkin lymphoma, non-Hodgkin lymphoma, and multiple myeloma.** *Adults:* 150 to 200 mg/m² I.V. by slow infusion as single dose, repeat every 6 weeks; or 75 to 100 mg/m² I.V. by slow infusion daily for 2 days; repeat every 6 weeks. Don't repeat dose until platelet count is above 100,000/mm³ and WBC count is above 4,000/mm³.

▨ **Adjust-a-dose:** Reduce dosage by 30% when WBC count is 2,000 to 3,000/mm³ and platelet count is 25,000 to 75,000/mm³. Reduce dosage by 50% when WBC count is less than 2,000/mm³ and platelet count is less than 25,000/mm³.

▶ **Recurrent glioblastoma multiforme (adjunct to surgery); newly diagnosed high-grade malignant glioma patients (adjunct to surgery and radiation).** *Adults:* 8 wafers implanted into resection cavity as size of cavity allows.

▶ **Brain‡, breast‡, GI tract‡, lung‡, and hepatic cancer‡; malignant melanomas‡.** *Adults:* 75 to 100 mg/m² I.V. by slow infusion daily for 2 days; repeat every 6 weeks if platelet count is above 100,000/mm³ and WBC count is above 4,000/mm³.

▼ I.V. administration

• To reconstitute, dissolve 100 mg of drug in 3 ml of absolute alcohol provided by manufac-

turer. Dilute solution with 27 ml of sterile water for injection. Resulting solution contains 3.3 mg of drug/ml in 10% alcohol. Dilute in normal saline solution or D_5W for I.V. infusion.
• If powder liquefies or appears oily, discard drug because decomposition has occurred.
• Give only in glass containers. Solution is unstable in plastic I.V. bags.
• Give at least 250 ml over 1 to 2 hours. To reduce pain of infusion, dilute further or slow infusion rate.
• Avoid contact with skin because drug will cause brown stain. If drug contacts skin, wash it off thoroughly.
• Store unopened vials of the dry powder in refrigerator. After reconstitution, drug is stable for 8 hours at room temperature. Protect from light. May decompose at temperatures above 80° F (27° C).
⊗ **Incompatibilities**
Sodium bicarbonate. Don't mix with other drugs.

Contraindications and cautions

• Contraindicated in patients hypersensitive to drug.
🜲 **Lifespan:** In pregnant or breast-feeding women, drug is contraindicated. In children, safety and effectiveness haven't been established.

Adverse reactions

CNS: ataxia, *brain edema,* drowsiness, *seizures.*
CV: facial flushing.
EENT: ocular toxicities.
GI: anorexia, diarrhea, dysphagia, esophagitis, nausea, vomiting.
GU: *nephrotoxicity,* renal impairment.
Hematologic: *acute leukemia or bone marrow dysplasia* (may occur after long-term use), *cumulative bone marrow suppression* (delayed 4 to 6 weeks, lasting 1 to 2 weeks), *leukopenia, thrombocytopenia.*
Hepatic: *hepatotoxicity.*
Metabolic: hyperuricemia (in lymphoma patients with rapid cell lysis).
Respiratory: *pulmonary fibrosis.*
Skin: hyperpigmentation (if drug contacts skin).
Other: *intense pain* (at infusion site from venous spasm).

Interactions

Drug-drug. *Anticoagulants, aspirin, NSAIDs:* May increase risk of bleeding. Avoid use together.
Cimetidine: May increase carmustine's bone marrow toxicity. Avoid use together.
Digoxin, phenytoin: May reduce levels of these drugs. Use together cautiously; monitor levels.
Mitomycin: May increase corneal and conjunctival damage with high doses. Monitor patient.
Myelosuppressives: May increase risk of myelosuppression. Monitor patient's CBC periodically.

Effects on lab test results

• May increase urine urea, AST, bilirubin, and alkaline phosphatase levels. May decrease hemoglobin level and hematocrit.
• May decrease WBC and platelet counts.

Pharmacokinetics

Absorption: Given I.V.
Distribution: Rapidly into CSF.
Metabolism: Extensively in liver.
Excretion: 60% to 70% in urine within 96 hours, 6% to 10% as carbon dioxide by lungs, and 1% in feces. *Half-life:* 15 to 30 minutes.

Route	Onset	Peak	Duration
I.V., wafer	Unknown	Unknown	Unknown

Action

Chemical effect: Inhibits enzymatic reactions involved with DNA synthesis, cross-links strands of cellular DNA, and interferes with RNA transcription, causing growth imbalance that leads to cell death.
Therapeutic effect: Kills selected cancer cells.

Available forms

Injection: 100-mg vial (lyophilized), with 3-ml vial of absolute alcohol supplied as diluent
Wafer: 7.7 mg

NURSING PROCESS

🔏 **Assessment**
• Assess patient's neoplastic disorder before therapy and regularly thereafter.
• Obtain baseline pulmonary function tests before starting therapy because pulmonary toxicity appears to be dose related. Evaluate results of

liver, renal, and pulmonary function tests periodically thereafter.
• Monitor CBC and uric acid levels.
• Be alert for adverse reactions and drug interactions.
• Assess patient's and family's knowledge of drug therapy.

Nursing diagnoses
• Ineffective health maintenance related to neoplastic disease
• Risk for injury related to drug-induced adverse reactions
• Deficient knowledge related to drug therapy

▶ Planning and implementation
• Preparing and giving drug has carcinogenic, mutagenic, and teratogenic risks. Follow facility policy to reduce risks.
• To reduce nausea, give antiemetic before giving drug.
• Unopened foil packs containing wafers are stable at room temperature for 6 hours. Store below –4° F (–20° C).
• If handling wafer in operating room, use double gloves.
• Allopurinol may be used with adequate hydration to prevent hyperuricemia and uric acid nephropathy.

Patient teaching
• Warn patient to watch for signs of infection (fever, sore throat, fatigue) and bleeding (easy bruising, nosebleed, bleeding gums, melena). Tell patient to take temperature daily.
• Instruct patient to avoid OTC products containing aspirin.
• Advise breast-feeding women to stop breast-feeding because of toxicity to infant.
• Advise women of childbearing age to avoid pregnancy during therapy and to consult prescriber before becoming pregnant.

✓ Evaluation
• Patient shows positive response to drug therapy as shown by follow-up diagnostic studies.
• Patient doesn't experience injury from drug-induced adverse reactions.
• Patient and family state understanding of drug therapy.

carvedilol
(kar-VAY-deh-lol)
Coreg, Coreg CR

Pharmacologic class: alpha$_1$ and beta blocker
Therapeutic class: antihypertensive, adjunct treatment for heart failure
Pregnancy risk category: C

Indications and dosages

▶ **Hypertension.** *Adults:* Dosage highly individualized. Initially, 6.25 mg P.O. b.i.d. with food. Obtain a standing blood pressure 1 hour after initial dose. If tolerated, continue dosage for 7 to 14 days. May increase to 12.5 mg P.O. b.i.d. for 7 to 14 days, monitor blood pressure as above. Maximum dosage, 25 mg P.O. b.i.d. as tolerated.

▶ **Mild to severe heart failure.** *Adults:* Individualize and adjust dosage carefully. Initially, 3.125 mg P.O. b.i.d. with food for 2 weeks; if tolerated, increase to 6.25 mg P.O. b.i.d. Double dose every 2 weeks as tolerated. At start of new dose, observe patient for dizziness or light-headedness for 1 hour. Maximum dosage for patients weighing less than 85 kg (187 lb) is 25 mg P.O. b.i.d.; for those weighing more than 85 kg, maximum dosage is 50 mg P.O. b.i.d.

▶ **Left ventricular dysfunction after MI.** *Adults:* Individualize dosage. Start therapy after patient is hemodynamically stable and fluid retention has been minimized. Initially, 6.25 mg P.O. b.i.d. with food. Increase after 3 to 10 days to 12.5 mg b.i.d., then again to a target dose of 25 mg b.i.d. Or, start with 3.25 mg b.i.d. May adjust dosage more slowly. Monitor blood pressure; observe patient for light-headedness with each dosage change.

⚠ Adjust-a-dose: In patients with pulse rate below 55 beats/minute, reduce dosage.
For patients switching to extended-release from, use the following table:

Daily dose, immediate-release	Daily dose, extended-release
6.25 mg	10 mg
12.5 mg	20 mg
25 mg	40 mg
50 mg	80 mg

Contraindications and cautions

• Contraindicated in patients hypersensitive to drug and in those with New York Heart Association class IV decompensated heart failure requiring I.V. inotropic therapy, bronchial asthma or related bronchospastic conditions, second- or third-degree AV block, sick sinus syndrome (unless a permanent pacemaker is in place), cardiogenic shock, or severe bradycardia.

• Drug isn't recommended for patients with symptomatic hepatic impairment.

• Use cautiously in hypertensive patients with left ventricular failure, perioperative patients who receive anesthetics that depress myocardial function, patients with diabetes who receive insulin or oral antidiabetics, and patients subject to spontaneous hypoglycemia. Also use cautiously in patients with thyroid disease, pheochromocytoma, Prinzmetal variant angina, bronchospastic disease, or peripheral vascular disease.

⚠ **Lifespan:** In pregnant women, use only if benefits outweigh risks to the fetus. Women should stop breast-feeding during therapy. In children, safety and effectiveness haven't been established. In elderly patients, drug levels are about 50% higher than in other adults. Monitor these patients closely.

Adverse reactions

CNS: asthenia, depression, *dizziness,* fatigue, fever, headache, hypesthesia, insomnia, pain, paresthesia, somnolence, **stroke,** syncope, vertigo.

CV: angina pectoris, *AV block, bradycardia,* edema, fluid overload, hypertension, *hypotension,* hypovolemia, orthostatic hypotension, palpitations, peripheral edema, peripheral vascular disorder.

EENT: abnormal vision, blurred vision, pharyngitis, rhinitis, sinusitis.

GI: abdominal pain, *diarrhea,* dyspepsia, melena, nausea, periodontitis, vomiting.

GU: abnormal renal function, albuminuria, hematuria, impotence, UTI.

Hematologic: anemia, purpura, *thrombocytopenia.*

Metabolic: diabetes mellitus, glycosuria, gout, hypercholesterolemia, *hyperglycemia,* **hyperkalemia,** hypertriglyceridemia, hyperuricemia, hypervolemia, *hypoglycemia,* hyponatremia, *weight gain,* weight loss.

Musculoskeletal: arthralgia, arthritis, back pain, hypotonia, muscle cramps.

Respiratory: bronchitis, cough, crackles, dyspnea, *lung edema, upper respiratory tract infection.*

Other: flulike symptoms, hypersensitivity reactions, infection, injury, viral infection.

Interactions

Drug-drug. *Calcium channel blockers:* May cause isolated conduction disturbances. Monitor patient's heart rhythm and blood pressure.

Catecholamine-depleting drugs (such as MAO inhibitors, reserpine): May cause bradycardia or severe hypotension. Monitor patient closely.

Cimetidine: May increase bioavailability of carvedilol. Monitor vital signs carefully.

Clonidine: May increase blood pressure and heart rate-lowering effects. Monitor vital signs closely.

Digoxin: May increase digoxin level by about 15% during therapy. Monitor digoxin level and vital signs carefully.

Fluoxetine, paroxetine, propafenone, quinidine: May increase level of R (+) enantiomer of carvedilol. Monitor patient for hypotension and dizziness.

Insulin, oral antidiabetics: May enhance hypoglycemic properties. Monitor glucose level.

Rifampin: May reduce level of carvedilol by 70%. Monitor vital signs closely.

Drug-food. *Any food:* Delays carvedilol absorption but doesn't alter extent of bioavailability. Advise patient to take drug with food to minimize orthostatic effects.

Effects on lab test results

• May increase creatinine, BUN, ALT, AST, GGT, cholesterol, triglyceride, alkaline phosphatase, sodium, uric acid, potassium, and nonprotein nitrogen levels. May increase or decrease glucose level.

• May decrease PT, INR, and platelet counts.

Pharmacokinetics

Absorption: Rapidly and extensively with absolute bioavailability of 25% to 35% because of significant first-pass metabolism.

Distribution: Extensively into extravascular tissues. About 98% protein-bound.

Metabolism: Mainly by aromatic ring oxidation and glucuronidation.

Excretion: Metabolites are excreted mainly via bile in feces. Less than 2% excreted unchanged in urine. *Half-life:* 7 to 10 hours.

Route	Onset	Peak	Duration
P.O.	Unknown	1–2 hr	7–10 hr

Action

Chemical effect: Causes significant reductions in systemic blood pressure, pulmonary arterial pressure, pulmonary capillary wedge pressure, and heart rate.
Therapeutic effect: Lowers blood pressure and heart rate.

Available forms

Tablets: 3.125 mg, 6.25 mg, 12.5 mg, 25 mg
Tablets (extended-release): 10 mg, 20 mg, 40 mg, 80 mg

NURSING PROCESS

🔖 Assessment

• Monitor patient for decreased PT and increased alkaline phosphatase, BUN, ALT, and AST levels.
• Assess patient with heart failure for worsened condition, renal impairment, or fluid retention; add or increase diuretics p.r.n.
• Monitor patient with diabetes closely because drug may mask signs of hypoglycemia or worsen hyperglycemia.
• Monitor elderly patients carefully because drug level is about 50% higher in elderly patients than in younger patients.
• Observe patient for dizziness or lightheadedness for 1 hour after each dosage change.
• Assess patient's and family's knowledge of drug therapy.

⊕ Nursing diagnoses

• Ineffective health maintenance related to underlying disorder
• Ineffective cerebral tissue perfusion secondary to therapeutic action of drug
• Deficient knowledge related to drug therapy

⟫ Planning and implementation

• Before therapy begins, stabilize dose of digoxin, diuretics, and ACE inhibitors.
⚠ ALERT: Patient taking a beta blocker who has a history of anaphylactic reaction to several allergens may be more reactive to repeated chal-

lenges (accidental, diagnostic, or therapeutic). Such a patient may be unresponsive to the doses of epinephrine typically used to treat allergic reactions.
• Give drug with food to reduce risk of orthostatic hypotension.
• If pulse drops below 55 beats/minute, notify prescriber and reduce the dose.
⚠ ALERT: Don't confuse carvedilol with captopril or carteolol.

Patient teaching

• Tell patient not to interrupt or stop taking the drug without medical approval. Drug should be withdrawn gradually over 1 to 2 weeks.
• Advise patient with heart failure to call prescriber about weight gain or shortness of breath.
• Inform patient that he may develop low blood pressure when standing. If he's dizzy or faint, advise him to sit or lie down.
• Warn patient not to drive or perform hazardous tasks until the drug's CNS effects are known.
• Tell patient to notify prescriber about dizziness or faintness. Dose may need to be adjusted.
• Advise patient with diabetes to promptly report changes in glucose level.
• Inform patient who wears contact lenses that decreased lacrimation may occur.

✓ Evaluation

• Patient responds well to therapy.
• Patient doesn't experience dizziness or lightheadedness.
• Patient and family state understanding of drug therapy.

caspofungin acetate

(kas-poh-FUN-jin AS-ih-tayt)
Cancidas

Pharmacologic class: echinocandin
Therapeutic class: antifungal
Pregnancy risk category: C

Indications and dosages

▶ **Invasive aspergillosis in patients refractory to or intolerant of other drugs, such as amphotericin B, lipid formulations of amphotericin B, itraconazole.** *Adults:* A single 70-mg loading dose I.V. on day 1, followed by 50 mg daily. Duration of therapy based on severity of

patient's underlying disease, recovery from immunosuppression, and response.

▶ **Candidemia and *Candida* infections including intra-abdominal abscesses, peritonitis, and pleural space infections.** *Adults:* Give a single 70-mg loading dose I.V. on day 1, followed by 50 mg daily thereafter. Duration of therapy is based on response. In general, continue antifungal therapy for at least 14 days after the last positive culture. Patients with persistent neutropenia may warrant a longer course of therapy while neutropenia resolves.

▶ **Esophageal candidiasis.** *Adults:* 50 mg I.V. daily. Because of the risk of relapse of oropharyngeal candidiasis in patients with HIV infections, suppressive oral therapy could be considered.

▶ **Empirical therapy for presumed fungal infections in febrile, neutropenic patients.** *Adults:* A single 70-mg loading dose I.V. on day 1, followed by 50 mg daily thereafter. Duration of therapy based on response. Continue empirical therapy until neutropenia resolves. Treat patients found to have a fungal infection for a minimum of 14 days; continue treatment for at least 7 days after both neutropenia and clinical symptoms are resolved. If the 50-mg dose is well tolerated but doesn't provide an adequate response, increase the daily dose to 70 mg.

❑ **Adjust-a-dose:** For patients with moderate hepatic impairment and a Child-Pugh score of 7 to 9, give 35 mg daily after initial 70-mg loading dose.

▼ I.V. administration

• Let refrigerated vial warm to room temperature before diluting.
• Dilute all doses (70 mg, 50 mg, 35 mg) in 250 ml of normal saline solution. In patients with fluid restrictions, dilute 50-mg and 35-mg doses in 100 ml of normal saline solution.
• Give by slow I.V. infusion over about 1 hour; don't give by I.V. bolus injection.
• Use reconstituted vials within 1 hour or discard.
• Diluted solutions may be stored at 77° F (25° C) for up to 24 hours, or at 36° F to 46° F (2° C to 8° C) for 48 hours.
⊗ **Incompatibilities**
Dextrose solutions, other I.V. drugs.

Contraindications and cautions

• Contraindicated in patients hypersensitive to the drug or any of its components.
⚕ **Lifespan:** In pregnant women, use only when potential benefits to the mother outweigh risks to the fetus. In breast-feeding women, use cautiously because it isn't known whether drug appears in breast milk. In children, safety and effectiveness haven't been established.

Adverse reactions

CNS: *chills, fever, headache,* paresthesia.
CV: peripheral edema, *phlebitis,* swelling, tachycardia, *thrombophlebitis.*
GI: abdominal pain, anorexia, diarrhea, nausea, vomiting.
GU: hematuria, proteinuria.
Hematologic: anemia, eosinophilia.
Hepatic: hepatic dysfunction.
Metabolic: hypercalcemia.
Musculoskeletal: myalgia, pain.
Respiratory: *tachypnea.*
Skin: *anaphylaxis,* histamine-mediated symptoms (rash, facial swelling, phlebitis, pruritus, sensation of warmth, erythema, sweating), *infusion site complication.*

Interactions

Drug-drug. *Carbamazepine, dexamethasone, efavirenz, nelfinavir, nevirapine, phenytoin, rifampin:* May decrease caspofungin level. Consider increasing caspofungin dosage to 70 mg daily if patient doesn't respond to lower dosage.
Cyclosporine: May significantly increase AST and ALT levels and bioavailability of caspofungin. Avoid using together unless potential benefit outweighs risk.
Tacrolimus: May decrease tacrolimus level. Monitor tacrolimus level, and adjust dosage accordingly.

Effects on lab test results

• May increase ALT, AST, alkaline phosphatase, bilirubin, creatinine, and urine protein levels. May decrease potassium, magnesium, and hemoglobin levels and hematocrit.
• May increase eosinophil and urine RBC counts.

Pharmacokinetics

Absorption: Rapid into plasma; slower into tissue.

Reactions may be *common,* uncommon, *life-threatening,* or COMMON AND LIFE-THREATENING.

Distribution: 97% bound to albumin.
Metabolism: Slowly in the tissues and liver.
Excretion: 35% of drug and metabolites in feces and 41% in urine. *Half-life:* 9 to 11 hours.

Route	Onset	Peak	Duration
I.V.	Immediate	Unknown	36–48 hr

Action

Chemical effect: Inhibits synthesis of beta (1, 3)-D-glucan, an integral component of the cell walls of susceptible filamentous fungi that isn't found in mammal cells.
Therapeutic effect: Prevents fungi formation.

Available forms

Lyophilized powder for injection: 50-mg, 70-mg single-use vials

NURSING PROCESS

🔲 Assessment
• Assess patient's hepatic function before starting therapy.
• Observe patient for histamine-mediated reactions (rash, facial swelling, pruritus, sensation of warmth, sweating).
• Monitor I.V. site carefully for phlebitis.
• Monitor patient's liver function test results carefully during therapy.
• Assess patient's and family's knowledge of drug therapy.

🔲 Nursing diagnoses
• Risk for infection and impaired skin integrity related to adverse effects of I.V. drug administration
• Ineffective health maintenance related to underlying disease process and immunocompromised state
• Deficient knowledge related to drug therapy

🔲 Planning and implementation
• An increase in dose to 70 mg daily hasn't been studied but may be well tolerated.
• A long course of therapy hasn't been studied but may be well tolerated.
• Adjust dose in a patient with moderate hepatic insufficiency.
Patient teaching
• Instruct patient to report signs and symptoms of phlebitis.

• Tell patient to report any adverse events during drug therapy.

☑ Evaluation
• Patient has no adverse reactions during drug therapy.
• Patient responds positively to antifungal drug therapy.
• Patient and family state understanding of drug therapy.

cefadroxil monohydrate
(seh-fuh-DROKS-il mon-oh-HIGH-drayt)
Duricef

Pharmacologic class: first-generation cephalosporin
Therapeutic class: antibiotic
Pregnancy risk category: B

Indications and dosages

▶ **UTI caused by** *Escherichia coli, Proteus mirabilis,* **and** *Klebsiella;* **skin and soft-tissue infections; and streptococcal pharyngitis.**
Adults: 1 to 2 g P.O. daily, depending on infection treated, usually as a single dose or in two divided doses.
Children: 30 mg/kg P.O. daily in two divided doses. Course of therapy is usually at least 10 days.
🔲 **Adjust-a-dose:** For adults with renal impairment, give initial dosage of 1 g P.O. daily. Reduce maintenance dosage as follows: If creatinine clearance is 25 to 50 ml/minute, give 500 mg every 12 hours. If creatinine clearance is 10 to 25 ml/minute, give 500 mg every 24 hours. If creatinine clearance is less than 10 ml/minute, give 500 mg every 36 hours.

Contraindications and cautions

• Contraindicated in patients hypersensitive to drug or other cephalosporins.
• Use cautiously in patients with renal impairment or a history of sensitivity to penicillin.
🔲 **Lifespan:** In pregnant or breast-feeding women, use cautiously.

Adverse reactions

CNS: dizziness, headache, malaise, paresthesia, *seizures.*

GI: abdominal cramps, anal pruritus, anorexia, diarrhea, dyspepsia, glossitis, oral candidiasis, *pseudomembranous colitis,* nausea, tenesmus, vomiting.
GU: candidiasis, genital pruritus.
Hematologic: *agranulocytosis,* anemia, eosinophilia, *leukopenia, thrombocytopenia, transient neutropenia.*
Respiratory: dyspnea.
Skin: erythematous and maculopapular rashes.
Other: hypersensitivity reactions (serum sickness, *anaphylaxis*).

Interactions

Drug-drug. *Probenecid:* May inhibit excretion and increase level of cefadroxil. Monitor patient.

Effects on lab test results

- May increase ALT, AST, alkaline phosphatase, bilirubin, GGT, and LDH levels. May decrease hemoglobin level and hematocrit.
- May increase eosinophil count. May decrease neutrophil, WBC, granulocyte, and platelet counts.
- About 40% to 75% of patients receiving cephalosporins show false-positive direct Coombs tests.
- May cause false-positive urine glucose determinations with copper sulfate tests (Clinitest).

Pharmacokinetics

Absorption: Rapid and complete.
Distribution: Wide. CSF penetration is poor. 20% protein-bound.
Metabolism: None.
Excretion: Mainly unchanged in urine. *Half-life:* About 1 to 2 hours.

Route	Onset	Peak	Duration
P.O.	Unknown	1–2 hr	6–9 hr

Action

Chemical effect: Inhibits cell-wall synthesis, promoting osmotic instability; usually bactericidal.
Therapeutic effect: Hinders or kills susceptible bacteria.

Available forms

Capsules: 500 mg
Oral suspension: 125 mg/5 ml, 250 mg/5 ml, 500 mg/5 ml
Tablets: 1 g

NURSING PROCESS

Assessment
- Assess patient's infection before therapy and regularly thereafter.
- Before giving first dose, obtain specimen for culture and sensitivity tests. Begin therapy pending test results.
- Be alert for adverse reactions and drug interactions.
- If adverse GI reactions occur, monitor patient's hydration.
- Assess patient's and family's knowledge of drug therapy.

Nursing diagnoses
- Ineffective protection related to bacteria susceptible to drug
- Risk for deficient fluid volume related to drug-induced adverse GI reactions
- Deficient knowledge related to drug therapy

Planning and implementation
- Drug's half-life permits once- or twice-daily use.
- If creatinine clearance is less than 50 ml/minute, expect prescriber to lengthen dosage interval to prevent drug accumulation.
- Store reconstituted suspension in refrigerator. Keep container tightly closed and shake well before using.
- **ALERT:** Don't confuse with other cephalosporins with similar-sounding names.

Patient teaching
- Tell patient to take drug exactly as prescribed, even after he feels better.
- Advise patient to take drug with food or milk to lessen GI discomfort.
- Tell patient to call prescriber if rash develops.
- Inform patient using oral suspension to shake it well before using and to refrigerate mixture in tightly closed container.

Evaluation
- Patient is free from infection.
- Patient maintains adequate hydration.
- Patient and family state understanding of drug therapy.

Reactions may be *common,* uncommon, *life-threatening*, or COMMON AND LIFE-THREATENING.

cefazolin sodium
(sef-EH-zoh-lin SOH-dee-um)

Pharmacologic class: first-generation cephalosporin
Therapeutic class: antibiotic
Pregnancy risk category: B

Indications and dosages

▶ **Serious infections of respiratory, biliary, and GU tracts; skin, soft-tissue, bone, and joint infections; septicemia; endocarditis caused by** *Escherichia coli, Enterobacteriaceae gonococci, Haemophilus influenzae, Klebsiella, Proteus mirabilis, Staphylococcus aureus, Streptococcus pneumoniae,* **and group A beta-hemolytic streptococci.** *Adults:* 250 mg I.V. or I.M. every 8 hours to 1 g every 6 hours. Maximum, 12 g daily in life-threatening situations.
Children and infants older than 1 month: 25 to 100 mg/kg daily I.V. or I.M. in three or four divided doses.
▶ **Perioperative prophylaxis in contaminated surgery.** *Adults:* 1 g I.V. or I.M. 30 to 60 minutes before surgery; then 0.5 to 1 g I.V. or I.M. every 6 to 8 hours for 24 hours. In operations lasting longer than 2 hours, another 0.5- to 1-g dose may be given intraoperatively. In cases where infection would be devastating, prophylaxis may continue for 3 to 5 days.
🔲 **Adjust-a-dose:** For patients with renal impairment, after initial dose, adjust dosage as follows. If creatinine clearance is 35 to 54 ml/minute, give full dose every 8 hours; if clearance is 11 to 34 ml/minute, give 50% of usual dose every 12 hours; if clearance is less than 10 ml/minute, give 50% of usual dose every 18 to 24 hours.

▼ I.V. administration

• Reconstitute with sterile water, bacteriostatic water, or normal saline solution as follows: 2 ml to 500-mg vial to yield 225 mg/ml; or 2.5 ml to 1-g vial to yield 330 mg/ml. Shake well until dissolved.
• For direct injection, further dilute with 5 ml of sterile water. Inject into large vein or into tubing of free-flowing I.V. solution over 3 to 5 minutes. For intermittent infusion, add reconstituted drug to 50 to 100 ml of compatible solution or use premixed solution. Give premixed frozen solutions of drug in D_5W only by intermittent or continuous I.V. infusion.
• If I.V. therapy lasts longer than 3 days, alternate injection sites. Use of small I.V. needles in larger veins may be preferable.
• Reconstituted drug is stable for 24 hours at room temperature and 96 hours if refrigerated.
⊗ **Incompatibilities**
Aminoglycosides, amiodarone, amobarbital, ascorbic acid injection, bleomycin, calcium gluconate, cimetidine, colistimethate, hydrocortisone, idarubicin, lidocaine, norepinephrine, oxytetracycline, pentobarbital sodium, polymyxin B, ranitidine, tetracycline, theophylline, vitamin B complex with C.

Contraindications and cautions

• Contraindicated in patients hypersensitive to other cephalosporins.
• Use cautiously in patients with a history of sensitivity to penicillin because of cross-allergic reaction, and in patients with renal impairment.
🕊 **Lifespan:** In pregnant and breast-feeding women, use cautiously.

Adverse reactions

CNS: dizziness, headache, malaise, paresthesia.
GI: abdominal cramps, anal pruritus, anorexia, *diarrhea,* dyspepsia, glossitis, nausea, oral candidiasis, *pseudomembranous colitis,* vomiting, tenesmus.
GU: genital pruritus and candidiasis, vaginitis.
Hematologic: anemia, eosinophilia, *leukopenia, thrombocytopenia, transient neutropenia.*
Respiratory: dyspnea.
Skin: injection site reactions (pain, induration, abscess, tissue sloughing), *maculopapular and erythematous rashes, Stevens-Johnson syndrome, urticaria.*
Other: hypersensitivity reactions (*anaphylaxis,* serum sickness).

Interactions

Drug-drug. *Probenecid:* May inhibit excretion and increase level of cefazolin. Monitor patient.

Effects on lab test results

• May increase ALT, AST, alkaline phosphatase, bilirubin, GGT, and LDH levels.
• May increase eosinophil count. May decrease neutrophil, WBC, and platelet counts.

• May cause false-positive urine glucose determinations with copper sulfate tests (Clinitest).

Pharmacokinetics
Absorption: Unknown after I.M. use.
Distribution: Wide. CSF penetration is poor. 74% to 86% protein-bound.
Metabolism: None.
Excretion: Mainly in urine. *Half-life:* About 1 to 2 hours.

Route	Onset	Peak	Duration
I.V.	Immediate	Immediate	Unknown
I.M.	Unknown	1–2 hr	Unknown

Action
Chemical effect: Inhibits cell-wall synthesis, promoting osmotic instability; usually bactericidal.
Therapeutic effect: Hinders or kills susceptible bacteria.

Available forms
Infusion: 500 mg/50 ml, 1 g/50 ml
Powder for injection: 500 mg, 1 g

NURSING PROCESS

🔲 Assessment
• Assess patient's infection before therapy and regularly thereafter.
• Before giving first dose, obtain specimen for culture and sensitivity tests. Begin therapy pending test results.
• Before giving first dose, ask patient about previous reactions to cephalosporins or penicillin.
• If adverse GI reactions occur, monitor patient's hydration.
• Assess patient's and family's knowledge of drug therapy.

🔷 Nursing diagnoses
• Ineffective protection related to bacteria susceptible to drug
• Risk for deficient fluid volume related to drug-induced adverse GI reactions
• Deficient knowledge related to drug therapy

▷ Planning and implementation
• Because of long duration of effect, most infections can be treated with every-8-hour use.
• After reconstitution, inject I.M. drug without further dilution (not as painful as other cephalo-

sporins). Inject deep into large muscle mass, such as gluteus maximus or lateral aspect of thigh.
⚠ **ALERT:** Don't confuse with other cephalosporins with similar-sounding names.
Patient teaching
• Tell patient to report adverse reactions.

✅ Evaluation
• Patient is free from infection.
• Patient maintains adequate hydration.
• Patient and family state understanding of drug therapy.

cefdinir
(SEF-dih-neer)
Omnicef

Pharmacologic class: third-generation cephalosporin
Therapeutic class: antibiotic
Pregnancy risk category: B

Indications and dosages
▶ **Mild to moderate infections caused by susceptible strains of microorganisms for conditions of community-acquired pneumonia and uncomplicated skin and skin-structure infections.** *Adults and children older than age 12:* Give 300 mg P.O. every 12 hours for 10 days. *Children ages 6 months to 12 years:* For uncomplicated skin and skin-structure infections, 7 mg/kg P.O. every 12 hours for 10 days; maximum daily dosage, 600 mg.
▶ **Acute maxillary sinusitis.** *Adults and children older than age 12:* Give 300 mg P.O. every 12 hours for 10 days or 600 mg P.O. every 24 hours for 10 days.
Children ages 6 months to 12 years: 7 mg/kg P.O. every 12 hours for 10 days or 14 mg/kg P.O. every 24 hours for 10 days, up to a maximum dose of 600 mg daily.
▶ **Pharyngitis; tonsillitis; acute exacerbations of chronic bronchitis; acute bacterial otitis media.** *Adults and children older than age 12:* Give 300 mg P.O. every 12 hours for 5 to 10 days or 600 mg P.O. every 24 hours for 10 days.
Children ages 6 months to 12 years: 7 mg/kg P.O. every 12 hours for 5 to 10 days or 14 mg/

kg P.O. every 24 hours for 10 days, up to a maximum dosage of 600 mg daily.

Adjust-a-dose: For patients with renal impairment, if creatinine clearance is less than 30 ml/minute, reduce adult dosage to 300 mg P.O. once daily; for children, reduce to 7 mg/kg up to 300 mg P.O. once daily. In patients receiving long-term hemodialysis, dosage is 300 mg or 7 mg/kg P.O. at end of each dialysis session and subsequently every other day.

Contraindications and cautions

• Contraindicated in patients hypersensitive to cephalosporins.
• Use cautiously in patients hypersensitive to penicillin because of risk of cross-sensitivity with other beta-lactam antibiotics. Also use cautiously in patients with history of colitis or renal impairment.
☀ Lifespan: In breast-feeding women, use cautiously. In children younger than age 6 months, safety and effectiveness haven't been established.

Adverse reactions

CNS: headache.
GI: abdominal pain, *diarrhea,* nausea, vomiting.
GU: vaginal candidiasis, vaginitis.
Skin: rash.

Interactions

Drug-drug. *Antacids containing aluminum or magnesium, iron supplements, multivitamins containing iron:* May decrease cefdinir's absorption and bioavailability. Give such preparations 2 hours before or after cefdinir dose.
Probenecid: May inhibit the renal excretion of cefdinir. Monitor patient.

Effects on lab test results

• May increase GGT, alkaline phosphatase, and urine protein levels.
• May increase RBC count.

Pharmacokinetics

Absorption: Bioavailability of drug is about 21% after 300-mg capsule dose, 16% after 600-mg capsule dose, and 25% for suspension.
Distribution: 60% to 70% protein-bound.
Metabolism: Not appreciably metabolized; activity results mainly from parent drug.

Excretion: Mainly by renal excretion. *Half-life:* 1¾ hours.

Route	Onset	Peak	Duration
P.O.	Unknown	2–4 hr	Unknown

Action

Chemical effect: Kills bacteria by inhibiting cell-wall synthesis.
Therapeutic effect: Is stable in the presence of some beta-lactamase enzymes, causing some microorganisms resistant to penicillins and cephalosporins to be susceptible to this drug.

Available forms

Capsules: 300 mg
Suspension: 125 mg/5 ml, 250 mg/5 ml

NURSING PROCESS

Assessment
• Before giving first dose, obtain specimen for culture and sensitivity tests. Begin therapy pending test results.
• Before giving first dose, ask patient about previous reactions to cephalosporins or penicillin.
• Monitor patient for symptoms of superinfection.
• Assess patient with diarrhea carefully because pseudomembranous colitis has been reported with drug.
• Assess patient's and family's knowledge of drug therapy.

Nursing diagnoses
• Ineffective protection related to susceptible bacteria
• Risk for deficient fluid volume related to drug-induced adverse GI reactions
• Deficient knowledge related to drug therapy

Planning and implementation
• If allergic reaction is suspected, notify prescriber; stop drug and give emergency care.
⚠ ALERT: Don't confuse with other cephalosporins with similar-sounding names.
Patient teaching
• If patient takes an antacid or iron supplement, instruct him to take it 2 hours before or after cefdinir.
• Inform patient with diabetes that each teaspoon of suspension contains 2.86 g of sucrose.

• Tell patient that drug may be taken with or without food.
• Advise patient to report severe diarrhea or diarrhea accompanied by abdominal pain.
• Tell patient to promptly report adverse reactions or symptoms of superinfection.

☑ Evaluation
• Patient is free from infection.
• Patient maintains adequate hydration.
• Patient and family state understanding of drug therapy.

cefditoren pivoxil
(sef-da-TOR-en pa-VOX-ill)
Spectracef

Pharmacologic class: semisynthetic third-generation cephalosporin
Therapeutic class: antibiotic
Pregnancy risk category: B

Indications and dosages

▶ **Acute bacterial exacerbation of chronic bronchitis or community-acquired pneumonia caused by** *Haemophilus influenzae,* *Haemophilus parainfluenzae, Streptococcus pneumoniae* **(penicillin-susceptible strains only), or** *Moraxella catarrhalis. Adults and children age 12 and older:* 400 mg P.O. b.i.d. with meals for 10 days if treating bronchitis, and 14 days if treating pneumonia.
▶ **Pharyngitis, tonsillitis, and uncomplicated skin and skin-structure infections caused by** *Streptococcus pyogenes. Adults and children age 12 and older:* 200 mg P.O. b.i.d. with meals for 10 days.
Adjust-a-dose: For patients with renal impairment, if creatinine clearance is 30 to 49 ml/minute, don't give more than 200 mg b.i.d. If creatinine clearance is less than 30 ml/minute, give 200 mg daily.

Contraindications and cautions

• Contraindicated in patients hypersensitive to drug, other cephalosporins, and penicillins. Also contraindicated in patients with carnitine deficiency or inborn errors of metabolism that may result in significant carnitine deficiency. Because tablets contain sodium caseinate, a milk protein, don't give them to patients hypersensitive to milk protein (distinct from those with lactose intolerance).
• Use cautiously in patients with renal impairment. Drug is dialyzable.
• Not recommended for prolonged antibiotic therapy.
⚞ Lifespan: In breast-feeding women, use cautiously because cephalosporins appear in breast milk. In children younger than age 12, safety and effectiveness haven't been established.

Adverse reactions

CNS: headache.
GI: abdominal pain, *colitis, diarrhea,* dyspepsia, hepatic dysfunction (including cholestasis), nausea, vomiting.
GU: hematuria, **nephrotoxicity,** vaginal candidiasis.
Hematologic: anemia.
Metabolic: hyperglycemia.
Skin: *Stevens-Johnson syndrome, toxic epidermal necrolysis.*
Other: *hypersensitivity reactions* (including serum sickness, rash, fever, *anaphylaxis*).

Interactions

Drug-drug. *Aluminum antacids, H_2-receptor antagonists, magnesium:* May reduce cefditoren absorption. Avoid use together. If used together, separate doses.
Oral anticoagulants: May increase bleeding time. Monitor PT and patient closely for unusual bleeding or bruising.
Probenecid: May increase cefditoren level. Avoid use together.
Drug-food. *Moderate- to high-fat meals:* May increase drug bioavailability. Advise patient to take drug with meals.

Effects on lab test results

• May increase liver enzyme levels. May decrease carnitine and hemoglobin levels and hematocrit.
• May decrease PT.
• May cause a false-positive direct Coombs test result and false-positive reaction for glucose in urine using copper reduction tests (those involving Benedict's solution, Fehling's solution, or Clinitest tablets).

Pharmacokinetics

Absorption: From the GI tract and hydrolyzed by esterases to cefditoren.
Distribution: Wide; based on volume of distribution. CSF penetration is unknown. About 88% protein-bound.
Metabolism: Not appreciably metabolized.
Excretion: Unchanged mainly in urine by glomerular filtration and tubular secretion. *Half-life:* 1½ to 2 hours in patients with normal renal function.

Route	Onset	Peak	Duration
P.O.	Unknown	1½–3 hr	Unknown

Action

Chemical effect: Mainly bactericidal. Drug acts by adhering to bacterial penicillin-binding proteins, thereby inhibiting cell-wall synthesis. Active against many gram-positive and gram-negative organisms.
Therapeutic effect: Kills susceptible bacteria.

Available forms

Tablets: 200 mg

NURSING PROCESS

Assessment

• Assess patient's history for hypersensitivity to cefditoren, cephalosporins, penicillins, or other contraindications for drug therapy.
• Monitor patient for overgrowth or recurrence of resistant organisms with prolonged or repeated drug therapy.
• Because cefditoren has been linked to *Clostridium difficile*–related colitis, monitor patient for diarrhea during therapy.
• Monitor patient for hypersensitivity reactions during therapy, as well as for any unusual bleeding or bruising.
• Assess patient's and family's knowledge of drug therapy.

Nursing diagnoses

• Noncompliance related to completion of 10-day antibiotic regimen
• Risk for infection with nonsusceptible bacteria or fungi related to prolonged or repeated drug therapy
• Deficient knowledge related to cephalosporin therapy

Planning and implementation

• Give drug with a meal to increase its bioavailability.
• If patient develops diarrhea after receiving cefditoren, keep in mind that this drug may cause pseudomembranous colitis. Notify prescriber immediately because colitis may be fatal.
• If patient needs prolonged therapy, use a different drug.
• Signs and symptoms of overdose may include nausea, vomiting, epigastric distress, diarrhea, and seizures. Treat symptoms and provide supportive therapy.
• If hypersensitivity or allergic reaction occurs, stop drug and provide emergency care.
⊛ **ALERT:** Don't confuse drug with other cephalosporins with similar-sounding names.

Patient teaching

• Instruct patient to take drug with food to increase its absorption.
• Caution patient not to take drug with an H_2 antagonist or an antacid because it may reduce cefditoren absorption. If an H_2 antagonist or antacid must be used, instruct the patient to take it 2 hours before or after cefditoren.
• Explain to patient the importance of taking drug for the prescribed duration, despite feeling better, to prevent any future drug resistance.
• Instruct patient to immediately stop taking drug and call prescriber if any adverse reactions develop, such as rash, hives, difficulty breathing, unusual bleeding or bruising, or diarrhea.
• Encourage patient to contact prescriber if signs and symptoms of infection don't improve after several days of therapy.
• Urge patient not to miss any doses. However, if patient misses a dose, instruct him to take the missed dose as soon as he remembers and to wait 12 hours before taking the next dose. Tell him not to double the dose.

Evaluation

• Patient completes prescribed 10-day therapy.
• Patient doesn't experience any adverse reactions during drug therapy.
• Patient and family state understanding of drug therapy and importance of completing entire drug regimen as prescribed.

cefixime

(sef-IKS-eem)
Suprax

Pharmacologic class: third-generation cephalosporin
Therapeutic class: antibiotic
Pregnancy risk category: B

Indications and dosages

▶ **Uncomplicated UTIs caused by** *Escherichia coli* **and** *Proteus mirabilis;* **otitis media caused by** *Haemophilus influenzae* **(beta-lactamase–positive and –negative strains),** *Moraxella catarrhalis,* **and** *Streptococcus pyogenes;* **pharyngitis and tonsillitis caused by** *S. pyogenes;* **acute bronchitis and acute exacerbations of chronic bronchitis caused by** *Streptococcus pneumoniae* **and** *H. influenzae* **(beta-lactamase–positive and –negative strains).**
Adults and children older than age 12 weighing more than 50 kg (110 lb): 400 mg P.O. daily or 200 mg every 12 hours.
Children age 6 months to 12 years: 8 mg/kg P.O. daily in one or two divided doses.
▶ **Uncomplicated gonorrhea caused by** *Neisseria gonorrhoeae. Adults:* 400 mg P.O. as single dose.
▶ **Disseminated gonococcal infections‡.**
Adults: 400 mg P.O. b.i.d. after initial therapy with I.M. or I.V. antibiotics for a total of 7 days of therapy.
⬧ Adjust-a dose: For patients with creatinine clearance of 21 to 60 ml/minute or who are receiving hemodialysis, give 75% of standard dose. For patients with creatinine clearance of 20 ml/minute or less, or who are receiving continuous ambulatory peritoneal dialysis, give 50% of standard dose.

Contraindications and cautions

• Contraindicated in patients hypersensitive to drug, other cephalosporins, or beta-lactam antibiotics.
• Use cautiously in patients with renal dysfunction or history of sensitivity to penicillin.
⚜ Lifespan: Use cautiously in pregnant or breast-feeding women.

Adverse reactions

CNS: dizziness, fatigue, headache, insomnia, malaise, nervousness, somnolence.
GI: abdominal pain, *diarrhea,* dyspepsia, flatulence, loose stools, nausea, *pseudomembranous colitis,* vomiting.
GU: genital candidiasis, genital pruritus, vaginitis.
Hematologic: eosinophilia, *leukopenia, thrombocytopenia.*
Hepatic: *hepatitis,* jaundice.
Skin: pruritus, rash, *Stevens-Johnson syndrome,* urticaria.
Other: drug fever, *hypersensitivity reactions* (serum sickness, *anaphylaxis*).

Interactions

Drug-drug. *Nifedipine:* May increase cefixime level. Avoid use together.
Probenecid: May inhibit excretion and increase level of cefixime. Monitor patient.
Salicylates: May displace cefixime from protein-binding sites. Significance is unknown.

Effects on lab test results

• May increase BUN, creatinine, ALT, AST, alkaline phosphatase, bilirubin, GGT, and LDH levels.
• May increase eosinophil count. May decrease platelet and WBC counts.
• May cause false-positive results in urine glucose tests that use copper sulfate (Clinitest).

Pharmacokinetics

Absorption: Good.
Distribution: Wide. Enters CSF in patients with inflamed meninges. 65% protein-bound.
Metabolism: 50% of drug.
Excretion: Mainly in urine. *Half-life:* 3 to 4 hours.

Route	Onset	Peak	Duration
P.O.	Unknown	2–6 hr	Unknown

Action

Chemical effect: Inhibits cell-wall synthesis, promoting osmotic instability; usually bactericidal.
Therapeutic effect: Hinders or kills bacteria, including *H. influenzae, M. catarrhalis, S. pyogenes, S. pneumoniae, E. coli,* and *P. mirabilis.*

Reactions may be *common,* uncommon, *life-threatening,* or **COMMON AND LIFE-THREATENING.**

Available forms

Oral suspension: 100 mg/5 ml (after reconstitution), 200 mg/5 ml (after reconstitution)

NURSING PROCESS

�� Assessment
• Assess patient's infection before therapy and regularly thereafter.
• Before giving first dose, obtain specimen for culture and sensitivity tests. Begin therapy pending test results.
• Before giving first dose, ask patient about previous reactions to cephalosporins or penicillin.
• Be alert for adverse reactions and drug interactions.
• If adverse GI reactions occur, monitor patient's hydration.
• Assess patient's and family's knowledge of drug therapy.

�� Nursing diagnoses
• Ineffective protection related to bacteria susceptible to drug
• Risk for deficient fluid volume related to drug-induced adverse GI reactions
• Deficient knowledge related to drug therapy

�� Planning and implementation
• To prepare oral suspension, add required amount of water to powder in two portions. Shake well after each addition. After mixing, suspension is stable for 14 days (no need to refrigerate). Keep tightly closed. Shake well before using.
� **ALERT:** Don't confuse with other cephalosporins with similar-sounding names.
Patient teaching
• Tell patient to take drug exactly as prescribed, even after he feels better.
• Tell patient to call prescriber if rash develops.
• Teach patient how to store drug.

�� Evaluation
• Patient is free from infection.
• Patient maintains adequate hydration.
• Patient and family state understanding of drug therapy.

---

cefotaxime sodium
(sef-oh-TAKS-eem SOH-dee-um)
Claforan

Pharmacologic class: third-generation cephalosporin
Therapeutic class: antibiotic
Pregnancy risk category: B

Indications and dosages

▶ **Perioperative prophylaxis in contaminated surgery.** *Adults:* 1 g I.V. or I.M. 30 to 90 minutes before surgery. In patients undergoing cesarean birth, give dose as soon as umbilical cord is clamped, followed by 1 g I.V. or I.M. 6 and 12 hours later.
▶ **Gonococcal urethritis or cervicitis; rectal gonorrhea in women or girls:** 0.5 g I.M. as a single dose.
▶ **Rectal gonorrhea.** *Men and boys:* 1 g I.M. as a single dose.
▶ **Serious infections of lower respiratory and urinary tracts, CNS, skin, bone, and joints; gynecologic and intra-abdominal infections; bacteremia; and septicemia.** Susceptible microorganisms include streptococci (including *Streptococcus pneumoniae* and *Streptococcus pyogenes*), *Staphylococcus aureus* (penicillinase- and non–penicillinase-producing), *Staphylococcus epidermidis, Escherichia coli, Klebsiella, Haemophilus influenzae, Enterobacter, Proteus,* and *Peptostreptococcus.*
Pelvic inflammatory disease‡. *Adults:* Usual dosage is 1 g I.V. or I.M. every 6 to 12 hours. Up to 12 g daily can be given in life-threatening infections.
Children weighing at least 50 kg (110 lb): Usual adult dose but don't exceed 12 g daily.
Children ages 1 month to 12 years weighing less than 50 kg: Give 50 to 180 mg/kg I.V. or I.M. daily in four to six divided doses.
Neonates ages 1 to 4 weeks: Give 50 mg/kg I.V. every 8 hours.
Neonates up to age 1 week: Give 50 mg/kg I.V. every 12 hours.
▶ **Disseminated gonococcal infection‡.**
Adults: 1 g I.V. every 8 hours.
Neonates and infants: 25 to 50 mg/kg I.V. every 8 to 12 hours for 7 days, or 50 to 100 mg/kg I.M or I.V. every 12 hours for 7 days.

▶ **Gonococcal ophthalmia‡.** *Adults:* 500 mg I.V. q.i.d.
Neonates: 100 mg I.V. or I.M. for one dose; may continue until ocular cultures are negative at 48 to 72 hours.

▶ **Gonorrheal meningitis or arthritis‡.**
Neonates and infants: 25 to 50 mg/kg I.V. every 8 to 12 hours for 10 to 14 days. Or 50 to 100 mg/kg I.M. or I.V. every 12 hours for 10 to 14 days.

▧ **Adjust-a-dose:** For patients with renal impairment, if creatinine clearance is less than 20 ml/minute, give half the usual dose at the usual interval.

▼ I.V. administration

• Reconstitute infusion vials with 50 to 100 ml D_5W or normal saline solution.
• For direct injection, reconstitute 500-mg, 1-g, or 2-g vials with 10-ml sterile water for injection. Solutions containing 1 g/14 ml are isotonic.
• Inject drug into large vein or into tubing of free-flowing I.V. solution over 3 to 5 minutes.
• Infuse drug over 20 to 30 minutes. Interrupt flow of primary I.V. solution during infusion.
⊗ **Incompatibilities**
Allopurinol, aminoglycosides, aminophylline, azithromycin, doxapram, filgrastim, fluconazole, hetastarch, pentamidine isethionate, sodium bicarbonate injection, vancomycin.

Contraindications and cautions

• Contraindicated in patients hypersensitive to drug or other cephalosporins.
• Use cautiously in patients with history of sensitivity to penicillin and in patients with renal impairment.
⚖ **Lifespan:** In pregnant or breast-feeding women, use cautiously.

Adverse reactions

CNS: dizziness, fever, headache, malaise, paresthesia.
GI: abdominal cramps, anal pruritus, anorexia, *diarrhea,* dyspepsia, glossitis, nausea, oral candidiasis, *pseudomembranous colitis,* tenesmus, vomiting.
GU: candidiasis, pruritus.
Hematologic: *agranulocytosis,* eosinophilia, hemolytic anemia, *thrombocytopenia, transient neutropenia.*
Respiratory: dyspnea.

Skin: maculopapular and erythematous rashes, urticaria.
Other: hypersensitivity reactions (serum sickness, *anaphylaxis*); pain, induration, sterile abscesses, warmth, tissue sloughing at injection site; phlebitis, thrombophlebitis with I.V. injection.

Interactions

Drug-drug. *Aminoglycosides:* May increase risk of nephrotoxicity. Monitor renal function closely.
Probenecid: May inhibit excretion and increase level of cefotaxime. Use together cautiously.

Effects on lab test results

• May increase ALT, AST, alkaline phosphatase, bilirubin, GGT, and LDH levels. May decrease hemoglobin level and hematocrit.
• May increase eosinophil count. May decrease neutrophil, platelet, and granulocyte counts.
• May cause false-positive urine glucose determinations with copper sulfate tests (Clinitest).

Pharmacokinetics

Absorption: Unknown after I.M. use.
Distribution: Wide. Adequate CSF penetration when meninges are inflamed. 13% to 38% protein-bound.
Metabolism: Partially to active metabolite.
Excretion: Mainly in urine. *Half-life:* 1 to 2 hours.

Route	Onset	Peak	Duration
I.V.	Immediate	Immediate	8–12 hr
I.M.	Unknown	30 min	8–12 hr

Action

Chemical effect: Inhibits cell-wall synthesis, promoting osmotic instability; usually bactericidal.
Therapeutic effect: Hinders or kills susceptible bacteria.

Available forms

Infusion: 1 g, 2 g
Injection: 500 mg, 1 g, 2 g

NURSING PROCESS

▨ **Assessment**
• Assess patient's infection before therapy and regularly thereafter.

Reactions may be *common,* uncommon, *life-threatening*, or COMMON AND LIFE-THREATENING.

• Before giving first dose, obtain specimen for culture and sensitivity tests. Begin therapy pending test results.
• Before giving first dose, ask patient about previous reactions to cephalosporins or penicillin.
• Be alert for adverse reactions and drug interactions.
• If adverse GI reactions occur, monitor patient's hydration.
• Assess patient's and family's knowledge of drug therapy.

✦ Nursing diagnoses
• Ineffective protection related to bacteria susceptible to drug
• Risk for deficient fluid volume related to drug-induced adverse GI reactions
• Deficient knowledge related to drug therapy

▶ Planning and implementation
• For I.M. use, inject deep into large muscle mass, such as gluteus maximus or lateral aspect of thigh.
⚡ **ALERT:** Don't confuse with other cephalosporins with similar-sounding names.
Patient teaching
• Tell patient to report adverse reactions.
• Teach patient to report decrease in urinary output. May have to decrease total daily dose.

✅ Evaluation
• Patient is free from infection.
• Patient maintains adequate hydration.
• Patient and family state understanding of drug therapy.

cefoxitin sodium
(sef-OKS-ih-tin SOH-dee-um)
Mefoxin

Pharmacologic class: second-generation cephalosporin
Therapeutic class: antibiotic
Pregnancy risk category: B

Indications and dosages

▶ **Serious infections of respiratory and GU tracts; skin, soft-tissue, bone, and joint infections; bloodstream and intra-abdominal infections caused by susceptible *Escherichia coli* and other coliform bacteria, *Staphylococ-***

cus aureus **(penicillinase- and non–penicillinase-producing),** *Staphylococcus epidermidis,* **streptococci,** *Klebsiella, Haemophilus influenzae,* **and** *Bacteroides,* **including** *B. fragilis;* **and perioperative prophylaxis.** *Adults:* 1 to 2 g I.V. every 6 to 8 hours for uncomplicated forms of infection. In life-threatening infections, up to 12 g daily.
Children and infants age 3 months and older: 80 to 160 mg/kg I.V. daily in four to six equally divided doses. Maximum daily dose is 12 g.
▶ **Prophylactic use in surgery.** *Adults:* 2 g I.V. 30 to 60 minutes before surgery; then 2 g I.V. every 6 hours for 24 hours. If used in cesarean birth give 2 g I.V. as soon as cord is clamped. Or, if a three-dose regimen is used, give 2 g I.V. as soon as cord is clamped, then 2 g I.V. 4 and 8 hours after first dose.
Children older than age 3 months: 30 to 40 mg/kg I.V. 30 to 60 minutes before surgery; then 30 to 40 mg/kg every 6 hours for 24 hours.
📎 **Adjust-a-dose:** For patients with renal impairment, if creatinine clearance is 30 to 50 ml/minute, give 1 to 2 g every 8 to 12 hours; if clearance is 10 to 29 ml/minute, give 1 to 2 g every 12 to 24 hours; and if clearance is 5 to 10 ml/minute, give 500 mg to 1 g every 12 to 24 hours. If clearance is less than 5 ml/minute, give 500 mg to 1 g every 24 to 48 hours. For hemodialysis patients, give loading dose of 1 to 2 g after each session, and maintenance dose as indicated above.

▽ I.V. administration
• Reconstitute 1 g with at least 10 ml of sterile water for injection and 2 g with 10 to 20 ml of sterile water for injection. Solutions of D_5W and normal saline solution for injection also can be used.
• For direct injection, inject reconstituted drug into large vein or into tubing of free-flowing I.V. solution over 3 to 5 minutes.
• For intermittent infusion, add reconstituted drug to 50 or 100 ml D_5W, $D_{10}W$, or normal saline solution for injection. Interrupt flow of primary I.V. solution during infusion.
• Assess I.V. site often for thrombophlebitis.
• After reconstitution, drug may be stored for 24 hours at room temperature or refrigerated for 1 week.
⊗ **Incompatibilities**
Aminoglycosides, filgrastim, hetastarch, pentamidine isethionate, ranitidine.

Contraindications and cautions

- Contraindicated in patients hypersensitive to drug or other cephalosporins.
- Use cautiously in patients with history of sensitivity to penicillin and in patients with renal impairment.

⚠ **Lifespan:** In pregnant or breast-feeding women, use cautiously.

Adverse reactions

CNS: fever.
CV: hypotension, *phlebitis, thrombophlebitis* with I.V. injection.
GI: *diarrhea, pseudomembranous colitis.*
GU: *acute renal failure.*
Hematologic: eosinophilia, hemolytic anemia, *thrombocytopenia, transient neutropenia.*
Respiratory: dyspnea.
Skin: *erythematous and maculopapular rashes, urticaria.*
Other: hypersensitivity reactions (*anaphylaxis,* serum sickness).

Interactions

Drug-drug. *Nephrotoxic drugs:* May increase risk of nephrotoxicity. Monitor renal function closely.
Probenecid: May inhibit excretion and increase level of cefoxitin. Sometimes used for this effect.

Effects on lab test results

- May increase ALT, AST, alkaline phosphatase, bilirubin, and LDH levels. May decrease hemoglobin level and hematocrit.
- May increase eosinophil count. May decrease neutrophil and platelet counts.
- May cause false-positive urine glucose determinations with copper sulfate tests (Clinitest).

Pharmacokinetics

Absorption: Unknown.
Distribution: Wide. CSF penetration is poor. 50% to 80% protein-bound.
Metabolism: Insignificant, about 2%.
Excretion: Mainly in urine. *Half-life:* About ½ to 1 hour.

Route	Onset	Peak	Duration
I.V.	Immediate	Immediate	Unknown

Action

Chemical effect: Inhibits cell-wall synthesis, promoting osmotic instability; usually bactericidal.
Therapeutic effect: Hinders or kills susceptible bacteria.

Available forms

Infusion: 1 g, 2 g
Injection: 1 g, 2 g

NURSING PROCESS

⚗ Assessment

- Assess patient's infection before therapy and regularly thereafter.
- Before giving first dose, obtain specimen for culture and sensitivity tests. Begin therapy pending test results.
- Before giving first dose, ask patient about previous reactions to cephalosporins or penicillin.
- Be alert for adverse reactions and drug interactions.
- If adverse GI reactions occur, monitor patient's hydration.
- Assess patient's and family's knowledge of drug therapy.

⊕ Nursing diagnoses

- Ineffective protection related to bacteria susceptible to drug
- Risk for deficient fluid volume related to drug-induced adverse GI reactions
- Deficient knowledge related to drug therapy

▶ Planning and implementation

- Patients with renal impairment need dosage adjustment.

⊛ **ALERT:** Don't confuse with other cephalosporins with similar-sounding names.

Patient teaching
- Tell patient to report adverse reactions and signs and symptoms of superinfection promptly.
- Instruct patient to notify prescriber if he has loose stools or diarrhea.

✓ Evaluation

- Patient is free from infection.
- Patient maintains adequate hydration.
- Patient and family state understanding of drug therapy.

cefpodoxime proxetil
(sef-poh-DOKS-eem PROKS-eh-til)
Vantin

Pharmacologic class: third-generation cephalosporin
Therapeutic class: antibiotic
Pregnancy risk category: B

Indications and dosages

▶ **Acute, community-acquired pneumonia caused by non–beta-lactamase–producing strains of *Haemophilus influenzae* or *Streptococcus pneumoniae*.** *Adults and children age 12 and older:* 200 mg P.O. every 12 hours for 14 days.

▶ **Acute bacterial exacerbation of chronic bronchitis caused by *S. pneumoniae, H. influenzae* (non–beta-lactamase–producing strains), or *Moraxella catarrhalis*.** *Adults and children age 12 and older:* 200 mg P.O. every 12 hours for 10 days.

▶ **Uncomplicated gonorrhea in men and women; rectal gonococcal infections in women.** *Adults and children age 12 and older:* 200 mg P.O. as single dose. Follow with doxycycline 100 mg P.O. b.i.d. for 7 days.

▶ **Uncomplicated skin and skin-structure infections caused by *Staphylococcus aureus* or *Streptococcus pyogenes*.** *Adults and children age 12 and older:* 400 mg P.O. every 12 hours for 7 to 14 days.

▶ **Acute otitis media caused by *S. pneumoniae, H. influenzae*, or *M. catarrhalis*.** *Children ages 2 months to 12 years:* 5 mg/kg (not to exceed 200 mg) P.O. every 12 hours for 5 days.

▶ **Pharyngitis or tonsillitis caused by *S. pyogenes*.** *Adults and children age 12 and older:* 100 mg P.O. every 12 hours for 5 to 10 days. *Children ages 2 months to 12 years:* 5 mg/kg (not to exceed 100 mg) P.O. every 12 hours for 10 days.

▶ **Uncomplicated UTIs caused by *Escherichia coli, Klebsiella pneumoniae, Proteus mirabilis*, or *Staphylococcus saprophyticus*.** *Adults and children age 12 and older:* 100 mg P.O. every 12 hours for 7 days.

▶ **Mild to moderate acute maxillary sinusitis caused by *H. influenzae, S. pneumoniae*, or *M. catarrhalis*.** *Adults and children age 12 and older:* 200 mg P.O. every 12 hours for 10 days.

Children ages 2 months to 12 years: 5 mg/kg P.O. every 12 hours for 10 days; maximum dosage is 200 mg.

⚠ **Adjust-a-dose:** For patients with renal impairment, if creatinine clearance is less than 30 ml/minute, increase dosage interval to every 24 hours. For patients undergoing dialysis, give dose three times weekly, after dialysis.

Contraindications and cautions

• Contraindicated in patients hypersensitive to drug or other cephalosporins.
• Use cautiously in patients with history of hypersensitivity to penicillin (risk of cross-sensitivity) and in patients receiving nephrotoxic drugs (other cephalosporins have had nephrotoxic potential).
⚠ **Lifespan:** In pregnant or breast-feeding women, use cautiously.

Adverse reactions

CNS: headache.
GI: abdominal pain, *diarrhea*, nausea, vomiting.
GU: vaginal fungal infections.
Skin: rash.
Other: hypersensitivity reactions *(anaphylaxis)*.

Interactions

Drug-drug. *Antacids, H$_2$-receptor antagonists:* May decrease cefpodoxime absorption. Avoid use together.
Probenecid: May decrease cefpodoxime excretion. Monitor patient for toxicity.
Drug-food. *Any food:* May increase absorption of tablets. Give tablet form with food. Oral suspension isn't affected by food.

Effects on lab test results

• May increase BUN, creatinine, AST, ALT, GGT, alkaline phosphatase, bilirubin, and LDH levels. May decrease albumin, potassium, sodium, and hemoglobin levels and hematocrit. May increase or decrease glucose level.
• May increase eosinophil, WBC, granulocyte, lymphocyte, basophil, and platelet counts. May prolong PT and PTT.
• May cause false-positive urine glucose determinations with copper sulfate tests (Clinitest). May cause positive Coombs' test.

Pharmacokinetics

Absorption: From GI tract.
Distribution: Widely into most body tissues and fluids except CSF.
Metabolism: Drug is de-esterified to its active metabolite, cefpodoxime.
Excretion: Mainly in urine. *Half-life:* 2 to 3 hours.

Route	Onset	Peak	Duration
P.O.	Unknown	2–3 hr	Unknown

Action

Chemical effect: Inhibits cell-wall synthesis, promoting osmotic instability; usually bactericidal.
Therapeutic effect: Hinders or kills susceptible bacteria.

Available forms

Oral suspension: 50 mg/5 ml, 100 mg/5 ml in 100-ml bottles
Tablets (film-coated): 100 mg, 200 mg

NURSING PROCESS

⚡ Assessment
• Assess patient's infection before therapy and regularly thereafter.
• Before giving first dose, obtain specimen for culture and sensitivity tests. Begin therapy pending test results.
• Before giving first dose, ask patient about previous reactions to cephalosporins or penicillin.
• Be alert for adverse reactions and drug interactions.
• If adverse GI reactions occur, monitor patient's hydration.
• Assess patient's and family's knowledge of drug therapy.

⊕ Nursing diagnoses
• Ineffective protection related to bacteria susceptible to drug
• Risk for deficient fluid volume related to drug-induced adverse GI reactions
• Deficient knowledge related to drug therapy

▶ Planning and implementation
• Give tablets with food to minimize adverse GI reactions and increase absorption.
• Oral suspension may be given without regard to food; shake well before using.

• Store suspension in refrigerator (36° to 46° F [2° to 8° C]). Discard unused portion after 14 days.
• Ⓢ **ALERT:** Don't confuse with other cephalosporins with similar-sounding names.

Patient teaching
• Advise patient to take tablets with meals to minimize GI adverse effects. Tell patient that oral suspension may be given without regard to food.
• Tell patient to take drug exactly as prescribed, even after he feels better.
• Instruct patient to notify prescriber if rash develops.
• Teach patient how to store drug.
• Instruct patient to notify prescriber about a reduction in urinary output, especially if patient takes a diuretic.

✓ Evaluation
• Patient is free from infection.
• Patient maintains adequate hydration.
• Patient and family state understanding of drug therapy.

cefprozil
(SEF-pruh-zil)
Cefzil

Pharmacologic class: second-generation cephalosporin
Therapeutic class: antibiotic
Pregnancy risk category: B

Indications and dosages

▶ **Pharyngitis or tonsillitis caused by *Streptococcus pyogenes*.** *Adults and children older than age 12:* Give 500 mg P.O. daily for 10 days. *Children ages 2 to 12:* Give 7.5 mg/kg P.O. every 12 hours for 10 days.
▶ **Otitis media caused by *Streptococcus pneumoniae*, *Haemophilus influenzae*, or *Moraxella catarrhalis*.** *Infants and children ages 6 months to 12 years:* 15 mg/kg P.O. every 12 hours for 10 days.
▶ **Secondary bacterial infections of acute bronchitis and acute bacterial exacerbation of chronic bronchitis caused by *S. pneumoniae*, *H. influenzae*, and *M. catarrhalis*.** *Adults and children older than age 12:* Give 500 mg P.O. every 12 hours for 10 days.

▶ **Uncomplicated skin and skin-structure infections caused by *Staphylococcus aureus* or *S. pyogenes*.** *Adults and children older than age 12:* Give 250 mg P.O. b.i.d., or 500 mg daily to b.i.d. for 10 days.
Children ages 2 to 12: Give 20 mg/kg P.O. every 24 hours for 10 days. Maximum dose is 1 g P.O. daily.

▶ **Acute sinusitis caused by *S. pneumoniae*, *H. influenzae*, and *M. catarrhalis*.** *Adults and children older than age 12:* Give 250 mg or 500 mg P.O. every 12 hours for 10 days.
Children ages 6 months to 12 years: 7.5 mg/kg P.O. every 12 hours or 15 mg/kg P.O. daily for 10 days.

Adjust-a-dose: For patients with renal impairment, if creatinine clearance is less than 30 ml/minute, give 50% of usual dose.

Contraindications and cautions

• Contraindicated in patients hypersensitive to drug or other cephalosporins.
• Use cautiously in patients with history of sensitivity to penicillin and patients with hepatic or renal impairment.
Lifespan: In pregnant and breast-feeding women, use cautiously. Don't give children more than the recommended adult dose.

Adverse reactions

CNS: dizziness, headache, hyperactivity, insomnia, nervousness.
GI: abdominal pain, diarrhea, *nausea,* vomiting.
GU: genital pruritus, vaginitis.
Hematologic: eosinophilia.
Skin: rash, urticaria.
Other: *hypersensitivity reactions (**anaphylaxis,** serum sickness),* superinfection.

Interactions

Drug-drug. *Aminoglycosides:* May increase risk of nephrotoxicity. Monitor patient closely.
Probenecid: May inhibit excretion and increase level of cefprozil. Monitor patient.

Effects on lab test results

• May increase BUN, creatinine, ALT, AST, alkaline phosphatase, bilirubin, and LDH levels.
• May increase eosinophil count. May decrease WBC, leukocyte, and platelet counts.
• May cause false-positive results in urine glucose tests that use copper sulfate (Clinitest).

Pharmacokinetics

Absorption: About 95% from GI tract.
Distribution: About 35% protein-bound. Distributed into various body tissues and fluids.
Metabolism: Probably by the liver.
Excretion: Mainly in urine. *Half-life:* 1¼ hours in patients with normal renal function; 2 hours in patients with impaired hepatic function; and 5¼ to 6 hours in patients with end-stage renal disease.

Route	Onset	Peak	Duration
P.O.	Unknown	Unknown	Unknown

Action

Chemical effect: Inhibits cell-wall synthesis, promoting osmotic instability; usually bactericidal.
Therapeutic effect: Hinders or kills susceptible bacteria.

Available forms

Oral suspension: 125 mg/5 ml, 250 mg/5 ml
Tablets: 250 mg, 500 mg

NURSING PROCESS

Assessment
• Assess patient's infection before therapy and regularly thereafter.
• Before giving first dose, obtain specimen for culture and sensitivity tests. Begin therapy pending test results.
• Before giving first dose, ask patient about previous reactions to cephalosporins or penicillin.
• Be alert for adverse reactions and drug interactions.
• If adverse GI reactions occur, monitor patient's hydration.
• Monitor patient's renal function.
• Assess patient's and family's knowledge of drug therapy.

Nursing diagnoses
• Ineffective protection related to bacteria susceptible to drug
• Risk for deficient fluid volume related to drug-induced adverse GI reactions
• Deficient knowledge related to drug therapy

Planning and implementation
• Give drug after hemodialysis is completed because procedure removes drug.

• Refrigerate reconstituted suspension (stable for 14 days). Keep tightly closed, and shake well before using.

⑤ ALERT: Don't confuse with other cephalosporins with similar-sounding names.

Patient teaching
• Tell patient to shake suspension well before measuring dose.
• Advise patient to take drug as prescribed, even after he feels better.
• Inform patient that oral suspensions are bubble-gum flavor to improve palatability and promote compliance in children. Tell him to refrigerate reconstituted suspension and to discard any unused portion after 14 days.
• Advise elderly patients also receiving diuretic therapy to notify prescriber of decreased urine output.

☑ Evaluation
• Patient is free from infection.
• Patient maintains adequate hydration.
• Patient and family state understanding of drug therapy.

ceftazidime
(sef-TAZ-ih-deem)
Ceptaz, Fortaz, Tazicef, Tazidime

Pharmacologic class: third-generation cephalosporin
Therapeutic class: antibiotic
Pregnancy risk category: B

Indications and dosages

▶ **Serious infections of lower respiratory and urinary tracts; gynecologic, intra-abdominal, CNS, and skin infections; bacteremia; and septicemia. Among susceptible microorganisms are streptococci (including *Streptococcus pneumoniae* and *Streptococcus pyogenes*), *Staphylococcus aureus, Escherichia coli, Klebsiella, Proteus, Enterobacter, Haemophilus influenzae, Pseudomonas,* and some strains of *Bacteroides*.** *Adults and children older than age 12:* Give 1 g I.V. or I.M. every 8 to 12 hours; maximum 6 g daily for life-threatening infections.
Children ages 1 month to 12 years: 30 to 50 mg/kg I.V. every 8 hours. Maximum 6 g daily.

Neonates age 4 weeks or younger: 30 mg/kg I.V. every 12 hours.
▶ **Uncomplicated UTI.** *Adults:* 250 mg I.V. or I.M. every 12 hours.
▶ **Complicated UTI.** *Adults:* 500 mg I.V. or I.M. every 8 to 12 hours.
▶ **Uncomplicated pneumonia or mild skin and skin-structure infection.** *Adults:* 0.5 to 1 g I.V. or I.M. every 8 hours.
▶ **Bone and joint infection.** *Adults:* 2 g I.V. every 12 hours.
▶ **Empiric therapy in febrile neutropenic patients‡.** *Adults:* 100 mg/kg I.V. daily in three divided doses; or 2 g I.V. every 8 hours either alone or with an aminoglycoside, such as amikacin.

⑤ Adjust-a-dose: For patients with renal impairment, if creatinine clearance is 31 to 50 ml/minute, give 1 g every 12 hours; if clearance is 16 to 30 ml/minute, give 1 g every 24 hours; if clearance is 6 to 15 ml/minute, give 500 mg every 24 hours; if clearance is less than 5 ml/minute, give 500 mg every 48 hours. Drug is removed by hemodialysis; give a supplemental dose of drug after each dialysis session.

▼ I.V. administration

• Reconstitute solutions containing sodium carbonate with sterile water for injection. Add 5 ml to 500-mg vial or 10 ml to 1- or 2-g vial. Shake well to dissolve drug.
• Carbon dioxide is released during dissolution, and positive pressure will develop in vial. Don't add air to the vial when removing dose.
• Reconstitute solutions containing arginine with 10 ml sterile water for injection; this formulation won't release gas bubbles.
• Infuse drug over 15 to 30 minutes.
⊗ Incompatibilities
Aminoglycosides, aminophylline, amiodarone, amphotericin B cholesteryl sulfate complex, azithromycin, clarithromycin, fluconazole, idarubicin, midazolam, pentamidine isethionate, ranitidine hydrochloride, sargramostim, sodium bicarbonate solutions, vancomycin.

Contraindications and cautions

• Contraindicated in patients hypersensitive to drug or other cephalosporins.
• Use cautiously in patients with history of sensitivity to penicillin and in patients with renal impairment.

C

▲ **Lifespan:** In pregnant and breast-feeding women, use cautiously. In children age 12 and younger, safety and effectiveness haven't been established.

Adverse reactions

CNS: dizziness, fever, headache, *seizures.*
GI: abdominal cramps, diarrhea, dysgeusia, nausea, *pseudomembranous colitis,* vomiting.
GU: candidiasis, genital pruritus.
Hematologic: *agranulocytosis,* eosinophilia, *leukopenia, thrombocytosis.*
Respiratory: dyspnea.
Skin: *maculopapular and erythematous rashes, urticaria.*
Other: hypersensitivity reactions (serum sickness, *anaphylaxis*); *pain, induration, sterile abscesses, tissue sloughing at injection site; phlebitis, thrombophlebitis with I.V. injection.*

Interactions

Drug-drug. *Chloramphenicol:* May have an antagonistic effect. Avoid use together.

Effects on lab test results

• May increase ALT, AST, alkaline phosphatase, bilirubin, and LDH levels. May decrease hemoglobin level and hematocrit.
• May increase eosinophil count. May decrease WBC and granulocyte counts. May increase or decrease platelet count.
• May cause false-positive urine glucose determinations with copper sulfate tests (Clinitest).

Pharmacokinetics

Absorption: Unknown with I.M. use.
Distribution: Wide, including CSF (unlike most other cephalosporins). 5% to 24% protein-bound.
Metabolism: None.
Excretion: Mainly in urine. *Half-life:* About 1½ to 2 hours.

Route	Onset	Peak	Duration
I.V.	Immediate	Immediate	Unknown
I.M.	Unknown	≤ 1 hr	Unknown

Action

Chemical effect: Inhibits cell-wall synthesis, promoting osmotic instability; usually bactericidal.

Therapeutic effect: Hinders or kills susceptible bacteria.

Available forms

Infusion: 1 g, 2 g in 50-ml and 100-ml vials (premixed)
Injection (with arginine): 1 g, 2 g
Injection (with sodium carbonate): 500 mg, 1 g, 2 g

NURSING PROCESS

🔖 Assessment

• Assess patient's infection before therapy and regularly thereafter.
• Before giving first dose, obtain specimen for culture and sensitivity tests. Begin therapy pending test results.
• Before giving first dose, ask patient about previous reactions to cephalosporins or penicillin.
• Be alert for adverse reactions and drug interactions.
• If adverse GI reactions occur, monitor patient's hydration.
• Assess patient's and family's knowledge of drug therapy.

🔷 Nursing diagnoses

• Ineffective protection related to bacteria susceptible to drug
• Risk for deficient fluid volume related to drug-induced adverse GI reactions
• Deficient knowledge related to drug therapy

▶ Planning and implementation

• Inject deep into large muscle mass, such as gluteus maximus or lateral aspect of thigh.
🔔 **ALERT:** Commercially available forms contain either sodium carbonate (Fortaz, Tazicef, Tazidime) or arginine (Ceptaz) to facilitate dissolution of drug.
🔔 **ALERT:** Don't confuse with other cephalosporins with similar-sounding names.
Patient teaching
• Tell patient to report adverse reactions.
• Instruct patient to immediately report to prescriber any change in urinary output. Dose may need to be reduced to compensate for decreased excretion.

☑ Evaluation

• Patient is free from infection.
• Patient maintains adequate hydration.

• Patient and family state understanding of drug therapy.

ceftibuten
(sef-tih-BY00-tin)
Cedax

Pharmacologic class: third-generation cephalosporin
Therapeutic class: antibiotic
Pregnancy risk category: B

Indications and dosages

▶ **Acute bacterial exacerbation of chronic bronchitis caused by** *Haemophilus influenzae, Moraxella catarrhalis,* **or penicillin-susceptible strains of** *Streptococcus pneumoniae. Adults and children age 12 and older:* 400 mg P.O. daily for 10 days.
▶ **Pharyngitis and tonsillitis caused by** *Streptococcus pyogenes,* **acute bacterial otitis media caused by** *H. influenzae, M. catarrhalis,* **or** *S. pyogenes. Adults and children age 12 and older:* 400 mg P.O. daily for 10 days.
Children younger than age 12: Give 9 mg/kg P.O. daily for 10 days. Maximum daily dose is 400 mg.
Children weighing more than 45 kg (99 lb): Give 400 mg oral suspension P.O. daily for 10 days.
Children older than age 6 months and weighing 45 kg or less: 9 mg/kg oral suspension P.O. daily for 10 days. Maximum daily dose is 400 mg.
☒ **Adjust-a-dose:** For patients with renal impairment, if creatinine clearance is 30 to 49 ml/minute, give 4.5 mg/kg or 200 mg P.O. every 24 hours; if creatinine clearance is 5 to 29 ml/minute, give 2.25 mg/kg or 100 mg P.O. every 24 hours. For patients undergoing hemodialysis, give 400 mg P.O. as a single dose at the end of each dialysis session.

Contraindications and cautions

• Contraindicated in patients hypersensitive to cephalosporins.
• Use cautiously in patients with history of hypersensitivity to penicillin and in patients with GI disease or renal impairment.
☙ **Lifespan:** In pregnant women, use cautiously. In breast-feeding women, use cautiously; it isn't known if drug appears in breast milk. In

elderly patients, use cautiously. Monitor their renal function, and adjust dosage as needed.

Adverse reactions

CNS: aphasia, dizziness, headache, psychosis.
GI: abdominal pain, diarrhea, dyspepsia, loose stools, nausea, *pseudomembranous colitis,* vomiting.
GU: renal dysfunction, *toxic nephropathy.*
Hematologic: *agranulocytosis, aplastic anemia,* hemolytic anemia, *hemorrhage, neutropenia, pancytopenia.*
Hepatic: hepatic cholestasis.
Skin: *Stevens-Johnson syndrome.*
Other: allergic reaction, *anaphylaxis,* drug fever.

Interactions

Drug-food. *Any food:* May decrease bioavailability of drug. Give drug 2 hours before or 1 hour after a meal.

Effects on lab test results

• May increase ALT, AST, alkaline phosphatase, bilirubin, and BUN and creatinine levels. May decrease hemoglobin level and hematocrit.
• May increase eosinophil count. May decrease leukocyte count. May increase or decrease platelet count.

Pharmacokinetics

Absorption: Rapid.
Distribution: 65% protein-bound.
Metabolism: By the kidneys.
Excretion: Mainly in urine. *Half-life:* 2 to 2½ hours.

Route	Onset	Peak	Duration
P.O.	Unknown	2–4 hr	Unknown

Action

Chemical effect: Exerts bacterial action by binding to essential target proteins of the bacterial cell wall, thus inhibiting cell-wall synthesis.
Therapeutic effect: Hinders or kills susceptible bacteria.

Available forms

Capsules: 400 mg
Oral suspension: 90 mg/5 ml

NURSING PROCESS

Assessment
- Before giving first dose, obtain specimen for culture and sensitivity tests. Begin therapy pending test results.
- Monitor patient for superinfection.
- Obtain specimen for *Clostridium difficile* in patient who develops diarrhea after therapy.
- Assess patient's and family's knowledge of drug therapy.

Nursing diagnoses
- Ineffective protection related to bacteria susceptible to drug
- Deficient knowledge related to drug therapy

Planning and implementation
- To prepare oral suspension, tap bottle to loosen powder. Follow chart supplied by manufacturer for mixing instructions. Suspension is stable for 14 days if refrigerated.
- Shake suspension well before use.
- If allergic reaction occurs, stop drug and notify prescriber.
- **ALERT:** Don't confuse with other cephalosporins with similar-sounding names.

Patient teaching
- Tell patient to take drug as prescribed, even if he feels better.
- Tell patient to take drug at least 2 hours before or 1 hour after a meal.
- Instruct patient using oral suspension to shake bottle before use.
- Tell patient to store oral suspension in the refrigerator, with lid tightly closed, and to discard unused drug after 14 days.
- Warn breast-feeding woman that it's unclear whether drug appears in breast milk.
- Tell patient with diabetes that suspension has 1 g sucrose per teaspoon.

Evaluation
- Patient is free from infection.
- Patient and family state understanding of drug therapy.

ceftizoxime sodium
(sef-tih-ZOKS-eem SOH-dee-um)
Cefizox

Pharmacologic class: third-generation cephalosporin
Therapeutic class: antibiotic
Pregnancy risk category: B

Indications and dosages

▶ **Serious infections of lower respiratory and urinary tracts, gynecologic infections, bacteremia, septicemia, meningitis, intra-abdominal infections, bone and joint infections, and skin infections. Among susceptible microorganisms are *Streptococcus pneumoniae*, *Streptococcus pyogenes*, *Staphylococcus aureus* (penicillinase- and non–penicillinase-producing), *Staphylococcus epidermidis*, *Escherichia coli*, *Klebsiella*, *Haemophilus influenzae*, *Enterobacter*, *Proteus*, some *Pseudomonas*, and *Peptostreptococcus*.** *Adults:* 1 to 2 g I.V. or I.M. every 8 to 12 hours. In life-threatening infections, 3 to 4 g I.V. every 8 hours.
Children older than age 6 months: 50 mg/kg I.V. every 6 to 8 hours. For serious infections, up to 200 mg/kg daily in divided doses may be used. Maximum, 12 g daily.
Adjust-a-dose: For patients with renal impairment, if creatinine clearance is 50 to 79 ml/minute, give 500 mg every 8 hours for less severe infections or 750 mg to 1.5 g every 8 hours for life-threatening infections. If clearance is 5 to 49 ml/minute, give 250 to 500 mg every 12 hours for less severe infections or 500 mg to 1 g every 12 hours for life-threatening infections. If clearance is less than 5 ml/minute or patient undergoes hemodialysis, give 500 mg every 48 hours or 250 every 24 hours for less severe infections or 500 mg to 1 g every 48 hours or 500 mg every 24 hours for life-threatening infections.

I.V. administration
- To reconstitute powder, add 5 ml sterile water to 500-mg vial, 10 ml to 1-g vial, or 20 ml to 2-g vial. Reconstitute piggyback vials with 50 to 100 ml of normal saline solution or D$_5$W. Shake vial well.

• Inject directly into vein over 3 to 5 minutes or slowly into I.V. tubing with free-flowing compatible solution.
• Give intermittent infusion over 15 to 30 minutes.
• After reconstitution or dilution, solutions are stable for 1 day at room temperature and 4 days if refrigerated.
⊗ **Incompatibilities**
Aminoglycosides.

Contraindications and cautions

• Contraindicated in patients hypersensitive to drug or other cephalosporins.
• Use cautiously in patients with history of sensitivity to penicillin and in patients with renal impairment.
⚖ **Lifespan:** In pregnant and breast-feeding women, use cautiously. In infants younger than age 6 months, safety and effectiveness haven't been established.

Adverse reactions

CNS: dizziness, fever, headache, malaise, paresthesia.
GI: abdominal cramps, anal pruritus, anorexia, diarrhea, dyspepsia, glossitis, nausea, *pseudomembranous colitis,* tenesmus, vomiting.
GU: candidiasis, pruritus.
Hematologic: eosinophilia, hemolytic anemia, *thrombocytopenia, transient neutropenia.*
Respiratory: dyspnea.
Skin: *erythematous and maculopapular rashes, urticaria.*
Other: hypersensitivity reactions (*anaphylaxis,* serum sickness); induration, sterile abscesses, tissue sloughing at injection site; phlebitis, thrombophlebitis with I.V. injection.

Interactions

Drug-drug. *Probenecid:* May inhibit excretion and increase level of ceftizoxime. Sometimes used for this effect.

Effects on lab test results

• May increase BUN, creatinine, ALT, AST, alkaline phosphatase, bilirubin, GGT, and LDH levels. May decrease albumin, protein, and hemoglobin levels and hematocrit.
• May increase eosinophil count. May decrease PT and RBC, WBC, platelet, granulocyte, and neutrophil counts.

• May cause false-positive urine glucose determinations with copper sulfate tests (Clinitest).

Pharmacokinetics

Absorption: Unknown with I.M. use.
Distribution: Wide. Unlike many other cephalosporins, ceftizoxime has good CSF penetration and achieves adequate level in inflamed meninges. 28% to 31% protein-bound.
Metabolism: None.
Excretion: Mainly in urine. *Half-life:* About 1½ to 2 hours.

Route	Onset	Peak	Duration
I.V.	Immediate	Immediate	Unknown
I.M.	Unknown	½–1½ hr	Unknown

Action

Chemical effect: Inhibits cell-wall synthesis, promoting osmotic instability; usually bactericidal.
Therapeutic effect: Hinders or kills susceptible bacteria.

Available forms

Infusion: 1 g, 2 g in 100-mg vials or in 50 ml of D_5W
Injection: 500 mg, 1 g, 2 g

NURSING PROCESS

⚕ Assessment

• Assess patient's infection before therapy and regularly thereafter.
• Before giving first dose, obtain specimen for culture and sensitivity tests. Begin therapy pending test results.
• Before giving first dose, ask patient about previous reactions to cephalosporins or penicillin.
• Be alert for adverse reactions and drug interactions.
• If adverse GI reactions occur, monitor patient's hydration.
• Assess patient's and family's knowledge of drug therapy.

⊕ Nursing diagnoses

• Ineffective protection related to bacteria susceptible to drug
• Risk for deficient fluid volume related to drug-induced adverse GI reactions
• Deficient knowledge related to drug therapy

Reactions may be *common*, uncommon, *life-threatening*, or COMMON AND LIFE-THREATENING.

▶ Planning and implementation
• Inject I.M. dose deep into large muscle mass, such as gluteus maximus or lateral aspect of thigh. Divide doses of 2 g or more, and give divided doses at two different sites.
⑤ ALERT: Don't confuse drug with other cephalosporins that have similar-sounding names.
Patient teaching
• Tell patient to report adverse reactions and signs and symptoms of superinfection promptly.
• Instruct patient to report discomfort at the I.V. site.
• Tell patient to notify prescriber if loose stools or diarrhea occur.

☑ Evaluation
• Patient is free from infection.
• Patient maintains adequate hydration.
• Patient and family state understanding of drug therapy.

ceftriaxone sodium
(sef-trigh-AKS-ohn SOH-dee-um)
Rocephin

Pharmacologic class: third-generation cephalosporin
Therapeutic class: antibiotic
Pregnancy risk category: B

Indications and dosages
▶ **Uncomplicated gonococcal vulvovaginitis.**
Adults and children older than age 12 or weighing more than 45 kg (99 lb): 125 to 250 mg I.M. as single dose, followed by either 100 mg of doxycycline P.O. every 12 hours for 7 days, or a single oral dose of azithromycin 1 g.
Children younger than age 12 or weighing less than 45 kg: 125 mg I.M. as a single dose.
▶ **Serious infections of lower respiratory and urinary tracts; gynecologic, bone, joint, intra-abdominal, and skin infections; bacteremia; and septicemia caused by susceptible microorganisms such as *Streptococcus pneumoniae, Streptococcus pyogenes, Staphylococcus aureus, Staphylococcus epidermidis, Escherichia coli, Klebsiella, Haemophilus influenzae, Neisseria meningitides, Neisseria gonorrhoeae, Enterobacter, Proteus, Pseudomonas, Peptostreptococcus,* and *Serratia marcescens.*** *Adults and children older than age*

12: Give 1 to 2 g I.V. or I.M. daily or in equally divided doses; maximum 4 g daily for 4 to 14 days depending on severity of infection.
Children age 12 and younger: 50 to 75 mg/kg, maximum 2 g daily, given in divided doses every 12 hours.
▶ **Meningitis.** *Adults and children:* Initially, 100 mg/kg I.M. or I.V. (maximum 4 g); thereafter, 100 mg/kg I.M. or I.V. given once daily or in divided doses every 12 hours. Maximum, 4 g, for 7 to 14 days.
▶ **Preoperative prophylaxis.** *Adults:* 1 g I.V. as single dose 30 minutes to 2 hours before surgery.
▶ **Acute bacterial otitis media.** *Children:* 50 mg/kg I.M. as a single dose; maximum I.M. dose is 1 g.
▶ **Persisting or relapsing otitis media in children‡.** *Children and infants age 3 months and older:* 50 mg/kg I.M daily for 3 days.
▶ **Sexually transmitted epididymitis, pelvic inflammatory disease‡.** *Adults:* 250 mg I.M. as a single dose; follow up with other antibiotics.
▶ **Anti-infectives for sexual assault victims‡.** *Adults:* 125 mg I.M. as a single dose given with other antibiotics.
▶ **Lyme disease‡.** *Adults:* 2 g I.V. daily for 14 to 28 days.

▼ I.V. administration
• Reconstitute with sterile water for injection, normal saline solution for injection, D_5W or $D_{10}W$ injection, or combination of saline solution and dextrose injection and other compatible solutions.
• Reconstitute by adding 2.4 ml of diluent to 250-mg vial, 4.8 ml to 500-mg vial, 9.6 ml to 1-g vial, and 19.2 ml to 2-g vial. All reconstituted solutions yield concentration that averages 100 mg/ml.
⑤ ALERT: In full-term and preterm neonates, drug may fatally precipitate in the lungs and kidneys when used with calcium or solutions or products containing calcium. Don't mix or administer simultaneously with calcium-containing solutions or products, and don't give calcium-containing solutions or products within 48 hours of the last ceftriazone dose.
• After reconstitution, dilute further to desired concentration for intermittent infusion.
• Dilutions are stable for 24 hours at room temperature.

⊗ Incompatibilities

Aminoglycosides, aminophylline, azithromycin, clindamycin phosphate, filgrastim, fluconazole, labetalol, lidocaine hydrochloride, pentamidine isethionate, theophylline, vancomycin, vinorelbine tartrate.

Contraindications and cautions

• Contraindicated in patients hypersensitive to drug or other cephalosporins.
• Use cautiously in patients with history of sensitivity to penicillin.
⚖ Lifespan: In pregnant and breast-feeding women, use cautiously. In hyperbilirubinemic neonates, especially if preterm, do not give drug.

Adverse reactions

CNS: dizziness, fever, headache.
GI: diarrhea, dysgeusia, nausea, *pseudomembranous colitis,* vomiting.
GU: genital pruritus and candidiasis.
Hematologic: eosinophilia, *leukopenia, thrombocytosis.*
Skin: pain, induration, and tenderness at injection site; phlebitis; *rash.*
Other: hypersensitivity reactions (serum sickness, *anaphylaxis*).

Interactions

Drug-drug. *Aminoglycosides:* May have additive effect. Monitor drug level and adjust dosage as needed.
Calcium, products containing calcium: May cause fatal precipitate. Don't give solutions or products containing calcium within 48 hours of the last ceftriaxone dose.
Probenecid: May shorten half-life of ceftriaxone in large doses. Avoid use together.
Quinolones: May have synergistic effect against *S. pneumoniae.* Use together against this organism is recommended.
Drug-lifestyle. *Alcohol use:* May cause disulfiram-like reaction. Discourage use together.

Effects on lab test results

• May increase BUN, ALT, AST, alkaline phosphatase, bilirubin, and LDH levels.
• May increase eosinophil and platelet counts. May decrease WBC count.
• May cause false-positive urine glucose determinations with copper sulfate tests (Clinitest).

Pharmacokinetics

Absorption: Unknown.
Distribution: Wide. Unlike many other cephalosporins, ceftriaxone has good CSF penetration. 58% to 96% protein-bound.
Metabolism: Partial.
Excretion: Mainly in urine, minimally in bile.
Half-life: About 5½ to 11 hours.

Route	Onset	Peak	Duration
I.V.	Immediate	Immediate	Unknown
I.M.	Unknown	1½–4 hr	Unknown

Action

Chemical effect: Inhibits cell-wall synthesis, promoting osmotic instability; usually bactericidal.
Therapeutic effect: Hinders or kills susceptible bacteria.

Available forms

Infusion: 1 g, 2 g
Injection: 250 mg, 500 mg, 1 g, 2 g

NURSING PROCESS

⚱ Assessment

• Assess patient's infection before therapy and regularly thereafter.
• Before giving first dose, obtain specimen for culture and sensitivity tests. Begin therapy pending test results.
• Before giving first dose, ask patient about previous reactions to cephalosporins or penicillin.
• Be alert for adverse reactions and drug interactions.
• If adverse GI reactions occur, monitor patient's hydration.
• Assess patient's and family's knowledge of drug therapy.

⊕ Nursing diagnoses

• Ineffective protection related to bacteria susceptible to drug
• Risk for deficient fluid volume related to drug-induced adverse GI reactions
• Deficient knowledge related to drug therapy

▷ Planning and implementation

• Inject deep into large muscle mass, such as gluteus maximus or lateral aspect of thigh. As needed, use lidocaine 1% without epinephrine to dilute for I.M. use.

Reactions may be *common*, uncommon, *life-threatening*, or COMMON AND LIFE-THREATENING.

⚠ **ALERT:** Don't confuse with other cephalosporins with similar-sounding names.

Patient teaching
- Tell patient to promptly report adverse reactions and signs and symptoms of superinfection.
- Instruct patient to report pain at the I.V. site.
- Tell patient to notify prescriber if loose stools or diarrhea occur.

☑ **Evaluation**
- Patient is free from infection.
- Patient maintains adequate hydration.
- Patient and family state understanding of drug therapy.

cefuroxime axetil
(sef-yoor-OKS-eem AKS-eh-til)
Ceftin

cefuroxime sodium
Zinacef

Pharmacologic class: second-generation cephalosporin
Therapeutic class: antibiotic
Pregnancy risk category: B

Indications and dosages

▶ **Serious lower respiratory tract infection, UTI, skin or skin-structure infections, bone or joint infection, septicemia, meningitis, and gonorrhea.** *Adults and children age 13 and older:* 750 mg to 1.5 g cefuroxime sodium I.M. or I.V. every 8 hours for 5 to 10 days. For life-threatening infections and infections caused by less susceptible organisms, 1.5 g I.M. or I.V. every 6 hours; for bacterial meningitis, up to 3 g I.V. every 8 hours.
Children ages 3 months to 12 years: 50 to 100 mg/kg/day cefuroxime sodium I.M. or I.V. in equally divided doses every 6 to 8 hours. For more severe or serious infections, use 100 mg/kg/day, not to exceed maximum adult dosage. For bacterial meningitis, 200 to 240 mg/kg cefuroxime sodium I.V. in divided doses every 6 to 8 hours.

▶ **Perioperative prevention.** *Adults:* 1.5 g I.V. 30 to 60 minutes before surgery; in lengthy operations, 750 mg I.V. or I.M. every 8 hours. For open-heart surgery, 1.5 g I.V. at induction of anesthesia and then every 12 hours for a total dose of 6 g.

▶ **Bacterial exacerbations of chronic bronchitis or secondary bacterial infection of acute bronchitis.** *Adults:* 250 or 500 mg P.O. b.i.d. for 10 days (chronic bronchitis) or 5 to 10 days (acute bronchitis).

▶ **Acute bacterial maxillary sinusitis.** *Adults and children age 13 and older:* 250 mg P.O. b.i.d. for 10 days.
Children ages 3 months to 12 years: 30 mg/kg/day oral suspension divided b.i.d. for 10 days.

▶ **Pharyngitis and tonsillitis.** *Adults and children age 13 and older:* 250 mg P.O. b.i.d. for 10 days.
Children ages 3 months to 12 years: 125 mg P.O. b.i.d. for 10 days. For children who can't swallow tablets whole, give 20 mg/kg daily of oral suspension divided b.i.d. for 10 days. Maximum daily dose for suspension is 500 mg.

▶ **Otitis media.** *Children ages 3 months to 12 years:* 250 mg P.O. b.i.d. for 10 days. For children who can't swallow tablets whole, give 30 mg/kg/day of oral suspension divided b.i.d. for 10 days. Maximum daily dose for suspension is 1,000 mg.

▶ **Uncomplicated skin and skin-structure infection.** *Adults and children age 13 and older:* 250 mg or 500 mg P.O. b.i.d. for 10 days.

▶ **Uncomplicated UTI.** *Adults:* 250 mg P.O. b.i.d. for 7 to 10 days.

▶ **Uncomplicated gonorrhea.** *Adults:* 1.5 g I.M. with 1 g probenecid P.O. for one dose. Or, 1 g P.O. as a single dose.

▶ **Early Lyme disease.** *Adults and children age 13 and older:* 500 mg P.O. b.i.d. for 20 days.

▶ **Impetigo.** *Children ages 3 months to 12 years:* 30 mg/kg/day of oral suspension divided b.i.d. for 10 days. Maximum daily dose, 1,000 mg.

📋 **Adjust-a-dose:** In adults with creatinine clearance of 10 to 20 ml/minute, give 750 mg I.M. or I.V. every 12 hours; if creatinine clearance is less than 10 ml/minute, give 750 mg I.M. or I.V. every 24 hours.

▽ I.V. administration

- For each 750-mg vial of Zinacef, reconstitute with 8 ml sterile water for injection; for each 1.5-g vial, reconstitute with 16 ml. In each case, withdraw entire contents of vial for dose.

- For direct injection, inject into large vein or into tubing of free-flowing I.V. solution over 3 to 5 minutes.
- For intermittent infusion, add reconstituted drug to 100 ml D₅W, normal saline solution for injection, or other compatible I.V. solution. Infuse over 15 to 60 minutes.

⊗ **Incompatibilities**
Aminoglycosides, ciprofloxacin, clarithromycin, filgrastim, fluconazole, midazolam, ranitidine, sodium bicarbonate injection, vinorelbine tartrate.

Contraindications and cautions

- Contraindicated in patients hypersensitive to drug or other cephalosporins.
- Use cautiously in patients with history of sensitivity to penicillin and in patients with renal impairment.

☀ **Lifespan:** In pregnant and breast-feeding women, use cautiously. In infants younger than age 3 months, safety and effectiveness haven't been established.

Adverse reactions

CNS: dizziness, headache, malaise, paresthesia.
GI: abdominal cramps, anal pruritus, anorexia, diarrhea, dyspepsia, glossitis, nausea, *pseudomembranous colitis,* tenesmus, vomiting.
GU: candidiasis, pruritus.
Hematologic: eosinophilia, hemolytic anemia, *thrombocytopenia, transient neutropenia.*
Respiratory: dyspnea.
Skin: *erythematous and maculopapular rashes,* urticaria.
Other: hypersensitivity reactions (*anaphylaxis,* serum sickness); pain, induration, sterile abscesses, warmth, tissue sloughing at injection site; phlebitis, thrombophlebitis with I.V. injection.

Interactions

Drug-drug. *Diuretics:* May increase risk of adverse renal reactions. Monitor renal function closely.
Probenecid: May inhibit excretion and increase level of cefuroxime. Sometimes used for this effect.
Drug-food. *Any food:* May increase drug absorption and bioavailability of suspension. Give suspension with food. Tablets may be given without regard to food.

Effects on lab test results

- May increase ALT, AST, alkaline phosphatase, bilirubin, and LDH levels. May decrease hemoglobin level and hematocrit.
- May increase eosinophil count, PT, and INR. May decrease neutrophil and platelet counts.
- May cause false-positive urine glucose determinations with copper sulfate tests (Clinitest).

Pharmacokinetics

Absorption: 37% to 52% of oral cefuroxime axetil reaches systemic circulation. Food appears to enhance absorption. Cefuroxime sodium isn't well absorbed from GI tract; absorption after I.M. use is unknown.
Distribution: Wide. CSF penetration is greater than that of most first- and second-generation cephalosporins and achieves adequate therapeutic level in inflamed meninges. 33% to 50% protein-bound.
Metabolism: None.
Excretion: Mainly in urine. *Half-life:* 1 to 2 hours.

Route	Onset	Peak	Duration
P.O.	Unknown	2–3 hr	Unknown
I.V.	Unknown	Immediate	Unknown
I.M.	Unknown	15–60 min	Unknown

Action

Chemical effect: Inhibits cell-wall synthesis, promoting osmotic instability; usually bactericidal.
Therapeutic effect: Hinders or kills susceptible bacteria, including many gram-positive organisms and enteric gram-negative bacilli.

Available forms

cefuroxime axetil
Suspension: 125 mg/5 ml, 250 mg/5 ml
Tablets: 125 mg, 250 mg, 500 mg
cefuroxime sodium
Infusion: 750 mg, 1.5 g premixed, frozen solution
Injection: 750 mg, 1.5 g

NURSING PROCESS

📖 **Assessment**
- Assess patient's infection before therapy and regularly thereafter.

- Before giving first dose, obtain specimen for culture and sensitivity tests. Begin therapy pending test results.
- Before giving first dose, ask patient about previous reactions to cephalosporins or penicillin.
- Be alert for adverse reactions and drug interactions.
- If adverse GI reactions occur, monitor patient's hydration.
- Assess patient's and family's knowledge of drug therapy.

✣ Nursing diagnoses
- Ineffective protection related to bacteria susceptible to drug
- Risk for deficient fluid volume related to drug-induced adverse GI reactions
- Deficient knowledge related to drug therapy

▷ Planning and implementation
- Food enhances absorption of cefuroxime axetil.
- Cefuroxime axetil is available only in tablet form, which may be crushed for patients who can't swallow tablets. Tablets may be dissolved in small amounts of apple, orange, or grape juice or chocolate milk. However, drug has bitter taste that's difficult to mask, even with food.
- ⚠ **ALERT:** Cefuroxime tablets and oral suspensions aren't bioequivalent and can't be substituted on a milligram-for-milligram basis.
- Inject deep into large muscle mass, such as gluteus maximus or lateral aspect of thigh. Before I.M. injection, aspirate to avoid injection into a blood vessel.
- Cefuroxime isn't considered the drug of choice for meningitis or gonorrhea infections.
- ⚠ **ALERT:** Don't confuse with other cephalosporins with similar-sounding names.

Patient teaching
- Instruct patient to take drug exactly as prescribed, even after he feels better.
- Advise patient to take oral suspension with food to enhance absorption; tablets may be taken without regard to meals. Explain that tablets may be crushed, but drug has bitter taste that's difficult to mask, even with food.
- Tell patient to report adverse reactions.

✓ Evaluation
- Patient is free from infection.
- Patient maintains adequate hydration.

- Patient and family state understanding of drug therapy.

celecoxib
(seh-leh-COKS-ib)
Celebrex✒

Pharmacologic class: cyclooxygenase-2 (COX-2) inhibitor
Therapeutic class: anti-inflammatory
Pregnancy risk category: C (D in third trimester)

Indications and dosages
▶ **Relief of signs and symptoms of osteoarthritis.** *Adults:* 200 mg P.O. daily as a single dose or divided equally b.i.d.
▶ **Relief of signs and symptoms of rheumatoid arthritis.** *Adults:* 100 to 200 mg P.O. b.i.d.
▶ **Relief of signs and symptoms of juvenile rheumatoid arthritis.** *Children age 2 and older weighing 10 to 25 kg (22 to 55 lb):* 50-mg capsule P.O. b.i.d.
Children age 2 and older weighing more than 25 kg: 100-mg capsule P.O. b.i.d.
▶ **Relief of signs and symptoms of ankylosing spondylitis.** *Adults:* 200 mg P.O. once daily or divided b.i.d. If no response after 6 weeks, may increase to 400 mg daily. If no response after 6 more weeks, consider different treatment.
▶ **Adjunct to familial adenomatous polyposis to reduce the number of adenomatous colorectal polyps.** *Adults:* 400 mg P.O. b.i.d. with food for up to 6 months.
▶ **Acute pain and primary dysmenorrhea.** *Adults:* Initially, give 400 mg P.O., followed by an additional 200-mg dose on the first day, if needed. On subsequent days, 200 mg P.O. b.i.d. p.r.n.
🔲 **Adjust-a-dose:** For patients with moderate hepatic impairment, reduce dose by 50%; don't use in patients with severe hepatic impairment (Child-Pugh class B). For elderly patients who weigh less than 50 kg (110 lb), use the lowest recommended dose.

Contraindications and cautions
- Contraindicated in patients hypersensitive to drug, sulfonamides, aspirin or other NSAIDs; patients with severe hepatic or renal impair-

ment; and patients with perioperative pain after coronary artery bypass graft surgery.

• Use cautiously in patients with known or suspected history of poor CYP2C9 metabolism and in patients with history of ulcers, GI bleeding, dehydration, anemia, symptomatic liver disease, hypertension, edema, heart failure, or asthma. Also use cautiously in patients who smoke or drink alcohol frequently, take oral corticosteroids or anticoagulants, or are at a high risk for CV complications, such as those who have recently had heart surgery.

☀ **Lifespan:** In women in third trimester of pregnancy, avoid use. In elderly and debilitated patients, use cautiously because of increased risk of GI bleeding and acute renal impairment.

Adverse reactions

CNS: dizziness, *headache,* insomnia, **stroke.**
CV: hypertension, *MI,* peripheral edema.
EENT: pharyngitis, rhinitis, sinusitis.
GI: *abdominal pain,* diarrhea, *dyspepsia,* flatulence, *nausea,* **GI bleeding.**
Metabolic: hyperchloremia, hypophosphatemia.
Musculoskeletal: back pain.
Respiratory: upper respiratory tract infection.
Skin: *erythema multiforme, exfoliative dermatitis,* rash, **Stevens-Johnson syndrome, toxic epidermal necrolysis.**
Other: accidental injury.

Interactions

Drug-drug. *ACE inhibitors:* May decrease antihypertensive effects. Monitor patient's blood pressure.
Aluminum- and magnesium-containing antacids: May decrease celecoxib level. Separate doses.
Aspirin: May increase risk of ulcers; low aspirin dosages can be used safely to prevent CV events. Monitor patient for GI bleeding.
Diuretics: May decrease sodium excretion of diuretics, leading to sodium retention. Monitor patient for swelling and increased blood pressure.
Fluconazole: May increase celecoxib level. Use lowest effective dose.
Lithium: May increase lithium level. Monitor lithium level.
Warfarin: May increase PT. Monitor PT and INR, and check for bleeding.

Drug-herb. *Dong quai, feverfew, garlic, ginger, ginkgo, horse chestnut, red clover:* May increase the risk of bleeding. Discourage use together.
Drug-lifestyle. *Chronic alcohol use, smoking:* May increase risk of GI irritation or bleeding. Check for evidence of bleeding, and discourage use together.

Effects on lab test results

• May increase BUN, ALT, AST, and chloride levels. May decrease phosphate level.

Pharmacokinetics

Absorption: Level peaks in about 3 hours. If patient receives multiple doses, expect steady-state level within 5 days. Elderly patients have higher level than younger adults.
Distribution: Extensive. Highly protein-bound, mainly to albumin.
Metabolism: By CYP2C9. No active metabolites have been identified.
Excretion: Mainly through hepatic metabolism, with less than 3% as unchanged drug in urine and feces. *Half-life:* 11 hours.

Route	Onset	Peak	Duration
P.O.	Unknown	3 hr	Unknown

Action

Chemical effect: May selectively inhibit COX-2, decreasing prostaglandin synthesis.
Therapeutic effect: Relieves pain and inflammation in joints and smooth muscle tissue.

Available forms

Capsules: 50 mg, 100 mg, 200 mg, 400 mg

NURSING PROCESS

☑ Assessment

• Assess patient for appropriateness of therapy. Drug must be used cautiously in patients with history of ulcers or GI bleeding, advanced renal disease, dehydration, anemia, symptomatic liver disease, hypertension, edema, heart failure, or asthma.
⚠ ALERT: Obtain accurate list of patient's allergies. Patients may be allergic to celecoxib if they're allergic and have had anaphylactic reactions to sulfonamides, aspirin, or other NSAIDs.
• Assess patient for risk factors for GI bleeding, including corticosteroid or anticoagulant ther-

apy, long-term NSAID therapy, smoking, alcoholism, older age, and poor overall health. Patients with a history of ulcers or GI bleeding are at higher risk for GI bleeding while taking NSAIDs such as celecoxib.

• Monitor patient for evidence of overt and occult bleeding.

⊛ **ALERT:** Assess patient's CV status, CV risk factors, and history, particularly for recent heart surgery, MI, or stroke, before starting therapy. NSAIDs may increase the risk of serious thrombotic events; the risk increases with duration of use and may be higher in patients with CV disease or risk factors for it.

• Monitor patient for signs and symptoms of liver toxicity. Celecoxib may be hepatotoxic.

• Assess patient's and family's knowledge of drug therapy.

🔯 Nursing diagnoses
• Acute pain related to underlying condition
• Risk for injury related to drug-induced adverse reactions
• Deficient knowledge related to drug therapy

▶ Planning and implementation
⊛ **ALERT:** Use cautiously in patients at a high risk for CV complications and in those taking the drug long term because such use may increase risk of MI and stroke.

• Although drug can be given with or without food, food may decrease GI upset.

• Before therapy, rehydrate patient.

• Although celecoxib may be used with low-dose aspirin, the combination may increase the risk of GI bleeding.

• NSAIDs such as celecoxib can cause fluid retention. Closely monitor patient who has hypertension, edema, or heart failure while taking this drug.

⊛ **ALERT:** Don't confuse Celebrex with Cerebyx or Celexa.

Patient teaching
• Instruct patient to immediately report to prescriber signs of GI bleeding (such as bloody vomitus, blood in urine or stool, and black, tarry stools).

⊛ **ALERT:** Advise patient to immediately report rash, unexplained weight gain, or edema to prescriber.

• Tell woman to notify prescriber if she becomes pregnant or is planning to become pregnant while taking this drug.

• Instruct patient to take drug with food if stomach upset occurs.

• Advise patient that all NSAIDs, including celecoxib, may adversely affect the liver. Signs and symptoms of liver toxicity include nausea, fatigue, lethargy, itching, jaundice, right upper quadrant tenderness, and flulike syndrome. Advise patient to stop therapy and seek immediate medical advice if he has any of these signs or symptoms.

• Inform patient that it may take several days before he feels consistent pain relief.

☑ Evaluation
• Patient is free from pain.
• Patient doesn't experience injury as a result of drug-induced adverse reactions.
• Patient and family state understanding of drug therapy.

cephalexin
(sef-uh-LEK-sin)
Apo-Cephalex ♦ , Keflex, Novo-Lexin ♦

Pharmacologic class: first-generation cephalosporin
Therapeutic class: antibiotic
Pregnancy risk category: B

Indications and dosages

▶ **Respiratory tract, GI tract, skin, soft-tissue, bone, and joint infections and otitis media caused by** *Escherichia coli* **and other coliform bacteria, group A beta-hemolytic streptococci,** *Haemophilus influenzae, Klebsiella, Moraxella catarrhalis, Proteus mirabilis, Streptococcus pneumoniae,* **and staphylococci.** *Adults:* 250 mg to 1 g P.O. every 6 hours or 500 mg every 12 hours; maximum, 4 g daily.
Children: 25 to 50 mg/kg P.O. in divided doses, maximum 4 g daily.

▧ **Adjust-a-dose:** For patients with renal impairment, if creatinine clearance is 11 to 40 ml/minute, give 500 mg every 8 to 12 hours; if clearance is 5 to 10 ml/minute, give 250 mg every 12 hours; if clearance is less than 5 ml/minute, give 250 mg every 12 to 24 hours.

Contraindications and cautions

• Contraindicated in patients hypersensitive to cephalosporins.
• Use cautiously in patients hypersensitive to penicillin and in patients with renal impairment.
☀ **Lifespan:** In pregnant and breast-feeding women, use cautiously.

Adverse reactions

CNS: dizziness, headache, malaise, paresthesia.
GI: abdominal cramps, anal pruritus, *anorexia, diarrhea,* dyspepsia, glossitis, *nausea,* oral candidiasis, *pseudomembranous colitis,* tenesmus, vomiting.
GU: candidiasis, genital pruritus, vaginitis.
Hematologic: anemia, eosinophilia, *thrombocytopenia, transient neutropenia.*
Respiratory: dyspnea.
Skin: maculopapular and erythematous rashes, urticaria.
Other: hypersensitivity reactions (*anaphylaxis,* serum sickness).

Interactions

Drug-drug. *Probenecid:* May increase cephalosporin level. Sometimes used for this effect.

Effects on lab test results

• May increase ALT, AST, alkaline phosphatase, bilirubin, and LDH levels. May decrease hemoglobin level and hematocrit.
• May increase eosinophil count. May decrease neutrophil and platelet counts.
• May cause false-positive urine glucose determinations with copper sulfate tests (Clinitest).

Pharmacokinetics

Absorption: Rapid and complete. Food delays but doesn't prevent complete absorption.
Distribution: Wide; CSF penetration is poor. 6% to 15% protein-bound.
Metabolism: None.
Excretion: Mainly unchanged in urine. *Half-life:* 30 minutes to 1 hour.

Route	Onset	Peak	Duration
P.O.	Unknown	≤1 hr	Unknown

Action

Chemical effect: Inhibits cell-wall synthesis, promoting osmotic instability; usually bactericidal.

Therapeutic effect: Hinders or kills susceptible bacteria.

Available forms

Capsules: 250 mg, 333 mg, 500 mg, 750 mg
Oral suspension: 125 mg/5 ml, 250 mg/5 ml
Tablets: 250 mg, 500 mg

NURSING PROCESS

📊 Assessment

• Assess patient's infection before therapy and regularly thereafter.
• Before giving first dose, obtain specimen for culture and sensitivity tests. Begin therapy pending test results.
• Before giving first dose, ask patient about previous reactions to cephalosporins or penicillin.
• Be alert for adverse reactions and drug interactions.
• If adverse GI reactions occur, monitor patient's hydration.
• Assess patient's and family's knowledge of drug therapy.

🔲 Nursing diagnoses

• Ineffective protection related to bacteria susceptible to drug
• Risk for deficient fluid volume related to drug-induced adverse GI reactions
• Deficient knowledge related to drug therapy

▶ Planning and implementation

• To prepare oral suspension, first add required amount of water to powder in two portions. Shake well after each addition. After mixing, store in refrigerator (stable for 14 days without significant loss of potency). Keep tightly closed, and shake well before using.
• To minimize adverse GI reactions, give drug with food or milk.
• Treat group A beta-hemolytic streptococcal infections for at least 10 days.
• If giving more than 4 g daily, give initial treatment with a parenteral cephalosporin; switch to oral form when patient is stable.
• ⚠ **ALERT:** Don't confuse with other cephalosporins with similar-sounding names.
Patient teaching
• Inform patient that drug may be taken with meals.
• Instruct patient to take drug exactly as prescribed, even after he feels better.

Reactions may be *common,* uncommon, *life-threatening,* or **COMMON AND LIFE-THREATENING.**

- Tell patient to call prescriber if rash develops.
- Teach patient how to store drug.

☑ Evaluation
- Patient is free from infection.
- Patient maintains adequate hydration.
- Patient and family state understanding of drug therapy.

---

cetuximab
(seh-TUX-eh-mab)
Erbitux

Pharmacologic class: recombinant monoclonal antibody
Therapeutic class: epidermal growth factor receptor (EGFR) antagonist
Pregnancy risk category: C

Indications and dosages

▶ **Epidermal growth factor–expressing metastatic colorectal cancer, as monotherapy in patients intolerant of irinotecan-based chemotherapy or with irinotecan in patients refractory to irinotecan therapy alone.**
Adults: Initial loading dose, 400 mg/m^2 I.V. over 2 hours (maximum, 5 ml/minute), alone or with irinotecan. Maintenance dosage, 250 mg/m^2 I.V. weekly over 1 hour (maximum, 5 ml/minute). Premedicate with an H_1 antagonist (such as 50 mg of diphenhydramine I.V.).

▶ **Squamous cell carcinoma of the head and neck.** *Adults:* Premedicate with an H_1 antagonist. Then loading dose of 400 mg/m^2 I.V. over 2 hours (maximum rate, 5 ml/minute) followed by weekly maintenance dose of 250 mg/m^2 I.V. over 1 hour. If used with radiation therapy, begin cetuximab 1 week before radiation starts and continue throughout radiation therapy (6 to 7 weeks). If used as monotherapy for recurrent or metastatic disease after failure of platinum-based therapy, continue treatment until disease progresses or unacceptable toxicity occurs.

⛏ Adjust-a-dose: If patient develops a grade 1 or 2 infusion reaction, permanently reduce infusion rate by 50%. If patient develops a grade 3 or 4 reaction, stop drug immediately and permanently.

▼ I.V. administration
- Solution should be clear and colorless and may contain a small amount of particulates.
- Don't shake or dilute.
- Give by infusion pump or syringe pump. Piggyback into the patient's infusion line.
- Don't give drug by I.V. push or bolus.
- Give drug through a low–protein-binding 0.22-micrometer in-line filter.
- Flush line with normal saline solution at the end of the infusion.
- Monitor patient for 1 hour after the infusion.
- If patient develops a severe acneiform rash, follow these guidelines: The first time, delay infusion 1 to 2 weeks. If the patient improves, continue at 250 mg/m^2. If the patient doesn't improve, stop the drug. The second time, delay infusion 1 to 2 weeks. If the patient improves, reduce dose to 200 mg/m^2. If the patient doesn't improve, stop the drug. The third time, delay infusion 1 to 2 weeks. If the patient improves, reduce dose to 150 mg/m^2. If the patient doesn't improve, stop the drug. The fourth time, stop the drug permanently.
- Store vials at 36° to 46° F (2° to 8° C). Don't freeze. Solution in infusion container is stable up to 12 hours in refrigerator and up to 8 hours at room temperature (68° to 77° F [20° to 25° C]).

⊗ **Incompatibilities**
Don't dilute cetuximab with other solutions.

Contraindications and cautions
- Use cautiously in patients hypersensitive to drug, its components, or murine proteins. Also, use cautiously in combination therapy with radiation in patients with a history of coronary artery disease, arrhythmias, or heart failure.

⚖ **Lifespan:** It isn't known whether drug can harm fetus, so give drug to a pregnant woman only if potential benefits justify risks to fetus. Before therapy starts, caution mother about risks to fetus. Urge women to stop breast-feeding while receiving drug and for 60 days after the last dose. In children, safety and effectiveness haven't been established.

Adverse reactions
CNS: *asthenia, fever,* depression, headache, insomnia, *pain.*
CV: *cardiopulmonary arrest,* edema.
EENT: conjunctivitis.

GI: *abdominal pain,* anorexia, *constipation, diarrhea,* dyspepsia, *dysphagia, mucositis, nausea,* stomatitis, *vomiting, xerostomia.*
GU: *acute renal failure.*
Hematologic: *anemia,* LEUKOPENIA.
Metabolic: dehydration, *weight loss.*
Musculoskeletal: *back pain.*
Respiratory: *bronchospasm,* cough, dyspnea, hoarseness, *pulmonary embolus,* stridor.
Skin: *acneiform rash,* alopecia, maculopapular rash, nail disorder, pruritus, *radiation dermatitis.*
Other: infection, *infusion reaction, sepsis.*

Interactions

Drug-lifestyle. *Sun exposure:* May worsen skin reactions. Urge patient to take precautions.

Effects on lab test results

None reported.

Pharmacokinetics

Absorption: Given I.V.
Distribution: Binds to EGFR, which is expressed in many normal epithelial tissues, such as skin and hair follicles, and in many cancers.
Metabolism: Unknown.
Excretion: Unknown. *Half-life:* 5 days.

Route	Onset	Peak	Duration
I.V.	Unknown	Unknown	Unknown

Action

Chemical effect: Binds to the EGFR on normal and tumor cells, keeping epidermal growth factor from binding, which inhibits cell growth, causes cell death, and decreases growth factor production.
Therapeutic effect: Inhibits tumor cells that overexpress EGFR in colorectal cancer patients.

Available forms

Injection: 2 mg/ml in 50-ml vial

NURSING PROCESS

Assessment

ALERT: Assess patient for signs and symptoms of severe infusion reactions, including acute airway obstruction, urticaria, and hypotension, usually with the first infusion and despite premedication. If a severe infusion reaction occurs, immediately stop giving the drug and treat symptoms. Treat mild to moderate infusion reactions by cutting infusion rate in half and continuing antihistamines.

• Monitor patient for infusion reactions for 1 hour after the infusion.
• Assess patient for acute onset or worsening of pulmonary symptoms. If interstitial lung disease is confirmed, stop the drug.
• Monitor patient for skin toxicity, which starts most often during the first 2 weeks of therapy. Give topical and oral antibiotics.
• Assess hematologic and renal function studies before therapy and periodically thereafter.
• Patients receiving cetuximab with radiation therapy need close monitoring of their electrolytes—particularly magnesium, potassium, and calcium—during and after therapy.
• Assess patient's and family's knowledge of drug therapy.

Nursing diagnoses

• Risk for injury related to drug infusion reaction
• Impaired skin integrity related to dermatologic toxicity
• Deficient knowledge related to cetuximab therapy

Planning and implementation

• To reduce risk of pulmonary drug reactions, premedicate with 50 mg diphenhydramine I.V.
• Keep epinephrine, corticosteroids, I.V. antihistamines, bronchodilators, and oxygen available to treat severe infusion reactions.
Patient teaching
• Tell patient to promptly report adverse reactions.
• Inform patient that skin reactions may occur, typically during the first 2 weeks.
• Advise patient to avoid prolonged or unprotected sun exposure, which can worsen adverse skin reactions.

Evaluation

• Patient doesn't experience a drug infusion reaction.
• Patient doesn't develop dermatologic toxicity.
• Patient and family state understanding of drug therapy.

chloral hydrate
(KLOR-ul HIGH-drayt)
Aquachloral Supprettes, Somnote

Pharmacologic class: general CNS depressant
Therapeutic class: sedative-hypnotic
Pregnancy risk category: C
Controlled substance schedule: IV

Indications and dosages

▶ **Sedation.** *Adults:* 250 mg P.O. or P.R. t.i.d. after meals. Maximum dosage, 2 g.
Children: 8 mg/kg P.O. or P.R. t.i.d.; maximum 500 mg per dose daily; doses may be divided.
▶ **Insomnia.** *Adults:* 500 mg to 1 g P.O. or P.R. 15 to 30 minutes before bedtime.
Children: 50 mg/kg P.O. or P.R. 15 to 30 minutes before bedtime; maximum single dose, 1 g.
▶ **Preoperative use.** *Adults:* 500 mg to 1 g P.O. or P.R. 30 minutes before surgery.
▶ **Premedication for EEG.** *Children:* 20 to 25 mg/kg P.O. or P.R.
▶ **Alcohol withdrawal.** *Adults:* 500 mg to 1 g P.O. or P.R.; repeat at 6-hour intervals, p.r.n. Maximum, 2 g daily.

Contraindications and cautions

• Contraindicated in patients hypersensitive to drug and in those with hepatic or renal impairment. Oral administration contraindicated in patients with gastric disorders.
• Use cautiously in patients with severe cardiac disease and in patients with mental depression, suicidal tendencies, or history of drug abuse.
⚠ **Lifespan:** In breast-feeding women, avoid use because small amounts of drug appear in breast milk and may cause drowsiness in infants.

Adverse reactions

CNS: ataxia, dizziness, drowsiness, hangover, nightmares, paradoxical excitement.
GI: diarrhea, flatulence, nausea, vomiting.
Hematologic: eosinophilia, *leukopenia.*
Other: hypersensitivity reactions.

Interactions

Drug-drug. *Alkaline solutions:* May be incompatible with aqueous solutions of chloral hydrate. Don't mix together.

CNS depressants, including opioid analgesics: May cause excessive CNS depression or vasodilation reaction. Use together cautiously.
Furosemide I.V.: May cause sweating, flushing, variable blood pressure, and uneasiness. Use together cautiously or use different hypnotic drug.
Oral anticoagulants: May increase risk of bleeding. Monitor patient closely.
Phenytoin: May decrease phenytoin level. Monitor level closely.
Drug-lifestyle. *Alcohol use:* May react synergistically, increasing CNS depression, or may cause a disulfiram-like reaction (rarely). Strongly discourage alcohol use.

Effects on lab test results

• May increase BUN level.
• May increase eosinophil count. May decrease WBC count.
• May interfere with fluorometric tests for urine catecholamines and Reddy-Jenkins-Thorn test for urine 17-hydroxycorticosteroids. May cause false-positive tests for urine glucose in copper sulfate tests (Clinitest).

Pharmacokinetics

Absorption: Good.
Distribution: Throughout body tissue and fluids; trichloroethanol (the active metabolite) is 35% to 41% protein-bound.
Metabolism: Rapid and nearly complete in liver and erythrocytes to trichloroethanol; then again in liver and kidneys to trichloroacetic acid and other inactive metabolites.
Excretion: Inactive metabolites mainly in urine, minimally in bile. *Half-life:* 8 to 10 hours for trichloroethanol.

Route	Onset	Peak	Duration
P.O.	≤ 30 min	Unknown	4–8 hr
P.R.	Unknown	Unknown	4–8 hr

Action

Chemical effect: Unknown; sedative effects may be caused by trichloroethanol.
Therapeutic effect: Promotes sleep and calmness.

Available forms

Capsules: 500 mg
Suppositories: 324 mg, 648 mg
Syrup: 250 mg/5 ml, 500 mg/5 ml

NURSING PROCESS

🗒 Assessment
• Assess patient's underlying condition.
• Evaluate drug's effectiveness.
• Be alert for adverse reactions and drug interactions.
• Assess patient's and family's knowledge of drug therapy.

⊕ Nursing diagnoses
• Insomnia related to patient's underlying condition
• Risk for trauma related to adverse CNS reactions
• Deficient knowledge related to drug therapy

▶ Planning and implementation
⚠ **ALERT:** Oral liquid form comes in two strengths; double-check dose, especially when giving to children. Fatal overdose may occur.
• To minimize unpleasant taste and stomach irritation, dilute or give drug with liquid and after meals.
• Store rectal suppositories in refrigerator.
• Don't use for long-term therapy because drug loses its effectiveness in promoting sleep after 14 days of continued use. Long-term use may also cause drug dependence, and patient may experience withdrawal symptoms if drug is suddenly stopped.
⚠ **ALERT:** Some products may contain tartrazine, which may cause hypersensitivity reactions in susceptible people.
Patient teaching
• Warn patient about performing activities that require mental alertness or physical coordination. For inpatients, particularly elderly patients, supervise walking and raise bed rails.
• Tell patient to store capsules or syrup in dark container and to store suppositories in refrigerator.
• Explain that drug may cause morning hangover. Encourage patient to report severe hangover or feelings of oversedation so that prescriber can adjust the dosage or change drug.

✓ Evaluation
• Patient states drug effectively induced sleep.
• Patient's safety is maintained.
• Patient and family state understanding of drug therapy.

HIGH ALERT!

chlorambucil
(klor-AM-byoo-sil)
Leukeran

Pharmacologic class: alkylating drug
Therapeutic class: antineoplastic
Pregnancy risk category: D

Indications and dosages

▶ **Chronic lymphocytic leukemia; malignant lymphomas, including lymphosarcoma, giant follicular lymphoma, non-Hodgkin lymphoma, Hodgkin lymphoma, autoimmune hemolytic anemia‡, nephrotic syndrome‡, polycythemia vera‡, and ovarian neoplasms‡.**
Adults: 0.1 to 0.2 mg/kg P.O. daily for 3 to 6 weeks; then adjust for maintenance (usually 4 to 10 mg daily).
Children: 0.1 to 0.2 mg/kg or 3 to 6 mg/m^2 P.O. as a single dose. Reduce initial dose if given within 4 weeks after a full course of radiation therapy or myelosuppressive drugs or if pretreatment leukocyte or platelet counts are depressed from bone marrow disease.
▶ **Macroglobulinemia‡.** *Adults:* 2 to 10 mg P.O. daily. Or 8 mg/m^2 for 10 days with prednisone 30 mg/m^2 daily; repeat cycle every 6 to 8 weeks as needed.
▶ **Metastatic trophoblastic neoplasia‡.**
Adults: 6 to 10 mg P.O. daily for 5 days; repeat every 1 to 2 weeks.
▶ **Idiopathic uveitis‡.** *Adults:* 6 to 12 mg P.O. daily for 1 year.
▶ **Rheumatoid arthritis‡.** *Adults:* 0.1 to 0.3 mg/kg P.O. daily.

Contraindications and cautions

• Contraindicated in patients hypersensitive or resistant to previous therapy (those hypersensitive to other alkylating drugs also may be hypersensitive to chlorambucil).
• Use cautiously in patients with history of head trauma or seizures and in patients receiving other drugs that lower seizure threshold.
⚕ **Lifespan:** In pregnant women, use cautiously, if at all, because drug may harm fetus. In breast-feeding women, drug is contraindicated. In children, safety and effectiveness haven't been established, and potential benefits must be weighed against risks.

Reactions may be *common*, uncommon, *life-threatening*, or COMMON AND LIFE-THREATENING.

Adverse reactions

CNS: *seizures.*
GI: *nausea, stomatitis, vomiting.*
GU: *azoospermia, infertility.*
Hematologic: *anemia,* **myelosuppression** (usually moderate, gradual, and rapidly reversible), **neutropenia** (delayed up to 3 weeks, lasting up to 10 days after last dose), **thrombocytopenia.**
Hepatic: *hepatotoxicity.*
Metabolic: hyperuricemia.
Respiratory: interstitial pneumonitis, ***pulmonary fibrosis.***
Skin: exfoliative dermatitis, rash, ***Stevens-Johnson syndrome.***
Other: *allergic febrile reaction.*

Interactions

Drug-drug. *Anticoagulants, aspirin:* May increase risk of bleeding. Avoid use together. If drugs must be used together, monitor patient's coagulation studies.

Effects on lab test results

• May increase AST, ALT, alkaline phosphatase, and blood and urine uric acid levels. May decrease hemoglobin level and hematocrit.
• May decrease neutrophil, platelet, WBC, granulocyte, and RBC counts.

Pharmacokinetics

Absorption: Good.
Distribution: Highly bound to proteins.
Metabolism: Main metabolite, phenylacetic acid mustard, also has cytotoxic activity.
Excretion: In urine. *Half-life:* 2 hours for parent compound; 2½ hours for phenylacetic acid metabolite.

Route	Onset	Peak	Duration
P.O.	3–4 wk	1 hr	Unknown

Action

Chemical effect: Cross-links strands of cellular DNA and interferes with RNA transcription, causing growth imbalance that leads to cell death.
Therapeutic effect: Kills selected cancer cells.

Available forms

Tablets: 2 mg

⬛ Assessment

• Assess patient's underlying neoplastic disorder before and regularly during therapy.
• Monitor CBC and uric acid level.
• Be alert for adverse reactions and drug interactions.
• Assess patient's and family's knowledge of drug therapy.

⬤ Nursing diagnoses

• Ineffective health maintenance related to presence of neoplastic disease
• Ineffective protection related to drug-induced hematologic adverse reactions
• Deficient knowledge related to drug therapy

▶ Planning and implementation

• Dosage is based on patient's response.
• Drug-related nausea and vomiting usually can be controlled with antiemetics.
• Allopurinol may be used with adequate hydration to prevent hyperuricemia with resulting uric acid nephropathy.
• Follow institutional policy for infection control in immunocompromised patients if WBC count falls below 2,000/mm³ or granulocyte count falls below 1,000/mm³. Severe neutropenia is reversible up to cumulative dosage of 6.5 mg/kg in single course.

Patient teaching
• Warn patient to watch for signs of infection (fever, sore throat, fatigue) and bleeding (easy bruising, nosebleed, bleeding gums, melena). Tell him to take temperature daily.
• Instruct patient to avoid OTC products that contain aspirin.
• Tell patient to take drug 1 hour before breakfast and 2 hours after evening meal if he's bothered by nausea and vomiting.
• Instruct patient to maintain fluid intake of 2,400 to 3,000 ml daily, if not contraindicated.
• Tell patient to use contraceptive measures while using this drug.

✔ Evaluation

• Patient shows improvement in underlying neoplastic condition on follow-up diagnostic tests.
• Patient remains infection free and doesn't bleed abnormally.

• Patient and family state understanding of drug therapy.

HIGH ALERT!

chlordiazepoxide hydrochloride
(klor-digh-eh-zuh-POKS-ighd high-droh-KLOR-ighd)
Librium

Pharmacologic class: benzodiazepine
Therapeutic class: anxiolytic, sedative-hypnotic
Pregnancy risk category: D
Controlled substance schedule: IV

Indications and dosages

▶ **Mild to moderate anxiety.** *Adults:* 5 to 10 mg P.O. t.i.d. or q.i.d.
Children age 6 and older: 5 mg P.O. b.i.d. to q.i.d. Maximum dosage, 10 mg P.O. b.i.d. or t.i.d.
▶ **Severe anxiety.** *Adults:* 20 to 25 mg P.O. t.i.d. or q.i.d. Or 50 to 100 mg I.V. or I.M. initially, followed by 25 to 50 mg I.V. 3 or 4 times daily p.r.n.
Elderly patients: 5 mg P.O. b.i.d. to q.i.d.
▶ **Withdrawal symptoms of acute alcoholism.** *Adults:* 50 to 100 mg P.O., I.V., or I.M. Repeat in 2 to 4 hours, p.r.n. Maximum dosage is 300 mg daily.
▶ **Preoperative apprehension and anxiety.** *Adults:* 5 to 10 mg P.O. t.i.d. or q.i.d. on day preceding surgery. Or 50 to 100 mg I.M. 1 hour before surgery.

▼ I.V. administration

• Make sure equipment and staff needed for emergency airway management are available.
• Don't give packaged diluent I.V. because air bubbles may form.
• Use 5 ml normal saline solution or sterile water for injection as diluent for an ampule containing 100 mg of drug. Give slowly over 1 minute.
• Monitor respirations every 5 to 15 minutes after use and before each repeated dose.
⊗ **Incompatibilities**
Other I.V. drugs.

Contraindications and cautions

• Contraindicated in patients hypersensitive to drug.

• Use cautiously in patients with mental depression, porphyria, or hepatic or renal disease. In debilitated patients, use cautiously and at a reduced dosage.
⚘ **Lifespan:** In pregnant women, drug is contraindicated. Breast-feeding women shouldn't use drug because of risk of adverse effects in infant. In children younger than age 6, safety and effectiveness haven't been established. In children younger than age 12, parenteral use isn't recommended. In elderly patients, use smallest effective dose to avoid ataxia and oversedation.

Adverse reactions

CNS: confusion, drowsiness, fainting, hangover, lethargy, psychosis, restlessness, *suicidal tendencies.*
CV: *thrombophlebitis,* transient hypotension.
EENT: visual disturbances.
GI: abdominal discomfort, constipation, nausea, vomiting.
GU: incontinence, menstrual irregularities, urine retention.
Hematologic: *agranulocytosis.*
Skin: pain at injection site, swelling.

Interactions

Drug-drug. *Cimetidine:* May increase sedation. Monitor patient carefully.
CNS depressants: May increase CNS depression. Avoid use together.
Digoxin: May increase digoxin level and risk of toxicity. Monitor patient closely; monitor level.
Fluconazole, itraconazole, ketoconazole, miconazole: May increase and prolong levels, CNS depression, and psychomotor impairment. Avoid use together.
Drug-herb. *Kava:* May lead to excessive sedation. Discourage use together.
Drug-lifestyle. *Alcohol use:* May cause additive CNS effects. Strongly discourage alcohol use.
Smoking: May increase clearance of drug. Monitor patient for lack of effectiveness.

Effects on lab test results

• May increase liver function test values. May decrease granulocyte count.
• May cause false-positive reaction in Gravindex pregnancy test. May interfere with certain tests for urine 17-ketosteroids.

Pharmacokinetics

Absorption: Good with P.O. use.

Reactions may be *common,* uncommon, *life-threatening,* or COMMON AND LIFE-THREATENING.

Distribution: Wide. 80% to 90% protein-bound.
Metabolism: In liver to several active metabolites.
Excretion: Most metabolites in urine. *Half-life:* 5 to 30 hours.

Route	Onset	Peak	Duration
P.O., I.V.	Unknown	½–4 hr	Unknown
I.M.	¼–½ hr	½–4 hr	Unknown

Action

Chemical effect: May potentiate the effects of GABA in brain and suppress the spread of seizure activity produced by epileptogenic foci in the cortex, thalamus, and limbic structures.
Therapeutic effect: Relieves anxiety and promotes sleep and calmness.

Available forms

Capsules: 5 mg, 10 mg, 25 mg
Powder for injection: 100 mg/ampule

NURSING PROCESS

Assessment
• Assess patient's underlying condition before and regularly during therapy.
• Monitor liver, renal, and hematopoietic function studies periodically in patients receiving repeated or prolonged therapy.
• Monitor patient for abuse and addiction.
• Be alert for adverse reactions and drug interactions.
• Assess patient's and family's knowledge of drug therapy.

Nursing diagnoses
• Anxiety related to patient's underlying condition
• Risk for injury related to drug-induced CNS reactions
• Deficient knowledge related to drug therapy

Planning and implementation
• Don't give drug regularly for everyday stress.
• Make sure patient has swallowed tablets before you leave the bedside.
• **ALERT:** The 5-mg and 25-mg unit-dose capsules may appear similar in color when viewed through the package. Verify contents, and read label carefully.

• When using I.M., add 2 ml of diluent to powder and agitate gently until clear. Use immediately. I.M. form may be erratically absorbed.
• Recommended for I.M. use only, but may be given I.V.
• Injectable form comes in two types of ampules: as diluent and as powdered drug. Read directions carefully.
• Don't mix injectable form with any other parenteral drug.
• Refrigerate powder and keep away from light; mix just before use and discard remainder.
• Don't stop drug abruptly after long-term use because withdrawal symptoms may occur.
Patient teaching
• Warn patient to avoid hazardous activities that require alertness and good psychomotor coordination until CNS effects of drug are known.
• Tell patient to avoid alcohol while taking drug.
• Warn patient to take this drug only as directed and not to stop taking it without prescriber's approval. Inform patient of drug's potential for dependence if taken longer than directed.

Evaluation
• Patient says he's less anxious.
• Patient's safety is maintained.
• Patient and family state understanding of drug therapy.

chloroquine phosphate
(KLOR-oh-kwin FOS-fayt)
Aralen Phosphate

Pharmacologic class: 4-amino-quinoline
Therapeutic class: antimalarial, amebicide
Pregnancy risk category: C

Indications and dosages

▶ **Acute malarial attacks caused by** *Plasmodium vivax, P. malariae, P. ovale,* **and susceptible strains of** *P. falciparum. Adults:* 1 g (600-mg base) P.O. followed by 500 mg (300-mg base) P.O. after 6 to 8 hours; for next 2 days, a single dose of 500 mg (300-mg base) P.O.
Children: Initially, 10 mg (base)/kg P.O.; then 5 mg (base)/kg at 6, 24, and 48 hours (don't exceed adult dosage).
▶ **Malaria prophylaxis.** *Adults:* 500 mg (300-mg base) P.O. on the same day once week-

ly, beginning 2 weeks before exposure. Continue for 4 weeks after leaving endemic area. *Children:* 5 mg (base)/kg P.O. on the same day once weekly (not to exceed adult dosage), beginning 2 weeks before exposure.

▶ **Extraintestinal amebiasis.** *Adults:* 1 g (600-mg base) P.O. daily for 2 days; then 500 mg (300-mg base) daily for at least 2 to 3 weeks. Therapy usually is combined with intestinal amebicide.

▶ **Rheumatoid arthritis‡.** *Adults:* 250 mg P.O. with evening meal.

▶ **Lupus erythematosus‡.** *Adults:* 250 mg P.O. daily with evening meal; reduce dosage gradually over several months when lesions regress.

Contraindications and cautions

• Contraindicated in patients hypersensitive to drug and in patients with retinal changes, visual field changes, or porphyria.

• Use cautiously in patients with severe GI, neurologic, or blood disorders. Also use cautiously in patients with hepatic disease or alcoholism (drug concentrates in liver), and in those with G6PD deficiency or psoriasis (drug may exacerbate these conditions).

⚜ **Lifespan:** In pregnant women, don't use except in women who may have been exposed to active malaria because fetal risks of malaria outweigh risks of drug. Warn pregnant women or those planning to become pregnant to avoid exposure to malaria. Breast-feeding women should stop breast-feeding or stop the drug.

Adverse reactions

CNS: dizziness, fatigue, irritability, mild and transient headache, neuromyopathy, nightmares, psychic stimulation, *seizures.*
CV: ECG changes, hypotension.
EENT: ototoxicity (with prolonged high doses), *visual disturbances* (blurred vision; trouble focusing; reversible corneal changes; typically irreversible, sometimes progressive or delayed retinal changes, such as narrowing of arterioles; macular lesions; pallor of optic disk; optic atrophy; patchy retinal pigmentation, typically leading to blindness).
GI: abdominal cramps, anorexia, diarrhea, nausea, stomatitis, vomiting.
Hematologic: *agranulocytosis, aplastic anemia,* hemolytic anemia, *thrombocytopenia.*

Skin: lichen planus eruptions, pleomorphic skin eruptions, pruritus, skin and mucosal pigment changes.

Interactions

Drug-drug. *Aluminum salts, kaolin, magnesium:* May decrease GI absorption. Separate doses.
Cimetidine: May decrease hepatic metabolism of chloroquine. Monitor patient for toxicity.
Drug-lifestyle. *Sun exposure:* May worsen drug-induced dermatoses. Tell patient to avoid excessive sun exposure and to wear protective clothing and sunblock.

Effects on lab test results

• May decrease hemoglobin level and hematocrit.
• May decrease granulocyte and platelet counts.

Pharmacokinetics

Absorption: Quick and almost complete.
Distribution: In liver, spleen, kidneys, heart, and brain and is strongly bound in melanin-containing cells.
Metabolism: 30%.
Excretion: 70% unchanged in urine; unabsorbed drug in feces. Small amounts of drug may be present in urine for months after drug is stopped. Renal excretion is enhanced by urine acidification. *Half-life:* 1 to 2 months.

Route	Onset	Peak	Duration
P.O.	Unknown	1–3 hr	Unknown

Action

Chemical effect: May bind to and alter properties of DNA in susceptible parasites.
Therapeutic effect: Prevents or eradicates malarial infections; eradicates amebiasis.

Available forms

Tablets: 250 mg (150-mg base), 500 mg (300-mg base)

NURSING PROCESS

🔞 **Assessment**
• Assess patient's infection before and regularly during therapy.
• Make sure baseline and periodic ophthalmic examinations are performed. After long-term use, check periodically for ocular muscle weakness.

Reactions may be *common*, uncommon, *life-threatening*, or COMMON AND LIFE-THREATENING.

- Assist patient with obtaining audiometric examinations before, during, and after therapy, especially long-term therapy.
- Monitor CBC and liver function studies periodically during long-term therapy.
- Be alert for adverse reactions and drug interactions.
- Assess patient for potential overdose, which can quickly lead to toxic symptoms: headache, drowsiness, visual disturbances, CV collapse, and seizures, followed by cardiopulmonary arrest. Children are highly susceptible to toxicity.
- Assess patient's and family's knowledge of drug therapy.

Nursing diagnoses
- Ineffective protection related to presence of organisms susceptible to drug
- Disturbed sensory perception (visual or auditory) related to adverse reactions to drug
- Deficient knowledge related to drug therapy

Planning and implementation
- Give drug at same time of same day each week.
- **ALERT:** Give missed doses as soon as possible. To avoid doubling doses in regimens requiring more than one dose per day, give missed dose within 1 hour of scheduled time or omit dose altogether.
- Give drug with milk or meals to minimize GI distress. Tablets may be crushed and mixed with food or chocolate syrup for patients who have trouble swallowing; however, drug has bitter taste and patients may find mixture unpleasant. Crushed tablets may be placed inside empty gelatin capsules, which are easier to swallow.
- Store drug in amber-colored containers to protect from light.
- Begin prophylactic antimalarial therapy 2 weeks before exposure and continue for 4 weeks after patient leaves endemic area.
- Monitor patient's weight for significant changes because dose is based on weight.
- If patient develops severe blood disorder not attributable to disease, notify prescriber and stop drug.

Patient teaching
- Tell patient to take drug with food at same time on same day each week.

- Instruct patient to avoid excessive sun exposure to avoid worsening drug-induced dermatoses.
- Tell patient to report blurred vision, increased sensitivity to light, trouble hearing, ringing in the ears, and muscle weakness.
- Warn patient to avoid alcohol while taking drug.
- Teach patient how to take missed doses.

Evaluation
- Patient is free from infection.
- Patient maintains normal visual and auditory function.
- Patient and family state understanding of drug therapy.

chlorothiazide
(klor-oh-THIGH-uh-zighd)
Diuril

chlorothiazide sodium
Diuril Sodium Intravenous

Pharmacologic class: diuretic
Therapeutic class: thiazide diuretic, antihypertensive
Pregnancy risk category: C

Indications and dosages
▶ **Edema, hypertension.** *Adults:* 500 mg to 1 g P.O. or I.V. daily or in divided doses.
▶ **Diuresis, hypertension.** *Children and infants age 6 months and older:* 10 to 20 mg/kg P.O. daily in divided doses, not to exceed 375 mg daily.
Infants age 6 months and younger: May require 30 mg/kg P.O. daily in two divided doses.

I.V. administration
- Reconstitute 500 mg with 18 ml sterile water for injection.
- Inject reconstituted drug directly into vein; through I.V. line containing free-flowing, compatible solution; or through intermittent infusion device. Compatible solutions include dextrose and saline.
- Monitor the patient for signs and symptoms of I.V. infiltration.
- Avoid simultaneous administration with whole blood and its derivatives.

• If hypersensitivity reactions occur, stop drug and notify prescriber.
• Store reconstituted solutions at room temperature up to 24 hours.

⊗ **Incompatibilities**
Amikacin; chlorpromazine; codeine; hydralazine; insulin (regular); Ionosol B, D, or K and invert sugar 10%; Ionosol B or D-CM and dextrose 5%; Ionosol PSL; levorphanol; methadone; morphine; norepinephrine; Normosol-M (900 calories); Normosol-M in dextrose 5%; Normosol-R in dextrose 5%; polymyxin B; procaine; prochlorperazine; promazine; promethazine hydrochloride; streptomycin; triflupromazine; vancomycin; vitamin B complex with C; whole blood and its derivatives.

Contraindications and cautions

• Contraindicated in patients hypersensitive to other thiazides or other sulfonamide-derived drugs and in patients with anuria.
• Use cautiously in patients with severe renal disease or impaired hepatic function.

⚘ **Lifespan:** In pregnant or breast-feeding women, safety and effectiveness haven't been established. In children, I.V. use isn't recommended.

Adverse reactions

CV: orthostatic hypotension.
GI: anorexia, nausea, *pancreatitis.*
GU: frequent urination, impotence, nocturia, polyuria, *renal impairment.*
Hematologic: *agranulocytosis, aplastic anemia, leukopenia, thrombocytopenia.*
Hepatic: *hepatic encephalopathy.*
Metabolic: asymptomatic hyperuricemia; fluid and electrolyte imbalances, including hyperkalemia, dilutional hypochloremia and hyponatremia, and metabolic alkalosis; gout; hyperglycemia; hypokalemia; and impaired glucose tolerance.
Skin: dermatitis, photosensitivity, rash.
Other: hypersensitivity reaction.

Interactions

Drug-drug. *Barbiturates, opioids:* May increase risk of orthostatic hypotension. Monitor blood pressure closely.
Bumetanide, chlorthalidone, ethacrynic acid, furosemide, hydrochlorothiazide, indapamide, metolazone, torsemide: May cause excessive diuretic response and serious electrolyte abnormalities or dehydration. Adjust doses carefully while monitoring the patient closely.
Cholestyramine, colestipol: May decrease intestinal absorption of thiazides. Separate doses.
Diazoxide: May increase antihypertensive, hyperglycemic, and hyperuricemic effects. Use together cautiously.
Digoxin: May increase risk of digitalis toxicity from chlorothiazide-induced hypokalemia. Monitor potassium and digitalis levels.
Lithium: May decrease lithium clearance, increasing risk of lithium toxicity. Monitor lithium level.
NSAIDs: May increase risk of NSAID-induced renal impairment. Monitor patient for this reaction.
Drug-herb. *Licorice root:* May worsen the potassium depletion caused by thiazides. Avoid use together.
Drug-lifestyle. *Alcohol use:* May increase orthostatic hypotension. Monitor patient closely and place patient on fall precautions.

Effects on lab test results

• May increase uric acid, glucose, and calcium levels. May decrease potassium, sodium, chloride, and hemoglobin levels and hematocrit.
• May decrease granulocyte, WBC, and platelet counts.

Pharmacokinetics

Absorption: Incomplete and variable.
Distribution: Unknown.
Metabolism: None.
Excretion: Unchanged in urine. *Half-life:* 1 to 2 hours.

Route	Onset	Peak	Duration
P.O.	≤ 2 hr	4 hr	6–12 hr
I.V.	≤ 15 min	30 min	6–12 hr

Action

Chemical effect: Increases sodium and water excretion by inhibiting sodium reabsorption in nephron's cortical diluting site.
Therapeutic effect: Promotes sodium and water excretion.

Available forms

Injection: 500-mg vial
Oral suspension: 250 mg/5 ml
Tablets: 250 mg, 500 mg

NURSING PROCESS

⚡ Assessment

• Assess patient's underlying condition before therapy and regularly thereafter.
• Monitor the drug's effectiveness by regularly checking blood pressure, fluid intake, urine output, blood pressure, and weight.
• Expect therapeutic response to be delayed several days in patients with hypertension.
• Monitor electrolyte and glucose levels.
• Monitor creatinine and BUN levels regularly. If they're more than twice normal, drug isn't as effective.
• Monitor blood uric acid level, especially in patients with history of gout.
• Be alert for adverse reactions and drug interactions.
• Assess patient's and family's knowledge of drug therapy.

⊕ Nursing diagnoses

• Excessive fluid volume related to patient's underlying condition
• Impaired urinary elimination related to drug therapy
• Deficient knowledge related to drug therapy

▶ Planning and implementation

• To prevent nocturia, give drug in the morning.
• Many patients with edema respond to intermittent therapy. Intermittent use reduces the risk of excessive response and electrolyte imbalances.
⊛ **ALERT:** Never inject I.M. or subcutaneously.
• Drug may be used with potassium-sparing diuretic to prevent potassium loss.
• Stop thiazides and thiazide-like diuretics before parathyroid function tests are performed.
Patient teaching
• Teach patient and family to identify and report signs of hypersensitivity and hypokalemia.
• Teach patient to monitor fluid intake and output and daily weight.
• Instruct patient to avoid high-sodium foods and to choose high-potassium foods.
• Tell patient to take drug in the morning to avoid nocturia.
• Advise patient to avoid sudden posture changes and to rise slowly to avoid orthostatic hypotension.
• Advise patient to use sunblock in order to prevent photosensitivity reactions.

• Teach patient the importance of periodic laboratory tests to detect electrolyte imbalances.

✅ Evaluation

• Patient is free from edema.
• Patient adjusts lifestyle to cope with altered patterns of urine elimination.
• Patient and family state understanding of drug therapy.

chlorpromazine hydrochloride

(klor-PROH-meh-zeen high-droh-KLOR-ighd)
Largactil ◆ , Thorazine

Pharmacologic class: aliphatic phenothiazine
Therapeutic class: antipsychotic, antiemetic
Pregnancy risk category: C

Indications and dosages

▶ **Psychosis.** *Adults:* Initially, 30 to 75 mg P.O. daily in two to four divided doses. Increase dosage by 20 to 50 mg twice weekly until symptoms are controlled. Some patients may need up to 800 mg daily. Or, for prompt control of severe symptoms, 25 mg I.M., followed by 25 to 50 mg I.M. in 1 hour if needed, then gradually increase dosage every 4 to 6 hours to maximum of 400 mg/dose. Switch to P.O. use as soon as symptoms are controlled.
Children age 6 months and older: 0.55 mg/kg P.O. every 4 to 6 hours or I.M. every 6 to 8 hours. Or 1.1 mg/kg P.R. every 6 to 8 hours. Maximum I.M. dose in children younger than age 5 or weighing less than 22.7 kg (50 lb) is 40 mg. Maximum I.M. dose in children ages 5 to 12 or weighing 22.7 to 45.5 kg (100 lb) is 75 mg.
▶ **Nausea and vomiting.** *Adults:* 10 to 25 mg P.O. every 4 to 6 hours, p.r.n. Or 50 to 100 mg P.R. every 6 to 8 hours, p.r.n. Or, 25 mg I.M. If no hypotension occurs, give 25 to 50 mg I.M. every 3 to 4 hours p.r.n. until vomiting stops.
Children and infants age 6 months and older: 0.55 mg/kg P.O. every 4 to 6 hours or I.M. every 6 to 8 hours. Or 1.1 mg/kg P.R. every 6 to 8 hours. Maximum I.M. dose in children younger than age 5 or weighing less than 22.7 kg is 40 mg. Maximum I.M. dose in children ages 5 to 12 or weighing 22.7 to 45.5 kg is 75 mg.
▶ **Intractable hiccups, acute intermittent porphyria.** *Adults:* 25 to 50 mg P.O. t.i.d. or

q.i.d. If symptoms persist for 2 to 3 days, 25 to 50 mg I.M. If symptoms still persist, 25 to 50 mg diluted in 500 to 1,000 ml normal saline solution and infused slowly, while patient lies supine.

▶ **Adjunct treatment of tetanus.** *Adults:* 25 to 50 mg I.V. or I.M. t.i.d. or q.i.d., usually with barbiturates.

Children and infants age 6 months and older: 0.5 mg/kg I.M. or I.V. every 6 to 8 hours. Maximum parenteral dosage in children weighing less than 22.7 kg is 40 mg daily; in children weighing 22.7 to 45.5 kg, 75 mg daily, except in severe cases.

▶ **To relieve apprehension and nervousness before surgery and to control acute nausea and vomiting during surgery.** *Adults:* Preoperatively, 25 to 50 mg P.O. 2 to 3 hours before surgery or 12.5 to 25 mg I.M. 1 to 2 hours before surgery. To control acute nausea and vomiting during surgery, 12.5 mg I.M.; repeat after 30 minutes if needed or fractional 2-mg doses I.V. at 2-minute intervals; maximum dose, 25 mg. Postoperatively, 10 to 25 mg P.O. every 4 to 6 hours or 12.5 mg to 25 mg I.M.; repeat in 1 hour if needed.

Children and infants age 6 months and older: Preoperatively, 0.5 mg/kg P.O. 2 to 3 hours before surgery or I.M. 1 to 2 hours before surgery. To control acute nausea and vomiting during surgery, 0.25 mg/kg I.M. repeated after 30 minutes, if needed or fractional 1-mg doses I.V. at 2-minute intervals, maximum dose, 0.25 mg/kg. May repeat fractional I.V. regimen in 30 minutes, if needed; postoperatively, 0.55 mg/kg P.O. every 4 to 6 hours or 0.55 mg/kg I.M.; repeat in 1 hour if needed and hypotension doesn't occur.

▼ I.V. administration

• Drug is compatible with most common I.V. solutions, including D_5W, Ringer's injection, lactated Ringer's injection, and normal saline solution for injection.

• For direct injection, drug may be diluted with normal saline solution for injection and injected into large vein or through tubing of free-flowing I.V. solution.

• Don't exceed 1 mg/minute for adults or 0.5 mg/minute for children.

• For I.V. infusion, dilute with 500 or 1,000 ml normal saline solution and infuse slowly, while patient lies supine.

⊗ Incompatibilities

Aminophylline, amphotericin B, ampicillin, chloramphenicol sodium succinate, chlorothiazide, cimetidine, dimenhydrinate, furosemide, heparin sodium, linezolid, melphalan, methohexital, paclitaxel, penicillin, pentobarbital, phenobarbital, solutions having a pH of 4 to 5, thiopental.

Contraindications and cautions

• Contraindicated in patients hypersensitive to drug and in patients with CNS depression, bone marrow suppression, subcortical damage, and coma.

• Use cautiously in debilitated patients and in those with hepatic or renal disease, severe CV disease (may cause sudden drop in blood pressure); exposure to extreme heat or cold (including antipyretic therapy); exposure to organophosphate insecticides, respiratory disorders, hypocalcemia, seizure disorders; severe reactions to insulin or electroconvulsive therapy; glaucoma; or prostatic hyperplasia.

🎋 **Lifespan:** In pregnant or breast-feeding women, drug isn't recommended. In acutely ill or dehydrated children, use cautiously. In elderly patients, use cautiously.

Adverse reactions

CNS: dizziness, extrapyramidal reactions, *neuroleptic malignant syndrome,* pseudoparkinsonism, sedation, *seizures,* tardive dyskinesia.
CV: ECG changes, *orthostatic hypotension,* tachycardia.
EENT: blurred vision, ocular changes.
GI: constipation, dry mouth.
GU: *erectile dysfunction,* inhibited ejaculation, menstrual irregularities, urine retention.
Hematologic: *agranulocytosis, aplastic anemia, hyperprolactinemia, thrombocytopenia, transient leukopenia.*
Hepatic: cholestatic jaundice.
Skin: mild photosensitivity.
Other: allergic reactions, gynecomastia, I.M. injection site pain, sterile abscess.

Interactions

Drug-drug. *Antacids:* May inhibit absorption of oral phenothiazines. Separate antacid and phenothiazine doses by at least 2 hours.
Anticholinergics, including antidepressants and antiparkinsonians: May increase anticholinergic

---

Reactions may be *common,* uncommon, *life-threatening,* or COMMON AND LIFE-THREATENING.

C

activity and aggravate parkinsonian symptoms. Use with caution.

Barbiturates, lithium: May decrease phenothiazine effect. Observe patient.

Centrally acting antihypertensives: May decrease antihypertensive effect. Monitor patient's blood pressure carefully.

CNS depressants: May increase CNS depression. Avoid use together.

Meperidine: May cause excessive sedation and hypotension. Don't use together.

Propranolol: May increase propranolol and chlorpromazine levels. Monitor patient.

Warfarin: May decrease effect of oral anticoagulants. Monitor PT and INR.

Drug-herb. *Dong quai, St. John's wort:* May increase risk of photosensitivity. Discourage prolonged or unprotected exposure to sunlight.

Kava: May increase the risk or severity of dystonic reactions. Discourage use together.

Yohimbe: May increase risk of toxicity. Discourage use together.

Drug-lifestyle. *Alcohol use:* May increase CNS depression, particularly psychomotor skills. Strongly discourage alcohol use.

Sun exposure: May increase photosensitivity. Discourage prolonged or unprotected exposure to sun.

Effects on lab test results

- May increase CK, GGT, and prolactin levels. May decrease hemoglobin level and hematocrit.
- May increase eosinophil count. May decrease WBC, granulocyte, and platelet counts.

Pharmacokinetics

Absorption: Erratic and variable with oral use; rapid with I.M. use.

Distribution: Wide; level usually is higher in CNS than plasma. 91% to 99% protein-bound.

Metabolism: Extensive. Forms 10 to 12 metabolites, and some are pharmacologically active.

Excretion: Most of drug as metabolites in urine; some in feces. Drug may undergo enterohepatic circulation. *Half-life:* 20 to 24 hours.

Route	Onset	Peak	Duration
P.O.	30–60 min	1–4 hr	4–6 hr
P.O. controlled-release	30–60 min	1–4 hr	10–12 hr
I.V., I.M.	Unknown	Unknown	Unknown
P.R.	>1 hr	1–4 hr	3–4 hr

Action

Chemical effect: May block postsynaptic dopamine receptors in brain and inhibit medullary chemoreceptor trigger zone.

Therapeutic effect: Relieves nausea and vomiting, hiccups, signs and symptoms of psychosis, acute intermittent porphyria, and tetanus. Produces calmness and sleep preoperatively.

Available forms

Capsules (controlled-release): 30 mg, 75 mg, 150 mg
Injection: 25 mg/ml
Oral concentrate: 30 mg/ml, 100 mg/ml
Suppositories: 25 mg, 100 mg
Syrup: 10 mg/5 ml
Tablets: 10 mg, 25 mg, 50 mg, 100 mg, 200 mg

NURSING PROCESS

Assessment

- Assess patient's underlying condition before therapy and regularly thereafter.
- Be alert for adverse reactions and drug interactions.
- Monitor blood pressure regularly. Watch for orthostatic hypotension, especially with parenteral use. Monitor blood pressure before and after I.M. use.
- Monitor patient for tardive dyskinesia, which may occur after prolonged use. It may not appear until months or years later and may disappear spontaneously or persist for life despite stopping drug.
- Watch for symptoms of neuroleptic malignant syndrome. It's rare, but commonly fatal. It isn't necessarily related to length of drug use or type of neuroleptic, but more than 60% of affected patients are men.
- Monitor therapy with weekly bilirubin tests during the first month, periodic blood tests (CBC and liver function), and ophthalmic tests (long-term use).
- Assess patient's and family's knowledge of drug therapy.

Nursing diagnoses

- Ineffective health maintenance related to patient's underlying condition
- Impaired physical mobility related to drug-induced extrapyramidal reactions
- Deficient knowledge related to drug therapy

>> Planning and implementation

⊛ **ALERT:** Wear gloves when preparing solutions, and prevent contact with skin and clothing. Oral liquid and parenteral forms can cause contact dermatitis.

• Slight yellowing of injection or concentrate is common; potency isn't affected. Discard very discolored solutions.

• Protect liquid concentrate from light.

• Dilute liquid forms with fruit juice, milk, or semisolid food just before giving.

• Don't give chlorpromazine oral solution and carbamazepine oral solutions together. Mixing causes orange, rubbery precipitate with unknown effect on bioavailability of either drug.

• Shake syrup before giving.

• Don't crush controlled-release form.

• Give deep I.M. only in upper outer quadrant of buttocks. Massage slowly afterward to prevent sterile abscess. Injection stings.

• Store suppositories in cool place.

• Keep patient supine for 1 hour after parenteral delivery, and advise him to get up slowly.

• Don't stop drug abruptly unless required by severe adverse reactions. After abruptly stopping long-term therapy, the patient may experience gastritis, nausea, vomiting, dizziness, and tremors.

• If patient develops jaundice; symptoms of blood dyscrasia (fever, sore throat, infection, cellulitis, weakness); extrapyramidal reactions that last longer than a few hours, or if a pregnant woman or a child develops extrapyramidal reaction, stop drug and notify prescriber.

• Dystonic reactions may often be treated with diphenhydramine or an antiparkinsonian drug.

⊛ **ALERT:** Don't confuse chlorpromazine with chlorpropamide or clomipramine.

Patient teaching

• Warn patient to avoid activities that require alertness or good psychomotor coordination until CNS effects of drug are known. Drowsiness and dizziness usually subside after first few weeks.

• Instruct patient to avoid alcohol while taking drug.

• Tell patient to notify prescriber about urine retention or constipation.

• Urge patient to use sunblock and wear protective clothing to avoid photosensitivity reactions. Chlorpromazine causes higher risk of photosensitivity than other drugs in its class.

• Instruct patient to use sugarless gum or hard candy to relieve dry mouth.

• Caution patient not to stop taking drug suddenly but to take it exactly as prescribed and not to double doses to compensate for missed ones.

• Tell patient which fluids are appropriate for diluting concentrate, and show dropper technique for measuring dose. Warn patient to avoid spilling liquid on skin because it may cause rash and irritation.

• Advise patient that injection stings.

☑ Evaluation

• Patient has fewer signs and symptoms.

• Patient maintains physical mobility throughout drug therapy.

• Patient and family state understanding of drug therapy.

cholestyramine
(koh-leh-STIGH-ruh-meen)
Prevalite, Questran, Questran Light

Pharmacologic class: anion exchange resin
Therapeutic class: antilipemic, bile acid sequestrant
Pregnancy risk category: C

Indications and dosages

▶ **Primary hyperlipidemia or pruritus caused by partial bile obstruction; adjunct for reduction of elevated cholesterol level in patients with primary hypercholesterolemia.**
Adults: 4 g P.O. t.i.d. before meals. Maintenance dosage is 4 g t.i.d. before meals or q.i.d. before meals and at bedtime. Maximum, 24 g daily.
Children: 240 mg/kg daily in two or three divided doses. Maximum, 8 g daily.

Contraindications and cautions

• Contraindicated in patients hypersensitive to bile-acid sequestering resins and in patients with complete biliary obstruction.

• Use cautiously in patients at risk for constipation and in those with conditions aggravated by constipation, such as severe, symptomatic coronary artery disease.

☀ **Lifespan:** In pregnant and breast-feeding women, use cautiously because of interference with fat-soluble vitamin absorption.

Adverse reactions

GI: *abdominal discomfort, constipation,* fecal impaction, flatulence, hemorrhoids, *nausea,* steatorrhea, vomiting.
Metabolic: folic acid deficiency; **hyperchloremic acidosis** (with long-term use or very high dosage); vitamin A, D, E, and K deficiency.
Skin: irritation of skin, tongue, and perianal area; rash.

Interactions

Drug-drug. *Acetaminophen, beta blockers, corticosteroids, digoxin, fat-soluble vitamins (A, D, E, and K), iron preparations, thiazide diuretics, thyroid hormones, warfarin and other coumarin derivatives:* May reduce absorption of these drugs. Give at least 1 hour before or 4 to 6 hours after cholestyramine.

Effects on lab test results

• May increase alkaline phosphatase and chloride levels. May decrease cholesterol; vitamins A, D, E, and K; folic acid; and hemoglobin levels and hematocrit.

Pharmacokinetics

Absorption: Not absorbed.
Distribution: None.
Metabolism: None.
Excretion: Insoluble drug with bile acid complex in feces. *Half-life:* Unknown.

Route	Onset	Peak	Duration
P.O.	1–2 wk	Unknown	2–4 wk

Action

Chemical effect: Combines with bile acid to form insoluble compound that's excreted. The liver must synthesize new bile acid from cholesterol, which reduces LDL cholesterol levels. Excretion of excess bile acids may decrease pruritus associated with partial cholestasis.
Therapeutic effect: Reduces cholesterol level and pruritus.

Available forms

Powder: 210-, 231-, 239-, 378-g cans; 5-, 5.7-, 9-g single-dose packets (4 g of cholestyramine resin in each scoop of powder or single-dose packet)

Assessment
• Assess patient's cholesterol level and pruritus before therapy.
• Monitor drug effectiveness by checking cholesterol and triglyceride levels in 4 weeks and every 3 to 6 months thereafter; also, ask patient whether pruritus has diminished or abated.
• Be alert for adverse reactions and drug interactions.
• Monitor patient for fat-soluble vitamin deficiency because long-term use may be linked to deficiency of vitamins A, D, E, and K and folic acid.
• Assess patient's and family's knowledge of drug therapy.

Nursing diagnoses
• Risk for injury related to elevated cholesterol level
• Constipation related to drug-induced adverse GI reactions
• Deficient knowledge related to drug therapy

Planning and implementation
• To mix powder, sprinkle on surface of preferred beverage or wet food (soup, applesauce, crushed pineapple). Let stand a few minutes; then stir to obtain uniform suspension. Mixing with carbonated beverages may cause excess foaming. Use large glass, and mix slowly.
• Give drug before meals and at bedtime.
• If therapy is stopped, lower the dose of digoxin to avoid toxicity.
• If severe constipation develops, lower the dose, add stool softener, increase fiber, and give a laxative if needed; or stop drug.
• Give all other drugs at least 1 hour before or 4 to 6 hours after cholestyramine to avoid blocking their absorption.
• Cholestyramine light contains 28.1 mg of phenylalanine per 6.4-g dose.
Patient teaching
• Instruct patient never to take drug in its dry form; esophageal irritation or severe constipation may result. Tell the patient to sprinkle powder on surface of preferred beverage in a large glass; to let mixture stand a few minutes; then to stir thoroughly. The best diluents are water, milk, and juice (especially pulpy fruit juice). Tell him that mixing with carbonated beverages

could cause excess foaming. Tell him to swirl small additional amount of liquid in same glass and then to drink it all to make sure he took the whole dose.

• Advise patient to take all other drugs at least 1 hour before or 4 to 6 hours after cholestyramine to avoid blocking their absorption.

• Teach patient about proper dietary management of serum lipids (restricting total fat and cholesterol intake), as well as measures to control other cardiac disease risk factors.

• When appropriate, recommend weight control, exercise, and smoking-cessation programs.

☑ Evaluation

• Patient's cholesterol level is normal with drug therapy.

• Patient maintains normal bowel patterns throughout drug therapy.

• Patient and family state understanding of drug therapy.

✳ New Drug

ciclesonide
(sigh-CLEH-so-nighd)
Omnaris

Pharmacologic class: nonhalogenated glucocorticoid
Therapeutic class: anti-inflammatory
Pregnancy risk category: C

Indications and dosages

▶ **Nasal symptoms associated with seasonal and perennial allergic rhinitis.** *Adults and children age 12 and older:* Two sprays in each nostril once daily, totaling 200 mcg/day.

Contraindications and cautions

• Contraindicated in patients who are hypersensitive to the drug or its components and in patients who have had recent nasal septal ulcers, nasal surgery, or nasal trauma, until healing has occurred.

• Use cautiously in patients who have changed from systemic to inhaled corticosteroids because signs of renal insufficiency or steroid withdrawal (pain, lassitude, depression), or acute worsening of their symptoms may occur.

• Use cautiously in immunosuppressed patients or in those with wounds, because corticosteroids suppress the immune system.

⚕ **Lifespan:** In pregnant women, use drug only if benefit to the mother outweighs risk to the fetus. Infants born to mothers taking the drug during pregnancy may develop hypoadrenalism; monitor infant closely. In breast-feeding women, use drug cautiously. It isn't known if drug appears in breast milk but other corticosteroids do appear in breast milk. In children older than age 12, use drug cautiously because it may slow growth rate. In children younger than age 12, safety and effectiveness haven't been established. Drug may cause a decline in growth velocity. The potential to regain growth after stopping drug hasn't been studied; risks versus benefits should be weighed. If deemed beneficial, growth should be monitored closely, and the lowest dosage possible should be used.

Adverse reactions

CNS: headache.
EENT: epistaxis, nasopharyngitis, ear pain, nasal discomfort.
Metabolic: growth retardation.

Interactions

None significant.

Effects on lab test results

None reported.

Pharmacokinetics

Absorption: Absorbed intranasally. Drug isn't absorbed from the GI tract, but its metabolite may be detectable in serum.
Distribution: More than 99% bound to plasma proteins.
Metabolism: In the liver, by CYP3A4 and CYP2D6 isoenzymes.
Excretion: After I.V. administration, 66% eliminated through bile and 20% in urine. *Half-life:* Unknown.

Route	Onset	Peak	Duration
Intranasally	1–2 days	1–5 wk	Unknown

Action

Chemical effect: Hydrolyzed by the nasal mucosa to a biologically active metabolite with anti-inflammatory properties that inhibits mast cells, eosinophils, neutrophils, leukotrienes, and cytokines.
Therapeutic effect: Decreases nasal inflammation caused by allergies.

Available forms

Nasal suspension: 50 mcg/metered spray

NURSING PROCESS

⚡ Assessment
• Obtain history of patient's condition before therapy, and reassess regularly thereafter.
• Assess for adverse reactions.
• Assess patient's and family's knowledge of drug therapy.

⊕ Nursing diagnoses
• Ineffective health maintenance related to allergy-induced nasal congestion
• Risk of injury related to drug-induced adverse reactions
• Deficient knowledge related to drug therapy

▷ Planning and implementation
• Monitor patient switching from systemic to inhaled corticosteroid; acute worsening of symptoms and other withdrawal side effects could occur.
• Monitor children for decline in growth rate. The potential to regain growth after discontinuing drug hasn't been studied.
• Monitor patient for nasal side effects.
• Warn patient taking immunosuppressants to avoid exposure to people with active infections.
Patient teaching
• Teach patient how to properly use inhaler. Tell him to read the package insert to ensure proper use.
• Tell patient to contact his prescriber if he has no relief from symptoms after 1 week.
• Advise patient to use drug every day.
• Warn patient to avoid exposure to people with infections (such as chickenpox or measles) because of the immunosuppressant effect of corticosteroids.

✔ Evaluation
• Patient's nasal congestion subsides.
• Patient is free from adverse reactions.
• Patient and family state understanding of drug therapy.

cidofovir
(sigh-doh-FOH-veer)
Vistide

Pharmacologic class: inhibitor of viral DNA synthesis
Therapeutic class: antiviral
Pregnancy risk category: C

Indications and dosages

▶ **CMV retinitis in patients with AIDS.**
Adults: 5 mg/kg I.V. infused over 1 hour once weekly for 2 consecutive weeks, followed by maintenance dosage of 5 mg/kg I.V. infused over 1 hour once every 2 weeks. Probenecid and prehydration with normal saline solution I.V. must be given at the same time and may reduce risk of nephrotoxicity.

⊠ **Adjust-a-dose:** For patients with renal impairment, if creatinine level increases 0.3 to 0.4 mg/dl above baseline, reduce dose to 3 mg/kg at same rate and frequency. If creatinine level increases 0.5 mg/dl or more above baseline, or if patient develops 3+ proteinuria, stop drug.

▽ I.V. administration

• Because of the mutagenic properties of drug, prepare in a class II laminar flow biological safety cabinet. Wear surgical gloves and a closed front surgical gown with knit cuffs.
• If drug contacts skin or membranes, wash and flush thoroughly with water. Place excess drug and all other materials used in the admixture preparation and administration in a leak-proof, puncture-proof container. Dispose of by high temperature.
• To prepare drug for infusion, remove it from vial using syringe, and transfer dose to an infusion bag containing 100 ml normal saline solution.
• Compatibility with Ringer's solution, lactated Ringer's solution, or bacteriostatic infusion fluids hasn't been evaluated.
• Infuse entire volume I.V. at constant rate over 1 hour. Use a standard infusion pump. Because of the risk of increased nephrotoxicity, don't exceed recommended dose, frequency, or rate of administration.
• Give admixtures for infusion within 24 hours of preparation.

• If admixtures aren't used immediately, they may be refrigerated at 36° to 46° F (2° to 8° C) for longer than 24 hours. Let drug reach room temperature before use.
⊗ **Incompatibilities**
Don't add other drugs or supplements to admixture.

Contraindications and cautions

• Contraindicated in patients hypersensitive to drug and in those with history of severe hypersensitivity to probenecid or other sulfa-containing drugs.
• Use cautiously in patients with renal impairment.
⚘ **Lifespan:** In pregnancy, use only if potential benefits to mother outweigh risks to fetus. In women who are breast-feeding, use cautiously. It isn't known whether drug appears in breast milk. In children, safety and effectiveness haven't been studied.

Adverse reactions

CNS: abnormal gait, amnesia, anxiety, *asthenia,* confusion, depression, dizziness, *fever,* hallucinations, *headache,* insomnia, malaise, neuropathy, paresthesia, **seizures,** somnolence, syncope.
CV: facial edema, hypotension, orthostatic hypotension, pallor, tachycardia, vasodilation.
EENT: abnormal vision, amblyopia, conjunctivitis, eye disorders, iritis, *ocular hypotony,* pharyngitis, retinal detachment, rhinitis, sinusitis, uveitis.
GI: *abdominal pain, anorexia,* aphthous stomatitis, colitis, constipation, *diarrhea,* dry mouth, dyspepsia, dysphagia, flatulence, gastritis, melena, mouth ulcerations, *nausea,* oral candidiasis, taste disturbance, tongue discoloration, rectal disorders, stomatitis, *vomiting.*
GU: glycosuria, hematuria, **nephrotoxicity,** *proteinuria,* urinary incontinence, UTI.
Hematologic: *anemia,* **neutropenia, thrombocytopenia.**
Hepatic: hepatomegaly.
Metabolic: decreased bicarbonate level, fluid imbalance, hyperglycemia, hyperlipidemia, **hyperkalemia,** hypocalcemia, hypokalemia, weight loss.
Musculoskeletal: arthralgia; myalgia; myasthenia; pain in back, chest, or neck.
Respiratory: *asthma,* bronchitis, cough, *dyspnea,* hiccups, increased sputum, lung disorders, pneumonia.

Skin: acne, *alopecia,* dry skin, pruritus, *rash,* skin discoloration, sweating, urticaria.
Other: allergic reactions, *chills,* herpes simplex, *infections,* **sarcoma, sepsis.**

Interactions

Drug-drug. *Nephrotoxic drugs (such as aminoglycosides, amphotericin B, foscarnet, I.V. pentamidine):* May increase nephrotoxicity. Use together is contraindicated.
Probenecid: Interacts with metabolism or renal tubular excretion of many drugs. May be used with drug to decrease nephrotoxicity.

Effects on lab test results

• May increase BUN, creatinine, urine glucose, protein, alkaline phosphatase, ALT, AST, and LDH levels. May decrease calcium, bicarbonate, and hemoglobin levels and hematocrit. May increase or decrease potassium level.
• May decrease neutrophil and platelet counts.

Pharmacokinetics

Absorption: Given I.V.
Distribution: Less than 6% protein-bound.
Metabolism: Mainly by kidneys.
Excretion: By renal tubular secretion. *Half-life:* Unknown.

Route	Onset	Peak	Duration
I.V.	Unknown	Unknown	Unknown

Action

Chemical effect: Selective inhibition of CMV DNA polymerase; inhibits DNA viral synthesis.
Therapeutic effect: Reduces CMV replication.

Available forms

Injection: 75 mg/ml in 5-ml ampule

NURSING PROCESS

☰ **Assessment**
• Before each dose, check WBC and neutrophil counts, with differential, and renal function.
• Monitor intraocular pressure, visual acuity, and ocular symptoms periodically.
⚠ **ALERT:** Don't use drug in patients with baseline creatinine level above 1.5 mg/dl or calculated creatinine clearance of 55 ml/minute or less unless potential benefits outweigh risks. Monitor creatinine and urine protein within 48 hours

before each dose and adjust dosage according to renal function.
- Assess patient's and family's knowledge of drug therapy.

✚ Nursing diagnoses
- Ineffective protection related to presence of virus
- Deficient knowledge related to drug therapy

▶ Planning and implementation
- Give 1 L normal saline solution, usually over 1- to 2-hour period, immediately before each cidofovir infusion.
- Give probenecid with each cidofovir infusion.
Patient teaching
- Inform patient that drug doesn't cure CMV retinitis and that regular ophthalmologic follow-up examinations are needed.
- Explain that close monitoring of renal function is critical.
- Tell patient to take probenecid with food to reduce drug-related nausea and vomiting.
- Advise men to use condoms during and for 3 months after drug therapy. Advise women of childbearing potential to use contraception during and for 1 month after therapy.

☑ Evaluation
- Patient's infection is eradicated.
- Patient and family state understanding of drug therapy.

---

cilostazol
(sil-OS-tah-zol)
Pletal

Pharmacologic class: phosphodiesterase III inhibitor
Therapeutic class: antiplatelet, arterial vasodilator
Pregnancy risk category: C

Indications and dosages
▶ **To reduce symptoms of intermittent claudication.** *Adults:* 100 mg P.O. b.i.d. taken at least 30 minutes before or 2 hours after breakfast and dinner.
▧ **Adjust-a-dose:** If used with CYP3A4- or CYP2C19-inhibiting drugs, decrease dosage to

50 mg P.O. b.i.d. because cilostazol level may be increased.

Contraindications and cautions
- Contraindicated in patients hypersensitive to drug or its components and in those with heart failure.
- Use cautiously in patients with severe underlying heart disease and with other drugs that have antiplatelet activity.
☀ **Lifespan:** In breast-feeding women, avoid use. In children, safety and effectiveness haven't been established.

Adverse reactions
CNS: *dizziness, headache,* vertigo.
CV: *palpitations,* peripheral edema, tachycardia.
EENT: *pharyngitis, rhinitis.*
GI: abdominal pain, *abnormal stools, diarrhea,* dyspepsia, flatulence, nausea.
Musculoskeletal: back pain, myalgia.
Respiratory: increased cough.
Other: *infection.*

Interactions
Drug-drug. *Diltiazem:* May increase cilostazol level. Reduce cilostazol dosage to 50 mg b.i.d. *Erythromycin, other macrolides:* May increase levels of cilostazol and one of the metabolites. Reduce cilostazol dosage to 50 mg b.i.d. *Omeprazole:* May increase level of active cilostazol metabolite. Reduce cilostazol dosage to 50 mg b.i.d.
Strong inhibitors of CYP3A4, such as fluconazole, fluoxetine, fluvoxamine, itraconazole, ketoconazole, miconazole, nefazodone, sertraline: May increase levels of cilostazol and its metabolites. Reduce cilostazol dosage to 50 mg b.i.d.
Drug-food. *Grapefruit juice:* May increase cilostazol level. Tell patient to avoid grapefruit juice during therapy.
Drug-lifestyle. *Smoking:* May decrease cilostazol exposure by about 20%. Monitor patient closely and discourage patient from smoking.

Effects on lab test results
- May increase HDL level. May decrease triglyceride level.

Pharmacokinetics

Absorption: Increases by 90% when given with a high-fat meal. Absolute bioavailability is unknown.
Distribution: Highly protein-bound, mainly to albumin.
Metabolism: Extensive, mainly by CYP3A4. There are two active metabolites, one of which accounts for at least 50% of activity.
Excretion: 74% through urine. 20% in feces.
Half-life: 11 to 13 hours.

Route	Onset	Peak	Duration
P.O.	Unknown	2–4 hr	Unknown

Action

Chemical effect: Drug is thought to inhibit the enzyme phosphodiesterase III, causing an increase of cAMP in platelets and blood vessels, thus inhibiting platelet aggregation. Drug also has a vasodilating effect that's greatest in the femoral vascular beds.
Therapeutic effect: Reduces symptoms of intermittent claudication.

Available forms

Tablets: 50 mg, 100 mg

NURSING PROCESS

☘ Assessment
• Assess patient's underlying condition and pain level before therapy and regularly thereafter.
• Before therapy starts, make sure patient has a thorough physical examination for signs and symptoms of heart failure.
• Be alert for adverse reactions and drug interactions.
• Assess patient's and family's knowledge of drug therapy.

✛ Nursing diagnoses
• Acute pain related to underlying disease
• Ineffective peripheral tissue perfusion secondary to underlying disease
• Deficient knowledge related to drug therapy

▶ Planning and implementation
• Beneficial effects may not appear for up to 12 weeks.
• Dose can be reduced or drug stopped without rebound effects, such as platelet hyperaggrega-

bility. Notify prescriber of coagulation study results.
• Monitor heart rate and CV condition regularly for evidence of heart failure or tachyarrhythmias.

Patient teaching
• Advise patient to read the patient package insert carefully before starting therapy.
• Instruct patient to take cilostazol on an empty stomach, at least 30 minutes before or 2 hours after breakfast and dinner.
• Tell patient that the beneficial effect of drug on intermittent claudication isn't likely to be noticed for 2 to 4 weeks and that it may take as long as 12 weeks.
• Instruct patient not to drink grapefruit juice while taking drug.
• Inform patient that CV risk is unknown in patients who use the drug on a long-term basis and in patients who have severe underlying heart disease.
• Tell patient that drug may cause dizziness. Warn patient not to drive or perform other activities that require alertness until response to drug is known.

☑ Evaluation
• Patient experiences a decrease in pain.
• Patient has adequate tissue perfusion.
• Patient and family state understanding of drug therapy.

cimetidine
(sih-MEH-tih-deen)
Tagamet, Tagamet HB†

Pharmacologic class: H$_2$-receptor antagonist
Therapeutic class: antiulcerative
Pregnancy risk category: B

Indications and dosages

▶ **Duodenal ulcer (short-term therapy).**
Adults and children age 16 and older: 800 mg P.O. at bedtime. Or 400 mg P.O. b.i.d. or 300 mg q.i.d., with meals and at bedtime. Therapy continues for 4 to 6 weeks unless endoscopy shows healing. For maintenance therapy, 400 mg at bedtime.
▶ **Active benign gastric ulceration.** *Adults:* 800 mg P.O. at bedtime, or 300 mg P.O. q.i.d., with meals and at bedtime, for up to 8 weeks.

Reactions may be *common*, uncommon, *life-threatening*, or COMMON AND LIFE-THREATENING.

► **Pathologic hypersecretory conditions (such as Zollinger-Ellison syndrome, systemic mastocytosis, and multiple endocrine adenomas).** *Adults and children age 16 and older:* 300 mg P.O. q.i.d. with meals and at bedtime; adjust to patient's needs. Maximum oral daily dosage is 2,400 mg.

► **Gastroesophageal reflux disease.** *Adults:* 800 mg P.O. b.i.d. or 400 mg q.i.d. before meals and at bedtime for up to 12 weeks.

► **Heartburn.** *Adults:* 200 mg Tagamet HB† P.O. with water as symptoms occur, or as directed, up to b.i.d. Maximum, 400 mg daily. Don't give daily for longer than 2 weeks.

► **To prevent upper GI bleeding in critically ill patients.** *Adults:* 50 mg/hour by continuous I.V. infusion for up to 7 days.

Adjust-a-dose: For patients with renal impairment, if creatinine clearance is less than 30 ml/ minute, give 25 mg/hour by continuous I.V. infusion.

► **Hospitalized patients with intractable ulcers or hypersecretory conditions or patients who can't take oral drugs.** *Adults:* 300 mg I.M. every 6 to 8 hours. Or 300 mg diluted to 20 ml with normal saline solution or other compatible solution by I.V. push over 5 minutes every 6 to 8 hours. Or 300 mg diluted in 50 ml D₅W or other compatible solution by I.V. infusion over 15 to 20 minutes every 6 to 8 hours. To increase dosage, give 300-mg doses more frequently to maximum daily dosage of 2,400 mg. Or, 37.5 mg/hour (900 mg/day) I.V. continuous infusion diluted in 100 to 1,000 ml of compatible solution.

► **Active upper GI bleeding, peptic esophagitis, stress ulcers‡.** *Adults:* 1 to 2 g I.V. or P.O. daily in four divided doses.

Adjust-a-dose: For patients with creatinine clearance less than 30 ml/minute, decrease dosage to 300 mg P.O. or I.V. every 12 hours. If patient also has liver impairment, may need to further reduce dosage. May increase cautiously to every 8 hours based on patient response.

▼ I.V. administration

• Dilute I.V. solutions with normal saline solution, D₅W, dextrose 10% in water, combinations of them, lactated Ringer's solution, or 5% sodium bicarbonate injection. Don't dilute with sterile water for injection. Cimetidine may be added to total parenteral nutrition solutions with or without fat emulsion.

• Direct injection requires dilution of drug in 20 ml of compatible solution. Give direct injection over at least 5 minutes. Rapid I.V. injection may result in arrhythmias and hypotension.

• Infuse drug over at least 30 minutes to minimize risk of adverse cardiac effects. If giving continuous I.V. infusion, use infusion pump if giving a total volume of 250 ml over 24 hours or less.

• In children younger than age 16, dosages of 20 to 40 mg/kg are seldom used.

⊗ **Incompatibilities**
Allopurinol, amphotericin B, barbiturates, cefepime, chlorpromazine, combination atropine sulfate and pentobarbital sodium, indomethacin sodium trihydrate, pentobarbital sodium, warfarin.

Contraindications and cautions

• Contraindicated in patients hypersensitive to drug.
• Use cautiously in debilitated patients because they may be more susceptible to drug-induced confusion.

Lifespan: In pregnant women, use cautiously. In breast-feeding women, drug is contraindicated. In patients younger than age 16, experience with drug is limited, and drug should only be used when anticipated benefits outweigh the risks. In elderly patients, use cautiously.

Adverse reactions

CNS: confusion, dizziness, headaches, peripheral neuropathy.
CV: *bradycardia.*
GI: mild and transient diarrhea.
Hematologic: *agranulocytosis, aplastic anemia, neutropenia, thrombocytopenia.*
Hepatic: jaundice.
Musculoskeletal: muscle pain.
Skin: acnelike rash, urticaria.
Other: hypersensitivity reactions, mild gynecomastia (if taken longer than 1 month).

Interactions

Drug-drug. *Antacids:* May interfere with cimetidine absorption. Separate administration by at least 1 hour.
Calcium channel blockers, carbamazepine, labetalol, pentoxifylline, phenytoin, some benzodiazepines, sulfonylureas, tacrine, theophylline, valproic acid, warfarin: May inhibit hepatic mi-

crosomal enzyme metabolism of these drugs. Monitor levels of these drugs.

Lidocaine (I.V.): May decrease clearance of lidocaine, increasing the risk of toxicity. Consider using a different H_2 antagonist. Monitor lidocaine level closely.

Metoprolol, propranolol, timolol: May increase the pharmacologic effects of beta blocker. Consider using another H_2 antagonist or decrease the dose of beta blocker.

Procainamide: May increase procainamide level. Use cautiously. Monitor procainamide level closely, and adjust the dosage as needed.

Drug-herb. *Pennyroyal:* May change the rate at which toxic metabolites of pennyroyal form. Discourage use together.

Yerba maté: May decrease clearance of yerba maté methylxanthines and cause toxicity. Tell patient to use together cautiously.

Effects on lab test results

● May increase creatinine, alkaline phosphatase, AST, and ALT levels. May decrease hemoglobin level and hematocrit.
● May decrease neutrophil, granulocyte, leukocyte, and platelet counts.

Pharmacokinetics

Absorption: 60% to 75% of oral amount. Rate, but not extent, may be affected by food. Unknown after I.M. use.
Distribution: To many body tissues. 15% to 20% protein-bound.
Metabolism: 30% to 40%.
Excretion: Mainly in urine (48% of oral dose, 75% of parenteral dose); 10% of oral dose in feces. *Half-life:* 2 hours.

Route	Onset	Peak	Duration
P.O.	Unknown	45–90 min	4–5 hr
I.V.	Unknown	Immediate	Unknown
I.M.	Unknown	Unknown	Unknown

Action

Chemical effect: Competitively inhibits action of H_2 at receptor sites of parietal cells, decreasing gastric acid secretion.
Therapeutic effect: Lessens upper GI irritation caused by increased gastric acid secretion.

Available forms

Injection: 150 mg/ml; 300 mg in 50 ml normal saline solution for injection

Oral liquid: 300 mg/5 ml
Tablets: 200 mg‡, 300 mg, 400 mg, 800 mg

NURSING PROCESS

Assessment
● Assess patient's underlying upper GI condition before and regularly throughout therapy.
● Be alert for adverse reactions and drug interactions.
● Identify tablet strength when obtaining drug history.
● Monitor patient's CV condition during I.V. use because drug can cause profound bradycardia and other cardiotoxic effects when given too rapidly.
● Assess patient's and family's knowledge of drug therapy.

Nursing diagnoses
● Impaired tissue integrity related to patient's underlying condition
● Diarrhea related to drug-induced adverse reaction
● Deficient knowledge related to drug therapy

Planning and implementation
● Give tablets with meals to ensure more consistent therapeutic effect.
● I.M. administration may be painful.
● Hemodialysis reduces level of drug. Schedule dose at end of hemodialysis. Lower dose in patients with renal impairment.
● Cimetidine shouldn't be used for self-medication (Tagamet HB†) in children younger than age 12 unless directed by a physician.
● **ALERT:** Don't confuse cimetidine with simethicone.

Patient teaching
● Remind patient taking drug once daily to take it at bedtime for best results.
● Instruct patient to take drug as directed and to continue taking it even after pain subsides, to allow for adequate healing.
● Remind patient not to take antacid within 1 hour of taking drug.
● Because of high potential for drug interactions, advise patient to tell prescriber if he's taking other drugs.
● Urge patient to avoid cigarette smoking because it may increase gastric acid secretion and worsen disease.

• Instruct patient to immediately report black tarry stools, diarrhea, confusion, or rash.

☑ **Evaluation**
• Patient experiences decrease in or relief of upper GI symptoms with drug therapy.
• Patient maintains normal bowel habits throughout drug therapy.
• Patient and family state understanding of drug therapy.

cinacalcet hydrochloride
(sin-uh-KAL-seht high-droh-KLOR-ighd)
Sensipar

Pharmacologic class: calcimimetic
Therapeutic class: hyperparathyroidism drug
Pregnancy risk category: C

Indications and dosages

▶ **Secondary hyperparathyroidism in patients with chronic kidney disease on dialysis.**
Adults: Initially, 30 mg P.O. once daily; adjust no more than every 2 to 4 weeks through sequential doses of 60 mg, 90 mg, 120 mg, and 180 mg P.O. once daily, to reach target range of 150 to 300 picograms (pg)/ml of intact parathyroid hormone (iPTH).

▶ **Hypercalcemia in patients with parathyroid carcinoma.** *Adults:* Initially, 30 mg P.O. b.i.d.; adjust every 2 to 4 weeks through sequential doses of 60 mg, and 90 mg P.O. b.i.d., and 90 mg P.O. t.i.d. or q.i.d. daily p.r.n. to normalize calcium level.

Contraindications and cautions

• Contraindicated in patients hypersensitive to drug or any of its components and in patients with calcium level below 8.4 mg/dl.
• Use cautiously in patients with a history of a seizure disorder and patients with moderate to severe hepatic impairment.
⚘ **Lifespan:** In women who are breast-feeding, use cautiously. It's not known if drug appears in breast milk. In children, safety and effectiveness haven't been established.

Adverse reactions

CNS: asthenia, *dizziness.*
CV: chest pain, hypertension.
GI: anorexia, diarrhea, nausea, vomiting.

Musculoskeletal: *myalgia.*
Other: dialysis venous access site infection.

Interactions

Drug-drug. *Drugs metabolized mainly by CYP2D6 with a narrow therapeutic index (such as flecainide, thioridazine, most tricyclic antidepressants, vinblastine):* May strongly inhibit CYP2D6. Adjust dosages of these drugs as needed.
Drugs that strongly inhibit CYP3A4 (such as erythromycin, itraconazole, ketoconazole): May increase cinacalcet level. If patient starts or stops therapy with one of these drugs, monitor parathyroid hormone (PTH) and calcium level closely, and adjust cinacalcet dosage as needed.
Drug-food. *Food:* May increase level of drug. Give with food or shortly after a meal.

Effects on lab test results

• May decrease calcium, phosphorus, and testosterone levels.

Pharmacokinetics

Absorption: Increases when drug is given with meals. Level peaks in about 2 to 6 hours.
Distribution: High volume. Drug reaches steady-state drug level within 7 days. 93% to 97% protein-bound.
Metabolism: Mainly by CYP3A4, CYP2D6, and CYP1A2.
Excretion: 80% in urine, 15% in feces. *Half-life:* 30 to 40 hours.

Route	Onset	Peak	Duration
P.O.	Unknown	2–6 hr	Unknown

Action

Chemical effect: Increases the sensitivity of calcium-sensing receptor to extracellular calcium.
Therapeutic effect: Decreases iPTH and calcium levels.

Available forms

Tablets: 30 mg, 60 mg, 90 mg

NURSING PROCESS

📝 **Assessment**
🔔 **ALERT:** Monitor calcium level closely, especially if patient has a history of seizures, be-

cause a decreased calcium level lowers the threshold for seizures.
- Measure calcium level within 1 week of starting therapy or adjusting dose. Once the maintenance dosage has been established, measure calcium level monthly in patients with chronic kidney disease on dialysis and every 2 months in patients with parathyroid carcinoma.
- Watch carefully for evidence of hypocalcemia, such as paresthesias, myalgias, cramping, tetany, and seizures.
- Measure iPTH 1 to 4 weeks after therapy starts or dosage is changed. Once the maintenance dosage is established, monitor PTH every 1 to 3 months. Keep level at 150 to 300 pg/ml in patients with chronic kidney disease on dialysis.
- Assess patient's and family's knowledge of drug therapy.

Nursing diagnoses
- Risk for injury related to drug-induced hypocalcemia
- Noncompliance related to GI adverse effects of drug
- Deficient knowledge related to drug therapy

Planning and implementation
- In patient with moderate to severe hepatic impairment, adjust dose based on PTH and calcium level. Monitor patient closely.
- Give drug alone or with vitamin D sterols, phosphate binders, or both.
- If calcium level is 7.5 to 8.4 mg/dl or patient develops symptoms of hypocalcemia, give phosphate binders containing calcium, vitamin D sterols, or both to raise level. If level is below 7.5 mg/dl or hypocalcemia symptoms persist, and the vitamin D dose has reached the maximum, withhold drug until level reaches 8 mg/dl, hypocalcemia symptoms resolve, or both. Resume with the next lowest dose.
- A dynamic bone disease may develop if iPTH levels are suppressed below 100 pg/ml. If this occurs, reduce the dosage of drug or vitamin D sterols, or stop therapy.
- **ALERT:** Drug isn't approved for patients with chronic kidney disease who aren't on dialysis because they have an increased risk of hypocalcemia.

Patient teaching
- Tell patient to take tablets whole, with food or shortly after a meal.

- Advise patient to report adverse reactions and signs of hypocalcemia, which include paresthesias, muscle weakness, muscle cramping, and muscle spasm.

Evaluation
- Patient doesn't develop hypocalcemia.
- Patient doesn't experience GI adverse effects.
- Patient and family state understanding of drug therapy.

ciprofloxacin
(sih-proh-FLOKS-uh-sin)
Cipro◆, Cipro I.V., Cipro XR

Pharmacologic class: fluoroquinolone
Therapeutic class: antibiotic
Pregnancy risk category: C

Indications and dosages
▶ **Mild to moderate UTI.** *Adults:* 250 mg P.O. or 200 mg I.V., every 12 hours for 7 to 14 days.
▶ **Severe or complicated UTI; mild to moderate bone and joint infections; mild to moderate respiratory tract infections; mild to moderate skin and skin-structure infections; infectious diarrhea; intra-abdominal infection.** *Adults:* 500 mg P.O. or 400 mg I.V., every 12 hours for 7 to 14 days; mild to moderate joint infections may require 4 to 6 weeks.
▶ **Severe or complicated bone or joint infections; severe respiratory tract infections; severe skin and skin-structure infections.** *Adults:* 750 mg P.O. every 12 hours. Or, 400 mg I.V. every 8 hours for 7 to 14 days. Bone and joint infections may require 4 to 6 weeks.
▶ **Mild to moderate acute sinusitis caused by** *Haemophilus influenzae, Streptococcus pneumoniae,* or *Moraxella catarrhalis;* **mild to moderate chronic bacterial prostatitis caused by** *Escherichia coli* or *Proteus mirabilis.* *Adults:* 500 mg P.O. every 12 hours or 400 mg I.V. infusion every 12 hours for 10 days.
▶ **Febrile neutropenia.** *Adults:* 400 mg I.V. every 8 hours for 7 to 14 days given in conjunction with piperacillin sodium (50 mg/kg I.V. every 4 hours, not to exceed 24 g daily).
▶ **Inhalation anthrax (postexposure).** *Adults:* 400 mg I.V. every 12 hours initially until susceptibility tests are known, then switch to 500 mg P.O. b.i.d. when patient's condition improves.

C

Children: 10 mg/kg I.V. every 12 hours, then switch to 15 mg/kg P.O. every 12 hours when patient's condition improves. Don't exceed 800 mg I.V. daily or 1 g P.O. daily.
For all patients: Also use one or two additional antimicrobials. Treat for a total of 60 days (I.V. and P.O. combined).

▶ **Acute uncomplicated cystitis.** *Women:* 100 or 250 mg P.O. every 12 hours for 3 days.

▶ **Cutaneous anthrax‡.** *Adults:* 500 mg P.O. b.i.d. for 60 days.
Children: 10 to 15 mg/kg every 12 hours, not to exceed 1 g daily, for 60 days.

▶ **Uncomplicated urethral, endocervical, rectal‡, or pharyngeal‡ gonorrhea.** *Adults:* 500 mg P.O. as a single dose (with other anti-infectives, if chlamydial infection isn't ruled out).

▶ *Neisseria meningitidis* **in nasal passages‡.** *Adults:* 500 to 750 mg P.O. as a single dose, or 250 mg P.O. b.i.d. for 2 days, or 500 mg P.O. b.i.d. for 5 days.

▓ **Adjust-a-dose:** In patients with renal impairment, for all indications above, if creatinine clearance is 30 to 50 ml/minute, give 250 to 500 mg P.O. every 12 hours or the usual I.V. dose; if creatinine clearance is 5 to 29 ml/minute, give 250 to 500 mg every 18 hours or 200 to 400 mg I.V. every 18 to 24 hours. If patient is on hemodialysis, give 250 to 500 mg P.O. every 24 hours after dialysis.

▶ **UTI.** *Adults:* If uncomplicated, 500 mg (extended-release) P.O. once daily for 3 days. If complicated, 1 g (extended-release) P.O. once daily for 3 days.

▓ **Adjust-a-dose:** For patients with renal impairment, if creatinine clearance is less than 30 ml/minute, give 500 mg (extended-release) P.O. daily. For dialysis patients, give dose after dialysis session.

▽ I.V. administration

• Dilute drug using D_5W or normal saline solution for injection to final concentration of 1 or 2 mg/ml. Infuse over 1 hour into large vein.
• If giving drug through a Y-type set, stop the other I.V. solution during infusion.
⊗ **Incompatibilities**
Aminophylline, ampicillin-sulbactam, azithromycin, cefepime, clindamycin phosphate, dexamethasone sodium phosphate, furosemide, heparin sodium, methylprednisolone sodium succinate, phenytoin sodium.

Contraindications and cautions

• Contraindicated in patients hypersensitive to fluoroquinolones.
• Use cautiously in patients with CNS disorders, such as severe cerebral arteriosclerosis or seizure disorders, and in those at increased risk for seizures. May cause CNS stimulation.
• Immunocompromised patients may receive the usual dose and regimen for anthrax.
⚖ **Lifespan:** In pregnant women, use cautiously. Pregnant women may receive the usual dose and regimen for anthrax. In breast-feeding women, drug is contraindicated because it appears in breast milk. In children, safety and effectiveness for indications other than anthrax haven't been established. In children younger than age 18, avoid use of Cipro XR because its safety and effectiveness haven't been established.

Adverse reactions

CNS: confusion, hallucinations, headache, light-headedness, paresthesia, restlessness, *seizures,* tremor.
CV: thrombophlebitis.
GI: abdominal pain or discomfort, *diarrhea, nausea,* oral candidiasis, vomiting.
GU: crystalluria, interstitial nephritis.
Hematologic: eosinophilia, *leukopenia, neutropenia, thrombocytopenia.*
Musculoskeletal: achiness, arthralgia, joint inflammation, joint or back pain, joint stiffness, neck or chest pain.
Skin: photosensitivity, rash, *Stevens-Johnson syndrome.*
Other: burning, erythema, pruritus, swelling with I.V. use.

Interactions

Drug-drug. *Aluminum hydroxide, aluminum-magnesium hydroxide, calcium carbonate, magnesium hydroxide:* May decrease effects of ciprofloxacin. Give antacid at least 6 hours before or 2 hours after ciprofloxacin.
Iron salts: May decrease absorption of ciprofloxacin, reducing anti-infective response. Give at least 2 hours apart.
Probenecid: May elevate level of ciprofloxacin. Monitor patient for toxicity.
Sucralfate: May decrease absorption of ciprofloxacin, reducing anti-infective response. Give at least 6 hours apart.
Theophylline: May increase theophylline level and prolong theophylline half-life. Monitor lev-

el of theophylline and observe patient for adverse effects.

Tizanidine: May increase plasma level of tizanidine and cause low blood pressure, somnolence, dizziness, and slowed psychomotor skills. Avoid use together.

Warfarin: May enhance anticoagulant effects. Monitor PT closely.

Drug-herb. *Yerba maté:* May decrease clearance of yerba maté methylxanthines and cause toxicity. Discourage use together.

Drug-food. *Orange juice fortified with calcium:* May decrease absorption of drug, reducing effects. Advise patient to avoid taking drug with calcium-fortified orange juice.

Drug-lifestyle. *Caffeine:* May increase effects of caffeine. Monitor patient.

Effects on lab test results

• May increase BUN, creatinine, ALT, AST, alkaline phosphatase, bilirubin, LDH, and GGT levels.
• May increase eosinophil count. May decrease WBC, neutrophil, and platelet counts.

Pharmacokinetics

Absorption: About 70%. Food delays rate but not extent; 35% of Cipro XR is an immediate-release form, whereas 65% is a slow-release matrix.

Distribution: 20% to 40% protein-bound. CSF level is only 10% of this level.

Metabolism: May be hepatic. Four metabolites have been identified; each has less antimicrobial activity than parent compound.

Excretion: Mainly renal. *Half-life:* 4 hours. *Half-life of Cipro XR:* 6 hours in adults with normal renal function.

Route	Onset	Peak	Duration
P.O.	Unknown	1–2 hr	Unknown
P.O. extended-release	Unknown	1–4 hr	Unknown
I.V.	Immediate	Immediate	Unknown

Action

Chemical effect: Unknown. Bactericidal effects may result from inhibition of bacterial DNA gyrase and prevention of replication in susceptible bacteria.

Therapeutic effect: Kills susceptible bacteria.

Available forms

Infusion (premixed): 200 mg in 100 ml D_5W, 400 mg in 200 ml D_5W
Injection: 200 mg, 400 mg
Oral suspension: 250 mg/5 ml; 500 mg/5 ml
Tablets: 100 mg, 250 mg, 500 mg, 750 mg
Tablets (extended-release, film-coated): 500 mg, 1,000 mg

NURSING PROCESS

⚕ Assessment

• Assess patient's infection before therapy and regularly throughout.
• Before giving first dose, obtain specimen for culture and sensitivity tests. Begin therapy pending results.
• Be alert for adverse reactions and drug interactions.
• If adverse GI reactions occur, monitor patient's hydration.
• Assess patient's and family's knowledge of drug therapy.

⊕ Nursing diagnoses

• Ineffective protection related to presence of bacteria
• Risk for deficient fluid volume related to drug-induced adverse GI reactions
• Deficient knowledge related to drug therapy

▷ Planning and implementation

• Give oral form 2 hours after meal or 2 hours before or 6 hours after taking antacids, sucralfate, or products that contain iron (such as vitamins with mineral supplements). Food doesn't affect absorption but may delay peak level.
• If patient has an NG tube don't use oral suspension because the microcapsules may occlude the tube.
• Reduce dose in patients with renal impairment.
• Have patient drink plenty of fluids to reduce risk of crystalluria.
• Additional antimicrobials for anthrax multidrug regimen can include rifampin, vancomycin, penicillin, ampicillin, chloramphenicol, imipenem, clindamycin, and clarithromycin.
• Steroids may be considered as adjunctive therapy for anthrax patients with severe edema and for meningitis, based on experience with bacterial meningitis of other etiologies.
• Ciprofloxacin and doxycycline are first-line therapy for anthrax. Amoxicillin 500 mg P.O.

---

t.i.d. for adults and 80 mg/kg daily divided every 8 hours for children is an option for completion of therapy after improvement.
• Follow current Centers for Disease Control and Prevention recommendations for anthrax.

Patient teaching
• Tell patient to take drug 2 hours after meal and to take prescribed antacids at least 2 hours after taking drug.
• Advise patient not to crush, split, or chew the extended-release tablets, but to swallow them whole.
• Advise patient to drink plenty of fluids to reduce risk of crystalluria.
• Warn patient to avoid hazardous tasks that require alertness, such as driving, until CNS effects of drug are known.
• Advise patient to avoid caffeine while taking drug because of potential for cumulative caffeine effects.
• Advise patient that hypersensitivity reactions may occur even after first dose. If he notices rash or other allergic reaction, tell him to stop taking the drug and notify prescriber immediately.
• Instruct patient either to stop breast-feeding or request a different drug.

☑ Evaluation
• Patient is free from infection.
• Patient maintains adequate hydration throughout drug therapy.
• Patient and family state understanding of drug therapy.

HIGH ALERT!

cisplatin (cis-platinum)
(sis-PLAH-tin)
Platinol-AQ

Pharmacologic class: alkylating drug
Therapeutic class: antineoplastic
Pregnancy risk category: D

Indications and dosages

▶ **Adjunct therapy in metastatic testicular cancer.** *Adults:* 20 mg/m² I.V. daily for 5 days. Repeat every 3 weeks for three cycles or longer.
▶ **Adjunct therapy in metastatic ovarian cancer.** *Adults:* 100 mg/m² I.V.; repeat every 4 weeks. Or 75 to 100 mg/m² I.V. once every 4 weeks with cyclophosphamide.

▶ **Advanced bladder cancer.** *Adults:* 50 to 70 mg/m² I.V. every 3 to 4 weeks. Give 50 mg/m² every 4 weeks to patients who have received other antineoplastics or radiation therapy.
▶ **Head and neck cancer‡.** *Adults:* 80 to 120 mg/m² I.V. once every 3 weeks.
▶ **Metastatic or recurrent cervical cancer‡.** *Adults:* 50 mg/m² I.V. once every 3 weeks.
▶ **Invasive cervical cancer‡.** *Adults:* 40 to 75 mg/m² I.V. weekly or daily with radiation therapy.
▶ **Non–small-cell lung cancer‡.** *Adults:* 75 to 100 mg/m² I.V. every 3 to 4 weeks with other drugs.
▶ **Brain tumor‡.** *Children:* 60 mg/m² I.V. for 2 days every 3 to 4 weeks.
▶ **Osteogenic sarcoma or neuroblastoma‡.** *Children:* 90 mg/m² I.V. every 3 weeks.
▶ **Advanced esophageal cancer‡.** *Adults:* 50 to 120 mg/m² I.V. every 3 to 4 weeks when used alone, or 75 to 100 mg/m² I.V. every 3 to 4 weeks when used with other chemotherapy.

▽ I.V. administration
• Preparing and giving drug are linked to carcinogenic, mutagenic, and teratogenic risks. Follow facility policy to reduce risks.
• Reconstitute powder using sterile water for injection. Add 10 ml to 10-mg vial or 50 ml to 50-mg vial to make a solution containing 1 mg/ml. Further dilute with D₅W in one-third normal saline solution for injection or dextrose 5% in half-normal saline solution for injection. Solutions are stable for 20 hours at room temperature. Don't refrigerate.
• Infusions are most stable in chloride-containing solutions (such as normal, half-normal, and quarter-normal saline solution). Don't use D₅W alone.
• To prevent hypokalemia, potassium chloride (10 to 20 mEq/L) is commonly added to I.V. fluids before and after therapy. Magnesium sulfate may be added to prevent hypomagnesemia.
• Hydrate patient with normal saline solution before giving drug. Maintain urine output of at least 100 ml/hour for 4 consecutive hours before therapy and for 24 hours after therapy. Prehydration and diuresis may reduce renal toxicity and ototoxicity significantly.
• Give mannitol or furosemide boluses or infusions before and with infusion to maintain diureses of 100 to 400 ml/hour during and for

24 hours after therapy. I.V. infusion in 2 L dextrose 5% in half-normal saline solution or dextrose 5% in 0.33% sodium chloride solution with 37.5 g mannitol over 6 to 8 hours is recommended.

• Do not use needles or I.V. sets containing aluminum because drug may precipitate.

⊗ **Incompatibilities**

Amifostine, cefepime, D₅W, fluorouracil, mesna, 0.1% sodium chloride solution, piperacillin sodium with tazobactam sodium, sodium bicarbonate, sodium bisulfate, sodium thiosulfate, solutions with a chloride content less than 2%, thiotepa. Don't use needles or I.V. administration sets that contain aluminum because it will displace platinum, causing loss of potency and formation of black precipitate.

Contraindications and cautions

• Contraindicated in patients hypersensitive to drug or other platinum-containing compounds. Also contraindicated in patients with severe renal disease, hearing impairment, or myelosuppression.

※ **Lifespan:** In pregnant women, use cautiously and only when absolutely needed because fetal harm may occur. In breast-feeding women, drug isn't recommended. In children, safety and effectiveness haven't been established.

Adverse reactions

CNS: *peripheral neuritis, seizures.*
EENT: *hearing loss, tinnitus.*
GI: diarrhea, loss of taste, metallic taste, *nausea and vomiting beginning 1 to 4 hours after dose and lasting 24 hours.*
GU: NEPHROTOXICITY.
Hematologic: anemia, *leukopenia,* MILD MYELOSUPPRESSION, nadirs in circulating platelet and WBC counts on days 18 to 23 with recovery by day 39, *thrombocytopenia.*
Metabolic: hypocalcemia, hypokalemia, *hypomagnesemia.*
Other: *anaphylactoid reaction.*

Interactions

Drug-drug. *Aminoglycoside antibiotics:* May cause additive nephrotoxicity. Monitor renal function studies carefully.
Bumetanide, furosemide: May cause additive ototoxicity. Avoid use together.
Phenytoin: May decrease phenytoin level. Monitor level.

Effects on lab test results

• May increase uric acid, liver enzyme, and bilirubin levels. May decrease magnesium, potassium, calcium, sodium, phosphate, and hemoglobin levels and hematocrit.
• May decrease WBC, RBC, and platelet counts.

Pharmacokinetics

Absorption: Given I.V.
Distribution: Wide, with highest level in kidneys, liver, and prostate. Doesn't readily cross blood–brain barrier. Extensively and irreversibly bound to plasma and tissue proteins.
Metabolism: Unknown.
Excretion: Mainly unchanged in urine. *Half-life:* Initial phase, 25 to 79 minutes; terminal phase, 58 to 78 hours.

Route	Onset	Peak	Duration
I.V.	Unknown	Immediate	Several days

Action

Chemical effect: Probably cross-links strands of cellular DNA and interferes with RNA transcription, causing imbalance of growth that leads to cell death.
Therapeutic effect: Kills selected cancer cells.

Available forms

Injection: 1 mg/ml

NURSING PROCESS

⚗ Assessment

• Assess patient's underlying neoplastic disease before and regularly throughout therapy.
• Monitor CBC, electrolyte levels (especially potassium and magnesium), platelet count, and renal function studies before initial and subsequent dosages.
• To detect permanent hearing loss, obtain audiometry test results before initial dose and subsequent courses.
• Be alert for adverse reactions and drug interactions.
• Assess patient's and family's knowledge of drug therapy.

⊕ Nursing diagnoses

• Ineffective health maintenance related to presence of neoplastic disease

---

- Ineffective protection related to drug-induced adverse reactions
- Deficient knowledge related to drug therapy

▶ Planning and implementation

- Renal toxicity is cumulative. Renal function must return to normal before next dose can be given.
- Don't repeat dose unless platelet count exceeds 100,000/mm³, WBC count exceeds 4,000/mm³, creatinine level is less than 1.5 mg/dl, or BUN level is less than 25 mg/dl.
- I.V. sodium thiosulfate may be used to minimize toxicity. Check current protocol.
- Nausea and vomiting may be severe and protracted (up to 24 hours). Provide I.V. hydration until patient can tolerate adequate oral intake.
- Antiemetics, such as ondansetron, granisetron, and high-dose metoclopramide, may be used to prevent and treat nausea and vomiting. Metoclopramide may be combined with dexamethasone and antihistamines, or ondansetron or granisetron with dexamethasone.
- Delayed-onset vomiting (3 to 5 days after therapy) may occur. Patients may need prolonged antiemetic treatment.
- Immediately give epinephrine, corticosteroids, or antihistamines for anaphylactoid reactions.
- Ⓢ **ALERT:** Don't confuse cisplatin with carboplatin.

Patient teaching

- Warn patient to watch for signs of infection (fever, sore throat, fatigue) and bleeding (easy bruising, nosebleeds, bleeding gums, melena). Tell him to take his temperature daily.
- Tell patient to immediately report tinnitus.
- Instruct patient to avoid OTC products that contain aspirin.
- Teach patient to record intake and output on daily basis and to report edema or decrease in urine output.
- Encourage patient to notify prescriber if any concerns arise during therapy.

☑ Evaluation

- Patient has positive response to cisplatin therapy according to follow-up diagnostic studies.
- Patient doesn't have permanent injury from drug-induced adverse reactions.
- Patient and family state understanding of drug therapy.

citalopram hydrobromide

(sih-TAL-oh-pram high-droh-BROH-mighd)
Celexa◆

Pharmacologic class: SSRI
Therapeutic class: antidepressant
Pregnancy risk category: C

Indications and dosages

▶ **Depression.** *Adults:* Initially, 20 mg P.O. once daily, increasing to maximum dosage of 40 mg daily after no less than 1 week.
▶ **Panic disorder‡.** *Adults:* 20 to 30 mg P.O. once daily.
▯ **Adjust-a-dose:** For elderly patients and patients with hepatic impairment, give 20 mg P.O. once daily. Increase to 40 mg daily only for patients not responding to therapy.

Contraindications and cautions

- Contraindicated within 14 days of MAO inhibitor therapy. Also contraindicated in patients hypersensitive to drug, any of its components, or escitalopram. Contraindicated in patients taking pimozide.
- Use cautiously in patients with history of mania, seizures, suicidal ideation, hepatic impairment, or renal impairment.
- ⚘ **Lifespan:** In breast-feeding women, avoid drug because it appears in breast milk and may cause serious adverse reactions in infants. Drug isn't approved for pediatric use and shouldn't be used in children and adolescents younger than age 18 for major depressive disorder because of possible increased risk of suicidal behavior. In elderly patients, reduce dosage.

Adverse reactions

CNS: agitation, amnesia, anxiety, apathy, confusion, depression, dizziness, fatigue, fever, impaired concentration, insomnia, migraine, paresthesia, *somnolence, suicide attempt,* tremor.
CV: hypotension, orthostatic hypotension, tachycardia.
EENT: abnormal accommodation, rhinitis, sinusitis.
GI: abdominal pain, anorexia, diarrhea, dry mouth, dyspepsia, flatulence, increased appetite, increased saliva, nausea, taste disturbance, vomiting, weight changes.

GU: amenorrhea, dysmenorrhea, ejaculation disorder, impotence, polyuria.
Musculoskeletal: arthralgia, myalgia.
Respiratory: cough, upper respiratory tract infection.
Skin: increased sweating, pruritus, rash.
Other: decreased libido, yawning.

Interactions

Drug-drug. *Carbamazepine:* May increase citalopram clearance. Monitor patient for effects.
CNS drugs: May increase CNS effects. Use together cautiously.
Drugs that inhibit CYP3A4 (such as fluconazole) and CYP2C19 (such as omeprazole): May decrease citalopram clearance. Monitor patient for toxicity.
Imipramine, other tricyclic antidepressants: May increase level of imipramine metabolite desipramine by about 50%. Use together cautiously.
Lithium: May enhance serotonergic effect of citalopram. Use cautiously and monitor lithium level.
Phenelzine, selegiline, tranylcypromine: May cause serotonin syndrome, including CNS irritability, shivering, and altered consciousness. Don't give together. Wait at least 2 weeks after stopping an MAO inhibitor before giving any SSRI.
SSNRIs, sumatriptan and other triptans: May cause serotonin syndrome (weakness, hyperreflexia, incoordination). Monitor patient closely.
Warfarin: PT increases by 5%. Monitor patient carefully; monitor PT and INR.
Drug-herb. *St. John's wort:* May raise serotonin level, causing serotonin syndrome. Discourage use together.
Drug-lifestyle. *Alcohol use:* May increase CNS effects. Discourage use together.

Effects on lab test results

• May increase liver function test values.

Pharmacokinetics

Absorption: Absolute bioavailability is 80%.
Distribution: Wide. About 80% protein-bound.
Metabolism: Mainly by the liver.
Excretion: 10% is recovered in urine. *Half-life:* 35 hours.

Route	Onset	Peak	Duration
P.O.	Unknown	4 hr	Unknown

Action

Chemical effect: May enhance serotonergic activity in CNS by inhibiting neuronal reuptake of serotonin.
Therapeutic effect: Relieves depression.

Available forms

Oral solution: 10 mg/5 ml
Tablets: 10 mg, 20 mg, 40 mg
Tablets (orally-disintegrating): 10 mg, 20 mg, 40 mg

NURSING PROCESS

Assessment
• Assess patient's underlying condition before therapy and regularly thereafter.
• Check vital signs regularly for decreased blood pressure or tachycardia.
• Closely supervise high-risk patients at start of drug therapy.
ALERT: Monitor patient for suicidal thinking and behavior, expecially in young adults ages 18 to 24 during the first 2 months of treatment.
• Assess patient's and family's knowledge of drug therapy.

Nursing diagnoses
• Risk for injury related to patient's underlying condition
• Ineffective coping related to patient's underlying condition
• Deficient knowledge related to drug therapy

Planning and implementation
ALERT: Don't start citalopram therapy within 14 days of MAO inhibitor therapy.
• For patient with hepatic impairment, reduce dosage.
• May increase risk of suicide in adolescents.
• Don't stop drug abruptly.
ALERT: Don't confuse Celexa with Celebrex, Cerebyx, or Concerta.
Patient teaching
• Urge patient to continue therapy as prescribed even if he improves within 1 to 4 weeks.
• Instruct patient to exercise caution when operating hazardous machinery, including automobiles, because psychoactive drugs can impair judgment, thinking, and motor skills.

- Warn patient that drug may cause photosensitivity; advise patient to take protective measures until tolerance is determined.
- Advise patient to consult prescriber before taking other prescription drugs, OTC medicines, or herbal remedies.
- Tell patient to let orally disintegrating tablet dissolve on the tongue and then swallow, with or without water. Urge patient not to cut, crush, or chew orally disintegrating tablets.
- ⊛ **ALERT:** If patient wishes to switch from an SSRI to St. John's wort, tell him to wait a few weeks for the SSRI to leave his system before he starts the herb. Urge him to ask his prescriber for advice.
- Warn patient not to consume alcohol during therapy.
- Advise patient and his family to immediately report changes in mood or behavior, especially suicidal thinking, to his health care provider.
- Instruct woman of childbearing age to use birth control during therapy and to notify prescriber immediately if she suspects pregnancy.

☑ **Evaluation**
- Patient's safety is maintained.
- Patient's condition is improved with drug.
- Patient and family state understanding of drug therapy.

clarithromycin
(klah-rith-roh-MIGH-sin)
Biaxin, Biaxin XL

Pharmacologic class: macrolide
Therapeutic class: antibiotic
Pregnancy risk category: C

Indications and dosages

▶ **Pharyngitis or tonsillitis caused by _Streptococcus pyogenes_.** _Adults:_ 250 mg P.O. every 12 hours for 10 days.
Children: 7.5 mg/kg P.O., every 12 hours for 10 days.
▶ **Acute maxillary sinusitis caused by _Streptococcus pneumoniae, Haemophilus influenzae,_ or _Moraxella catarrhalis_.** _Adults:_ 500 mg P.O. every 12 hours for 14 days. Or, two 500-mg or one 1,000 mg extended-release tablets P.O. daily for 14 days.

Children: 7.5 mg/kg P.O. daily every 12 hours for 10 days.
▶ **Acute exacerbation of chronic bronchitis caused by _M. catarrhalis, S. pneumoniae, H. influenzae,_ or _Haemophilus parainfluenzae_.** _Adults:_ 250 mg P.O. every 12 hours for 7 to 14 days (for _M. catarrhalis_ and _S. pneumoniae_), or 500 mg P.O. every 12 hours for 7 days for _H. parainfluenzae_ (up to 14 days for _H. influenzae_). Or two 500-mg or one 1,000 mg extended-release tablets P.O. daily for 7 days.
▶ **Uncomplicated skin and skin-structure infections caused by _Staphylococcus aureus_ or _S. pyogenes_.** _Adults:_ 250 mg P.O. every 12 hours for 7 to 14 days.
▶ **Prophylaxis and treatment of disseminated infection from _Mycobacterium avium_ complex.** _Adults:_ 500 mg P.O. b.i.d.
Children: 7.5 mg/kg, up to 500 mg, P.O. b.i.d.
▶ **Acute otitis media caused by _H. influenzae, M. catarrhalis,_ or _S. pneumoniae_.** _Children:_ 7.5 mg/kg, up to 500 mg, P.O. every 12 hours.
▶ **_Helicobacter pylori_ eradication to reduce risk of duodenal ulcer recurrence.** _Adults:_ For triple therapy, 500 mg clarithromycin with 30 mg lansoprazole and 1 g amoxicillin, all given P.O. every 12 hours for 10 to 14 days; or 500 mg clarithromycin with 20 mg omeprazole and 1 g amoxicillin, all given P.O. every 12 hours for 10 days; or clarithromycin 500 mg with 20 mg rabeprazole and 1 g amoxicillin, all given P.O. every 12 hours for 7 days. For dual therapy, 500 mg clarithromycin every 8 hours and 40 mg omeprazole once daily P.O. for 14 days.
▶ **Community-acquired pneumonia from _Chlamydia pneumoniae, Mycoplasma pneumoniae, S. pneumoniae, H. influenzae, H. parainfluenzae, M. catarrhalis_.** _Adults:_ 250 mg P.O. every 12 hours for 7 to 14 days (for _H. influenzae,_ 7 days). Or two 500-mg or one 1,000 mg extended-release tablets P.O. daily for 7 days for all listed organisms. Don't use conventional tablets to treat pneumonia caused by _H. parainfluenzae_ or _M. catarrhalis._
Children: 7.5 mg/kg P.O. every 12 hours for 10 days (for _C. pneumoniae, M. pneumoniae,_ or _S. pneumoniae_ only).
▶ **Lyme disease‡.** _Adults:_ 500 mg P.O. b.i.d. for 14 to 21 days.
Children: 7.5 mg/kg P.O., up to 500 mg, b.i.d. for 14 to 21 days

Adjust-a-dose: For patients with renal impairment, if creatinine clearance is less than 30 ml/minute, reduce dose by 50% or double frequency interval.

Contraindications and cautions

• Contraindicated in patients hypersensitive to drug and other macrolides. Use with pimozide, cisapride, or other drugs that prolong QT interval or may cause ventricular arrhythmias is contraindicated.

• Use cautiously in patients with hepatic or renal impairment.

Lifespan: In pregnant or breast-feeding women, use cautiously. In infants younger than age 6 months, safety and effectiveness haven't been established.

Adverse reactions

CNS: headache.
CV: *ventricular arrhythmias.*
GI: abdominal pain or discomfort, abnormal taste, diarrhea, dyspepsia, nausea, *pseudomembranous colitis,* vomiting (pediatric).
Hematologic: coagulation abnormalities, *leukopenia.*
Skin: rash (pediatric), *Stevens-Johnson syndrome, toxic epidermal necrolysis.*

Interactions

Drug-drug. *Alprazolam, midazolam, triazolam:* May increase adverse CNS effects. Assess patient carefully.
Carbamazepine: May inhibit metabolism of carbamazepine and increase level and risk of toxicity. Avoid use together.
Digoxin, theophylline: May increase levels of these drugs; dosage may be reduced at start of clarithromycin therapy. Monitor patient for toxicity.
Dihydroergotamine, ergotamine: May increase risk of acute ergot toxicity with severe peripheral vasospasm and dysesthesia. Monitor patient closely.
Drugs metabolized by the CYP3A system (alfentanil, bromocriptine, cilostazol, cyclosporine, disopyramide, hexobarbital, HMG-CoA reductase inhibitors, methylprednisolone, phenytoin, quinidine, rifabutin, rifampin, sildenafil, tacrolimus, valproate): May decrease clearance of these drugs, increasing risk of toxicity. Monitor drug levels and effects closely.

Fluconazole: May increase clarithromycin level. Monitor patient.
Ritonavir: May prolong absorption of clarithromycin. Don't adjust dosage in patients with normal renal function; if creatinine clearance is 30 to 60 ml/minute, give 50% of clarithromycin dose; if less than 30 ml/minute, give 25% of clarithromycin dose.
Warfarin: May increase bleeding times. Monitor PT and INR.
Zidovudine: May alter zidovudine level. Monitor patient closely for effectiveness of both drugs.

Effects on lab test results

• May increase AST, ALT, GGT, alkaline phosphatase, LDH, total bilirubin, creatinine, and BUN levels.

• May increase PT and INR. May decrease WBC counts.

Pharmacokinetics

Absorption: Rapid.
Distribution: Wide. 40% to 70% protein-bound.
Metabolism: Extensive. Major metabolite has significant antimicrobial activity.
Excretion: In urine and feces. *Half-life:* 5 to 6 hours with 250 mg every 12 hours; 7 hours with 500 mg every 12 hours.

Route	Onset	Peak	Duration
P.O.	Unknown	2–3 hr	Unknown
P.O. extended-release	Unknown	5–6 hr	Unknown

Action

Chemical effect: Binds to 50S subunit of bacterial ribosomes, blocking protein synthesis; bacteriostatic or bactericidal, depending on concentration.
Therapeutic effect: Hinders or kills susceptible bacteria.

Available forms

Suspension: 125 mg/5 ml, 250 mg/5 ml
Tablets: 250 mg, 500 mg
Tablets (extended-release): 500 mg, 1,000 mg

NURSING PROCESS

Assessment

• Assess patient's infection before and regularly throughout therapy.

- Obtain urine specimen for culture and sensitivity tests before giving the first dose. Begin therapy pending results.
- Be alert for adverse reactions and drug interactions.
- If adverse GI reactions occur, monitor patient's hydration.
- Assess patient's and family's knowledge of drug therapy.

💠 Nursing diagnoses
- Ineffective protection related to presence of bacteria susceptible to drug
- Risk for deficient fluid volume related to drug-induced adverse GI reactions
- Deficient knowledge related to drug therapy

▷ Planning and implementation
- Give drug with or without food. It may be taken with milk.
- Don't refrigerate oral suspension after reconstitution. Discard unused portion after 14 days.
- 🛑 **ALERT:** Don't confuse or interchange Biaxin XL (extended-release) with Biaxin (immediate release).

Patient teaching
- Tell patient to complete therapy as prescribed, even after he feels better.
- Urge patient to notify prescriber about all prescription and OTC medications taken, and to immediately report any adverse reactions.
- Instruct patient to report persistent diarrhea to prescriber, even if it occurs a month after antibiotic therapy has ended.
- Tell patient not to chew or crush extended-release tablets.

☑ Evaluation
- Patient is free from infection.
- Patient maintains adequate hydration throughout drug therapy.
- Patient and family state understanding of drug therapy.

clindamycin hydrochloride
(klin-duh-MIGH-sin high-droh-KLOR-ighd)
Cleocin, Dalacin C ♦

clindamycin palmitate hydrochloride
Cleocin Pediatric

clindamycin phosphate
Cleocin T, Clindagel, ClindaMax, ClindaMax Lotion, Clindesse, Clindets, Evoclin Foam

Pharmacologic class: lincomycin derivative
Therapeutic class: antibiotic
Pregnancy risk category: B

Indications and dosages

▶ **Infections caused by sensitive staphylococci, streptococci, pneumococci, *Bacteroides, Fusobacterium, Clostridium perfringens,* and other sensitive aerobic and anaerobic organisms.** *Adults:* 150 to 450 mg P.O. every 6 hours. Or 600 to 2,700 mg I.M. or I.V. daily divided into two to four doses. Don't exceed 600 mg in one I.M. dose. Don't give more than 1.2 g I.V. in a 1-hour period. Maximum adult I.V. dosage is 4.8 g daily.

Children ages 1 month to 16 years: 8 to 25 mg/kg P.O. daily in three or four equally divided doses. Or 20 to 40 mg/kg I.M. or I.V. daily, in three or four equally divided doses, or 350 to 450 mg/m² daily.

Neonates younger than age 1 month: 15 to 20 mg/kg I.V. daily in three or four equally divided doses.

▶ **Endocarditis prophylaxis for dental procedures in patients allergic to penicillin.** *Adults:* 600 mg P.O. 1 hour before procedure or 600 mg I.V. 30 minutes before procedure.

Children ages 1 month to 16 years: 20 mg/kg P.O. 1 hour before procedure or 20 mg/kg I.V. 30 minutes before procedure (not to exceed adult dosage).

▶ **Acne vulgaris.** *Adults:* Apply a thin film of topical suspension, gel, or lotion to affected areas b.i.d. Or apply foam to skin once daily after washing with mild soap and water. Cover affected areas completely and massage in until foam disappears. Or, 150 mg P.O. b.i.d.‡

▶ **Bacterial vaginosis.** *Adults:* One applicatorful intravaginally at bedtime daily for 3 to

7 days per prescriber instructions. Or, 1 suppository intravaginally at bedtime daily for 3 days.

▶ **Pneumocystis jiroveci (carinii) pneumonia‡.** *Adults:* 600 mg I.V. every 6 hours. Or 300 to 450 mg P.O. q.i.d. With primaquine, give 30 mg P.O. daily for 21 days.

▶ **Toxoplasmosis (cerebral or ocular) in immunocompromised patients‡.** *Adults:* 300 to 450 mg P.O. every 6 to 8 hours with pyrimethamine (25 to 75 mg once daily) and leucovorin (10 to 25 mg once daily).
Infants and children age 16 and younger: 20 to 30 mg/kg P.O. daily in four divided doses with oral pyrimethamine (1 mg/kg daily) and oral leucovorin (5 mg once every 3 days).

▽ I.V. administration

• For I.V. infusion, dilute each 300 mg in 50 ml solution.
• Give no faster than 30 mg/minute (over 10 to 60 minutes). Never give undiluted as bolus.
• Check I.V. site daily for phlebitis and irritation.

⊗ Incompatibilities
Allopurinol; aminophylline; ampicillin; azithromycin; barbiturates; calcium gluconate; ceftriaxone; ciprofloxacin hydrochloride; filgrastim; fluconazole; idarubicin; magnesium sulfate; phenytoin sodium; rubber closures, such as those on I.V. tubing; tobramycin sulfate.

Contraindications and cautions

• Contraindicated in patients hypersensitive to drug or lincomycin.
• Use cautiously in patients with renal or hepatic disease, asthma, history of GI disease, or significant allergies.
• **Lifespan:** Breast-feeding women should stop breast-feeding. In neonates, use cautiously.

Adverse reactions

CV: thrombophlebitis.
EENT: pharyngitis.
GI: abdominal pain, anorexia, *bloody or tarry stools,* constipation, *diarrhea, dysphagia,* esophagitis, flatulence, *nausea,* **pseudomembranous colitis,** unpleasant or bitter taste, vomiting.
GU: UTI, vaginal discharge.
Hematologic: eosinophilia, ***thrombocytopenia, transient leukopenia.***
Skin: maculopapular rash, urticaria.
Other: *anaphylaxis;* erythema, pain (I.V. use); *induration, pain, sterile abscess* (I.M. use).

Interactions

Drug-drug. *Erythromycin:* May block clindamycin site of action. Avoid use together.
Kaolin: May decrease absorption of oral clindamycin. Separate doses.
Neuromuscular blockers: May potentiate neuromuscular blockade. Monitor patient closely.

Effects on lab test results

• May increase bilirubin, AST, alkaline phosphatase, and CK levels.
• May increase eosinophil count. May decrease WBC and platelet counts.

Pharmacokinetics

Absorption: Rapid and almost complete when given P.O. Good after I.M. administration. Minimal vaginal absorption.
Distribution: Widely to most body tissues and fluids (except CSF). Drug is about 93% protein-bound.
Metabolism: Partially, to inactive metabolites.
Excretion: 10% unchanged in urine; rest as inactive metabolites. *Half-life:* 2½ to 3 hours; 1½ to 2½ hours for cream.

Route	Onset	Peak	Duration
P.O.	Unknown	45–60 min	Unknown
I.V.	Immediate	Immediate	Unknown
I.M.	Unknown	3 hr	Unknown
Topical	Unknown	Unknown	Unknown
Vaginal	Unknown	10–14 hr	20–24 hr

Action

Chemical effect: Inhibits bacterial protein synthesis by binding to 50S subunit of ribosome.
Therapeutic effect: Hinders or kills susceptible bacteria.

Available forms

clindamycin hydrochloride
Capsules: 75 mg, 150 mg, 300 mg
clindamycin palmitate hydrochloride
Oral solution: 75 mg/5 ml
clindamycin phosphate
Foam, topical: 1%
Gel, lotion, topical suspension: 1%
Injection: 150 mg/ml
Vaginal cream: 2%
Vaginal suppository: 100 mg

NURSING PROCESS

Assessment
• Assess patient's infection before and regularly throughout therapy.
• Before giving first dose, obtain specimen for culture and sensitivity tests. Begin therapy pending results.
• Monitor renal, hepatic, and hematopoietic functions during prolonged therapy.
• Be alert for adverse reactions and drug interactions.
• If adverse GI reactions occur, monitor patient's hydration.
• Assess patient's and family's knowledge of drug therapy.

Nursing diagnoses
• Ineffective protection related to presence of bacteria susceptible to drug
• Risk for deficient fluid volume related to drug-induced adverse GI reactions
• Deficient knowledge related to drug therapy

Planning and implementation
• Don't refrigerate reconstituted oral solution because it will thicken. Drug is stable for 2 weeks at room temperature.
• Give capsule form with full glass of water to prevent dysphagia.
• For I.M. injection, inject deeply. Rotate sites. Warn patient that I.M. injection may be painful. Doses over 600 mg per injection aren't recommended.
• I.M. injection may raise CK in response to muscle irritation.
ALERT: Don't give opioid antidiarrheals to treat drug-induced diarrhea; they may prolong and worsen diarrhea.
ALERT: Because of a link to severe and even fatal colitis, give clindamycin only for serious infections.
Patient teaching
• Teach patient how to store oral solution.
• Tell patient to take entire amount prescribed even after he feels better.
• Warn patient that I.M. injection may be painful.
ALERT: Inform patient that vaginal cream contains mineral oil, which may weaken the rubber latex of condoms or contraceptive diaphragms. Tell patient not to rely on such products while taking drug and for 5 days afterward. Contra-

ceptive and sexually transmitted disease protection may be impaired.
• Instruct patient to report diarrhea and to avoid self-treatment because of the risk of life-threatening pseudomembranous colitis.
• Tell patient receiving drug I.V. to report discomfort at infusion site.

Evaluation
• Patient is free from infection after drug therapy.
• Patient maintains adequate hydration during drug therapy.
• Patient and family state understanding of drug therapy.

clobetasol propionate
(kloh-BAY-tah-sol PRO-pee-uh-nayt)
Cormax, Dermovate*, Embeline E, Olux, Temovate, Temovate Emollient

Pharmacologic class: topical corticosteroid
Therapeutic class: anti-inflammatory
Pregnancy risk category: C

Indications and dosages
▶ **Inflammation and pruritus from moderate to severe corticosteroid-responsive dermatoses.** *Adults:* Apply a thin layer to affected skin areas b.i.d., once in the morning and once at night. Limit therapy to 14 days, with no more than 50 g cream or ointment or 50 ml lotion (25 mg total) weekly.
▶ **Inflammation and pruritus from moderate to severe corticosteroid-responsive dermatoses of the scalp; short-term topical therapy for mild to moderate plaque-type psoriasis of nonscalp regions, excluding the face and intertriginous areas.** *Adults:* Apply a small amount of Olux foam, up to a maximum of a golf ball–sized dollop, to affected skin b.i.d., once in the morning and once at night. Limit therapy to 14 days, with no more than 50 g of foam weekly.

Contraindications and cautions
• Contraindicated in patients hypersensitive to corticosteroids. Also contraindicated for acne, rosacea, perioral dermatitis, or as monotherapy for widespread plaque psoriasis.

- Use caution when applying drug to face, groin, or axillae because these areas are at an increased risk for atrophic changes.
- Use cautiously in patients with glaucoma and diabetes.
- ☀ **Lifespan:** In pregnant women, avoid use because of possibility of teratogenic effects. In breast-feeding women, use cautiously and avoid applying to breasts because it's unknown whether drug appears in breast milk. In patients younger than age 12, drug isn't recommended. In elderly patients, begin at the low end of the dosage range and adjust carefully.

Adverse reactions

GU: glucosuria.
Metabolic: hyperglycemia.
Skin: burning and stinging sensation, pruritus, irritation, dryness and cracking, erythema, folliculitis, perioral dermatitis, allergic contact dermatitis, hypopigmentation, hypertrichosis, acneiform eruptions, skin atrophy, telangiectasia (dilatation of capillaries), striae.
Other: *hypothalamic-pituitary-adrenal axis suppression,* Cushing syndrome, numbness of fingers.

Interactions

None reported.

Effects on lab test results

- May increase glucose level.
- May cause false-positive results with adrenocorticotropic hormone (ACTH) stimulation, a.m. cortisol, and urine-free cortisol tests.

Pharmacokinetics

Absorption: Variable, mainly by skin. Increases in areas of skin damage, inflammation, or occlusion. Small amount is systemic.
Distribution: Throughout the local skin. Any drug absorbed systemically is rapidly removed from the blood and goes to muscle, liver, skin, intestines, and kidneys.
Metabolism: Mainly in skin. Small amount in liver to inactive compounds.
Excretion: Drug and active metabolites, in the liver and bile. Inactive metabolites, by the kidneys, mainly as glucuronides and sulfates but also as unconjugated products. Small amounts of the metabolites are also in urine and feces.
Half-life: Unknown.

Route	Onset	Peak	Duration
Topical	Unknown	Unknown	Unknown

Action

Chemical effect: Unknown. Drug is a high-potency group I fluorinated corticosteroid usually reserved for severe dermatoses that haven't responded to a less potent formulation.
Therapeutic effect: Decreases inflammation and itching.

Available forms

Cream, foam, gel, lotion, ointment, shampoo, solution, spray: 0.05%

NURSING PROCESS

℞ Assessment
- Assess patient before and during therapy. Topical corticosteroid therapy may adversely affect and worsen symptoms in patients with diabetes or glaucoma.
- Monitor patient for adverse effects of corticosteroid therapy.
- If applied to face, groin, or axillae, observe often for skin atrophy.
- During long-term use, obtain ACTH stimulation, a.m. cortisol, and urine-free cortisol tests to monitor patient for hypothalamic-pituitary-adrenal (HPA) axis suppression.
- Assess patient's and family's knowledge of drug therapy.

Nursing diagnoses
- Risk for infection related to prolonged and very potent corticosteroid therapy
- Impaired skin integrity related to underlying skin disease process
- Situational low self-esteem from underlying skin disease process
- Deficient knowledge related to topical corticosteroid therapy

▶ Planning and implementation
- When applying foam to the scalp, move hair away from the affected area so that the foam can be applied to each affected area.
- Don't use longer than 2 weeks.
- Drug is for external use only. Avoid rubbing eyes during and after application. If drug gets into the eyes, flush affected eye with copious amounts of water.

• Don't dispense directly onto hand because cream and foam will begin to melt immediately upon contact with warm skin. When using foam, invert can and dispense foam into can cap or directly onto the lesion.

• Apply sparingly in light film; then massage into skin gently until foam disappears.

• Don't use occlusive dressings or bandages. Don't cover or wrap treated area unless instructed by prescriber.

• If skin infection develops, give antifungal or antibacterial drugs. If infection doesn't respond promptly, stop drug until infection is under control.

• If irritation, skin infection, striae, or atrophy occurs, stop drug and notify prescriber.

• Drug can suppress HPA axis at doses as low as 2 g daily. If HPA axis suppression occurs, stop giving the drug, reduce the dosage, or substitute a less potent steroid.

• If no improvement occurs within 2 weeks, reassess diagnoses.

• Don't refrigerate. Store drug at room temperature.

Patient teaching

• Advise patient that drug is for external use only and to avoid contact with eyes.

• Instruct patient to use medication only as prescribed.

• Teach patient proper application of the topical steroid to affected area. Explain that occlusive dressings aren't recommended and may increase absorption and skin atrophy.

• Inform patient of potential adverse reactions and of signs and symptoms of infection and impaired healing. Urge patient to immediately notify prescriber if any occur.

• Warn patient not to use drug for longer than 14 days.

• Caution patient that foam formulation is flammable and to avoid flames or smoking during and immediately after application.

• Instruct patients using Olux foam that the contents are under pressure and container shouldn't be punctured or incinerated. Also, tell patient not to expose to heat or store at temperatures above 120° F (49° C).

✓ Evaluation

• Patient doesn't suffer from any infection caused by drug therapy.

• Patient is relieved of symptoms and remains free from any adverse effects of drug therapy.

• Patient's self-esteem increases as patient's skin improves.

• Patient and family state understanding of drug therapy.

HIGH ALERT!

clofarabine
(kloh-FAR-uh-been)
Clolar

Pharmacologic class: purine nucleoside antimetabolite
Therapeutic class: antineoplastic
Pregnancy risk category: D

Indications and dosages

▶ **Relapsed or refractory acute lymphoblastic leukemia after at least two previous regimens.** *Children ages 1 to 21:* Give 52 mg/m² by I.V. infusion over 2 hours daily for 5 consecutive days. Repeat about every 2 to 6 weeks based on recovery or return to baseline of organ function. May also administer hydrocortisone 100 mg/m² I.V. on days 1 to 3 of cycle to help prevent capillary leak syndrome.

▼ I.V. administration

• Draw up the calculated dose through a 0.2-micron syringe filter and further dilute with D₅W or normal saline solution before infusion.

• Infuse drug within 24 hours of preparing it.

• Give over 2 hours with I.V. fluids.

• Store undiluted vials and resulting infusion solution at room temperature.

⊗ **Incompatibilities**
Don't give drug with other drugs through the same I.V. line.

Contraindications and cautions

• There are no known contraindications.

• Use very cautiously in patients with hepatic or renal dysfunction.

⚜ **Lifespan:** In pregnant women, drug may cause fetal harm. Women of childbearing potential should avoid becoming pregnant while receiving this drug. It isn't known whether drug appears in breast milk. Women shouldn't breastfeed while receiving drug.

Adverse reactions

CNS: *anxiety, depression, dizziness, fatigue, headache, irritability, lethargy, pain, somnolence, tremor.*

CV: *edema, flushing, hypertension, hypotension, left ventricular systolic dysfunction, pericardial effusion, tachycardia.*

EENT: *epistaxis, mucosal inflammation, sore throat.*

GI: *abdominal pain, anorexia, constipation, decreased appetite, decreased weight, diarrhea, gingival bleeding, oral candidiasis, nausea, vomiting.*

GU: *hematuria.*

Hematologic: ***bone marrow suppression,*** FEBRILE NEUTROPENIA, NEUTROPENIA.

Hepatic: *hepatomegaly, jaundice.*

Musculoskeletal: *arthralgia, back pain, limb pain, myalgia.*

Respiratory: *pneumonia, cough, dyspnea, pleural effusion,* RESPIRATORY DISTRESS.

Skin: *contusion, dermatitis, dry skin, erythema, hand-foot syndrome, petechiae, pruritus.*

Other: BACTEREMIA, ***capillary leak syndrome,*** *cellulitis, herpes simplex, injection site pain, pyrexia, rigors,* SEPSIS, *staphylococcal infections,* ***systemic inflammatory response syndrome,*** *transfusion reaction.*

Interactions

Drug-drug. *Blood pressure or cardiac drugs:* May increase the risk of adverse effects. Monitor patient closely.

Hepatotoxic drugs: May increase the risk of hepatic toxicity. Avoid use together.

Nephrotoxic drugs: May decrease excretion of clofarabine. Avoid use during the 5 days of clofarabine treatment.

Effects on lab test results

• May increase ALT, AST, bilirubin, creatinine, and hemoglobin levels and hematocrit.
• May decrease WBC counts and platelet counts.

Pharmacokinetics

Absorption: Given I.V.
Distribution: 47% bound to plasma proteins, mainly albumin.
Metabolism: Limited hepatic metabolism.
Excretion: 49% to 60% in urine unchanged.
Elimination half-life: about 5¼ hours.

Route	Onset	Peak	Duration
I.V.	Unknown	Unknown	Unknown

Action

Chemical effect: Inhibits DNA synthesis and repair and disrupts integrity of mitochondrial membranes, leading to programmed cell death.
Therapeutic effect: Kills selected cancer cells.

Available forms

Injection: 1 mg/ml in 20-ml vials

NURSING PROCESS

🗹 Assessment
• Assess patient's underlying condition before therapy and regularly throughout therapy.
• Assess patient for signs and symptoms of tumor lysis syndrome, cytokine release (tachypnea, tachycardia, hypotension, pulmonary edema) that could develop into systemic inflammatory response syndrome, capillary leak syndrome, and organ dysfunction.
• Monitor patient's respiratory status and blood pressure closely during treatment.
• Obtain CBC and platelet counts, and monitor hepatic and renal function regularly during treatment.
• Assess patient's and family's knowledge of drug therapy.

⊕ Nursing diagnoses
• Ineffective health maintenance related to underlying condition
• Risk for injury related to drug-induced adverse hematologic reactions
• Deficient knowledge related to drug therapy

▶ Planning and implementation
• Monitor the patient for dehydration. Give I.V. fluids continuously during the 5-day treatment period.
• If you suspect hyperuricemia, give allopurinol.
• If the patient has signs and symptoms of systemic inflammatory response syndrome or capillary leak syndrome, stop drug immediately.
• If hypotension develops, stop the drug. If it resolves without treatment, restart clofarabine at a lower dose.

Patient teaching
- Tell patient and caregiver that adverse effects are common. The patient will need close monitoring during treatment.
- Tell patient and caregiver to report dizziness, light-headedness, fainting, decreased urine output, bruising, flulike symptoms, and infection immediately.
- Urge patient and caregiver to report yellowing of skin or eyes, darkened urine, or abdominal pain.
- Tell a patient of childbearing potential to avoid pregnancy and breast-feeding during therapy.

☑ Evaluation
- Patient demonstrates positive response to drug therapy.
- Patient doesn't experience injury as a result of drug therapy.
- Patient and family state understanding of drug therapy.

clomiphene citrate
(KLOH-meh-feen SIGH-trayt)
Clomid, Milophene, Serophene

Pharmacologic class: chlorotrianisene derivative
Therapeutic class: ovulation stimulant
Pregnancy risk category: X

Indications and dosages

▶ **To induce ovulation.** *Women:* 50 mg P.O. daily for 5 days starting on day 5 of menstrual cycle if bleeding occurs (first day of menstrual flow is day 1), or at any time if woman hasn't had recent uterine bleeding. If ovulation doesn't occur, may increase dosage to 100 mg P.O. daily for 5 days as soon as 30 days after previous course. Repeat until conception occurs or until three courses of therapy are completed.
▶ **Infertility‡.** *Men:* 50 to 400 mg P.O. daily for 2 to 12 months.

Contraindications and cautions

- Contraindicated in patients with undiagnosed abnormal genital bleeding, ovarian cyst not caused by polycystic ovarian syndrome, hepatic disease or dysfunction, uncontrolled thyroid or

adrenal dysfunction, or organic intracranial lesion (such as pituitary tumor).
⚥ **Lifespan:** In pregnant women, drug is contraindicated.

Adverse reactions

CNS: depression, dizziness, fatigue, headache, insomnia, light-headedness, restlessness, tension, *vasomotor flushes.*
CV: hypertension.
EENT: blurred vision, diplopia, photophobia, scotoma.
GI: bloating, distention, nausea, vomiting.
GU: *ovarian enlargement and cyst formation,* which regress spontaneously when drug is stopped; urinary frequency and polyuria.
Metabolic: *hyperglycemia,* increased appetite, weight gain.
Skin: dermatitis, rash, reversible alopecia, urticaria.
Other: breast discomfort.

Interactions

None significant.

Effects on lab test results

- May increase blood glucose level.

Pharmacokinetics

Absorption: Good.
Distribution: May undergo enterohepatic recirculation or may be stored in fat.
Metabolism: By liver.
Excretion: Mainly in feces via biliary elimination. *Half-life:* 5 days.

Route	Onset	Peak	Duration
P.O.	Unknown	Unknown	Unknown

Action

Chemical effect: May stimulate release of pituitary gonadotropins, follicle-stimulating hormone, and luteinizing hormone, resulting in maturation of ovarian follicle, ovulation, and development of corpus luteum.
Therapeutic effect: Induces ovulation.

Available forms

Tablets: 50 mg

NURSING PROCESS

⚖ Assessment
- Assess patient's underlying condition before therapy and regularly thereafter.
- Monitor drug's effectiveness by assessing ovulation through biphasic body temperature measurement, postovulatory pregnanediol level in urine, estrogen excretion, and changes in endometrial tissues.
- Be alert for adverse reactions.
- Assess patient's and family's knowledge of drug therapy.

🔲 Nursing diagnoses
- Excess fluid volume related to drug-induced fluid retention
- Sexual dysfunction related to underlying condition
- Deficient knowledge related to drug therapy

▶ Planning and implementation
- Prepare administration instructions for patient: Begin daily dose on fifth day of menstrual flow and take for 5 consecutive days.
- Don't give more than three courses of therapy to attempt conception.

Patient teaching
- Tell patient about risk of multiple births and that risk increases with larger doses.
- Teach patient how to take and chart basal body temperature and to ascertain whether ovulation has occurred.
- Reassure woman that ovulation typically occurs after first course of therapy. If pregnancy doesn't occur, course of therapy may be repeated twice.
- ⏺ ALERT: Advise woman to stop taking drug and to contact prescriber immediately if pregnancy is suspected, because drug may have teratogenic effect on fetus.
- Advise woman to stop taking drug and to contact prescriber immediately if abdominal symptoms or pain occur; they may indicate ovarian enlargement or ovarian cyst.
- Tell patient to immediately report signs of impending visual toxicity, such as blurred vision, diplopia, scotoma, or photophobia.
- Warn patient to avoid hazardous activities until the drug's CNS effects are known; drug may cause dizziness or visual disturbances.

☑ Evaluation
- Patient is free from fluid retention at end of therapy.
- Woman ovulates with drug therapy.
- Patient and family state understanding of drug therapy.

clomipramine hydrochloride
(kloh-MIH-pruh-meen high-droh-KLOR-ighd)
Anafranil

Pharmacologic class: tricyclic antidepressant (TCA)
Therapeutic class: obsessive-compulsive disorder (OCD) drug
Pregnancy risk category: C

Indications and dosages

▶ **OCD.** *Adults:* Initially, 25 mg P.O. daily in divided doses with meals, gradually increase to 100 mg daily during first 2 weeks. Then increase, if needed, to maximum dosage of 250 mg daily in divided doses with meals. After adjusting dosage, give total daily dosage at bedtime.
Children ages 10 to 18: Initially, 12.5 mg P.O. b.i.d. with meals, gradually increase to daily maximum of 3 mg/kg or 100 mg P.O., whichever is smaller. After adjusting dosage, give total daily dosage at bedtime. Reassess and adjust periodically.
▶ **Panic disorder‡.** *Adults:* 12.5 to 150 mg (maximum, 200 mg) daily.

Contraindications and cautions

- Contraindicated in patients hypersensitive to drug or other TCAs, in patients in acute recovery period after MI, and within 14 days of MAO inhibitor therapy.
- Use cautiously in patients with history of seizure disorders or with brain damage; in those receiving other seizure-threshold–lowering drugs; in patients at risk for suicide; in patients with history of urine retention or angle-closure glaucoma, increased intraocular pressure, CV disease, impaired hepatic or renal function, or hyperthyroidism; in patients with tumors of the adrenal medulla; in patients receiving thyroid drug or electroconvulsive therapy; and in those undergoing elective surgery.

C

⚘ **Lifespan:** In pregnant and breast-feeding women, use cautiously. Young adults ages 18 to 24 may be at risk for suicidal thinking and behavior during the first 2 months of treatment.

Adverse reactions

CNS: aggressiveness, asthenia, dizziness, EEG changes, extrapyramidal reactions, fatigue, headache, insomnia, nervousness, myoclonus, *seizures,* somnolence, tremors.
CV: orthostatic hypotension, palpitations, tachycardia.
EENT: abnormal vision, laryngitis, otitis media in children, pharyngitis, rhinitis.
GI: abdominal pain, anorexia, constipation, diarrhea, dry mouth, dyspepsia, eructation, *nausea.*
GU: dysmenorrhea, impaired ejaculation, impotence, urinary hesitancy, UTI.
Hematologic: anemia, bone marrow suppression.
Metabolic: increased appetite, *weight gain.*
Musculoskeletal: *myalgia.*
Skin: *diaphoresis,* dry skin, photosensitivity, pruritus, rash.
Other: altered libido.

Interactions

Drug-drug. *Barbiturates:* May decrease TCA level. Monitor patient for decreased antidepressant effect.
Cimetidine, methylphenidate: May increase TCA level. Monitor patient for increased antidepressant effect.
Clonidine: May cause loss of blood pressure control and potentially life-threatening elevations in blood pressure. Avoid use together.
CNS depressants: May enhance CNS depression. Avoid use together.
Epinephrine, norepinephrine: May increase hypertensive effect. Use with caution, and monitor blood pressure.
MAO inhibitors: May cause hyperpyretic crisis, seizures, coma, or death. Don't use together or within 14 days of each other.
Drug-herb. *St. John's wort:* May raise serotonin level, causing serotonin syndrome. Discourage use together.
Drug-lifestyle. *Alcohol use:* May increase CNS depression. Discourage use together.
Smoking: May increase metabolism and decrease effectiveness. Discourage smoking.

Sun exposure: May cause photosensitivity. Urge patient to avoid sun exposure and to wear protective clothing and sunblock.

Effects on lab test results

• May decrease hemoglobin level and hematocrit.

Pharmacokinetics

Absorption: Good, but extensive first-pass metabolism limits bioavailability to about 50%.
Distribution: Into lipophilic tissues. About 98% protein-bound.
Metabolism: Mainly hepatic with several metabolites.
Excretion: 66% in urine; remainder in feces.
Half-life: Parent compound, 32 hours; active metabolite, 69 hours.

Route	Onset	Peak	Duration
P.O.	≥ 2 wk	Unknown	Unknown

Action

Chemical effect: Selectively inhibits serotonin reuptake.
Therapeutic effect: Reduces OCD behaviors.

Available forms

Capsules: 25 mg, 50 mg, 75 mg

NURSING PROCESS

⟁ **Assessment**
• Assess patient's underlying condition before therapy and regularly thereafter.
• Assess patient's and family's knowledge of drug therapy.

⊞ **Nursing diagnoses**
• Ineffective coping related to patient's underlying condition
• Risk for injury related to drug-induced adverse reactions
• Deficient knowledge related to drug therapy

▶ **Planning and implementation**
• During dosage adjustment, divide dose and give with meals to minimize GI effects. After dosage adjustment, give total daily dosage at bedtime.
• Don't abruptly stop giving the drug.

• Because hypertensive episodes may occur during surgery, taper off drug several days before surgery.

⊛ ALERT: Don't confuse clomipramine with chlorpromazine or clomiphene; don't confuse Anafranil with enalapril, nafarelin, or alfentanil.

Patient teaching

• Warn patient to avoid hazardous activities requiring alertness and good psychomotor coordination, especially during dosage adjustment. Daytime sedation and dizziness may occur.

• Tell patient to avoid alcohol while taking drug.

• Warn patient not to abruptly stop taking drug.

• Tell patient and his family to immediately report changes in mood or behavior, especially suicidal thinking, to his health care provider.

• Advise patient to use sunblock, wear protective clothing, and avoid prolonged exposure to strong sunlight.

☑ Evaluation

• Patient's behavior and communication indicate improvement of obsessive-compulsive pattern.

• Patient doesn't experience injury from drug-induced adverse CNS reactions.

• Patient and family state understanding of drug therapy.

HIGH ALERT!

clonazepam
(kloh-NEH-zuh-pam)
Klonopin, Rivotril ◆

Pharmacologic class: benzodiazepine
Therapeutic class: anticonvulsant, anxiolytic
Pregnancy risk category: D
Controlled substance schedule: IV

Indications and dosages

▶ **Lennox-Gastaut syndrome; atypical absence seizures; akinetic and myoclonic seizures.** *Adults:* Initially, not to exceed 1.5 mg P.O. t.i.d. May increase by 0.5 to 1 mg every 3 days until seizures are controlled. If given in unequal doses, give largest dose at bedtime. Maximum daily dose is 20 mg.
Children age 10 and younger or weighing 30 kg (66 lb) or less: Initially, 0.01 to 0.03 mg/kg P.O. daily (maximum, 0.05 mg/kg daily) in two or three divided doses. Increase by 0.25 to 0.5 mg

every third day to maximum maintenance dosage of 0.1 to 0.2 mg/kg daily as needed.

▶ **Panic disorder.** *Adults:* Initially, 0.25 mg P.O. b.i.d.; increase to target dose of 1 mg daily after 3 days. Some patients may benefit from doses up to maximum of 4 mg daily. To achieve 4 mg daily, increase dosage in increments of 0.125 to 0.25 mg b.i.d. every 3 days as tolerated until panic disorder is controlled. Stop drug gradually by decreases of 0.125 mg b.i.d. every 3 days until stopped.

▶ **Restless legs syndrome; adjunct in schizophrenia‡.** *Adults:* 0.5 to 2 mg P.O. at bedtime.

▶ **Parkinsonian dysarthria‡.** *Adults:* 0.25 to 0.5 mg P.O. daily.

▶ **Acute manic episodes‡.** *Adults:* 0.75 to 16 mg P.O. daily.

▶ **Multifocal tic disorders‡.** *Adults:* 1.5 to 12 mg P.O. daily.

▶ **Neuralgia‡.** *Adults:* 2 to 4 mg P.O. daily.

Contraindications and cautions

• Contraindicated in patients hypersensitive to benzodiazepines and in those with acute angle-closure glaucoma or significant hepatic disease.

• Use cautiously in patients with mixed type of seizure because drug may precipitate generalized tonic-clonic seizures. Also, use cautiously in patients with chronic respiratory disease, or open-angle glaucoma not well controlled.

⚘ Lifespan: In pregnant women, use only when benefits to mother outweigh risks to fetus. Breast-feeding women should stop breast-feeding because drug appears in breast milk. In children, use cautiously. In elderly patients, use cautiously and start with low doses because of possible reduced hepatic and renal function.

Adverse reactions

CNS: agitation, *ataxia, behavioral disturbances* (especially in children), confusion, *drowsiness,* migraine, nightmares, psychosis, sleep disorders, slurred speech, **suicidal ideation,** tremor, vertigo.
EENT: abnormal eye movements, diplopia, earache, *increased salivation,* nystagmus, otitis, rhinitis, sinusitis, sore gums.
CV: chest pain, facial and ankle edema, palpitations, postural hypotension, thrombophlebitis.
GI: abnormal thirst, appetite changes, constipation, diarrhea, gastritis, nausea.
GU: dysuria, enuresis, nocturia, urine retention.

Reactions may be *common*, uncommon, *life-threatening*, or COMMON AND LIFE-THREATENING.

Hematologic: eosinophilia, *leukopenia, thrombocytopenia.*
Metabolic: change in appetite.
Musculoskeletal: muscle weakness, pain.
Respiratory: *respiratory depression,* upper respiratory tract infection.
Skin: acne flare, alopecia, contact dermatitis, flushing, rash.

Interactions

Drug-drug. *CNS depressants:* May increase CNS depression. Monitor patient closely.
Fluconazole, itraconazole, ketoconazole, miconazole: May increase and prolong levels, CNS depression, and psychomotor impairment. Don't use together.
Drug-herb. *Catnip, kava, lady's slipper, lemon balm, passion flower, sassafras, skullcap, valerian:* May enhance sedative effects of clonazepam. Discourage use together.
Drug-lifestyle. *Alcohol use:* May cause additive CNS effects. Strongly discourage alcohol use.

Effects on lab test results

• May increase liver function test values and eosinophil count. May decrease WBC and platelet counts.

Pharmacokinetics

Absorption: Good.
Distribution: Wide. 85% protein-bound.
Metabolism: By liver to several metabolites.
Excretion: In urine. *Half-life:* 18 to 50 hours.

Route	Onset	Peak	Duration
P.O.	Unknown	1–2 hr	Unknown

Action

Chemical effect: May act by facilitating effects of inhibitory neurotransmitter GABA.
Therapeutic effect: Prevents or stops seizure activity.

Available forms

Tablets: 0.5 mg, 1 mg, 2 mg
Tablets (orally-disintegrating): 0.125 mg, 0.25 mg, 0.5 mg, 1 mg, 2 mg

NURSING PROCESS

Assessment
• Assess patient's seizure condition before therapy and regularly thereafter.

• Monitor clonazepam level. Therapeutic level for anticonvulsant effects has been reported to be 20 to 80 nanograms/ml.
• Monitor CBC and liver function tests.
• Be alert for adverse reactions and drug interactions.
• Assess patient's and family's knowledge of drug therapy.

Nursing diagnoses
• Risk for injury related to potential for seizure activity
• Activity intolerance related to drug-induced sedation
• Deficient knowledge related to drug therapy

Planning and implementation
• Increase dosage gradually.
ALERT: Never stop drug abruptly because seizures may worsen. Follow weaning protocol for safety.
• Withdrawal symptoms are similar to those of barbiturates (insomnia, dysphoria; then abdominal and muscle cramps, tremor, behavioral disorder; progressing to hallucinations, psychosis, convulsions).
• If adverse reactions develop, immediately call prescriber.
• Maintain seizure precautions.
ALERT: Don't confuse Klonopin or clonazepam with clonidine, clozapine, or clomiphene.
Patient teaching
• Advise patient to avoid driving or other potentially hazardous activities until drug's CNS effects are known.
• Instruct parents to monitor child's school performance because drug may interfere with attentiveness.
• For orally disintegrating tablets, instruct patient to peel back the foil blister pouch using dry hands and to place tablet in mouth immediately. The tablet disintegrates rapidly in saliva.
• Instruct patient or family to notify prescriber if oversedation or other adverse reaction develops or questions arise about therapy.
• Advise patients with panic disorder to continue psychotherapeutic interventions in addition to drug therapy.

Evaluation
• Patient is free from seizure activity during drug therapy.
• Patient can meet daily activity needs.

• Patient and family state understanding of drug therapy.

---

clonidine hydrochloride
(KLON-uh-deen high-droh-KLOR-ighd)
Catapres, Catapres-TTS, Dixarit ♦ , Duraclon

Pharmacologic class: centrally acting sympatholytic
Therapeutic class: antihypertensive
Pregnancy risk category: C

Indications and dosages

▶ **Essential, renal, and malignant hypertension.** *Adults:* Initially, 0.1 mg P.O. b.i.d. Then, increase by 0.1 to 0.2 mg daily every week. Usual dosage range is 0.1 to 0.3 mg b.i.d.; infrequently, dosages as high as 2.4 mg daily are used. Or transdermal patch applied to nonhairy area of intact skin on upper arm or torso every 7 days. Start with 0.1-mg system and adjust after 1 to 2 weeks with another 0.1-mg system or larger system if increases are needed to maintain normal blood pressure.

▶ **Severe pain.** *Adults:* Starting dosage for continuous epidural infusion is 30 mcg/hour. Adjust according to patient's response.

▶ **Prophylaxis for vascular headache‡.** *Adults:* 0.025 mg P.O. b.i.d. to q.i.d., up to 0.15 mg P.O. daily in divided doses.

▶ **Adjunctive therapy for nicotine withdrawal‡.** *Adults:* Initially, 0.1 mg P.O. b.i.d., then gradually increase dose by 0.1 mg daily every week, up to 0.75 mg P.O. daily, as tolerated. Alternatively, apply transdermal patch (0.1 to 0.2 mg/24 hours) and replace weekly for the first 2 or 3 weeks after smoking cessation.

▶ **Adjunct in opioid withdrawal‡.** *Adults:* 5 to 17 mcg/kg P.O. daily in divided doses for up to 10 days. Adjust dosage to avoid hypotension and excessive sedation, and slowly withdraw drug.

▶ **Adjunct in menopausal symptoms‡.** *Adults:* 0.025 to 0.2 mg P.O. b.i.d. Or apply transdermal patch (0.1 mg/24 hours) and replace weekly.

▶ **Dysmenorrhea‡.** *Adults:* 0.025 mg P.O. b.i.d. for 14 days before onset of menses and during menses.

▶ **Ulcerative colitis‡.** *Adults:* 0.3 mg P.O. t.i.d.

▶ **Diabetic diarrhea‡.** *Adults:* 0.15 to 1.2 mg P.O. daily. Or 1 to 2 patches every week (0.3 mg/24 hours).

▶ **Attention deficit hyperactivity disorder‡.** *Children:* Initially, 0.05 mg P.O. at bedtime. Increase cautiously over 2 to 4 weeks to reach maintenance dosage of 0.05 to 0.4 mg daily depending on the patient's weight and tolerance. May also use 5 mcg/kg P.O. daily for 8 weeks.

Contraindications and cautions

• Contraindicated in patients hypersensitive to drug. Transdermal form is contraindicated in patients hypersensitive to any component of adhesive layer. Injectable form is contraindicated in patients receiving anticoagulation therapy and patients with a bleeding diathesis or injection-site infection.

• Use cautiously in patient with severe coronary insufficiency, recent MI, cerebrovascular disease, and chronic renal or hepatic impairment.

⚖ **Lifespan:** In pregnant women, safety and effectiveness haven't been established. In breast-feeding women, use cautiously. In children, safety and effectiveness haven't been established. In children with severe intractable pain from malignancy that is unresponsive to epidural or spinal opioids or other conventional analgesic techniques, injectable form is restricted.

Adverse reactions

CNS: *anxiety, confusion, dizziness, drowsiness,* fatigue, headache, nervousness, sedation, *somnolence,* vivid dreams.
CV: *bradycardia, hypotension,* orthostatic hypotension, *severe rebound hypertension.*
GI: *constipation, dry mouth, nausea, vomiting.*
GU: urine retention, impotence, UTI.
Metabolic: transient glucose intolerance.
Skin: *pruritus and dermatitis* with transdermal patch.

Interactions

Drug-drug. *Amitriptyline, amoxapine, clomipramine, desipramine, doxepin, imipramine, nortriptyline, protriptyline, trimipramine:* May cause loss of blood pressure control with potentially life-threatening elevations in blood pressure. Don't use together.
Beta blockers, such as propranolol: May cause severe rebound hypertension. Monitor patient carefully.

CNS depressants: May enhance CNS depression. Use together cautiously.
MAO inhibitors: May decrease antihypertensive effect. Use together cautiously.
Drug-herb. *Capsicum, yohimbe:* May reduce antihypertensive effectiveness. Discourage use together.

Effects on lab test results

• May increase glucose and CK levels.

Pharmacokinetics

Absorption: Good.
Distribution: Wide.
Metabolism: Nearly 50% is transformed to inactive metabolites.
Excretion: 65% in urine; 20% in feces. *Half-life:* 6 to 20 hours.

Route	Onset	Peak	Duration
P.O.	15–30 min	1½–2½ hr	6–8 hr
Epidural	Immediate	19 min	Unknown
Transdermal	2–3 days	2–3 days	Several days

Action

Chemical effect: May inhibit central vasomotor centers, decreasing sympathetic outflow to heart, kidneys, and peripheral vasculature, resulting in decreased peripheral vascular resistance, decreased systolic and diastolic blood pressure, and decreased heart rate. Produces analgesia by mimicking the activation of descending pain-suppressing pathways arising from supraspinal control centers. Also inhibits the release of substance P, an inflammatory neuropeptide.
Therapeutic effect: Lowers blood pressure and decreases neurogenic pain.

Available forms

Injectable: 100 mcg/ml, 500 mcg/ml
Tablets: 0.025 mg, 0.1 mg, 0.2 mg, 0.3 mg
Transdermal: TTS-1 (releases 0.1 mg/24 hours), TTS-2 (releases 0.2 mg/24 hours), TTS-3 (releases 0.3 mg/24 hours)

NURSING PROCESS

Assessment

• Assess patient's blood pressure before therapy and regularly thereafter.
• Antihypertensive effects of transdermal clonidine may take 2 to 3 days to become apparent.

Oral antihypertensive therapy may have to be continued in interim.
• Be alert for adverse reactions and drug interactions.
• Observe patient for tolerance to drug's therapeutic effects; increase dosage if needed.
• Periodic eye examinations are recommended.
• Monitor site of transdermal patch for dermatitis. Ask patient about pruritus.
• Assess patient's and family's knowledge of drug therapy.

Nursing diagnoses

• Risk for injury related to presence of hypertension
• Ineffective protection related to severe rebound hypertension caused by abrupt cessation of drug
• Deficient knowledge related to drug therapy

Planning and implementation

• Drug may be given to lower blood pressure rapidly in some hypertensive emergency situations.
• Adjust dosage to patient's blood pressure and tolerance.
• Give last dose of day at bedtime.
• Epidural clonidine is more likely to be effective in patients with neuropathic pain than somatic or visceral pain.
ALERT: Injection form is for epidural use only. The 500-mcg/ml dose must be diluted in normal saline for injection to provide a final concentration of 100 mcg/ml.
• When giving by epidural route, carefully monitor infusion pump and inspect catheter tubing for obstruction or dislodgement. Monitor access site for signs of infection or inflammation.
• Monitor patient closely, especially during the first few days of therapy. Respiratory depression or deep sedation may occur.
• To improve adherence of patch, apply adhesive overlay. Place patch at different site each week.
• Remove transdermal patch before defibrillation to prevent arcing.
• When stopping therapy in patients receiving both clonidine and beta blocker, gradually withdraw beta blocker first to minimize adverse reactions.
• Don't stop giving clonidine before surgery.

⚛ **ALERT:** Don't confuse clonidine with quinidine, with clozapine, Klonopin, clonazepam, or clomiphene; or Catapres with Cetapred or Combipres.

Patient teaching

• Advise patient not to stop drug abruptly because doing so may cause severe rebound hypertension. Explain that dose must be reduced gradually over 2 to 4 days.

• Tell patient to take the last daily dose immediately before bedtime.

• Reassure patient that transdermal patch usually adheres despite showering and other routine daily activities. Teach him how to use adhesive overlay to improve skin adherence. Also tell patient to place patch at different site each week.

• Caution patient that drug can cause drowsiness, but that he will develop tolerance to this adverse effect.

• Urge patient to rise slowly and avoid sudden position changes to reduce orthostatic hypotension.

✔ **Evaluation**

• Patient's blood pressure is normal with drug therapy.

• Patient understands not to stop drug abruptly.

• Patient and family state understanding of drug therapy.

clopidogrel bisulfate
(kloh-PIH-doh-grel bigh-SUL-fayt)
Plavix

Pharmacologic class: inhibitor of adenosine diphosphate (ADP)–induced platelet aggregation
Therapeutic class: antiplatelet
Pregnancy risk category: B

Indications and dosages

▶ **Reduce atherosclerotic events in patients with atherosclerosis documented by recent stroke, MI, or peripheral arterial disease.**
Adults: 75 mg P.O. daily.

▶ **Reduce atherosclerotic events in patients with acute coronary syndrome (unstable angina, non–ST-segment elevation MI), including those managed medically and those who are to be managed with percutaneous coronary intervention (with or without stent)**

or coronary artery bypass graft. *Adults:* Start with a single 300-mg P.O. loading dose, then continue at 75 mg P.O. once daily. Also, give 75 to 325 mg aspirin once daily during therapy.

▶ **ST-segment elevation acute MI.** *Adults:* 75 mg P.O. once daily with aspirin, with or without thrombolytics. An optional 300-mg loading dose may be given.

Contraindications and cautions

• Contraindicated in patients hypersensitive to drug or any of its components, and in those with pathologic bleeding, such as peptic ulcer or intracranial hemorrhage.

• Use cautiously in patients with hepatic impairment and in those at risk for increased bleeding from trauma, surgery, or other conditions.

⚖ **Lifespan:** In breast-feeding women, drug is contraindicated. In children, safety and effectiveness haven't been established.

Adverse reactions

CNS: depression, dizziness, fatigue, headache, pain.
CV: chest pain, edema, hypertension.
EENT: epistaxis, rhinitis.
GI: abdominal pain, constipation, diarrhea, dyspepsia, gastritis, *hemorrhage,* ulcers.
GU: UTI.
Hematologic: purpura.
Musculoskeletal: arthralgia, back pain.
Respiratory: bronchitis, cough, dyspnea, upper respiratory tract infection.
Skin: rash, pruritus.
Other: flulike symptoms.

Interactions

Drug-drug. *Aspirin, NSAIDs:* May increase risk of GI bleeding. Monitor patient for signs of GI bleeding, such as abdominal pain or blood in vomitus or stool.
Heparin, warfarin: Safety hasn't been established. Use together cautiously, and monitor patient for bleeding.
Drug-herb. *Dong quai, feverfew, garlic, ginger, horse chestnut, red clover:* May increase risk of bleeding. Monitor patient closely.

Effects on lab test results

• May decrease platelet count.

Pharmacokinetics

Absorption: At least 50% and rapid.

Distribution: 94% to 98% protein-bound.
Metabolism: Extensive.
Excretion: 50% in urine and 46% in feces.
Half-life: 8 hours.

Route	Onset	Peak	Duration
P.O.	2 hr	Unknown	5 days

Action

Chemical effect: Inhibits binding of ADP to its platelet receptor, which inhibits ADP-mediated activation and subsequent platelet aggregation. Because drug acts by irreversibly modifying the platelet ADP receptor, platelets exposed to drug are affected for their lifespan.
Therapeutic effect: Prevents clot formation.

Available forms

Tablets: 75 mg

NURSING PROCESS

Assessment
• Assess current use of OTC drugs, such as aspirin or NSAIDs, and herbal remedies.
• Assess patient for increased bleeding or bruising tendencies before and during drug therapy.
• Assess patient's and family's knowledge of drug therapy.

Nursing diagnoses
• Risk for injury related to potential for atherosclerotic events from underlying condition
• Ineffective protection related to increased risk of bleeding
• Deficient knowledge related to drug therapy

Planning and implementation
• Five days after stopping drug, expect platelet aggregation to return to normal.
• Don't give drug to a patient with hepatic impairment or an increased risk of bleeding from trauma, surgery, or other pathologic conditions.
⊛ **ALERT:** Don't confuse Plavix with Paxil.
Patient teaching
• Tell patient it may take longer than usual to stop bleeding. Urge him to refrain from activities that increase the risk of trauma and bleeding.
• Instruct patient to notify prescriber about unusual bleeding or bruising.
• Tell patient to inform prescriber or dentist that he's taking drug before having surgery or starting new drug therapy.

• Inform patient that drug may be taken with or without food.

Evaluation
• Patient has less risk of stroke, MI, and vascular death.
• Patient states appropriate bleeding precautions to take.
• Patient and family state understanding of drug therapy.

HIGH ALERT!

clozapine
(KLOH-zuh-peen)
Clozaril, FazaClo

Pharmacologic class: tricyclic dibenzodiazepine derivative
Therapeutic class: antipsychotic
Pregnancy risk category: B

Indications and dosages

▶ **Schizophrenia in severely ill patients unresponsive to other therapies; reduction in risk of recurrent suicidal behavior in schizophrenia or schizoaffective disorder.** *Adults:* Initially, 12.5 mg P.O. once daily or b.i.d.; increase by 25 to 50 mg daily (if tolerated) to 300 to 450 mg daily by end of 2 weeks. Base dosage on response, patient tolerance, and adverse reactions. Don't increase subsequent doses more than once or twice weekly, and don't exceed 100 mg. Many patients respond to 300 to 600 mg daily, but some may need as much as 900 mg daily. Maximum, 900 mg daily.
🚫 **Adjust-a-dose:** In elderly patients, use lowest recommended dose when starting therapy.

Contraindications and cautions

• Contraindicated in patients taking drugs that suppress bone marrow function and in those with paralytic ileus, uncontrolled epilepsy, history of drug-induced agranulocytosis, myelosuppressive disorders, severe CNS depression or coma, paralytic ileus, or WBC count less than 3,500/mm3.
• Use cautiously in patients with prostatic hyperplasia, urinary retention, or angle-closure glaucoma because clozapine has potent anticholinergic effects. Also use cautiously in patients receiving general anesthesia and in those with hepatic, renal, or cardiac disease.

♨ **Lifespan:** In pregnant women, use cautiously. In breast-feeding women, drug is contraindicated. In children younger than age 12, safety and effectiveness haven't been established. In elderly patients, use cautiously and at lowest recommended dose.

Adverse reactions

CNS: agitation, akathisia, anxiety, ataxia, confusion, depression, disturbed sleep or nightmares, *dizziness, drowsiness,* fatigue, fever, headache, hyperkinesia, hypokinesia or akinesia, insomnia, myoclonus, rigidity, *sedation, seizures,* slurred speech, *syncope,* tremor, *vertigo,* weakness.
CV: *cardiomyopathy,* chest pain, ECG changes, hypertension, hypotension, orthostatic hypotension, tachycardia.
GI: constipation, dry mouth, *excessive salivation,* heartburn, nausea, vomiting.
GU: abnormal ejaculation, incontinence, urinary frequency, urinary urgency, urine retention.
Hematologic: *agranulocytosis, leukopenia.*
Metabolic: hypercholesterolemia, hypertriglyceridemia, *severe hyperglycemia,* weight gain.
Musculoskeletal: muscle pain or spasm, muscle weakness.
Skin: rash.

Interactions

Drug-drug. *Anticholinergics:* May increase anticholinergic effects of clozapine. Avoid use together.
Antihypertensives: May increase hypotensive effects. Monitor blood pressure.
Bone marrow suppressants: May increase bone marrow toxicity. Don't use together.
Citalopram: May significantly increase clozapine level and adverse effects. Avoid use together.
Digoxin, warfarin, other highly protein-bound drugs: May increase levels of these drugs. Monitor patient closely for adverse reactions.
Psychoactive drugs: May produce additive effects. Use together cautiously.
Drug-herb. *St. John's wort:* May reduce drug level, causing a loss of symptom control in patients taking an antipsychotic. Discourage use together.
Drug-food. *Caffeine:* May increase clozapine level. Large fluctuations in caffeine consumption may affect therapeutic response to drug. Advise patient to limit caffeine.

Drug-lifestyle. *Alcohol use:* May increase CNS depression. Discourage use together.
Smoking: May increase metabolism of drug and decrease its effectiveness. Discourage smoking.

Effects on lab test results

• May increase ALT, AST, LDH, and alkaline phosphatase levels. May increase or decrease glucose level.
• May decrease WBC and granulocyte counts.

Pharmacokinetics

Absorption: Rapid.
Distribution: 95% protein-bound.
Metabolism: Extensive.
Excretion: 50% of drug appears in urine and 30% in feces, mostly as metabolites. *Half-life:* Appears proportional to dose and may range from 8 to 12 hours.

Route	Onset	Peak	Duration
P.O.	Unknown	2½ hr	4–12 hr
P.O. orally disintegrating	Unknown	2½ hr	Unknown

Action

Chemical effect: Unknown. Binds to dopaminergic receptors (both D1 and D2) in limbic system of CNS and may interfere with adrenergic, cholinergic, histaminergic, and serotoninergic receptors.
Therapeutic effect: Relieves psychotic signs and symptoms.

Available forms

Tablets: 12.5 mg, 25 mg, 50mg, 100 mg, 200 mg
Tablets (orally-disintegrating): 12.5 mg, 50 mg, 25 mg, 100 mg

NURSING PROCESS

🔲 **Assessment**

• Assess patient's psychotic condition before therapy and regularly thereafter.
• Monitor patient's baseline WBC and differential counts before therapy and weekly thereafter.
• Be alert for adverse reactions and drug interactions.
• Assess patient for risk factors of diabetes, and obtain baseline fasting blood glucose level. Routinely reassess patient for signs and symp-

toms of hyperglycemia, and obtain repeat laboratory work.
• After stopping drug, monitor WBC counts weekly for at least 4 weeks, and monitor patient closely for recurrence of psychotic symptoms.
• Assess patient's and family's knowledge of drug therapy.

✛ Nursing diagnoses
• Disturbed thought processes related to patient's underlying condition
• Risk for infection related to potential for drug-induced agranulocytosis
• Deficient knowledge related to drug therapy

➤ Planning and implementation
• Drug carries significant risk of agranulocytosis. If possible, give at least two trials of a standard antipsychotic before giving this drug.
• Before starting treatment, patient must have a baseline WBC count of at least 3,500/mm³ and baseline ANC of at least 2,000/mm³. During the first 6 months of therapy, monitor patient weekly. If WBC count and ANC remain acceptable (WBC count at least 3,500/mm³ and ANC at least 2,000/mm³) for the first 6 months of continuous therapy, reduce monitoring to every other week. After 6 more months of continuous therapy, monitoring may be reduced to monthly. If therapy stops, return to weekly monitoring of WBC count and ANC for at least 4 weeks.
⚕ ALERT: Watch for signs and symptoms of cardiomyopathy, including exertional dyspnea, fatigue, orthopnea, paroxysmal nocturnal dyspnea, and peripheral edema, and report them immediately.
⚕ ALERT: Drug may increase risk of fatal myocarditis, especially during, but not limited to, the first month of therapy. In patients for whom myocarditis is suspected (unexplained fatigue, dyspnea, tachypnea, chest pain, tachycardia, fever, palpitations, and other signs of heart failure or ECG abnormalities, such as ST-segment and T-wave abnormalities or arrhythmias), stop therapy immediately and don't rechallenge.
⚕ ALERT: If drug must be stopped, withdraw gradually over a 1- to 2-week period. However, changes in patient's medical condition (including development of leukopenia) may require abruptly stopping the drug. Abruptly stopping long-term therapy may cause a sudden recurrence of psychotic symptoms.

• If therapy is restarted, even after a lapse as short as 2 days, start at 12.5 mg P.O. daily, and then follow usual guidelines for dosage increase. Re-exposure to drug may increase the risk and severity of adverse reactions. If therapy was stopped because WBC counts were below 2,000/mm³ or granulocyte counts were below 1,000/mm³, don't restart therapy.
⚕ ALERT: If dose has been set for a patient already taking St. John's wort, stopping the herb could increase drug level and cause dangerous toxic symptoms.
• Severe hypoglycemia may occur in a patient without a history of hypoglycemia. Drug may also cause hyperglycemia. Monitor diabetic patient regularly.
• Give patient no more than a 1-week supply of the drug.
• Orally disintegrating tablets contain phenylalanine.

Patient teaching
• Warn patient about risk of agranulocytosis. Tell him drug is available only through special monitoring program that requires weekly blood tests to check for agranulocytosis. Advise patient to report flulike symptoms, fever, sore throat, lethargy, malaise, or other signs of infection.
• Explain that patient should avoid activities that require alertness and good psychomotor coordination during therapy.
• Tell patient to rise slowly to avoid orthostatic hypotension.
• Advise patient to check with prescriber before taking OTC medicines, herbal remedies, or alcohol.
• Teach patient signs and symptoms of hyperglycemia (increased thirst and urination, increased appetite, weakness) and risks of diabetes, which may not resolve when drug is stopped.
• Recommend ice chips or sugarless candy or gum to help relieve dry mouth.
• Tell patient to store orally disintegrating tablets in blister pack, to immediately place in his mouth after opening pack, and to let tablet dissolve and then swallow it. There's no need for water.
• Inform patient that if 25-mg orally disintegrating tablet is used for the initial 12.5 mg dose, he should discard the other half of the tablet, not save it.

✔ Evaluation
• Patient demonstrates reduction in psychotic symptoms with drug therapy.

- Patient doesn't develop infection throughout drug therapy.
- Patient and family state understanding of drug therapy.

HIGH ALERT!

codeine phosphate
(KOH-deen FOS-fayt)

codeine sulfate

Pharmacologic class: opioid
Therapeutic class: analgesic, antitussive
Pregnancy risk category: C
Controlled substance schedule: II

Indications and dosages

▶ **Mild-to-moderate pain.** *Adults:* 15 to 60 mg P.O. or 15 to 60 mg codeine phosphate by subcutaneous, I.M., or I.V. route every 4 to 6 hours, p.r.n.
Children older than age 1: Give 0.5 mg/kg P.O., I.M., or subcutaneously every 4 hours, p.r.n.
▶ **Nonproductive cough.** *Adults:* 10 to 20 mg P.O. every 4 to 6 hours. Maximum daily dosage is 120 mg.
Children ages 6 to 12: Give 5 to 10 mg P.O. every 4 to 6 hours. Maximum daily dosage is 60 mg.
Children ages 2 to 6: Give 2.5 to 5 mg P.O. every 4 to 6 hours. Maximum daily dosage is 30 mg.

▼ I.V. administration

- Keep opioid antagonist (naloxone) and resuscitative equipment available.
- Give drug very slowly by direct injection into large vein.
- Don't give drug to children by I.V. route.
⊗ **Incompatibilities**
Aminophylline, ammonium chloride, amobarbital, bromides, chlorothiazide, heparin, iodides, pentobarbital, phenobarbital, phenytoin, salts of heavy metals, sodium bicarbonate, sodium iodide, thiopental. Don't mix with other drugs.

Contraindications and cautions

- Contraindicated in patients hypersensitive to drug.
- Use cautiously in debilitated patients and in patients with head injury, increased intracranial pressure, increased CSF pressure, hepatic or re-

nal disease, hypothyroidism, Addison disease, acute alcoholism or other drug dependencies, seizures, severe CNS depression, bronchial asthma, COPD, respiratory depression, and shock.
✦ **Lifespan:** In pregnant and breast-feeding women, use cautiously. In children, use cautiously. In elderly patients, use cautiously.

Adverse reactions

CNS: *clouded sensorium, dizziness, euphoria, sedation, **seizures.***
CV: *bradycardia,* flushing, *hypotension.*
GI: *constipation, dry mouth,* ileus, *nausea, vomiting.*
GU: urine retention.
Respiratory: *respiratory depression.*
Skin: pruritus.
Other: physical dependence.

Interactions

Drug-drug. *CNS depressants, general anesthetics, hypnotics, MAO inhibitors, other opioid analgesics, sedatives, tranquilizers, tricyclic antidepressants:* May have additive effects. Use together cautiously. Monitor patient response.
Drug-lifestyle. *Alcohol use:* May have additive effects. Discourage use together.

Effects on lab test results

- May increase amylase and lipase levels.

Pharmacokinetics

Absorption: Good. Two-thirds as potent orally as parenterally.
Distribution: Wide.
Metabolism: Mainly in liver.
Excretion: Mainly in urine. *Half-life:* 2½ to 4 hours.

Route	Onset	Peak	Duration
P.O.	10–30 min	1–2 hr	4–6 hr
I.V.	Immediate	Immediate	4–6 hr
I.M.	10–30 min	½–2 hr	4–6 hr
SubQ	10–30 min	Unknown	4–6 hr

Action

Chemical effect: Binds with opiate receptors in CNS, altering perception of and emotional response to pain through unknown mechanism. Also suppresses cough reflex by direct action on cough center in medulla.
Therapeutic effect: Relieves pain and cough.

Available forms

codeine phosphate
Injection: 15 mg/ml, 30 mg/ml
Oral solution: 15 mg/5 ml
Soluble tablets: 30 mg, 60 mg
codeine sulfate
Tablets: 15 mg, 30 mg, 60 mg

NURSING PROCESS

Assessment
• Assess patient's pain or cough before and after drug therapy.
• Be alert for adverse reactions and drug interactions.
• Assess patient's and family's knowledge of drug therapy.

Nursing diagnoses
• Acute pain related to patient's underlying condition
• Fatigue related to presence of cough
• Deficient knowledge related to drug therapy

Planning and implementation
ALERT: Breast-feeding while taking codeine can cause overdose in the baby. The smallest amount of codeine should be prescribed for the shortest time possible. Breastfed babies of women who are ultra-rapid metabolizers are at greatest risk.
• For full analgesic effect, give drug before patient has intense pain.
ALERT: Codeine is metabolized to morphine by CYP2D6; this gene may be absent in up to 7% of the population who experience reduced analgesic effect.
• Don't use drug when cough is valuable diagnostic sign or is beneficial (as after thoracic surgery).
• Give drug with food or milk to minimize adverse GI reactions.
• Don't inject discolored solution.
• Codeine is often prescribed with aspirin or acetaminophen to increase pain relief.
• Abuse potential is much lower for codeine than for morphine.
• If pain or cough isn't relieved, notify prescriber.
ALERT: Don't confuse codeine with Cardene, Lodine, or Cordran.

Patient teaching
• Tell a woman who's breastfeeding to watch her baby for signs and symptoms of overdose (increased sleepiness, difficulty nursing, difficulty breathing, limpness).
• Instruct patient to monitor bowel movements while increasing dietary fiber, fruit, and fluids if possible. Begin stimulant laxative promptly if stool hardens. Patient should notify prescriber of first missed bowel movement and secure instructions for laxative use.
• Advise patient to take oral drug with milk or meals to minimize GI distress.
• Urge patient to ask for or take drug (if at home) before pain becomes severe.
• Warn ambulatory patient that he may feel dizzy when getting out of bed or walking. Tell outpatient to avoid driving and other hazardous activities until drug's CNS effects are known.
• Tell patient to report adverse drug reactions.

Evaluation
• Patient is free of pain after drug administration.
• Patient's cough is suppressed after drug administration.
• Patient and family state understanding of drug therapy.

colchicine
(KOHL-chih-seen)

Pharmacologic class: *Colchicum autumnale* alkaloid
Therapeutic class: antigout drug
Pregnancy risk category: C (P.O.), D (I.V.)

Indications and dosages

▶ **To prevent acute gout attacks as prophylactic or maintenance therapy.** *Adults:* 0.6 mg P.O. daily. Give drug 3 to 4 days per week to patients who normally have one attack per year or fewer; give drug daily to patients who have more than one attack per year. In severe cases, 1.2 to 1.8 mg daily.

▶ **To prevent gout attacks in patients undergoing surgery.** *Adults:* 0.6 mg P.O. t.i.d. 3 days before and 3 days after surgery.

▶ **Acute gout, acute gouty arthritis.** *Adults:* Initially, 1.2 mg P.O.; then 0.6 mg every 1 to 2 hours until pain is relieved; nausea, vomiting,

or diarrhea ensues; or a maximum dose of 8 mg is reached. Or 2 mg I.V. followed by 0.5 mg I.V. every 6 hours if needed. Or an initial dose of 1 mg I.V. followed by 0.5 mg once or twice daily if needed. Some prescribers prefer to give a single injection of 3 mg I.V. Don't give more than 4 mg for total I.V. dosage over 24 hours (one course). Don't give any further drug (I.V. or P.O.) for 7 days or more.

▶ **Familial Mediterranean fever‡.** *Adults:* 1 to 2 mg P.O. daily in divided doses.

▶ **Hepatic cirrhosis‡.** *Adults:* 1 mg P.O. 5 days weekly.

▶ **Primary biliary cirrhosis‡.** *Adults:* 0.6 mg P.O. b.i.d.

▶ **Behçet disease‡.** *Adults:* 0.5 to 1.5 mg P.O. daily.

▶ **Scleroderma‡.** *Adults:* 1 mg P.O. daily.

▶ **Sweet syndrome‡.** *Adults:* 0.5 mg P.O. once daily to t.i.d.

⑤ Adjust-a-dose: For patients with hepatic impairment or creatinine clearance of 10 to 50 ml/ minute, decrease dosage by 50%.

▼ I.V. administration

• Don't dilute injection with D_5W injection or other fluids that might change pH of solution. If lower concentration is needed, dilute with normal saline solution or sterile water for injection.
• Preferably, inject into tubing of free-flowing I.V. solution. If diluted solution becomes turbid, don't inject.
• Give drug by slow I.V. push over 2 to 5 minutes. Monitor patient for signs of extravasation.

⊗ **Incompatibilities**
Dextrose 5% injection, bacteriostatic normal saline injection.

Contraindications and cautions

• Contraindicated in patients with serious cardiac disease, renal disease, or GI disorders.
• Use cautiously in debilitated patients, and in patients with early evidence of cardiac, renal, or GI disease.
☀ **Lifespan:** In pregnant women, use cautiously if at all because fetal harm may occur. In breast-feeding women and in children, safety and effectiveness haven't been established. In elderly patients, use cautiously.

Adverse reactions

CNS: peripheral neuritis.

GI: *abdominal pain, diarrhea, nausea, vomiting.*
Hematologic: *agranulocytosis* (with prolonged use), *aplastic anemia,* nonthrombocytopenic purpura, *thrombocytopenia.*
Hepatic: *hepatic necrosis.*
Skin: alopecia, dermatitis, urticaria.
Other: *anaphylaxis,* hypersensitivity reactions, severe local irritation (if extravasation occurs).

Interactions

Drug-drug. *Loop diuretics:* May decrease effectiveness of colchicine prophylaxis. Avoid use together.
Phenylbutazone: May increase risk of leukopenia or thrombocytopenia. Don't use together.
Vitamin B_{12}: May impair absorption of vitamin B_{12}. Avoid use together.
Drug-lifestyle. *Alcohol use:* May impair effectiveness of drug prophylaxis. Discourage use together.

Effects on lab test results

• May increase alkaline phosphatase, AST, and ALT levels. May decrease carotene, cholesterol, and hemoglobin levels and hematocrit.
• May decrease platelet and granulocyte counts.
• May cause false-positive results in urine tests for hemoglobin and erythrocytes. May interfere with urinary determinations of 17-hydroxycorticosteroids using the Reddy-Jenkins-Thorn test.

Pharmacokinetics

Absorption: Rapid. Unchanged drug may be reabsorbed from intestine by biliary processes.
Distribution: Rapid. Concentrated in leukocytes and distributed into kidneys, liver, spleen, and intestinal tract, but absent in heart, skeletal muscle, and brain.
Metabolism: Partially in liver and also slowly in other tissues.
Excretion: Mainly in feces, with lesser amounts in urine. *Half-life:* 1 to 10½ hours.

Route	Onset	Peak	Duration
P.O.	≤ 12 hr	½–2 hr	Unknown
I.V.	6–12 hr	½–2 hr	Unknown

Action

Chemical effect: May decrease WBC motility, phagocytosis, and lactic acid production, decreasing urate crystal deposits and reducing inflammation. As antiosteolytic drug, apparently

---

Reactions may be *common*, uncommon, *life-threatening*, or COMMON AND LIFE-THREATENING.

inhibits mitosis of osteoprogenitor cells and decreases osteoclast activity.
Therapeutic effect: Relieves gout signs and symptoms.

Available forms

Injection: 0.5 mg/ml
Tablets: 0.6 mg (1/100 grain) as sugar-coated granules

NURSING PROCESS

Assessment

• Assess patient's underlying condition before therapy and regularly thereafter.
• Before therapy, obtain baseline laboratory studies, including CBC and uric acid level. Repeat regularly.
• Be alert for adverse reactions and drug interactions.
• Assess patient's and family's knowledge of drug therapy.

Nursing diagnoses

• Acute pain related to presence of gout
• Ineffective protection related to drug-induced hematologic adverse reactions
• Deficient knowledge related to drug therapy

Planning and implementation

• Give oral form of drug with meals to reduce GI effects. May be used with uricosurics.
• **ALERT:** After a full course of 4 mg I.V., don't give drug by any other route for at least 7 days. Drug is toxic and death can result from overdose.
• Don't give I.M. or subcutaneously because severe local irritation occurs.
• Store drug in tightly closed, light-resistant container.
• Stop drug as soon as gout pain is relieved or at first sign of GI symptoms.
• Force fluids to maintain output at 2,000 ml daily.
Patient teaching
• Teach patient how to take drug.
• Advise patient to report rash, sore throat, fever, unusual bleeding, bruising, fatigue, weakness, numbness, or tingling.
• Tell patient when to stop drug.
• Urge patient not to drink alcohol during drug therapy because it may inhibit drug action.

• Advise patient to avoid all aspirin-containing drugs because they may precipitate gout.

Evaluation

• Patient becomes pain free after drug therapy.
• Patient's CBC and platelet counts remain normal throughout drug therapy.
• Patient and family state understanding of drug therapy.

colesevelam hydrochloride
(koh-leh-SEV-eh-lam high-droh-KLOR-ighd)
WelChol

Pharmacologic class: polymeric bile acid sequestrant
Therapeutic class: antilipemic
Pregnancy risk category: B

Indications and dosages

▶ **Reduction of elevated LDL cholesterol level in patients with primary hypercholesterolemia (Frederickson Type IIa). May be given either alone or with an HMG-CoA reductase inhibitor.** *Adults:* If given alone, give 3 tablets (1,875 mg) P.O. twice daily with meals and liquid or 6 tablets (3,750 mg) once daily with a meal and liquid. Maximum dose is 7 tablets (4,375 mg). If given with an HMG-CoA reductase inhibitor (atorvastatin, fluvastatin, lovastatin, pravastatin, simvastatin), recommended dose is 4 to 6 tablets P.O. daily.

Contraindications and cautions

• Contraindicated in patients hypersensitive to drug or any of its components and in patients with bowel obstruction.
• Use cautiously in patients susceptible to vitamin K deficiency or deficiencies of fat-soluble vitamins. Also use cautiously in patients with dysphagia, swallowing disorders, severe GI motility disorders, and major GI tract surgery. Use cautiously in patients with triglyceride levels above 300 mg/dl because effects aren't known.
• **Lifespan:** In pregnant women, use only if clearly needed for risk of fat-soluble vitamin deficiency. In breast-feeding women, use cautiously; drug probably doesn't appear in breast milk because of lack of systemic absorption. In children, safety and effectiveness haven't been established.

Adverse reactions

CNS: asthenia, headache, pain.
EENT: pharyngitis, rhinitis, sinusitis.
GI: abdominal pain, *constipation,* diarrhea, *dyspepsia, flatulence,* nausea.
Musculoskeletal: back pain, myalgia.
Respiratory: increased cough.
Other: accidental injury, flulike syndrome, *infection.*

Interactions

None reported.

Effects on lab test results

• May increase HDL cholesterol and triglyceride levels. May decrease total cholesterol, LDL cholesterol, and apolipoprotein B levels.

Pharmacokinetics

Absorption: Not absorbed.
Distribution: None.
Metabolism: None.
Excretion: Mainly in feces as a complex bound to bile acids. Less than 0.05% of drug in urine.
Half-life: Unknown.

Route	Onset	Peak	Duration
P.O.	Unknown	2 wk	Unknown

Action

Chemical effect: Binds to bile acids in the intestines and forms a nonabsorbable complex that's eliminated in feces. Partial removal of bile acids from the enterohepatic circulation results in an increased conversion of cholesterol to bile acids in the liver in an attempt to restore the depleted bile acids. The resulting increase in cholesterol causes systemic clearance of circulating LDL level.
Therapeutic effect: Lowers LDL and total cholesterol levels.

Available forms

Tablets: 625 mg

NURSING PROCESS

⚖ Assessment

• Rule out secondary causes of hypercholesterolemia before starting drug, such as poorly controlled diabetes, hypothyroidism, nephrotic syndrome, dysproteinemias, obstructive liver disease, other drug therapy, and alcoholism.

• Monitor total cholesterol, LDL, and triglyceride levels before and periodically during therapy.
• Monitor patient's bowel habits. If severe constipation develops, lower the dose and add a stool softener, or stop giving the drug.
• Assess patient's compliance with restricted diet and exercise program adjunctive to antilipemic therapy.
• Evaluate patient's and family's knowledge of drug therapy and importance of diet and exercise regimen.

⊕ Nursing diagnoses

• Imbalanced nutrition: more than body requirements of saturated fat and cholesterol related to dietary intake and lack of exercise program
• Risk for constipation related to drug-induced adverse gastrointestinal reactions
• Risk for injury related to presence of elevated LDL cholesterol level
• Deficient knowledge related to antilipemic drug therapy

▶ Planning and implementation

• Give drug with a meal and a liquid.
• If given with an HMG-CoA reductase inhibitor, separate HMG-CoA reductase inhibitor and colesevelam.
• Store drug at room temperature but protect from moisture.

Patient teaching
• Instruct patient to take drug with a meal and a liquid.
• Teach patient to monitor bowel habits. Encourage a diet high in fiber and fluids. Instruct patient to notify prescriber promptly if severe constipation develops.
• Urge patient to follow prescribed diet that's restricted in saturated fat and cholesterol and high in vegetables and fiber. Also discuss and encourage an appropriate exercise program.
• Discuss with patient the importance of regularly monitoring lipid levels.
• Tell patient to notify prescriber if she's pregnant or breast-feeding.

✔ Evaluation

• Patient begins a balanced diet and exercise regimen that's approved by prescriber.
• Patient doesn't suffer adverse GI effect from drug therapy.

Reactions may be *common,* uncommon, *life-threatening,* or **COMMON AND LIFE-THREATENING.**

- Patient's LDL cholesterol and total cholesterol levels are within normal limits.
- Patient and family state understanding of drug therapy.

conivaptan hydrochloride
(kahn-nih-VAPP-tan high-droh-KLOR-ighd)
Vaprisol

Pharmacologic class: arginine vasopressin receptor antagonist
Therapeutic class: hyponatremic drug
Pregnancy risk category: C

Indications and dosages

▶ **Euvolemic hyponatremia (as from SIADH, hypothyroidism, adrenal insufficiency, pulmonary disorders) in hospitalized patients.**
Adults: Loading dose of 20 mg I.V. over 30 minutes; then 20 mg I.V. by continuous infusion over 24 hours for 1 to 3 days. If sodium level doesn't rise at desired rate, increase to 40 mg/day by continuous infusion. Don't exceed 4 days of treatment after loading dose.
Adjust-a-dose: If serum sodium level rises more than 12 mEq/L in 24 hours, stop infusion. If hyponatremia persists or recurs and the patient has had no adverse neurologic effects from the rapid rise in sodium level, restart infusion at a reduced dose.

If patient develops hypotension or hypovolemia, stop infusion. Monitor vital signs and volume status often. If hyponatremia persists once the patient is no longer hypotensive and volume status returns to normal, restart infusion at a reduced dose.

▼ I.V. administration

- Dilute only with D$_5$W.
- For the loading dose, add 20 mg to 100 ml of D$_5$W. Gently invert bag to ensure complete mixing. Infuse over 30 minutes.
- For continuous infusion, add 40 mg to 250 ml of D$_5$W. Gently invert bag to ensure complete mixing. Infuse over 24 hours.
- Give via a large vein, and change infusion site every 24 hours.
- Solution is stable for 24 hours at room temperature.

⊗ **Incompatibilities**
Lactated Ringer's solution, normal saline solution. Don't mix or infuse with other I.V. drugs.

Contraindications and cautions

- Contraindicated in patients with hypovolemic hyponatremia, patients hypersensitive to drug or its components, and patients taking potent CYP3A4 inhibitors, such as clarithromycin, indinavir, itraconazole, ketoconazole, or ritonavir.
- Use cautiously in hyponatremic patients with underlying heart failure and patients with hepatic or renal impairment.
- **Lifespan:** In pregnant women, safety hasn't been established; use only if benefit to mother outweighs risk to fetus. Patient shouldn't breast-feed during therapy. In children, safety hasn't been established.

Adverse reactions

CNS: confusion, fever, *headache*, insomnia.
CV: atrial fibrillation, hypertension, hypotension, orthostatic hypotension.
GI: constipation, diarrhea, dry mouth, nausea, oral candidiasis, *vomiting*.
GU: frequency, hematuria, polyuria, UTI.
Hematologic: anemia.
Metabolic: dehydration, hyperglycemia, *hypoglycemia, hypokalemia, hypomagnesemia,* hyponatremia.
Respiratory: pneumonia.
Skin: erythema.
Other: *infusion site reactions, thirst.*

Interactions

Drug-drug. *Amlodipine:* May increase amlodipine level and half-life. Monitor blood pressure.
Digoxin: May increase digoxin level. Monitor patient, and adjust digoxin dosage as needed.
Midazolam: May increase midazolam level. Monitor patient for respiratory depression and hypotension.
Potent CYP3A4 inhibitors (clarithromycin, indinavir, itraconazole, ketoconazole, ritonavir): May cause serious increases in serum levels and toxic effects. This combination is contraindicated.
Simvastatin: May increase simvastatin level. Monitor patient for evidence of rhabdomyolysis, including muscle pain, weakness, and tenderness.

Effects on lab test results

• May decrease potassium, magnesium, sodium, and hemoglobin levels and hematocrit. May increase or decrease blood glucose level.

Pharmacokinetics

Absorption: Given I.V.
Distribution: 99% protein-bound.
Metabolism: Mainly via CYP3A4 to four metabolites.
Excretion: 83% in feces; 12% in urine. *Half-life:* 5 hours.

Route	Onset	Peak	Duration
I.V.	Unknown	2–4 hr	12 hr

Action

Chemical effect: Increases the amount of free water eliminated by the kidneys by antagonizing V_{1A} and V_2 receptors in renal collecting ducts, inhibiting inappropriate or excessive arginine vasopressin (antidiuretic hormone) secretion.
Therapeutic effect: Increased net fluid loss, increased urine output, and decreased urine osmolality causing normalization of serum sodium levels.

Available forms

Injection: 20 mg/4 ml

NURSING PROCESS

⚗ Assessment

• Check serum sodium level and neurologic status regularly during therapy.
• Assess patient for infusion site reactions.
• Monitor patient for orthostatic hypotension during drug therapy.
• Assess patient's and family's knowledge of drug therapy.

🔁 Nursing diagnoses

• Risk for deficient fluid volume related to excessive diuresis
• Risk for injury related to drug-induced orthostatic hypotension
• Deficient knowledge related to drug therapy

▶ Planning and implementation

• Drug may cause significant infusion site reactions, even with proper dilution and administration. Rotate infusion site every 24 hours to reduce risk of reaction.

⚠ ALERT: Rapid correction of serum sodium level may cause osmotic demyelination syndrome. Monitor patient's serum sodium level and volume status.
• Adverse effects, including hypotension and thirst, are more common at higher doses. Monitor vital signs, and treat symptomatically if overdose occurs.

Patient teaching
• Inform patient that the infusion will be given for a maximum of 4 days after the loading dose.
• Inform patient that low blood pressure may cause him to feel dizzy or faint when rising from a sitting or lying position. Advise him to change positions slowly and to sit or lie down if needed.
• Advise patient to promptly report signs and symptoms of hypoglycemia, such as feeling shaky, nervous, tired, sweaty, cold, hungry, confused, or irritable.
• Emphasize the importance of reporting an unusually fast heartbeat or weakness.
• Tell patient that analgesics and moist heating pads can be used to treat pain and inflammation at the infusion site.

✔ Evaluation

• Patient maintains adequate fluid volume.
• Patient maintains safety during drug therapy.
• Patient and family state understanding of drug therapy.

co-trimoxazole (sulfamethoxazole and trimethoprim)
(koh-trigh-MOX-uh-zohl)
Apo-Sulfatrim ♦ , Apo-Sulfatrim DS ♦ , Bactrim*, Bactrim DS, Bactrim I.V., Cotrim, Cotrim DS, Novo-Trimel ♦ , Novo-Trimel D.S. ♦ , Nu-Cotrimox ♦ , Septra*, Septra DS, Septra-I.V., SMZ-TMP

Pharmacologic class: sulfonamide and folate antagonist
Therapeutic class: antibiotic
Pregnancy risk category: C (X at term)

Indications and dosages

▶ **UTI, shigellosis.** *Adults:* 160 mg trimethoprim and 800 mg sulfamethoxazole (double-

strength tablet) P.O. every 12 hours for 10 to 14 days in UTIs and for 5 days in shigellosis. If indicated, I.V. infusion is given at 8 to 10 mg/kg daily (based on trimethoprim component) in two to four divided doses every 6, 8, or 12 hours for up to 14 days. Maximum trimethoprim dosage is 960 mg daily.

Children age 2 months and older: 8 mg/kg trimethoprim and 40 mg/kg sulfamethoxazole P.O. daily, in two divided doses every 12 hours (10 days for UTI; 5 days for shigellosis). If indicated, I.V. infusion is given at 8 to 10 mg/kg daily (based on trimethoprim component) in two to four divided doses every 6, 8, or 12 hours. Don't exceed adult dose.

Ŝ Adjust-a-dose: In patients with impaired renal function, if creatinine clearance is 15 to 30 ml/minute, reduce dosage by 50%. Don't use if creatinine clearance is less than 15 ml/minute.

▶ **Otitis media in patients with penicillin allergy or penicillin-resistant infection.** *Children and infants age 2 months and older:* 8 mg/kg daily (based on trimethoprim component) P.O., in two divided doses every 12 hours for 10 days.

▶ **Pneumocystis jiroveci (carinii) pneumonia.** *Adults, children, and infants age 2 months and older:* 20 mg/kg trimethoprim and 100 mg/kg sulfamethoxazole P.O. daily, in equally divided doses every 6 hours for 14 to 21 days. If indicated, I.V. infusion may be given 15 to 20 mg/kg daily (based on trimethoprim component) in three or four divided doses every 6 to 8 hours for up to 14 days.

▶ **Chronic bronchitis.** *Adults:* 160 mg trimethoprim and 800 mg sulfamethoxazole P.O. every 12 hours for 10 to 14 days.

▶ **Traveler's diarrhea.** *Adults:* 160 mg trimethoprim and 800 mg sulfamethoxazole P.O. b.i.d. for 3 to 5 days. Some patients may require 2 days of therapy or less.

▶ **UTI in men with prostatitis‡.** *Adults:* 160 mg trimethoprim and 800 mg sulfamethoxazole P.O. b.i.d. for 3 to 6 months.

▶ **Prophylaxis of chronic UTI‡.** *Adults:* 40 mg trimethoprim and 200 mg sulfamethoxazole or 80 mg trimethoprim and 400 mg sulfamethoxazole P.O. daily or three times weekly for 3 to 6 months.

▶ **Septic agranulocytosis‡.** *Adults:* 2.5 mg/kg I.V. q.i.d.; for prophylaxis, 80 to 160 mg b.i.d.

▶ **Nocardia infection‡.** *Adults:* 640 (as trimethoprim component) daily for 7 months.

▶ **Pharyngeal gonococcal infection‡.** *Adults:* 720 mg P.O. (as trimethoprim component) daily for 5 days.

▶ **Chancroid‡.** *Adults:* 160 mg P.O. b.i.d. (as trimethoprim component) for 7 days.

▶ **Pertussis‡.** *Adults:* 320 mg P.O. daily (as trimethoprim component) in two divided doses. *Children:* 40 mg/kg P.O. daily in two divided doses.

▶ **Cholera‡.** *Adults:* 160 mg P.O. b.i.d. (as trimethoprim component) for 3 days.

Ŝ Adjust-a-dose: For patients with renal impairment, if creatinine clearance is 15 to 30 ml/minute, reduce daily dose by 50%. Don't use if creatinine clearance is less than 15 ml/minute.

▼ I.V. administration

• Dilute contents of 5-ml ampule of drug in 125 ml D_5W before giving. If patient is on a fluid restriction, dilute 5 ml of drug in 75 ml D_5W.
• Infuse slowly over 60 to 90 minutes. Don't give by rapid infusion or bolus injection.
• Don't refrigerate. Use within 6 hours if diluted in 125 ml and within 2 hours if diluted in 75 ml. If cloudiness or evidence of crystallization is noted after mixing, discard solution.

⊗ **Incompatibilities**
All I.V. solutions except D_5W, other I.V. drugs.

Contraindications and cautions

• Contraindicated in patients with megaloblastic anemia caused by folate deficiency, porphyria, severe renal impairment (creatinine clearance less than 15 ml/minute), or hypersensitivity to trimethoprim or sulfonamides.
• Use cautiously and reduce dose in patient with hepatic impairment, a creatinine clearance of 15 to 30 ml/minute, severe allergy or bronchial asthma, G6PD deficiency, or blood dyscrasia.

☀ **Lifespan:** In pregnant women at term and in breast-feeding women, drug is contraindicated. In infants younger than age 2 months, safety and effectiveness haven't been established.

Adverse reactions

CNS: ataxia, fatigue, hallucinations, headache, insomnia, mental depression, nervousness, *seizures,* vertigo.
CV: thrombophlebitis.
GI: abdominal pain, anorexia, *diarrhea, nausea, stomatitis, vomiting.*
GU: crystalluria, hematuria, *toxic nephrosis with oliguria and anuria.*
Hematologic: *agranulocytosis, aplastic anemia,* hemolytic anemia, *leukopenia,* megaloblastic anemia, *thrombocytopenia.*
Hepatic: *hepatic necrosis,* jaundice.
Musculoskeletal: muscle weakness.
Skin: *epidermal necrolysis, erythema multiforme,* exfoliative dermatitis, generalized skin eruption, photosensitivity, pruritus, *Stevens-Johnson syndrome,* urticaria.
Other: *hypersensitivity reactions (anaphylaxis,* drug fever, serum sickness).

Interactions

Drug-drug. *Hormonal contraceptives:* May decrease contraceptive effectiveness and increase risk of breakthrough bleeding. Suggest nonhormonal contraception.
Oral anticoagulants: May increase anticoagulant effect. Monitor patient for bleeding.
Oral antidiabetics: May increase hypoglycemic effect. Monitor glucose level.
Phenytoin: May inhibit hepatic metabolism of phenytoin. Monitor phenytoin level.
Drug-herb. *Dong quai, St. John's wort:* May increase risk of photosensitivity. Advise patient to avoid unprotected exposure to sunlight.
Drug-lifestyle. *Sun exposure:* May cause photosensitivity reactions. Urge patient to avoid sun exposure and wear protective clothing and sunblock.

Effects on lab test results

• May increase BUN, creatinine, aminotransferase, and bilirubin levels. May decrease hemoglobin level and hematocrit.
• May decrease granulocyte, platelet, and WBC counts.

Pharmacokinetics

Absorption: Good.
Distribution: Wide (including middle ear fluid, prostatic fluid, bile, aqueous humor, and CSF). Protein-binding is 44% for trimethoprim, 70% for sulfamethoxazole.
Metabolism: By liver.
Excretion: Mainly in urine. *Half-life:* Trimethoprim, 8 to 11 hours; sulfamethoxazole, 10 to 13 hours.

Route	Onset	Peak	Duration
P.O.	Unknown	1–4 hr	Unknown
I.V.	Immediate	Immediate	Unknown

Action

Chemical effect: Sulfamethoxazole inhibits formation of dihydrofolic acid from PABA; trimethoprim inhibits dihydrofolate reductase. Both decrease bacterial folic acid synthesis.
Therapeutic effect: Inhibits susceptible bacteria.

Available forms

Injection: 16 mg trimethoprim and 80 mg/ml sulfamethoxazole (5 ml/ampule)
Oral suspension: trimethoprim 40 mg and sulfamethoxazole 200 mg/5 ml
Tablets: 80 mg trimethoprim and 400 mg sulfamethoxazole; 160 mg trimethoprim and 800 mg sulfamethoxazole

NURSING PROCESS

Assessment
• Assess patient's infection before therapy and regularly thereafter.
• Before giving first dose, obtain specimen for culture and sensitivity tests. Begin therapy pending results.
• Be alert for adverse reactions and drug interactions.
• If adverse GI reaction occurs, monitor patient's hydration.
• Monitor intake and output. Make sure urine output is at least 1,500 ml daily to ensure proper hydration. Inadequate urine output can lead to crystalluria or tubular deposits of drug.
• Assess patient's and family's knowledge of drug therapy.

Nursing diagnoses
• Ineffective protection related to presence of bacteria susceptible to drug
• Risk for deficient fluid volume related to drug-induced adverse GI reactions
• Deficient knowledge related to drug therapy

▶ Planning and implementation

- For maximum absorption, give drug with full glass of water at least 1 hour before or 2 hours after meals. Shake oral suspension thoroughly before giving.
- Never give I.M.
- ⓢ **ALERT:** Double-check dosage, which may be written as trimethoprim component.
- Note that DS in product name means double strength.
- ⓢ **ALERT:** Adverse reactions, especially hypersensitivity reactions, rash, and fever, occur more frequently in patients with AIDS.

Patient teaching
- Tell patient to take entire amount of drug exactly as prescribed, even if he feels better.
- Tell patient to take drug with full glass of water and to drink at least 3 to 4 L of water daily.
- Advise patient to avoid exposure to direct sunlight because of risk of photosensitivity reaction.
- Tell patient to report signs of rash, sore throat, fever, or mouth sores because drug may need to be stopped.

☑ Evaluation

- Patient is free from infection after drug therapy.
- Patient maintains adequate hydration after drug therapy.
- Patient and family state understanding of drug therapy.

---

cyanocobalamin (vitamin B₁₂)
(sigh-an-oh-koh-BAH-luh-meen)
Anacobin ◆, Bedoz ◆, Big Shot B-12, Crystamine, Crysti 1000, Cyanoject, Cyomin, Nascobal

hydroxocobalamin (vitamin B₁₂)
Cyanokit, Hydro-Cobex, LA-12

Pharmacologic class: water-soluble vitamin
Therapeutic class: vitamin, nutrition supplement
Pregnancy risk category: A (C if used in doses above RDA)

Indications and dosages

▶ **RDA for cyanocobalamin.** *Adults and children ages 11 and older:* Give 2 mcg.
Pregnant women: Give 2.2 mcg.

Breast-feeding women: Give 2.6 mcg.
Children ages 7 to 10: Give 1.4 mcg.
Children ages 4 to 6: Give 1 mcg.
Children ages 1 to 3: Give 0.7 mcg.
Infants ages 6 months to 1 year: Give 0.5 mcg.
Neonates and infants younger than age 6 months: Give 0.3 mcg.

▶ **Vitamin B₁₂ deficiency caused by inadequate diet, subtotal gastrectomy, or any other condition, disorder, or disease except malabsorption related to pernicious anemia or other GI disease.** *Adults:* 30 mcg hydroxocobalamin I.M. daily for 5 to 10 days, depending on severity of deficiency. Maintenance dosage is 100 to 200 mcg I.M. once monthly. Or 500 mcg intranasally once weekly. For subsequent prophylaxis, advise adequate nutrition and daily RDA vitamin B₁₂ supplements.
Children: 1 to 5 mg hydroxocobalamin spread over 2 or more weeks in doses of 100 mcg I.M., depending on severity of deficiency. Maintenance dosage is 30 to 50 mcg I.M. monthly. For subsequent prophylaxis, advise adequate nutrition and daily RDA vitamin B₁₂ supplements.

▶ **Pernicious anemia or vitamin B₁₂ malabsorption.** *Adults:* Initially, 100 mcg cyanocobalamin I.M. or subcutaneously daily for 6 to 7 days; then 100 mcg I.M. or subcutaneously once monthly.
Children: 30 to 50 mcg I.M. or subcutaneously daily over 2 or more weeks; then 100 mcg I.M. or subcutaneously monthly for life.

▶ **Maintenance treatment for remission of pernicious anemia following I.M. vitamin B₁₂ therapy in patients with no nervous system involvement; dietary deficiency, malabsorption disorders, inadequate secretion of intrinsic factor.** *Adults:* Initially, 1 spray in one nostril once weekly. Give at least 1 hour before or 1 hour after ingestion of hot foods or liquids.

▶ **Methylmalonic aciduria.** *Neonates:* 1,000 mcg cyanocobalamin I.M. daily.

▶ **Schilling test flushing dose.** *Adults and children:* 1,000 mcg hydroxocobalamin I.M. as a single dose.

◢ **NEW INDICATION: Cyanide poisoning.** *Adults:* Initially, 5 g I.V. over 15 minutes. May give another 5-g dose over 15 minutes to 2 hours based on severity of poisoning and patient's condition.

▽ I.V. administration

- Add 100 ml normal saline solution to each vial. If normal saline solution isn't available, use lactated Ringer's or 5% dextrose solution.
- With vial in upright position, fill to the line. Then rotate vial for 30 seconds to mix solution. Don't shake.
- Inspect the solution. It should be dark red and contain no particulate matter. If otherwise, don't use.
- Infuse the solution over 7.5 minutes.
- Repeat this process for the second vial.
- Store dry vials at room temperature. Reconstituted solution is stable 6 hours at temperatures below 104° F (40° C).

⊗ **Incompatibilities**

Don't give through same I.V. line with diazepam, dobutamine, dopamine, fentanyl, nitroglycerin, pentobarbital, propofol, or thiopental because particles may form. Don't give through same I.V. line with sodium thiosulfate, sodium nitrite, or ascorbic acid because these drugs are chemically incompatible. Effect of giving more than one cyanide antidote isn't known. Give through separate lines.

Give blood products through separate lines; don't administer simultaneously.

Contraindications and cautions

- Contraindicated in patients with early Leber disease or hypersensitivity to vitamin B_{12} or cobalt.
- Use cautiously in anemic patients with cardiac, pulmonary, or hypertensive disease and in those with severe vitamin B_{12}–dependent deficiencies.

☀ **Lifespan:** In premature infants, use cautiously because some products contain benzyl alcohol, which may cause gasping syndrome. High dose hydroxocobalamin: Use during pregnancy only if potential benefit to mother outweighs risk to fetus. It isn't known if drug appears in breast milk. In children, safety and effectiveness haven't been established.

Adverse reactions

CV: *heart failure, peripheral vascular thrombosis.*
GI: transient diarrhea.
Respiratory: *pulmonary edema.*
Skin: itching, transitory exanthema, urticaria.
Other: *anaphylactoid reactions, anaphylaxis* (with parenteral use); burning, pain (at subcutaneous or I.M. injection sites).

Hydroxocobalamin
CNS: dizziness, headache, memory impairment, restlessness.
CV: chest discomfort, *ECG abnormalities,* edema, flushing, *hypertension,* increased heart rate, ventricular extrasystoles.
EENT: dry throat, eye irritation and redness, swelling, throat tightness.
GI: abdominal discomfort, diarrhea, dyspepsia, dysphagia, hematochezia, nausea, vomiting.
GU: *chromaturia* (red urine).
Respiratory: dyspnea, pleural effusion.
Skin: *erythema,* infusion site reaction, pruritus, *rash.*

Interactions

Drug-drug. *Aminoglycosides, chloramphenicol, colchicine, para-aminosalicylic acid and salts:* May cause malabsorption of vitamin B_{12}. Don't use together.
Drug-lifestyle. *Alcohol use:* May cause malabsorption of vitamin B_{12}. Discourage use together.
Sun exposure: May lead to photosensitivity reaction with hydrocobalamin. Tell patient to avoid direct sunlight while skin is discolored.

Effects on lab test results

- May decrease potassium level.
- May cause false-positive results for intrinsic factor antibody test.

Hydroxocobalamin
- May increase blood creatinine, triglyceride, cholesterol, total protein, glucose, albumin, alkaline phosphatase, and bilirubin levels; urine glucose, protein, ketones, bilirubin, urobilinogen, and nitrite levels; and hemoglobin level. May decrease ALT and amylase levels.
- May increase urine pH and RBC, WBC, and basophil counts.
- May increase or decrease aPTT, PT, and phosphate, uric acid, AST, CK, creatine kinase MB, and LDH levels.

Pharmacokinetics

Absorption: After oral use, irregular and dependent on sufficient intrinsic factor and calcium. After intranasal, I.M., and subcutaneous use, rapid. Vitamin B_{12} is protein-bound.
Distribution: Into liver, bone marrow, and other tissues.
Metabolism: In liver.

Reactions may be *common,* uncommon, *life-threatening,* or COMMON AND LIFE-THREATENING.

Excretion: Amount of vitamin B_{12} needed by body is reabsorbed; excess in urine. *Half-life:* 6 days.

Route	Onset	Peak	Duration
P.O.	Unknown	8–12 hr	Unknown
I.M.	Unknown	60 min	Unknown
I.V.	Rapid	Unknown	Unknown
SubQ	Unknown	Unknown	Unknown
Intranasal	Unknown	1–2 hr	Unknown

Action

Chemical effect: Acts as a coenzyme that stimulates metabolic functions. Needed for cell replication, hematopoiesis, and nucleoprotein and myelin synthesis.

As antidote, hydroxocobalamin binds cyanide ions forming cyanocobalamin which is excreted in urine.

Therapeutic effect: Increases vitamin B_{12} level. Removes cyanide from the body.

Available forms

cyanocobalamin
Injection: 100 mcg/ml, 1,000 mcg/ml
Intranasal: 500 mcg/0.1 ml
Tablets: 25 mcg†, 50 mcg†, 100 mcg†, 250 mcg†, 500 mcg†, 1,000 mcg†
hydroxocobalamin
Injection: 1,000 mcg/ml, Cyanokit 2 g vial, two vials per kit

NURSING PROCESS

Assessment

• Assess patient's vitamin B_{12} deficiency before therapy.
• Determine reticulocyte count, hematocrit, and B_{12}, iron, and folate levels before therapy starts.
• Monitor drug's effectiveness by assessing patient for improvement in signs and symptoms of vitamin B_{12} deficiency. Also, monitor reticulocyte count, hematocrit, and B_{12}, iron, and folate levels between fifth and seventh day of therapy and periodically thereafter.
• Infection, tumors, and renal, hepatic, or other debilitating diseases may reduce therapeutic response.
• Closely monitor potassium level for first 48 hours. Be alert for adverse reactions and drug interactions.

• Assess patient's and family's knowledge of drug therapy.
Hydroxocobalamin
• Assess if patient is hypersensitive to hydroxocobalamin or cyanocobalamine.
• Assess baseline vital signs.
• Assess kidney and liver studies. Safety and efficacy haven't been established in patients with renal or hepatic impairment.

Nursing diagnoses

• Ineffective health maintenance related to underlying vitamin B_{12} deficiency or cyanide poisoning
• Risk for injury related to parenteral administration and drug-induced hypersensitivity reactions
• Deficient knowledge related to drug therapy

Planning and implementation

• Don't mix parenteral liquids in same syringe with other drugs.
• Drug is physically incompatible with dextrose solutions, alkaline or strongly acidic solutions, oxidizing or reducing drugs, heavy metals, chlorpromazine, phytonadione, prochlorperazine, and many other drugs.
• Hydroxocobalamin is approved for I.M. or deep subcutaneous use only. Its only advantage over cyanocobalamin is its longer duration.
• Don't give large oral doses of vitamin B routinely because drug is lost through excretion.
• Protect vitamin from light. Don't refrigerate or freeze.
• Give potassium supplement, if needed.
• For intranasal form, prime the nasal device before first use. Repriming between doses isn't needed if the unit is upright.
• Give intranasal spray to one nostril weekly, at least 1 hour before or 1 hour after ingestion of hot foods or liquids.
• Hydroxocobalamin's deep red color may affect the results of many laboratory tests, including those involving urine, blood chemistry, hematology, and coagulation.
• Obtaining a serum sample to test for cyanide poisoning before treatment isn't required but may be helpful for documentation.
• Monitor patient's blood pressure during and after I.V. infusion.
• Photosensitivity reactions are possible with high doses of hydroxocobalamin.

• Because the drug is cleared unchanged in the kidney, oxalate crystals may occur.

Patient teaching

• Stress need for patient with pernicious anemia to return for monthly injections. Although total body stores may last 3 to 6 years, anemia will recur without monthly therapy.

• Emphasize importance of well-balanced diet.

• Tell patient to store oral tablets in tightly closed container at room temperature.

Hydroxocobalamine

• Explain that skin may turn red for up to 2 weeks after infusion and may increase the risk of photosensitivity. Urge patient to avoid direct sun while skin is discolored.

• Inform patient that urine may be red for up to 5 weeks after infusion.

• Tell patient that an acnelike rash appears in some people 7 to 28 days after infusion and usually resolves without treatment in a few weeks.

• If patient was breast-feeding, instruct her to consult prescriber about whether to resume after the infusion.

• Urge patient to disclose a history of hypertension because blood pressure may increase during infusion.

• Tell patient that the result of some blood and urine tests may be altered for several days after infusion.

☑ **Evaluation**

• Patient responds positively to drug therapy.

• Patient doesn't experience hypersensitivity reactions following parenteral administration of drug.

• Patient and family state understanding of drug therapy.

cyclobenzaprine hydrochloride
(sigh-kloh-BEN-zah-preen high-droh-KLOR-ighd)
Amrix, Flexeril

Pharmacologic class: tricyclic antidepressant derivative
Therapeutic class: skeletal muscle relaxant
Pregnancy risk category: B

Indications and dosages

▶ **Adjunct to rest and physical therapy for relief of muscle spasm associated with acute, painful musculoskeletal conditions.** *Adults*

and children age 15 and older: 5 mg P.O. t.i.d. May increase to 10 mg P.O. t.i.d. Usual daily dose, 30 mg. Or, 15 mg P.O. extended-release tablet once daily. Usual daily maximum, 30 mg. Don't use for periods longer than 3 weeks.

◹ **Adjust-a-dose:** In elderly patients and in patients with mild hepatic impairment, start with 5 mg and increase slowly. In patients with moderate to severe hepatic impairment, drug isn't recommended.

▶ **Fibrositis‡.** *Adults:* 10 to 40 mg P.O. daily.

Contraindications and cautions

• Contraindicated in patients hypersensitive to drug; in patients in the acute recovery phase of MI; in patients with hyperthyroidism, heart block, arrhythmias, conduction disturbances, or heart failure. Also contraindicated within 14 days of MAO inhibitor therapy.

• Use cautiously in debilitated patients and in patients with history of urine retention, acute angle-closure glaucoma, or increased intraocular pressure. Also use cautiously in patients taking anticholinergics.

✦ **Lifespan:** In pregnant and breast-feeding women, and in children younger than age 15, safety and effectiveness haven't been established. In elderly patients, use cautiously.

Adverse reactions

CNS: depression, *dizziness, drowsiness,* euphoria, headache, insomnia, nightmares, paresthesia, *seizures,* visual disturbances, weakness.
CV: *arrhythmias,* tachycardia.
EENT: blurred vision.
GI: abdominal pain, abnormal taste, constipation, *dry mouth,* dyspepsia.
GU: urine retention.
Skin: pruritus, rash, urticaria.

Interactions

Drug-drug. *Anticholinergics:* May have additive anticholinergic effects. Avoid use together.
CNS depressants: May cause additive CNS depression. Avoid use together.
MAO inhibitors: May worsen CNS depression or anticholinergic effects. Don't give within 14 days after stopping an MAO inhibitor.
Drug-lifestyle. *Alcohol use:* May cause additive CNS depression. Discourage use together.

Effects on lab test results

None reported.

Reactions may be *common*, uncommon, *life-threatening*, or COMMON AND LIFE-THREATENING.

Pharmacokinetics

Absorption: Almost complete.
Distribution: 93% protein-bound.
Metabolism: During first pass, drug and metabolites undergo enterohepatic recycling.
Excretion: Mainly in urine as conjugated metabolites; also in feces via bile as unchanged drug. *Half-life:* 1 to 3 days.

Route	Onset	Peak	Duration
P.O.	≤1 hr	3–8 hr	12–24 hr

Action

Chemical effect: Unknown.
Therapeutic effect: Relieves muscle spasms.

Available forms

Capsules (extended released): 15 mg, 30 mg
Tablets: 5 mg, 7.5 mg, 10 mg

NURSING PROCESS

🔲 Assessment
• Assess patient's underlying condition before therapy.
• Monitor the drug's effectiveness by assessing severity and frequency of the patient's muscle spasms.
• If drug is stopped abruptly after long-term use, watch for nausea, headache, and malaise.
• Assess patient's and family's knowledge of drug therapy.

🔲 Nursing diagnoses
• Acute pain related to presence of muscle spasms
• Risk for injury related to potential for drug-induced CNS adverse reactions
• Deficient knowledge related to drug therapy

🔲 Planning and implementation
🛈 **ALERT:** Watch for symptoms of overdose, including cardiac toxicity. If you suspect toxicity, keep physostigmine available, and notify prescriber immediately.
• Don't give drug with other CNS depressants.
• With high doses, watch for adverse reactions similar to those of other TCAs.
🛈 **ALERT:** Don't confuse cyclobenzaprine with cyproheptadine.
Patient teaching
• Advise patient to report urinary hesitancy or urine retention. If constipation occurs, tell pa-

tient to increase fluid intake and suggest use of a stool softener.
• Caution patient not to split generic 10-mg tablets because the active ingredient may not split evenly.
• Warn patient to avoid activities that require alertness until drug's CNS effects are known.
• Warn patient to avoid using alcohol or other CNS depressants.
• Suggest sugarless chewing gum or hard candy to relieve dry mouth.

🔲 Evaluation
• Patient is free from pain with drug therapy.
• Patient doesn't experience injury as a result of drug-induced adverse CNS reactions.
• Patient and family state understanding of drug therapy.

HIGH ALERT!

cyclophosphamide
(sigh-kloh-FOS-fuh-mighd)
Cytoxan, Cytoxan Lyophilized, Neosar, Procytox ◆

Pharmacologic class: alkylating drug
Therapeutic class: antineoplastic
Pregnancy risk category: D

Indications and dosages

▶ **Breast, head, neck, prostate, lung, and ovarian cancers; Hodgkin lymphoma; chronic lymphocytic leukemia; chronic myelocytic leukemia; acute lymphoblastic leukemia; acute myelocytic leukemia; neuroblastoma; retinoblastoma; malignant lymphoma; multiple myeloma; mycosis fungoides; sarcoma.**
Adults and children: Initially, 40 to 50 mg/kg I.V. in divided doses over 2 to 5 days. Or 10 to 15 mg/kg I.V. every 7 to 10 days, 3 to 5 mg/kg I.V. twice weekly, or 1 to 5 mg/kg P.O. daily, based on patient tolerance. Adjust dosage according to evidence of antitumor activity or leukopenia.
▶ **"Minimal change" nephrotic syndrome.**
Children: 2.5 to 3 mg/kg P.O. daily for 60 to 90 days.
▶ **Polymyositis ‡.** *Adults:* 500 mg I.V. over 1 hour every 1 to 3 weeks, alone or with corticosteroids.
▶ **Rheumatoid arthritis‡.** *Adults:* 1.5 to 3 mg/kg P.O. daily.

▶ **Wegener granulomatosis‡.** *Adults:* 1 to 2 mg/kg P.O. daily (usually given with prednisone).

▼ I.V. administration

• Preparing and giving I.V. form of drug cause carcinogenic, mutagenic, and teratogenic risks. Follow facility policy to reduce risks.

• Reconstitute powder using sterile water for injection or bacteriostatic water for injection that contains only parabens. For nonlyophilized product, add 5 ml to 100-mg vial, 10 ml to 200-mg vial, 25 ml to 500-mg vial, 50 ml to 1-g vial, or 100 ml to 2-g vial to produce solution containing 20 mg/ml. Shake to dissolve. Shaking may take up to 6 minutes because it may be difficult to completely dissolve drug. Lyophilized preparation is much easier to reconstitute. Check package insert for quantity of diluent needed to reconstitute drug.

• Check reconstituted solution for small particles. Filter solution if needed.

• Give by direct I.V. injection or infusion. For I.V. infusion, further dilute with D_5W, dextrose 5% in normal saline solution, dextrose 5% in Ringer's injection, lactated Ringer's injection, sodium lactate injection, or half-normal saline solution for injection.

• Reconstituted solution is stable for 6 days refrigerated or 24 hours at room temperature. However, use stored solutions cautiously because drug contains no preservatives.

⊗ **Incompatibilities**
None known.

Contraindications and cautions

• Contraindicated in patients with severe bone marrow depression.

• Use cautiously in patients who have recently undergone radiation therapy or chemotherapy and in patients with leukopenia, thrombocytopenia, malignant cell infiltration of bone marrow, or hepatic or renal disease.

🔥 **Lifespan:** In pregnant women, use cautiously, if at all, because fetal harm may occur. In breast-feeding women, drug is contraindicated.

Adverse reactions

CV: *cardiotoxicity* (with very high doses and with doxorubicin).
GI: anorexia, mucositis, nausea and vomiting beginning within 6 hours, stomatitis.

GU: bladder fibrosis, gonadal suppression (may be irreversible), sterile hemorrhagic cystitis.
Hematologic: *anemia; leukopenia,* nadir between days 8 and 15, recovery in 17 to 28 days; *thrombocytopenia.*
Metabolic: hyperuricemia.
Respiratory: *pulmonary fibrosis* (with high doses).
Skin: reversible alopecia in 50% of patients, especially with high doses.
Other: *anaphylaxis, secondary malignancies,* SIADH (with high doses), sterility.

Interactions

Drug-drug. *Barbiturates:* May increase drug effect and cyclophosphamide toxicity by inducing hepatic enzymes. Avoid use together.
Cardiotoxic drugs: May cause additive adverse cardiac effects. Avoid use together.
Chloramphenicol, corticosteroids: May reduce activity of cyclophosphamide. Use cautiously and monitor patient.
Digoxin: May decrease digoxin level. Monitor level closely and adjust dosage as needed.
Succinylcholine: May prolong neuromuscular blockade. Avoid use together.

Effects on lab test results

• May increase uric acid level. May decrease pseudocholinesterase and hemoglobin levels and hematocrit.

• May decrease WBC, RBC, and platelet counts.

Pharmacokinetics

Absorption: Almost complete with doses of 100 mg or less. Higher doses are 75% absorbed.
Distribution: Throughout body, with minimal amounts in saliva, sweat, and synovial fluid. Active metabolites are about 50% protein-bound.
Metabolism: Metabolized to its active form by hepatic microsomal enzymes.
Excretion: Mainly in urine, with 5% to 30% as unchanged drug. *Half-life:* 3 to 12 hours.

Route	Onset	Peak	Duration
P.O., I.V.	Unknown	1 hr	Unknown

Action

Chemical effect: Cross-links strands of cellular DNA and interferes with RNA transcription,

---

causing imbalance of growth that leads to cell death.

Therapeutic effect: Kills specific types of cancer cells; improves renal function in mild nephrotic syndrome in children.

Available forms

Injection: 100-mg, 200-mg, 500-mg, 1-g, 2-g vials
Tablets: 25 mg, 50 mg

NURSING PROCESS

⚡ Assessment
• Assess patient's underlying condition before and regularly during therapy.
• Monitor CBC, uric acid level, and renal and liver function tests.
• If corticosteroid therapy is stopped, monitor patient for cyclophosphamide toxicity.
• Be alert for adverse reactions and drug interactions.
• Assess patient's and family's knowledge of drug therapy.

🔷 Nursing diagnoses
• Ineffective health maintenance related to underlying condition
• Risk for injury related to drug-induced adverse reactions
• Deficient knowledge related to drug therapy

▶ Planning and implementation
• Tablets are used for children with "minimal change" nephrotic syndrome, not to treat neoplastic disease.
• To prevent hyperuricemia with resulting uric acid nephropathy, allopurinol may be used with adequate hydration.
Patient teaching
• Warn patient that alopecia is likely to occur but is reversible.
• Warn patient to watch for evidence of infection (fever, sore throat, fatigue) and bleeding (easy bruising, nosebleeds, bleeding gums, melena) and to take temperature daily.
• Instruct patient to avoid OTC products that contain aspirin.
• Encourage patient to void every 1 to 2 hours while awake and to drink at least 3 L of fluid daily to minimize risk of hemorrhagic cystitis. Tell patient not to take drug at bedtime because infrequent urination during night may increase

possibility of cystitis. If cystitis occurs, tell patient to stop drug and notify prescriber. Cystitis can occur months after therapy ends. Mesna may be given to lower risk and severity of bladder toxicity.
• Advise both men and women to practice contraception while taking drug and for 4 months after because drug is potentially teratogenic.
• Advise women of childbearing age to avoid becoming pregnant during therapy. Also recommend consulting with prescriber before becoming pregnant.

☑ Evaluation
• Patient shows positive response to drug therapy.
• Patient doesn't experience injury as a result of drug-induced adverse reactions.
• Patient and family state understanding of drug therapy.

cycloserine
(sigh-kloh-SER-een)
Seromycin

Pharmacologic class: isoxazoline, D-alanine analogue
Therapeutic class: antituberculotic
Pregnancy risk category: C

Indications and dosages

▶ **Adjunct in pulmonary or extrapulmonary tuberculosis.** *Adults:* Initially, 250 mg P.O. every 12 hours for 2 weeks; then, if level is below 25 to 30 mcg/ml and no toxicity has developed, 250 mg every 8 hours for 2 weeks. If optimum blood level isn't achieved and no toxicity has developed, increase to 250 mg every 6 hours. Maximum, 1 g daily. If CNS toxicity occurs, stop drug for 1 week and then resume at 250 mg daily for 2 weeks. If no serious toxic effects occur, increase by 250-mg increments every 10 days until level is 25 to 30 mcg/ml, or maximum is reached.

Contraindications and cautions

• Contraindicated in patients hypersensitive to drug, patients who consume excessive amounts of alcohol, and patients with seizure disorders,

depression, severe anxiety, psychosis, or severe renal insufficiency.

● Use cautiously in patients with renal impairment, and reduce dosage.

⚜ **Lifespan:** In pregnant and breast-feeding women, use cautiously. In children, safety and effectiveness haven't been established.

Adverse reactions

CNS: *coma,* confusion, *depression,* drowsiness, dysarthria, *hallucinations,* headache, hyperirritability, hyperreflexia, memory loss, *nervousness,* paresis, paresthesia, **seizures, suicidal tendencies** and other psychotic symptoms, tremor, vertigo.

Other: hypersensitivity reactions (allergic dermatitis).

Interactions

Drug-drug. *Ethionamide, isoniazid:* May increase risk of CNS toxicity (seizures, dizziness, or drowsiness). Monitor patient closely.

Phenytoin: May increase phenytoin level. Adjust phenytoin dosage p.r.n.

Drug-lifestyle. *Alcohol use:* May increase risk of CNS toxicity. Advise patient to refrain from alcohol consumption during therapy.

Effects on lab test results

● May increase transaminase level.

Pharmacokinetics

Absorption: About 80%.

Distribution: Widely into body tissues and fluids, including CSF. Doesn't bind to proteins.

Metabolism: Possibly partial.

Excretion: Mainly in urine. *Half-life:* 10 hours.

Route	Onset	Peak	Duration
P.O.	Unknown	3–4 hr	Unknown

Action

Chemical effect: Inhibits cell-wall biosynthesis by interfering with bacterial use of amino acids (bacteriostatic).

Therapeutic effect: Aids in eradicating tuberculosis.

Available forms

Capsules: 250 mg

NURSING PROCESS

⬛ Assessment

● Assess patient's underlying condition before therapy.

● Obtain specimen for culture and sensitivity tests before therapy begins and periodically thereafter to detect resistance.

● Monitor drug's effectiveness by evaluating culture and sensitivity results; watch for improvement in patient's underlying condition.

● Monitor cycloserine level periodically, especially in patients receiving high doses (more than 500 mg daily) because toxic reactions may occur with blood level above 30 mcg/ml.

● Monitor results of hematologic tests and renal and liver function studies.

● Be alert for adverse reactions and drug interactions.

● Assess patient's and family's knowledge of drug therapy.

⬛ Nursing diagnoses

● Ineffective health maintenance related to presence of tuberculosis

● Risk for injury related to drug-induced CNS adverse reactions

● Deficient knowledge related to drug therapy

▶ Planning and implementation

● Always give with other antituberculotics to prevent development of resistant organisms. Drug is considered second-line treatment for tuberculosis.

● Adjust dosage according to level, toxicity, or effectiveness.

● Give pyridoxine, anticonvulsants, tranquilizers, or sedatives to relieve adverse reactions.

● Pyridoxine may prevent neurotoxicity.

⚠ **ALERT:** Don't confuse cycloserine with cyclophosphamide or cyclosporine.

Patient teaching

● Warn patient to avoid alcohol, which may cause serious neurologic reactions.

● Instruct patient to take drug exactly as prescribed, and warn against stopping drug without prescriber's approval.

● Stress importance of having laboratory studies done to monitor drug effectiveness and toxicity.

✔ Evaluation

● Patient maintains health after drug therapy.

Reactions may be *common,* uncommon, *life-threatening,* or COMMON AND LIFE-THREATENING.

- Patient has no injury as a result of drug-induced adverse reactions.
- Patient and family state understanding of drug therapy.

cyclosporine (cyclosporin)
(sigh-kloh-SPOOR-een)
Sandimmune

cyclosporine, modified
Gengraf, Neoral

Pharmacologic class: polypeptide antibiotic
Therapeutic class: immunosuppressant
Pregnancy risk category: C

Indications and dosages

▶ **To prevent organ rejection in kidney, liver, or heart transplantation.** *Adults and children:* 15 mg/kg P.O. 4 to 12 hours before transplantation and continued daily postoperatively for 1 to 2 weeks. Reduce dosage by 5% each week to maintenance level of 5 to 10 mg/kg daily. Or 5 to 6 mg/kg I.V. concentrate 4 to 12 hours before transplantation. Postoperatively, repeat dosage daily until patient can tolerate P.O. forms. When converting from Sandimmune to Neoral or Gengraf, use same daily dose as previously used for Sandimmune. Monitor level every 4 to 7 days after converting, and monitor blood pressure and creatinine level every 2 weeks during the first 2 months.
▶ **Severe, active rheumatoid arthritis that hasn't adequately responded to methotrexate.** *Adults:* 1.25 mg/kg Gengraf or Neoral P.O. b.i.d. Increase dosage by 0.5 to 0.75 mg/kg daily after 8 weeks and again after 12 weeks to a maximum of 4 mg/kg daily. If no response is seen after 16 weeks, stop therapy.
▶ **Recalcitrant plaque psoriasis that isn't adequately responsive to at least one systemic therapy or in patients for whom other systemic therapy is contraindicated or isn't tolerated.** *Adults:* Initially, 2.5 mg/kg Gengraf or Neoral P.O. daily divided b.i.d. Maintain initial dose for 4 weeks. Increase by 0.5 mg/kg daily to a maximum of 4 mg/kg daily at 2-week intervals, if needed.
◪ **Adjust-a-dose:** In patients with rheumatoid arthritis or plaque psoriasis, decrease dose by 25% to 50% at any time to control adverse

events (such as hypertension), elevated serum creatinine level (25% or more above baseline), or clinically significant laboratory abnormalities.

▼ I.V. administration
- Give drug I.V. to patients who can't tolerate oral drugs.
- Dilute each milliliter of concentrate in 20 to 100 ml of D$_5$W or normal saline solution for injection. Dilute immediately before infusion; infuse over 2 to 6 hours.
- Give I.V. concentrate at one-third oral dose and dilute before use.
- Protect I.V. solution from light.
⊗ **Incompatibilities**
None reported.

Contraindications and cautions
- Contraindicated in patients hypersensitive to drug or to polyoxyethylated castor oil (found in injectable form). Neoral and Gengraf are contraindicated in patients with psoriasis or rheumatoid arthritis who also have renal impairment, uncontrolled hypertension, or malignancies.
▒ **Lifespan:** In pregnant women, use cautiously. In breast-feeding women, safety and effectiveness haven't been established.

Adverse reactions
CNS: headache, *seizures, tremor.*
CV: flushing, hypertension.
EENT: sinusitis.
GI: diarrhea, *gum hyperplasia,* nausea, oral thrush, vomiting.
GU: NEPHROTOXICITY.
Hematologic: anemia, LEUKOPENIA, THROMBOCYTOPENIA.
Hepatic: *hepatotoxicity.*
Skin: acne, *hirsutism.*
Other: *anaphylaxis,* infections.

Interactions
Drug-drug. *Aminoglycosides, amphotericin B, co-trimoxazole, NSAIDs:* May increase risk of nephrotoxicity. Monitor patient for toxicity.
Amphotericin B, cilastatin, cimetidine, diltiazem, erythromycin, imipenem, ketoconazole, metoclopramide, prednisolone: May increase level of cyclosporine. Monitor patient for increased toxicity.
Azathioprine, corticosteroids, cyclophosphamide, verapamil: May increase immunosuppression. Monitor patient closely for infection.

Carbamazepine, isoniazid, phenobarbital, phenytoin, rifampin: May decrease immunosuppressant effect. Increase cyclosporine dosage.
Vaccines: May decrease immune response. Postpone routine immunization.
Drug-herb. *Pill-bearing spurge:* May inhibit CYP3A enzymes affecting drug metabolism. Discourage use together.
St. John's wort: May significantly lower drug level and contribute to organ rejection. Discourage use together.
Drug-food. *Grapefruit:* May increase drug level and cause toxicity. Discourage use together.

Effects on lab test results

• May increase BUN, creatinine, LDL, bilirubin, AST, ALT, and glucose levels. May decrease hemoglobin level and hematocrit.
• May decrease WBC and platelet counts.

Pharmacokinetics

Absorption: Varies widely. Only 30% of Sandimmune oral dose reaches systemic circulation, while 60% of Neoral reaches systemic circulation. Gengraf absorption is 10% to 89%, depending on patient population.
Distribution: Wide. 90% protein-bound.
Metabolism: Extensive, in liver.
Excretion: Mainly in feces. *Half-life:* 10 to 27 hours.

Route	Onset	Peak	Duration
P.O.	Unknown	1½–3 hr	Unknown
I.V.	Unknown	Unknown	Unknown

Action

Chemical effect: Inhibits proliferation of T lymphocytes.
Therapeutic effect: Prevents organ rejection.

Available forms

Capsules: 25 mg, 100 mg
Capsules for microemulsion: 25 mg, 100 mg
Injection: 50 mg/ml
Oral solution: 100 mg/ml

NURSING PROCESS

🕮 Assessment

• Assess patient's organ transplant before therapy.
• Monitor drug effectiveness by evaluating patient for signs and symptoms of organ rejection.

• Check drug level at regular intervals.
• Monitor BUN and creatinine levels because nephrotoxicity may develop 2 to 3 months after transplant surgery and require reducing the dose.
• Monitor liver function tests for hepatotoxicity, which usually occurs during first month after transplant.
• Monitor CBC and platelet counts regularly.
• Be alert for adverse reactions and drug interactions.
• Assess patient's and family's knowledge of drug therapy.

✛ Nursing diagnoses

• Risk for injury related to potential for organ rejection
• Ineffective protection related to drug-induced immunosuppression
• Deficient knowledge related to drug therapy

▶ Planning and implementation

• Don't give psoralen plus ultraviolet A or ultraviolet B therapy, methotrexate, other immunosuppressants, coal tar, or radiation therapy to psoriasis patient taking Neoral or Gengraf.
• Always give drug with adrenal corticosteroids.
• Measure oral dose carefully in oral syringe. To increase palatability of conventional oral solution, mix with whole milk, chocolate milk, or fruit juice (except grapefruit juice). Modified oral solution (Gengraf or Neoral) is less palatable when mixed with milk; to increase its palatability, mix with room-temperature orange or apple juice. Use glass container to minimize adherence to container walls.
• Give drug with meals to minimize GI distress.
• **⚠ ALERT:** Sandimmune isn't bioequivalent with Neoral or Gengraf. When converting from Sandimmune to either of these drugs, increase monitoring to detect inadequate doses. Gengraf is bioequivalent to and interchangeable with Neoral capsules.
• Before giving drug to patient with rheumatoid arthritis, measure blood pressure at least twice and obtain two creatinine levels to estimate baseline. Evaluate patient's blood pressure and creatinine level every 2 weeks during first 3 months, then monthly if patient is stable. Monitor blood pressure and creatinine level after an increase in NSAID dosage or introduction of a new NSAID. If hypertension occurs, decrease dosage of Gengraf or Neoral by 25% to 50%. If

hypertension persists, decrease dosage further or control blood pressure with antihypertensives.

• If patient also receives methotrexate, monitor CBC and liver function tests monthly.

• For patient with psoriasis, watch for occult infection and tumors before and during therapy.

• Before starting therapy in psoriasis patient, take blood pressure at least twice and obtain two creatinine levels. Also, obtain CBC and BUN, magnesium, uric acid, potassium, and lipid levels. Evaluate blood pressure, CBC, uric acid, creatinine, BUN, potassium, lipid, and magnesium levels every 2 weeks for the first 3 months, then monthly if patient is stable, or more frequently when adjusting dose. Reduce dose by 25% to 50% in case of significant abnormality.

• Monitor blood pressure and creatinine level after an increase in NSAID dosage or introduction of a new NSAID.

⊛ **ALERT:** Don't confuse cyclosporine with cyclophosphamide or cycloserine.

⊛ **ALERT:** Don't confuse Sandimmune with Sandoglobulin or Sandostatin.

Patient teaching

• Encourage patient to take drug at the same time each day.

• Advise patient to take Neoral or Gengraf on an empty stomach and not to mix with grapefruit juice.

• Advise patient to take drug with meals if it causes nausea.

• Tell patient not to stop taking drug without prescriber's approval.

• Instruct patient to swish and swallow nystatin four times daily to prevent oral thrush.

• Instruct patient on infection control and bleeding precautions, as indicated by CBC and platelet count results.

☑ **Evaluation**

• Patient doesn't experience organ rejection while taking drug.

• Patient is free from infection and serious bleeding episodes throughout drug therapy.

• Patient and family state understanding of drug therapy.

HIGH ALERT!

cytarabine (ara-C, cytosine arabinoside)
(sigh-TAR-uh-been)
Cytosar ◆ , Tarabine PFS

Pharmacologic class: antimetabolite
Therapeutic class: antineoplastic
Pregnancy risk category: D

Indications and dosages

▶ **Acute nonlymphocytic leukemia.** *Adults and children:* 100 mg/m²/day by continuous I.V. infusion (days 1 to 7) or 100 mg/m² I.V. every 12 hours (days 1 to 7). Give with other anticancer drugs.

▶ **Acute lymphocytic leukemia.** Consult literature for current recommendations.

▶ **Refractory acute leukemia.** *Adults and children:* 3 g/m² I.V. over 2 hours every 12 hours for 4 to 12 doses (repeated at 2- to 3-week intervals).

▶ **Meningeal leukemia.** *Adults and children:* Highly variable from 5 to 75 mg/m² intrathecally. Frequency also varies from once a day for 4 days to once every 4 days. Most common dosage is 30 mg/m², every 4 days until CSF is normal, followed by one more dose.

◼ **NEW INDICATION: Lymphomatous meningitis.** *Adults:* For induction, give 50 mg intrathecally every 14 days for two doses (weeks 1 and 3); then, for consolidation therapy, give 50 mg intrathecally every 14 days for three doses (weeks 5, 7, and 9) followed by one additional dose at week 13. Maintenance dosage, 50 mg intrathecally every 28 days for four doses (weeks 17, 21, 25, and 29).

◧ **Adjust-a-dose:** For patients with neurotoxicity, reduce dose to 25 mg. If neurotoxicity persists, discontinue therapy.

▽ I.V. administration

• Preparing and giving I.V. form are linked to carcinogenic, mutagenic, and teratogenic risks. Follow facility policy to reduce risks.

• To reduce nausea, give antiemetic before drug. Nausea and vomiting are more frequent when large doses are given rapidly by I.V. push. These reactions are less frequent when given by infusion. Dizziness may occur with rapid infusion.

• Reconstitute drug using provided diluent, which is bacteriostatic water for injection containing benzyl alcohol. Avoid this diluent when preparing drug for neonates or for intrathecal use. Reconstitute 100-mg vial with 5 ml of diluent or 500-mg vial with 10 ml of diluent. Reconstituted solution is stable for 48 hours. Discard cloudy reconstituted solution.

• For I.V. infusion, further dilute using normal saline solution for injection, D₅W, or sterile water for injection.

⊗ **Incompatibilities**
Allopurinol sodium, fluorouracil, ganciclovir sodium, heparin sodium, insulin (regular), methylprednisolone sodium succinate, nafcillin, oxacillin, penicillin.

Contraindications and cautions

• Contraindicated in patients hypersensitive to drug.
• Use cautiously in patients with hepatic disease.

⚠ **Lifespan:** In pregnant women, drug isn't recommended because fetal harm may occur. In breast-feeding women, drug is contraindicated.

Adverse reactions

CNS: neurotoxicity, including ataxia and cerebellar dysfunction (with high doses).
EENT: keratitis, nystagmus.
GI: *anal ulceration, anorexia, constipation,* diarrhea, *nausea, vomiting,* dysphagia, projectile vomiting from large I.V. dose given rapidly, reddened area at juncture of lips followed by sore mouth and oral ulcers in 5 to 10 days.
GU: urate nephropathy.
Hematologic: anemia; *leukopenia,* with initial WBC count nadir 7 to 9 days after drug is stopped and second (more severe) nadir 15 to 24 days after drug is stopped; reticulocytopenia; *thrombocytopenia,* with platelet count nadir occurring on day 10; *megaloblastosis.*
Hepatic: *hepatotoxicity* (usually mild and reversible).
Metabolic: hyperuricemia.
Skin: rash.
Other: *anaphylaxis,* flulike syndrome.

Interactions

Drug-drug. *Digoxin:* May decrease digoxin level. Monitor digoxin level.

Flucytosine: May decrease flucytosine activity. Monitor patient closely.
Gentamicin: May decrease activity against *Klebsiella pneumoniae.* Avoid use together.

Effects on lab test results

• May increase uric acid level. May decrease hemoglobin level and hematocrit.
• May increase megaloblasts. May decrease WBC, RBC, platelet, and reticulocyte counts.

Pharmacokinetics

Absorption: Good.
Distribution: Rapid and wide. 13% protein-bound. Drug penetrates the blood–brain barrier only slightly after rapid I.V. dose; however, when drug is given by continuous I.V. infusion, CSF level reaches 40% to 60% of plasma level.
Metabolism: Mainly in liver but also in kidneys, GI mucosa, and granulocytes.
Excretion: In urine. Less than 10% of dose as unchanged drug in urine. *Half-life:* Initial, 8 minutes; terminal, 1 to 3 hours; in CSF, 2 hours.

Route	Onset	Peak	Duration
I.V., intrathecal	Unknown	Unknown	Unknown
SubQ	Unknown	20–60 min	Unknown

Action

Chemical effect: Inhibits DNA synthesis.
Therapeutic effect: Kills selected cancer cells.

Available forms

Injection: 100-mg, 500-mg, 1-g, 2-g vials

NURSING PROCESS

Assessment
• Assess patient's underlying condition before and regularly throughout therapy.
• Monitor uric acid level, hepatic and renal function studies, and CBC.
• Be alert for adverse reactions and drug interactions.
• If patient receives high doses, watch for neurotoxicity, which may first appear as nystagmus but can progress to ataxia and cerebellar dysfunction.
• Assess patient's and family's knowledge of drug therapy.

⊕ Nursing diagnoses

- Ineffective health maintenance related to underlying condition
- Risk for injury related to drug-induced adverse hematologic reactions
- Deficient knowledge related to drug therapy

❯ Planning and implementation

- When giving intrathecally, use preservative-free normal saline solution. Add 5 ml to 100-mg vial or 10 ml to 500-mg vial. Use immediately after reconstitution. Discard unused drug.
- Maintain high fluid intake and give allopurinol to avoid urate nephropathy in leukemia induction therapy.
- If granulocyte count is below 1,000/mm^3 or if platelet count is below 50,000/mm^3, modify or stop therapy.
- Corticosteroid eyedrops are prescribed to prevent drug-induced keratitis.
- Potential benefit must be judged against known adverse effects.

Patient teaching
- Warn patient to watch for signs of infection (fever, sore throat, fatigue) and bleeding (easy bruising, nosebleeds, bleeding gums, melena). Tell patient to take temperature daily.
- Instruct patient on infection control and bleeding precautions.
- Advise woman of childbearing age to avoid becoming pregnant during therapy. Also recommend consulting with prescriber before becoming pregnant.
- Encourage patient to drink at least 3 L of fluids daily.
- Instruct patient about need for frequent oral hygiene.

☑ Evaluation

- Patient demonstrates positive response to drug therapy.
- Patient doesn't experience injury as result of drug therapy.
- Patient and family state understanding of drug therapy.

cytomegalovirus immune globulin, intravenous (CMV-IGIV)

(sigh-toh-MEH-gah-loh-VIGH-rus ih-MYOON GLOH-byoo-lin)
CytoGam

Pharmacologic class: immune globulin
Therapeutic class: immune serum
Pregnancy risk category: C

Indications and dosages

▶ **To attenuate primary CMV disease in seronegative kidney transplant recipients who receive kidney from a CMV seropositive donor.** *Adults:* Give I.V. based on time after transplantation:
- Within 72 hours, 150 mg/kg
- 2 weeks after, 100 mg/kg
- 4 weeks after, 100 mg/kg
- 6 weeks after, 100 mg/kg
- 8 weeks after, 100 mg/kg
- 12 weeks after, 50 mg/kg
- 16 weeks after, 50 mg/kg.

Give first dose at 15 mg/kg/hour. If no adverse reactions occur after 30 minutes, increase to 30 mg/kg/hour. If no adverse reactions occur after another 30 minutes, increase to 60 mg/kg/hour. Don't exceed 75 ml/hour. Subsequent doses may be given at 15 mg/kg/hour for 15 minutes, increasing at 15-minute intervals in stepwise fashion to 60 mg/kg/hour. Don't exceed 75 ml/hour. Monitor patient closely during and after rate change.

▶ **Prophylaxis of CMV disease related to lung, liver, pancreas, and heart transplants.** *Adults:* Use with ganciclovir in organ transplants from CMV seropositive donors into seronegative recipients. Maximum total dose per infusion is 150 mg/kg I.V. Give as follows based on time after transplantation:
- Within 72 hours, 150 mg/kg
- 2 weeks after, 150 mg/kg
- 4 weeks after, 150 mg/kg
- 6 weeks after, 150 mg/kg
- 8 weeks after, 150 mg/kg
- 12 weeks after, 100 mg/kg
- 16 weeks after, 100 mg/kg.

Give first dose at 15 mg/kg/hour. If no adverse reactions occur after 30 minutes, increase to 30 mg/kg/hour. If no adverse reactions occur after another 30 minutes, increase to 60 mg/kg/

hour. (Don't exceed 75 ml/hour.) Later doses may be given at 15 mg/kg/hour for 15 minutes, increasing every 15 minutes in a stepwise fashion to a maximum of 60 mg/kg/hour. (Don't exceed 75 ml/hour.) Monitor patient closely during and after each rate change.

▼ I.V. administration

• Remove tab portion of vial cap and clean rubber stopper with 70% alcohol or equivalent. Don't shake vial; avoid foaming. Don't infuse if the solution has color or particulate matter or is turbid. Don't predilute.
• Give through separate I.V. line using constant infusion pump. Filters aren't needed. If unable to give through separate line, piggyback into existing line of saline solution injection or one of the following dextrose solutions with or without saline solution: dextrose 2.5% in water, D_5W, dextrose 10% in water, or dextrose 20% in water. Don't dilute more than 1:2 with any of these solutions.
• Begin infusion within 6 hours of entering vial; finish within 12 hours.
• Refrigerate drug at 36° to 46° F (2° to 8° C).
⊗ **Incompatibilities**
Other I.V. drugs.

Contraindications and cautions

• Contraindicated in patients with selective immunoglobulin (Ig)A deficiency or history of sensitivity to other human immunoglobulin preparations.
☀ **Lifespan:** In pregnant women, use cautiously. In breast-feeding women and in children, safety and effectiveness haven't been established.

Adverse reactions

CNS: fever.
CV: flushing, hypotension.
GI: nausea, vomiting.
Musculoskeletal: back pain, muscle cramps.
Respiratory: wheezing.
Other: *anaphylaxis,* chills.

Interactions

Drug-drug. *Live-virus vaccines:* May interfere with immune response to live-virus vaccines. Defer vaccination for at least 3 months.

Effects on lab test results

None reported.

Pharmacokinetics

Absorption: Given I.V.
Distribution: Unknown.
Metabolism: Unknown.
Excretion: Unknown. *Half-life:* Immediately after transplantation, 8 days; 60 or more days after transplantation, 13 to 15 days.

Route	Onset	Peak	Duration
I.V.	Unknown	Unknown	Unknown

Action

Chemical effect: Supplies relatively high concentration of IgG antibodies against CMV. Increasing these antibody levels in CMV-exposed patients may reduce risk of serious CMV disease.
Therapeutic effect: Provides passive immunity to CMV.

Available forms

Solution for injection: 50 ± 10 mg protein/ml

NURSING PROCESS

📋 Assessment

• Assess patient's underlying condition before therapy starts.
• Take vital signs before starting therapy, mid-infusion, post-infusion, and before any increase in infusion rate.
• Monitor drug's effectiveness by evaluating kidney function.
• Be alert for adverse reactions and drug interactions.
• Assess patient's and family's knowledge of drug therapy.

⊕ Nursing diagnoses

• Risk for injury related to potential for organ rejection
• Decreased cardiac output related to drug-induced hypotension
• Deficient knowledge related to drug therapy

▶ Planning and implementation

• If patient develops anaphylaxis or if blood pressure drops, stop infusion, notify prescriber, and give CPR and drugs, such as diphenhydramine and epinephrine.
Patient teaching
• Teach patient about drug therapy.

- Instruct patient to notify prescriber immediately if adverse reactions develop.

☑ **Evaluation**
- Patient doesn't reject transplanted kidney during drug therapy.
- Patient maintains normal cardiac output throughout drug therapy.
- Patient and family state understanding of drug therapy.

HIGH ALERT!

dacarbazine
(deh-KAR-buh-zeen)
DTIC-Dome ◆

Pharmacologic class: alkylating drug
Therapeutic class: antineoplastic
Pregnancy risk category: C

Indications and dosages

▶ **Metastatic malignant melanoma.** *Adults:*
2 to 4.5 mg/kg I.V. daily for 10 days; then every 4 weeks, as tolerated. Or, 250 mg/m² I.V. daily for 5 days; repeat at 3-week intervals.
▶ **Hodgkin lymphoma.** *Adults:* 150 mg/m² I.V. daily (with other drugs) for 5 days; repeat every 4 weeks. Or, 375 mg/m² on first day of combined regimen; repeat every 15 days.

▼ I.V. administration

- Preparing and giving drug raises risk of carcinogenic, mutagenic, and teratogenic effects. Follow facility policy to reduce risks.
- Reconstitute drug with sterile water for injection. Add 9.9 ml to 100-mg vial or 19.7 ml to 200-mg vial. Solution should be colorless to clear yellow. For infusion, further dilute, using up to 250 ml of normal saline solution or D₅W. Infuse over 30 minutes.
- During infusion, protect bag from direct sunlight to avoid drug breakdown. Dilute solution further or slow infusion to decrease pain at infusion site.
- If infiltration occurs, stop infusion immediately, apply ice to area for 24 to 48 hours, and notify prescriber.

- Reconstituted solutions are stable for 8 hours at room temperature under normal lighting conditions and up to 3 days if refrigerated. Diluted solutions are stable for 8 hours at room temperature under normal light and up to 24 hours if refrigerated. If solutions turn pink, this is a sign of decomposition; discard drug.
⊗ **Incompatibilities**
Allopurinol sodium, cefepime, hydrocortisone sodium succinate, piperacillin with tazobactam.

Contraindications and cautions

- Contraindicated in patients hypersensitive to drug.
- Use cautiously in impaired bone marrow function.
⚠ **Lifespan:** In pregnant women, use cautiously and only when absolutely needed because fetal harm may occur. In breast-feeding women, drug is contraindicated. In children, safety and effectiveness haven't been established.

Adverse reactions

GI: *anorexia, severe nausea and vomiting.*
Hematologic: *leukopenia, thrombocytopenia* (nadir at 3 to 4 weeks).
Hepatic: *hepatotoxicity.*
Metabolic: hyperuricemia.
Skin: alopecia, phototoxicity.
Other: *anaphylaxis, flulike symptoms,* severe pain with concentrated solution or extravasation, tissue damage.

Interactions

Drug-drug. *Allopurinol:* May have additive hypouricemic effects. Monitor patient closely.
Anticoagulants, aspirin: May increase risk of bleeding. Avoid use together.
Bone marrow suppressants: May increase toxicity. Monitor hematologic studies closely.
Phenobarbital, phenytoin, and other drugs that induce hepatic metabolism: May increase dacarbazine metabolism. Adjust dosage.
Drug-lifestyle. *Sun exposure:* May cause photosensitivity reactions, especially during the first 2 days of therapy. Advise patient to avoid prolonged sun exposure and to wear protective clothing and sunblock.

Effects on lab test results

- May increase BUN and liver enzyme levels.
- May decrease WBC, RBC, and platelet counts.

Pharmacokinetics

Absorption: Given I.V.
Distribution: May localize in body tissues, especially the liver. Minimally protein-bound.
Metabolism: Rapid to several compounds, some of which may be active.
Excretion: About 30% to 45% in urine. *Half-life:* Initial, 19 minutes; terminal, 5 hours.

Route	Onset	Peak	Duration
I.V.	Unknown	Unknown	Unknown

Action

Chemical effect: May cross-link strands of cellular DNA and interfere with RNA transcription, causing imbalance of growth that leads to cell death.
Therapeutic effect: Kills selected cancer cells.

Available forms

Injection: 100-mg, 200-mg, 500-mg, 600-mg ♦ vials

NURSING PROCESS

⚖ Assessment

• Obtain history of patient's underlying disease before therapy, and reassess regularly throughout therapy.
• Monitor CBC and platelet count.
• **ALERT:** Monitor liver function closely because toxicity is possible.
• Look for adverse reactions and drug interactions.
• Assess patient's and family's knowledge of drug therapy.

Nursing diagnoses

• Ineffective health maintenance related to presence of neoplastic disease
• Risk for injury related to risk of drug-induced adverse reactions
• Deficient knowledge related to drug therapy

Planning and implementation

• For Hodgkin lymphoma, drug usually is given with other antineoplastic drugs.
• To help decrease nausea, give antiemetics before use. Nausea and vomiting may subside after several doses.
• To prevent bleeding, avoid all I.M. injections when platelet count is below 50,000/mm^3.

• Use blood transfusions to combat anemia. Patient may receive injections of RBC colony-stimulating factors to promote RBC production and decrease need for blood transfusions.
• **ALERT:** Don't confuse dacarbazine with Dicarbosil, carbamazepine, or procarbazine.

Patient teaching

• Warn patient to watch for signs of infection (fever, sore throat, fatigue) and bleeding (easy bruising, nosebleeds, bleeding gums, melena). Tell patient to take temperature daily.
• Instruct patient to avoid OTC products containing aspirin.
• Advise patient to avoid sunlight and sunlamps for first 2 days after therapy.
• Reassure patient that flulike symptoms may be treated with mild antipyretics, such as acetaminophen.

✓ Evaluation

• Patient has positive response to therapy, as shown on follow-up diagnostic studies and overall physical condition.
• Patient has no injury from drug-induced adverse reactions.
• Patient and family state understanding of drug therapy.

daclizumab
(da-KLIZ-yoo-mab)
Zenapax

Pharmacologic class: humanized immunoglobulin G1 monoclonal antibody
Therapeutic class: immunosuppressant
Pregnancy risk category: C

Indications and dosages

▶ **To prevent acute organ rejection in renal transplant patients receiving an immunosuppressive regimen that includes cyclosporine and corticosteroids.** *Adults:* 1 mg/kg I.V. Standard course of therapy is five doses. Give first dose no more than 24 hours before transplantation; give remaining four doses at 14-day intervals.

▽ I.V. administration

• Don't give drug in a direct I.V. injection. Dilute in 50 ml of sterile normal saline solution before administration. To avoid foaming, don't

shake. Inspect for particulates and discoloration before use.
- Infuse over 15 minutes via a central or peripheral line. Don't add or infuse other drugs simultaneously through the same line.
- Drug may be refrigerated at 36° to 46° F (2° to 8° C) for 24 hours and is stable at room temperature for 4 hours. Discard solution if not used within 24 hours.
- Protect undiluted solution from direct light.
⊗ **Incompatibilities**
Other drugs infused through same I.V. line.

Contraindications and cautions

- Contraindicated in patients hypersensitive to drug or any of its components.
⚘ **Lifespan:** In pregnant or breast-feeding women, use cautiously. Tell women of childbearing age to use contraception before, during, and for 4 months after drug therapy.

Adverse reactions

CNS: *anxiety,* depression, dizziness, fatigue, fever, generalized weakness, headache, insomnia, pain, prickly sensation, tremors.
CV: aggravated hypertension, chest pain, edema, fluid overload, hypertension, hypotension, tachycardia.
EENT: blurred vision, pharyngitis, rhinitis.
GI: abdominal distention, *abdominal pain, constipation, diarrhea, dyspepsia,* epigastric pain, flatulence, gastritis, hemorrhoids, *nausea, pyrosis,* vomiting.
GU: dysuria, hydronephrosis, lymphocele, *oliguria,* renal damage, renal insufficiency, *renal tubular necrosis,* urinary tract bleeding, urinary tract disorder, urine retention.
Hematologic: *bleeding.*
Metabolic: dehydration, *diabetes mellitus.*
Musculoskeletal: arthralgia, leg cramps, musculoskeletal or back pain, myalgia.
Respiratory: abnormal breath sounds, atelectasis, congestion, coughing, crackles, dyspnea, *hypoxia,* pleural effusion, *pulmonary edema.*
Skin: acne, cellulitis, hirsutism, impaired wound healing without infection, *increased sweating,* night sweats, *pruritus, rash,* wound infections.
Other: *anaphylaxis,* limb edema, *severe infection,* shivering.

Interactions

Drug-drug. *Corticosteroids, cyclosporine, mycophenolate mofetil:* May increase mortality.

Monitor patient closely for lymphoproliferative disorders and opportunistic infections.

Effect on lab test results
- May increase BUN and creatinine levels.

Pharmacokinetics
Absorption: Given I.V.
Distribution: Unknown.
Metabolism: Unknown.
Excretion: Unknown. *Half-life:* 20 days.

Route	Onset	Peak	Duration
I.V.	Unknown	Unknown	Unknown

Action
Chemical effect: Inhibits interleukin-2 (IL-2) binding to prevent IL-2 from activating lymphocytes. Once in circulation, drug impairs response of immune system.
Therapeutic effect: Prevents organ rejection.

Available forms
Injection: 25 mg/5 ml

NURSING PROCESS

Assessment
- Obtain history of patient's underlying condition before therapy, and reassess regularly.
- Check for opportunistic infections.
ALERT: Monitor patient for severe, acute hypersensitivity reactions when giving each dose (includes anaphylaxis, hypotension, bronchospasm, loss of consciousness, injection site reactions, edema, and arrhythmias). Stop drug if severe reaction occurs.
- Assess patient's and family's knowledge of drug therapy.

Nursing diagnoses
- Risk for injury related to potential for organ rejection
- Ineffective protection related to drug-induced immunosuppression
- Deficient knowledge related to drug therapy

Planning and implementation
- Use only with a prescriber experienced in immunosuppressant therapy and management of organ transplantation.
ALERT: Using daclizumab as part of an immunosuppressive regimen that includes cyclo-

sporine, mycophenolate mofetil, and corticosteroids may increase the patient's risk of death.

Patient teaching

• Tell patient to consult prescriber before taking other drugs during therapy.

• Advise patient to take precautions against infection.

• Inform patient that neither he nor any household member should receive vaccinations unless medically approved.

• Tell patient to immediately report wounds that fail to heal, unusual bruising or bleeding, or fever.

• Advise patient to drink plenty of fluids during therapy and to report painful urination, blood in the urine, or a decrease in urine output.

• Instruct women of childbearing age to use effective contraception before starting therapy, during therapy, and to continue until 4 months after completing therapy.

☑ **Evaluation**

• Patient doesn't experience organ rejection while taking drug.

• Patient is free from infection and serious bleeding episodes throughout drug therapy.

• Patient and family state understanding of drug therapy.

HIGH ALERT!

dalteparin sodium

(dal-TEH-peh-rin SOH-dee-um)
Fragmin

Pharmacologic class: low–molecular-weight heparin
Therapeutic class: anticoagulant
Pregnancy risk category: B

Indications and dosages

▶ **Prevention of deep vein thrombosis (DVT) in patients undergoing abdominal surgery who are at risk for thromboembolic complications.** *Adults:* 2,500 international units subcutaneously daily, starting 1 to 2 hours before surgery and repeated once daily for 5 to 10 days postoperatively. In abdominal surgery patients at high risk for thromboembolic complications (such as those with malignant disease), 5,000 international units subcutaneously daily starting on the evening before surgery and repeated once daily for 5 to 10 days postopera-

tively. Or, 2,500 international units subcutaneously within 1 to 2 hours before surgery, followed 12 hours later by a second dose of 2,500 international units subcutaneously and then 5,000 international units subcutaneously once daily for 5 to 10 days postoperatively.

▶ **Prevention of DVT in patients undergoing hip replacement surgery.** *Adults:* 2,500 international units subcutaneously within 2 hours before surgery and second dose 2,500 international units subcutaneously in the evening following surgery (at least 6 hours after first dose). If surgery is performed in the evening, omit second dose on day of surgery. Starting on first postoperative day, give 5,000 international units subcutaneously once daily for 5 to 10 days. Or, 5,000 international units subcutaneously on the evening before surgery, followed by 5,000 international units subcutaneously once daily starting in the evening of surgery for 5 to 10 days postoperatively. If the initial dose is scheduled after surgery, give 2,500 international units subcutaneously 4 to 8 hours following surgery, provided hemostasis has been achieved. Then begin 5,000 international units subcutaneously once daily, allowing at least 6 hours between the initial post-operative dose and the second dose.

▶ **To decrease risk of thromboembolism in patients with severely restricted mobility during acute illness.** *Adults:* 5,000 international units subcutaneously daily for 12 to 14 days.

▶ **Unstable angina, non–ST-segment elevation MI.** *Adults:* 120 international units/kg up to 10,000 international units subcutaneously every 12 hours with oral aspirin (75 to 165 mg/day) therapy. Continue until patient is stable. Usual duration of treatment is 5 to 8 days.

◆ **NEW INDICATION: Symptomatic venous thromboembolism in cancer patients.** *Adults:* Initially, 200 international units/kg (maximum, 18,000 international units) subcutaneously daily for 30 days; then, 150 international units/kg (maximum, 18,000 international units) subcutaneously daily months 2 through 6.

◩ **Adjust-a-dose:** In patients with platelet count 50,000 to 100,000/mm³, reduce dose by 2,500 international units until platelet count exceeds 100,000/mm³. In patients with platelet count less than 50,000/mm³, discontinue drug until platelet count exceeds 50,000/mm³.

• For patients with creatinine clearance 30 ml/minute or less, monitor anti-Xa levels to determine the appropriate dose. Target anti-Xa range

---

is 0.5 to 1.5 international units/ml. Draw anti-Xa 4 to 6 hours after dose and only after the patient has received 3 to 4 doses.

Contraindications and cautions

• Contraindicated in patients hypersensitive to drug, heparin, or pork products, and in those with major bleeding or thrombocytopenia with positive in vitro tests for antiplatelet antibody in presence of drug.
• Use cautiously in patients with a history of heparin-induced thrombocytopenia; in patients with an increased risk of hemorrhage, such as those with severe uncontrolled hypertension, bacterial endocarditis, congenital or acquired bleeding disorders, active ulceration, angiodysplastic GI disease, or hemorrhagic stroke; and in those who recently underwent brain, spinal, or ophthalmologic surgery.
• Also use cautiously in patients with bleeding diathesis, thrombocytopenia, platelet defects, severe liver or kidney insufficiency, hypertensive or diabetic retinopathy, or recent GI bleeding.
Lifespan: In pregnant and breast-feeding women, use cautiously. In children, safety and effectiveness haven't been established.

Adverse reactions

CNS: fever.
Hematologic: bleeding complications, ***hemorrhage, thrombocytopenia.***
Skin: ecchymosis, pruritus, rash.
Other: ***anaphylaxis,*** *hematoma at injection site* (when given with heparin), pain at injection site.

Interactions

Drug-drug. *Antiplatelet drugs, oral anticoagulants:* May increase risk of bleeding. Use together cautiously; monitor patient for bleeding.

Effects on lab test results

• May increase ALT and AST levels.
• May decrease platelet count.

Pharmacokinetics

Absorption: Absolute bioavailability of anti-factor Xa is 87%.
Distribution: Volume is 40 to 60 ml/kg.
Metabolism: Unknown.
Excretion: In urine. *Half-life:* 3 to 5 hours.

Route	Onset	Peak	Duration
SubQ	Unknown	4 hr	Unknown

Action

Chemical effect: Enhances inhibition of factor Xa and thrombin by antithrombin.
Therapeutic effect: Prevents DVT.

Available forms

Multidose vial: 10,000 anti-factor Xa international units/ml, 25,000 anti-factor international units/ml
Syringe: 2,500 anti-factor Xa international units/0.2 ml; 5,000 anti-factor Xa international units/0.2 ml; 7,500 anti-factor Xa international units/0.3 ml; 10,000 anti-factor Xa international units/0.4 ml; 10,000 anti-factor Xa international units/1 ml; 12,500 anti-factor Xa international units/0.5 ml; 15,000 anti-factor Xa international units/0.6 ml; 18,000 anti-factor Xa international units/0.72 ml

NURSING PROCESS

Assessment
• Obtain history of patient's underlying condition before starting therapy.
• Those at risk for DVT include obese patients older than age 40 who are having surgery under general anesthesia that lasts longer than 30 minutes. Other risk factors include cancer and a history of DVT or pulmonary embolism.
• Monitor effectiveness by assessing patient for evidence of DVT.
• Perform routine CBCs (including platelet count) and fecal occult blood tests.
ALERT: Low–molecular-weight heparins used during neuraxial anesthesia or spinal puncture increase risk of epidural or spinal hematoma. Monitor patient closely for neurologic impairment.
• Look for adverse reactions and drug interactions.
• Assess patient's and family's knowledge of drug therapy.

Nursing diagnoses
• Risk for injury related to risk of DVT as result of underlying condition
• Ineffective protection related to drug-induced adverse hematologic reactions
• Deficient knowledge related to drug therapy

Planning and implementation
• Place patient in sitting or supine position when giving drug. Give by deep subcutaneous injection. Injection sites include U-shaped area below

navel, upper outer side of thigh, and upper outer quadrangle of buttock. Rotate sites daily.

⊛ **ALERT:** Drug should never be given I.M. or I.V.

• Don't mix with other injections or infusions unless specific compatibility data are available that support such mixing.

⊛ **ALERT:** Drug isn't interchangeable unit for unit with unfractionated heparin or other low–molecular-weight heparin derivatives.

• Stop drug and notify prescriber if a thrombo-embolism occurs despite therapy.

Patient teaching

• Instruct patient and family to immediately notify the prescriber if signs of bleeding occur.

• Tell patient to avoid OTC medications containing aspirin or other salicylates.

☑ **Evaluation**

• Patient doesn't develop DVT.

• Patient maintains stable hematologic function.

• Patient and family state understanding of drug therapy.

dantrolene sodium

(DAN-troh-leen SOH-dee-um)
Dantrium, Dantrium Intravenous

Pharmacologic class: hydantoin derivative
Therapeutic class: skeletal muscle relaxant
Pregnancy risk category: C

Indications and dosages

▶ **Spasticity and sequelae from severe chronic disorders (such as multiple sclerosis, cerebral palsy, spinal cord injury, stroke).** *Adults:* 25 mg P.O. daily. Increase in 25-mg increments up to 100 mg b.i.d. to q.i.d. Maximum, 400 mg daily. Maintain each dosage level for 4 to 7 days to determine response.
Children: Initially, 0.5 mg/kg P.O. b.i.d., increase to t.i.d. and then to q.i.d. Increase dosage as needed by 0.5 mg/kg daily to 3 mg/kg b.i.d. to q.i.d. Maximum, 100 mg q.i.d.

▶ **To manage malignant hyperthermic crisis.** *Adults and children:* 1 mg/kg I.V. initially, then repeat as needed up to a total dosage of 10 mg/kg.

▶ **To prevent or lessen malignant hyperthermia in susceptible patients who need surgery.** *Adults:* 4 to 8 mg/kg P.O. daily in three or four

divided doses for 1 or 2 days before procedure. Final dose 3 to 4 hours before procedure. Or 2.5 mg/kg I.V. infused over 1 hour about 1 hour before anesthesia. Additional doses, which must be individualized, may be given intraoperatively.

▶ **To prevent recurrence of malignant hyperthermia.** *Adults:* 4 to 8 mg/kg P.O. daily in four divided doses for up to 3 days after hyperthermic crisis.

▶ **To reduce succinylcholine-induced muscle fasciculations and postoperative muscle pain‡.** *Adults weighing less than 45 kg (99 lb):* 100 mg P.O. 2 hours before succinylcholine. *Adults weighing more than 45 kg:* 150 mg P.O. 2 hours before succinylcholine.

▽ I.V. administration

• Give as soon as malignant hyperthermia reaction is recognized.

• Reconstitute each vial with 60 ml of sterile water for injection, and shake vial until clear. Don't use diluent that contains bacteriostatic agent.

• Protect contents from light and use within 6 hours.

• Monitor patient for extravasation.

⊗ **Incompatibilities**
D_5W, normal saline solution, other I.V. drugs mixed in a syringe.

Contraindications and cautions

• Contraindicated in patients whose spasticity is used to maintain motor function and in patients with upper motor neuron disorders, spasms from rheumatic disorders, or active hepatic disease.

• Use cautiously in women, and in patients with hepatic disease or severely impaired cardiac or pulmonary function.

⚖ **Lifespan:** In pregnant women and patients older than age 35, use cautiously. In breastfeeding women, drug is contraindicated.

Adverse reactions

CNS: confusion, *dizziness, drowsiness,* fever, hallucinations, headache, insomnia, lightheadedness, *malaise,* nervousness, *seizures.*
CV: blood pressure changes, tachycardia.
EENT: auditory or visual disturbances, excessive tearing.
GI: anorexia, *bleeding,* constipation, cramping, drooling, dysphagia, metallic taste, severe diarrhea.

GU: crystalluria, difficulty achieving erection, dysuria, hematuria, incontinence, nocturia, urinary frequency.
Hepatic: *hepatitis.*
Musculoskeletal: *muscle weakness,* myalgia.
Respiratory: pleural effusion.
Skin: abnormal hair growth, diaphoresis, eczematous eruption, photosensitivity, pruritus, urticaria.
Other: chills.

Interactions

Drug-drug. *CNS depressants:* May increase CNS depression. Avoid use together.
Estrogens: May increase risk of hepatotoxicity. Use together cautiously.
I.V. verapamil: May cause CV collapse when used together in anesthetized patients. Manufacturer recommends stopping verapamil before giving I.V. dantrolene based on animal studies.
Drug-lifestyle. *Alcohol use:* May increase CNS depression. Avoid use together.
Sun exposure: Photosensitivity may occur. Urge patient to avoid prolonged and unprotected sun exposure.

Effects on lab test results

• May increase BUN, ALT, AST, and bilirubin levels.

Pharmacokinetics

Absorption: 35% of P.O. dose.
Distribution: Substantially protein-bound, mainly to albumin.
Metabolism: In liver to its less active 5-hydroxy derivatives and to its amino derivative by reductive pathways.
Excretion: In urine as metabolites. *Half-life:* P.O., 9 hours; I.V., 4 to 8 hours.

Route	Onset	Peak	Duration
P.O.	≤ 1 wk	5 hr	Unknown
I.V.	Unknown	Unknown	Unknown

Action

Chemical effect: Acts directly on skeletal muscle to interfere with intracellular calcium movement.
Therapeutic effect: Relieves muscle spasms.

Available forms

Capsules: 25 mg, 50 mg, 100 mg
Injection: 20 mg/vial

Assessment

• Obtain history of patient's disorder before therapy.
• Obtain liver function tests at start of therapy.
• Monitor effectiveness by evaluating severity of spasticity.
• Be alert for adverse reactions and drug interactions.
• Assess patient's and family's knowledge of drug therapy.

Nursing diagnoses

• Acute pain related to presence of spasticity
• Risk for injury related to drug-induced adverse reactions
• Deficient knowledge related to drug therapy

▶ Planning and implementation

• For optimum drug effect, divide daily dose into four doses.
• Give drug with meals or milk to prevent GI distress.
• Prepare oral suspension for each dose by dissolving capsule contents in juice or other suitable liquid. For multiple doses, use acid vehicle, such as citric acid in USP syrup. Refrigerate, and use within several days.
• Amount of relief determines whether dose can be reduced.
• If hepatitis, severe diarrhea, severe weakness, or sensitivity reaction occurs, don't give the drug, and immediately notify prescriber.
⑤ **ALERT:** Don't confuse Dantrium with Daraprim.
Patient teaching
• Tell patient to use caution when eating to avoid choking. Some patients may have trouble swallowing during therapy.
• Warn patient to avoid hazardous activities until the drug's full CNS effects are known.
• Advise patient to avoid combining dantrolene with alcohol or other CNS depressants.
• Tell patient to use sunblock and wear protective clothing, to report GI problems immediately, and to follow prescriber's orders regarding rest and physical therapy.

Evaluation

• Patient states that pain from muscle spasticity has lessened.

• Patient has no injury from drug-induced adverse reactions.
• Patient and family state understanding of drug therapy.

daptomycin
(dapp-toh-MY-sin)
Cubicin

Pharmacologic class: cyclic lipopeptide antibacterial
Therapeutic class: antibiotic
Pregnancy risk category: B

Indications and dosages

▶ **Complicated skin and skin-structure infections caused by susceptible strains of** *Staphylococcus aureus* **(including methicillin-resistant strains),** *Streptococcus pyogenes,* *Streptococcus agalactiae, Streptococcus dysgalactiae,* **and** *Enterococcus faecalis* **(vancomycin-susceptible strains only).** *Adults:* 4 mg/kg by I.V. infusion over 30 minutes every 24 hours for 7 to 14 days.

▶ **Bacteremia caused by** *S. aureus* **(including right-sided endocarditis caused by methicillin-susceptible and methicillin-resistant strains).** *Adults:* 6 mg/kg I.V. over 30 minutes every 24 hours for at least 2 to 6 weeks.

Adjust-a-dose: In patients with infections of skin or skin structure whose creatinine clearance is less than 30 ml/minute (including those receiving hemodialysis or continuous ambulatory peritoneal dialysis), give 4 mg/kg I.V. every 48 hours. For bacteremic patients with a clearance less than 30 ml/minute, give 6 mg/kg I.V. every 48 hours. When possible, give drug after hemodialysis.

I.V. administration

• Reconstitute 500-mg vial with 10 ml of normal saline solution. Further dilute admixture with normal saline solution. Vials are for single use. Discard excess.
• Compatible with normal saline solution and lactated Ringer's injection. Flush line also used for other drugs with compatible fluids.
• For intermittent infusion, give drug over 30 minutes.
• Refrigerate vials at 36° to 46° F (2° to 8° C). Reconstituted and diluted solutions are stable

12 hours at room temperature or 48 hours at 36° to 46° F.
⊗ **Incompatibilities**
Dextrose-containing solutions. Any other I.V. drugs and solutions.

Contraindications and cautions

• Contraindicated in patients hypersensitive to drug or any of its components.
• Use cautiously in those with renal insufficiency.
Lifespan: In pregnant women, use cautiously. In breast-feeding women, use cautiously because it's unknown if drug appears in breast milk. In children, safety and effectiveness haven't been established. In patients older than age 65, use cautiously because drug may be less effective and cause more adverse reactions.

Adverse reactions

CNS: anxiety, confusion, dizziness, fever, headache, insomnia.
CV: chest pain, edema, *heart failure,* hypertension, hypotension.
EENT: sore throat.
GI: abdominal pain, constipation, decreased appetite, diarrhea, nausea, *pseudomembranous colitis,* vomiting.
GU: *renal failure,* UTI.
Hematologic: anemia.
Metabolic: hyperglycemia, *hypoglycemia,* hypokalemia.
Musculoskeletal: limb and back pain.
Respiratory: cough, dyspnea.
Skin: cellulitis, pruritus, rash.
Other: fungal infections, injection site reactions.

Interactions

Drug-drug. *HMG-CoA reductase inhibitors:* May increase risk of myopathy. Consider stopping these drugs while giving daptomycin.
Tobramycin: May affect levels of both drugs. Use together cautiously.
Warfarin: May alter anticoagulant activity. Monitor PT and INR for the first several days of daptomycin therapy.

Effects on lab test results

• May increase CPK and alkaline phosphatase levels. May decrease potassium and hemoglobin levels and hematocrit. May increase or decrease glucose level.
• May increase liver function test values.

Pharmacokinetics

Absorption: Given I.V.
Distribution: 92% protein-bound, mainly to albumin.
Metabolism: Unknown.
Excretion: Mainly by kidneys. *Half-life:* About 8 hours.

Route	Onset	Peak	Duration
I.V.	Rapid	< 1 hr	Unknown

Action

Chemical effect: Binds to and depolarizes bacterial membranes to inhibit protein, DNA, and RNA synthesis.
Therapeutic effect: Kills bacteria in susceptible organisms.

Available forms

Powder for injection: 500-mg vial

NURSING PROCESS

✍ Assessment
• Monitor CBC and renal and liver function tests periodically.
• Monitor patient for superinfection because drug may cause overgrowth of nonsusceptible organisms.
• Watch for evidence of pseudomembranous colitis, and treat accordingly.
• Assess patient's and family's knowledge of drug therapy.

Nursing diagnoses
• Risk for infection related to bacteria
• Impaired urinary elimination related to daptomycin-induced renal impairment
• Deficient knowledge related to drug therapy

➤ Planning and implementation
• Obtain specimen for culture and sensitivity tests before giving the first dose. Begin therapy pending test results.
• **ALERT:** Because drug may increase the risk of myopathy, monitor CPK level weekly. If it rises, check it more often. Stop giving drug to a patient with evidence of myopathy and CPK level that exceeds 1,000 units/L. Also stop giving the drug to a patient with CPK level more than 10 times the upper limit of normal, even if he is asymptomatic of myopathy. Consider stopping

all other drugs linked with myopathy (such as HMG-CoA reductase inhibitors).
Patient teaching
• Advise patient to immediately report muscle weakness and infusion site irritation.
• Tell patient to report severe diarrhea, rash, and infection.
• Inform patient about adverse reactions.

✓ Evaluation
• Patient's infection is eradicated.
• Patient's renal function test values remain unchanged.
• Patient and family state understanding of drug therapy.

HIGH ALERT!

darbepoetin alfa
(dar-beh-POE-eh-tin AL-fah)
Aranesp

Pharmacologic class: hematopoietic
Therapeutic class: antianemic
Pregnancy risk category: C

Indications and dosages

• Give the lowest dose that will gradually increase hemoglobin to a level where blood transfusion isn't necessary.
▶ **Anemia from chronic renal failure.** *Adults:* 0.45 mcg/kg I.V. or subcutaneously once weekly. The I.V. route is preferred for patients undergoing dialysis. Adjust dosage so hemoglobin level doesn't exceed 12 g/dl. Don't increase dose more often than once a month.
Adults and children older than age 1 who are converting from epoetin alfa: Base starting dose on the previous epoetin alfa dose, as shown in the table.

Previous epoetin alfa dose (units/wk)	Darbepoetin alfa dose (mcg/wk)	
	Adults	**Children**
< 1,500	6.25	Unknown
1,500–2,499	6.25	6.25
2,500–4,999	12.5	10
5,000–10,999	25	20
11,000–17,999	40	40
18,000–33,999	60	60
34,000–89,999	100	100
≥ 90,000	200	200

Give darbepoetin alfa less often than epoetin alfa. If patient was receiving epoetin alfa two to three times weekly, give darbepoetin alfa once weekly. If patient was receiving epoetin alfa once weekly, give darbepoetin alfa once every 2 weeks.

☒ Adjust-a-dose: If increasing hemoglobin level approaches 12 g/dl, reduce dose by 25%. If level continues to increase, withhold dose until it begins to decrease; then restart drug at a dose 25% below the previous dose. If hemoglobin level increases more than 1 g/dl in 2 weeks, decrease dose by 25%. If it increases less than 1 g/dl over 4 weeks and iron stores are adequate, increase dose by 25% of previous dose. Make further increases at 4-week intervals until target hemoglobin level is reached. Patients who don't need dialysis may need lower maintenance doses.

▶ **Anemia from chemotherapy in patients with nonmyeloid malignancies.** *Adults:* 2.25 mcg/kg subcutaneously once weekly or 500 mcg subcutaneously once every 3 weeks.

☒ Adjust-a-dose: For either dosage schedule, adjust dose to keep hemoglobin level below 12 g/dl. If hemoglobin level exceeds 13 g/dl, hold drug until it drops to 12 g/dl; then resume at 40% of previous dose. If hemoglobin level increases more than 1 g/dl in 2 weeks or it exceeds 11 g/dl, reduce dose by 40%. If patient receives drug once weekly and hemoglobin level increases less than 1 g/dl in 6 weeks, increase dose to 4.5 mcg/kg.

▽ I.V. administration

• Don't shake drug because doing so can denature it.
• Drug is provided in single-dose vials without a preservative. Don't pool or retain unused portions.
• If drug has particulate matter or is discolored, don't use.
• Give undiluted by I.V. injection.
• Store drug in refrigerator; don't freeze. Protect drug from light.
⊗ **Incompatibilities**
Other I.V. drugs and solutions.

Contraindications and cautions

• Contraindicated in patients hypersensitive to drug or any of its components and in patients with uncontrolled hypertension.

• Use cautiously in patients with underlying hematologic disease, such as hemolytic anemia, sickle cell anemia, thalassemia, or porphyria, because safety and effectiveness haven't been established.
⚖ **Lifespan:** In pregnant women, safety and effectiveness haven't been established. In breastfeeding women, use cautiously because it's unknown whether drug appears in breast milk. In children with chronic renal failure, use as initial treatment to correct anemia hasn't been studied. Elderly patients may have greater sensitivity to the drug.

Adverse reactions

CNS: asthenia, dizziness, fatigue, fever, headache, *seizures, stroke, TIA.*
CV: *acute MI,* angina, CARDIAC ARREST, CARDIAC ARRHYTHMIA, chest pain, *edema,* fluid overload, *heart failure, hypertension, hypotension, thrombosis.*
GI: abdominal pain, constipation, diarrhea, nausea, vomiting.
Metabolic: dehydration.
Musculoskeletal: arthralgia, back pain, limb pain, myalgia.
Respiratory: bronchitis, cough, dyspnea, pneumonia, *pulmonary embolism,* upper respiratory tract infection.
Skin: *hemorrhage at access site,* pruritus, rash.
Other: flulike symptoms, *infection.*

Interactions

None reported.

Effects on lab test results

• May increase hemoglobin level and hematocrit. May decrease ferritin level.
• May increase RBC count.

Pharmacokinetics

Absorption: Slow and rate limiting. Bioavailability ranges from 30% to 50% (mean: 37%).
Distribution: Mostly to vascular space.
Metabolism: Unknown.
Excretion: Steady-state levels occur within 4 weeks. *Half-life:* 21 hours (I.V.); 49 hours (subcutaneous).

Route	Onset	Peak	Duration
I.V.	Unknown	Unknown	21 hr
SubQ	Unknown	34 hr	49 hr

Reactions may be *common,* uncommon, *life-threatening*, or COMMON AND LIFE-THREATENING.

Action

Chemical effect: Stimulates erythropoiesis the same way as endogenous erythropoietin produced by the kidneys. In a healthy patient, erythropoiesis increases the number of RBCs.
Therapeutic effect: Corrects anemia in patients with chronic renal failure.

Available forms

Injection (in albumin or polycarbonate solutions): 25 mcg/0.42 ml, 40 mcg/0.4 ml, 60 mcg/0.3 ml, 100 mcg/0.5 ml; 150 mcg/0.3 ml, 200 mcg/0.4 ml, 300 mcg/0.6 ml, 500 mcg/ml in single-dose syringes or auto injectors; 25 mcg/ml, 40 mcg/ml, 60 mcg/ml, 100 mcg/ml, 150 mcg/0.75 ml, 200 mcg/ml, 300 mcg/ml, 500 mcg/ml in single-dose vials

NURSING PROCESS

Assessment
• Drug may increase blood pressure. Blood pressure should be controlled before starting therapy. Obtain baseline blood pressure before therapy, and carefully monitor and control patient's blood pressure during therapy.
• Monitor renal function and electrolytes in predialysis patients.
ALERT: Hemoglobin level may not increase until 2 to 6 weeks after therapy starts. Monitor level weekly until stabilized. Don't exceed the target level of 12 g/dl in patients with chronic renal impairment.
• May increase the risk for serious cardiovascular events, including death when given to a target hemoglobin greater than 12 g/dl. Monitor hemoglobin level closely. Hemoglobin shouldn't exceed 12 g/dl and the rate of hemoglobin increase shouldn't exceed 1 g/dl in 2 weeks.
• Patient may have seizures. Follow patient closely, especially during the first several months of therapy.

Nursing diagnoses
• Risk for injury related to drug-induced adverse cardiac events
• Fatigue related to underlying anemia
• Deficient knowledge related to darbepoetin alfa therapy

Planning and implementation
ALERT: Hemoglobin levels of 12 g/dl or greater achieved with erythropoiesis-stimulating

agents are associated with increased risk of tumor growth and shortened survival in cancer patients, and serious CV events in patients with chronic kidney failure.
ALERT: If hemoglobin level increases 1 g/dl in any 2-week period, decrease dose. Any increase greater than 1 g/dl within a 2-week period will increase the risk of adverse CV reactions, such as seizures, stroke, exacerbation of hypertension, heart failure, acute MI, fluid overload, edema, or vascular thrombosis, infarction, or ischemia. If symptoms occur, decrease drug dose by 25%.
ALERT: If patient suddenly loses response to drug and has severe anemia and a low reticulocyte count, withhold drug and test patient for antierythropoietin antibodies. If they're present, stop treatment. Don't switch to another erythropoietic protein because a cross reaction is possible.
• Monitor iron level before and during therapy. If ferritin level is less than 100 mcg/L and transferrin saturation is less than 20%, provide supplemental iron.
• Serious allergic reactions, including rash and urticaria, may occur. If an anaphylactic reaction occurs, stop giving drug and provide appropriate therapy.
• The maximum safe dose isn't known. Although doses greater than 3 mcg/kg/week for up to 28 weeks can be given, an excessive rise or rate of rise of hemoglobin level leads to adverse reactions. If patient has polycythemia, don't give drug.
• If patient doesn't respond to therapy, reevaluate patient for other etiologies that may inhibit erythropoiesis, such as folic acid or vitamin B_{12} deficiencies, infections, inflammatory or malignant processes, osteofibrosis cystica, occult blood loss, hemolysis, severe aluminum toxicity, and bone marrow fibrosis.
Patient teaching
• Teach patient how to give drug properly, including how to use and dispose of needles.
• Advise patient of adverse effects and allergic reactions.
• Inform patient of need to frequently monitor blood pressure, hemoglobin level, and hematocrit. Advise him to comply with antihypertensive therapy and dietary restrictions to keep blood pressure under control. Uncontrolled blood pressure is believed to cause seizures and hypertensive encephalopathy in patients with chronic renal impairment.

☑ Evaluation

- Patient's hemoglobin level increases to no more than 12 g/dl.
- Patient's blood pressure remains adequately controlled, and patient doesn't suffer any adverse reactions related to drug therapy.
- Patient and family state understanding of drug therapy.

darifenacin
(dayr-ee-FEN-uh-sin)
Enablex⟁

Pharmacologic class: muscarinic receptor antagonist
Therapeutic class: anticholinergic
Pregnancy risk category: C

Indications and dosages

▶ **Symptoms of urge incontinence, urgency, and frequency from an overactive urinary bladder.** *Adults:* Initially, 7.5 mg P.O. once daily. If needed, may increase to 15 mg P.O. once daily after 2 weeks.
🔲 **Adjust-a-dose:** If patient has moderate hepatic impairment (Child-Pugh class B) or takes a potent CYP3A4 inhibitor (such as clarithromycin, itraconazole, ketoconazole, nefazodone, nelfinavir, or ritonavir), don't exceed 7.5 mg P.O. once daily.

Contraindications and cautions

- Contraindicated in patients hypersensitive to drug or its ingredients. Also contraindicated in patients with or at risk for urine retention, gastric retention, or uncontrolled narrow-angle glaucoma. Avoid use in patients with severe hepatic impairment (Child-Pugh C).
- Use cautiously in patients with bladder outflow obstruction, decreased GI motility, GI obstruction, ulcerative colitis, myasthenia gravis, severe constipation, controlled narrow-angle glaucoma, or moderate hepatic impairment (Child-Pugh B).
🔥 **Lifespan:** In pregnant women, use only if benefit to mother outweighs risk to fetus. In breast-feeding women, use cautiously; it isn't known if drug appears in breast milk. In children, safety and effectiveness haven't been established.

Adverse reactions

CNS: asthenia, dizziness.
CV: hypertension.
EENT: abnormal vision, dry eyes, pharyngitis, rhinitis, sinusitis.
GI: abdominal pain, *constipation,* diarrhea, *dry mouth,* dyspepsia, nausea, vomiting.
GU: urinary tract disorder, UTI, vaginitis.
Metabolic: weight gain.
Musculoskeletal: arthralgia, back pain.
Respiratory: bronchitis.
Skin: dry skin, pruritus, rash.
Other: accidental injury, flulike symptoms, pain, peripheral edema.

Interactions

Drug-drug. *Anticholinergics:* May increase anticholinergic effects, such as dry mouth, blurred vision, and constipation. Monitor patient closely.
Digoxin: May increase digoxin level. Monitor digoxin level.
Drugs metabolized by CYP2D6 (such as flecainide, thioridazine, tricyclic antidepressants): May increase levels of these drugs. Use together cautiously.
Drugs that are potent CYP3A4 inhibitors (such as clarithromycin, itraconazole, ketoconazole, nefazodone, nelfinavir, ritonavir): May increase darifenacin levels. Maximum darifenacin dose is 7.5 mg P.O. daily.
Midazolam: May increase midazolam level. Monitor patient carefully.
Drug-lifestyle. *Hot weather:* May cause heat prostration from decreased sweating. Advise caution.

Effects on lab test results

None reported.

Pharmacokinetics

Absorption: Level peaks 7 hours after multiple doses.
Distribution: 98% bound to plasma proteins, mainly to alpha$_1$-acid glycoprotein.
Metabolism: Extensive, in liver (CYP2D6, CYP3A4).
Excretion: 60% in urine, 40% in feces; 3% unchanged. *Half-life:* 13 to 19 hours.

Route	Onset	Peak	Duration
P.O.	Unknown	7 hr	Unknown

Action

Chemical effect: Antagonizes muscarinic (M3) receptors, increasing bladder capacity and decreasing unstable detrusor contractions.
Therapeutic effect: Relieves symptoms of overactive bladder.

Available forms

Tablets (extended-release): 7.5 mg, 15 mg

NURSING PROCESS

Assessment
• Assess bladder function before therapy starts.
• Monitor drug effects.
• If patient has bladder outlet obstruction, watch for urine retention.
• Assess patient for decreased gastric motility and constipation.
• Assess patient's and family's knowledge of drug therapy.

Nursing diagnoses
• Impaired urinary elimination related to underlying medical condition
• Risk for injury related to drug-induced adverse effects
• Deficient knowledge related to drug therapy

Planning and implementation
• If patient has a UTI, give antibiotics.
• Reduce GI distress by giving drug with food.
• If patient develops urine retention, notify physician and prepare for urinary catheterization.
Patient teaching
• Tell patient to swallow tablet whole with plenty of liquid; caution against crushing or chewing the tablets.
• Inform patient that drug may be taken with or without food.
• Explain that drug may cause blurred vision. Tell patient to use caution, especially when performing hazardous tasks, until drug effects are known.
• Tell patient to report blurred vision, constipation, and urine retention.
• Discourage use of other drugs that may cause dry mouth, constipation, urine retention, or blurred vision.
• Tell patient that drug decreases sweating. Advise caution in hot environments and during strenuous activity.

Evaluation
• Patient experiences improved bladder function with drug therapy.
• Patient sustains no injuries from drug-induced effects.
• Patient and family state understanding of drug therapy.

darunavir ethanolate
(duh-ROO-nah-veer eh-THAH-nuh-layt)
Prezista

Pharmacologic class: protease inhibitor
Therapeutic class: antiretroviral
Pregnancy risk category: B

Indications and dosages

▶ **HIV infection in antiretroviral treatment–experienced patients, with ritonavir and other antiretrovirals.** *Adults:* 600 mg P.O. b.i.d., given with ritonavir 100 mg P.O. b.i.d. and food.

Contraindications and cautions

• Contraindicated in patients hypersensitive to drug or its components and in patient taking drugs metabolized by CYP3A, such as astemizole, dihydroergotamine, ergonovine, ergotamine, methylergonovine, midazolam, pimozide, terfenadine, and triazolam.
• Use cautiously in patients with liver or renal impairment, diabetes mellitus, hemophilia, sulfonamide allergy, or a history of opportunistic infections.
Lifespan: In pregnant women, use only if potential benefits to mother justify risk to fetus. HIV-infected mothers shouldn't breast-feed to avoid transmitting HIV to their infants. In children, safety and efficacy haven't been established. In elderly patients, use cautiously because these patients are more likely to have decreased hepatic function.

Adverse reactions

CNS: altered mood, anxiety, asthenia, confusion, disorientation, fatigue, *headache,* hypoesthesia, irritability, memory impairment, nightmares, paresthesia, peripheral neuropathy, somnolence, transient ischemic attack, vertigo.
CV: hypertension, *MI,* tachycardia.
EENT: *nasopharyngitis.*

GI: abdominal distension, abdominal pain, anorexia, constipation, *diarrhea,* dry mouth, dyspepsia, flatulence, *nausea,* polydipsia, vomiting.
GU: *acute renal failure,* renal insufficiency, nephrolithiasis, polyuria.
Hematologic: LEUKOPENIA, *neutropenia, thrombocytopenia.*
Metabolic: decreased appetite, diabetes mellitus, hypercholesterolemia, hyperlipidemia, hypernatremia, hyperuricemia, hyponatremia, obesity.
Musculoskeletal: arthralgia, limb pain, myalgia, osteopenia, osteoporosis.
Respiratory: cough, dyspnea, hiccups.
Skin: allergic dermatitis, alopecia, dermatitis medicamentosa, eczema, *erythema multiforme,* folliculitis, increased sweating, inflammation, lipoatrophy, maculopapular rash, night sweats, *Stevens-Johnson syndrome,* toxic skin eruption.
Other: fat redistribution, gynecomastia, hyperthermia, peripheral edema, pyrexia, rigors.

Interactions

Drug-drug. *Amiodarone, bepridil, cyclosporine, felodipine, fluticasone, lidocaine, nicardipine, nifedipine, quinidine, rifabutin, sildenafil, sirolimus, tacrolimus, tadalafil, trazodone, vardenafil:* May increase levels of these drugs and risk of adverse reactions. Use caution, and monitor patient carefully.
Astemizole, cisapride, ergot derivatives, midazolam, pimozide, terfenadine, triazolam: May cause serious or life-threatening reactions. Use together is contraindicated.
Atorvastatin, pravastatin: May increase levels of these drugs. Start at the lowest dose, and monitor patient carefully.
Clarithromycin: May increase clarithromycin level. Reduce clarithromycin dose in patients with renal impairment.
CYP3A inducers (carbamazepine, dexamethasone, phenobarbital, phenytoin, rifabutin, rifampin), efavirenz, lopinavir, saquinavir: May increase darunavir clearance and decrease darunavir level. Avoid use together.
Ethinyl estradiol, norethindrone: May decrease estrogen level. Recommend alternative or additional contraception.
Itraconazole, ketoconazole: May increase levels of these drugs and darunavir. Don't exceed 200 mg of itraconazole or ketoconazole daily.

Lovastatin, simvastatin: May increase risk of myopathy, including rhabdomyolysis. Use caution.
Methadone: May decrease methadone level. Monitor patient for opioid abstinence syndrome, and consider increasing methadone dosage.
Rifabutin: May decrease darunavir level. If used together, give rifabutin as 150 mg every other day.
SSRIs (paroxetine, sertraline): May decrease levels of these drugs. Adjust dosage carefully based on antidepressant response.
Trazodone: May increase trazodone level and risk of toxicity. Decrease trazodone dosage.
Warfarin: May decrease warfarin level. Monitor patient carefully.
Drug-food. *Food:* Increases darunavir absorption, which is needed for adequate therapeutic effect. Always give with food.
Drug-herb. *St. John's wort:* May decrease darunavir level significantly. Discourage use together.

Effects on lab test results

● May increase AST, ALT, GGT, alkaline phosphatase, bilirubin, pancreatic amylase, pancreatic lipase, cholesterol, triglyceride, and uric acid levels. May decrease albumin, bicarbonate, and calcium levels. May increase or decrease sodium and glucose levels.
● May decrease WBC, neutrophil, lymphocyte, and platelet counts.

Pharmacokinetics

Absorption: Greater when taken with ritonavir and food.
Distribution: About 95% bound to plasma proteins.
Metabolism: Metabolized extensively in the liver by CYP3A.
Excretion: Mainly in feces, with a small amount in urine. *Half-life:* About 15 hours when combined with ritonavir.

Route	Onset	Peak	Duration
P.O.	Unknown	2½–4 hr	Unknown

Action

Chemical effect: Drug binds to the protease-active site and selectively inhibits enzyme activity. This inhibition prevents cleavage of viral

polyproteins, resulting in the formation of immature noninfectious viral particles.
Therapeutic effect: Treats HIV infection.

Available forms

Tablets: 300 mg

NURSING PROCESS

⚖ Assessment

• Assess patient for appropriateness of drug therapy.
• Because drug may interact with other drugs, obtain patient's complete drug history.
• Monitor patient for diarrhea, nausea, headache, and signs and symptoms of a common cold. If patient develops a rash, report it to prescriber.
• Find out whether patient is pregnant or plans to become pregnant.
• Assess patient's and family's knowledge about drug therapy.

⊕ Nursing diagnoses

• Risk for infection secondary to presence of HIV
• Ineffective coping related to HIV infection
• Deficient knowledge related to drug therapy

❯ Planning and implementation

• Always give drug with ritonavir and food.
• Drug may cause spontaneous bleeding in some patients with hemophilia. Monitor patient closely.
• Patients with hepatic impairment, diabetes mellitus, sulfonamide allergy, or hemophilia must be monitored closely while taking this drug.
• To monitor maternal-fetal outcome of a pregnant woman exposed to this drug, the prescriber is encouraged to register woman in the Antiretroviral Pregnancy Registry by calling 1-800-258-4263.

Patient teaching

• Explain that many drugs interact with darunavir; advise patient to report all drugs he takes, including OTC products.
• ⊕ **ALERT:** Instruct patient to take darunavir and ritonavir at the same time every day, with food.
• Advise patient to swallow the tablet whole and not to chew it.
• Tell patient that darunavir doesn't cure HIV infection or AIDS and doesn't reduce the risk of passing HIV to others.
• Explain that opportunistic infections and other complications of HIV infection may still develop.

• If patient misses a dose by more than 6 hours, tell him to wait and take the next dose at the regularly scheduled time. If he remembers within 6 hours, tell him to take the missed dose immediately.

☑ Evaluation

• Patient has reduced signs and symptoms of infection.
• Patient demonstrates adequate coping mechanisms.
• Patient and family state understanding of drug therapy.

dasatinib
(duh-SAH-tih-nib)
Sprycel⬦

Pharmacologic class: protein-tyrosine kinase inhibitor
Therapeutic class: antineoplastic
Pregnancy risk category: D

Indications and dosages

❯ **Accelerated, myeloid, or lymphoid blast phase of chronic myeloid leukemia with resistance or intolerance to earlier treatment, including imatinib; Philadelphia chromosome–positive acute lymphoblastic leukemia with resistance or tolerance to previous therapy.** *Adults:* 70 mg P.O. b.i.d. in the morning and evening with or without food. If patient tolerates this dose but fails to respond, may increase to 90 or 100 mg b.i.d. Continue until disease progresses or intolerable adverse effects occur.

❯ **Chronic phase of chronic myeloid leukemia with resistance or intolerance to earlier treatment, including imatinib.** *Adults:* 100 mg P.O. daily. May increase to 140 mg daily.
▨ **Adjust-a-dose:** If patient has hematologic toxicity, consider reducing dose or interrupting or stopping therapy. If patient has severe, nonhematologic toxicity, hold dose until condition resolves; then resume at previous or reduced dose.

Contraindications and cautions

• No known contraindications.
• Use cautiously in patients receiving antiarrhythmics, antiplatelets, or anticoagulants; pa-

tients receiving cumulative high-dose anthracycline therapy; patients with a prolonged QT interval or risk of prolonged QT interval (those with hypokalemia, hypomagnesemia, or current use of drugs that prolong the QT interval); patients with liver impairment; and patients who are lactose intolerant.

⚠ **Lifespan:** In pregnant women, drug may cause fetal harm. Mothers shouldn't breast-feed during treatment. In children, safety and efficacy haven't been established. Elderly patients may be more sensitive to drug's effects.

Adverse reactions

CNS: anxiety, *asthenia*, **bleeding**, *chills*, confusion, depression, *dizziness, fatigue, headache,* insomnia, malaise, *neuropathy,* **pyrexia, seizures,** somnolence, syncope, tremor, vertigo.
CV: arrhythmias, cardiac dysfunction, *chest pain,* edema, **heart failure, hemorrhage,** hypertension, hypotension, pericardial effusion.
EENT: conjunctivitis, dry eyes, dysgeusia, *mucositis, stomatitis,* tinnitus.
GI: *abdominal distention and pain, anorexia,* anal fissure, **bleeding,** colitis, *constipation, diarrhea,* dyspepsia, dysphagia, *nausea, vomiting.*
GU: renal failure, urinary frequency.
Hematologic: anemia, *febrile neutropenia,* **pancytopenia, thrombocytopenia.**
Hepatic: cholecystitis, cholestasis, **hepatitis.**
Metabolic: hyperuricemia, *weight loss or gain.*
Musculoskeletal: arthralgia, inflammation, *myalgia,* muscle stiffness, *pain.*
Respiratory: asthma, *cough, dyspnea, pleural effusion, pneumonia,* **pulmonary edema** and *hypertension, upper respiratory tract infection.*
Skin: acne, alopecia, dry skin, nail or pigment disorders, *pruritus, rash,* sweating.
Other: ascites, gynecomastia, herpes infection, *infection,* **tumor lysis syndrome.**

Interactions

Drug-drug. *Antacids:* May decrease dasatinib absorption. Give antacid 2 hours before or 2 hours after dasatinib.
CYP3A4 inducers (carbamazepine, dexamethasone, phenobarbital, phenytoin, rifampicin): May decrease dasatinib level. Avoid use together, or increase dasatinib dose in 20-mg increments.
CYP3A4 inhibitors (atazanavir, clarithromycin, erythromycin, indinavir, itraconazole, ketoconazole, nefazodone, nelfinavir, ritonavir,

saquinavir, telithromycin): May increase dasatinib level and toxicity. Avoid use together; if it can't be avoided, monitor patient closely. Dasatinib dose may be decreased 20 to 40 mg daily.
CYP3A4 substrates (cyclosporine, ergot alkaloids, fentanyl, pimozide, quinidine, sirolimus, tacrolimus): May alter levels of these drugs. Use cautiously together, and monitor patient.
H₂-blockers, proton pump inhibitors: May decrease dasatinib level because of gastric acid suppression. Avoid use together. Consider antacids as an alternative.
Drug-herb. *St. John's wort:* May decrease dasatinib level. Discourage use together.

Effects on lab test results

● May increase uric acid, bilirubin, creatinine, AST, ALT, CPK, and troponin levels. May decrease phosphate and calcium levels.
● May decrease RBC, platelet, and neutrophil counts.

Pharmacokinetics

Absorption: Well absorbed. Absorption is pH dependent.
Distribution: 96% protein-bound.
Metabolism: Mainly by CYP3A4.
Excretion: Mainly in feces as metabolites.
Half-life: 3 to 5 hours.

Route	Onset	Peak	Duration
P.O.	Unknown	½–6 hr	Unknown

Action

Chemical effect: Reduces leukemic cell growth by inhibiting tyrosine kinase BRC-ABL.
Therapeutic effect: Helps bone marrow to resume production of normal red cells, white cells, and platelets.

Available forms

Tablets: 20 mg, 50 mg, 70 mg

NURSING PROCESS

▧ Assessment
● Ask patient if he is lactose intolerant because drug contains lactose.
● Monitor CBC weekly for the first 2 months of treatment, then monthly thereafter, or as clinically indicated.

D

• If patient develops dyspnea or a dry cough, notify prescriber. Obtain a chest X-ray and give oxygen, diuretics, and steroids, as indicated.
• Monitor patient for easy bruising or bleeding, and report it to the prescriber.
• Assess patient's and family's knowledge of drug therapy.

🔆 Nursing diagnoses
• Ineffective breathing pattern related to pulmonary edema and fluid retention
• Risk for infection related to drug's adverse reaction
• Deficient knowledge related to drug therapy

▶ Planning and implementation
🔆 ALERT: Don't crush or cut tablets. If tablet is crushed or broken, wear chemotherapy gloves to dispose of it. Pregnant women shouldn't handle broken tablets.
• Obtain patient's baseline weight, and check regularly for swelling or weight gain.
• Correct electrolyte imbalances, especially of potassium and magnesium, before treatment.
Patient teaching
• Tell patient to take tablets at about the same time each day.
• Caution patient not to crush or cut the tablets.
• Warn women of childbearing potential to use reliable contraception during treatment. A man who takes this drug should use condoms to avoid impregnating his partner.
• Tell patient to report weight gain, swelling, and shortness of breath.
• Advise patient to notify prescriber immediately about easy or unusual bruising.

✅ Evaluation
• Patient maintains adequate respiratory function.
• Patient is free from infection.
• Patient and family state understanding of drug therapy.

HIGH ALERT!

daunorubicin citrate liposomal
(daw-noh-ROO-buh-sin SIH-trayt li-poh-SOE-mul)
DaunoXome

Pharmacologic class: anthracycline
Therapeutic class: antineoplastic
Pregnancy risk category: D

Indications and dosages
▶ **First-line cytotoxic therapy for advanced HIV-related Kaposi sarcoma.** *Adults:* 40 mg/m² I.V. over 60 minutes once every 2 weeks. Continue therapy unless patient shows signs of progressive disease or until drug has to be stopped from other complications of HIV.
🔆 **Adjust-a-dose:** For patients with renal or hepatic impairment, if bilirubin is 1.2 to 3 mg/dl, give ¾ of normal dose; if bilirubin or creatinine level is greater than 3 mg/dl, give ½ of normal dose.

▼ I.V. administration
• Preparing and giving drug raises carcinogenic, mutagenic, and teratogenic risks. Follow facility policy to reduce risks.
• Dilute drug with D_5W only. Withdraw the calculated volume of drug from the vial, and transfer it into an equivalent amount of D_5W to yield 1 mg/ml.
• After dilution, immediately give I.V. over 60 minutes. If unable to use drug immediately, refrigerate at 36° to 46° F (2° to 8° C) for a maximum of 6 hours.
• Don't use in-line filters for I.V. infusion.
• Because local tissue necrosis may occur, monitor I.V. site closely to avoid extravasation. If extravasation occurs, stop I.V., apply ice, and notify prescriber.
• Monitor patient for adverse reactions. A triad of back pain, flushing, and chest tightness may occur within the first 5 minutes of the infusion. These symptoms subside after stopping the infusion and typically don't recur when the infusion resumes at a slower rate.
• Follow facility policy for handling and disposing of antineoplastics.
⊗ **Incompatibilities**
Bacteriostatic agents, other I.V. drugs, saline and other solutions.

Contraindications and cautions
• Contraindicated in patients hypersensitive to drug or any of its components.
• Use cautiously in patients with myelosuppression, cardiac disease, previous radiotherapy involving the heart, previous anthracycline use (doxorubicin greater than 300 mg/m² or equivalent), or hepatic or renal impairment.
🔆 **Lifespan:** In pregnant women, avoid use because the drug may harm the fetus. In children

---

and the elderly, safety and effectiveness haven't been established.

Adverse reactions

CNS: abnormal gait, abnormal thinking, amnesia, anxiety, ataxia, confusion, depression, dizziness, emotional lability, *fatigue, fever,* hallucinations, *headache,* hyperkinesia, hypertonia, insomnia, malaise, meningitis, *neuropathy, seizures,* somnolence, syncope, tremor.
CV: angina pectoris, *arrhythmias, cardiac arrest, cardiac tamponade, cardiomyopathy,* chest pain, edema, flushing, hypertension, *MI,* palpitations, *pericardial effusion, pulmonary hypertension,* tachycardia.
EENT: abnormal vision, conjunctivitis, deafness, dry mouth, earache, eye pain, gingival bleeding, *rhinitis,* sinusitis, taste disturbance, tinnitus, tooth caries.
GI: *abdominal pain, anorexia,* constipation, *diarrhea,* dysphagia, gastritis, *hemorrhage,* hemorrhoids, increased appetite, melena, *nausea,* stomatitis, tenesmus, vomiting.
GU: dysuria, nocturia, polyuria.
Hematologic: NEUTROPENIA, splenomegaly.
Hepatic: hepatomegaly.
Metabolic: dehydration.
Musculoskeletal: arthralgia, *back pain,* myalgia, *rigors.*
Respiratory: *cough, dyspnea,* hemoptysis, hiccups, increased sputum, pulmonary infiltration.
Skin: alopecia, dry skin, folliculitis, increased sweating, pruritus, seborrhea.
Other: *allergic reactions,* flulike symptoms, injection site inflammation, lymphadenopathy, *opportunistic infections,* thirst.

Interactions

None reported.

Effect on lab test results

• May decrease neutrophil and platelet counts.

Pharmacokinetics

Absorption: Given I.V.
Distribution: Probably mainly in vascular fluid volume.
Metabolism: By the liver into active metabolites.
Excretion: Unknown. *Half-life:* 4½ hours.

Route	Onset	Peak	Duration
I.V.	Unknown	Unknown	Unknown

Action

Chemical effect: Exerts cytotoxic effects by intercalating between DNA base pairs and uncoiling the DNA helix. This inhibits DNA synthesis and DNA-dependent RNA synthesis. Also inhibits polymerase activity. The liposomal preparation maximizes the selectivity of daunorubicin for solid tumors in situ.
Therapeutic effect: Decreases tumor growth for advanced HIV-related Kaposi sarcoma.

Available forms

Injection: 2 mg/ml (equivalent to 50 mg daunorubicin base)

NURSING PROCESS

Assessment
• Obtain history of patient's underlying condition before therapy, and reassess regularly thereafter.
• Obtain hepatic and renal studies before therapy.
• Monitor cardiac function regularly, especially immediately before giving a dose, because of the risk of cardiac toxicity and heart failure. Determine left ventricular ejection fraction at a total cumulative dose of 320 mg/m^2 and every 160 mg/m^2 thereafter.
• Monitor patient closely for signs of opportunistic infections.
• Be alert for adverse reactions and drug interactions.
• Assess patient's and family's knowledge of drug therapy.

Nursing diagnoses
• Risk for injury related to drug-induced adverse reactions
• Risk for infection related to myelosuppression
• Deficient knowledge related to drug therapy

Planning and implementation
• Drug causes less nausea, vomiting, alopecia, neutropenia, thrombocytopenia, and potentially less cardiotoxicity than conventional daunorubicin.
• Give only under the supervision of a prescriber specializing in cancer chemotherapy.

Reactions may be *common,* uncommon, *life-threatening,* or COMMON AND LIFE-THREATENING.

• Monitor hematology closely because severe myelosuppression may occur. Obtain and check blood counts before each dose. If absolute granulocyte count is less than 750 cells/mm³, withhold drug.

⊛ **ALERT:** Drug has unique kinetic properties that are different from the conventional daunorubicin hydrochloride. Don't substitute or interchange the drugs on a milligram-to-milligram basis.

Patient teaching
• Inform patient that alopecia may occur, but that it's usually reversible.
• Tell patient to notify prescriber about sore throat, fever, or other signs of infection. Tell patient to avoid exposure to people with infections.
• Advise patient to report suspected or known pregnancy during therapy.
• Tell patient to report back pain, flushing, and chest tightness during the infusion.

☑ Evaluation
• Patient has no injury as a result of drug-induced adverse reactions.
• Patient remains free of infection.
• Patient and family state understanding of drug therapy.

HIGH ALERT!

daunorubicin hydrochloride
(daw-noh-ROO-buh-sin hy-droh-KLOR-ighd)
Cerubidine

Pharmacologic class: anthracycline antineoplastic
Therapeutic class: antineoplastic
Pregnancy risk category: D

Indications and dosages

▶ **To induce remission in acute nonlymphocytic (myelogenous, monocytic, erythroid) leukemia.** *Adults younger than age 60:* When given with other drugs, 45 mg/m² I.V. daily on days 1, 2, and 3 of first course and on days 1 and 2 of subsequent courses with cytarabine infusions.
Adults age 60 or older: When given with other drugs, 30 mg/m² I.V. daily on days 1, 2, and 3 of first course and on days 1 and 2 of subsequent courses with cytarabine infusions.
▶ **To induce remission in acute lymphocytic leukemia.** *Adults:* 45 mg/m² I.V. daily on days

1, 2, and 3 of courses containing vincristine, prednisone, and L-asparaginase.
Children age 2 and older: 25 mg/m² I.V. on day 1 every week for up to 6 weeks, if needed. Give with courses containing vincristine and prednisone.
Children younger than age 2 or with body surface area smaller than 0.5 m²: Calculate dose based on body weight (1 mg/kg).
⬛ **Adjust-a-dose:** For patients with impaired hepatic or renal function, reduce dosage as follows: If bilirubin level is 1.2 to 3 mg/dl, give 75% of normal dose; if bilirubin or creatinine level exceeds 3 mg/dl, give 50% of the normal dose.

▼ I.V. administration

• Preparing and giving drug raises carcinogenic, mutagenic, and teratogenic risks. Follow institutional policy to reduce risks.
• Reconstitute drug using 4 ml of sterile water for injection to produce a 5-mg/ml solution.
• Withdraw desired dose into syringe containing 10 to 15 ml of normal saline solution for injection. Over 2 to 3 minutes, inject into I.V. line containing free-flowing D₅W or normal saline solution.
• Monitor I.V. site for extravasation. If it occurs, stop I.V. injection immediately, notify prescriber, and apply ice to area for 24 to 48 hours.
• Don't inject with dexamethasone or heparin because a precipitate may form.
• Reconstituted undiluted solution is stable 24 hours at room temperature, 48 hours if refrigerated.
⊗ **Incompatibilities**
Other I.V. drugs.

Contraindications and cautions

• Use cautiously in patients with myelosuppression and in those with impaired cardiac, renal, or hepatic function.
⚖ **Lifespan:** In pregnant women, avoid use because of potential fetal abnormality or death. Women of childbearing age should avoid becoming pregnant while on drug. Males being treated have increased risk of fertility impairment. Breast-feeding isn't recommended during therapy because of possible increased risk of breast tumors. In children and the elderly, cardiotoxicity may be more frequent and occur at lower cumulative doses.

Adverse reactions

CNS: fever.
CV: *arrhythmias,* ECG changes, *irreversible cardiomyopathy,* myocarditis, *pericarditis.*
GI: anorexia, diarrhea, esophagitis, nausea, stomatitis, vomiting.
GU: red urine.
Hematologic: *bone marrow suppression.*
Hepatic: *hepatotoxicity.*
Metabolic: hyperuricemia.
Skin: *generalized alopecia,* pigmentation of fingernails and toenails, rash, *tissue sloughing with extravasation.*
Other: *anaphylaxis,* chills, severe cellulitis.

Interactions

Drug-drug. *Bone marrow suppressants:* May increase risk of myelosuppression. Monitor patient closely.
Cyclophosphamide: May increase risk of cardiotoxicity. Monitor patient closely.
Doxorubicin: May increase risk of cardiotoxicity. Monitor patient closely.
Hepatotoxic drugs: May increase risk of hepatotoxicity. Monitor hepatic function closely.

Effect on lab test results

• May increase uric acid level.

Pharmacokinetics

Absorption: Given I.V. only.
Distribution: Wide. Drug doesn't cross blood–brain barrier.
Metabolism: Extensive. One of metabolites has cytotoxic activity.
Excretion: Mainly in bile, with small portion in urine. *Half-life:* Initial, 45 minutes; terminal, 18½ hours.

Route	Onset	Peak	Duration
I.V.	Unknown	Unknown	Unknown

Action

Chemical effect: May interfere with DNA-dependent RNA synthesis by intercalation.
Therapeutic effect: Kills selected cancer cells.

Available forms

Injection: 20 mg/vial, 50 mg/vial

NURSING PROCESS

Assessment

• Obtain history of patient's underlying disease before therapy, and reassess regularly throughout therapy.
• Check ECG before therapy.
• Monitor CBC and liver function tests; monitor ECG every month (or more frequently if needed) during therapy.
• Monitor pulse rate closely.
• Look for adverse reactions and drug interactions.
• Monitor patient for nausea and vomiting, which may be severe and may last 24 to 48 hours. Monitor patient's hydration during episodes of nausea and vomiting.
• Assess patient's and family's knowledge of drug therapy.

Nursing diagnoses

• Risk for injury related to presence of neoplastic disease
• Risk for deficient fluid volume related to drug-induced nausea and vomiting
• Deficient knowledge related to drug therapy

Planning and implementation

ALERT: Never give drug by I.M. or subcutaneous route.
• Limit cumulative dose to 400 to 550 mg/m² (400 mg/m² if patient receives or has received cyclophosphamide or radiation therapy to cardiac area).
ALERT: Color is similar to that of doxorubicin. Don't confuse these two drugs.
• If signs of heart failure or cardiomyopathy develop, stop giving the drug and immediately notify the prescriber.
ALERT: The risk of myocardial toxicity increases after a total cumulative dose higher than 400 to 550 mg/m² in adults, 300 mg/m² in children older than age 2, and 10 mg/kg in children younger than age 2.
• Give antiemetics to help control nausea and vomiting.
Patient teaching
• Warn patient to watch for signs of infection and bleeding.
• Advise patient that red urine for 1 to 2 days is normal and doesn't indicate blood in urine.
• Inform patient that alopecia may occur, but that it's usually reversible.

Reactions may be *common,* uncommon, *life-threatening,* or COMMON AND LIFE-THREATENING.

• Advise women of childbearing age to avoid becoming pregnant during therapy.
• Instruct patient about need for protective measures, including conservation of energy, balanced diet, adequate rest, personal hygiene, clean environment, and avoidance of people with infections.

☑ **Evaluation**
• Patient shows positive response to therapy as shown by reports of follow-up diagnostic tests and improved physical condition.
• Patient maintains adequate hydration throughout therapy.
• Patient and family state understanding of drug therapy.

delavirdine mesylate
(deh-luh-VEER-deen MES-ih-layt)
Rescriptor

Pharmacologic class: nonnucleoside reverse transcriptase inhibitor
Therapeutic class: antiretroviral
Pregnancy risk category: C

Indications and dosages

▶ **HIV-1 infection.** *Adults:* 400 mg P.O. t.i.d. with other appropriate antiretrovirals.

Contraindications and cautions

• Contraindicated in patients hypersensitive to drug or any of its components.
• Use cautiously in patients with impaired hepatic function.
⚠ **Lifespan:** In pregnant women, use only if potential benefits to the woman outweigh risks to the fetus. Breast-feeding women can transmit HIV to their infants. In children younger than age 16, safety and effectiveness haven't been established.

Adverse reactions

CNS: anxiety, *asthenia*, depression, *fatigue*, fever, *headache*, insomnia, pain.
EENT: pharyngitis, sinusitis.
GI: abdominal pain (generalized or localized), diarrhea, nausea, vomiting.
Respiratory: bronchitis, cough, upper respiratory tract infection.

Skin: *rash.*
Other: flulike symptoms.

Interactions

Drug-drug. *Amphetamines, antihistamines (nonsedating), benzodiazepines, calcium channel blockers, clarithromycin, dapsone, ergot alkaloids, indinavir, quinidine, rifabutin, sedative hypnotics, warfarin:* May increase or prolong therapeutic and adverse effects of these drugs. Avoid use together; however, reduced doses of indinavir and clarithromycin may be used.
Antacids: May reduce absorption of delavirdine. Separate doses by at least 1 hour.
Carbamazepine, phenobarbital, phenytoin: May decrease delavirdine level; use together cautiously.
Clarithromycin, fluoxetine, ketoconazole: May cause a 50% increase in delavirdine bioavailability. Monitor patient. Reduce dose of clarithromycin.
Didanosine: May decrease absorption of both drugs by 20%. Separate doses by at least 1 hour.
H$_2$-receptor antagonists: May increase gastric pH, reducing absorption of delavirdine. Longterm use together isn't recommended.
HMG-CoA reductase inhibitors, such as atorvastatin, lovastatin, and simvastatin: May increase levels of these drugs, raising risk for myopathy, including rhabdomyolysis. Avoid use together.
Rifabutin, rifampin: May decrease delavirdine levels. Rifabutin levels are increased by 100%. Avoid use together.
Saquinavir: May increase bioavailability of saquinavir fivefold. Monitor AST and ALT levels frequently when used together.
Sildenafil: May increase sildenafil level and risk of hypotension, visual changes, and priapism. Tell patient not to exceed 25 mg of sildenafil in a 48-hour period.

Effects on lab test results

• May increase ALT, GGT, amylase, bilirubin, and AST levels. May decrease hemoglobin level and hematocrit. May increase or decrease glucose level.
• May increase PT, PTT, and eosinophil count. May decrease granulocyte, neutrophil, WBC, RBC, and platelet counts.

Pharmacokinetics

Absorption: Rapid.
Distribution: 98% protein-bound.

Metabolism: Extensive, to inactive metabolites. Mainly in liver by cytochrome P-450 enzyme systems.
Excretion: 51% in the urine (less than 5% unchanged), 44% in the feces. *Half-life:* About 5¾ hours.

Route	Onset	Peak	Duration
P.O.	Unknown	1 hr	Unknown

Action

Chemical effect: Drug binds directly to reverse transcriptase and blocks RNA- and DNA-dependent DNA polymerase activities.
Therapeutic effect: Inhibits HIV replication.

Available forms

Tablets: 100 mg, 200 mg

NURSING PROCESS

🔖 Assessment
● Assess patient's underlying condition before therapy and regularly thereafter.
● Be alert for adverse reactions and drug interactions.
● Monitor patient for drug-induced rash.
● Assess patient's and family's knowledge of drug therapy.

🔲 Nursing diagnoses
● Risk for impaired skin integrity related to potential adverse effects of medication
● Risk for infection related to patient's underlying condition
● Deficient knowledge related to drug therapy

▶ Planning and implementation
● If rash develops, give diphenhydramine, hydroxyzine, or topical corticosteroids to relieve symptoms.
● Resistance develops rapidly when drug is used as monotherapy. Always give with appropriate antiretroviral therapy.
● If patient has trouble swallowing pills, add tablets to at least 3 oz (90 ml) of water, let stand for a few minutes, then stir well. Have patient drink promptly, rinse the glass, and swallow the rinse to make sure entire dose is consumed.
Patient teaching
● Tell patient to stop taking the drug and to call prescriber if he develops a severe rash or rash accompanied by symptoms such as fever, blis-

tering, oral lesions, conjunctivitis, swelling, or muscle or joint aches.
● Tell patient that drug doesn't cure HIV-1 infection and that he may continue to acquire illnesses related to HIV-1 infection.
● Urge patient to remain under medical supervision when taking drug because long-term effects aren't known.
● Advise patient to take drug as prescribed and not to alter doses without prescriber's approval. If a dose is missed, tell him to take the next dose as soon as possible but not to double the next dose.
● Inform patient that drug may be taken with or without food.
● Tell patient with achlorhydria to take drug with an acidic beverage, such as orange or cranberry juice.
● Advise patient taking sildenafil of increased risk for sildenafil-associated adverse events, including hypotension, vision changes, and priapism. Tell him to promptly report any symptoms to prescriber. Tell him not to exceed 25 mg of sildenafil in a 48-hour period.
● Advise patient to report use of other prescription drugs, OTC medicines, or herbal remedies.

✅ Evaluation
● Patient's skin integrity is maintained.
● Patient is free from opportunistic infections.
● Patient and family state understanding of drug therapy.

desipramine hydrochloride
(deh-SIP-rah-meen high-droh-KLOR-ighd)
Norpramin

Pharmacologic class: tricyclic antidepressant (TCA)
Therapeutic class: antidepressant
Pregnancy risk category: C

Indications and dosages
▶ **Depression.** *Adults:* Initially, 100 to 200 mg P.O. daily in divided doses; increase to maximum, 300 mg daily. Or, entire dose can be given at bedtime.
Elderly patients and adolescents: 25 to 100 mg P.O. daily in divided doses; increase gradually to maximum, 150 mg daily, if needed.

Contraindications and cautions

• Contraindicated in patients hypersensitive to drug or any of its components, in those in acute recovery phase of MI, and within 14 days of MAO inhibitor therapy.
• Use cautiously in patients taking thyroid medication and in those with CV disease, seizure disorder, glaucoma, thyroid disorder, or history of urine retention.
⚕ Lifespan: In pregnant and breast-feeding women, use cautiously. In children younger than age 12, use is contraindicated.

Adverse reactions

CNS: confusion, *dizziness, drowsiness,* EEG changes, excitation, extrapyramidal reactions, headache, nervousness, **seizures, suicidal thinking and behavior in adolescents,** tremors, weakness.
CV: ECG changes, hypertension, orthostatic hypotension, tachycardia.
EENT: *blurred vision,* mydriasis, tinnitus.
GI: anorexia, *constipation, dry mouth,* nausea, paralytic ileus, vomiting.
GU: urine retention.
Skin: *diaphoresis,* photosensitivity, rash, urticaria.
Other: hypersensitivity reaction, **sudden death.**

Interactions

Drug-drug. *Anticholinergics:* May enhance anticholinergic effects. Monitor patient closely.
Barbiturates, CNS depressants: May enhance CNS depression. Avoid use together.
Cimetidine, methylphenidate: May increase desipramine levels. Monitor patient for adverse reactions.
Clonidine: May cause loss of blood pressure control with potentially life-threatening elevations in blood pressure. Don't use together.
Epinephrine, norepinephrine: May increase hypertensive effect. Use together cautiously.
MAO inhibitors: May cause severe excitation, hyperpyrexia, or seizures, usually with high dosage. Contraindicated within 14 days of MAO inhibitor therapy.
SSRIs: May inhibit the metabolism of TCAs, causing toxicity. Symptoms of TCA toxicity may persist for several weeks after stopping SSRI. At least 5 weeks may be needed when switching from fluoxetine to a tricyclic antidepressant because of the long half-life of the active and parent metabolite.

Drug-lifestyle. *Alcohol use:* May enhance CNS depression. Discourage use together.
Smoking: May lower desipramine level. Monitor patient for lack of effect; encourage smoking cessation.
Sun exposure: May increase risk of photosensitivity. Advise against unprotected or prolonged sun exposure.

Effects on lab test results

• May increase or decrease glucose level.
• May increase liver function test values.

Pharmacokinetics

Absorption: Rapid.
Distribution: Wide, including CNS. 90% protein-bound.
Metabolism: By the liver; significant first-pass effect may explain different levels in patients taking same dosage.
Excretion: Mainly in urine. *Half-life:* Unknown.

Route	Onset	Peak	Duration
P.O.	2–4 wk	4–6 hr	Unknown

Action

Chemical effect: May increase amount of norepinephrine, serotonin, or both in the CNS by blocking their reuptake by neurons.
Therapeutic effect: Relieves depression.

Available forms

Tablets: 10 mg, 25 mg, 50 mg, 75 mg, 100 mg, 150 mg

NURSING PROCESS

Assessment
• Obtain history of patient's depression before therapy, and reassess regularly.
• Be alert for adverse reactions and drug interactions.
• Assess patient's and family's knowledge of drug therapy.

Nursing diagnoses
• Ineffective coping related to depression
• Risk for injury related to drug-induced adverse reactions
• Deficient knowledge related to drug therapy

▷ Planning and implementation

⊕ **ALERT:** Short-term studies in children and adolescents with major depressive disorder and other psychiatric disorders have shown an increased risk of suicidal thinking and behavior.

⊕ **ALERT:** Drug may increase the risk of suicidal thinking and behavior in young adults ages 18 to 24 during the first two months of treatment. Monitor closely. Observe for clinical worsening, suicidality, or unusual behavior changes.

• Don't abruptly stop giving the drug. Abruptly stopping long-term therapy may cause nausea, headache, and malaise.

• Because drug produces fewer anticholinergic effects than other TCAs, it's prescribed often for patients with cardiac problems.

• Because hypertensive episodes may occur during surgery, stop drug gradually several days before surgery.

⊕ **ALERT:** This drug may cause sudden death in children, although the cause isn't clearly defined.

• If signs of psychosis occur or increase, reduce dosage.

Patient teaching

• Advise parents, caregivers, and family to closely observe adolescents and young adults for suicidality, behavior changes, or worsening of depression and report to prescriber immediately.

• Warn patient to avoid hazardous activities until the drug's CNS effects are known. Drowsiness and dizziness usually subside after a few weeks.

• Tell patient to avoid alcohol during therapy because it may antagonize drug effects.

• Warn patient not to abruptly stop taking the drug.

• Advise patient to consult prescriber before taking other prescription drugs, OTC medications, or herbal remedies.

• Instruct patient to use sunblock, wear protective clothing, and avoid prolonged exposure to strong sunlight.

☑ Evaluation

• Patient behavior and communication indicate improvement of depression.

• Patient has no injury as a result of drug-induced adverse reactions.

• Patient and family state understanding of drug therapy.

desloratadine
(des-lor-AT-ah-deen)
Clarinex✒, Clarinex RediTabs

Pharmacologic class: selective H_1-receptor antagonist
Therapeutic class: antihistamine
Pregnancy risk category: C

Indications and dosages

▶ **Perennial allergic rhinitis; chronic idiopathic urticaria.** *Adults and children age 12 and older:* 5 mg P.O. using tablets, RediTabs, or syrup.
Children ages 6 to 11 years: 2.5 mg (5 ml) syrup P.O. daily or one 2.5-mg RediTab P.O. once daily.
Children ages 1 to 5 years: 1.25 mg (2.5 ml) syrup P.O. daily.
Children ages 6 to 11 months: 1 mg (2 ml) syrup P.O. daily.
▶ **Seasonal allergic rhinitis.** *Adults and children age 12 and older:* 5 mg P.O. daily using tablets, RediTabs, or syrup.
Children ages 6 to 11: Give 2.5 mg (5 ml) syrup P.O. daily or one 2.5-mg RediTab P.O. once daily.
Children ages 2 to 5: Give 1.25 mg (2.5 ml) syrup P.O. daily.
⧅ **Adjust-a-dose:** In patients with hepatic or renal impairment, start with 5 mg P.O. every other day.

Contraindications and cautions

• Contraindicated in patients hypersensitive to drug or any of its components, or loratadine. Drug can't be eliminated by hemodialysis.
⚞ **Lifespan:** Breast-feeding women should stop nursing or stop taking the drug because drug appears in breast milk. In children younger than age 6 months, safety and effectiveness haven't been established. In elderly patients, use cautiously because they may have decreased hepatic, renal, or cardiac function or other diseases and may be taking other drugs.

Adverse reactions

CNS: dizziness, fatigue, *fever, headache,* somnolence.
CV: tachycardia.
EENT: pharyngitis, sore throat.

Reactions may be *common,* uncommon, *life-threatening,* or COMMON AND LIFE-THREATENING.

GI: *diarrhea,* dry mouth, dyspepsia, nausea.
GU: dysmenorrhea.
Musculoskeletal: myalgia.
Respiratory: upper respiratory tract infection.

Interactions

None reported.

Effect on lab test results

• May increase liver enzyme and bilirubin levels.

Pharmacokinetics

Absorption: Readily absorbed in plasma.
Doesn't cross the blood–brain barrier. All forms
equal in pharmacokinetics.
Distribution: 82% to 87% protein-bound. Active metabolite is 85% to 89% protein-bound.
Metabolism: Extensive, to inactive metabolite.
Excretion: Equal in urine and feces, mainly as
metabolites. *Half-life:* 27 hours.

Route	Onset	Peak	Duration
P.O.	1 hr	3 hr	Unknown

Action

Chemical effect: Inhibits histamine release
from human mast cells in vitro.
Therapeutic effect: Relieves allergy symptoms.

Available forms

Syrup: 0.5 mg/ml
Tablets: 5 mg
Tablets (orally-disintegrating): 2.5 mg, 5 mg

NURSING PROCESS

☑ Assessment
• Assess patient's condition before therapy and
regularly thereafter.
• Be alert for adverse reactions.
• Assess patient's and family's knowledge of
drug therapy.

✤ Nursing diagnoses
• Ineffective health maintenance related to underlying allergic condition
• Fatigue related to drug-induced reaction
• Deficient knowledge related to drug therapy

▶ Planning and implementation
• Drug may be taken with or without food.

• Overdose may cause somnolence and increased heart rate. If these symptoms occur,
consider removing unabsorbed drug through
standard measures; treat symptoms and provide
supportive therapy.

Patient teaching
• Inform phenylketonuric patients that RediTabs
contain phenylalanine.
• Advise patient not to exceed prescribed
dosage. Doses of more than 5 mg don't increase
effectiveness and may cause somnolence.
• Tell patient to report adverse effects.
• Store all forms at room temperature, not to exceed 86° F (30° C), and avoid exposure to light
and moisture.
• Inform patient that orally disintegrating tablet
may be taken with or without water.
• Instruct patient to remove a tablet from the
blister pack and immediately place it on his
tongue. The tablet will dissolve.
• Teach parents to use properly calibrated 5- to
10-ml dropper or syringe for syrup administration, not household measuring devices.

☑ Evaluation
• Patient's allergic symptoms are relieved.
• Patient doesn't suffer any drug-induced adverse effects.
• Patient and family state understanding of drug
therapy.

desmopressin acetate
(dez-moh-PREH-sin AS-ih-tayt)
DDAVP, Minirin, Stimate

Pharmacologic class: posterior pituitary hormone
Therapeutic class: antidiuretic, hemostatic
Pregnancy risk category: B

Indications and dosages

▶ **Nonnephrogenic diabetes insipidus, temporary polyuria, and polydipsia from pituitary trauma.** *Adults:* 10 to 40 mcg intranasally
daily in one to three divided doses. Adjust
morning and evening doses separately for adequate diurnal rhythm of water turnover. Or
0.05 mg P.O. b.i.d. Adjust each dose separately
for an adequate diurnal rhythm of water turnover. Increase or decrease total oral daily dosage
as needed to achieve desired response. Dosage

may range from 0.1 to 1.2 mg, divided into two or three daily doses. Start oral therapy 12 hours after last intranasal dose. Or, give 2 to 4 mcg I.V. or subcutaneously daily, usually in two equally divided doses.

Children ages 3 months to 12 years: 0.05 to 0.3 ml intranasally daily in one or two doses.

Children age 4 and older: Begin with 0.05 mg oral form P.O. b.i.d. Adjust each dose separately for an adequate diurnal rhythm of water turnover. Increase or decrease total oral daily dosage to achieve desired response. Dosages may range from 0.1 to 1.2 mg, divided into two or three daily doses. Start oral therapy 12 hours after the last intranasal dose.

Children younger than age 4: Adjust dosage of oral form individually to prevent an excessive decrease in blood osmolality.

▶ **Hemophilia A and von Willebrand disease.** *Adults and children:* 0.3 mcg/kg diluted in normal saline solution and infused I.V. over 15 to 30 minutes. May repeat dose, if needed, based on laboratory response and patient's condition. Intranasal dose is 1 spray (of solution containing 1.5 mg/ml) into each nostril to provide total of 300 mcg.

Adults and children weighing less than 50 kg (110 lb): 1 spray into a single nostril (150 mcg).

▶ **Primary nocturnal enuresis.** *Children age 6 and older:* 0.2 mg P.O. at bedtime. Adjust dosage up to 0.6 mg P.O. to achieve desired response.

▼ I.V. administration

- For adults and children weighing more than 10 kg (22 lb), dilute with 50 ml sterile physiologic saline solution. For children weighing 10 kg or less, use 10 ml of diluent.
- Inspect for particulate matter and discoloration before infusing drug.
- Monitor blood pressure and pulse during infusion.

⊗ **Incompatibilities**
None reported.

Contraindications and cautions

- Contraindicated in patients hypersensitive to drug (or any of its components), and in those with type IIB von Willebrand disease.
- Intranasal form contraindicated in hyponatremic patients and those with a history of hyponatremia.

- Use cautiously in patients with coronary artery insufficiency or hypertensive CV disease and in those with conditions linked to fluid and electrolyte imbalance, such as cystic fibrosis, because these patients are prone to hyponatremia.
- Use cautiously in patients at risk for water intoxication with hyponatremia.

⚖ **Lifespan:** In pregnant and breast-feeding women, use cautiously. In infants younger than age 3 months, use of drug isn't recommended because of their increased tendency to develop fluid imbalance. In children younger than age 12, safety of parenteral form of drug hasn't been established for management of diabetes insipidus.

Adverse reactions

CNS: headache.
CV: slight rise in blood pressure.
EENT: epistaxis, nasal congestion, rhinitis, sore throat.
GI: abdominal cramps, nausea.
GU: vulvar pain.
Respiratory: cough.
Other: flushing, local erythema, swelling or burning after injection.

Interactions

Drug-drug. *Carbamazepine, chlorpropamide:* May potentiate effects of desmopressin. Monitor patient.
Demeclocycline, epinephrine, heparin, lithium: May decrease response to desmopressin. Monitor patient closely.
Vasopressors: May potentiate pressor effect of these drugs. Use large intranasal or parenteral doses cautiously.
Drug-lifestyle. *Alcohol use:* May increase risk of adverse effects. Discourage use together.

Effects on lab test results

None reported.

Pharmacokinetics

Absorption: After intranasal use, 10% to 20% by nasal mucosa. After subcutaneous use, unknown. After P.O. use, minimal.
Distribution: Unknown.
Metabolism: Unknown.
Excretion: Unknown. *Half-life (injection):* Fast phase, about 8 minutes; slow phase, 75.5 min-

utes. *Half-life (intranasal):* About 3½ hours. *Half-life (oral):* 1½ to 2½ hours.

Route	Onset	Peak	Duration
P.O.	1 hr	4–7 hr	8–12 hr
I.V.	15–30 min	½–2 hr	4–12 hr
SubQ	Unknown	Unknown	Unknown
Intranasal	≤1 hr	1–5 hr	8–12 hr

Action

Chemical effect: Increases flow of adenosine monophosphate and water through the kidneys, promoting reabsorption of water and producing concentrated urine (ADH effect). Releases factor VIII from plasma.
Therapeutic effect: Decreases diuresis and promotes clotting.

Available forms

Injection: 4 mcg/ml
Nasal solution: 0.1 mg/ml, 1.5 mg/ml
Nasal spray: 0.1 mg/ml (10 mcg/spray)
Tablets: 0.1 mg, 0.2 mg

NURSING PROCESS

⚕ Assessment

• Obtain history of patient's underlying condition before therapy.
• Monitor effectiveness for diabetes insipidus or relief of symptoms of other disorders by checking patient's fluid intake and output, serum and urine osmolality, and urine specific gravity.
• Be alert for adverse reactions and drug interactions.
• Monitor patient carefully for hypertension during high-dose therapy.
• Assess patient's and family's knowledge of drug therapy.

⊕ Nursing diagnoses

• Deficient fluid volume related to underlying condition
• Acute pain related to drug-induced headache
• Deficient knowledge related to drug therapy

▷ Planning and implementation

• When giving drug subcutaneously, rotate injection sites.
• Follow manufacturer's instructions exactly for intranasal administration.
• Ensure nasal passages are intact, clean, and free of obstruction before intranasal use.

• Intranasal use can cause changes in nasal mucosa, resulting in erratic, unreliable absorption. Report worsening condition to prescriber, who may prescribe injectable DDAVP.
⑤ **ALERT:** Use of tablets should be interrupted during acute illness that might result in fluid or electrolyte imbalance.
• Don't use drug to treat severe cases of von Willebrand disease or hemophilia A with factor VIII levels of 0% to 5%.
• Patients may be switched from intranasal to subcutaneous form, such as during episodes of rhinorrhea. Give ¹⁄₁₀ or ¼ of their usual nasal dose subcutaneously.
• When drug is used to treat diabetes insipidus, adjust dosage according to patient's fluid output. Adjust morning and evening doses separately for adequate diurnal rhythm of water turnover.
⑤ **ALERT:** Don't confuse desmopressin with vasopressin.

Patient teaching

• Instruct patient to clear nasal passages before using intranasal form of the drug.
• Patient may have trouble measuring and inhaling drug into nostrils. Teach patient and caregiver correct way to give drug.
• Advise patient to report conditions such as nasal congestion, allergic rhinitis, or upper respiratory tract infection because dose adjustment may be required.
• Teach patient using subcutaneous desmopressin to rotate injection sites to avoid tissue damage.
• Warn patient to drink only enough water to satisfy thirst.
• Inform patient that when treating hemophilia A and von Willebrand disease, giving desmopressin may avoid hazards of using blood products.
• Advise patient to wear or carry medical identification indicating use of drug.

☑ Evaluation

• Patient achieves normal fluid and electrolyte balance.
• Patient states that headache is relieved with mild analgesic.
• Patient and family state understanding of drug therapy.

dexamethasone

(deks-ah-METH-uh-sohn)
**Dexamethasone Intensol*, Dexasone ♦,
Dexpak, Oradexon ♦**

dexamethasone sodium phosphate

Pharmacologic class: glucocorticoid
Therapeutic class: anti-inflammatory, immuno-suppressant
Pregnancy risk category: NR

Indications and dosages

▶ **Cerebral edema.** *Adults:* Initially, 10 mg dexamethasone sodium phosphate I.V. Then 4 mg I.M. every 6 hours until symptoms subside (usually 2 to 4 days). Then taper down over 5 to 7 days.

▶ **Inflammatory conditions, allergic reactions, neoplasias.** *Adults:* 4 mg dexamethasone sodium phosphate I.M. as a single dose. Continue maintenance therapy with dexamethasone tablets, 1.5 mg P.O. b.i.d. for 2 days; then 0.75 mg P.O. b.i.d. for 1 day; then 0.75 mg P.O. once daily for 2 days; then stop drug.

▶ **Shock.** *Adults:* 1 to 6 mg/kg dexamethasone sodium phosphate I.V. as single dose or 40 mg I.V. every 2 to 6 hours, as needed. Or 20 mg I.V. as a single dose, followed by continuous infusion of 3 mg/kg every 24 hours. Limit high-dose therapy to 48 to 72 hours.

▶ **Suppression test for Cushing syndrome.** *Adults:* After determining baseline 24-hour urine levels of 17-hydroxycorticosteroids, 0.5 mg P.O. every 6 hours for 48 hours; perform 24-hour urine collection to determine 17-hydroxycorticosteroid excretion again during second 24 hours of dexamethasone administration. Or 1 mg P.O. as a single dose at 11 PM. Draw blood for cortisol level at 8 AM the following day.

▶ **Tuberculous meningitis.** *Adults:* 8 to 12 mg (phosphate) I.M. daily tapered over 6 to 8 weeks.

▶ **Bacterial meningitis‡.** *Adults, infants, and children:* 0.15 mg/kg (phosphate) I.V. q.i.d. for the first 2 to 4 days of anti-infective therapy.

▶ **To prevent hyaline membrane disease in preterm infants‡.** *Adults:* 4 mg dexamethasone sodium phosphate I.M. t.i.d. to mother for 2 days before delivery.

▶ **To prevent chemotherapy-induced nausea and vomiting‡.** *Adults:* 10 to 20 mg I.V. before giving chemotherapy. Additional doses (individualized for each patient and usually lower than initial dose) may be given I.V. or P.O. for 24 to 72 hours following cancer chemotherapy.

▼ I.V. administration

● When giving as direct injection, inject undiluted over at least 1 minute.
● When giving as intermittent or continuous infusion, dilute solution in normal saline solution or D₅W. For continuous infusion, change solution every 24 hours.
⊗ **Incompatibilities**
Ciprofloxacin, daunorubicin, diphenhydramine, doxapram, doxorubicin, glycopyrrolate, idarubicin, midazolam, vancomycin.

Contraindications and cautions

● Contraindicated in patients hypersensitive to drug or any of its components and in those with systemic fungal infections.
● Use cautiously in patients with seizures, emotional instability, psychotic tendencies, recent MI, thromboembolic disorders, heart failure, hypertension, GI ulcer, diverticulitis, nonspecific ulcerative colitis, recent intestinal anastomoses, renal disease, ocular herpes simplex, cirrhosis, diabetes mellitus, hypothyroidism, myasthenia gravis, osteoporosis, or tuberculosis. Because some forms contain sulfite preservatives, use cautiously in patients sensitive to sulfites.
🕯 **Lifespan:** In pregnant women, use cautiously. In breast-feeding women, drug isn't recommended. In children, long-term use of drug may delay growth and maturation.

Adverse reactions

CNS: *euphoria, insomnia,* pseudotumor cerebri, psychotic behavior, *seizures,* headache, vertigo.
CV: *arrhythmias,* edema, *heart failure,* hypertension, *thromboembolism.*
EENT: cataracts, glaucoma.
GI: GI irritation, increased appetite, *pancreatitis, peptic ulceration.*
GU: menstrual irregularities.
Metabolic: carbohydrate intolerance, hyperglycemia, hypokalemia, negative nitrogen balance caused by protein catabolism.
Musculoskeletal: growth suppression in children, muscle weakness, osteoporosis.

Reactions may be *common,* uncommon, *life-threatening,* or **COMMON AND LIFE-THREATENING.**

Skin: acne, allergic dermatitis, angioneurotic edema, atrophy at I.M. injection sites, delayed wound healing, hirsutism, skin eruptions, thin fragile skin, urticaria.

Other: *acute adrenal insufficiency* (may follow abrupt withdrawal after long-term therapy or such increased stress as infection, surgery, or trauma), cushingoid state (moonface, buffalo hump, central obesity), susceptibility to infections.

Interactions

Drug-drug. *Antidiabetics, including insulin:* May decrease corticosteroid response. May need dosage adjustment.

Aspirin, indomethacin, other NSAIDs: May increase risk of GI distress and bleeding. Give together cautiously.

Barbiturates, phenytoin, rifampin: May decrease corticosteroid effect. Increase corticosteroid dosage.

Digoxin: May increase risk of arrhythmia from hypokalemia. May need dosage adjustment.

Oral anticoagulants: May alter dosage requirements. Monitor PT and INR closely.

Potassium-depleting drugs: May enhance potassium-wasting effects of dexamethasone. Monitor potassium level.

Salicylates: May decrease salicylate level. Monitor patient for lack of therapeutic effects.

Skin-test antigens: May decrease response of skin-test antigens. Defer skin testing until therapy is completed.

Toxoids, vaccines: May decrease antibody response and increase risk of neurologic complications. Avoid use together.

Drug-lifestyle. *Alcohol use:* May increase risk of gastric irritation and GI ulceration. Discourage use together.

Effects on lab test results

• May increase glucose and cholesterol levels. May decrease potassium, calcium, T_3, and T_4 levels.

• May cause false negative dexamethasone suppression test in patients taking indomethacin.

Pharmacokinetics

Absorption: For P.O. use, good. For injections, depends on location.

Distribution: To muscle, liver, skin, intestines, and kidneys. Bound weakly to transcortin and albumin. Only unbound portion is active.

Metabolism: In liver to inactive glucuronide and sulfate metabolites.

Excretion: Inactive metabolites and small amounts of unmetabolized drug by kidneys. Insignificant in feces. *Half-life:* About 1 to 2 days.

Route	Onset	Peak	Duration
P.O.	1–2 hr	1–2 hr	2½ days
I.V., I.M.	≤ 1 hr	1 hr	2 days–3 wk

Action

Chemical effect: May stabilize leukocyte lysosomal membranes; stimulate bone marrow; and influence protein, fat, and carbohydrate metabolism.

Therapeutic effect: Relieves cerebral edema, reduces inflammation and immune response, and reverses shock.

Available forms

dexamethasone
Elixir: 0.5 mg/5 ml
Oral solution: 0.5 mg/5 ml, 1 mg/ml
Tablets: 0.25 mg, 0.5 mg, 0.75 mg, 1 mg, 1.5 mg, 2 mg, 4 mg, 6 mg
dexamethasone sodium phosphate
Injection: 4 mg/ml, 10 mg/ml, 20 mg/ml, 24 mg/ml

NURSING PROCESS

Assessment
• Obtain history of patient's underlying condition before therapy.
• Monitor patient's weight, blood pressure, glucose level, and electrolyte levels.
• Look for adverse reactions and drug interactions. Most adverse reactions to corticosteroids are dosage-dependent.
• Watch for depression or psychotic episodes, especially in high-dose therapy.
• Assess patient's and family's knowledge of drug therapy.

Nursing diagnoses
• Ineffective health maintenance related to underlying condition
• Risk for injury related to drug-induced adverse reactions
• Deficient knowledge related to drug therapy

▶ Planning and implementation

● For better results and less toxicity, give once-daily dose in the morning.

● Give with food when possible.

● Give I.M. deep into gluteal muscle. Rotate injection sites to prevent muscle atrophy.

● If possible, avoid giving drug subcutaneously because atrophy and sterile abscesses may occur.

● Always adjust to lowest effective dose.

● Corticosteroids may mask signs of infection and new infections may arise during their use.

⑤ **ALERT:** When stopping drug after long-term use, reduce dosage gradually. Stopping drug abruptly may cause rebound inflammation, fatigue, weakness, arthralgia, fever, dizziness, lethargy, depression, fainting, orthostatic hypotension, dyspnea, anorexia, or hypoglycemia, or may be fatal.

⑤ **ALERT:** Give patient low-sodium diet high in potassium and protein. Also, give potassium supplements as directed.

● If patient's stress level (physical or psychological) increases, notify prescriber and increase dose.

● If patient has adverse reaction, notify prescriber, treat symptoms, and provide supportive therapy.

⑤ **ALERT:** Don't confuse dexamethasone with desoximetasone.

Patient teaching

● Tell patient not to abruptly stop taking the drug because this may be fatal.

● Teach patient the early signs of adrenal insufficiency (fatigue, muscle weakness, joint pain, fever, anorexia, nausea, dyspnea, dizziness, and fainting).

● Instruct patient to wear or carry medical identification that indicates need for supplemental systemic glucocorticoids during stress, especially as dose is decreased.

● Warn patient receiving long-term therapy about cushingoid symptoms and the need to notify prescriber about sudden weight gain or swelling.

● Warn patient about easy bruising.

● Advise patient receiving long-term therapy to consider exercise or physical therapy. Give vitamin D or calcium supplements.

● Advise patient receiving long-term therapy to have periodic ophthalmologic examinations.

☑ Evaluation

● Patient's condition improves with drug therapy.

● Patient has no injury as a result of drug therapy.

● Patient and family state understanding of drug therapy.

HIGH ALERT!

dexmedetomidine hydrochloride
(dex-meh-dih-TOE-mih-deen high-droh-KLOR-ighd)
Precedex

Pharmacologic class: selective alpha$_2$-adrenoreceptor agonist with sedative properties
Therapeutic class: sedative
Pregnancy risk category: C

Indications and dosages

▶ **Sedation of initially intubated and mechanically ventilated patients in the ICU.**
Adults: Loading infusion of 1 mcg/kg I.V. over 10 minutes; then a maintenance infusion of 0.2 to 0.7 mcg/kg/hour for up to 24 hours; adjust to achieve the desired level of sedation.

🔁 **Adjust-a-dose:** In elderly patients and those with renal or hepatic failure, reduce dosage.

▼ I.V. administration

● Dilute in normal saline solution. To prepare the infusion, withdraw 2 ml of drug and add to 48 ml of normal saline injection to a total of 50 ml. Shake gently to mix well.

● Don't give through the same I.V. line with blood or plasma because physical compatibility hasn't been established.

● Administer using a controlled infusion device.

● Infusion is compatible with lactated Ringer's solution, D$_5$W, normal saline solution, 20% mannitol, many anesthetic agents, atropine sulfate, morphine sulfate, and plasma substitute.

● Don't give infusion for longer than 24 hours.

⊗ **Incompatibilities**
Amphotericin B, blood, diazepam, plasma.

Contraindications and cautions

● Contraindicated in patients with hypersensitivity to dexmedetomidine.

● Use cautiously in patients with chronic hypertension, diabetes mellitus, advanced heart block, or renal or hepatic impairment.

⚜ **Lifespan:** In pregnant women, use only if potential benefits to the woman outweigh risks to the fetus because drug may be toxic to fetus. In breast-feeding women, use cautiously. In children, use isn't recommended. In elderly patients, use cautiously.

Reactions may be *common*, uncommon, *life-threatening*, or COMMON AND LIFE-THREATENING.

Adverse reactions

CNS: pain, fever.
CV: *arrhythmias, bradycardia,* hypotension, hypertension.
GI: *nausea,* thirst.
GU: oliguria.
Hematologic: anemia, leukocytosis.
Respiratory: *hypoxia,* pleural effusion, *pulmonary edema.*
Other: infection.

Interactions

Drug-drug. *Anesthetics, hypnotics, opioids, sedatives:* May enhance effects. May need to reduce dexmedetomidine dose.

Effects on lab test results

- May decrease hemoglobin level and hematocrit.
- May increase WBC count.

Pharmacokinetics

Absorption: Given I.V.
Distribution: Rapid and wide. 94% protein-bound.
Metabolism: Almost complete.
Excretion: 95% in urine and 4% in feces. *Half-life:* About 2 hours.

Route	Onset	Peak	Duration
I.V.	Unknown	Unknown	Unknown

Action

Chemical effect: Selectively stimulates alpha$_2$-adrenoceptors in the CNS.
Therapeutic effect: Produces sedation of initially intubated and mechanically ventilated patients.

Available forms

Injection: 100 mcg/ml in 2-ml vials

NURSING PROCESS

Assessment

- Assess renal and hepatic function before administration, particularly in elderly patients.
- Assess patient's response to drug. Some patients may stir and be alert when stimulated. This doesn't necessarily indicate lack of effectiveness.

- Look for adverse reactions and drug interactions.
- Assess patient's and family's knowledge of drug therapy.

Nursing diagnoses

- Risk for injury related to drug-induced adverse reactions
- Impaired spontaneous ventilation related to underlying disease process
- Deficient knowledge related to drug therapy

Planning and implementation

ALERT: Use a controlled infusion device at the rate calculated for patient's body weight.
- Continuously monitor cardiac condition.
- Drug may be continuously infused in mechanically ventilated patients before, during, and after extubation. Drug doesn't need to be stopped before extubation.

Patient teaching
- Tell patient that he'll be sedated while the drug is given, but that he may wake when stimulated.
- Tell patient that he'll be closely monitored and attended while sedated.

Evaluation

- Patient has no injury as a result of drug-induced adverse reactions.
- Patient regains spontaneous ventilation.
- Patient and family state understanding of drug therapy.

dexmethylphenidate hydrochloride

(dex-meth-il-FEN-uh-date high-droh-KLOR-ighd)
Focalin, Focalin XR

Pharmacologic class: CNS stimulant
Therapeutic class: CNS stimulant
Pregnancy risk category: C
Controlled substance schedule: II

Indications and dosages

▶ **Attention deficit hyperactivity disorder (ADHD).**
Immediate-release tablets
Children age 6 and older: For patients who aren't taking racemic methylphenidate or who

are taking another stimulant, start with 2.5 mg P.O.b.i.d., at least 4 hours apart. For patients who are being switched from methylphenidate, start with one-half of the current methylphenidate dosage. Additionally, adjust doagse weekly in increments of 2.5 to 5 mg daily to maximum of 20 mg daily in two divided doses.

Extended-release capsules

Adults: If patient takes neither dexmethylphenidate nor methylphenidate or takes a stimulant other than methylphenidate, 10 mg P.O. once daily in the morning. May adjust by 10 mg weekly. If patient takes methylphenidate, start with half the total daily methylphenidate dose. If patient takes immediate-release dexmethylphenidate, may switch to same daily dose of extended-release form. Maximum, 20 mg daily.

Children age 6 and older: If patient takes neither dexmethylphenidate nor methylphenidate, or takes a stimulant other than methylphenidate, 5 mg P.O. once daily in the morning. May adjust by 5 mg weekly. If patient takes methylphenidate, start with half the total daily methylphenidate dose. If patient takes immediate-release dexmethylphenidate, may switch to same daily dose of extended-release form. Maximum, 20 mg daily.

Contraindications and cautions

• Contraindicated in patients hypersensitive to drug or any of its components. Also contraindicated in patients with severe anxiety, tension, agitation, or glaucoma and in those who have motor tics or a family history or diagnosis of Tourette syndrome. Also contraindicated within 14 days of MAO inhibitor therapy because hypertensive crisis may occur. Don't use to treat severe depression or to prevent or treat normal fatigue states. Don't use drug in children or adolescents with structural cardiac abnormalities or other serious heart problems.

• Use cautiously in patients with a history of seizures, drug abuse, alcoholism, psychiatric illness, bipolar disorder, depression, or family history of suicide. Also use cautiously in patients whose underlying condition may be worsened by an increase in blood pressure or heart rate (such as those with hypertension, heart failure, recent MI).

⚠ Lifespan: In pregnant women, use only if the potential benefits to the woman outweigh the risks to the fetus. In breast-feeding women, use cautiously because it's unknown if drug appears in breast milk. In children younger than age 6, don't use.

Adverse reactions

CNS: blurred vision, fever, insomnia, nervousness, psychosis, dizziness, drowsiness.
CV: hypertension, tachycardia, angina, *arrhythmia.*
GI: *abdominal pain,* anorexia, nausea.
Hematologic: anemia, *leukopenia.*
Hepatic: abnormal liver function.
Metabolic: weight loss.
Musculoskeletal: arthralgia, growth suppression, twitching (motor or vocal tics).
Skin: scalp hair loss.

Interactions

Drug-drug. *Anticoagulants, anticonvulsants, SSRIs, tricyclic antidepressants:* May inhibit metabolism of these drugs. May need to decrease dosage of these drugs; monitor drug levels.
Antihypertensives: May decrease effectiveness of these drugs. Use together cautiously; monitor blood pressure.
Clonidine, other centrally acting alpha$_2$ agonists: May cause serious adverse effects. Use together cautiously.
MAO inhibitors: May increase risk of hypertensive crisis. Avoid use within 14 days of using MAO inhibitors.

Effects on lab test results

• May decrease hemoglobin level and hematocrit.
• May increase liver function test values. May decrease WBC count.

Pharmacokinetics

Absorption: Food delays rate of peak level but doesn't affect the amount absorbed.
Distribution: Rapid.
Metabolism: Extensive via de-esterification. Doesn't inhibit the cytochrome P-450 system. No active metabolites.
Excretion: 90% in urine. *Half-life:* About 2 hours.

Route	Onset	Peak	Duration
P.O.			
immediate-release	Unknown	1–1½ hr	Unknown
extended-release	Unknown	1–4 hr; 4½–7 hr	Unknown

Action

Chemical effect: May block presynaptic reuptake of norepinephrine and dopamine and increase the release of these neurotransmitters.
Therapeutic effect: Increases attention span and decreases hyperactivity and impulsiveness related to ADHD.

Available forms

Capsules (extended-release): 5 mg, 10 mg, 15 mg, 20 mg
Tablets: 2.5 mg, 5 mg, 10 mg

NURSING PROCESS

Assessment
• Diagnosis must be based on complete history and evaluation of the child in consultation with psychological, educational, and social specialists.
• Obtain a detailed patient history, including a family history for mental disorders, family suicide, ventricular arrhythmias, or sudden death.
• Monitor blood pressure and pulse routinely during drug therapy.
• Monitor for growth retardation in children.
• Look for adverse reactions.
• Check CBC with differential and platelet counts during long-term use.

Nursing diagnoses
• Ineffective health maintenance related to underlying condition
• Compromised family coping because of patient's underlying hyperactivity condition
• Deficient knowledge of drug therapy

Planning and implementation
• Drug is meant to be an adjunct to comprehensive therapy program that includes psychological, educational, and social support.
• Drug contains only the active isomer required to effectively manage the symptoms of ADHD, at half the dose of Ritalin.

• Growth may be suppressed with long-term stimulant use. Monitor children for growth and weight gain. If growth is suppressed or if weight gain is lower than expected, stop giving the drug.
• If symptoms are aggravated or adverse reactions occur, reduce dosage or stop drug.
• If seizures occur, stop giving the drug.
• Symptoms of overdose include vomiting, agitation, tremors, hyperreflexia, muscle twitching, convulsions, euphoria, confusion, hallucinations, delirium, sweating, flushing, headache, hyperpyrexia, tachycardia, palpitations, cardiac arrhythmias, hypertension, mydriasis, and dry mucous membranes. Give supportive care and protection against self-injury and additional overstimulation.
• Stop drug if symptoms don't improve after 1 month.

Patient teaching
ALERT: Warn patient that misuse of amphetamines can cause serious adverse cardiovascular events, including sudden death.
• Caution patient that drug may cause blurred vision or trouble focusing. Urge patient to use caution during activities that require a clear visual field.
• Inform parents that children may show increased aggression or hostility. Urge them to report worsening behavior.
• Advise parents to monitor child's height and weight and to tell prescriber if they suspect any growth suppression.
• If patient can't swallow capsules, tell him to empty the contents onto a spoonful of applesauce and eat immediately.
ALERT: Tell patient or parent not to cut, crush, or chew contents of extended-release capsules.
• Advise patient to take drug at the same time every day at the prescribed dose. Tell patient to report any adverse reactions to prescriber immediately.

Evaluation
• Patient responds positively to drug therapy.
• Patient and family are effectively coping with patient's underlying condition.
• Patient and family state understanding of drug therapy.

dextran, high–molecular-weight (dextran 70, dextran 75)

(DEKS-tran, high moh-LEH-kyoo-ler wayt)
Dextran 70, Dextran 75, Gentran 70, Macrodex

Pharmacologic class: glucose polymer
Therapeutic class: plasma volume expander
Pregnancy risk category: C

Indications and dosages

▶ **Plasma expander.** *Adults:* 30 g (500 ml of 6% solution) I.V. In emergencies, may give 1.2 to 2.4 g (20 to 40 ml)/minute. In normovolemic or nearly normovolemic patients, don't infuse faster than 240 mg (4 ml)/minute. Don't give more than 1.2 g/kg during the first 24 hours of therapy. Actual dosage depends on amount of fluid loss and resulting hemoconcentration and must be determined for each patient.
Children:‡ Don't exceed total dosage of 20 ml/kg.

▼ I.V. administration

• Use D₅W instead of normal saline solution because drug is hazardous for patients with heart failure, especially when given in normal saline solution.
• Give 20 ml of dextran 1 (containing 150 mg/ml) I.V. over 60 seconds 1 to 2 minutes before I.V. infusion of dextran, to protect against drug-induced anaphylaxis.
• Observe patient closely during early phase of infusion, when most anaphylactic reactions occur.
• Store drug at constant 77° F (25° C). Precipitate may form in storage. Heat to dissolve.
⊗ **Incompatibilities**
Any other I.V. drug added to a bottle of dextran, ascorbic acid, phytonadione, promethazine, protein hydrolysate.

Contraindications and cautions

• Contraindicated in patients hypersensitive to drug and in those with marked hemostatic defects, marked cardiac decompensation, renal disease with severe oliguria or anuria, hypervolemic conditions, or severe bleeding disorders.
• Use cautiously in patients with active hemorrhage, thrombocytopenia, impaired renal clearance, chronic liver disease, or abdominal conditions, and in patients undergoing bowel surgery.
⚘ **Lifespan:** In pregnant women, use cautiously. Breast-feeding women should stop nursing or stop the drug. In children, safety and effectiveness haven't been established.

Adverse reactions

CNS: fever.
CV: fluid overload, thrombophlebitis.
EENT: nasal congestion.
GI: nausea, vomiting.
GU: *anuria,* increased specific gravity and viscosity of urine, oliguria, *tubular stasis and blocking.*
Musculoskeletal: arthralgia.
Skin: urticaria.
Other: *anaphylaxis,* hypersensitivity reactions.

Interactions

Drug-drug. *Abciximab, aspirin, heparin, thrombolytics, warfarin:* May increase bleeding. Use together cautiously; monitor patient for bleeding.

Effects on lab test results

• May increase ALT and AST levels. May decrease hemoglobin level and hematocrit.
• May increase bleeding time.

Pharmacokinetics

Absorption: Given I.V.
Distribution: Throughout vascular system.
Metabolism: Drug molecules with molecular weights above 50,000 are degraded to glucose at rate of about 70 to 90 mg/kg/day.
Excretion: Drug molecules with molecular weights below 50,000 in urine. *Half-life:* Unknown.

Route	Onset	Peak	Duration
I.V.	Immediate	Immediate	Unknown

Action

Chemical effect: Expands plasma volume by way of colloidal osmotic effect, drawing fluid from interstitial to intravascular space, providing fluid replacement.
Therapeutic effect: Expands plasma volume.

Reactions may be *common,* uncommon, *life-threatening*, or COMMON AND LIFE-THREATENING.

Available forms

Injection: Dextran 70 in normal saline solution or D_5W; 6% dextran 75 in normal saline solution or D_5W

NURSING PROCESS

⚡ Assessment
• Obtain history of patient's underlying condition and hydration before therapy, and reassess regularly. Frequently assess vital signs, fluid intake and output, and urine or serum osmolarity levels.
• Be alert for adverse reactions.
• Watch for circulatory overload and rise in central venous pressure. Plasma expansion is slightly greater than volume infused.
• Monitor hemoglobin level and hematocrit.
• Assess patient's and family's knowledge of drug therapy.

⊕ Nursing diagnoses
• Decreased cardiac output related to underlying condition
• Risk for injury related to potential for drug-induced hypersensitivity reaction
• Deficient knowledge related to drug therapy

▶ Planning and implementation
• May significantly suppress platelet function with doses of 15 ml/kg or more than 1 L.
• If oliguria or anuria occurs or isn't relieved by infusion, stop dextran and give loop diuretic.
• If hematocrit values fall below 30% by volume, notify prescriber.
• Drug may interfere with analyses of blood grouping, crossmatching, and bilirubin, glucose, and protein levels.
• ⊛ **ALERT:** Low– and high–molecular-weight dextrans aren't interchangeable. Verify preparation before use.

Patient teaching
• Inform patient or family about drug therapy.
• Instruct patient to notify prescriber if adverse reactions, such as itching, occur.

✔ Evaluation
• Patient's vital signs and urine output return to normal.
• Patient doesn't develop hypersensitivity reaction to drug.
• Patient and family state understanding of drug therapy.

dextran, low–molecular-weight (dextran 40)
(DEKS-tran, LOH moh-LEH-kyoo-ler wayt)
Dextran 40, Gentran 40, 10% LMD, Rheomacrodex

Pharmacologic class: glucose polymer
Therapeutic class: plasma volume expander
Pregnancy risk category: C

Indications and dosages

▶ **Plasma volume expansion.** *Adults:* Dosage by I.V. infusion depends on amount of fluid loss. Initially, 10 ml/kg of dextran infused rapidly with central venous pressure monitoring; remainder of dose given slowly. Total dosage not to exceed 20 ml/kg in the first 24 hours. If therapy is continued longer than 24 hours, don't exceed 10 ml/kg daily. Continue for no longer than 5 days.
▶ **To prevent venous thrombosis.** *Adults:* 10 ml/kg (500 to 1,000 ml) I.V. on day of procedure; 500 ml on days 2 and 3.
▶ **Hemodiluent in extracorporeal circulation.** *Adults:* 10 to 20 ml/kg added to perfusion circuit. Total dosage not to exceed 20 ml/kg.

▽ I.V. administration

• Use D_5W solution instead of normal saline solution because drug is hazardous for patients with heart failure, especially when given in normal saline solution.
• Prescriber may order dextran 1, a dextran adjunct, to protect against drug-induced anaphylaxis. Give 20 ml of dextran 1 (containing 150 mg/ml) I.V. over 60 seconds, 1 to 2 minutes before I.V. infusion of dextran.
• Observe patient closely during early phase of infusion, when most anaphylactic reactions occur.
• Store at constant 77° F (25° C). Precipitate may form during storage. Heat to dissolve.
• Discard partially used containers.
⊗ **Incompatibilities**
Any other I.V. drug added to a bottle of dextran, ascorbic acid, phytonadione, promethazine, protein hydrolysate.

Contraindications and cautions

• Contraindicated in patients hypersensitive to drug and in those with marked hemostatic de-

fects, marked cardiac decompensation, and renal disease with severe oliguria or anuria.
• Use cautiously in patients with active hemorrhage, thrombocytopenia, or diabetes mellitus.
❇ **Lifespan:** In pregnant women, use cautiously. Breast-feeding women should stop breast-feeding or not use the drug. In children, safety and effectiveness haven't been established.

Adverse reactions

CV: thrombophlebitis.
GI: nausea, vomiting.
GU: increased urine viscosity, *tubular stasis and blocking.*
Hematologic: anemia.
Skin: urticaria.
Other: *anaphylaxis,* hypersensitivity reactions.

Interactions

None significant.

Effects on lab test results

• May increase ALT and AST levels. May decrease hemoglobin level and hematocrit.
• May increase bleeding time.

Pharmacokinetics

Absorption: Given I.V.
Distribution: Throughout vascular system.
Metabolism: Drug molecules with molecular weights above 50,000 are degraded to glucose at about 70 to 90 mg/kg/day.
Excretion: By kidneys for drug molecules with molecular weights below 50,000. *Half-life:* Unknown.

Route	Onset	Peak	Duration
I.V.	Immediate	Immediate	≤ 3 hr

Action

Chemical effect: Expands plasma volume by colloidal osmotic effect, drawing fluid from interstitial to intravascular space, providing fluid replacement.
Therapeutic effect: Expands plasma volume.

Available forms

Injection: 10% dextran 40 in D_5W or normal saline solution

NURSING PROCESS

✍ Assessment

• Obtain history of patient's underlying condition and hydration before therapy, and reassess regularly. Frequently assess vital signs, fluid intake and output, and urine or serum osmolarity levels.
• Be alert for adverse reactions.
• Watch for circulatory overload and rise in central venous pressure. Plasma expansion is slightly greater than volume infused.
• Check hemoglobin level and hematocrit.
• Assess patient's and family's knowledge of drug therapy.

🔱 Nursing diagnoses

• Decreased cardiac output related to underlying condition
• Risk for injury related to potential for drug-induced hypersensitivity reaction
• Deficient knowledge related to drug therapy

➤ Planning and implementation

• If oliguria or anuria occurs or isn't relieved by infusion, stop dextran and give loop diuretic.
• If hematocrit falls below 30% by volume, notify prescriber.
• Drug may interfere with analyses of blood grouping, crossmatching, and bilirubin, glucose, and protein levels.
🛇 **ALERT:** Low– and high–molecular-weight dextrans aren't interchangeable. Verify preparation before use.

Patient teaching
• Tell patient and family about therapy.
• Instruct patient to notify prescriber if adverse reactions, such as itching, occur.

✅ Evaluation

• Patient's vital signs and urine output return to normal.
• Patient has no hypersensitivity reaction to drug.
• Patient and family state understanding of drug therapy.

dextroamphetamine sulfate

(deks-troh-am-FET-uh-meen SUL-fayt)
Dexedrine*, Dexedrine Spansule, DextroStat

Pharmacologic class: amphetamine
Therapeutic class: CNS stimulant
Pregnancy risk category: C
Controlled substance schedule: II

Indications and dosages

▶ **Narcolepsy.** *Adults:* 5 to 60 mg P.O. daily in divided doses.
Children age 12 and older: 10 mg P.O. daily; increase by 10-mg increments weekly until desired response occurs or adult dose is reached.
Children ages 6 to 11: Give 5 mg P.O. daily; increase by 5-mg increments weekly until desired response occurs. Give first dose on awakening, additional doses (one or two) at intervals of 4 to 6 hours.
▶ **Attention deficit hyperactivity disorder.**
Children age 6 and older: 5 mg P.O. once daily or b.i.d.; increase by 5-mg increments weekly, as needed.
Children ages 3 to 5: Give 2.5 mg P.O. daily; increase by 2.5-mg increments weekly, as needed. In rare cases, more than 40 mg daily is needed.

Contraindications and cautions

• Contraindicated in patients hypersensitive to sympathomimetic amines and those with idiosyncratic reactions to them; within 14 days of MAO inhibitor use; and in those with hyperthyroidism, glaucoma, advanced arteriosclerosis, or a history of drug abuse.
• Don't use in children or adolescents with structural cardiac abnormalities or other serious heart problems.
• Use cautiously in patients whose underlying condition may be worsened by an increase in blood pressure or heart rate (pre-existing hypertension, heart failure, recent MI); patients with a psychiatric illness, bipolar disorder, depression, or family history of suicide; those with a seizure disorder or in patients with motor and phonic tics, Tourette syndrome, and agitated states.
⚜ Lifespan: In pregnant women, use cautiously. In breast-feeding women, safety and effec-

tiveness haven't been established. Because growth stunting may occur, monitor children on long-term therapy carefully.

Adverse reactions

CNS: dizziness, dysphoria, headache, *insomnia,* overstimulation, *restlessness,* tremors.
CV: *arrhythmias,* hypertension, palpitations, tachycardia, *cardiomyopathy.*
GI: anorexia, constipation, diarrhea, dry mouth, other GI disturbances, unpleasant taste, weight loss.
GU: impotence.
Skin: urticaria.
Other: altered libido, chills.

Interactions

Drug-drug. *Acetazolamide, alkalizing drugs, antacids, sodium bicarbonate:* May increase renal reabsorption. Monitor patient for enhanced amphetamine effects.
Acidifying drugs, ammonium chloride, ascorbic acid: May decrease level and increase renal clearance of dextroamphetamine. Monitor patient for decreased amphetamine effects.
Adrenergic blockers: May be inhibited by amphetamines. Avoid use together.
Antihistamines: May counteract sedative effects of antihistamines. Monitor patient for loss of therapeutic effects.
Chlorpromazine: May inhibit central stimulant effects of amphetamines, and may be used to treat amphetamine poisoning. Monitor patient closely.
Haloperidol, phenothiazines, tricyclic antidepressants: May decrease amphetamine effect. Increase dosage as needed.
Insulin, oral antidiabetics: May decrease antidiabetic requirement. Monitor glucose levels.
Lithium carbonate: May inhibit antiobesity and stimulating effects of amphetamines. Monitor patient closely.
MAO inhibitors: May cause severe hypertension; possibly hypertensive crisis. Don't use within 14 days of MAO inhibitor therapy.
Meperidine: Amphetamines may potentiate analgesic effect. Use together cautiously.
Methenamine: May increase urinary excretion and reduces effectiveness of amphetamines. Monitor effects.
Norepinephrine: May enhance adrenergic effect of norepinephrine. Monitor patient closely.

Phenobarbital, phenytoin: May delay absorption of dextroamphetamine. Monitor patient closely.

Propoxyphene: In cases of propoxyphene overdose, amphetamine CNS stimulation may be potentiated and fatal seizures can occur. Don't use together.

Drug-food. *Caffeine:* May increase amphetamine and related amine effects. Monitor patient closely.

Effect on lab test results

• May increase corticosteroid level.

Pharmacokinetics

Absorption: Rapid; for sustained-release capsules, more slowly.
Distribution: Wide.
Metabolism: Unknown.
Excretion: In urine. *Half-life:* 10 to 12 hours.

Route	Onset	Peak	Duration
P.O.	Unknown	Unknown	Unknown

Action

Chemical effect: Unknown; probably promotes nerve impulse transmission by releasing stored norepinephrine from nerve terminals in brain. Main sites of activity appear to be the cerebral cortex and reticular activating system.
Therapeutic effect: Helps prevent sleep and calms hyperactive children.

Available forms

Capsules (sustained-release): 5 mg, 10 mg, 15 mg
Tablets: 5 mg, 10 mg

NURSING PROCESS

Assessment

• Obtain history of patient's underlying condition before therapy, and reassess regularly throughout therapy.
• Obtain a detailed patient history, including a family history for mental disorders, family suicide, ventricular arrhythmias, or sudden death.
• Monitor for growth retardation in children.
• Be alert for adverse reactions and drug interactions.
• Monitor sleeping pattern, and observe patient for signs of excessive stimulation.

• Assess patient's and family's knowledge of drug therapy.

Nursing diagnoses

• Ineffective health maintenance related to underlying condition
• Insomnia related to adverse effect of drug
• Deficient knowledge related to drug therapy

Planning and implementation

• Give at least 6 hours before bedtime to avoid sleep interference.
• Prolonged use may cause psychological dependence or habituation, especially in patients with history of drug addiction. After prolonged use, reduce dose gradually to prevent acute rebound depression.

Patient teaching
ALERT: Warn patient that misuse of amphetamines can cause serious adverse cardiovascular events, including sudden death.
• Warn patient that drug may cause blurred vision or trouble focusing. Urge patient to use caution during activities that require a clear visual field.
• Tell parents that children may show increased aggression or hostility. Urge them to report worsening behavior.
• Tell patient to avoid drinks containing caffeine, which increases the effects of amphetamines and related amines.
• Inform patient that fatigue may result as drug effects wear off.
• Instruct patient to report signs of excessive stimulation.
• Inform patient that when tolerance to anorexigenic effect develops, he should stop the drug, not increase the dose. Tell him to report decreased effectiveness of drug. Warn patient against stopping drug abruptly.

Evaluation

• Patient shows improvement in underlying condition.
• Patient can sleep without difficulty.
• Patient and family state understanding of drug therapy.

HIGH ALERT!

diazepam
(digh-AZ-uh-pam)
Diastat, Diazemuls ♦, Diazepam Intensol, Novo-Dipam ♦, Valium⁄, Vivol ♦

Pharmacologic class: benzodiazepine
Therapeutic class: anxiolytic, skeletal muscle relaxant, anticonvulsant, sedative-hypnotic
Pregnancy risk category: D
Controlled substance schedule: IV

Indications and dosages

▶ **Anxiety.** *Adults:* Depending on severity, 2 to 10 mg P.O. b.i.d. to q.i.d. Or, 2 to 10 mg I.M. or I.V. every 3 to 4 hours, if needed.
Elderly patients: 2 to 2.5 mg P.O. once or twice daily; increase gradually, as needed.
Children age 6 months and older: 1 to 2.5 mg P.O. t.i.d. or q.i.d.; increase gradually, as needed and tolerated.

▶ **Acute alcohol withdrawal.** *Adults:* 10 mg P.O. t.i.d. or q.i.d. for the first 24 hours and reduce to 5 mg P.O. t.i.d. or q.i.d., as appropriate. Or, initially, 10 mg I.M. or I.V.; then 5 to 10 mg I.M. or I.V. in 3 to 4 hours, if needed.

▶ **Before endoscopic procedures.** *Adults:* Titrate I.V. dosage to desired sedative response (up to 20 mg). Or 5 to 10 mg I.M. 30 minutes before procedure.

▶ **Muscle spasm.** *Adults:* 2 to 10 mg P.O. b.i.d. to q.i.d. daily. Or 5 to 10 mg I.M. or I.V. initially; then 5 to 10 mg I.M. or I.V. in 3 to 4 hours, p.r.n. For tetanus, larger doses may be required.
Elderly patients: 2 to 2.5 mg I.M. or I.V. once or twice daily; increase as needed.
Children age 5 and older: 5 to 10 mg I.M. or I.V. every 3 to 4 hours, p.r.n.
Infants older than age 30 days and children younger than age 5: Give 1 to 2 mg I.M. or I.V. slowly repeated every 3 to 4 hours, as needed.

▶ **Preoperative sedation.** *Adults:* 10 mg I.M. (preferred) or I.V. before surgery.

▶ **Cardioversion.** *Adults:* 5 to 15 mg I.V. 5 to 10 minutes before procedure.

▶ **Adjunct in seizure disorders.** *Adults:* 2 to 10 mg P.O. b.i.d. to q.i.d.
Elderly patients: 2 to 2.5 mg P.O. once or twice daily; increase as needed.
Children and infants age 6 months and older: 1 to 2.5 mg P.O. t.i.d. or q.i.d. initially; increase as tolerated and needed.

▶ **Status epilepticus.** *Adults:* 5 to 10 mg I.V. (preferred) or I.M. initially. Repeat every 10 to 15 minutes, p.r.n, to maximum, 30 mg. Repeat in 2 to 4 hours, if needed.
Children age 5 and older: 1 mg I.V. every 2 to 5 minutes to maximum, 10 mg. Repeat in 2 to 4 hours, if needed.
Infants older than age 30 days and children younger than age 5: Give 0.2 to 0.5 mg I.V. slowly every 2 to 5 minutes to maximum, 5 mg. Repeat in 2 to 4 hours, if needed.

▶ **To control acute repetitive seizure activity in patients already taking anticonvulsants.**
Adults and children age 12 and older: 0.2 mg/kg P.R. using applicator. A second dose may be given 4 to 12 hours after the first dose, if needed.
Children ages 6 to 11: Give 0.3 mg/kg P.R. using applicator. A second dose may be given 4 to 12 hours after the first dose, if needed.
Children ages 2 to 5: Give 0.5 mg/kg P.R. using applicator. A second dose may be given 4 to 12 hours after the first dose, if needed.

▼ I.V. administration

• Give drug no faster than 5 mg/minute.
• Inject drug directly into vein. If this is impossible, inject slowly through infusion tubing as near to venous insertion site as possible. Watch closely for phlebitis at injection site.
• To avoid extravasation, don't inject into small veins.
• Monitor respirations every 5 to 15 minutes and before each I.V. dose. Have emergency resuscitation equipment and oxygen at bedside when giving drug I.V.
⊗ **Incompatibilities**
All other I.V. drugs, most I.V. solutions.

Contraindications and cautions

• Contraindicated in patients hypersensitive to drug or any of its components and in those with angle-closure glaucoma, shock, coma, or acute alcohol intoxication (parenteral form).
• Use cautiously in patients with hepatic or renal impairment, depression, or chronic open-angle glaucoma.
⚘ **Lifespan:** In pregnant women (especially during the first trimester) and in breast-feeding women, avoid using the drug. In infants younger than age 6 months, oral form of drug is contraindicated. Safety and efficacy of parenteral form in neonates younger than 30 days haven't been

established. In elderly and debilitated patients, use cautiously and give smallest effective dose because these patients may be more susceptible to adverse CNS effects of drug.

Adverse reactions

CNS: anterograde amnesia, *ataxia,* depression, *drowsiness,* fainting, *hangover,* headache, insomnia, *lethargy, pain,* psychosis, restlessness, slurred speech, tremors.
CV: *bradycardia, CV collapse,* transient hypotension.
EENT: blurred vision, diplopia, nystagmus.
GI: abdominal discomfort, constipation, nausea, vomiting.
GU: incontinence, urine retention.
Respiratory: *respiratory depression.*
Skin: desquamation, rash, urticaria.
Other: *acute withdrawal syndrome* after stopping drug suddenly in physically dependent person, *phlebitis at injection site,* physical or psychological dependence.

Interactions

Drug-drug. *Cimetidine:* May increase sedation. Monitor patient carefully.
CNS depressants: May increase CNS depression. Avoid use together.
Digoxin: May increase digoxin level and toxicity. Monitor digoxin level.
Diltiazem: May increase CNS depression and prolong effects of diazepam. Use lower dose of diazepam.
Fluconazole, itraconazole, ketoconazole, miconazole: May increase and prolong diazepam level, CNS depression, and psychomotor impairment. Don't use together.
Phenobarbital: May increase effects of both drugs. Use together cautiously.
Phenytoin: May increase level of phenytoin. Monitor patient for toxicity.
Ranitidine: May decrease absorption. Monitor patient for decreased effect.
Drug-herb. *Kava, sassafras, valerian:* Sedative effects may be enhanced. Discourage use together.
St. John's wort: May decrease drug effects. Discourage use together.
Drug-food. *Grapefruit juice:* May increase sedative effects. Advise patient to take with a beverage other than grapefruit juice.

Drug-lifestyle. *Alcohol use:* May cause additive CNS effects. Strongly discourage use of alcohol with these drugs.
Smoking: May increase benzodiazepine clearance. Monitor patient for lack of drug effect.

Effects on lab test results

• May increase liver function test values. May decrease neutrophil count.

Pharmacokinetics

Absorption: For I.M. use, erratic.
Distribution: Wide. About 85% to 95% bound to plasma protein.
Metabolism: In liver to active metabolite, desmethyldiazepam.
Excretion: Most metabolites in urine, with small amount in feces. *Half-life:* About 1 to 12 days.

Route	Onset	Peak	Duration
P.O.	30 min	½–2 hr	3–8 hr
I.V.	1–5 min	≤ 15 min	15–60 min
I.M.	Unknown	2 hr	Unknown
P.R.	Unknown	1–5 hr	Unknown

Action

Chemical effect: May depress CNS at limbic and subcortical levels of brain; suppresses spread of seizure activity produced by epileptogenic foci in cortex, thalamus, and limbic system.
Therapeutic effect: Relieves anxiety, muscle spasms, and seizures (parenteral form); promotes calmness and sleep.

Available forms

Injection: 5 mg/ml
Oral solution: 5 mg/ml, 5 mg/5 ml
Rectal gel: 2.5 mg*, 5 mg*, 10 mg*, 15 mg*, 20 mg*
Sterile emulsion for injection: 5 mg/ml*
Tablets: 2 mg, 5 mg, 10 mg

NURSING PROCESS

✍ Assessment

• Obtain history of patient's underlying condition before therapy, and reassess regularly thereafter.
• Periodically monitor liver, kidney, and hematopoietic function studies in patient receiving repeated or prolonged therapy.
• Look for adverse reactions and drug interactions.

- Assess patient's and family's knowledge of drug therapy.

🔶 Nursing diagnoses
- Ineffective health maintenance related to underlying condition
- Risk for injury related to drug-induced adverse CNS reactions
- Deficient knowledge related to drug therapy

▶ Planning and implementation
- When oral concentrate solution is used, dilute dose just before giving. Use water, juice, or carbonated beverages, or mix with semisolid food such as applesauce or pudding.
- Avoid P.R. use of Diastat for more than 5 episodes per month or one episode every 5 days.
- ⓘ ALERT: Drug should be given only by caregivers who can distinguish the distinct cluster of seizures or events from the patient's ordinary seizure activity, who can give the drug competently, who understand which seizure characteristics can be treated with drug, and who can monitor the patient's response and recognize when immediate professional help is needed.
- Give drug I.M. only when giving I.V. or P.O. isn't possible because absorption is variable and injection is painful.
- Don't mix injectable form with other drugs because diazepam is incompatible with most drugs.
- Don't store parenteral solution in plastic syringes.
- Parenteral emulsion—a stabilized oil-in-water emulsion—should appear milky white and uniform. Avoid mixing with any other drugs or solutions, and avoid infusion sets or containers made from polyvinyl chloride. If diluting, mix drug with I.V. fat emulsion. Use admixture within 6 hours.
- Possibility of abuse and addiction exists. Don't withdraw drug abruptly after long-term use. Withdrawal symptoms may occur.
- ⓘ ALERT: Don't confuse diazepam with diazoxide.

Patient teaching
- Warn patient to avoid hazardous activities until the drug's CNS effects are known.
- Tell patient to avoid using alcohol during therapy.
- Warn patient to take drug only as directed and not to stop it without prescriber's approval.

- Warn patient about risk of physical and psychological dependence.

☑ Evaluation
- Patient shows improvement in underlying condition.
- Patient has no injury as result of drug-induced adverse CNS reactions.
- Patient and family state understanding of drug therapy.

diclofenac epolamine
(digh-KLOH-fen-ek)
Flector Patch

diclofenac potassium
Cataflam

diclofenac sodium
Novo-Difenac ◆ , Nu-Diclo ◆ , Pennsaid ◆ , Solaraze, Voltaren, Voltaren SR ◆ , Voltaren-XR

Pharmacologic class: NSAID
Therapeutic class: antiarthritic, anti-inflammatory
Pregnancy risk category: B

Indications and dosages
▶ **Ankylosing spondylitis.** *Adults:* 25-mg delayed-release tablets P.O. q.i.d. (may give another 25 mg at bedtime, if needed). Or, 50 mg potassium form P.O. b.i.d.
▶ **Osteoarthritis.** *Adults:* 50-mg immediate- or delayed-release tablets P.O. b.i.d. or t.i.d. Or, 75 mg P.O. b.i.d. Or, 100-mg extended-release tablets P.O. daily. Or, using dosing card to measure gel, apply 4 g to affected foot, knee, or ankle q.i.d.; massage into skin ensuring application to entire joint. Don't apply more than 16 g/day to lower limbs. For elbows, wrists, and hands, apply 2 g to affected joint q.i.d. Don't apply more than 8 g/day to upper limbs. Don't exceed 32 g per day total.
▶ **Rheumatoid arthritis.** *Adults:* 50-mg immediate- or delayed-release tablets P.O. t.i.d. or q.i.d. Or, 75 mg P.O. b.i.d. Or 50 to 100 mg P.R. (where available) at bedtime as substitute for last P.O. dose of day. Not to exceed 225 mg daily. Or 100-mg extended-release tablets P.O. daily or b.i.d.

▶ **Analgesia and primary dysmenorrhea.**
Adults: 50 mg potassium form P.O. t.i.d. If needed, 100 mg may be given for first dose only. Maximum total daily dose is 150 mg.
▶ **Actinic keratosis.** *Adults:* Apply gel to lesion b.i.d.
▶ **Acute pain associated with minor strains, sprains, and contusions.** *Adults:* 1 patch to the painful area b.i.d.
▶ **Postoperative ocular inflammation.** *Adults:* Instill 1 drop q.i.d., beginning 24 hours after surgery for 2 weeks.
▶ **Ocular pain and photophobia.** *Adults:* Instill 1 or 2 drops q.i.d. for up to 3 days.

Contraindications and cautions

● Contraindicated in patients hypersensitive to drug or any of its components and in those with hepatic porphyria or a history of asthma, urticaria, or other allergic reactions after taking aspirin or other NSAIDs. Also contraindicated for treatment of perioperative pain in patients undergoing CABG surgery.
● Use cautiously in patients with history of peptic ulcer disease, hepatic dysfunction, cardiac disease, hypertension, conditions that cause fluid retention, or impaired kidney function.
⚖ **Lifespan:** For women in late pregnancy or who are breast-feeding, drug isn't recommended. In children, safety and effectiveness haven't been established.

Adverse reactions

CNS: anxiety, depression, dizziness, drowsiness, headache, insomnia, irritability, migraine, myoclonus.
CV: edema, fluid retention, *heart failure,* hypertension.
EENT: blurred vision, epistaxis, eye pain, *laryngeal edema,* night blindness, reversible hearing loss, swelling of lips and tongue, tinnitus.
GI: abdominal distention, *abdominal pain or cramps,* appetite change, *bleeding,* bloody diarrhea, colitis, *constipation, diarrhea,* flatulence, *indigestion,* melena, *nausea,* peptic ulceration, taste disorder.
GU: *acute renal failure,* azotemia, *fluid retention,* interstitial nephritis, nephrotic syndrome, *oliguria,* papillary necrosis, proteinuria.
Hepatic: *hepatitis, hepatotoxicity,* jaundice.
Metabolic: hyperglycemia, *hypoglycemia.*
Musculoskeletal: back, leg, or joint pain.

Respiratory: *asthma.*
Skin: allergic purpura, alopecia, bullous eruption, dermatitis, eczema, photosensitivity, pruritus, rash, *Stevens-Johnson syndrome,* urticaria.
Other: *anaphylaxis, angioedema.*

Interactions

Drug-drug. *Anticoagulants, including warfarin:* May increase risk of bleeding. Monitor patient closely for bleeding.
Aspirin: May increase risk of bleeding. Don't use together.
Beta blockers: Antihypertensive effect of beta blocker may be blunted. Monitor blood pressure closely.
Cyclosporine, digoxin, lithium, methotrexate: May reduce renal clearance of these drugs and increase risk of toxicity. Monitor patient closely; monitor drug levels if appropriate.
Diuretics: May decrease diuretic effectiveness. Monitor patient for fluid retention.
Insulin, oral antidiabetics: May alter antidiabetic requirement. Monitor glucose level.
Potassium-sparing diuretics: May enhance potassium retention and increases potassium levels. Monitor patient for hyperkalemia.
Drug-herb. *Dong quai, feverfew, garlic, ginger, horse chestnut, red clover:* May increase risk of bleeding. Discourage use together.
St. John's wort: May increase risk of photosensitivity. Advise against unprotected and prolonged exposure to sunlight.
Drug-lifestyle. *Sun exposure:* May cause photosensitivity reactions. Urge patient to wear protective clothing and sunblock.

Effects on lab test results

● May increase ALT, AST, alkaline phosphatase, bilirubin, BUN, creatinine, and LDH levels.
● May increase or decrease glucose level.

Pharmacokinetics

Absorption: Rapid and almost complete. Delayed by food.
Distribution: Almost 100% protein-bound.
Metabolism: Undergoes first-pass metabolism, with 60% of unchanged drug reaching systemic circulation.
Excretion: About 40% to 60% in urine; balance in bile. *Half-life:* 1 to 2 hours; 12 hours (transdermal patch).

Reactions may be *common,* uncommon, *life-threatening,* or COMMON AND LIFE-THREATENING.

Route	Onset	Peak	Duration
P.O., P.R.	30 min	Unknown	8 hr
P.O. enteric-coated	30 min	2–3 hr	8 hr
Topical	Unknown	Unknown	Unknown
Transdermal	Unknown	10–20 hr	Unknown

Action

Chemical effect: Produces anti-inflammatory, analgesic, and antipyretic effects, possibly by inhibiting prostaglandin synthesis.

Therapeutic effect: Relieves inflammation, pain, and fever.

Available forms

diclofenac epolamine
Topical patch: 180 mg
diclofenac potassium
Tablets: 50 mg
diclofenac sodium
Gel: 1%, 1.5% ◆, 3%
Ophthalmic solution: 0.1%
Suppositories: 50 mg ◆, 100 mg ◆
Tablets (delayed-release, enteric-coated): 25 mg, 50 mg, 75 mg
Tablets (extended-release): 100 mg ◆

NURSING PROCESS

Assessment
- Obtain history of patient's underlying condition before therapy.
- Monitor effectiveness by assessing patient for pain relief.
- Liver enzyme level may elevate. Monitor transaminase level, especially ALT level, periodically in a patient undergoing long-term therapy. Take first level within the first 8 weeks of therapy.
- Look for adverse reactions and drug interactions.
- Assess patient's and family's knowledge of drug therapy.

Nursing diagnoses
- Acute pain related to underlying condition
- Risk for injury related to drug-induced adverse reactions
- Deficient knowledge related to drug therapy

Planning and implementation

ALERT: NSAIDs may cause an increased risk of serious or fatal CV thrombotic events, including MI and stroke.

ALERT: NSAIDs increase the risk of serious GI adverse events, including inflammation, bleeding, ulceration, and perforation, which can be fatal.

- If drug causes GI distress. Give with milk or food.
- Notify prescriber immediately if patient develops signs of GI bleeding, hepatotoxicity, or other adverse reactions.
- The sodium and potassium preparations may not be bioequivalent.
- Rectal preparation isn't commercially available in the United States. Elsewhere, it may be substituted for the last oral dose of the day to decrease GI distress if can't take with food.
- The patch shouldn't be applied to non-intact skin or worn when bathing or showering.

Patient teaching
- Tell patient to take drug with milk or food to minimize GI distress.
- Instruct patient not to crush, break, or chew enteric-coated tablets.
- Tell patient not to apply patch to damaged or non-intact skin.
- Advise patient to remove patch before bathing or showering.
- Tell patient to avoid bathing or showering for 1 hour after applying gel and to wait at least 10 minutes before covering area with clothing.
- Instruct patient to wash his hands after applying gel, unless the hands are being treated.
- Teach patient signs and symptoms of GI bleeding, and tell him to contact prescriber immediately if they occur.
- Teach patient signs and symptoms of hepatotoxicity, including nausea, fatigue, lethargy, pruritus, jaundice, right upper quadrant tenderness, and flulike symptoms. Tell him to contact prescriber immediately if these symptoms appear.

Evaluation
- Patient is free from pain.
- Patient has no injury as result of drug-induced adverse reactions.
- Patient and family state understanding of drug therapy.

dicyclomine hydrochloride
(digh-SIGH-kloh-meen high-droh-KLOR-ighd)
Bentyl, Bentylol ♦, Byclomine, Dibent,
Dilomine, Di-Spaz, Formulex ♦, Lomine ♦,
Or-Tyl

Pharmacologic class: anticholinergic
Therapeutic class: antimuscarinic, GI antispasmodic
Pregnancy risk category: B

Indications and dosages

▶ **Irritable bowel syndrome and other functional GI disorders.** *Adults:* Initially, 20 mg P.O. q.i.d.; increase to 40 mg q.i.d. Or 80 mg I.M. daily in four divided doses.
Children age 2 and older: 10 mg P.O. t.i.d. or q.i.d.
Infants ages 6 months to 2 years: 5 to 10 mg P.O. t.i.d. or q.i.d.
▶ **Colic‡.** *Infants age 6 months and older:* 5 to 10 mg P.O. t.i.d. or q.i.d. Adjust dosage according to patient's needs and response.

Contraindications and cautions

• Contraindicated in patients hypersensitive to anticholinergics and in those with obstructive uropathy, obstructive disease of GI tract, reflux esophagitis, severe ulcerative colitis, myasthenia gravis, unstable CV status in acute hemorrhage, or glaucoma.
• Use cautiously in patients with autonomic neuropathy, hyperthyroidism, coronary artery disease, arrhythmias, heart failure, hypertension, hiatal hernia, hepatic or renal disease, prostatic hypertrophy, or ulcerative colitis.
⚠ Lifespan: In pregnant women, use cautiously. In breast-feeding women and in infants younger than age 6 months, drug is contraindicated.

Adverse reactions

CNS: *dizziness;* drowsiness; fever; *headache;* insomnia; nervousness, confusion, and excitement in elderly patients.
CV: *palpitations,* tachycardia.
EENT: blurred vision, increased intraocular pressure, mydriasis.
GI: abdominal distention, *constipation, dry mouth,* heartburn, nausea, paralytic ileus, vomiting.

GU: impotence, urinary hesitancy, urine retention.
Skin: decreased sweating or possibly anhidrosis, other dermal changes, urticaria.
Other: allergic reactions.

Interactions

Drug-drug. *Amantadine, antihistamines, antiparkinsonians, disopyramide, glutethimide, MAO inhibitors, meperidine, phenothiazines, procainamide, quinidine, tricyclic antidepressants:* May cause additive adverse effects. Avoid use together.
Antacids: May decrease absorption of oral anticholinergics. Separate doses by 2 to 3 hours.
Ketoconazole: May interfere with ketoconazole absorption. Give at least 2 hours after ketoconazole.

Effects on lab test results

None reported.

Pharmacokinetics

Absorption: 67% of P.O. dose.
Distribution: Extensive in tissue.
Metabolism: Unknown.
Excretion: 80% of P.O. dose in urine and 10% in feces. *Half-life:* Initial, about 2 hours; secondary, 9 to 10 hours.

Route	Onset	Peak	Duration
P.O.	Unknown	1–1½ hr	Unknown
I.M.	Unknown	Unknown	Unknown

Action

Chemical effect: Appears to exert nonspecific, indirect spasmolytic action on smooth muscle. Also possesses local anesthetic properties that may be partly responsible for spasmolysis.
Therapeutic effect: Relieves GI spasms.

Available forms

Capsules: 10 mg, 20 mg
Injection: 10 mg/ml
Syrup: 10 mg/5 ml
Tablets: 20 mg

NURSING PROCESS

Assessment
• Obtain history of patient's underlying condition before therapy.

- Monitor the drug's effectiveness by regularly assessing patient for pain relief and improvement of underlying condition.
- Look for adverse reactions and drug interactions.
- Assess patient's and family's knowledge of drug therapy.

🔲 Nursing diagnoses
- Acute pain related to underlying condition
- Risk for injury related to drug-induced adverse CNS reactions
- Deficient knowledge related to drug therapy

▷ Planning and implementation
- Drug is synthetic tertiary derivative that may cause atropine-like adverse reactions. Overdose may cause curare-like effects, such as respiratory paralysis.
- High environmental temperatures may induce heatstroke during drug use. If symptoms occur, stop giving the drug.
- Give 30 to 60 minutes before meals and at bedtime. Bedtime dose can be larger; give at least 2 hours after last meal of the day.
- ⓘ **ALERT:** Don't give drug subcutaneously or I.V.
- Adjust dosage according to patient's needs and response. Up to 40 mg P.O. q.i.d. may be used in adults, but safety and effectiveness for more than 2 weeks haven't been established.
- ⓘ **ALERT:** The dicyclomine label may be misleading. The ampule label reads 10 mg/ml, but doesn't indicate that the ampule contains 2 ml of solution (20 mg of drug).
- ⓘ **ALERT:** Don't confuse dicyclomine with dyclonine or doxycycline; don't confuse Bentyl with Aventyl or Benadryl.

Patient teaching
- Instruct patient to refrain from driving and performing other hazardous activities if he's drowsy or dizzy or has blurred vision.
- Tell him to drink plenty of fluids to help prevent constipation.
- Urge patient to report rash or skin eruption.
- Tell patient to use sugarless gum or hard candy to relieve dry mouth.

✔ Evaluation
- Patient is free from pain.
- Patient doesn't experience injury as a result of drug-induced adverse CNS reactions.
- Patient and family state understanding of drug therapy.

didanosine (ddI)
(digh-DAN-uh-zeen)
Videx, Videx EC

Pharmacologic class: nucleoside reverse transcriptase inhibitor
Therapeutic class: antiretroviral
Pregnancy risk category: B

Indications and dosages

▶ **HIV infection.** *Adults weighing 60 kg (132 lb) and more:* 200 mg tablet or 250 mg powder form P.O. b.i.d., or 400 mg delayed-release form P.O. daily.
Adults weighing less than 60 kg: 125 mg tablet or 167 mg powder form P.O. b.i.d. or 250 mg delayed-release form P.O. daily.
Children older than age 8 months: 120 mg/m² P.O. b.i.d.
Children ages 2 weeks to 8 months: 100 mg/m² P.O. b.i.d.
🔲 **Adjust-a-dose:** In adults who weigh 60 kg or more with creatinine clearance of 30 to 59 ml/minute, give 200 mg once daily. For clearance of 10 to 29 ml/minute, give 125-mg delayed-release capsule once daily. For clearance less than 10 ml/minute, give 125-mg delayed-release capsule once daily.
   In adults who weigh less than 60 kg and have a clearance of 10 to 59 ml/minute, give 125-mg delayed-release capsule once daily. For clearance less than 10 ml/minute or patients on dialysis, give alternate form. No additional dose is needed after hemodialysis.
▶ **Postexposure prevention following occupational or nonoccupational exposure to HIV, with other antiretrovirals‡.** *Adults weighing 60 kg or more:* 400 mg P.O. once daily or divided b.i.d. for 4 weeks.
Adults weighing less than 60 kg: 250 mg P.O. once daily or divided b.i.d. for 4 weeks.

Contraindications and cautions

- Contraindicated in patients hypersensitive to drug or any of its components.
- Use cautiously in patients with a history of pancreatitis and in patients with peripheral neuropathy, renal or hepatic impairment, or hyperuricemia.

⚖ **Lifespan:** In pregnant women, use cautiously. In breast-feeding women, drug isn't recommended.

Adverse reactions

CNS: abnormal thinking, asthenia, anxiety, confusion, depression, *dizziness, fever, headache,* hypertonia, insomnia, nervousness, pain, *peripheral neuropathy,* **seizures,** twitching.

CV: edema, **heart failure,** hyperlipidemia, hypertension.

GI: abdominal pain, diarrhea, dry mouth, dyspepsia, flatulence, nausea, **pancreatitis,** vomiting.

Hematologic: anemia, **leukopenia, thrombocytopenia.**

Hepatic: **hepatic failure,** liver abnormalities, **severe hepatomegaly.**

Metabolic: lactic acidosis.

Musculoskeletal: arthritis, myalgia, myopathy, **rhabdomyolysis.**

Respiratory: cough, dyspnea, pneumonia.

Skin: alopecia, pruritus, rash.

Other: **anaphylactoid reaction,** chills, infection, sarcoma.

Interactions

Drug-drug. *Amprenavir, delavirdine, indinavir, nelfinavir, ritonavir, saquinavir:* May alter pharmacokinetics. Separate doses.

Antacids containing magnesium or aluminum hydroxides: Enhances adverse effects of antacid component (including diarrhea or constipation). Avoid use together.

Dapsone, ketoconazole, drugs that require gastric acid for adequate absorption: May decrease absorption from buffering action. Give these drugs 2 hours before didanosine.

Fluoroquinolones, tetracyclines: May decrease absorption because of buffers in didanosine antacids in pediatric solution. Monitor patient for decreased effectiveness.

Itraconazole: May decrease levels of itraconazole. Avoid use together.

Tenofovir: May cause high rate of early virologic failure and emerging resistance. Don't use together. Switch patients currently on this regimen to eliminate tenofovir.

Drug-food. *Any food:* May increase rate of absorption. Give drug on an empty stomach.

Drug-herb. *St. John's wort:* May decrease drug levels, decreasing therapeutic effect. Discourage use together.

Effects on lab test results

• May increase uric acid, AST, ALT, alkaline phosphatase, and bilirubin levels. May decrease hemoglobin level and hematocrit.

• May decrease WBC, granulocyte, and platelet counts.

Pharmacokinetics

Absorption: Rapid. Commercially available forms contain buffers to raise stomach pH. Bioavailability averages 33%. Food decreases absorption by 50%.

Distribution: Wide. Drug penetration into CNS varies, but CSF levels average 46% of concurrent plasma levels in children and 21% in adults.

Metabolism: Probably similar to that of endogenous purines.

Excretion: In urine. *Half-life:* 48 minutes; half-life increases as creatinine clearance decreases.

Route	Onset	Peak	Duration
P.O.	Unknown	30–60 min	Unknown

Action

Chemical effect: Unknown; appears to inhibit replication of HIV by preventing DNA replication.

Therapeutic effect: Inhibits replication of HIV.

Available forms

Capsules (delayed-release): 125 mg, 200 mg, 250 mg, 400 mg

Powder for oral solution (pediatric): 10 mg/ml in 2- and 4-g bottles

NURSING PROCESS

📋 **Assessment**

• Obtain history of patient's underlying condition before therapy, and reassess regularly thereafter.

• Be alert for adverse reactions and drug interactions.

• Assess patient's and family's knowledge of drug therapy.

⊕ **Nursing diagnoses**

• Ineffective protection related to presence of HIV infection

• Diarrhea related to drug-induced adverse effect on bowel

• Deficient knowledge related to drug therapy

Reactions may be *common*, uncommon, *life-threatening*, or COMMON AND LIFE-THREATENING.

▶ Planning and implementation
• Give drug on empty stomach at least 30 minutes before or 2 hours after meals, regardless of dosage form used, because giving drug with meals can decrease absorption by 50%.
• Pharmacist must prepare pediatric powder for oral solution to a final concentration of 10 mg/ml. The solution is stable for 30 days if refrigerated. Shake well before measuring dose.
• If pancreatitis is suspected, stop drug and don't continue until pancreatitis is ruled out.

Patient teaching
• Tell patient to take drug on an empty stomach and to drink at least 1 oz (30 ml) water with each dose.
• Instruct patient not to crush or break capsules.
• Explain the importance of complying with drug regimen for treatment of HIV infection.
• Warn patient about adverse CNS reactions, and tell patient to take safety precautions.
• Tell patient to notify prescriber if adverse GI reaction occurs.

☑ Evaluation
• Patient improves with therapy.
• Patient regains normal bowel pattern.
• Patient and family state understanding of drug therapy.

diflunisal
(digh-FLOO-neh-sol)
Dolobid

Pharmacologic class: NSAID
Therapeutic class: analgesic, anti-inflammatory
Pregnancy risk category: C

Indications and dosages
▶ **Mild to moderate pain.** *Adults:* Initially, 500 mg to 1 g P.O., followed by 250 to 500 mg every 8 to 12 hours.
▶ **Osteoarthritis, rheumatoid arthritis.**
Adults: 500 mg to 1 g P.O. daily in two divided doses, usually every 12 hours. Maximum, 1,500 mg daily.
⚠ **Adjust-a-dose:** For patients older than age 65, give half the usual adult dose.

Contraindications and cautions
• Contraindicated in patients hypersensitive to drug or any of its components and in those who develop acute asthmatic attacks, urticaria, or rhinitis after taking aspirin or other NSAIDs.
• Use cautiously in patients with GI bleeding, history of peptic ulcer disease, renal impairment, compromised cardiac function, hypertension, or other conditions predisposing patient to fluid retention.
⚠ **Lifespan:** In breast-feeding women, drug isn't recommended. In children and teenagers with chickenpox or flulike illness, salicylates aren't recommended because of epidemiologic connection to Reye syndrome.

Adverse reactions
CNS: *dizziness,* fatigue, *headache,* insomnia, somnolence.
EENT: *tinnitus,* visual disturbances.
GI: constipation, *diarrhea, dyspepsia,* flatulence, *GI pain, nausea,* vomiting.
GU: hematuria, interstitial nephritis, renal impairment.
Skin: *erythema multiforme,* pruritus, rash, *Stevens-Johnson syndrome,* stomatitis, sweating.
Other: dry mucous membranes.

Interactions
Drug-drug. *Acetaminophen, hydrochlorothiazide, indomethacin, lithium:* May substantially increase levels of these drugs, increasing risk of toxicity. Avoid use together, or monitor patient closely.
Antacids: May decrease diflunisal level. Monitor patient for decreased therapeutic effect.
Aspirin: May increase adverse effects. Monitor patient closely.
Cyclosporine: May increase nephrotoxicity of cyclosporine. Avoid use together.
Methotrexate: May increase toxicity of methotrexate. Avoid use together.
Oral anticoagulants, thrombolytics: May enhance effects of these drugs. Use together cautiously.
Sulindac: May decrease level of sulindac's active metabolite. Monitor patient for decreased effect.
Drug-herb. *Dong quai, feverfew, garlic, ginger, horse chestnut, red clover:* May increase risk of bleeding. Discourage use together.

Effect on lab test results
• May falsely elevate salicylate levels.

Pharmacokinetics
Absorption: Rapid and complete.
Distribution: Highly protein-bound.
Metabolism: In liver.
Excretion: In urine. *Half-life:* 8 to 12 hours.

Route	Onset	Peak	Duration
P.O.	1 hr	2–3 hr	8–12 hr

Action
Chemical effect: May inhibit prostaglandin synthesis.
Therapeutic effect: Relieves inflammation and pain; reduces body temperature.

Available forms
Tablets: 250 mg, 500 mg

NURSING PROCESS

⚡ Assessment
• Obtain history of patient's underlying condition before therapy, and reassess regularly thereafter.
• Look for adverse reactions and drug interactions.
• Assess patient's and family's knowledge of drug therapy.

⊕ Nursing diagnoses
• Acute pain related to underlying condition
• Risk for deficient fluid volume related to drug-induced adverse reactions
• Deficient knowledge related to drug therapy

▶ Planning and implementation
• Give drug with milk or food to minimize adverse GI reactions.
• **ALERT:** Don't confuse Dolobid with Slo-bid.
Patient teaching
• Advise patient to take with water, milk, or meals.
• Warn patient to avoid drug interactions by checking with prescriber or pharmacist before taking OTC drugs or herbal remedies, such as those containing aspirin or salicylates.

✓ Evaluation
• Patient is free from pain.

• Patient maintains adequate hydration throughout therapy.
• Patient and family state understanding of drug therapy.

HIGH ALERT!

digoxin
(dih-JOKS-in)
Digitek, Digoxin, Lanoxicaps, Lanoxin*

Pharmacologic class: cardiac glycoside
Therapeutic class: antiarrhythmic, inotropic
Pregnancy risk category: C

Indications and dosages

▶ **Heart failure, paroxysmal supraventricular tachycardia, atrial fibrillation and flutter.**
Tablets, elixir
Adults: For rapid digitalization, give 0.75 to 1.25 mg P.O. over 24 hours in two or more divided doses every 6 to 8 hours. For slow digitalization, give 0.125 to 0.5 mg daily for 5 to 7 days. Maintenance dose is 0.125 to 0.5 mg daily.
Children age 10 and older: 10 to 15 mcg/kg P.O. over 24 hours in two or more divided doses every 6 to 8 hours. Maintenance dose is 25% to 35% of total digitalizing dose.
Children ages 5 to 10: Give 20 to 35 mcg/kg P.O. over 24 hours in two or more divided doses every 6 to 8 hours. Maintenance dose is 25% to 35% of total digitalizing dose.
Children ages 2 to 5: Give 30 to 40 mcg/kg P.O. over 24 hours in two or more divided doses every 6 to 8 hours. Maintenance dose is 25% to 35% of total digitalizing dose.
Infants ages 1 month to 2 years: 35 to 60 mcg/kg P.O. over 24 hours in two or more divided doses every 6 to 8 hours. Maintenance dose is 25% to 35% of total digitalizing dose.
Neonates: 25 to 35 mcg/kg P.O. over 24 hours in two or more divided doses every 6 to 8 hours. Maintenance dose is 25% to 35% of total digitalizing dose.
Preterm infants: 20 to 30 mcg/kg P.O. over 24 hours in two or more divided doses every 6 to 8 hours. Maintenance dose is 20% to 30% of total digitalizing dose.
Capsules
Adults: For rapid digitalization, give 0.4 to 0.6 mg P.O. initially, followed by 0.1 to 0.3 mg every 6 to 8 hours, as needed and tolerated, for

24 hours. For slow digitalization, give 0.05 to 0.35 mg daily in two divided doses for 7 to 22 days until therapeutic levels are reached. Maintenance dose is 0.05 to 0.35 mg daily in one or two divided doses.

Adjust-a-dose: In children, digitalizing dose is based on child's age and is given in three or more divided doses over the first 24 hours. First dose is 50% of the total dose; subsequent doses are given every 4 to 8 hours as needed and tolerated.

Children age 10 and older: For rapid digitalization, give 8 to 12 mcg/kg P.O. over 24 hours, divided as above. Maintenance dose is 25% to 35% of total digitalizing dose, given daily as a single dose.

Children ages 5 to 10: For rapid digitalization, give 15 to 30 mcg/kg P.O. over 24 hours, divided as above. Maintenance dose is 25% to 35% of total digitalizing dose, divided and given in two or three equal portions daily.

Children ages 2 to 5: For rapid digitalization, give 25 to 35 mcg/kg P.O. over 24 hours, divided as above. Maintenance dose is 25% to 35% of total digitalizing dose, divided and given in two or three equal portions daily.

Injection

Adults: For rapid digitalization, give 0.4 to 0.6 mg I.V. initially, followed by 0.1 to 0.3 mg I.V. every 4 to 8 hours, as needed and tolerated, for 24 hours. For slow digitalization, give appropriate daily maintenance dose for 7 to 22 days as needed until therapeutic levels are reached. Maintenance dose is 0.125 to 0.5 mg I.V. daily in one or two divided doses.

Children: Digitalizing dose is based on child's age and is given in three or more divided doses over the first 24 hours. First dose is 50% of total dose; subsequent doses are given every 4 to 8 hours as needed and tolerated.

Children age 10 and older: For rapid digitalization, give 8 to 12 mcg/kg I.V. over 24 hours, divided as above. Maintenance dose is 25% to 35% of total digitalizing dose, given daily as a single dose.

Children ages 5 to 10: For rapid digitalization, give 15 to 30 mcg/kg I.V. over 24 hours, divided as above. Maintenance dose is 25% to 35% of total digitalizing dose, divided and given in two or three equal portions daily.

Children ages 2 to 5: For rapid digitalization, give 25 to 35 mcg/kg I.V. over 24 hours, divided as above. Maintenance dose is 25% to 35% of

total digitalizing dose, divided and given in two or three equal portions daily.

Infants ages 1 month to 2 years: For rapid digitalization, give 30 to 50 mcg/kg I.V. over 24 hours, divided as above. Maintenance dose is 25% to 35% of total digitalizing dose, divided and given in two or three equal portions daily.

Neonates: For rapid digitalization, give 20 to 30 mcg/kg I.V. over 24 hours, divided as above. Maintenance dose is 25% to 35% of the total digitalizing dose, divided and given in two or three equal portions daily.

Preterm infants: For rapid digitalization, give 15 to 25 mcg/kg I.V. over 24 hours, divided as above. Maintenance dose is 20% to 30% of the total digitalizing dose, divided and given in two or three equal portions daily.

Adjust-a-dose: In all dosage forms, give smaller loading and maintenance doses to patients with impaired renal function.

For patients with renal impairment, decrease dosage. For patients with hyperthyroidism, may need to increase dosage.

I.V. administration

• Dilute fourfold with D_5W, normal saline solution, or sterile water for injection to reduce the chance of precipitation.
• Infuse drug slowly over at least 5 minutes.
• Protect prepared drug from light.
⊗ **Incompatibilities**
Amiodarone, dobutamine, doxapram, drugs or solutions given through the same I.V. line, fluconazole, foscarnet, other I.V. drugs, propofol.

Contraindications and cautions

• Contraindicated in patients hypersensitive to the drug or any of its components and in those with digoxin-induced toxicity, ventricular fibrillation, or ventricular tachycardia unless caused by heart failure.
• Use cautiously in patients with acute MI, incomplete AV block, sinus bradycardia, PVCs, chronic constrictive pericarditis, hypertrophic cardiomyopathy, renal insufficiency, severe pulmonary disease, or hypothyroidism.
Lifespan: In pregnant women, use cautiously. In breast-feeding women, use cautiously; it's unknown if the drug appears in breast milk. In elderly patients, use cautiously.

Adverse reactions

CNS: agitation, dizziness, fatigue, generalized muscle weakness, hallucinations, headache, malaise, paresthesia, stupor, vertigo.
CV: *arrhythmias, heart failure,* hypotension.
EENT: blurred vision, diplopia, light flashes, photophobia, yellow-green halos around visual images.
GI: anorexia, diarrhea, nausea, vomiting.

Interactions

Drug-drug. *Amiloride:* May inhibit digoxin effect and increase digoxin excretion. Monitor patient for altered digoxin effect.
Amiodarone, diltiazem, nifedipine, quinidine, rifampin, verapamil: May increase digoxin level. Monitor patient for digoxin toxicity.
Amphotericin B, carbenicillin, corticosteroids, diuretics (including loop diuretics, chlorthalidone, metolazone, and thiazides), ticarcillin: May decrease potassium level, predisposing patient to digoxin toxicity. Monitor potassium levels.
Antacids, kaolin-pectin: May decrease digoxin absorption. Schedule doses as far as possible from P.O. digoxin administration.
Cholestyramine, colestipol, metoclopramide: May decrease absorption of P.O. digoxin. Monitor patient for decreased effect and low blood levels. Increase dosage.
Parenteral calcium, thiazides: May increase calcium level and decrease magnesium level, predisposing patient to digoxin toxicity. Monitor calcium and magnesium levels.
Drug-herb. *Betel palm, fumitory, goldenseal, lily of the valley, motherwort, rue, shepherd's purse:* May increase cardiac effect. Discourage use together.
Horsetail, licorice: May deplete potassium stores, leading to digoxin toxicity. Monitor potassium level closely.
Oleander, Siberian ginseng, squill: May enhance toxicity. Discourage use together.
St. John's wort: May reduce therapeutic effect of digoxin, requiring an increased dosage. Monitor patient for loss of therapeutic effect, and advise patient to avoid this herb.
Drug-lifestyle. *Alcohol use:* May increase CNS effects. Discourage use together.

Effects on lab test results

None reported.

Pharmacokinetics

Absorption: For tablet or elixir, 60% to 85%. For capsule, 90% to 100%.
Distribution: Wide. About 20% to 30% bound to plasma proteins.
Metabolism: Small amount in liver and gut by bacteria. This varies and may be substantial in some patients. Drug undergoes some enterohepatic recirculation (also variable). Metabolites have minimal cardiac activity.
Excretion: Mostly by kidneys as unchanged drug, although a substantial amount of metabolized or reduced drug may be excreted. In patients with renal impairment, biliary excretion is most important. *Half-life:* 30 to 40 hours.

Route	Onset	Peak	Duration
P.O.	30 min–2 hr	2–6 hr	3–4 days
I.V.	5–30 min	1–4 hr	3–4 days

Action

Chemical effect: Inhibits sodium-potassium-activated adenosine triphosphatase, thereby promoting movement of calcium from extracellular to intracellular cytoplasm and strengthening myocardial contraction. Also acts on CNS to enhance vagal tone, slowing conduction through SA and AV nodes and providing antiarrhythmic effect.
Therapeutic effect: Strengthens myocardial contractions and slows conduction through SA and AV nodes.

Available forms

Capsules: 0.05 mg, 0.1 mg, 0.2 mg
Elixir: 0.05 mg/ml
Injection: 0.05 mg/ml, 0.1 mg/ml (pediatric), 0.25 mg/ml
Tablets: 0.125 mg, 0.25 mg

NURSING PROCESS

Assessment
- Obtain history of patient's underlying condition before therapy.
- Monitor effectiveness by taking apical pulse for 1 full minute before giving a dose. Evaluate ECG, and regularly assess patient's cardiopulmonary condition for signs of improvement.
- Monitor drug level. Therapeutic level ranges from 0.5 to 2 nanograms/ml. Take level 8 hours after last P.O. dose.
- Monitor potassium level carefully.

• Look for adverse reactions and drug interactions. In children, arrhythmias are the earliest and most frequent manifestation of excessive dosing.
• Assess patient's and family's knowledge of drug therapy.

🔱 Nursing diagnoses
• Decreased cardiac output related to underlying condition
• Ineffective protection related to digoxin toxicity caused by drug
• Deficient knowledge related to drug therapy

▶ Planning and implementation
• Adjust dosages as needed. Hypothyroid patients are extremely sensitive to drug, and hyperthyroid patients may need a larger dosage. Reduce the dosage in patients with renal impairment.
• Before giving loading dose, obtain baseline heart rate and rhythm, blood pressure, and electrolyte levels, and question patient about use of drug within the previous 2 to 3 weeks.
• Loading dose is always divided over first 24 hours unless patient's condition indicates otherwise.
• Before giving drug, take apical pulse for 1 full minute. Record and report to prescriber significant changes (sudden increase or decrease in pulse rate, pulse deficit, irregular beats, and regularization of previously irregular rhythm). If these changes occur, check blood pressure and obtain 12-lead ECG.
• ⚠ ALERT: If pulse rate slows to 60 beats/minute or less, withhold drug and notify prescriber.
• Reduce dosage by 20% to 25% when changing from tablets or elixir to liquid-filled capsules or injection because the new forms are better absorbed.
• For digoxin toxicity, give drugs that bind drug in intestine (for example, colestipol or cholestyramine). Treat arrhythmias with phenytoin I.V. or lidocaine I.V., and treat potentially life-threatening toxicity with specific antigen-binding fragments (such as digoxin immune Fab).
• Withhold drug for 1 to 2 days before elective cardioversion. Adjust dose after cardioversion.
• ⚠ ALERT: Be careful when calculating doses. A tenfold miscalculation of a child's dose can easily occur.
• ⚠ ALERT: Don't confuse digoxin with doxepin.

Patient teaching
• Instruct patient and caregiver about drug action, dosage regimen, pulse taking, reportable signs, and follow-up plans.
• Instruct patient not to substitute one brand of digoxin for another.
• Tell patient to eat potassium-rich foods.

☑ Evaluation
• Patient has adequate cardiac output.
• Patient has no digoxin toxicity.
• Patient and family state understanding of drug therapy.

digoxin immune Fab (ovine)
(dih-JOKS-in ih-MYOON Fab)
Digibind, DigiFab

Pharmacologic class: antibody fragment
Therapeutic class: cardiac glycoside antidote
Pregnancy risk category: C

Indications and dosages

▶ **Life-threatening digoxin toxicity.** *Adults and children:* Dosage based on ingested amount or level of digoxin. When calculating amount of antidote, round up to the nearest whole number.
　For digoxin tablets, find the number of antidote vials by multiplying the ingested amount by 0.8 and dividing answer by 0.5. For example, if patient takes 25 tablets of 0.25-mg digoxin, the ingested amount is 6.25 mg. Multiply 6.25 mg by 0.8 and divide answer by 0.5 to obtain 10 vials of antidote.
　For digoxin capsules, find the number of antidote vials by dividing the ingested dose in mg by 0.5. For example, if patient takes 50 of 0.2-mg capsules, the ingested amount is 10 mg. Divide 10 mg by 0.5 to obtain 20 vials of antidote.
　If the digoxin level is known, determine the number of antidote vials as follows: multiply the digoxin level in nanograms/ml by patient's weight in kg, divide by 100. For example, if digoxin is 4 nanograms/ml, and patient weighs 60 kg, multiply together to obtain 240. Divide by 100 to obtain 2.4 vials; then round up to 3 vials.
▶ **Acute toxicity or if estimated ingested amount or digoxin level is unknown.** *Adults and children:* Consider giving 10 vials of digoxin immune Fab and observing patient's re-

sponse. Follow with another 10 vials. Dose is effective in most life-threatening ingestions in adults and children but may cause volume overload in young children.

▽ I.V. administration

• Reconstitute with 4 ml of sterile water for injection. For infusion, further dilute solution with normal saline. For children or other patients who need small doses, reconstitute Digibind in 38-mg vial with 34 ml of normal saline for 1 mg/ml concentration; reconstitute DigiFab in 40-mg vial with 36 ml of normal saline for 1 mg/ml concentration.
• Infuse over 30 minutes. If cardiac arrest is imminent, give as a bolus injection. Infuse via a 0.22-micron membrane filter to ensure no undissolved particulate matter is infused.
• Use reconstituted solution promptly. If not used immediately, refrigerate for up to 4 hours.
⊗ **Incompatibilities**
None reported.

Contraindications and cautions

• Use cautiously in patients allergic to ovine proteins. In these high-risk patients, perform skin test because drug is derived from digoxin-specific antibody fragments obtained from immunized sheep.
🔆 **Lifespan:** In pregnant women, use cautiously. In breast-feeding women, use cautiously; it's unknown if the drug appears in breast milk.

Adverse reactions

CV: *heart failure, rapid ventricular rate.*
Metabolic: hypokalemia.
Other: *anaphylaxis,* hypersensitivity reactions.

Interactions

None reported.

Effect on lab test results

• May decrease potassium level.

Pharmacokinetics

Absorption: Given I.V.
Distribution: Unknown.
Metabolism: Unknown.
Excretion: In urine. *Half-life:* 15 to 20 hours.

Route	Onset	Peak	Duration
I.V.	Varies	End of dose	2–6 hr

Action

Chemical effect: Binds molecules of digoxin, making them unavailable for binding at site of action on cells.
Therapeutic effect: Reverses digoxin toxicity.

Available forms

Injection: 38-mg vial (Digibind) and 40-mg vial (DigiFab)

NURSING PROCESS

🔖 Assessment
• Obtain history of patient's digoxin intoxication before therapy.
• Monitor effectiveness by watching for decreased signs and symptoms of digoxin toxicity. In most patients, signs of digoxin toxicity disappear within a few hours.
• Because drug interferes with digoxin immunoassay measurements, standard digoxin levels are misleading until drug is cleared from body (about 2 days).
• Watch for adverse reactions.
• Assess patient's and family's knowledge of drug therapy.

🔲 Nursing diagnoses
• Ineffective health maintenance related to digoxin intoxication
• Decreased cardiac output related to drug-induced heart failure
• Deficient knowledge related to drug therapy

▷ Planning and implementation
• Drug is used only for life-threatening overdose in patients with shock or cardiac arrest; ventricular arrhythmias, such as ventricular tachycardia or fibrillation; progressive bradycardia, such as severe sinus bradycardia; or second- or third-degree AV block not responsive to atropine.
• Give oxygen. Keep resuscitation equipment nearby.
Patient teaching
• Instruct patient to report respiratory difficulty, chest pain, or dizziness immediately.

✅ Evaluation
• Patient exhibits improved health with alleviation of digoxin toxicity.

- Patient demonstrates adequate cardiac output through normal vital signs and urine output and clear mental condition.
- Patient and family state understanding of drug therapy.

diltiazem hydrochloride

(dil-TIGH-uh-zem high-droh-KLOR-ighd)
Cardizem⊘, Cardizem CD⊘, Cardizem LA⊘, Cartia XT, Dilacor XR, Dilt-XR, Diltia XT, Taztia XT, Tiazac

Pharmacologic class: calcium channel blocker
Therapeutic class: antianginal, antihypertensive
Pregnancy risk category: C

Indications and dosages

▶ **Vasospastic angina (Prinzmetal [variant] angina), classic chronic stable angina pectoris.** *Adults:* 30 mg P.O. t.i.d. or q.i.d. before meals and at bedtime. Increase dosage gradually to maximum, 360 mg daily in divided doses. Or 120- to 180-mg extended-release capsules P.O. once daily. Adjust dosage up to 480 mg once daily.

▶ **Chronic stable angina.** *Adults:* Initially, 180 mg (Cardizem LA, Cardizem CD, or extended-release capsules) once daily in the morning or evening. May increase at intervals of 1 to 2 weeks if needed to maximum 360 mg.

▶ **Hypertension.** *Adults:* Initially, 180- to 240-mg extended-release capsules daily. Adjust dosage as needed. As monotherapy, 120 to 240 mg Cardizem LA P.O. once daily at the same time each day, either in the morning or at bedtime. Adjust dosage about every 14 days. Maximum, 540 mg daily.

▶ **Atrial fibrillation or flutter; paroxysmal supraventricular tachycardia.** *Adults:* 0.25 mg/kg as I.V. bolus injection over 2 minutes. If response is inadequate, 0.35 mg/kg I.V. after 15 minutes, followed with continuous infusion of 10 mg/hour. May increase in increments of 5 mg/hour. Maximum, 15 mg/hour.

▽ I.V. administration

- For direct I.V. injection, no dilution of 5 mg/ml injection is needed.
- For continuous I.V. infusion, add 5 mg/ml injection to 100, 200, or 500 ml of normal saline

solution, D_5W, or 5% dextrose and half-normal saline solution to produce a final concentration of 1, 0.83, or 0.45 mg/ml, respectively.
- Reconstitute drug in monovials and store up to 24 hours in PVC bag as directed.
- For direct injection or continuous infusion, give slowly while continuously monitoring ECG and blood pressure.
- Don't give reconstituted solutions stored longer than 24 hours or those with discoloration or visible particulate matter.

⊗ **Incompatibilities**
Acetazolamide, acyclovir, aminophylline, ampicillin, cefoperazone, diazepam, furosemide, heparin, hydrocortisone, insulin, methylprednisolone, nafcillin, phenytoin, rifampin, sodium bicarbonate, thiopental.

Contraindications and cautions

- Contraindicated in patients hypersensitive to drug and in those with sick sinus syndrome, second- or third-degree AV block without artificial pacemaker, hypotension (systolic blood pressure below 90 mm Hg), acute MI, or pulmonary congestion (documented by X-ray).
- Use cautiously in patients with heart failure and those with impaired liver or kidney function.
🕭 **Lifespan:** In pregnant women, use cautiously. Women who are breast-feeding should stop breast-feeding or not use this drug. In children, safety and effectiveness haven't been established. In elderly patients, use cautiously.

Adverse reactions

CNS: asthenia, dizziness, *headache,* insomnia, somnolence.
CV: abnormal ECG, *arrhythmias, AV block, bradycardia,* conduction abnormalities, *edema,* flushing, *heart failure,* hypotension.
GI: abdominal discomfort, constipation, diarrhea, nausea, vomiting.
GU: nocturia, polyuria.
Skin: photosensitivity, pruritus, rash.

Interactions

Drug-drug. *Anesthetics:* May potentiate effects. Monitor patient.
Carbamazepine: May cause increased carbamazepine levels. Monitor levels and adjust dosage as needed.
Cimetidine: May inhibit diltiazem metabolism. Monitor patient for toxicity.

Cyclosporine: May increase cyclosporine levels by decreasing its metabolism, leading to increased risk of cyclosporine toxicity. Avoid use together.

Diazepam, midazolam, triazolam: May increase CNS depression and prolong effects of these drugs. Use lower dose of these benzodiazepines.

Digoxin: May increase levels of digoxin. Monitor patient and digoxin levels.

Propranolol, other beta blockers: May precipitate heart failure or prolong cardiac conduction time. Use together cautiously.

Quinidine: May cause increased quinidine effects. Use together cautiously.

Drug-lifestyle. *Sun exposure:* May cause photosensitivity reactions. Advise patient to avoid unprotected or prolonged sun exposure.

Effect on lab test results

- May cause transient increase in liver enzyme levels.

Pharmacokinetics

Absorption: 80%. 40% of drug enters systemic circulation because of significant first-pass effect in liver.

Distribution: 70% to 85% of circulating drug is bound to plasma proteins.

Metabolism: In liver.

Excretion: 35% in urine and 65% in bile as unchanged drug and inactive and active metabolites. *Half-life:* 2 to 11 hours.

Route	Onset	Peak	Duration
P.O.	30 min–4 hr	2–18 hr	6–24 hr
I.V.			
bolus	3 min	Immediate	1–3 hr
infusion	3 min	Immediate	< 10 hr

Action

Chemical effect: Inhibits calcium ion influx across cardiac and smooth muscle cells, decreasing myocardial contractility and oxygen demand; also dilates coronary arteries and arterioles.

Therapeutic effect: Relieves anginal pain, lowers blood pressure, and restores normal sinus rhythm.

Available forms

Capsules (extended-release): 60 mg, 90 mg, 120 mg, 180 mg, 240 mg, 300 mg, 360 mg, 420 mg

Injection: 5 mg/ml (25 mg and 50 mg)
Tablets: 30 mg, 60 mg, 90 mg, 120 mg

NURSING PROCESS

Assessment

- Obtain history of patient's underlying condition before therapy, and reassess regularly thereafter.
- Monitor blood pressure when therapy starts and when dosage changes.
- Monitor patient's ECG and heart rate and rhythm regularly.
- Be alert for adverse reactions and drug interactions.
- Assess patient's and family's knowledge of drug therapy.

Nursing diagnoses

- Ineffective health maintenance related to underlying condition
- Decreased cardiac output related to drug-induced adverse reactions
- Deficient knowledge related to drug therapy

Planning and implementation

- Give tablets before meals and at bedtime.
- Patients controlled on diltiazem alone or with other medications may be switched to Cardizem LA tablets once a day at the nearest equivalent total daily dose.
- **ALERT:** If systolic blood pressure is below 90 mm Hg or heart rate is below 60 beats/minute, don't give the dose and notify prescriber.
- Assist patient with ambulation during start of therapy because dizziness may occur.
- To minimize edema, restrict the patient's fluid and sodium intake.

Patient teaching
- If nitrate therapy is prescribed during adjustment of diltiazem dosage, urge patient compliance. Tell patient that S.L. nitroglycerin may be taken p.r.n. and as directed when angina is acute.
- Instruct patient to call prescriber if he experiences chest pain, shortness of breath, dizziness, palpitations, or swelling of the limbs.
- Tell patient to swallow extended-release capsules whole and not to open, crush, or chew them.
- Instruct patient to take drug exactly as prescribed, even when feeling better.

Reactions may be *common,* uncommon, *life-threatening,* or COMMON AND LIFE-THREATENING.

• Advise patient to minimize exposure to direct sunlight and to take precautions when in sun because of drug-induced photosensitivity.
• Instruct patient to limit fluid and sodium intake to minimize edema.

☑ **Evaluation**
• Patient exhibits improvement in underlying condition.
• Patient maintains adequate cardiac output throughout therapy.
• Patient and family state understanding of drug therapy.

diphenhydramine hydrochloride
(digh-fen-HIGH-drah-meen high-droh-KLOR-ighd)
Allerdryl ◆ †, AllerMax Caplets†, Banophen†, Banophen Caplets†, Beldin†, Benadryl†, Benadryl 25†, Benadryl Kapseals, Benylin Cough†, Bydramine Cough†, Compoz†, Diphenadryl†, Diphen Cough†, Diphenhist†, Diphenhist Captabs†, Genahist†, Hyrexin-50, Nytol Maximum Strength†, Nytol with DPH†, Sleep-Eze 3†, Sominex Nighttime Sleep Aid†, Tusstat†, Twilite Caplets†, Uni-Bent Cough†

Pharmacologic class: nonselective ethanolamine derivative antihistamine
Therapeutic class: antihistamine (H_1-receptor antagonist), antitussive, sleep aid
Pregnancy risk category: B

Indications and dosages

▶ **Rhinitis, allergy symptoms, motion sickness, Parkinson disease.** *Adults and children age 12 and older:* 25 to 50 mg P.O. t.i.d. or q.i.d. Or 10 to 50 mg deep I.M. or I.V. Maximum I.M. or I.V. dosage, 400 mg daily.
Children younger than age 12: Give 5 mg/kg daily P.O., deep I.M., or I.V. in divided doses q.i.d. Maximum, 300 mg daily.
▶ **Sedation.** *Adults:* 25 to 50 mg P.O. or deep I.M., p.r.n.
▶ **Nighttime sleep aid.** *Adults:* 50 mg P.O. at bedtime.
▶ **Nonproductive cough.** *Adults:* 25 mg P.O. every 4 to 6 hours (up to 150 mg daily).
Children ages 6 to 11: Give 12.5 mg P.O. every 4 to 6 hours (up to 75 mg daily).

Children ages 2 to 5: Give 6.25 mg P.O. every 4 to 6 hours (up to 25 mg daily).

▼ I.V. administration
• Make sure I.V. site is patent, and monitor it for irritation.
• Don't give I.V. drug faster than 25 mg/minute.
⊗ **Incompatibilities**
Allopurinol, amobarbital, amphotericin B, cefepime, dexamethasone, foscarnet, haloperidol lactate, pentobarbital, phenytoin, phenobarbital, thiopental.

Contraindications and cautions
• Contraindicated in patients hypersensitive to drug and in patients having acute asthma attacks.
• Use cautiously in patients with CV disease, hypertension, angle-closure glaucoma, increased intraocular pressure, stenosing peptic ulcer, pyloroduodenal and bladder-neck obstruction, prostatic hyperplasia, hyperthyroidism, asthma, or COPD.
⚘ **Lifespan:** In pregnant women, use cautiously. In neonates, preterm neonates, and breastfeeding women, drug is contraindicated. In children younger than age 12, safety and effectiveness as a nighttime sleep aid haven't been established. Children younger than age 6 should use only when directed by prescriber. Age restrictions for topical preparations vary depending on drug's formulation and manufacturer.

Adverse reactions
CNS: confusion, *dizziness, drowsiness,* fatigue, headache, incoordination, insomnia, nervousness, restlessness, *sedation, seizures, sleepiness,* tremor, vertigo.
CV: hypotension, palpitations, tachycardia.
EENT: blurred vision, diplopia, nasal congestion, tinnitus.
GI: anorexia, constipation, diarrhea, *dry mouth, epigastric distress, nausea,* vomiting.
GU: dysuria, urinary frequency, urine retention.
Hematologic: *agranulocytosis,* hemolytic anemia, *thrombocytopenia.*
Respiratory: thickening of bronchial secretions.
Skin: photosensitivity, rash, urticaria.
Other: *anaphylactic shock.*

Interactions

Drug-drug. *CNS depressants:* May increase sedation. Use together cautiously; monitor patient for increased sedation.

MAO inhibitors: May increase anticholinergic effects. Don't use together.

Other products containing diphenhydramine, including topical forms: May increase risk of adverse reactions. Avoid use together.

Drug-lifestyle. *Alcohol use:* May increase adverse CNS effects. Discourage use together.

Sun exposure: May cause photosensitivity reactions. Urge patient to wear protective clothing and sunblock.

Effects on lab test results

- May decrease hemoglobin level and hematocrit.
- May decrease platelet and granulocyte counts.

Pharmacokinetics

Absorption: Good after P.O. use.
Distribution: Wide, including CNS. About 82% protein-bound.
Metabolism: In liver.
Excretion: Drug and metabolites mainly in urine. *Half-life:* About 3½ hours.

Route	Onset	Peak	Duration
P.O.	≤15 min	1–4 hr	6–8 hr
I.V.	Immediate	1–4 hr	6–8 hr
I.M.	Unknown	1–4 hr	6–8 hr

Action

Chemical effect: Competes with histamine for H_1-receptor sites on effector cells. Prevents but doesn't reverse histamine-mediated responses, particularly histamine's effects on smooth muscle of bronchial tubes, GI tract, uterus, and blood vessels. Provides local anesthesia by preventing initiation and transmission of nerve impulses, and suppresses cough reflex by direct effect in medulla of brain.

Therapeutic effect: Relieves allergy symptoms, motion sickness, and cough; improves voluntary movement; and promotes sleep and calmness.

Available forms

Capsules: 25 mg†, 50 mg†
Elixir: 12.5 mg/5 ml*†
Injection: 10 mg/ml, 50 mg/ml
Syrup: 12.5 mg/5 ml†, 6.25 mg/5 ml†

Tablets: 25 mg†, 50 mg†
Tablets (chewable): 12.5 mg†

NURSING PROCESS

Assessment

- Obtain history of patient's underlying condition before therapy, and reassess regularly thereafter.
- Be alert for adverse reactions and drug interactions.
- Assess patient's and family's knowledge of drug therapy.

Nursing diagnoses

- Ineffective health maintenance related to underlying condition
- Risk for injury related to drug-induced adverse CNS reactions
- Deficient knowledge related to drug therapy

Planning and implementation

- Reduce GI distress by giving drug with food or milk.
- Alternate injection sites to prevent irritation. Give I.M. injection deep into large muscle.
- If tolerance is observed, notify prescriber because another antihistamine may need to be substituted.
- **ALERT:** Don't confuse diphenhydramine with dicyclomine, or Benadryl with Bentyl or Benylin.

Patient teaching
- Instruct patient to take drug 30 minutes before travel, to prevent motion sickness.
- Warn patient to avoid alcohol and to refrain from driving or performing other hazardous activities that require alertness.
- Tell patient that coffee or tea may reduce drowsiness.
- Inform patient that ice chips, sugarless gum, or hard candy may relieve dry mouth.
- Advise patient to stop taking the drug 4 days before allergy skin tests to preserve test accuracy.
- Tell patient to notify prescriber if tolerance develops because different antihistamine may need to be prescribed.
- Warn patient that he may be photosensitive. Advise use of sunblock or protective clothing.
- Warn patient to avoid using other products containing diphenhydramine, including topical forms, because of risk of adverse reactions.

☑ Evaluation
- Patient shows improvement in underlying condition.
- Patient has no injury as result of therapy.
- Patient and family state understanding of drug therapy.

diphenoxylate hydrochloride and atropine sulfate
(digh-fen-OKS-ul-ayt high-droh-KLOR-ighd and AH-troh-peen SUL-fayt)
Logen, Lomanate, Lomotil*, Lonox

Pharmacologic class: opioid
Therapeutic class: antidiarrheal
Pregnancy risk category: C
Controlled substance schedule: V

Indications and dosages

▶ **Acute, nonspecific diarrhea.** *Adults:* Initially, 5 mg P.O. q.i.d.; then reduce dosage as soon as initial control is achieved. Maximum, 20 mg P.O. daily.
Children ages 2 to 12: Give 0.3 to 0.4 mg/kg liquid form P.O. daily in four divided doses. Maintenance dosage may be as low as 25% of initial dosage. Maximum, 20 mg P.O. daily.

Contraindications and cautions

- Contraindicated in patients hypersensitive to drug or any of its components and in those with acute diarrhea from poison (until toxic material is eliminated), acute diarrhea caused by organisms that penetrate the intestinal mucosa, or diarrhea from antibiotic-induced pseudomembranous enterocolitis. Also contraindicated in jaundiced patients.
- Use cautiously in patients with hepatic disease, opioid dependence, or acute ulcerative colitis. If abdominal distention or other signs of toxic megacolon develop, stop therapy immediately and notify prescriber.
- ☀ **Lifespan:** In pregnant women, use cautiously. In breast-feeding women, drug isn't recommended. In children ages 2 to 12, use cautiously and in liquid form only. In children younger than age 2, drug is contraindicated.

Adverse reactions
CNS: confusion, depression, *dizziness,* drowsiness, euphoria, headache, lethargy, malaise, numbness in limbs, restlessness, *sedation.*
CV: tachycardia.
EENT: mydriasis.
GI: abdominal discomfort or distention, anorexia, *dry mouth,* fluid retention in bowel, nausea, *pancreatitis,* paralytic ileus, vomiting.
GU: urine retention.
Respiratory: *respiratory depression.*
Skin: pruritus, rash.
Other: *angioedema, anaphylaxis,* possible physical dependence with long-term use.

Interactions
Drug-drug. *Barbiturates, CNS depressants, opioids, tranquilizers:* May increase CNS depression. Monitor patient closely for increased sedation.
MAO inhibitors: May cause a hypertensive crisis. Don't use together.
Drug-lifestyle. *Alcohol use:* May increase CNS depression. Discourage use together.

Effects on lab test results
None reported.

Pharmacokinetics
Absorption: 90%.
Distribution: Unknown.
Metabolism: Extensive.
Excretion: Metabolites mainly in feces with lesser amounts in urine. *Half-life:* Diphenoxylate, 2½ hours; its major metabolite, diphenoxylic acid, 4½ hours; atropine, 2½ hours.

Route	Onset	Peak	Duration
P.O.	45–60 min	2 hr	3–4 hr

Action
Chemical effect: Unknown; probably increases smooth-muscle tone in GI tract, inhibits motility and propulsion, and diminishes secretions.
Therapeutic effect: Relieves diarrhea.

Available forms
Liquid: 2.5 mg/5 ml (with atropine sulfate 0.025 mg/5 ml)*
Tablets: 2.5 mg (with atropine sulfate 0.025 mg)

NURSING PROCESS

Assessment
• Assess patient's diarrhea before and regularly during therapy.
• Be alert for adverse reactions and drug interactions.
• Assess patient's and family's knowledge of drug therapy.

Nursing diagnoses
• Diarrhea related to underlying condition
• Ineffective breathing pattern related to drug-induced respiratory depression
• Deficient knowledge related to drug therapy

Planning and implementation
• Fluid retention in the bowel may mask depletion of extracellular fluid and electrolytes, especially in young children with acute gastroenteritis. Correct fluid and electrolyte disturbances before starting therapy. Dehydration may increase risk of delayed toxicity.
• A 2.5-mg dose is as effective as 5 ml of camphorated opium tincture.
• Drug isn't indicated for treating antibiotic-induced diarrhea.
• Drug is unlikely to be effective if patient doesn't respond within 48 hours.
• Risk of physical dependence increases with high dosage and long-term use. Atropine sulfate helps discourage abuse.
• Use naloxone to treat respiratory depression caused by overdose.
• **ALERT:** Don't confuse Lomotil (diphenoxylate hydrochloride and atropine sulfate) with Lamictal (lamotrigine).
Patient teaching
• Tell patient not to exceed prescribed dosage.
• Warn patient not to use drug to treat acute diarrhea for longer than 2 days. Encourage him to seek medical attention if diarrhea persists.
• Advise patient to avoid hazardous activities, such as driving, until CNS effects of drug are known.

Evaluation
• Patient regains normal bowel pattern.
• Patient maintains normal breathing pattern throughout therapy.
• Patient and family state understanding of drug therapy.

dipyridamole
(digh-peer-IH-duh-mohl)
Persantine

Pharmacologic class: pyrimidine analogue
Therapeutic class: coronary vasodilator, platelet aggregation inhibitor
Pregnancy risk category: B

Indications and dosages
▶ **To inhibit platelet adhesion in prosthetic heart valves.** *Adults:* 75 to 100 mg P.O. q.i.d. (with warfarin or aspirin).
▶ **Alternative to exercise in evaluation of coronary artery disease during thallium-201 myocardial perfusion scintigraphy.** *Adults:* 0.57 mg/kg as I.V. infusion at constant rate over 4 minutes (0.142 mg/kg/minute).
▶ **Chronic angina pectoris‡.** *Adults:* 50 mg P.O. t.i.d. at least 1 hour before meals; 2 to 3 months of therapy may be required to achieve therapeutic response.
▶ **To prevent thromboembolic complications in patients with thromboembolic disorders other than prosthetic heart valves‡.** *Adults:* 150 to 400 mg P.O. daily (with warfarin or aspirin).

I.V. administration
• If giving drug as a diagnostic agent, dilute in half-normal or normal saline solution or D_5W in at least a 1:2 ratio for total volume of 20 to 50 ml.
• Inject thallium-201 within 5 minutes of completing 4-minute infusion.
• Avoid freezing and protect from direct light.
⊗ **Incompatibilities**
Other I.V. drugs.

Contraindications and cautions
• Use cautiously in patients with hypotension.
Lifespan: In pregnant women, use cautiously. In breast-feeding women and in children, safety and effectiveness haven't been established.

Adverse reactions
CNS: *dizziness, headache,* weakness.
CV: blood pressure lability, chest pain, ECG abnormalities, fainting, flushing, hypertension (with I.V. infusion), hypotension.

GI: abdominal distress, diarrhea, nausea, vomiting.
Skin: irritation (with undiluted injection), pruritus, rash.

Interactions

Drug-drug. *Heparin:* May increase bleeding. Monitor patient closely for increased bleeding; monitor PTT.
Theophylline: May prevent coronary vasodilation by I.V. dipyridamole. Avoid use together.
Drug-herb. *Dong quai, feverfew, garlic, ginger, horse chestnut, red clover:* May increase risk of bleeding. Discourage use together.

Effects on lab test results

None reported.

Pharmacokinetics

Absorption: Variable and slow; 27% to 59%.
Distribution: Wide. 91% to 97% protein-bound.
Metabolism: By liver.
Excretion: By way of biliary excretion of glucuronide conjugates. Some dipyridamole and conjugates may undergo enterohepatic circulation and fecal excretion; small amount in urine.
Half-life: 10 to 12 hours.

Route	Onset	Peak	Duration
P.O.	Unknown	45–150 min	Unknown
I.V.	Unknown	2 min after therapy	Unknown
I.M.	Unknown	Unknown	Unknown

Action

Chemical effect: May involve its ability to increase adenosine, which is a coronary vasodilator and platelet aggregation inhibitor.
Therapeutic effect: Dilates coronary arteries and helps prevent clotting.

Available forms

Injection: 10 mg/2 ml
Tablets: 25 mg, 50 mg, 75 mg

NURSING PROCESS

☞ Assessment
• Obtain history of patient's underlying condition before therapy, and reassess regularly thereafter.

• Be alert for adverse reactions and drug interactions.
• Assess patient's and family's knowledge of drug therapy.

⊕ Nursing diagnoses
• Ineffective cardiopulmonary tissue perfusion related to underlying condition
• Acute pain related to drug-induced headache
• Deficient knowledge related to drug therapy

⊳ Planning and implementation
• Give drug 1 hour before meals. If patient develops adverse GI reactions, give drug with meals.
• The value of dipyridamole as part of an antithrombotic regimen is controversial; its use may not provide significantly better results than aspirin alone.
⚠ ALERT: Don't confuse dipyridamole with disopyramide, or Persantine with Periactin.
Patient teaching
• Instruct patient when to take drug.
• Tell patient to have his blood pressure checked frequently.
• Advise patient to take mild analgesic if headache occurs.
• Instruct patient to notify prescriber if chest pain occurs.

☑ Evaluation
• Patient maintains adequate tissue perfusion and cellular oxygenation.
• Patient obtains relief from drug-induced headache with use of mild analgesic.
• Patient and family state understanding of drug therapy.

disopyramide
(digh-so-PEER-uh-mighd)
Rythmodan ◆

disopyramide phosphate
Norpace, Norpace CR, Rythmodan LA ◆

Pharmacologic class: pyridine derivative
Therapeutic class: antiarrhythmic
Pregnancy risk category: C

Indications and dosages

▶ **Symptomatic PVCs (unifocal, multifocal, or coupled), ventricular tachycardia not se-**

vere enough to require cardioversion. *Adults:* For parenteral use, initially give 2 mg/kg I.V. slowly (over at least 15 minutes). Give drug until arrhythmia is gone or patient has received 150 mg. If conversion is successful but arrhythmia returns, repeat dosage. Don't exceed total I.V. dosage of 300 mg in first hour. Follow with I.V. infusion of 0.4 mg/kg/hour (usually 20 to 30 mg/hour) to maximum, 800 mg daily.

Adults weighing more than 50 kg (110 lb): Initial loading dose is 300 mg P.O. for rapid control of ventricular arrhythmia. Follow with 150 mg every 6 hours or 300 mg every 12 hours with controlled-release capsules.

Adults weighing 50 kg or less: Initial loading dose is 200 mg P.O., then 100 mg P.O. every 6 hours as conventional capsules or 200 mg P.O. every 12 hours with controlled-release capsules.

Children ages 12 to 18: Give 6 to 15 mg/kg P.O. daily, divided into equal amounts and given every 6 hours.

Children ages 4 to 12: Give 10 to 15 mg/kg P.O. daily, divided into equal amounts and given every 6 hours.

Children ages 1 to 4: Give 10 to 20 mg/kg P.O. daily, divided into equal amounts and given every 6 hours.

Children younger than age 1: Give 10 to 30 mg/kg P.O. daily, divided into equal amounts and given every 6 hours.

☒ Adjust-a-dose: For patients with renal impairment, if creatinine clearance is 30 to 40 ml/minute, give 100 mg every 8 hours. If creatinine clearance is 15 to 30 ml/minute, give 100 mg every 12 hours. If creatinine clearance is less than 15 ml/minute, give 100 mg every 24 hours.

▼ I.V. administration

• Add 200 mg to 500 ml of compatible solution, such as normal saline solution or D₅W.
• Use an infusion pump. Don't mix with other drugs.
• Give slowly over at least 15 minutes.
• Switch to P.O. therapy as soon as possible.
⊗ **Incompatibilities**
Other I.V. drugs.

Contraindications and cautions

• Contraindicated in patients hypersensitive to the drug or any of its components and in those with cardiogenic shock or second- or third-

degree heart block without an artificial pacemaker.
• Use cautiously or avoid using, if possible, in patients with heart failure.
• Use cautiously in patients with underlying conduction abnormalities, urinary tract diseases (especially prostatic hypertrophy), hepatic or renal impairment, myasthenia gravis, or acute angle-closure glaucoma.

⚖ Lifespan: In pregnant women, use cautiously. In breast-feeding women, drug isn't recommended.

Adverse reactions

CNS: *acute psychosis,* agitation, depression, dizziness, fatigue, headache, syncope.
CV: *arrhythmias,* chest pain, edema, **heart block, heart failure,** hypotension.
EENT: blurred vision, dry eyes, dry nose.
GI: abdominal pain, anorexia, bloating, *constipation,* diarrhea, *dry mouth,* nausea, vomiting.
GU: *urinary hesitancy,* urine retention.
Hepatic: cholestatic jaundice.
Metabolic: weight gain.
Musculoskeletal: aches, muscle weakness, pain.
Respiratory: shortness of breath.
Skin: dermatosis, pruritus, rash.

Interactions

Drug-drug. *Antiarrhythmics:* May cause additive or antagonized antiarrhythmic effects. Monitor patient ECG closely.
Erythromycin: May increase disopyramide level, causing arrhythmias and prolonged QTc interval. Monitor ECG closely.
Phenytoin: May increase metabolism of disopyramide. Monitor patient for decreased antiarrhythmic effect.
Rifampin: May decrease disopyramide level. Monitor patient for decreased effectiveness.
Drug-herb. *Jimson weed:* May adversely affect CV function. Discourage use together.

Effects on lab test results

None reported.

Pharmacokinetics

Absorption: Rapid and good.
Distribution: Throughout extracellular fluid but not extensively bound to tissues. 50% to 65% protein-bound.

Metabolism: In liver.
Excretion: In urine. *Half-life:* 7 hours.

Route	Onset	Peak	Duration
P.O.	½–3½ hr	2–2½ hr	1½–8½ hr
I.V.	Unknown	Unknown	Unknown

Action

Chemical effect: May depress phase 0 and prolong action potential. All class I drugs have membrane-stabilizing effects.
Therapeutic effect: Restores normal sinus rhythm.

Available forms

disopyramide
Capsules: 100 mg ♦, 150 mg ♦
disopyramide phosphate
Capsules: 100 mg, 150 mg
Capsules (controlled-release): 100 mg, 150 mg
Injection: 10 mg/ml ♦
Tablets (sustained-release): 150 mg ♦

NURSING PROCESS

✏ Assessment
• Obtain history of patient's arrhythmia before therapy.
• Monitor drug effectiveness by assessing patient's ECG pattern and apical pulse rate.
• Be alert for adverse reactions and drug interactions.
• Assess patient's and family's knowledge of drug therapy.

✦ Nursing diagnoses
• Decreased cardiac output related to underlying arrhythmia
• Ineffective protection related to drug-induced proarrhythmias
• Deficient knowledge related to drug therapy

▶ Planning and implementation
• Correct electrolyte abnormalities before therapy begins.
• Check apical pulse before therapy. Notify prescriber if pulse rate is slower than 60 beats/minute or faster than 120 beats/minute.
• Don't use sustained- and controlled-release preparations for rapid control of ventricular arrhythmias, when therapeutic levels must be rapidly attained; in patients with cardiomyopathy

or suspected cardiac decompensation; or in those with severe renal impairment.
• For young children, pharmacist may prepare disopyramide suspension from 100-mg capsules using cherry syrup. Suspension should be dispensed in amber glass bottles and protected from light.
• If heart block develops, QRS complex widens by more than 25%, or QT interval is prolonged by more than 25% above baseline; stop the drug and notify the prescriber.

Patient teaching
• When switching patient from immediate- to sustained-release capsules, advise taking sustained-release capsule 6 hours after last immediate-release capsule.
• Teach patient importance of taking drug on time and exactly as prescribed. This may require use of alarm clock for night doses.
• Advise patient to use sugarless gum or hard candy to relieve dry mouth.
• Tell patient not to crush or chew extended-release tablets.

✓ Evaluation
• Patient's ECG reveals that arrhythmia has been corrected.
• Patient develops no new arrhythmias as result of therapy.
• Patient and family state understanding of drug therapy.

disulfiram
(digh-SUL-fih-ram)
Antabuse

Pharmacologic class: aldehyde dehydrogenase inhibitor
Therapeutic class: alcohol deterrent
Pregnancy risk category: C

Indications and dosages

▶ **Adjunct to manage alcohol dependence.**
Adults: 250 to 500 mg P.O. as single dose in morning for 1 to 2 weeks. If drowsiness occurs, give in the evening. Maintenance dosage is 125 to 500 mg P.O. daily (average dosage, 250 mg) until permanent self-control is established. Therapy may continue for months or years.

Contraindications and cautions

• Contraindicated during alcohol intoxication and within 12 hours of alcohol ingestion. Also contraindicated in patients hypersensitive to disulfiram or thiram derivatives used in pesticides and rubber vulcanization; patients with psychoses, myocardial disease, or coronary occlusion; and patients receiving metronidazole, paraldehyde, alcohol, or alcohol-containing preparations.

• Use cautiously in patients receiving phenytoin therapy and in patients with diabetes mellitus, hypothyroidism, seizure disorder, cerebral damage, nephritis, or hepatic cirrhosis or insufficiency.

⚖ Lifespan: In pregnant women, don't use. In breast-feeding women, use cautiously. In children, safety and effectiveness haven't been established.

Adverse reactions

CNS: delirium, depression, drowsiness, fatigue, headache, neuritis, peripheral neuritis, polyneuritis, psychotic reactions, restlessness.
EENT: optic neuritis.
GI: metallic or garlic aftertaste.
GU: impotence.
Hepatic: *hepatitis, hepatic failure.*
Skin: acneiform or allergic dermatitis.
Other: *disulfiram reaction.*

Interactions

Drug-drug. *Alfentanil:* May prolong duration of effect. Monitor patient closely.
Anticoagulants: May increase anticoagulant effect. Adjust dosage of anticoagulant accordingly; monitor patient for bleeding.
CNS depressants: May increase CNS depression. Use together cautiously.
Isoniazid: May cause ataxia or marked change in behavior. Avoid use together.
Metronidazole: May cause psychotic reaction. Avoid use together; wait for 2 weeks following disulfiram.
Midazolam: May increase plasma levels of midazolam. Use together cautiously.
Paraldehyde: May cause toxic level of acetaldehyde. Don't use together.
Phenytoin: May increase toxic effects of phenytoin. Monitor phenytoin levels closely and adjust dosage.

Tricyclic antidepressants, especially amitriptyline: May cause transient delirium. Monitor patient closely.
Drug-herb. *Passion flower, pill-bearing spurge, pokeweed, squaw vine, squill, sundew, sweet flag, tormentil, valerian, yarrow:* May cause disulfiram reaction if herb contains alcohol. Discourage use together.
Drug-food. *Caffeine:* May increase cardiovascular and CNS stimulant effects of caffeine. Advise against caffeine use.
Drug-lifestyle. *Alcohol use:* May cause disulfiram reaction, including flushing, tachycardia, bronchospasm, sweating, nausea, and vomiting. Death may also occur. Warn against any alcohol consumption.
Cocaine use: May increase adverse cardiovascular effects of cocaine. Inform patient of this interaction.

Effect on lab test results

• May increase cholesterol level.

Pharmacokinetics

Absorption: Complete.
Distribution: Highly lipid soluble and initially localized in fat.
Metabolism: Mostly oxidized in liver.
Excretion: Mainly in urine; 5% to 20% in feces. *Half-life:* Unknown.

Route	Onset	Peak	Duration
P.O.	1–2 hr	Unknown	< 14 days

Action

Chemical effect: Blocks oxidation of ethanol at acetaldehyde stage. Excess acetaldehyde produces highly unpleasant reaction in presence of even small amounts of ethanol.
Therapeutic effect: Deters alcohol consumption.

Available forms

Tablets: 250 mg, 500 mg

NURSING PROCESS

🔍 Assessment

• Obtain history of patient's alcoholism before therapy.
• Do a complete physical examination and laboratory studies, including CBC, chemistry panel, and transaminase determination before therapy.

Repeat physical examination and laboratory studies regularly.

• Monitor the drug's effectiveness by assessing patient's abstinence from alcohol.

• Measure blood alcohol level weekly.

• Be alert for adverse reactions and drug interactions. Disulfiram reaction is precipitated by alcohol use and may include flushing, throbbing headache, dyspnea, nausea, copious vomiting, diaphoresis, thirst, chest pain, palpitations, hyperventilation, hypotension, syncope, anxiety, weakness, blurred vision, and confusion. Severe reaction may cause respiratory depression, CV collapse, arrhythmias, MI, acute heart failure, seizures, unconsciousness, and death.

• Mild reactions may occur in sensitive patients with blood alcohol levels of 5 to 10 mg/dl; symptoms are fully developed at 50 mg/dl. At 125 to 150 mg/dl, patient typically is unconscious. Reaction may last from 30 minutes to several hours or as long as alcohol remains in blood.

• Assess patient's and family's knowledge of drug therapy.

⊕ Nursing diagnoses

• Ineffective health maintenance related to alcoholism

• Acute pain related to drug-induced headache

• Deficient knowledge related to drug therapy

❯ Planning and implementation

• Use only under close medical and nursing supervision. Only give drug to patient who hasn't used alcohol for at least 12 hours. Make sure that patient clearly understands consequences of therapy and gives permission for its use. Use drug only if patient is cooperative, well-motivated, and receiving supportive psychiatric therapy.

• Drug is usually given during the day, although it may be given at night if drowsiness occurs. Establish lowered maintenance dose until permanent self-control is practiced. Therapy may continue for months or years.

Patient teaching

• Caution patient's family that drug should never be given to the patient without his knowledge because severe reaction or death could result if the patient ingests alcohol.

• Warn patient to avoid all sources of alcohol (including, for example, sauces and cough syrups). Even external application of liniments, shaving lotion, and back-rub preparations may cause disulfiram reaction. Tell patient that alcohol reaction may occur as long as 2 weeks after single dose of disulfiram, and that the longer he remains on drug, the more sensitive he becomes to alcohol.

• Tell patient to wear or carry medical identification identifying him as a disulfiram user.

• Reassure patient that drug-induced adverse reactions (unrelated to alcohol use), such as drowsiness, fatigue, impotence, headache, peripheral neuritis, and metallic or garlic taste, subside after about 2 weeks of therapy.

☑ Evaluation

• Patient abstains from alcohol consumption.

• Patient's headache is relieved with mild analgesic therapy.

• Patient and family state understanding of drug therapy.

HIGH ALERT!

dobutamine hydrochloride
(doh-BY00-tuh-meen high-droh-KLOR-ighd)

Pharmacologic class: adrenergic, beta$_1$ agonist
Therapeutic class: inotropic drug
Pregnancy risk category: B

Indications and dosages

▶ **To increase cardiac output in short-term treatment of cardiac decompensation caused by depressed contractility, such as during refractory heart failure, and as adjunct in cardiac surgery.** *Adults:* 2 to 20 mcg/kg/minute I.V. infusion. Usual dosage range is 2.5 to 10 mcg/kg/minute. Rarely, rates up to 40 mcg/kg/minute may be needed; however, such doses may worsen ischemia.

▼ I.V. administration

• Dilute concentrate for injection to no more than 5 mg/ml. Compatible solutions include D$_5$W, half-normal saline solution injection, normal saline solution injection, and lactated Ringer's injection. The contents of one vial (250 mg) diluted with 1,000 ml of solution yield 250 mcg/ml; diluted with 500 ml, 500 mcg/ml; diluted with 250 ml, 1,000 mcg/ml.

• Oxidation of drug may slightly discolor admixtures containing dobutamine. This doesn't indicate significant loss of potency, provided drug is used within 24 hours of reconstitution.

• Don't mix with sodium bicarbonate injection because drug is incompatible with alkaline solutions.
• Don't give in same I.V. line with other drugs. Drug is incompatible with heparin, hydrocortisone sodium succinate, cefazolin, neutral cephalothin, penicillin, and ethacrynate sodium.
• Give drug using central venous catheter or large peripheral vein. Titrate infusion according to patient's condition per prescriber's guidelines. Use infusion pump.
• Watch for irritation and infiltration. Extravasation can cause inflammation, tissue damage, and necrosis. Change I.V. sites regularly to avoid phlebitis.
• Solutions remain stable for 24 hours.
⊗ **Incompatibilities**
Acyclovir, alkaline solutions, alteplase, aminophylline, bretylium, bumetanide, calcium chloride, calcium gluconate, cefepime, diazepam, digoxin, doxapram, furosemide, heparin, indomethacin, insulin, magnesium sulfate, midazolam, piperacillin with tazobactam, phenytoin, phytonadione, potassium chloride, sodium bicarbonate, thiopental, verapamil, warfarin.

Contraindications and cautions

• Contraindicated in patients hypersensitive to drug or any of its components and in those with idiopathic hypertrophic subaortic stenosis.
• Use cautiously in patients with history of hypertension. Drug may cause exaggerated pressor response.
⚱ **Lifespan:** In pregnant and breast-feeding women and in children, safety and effectiveness haven't been established.

Adverse reactions

CNS: headache.
CV: angina, *hypertension, hypotension, increased heart rate,* nonspecific chest pain, phlebitis, *PVCs.*
GI: nausea, vomiting.
Musculoskeletal: mild leg cramps or tingling sensation.
Respiratory: *asthma attacks,* shortness of breath.
Other: *anaphylaxis.*

Interactions

Drug-drug. *Beta blockers:* May antagonize dobutamine effects. Don't use together.

Bretylium: May potentiate action of vasopressors on adrenergic receptors; arrhythmias may result. Monitor ECG closely.
General anesthetics: May increase risk of ventricular arrhythmias. Monitor patient closely.
Guanethidine: May increase pressor response possibly causing severe hypertension. Monitor closely.
Oxytocic drugs: May cause severe persistent hypertension. Use with caution.
Tricyclic antidepressants: May potentiate the pressor response and cause arrhythmias. Use with caution.
Drug-herb. *Rue:* May increase inotropic potential. Monitor vital signs closely.

Effect on lab test results

• May decrease potassium level.

Pharmacokinetics

Absorption: Given I.V.
Distribution: Wide.
Metabolism: By liver.
Excretion: Mainly in urine with minor amounts in feces. *Half-life:* 2 minutes.

Route	Onset	Peak	Duration
I.V.	1–2 min	≤ 10 min	Unknown

Action

Chemical effect: Directly stimulates beta$_1$ receptors to increase myocardial contractility and stroke volume. Decreases peripheral vascular resistance (afterload), reduces ventricular filling pressure (preload), and may facilitate AV node conduction.
Therapeutic effect: Increases cardiac output.

Available forms

Injection: 12.5 mg/ml in 20-ml vials
Premixed: 0.5 mg/ml (125 mg or 250 mg) in D$_5$W, 1 mg/ml (250 mg or 500 mg) in D$_5$W 2 mg/ml (500 mg) in D$_5$W, 4 mg/ml (1,000 mg) in D$_5$W

NURSING PROCESS

Assessment
• Assess patient's condition before therapy and regularly thereafter.
• Continuously monitor ECG, blood pressure, pulmonary capillary wedge pressure, cardiac condition, and urine output.

- Monitor electrolyte level.
- Be alert for adverse reactions and drug interactions.
- Assess patient's and family's knowledge of drug therapy.

🌐 Nursing diagnoses

- Decreased cardiac output related to underlying condition
- Acute pain related to headache
- Deficient knowledge related to drug therapy

▶ Planning and implementation

- Before starting therapy, correct hypovolemia with plasma volume expanders.
- Give digoxin before giving this drug. Because drug increases AV node conduction, patients with atrial fibrillation may develop rapid ventricular rate.

ⓢ **ALERT:** Don't confuse dobutamine with dopamine.

Patient teaching

- Tell patient to report chest pain, shortness of breath, and headache.

✔ Evaluation

- Patient regains adequate cardiac output exhibited by stable vital signs, normal urine output, and clear mental condition.
- Patient's headache is relieved with analgesic administration.
- Patient and family state understanding of drug therapy.

HIGH ALERT!

docetaxel

(doks-uh-TAHKS-ul)

Taxotere

Pharmacologic class: taxoid antineoplastic
Therapeutic class: antineoplastic
Pregnancy risk category: D

Indications and dosages

▶ **Locally advanced or metastatic breast cancer for which prior chemotherapy has failed.**
Adults: 60 to 100 mg/m^2 I.V. over 1 hour every 3 weeks.

▶ **Locally advanced or metastatic non–small-cell lung cancer after failure of platinum-based chemotherapy.** *Adults:* 75 mg/m^2 I.V. over 1 hour every 3 weeks.

▶ **Unresectable, locally advanced, or metastatic non–small-cell lung cancer in patient who has not previously received chemotherapy for this condition with cisplatin.**
Adults: 75 mg/m^2 I.V. over 1 hour immediately followed by cisplatin 75 mg/m^2 I.V. over 30 to 60 minutes every 3 weeks.

▶ **Androgen-independent metastatic prostate cancer in combination with prednisone.** *Men:* 75 mg/m^2 I.V. as a 1-hour infusion every 3 weeks given with prednisone, 5 mg P.O. b.i.d. continuously. Premedicate with dexamethasone 8 mg P.O. at 12 hours, 3 hours, and 1 hour before the infusion.

▶ **Adjuvant post-surgery treatment of operable node-positive breast cancer.** *Adults:* 75 mg/m^2 I.V. as a 1-hour infusion given 1 hour after doxorubicin 50 mg/m^2 and cyclophosphamide 500 mg/m^2 every 3 weeks for 6 cycles. Patient's neutrophil count should be 1,500 cells/mm^3 or higher.

▶ **Advanced gastric adenocarcinoma, with cisplatin and fluorouracil (5–FU), in patients who haven't received chemotherapy for advanced disease.** *Adults:* Premedicate with antiemetics and hydration according to cisplatin recommendations. Give 75 mg/m^2 docetaxel I.V. over 1 hour, followed by cisplatin 75 mg/m^2 I.V. over 1 to 3 hours on day 1. Then give fluorouracil 750 mg/m^2 I.V. daily as a 24-hour continuous infusion for 5 days starting when cisplatin infusion ends. Repeat cycle every 3 weeks.

◢▪ **NEW INDICATION:** Induction treatment of inoperable locally advanced squamous cell cancer of the head and neck with cisplatin and fluorouracil (5-FU). *Adults:* 75 mg/m^2 I.V. infusion over 1 hour followed by cisplatin 75 mg/m^2 I.V. infusion over 1 hour, on day 1, followed by fluorouracil 750 mg/m^2 per day as a continuous I.V. infusion for 5 days. Repeat this regimen every 3 weeks for 4 cycles. Following chemotherapy, patients should receive radiotherapy. Premedicate with antiemetics and appropriate hydration before and after giving cisplatin.

◩ **Adjust-a-dose:** If patient develops hematologic, GI, or hepatic toxicities, reduce dose or stop treatment. In some cases, colony-stimulating factor may be helpful.

▼ I.V. administration

- Premedicate with oral corticosteroids for 3 days, starting 1 day before treatment to reduce fluid retention and hypersensitivity reactions.

• Wear gloves while preparing and giving drug. If solution contacts skin, wash immediately and thoroughly with soap and water. If drug contacts mucous membranes, flush thoroughly with water. Mark all waste materials with chemotherapy hazard labels.

• Prepare and store infusion solutions in bottles (glass or polypropylene) or plastic bags, and give through polyethylene-lined administration sets.

• Dilute drug with diluent supplied. Allow drug and diluent to stand at room temperature for 5 minutes before mixing. After adding diluent contents to vial, rotate vial gently for 15 seconds. Let solution stand for a few minutes for foam to dissipate.

• To prepare solution for infusion, withdraw required amount of premixed solution from vial and add it to 250 ml normal saline solution or D_5W to yield 0.3 to 0.9 mg/ml. Doses exceeding 240 mg need a larger volume of infusion solution to stay below 0.9 mg/ml of drug. Mix infusion thoroughly by manual rotation.

• Give drug as a 1-hour infusion; store unopened vials in the refrigerator.

• If solution isn't clear or if it contains precipitates, discard it. Use infusion solution within 8 hours.

⊗ **Incompatibilities**
None reported.

Contraindications and cautions

• Contraindicated in patients hypersensitive to drug or other drugs containing polysorbate 80 and in those with neutrophil counts below 1,500 cells/mm³.

• Don't give drug to patients with severe hepatic impairment, bilirubin level higher than the upper limits of normal (ULN) or with AST or ALT level higher than 1.5 times ULN and alkaline phosphatase level higher than 2.5 times ULN.

⚘ **Lifespan:** In pregnant and breast-feeding women, drug is contraindicated. In children younger than age 16, safety and effectiveness haven't been established.

Adverse reactions

CNS: *asthenia,* dysesthesia, pain, paresthesia, weakness.
CV: fluid retention, hypotension.
GI: diarrhea, nausea, stomatitis, vomiting.
Hematologic: *anemia,* FEBRILE NEUTROPENIA, LEUKOPENIA, MYELOSUPPRESSION, NEUTROPENIA, THROMBOCYTOPENIA.

Musculoskeletal: arthralgia, back pain, *myalgia.*
Respiratory: dyspnea.
Skin: *alopecia,* desquamation, flushing, nail pain, nail pigment changes, rash, skin eruptions.
Other: chest tightness, chills, drug fever, HYPERSENSITIVITY REACTIONS, infection, *septic and nonseptic death.*

Interactions

Drug-drug. *Drugs that are induced, inhibited, or metabolized by CYP3A4 (cyclosporin, ketoconazole, erythromycin, troleandomycin):* May modify docetaxel metabolism. Use together cautiously.

Effects on lab test results

• May increase ALT, AST, bilirubin, and alkaline phosphatase levels. May decrease hemoglobin level and hematocrit.

• May decrease WBC and platelet counts.

Pharmacokinetics

Absorption: Given I.V.
Distribution: 94% protein-bound.
Metabolism: Partly by liver.
Excretion: Mainly in feces. *Half-life:* About 12 hours.

Route	Onset	Peak	Duration
I.V.	Immediate	Unknown	Unknown

Action

Chemical effect: Disrupts the microtubular network essential for mitotic and interphase cellular functions.
Therapeutic effect: Inhibits mitosis, producing antineoplastic effect.

Available forms

Injection: 20 mg, 80 mg

NURSING PROCESS

▨ Assessment
• Monitor blood count often during therapy.
• Assess patient's and family's knowledge of drug therapy.

▣ Nursing diagnoses
• Ineffective health maintenance related to neoplastic disease
• Deficient knowledge related to drug therapy

Reactions may be *common,* uncommon, *life-threatening*, or COMMON AND LIFE-THREATENING.

D

⟫ Planning and implementation
- Don't give drug to patients with baseline neutrophil count less than 1,500/mm³.
- ⑤ **ALERT:** Don't confuse Taxotere with Taxol.

Patient teaching
- Warn patient that alopecia occurs in almost 80% of patients.
- Tell patient to promptly report sore throat, fever, unusual bruising or bleeding, or signs of fluid retention.

☑ Evaluation
- Patient shows positive response to drug.
- Patient and family state understanding of drug therapy.

---

docusate calcium (dioctyl calcium sulfosuccinate)
(DOK-yoo-sayt KAL-see-um)
DC Softgels†, Sulfolax†

docusate sodium (dioctyl sodium sulfosuccinate)
Colace†, Diocto†, Dioctyn†, Docu†, D-S-S†, ex-lax†, Phillips' Liqui-Gel†, Regulax SS†, Silace†, Sof-lax†

Pharmacologic class: surfactant
Therapeutic class: emollient laxative
Pregnancy risk category: C

Indications and dosages
▶ **Stool softener.** *Adults and children age 12 and older:* 50 to 360 mg P.O. daily until bowel movements are normal. Or give enema (where available). Dilute 1:24 with sterile water before administration, and give 100 to 150 ml (retention enema), 300 to 500 ml (evacuation enema), or 0.5 to 1.5 liters (flushing enema).
Children ages 6 to 12: Give 40 to 120 mg docusate sodium P.O. daily.
Children ages 3 to 6: Give 20 to 60 mg docusate sodium P.O. daily.
Children younger than age 3: Give 10 to 40 mg docusate sodium P.O. daily. Higher dosages used for initial therapy. Adjust dosage to individual response.
Adults and children: Usual dosage, 240 mg docusate calcium P.O. daily until bowel movements are normal.

Contraindications and cautions
- Contraindicated in patients hypersensitive to drug or any of its components and in those with intestinal obstruction, undiagnosed abdominal pain, signs of appendicitis, fecal impaction, or acute surgical abdomen.
- ⚖ **Lifespan:** In pregnant women, use cautiously.

Adverse reactions
CNS: fainting.
EENT: throat irritation.
GI: bitter taste, diarrhea, laxative dependence with long-term or excessive use, mild abdominal cramping.

Interactions
Drug-drug. *Mineral oil:* May increase mineral oil absorption and cause toxicity and lipoid pneumonia. Separate doses.

Effects on lab test results
None reported.

Pharmacokinetics
Absorption: Minimal.
Distribution: Mainly local.
Metabolism: None.
Excretion: In feces. *Half-life:* Unknown.

Route	Onset	Peak	Duration
P.O.	Varies	Varies	24–72 hr
P.R.	Unknown	Unknown	Unknown

Action
Chemical effect: Reduces surface tension of interfacing liquid contents of bowel. This detergent activity promotes incorporation of additional liquid into stool, thus forming softer mass.
Therapeutic effect: Softens stool.

Available forms
docusate calcium
Capsules: 240 mg†
docusate potassium
Capsules: 100 mg†, 240 mg†
docusate sodium
Capsules: 50 mg†, 60 mg†, 100 mg†, 240 mg†, 250 mg†
Oral liquid: 150 mg/15 ml†
Oral solution: 50 mg/ml†

Syrup: 20 mg/5 ml*†, 50 mg/15 ml†, 60 mg/15 ml†, 100 mg/30 ml†
Tablets: 100 mg†

Assessment
- Obtain history of patient's bowel patterns before therapy, and reassess regularly thereafter.
- Before giving drug for constipation, determine if patient has adequate fluid intake, exercise, and diet.
- Be alert for adverse reactions and drug interactions.
- Assess patient's and family's knowledge of drug therapy.

Nursing diagnoses
- Constipation related to underlying condition
- Diarrhea related to prolonged or excessive use of drug
- Deficient knowledge related to drug therapy

Planning and implementation
- Give liquid in milk, fruit juice, or infant formula to mask bitter taste.
- Drug is the laxative of choice for patients who shouldn't strain during defecation, including patients recovering from MI or rectal surgery, patients with a rectal or anal disease that makes passage of firm stool difficult, or patients with postpartum constipation.
- Store drug at 59° to 86° F (15° to 30° C), and protect liquid from light.
- If abdominal cramping occurs, stop drug and notify prescriber.
- Drug doesn't stimulate intestinal peristaltic movements.
- **ALERT:** Don't confuse Colace and Calan.

Patient teaching
- Teach patient about dietary sources of bulk, which include bran and other cereals, fresh fruit, and vegetables.
- Instruct patient to use only occasionally and not to use for longer than 1 week without prescriber's knowledge.
- Tell patient to stop taking the drug and to notify the prescriber if severe cramping occurs.

Evaluation
- Patient's constipation is relieved.
- Patient remains free from diarrhea during therapy.

- Patient and family state understanding of drug therapy.

dofetilide
(doh-FET-eh-lighd)
Tikosyn

Pharmacologic class: antiarrhythmic
Therapeutic class: class III antiarrhythmic
Pregnancy risk category: C

Indications and dosages
▶ **To maintain normal sinus rhythm in patients with symptomatic atrial fibrillation or atrial flutter for longer than 1 week who have been converted to normal sinus rhythm; to convert atrial fibrillation and atrial flutter to normal sinus rhythm.** *Adults:* Dosage is individualized and is based on creatinine clearance and QT interval, which must be obtained before first dose. (If pulse is less than 60 beats/minute, use QT interval.) Usual dosage is 500 mcg P.O. b.i.d. for patients with creatinine clearance above 60 ml/minute.
Adjust-a-dose: For patients with renal impairment, if creatinine clearance is 40 to 60 ml/minute, give 250 mcg P.O. b.i.d. If creatinine clearance is 20 to 39 ml/minute, give 125 mcg P.O. b.i.d. If creatinine clearance is less than 20 ml/minute, drug is contraindicated.
For patients who develop prolonged QT interval, adjust dosage or stop drug.

Contraindications and cautions
- Contraindicated in patients with congenital or acquired prolonged QT-interval syndromes. Also contraindicated in patients with baseline QTc interval greater than 440 msec (500 msec in patients with ventricular conduction abnormalities). Also contraindicated in patients with creatinine clearance below 20 ml/min and in patients hypersensitive to drug and in those receiving verapamil, cimetidine, hydrochlorothiazide (alone or with triamterene), trimethoprim (alone or with sulfamethoxazole), or ketoconazole.
- Use cautiously in patients with severe hepatic impairment.
- **Lifespan:** In pregnant women, use cautiously. In breast-feeding women, drug isn't recommended. In children, safety and effectiveness haven't been established.

Adverse reactions

CNS: anxiety, asthenia, *cerebral ischemia,* dizziness, *headache,* insomnia, migraine, paresthesia, *stroke,* syncope.
CV: angina, atrial fibrillation, *bradycardia,* bundle branch block, *cardiac arrest,* chest pain, edema, heart block, hypertension, *MI,* palpitations, peripheral edema, *torsades de pointes, ventricular fibrillation, ventricular tachycardia.*
EENT: facial paralysis.
GI: abdominal pain, diarrhea, nausea.
GU: UTI.
Hepatic: *liver damage.*
Musculoskeletal: arthralgia, back pain.
Respiratory: dyspnea, increased cough, respiratory tract infection.
Skin: rash, sweating.
Other: *angioedema,* flulike symptoms.

Interactions

Drug-drug. *Amiloride, metformin, triamterene:* May increase dofetilide level. Use together cautiously.
Cimetidine, ketoconazole, sulfamethoxazole, trimethoprim, verapamil: May increase dofetilide level. Don't use together.
Inhibitors of CYP3A4 (amiodarone, azole antifungals, cannabinoids, diltiazem, macrolide antibiotics, nefazodone, norfloxacin, protease inhibitors, quinine, serotonin reuptake inhibitors, zafirlukast): May decrease metabolism and increase dofetilide level. Use together cautiously; monitor patient for toxicity.
Inhibitors of renal cationic secretion (megestrol, prochlorperazine): May increase dofetilide level. Avoid use together.
Drug-food. *Grapefruit juice:* May decrease dofetilide's hepatic metabolism and increase its level. Avoid use together.

Effects on lab test results

None reported.

Pharmacokinetics

Absorption: More than 90%; levels peak at 2 to 3 hours. Steady-state levels are achieved in 2 to 3 days. Unaffected by food or antacid.
Distribution: Wide with a volume of distribution of 3 L/kg. 60% to 70% protein-bound.
Metabolism: Small, by the CYP3A4 isoenzyme in the liver.

Excretion: 80% in urine, of which 80% is unchanged drug while the rest is inactive or minimally active metabolites. *Half-life:* 10 hours.

Route	Onset	Peak	Duration
P.O.	Unknown	2–3 hr	Unknown

Action

Chemical effect: Prolongs repolarization without affecting conduction velocity by blocking the cardiac ion channel carrying potassium current.
Therapeutic effect: Converts atrial fibrillation and atrial flutter to normal sinus rhythm, and maintains normal rhythm.

Available forms

Capsules: 125 mcg (0.125 mg), 250 mcg (0.25 mg), 500 mcg (0.5 mg)

NURSING PROCESS

Assessment

• Obtain accurate medication list (prescription, OTC, and herbal) from patient before starting drug; stop antiarrhythmic under careful monitoring for at least 2 days before giving second antiarrhythmic. Don't give drug within 3 months of amiodarone unless level is below 0.3 mcg/ml.
• Assess patient's QTc interval, cardiac rhythm, creatinine clearance, and vital signs before starting medication. Prolongation of the QTc interval requires subsequent dosage adjustments or discontinuation. Continuous ECG monitoring is required for a minimum of 3 days for maintenance therapy, or 12 hours after conversion to normal sinus rhythm.
• Obtain potassium level before starting therapy and regularly thereafter. Hypokalemia and hypomagnesemia may occur when giving potassium-depleting diuretics, increasing the risk of torsades de pointes. Achieve and maintain normal potassium level.
• Monitor patient for prolonged diarrhea, sweating, and vomiting, and report any such symptoms to the prescriber because electrolyte imbalance may increase the risk of arrhythmias.
• Monitor renal function and QTc interval every 3 months.
• Assess patient's and family's knowledge of drug therapy.

⊕ Nursing diagnoses
- Decreased cardiac output related to underlying arrhythmia
- Risk for injury related to drug-induced adverse reactions
- Deficient knowledge related to drug therapy

▶ Planning and implementation
- Drug is distributed only to hospitals and other institutions with dosage and treatment initiation programs. Inpatient and outpatient discharge and refills of prescriptions are allowed only with confirmation that prescriber has access to these programs.
- If patient doesn't convert to normal sinus rhythm within 24 hours after starting drug, use electrical cardioversion.
- Drug must be given by specially certified prescriber in an acute care facility because of potentially high risk of torsades de pointes.
- If drug must be stopped to allow administration of other interacting drugs, allow washout period of at least 2 days before starting other drug.

Patient teaching
- Instruct patient to notify prescriber about any change in prescription drugs, OTC medications, or herbal remedies.
- Urge patient to immediately report excessive or prolonged diarrhea, sweating, vomiting, or loss of appetite or thirst to prescriber.
- Inform patient that dofetilide can be taken without regard to meals or antacids.
- Tell patient not to take drug with grapefruit juice.
- Warn patient not to use OTC Tagamet-HB for ulcers or heartburn. Explain that antacids and OTC acid reducers such as Zantac 75 mg, Pepcid, Axid, and Prevacid are acceptable.
- Instruct woman to notify prescriber about planned, suspected, or known pregnancy.
- Advise patient not to breast-feed while taking dofetilide.
- If patient misses a dose, tell him to skip it and wait for the next scheduled dose. Caution against doubling the dose.

☑ Evaluation
- Patient maintains normal sinus rhythm.
- Patient has no injury as a result of drug-induced adverse reactions.
- Patient and family state understanding of drug therapy.

dolasetron mesylate
(doh-LEH-seh-trohn MES-ih-layt)
Anzemet

Pharmacologic class: selective serotonin (5-HT₃) receptor antagonist
Therapeutic class: antiemetic
Pregnancy risk category: B

Indications and dosages
▶ **To prevent nausea and vomiting after cancer chemotherapy.** *Adults:* 100 mg P.O. given as a single dose 1 hour before chemotherapy. Or 1.8 mg/kg (or a fixed dose of 100 mg) as a single I.V. dose given 30 minutes before chemotherapy.
Children ages 2 to 16: Give 1.8 mg/kg P.O. 1 hour before chemotherapy. Or 1.8 mg/kg as single I.V. dose 30 minutes before chemotherapy. Injectable form can be mixed with apple juice and given P.O. Maximum dose, 100 mg.
▶ **To prevent postoperative nausea and vomiting.** *Adults:* 100 mg P.O. within 2 hours before surgery. Or 12.5 mg as single I.V. dose about 15 minutes before cessation of anesthesia.
Children ages 2 to 16: Give 1.2 mg/kg P.O. within 2 hours before surgery, to maximum, 100 mg. Or 0.35 mg/kg (up to 12.5 mg) as single I.V. dose about 15 minutes before cessation of anesthesia. Injectable form can be mixed with apple juice and given P.O.
▶ **Postoperative nausea and vomiting.** *Adults:* 12.5 mg as a single I.V. dose as soon as nausea or vomiting begins.
Children ages 2 to 16: Give 0.35 mg/kg to maximum, 12.5 mg, as a single I.V. dose as soon as nausea or vomiting begins.

▼ I.V. administration
- Drug can be injected as rapidly as 100 mg in 30 seconds, or diluted in 50 ml of compatible solution and infused over 15 minutes.
- If an arrhythmia develops, stop the drug and notify prescriber immediately.
- After dilution, solution is stable for 24 hours at room temperature or 48 hours if refrigerated.
⊗ **Incompatibilities**
Injection shouldn't be mixed with other drugs.

Contraindications and cautions

• Contraindicated in patients hypersensitive to drug or any of its components.
• Give cautiously to patients who have or may develop prolonged cardiac conduction intervals, such as those with electrolyte abnormalities, history of arrhythmias, and cumulative high-dose anthracycline therapy.
⚘ **Lifespan:** In breast-feeding women, use cautiously because it's unknown if drug appears in breast milk. In infants, drug isn't recommended.

Adverse reactions

CNS: dizziness, drowsiness, fatigue, fever, *headache.*
CV: *arrhythmias, bradycardia,* ECG changes, hypertension, hypotension, tachycardia.
GI: abdominal pain, anorexia, constipation, *diarrhea,* dyspepsia.
GU: oliguria, urine retention.
Skin: pruritus, rash.
Other: chills, pain at injection site.

Interactions

Drug-drug. *Drugs that induce cytochrome P-450 enzymes (such as rifampin):* May decrease hydrodolasetron level. Monitor patient for decreased effectiveness of drug.
Drugs that inhibit cytochrome P-450 enzymes (such as atenolol, cimetidine): May increase hydrodolasetron level. Monitor patient for adverse effects.
Drugs that prolong ECG intervals (such as antiarrhythmics): May increase risk of arrhythmia. Monitor patient closely.

Effect on lab test results

• May increase ALT and AST levels.

Pharmacokinetics

Absorption: Rapid for hydrodolasetron, an active metabolite that has an absolute bioavailability of 75%.
Distribution: Wide, with 69% to 77% bound to plasma protein.
Metabolism: Rapid and complete.
Excretion: Two-thirds of hydrodolasetron is in urine; rest in feces. *Half-life:* 8 hours.

Route	Onset	Peak	Duration
P.O.	Rapid	1 hr	8 hr
I.V.	Rapid	36 min	7 hr

Action

Chemical effect: Blocks the action of serotonin, thereby preventing serotonin from stimulating the vomiting reflex.
Therapeutic effect: Prevents nausea and vomiting.

Available forms

Injection: 20 mg/ml as 12.5 mg/0.625 ml-ampule or 100 mg/5 ml-vial
Tablets: 50 mg, 100 mg

NURSING PROCESS

⚡ Assessment

• Assess patient for history of nausea and vomiting related to chemotherapy or postoperative recovery.
• Be alert for adverse reactions and drug interactions.
• Monitor ECG carefully in patients who have or may develop prolonged cardiac conduction intervals.
• Assess patient's and family's knowledge of drug therapy.

🔆 Nursing diagnoses

• Imbalanced nutrition: less than body requirements, related to nausea and vomiting
• Risk for injury related to drug-induced adverse CNS reaction
• Deficient knowledge related to drug therapy

▶ Planning and implementation

• Injection for P.O. use is stable in apple juice for 2 hours at room temperature.
🔵 **ALERT:** Don't confuse Anzemet with Avandamet.
Patient teaching
• Tell patient about potential adverse effects.
• Instruct patient not to mix injection in juice for P.O. use until just before taking the dose.
• Tell patient to report nausea or vomiting.

✓ Evaluation

• Patient has no nausea and vomiting.
• Patient is free from injury.
• Patient and family state understanding of drug therapy.

donepezil hydrochloride
(doh-NEH-peh-zil high-droh-KLOR-ighd)
Aricept, Aricept ODT

Pharmacologic class: reversible inhibitor of acetylcholinesterase
Therapeutic class: psychotherapeutic drug for Alzheimer disease
Pregnancy risk category: C

Indications and dosages

▶ **Mild to moderate and severe dementia of the Alzheimer type.** *Adults:* Initially, 5 mg P.O. daily at bedtime. After 4 to 6 weeks, may increase dosage to 10 mg daily.

Contraindications and cautions

• Contraindicated in patients hypersensitive to drug or to piperidine derivatives.
• Use cautiously in patients with history of ulcer disease, CV disease, asthma or COPD, or urinary outflow impairment. Also use cautiously in patients currently taking NSAIDs.
⚜ **Lifespan:** In pregnant women, use only if benefits to the woman outweigh risks to the fetus. Breast-feeding women shouldn't nurse during therapy. In children, safety and effectiveness haven't been established.

Adverse reactions

CNS: abnormal crying, abnormal dreams, aggression, aphasia, ataxia, depression, dizziness, fatigue, *headache,* insomnia, irritability, nervousness, pain, paresthesia, restlessness, *seizures,* somnolence, syncope, tremor, vertigo.
CV: atrial fibrillation, chest pain, hypertension, hypotension, vasodilation.
EENT: blurred vision, cataracts, eye irritation, sore throat.
GI: anorexia, bloating, *diarrhea,* epigastric pain, fecal incontinence, *GI bleeding, nausea,* vomiting.
GU: frequent urination, nocturia, urinary incontinence.
Metabolic: dehydration, weight decrease.
Musculoskeletal: arthritis, bone fracture, muscle cramps, toothache.
Respiratory: bronchitis, dyspnea.
Skin: diaphoresis, ecchymosis, pruritus, urticaria.

Other: accident, hot flushes, increased libido, influenza.

Interactions

Drug-drug. *Anticholinergics:* May interfere with anticholinergic activity. Monitor patient for effects.
Bethanechol, succinylcholine: May have additive effects. Monitor patient closely.
Carbamazepine, dexamethasone, phenytoin, phenobarbital, rifampin: May increase rate of donepezil elimination. Monitor patient for effects.
Cholinomimetics, cholinesterase inhibitors: May have synergistic effect. Monitor patient closely.
NSAIDs: May increase gastric acid secretion. Monitor patient for occult bleeding.
Drug-herb. *Jaborandi tree, pill-bearing spurge:* May cause additive effect and increased risk of toxicity. Discourage use together.

Effects on lab test results

None reported.

Pharmacokinetics

Absorption: Good.
Distribution: 96% bound to plasma proteins, mainly to albumin.
Metabolism: Extensive.
Excretion: In urine and feces. *Half-life:* 70 hours.

Route	Onset	Peak	Duration
P.O.	Unknown	3–4 hr	Unknown

Action

Chemical effect: Reversibly inhibits acetylcholinesterase in the CNS, thereby increasing the acetylcholine level.
Therapeutic effect: Temporarily improves cognitive function in patients with Alzheimer disease.

Available forms

Tablets: 5 mg, 10 mg
Tablets (orally-disintegrating): 5 mg, 10 mg

NURSING PROCESS

📖 Assessment

• Monitor patient for symptoms of active or occult GI bleeding.
• Assess patient's and family's knowledge of drug therapy.

Reactions may be *common,* uncommon, *life-threatening*, or COMMON AND LIFE-THREATENING.

⊕ Nursing diagnoses
• Risk for injury related to adverse effects of drug
• Deficient knowledge related to drug therapy

▶ Planning and implementation
• Give drug at bedtime, with or without food.
• If cholinergic crisis (severe nausea, vomiting, salivation, sweating, bradycardia, hypotension, respiratory depression, convulsions, and collapse) occurs, treat with an anticholinergic such as atropine.

Patient teaching
• Explain that drug doesn't alter underlying degenerative disease but can alleviate symptoms.
• Tell caregiver to give drug in the evening, just before bedtime.
• Advise patient and caregiver to immediately report significant adverse effects or changes in overall health condition.
• Tell caregiver to inform health care team that patient is taking drug before patient receives anesthesia.

✔ Evaluation
• Patient remains free from injury.
• Patient and family state understanding of drug therapy.

HIGH ALERT!

dopamine hydrochloride
(DOH-puh-meen high-droh-KLOR-ighd)

Pharmacologic class: adrenergic
Therapeutic class: inotropic, vasopressor
Pregnancy risk category: C

Indications and dosages

▶ **To treat shock and correct hemodynamic imbalances; to improve perfusion to vital organs; to increase cardiac output; to correct hypotension.** *Adults and children:* Initially, 2 to 5 mcg/kg/minute by I.V. infusion. Adjust dosage to desired hemodynamic or renal response, increase by 1 to 4 mcg/kg/minute at 10- to 30-minute intervals.

▼ I.V. administration
• Dilute with D_5W, normal saline solution, or combination of D_5W and normal saline solution. Mix just before use.

• Use continuous infusion pump to regulate flow rate.
• Use central line or large vein, such as in antecubital fossa, to minimize risk of extravasation. If extravasation occurs, stop infusion immediately and call prescriber. Extravasation may require treatment by infiltration of area with 5 to 10 mg of phentolamine and 10 to 15 ml of normal saline solution.
• If solution is discolored, discard within 24 hours.

⊗ **Incompatibilities**
Acyclovir sodium, additives with a dopamine and dextrose solution, alteplase, amphotericin B, cefepime, furosemide, gentamicin, indomethacin sodium trihydrate, iron salts, insulin, oxidizing agents, penicillin G potassium, sodium bicarbonate or other alkaline solutions, thiopental.

Contraindications and cautions
• Contraindicated in patients with uncorrected tachyarrhythmias, pheochromocytoma, or ventricular fibrillation.
• Use cautiously in patients with occlusive vascular disease, cold injuries, diabetic endarteritis, and arterial embolism, and in those taking MAO inhibitors.
  ⚠ **Lifespan:** In pregnant women, use cautiously. In breast-feeding women, safety and effectiveness haven't been established.

Adverse reactions
CNS: headache, anxiety.
CV: anginal pain, *arrhythmias, bradycardia,* conduction disturbances, ectopic beats, hypertension, hypotension, palpitations, tachycardia, vasoconstriction, *widening of QRS complex.*
GI: nausea, vomiting.
GU: azotemia.
Respiratory: *asthma attacks,* dyspnea.
Skin: necrosis, piloerection, tissue sloughing with extravasation.
Other: *anaphylaxis.*

Interactions
Drug-drug. *Alpha and beta blockers:* May antagonize dopamine effects. Monitor patient for effect.
Ergot alkaloids: May increase blood pressure. Don't use together.

Inhaled anesthetics: May increase risk of arrhythmias or hypertension. Monitor vital signs and ECG closely.

Oxytocic drugs: May potentiate pressor effect, resulting in severe hypertension. Avoid use together, if possible.

Phenelzine, tranylcypromine: May cause severe headache, hypertension, fever, and hypertensive crisis. Avoid use together.

Phenytoin: May lower blood pressure in dopamine-stabilized patients. Monitor blood pressure carefully.

Tricyclic antidepressants: May decrease pressor response. Monitor patient closely.

Effects on lab test results

• May increase glucose and urea levels.

Pharmacokinetics

Absorption: Given I.V.
Distribution: Wide; doesn't cross blood–brain barrier.
Metabolism: To inactive compounds in liver, kidneys, and plasma.
Excretion: In urine, mainly as its metabolites.
Half-life: 2 minutes in adults; 5 to 11 minutes in neonates.

Route	Onset	Peak	Duration
I.V.	≤ 5 min	Unknown	≤ 10 min

Action

Chemical effect: Stimulates dopaminergic, beta-adrenergic, and alpha-adrenergic receptors of sympathetic nervous system.
Therapeutic effect: Increases cardiac output, blood pressure, and renal perfusion (in low doses).

Available forms

Injection: 40 mg/ml, 80 mg/ml, 160 mg/ml as concentrate for injection for I.V. infusion; 0.8 mg/ml (200 or 400 mg) in D₅W; 1.6 mg/ml (400 or 800 mg) in D₅W; 3.2 mg/ml (800 mg) in D₅W as parenteral injection for I.V. infusion

NURSING PROCESS

Assessment

• Obtain history of patient's underlying condition before therapy.
• During infusion, frequently monitor ECG, blood pressure, cardiac output, central venous pressure, pulmonary capillary wedge pressure, pulse rate, urine output, and color and temperature of limbs.

• Be alert for adverse reactions and drug interactions.

• Be aware that acidosis decreases effectiveness of dopamine.

• After drug is stopped, watch closely for sudden drop in blood pressure.

• Assess patient's and family's knowledge of drug therapy.

Nursing diagnoses

• Ineffective tissue perfusion (cerebral, cardiopulmonary, and renal) related to underlying condition

• Risk for injury related to drug-induced adverse reactions

• Deficient knowledge related to drug therapy

Planning and implementation

• Be aware that dosages of 0.5 to 2 mcg/kg/minute mainly stimulate dopamine receptors and dilate renal vasculature increasing urine output. Dosages of 2 to 10 mcg/kg/minute stimulate beta receptors for increased cardiac output. Higher dosages also stimulate alpha-adrenergic receptors, causing vasoconstriction and increased blood pressure. Most patients are satisfactorily maintained on dosages below 20 mcg/kg/minute.

• Drug isn't used to treat blood or fluid volume deficit. If deficit exists, replace fluid before giving vasopressors.

• Taper dosage slowly to evaluate stability of blood pressure.

• If patient receiving dopamine has disproportionate rise in diastolic pressure (a marked decrease in pulse pressure), decrease infusion rate, and watch carefully for further evidence of predominant vasoconstrictor activity, unless such effect is desired.

• If an adverse reaction develops, notify prescriber, who will reduce the dosage or stop the drug.

• If urine flow decreases without hypotension, notify prescriber and reduce dosage.

ALERT: Don't confuse dopamine with dobutamine.

Patient teaching

• Emphasize importance of reporting discomfort at I.V. site immediately.

• Explain to patient the need for drug therapy.

Reactions may be *common*, uncommon, *life-threatening*, or COMMON AND LIFE-THREATENING.

☑ Evaluation
• Patient regains adequate cerebral, cardiopulmonary, and renal tissue perfusion.
• Patient doesn't experience injury as result of drug-induced adverse reactions.
• Patient and family state understanding of drug therapy.

✳ New Drug

doripenem
(dor-eh-PEN-em)
Doribax

Pharmacologic class: carbapenem
Therapeutic class: antibiotic
Pregnancy risk category: B

Indications and dosages

▶ **Complicated intra-abdominal infections caused by** *Escherichia coli, Klebsiella pneumoniae, Pseudomonas aeruginosa, Bacteroides caccae, Bacteroides fragilis, Bacteroides thetaiotaomicron, Bacteroides uniformis, Bacteroides vulgatas, Streptococcus intermedius, Streptococcus constellatus,* **and** *Peptostreptococcus micros. Adults:* 500 mg I.V. every 8 hours for 5 to 14 days.
▶ **Complicated UTIs, including pyelonephritis caused by** *E. coli, K. pneumoniae, Proteus mirabilis, P. aeruginosa,* **and** *Acinetobacter baumannii. Adults:* 500 mg I.V. every 8 hours for 10 to 14 days.
🔂 **Adjust-a-dose:** In patients with creatinine clearance of 30 to 50 ml/minute give 250 mg I.V. every 8 hours; with creatinine clearance 11 to 29 ml/minute, give 250 mg I.V. every 12 hours.

▼ I.V. administration

• Dilute drug in single-use vial with sterile water for injection or normal saline for injection and shake gently to form a concentration of 50 mg/ml.
• Add reconstituted drug to normal saline or D_5W according to manufacturer's instructions for a final concentration of 4.5 mg/ml.
• Inspect solution for particulate matter and discoloration. Solution should be clear to slightly yellow.
• Give only by infusion over 1 hour.

• Solution prepared with normal saline may be stored at room temperature for 8 hours; D_5W for 4 hours.
⊗ **Incompatibilities**
Other I.V. drugs.

Contraindications and cautions

• Contraindicated in patients hypersensitive to drug, its components, or other beta-lactams.
• Use cautiously in those with moderate to severe renal impairment.
🚢 **Lifespan:** In pregnant women, drug hasn't been adequately studied. Use only if need outweighs risk to fetus. In breast-feeding women, it isn't known if drug is excreted in breast milk. Use cautiously. In children, safety and effectiveness haven't been established.

Adverse reactions

CNS: *headache,* seizure.
GI: *pseudomembranous colitis, nausea, diarrhea.*
GU: renal insufficiency or *failure.*
Hematologic: *anemia.*
Respiratory: interstitial pneumonia.
Skin: *skin reactions (Stevens-Johnson syndrome, toxic epidermal necrolysis),* phlebitis, pruritus, rash.
Other: *anaphylaxis,* infection.

Interactions

Drug-drug. *Probenecid:* Increases drug level. Avoid use together.
Valproic acid: May decrease valproic acid levels and cause seizures. Monitor valproic acid levels. May need to switch to another antibacterial or anticonvulsant if valproic acid levels can't be maintained.

Effects on lab test results

• May increase ALT, AST, transaminases, other hepatic enzyme levels.
• May decrease RBC count.

Pharmacokinetics

Absorption: Rapid.
Distribution: About 8% bound to plasma proteins. Penetrates retroperitoneal fluid, peritoneal exudates, gallbladder, bile, and urine.
Metabolism: Via dehydropeptidase-1.

Excretion: Unchanged in urine. *Half-life:* 1 hour.

Route	Onset	Peak	Duration
I.V.	Unknown	Unknown	Unknown

Action

Chemical effect: Inhibits bacteria cell wall biosynthesis by inactivating multiple penicillin-binding proteins causing cell death.
Therapeutic effect: Antibiotic.

Available forms

Injection: 500-mg vial

NURSING PROCESS

☆ Assessment

• Assess for history of anaphylaxis to beta-lactams (carbapenems, penicillins, cephalosporins). Use cautiously if drug is used in those with history of allergies; serious and fatal anaphylaxis and skin reactions have occurred. If reaction occurs, stop drug and use supportive measures such as oxygen, I.V. fluids, I.V. antihistamines, corticosteroids, pressor amines, and airway management.
• Culture organism before administration to make sure organism is susceptible to therapy; this will reduce the development of drug-resistant organisms.
• Assess patient's and family's knowledge of drug therapy.

⊕ Nursing diagnoses

• Risk for infection related to presence of susceptible bacterial infection
• Risk for deficient fluid volume related to drug-induced adverse GI reactions
• Deficient knowledge related to drug therapy

▷ Planning and implementation

• Monitor patient for psuedomembranous colitis, which can occur for up to 2 months after administration; treat with supportive measures (fluid and electrolyte therapy, protein supplementation, antibiotics, and surgical evaluation).
• Monitor renal function, especially in those with renal impairment and in the elderly.
• Report adverse reactions to Ortho-McNeil at 1-800-526-7736 or the FDA at 1-800-FDA-1088 or www.fda.gov/medwatch.

Patient teaching

• Tell patient to report serious adverse effects, such as dyspnea, skin reaction, pain at injection site, or diarrhea.
• Advise patient that severe and life-threatening diarrhea can occur for up to 2 months after drug is given. Report diarrhea to prescriber immediately.

☑ Evaluation

• Patient is free from infection.
• Patient doesn't experience adverse effects of therapy.
• Patient and family state understanding of drug therapy.

dorzolamide hydrochloride

(dor-ZOLE-uh-mighd high-droh-KLOR-ighd)
Trusopt

Pharmacologic class: carbonic anhydrase inhibitor, sulfonamide
Therapeutic class: antiglaucoma drug
Pregnancy risk category: C

Indications and dosages

▶ **Increased intraocular pressure (IOP) in patients with ocular hypertension or open-angle glaucoma.** *Adults and children:* Instill 1 drop in the conjunctival sac of affected eye t.i.d.

Contraindications and cautions

• Contraindicated in patients hypersensitive to drug or any of its components. Also contraindicated in those with renal impairment.
• Use cautiously in patients with impaired hepatic function.
⚘ **Lifespan:** In pregnant women, use only if potential benefits to the woman outweigh the risks to the fetus. In breast-feeding women, drug isn't recommended because it's unknown if it appears in breast milk. In elderly patients, use cautiously because they may have greater sensitivity to drug.

Adverse reactions

CNS: asthenia, dizziness, fatigue, headache, paresthesia.
EENT: blurred vision; dryness; eyelid crusting; iridocyclitis; lacrimation; ocular allergic reac-

tions, including conjunctivitis, itching, and lid reactions; ocular burning, stinging, and discomfort; ocular pain; photophobia; redness; superficial punctate keratitis; throat irritation; transient myopia.

GI: bitter taste, nausea.
GU: urolithiasis.
Respiratory: *bronchospasm,* dyspnea.
Skin: contact dermatitis, pruritus, rash, urticaria.
Other: *angioedema.*

Interactions

Drug-drug. *Oral carbonic anhydrase inhibitors:* May cause additive effects. Don't use together.
Topical beta blockers: May cause additive effects. Give drugs 10 minutes apart.

Effects on lab tests results

• May decrease potassium and pH levels.

Pharmacokinetics

Absorption: Systemic.
Distribution: 33% bound to plasma proteins. Accumulates in RBCs during regular therapy.
Metabolism: In the liver by cytochrome P-450 isoenzymes.
Excretion: Mainly unchanged in urine. *Half-life:* 4 months.

Route	Onset	Peak	Duration
Ophthalmic	1–2 hr	2–3 hr	8 hr

Action

Chemical effect: Inhibits carbonic anhydrase in the ciliary processes of the eye. This action reduces aqueous humor secretion, presumably by slowing the formation of bicarbonate ions with subsequent reduction in sodium and fluid transport.
Therapeutic effect: Reduces IOP.

Available forms

Ophthalmic solution: 2%

NURSING PROCESS

Assessment
• Assess patient before starting therapy.
• Because drug is a sulfonamide that is absorbed systemically, the adverse reactions caused by sulfonamides, such as Stevens-

Johnson syndrome, agranulocytosis, and aplastic anemia, may occur. Although these symptoms haven't been shown with this drug, monitor for them during therapy.
• Overdose may result in electrolyte imbalance, acidosis, and CNS effects. Monitor electrolyte levels (especially potassium) and pH levels. Provide supportive therapy for any overdose.
• Assess patient's and family's understanding of drug therapy.

Nursing diagnoses
• Risk for infection to the eyes related to inadvertent contamination of the multidose container
• Disturbed visual perception related to underlying ocular condition
• Deficient knowledge related to drug therapy

Planning and implementation
• If patient is wearing contact lenses, remove lenses before giving the drug. Contact lenses may be reinserted 15 minutes after the drug is given.
• Instruct patient not to blink after administration, just close eyes. Apply light finger pressure on lacrimal sac for 1 minute after instillation to minimize systemic absorption of drug.
• If more than one topical ophthalmic drug is being used, give drugs at least 10 minutes apart.
Patient teaching
• Teach patient how to instill drops properly. Advise him to wash hands before and after instilling solution, and warn him not to touch dropper or tip to eye or surrounding tissue, to prevent contamination to the dropper.
• If patient wears contact lenses, instruct him to remove them before instilling the drops and to reinsert them 15 minutes after instillation.
• Advise patient to report ocular reactions, particularly conjunctivitis and lid reactions, immediately to prescriber and to stop drug.

Evaluation
• Patient doesn't suffer from any infection related to drug administration.
• Patient's underlying condition is resolved with drug therapy.
• Patient and family state understanding of drug therapy.

doxapram hydrochloride

(DOKS-uh-prahm high-droh-KLOR-ighd)
Dopram

Pharmacologic class: analeptic
Therapeutic class: CNS and respiratory stimulant
Pregnancy risk category: B

Indications and dosages

▶ **Postanesthesia respiratory stimulation, drug-induced CNS depression, chronic pulmonary disease with acute hypercapnia.**
Adults: 0.5 to 1 mg/kg of body weight (up to 2 mg/kg in CNS depression) by I.V. injection or infusion. Repeat every 5 minutes, if needed. Maximum, 4 mg/kg, up to 3 g daily.
▶ **COPD.** *Adults:* 1 to 2 mg/minute by I.V. infusion. Maximum, 3 mg/minute for maximum duration of 2 hours.

▽ I.V. administration

• For I.V. infusion, add 250 mg of drug to 250 ml of 5% or 10% dextrose or normal saline solution injection; concentration equals 1 mg/ml.
• For acute hypercapnia related to COPD, add 400 mg of drug to 180 ml of dextrose or normal saline solution to equal 2 mg/ml. Infuse at 1 to 3 mg/minute.
• Give drug slowly because rapid infusion may cause hemolysis.
• Watch for irritation and infiltration.
⊗ **Incompatibilities**
Aminophylline, ascorbic acid, cefoperazone, cefotaxime, cefuroxime sodium, dexamethasone sodium phosphate, diazepam, digoxin, dobutamine, folic acid, furosemide, hydrocortisone sodium phosphate, hydrocortisone sodium succinate, ketamine, methylprednisolone sodium succinate, minocycline, thiopental, ticarcillin disodium.

Contraindications and cautions

• Contraindicated in patients with seizure disorders; head injury; CV disorders; frank, uncompensated heart failure; severe hypertension; stroke; respiratory failure or incompetence secondary to neuromuscular disorders, muscle paresis, flail chest, obstructed airway, pulmonary embolism, pneumothorax, restrictive respiratory disease, acute bronchial asthma, or dyspnea; or hypoxia not related to hypercapnia.
• Don't use in patients with severe hypotension. If sudden hypotension occurs, stop drug.
• Use cautiously in patients with bronchial asthma, severe tachycardia or arrhythmias, cerebral edema or increased CSF pressure, hyperthyroidism, pheochromocytoma, or metabolic disorders.
⚜ **Lifespan:** In pregnant women, use cautiously. In breast-feeding women and in children, safety and effectiveness haven't been established.

Adverse reactions

CNS: apprehension, bilateral Babinski signs, disorientation, dizziness, fever, *headache*, paresthesia, pupil dilation, **seizures.**
CV: *arrhythmias,* chest pain and tightness, depressed T waves, flushing, increased blood pressure, variations in heart rate.
EENT: *laryngospasm,* sneezing.
GI: diarrhea, nausea, urge to defecate, vomiting.
GU: bladder stimulation with incontinence, urine retention, albuminuria.
Musculoskeletal: muscle spasms.
Respiratory: *bronchospasm,* cough, dyspnea, hiccups, rebound hypoventilation.
Skin: diaphoresis, pruritus.

Interactions

Drug-drug. *MAO inhibitors, sympathomimetics:* May potentiate adverse CV effects. Use together cautiously.

Effects on lab test results

• May increase BUN and hemoglobin levels and hematocrit.
• May decrease erythrocyte, WBC, and RBC counts.

Pharmacokinetics

Absorption: Given I.V.
Distribution: Wide.
Metabolism: 99% by liver.
Excretion: In urine. *Half-life:* 2½ to 4 hours.

Route	Onset	Peak	Duration
I.V.	20–40 sec	1–2 min	5–12 min

Reactions may be *common*, uncommon, *life-threatening*, or COMMON AND LIFE-THREATENING.

Action

Chemical effect: Not clearly defined; acts either directly on central respiratory centers in medulla or indirectly on chemoreceptors.
Therapeutic effect: Stimulates respirations.

Available forms

Injection: 20 mg/ml (benzyl alcohol 0.9%)

NURSING PROCESS

☑ Assessment
• Obtain history of patient's underlying condition before beginning therapy.
• Assess blood pressure, heart rate, deep tendon reflexes, and arterial blood gases before giving drug, and monitor closely throughout therapy.
• Monitor the drug's effectiveness by observing patient for improvement in CNS and respiratory function.
• Be alert for adverse reactions and drug interactions.
• Assess patient's and family's knowledge of drug therapy.

⚙ Nursing diagnoses
• Ineffective breathing pattern related to underlying condition
• Risk for trauma related to potential for drug-induced seizure activity
• Deficient knowledge related to drug therapy

▷ Planning and implementation
• Don't use in patients with severe hypotension. If sudden hypotension occurs or dyspnea develops, stop giving the drug.
• Establish adequate airway before giving the drug. Prevent patient from aspirating vomitus by placing him on his side. Have suction equipment nearby.
• Drug is used only in surgical or emergency situations.
• If patient's arterial carbon dioxide or oxygen tension increases, or if mechanical ventilation is started, stop drug and notify prescriber.
⚠ **ALERT:** Don't confuse doxapram with doxorubicin, doxepin, doxacurium, or doxazosin.
Patient teaching
• If patient is alert, instruct him to report chest pain or tightness immediately.

☑ Evaluation
• Patient regains normal respiratory pattern.
• Patient has no seizures as result of therapy.
• Patient and family state understanding of drug therapy.

doxazosin mesylate
(doks-AY-zoh-sin MES-ih-layt)
Cardura

Pharmacologic class: alpha blocker
Therapeutic class: antihypertensive
Pregnancy risk category: C

Indications and dosages

▶ **Essential hypertension.** *Adults:* Initially, 1 mg P.O. daily. Increase to 2 mg daily, then 4 mg daily, then 8 mg. Maximum, 16 mg daily, but dosage above 4 mg daily increases risk of adverse reactions. To minimize adverse reactions, adjust dosage slowly (typically increase only every 2 weeks).
▶ **BPH.** *Adults:* Initially, 1 mg P.O. once daily, morning or evening; may increase to 2 mg and, thereafter, to 4 mg and to 8 mg once daily or as needed. Adjust dosage in 1- to 2-week intervals.

Contraindications and cautions

• Contraindicated in patients hypersensitive to drug and to quinazoline derivatives (including prazosin and terazosin).
• Use cautiously in patients with impaired liver function.
☀ **Lifespan:** In pregnant women, use cautiously. In breast-feeding women, drug isn't recommended because it appears in breast milk at levels about 20 times greater than those in maternal plasma. In children, safety and effectiveness haven't been established.

Adverse reactions

CNS: *asthenia, dizziness,* drowsiness, *headache,* pain, somnolence, vertigo.
CV: *arrhythmias,* edema, hypotension, palpitations, *orthostatic hypotension,* tachycardia.
EENT: abnormal vision, pharyngitis, rhinitis.
GI: constipation, diarrhea, nausea, vomiting.
Musculoskeletal: arthralgia, myalgia.
Respiratory: dyspnea.
Skin: pruritus, rash.

Interactions

Drug-drug. *Clonidine:* May decrease clonidine effects. Adjust dosage.
Drug-herb. *Butcher's broom:* May reduce drug effects. Discourage use together.

Effects on lab test results

• May decrease WBC and neutrophil counts.

Pharmacokinetics

Absorption: Good.
Distribution: 98% protein-bound.
Metabolism: Extensive.
Excretion: 63% in bile and feces; 9% in urine.
Half-life: 19 to 22 hours.

Route	Onset	Peak	Duration
P.O.	1–2 hr	2–6 hr	24 hr

Action

Chemical effect: Acts on peripheral vasculature to produce vasodilation.
Therapeutic effect: Lowers blood pressure.

Available forms

Tablets: 1 mg, 2 mg, 4 mg, 8 mg

NURSING PROCESS

✍ Assessment

• Obtain history of patient's blood pressure before beginning therapy, and reassess regularly thereafter.
• Determine effect on standing and supine blood pressure at 2 to 6 hours and 24 hours after giving the drug.
• Be alert for adverse reactions.
• Monitor patient's ECG for arrhythmias.
• Assess patient's and family's knowledge of drug therapy.

Nursing diagnoses

• Risk for injury related to presence of hypertension
• Decreased cardiac output related to drug-induced adverse CV reactions
• Deficient knowledge related to drug therapy

Planning and implementation

• Increase dosage gradually, with adjustments every 2 weeks for hypertension and every 1 to 2 weeks for BPH.

• If syncope occurs, place patient in recumbent position and provide supportive therapy. A transient hypotensive response isn't considered a contraindication to continued therapy.
⚠ ALERT: Don't confuse doxazosin with doxapram, doxorubicin, or doxepin. Don't confuse Cardura with Coumadin, K-Dur, Cardene, or Cordarone.

Patient teaching

• Advise patient that he's susceptible to a first-dose effect similar to that produced by other alpha blockers: marked orthostatic hypotension, accompanied by dizziness or syncope. Orthostatic hypotension is most common after first dose, but it can also occur when stopping therapy or adjusting dosage.
• Warn patient that dizziness or fainting may occur. Advise patient to refrain from driving and performing other hazardous activities until drug's adverse CNS effects are known.
• Stress importance of regular follow-up visits.

☑ Evaluation

• Patient's blood pressure becomes normal.
• Patient maintains adequate cardiac output throughout therapy.
• Patient and family state understanding of drug therapy.

doxepin hydrochloride
(DOKS-eh-pin high-droh-KLOR-ighd)
Sinequan

Pharmacologic class: tricyclic antidepressant
Therapeutic class: antidepressant
Pregnancy risk category: C

Indications and dosages

▶ **Depression, anxiety.** *Adults and children age 12 and older:* Initially, 25 to 75 mg P.O. daily in divided doses to maximum, 300 mg daily. Or, give entire maintenance dosage once daily. Maximum, 150 mg.
▣ Adjust-a-dose: In elderly or debilitated patients, adolescents, and those receiving other drugs (especially anticholinergics), reduce dosage.

Contraindications and cautions

• Contraindicated in patients hypersensitive to the drug or any of its components and in those with glaucoma or a tendency for urine retention.

🎖 Lifespan: In pregnant women and in children younger than age 12, safety and effectiveness haven't been established. In breast-feeding women, drug isn't recommended.

Adverse reactions

CNS: ataxia, confusion, *dizziness, drowsiness,* EEG changes, excitation, extrapyramidal reactions, hallucinations, headache, nervousness, paresthesia, *seizures, suicidal thinking,* tremors, weakness.

CV: ECG changes, hypertension, orthostatic hypotension, tachycardia.

EENT: *blurred vision,* mydriasis, tinnitus.

GI: anorexia, constipation, dry mouth, glossitis, nausea, vomiting.

GU: urine retention.

Hematologic: *bone marrow depression, including agranulocytosis, aplastic anemia, leukopenia, and thrombocytopenia;* eosinophilia.

Skin: *diaphoresis,* photosensitivity, rash, urticaria.

Other: hypersensitivity reaction.

Interactions

Drug-drug. *Barbiturates, CNS depressants:* May increase CNS depression. Avoid use together.

Cimetidine, fluoxetine, methylphenidate, sertraline: May increase doxepin level. Monitor patient for increased adverse reactions.

Clonidine: May cause loss of blood pressure control with potentially life-threatening elevations in blood pressure. Don't use together.

Epinephrine, norepinephrine: May increase hypertensive effect. Use cautiously; monitor blood pressure closely.

MAO inhibitors: May cause severe excitation, hyperpyrexia, or seizures, usually with high dosage. Avoid use together.

Drug-herb. *SAMe, St. John's wort, yohimbe:* May elevate serotonin level. Discourage use together.

Drug-food. *Carbonated beverages, grape juice:* May be incompatible. Avoid use together.

Drug-lifestyle. *Alcohol use:* May increase CNS depression. Discourage use together.

Sun exposure: May increase risk of photosensitivity reactions. Discourage unprotected or prolonged exposure to the sun.

Effects on lab test results

• May increase liver enzyme levels. May decrease hemoglobin level and hematocrit. May increase or decrease glucose level.

• May increase eosinophil count. May decrease RBC, WBC, granulocyte, and platelet counts.

Pharmacokinetics

Absorption: Rapid.

Distribution: Wide, including CNS. 90% protein-bound.

Metabolism: By liver. A significant first-pass effect may explain varying levels in patients with same dosage.

Excretion: Mainly in urine. *Half-life:* 6 to 8 hours.

Route	Onset	Peak	Duration
P.O.	Unknown	≤ 2 hr	Unknown

Action

Chemical effect: Unknown; increases amount of norepinephrine, serotonin, or both in CNS by blocking their reuptake by presynaptic neurons.

Therapeutic effect: Relieves depression and anxiety.

Available forms

Capsules: 10 mg, 25 mg, 50 mg, 75 mg, 100 mg, 150 mg

Oral concentrate: 10 mg/ml

NURSING PROCESS

🇷 Assessment

• Assess patient's depression or anxiety before and during therapy.

• Be alert for adverse reactions and drug interactions.

• Assess patient's and family's knowledge of drug therapy.

⊕ Nursing diagnoses

• Ineffective coping related to underlying condition

• Risk for injury related to drug-induced adverse CNS reactions

• Deficient knowledge related to drug therapy

▶ Planning and implementation
• Dilute oral concentrate with 120 ml of water, milk, or juice (except grape juice). Don't mix with carbonated beverages because they are incompatible.
• Don't stop long-term therapy abruptly; doing so can cause nausea, headache, and malaise, which don't indicate addiction.
• Stop drug gradually several days before surgery because hypertensive episodes may occur.
• If signs of psychosis occur or increase, notify prescriber and reduce dosage.
⚠ **ALERT:** Antidepressants may increase the risk of suicidal thinking and behavior in children and adolescents with major depressive disorder and other psychiatric disorders. Balance risk with patient's need for drug.
⚠ **ALERT:** May increase the risk of suicidal thinking and behavior in young adults ages 18 to 24 during the first 2 months of treatment. Monitor patient closely.
⚠ **ALERT:** Don't confuse doxepin with doxazosin, digoxin, doxapram, or Doxidan; don't confuse Sinequan with saquinavir.
Patient teaching
• Tell patient to dilute oral concentrate with 120 ml of water, milk, or juice (orange, grapefruit, tomato, prune, or pineapple). Drug is incompatible with carbonated beverages and grape juice.
• Advise patient to take full dose at bedtime, but warn him that he may have morning orthostatic hypotension.
• Warn patient to avoid hazardous activities that require alertness and good psychomotor coordination until the drug's CNS effects are known. Drowsiness and dizziness usually subside after a few weeks.
• Advise family to observe for suicidal thinking and behavior in children, adolescents, and young adults, and to report to prescriber immediately.
• Tell patient to avoid using alcohol while taking the drug.
• Warn patient not to stop drug therapy suddenly.
• Advise patient to consult prescriber before taking prescription drugs, OTC medications, or herbal remedies.
• Advise patient to use sunblock, wear protective clothing, and avoid prolonged exposure to strong sunlight.

☑ Evaluation
• Patient behavior and communication indicate improvement of depression or anxiety.
• Patient has no injury as result of drug-induced adverse CNS reactions.
• Patient and family state understanding of drug therapy.

doxercalciferol
(dox-er-kal-SIF-eh-rol)
Hectorol

Pharmacologic class: synthetic vitamin D analogue
Therapeutic class: parathyroid hormone antagonist
Pregnancy risk category: B

Indications and dosages
▶ **To reduce intact parathyroid hormone (iPTH) levels to manage secondary hyperparathyroidism in patients undergoing long-term renal dialysis.** *Adults:* Initially, 10 mcg P.O. three times weekly at dialysis. Adjust dosage as needed to lower iPTH level to 150 to 300 picograms per milliliter (pg/ml). Increase dosage by 2.5 mcg at 8-week intervals if iPTH level doesn't decline by 50% and fails to reach target range. Maximum, 20 mcg P.O. three times weekly. If iPTH level falls below 100 pg/ml, stop drug for 1 week and then resume at a dose that's at least 2.5 mcg lower than the last dose. Or, 4 mcg I.V. bolus three times weekly (about every other day) at the end of dialysis. Adjust dosage as needed to lower iPTH level to 150 to 300 pg/ml. Dosage may be increased by 1 to 2 mcg at 8-week intervals if iPTH level isn't decreased by 50% and fails to reach target range. Maximum, 18 mcg weekly. If iPTH level goes below 100 pg/ml, suspend drug for 1 week; then resume at a dosage that's at least 1 mcg P.O. lower than the last dose.
▶ **Secondary hyperparathyroidism in pre-dialysis patients with stage 3 or 4 chronic kidney disease.** *Adults:* 1 mcg P.O. daily. Adjust dosage as needed to lower blood iPTH level to target range. Target range for stage 3 is 35 to 70 pg/ml. Target range for stage 4 is 70 to 110 pg/ml. Increase dosage at 2-week intervals by 0.5 mcg if level is above 70 pg/ml (stage 3) or above 110 pg/ml (stage 4). If level falls be-

low 35 pg/ml for stage 3 or 70 pg/ml for stage 4, stop drug for 1 week, then resume at a dosage at least 0.5 mcg lower than the last dose. Maximum dose is 3.5 mcg daily.

▼ I.V. administration

- Administer by bolus injection.
- Store at a controlled room temperature.
- Protect from light.

⊗ **Incompatibilities**
None reported.

Contraindications and cautions

- Contraindicated in patients with a recent history of hypercalcemia, hyperphosphatemia, or vitamin D toxicity.
- Use cautiously in patients with hepatic insufficiency, and frequently monitor calcium, phosphorus, and iPTH levels in these patients.

⚇ **Lifespan:** In breast-feeding women, and in children younger than age 12, drug isn't recommended. In elderly patients, use cautiously because adverse CNS reactions, orthostatic hypotension, and GI and GU distresses are more likely to develop.

Adverse reactions

CNS: dizziness, headache, malaise, sleep disorder.
CV: *bradycardia,* edema.
GI: anorexia, constipation, dyspepsia, *nausea, vomiting.*
Metabolic: weight gain or loss.
Musculoskeletal: arthralgia.
Respiratory: *dyspnea.*
Skin: pruritus.
Other: abscess.

Interactions

Drug-drug. *Calcium-containing or non–aluminum-containing phosphate binders:* May cause hypercalcemia or hyperphosphatemia and decrease effectiveness of doxercalciferol. Use together cautiously, and adjust dosage of phosphate binders as directed.
Cholestyramine, mineral oil: May decrease intestinal absorption of doxercalciferol. Avoid use together.
Glutethimide, phenobarbital, and other enzyme inducers; phenytoin and other enzyme inhibitors: May affect doxercalciferol metabolism. Adjust dosage as directed.

Magnesium-containing antacids: May cause hypermagnesemia. Monitor patient for toxicity.
Orlistat: May interfere with intestinal absorption of vitamin D analogues. Give drug at least 2 hours before or 2 hours after Orlistat administration.
Vitamin D supplements: May cause additive effects and hypercalcemia. Monitor patient for toxicity.

Effects on lab test results

None reported.

Pharmacokinetics

Absorption: Good.
Distribution: Unknown.
Metabolism: To its active forms in the liver.
Excretion: Major metabolite attains peak levels at 11 to 12 hours after repeated doses. *Half-life:* 32 to 37 hours, with a range of up to 96 hours.

Route	Onset	Peak	Duration
P.O.	Unknown	11–12 hr	Unknown

Action

Chemical effect: Regulates calcium levels. Acts directly on the parathyroid glands to suppress PTH synthesis and secretion.
Therapeutic effect: Reduces elevated iPTH levels.

Available forms

Capsules: 0.5 mcg, 2.5 mcg
Injection: 4 mcg/2 ml

NURSING PROCESS

☘ Assessment
- Assess hepatic function before starting therapy.
- Monitor calcium, phosphorus, and iPTH levels. Monitor them more frequently in patients with hepatic insufficiency.
- Be alert for adverse reactions and drug interactions.
- Assess patient's and family's knowledge of drug therapy.

⊕ Nursing diagnoses
- Imbalanced nutrition: less than body requirements related to adverse GI effects
- Risk for injury related to adverse CNS effects
- Deficient knowledge related to drug therapy

⤷ Planning and implementation

• Give drug with dialysis (about every other day). Individualize doses based on intact PTH levels, with monitoring of calcium and phosphorus levels before therapy and weekly thereafter.

• If patient has hypercalcemia or hyperphosphatemia, or if the calcium level multiplied by the phosphorus level (Ca × P) is greater than 70, immediately stop doxercalciferol until these values decrease.

• Progressive hypercalcemia from vitamin D overdose may require emergency attention. Acute hypercalcemia may worsen arrhythmias and seizures and affect the action of digoxin. Chronic hypercalcemia can lead to vascular and soft-tissue calcification.

• Calcium-based or non–aluminum-containing phosphate binders and a low-phosphate diet are used to control phosphorus levels in patients undergoing dialysis. Adjust dosage of this drug and other therapies to maintain PTH suppression and calcium and phosphorus levels.

Patient teaching

• Inform patient that dosage will be adjusted over several months to achieve satisfactory PTH suppression.

• Tell patient to adhere to a low-phosphorus diet and to follow instructions regarding calcium supplements.

• Tell patient to obtain prescriber's approval before using OTC drugs, including antacids and vitamin preparations containing calcium or vitamin D.

• Inform patient that early signs and symptoms of hypercalcemia include weakness, headache, somnolence, nausea, vomiting, dry mouth, constipation, muscle pain, bone pain, and metallic taste. Late signs and symptoms include polyuria, polydipsia, anorexia, weight loss, nocturia, conjunctivitis, pancreatitis, photophobia, rhinorrhea, pruritus, hyperthermia, decreased libido, hypertension, and arrhythmias.

✓ Evaluation

• Patient has no nausea and vomiting.
• Patient remains free from injury.
• Patient and family state understanding of drug therapy.

HIGH ALERT!

doxorubicin hydrochloride
(doks-oh-ROO-bih-sin high-droh-KLOR-ighd)

Pharmacologic class: anthracycline antibiotic
Therapeutic class: antineoplastic
Pregnancy risk category: D

Indications and dosages

▶ **Bladder, breast, lung, ovarian, stomach, testicular, and thyroid cancers; Hodgkin lymphoma; acute lymphoblastic and myeloblastic leukemia; Wilms tumor; neuroblastoma; lymphoma; sarcoma.** *Adults:* 60 to 75 mg/m² I.V. as single dose every 3 weeks; or 30 mg/m² I.V. in single daily dose on days 1 through 3 of 4-week cycle. Or, 20 mg/m² I.V. once weekly. Maximum cumulative dose, 550 mg/m².

⧄ **Adjust-a-dose:** In elderly patients and those with myelosuppression or impaired cardiac or hepatic function, dosage may need adjustment.

If bilirubin level increases, decrease dosage: 50% of dosage when bilirubin level is 1.2 to 3 mg/dl; 25% of dosage when bilirubin level is greater than 3 mg/dl.

▽ I.V. administration

• Preparing and giving drug carry carcinogenic, mutagenic, and teratogenic risks. Follow facility policy to reduce risks.

• Reconstitute using preservative-free normal saline solution injection. Add 5 ml to 10-mg vial, 10 ml to 20-mg vial, or 25 ml to 50-mg vial. Shake vial, and allow drug to dissolve; final concentration is 2 mg/ml.

• Give by direct injection into I.V. line of free-flowing compatible I.V. solution containing D₅W or normal saline solution injection in no less than 3 minutes.

• Drug is a severe vesicant, and extravasation may cause tissue necrosis. To avoid extravasation, don't place I.V. line over joints or in limbs with poor venous or lymphatic drainage.

• If extravasation occurs, stop I.V. injection immediately, notify prescriber, and apply ice to area for 24 to 48 hours. Monitor area closely because extravasation reaction may be progressive. Early consultation with plastic surgeon may be advisable.

• If vein streaking occurs, slow administration rate. If welts occur, stop administration and notify prescriber.

• Refrigerated, reconstituted solution is stable for 48 hours; at room temperature, it's stable for 24 hours.

⊗ **Incompatibilities**

Allopurinol, aluminum, aminophylline, bacteriostatic diluents, cefepime, cephalothin, dexamethasone sodium phosphate, diazepam, fluorouracil, furosemide, ganciclovir, heparin sodium, hydrocortisone sodium succinate, piperacillin with tazobactam.

Contraindications and cautions

• Contraindicated in patients with marked myelosuppression induced by previous therapy with other antitumor drugs or radiotherapy and in those who have received lifetime cumulative dose of 550 mg/m^2.

⚱ **Lifespan:** In pregnant and breast-feeding women, drug isn't recommended. In children, safety and effectiveness haven't been established.

Adverse reactions

CV: *arrhythmias;* cardiac depression, seen in ECG changes, such as sinus tachycardia, T-wave flattening, ST-segment depression, voltage reduction; *irreversible cardiomyopathy.*
EENT: conjunctivitis.
GI: anorexia, diarrhea, esophagitis, *nausea, stomatitis, vomiting.*
GU: transient red urine.
Hematologic: *leukopenia* during days 10 through 15, with recovery by day 21; MYELO-SUPPRESSION; *thrombocytopenia.*
Skin: *complete alopecia;* facial flushing; *hyperpigmentation of nails, dermal creases,* or skin (especially in previously irradiated areas); urticaria.
Other: *anaphylaxis,* hyperuricemia, severe cellulitis or tissue sloughing if drug extravasates.

Interactions

Drug-drug. *Calcium channel blockers:* May potentiate cardiotoxic effects. Monitor patient closely.
Digoxin: May decrease digoxin level. Monitor patient closely.
Paclitaxel: May decrease doxorubicin clearance. Monitor patient for toxicity.
Phenobarbital: May increase doxorubicin clearance. Monitor patient closely.
Phenytoin: May decrease phenytoin level. Check level.

Progesterone: May enhance doxorubicin-induced neutropenia and thrombocytopenia. Monitor closely.
Streptozocin: May increase and prolong blood level of doxorubicin HCl. Dosage may need adjustment.
Drug-herb. *Green tea:* May enhance antitumor effects of drug. Urge patient to discuss with prescriber before using together.

Effects on lab test results

• May increase bilirubin, uric acid, and glucose levels. May decrease calcium and hemoglobin levels and hematocrit.
• May decrease WBC, neutrophil, and platelet counts.

Pharmacokinetics

Absorption: Given I.V.
Distribution: Wide; doesn't cross blood–brain barrier.
Metabolism: Extensive, by hepatic microsomal enzymes to several metabolites, one of which has cytotoxic activity.
Excretion: Mainly in bile, minimally in urine.
Half-life: Triphasic pattern of 12 minutes, about 3½ hours, and 30 to 40 hours.

Route	Onset	Peak	Duration
I.V.	Unknown	Unknown	Unknown

Action

Chemical effect: May interfere with DNA-dependent RNA synthesis by intercalation.
Therapeutic effect: Hinders or kills certain cancer cells.

Available forms

Injection (preservative-free): 2 mg/ml
Powder for injection: 10-mg, 20-mg, 50-mg, 100-mg, 150-mg vials

NURSING PROCESS

📝 Assessment

• Obtain history of patient's neoplastic disorder before therapy, and reassess regularly thereafter.
• Assess ECG before therapy.
• Monitor CBC and liver function tests; monitor ECG monthly during therapy.
• Be alert for adverse reactions and drug interactions.

- Assess patient's and family's knowledge of drug therapy.

⚕ Nursing diagnoses
- Ineffective health maintenance related to presence of neoplastic disease
- Decreased cardiac output related to drug-induced cardiotoxicity
- Deficient knowledge related to drug therapy

▶ Planning and implementation
- To reduce nausea, premedicate with antiemetic.
- If skin or mucosal contact occurs, immediately wash area with soap and water.
- In case of leak or spill, inactivate drug with 5% sodium hypochlorite solution (household bleach).
- Never give drug I.M. or subcutaneously.
- If tachycardia develops, stop giving the drug or slow infusion rate, and notify the prescriber.
- If signs of heart failure develop, stop drug immediately and notify prescriber. Limit cumulative dose to 550 mg/m² (400 mg/m² when patient also receives or has received cyclophosphamide or radiation therapy to cardiac area) to prevent heart failure.
- Alternate dosage schedule (once weekly) to lower the risk of cardiomyopathy.
- Provide adequate hydration. Alkalinizing urine or giving allopurinol may prevent or minimize uric acid nephropathy.
- Radiation may increase radiation-induced toxicity to the myocardium, mucosa, skin, and liver. Monitor patient.
- Report adverse reactions to prescriber and provide supportive care.
- **(❋) ALERT:** Avoid confusing doxorubicin and daunorubicin. Red color is similar.
- **(❋) ALERT:** Liposomal doxorubicin and conventional doxorubicin aren't interchangeable. Clearance of liposomal form is significantly less than conventional form. Decrease liposomal doxorubicin dose.

Patient teaching
- Warn patient to watch for signs of infection (fever, sore throat, fatigue) and bleeding (easy bruising, nosebleed, bleeding gums, melena). Have patient take temperature daily.
- Advise patient that orange to red urine for 1 to 2 days is normal and doesn't indicate presence of blood in urine.
- Tell patient that total alopecia may occur within 3 to 4 weeks. Hair may regrow 2 to 5 months after drug is stopped.

- Instruct patient to report symptoms of heart failure and other cardiac signs and symptoms promptly to prescriber.
- Tell patient to use safety precautions to prevent injury.

✅ Evaluation
- Patient exhibits positive response to therapy, as noted on improved follow-up studies.
- Patient maintains adequate cardiac output throughout therapy.
- Patient and family state understanding of drug therapy.

HIGH ALERT!

doxorubicin hydrochloride liposomal
(doks-oh-ROO-bih-sin high-droh-KLOR-ighd ly-puh-SOE-mul)
Doxil

Pharmacologic class: anthracycline antibiotic
Therapeutic class: antineoplastic
Pregnancy risk category: D

Indications and dosages

▶ **Metastatic ovarian cancer in women with disease refractory to paclitaxel- and platinum-based chemotherapy regimens.**
Women: 50 mg/m² (doxorubicin hydrochloride equivalent) I.V. at an initial infusion rate of 1 mg/minute once every 4 weeks for at least four courses. Continue as long as patient doesn't progress, shows no evidence of cardiotoxicity, and continues to tolerate treatment. If no infusion-related adverse events occur, increase infusion rate to complete administration over 1 hour.

▶ **AIDS-related Kaposi sarcoma in patients with disease that has progressed with previous combination chemotherapy or in patients who are intolerant to such therapy.** *Adults:* 20 mg/m² (doxorubicin hydrochloride equivalent) I.V. over 30 minutes, once every 3 weeks, for as long as patient responds satisfactorily and tolerates therapy.

⎹ Adjust-a-dose: For patients with impaired hepatic function, if bilirubin level is 1.2 to 3 mg/dl, give one-fourth of the normal dose; if bilirubin level is more than 3 mg/dl, give one-half of the normal dose. Consult package insert

---

for dosage modifications for hand-foot syndrome, hematologic toxicity, and stomatitis.

▽ I.V. administration

• Follow facility procedures for proper handling and disposal of antineoplastics.
• Dilute dose (maximum, 90 mg) in 250 ml of D_5W using aseptic technique.
• Carefully check label on the I.V. bag before giving drug. Accidentally substituting Doxil for conventional doxorubicin hydrochloride can cause severe adverse effects.
• Infuse I.V. over 30 to 60 minutes, depending on the dose. Don't use with in-line filters.
• Monitor patient carefully during infusion. Flushing, shortness of breath, facial swelling, headache, chills, back pain, tightness in the chest or throat, or hypotension may occur. These reactions resolve over several hours to a day once the infusion is stopped; they may also resolve by slowing the infusion rate.
• If extravasation occurs, stop infusion immediately and restart in another vein. Applying ice over the extravasation site for about 30 minutes may help to alleviate the local reaction.
• Refrigerate diluted solution at 36° to 46° F (2° to 8° C), and give within 24 hours.
⊗ **Incompatibilities**
Other I.V. drugs.

Contraindications and cautions

• Contraindicated in patients hypersensitive to the conventional form of doxorubicin hydrochloride or any component in the liposomal form. Also contraindicated in patients with marked myelosuppression or those who have received a lifetime cumulative dosage of 550 mg/m² (400 mg/m² if patient received radiotherapy to the mediastinal area or simultaneous therapy with other cardiotoxic drugs, such as cyclophosphamide).
• Use in patients with a history of CV disease only when the potential benefits of the drug outweigh the risks.
• Use cautiously in patients who have received another anthracycline.
⚕ **Lifespan:** In women of childbearing age, avoid pregnancy during therapy; don't start drug if patient is pregnant. In breast-feeding women, drug is contraindicated. In children, safety and effectiveness haven't been established. In elderly patients, use cautiously because they may have greater sensitivity to the drug.

Adverse reactions

CNS: anxiety, *asthenia,* depression, dizziness, emotional lability, fatigue, fever, headache, insomnia, malaise, paresthesia, somnolence.
CV: *arrhythmias, cardiomyopathy,* chest pain, *heart failure,* hypotension, *pericardial effusion,* peripheral edema, tachycardia.
EENT: conjunctivitis, mouth ulceration, mucous membrane disorder, optic neuritis, pharyngitis, retinitis, rhinitis.
GI: abdominal pain, anorexia, constipation, diarrhea, dyspepsia, dysphagia, enlarged abdomen, esophagitis, glossitis, *nausea,* oral candidiasis, *stomatitis,* taste disturbance, vomiting.
GU: albuminuria.
Hematologic: *anemia, leukopenia,* NEUTROPENIA, THROMBOCYTOPENIA.
Hepatic: hyperbilirubinemia.
Metabolic: dehydration, hyperglycemia, hypocalcemia, weight loss.
Musculoskeletal: back pain, myalgia.
Respiratory: dyspnea, increased cough, pneumonia.
Skin: *alopecia,* dry skin, exfoliative dermatitis, hand-foot syndrome, herpes zoster, pruritus, *rash,* skin discoloration, skin disorder, sweating.
Other: *allergic reaction,* chills, *infection,* infusion-related reactions, *sepsis.*

Interactions

No drug interactions have been reported; however, doxorubicin hydrochloride liposomal may interact with drugs known to interact with the conventional form of doxorubicin hydrochloride.

Effects on lab test results

• May increase bilirubin and glucose levels. May decrease calcium and hemoglobin levels and hematocrit.
• May increase PT. May decrease WBC, neutrophil, and platelet counts.

Pharmacokinetics

Absorption: Given I.V.
Distribution: Mostly to vascular fluid.
Metabolism: Doxorubicinol, the major metabolite, is detected at very low levels.
Excretion: Slow, in two phases. *Half-life:* 5 hours in the first phase, 55 hours in the second phase with doses of 10 to 20 mg/m².

Route	Onset	Peak	Duration
I.V.	Unknown	Unknown	Unknown

Action

Chemical effect: Doxil is doxorubicin hydrochloride encapsulated in liposomes that, because of their small size and persistence in circulation, can penetrate the altered vasculature of tumors. The mechanism of action of doxorubicin hydrochloride is probably related to its ability to bind DNA and inhibit nucleic acid synthesis.

Therapeutic effect: Hinders or kills certain cancer cells in patients with ovarian cancer or AIDS-related Kaposi sarcoma.

Available forms

Injection: 2 mg/ml, 20 mg/10 ml, 50 mg/30 ml

NURSING PROCESS

Assessment
• Obtain an accurate medication list from patient, including previous or current chemotherapeutic drugs.
• Evaluate patient's hepatic function before beginning therapy, and adjust dose accordingly.
• Monitor cardiac function closely by endomyocardial biopsy, echocardiography, or gated radionuclide scans. If results indicate that the patient may have cardiac injury, the benefit of continued therapy must be weighed against the risk of myocardial injury.
• Be alert for adverse reactions.
• Assess patient's and family's knowledge of drug therapy.

Nursing diagnoses
• Risk for infection related to myelosuppression
• Risk for injury related to drug-induced adverse reactions
• Deficient knowledge related to drug therapy

Planning and implementation
• Don't give drug I.M. or subcutaneously.
• **ALERT:** Don't substitute on a milligram-per-milligram basis with conventional doxorubicin hydrochloride.
• Drug may increase the toxicity of other antineoplastic therapies.
• Take into account any earlier or simultaneous therapy with related compounds, such as daunorubicin, when giving total dose. Heart failure and cardiomyopathy may occur after therapy stops.

• Monitor CBC, including platelets, before each dose and frequently throughout therapy. Leukopenia is usually transient. Hematologic toxicity may require dosage reduction or suspension or delay of therapy. Persistent severe myelosuppression may result in superinfection or hemorrhage. Patient may need granulocyte colony-stimulating factor (or granulocyte-macrophage colony-stimulating factor) to support blood counts.

Patient teaching
• Tell patient to notify prescriber about symptoms of hand-foot syndrome, such as tingling or burning, redness, flaking, bothersome swelling, small blisters, or small sores on the palms of hands or soles of feet.
• Advise patient to report symptoms of stomatitis, such as painful redness, swelling, or sores in the mouth.
• Advise patient to avoid exposure to people with infections. Tell patient to report fever of 100.5° F (38° C) or higher.
• Urge patient to report nausea, vomiting, tiredness, weakness, rash, or mild hair loss.
• Advise woman of childbearing age to avoid pregnancy during therapy.

Evaluation
• Patient has no infection.
• Patient has no injury as a result of drug-induced adverse reactions.
• Patient and family state understanding of drug therapy.

doxycycline
(docks-ih-SYE-kleen)
Oracea

doxycycline hyclate
Apo-Doxy◆, Doryx, Doxy-100, Doxy-200, Doxycin◆, Novo-Doxylin◆, Periostat, Vibramycin, Vibra-Tabs

doxycycline monohydrate
Adoxa, Monodox, Vibramycin

Pharmacologic class: tetracycline
Therapeutic class: antibiotic
Pregnancy risk category: D

Indications and dosages

▶ **Infections caused by sensitive gram-negative and gram-positive organisms, *Chlamydia, Mycoplasma, Rickettsia*, and organisms that cause trachoma.** *Adults and children weighing more than 45 kg (99 lb):* 100 mg P.O. every 12 hours on first day; then 100 mg P.O. daily. Or, 200 mg I.V. on first day in one or two infusions; then 100 to 200 mg I.V. daily. For severe infections, 100 mg P.O. every 12 hours may be used.

Children older than age 8 and weighing less than 45 kg: 4.4 mg/kg P.O. or I.V. daily in divided doses every 12 hours on first day, then 2.2 to 4.4 mg/kg daily.

▶ **Gonorrhea in patients allergic to penicillin.** *Adults:* 100 mg P.O. b.i.d. for 7 days. Or 300 mg P.O. initially; repeat dose in 1 hour.

▶ **Primary or secondary syphilis in patients allergic to penicillin.** *Adults and children older than age 8:* Give 100 mg P.O. b.i.d. for 2 weeks (early detection) or for 4 weeks (if more than 1 year's duration).

▶ **Uncomplicated urethral, endocervical, or rectal infection caused by *Chlamydia trachomatis* or *Ureaplasma urealyticum*.** *Adults:* 100 mg P.O. b.i.d. for at least 7 days.

▶ **To prevent malaria.** *Adults:* 100 mg P.O. daily.

Children older than age 8: Give 2 mg/kg P.O. once daily. Don't exceed adult dose. Begin 1 to 2 days before travel to malarious area and continue throughout travel and for 4 weeks thereafter.

▶ **Adjunct to scaling and root planing to promote attachment level gain and to reduce pocket depth in patients with adult periodontitis.** *Adults:* 20 mg Periostat P.O. b.i.d. more than 1 hour before or 2 hours after the morning and evening meals and after scaling and root planing. Effective for 9 months.

▶ **Adjunct to other antibiotics for inhalation, GI, and oropharyngeal anthrax.** *Adults:* 100 mg I.V. every 12 hours initially until susceptibility test results are known. Switch to 100 mg P.O. b.i.d. when appropriate. Treat for 60 days total.

Children older than age 8 and weighing more than 45 kg: 100 mg I.V. every 12 hours, then switch to 100 mg P.O. b.i.d. when appropriate. Treat for 60 days total.

Children older than age 8 and weighing 45 kg or less: 2.2 mg/kg I.V. every 12 hours, then switch to 2.2 mg/kg P.O. b.i.d. when appropriate. Treat for 60 days total.

Children age 8 and younger: 2.2 mg/kg I.V. every 12 hours, then switch to 2.2 mg/kg P.O. b.i.d. when appropriate. Treat for 60 days total.

▶ **Cutaneous anthrax.** *Adults:* 100 mg P.O. b.i.d. for 60 days.

Children older than age 8 and weighing more than 45 kg: 100 mg P.O. every 12 hours for 60 days.

Children older than age 8 and weighing 45 kg or less: 2.2 mg/kg P.O. every 12 hours for 60 days.

Children age 8 and younger: 2.2 mg/kg P.O. every 12 hours for 60 days.

▶ **Adjunct to severe acne.** *Adults:* 200 mg Adoxa P.O. on day 1 (give as 100 mg every 12 hours or 50 mg every 6 hours); follow with a maintenance dosage of 100 mg P.O. daily, or 50 mg P.O. b.i.d.

▶ **Inflammatory lesions (papules and pustules) of rosacea.** *Adults:* 40 mg P.O. once daily in the morning, 1 hour before or 2 hours after a meal, with a full glass of water.

▶ **To prevent traveler's diarrhea commonly caused by enterotoxigenic *Escherichia coli*‡.** *Adults:* 100 mg P.O. daily for up to 3 days.

▶ **To prevent sexually transmitted diseases in rape victims‡.** *Adults and adolescents:* 100 mg Adoxa P.O. b.i.d. for 7 days after a single 2-g oral dose of metronidazole is given with a single 125-mg I.M. dose of ceftriaxone.

▶ **Lyme disease‡.** *Adults and children older than age 9:* 100 mg Adoxa P.O. b.i.d. or t.i.d. for 10 to 30 days.

▶ **Pleural effusions related to cancer‡.** *Adults:* 500 mg of doxycycline diluted in 250 ml of normal saline solution and instilled into pleural space via chest tube.

▼ I.V. administration

- Reconstitute powder for injection with sterile water for injection. Use 10 ml in 100-mg vial and 20 ml in 200-mg vial. Dilute solution to 100 to 1,000 ml for I.V. infusion.
- Don't expose drug to light or heat. Protect it from sunlight during infusion.
- Don't infuse solutions that are more concentrated than 1 mg/ml.
- Depending on the dose, infusion lasts typically 1 to 4 hours. Complete infusion within 12 hours.
- Monitor I.V. infusion site for signs of thrombophlebitis.
- Monitor for infiltration or irritation.

• Reconstituted injectable solution is stable for 72 hours if refrigerated.

⊗ **Incompatibilities**
Allopurinol; drugs unstable in acidic solutions, such as barbiturates; erythromycin lactobionate; heparin; meropenem; nafcillin; penicillin G potassium; piperacillin with tazobactam; riboflavin; and sulfonamides.

Contraindications and cautions

• Contraindicated in patients hypersensitive to drug or other tetracyclines.
• Use cautiously in patients with impaired kidney or liver function.
🌡 **Lifespan:** In the first half of pregnancy, drug isn't recommended unless other options aren't available because of the risk of bone growth retardation and neural tube defects in the fetus. In breast-feeding women, avoid drug because of possible adverse effects on the infant. In children younger than age 8 and in the fetus during last half of pregnancy, these drugs may cause permanent tooth discoloration, enamel defects, and retarded bone growth. These effects are dose-limited; therefore, drug may be used for a short course (7 to 14 days) and not repeated. For anthrax in pregnant women, children younger than age 8, and immunocompromised patients, give the usual dose and regimen.

Adverse reactions

CNS: *intracranial hypertension (pseudotumor cerebri).*
CV: pericarditis, thrombophlebitis.
EENT: dysphagia, glossitis.
GI: anogenital inflammation, anorexia, *diarrhea,* enterocolitis, *epigastric distress,* nausea, oral candidiasis, vomiting.
Hematologic: eosinophilia, hemolytic anemia, *neutropenia, thrombocytopenia.*
Musculoskeletal: bone growth retardation if used in children younger than age 8.
Skin: increased pigmentation, maculopapular and erythematous rash, photosensitivity, urticaria.
Other: *anaphylaxis,* enamel defects, hypersensitivity reactions, permanent discoloration of teeth, superinfection.

Interactions

Drug-drug. *Antacids (including sodium bicarbonate) and laxatives containing aluminum, magnesium, or calcium; antidiarrheals:* May

decrease antibiotic absorption. Give antibiotic 1 hour before or 2 hours after these drugs.
Carbamazepine, phenobarbital: May decrease antibiotic effect. Avoid use together, if possible.
Digoxin: May increase digoxin levels. Monitor levels and signs of toxicity.
Ferrous sulfate and other iron products, zinc: May decrease antibiotic absorption. Give drug 3 hours after or 2 hours before iron.
Hormonal contraceptives: May decrease contraceptive effectiveness and increase risk of breakthrough bleeding. Recommend nonhormonal form of birth control.
Isotretinoin: May cause pseudotumor cerebri. Avoid concomitant use.
Methoxyflurane: May cause nephrotoxicity with tetracyclines. Avoid use together.
Oral anticoagulants: May increase anticoagulant effect. Monitor PT and INR, and adjust dosage.
Penicillins: May interfere with bactericidal action of penicillins. Avoid use together.
Drug-lifestyle. *Alcohol use:* May decrease antibiotic effect. Avoid use together.
Sun exposure: May cause photosensitivity reactions. Urge patient to avoid unprotected and prolonged sun exposure.

Effects on lab test results

• May increase BUN and liver enzyme levels. May decrease hemoglobin level and hematocrit.
• May increase eosinophil count. May decrease platelet, neutrophil, and WBC counts.
• May cause false-negative reading of glucose oxidase reagent (Diastix or Chemstrip uG). May cause false-positive reading of copper sulfate tests (Clinitest) with parenteral form.
• May falsely elevate urinary catecholamine levels.

Pharmacokinetics

Absorption: 90% to 100%.
Distribution: Wide, but poor in CSF. 25% to 93% protein-bound.
Metabolism: Insignificant; some hepatic degradation occurs.
Excretion: Mainly unchanged in urine; some in feces. *Half-life:* About 1 day after multiple doses.

Route	Onset	Peak	Duration
P.O.	Unknown	1½–4 hr	Unknown
I.V.	Immediate	Unknown	Unknown

Reactions may be *common,* uncommon, *life-threatening,* or COMMON AND LIFE-THREATENING.

Action

Chemical effect: May exert bacteriostatic effect by binding to 30S ribosomal subunit of microorganisms, thus inhibiting protein synthesis.
Therapeutic effect: Hinders bacterial growth.

Available forms

doxycycline calcium
Capsules: 40 mg
Syrup: 50 mg/5 ml
doxycycline hyclate
Capsules: 20 mg, 50 mg, 100 mg
Capsules (coated pellets): 75 mg, 100 mg
Injection: 100 mg, 200 mg
Tablets: 20 mg, 100 mg
doxycycline monohydrate
Capsules: 50 mg, 100 mg
Oral suspension: 25 mg/5 ml
Tablets: 50 mg, 75 mg, 100 mg

NURSING PROCESS

🗓 Assessment

• Obtain history of patient's infection before therapy, and reassess regularly thereafter.
• Obtain specimen for culture and sensitivity tests before giving the first dose. Begin therapy pending test results.
• Be alert for adverse reactions and drug interactions.
• If patient has adverse GI reactions, monitor his hydration.
• Assess patient's and family's knowledge of drug therapy.

🔱 Nursing diagnoses

• Ineffective protection related to presence of susceptible bacteria
• Risk for deficient fluid volume related to drug-induced adverse GI reactions
• Deficient knowledge related to drug therapy

▶ Planning and implementation

• Check expiration date. Outdated or deteriorated tetracyclines may cause reversible nephrotoxicity (Fanconi syndrome).
• If drug causes adverse GI reaction, may give with milk or food.
• Follow current Centers for Disease Control and Prevention recommendations for anthrax.
• Ciprofloxacin and doxycycline are first-line therapy for anthrax; 500 mg amoxicillin P.O. t.i.d. for adults and 80 mg/kg/day divided every

8 hours for children is an option for completing therapy after improvement.
• Cutaneous anthrax with signs of systemic involvement, extensive edema, or lesions on the head or neck requires I.V. therapy and a multidrug approach.
• Additional antimicrobials for anthrax multidrug regimens can include rifampin, vancomycin, penicillin, ampicillin, chloramphenicol, imipenem, clindamycin, and clarithromycin.
• Steroids may be considered as adjunctive therapy for anthrax patients with severe edema and for meningitis, based on experience with bacterial meningitis of other etiologies.
• If meningitis is suspected, doxycycline would be less optimal because of poor CNS penetration.
• Notify prescriber of adverse reactions. Some adverse reactions, such as superinfection, may necessitate substitution of another antibiotic.
⑤ **ALERT:** Don't confuse doxycycline with doxylamine or dicyclomine.

Patient teaching

• Tell patient to take entire amount of medication exactly as prescribed, even after he feels better.
• Instruct patient to take oral drug with milk or food but not with antacids if adverse GI reaction develops. Tell patient to take drug no less than 1 hour before bedtime to prevent irritation from esophageal reflux.
• Advise parent giving drug to a child that tablets may be crushed and mixed with low-fat milk, low-fat chocolate milk, regular (whole) chocolate milk, chocolate pudding, or apple juice mixed with sugar in equal proportions. Store mixtures in refrigerator, except apple juice mixture (which can be stored at room temperature), and discard after 24 hours.
• Tell patient to use sunscreen and avoid strong sunlight during therapy to prevent photosensitivity reactions.
• Stress good oral hygiene.
• Tell patient to check expiration dates and to discard outdated doxycycline because it may become toxic.
• Advise patient taking hormonal contraceptive to use alternative means of contraception within 1 week of therapy.

☑ Evaluation

• Patient is free from infection.

- Patient maintains adequate hydration throughout therapy.
- Patient and family state understanding of drug therapy.

dronabinol
(delta-9-tetrahydrocannabinol)

(droh-NAB-eh-nohl)
Marinol

Pharmacologic class: cannabinoid
Therapeutic class: antiemetic, appetite stimulant
Pregnancy risk category: C
Controlled substance schedule: III

Indications and dosages

▶ **Nausea and vomiting from chemotherapy.**
Adults: 5 mg/m^2 P.O. 1 to 3 hours before administration of chemotherapy. Then same dose every 2 to 4 hours after chemotherapy for total of four to six doses daily. If needed, increase dosage in increments of 2.5 mg/m^2 to maximum dose, 15 mg/m^2.
▶ **Anorexia and weight loss in patients with AIDS.** *Adults:* 2.5 mg P.O. b.i.d. before lunch and dinner, increase as needed to maximum, 20 mg daily.

Contraindications and cautions

- Contraindicated in patients hypersensitive to sesame oil or cannabinoids.
- Use cautiously in patients with heart disease, psychiatric illness, or history of drug abuse.
- **Lifespan:** In breast-feeding women, drug isn't recommended. In children, safety and effectiveness haven't been established. In elderly patients, use cautiously.

Adverse reactions

CNS: amnesia, asthenia, ataxia, confusion, depersonalization, disorientation, *dizziness, drowsiness, euphoria,* hallucinations, headache, muddled thinking, *paranoia, somnolence.*
CV: orthostatic hypotension, palpitations, tachycardia, vasodilation.
EENT: visual disturbances.
GI: abdominal pain, diarrhea, dry mouth, nausea, vomiting.

Interactions

Drug-drug. *CNS depressants, psychotomimetic substances, sedatives:* May have additive effects. Avoid use together.
Drug-lifestyle. *Alcohol use:* May have additive effects. Discourage use together.

Effects on lab test results

None reported.

Pharmacokinetics

Absorption: 95%.
Distribution: Rapid. 97% to 99% protein-bound.
Metabolism: Extensive.
Excretion: Mainly in feces. *Half-life:* 1 to 1½ days.

Route	Onset	Peak	Duration
P.O.	Unknown	2–4 hr	4–6 hr; ≥ 24 hours for appetite stimulation

Action

Chemical effect: Unknown.
Therapeutic effect: Relieves nausea and vomiting caused by chemotherapy and stimulates appetite.

Available forms

Capsules: 2.5 mg, 5 mg, 10 mg

NURSING PROCESS

⚡ Assessment
- Obtain history of patient's underlying condition before therapy.
- Monitor the drug's effectiveness by assessing for nausea, vomiting, or weight gain. Drug effects may persist for days after therapy ends.
- Be alert for adverse reactions and drug interactions.
- Drug is the principal active substance in *Cannabis sativa* (marijuana). It can produce physical and psychological dependence and has potential for abuse. Monitor patient for dependence.
- Monitor patient's hydration, weight, and nutrition regularly.
- Assess patient's and family's knowledge of drug therapy.

Reactions may be common, uncommon, *life-threatening*, or COMMON AND LIFE-THREATENING.

⊕ Nursing diagnoses
• Risk for deficient fluid volume related to nausea and vomiting from chemotherapy
• Disturbed thought processes related to drug-induced adverse CNS reactions
• Deficient knowledge related to drug therapy

▶ Planning and implementation
• Give drug only to patients who haven't responded satisfactorily to other antiemetics.
• Give drug 1 to 3 hours before chemotherapy starts and again 2 to 4 hours after chemotherapy.
Patient teaching
• Inform patient that drug may cause unusual changes in mood or other adverse behavioral effects.
• Caution patient to avoid hazardous activities until the drug's CNS effects are known.
• Warn family members to make sure patient is supervised by a responsible person during and immediately after therapy.

☑ Evaluation
• Patient maintains adequate hydration.
• Patient regains normal thought processes after effects of drug therapy have dissipated.
• Patient and family state understanding of drug therapy.

drotrecogin alfa (activated)
(droh-truh-KO-jin AL-fah)
Xigris

Pharmacologic class: recombinant protease of human activated protein C
Therapeutic class: antithrombotic
Pregnancy risk category: C

Indications and dosages
▶ **Reduction of mortality in patients with severe sepsis (sepsis from acute organ dysfunction).** *Adults:* 24 mcg/kg/hour I.V. infusion for a total of 96 hours.

▽ I.V. administration
• Reconstitute 5-mg vials with 2.5 ml sterile water for injection, USP, and 20-mg vials with 10 ml of sterile water for injection, USP. The resulting concentration is 2 mg/ml. Gently swirl each vial until powder is completely dissolved; avoid inverting or shaking the vial.

• If the reconstituted vial isn't used immediately, it may be held at controlled room temperature of 59° to 86° F (15° to 30° C) for up to 3 hours, or stored in a refrigerator at 36° to 46° F (2° to 8° C).
• Further dilute the reconstituted solution with sterile normal saline injection. Withdraw appropriate amount of reconstituted drug into a prepared infusion bag of sterile normal saline solution. When adding the drug, direct the stream to the side of the bag to minimize agitation of the solution.
• Gently invert the infusion bag to obtain a homogenous solution. Don't transport the infusion bag between locations using mechanical delivery systems.
• Inspect for particulate matter and discoloration before giving.
• Give drug within 12 hours of preparing solution for infusion. Don't freeze. Avoid heat and direct sunlight.
• For an I.V. pump, the solution of reconstituted drug is typically diluted into an infusion bag containing sterile normal saline solution to a final concentration between 100 mcg/ml and 200 mcg/ml.
• For a syringe pump, the reconstituted solution is typically diluted with sterile normal saline solution to a final concentration between 100 mcg/ml and 1,000 mcg/ml. When giving less than 200 mcg/ml at less than 5 ml/hour, the infusion set must be primed for about 15 minutes at a flow rate of about 5 ml/hour.
• Give via a dedicated I.V. line or lumen of a multilumen central venous catheter. The only other solutions that can be given through the same line are normal saline solution, lactated Ringer's injection, dextrose, or dextrose and saline mixtures.
⊗ **Incompatibilities**
Other I.V. drugs.

Contraindications and cautions
• Contraindicated in patients with active internal bleeding, hemorrhagic stroke within 3 months, intracranial or intraspinal surgery within 2 months, severe head trauma, trauma with an increased risk of life-threatening bleeding, an epidural catheter, intracranial neoplasm or mass lesion, or evidence of cerebral herniation. Drug is also contraindicated in patients hypersensitive to drotrecogin alfa (activated) or any of its components.

• Use cautiously in patients with a high risk of bleeding, such as those who are taking heparin (15 units/kg/hour or more); those with a platelet count less than 30,000 × 10⁶/L (even if platelet count increases after transfusions); those with an INR greater than 3; those who have experienced GI bleeding within 6 weeks; those who have had thrombolytic therapy within 3 days; those who have been given oral anticoagulants, glycoprotein IIb/IIIa inhibitors, aspirin (more than 650 mg/day) or other platelet inhibitors within 7 days; those who have had an ischemic stroke within 3 months; and those who have had intracranial arteriovenous malformation or aneurysm, bleeding diathesis, chronic severe hepatic disease, or any other condition in which bleeding constitutes a significant hazard or would be particularly difficult to manage because of its location.

• Use only after careful consideration of the risk versus benefit in patients with single-organ dysfunction and recent surgery because they may not be at high risk of death.

⚖ **Lifespan:** In pregnant women, drug should be used only if benefit to patient exceeds risk to the fetus. Breast-feeding women should stop nursing or stop taking the drug because it's unknown whether drug appears in breast milk. In children, safety and effectiveness haven't been established.

Adverse reactions

Hematologic: HEMORRHAGE.

Interactions

Drug-drug. *Drugs that affect hemostasis:* May increase risk of bleeding. Use together cautiously; monitor patient for bleeding.

Effects on lab test results

• May increase PTT and PT.
• May interfere with one-stage coagulation assays based on PTT (such as factors VIII, IX, and XI assays), causing inconclusive results.

Pharmacokinetics

Absorption: Given I.V.
Distribution: Steady-state levels within 2 hours.
Metabolism: Unknown.
Excretion: Unknown. *Half-life:* Unknown.

Route	Onset	Peak	Duration
I.V.	Rapid	Unknown	Unknown

Action

Chemical effect: Inhibits monocytes from producing human tumor necrosis factor, by blocking leukocyte from adhering to selectins, and by limiting the thrombin-induced inflammatory response.
Therapeutic effect: Prevents clots and blocks cell death.

Available forms

Injection: 5 mg, 20 mg

NURSING PROCESS

ᗌ Assessment
• Assess patient before starting and during drug therapy for risk of bleeding or contraindications.
• Monitor patient closely for bleeding. If significant bleeding occurs, immediately stop the infusion.
• Because drug may prolong PTT, it can't be used to reliably assess the condition of the coagulopathy during infusion. Because drug has minimal effect on PT, PT can be used instead.

⊞ Nursing diagnoses
• Risk for injury caused by increased bleeding potential related to drug therapy
• Deficient knowledge related to drug therapy

❯ Planning and implementation
• If the infusion is interrupted, restart at the baseline 24-mcg/kg/hour infusion rate. Dose escalation, bolus doses, and dose adjustment based on observation or laboratory parameters aren't recommended.
• Stop drug 2 hours before an invasive surgical procedure with a risk of bleeding. After hemostasis is reached, drug may be restarted 12 hours after major invasive procedures or surgery or immediately after uncomplicated, less-invasive procedures.
Patient teaching
• Inform patient of potential adverse reactions.
• Instruct patient to report signs of bleeding promptly.
• Advise patient that bleeding may occur for up to 28 days after therapy.

✓ Evaluation
• Patient doesn't experience any hemorrhaging during and 28 days after drug therapy.

Reactions may be *common*, uncommon, *life-threatening*, or COMMON AND LIFE-THREATENING.

• Patient and family state understanding of drug therapy.

duloxetine hydrochloride
(dull-OX-uh-teen high-droh-KLOR-idgh)
Cymbalta✐

Pharmacologic class: selective serotonin and norepinephrine reuptake inhibitor
Therapeutic class: antidepressant, central pain inhibitor
Pregnancy risk category: C

Indications and dosages

▶ **Major depressive disorder.** *Adults:* Initially, 20 mg P.O. b.i.d. to 60 mg P.O. once daily or in two divided doses. Maximum, 60 mg daily.
▶ **Neuropathic pain from diabetic peripheral neuropathy.** *Adults:* 60 mg P.O. once daily
◾ **NEW INDICATION: Generalized anxiety disorder.** *Adults:* 60 mg P.O. once daily. May start 30 mg P.O. once daily for 1 week, and then increase to 60 mg once daily.
◨ **Adjust-a-dose:** Patients with renal impairment may need a lower initial dose and gradual dose increases. In patients with creatinine clearance less than 30 ml/minute, don't give.

Contraindications and cautions

• Contraindicated in patients hypersensitive to drug or its ingredients, those taking MAO inhibitors, and those with uncontrolled narrow angle-closure glaucoma or with a creatinine clearance less than 30 ml/minute. Drug isn't recommended for patients with hepatic dysfunction, or end-stage renal disease or those who drink substantial amounts of alcohol.
• Use cautiously in patients with a history of mania or seizures and those with hypertension, controlled narrow angle-closure glaucoma, or conditions that slow gastric emptying.
⚘ **Lifespan:** In pregnant women, use during third trimester may cause complications for the neonate, including respiratory distress, cyanosis, apnea, seizures, vomiting, hypoglycemia, and hyperreflexia, that may require prolonged hospitalization, respiratory support, and tube feeding. Weigh potential benefit for the mother versus risks to the fetus. Breast-feeding women shouldn't use. Safety and effectiveness in children and adolescents haven't been established.

Adverse reactions

CNS: anxiety, asthenia, *dizziness, fatigue,* fever, *headache,* hypoesthesia, initial insomnia, *insomnia,* irritability, lethargy, nervousness, nightmares, restlessness, sleep disorder, *somnolence,* **suicidal ideation,** tremor.
CV: hot flushes, hypertension, increased heart rate.
EENT: blurred vision, nasopharyngitis, pharyngolaryngeal pain.
GI: *constipation, diarrhea, dry mouth,* dyspepsia, gastritis, nausea, vomiting.
GU: abnormal orgasm, abnormally increased frequency of urination, delayed or dysfunctional ejaculation, dysuria, erectile dysfunction, urinary hesitancy.
Metabolic: *decreased appetite,* **hypoglycemia,** increased appetite, weight gain or loss.
Musculoskeletal: muscle cramps, myalgia.
Respiratory: cough.
Skin: increased sweating, night sweats, pruritus, rash.
Other: decreased libido, rigors.

Interactions

Drug-drug. *CNS drugs:* May increase adverse effects. Use cautiously together.
CYP1A2 inhibitors (cimetidine, fluvoxamine, certain quinolones): May increase duloxetine level. Avoid use together.
CYP2D6 inhibitors (fluoxetine, paroxetine, quinidine): May increase duloxetine level. Use together cautiously.
Drugs that reduce gastric acidity: May cause breakdown of duloxetine's protective coating and early release of the drug. Monitor patient for effects.
MAO inhibitors: May cause hyperthermia, rigidity, myoclonus, autonomic instability, rapid fluctuations of vital signs, agitation, and eventually, delirium and coma. Wait at least 14 days after stopping an MAO inhibitor before starting duloxetine; wait at least 5 days after stopping duloxetine before starting an MAO inhibitor.
Thioridazine: May prolong the QT interval and increase the risk of serious ventricular arrhythmias and sudden death. Avoid use together.
Tricyclic antidepressants (amitriptyline, nortriptyline, imipramine): May increase levels of these drugs. Tricyclic antidepressant dose may need to be reduced and levels monitored closely.
Triptans: May cause serotonin syndrome (restlessness, hallucinations, loss of coordination,

tachycardia, labile blood pressure, fever, hyper-reflexia, nausea, vomiting, diarrhea). Use together cautiously.

Type 1C antiarrhythmics (flecainide, propafenone), phenothiazines (except thioridazine): May increase levels of these drugs. Use together cautiously.

Drug-lifestyle. *Alcohol use:* May increase the risk of liver damage. Discourage alcohol use.

Effects on lab test results

• May increase alkaline phosphatase, ALT, AST, bilirubin, and CK levels.

Pharmacokinetics

Absorption: Compared with the morning dose, the evening dose has a 3-hour delay in absorption and a one-third increase in clearance.
Distribution: More than 90% protein-bound to albumin and alpha$_1$-acid glycoprotein.
Metabolism: Numerous metabolites by the liver via CYP2D6 and CYP1A2.
Excretion: 70% in urine and 20% in feces as metabolites. *Half-life:* 12 hours.

Route	Onset	Peak	Duration
P.O.	Unknown	6 hr	Unknown

Action

Chemical effect: May inhibit serotonin and norepinephrine reuptake in the CNS.
Therapeutic effect: Relieves depression. Relieves neuropathic pain in patients with diabetic peripheral neuropathy.

Available forms

Capsules (delayed-release): 20 mg, 30 mg, 60 mg

NURSING PROCESS

☲ Assessment
• Monitor patient for worsening depression or suicidal behavior, especially during dosage initiation or changes.
• Monitor blood pressure periodically during therapy.
• Reassess patient periodically to determine whether therapy needs to continue.
• Assess patient's and family's knowledge of drug therapy.

⊞ Nursing diagnoses
• Disturbed thought processes related to presence of depression
• Chronic pain related to underlying disease process and neuropathic pain
• Deficient knowledge related to drug therapy

▶ Planning and implementation
• Monitor older patient for increased effect, and adjust dosage. Old and young adults respond similarly, but older patients may be more sensitive to drug effects.
• Decrease dosage gradually, and watch for symptoms such as dizziness, nausea, headache, paresthesia, vomiting, irritability, and nightmares. If symptoms occur, restart at previous dose and decrease even more gradually.
⚠ **ALERT:** Antidepressants may increase the risk of suicidal thinking and behavior in children and adolescents with major depressive disorder and other psychiatric disorders. Balance risk with patient's need for drug.
⚠ **ALERT:** May increase the risk of suicidal thinking and behavior in young adults ages 18 to 24 during the first 2 months of treatment. Monitor patient closely.
Patient teaching
⚠ **ALERT:** Warn families or caregivers to report signs of worsening depression (such as agitation, irritability, insomnia, hostility, impulsivity) or suicidal behavior to prescriber immediately.
• Tell patient to consult his prescriber or pharmacist if he plans to take other prescription or OTC drugs or an herbal or other dietary supplement.
• Instruct patient to swallow capsules whole and not to chew, crush, or open them because they have an enteric coating.
• Urge patient to avoid activities that are hazardous or require mental alertness until he knows the drug's effects.
• Warn against drinking substantial amounts of alcohol because of risk of severe liver toxicity.
• If patient takes drug for depression, explain that it may take 1 to 4 weeks to take effect.

☑ Evaluation
• Patient's behavior and communication indicate improved thought processes.
• Patient reports decreased pain.
• Patient and family state understanding of drug therapy.

dutasteride

(doo-TAS-teer-ighd)
Avodart

Pharmacologic class: 5-alpha-reductase enzyme inhibitor
Therapeutic class: BPH drug
Pregnancy risk category: X

Indications and dosages

▶ **BPH.** *Men:* 0.5 mg P.O. once daily.

Contraindications and cautions

• Contraindicated in patients hypersensitive to drug, its components, or other 5-alpha-reductase inhibitors.
• Use cautiously in patients with hepatic disease and in those taking long-term potent CYP3A4 inhibitors.
⚱ **Lifespan:** Contraindicated in women and children.

Adverse reactions

GU: decreased libido, ejaculation disorder, impotence.
Other: gynecomastia.

Interactions

Drug-drug. *CYP3A4 inhibitors (cimetidine, diltiazem, itraconazole, ketoconazole, macrolide antibiotics, protease inhibitors, ritonavir, verapamil):* May increase dutasteride level. Use together cautiously.

Effect on lab test results

• May decrease prostate-specific antigen (PSA) level.

Pharmacokinetics

Absorption: Bioavailability of about 60%.
Distribution: 99% bound to albumin and 96.6% bound to alpha$_1$-acid glycoprotein.
Metabolism: Extensive, by CYP3A4.
Excretion: Mainly in feces, 5% unchanged and 40% as metabolites, trace amounts in urine.
Half-life: 5 weeks.

Route	Onset	Peak	Duration
P.O.	Unknown	2–3 hr	Unknown

Action

Chemical effect: Inhibits conversion of testosterone to dihydrotestosterone, the androgen mainly responsible for initial development and later enlargement of the prostate gland.
Therapeutic effect: Resolves BPH.

Available forms

Capsules: 0.5 mg

D

NURSING PROCESS

📝 Assessment
• Before therapy, assess patient to rule out other urologic diseases.
• Carefully monitor patients with a large residual urine volume, severely diminished urine flow, or both, for obstructive uropathy.
• Perform digital rectal examinations and other evaluations for prostate cancer on patients with BPH before starting therapy, and reassess periodically thereafter.
• Be alert for adverse effects.
• Assess patient's and family's knowledge of drug therapy.

🔹 Nursing diagnoses
• Impaired urinary elimination related to underlying condition
• Sexual dysfunction related to adverse effects of medication
• Deficient knowledge related to drug therapy

▶ Planning and implementation
• Because drug may be absorbed through the skin, don't allow women who are or may become pregnant to handle the drug.
• If capsule leaks onto skin, wash the area immediately with soap and water.
• Patient shouldn't donate blood within 6 months of last dose.
• Establish new baseline PSA level in men treated for 3 to 6 months, and use it to assess potentially cancer-related changes in PSA level.
• To interpret PSA level in men treated for 6 months or more, double the PSA level for comparison with normal levels in untreated men.
Patient teaching
• Tell patient to swallow the capsule whole and to take with or without food.
• Inform patient that ejaculate volume may decrease, but sexual function will remain normal.

- Tell patient that pregnant women shouldn't handle drug. A boy born to a woman who was exposed to the drug during pregnancy may have abnormal sex organs.
- Tell patient not to donate blood within 6 months of his final dose.

☑ Evaluation

- Patient has normal urinary flow without urinary residual volume.
- Patient doesn't experience adverse effects.
- Patient and family state understanding of drug therapy.

✳ New Drug

HIGH ALERT!

eculizumab
(eck-u-LIZ-uh-mahb)
Soliris

Pharmacologic class: monoclonal IgG antibody
Therapeutic class: hemolysis inhibitor
Pregnancy risk category: C

Indications and dosages

▶ **To reduce hemolysis in patients with paroxysmal nocturnal hemoglobinuria (PNH).** *Adults:* 600 mg every 7 days for 4 weeks, 900 mg 7 days later, then 900 mg every 14 days thereafter. Meningococcal vaccine is required at least 2 weeks before giving drug. Revaccinate according to current medical guidelines.

▽ I.V. administration

- Patients and clinicians must be registered in the Soliris Safety Registry before start of treatment.
- Vials should be refrigerated and protected from light.
- Don't freeze or shake drug.
- For infusion, using a sterile syringe, transfer the required amount of drug to the infusion bag.
- Dilute to a final concentration of 5 mg/ml with normal or half-normal saline, D_5W, or

Ringer's solution to final volumes of 120 ml for 600 mg and 180 ml for 900 mg.
- Mix gently; solution should be clear and at room temperature before administration. Don't heat.
- Infuse over 35 minutes by gravity, syringe pump, or infusion pump.
- Monitor the patient for adverse reactions, including anaphylaxis or hypersensitivity, during and 1 hour after infusion; slow or stop the infusion if a reaction occurs.
- If the infusion is slowed, don't exceed 2 hours for total infusion time.
- The solution is preservative-free; discard unused portion.
- Reconstituted solution remains stable for 24 hours, refrigerated or at room temperature.
⊗ **Incompatibilities**
No known incompatibilities.

Contraindications and cautions

- Contraindicated in patients with severe *Neisseria meningitidis* infection or in patients who aren't vaccinated against *N. meningitidis*.
- Contraindicated in patients who are hypersensitive to the drug.

⚕ **Lifespan:** In pregnant women, use only if the potential benefits outweigh the risks. Drug may appear in breast milk. The risk of exposing infants to the drug should be weighed against the benefits of breast-feeding. In patients younger than age 18, safety and effectiveness of the drug are unknown.

Adverse reactions

CNS: headache, fatigue, fever.
EENT: nasopharyngitis, cough, sinusitis, respiratory tract infection, flulike symptoms.
GI: nausea, constipation.
Hematologic: anemia.
Musculoskeletal: back pain, myalgia, pain in arm or leg.
Other: meningococcal infection and *sepsis,* herpes simplex infection.

Interactions

No known interactions.

Effects on lab test results

- May increase LDH levels if hemolysis occurs or may decrease LDH levels if hemolysis declines.

Pharmacokinetics

Absorption: Given I.V.
Distribution: Volume of distribution is 7.7 L.
Metabolism: Unknown.
Excretion: Unknown. *Half-life:* About 11 days.

Route	Onset	Peak	Duration
I.V.	Immediate	Unknown	Unknown

Action

Chemical effect: A monoclonal antibody, it binds to complement protein C5 to reduce intravascular hemolysis.
Therapeutic effect: Reduction in hemolysis and LDH levels.

Available forms

Single-use vial: 300 mg (10 mg/ml)

NURSING PROCESS

⚗ Assessment
• Obtain history of patient's underlying condition before therapy.
• Monitor drug's effectiveness by checking LDH levels.
• Monitor hemoglobin.
• Monitor patient for any signs of infection.
• Be alert for adverse reactions.
• Assess patient's and family's knowledge of drug therapy.

🔧 Nursing diagnoses
• Risk for injury related to elevated LDL levels
• Risk for infection related to bacteria
• Deficient knowledge related to drug therapy

▶ Planning and implementation
• Give meningococcal vaccine at least 2 weeks before starting drug.
• Give infusion at indicated intervals but don't exceed total infusion time of 2 hours.
• **ALERT:** For 8 weeks after the drug is stopped, monitor the patient for hemolysis. Signs of hemolysis include LDH levels higher than pretreatment levels, more than 25% absolute decrease in PNH clone size within a week, hemoglobin lower than 5 g/dl, hemoglobin decrease of more than 4 g/dl in less than 7 days, angina, mental status change, 50% increase in creatinine level, and thrombosis.
• If hemolysis occurs, treatment may include blood transfusion, exchange transfusion, antico-agulation, corticosteroids, or restarting eculizumab.

Patient teaching
• Inform patient that the meningococcal vaccine is required at least 2 weeks before therapy; revaccination will also be required.
• Inform the patient to report moderate to severe headache with nausea or vomiting, a fever, or a stiff neck or back. Patients should also report immediately a fever higher than 103° F (39.5° C), fever with a rash, confusion, or weakness.
• Inform the patient that he will need to be in the Patient Safety Registry while receiving this drug. Patients will receive a Patient Safety Card, which should be carried at all times.
• Inform the patient that he will be monitored for at least 8 weeks after the drug is stopped.

✓ Evaluation
• Patient doesn't sustain injury as a result of hemolysis.
• Patient has no signs of infection.
• Patient and family state understanding of drug therapy.

edetate calcium disodium (calcium EDTA)
(ED-eh-tayt KAL-see-um digh-SOH-dee-um)
Calcium Disodium Versenate

Pharmacologic class: chelating drug
Therapeutic class: heavy metal antagonist
Pregnancy risk category: B

Indications and dosages

▶ **Acute lead encephalopathy or lead level above 70 mcg/dl.** *Adults and children:* 1.5 g/m^2 I.V. or I.M. daily in divided doses at 12-hour intervals for 3 to 5 days, usually with dimercaprol. Give a second course in 5 to 7 days.
▶ **Lead poisoning without encephalopathy, or asymptomatic patient with lead level between 20 mcg/dl and 70 mcg/dl.** *Children:* 1 g/m^2 I.V. or I.M. daily in divided doses for 5 days. Give second course after 2 to 4 days, as needed.
Adjust-a-dose: In patients with lead nephropathy, decrease dosage and frequency as follows. If creatinine level is 2 to 3 mg/dl, give 500 mg/m^2/day for 5 days. If serum creatinine

level is 3 to 4 mg/dl, give 500 mg/m²/day every 48 hours for three doses. If creatinine level exceeds 4 mg/dl, give 500 mg/m² once weekly.

▼ I.V. administration

• I.V. use may increase intracranial pressure. To treat lead encephalopathy, give by I.M. route instead.
• Dilute drug with 250 to 500 ml of D_5W or normal saline injection.
• Infuse half of daily dose over 1 hour in asymptomatic patients or over 2 hours in symptomatic patients. Give rest of infusion at least 6 hours later. Or give by slow infusion over 4 to 24 hours.

⊗ **Incompatibilities**
Amphotericin B, dextrose 10% in water, hydralazine hydrochloride, invert sugar 10% in normal saline solution, invert sugar 10% in water, lactated Ringer's solution, Ringer's injection, 1/6 M sodium lactate.

Contraindications and cautions

• Contraindicated in patients with anuria, acute renal disease, or hepatitis.
• Use cautiously and reduce dosage in patients with mild renal disease. Drug may cause life-threatening toxic effects.
☀ **Lifespan:** In pregnant and breast-feeding women, use cautiously.

Adverse reactions

CNS: fatigue, headache, numbness, paresthesia, sudden fever.
CV: *arrhythmias,* hypotension.
EENT: nasal congestion, sneezing.
GI: anorexia, cheilosis, nausea, vomiting.
GU: *acute necrosis of proximal tubules,* hematuria, *nephrotoxicity,* proteinuria.
Hematologic: anemia, transient bone marrow depression.
Metabolic: hypercalcemia, zinc deficiency.
Musculoskeletal: arthralgia, myalgia.
Skin: rash.
Other: allergic histamine-like reaction, chills, excessive thirst.

Interactions

Drug-drug. *Zinc insulin:* May interfere with action of insulin by binding with zinc. Monitor patient closely.
Zinc supplements: May decrease effectiveness of edetate calcium disodium and zinc supplements because of chelation. Withhold zinc supplements until therapy is complete.

Effects on lab test results

• May increase AST, ALT, and calcium levels. May decrease zinc and hemoglobin levels and hematocrit.

Pharmacokinetics

Absorption: Well absorbed after I.M. use.
Distribution: Mainly in extracellular fluid.
Metabolism: None.
Excretion: In urine. *Half-life:* 20 minutes to 1½ hours.

Route	Onset	Peak	Duration
I.V., I.M.	1 hr	1–2 days	Unknown

Action

Chemical effect: Forms stable, soluble complexes with metals, particularly lead.
Therapeutic effect: Abolishes effects of lead poisoning.

Available forms

Injection: 200 mg/ml

NURSING PROCESS

📋 Assessment
• Obtain history of patient's underlying condition before therapy.
• Monitor drug's effectiveness by checking lead level and watching for decreasing evidence of lead poisoning.
• Monitor fluid intake and output; conduct urinalysis, BUN, and ECG daily.
• Be alert for adverse reactions.
• Assess patient's and family's knowledge of drug therapy.

🔷 Nursing diagnoses
• Risk for injury related to lead poisoning
• Ineffective renal tissue perfusion related to drug-induced fatal nephrosis
• Deficient knowledge related to drug therapy

▶ Planning and implementation
• When giving I.M., add procaine hydrochloride to I.M. solution to minimize pain. Watch for local reactions.
• Use I.M. route for children and patients with lead encephalopathy.

- Force fluids to facilitate lead excretion, except in patients with lead encephalopathy.
- To avoid toxicity, use with dimercaprol.
- Apply ice or cold compresses to injection site to ease local reaction.

⊛ **ALERT:** Don't confuse edetate calcium disodium with edetate disodium, which is used to treat hypercalcemia.

Patient teaching

- Warn patient that some adverse reactions, such as fever, chills, thirst, and nasal congestion, may occur 4 to 8 hours after use.
- Encourage patient and family to identify and remove source of lead in home.

☑ **Evaluation**

- Patient sustains no injury as a result of lead poisoning.
- Patient has no signs of altered renal tissue perfusion.
- Patient and family state understanding of drug therapy.

edetate disodium
(ED-eh-tayt digh-SOH-dee-um)
Disodium EDTA, Endrate, Sodium Edetate

Pharmacologic class: chelating drug
Therapeutic class: heavy metal antagonist
Pregnancy risk category: C

Indications and dosages

▶ **Hypercalcemic crisis.** *Adults:* 50 mg/kg/day by slow I.V. infusion for 5 days; no drug for 2 days; then repeat course, as needed. Maximum, 3 g I.V. daily and 15 doses total.
Children: 40 to 70 mg/kg/day by slow I.V. infusion. Maximum, 70 mg/kg I.V. daily.
▶ **Digoxin-induced arrhythmias.** *Adults and children:* 15 mg/kg/hour I.V. daily. Maximum, 60 mg/kg I.V. daily.

▼ I.V. administration

- Don't give as a direct or intermittent injection.
- Keep I.V. calcium available to treat hypocalcemia.
- Dilute before use. For adults, add dose to 500 ml of D₅W or normal saline solution and give over 3 or more hours. For children, dilute to maximum of 30 mg/ml in D₅W or normal saline solution and give over 3 or more hours.

- Don't exceed prescribed dose or rate of administration.
- Avoid rapid I.V. infusion, which may result in profound hypocalcemia and lead to tetany, seizures, arrhythmias, and respiratory arrest.
- Extravasation can cause tissue damage and necrosis; watch for irritation and infiltration.
- Record I.V. site used and avoid repeated use of same site to decrease likelihood of thrombophlebitis.
- Keep patient in bed for 15 minutes after infusion to avoid orthostatic hypotension.

⊗ **Incompatibilities**
None reported.

Contraindications and cautions

- Contraindicated in patients hypersensitive to the drug or any of its components and in those with anuria, known or suspected hypocalcemia, significant renal disease, active or healed tubercular lesions, or a history of seizures or intracranial lesions.
- Use cautiously in patients with limited cardiac reserve, heart failure, or hypokalemia.

⚘ **Lifespan:** In pregnant and breast-feeding women, use cautiously.

Adverse reactions

CNS: circumoral paresthesia, numbness, headache.
CV: hypertension, orthostatic hypotension, thrombophlebitis.
GI: abdominal cramps, anorexia, diarrhea, nausea, vomiting.
GU: dysuria, *nephrotoxicity,* nocturia, polyuria, proteinuria, *renal failure,* renal insufficiency, *tubular necrosis,* urinary urgency.
Metabolic: hypocalcemia, *hypomagnesia.*
Skin: dermatitis, erythema.
Other: infusion site pain.

Interactions

Drug-drug. *Digoxin:* May reverse effects of digoxin overdose because of drop in calcium caused by edetate disodium. If hypercalcemia recurs, monitor patient closely for renewed digoxin toxicity.
Zinc insulins: May decrease glucose and chelate zinc in some insulin. Dosage adjustments of insulin may be required.

Effects on lab test results

• May increase uric acid level. May decrease calcium, magnesium, potassium, zinc, and hemoglobin levels and hematocrit.

Pharmacokinetics

Absorption: Administered I.V.
Distribution: Distributed widely throughout body but doesn't enter CSF in significant amounts.
Metabolism: None.
Excretion: In urine. *Half-life:* Unknown.

Route	Onset	Peak	Duration
I.V.	Unknown	Unknown	Unknown

Action

Chemical effect: Chelates with metals, such as calcium, to form stable, soluble complex.
Therapeutic effect: Lowers calcium level and stabilizes heart rhythm in emergency conditions.

Available forms

Injection: 150 mg/ml

NURSING PROCESS

Assessment
• Obtain history of patient's calcium level before therapy.
• Monitor drug's effectiveness by obtaining calcium level after each dose. If drug is used to treat digoxin-induced arrhythmias, evaluate patient's ECG often.
• Monitor kidney function tests often.
• Be alert for adverse reactions.
• Assess patient's and family's knowledge of drug therapy.

Nursing diagnoses
• Risk for injury related to hypercalcemia
• Ineffective protection related to drug-induced hypocalcemia
• Deficient knowledge related to drug therapy

Planning and implementation
• If generalized systemic reactions (fever, chills, back pain, emesis, muscle cramps, urinary urgency) occur 4 to 8 hours after infusion, report them to prescriber. Treatment is usually symptomatic. Effects usually subside within 12 hours.
• Other drugs for hypercalcemia are safer and more effective than edetate disodium.

⚠ ALERT: Don't confuse edetate disodium with edetate calcium disodium, which is used to treat lead toxicity.
Patient teaching
• Instruct patient to immediately report respiratory difficulty, dizziness, and muscle cramping.
• Advise patient to move from sitting or lying position slowly to avoid dizziness.
• Reassure patient that generalized systemic reaction usually subsides within 12 hours.
• If treating digoxin toxicity, instruct patient on correct usage of drug and required laboratory follow-up.

☑ Evaluation
• Patient sustains no injury as result of hypercalcemia.
• Patient's calcium level doesn't fall below normal after edetate disodium therapy.
• Patient and family state understanding of drug therapy.

efalizumab
(eh-fah-LEE-zoo-mab)
Raptiva

Pharmacologic class: immunosuppressant
Therapeutic class: antipsoriatic
Pregnancy risk category: C

Indications and dosages

▶ **Chronic moderate-to-severe plaque psoriasis when systemic therapy or phototherapy is appropriate.** *Adults:* Single dose of 0.7 mg/kg subcutaneously; follow with weekly doses of 1 mg/kg subcutaneously. Maximum single dose, 200 mg.

Contraindications and cautions

• Contraindicated in patients hypersensitive to drug or any of its components and in patients with significant infection.
• Contraindicated in patients with clinically important infections.
• Use cautiously in patients with chronic infection or a history of recurrent infection. Also use cautiously in patients with a history of or high risk for malignancy.
• Use cautiously in patients with thrombocytopenia.

⚕ **Lifespan:** In pregnant women, use cautiously; it isn't known whether drug harms fetus. Tell breast-feeding women to stop breast-feeding or to stop using the drug because risk to the infant is unknown. In children, safety and effectiveness haven't been established. In elderly patients, use cautiously because of his increased risk of infection.

Adverse reactions

CNS: fever, *headache,* pain, **stroke.**
GI: *nausea.*
Hematologic: *thrombocytopenia.*
Musculoskeletal: back pain, myalgia.
Skin: acne.
Other: chills, flulike symptoms, hypersensitivity reaction, *infection,* **malignancy.**

Interactions

Drug-drug. *Immunosuppressants:* May increase risk of infection and malignancy. Avoid use together.
Vaccines: May decrease or eliminate immune response to vaccine. Avoid use together.

Effects on lab test results

• May increase alkaline phosphatase level.
• May increase lymphocyte and leukocyte counts. May decrease platelet count.

Pharmacokinetics

Absorption: 50% bioavailable.
Distribution: Unknown.
Metabolism: Unknown.
Excretion: Unknown. *Half-life:* Unknown.

Route	Onset	Peak	Duration
SubQ	1–2 days	Unknown	25 days

Action

Chemical effect: Binds to a leukocyte function antigen and decreases its expression, thus inhibiting the action of T lymphocytes at sites of inflammation, including psoriatic skin.
Therapeutic effect: Decreases inflammation of psoriatic skin.

Available forms

Injection: 125-mg single-use vial

NURSING PROCESS

Assessment
• Watch for thrombocytopenia. Check patient's platelet count monthly before start of treatment, monthly until laboratory effects are stable, and then every 3 months.
• Monitor patient for worsening of psoriasis during or after therapy.
• Assess patient's and family's knowledge of drug therapy.

Nursing diagnoses
• Impaired skin integrity related to underlying condition
• Ineffective protection related to drug-induced thrombocytopenia
• Deficient knowledge related to drug therapy

Planning and implementation
• To reconstitute, inject 1.3 ml of sterile water for injection into the vial. Swirl gently to dissolve powder, which takes less than 5 minutes. Don't shake the vial.
• Reconstitute drug immediately before use.
• Don't use any other diluent besides sterile water, and use a vial only once.
• The reconstituted solution should be colorless to pale yellow and free of particulates. Don't use solution that contains particulates or is discolored.
• Use reconstituted solution immediately, or store it at room temperature and use within 8 hours.
• Rotate injection sites.
• Don't add other drugs to solution.
• Keep powder refrigerated, and protect vials from light.
• Stop drug if patient develops severe infection or malignancy.
• Don't give vaccines to patients taking this drug because the immune response may be inadequate.
• If patient becomes pregnant while taking the drug or within 6 weeks after stopping it, enroll her in the efalizumab Pregnancy Registry by calling 1-877-727-8482.
Patient teaching
• Tell patient to take drug exactly as prescribed.
• Explain that platelet counts will be monitored during therapy.

• Urge patient to immediately report evidence of severe thrombocytopenia, such as bleeding gums, bruising, or petechiae.
• Tell patient to report weight changes because dosage may need to be changed.
• Advise patient to report any newly diagnosed infection or malignancy.
• Tell patient to report worsening psoriasis.
• Caution patient to immediately report pregnancy or suspected pregnancy while taking drug or within 6 weeks of stopping drug.
• Encourage pregnant women to enroll in the efalizumab Pregnancy Registry.

☑ **Evaluation**
• Patient's underlying condition improves with drug therapy.
• Patient has no serious complications from drug-induced thrombocytopenia.
• Patient and family state understanding of drug therapy.

efavirenz
(eh-FAH-veer-enz)
Sustiva

Pharmacologic class: nonnucleoside reverse transcriptase inhibitor (NNRTI)
Therapeutic class: antiretroviral
Pregnancy risk category: D

Indications and dosages

▶ **HIV-1 infection.** *Adults:* 600 mg P.O. daily with a protease inhibitor or nucleoside analogue reverse transcriptase inhibitors.
Children age 3 and older who weigh 10 to less than 15 kg (22 to less than 33 lb): 200 mg P.O. daily.
Children who weigh 15 to less than 20 kg (33 to 44 lb): 250 mg P.O. daily.
Children who weigh 20 to less than 25 kg (44 to 55 lb): 300 mg P.O. daily.
Children who weigh 25 to less than 32.5 kg (55 to 72 lb): 350 mg P.O. daily.
Children who weigh 32.5 to less than 40 kg (72 to 88 lb): 400 mg P.O. daily.
Children who weigh 40 kg (88 lb) or more: 600 mg P.O. once daily.
🔧 **Adjust-a-dose:** For adults also taking voriconazole, increase voriconazole maintenance dosage to 400 mg every 12 hours and decrease the efavirenz (capsules) dose to 300 mg once daily.

Contraindications and cautions

• Contraindicated in patients hypersensitive to drug or any of its components and in those taking astemizole, bepridil, cisapride, midazolam, pimozide, triazolam or ergot derivatives.
• Use cautiously in patients with hepatic impairment or in those receiving hepatotoxic drugs.
🌟 **Lifespan:** In pregnant and breast-feeding women, drug is contraindicated. In children and elderly patients, use cautiously.

Adverse reactions

CNS: abnormal dreams or thinking, agitation, amnesia, confusion, depersonalization, depression, dizziness, euphoria, fatigue, hallucinations, headache, hypoesthesia, impaired concentration, insomnia, somnolence, nervousness, fever.
GI: abdominal pain, anorexia, constipation, diarrhea, dyspepsia, flatulence, malabsorption, nausea, vomiting.
GU: hematuria, renal calculi.
Skin: *erythema multiforme,* increased sweating, pruritus, rash, *Stevens-Johnson syndrome, toxic epidermal necrolysis.*
Other: gynecomastia.

Interactions

Drug-drug. *Amprenavir, atorvastatin, calcium channel blockers, indinavir, itraconazole, lopinavir, pravastatin, rifampin, simvastatin:* May decrease levels of these drugs. Consider alternative therapy or adjust dosages.
Bepridil, cisapride, pimozide: May cause life-threatening adverse events such as arrhythmias, prolonged sedation, or respiratory depression. Avoid use together.
Clarithromycin: May decrease clarithromycin level and increase level of main metabolite. Also increases risk of rash. Consider using azithromycin instead.
Drugs that induce the cytochrome P-450 enzyme system (such as phenobarbital, rifampin): May increase clearance of efavirenz, resulting in lower level. Avoid use together.
Ergot derivatives, midazolam, triazolam: May inhibit metabolism of these drugs through competition for the cytochrome P-450 enzyme system, possibly causing serious or life-threatening adverse events (such as arrhythmias, prolonged

sedation, or respiratory depression). Avoid use together.
Ethinyl estradiol: May increase level of ethinyl estradiol. Advise use of barrier contraception in addition to hormonal contraceptive.
Psychoactive drugs: May cause additive CNS effects. Avoid use together.
Rifabutin: May decrease rifabutin level. Increase dosage of rifabutin to 450 to 600 mg once daily or 600 mg two to three times a week.
Ritonavir: May increase levels of efavirenz and ritonavir. Monitor patient closely.
Saquinavir: May significantly decrease saquinavir level. Don't use with saquinavir as sole protease inhibitor.
Voriconazole: May significantly decrease voriconazole level while significantly increasing efavirenz level. Avoid use together.
Warfarin: May increase or decrease level and effects of warfarin. Monitor INR.
Drug-herb. *St. John's wort:* May decrease efavirenz level. Discourage use together.
Drug-food. *High-fat meals:* May increase absorption of drug, increasing risk of adverse effects. Instruct patient to maintain a low-fat diet.
Drug-lifestyle. *Alcohol use:* Enhances CNS effects. Discourage alcohol use.

Effects on lab test results
• May increase ALT, AST, amylase, and cholesterol levels.

Pharmacokinetics
Absorption: Steady-state levels reached in 6 to 10 days. Food increases amount of drug in body.
Distribution: Highly protein-bound, mainly to albumin.
Metabolism: Mainly by cytochrome P-450 system to metabolites that are inactive against HIV-1.
Excretion: Mainly in feces. *Half-life:* 40 to 76 hours.

Route	Onset	Peak	Duration
P.O.	Unknown	3–5 hr	Unknown

Action
Chemical effect: An NNRTI that inhibits the transcription of HIV-1 RNA to DNA, a critical step in the viral replication process.
Therapeutic effect: Lowers viral load of HIV in the blood and increases CD4+ lymphocytes.

Available forms
Capsules: 50 mg, 100 mg, 200 mg
Tablets: 600 mg

NURSING PROCESS

Assessment
• Monitor liver function test results in a patient with a history of hepatitis B or C and in those taking ritonavir.
• Monitor cholesterol level.
• Children may be more susceptible to adverse reactions, especially diarrhea, nausea, vomiting, and rash.
• Observe skin before starting drug and regularly thereafter for signs of rash.
• Assess patient's and family's knowledge of drug therapy.

Nursing diagnoses
• Risk for infection related to patient's underlying condition
• Risk for impaired skin integrity related to potential adverse effects of drug
• Deficient knowledge related to drug therapy

Planning and implementation
• Use drug with other antiretrovirals and not as monotherapy because resistant viruses emerge rapidly when it's used alone. Don't add it as a single drug to a failing regimen.
• Using drug with ritonavir may cause a higher occurrence of adverse effects, such as dizziness, nausea, paresthesia, and elevated liver enzyme levels.
• Rule out pregnancy before starting therapy in women of childbearing age.
• Give drug at bedtime on an empty stomach to decrease adverse effects.
Patient teaching
• Instruct patient to take drug on an empty stomach, preferably at bedtime, and to take it with water, juice, milk, or soda.
• Inform patient about need for scheduled blood tests to monitor liver function and cholesterol levels.
• Tell patient to use barrier contraception in addition to hormonal contraceptives, and to notify prescriber immediately if pregnancy is suspected. Drug is a known risk to the fetus.
• Inform patient that drug doesn't cure HIV infection and that it won't affect the complications of HIV. Explain that it doesn't reduce the risk of

HIV transmission through sexual contact or blood contamination.
- Instruct patient to take drug at the same time each day and always with other antiretrovirals.
- Tell patient to take drug exactly as prescribed and not to stop without medical approval.
- Inform patient that rash is the most common adverse effect. Tell patient to immediately report any rash or any other adverse effects. Rash may be serious in rare cases.
- Instruct patient to report use of other drugs.
- Advise patient that dizziness, difficulty sleeping or concentrating, drowsiness, or unusual dreams may occur during the first few days of therapy. Reassure patient that these symptoms typically resolve after 2 to 4 weeks and that it may help to take drug at bedtime.
- Tell patient not to use alcohol and not to drive or operate machinery until drug's effects are known.

☑ **Evaluation**
- Patient is free from opportunistic infections.
- Patient's skin integrity is maintained.
- Patient and family state understanding of drug therapy.

eletriptan hydrobromide
(el-eh-TRIP-tan high-dro-BRO-mighd)
Relpax

Pharmacologic class: serotonin receptor agonist
Therapeutic class: antimigraine
Pregnancy risk category: C

Indications and dosages

▶ **Acute migraine with or without aura.**
Adults: 20 to 40 mg P.O. at the first migraine symptom. If headache recurs after initial relief, repeat dose at least 2 hours later. Maximum, 80 mg daily.

Contraindications and cautions

- Contraindicated in patients hypersensitive to drug or any of its components and in those with severe hepatic impairment; ischemic heart disease, such as angina pectoris, a history of MI, or silent ischemia; coronary artery vasospasm, including Prinzmetal variant angina; and other CV conditions. Also contraindicated in patients with

cerebrovascular disorders, such as stroke or transient ischemic attack; peripheral vascular disease, including ischemic bowel disease; uncontrolled hypertension; or hemiplegic or basilar migraine.
- Avoid use within 24 hours of another serotonin agonist or an ergotamine-containing or ergot-type drug.
⚠ **Lifespan:** In pregnant women, use drug only when benefits outweigh risks to fetus. In breastfeeding women, use cautiously because drug appears in breast milk. In children, safety and effectiveness haven't been established. In elderly patients, use cautiously because they may have 15% lower drug clearance, the half-life of the drug is prolonged to about 6 hours, and these patients may develop higher blood pressure than younger patients.

Adverse reactions

CNS: *asthenia,* dizziness, headache, hypertonia, hypesthesia, pain, paresthesia, somnolence, vertigo.
CV: chest tightness, pain, and pressure; flushing; palpitations.
EENT: abnormal accommodation, abnormal vision, conjunctivitis, dry eyes, eye hemorrhage, *lacrimation disorder,* melanin toxicity, photophobia, transient corneal opacity.
GI: abdominal pain, discomfort, or cramps; dry mouth; dyspepsia; dysphagia; nausea.
Musculoskeletal: back pain.
Respiratory: pharyngitis.
Skin: increased sweating.
Other: chills.

Interactions

Drug-drug. *CYP3A4 inhibitors, such as clarithromycin, itraconazole, ketoconazole, nefazodone, nelfinavir, ritonavir, and troleandomycin:* May decrease eletriptan metabolism. Avoid use within 72 hours of these drugs.
Ergotamine-containing or ergot-type drugs, such as dihydroergotamine or methysergide; serotonin agonists: May prolong vasospastic reactions. Avoid use within 24 hours of these drugs.
Propranolol: May increase bioavailability of eletriptan. No dosage adjustment is needed.

Effects on lab test results

None reported.

Pharmacokinetics

Absorption: Oral bioavailability is 50%. Drug level peaks in 1½ to 2 hours.
Distribution: About 85% protein-bound.
Metabolism: Mainly by CYP3A4. The metabolite of eletriptan is active but without therapeutic effect.
Excretion: Clearance is 10% renal and 90% nonrenal. *Half-life:* About 4 hours.

Route	Onset	Peak	Duration
P.O.	½ hr	1½–2 hr	Unknown

Action

Chemical effect: Binds to serotonin receptors and may constrict intracranial blood vessels and inhibit proinflammatory neuropeptide release.
Therapeutic effect: Relieves migraine symptoms.

Available forms

Tablets: 20 mg, 40 mg

NURSING PROCESS

Assessment
• Obtain history of patient's underlying condition before therapy.
• Assess patient for medical history or risk factors for liver disease, heart disease, cerebrovascular disease, peripheral vascular disease, ischemic bowel, or uncontrolled hypertension.
• Be alert for adverse reactions.
• Assess patient's and family's knowledge of drug therapy.

Nursing diagnoses
• Acute pain related to migraine headaches
• Risk for injury related to adverse reactions
• Deficient knowledge related to drug therapy

Planning and implementation
• Use only in patients with a clear diagnosis of migraine, not for prevention.
• If first use produces no response, reconsider diagnosis; a second dose will probably not be effective if the first dose causes no response.
• The safety of treating more than three migraines in 30 days hasn't been established.
• **ALERT:** Serious cardiac events, including acute MI, arrhythmias, and death, occur rarely—usually within a few hours after use.

• Don't use in patient with risk factors for coronary artery disease, in a postmenopausal woman, or in a man older than age 40, unless patient is reasonably free of underlying CV disease. If drug must be used because of intractable migraine pain unresponsive to other drugs, give the first dose under medical supervision.
• Ocular effects, such as melanin-binding and toxicity, and corneal opacities, may occur with long-term use.

Patient teaching
• Instruct patient to take dose at the first sign of a migraine headache. If headache returns after the first dose, he may take a second dose after 2 hours. Caution patient not to take more than 80 mg in 24 hours.
• Warn patient to avoid driving and operating machinery if he feels dizzy or fatigued after taking drug.
• Tell patient to immediately report pain, tightness, heaviness, or pressure in the chest, throat, neck, or jaw.

Evaluation
• Patient experiences relief from migraine headache.
• Patient has no signs of adverse reaction to the drug.
• Patient and family state understanding of drug therapy and conditions that are contraindications for use of this drug.

emtricitabine
(em-trih-SIGH-tah-been)
Emtriva

Pharmacologic class: nucleoside reverse transcriptase inhibitor (NRTI)
Therapeutic class: antiretroviral
Pregnancy risk category: B

Indications and dosages

▶ **HIV-1 infection with other antiretrovirals.**
Adults: 200 mg capsule P.O. once daily or 240 mg (24 ml) oral solution P.O. once daily.
Children age 3 months to 17 years: For children who weigh more than 33 kg (73 lb) and can swallow intact capsule, give one 200-mg capsule P.O. once daily. Otherwise, give 6 mg/kg oral solution, up to a maximum dose of 240 mg once daily.

Children younger than age 3 months: 3 mg/kg oral solution P.O. once daily.

▧ Adjust-a-dose: For adults who have baseline creatinine clearance of 30 to 49 ml/minute, give 200-mg capsule every 48 hours or 120 mg oral solution every 24 hours. If creatinine clearance is 15 to 29 ml/minute, give 200-mg capsule every 72 hours or 80-mg oral solution every 24 hours. If clearance is less than 15 ml/minute (including patients requiring dialysis), give 200-mg capsule every 96 hours or 60-mg oral solution every 24 hours. If dose is scheduled on the day of hemodialysis, give it after dialysis. For children with renal insufficiency, there's no established dosage reduction. Consider reducing the dose and increasing the interval.

Contraindications and cautions

- Contraindicated in patients hypersensitive to drug or any of its components.
- Lactic acidosis and severe hepatomegaly with steatosis, including fatal cases, have been reported with the use of nucleoside analogues alone and in combination with other antiretrovirals.
- In patients with renal impairment, lower the dose and use drug cautiously.
- Drug isn't indicated for chronic hepatitis B virus infection, and safety and effectiveness of the drug haven't been established in patients infected with hepatitis B virus and HIV.

⚖ Lifespan: In pregnant women, use cautiously because there are no adequate and well-controlled studies in this group. Women should avoid breast-feeding to prevent transmitting HIV to infants.

Adverse reactions

CNS: *asthenia,* depression, *headache,* insomnia, neuritis, nightmares, paresthesia, peripheral neuropathy.
EENT: rhinitis.
GI: abdominal pain, *diarrhea,* dyspepsia, *nausea,* vomiting.
Hepatic: severe hepatomegaly, steatosis.
Metabolic: *lactic acidosis.*
Musculoskeletal: arthralgia, myalgia.
Respiratory: *cough.*
Skin: rash.

Interactions

None reported.

Effects on lab test results

- May increase ALT, AST, bilirubin, triglyceride, amylase, lipase, CK, and glucose levels.

Pharmacokinetics

Absorption: Rapid.
Distribution: At peak level, the mean plasma-to-blood ratio is about 1, and the mean semen-to-plasma ratio is about 4.
Metabolism: Not metabolized by cytochrome P-450 enzymes. Less than 15% undergoes oxidation and glucuronidation by the liver.
Excretion: Mainly in urine. *Half-life:* About 10 hours.

Route	Onset	Peak	Duration
P.O.	Unknown	1–2 hr	Unknown

Action

Chemical effect: Inhibits activity of HIV-1 reverse transcriptase by competing with natural substrate and being incorporated into new viral DNA chains, which results in their destruction.
Therapeutic effect: Helps block HIV replication.

Available forms

Capsules: 200 mg
Oral solution: 10 mg/ml

NURSING PROCESS

▧ Assessment
- Monitor liver and renal function tests.
- Assess all HIV-positive patients for chronic HBV infection before starting therapy.
- In a patient infected with both HBV and HIV, hepatitis B may worsen after therapy. Monitor patient closely for at least several months.
- Assess patient's and family's knowledge of drug therapy.

▧ Nursing diagnoses
- Risk for infection related to patient's underlying condition
- Disturbed body image related to redistribution of body fat due to antiretroviral therapy
- Deficient knowledge related to drug therapy

▧ Planning and implementation
- If patient develops symptoms of lactic acidosis or pronounced hepatotoxicity, stop drug.

- Drug may cause redistribution or accumulation of body fat, including central obesity, dorsocervical fat enlargement (buffalo hump), peripheral wasting, facial wasting, breast enlargement, and cushingoid appearance.
- Effects of higher doses aren't known; overdose can be treated with hemodialysis.

Patient teaching

- Tell patient that drug doesn't cure HIV infection and doesn't reduce the risk of transmitting HIV to others.
- Tell patient that drug must be taken for life.
- Stress importance of compliance and of planning compliance strategies in advance.
- Inform patient of potential adverse reactions, including lactic acidosis, hepatotoxicity, and redistribution or accumulation of body fat.
- Tell patient to contact prescriber immediately if she suspects she is pregnant.
- Instruct patient or family to refrigerate the oral solution. If it's stored at room temperature, they should use it within 3 months.

☑ Evaluation

- Patient remains free from opportunistic infection.
- Patient has no adverse drug effects.
- Patient and family state understanding of drug therapy.

enalaprilat
(eh-NAH-leh-prel-at)

enalapril maleate
Vasotec♦

Pharmacologic class: ACE inhibitor
Therapeutic class: antihypertensive
Pregnancy risk category: C (D in second and third trimesters)

Indications and dosages

▶ **Hypertension.** *Adults:* Initially 5 mg P.O. once daily; adjust according to response. Usual dosage range is 10 to 40 mg daily as single dose or two divided doses. Or 1.25 mg I.V. over 5 minutes every 6 hours.

⊠ Adjust-a-dose: For patient taking a diuretic, initially 2.5 mg P.O. once daily. Or 0.625 mg I.V. over 5 minutes, repeated in 1 hour, if needed, and followed by 1.25 mg I.V. every 6 hours.

In patients with creatinine clearance of 30 ml/minute or less, initial dose is 2.5 mg P.O. daily, increased gradually to maximum of 40 mg daily. Or give 0.625 mg I.V. and repeat in 1 hour if needed. Then give 1.25 mg I.V. every 6 hours. In hemodialysis patients, give 2.5 mg P.O. on dialysis days and adjust dosage on nondialysis days based on blood pressure. Or give 0.625 mg I.V. every 6 hours.

▶ **Heart failure.** *Adults:* Initially 2.5 mg P.O. daily. Increase dosage after a few days or weeks according to response. Range is 2.5 to 20 mg b.i.d.

⊠ Adjust-a-dose: In patients with hyponatremia (sodium level less than 130 mEq/L) or severe renal impairment (creatinine clearance 30 ml/minute or less), initial dose is 2.5 mg P.O. daily given under close supervision. Increase at intervals of 4 or more days to 2.5 mg b.i.d., then 5 mg b.i.d., to a maximum of 40 mg daily.

▶ **Asymptomatic left ventricular dysfunction.** *Adults:* 2.5 mg P.O. b.i.d.; adjust as tolerated to target of 20 mg P.O. daily in divided doses.

▼ I.V. administration

- Giving doses greater than 1.25 mg isn't more effective.
- Compatible solutions include D_5W, normal saline solution, dextrose 5% in lactated Ringer's solution, and D_5W in normal saline solution.
- Inject drug slowly over at least 5 minutes, or dilute in 50 ml of compatible solution and infuse over 15 minutes.

⊗ **Incompatibilities**
Amphotericin B, phenytoin sodium.

Contraindications and cautions

- Contraindicated in patients hypersensitive to drug or any of its components and in those with a history of angioedema from ACE inhibitor.
- Use cautiously in patients with renal impairment, especially those with bilateral renal artery stenosis or unilateral renal artery stenosis in a single functioning kidney.
- **☀ Lifespan:** In pregnant women, use only when benefits outweigh risks to the fetus. In second and third trimesters, ACE inhibitors may be harmful or fatal to fetus. In breast-feeding women and in children, safety hasn't been established.

Adverse reactions

CNS: asthenia, *dizziness, fatigue, headache,* syncope, vertigo.
CV: chest pain, *hypotension.*
GI: abdominal pain, diarrhea, nausea, vomiting.
GU: decreased renal function.
Hematologic: *agranulocytosis, neutropenia, thrombocytopenia.*
Metabolic: *hyperkalemia.*
Respiratory: dry, persistent, tickling, nonproductive cough; dyspnea.
Skin: rash.
Other: *angioedema.*

Interactions

Drug-drug. *Diuretics:* May cause excessive reduction of blood pressure. Monitor patient.
Insulin, oral antidiabetics: May increase risk of hypoglycemia, especially at start of enalapril therapy. Monitor patient and glucose levels closely.
Lithium: May increase risk of lithium toxicity. Monitor lithium level.
NSAIDs: May reduce antihypertensive effect. Monitor blood pressure.
Potassium supplements, potassium-sparing diuretics: May increase risk of hyperkalemia. Avoid these drugs unless hypokalemic blood levels are confirmed.
Drug-herb. *Licorice:* May cause sodium retention and increase blood pressure, interfering with ACE inhibitor effects. Discourage licorice intake during drug therapy.
Drug-lifestyle. *Alcohol use:* May produce additive hypotensive effect. Discourage use together.
Sun exposure: May increase risk of photosensitivity reaction. Urge patient to avoid unprotected or prolonged sun exposure.

Effects on lab test results

- May increase ALT, AST, bilirubin, BUN, creatinine, and potassium levels. May decrease sodium and hemoglobin levels and hematocrit.
- May decrease neutrophil, granulocyte, and platelet counts.

Pharmacokinetics

Absorption: About 60% of P.O. dose absorbed from GI tract.
Distribution: Unknown.
Metabolism: Metabolized extensively to active metabolite.

Excretion: About 94% in urine and feces as enalaprilat and enalapril. *Half-life:* 35 to 38 hours.

Route	Onset	Peak	Duration
P.O.	1 hr	4–6 hr	24 hr
I.V.	15 min	1–4 hr	6 hr

Action

Chemical effect: May inhibit ACE, preventing conversion of angiotensin I to angiotensin II, a potent vasoconstrictor. Reduced formation of angiotensin II decreases peripheral arterial resistance, thus decreasing aldosterone secretion.
Therapeutic effect: Lowers blood pressure.

Available forms

Injection: 1.25 mg/ml
Tablets: 2.5 mg, 5 mg, 10 mg, 20 mg

NURSING PROCESS

Assessment

- Obtain history of patient's blood pressure before starting therapy, and reassess regularly.
- Monitor CBC with differential counts before therapy, every 2 weeks for first 3 months of therapy, and periodically thereafter.
- Monitor potassium intake and level.
- Be alert for adverse reactions and drug interactions.
- Assess patient's and family's knowledge of drug therapy.

Nursing diagnoses

- Risk for injury related to presence of hypertension
- Risk for infection related to drug-induced adverse hematologic reactions
- Deficient knowledge related to drug therapy

Planning and implementation

- If patient has hypotension after first dose, adjust dosage as long as patient is under medical supervision.
- If CBC becomes abnormal or evidence of infection arises, notify prescriber immediately.
- If angioedema (including laryngeal edema) occurs, notify prescriber and stop drug immediately. Institute appropriate therapy (epinephrine solution 1:1,000 [0.3 to 0.5 ml] subcutaneously), and take measures to ensure patent airway.

Patient teaching

- Advise patient to report evidence of angioedema, such as breathing difficulty and swelling of face, eyes, lips, or tongue.
- Instruct patient to report signs of infection, such as fever and sore throat.
- Advise patient that light-headedness can occur, especially during first few days of therapy. Tell patient to rise slowly to minimize this effect and to report symptoms to prescriber. If patient experiences syncope, tell him to stop taking drug and to call prescriber immediately.
- Tell patient to use caution in hot weather and during exercise. Inadequate fluid intake, vomiting, diarrhea, and excessive perspiration can lead to light-headedness and syncope.
- Advise patient to avoid sodium substitutes; these products may contain potassium, which can cause hyperkalemia.
- Tell patient to notify prescriber if pregnancy occurs. Drug will probably need to be changed.

☑ Evaluation

- Patient's blood pressure becomes normal.
- Patient's CBC remains normal throughout therapy.
- Patient and family state understanding of drug therapy.

enfuvirtide
(ehn-FOO-ver-tighd)
Fuzeon

Pharmacologic class: fusion inhibitor
Therapeutic class: antiretroviral
Pregnancy risk category: B

Indications and dosages

▶ **HIV-1 infection, with other antiretrovirals, in patients with continued HIV-1 replication despite antiretroviral therapy.** *Adults:* 90 mg subcutaneously b.i.d., injected into the upper arm, anterior thigh, or abdomen.
Children ages 6 to 16: Give 2 mg/kg subcutaneously b.i.d.; maximum dose, 90 mg.

Contraindications and cautions

- Contraindicated in patients hypersensitive to drug or any of its components.
- ≋ **Lifespan:** In pregnant women, use only when benefits outweigh risks to the fetus.

Breast-feeding women should stop breast-feeding to prevent transmitting HIV to infants. In children younger than age 6, safety and effectiveness haven't been established.

Adverse reactions

CNS: anxiety, asthenia, depression, *insomnia,* peripheral neuropathy.
EENT: conjunctivitis, sinusitis, taste disturbance.
GI: abdominal pain, constipation, *diarrhea, nausea,* **pancreatitis.**
Hematologic: lymphadenopathy.
Metabolic: anorexia, weight decrease.
Musculoskeletal: myalgia.
Respiratory: *bacterial pneumonia,* cough.
Skin: *ecchymosis,* pruritus, skin papilloma.
Other: flulike illness, herpes simplex, influenza, *injection-site reactions.*

Interactions

None reported.

Effects on lab test results

- May increase triglyceride, amylase, lipase, ALT, AST, CK, and GGT levels. May decrease hemoglobin level and hematocrit.
- May decrease eosinophil count.

Pharmacokinetics

Absorption: Absorbed well after subcutaneous administration into arm, thigh, or abdomen.
Distribution: 92% protein-bound.
Metabolism: May undergo catabolism to its constituent amino acids; hydrolyzed to a metabolite detectable in plasma.
Excretion: Unknown. *Half-life:* 4 hours.

Route	Onset	Peak	Duration
SubQ	Unknown	4–8 hr	Unknown

Action

Chemical effect: Interferes with entry of HIV-1 into cells by inhibiting fusion of HIV-1 to cell membranes.
Therapeutic effect: Controls symptoms of HIV infection.

Available forms

Injection: 108-mg single-use vials (90 mg/ml after reconstitution)

NURSING PROCESS

⚡ Assessment

• Use drug only in patients who are HIV-positive.
• Assess patient for evidence of bacterial pneumonia.
• Observe injection site for local reaction.
• Assess patient's and family's knowledge of drug therapy.

⊕ Nursing diagnoses

• Risk for infection related to underlying condition
• Deficient knowledge related to drug therapy

▷ Planning and implementation

• Reconstitute vial with 1.1 ml sterile water for injection. Tap vial for 10 seconds, and then gently roll it between hands to prevent foaming. Let drug stand for up to 45 minutes to ensure reconstitution. Or gently roll vial between hands until product is completely dissolved. Then draw up correct dose and inject drug.
• If drug isn't used immediately after reconstitution, refrigerate in original vial and use within 24 hours. Don't inject drug until it's at room temperature.
• Store vials that haven't been reconstituted at room temperature.
• Vial is for single use; discard unused portion.
• Rotate injection sites. Don't inject into same site for two consecutive doses, and don't inject into moles, scar tissue, bruises, or the navel.
• Injection-site reactions (pain, discomfort, induration, erythema, pruritus, nodules, cysts, ecchymosis) are common and may require analgesics or rest.
• ⑤ ALERT: Monitor patient closely for bacterial pneumonia. Patients at high risk include those with a low initial CD4+ count or high initial viral load, those who use I.V. drugs or smoke, and those with a history of lung disease.
• Hypersensitivity may occur with the first dose or later doses. If symptoms occur, stop drug.
• Register pregnant women in the Antiretroviral Pregnancy Registry by phoning 1-800-258-4263.

Patient teaching
• Teach patient how to prepare and give drug and how to safely dispose of used needles and syringes.

• Tell patient to rotate injection sites and to watch for cellulitis or local infection.
• Urge patient to immediately report evidence of pneumonia, such as cough with fever, rapid breathing, or shortness of breath.
• Tell patient to stop taking drug and seek medical attention if evidence of hypersensitivity develops, such as rash, fever, nausea, vomiting, chills, rigors, and hypotension.
• Inform patient that drug doesn't cure HIV infection and that it must be taken with other antiretrovirals.
• Tell patient to inform prescriber if she's pregnant, plans to become pregnant, or is breast-feeding while taking this drug.
• Tell patient that drug may impair the ability to drive or operate machinery.

☑ Evaluation

• Patient is free from opportunistic infections.
• Patient and family state understanding of drug therapy.

HIGH ALERT!

enoxaparin sodium
(eh-NOKS-uh-pah-rin SOH-dee-um)
Lovenox

Pharmacologic class: low–molecular-weight heparin derivative
Therapeutic class: anticoagulant
Pregnancy risk category: B

Indications and dosages

▷ **To prevent deep vein thrombosis (DVT) following hip or knee replacement surgery.** *Adults:* 30 mg subcutaneously every 12 hours for 7 to 10 days. Initial dose given 12 to 24 hours after surgery, provided hemostasis has been established. Or, for hip replacement surgery, 40 mg subcutaneously once daily given initially 9 to 15 hours before surgery. May continue with 40 mg subcutaneously once daily or 30 mg subcutaneously every 12 hours for 3 weeks.
▷ **To prevent DVT following abdominal surgery.** *Adults:* 40 mg subcutaneously once daily for 7 to 10 days with initial dose given 2 hours before surgery.
▷ **To prevent ischemic complications of unstable angina and non–ST-segment elevation MI (NSTEMI).** *Adults:* 1 mg/kg subcutaneous-

ly every 12 hours for 2 to 8 days with oral aspirin therapy (100 to 325 mg daily).

▶ **Inpatient with acute DVT with or without pulmonary embolism.** *Adults:* 1 mg/kg subcutaneously every 12 hours. Or 1.5 mg/kg subcutaneously once daily (at same time every day) for 5 to 7 days until therapeutic oral anticoagulant effect (INR of 2 to 3) is achieved. Warfarin therapy usually starts within 72 hours of enoxaparin injection.

▶ **Outpatient with acute DVT and without pulmonary embolism.** *Adults:* 1 mg/kg subcutaneously every 12 hours for 5 to 7 days until INR of 2 to 3 is achieved. Warfarin therapy is usually started within 72 hours of the enoxaparin injection.

▶ **Immobile patients during an acute illness.** *Adults:* 40 mg subcutaneously given once daily for 6 to 11 days. Up to 14 days may be tolerated.

▪ **NEW INDICATION: Treatment of patients with acute ST-segment elevation myocardial infarction (STEMI).** *Adults younger than age 75:* Give 30 mg single I.V. bolus, plus 1 mg/kg subcutaneously followed by 1 mg/kg subcutaneously every 12 hours with daily aspirin. *Adults older than age 75:* 0.75 mg/kg subcutaneously every 12 hours.

◙ **Adjust-a-dose:** In patients with a creatinine clearance less than 30 ml/minute receiving drug as prophylaxis following abdominal surgery or hip or knee replacement surgery or during acute illness, decrease dosage to 30 mg subcutaneously daily. In patients with creatinine clearance less than 30 ml/minute receiving drug for acute DVT or prophylaxis of ischemic complications of unstable angina and NSTEMI, give 1 mg/kg subcutaneously daily.

In patient with acute STEMI and severe renal impairment, omit aspirin. If older than age 75 with severe renal impairment, give 1 mg/kg subcutaneously once daily, no bolus.

Contraindications and cautions

• Contraindicated in patients hypersensitive to drug or any of its components, to heparin, or to pork products; in those with active major bleeding or thrombocytopenia; and in those who have antiplatelet antibodies in presence of drug.
• In patients with prosthetic heart valves, don't give for thromboprophylaxis.
• Use cautiously in patients with postoperative indwelling epidural catheters and patients who have had epidural or spinal anesthesia. Epidural

and spinal hematomas may result in long-term or permanent paralysis. Also use cautiously in patients with a history of heparin-induced thrombocytopenia; in patients with conditions that increase their risk of hemorrhage (such as bacterial endocarditis); and in patients with congenital or acquired bleeding disorders, ulcer disease, angiodysplastic GI disease, hemorrhagic stroke, or recent spinal, eye, or brain surgery.

☀ **Lifespan:** In pregnant women, use cautiously, and only when benefits outweigh risks to fetus. In breast-feeding women, use cautiously because it's unknown if drug appears in breast milk. In children, safety and effectiveness haven't been established.

Adverse reactions

CNS: confusion, fever, pain.
CV: edema, peripheral edema.
GI: nausea.
Hematologic: anemia, *bleeding complications, hemorrhage, thrombocytopenia.*
Skin: ecchymosis; hematoma, irritation, pain, or erythema at injection site; rash; urticaria.
Other: *angioedema, anaphylaxis.*

Interactions

Drug-drug. *Anticoagulants, antiplatelet drugs, dipyridamole, NSAIDs, sulfinpyrazone:* May increase risk of bleeding. Don't use together.
Plicamycin, valproic acid: May cause hypoprothrombinemia and inhibit platelet aggregation. Monitor patient closely.

Effects on lab test results

• May increase ALT and AST levels. May decrease hemoglobin level and hematocrit.
• May decrease platelet count.

Pharmacokinetics

Absorption: Unknown.
Distribution: Unknown.
Metabolism: Unknown.
Excretion: Unknown. *Half-life:* 4½ hours.

Route	Onset	Peak	Duration
SubQ	Unknown	3–5 hr	< 12 hr

Action

Chemical effect: Accelerates formation of antithrombin IIIB–thrombin complex and deactivates thrombin, preventing conversion of fibrinogen to fibrin.

Therapeutic effect: Prevents pulmonary embolism and DVT.

Available forms

Ampules: 30 mg/0.3 ml
Syringes (prefilled, graduated): 60 mg/0.6 ml, 80 mg/0.8 ml, 100 mg/ml, 120 mg/0.8 ml, 150 mg/ml
Syringes (prefilled): 30 mg/0.3 ml, 40 mg/0.4 ml
Vial (multidose): 300 mg/3 ml (contains 15 mg/ml of benzyl alcohol)

NURSING PROCESS

☲ Assessment
• Obtain history of patient's coagulation parameters before starting therapy.
• Monitor drug's effectiveness by evaluating patient for evidence of pulmonary embolism or DVT.
• Monitor platelet counts regularly. Patient with normal coagulation doesn't require regular monitoring of PT, INR, or PTT.
• If patient has had spinal or epidural anesthesia, monitor neurologic condition often. If abnormalities are discovered, alert prescriber immediately.
• Be alert for adverse reactions and drug interactions.
• Assess patient's and family's knowledge of drug therapy.

⊕ Nursing diagnoses
• Risk for injury related to risk for pulmonary embolism or DVT after knee or hip replacement surgery
• Ineffective protection related to drug-induced bleeding complications
• Deficient knowledge related to drug therapy

▷ Planning and implementation
⊛ **ALERT:** To avoid drug loss, don't expel air bubble from 30- or 40-mg prefilled syringes.
⊛ **ALERT:** Never give drug I.M.
• Don't massage after subcutaneous injection. Rotate sites among the left and right anterolateral and the left and right posterolateral abdominal walls.
⊛ **ALERT:** Drug can't be used interchangeably (unit for unit) with unfractionated heparin or other low–molecular-weight heparins.

• Avoid excessive I.M. injections of other drugs to prevent or minimize hematomas. Don't give I.M. injections when patient is anticoagulated.
• To treat severe overdose, give protamine sulfate (a heparin antagonist) by slow I.V. infusion at concentration of 1% to equal dosage of enoxaparin injected.

Patient teaching
• Instruct patient and family to watch for signs of bleeding and to notify prescriber at once.
• Tell patient to avoid OTC drugs that contain aspirin or other salicylates.
• Tell pregnant women and women of childbearing potential about the potential hazard to fetus and mother if drug is used during pregnancy.

✓ Evaluation
• Patient doesn't develop pulmonary embolism or DVT.
• Patient has no bleeding complications during therapy.
• Patient and family state understanding of drug therapy.

entacapone
(en-TAK-uh-pohn)
Comtan

Pharmacologic class: COMT inhibitor
Therapeutic class: antiparkinsonian
Pregnancy risk category: C

Indications and dosages

▶ **Adjunct to levodopa and carbidopa in idiopathic Parkinson disease in patients who experience end-of-dose wearing-off.** *Adults:* 200 mg P.O. with each dose of levodopa and carbidopa up to eight times daily. Maximum, 1,600 mg daily. Reducing daily levodopa dose or extending interval between doses may optimize patient's response.

Contraindications and cautions
• Contraindicated in patients hypersensitive to the drug or any of its components.
• Use cautiously in patients with hepatic impairment, biliary obstruction, or orthostatic hypotension.
☀ **Lifespan:** In pregnant women, use drug only when benefits outweigh risks to the fetus. In

breast-feeding women, use cautiously because it's unknown if the drug appears in breast milk.

Adverse reactions

CNS: agitation, anxiety, asthenia, dizziness, *dyskinesia,* fatigue, hallucinations, *hyperkinesia,* hypokinesia, somnolence.
GI: abdominal pain, constipation, *diarrhea,* dry mouth, dyspepsia, flatulence, gastritis, *nausea,* taste perversion, vomiting.
GU: urine discoloration.
Hematologic: purpura.
Musculoskeletal: back pain, *rhabdomyolysis.*
Respiratory: dyspnea.
Skin: sweating.
Other: bacterial infection.

Interactions

Drug-drug. *Ampicillin, chloramphenicol, cholestyramine, erythromycin, probenecid, rifampin:* May block biliary excretion, resulting in higher levels of entacapone. Use cautiously.
CNS depressants: May have additive effects. Use cautiously.
Drugs metabolized by COMT, such as bitolterol, dobutamine, dopamine, epinephrine, isoetharine, isoproterenol, and norepinephrine: May increase levels of these drugs, which may increase heart rate, change blood pressure, or cause arrhythmias. Use cautiously.
Nonselective MAO inhibitors, such as phenelzine and tranylcypromine: May inhibit normal catecholamine metabolism. Don't use together.
Drug-lifestyle. *Alcohol use:* May cause additive CNS effects. Discourage use together.

Effects on lab test results

None reported.

Pharmacokinetics

Absorption: Rapid, with level peaking in about 1 hour. Food doesn't affect absorption.
Distribution: About 98% protein-bound, mainly to albumin. Doesn't distribute widely into tissues.
Metabolism: Almost completely metabolized by glucuronidation before elimination.
Excretion: About 10% in urine; the remainder in bile and feces. *Half-life:* About 30 to 45 minutes for first phase and 2½ hours for second phase.

Route	Onset	Peak	Duration
P.O.	1 hr	1 hr	6 hr

Action

Chemical effect: A reversible inhibitor of peripheral COMT, which is responsible for elimination of various catecholamines, including dopamine. Blocking this pathway when giving levodopa and carbidopa may result in higher levels of levodopa, which allows greater dopaminergic stimulation in the CNS and leads to a greater effect on parkinsonian symptoms.
Therapeutic effect: Controls idiopathic Parkinson disease signs and symptoms.

Available forms

Tablets: 200 mg

NURSING PROCESS

Assessment

• Assess hepatic and biliary function before starting therapy.
• Monitor blood pressure closely. Watch for orthostatic hypotension.
• Monitor patient for hallucinations.
• Assess patient's and family's knowledge of drug therapy.

Nursing diagnoses

• Impaired physical mobility related to presence of parkinsonism
• Disturbed thought processes related to drug-induced adverse reactions
• Deficient knowledge related to drug therapy

Planning and implementation

• Use with levodopa and carbidopa. Drug isn't effective when given as monotherapy.
• Drug may be given with immediate- or sustained-release levodopa and carbidopa and may be taken with or without food.
• Decrease levodopa and carbidopa dose or increase interval to avoid adverse effects.
• Drug may cause or worsen dyskinesia despite reduction of levodopa dosage.
• Watch for diarrhea, which usually begins 4 to 12 weeks after therapy starts but may begin as early as the first week or as late as many months after therapy starts.
• Stopping drug abruptly or lowering dosage abruptly could lead to sudden worsening of Parkinson disease; it also may lead to hyper-

pyrexia and confusion, a symptom complex resembling neuroleptic malignant syndrome. Taper dose, and monitor patient closely. Adjust other antiparkinson drugs as needed.
• Assess patient for urine discoloration.
• Rarely, rhabdomyolysis may occur with drug use.

Patient teaching
• Instruct patient not to crush or break tablet and to take it at same time as levodopa and carbidopa.
• Warn patient to avoid hazardous activities until drug's CNS effects are known.
• Advise patient not to consume alcohol.
• Instruct patient to use caution when standing after a prolonged period of sitting or lying down because dizziness may occur. This effect is more common early in therapy.
• Warn patient that hallucinations, dyskinesia, nausea, diarrhea, and urine discoloration may occur.
• Inform patient that abruptly stopping drug therapy can cause sudden severe symptoms.
• Advise female patient to notify prescriber if she's pregnant or breast-feeding or if she plans to become pregnant.

☑ Evaluation
• Patient has improved physical mobility.
• Patient maintains normal thought process.
• Patient and family state understanding of drug therapy.

entecavir
(ehn-TECK-ah-veer)
Baraclude

Pharmacologic class: guanosine nucleoside analogue
Therapeutic class: antiviral
Pregnancy risk category: C

Indications and dosages

▶ **Chronic hepatitis B infection in patients with active viral replication and either persistently increased aminotransferase levels or histologically active disease.** *Adults and adolescents age 16 and older who have had no previous nucleoside treatment:* 0.5 mg P.O. once daily on an empty stomach.

Adults and adolescents age 16 and older who have a history of viremia and are taking lamivudine or have resistance mutations: 1 mg P.O. once daily on an empty stomach.

⬛ **Adjust-a-dose:** *Patients with no previous nucleoside treatment:* If creatinine clearance is 30 to 49 ml/minute, give 0.25 mg P.O. once daily. If clearance is 10 to 29 ml/minute, give 0.15 mg P.O. once daily. If clearance is less than 10 ml/minute or patient is undergoing hemodialysis or continuous ambulatory peritoneal dialysis, give 0.05 mg P.O. once daily.

Patients with lamivudine resistance: If creatinine clearance is 30 to 49 ml/minute, give 0.5 mg P.O. once daily. If clearance is 10 to 29 ml/minute, give 0.3 mg P.O. once daily. If clearance is less than 10 ml/minute or patient is undergoing hemodialysis or continuous ambulatory peritoneal dialysis, give 0.1 mg P.O. once daily.

Contraindications and cautions

• Contraindicated in patients hypersensitive to drug or its components.
• Use cautiously in patients with renal impairment and after liver transplantation.
• Lactic acidosis and severe hepatomegaly with steatosis, including fatal cases, have been reported with the use of nucleoside analogues alone and in combination with other antiretrovirals.
• Potential for development of HIV resistance to nucleoside reverse transcriptase inhibitors if used to treat chronic hepatitis B in patients coinfected with HIV who are not also receiving highly active antiretroviral therapy.
⚖ **Lifespan:** In pregnant women, use only when benefits outweigh risks to fetus. In breast-feeding women, avoid use; it's unknown if drug appears in breast milk. In patients younger than age 16, safety and effectiveness haven't been established. In elderly patients, adjust dosage for age-related decreases in renal function.

Adverse reactions

CNS: dizziness, fatigue, headache.
GI: diarrhea, dyspepsia, nausea.
GU: glycosuria, hematuria.
Hepatic: hepatomegaly with steatosis.
Other: *lactic acidosis.*

Interactions

Drug-drug. *Cyclosporine, tacrolimus:* May further decrease renal function. Monitor renal function carefully.

Drugs that reduce renal function or compete for active tubular secretion: May increase levels of either drug. Monitor renal function, and watch for adverse effects.

Drug-food. *Food:* May delay absorption and decrease drug level. Give drug on an empty stomach, at least 2 hours before or after a meal.

Effects on lab test results

• May increase ALT, amylase, AST, blood glucose, creatinine, lipase, and total bilirubin levels.
• May decrease platelet count.

Pharmacokinetics

Absorption: Absorbed through the GI tract. Food delays and decreases absorption.
Distribution: Extensive in tissues. 13% bound to plasma proteins.
Metabolism: Drug isn't a substrate, inhibitor, or inducer of the cytochrome P-450 enzyme system.
Excretion: By kidneys, 62% to 73% unchanged. *Half-life:* 128 to 149 hours.

Route	Onset	Peak	Duration
P.O.	Unknown	½–1½ hr	Unknown

Action

Chemical effect: Inhibits hepatitis B virus polymerase and reduces viral DNA levels.
Therapeutic effect: Reduces symptoms of hepatitis B infection.

Available forms

Oral solution: 0.05 mg/ml
Tablets: 0.5 mg, 1 mg

NURSING PROCESS

⚗ Assessment

• Assess patient's condition before therapy and regularly thereafter.
• Monitor renal and liver function tests during therapy.
⊛ **ALERT:** Hepatitis B may worsen severely after entecavir therapy stops.

• Monitor hepatic function for several months in patients who stop therapy. If appropriate, restart therapy for hepatitis B.
• Assess patient's and family's knowledge of drug therapy.

☺ Nursing diagnoses

• Risk for injury related to development of lactic acidosis and severe hepatomegaly with steatosis secondary to drug therapy
• Ineffective therapeutic regimen management secondary to long-term drug therapy
• Deficient knowledge related to drug therapy

▶ Planning and implementation

⊛ **ALERT:** The drug may cause life-threatening lactic acidosis and severe hepatomegaly with steatosis.

• Register pregnant women in the Antiretroviral Pregnancy Registry by phoning 1-800-258-4263.
• The optimal duration of treatment hasn't been established.
Patient teaching
• Tell patient that drug should be taken on an empty stomach at least 2 hours before or after a meal.
• Caution against mixing or diluting oral solution with any other substances. Teach proper use of spoon used to measure dose.
• Advise patient to report new adverse effects or new therapy with another drug.
• Explain that drug doesn't reduce the risk of transmitting hepatitis B virus to others.
• Teach patient the signs and symptoms of lactic acidosis, such as muscle pain, weakness, dyspnea, GI distress, cold extremities, dizziness, and fast or irregular heartbeat.
• Teach patient the signs and symptoms of hepatotoxicity, such as jaundice, dark urine, light-colored stool, loss of appetite, nausea, and lower stomach pain.
• Warn patient not to stop drug abruptly.

✓ Evaluation

• Patient remains free from lactic acidosis and severe hepatomegaly with steatosis during therapy.
• Patient maintains therapeutic regimen as shown by improvement of hepatitis B viral infection.
• Patient and family state understanding of drug therapy.

HIGH ALERT!

ephedrine sulfate
(eh-FED-rihn SUL-fayt)

Pharmacologic class: adrenergic
Therapeutic class: bronchodilator, vasopressor
Pregnancy risk category: C

Indications and dosages

▶ **Hypotension.** *Adults:* 25 to 50 mg I.M. or subcutaneously, or 10 to 25 mg I.V. infusion, or 5 to 25 mg by slow I.V. bolus injection, p.r.n., up to maximum of 150 mg/24 hours.
Children: 3 mg/kg or 100 mg/m² subcutaneously or I.V. daily in four to six divided doses.
▶ **Bronchodilation.** *Adults and children older than age 12:* Give 25 to 50 mg P.O. every 3 to 4 hours p.r.n. For use as a bronchodilator, 12.5 to 25 mg P.O. every 4 hours. Maximum, 150 mg in 24 hours.
Children ages 2 to 12: Give 2 to 3 mg/kg or 100 mg/m² P.O. daily in four to six divided doses.

▽ I.V. administration

• Drug is compatible with most common I.V. solutions.
• For vasopressor action, use I.V. route initially. Give slowly until systolic blood pressure is 30 to 40 mm Hg below patient's normal systolic pressure or 80 to 100 mm Hg.
⊗ **Incompatibilities**
Fructose 10% in normal saline solution; hydrocortisone sodium succinate; Ionosol B, D-CM, and D solutions; pentobarbital sodium; phenobarbital sodium; thiopental.

Contraindications and cautions

• Contraindicated in patients hypersensitive to drug, to any of its components, or to other sympathomimetic drugs; in those with porphyria, severe coronary artery disease, arrhythmias, angle-closure glaucoma, psychoneurosis, angina pectoris, substantial organic heart disease, or CV disease; and in those taking MAO inhibitors.
• Use cautiously in patients with hypertension, hyperthyroidism, nervous or excitable states, diabetes, or prostatic hyperplasia.
⚐ **Lifespan:** In pregnant women, children, and older men, use cautiously. In breast-feeding women, drug is contraindicated.

Adverse reactions

CNS: *confusion, delirium, dizziness, euphoria, headache, insomnia, nervousness.*
CV: hypertension, *palpitations,* precordial pain, *tachycardia.*
GI: *anorexia, nausea, vomiting.*
GU: painful urination from visceral sphincter spasm, *urine retention.*
Musculoskeletal: muscle weakness.
Skin: diaphoresis.

Interactions

Drug-drug. *Acetazolamide:* May increase ephedrine level. Monitor patient for toxicity.
Alpha blockers: Doesn't counteract beta blocker effects, resulting in hypotension. Monitor blood pressure.
Antihypertensives: May decrease effects. Monitor blood pressure.
Beta blockers: Doesn't counteract alpha-adrenergic effects, resulting in hypertension. Monitor blood pressure.
Digoxin, general anesthetics (halogenated hydrocarbons): May increase risk of ventricular arrhythmias. Monitor patient closely.
Ergot alkaloids: May enhance vasoconstrictor activity. Monitor patient closely.
Guanadrel, guanethidine: May enhance pressor effects of ephedrine. Monitor patient closely.
MAO inhibitors: When given with sympathomimetics, may cause hypertensive crisis. Don't use together.
Methyldopa, reserpine: May inhibit effects of ephedrine. Use together cautiously.
Phenelzine, tranylcypromine: May cause severe headache, hypertension, fever, and hypertensive crisis. Avoid use together.
Tricyclic antidepressants: May decrease pressor response. Monitor patient's blood pressure closely.

Effects on lab test results

None reported.

Pharmacokinetics

Absorption: Rapid and complete after P.O., I.M., or subcutaneous use; unknown after I.V. use.
Distribution: Widely distributed throughout body.
Metabolism: Slow, in liver.

Reactions may be *common*, uncommon, *life-threatening*, or COMMON AND LIFE-THREATENING.

Excretion: Unchanged in urine. Rate of excretion depends on urine pH. *Half-life:* 3 to 6 hours.

Route	Onset	Peak	Duration
P.O.	15–60 min	Unknown	3–5 hr
I.V.	≤ 5 min	Unknown	1 hr
I.M.	10–20 min	Unknown	1 hr
SubQ	Unknown	Unknown	1 hr

Action

Chemical effect: Stimulates alpha and beta receptors; direct- and indirect-acting sympathomimetic.

Therapeutic effect: Raises blood pressure and causes bronchodilation.

Available forms

Capsules: 25 mg†, 50 mg
Injection: 25 mg/ml, 50 mg/ml
Tablets: 30 mg†

NURSING PROCESS

Assessment

• Obtain history of patient's underlying condition before starting therapy, and reassess regularly.
• Be alert for adverse reactions and drug interactions.
• Assess patient's and family's knowledge of drug therapy.

Nursing diagnoses

• Ineffective health maintenance related to underlying condition
• Risk for deficient fluid volume related to drug-induced adverse GI reactions
• Deficient knowledge related to drug therapy

Planning and implementation

• Hypoxia, hypercapnia, and acidosis, which may reduce drug effectiveness or increase adverse reactions, must be identified and corrected before or during ephedrine administration for shock.
• Volume deficit must be corrected before giving vasopressors. This drug isn't a substitute for blood or fluid volume replenishment.
• To prevent insomnia, avoid giving within 2 hours of bedtime.
• When effectiveness decreases, notify prescriber. Effectiveness decreases after 2 to

3 weeks, as tolerance develops. Drug isn't addictive.

Patient teaching

• Warn patient not to take OTC drugs that contain ephedrine without consulting prescriber.
• Advise patient to notify prescriber if effectiveness decreases and to adjust dosage as instructed.
• Instruct patient to notify prescriber if adverse reactions occur.
• Caution patient not to perform hazardous activities if adverse CNS reactions occur.

☑ Evaluation

• Patient shows improvement in underlying condition.
• Patient maintains adequate hydration throughout therapy.
• Patient and family state understanding of drug therapy.

`HIGH ALERT!`

epinephrine hydrochloride
(eh-pih-NEF-rin high-droh-KLOR-ighd)
Adrenalin Chloride, Ana-Guard, EpiPen Auto-Injector, EpiPen Jr. Auto-Injector

Pharmacologic class: adrenergic
Therapeutic class: bronchodilator, vasopressor, cardiac stimulant, topical antihemorrhagic
Pregnancy risk category: C

Indications and dosages

▶ **Bronchospasm, hypersensitivity reactions, anaphylaxis.** *Adults:* 0.1 to 0.5 ml of 1:1,000 subcutaneously or I.M.; repeat every 10 to 15 minutes, p.r.n. Or 1 to 2.5 ml of 1:10,000 injection I.V. slowly over 5 to 10 minutes.
Children: 0.01 ml (10 mcg) of 1:1,000/kg subcutaneously; repeat every 20 minutes to 4 hours, p.r.n.
▶ **Hemostasis.** *Adults:* 1:50,000 to 1:1,000 applied topically.
▶ **Prolonging local anesthetic effect.** *Adults and children:* Mix 1:500,000 to 1:50,000 with local anesthetic.
▶ **Restoring cardiac rhythm in cardiac arrest.** *Adults:* 1 to 10 ml of 1:10,000 solution by slow I.V., every 3 to 5 minutes, p.r.n. Or 2 to 25 ml with 10 ml normal saline solution or D_5W for injection via endotracheal tube. If no I.V. route or intratracheal route is available, give

drug intracardiac. Intracardiac dose is 0.3 to 0.5 mg (1:10,000 solution). Up to 5 mg may be given, especially in patients who don't respond to usual I.V. dose. After initial I.V. bolus administration, drug may be infused I.V. at 1 to 4 mcg/minute.

Children: 10 mcg/kg I.V., or 5 to 10 mcg (0.05 to 0.1 ml of 1:10,000)/kg intracardiac.

▼ I.V. administration

• Dosages in emergencies are controversial; some prescribers may use higher than usual dosages for cardiac resuscitation.

• Use D₅W, normal saline injection, lactated Ringer's injection, or combinations of dextrose in sodium chloride. Mix just before use.

• Give 1:10,000 dilution prepared by diluting 1 ml of commercially available 1:1,000 injection with 10 ml of water for injection or normal saline injection.

• In emergency situations, drug may be injected slowly as a dilute solution or infused slowly I.V. Injection may be repeated in 5 to 10 minutes, as needed.

• Follow peripheral administration with a 20-ml flush, and elevate the site for 10 to 20 seconds to ensure delivery to the central circulation.

• Discard solution after 24 hours or if solution is discolored or contains precipitate. Keep solution in light-resistant container, and don't remove before use.

⊗ **Incompatibilities**
Aminophylline; ampicillin sodium; cephapirin; furosemide; Ionosol D-CM, PSL, and T solutions with D₅W; mephentermine. Rapidly destroyed by alkaline solutions or oxidizing drugs, including halogens, nitrates, nitrites, permanganates, sodium bicarbonate, and salts of easily reducible metals, such as iron, copper, and zinc.

Contraindications and cautions

• Contraindicated in patients with angle-closure glaucoma, shock (other than anaphylactic shock), organic brain damage, cardiac dilation, arrhythmias, coronary insufficiency, or cerebral arteriosclerosis. Also contraindicated in patients receiving general anesthesia with halogenated hydrocarbons or cyclopropane and in patients in labor (may delay second stage).

• Some commercial products contain sulfites and are contraindicated in patients with sulfite allergies except when drug is used for serious allergic reactions or in other emergency situations.

• In conjunction with local anesthetics, epinephrine is contraindicated for use in fingers, toes, ears, nose, or genitalia.

• Use cautiously in patients with long-standing bronchial asthma or emphysema who have developed degenerative heart disease and in those with hyperthyroidism, CV disease, hypertension, psychoneurosis, or diabetes.

⚕ **Lifespan:** In pregnant women in labor, drug is contraindicated. In pregnant women not in labor, in children, and in elderly patients, use cautiously. Breast-feeding women should stop breast-feeding or stop taking the drug.

Adverse reactions

CNS: agitation, anxiety, *cerebral hemorrhage,* cold limbs, diaphoresis, disorientation, *drowsiness,* euphoria, fear, *headache,* increased rigidity and tremors in patients with Parkinson disease, *nervousness, stroke, tremors,* vertigo, weakness.
CV: anginal pain, ECG changes, *hypertension, palpitations, shock,* tachycardia, *ventricular fibrillation,* widened pulse pressure.
GI: nausea, vomiting.
Metabolic: glycosuria, hyperglycemia.
Respiratory: dyspnea.
Skin: pain, urticaria.
Other: hemorrhage at injection site, pallor.

Interactions

Drug-drug. *Alpha blockers:* May cause hypotension from unopposed beta blocker effects. Monitor blood pressure.
Antihistamines, thyroid hormones: May cause severe adverse cardiac effects when given with sympathomimetics. Avoid giving together.
Carteolol, nadolol, penbutolol, pindolol, propranolol, timolol: May cause an initial hypertensive episode followed by bradycardia. Stop the beta blocker 3 days before anticipated epinephrine use. Monitor blood pressure.
Digoxin, general anesthetics (halogenated hydrocarbons): May increase risk of ventricular arrhythmias. Monitor patient closely.
Doxapram, methylphenidate: May increase CNS stimulation or pressor effects. Monitor patient closely.
Ergot alkaloids: May increase vasoconstrictor activity. Monitor patient closely.
Guanadrel, guanethidine: May increase pressor effects of epinephrine. Monitor the patient closely.

Reactions may be *common,* uncommon, *life-threatening,* or COMMON AND LIFE-THREATENING.

Levodopa: May increase risk of cardiac arrhythmias. Monitor patient closely.
MAO inhibitors: May increase risk of hypertensive crisis. Don't use together.
Methyldopa: May increase pressor effects. Monitor patient closely.
Oxytoxic drugs: May cause persistent hypertension. Don't use together.
Tricyclic antidepressants: May increase the pressor response and cause arrhythmias. Use cautiously.

Effects on lab test results

• May increase BUN, glucose, and lactic acid levels.

Pharmacokinetics

Absorption: Well absorbed after subcutaneous or I.M. injection.
Distribution: Wide, throughout body.
Metabolism: Metabolized at sympathetic nerve endings, liver, and other tissues to inactive metabolites.
Excretion: In urine. *Half-life:* Unknown.

Route	Onset	Peak	Duration
I.V.	Immediate	≤ 5 min	1–4 hr
I.M.	Varies	Unknown	1–4 hr
SubQ	6–15 min	≤ 30 min	1–4 hr

Action

Chemical effect: Stimulates alpha and beta receptors in sympathetic nervous system.
Therapeutic effect: Relaxes bronchial smooth muscle, causes cardiac stimulation, relieves allergic signs and symptoms, helps stop local bleeding, and decreases pain sensation.

Available forms

Injection: 0.01 mg/ml (1:100,000), 0.1 mg/ml (1:10,000), 0.5 mg/ml (1:2,000), 1 mg/ml (1:1,000)
Nebulizer inhaler: 1% (1:100), 2.25% (racepinephrine)†
Parenteral: 5 mg/ml (1:200) parenteral suspension

NURSING PROCESS

Assessment
• Obtain history of patient's underlying condition before starting therapy; reassess regularly.

• When giving drug I.V., monitor blood pressure, heart rate, and ECG when therapy starts and frequently thereafter.
• Be alert for adverse reactions and drug interactions.
• Assess patient's and family's knowledge of drug therapy.

Nursing diagnoses
• Ineffective health maintenance related to underlying condition
• Decreased cardiac output related to drug-induced adverse CV effects
• Deficient knowledge related to drug therapy

Planning and implementation
ALERT: 1 mg of epinephrine is equal to 1 ml of 1:1,000 or 10 ml of 1:10,000.
• Epinephrine is drug of choice in emergency treatment of anaphylactic reaction.
• Avoid I.M. injection of parenteral suspension into buttocks. Gas gangrene may occur because epinephrine reduces oxygen tension of tissues, encouraging growth of contaminating organisms.
• Massage site after I.M. injection to counteract vasoconstriction. Repeated local injection can cause necrosis, resulting from vasoconstriction at injection site.
• Giving drug on time is important.
• If adverse reactions develop, notify prescriber, and adjust dosage or stop the drug. If patient's pulse increases by 20% or more when drug is given, notify prescriber.
• If blood pressure rises sharply, rapid-acting vasodilators, such as nitrites or alpha blockers, can be given to counteract marked pressor effect of large doses of epinephrine.
Patient teaching
• Tell patient to take drug exactly as prescribed and to take it around the clock.
• Instruct patient who has acute hypersensitivity reactions, such as to bee stings, to self-inject epinephrine at home.
• Tell patient to reduce intake of foods containing caffeine, such as coffee, colas, and chocolates, when taking bronchodilator.
• Instruct patient to contact prescriber immediately if he experiences fluttering of heart, rapid beating of heart, shortness of breath, or chest pain.
• Tell patient to obtain approval from prescriber before taking OTC medicines or herbal remedies.

• Show patient how to check pulse. Instruct him to check pulse before and after using bronchodilator and to call prescriber if pulse rate increases by more than 20 beats/minute.

☑ **Evaluation**
• Patient shows improvement in underlying condition.
• Patient maintains adequate cardiac output throughout therapy.
• Patient and family state understanding of drug therapy.

HIGH ALERT!

epirubicin hydrochloride
(ep-uh-ROO-bih-sin high-droh-KLOR-ighd)
Ellence

Pharmacologic class: anthracycline
Therapeutic class: antineoplastic
Pregnancy risk category: D

Indications and dosages

▶ **Adjuvant therapy for breast cancer with lymphnode metastasis after resection.**
Adults: 100 to 120 mg/m² I.V. infusion over 3 to 20 minutes via a free-flowing I.V. solution on day 1 of each cycle every 3 to 4 weeks; or divided equally in two doses on days 1 and 8 of each cycle. Maximum cumulative (lifetime) dosage is 900 mg/m².

⚠ **Adjust-a-dose:** Dosage change after the first cycle is based on toxicity. If patient has a platelet count below 50,000/mm³, absolute neutrophil count (ANC) below 250/mm³, neutropenic fever, or grade 3 or 4 nonhematologic toxicity, give 75% of day 1 dose in later cycles. Delay day 1 therapy in later cycles until platelet count is 100,000/mm³ or above, ANC is 1,500/mm³ or above, and nonhematologic toxicities recover to grade 1.

For patients receiving divided doses (days 1 and 8), give 75% of the day 1 dose on day 8 if platelet count is 75,000 to 100,000/mm³ and ANC is 1,000 to 1,499/mm³. If day 8 platelet count is below 75,000/mm³, ANC is below 1,000/mm³, or grade 3 or 4 nonhematologic toxicity occurs, skip the day 8 dose.

In patients with bone marrow impairment, start dose at 75 to 90 mg/m². Reduce dosage in patients with hepatic or severe renal impairment.

▼ I.V. administration
• Drug is a vesicant. Never give I.M. or subcutaneously. Always give through free-flowing I.V. solution of normal saline solution or D₅W over 3 to 20 minutes. Infuse initial doses over 15 to 20 minutes.
• Give prophylactic antibiotic therapy with trimethoprim and sulfamethoxazole or a fluoroquinolone to patients receiving 120 mg/m² dose.
• Give antiemetics before giving drug to reduce nausea and vomiting.
• Avoid veins over joints and limbs with compromised venous or lymphatic drainage.
• If burning or stinging occurs, immediately stop infusion and restart in another vein.
• Facial flushing and local erythematous streaking along the vein may indicate too-rapid administration.
• Discard unused solution in vial 24 hours after vial is penetrated.
⊗ **Incompatibilities**
Fluorouracil, heparin, other I.V. drugs.

Contraindications and cautions
• Contraindicated in patients hypersensitive to drug or its components, other anthracyclines, or anthracenediones. Also contraindicated in patients with baseline neutrophil count below 1,500/mm³, those with severe myocardial insufficiency or recent MI, those previously treated with anthracyclines to total cumulative dosages, and those with severe hepatic dysfunction.
• Use cautiously in patients with active or dormant cardiac disease, previous or simultaneous radiotherapy to the mediastinal and pericardial area, or previous therapy with other anthracyclines or anthracenediones. Also use cautiously with other cardiotoxic drugs.
⚘ **Lifespan:** In pregnant and breast-feeding women, drug is contraindicated. In children, safety and effectiveness haven't been established. In elderly patients, especially women older than age 70, use cautiously because of greater chance of toxicity.

Adverse reactions
CNS: fever, *lethargy.*
CV: ***cardiomyopathy, heart failure.***
EENT: *conjunctivitis, keratitis.*
GI: anorexia, *diarrhea, mucositis, nausea, vomiting.*
GU: *amenorrhea.*

Hematologic: *anemia,* LEUKOPENIA, NEU-
TROPENIA, THROMBOCYTOPENIA.
Skin: *alopecia,* itch, rash, skin changes.
Other: *hot flushes, infection, local toxicity.*

Interactions

Drug-drug. *Calcium channel blockers, other
cardioactive compounds:* May increase risk of
heart failure. Monitor cardiac function closely.
Cimetidine: May increase epirubicin level (by
50%) and decrease clearance. Avoid use together.
Cytotoxic drugs: May result in additive toxicities
(especially hematologic and GI). Monitor patient
closely.
Radiation therapy: May enhance effects. Monitor patient carefully.

Effects on lab test results

• May decrease hemoglobin level and hematocrit.
• May decrease WBC, neutrophil, and platelet
counts.

Pharmacokinetics

Absorption: Given I.V.
Distribution: Rapid and widely distributed into
tissues. About 77% protein-bound, mainly to albumin. Appears to concentrate in RBCs.
Metabolism: Extensive and rapid.
Excretion: Mostly biliary. *Half-life:* 31 to
35 hours.

Route	Onset	Peak	Duration
I.V.	Unknown	Unknown	Unknown

Action

Chemical effect: The precise mechanism of
drug's cytotoxic effects isn't completely known.
It's thought to form a complex with DNA by intercalation between nucleotide base pairs, thereby inhibiting DNA, RNA, and protein synthesis,
resulting in cytocidal activity. Drug may also interfere with replication and transcription of DNA.
Therapeutic effect: Kills certain cancer cells.

Available forms

Injection: 2 mg/ml

NURSING PROCESS

Assessment
• Obtain baseline total bilirubin, AST, creatinine, and CBC (including ANC). Evaluate car-

diac function by obtaining an ECG and measuring left ventricular ejection fraction (LVEF) before therapy.
• Monitor LVEF regularly during therapy, and
stop drug at first sign of cardiac impairment.
Monitor patient for early signs of cardiac toxicity, including sinus tachycardia, ECG abnormalities, tachyarrhythmias, bradycardia, AV block,
and bundle branch block.
• Obtain total and differential WBC, RBC, and
platelet counts before and during each therapy
cycle.
• Assess patient's and family's knowledge of
drug therapy.

Nursing diagnoses
• Risk for injury related to drug-induced ad-
verse reactions
• Risk for infection related to myelosuppression
• Deficient knowledge related to drug therapy

Planning and implementation
• Give drug under supervision of a prescriber
experienced in the use of cancer chemotherapy.
• Wear protective clothing (goggles, gown, disposable gloves) when handling this drug. Pregnant health care providers shouldn't handle this
drug because of risks to fetus.
• Cardiac toxicity may occur 2 to 3 months after
stopping drug, causing reduced LVEF, evidence
of heart failure (tachycardia, dyspnea, pulmonary edema, dependent edema, hepatomegaly,
ascites, pleural effusion, and gallop rhythm).
Delayed cardiac toxicity depends on the cumulative dosage of epirubicin. Don't exceed a cumulative dose of 900 mg/m².
• Monitor uric acid, potassium, calcium phosphate, and creatinine levels immediately after
initial chemotherapy in patients susceptible to
tumor lysis syndrome. Hydration, urine alkalinization, and prophylaxis with allopurinol may
prevent hyperuricemia and minimize complications of tumor lysis syndrome.
• Lowest WBC count usually occurs 10 to
14 days after drug administration and returns to
normal by day 21.
• Anthracycline-induced leukemia may occur.
• Giving drug after previous radiation therapy
may induce an inflammatory cell reaction at the
site of irradiation.
⚠ **ALERT:** Don't confuse epirubicin with other
anthracyclines, such as daunorubicin, doxorubicin, or idarubicin.

Patient teaching

- Advise patient to report nausea, vomiting, stomatitis, dehydration, fever, evidence of infection, symptoms of heart failure (tachycardia, dyspnea, edema), or injection-site pain.
- Inform patient of the risk of cardiac damage and drug-related leukemia.
- Tell women of childbearing age not to become pregnant. Tell men to use effective contraception.
- Advise women that irreversible amenorrhea or premature menopause may occur.
- Advise patient about probable hair loss. Tell patient that hair usually regrows 2 to 3 months after therapy is stopped.
- Advise patient that urine may appear red 1 to 2 days after administration of the drug.

☑ Evaluation

- Patient sustains no injury from drug-induced adverse reactions.
- Patient remains free from infection.
- Patient and family state understanding of drug therapy.

eplerenone

(eh-PLAIR-eh-nown)
Inspra

Pharmacologic class: aldosterone receptor antagonist
Therapeutic class: antihypertensive
Pregnancy risk category: B

Indications and dosages

▶ **Heart failure post-MI.** *Adults:* Initially 25 mg P.O. daily or every other day. Increase to 50 mg P.O. daily if needed within 4 weeks, according to potassium level.

⧅ Adjust-a-dose: In patients with potassium level less than 5 mEq/L, increase dosage from 25 mg every other day to 25 mg daily, or increase dosage from 25 mg daily to 50 mg daily. For potassium level of 5 to 5.4 mEq/L, no dosage adjustment needed. For potassium level of 5.5 to 5.9 mEq/L, decrease dosage from 50 mg daily to 25 mg daily, or decrease dosage from 25 mg daily to 25 mg every other day; or if dosage was 25 mg every other day, withhold drug. For potassium level greater than 6 mEq/L, withhold drug. May restart drug at 25 mg every

other day when potassium level is less than 5.5 mEq/L.

▶ **Hypertension.** *Adults:* 50 mg P.O. once daily alone or with other antihypertensives. If response is inadequate after 4 weeks, increase dosage to 50 mg P.O. b.i.d. Maximum, 100 mg daily.

⧅ Adjust-a-dose: For either indication, patients who also take a weak CYP3A4 inhibitor (such as erythromycin, verapamil, or fluconazole) need a reduced starting dose of 25 mg P.O. daily.

Contraindications and cautions

- Contraindicated in patients with potassium level greater than 5.5 mEq/L at start of treatment, type 2 diabetes with microalbuminuria, creatinine level greater than 2 mg/dl in men or greater than 1.8 mg/dl in women, or creatinine clearance less than 30 ml/minute (less than 50 ml/minute if patient is being treated for high blood pressure). Also contraindicated in patients treated simultaneously with potassium supplements, potassium-sparing diuretics (amiloride, spironolactone, or triamterene), or strong CYP3A4 inhibitors, such as ketoconazole, itraconazole, clarithromycin, nefazodone, nelfinavir, and ritonavir.
- Use cautiously in patients with mild to moderate hepatic impairment.

⚒ **Lifespan:** In pregnant women, use only if benefits outweigh risks to fetus. In breast-feeding women, use cautiously because it's unknown whether drug appears in breast milk. In children, safety and effectiveness haven't been established.

Adverse reactions

CNS: dizziness, fatigue.
GI: abdominal pain, diarrhea.
GU: abnormal vaginal bleeding, albuminuria.
Metabolic: *hyperkalemia.*
Respiratory: cough.
Other: flulike symptoms, gynecomastia.

Interactions

Drug-drug. *ACE inhibitors, angiotensin II receptor antagonists:* May increase risk of hyperkalemia. Use together cautiously.
Lithium: May increase risk of lithium toxicity. Monitor lithium level.
NSAIDs: May reduce the antihypertensive effect and cause severe hyperkalemia in patients with

renal impairment. Monitor blood pressure and potassium level.

Potassium supplements, potassium-sparing diuretics (amiloride, spironolactone, triamterene): May increase risk of hyperkalemia and sometimes fatal arrhythmias. Avoid use together.

Strong CYP3A4 inhibitors (clarithromycin, itraconazole, ketoconazole, nefazodone, nelfinavir, ritonavir, troleandomycin): May increase eplerenone level. Avoid use together.

Weak CYP3A4 inhibitors (erythromycin, fluconazole, saquinavir, verapamil): May increase eplerenone level. Reduce eplerenone starting dose to 25 mg P.O. once daily.

Drug-herb. *St. John's wort:* May decrease eplerenone level over time. Discourage use together.

Effects on lab test results

• May increase potassium, creatinine, BUN, triglyceride, cholesterol, ALT, and GGT levels. May decrease sodium level.

Pharmacokinetics

Absorption: Bioavailability of drug is unknown.
Distribution: About 50% protein-bound.
Metabolism: Mainly by CYP3A4.
Excretion: Mainly in urine. *Half-life:* 4 to 6 hours.

Route	Onset	Peak	Duration
P.O.	Unknown	1½ hr	Unknown

Action

Chemical effect: Binds to mineralocorticoid receptors and blocks aldosterone. Aldosterone may increase blood pressure through induction of sodium reabsorption and other mechanisms.
Therapeutic effect: Lowers blood pressure.

Available forms

Tablets: 25 mg, 50 mg

NURSING PROCESS

Assessment

• Obtain history of patient's underlying condition before starting therapy.
• Obtain patient's baseline blood pressure and potassium levels and reassess regularly.
• Assess patient's and family's knowledge of drug therapy.

Nursing diagnoses

• Ineffective health maintenance related to hypertension
• Risk for injury related to the presence of hypertension
• Deficient knowledge related to drug therapy

Planning and implementation

• Drug may be used alone or with other antihypertensives.
• The drug's full therapeutic effect occurs within 4 weeks.
• Monitor patient for signs and symptoms of hyperkalemia.
• Overdose may cause hypotension and hyperkalemia. Treat symptoms and provide support. Drug binds extensively to charcoal but can't be removed by hemodialysis.

ALERT: Don't confuse Inspra (eplerenone) with Spiriva (tiotropium bromide).

Patient teaching
• Tell patient drug can be taken with or without food.
• Advise patient to avoid potassium supplements and salt substitutes.
• Tell patient to report adverse reactions.

Evaluation

• Patient's blood pressure remains within normal limits.
• Patient's potassium remains within normal limits.
• Patient and family state understanding of drug therapy.

HIGH ALERT!

epoetin alfa (erythropoietin)
(ee-POH-eh-tin AL-fah)
Epogen, Procrit

Pharmacologic class: glycoprotein
Therapeutic class: hematopoietic
Pregnancy risk category: C

Indications and dosages

▶ **Anemia caused by chronic renal disease.**
Adults: Starting dosage is 50 to 100 units/kg I.V. or subcutaneously three times weekly. Maintenance dosage is highly individualized.
Infants and children ages 1 month to 16 years who are on dialysis: 50 units/kg I.V. or subcutaneously three times weekly. Maintenance

dosage is highly individualized to keep hemoglobin level in target range.

🚫 **Adjust-a-dose:** When target hemoglobin level approaches 12 g/dl or if it rises more than 1 g/dl in any 2-week period, reduce dosage. If hemoglobin level doesn't increase by 2 g/dl after 8 weeks of therapy and is below the target range, increase dosage.

▶ **Anemia from zidovudine therapy in HIV-infected patients.** *Adults:* 100 units/kg I.V. or subcutaneously three times weekly for 8 weeks or until target hemoglobin level is reached. If response isn't satisfactory after 8 weeks, increase dosage by 50 to 100 units/kg I.V. or subcutaneously three times weekly. After 4 to 8 weeks, further increase dosage in increments of 50 to 100 units/kg three times weekly, up to a maximum of 300 units/kg three times weekly. *Infants and children ages 8 months to 17 years‡:* 50 to 400 units/kg subcutaneously or I.V. two to three times weekly.

▶ **Anemia from cancer chemotherapy.** *Adults:* 150 units/kg subcutaneously three times weekly for 8 weeks or until target hemoglobin level is reached. If response isn't satisfactory after 8 weeks, increase dosage up to 300 units/kg subcutaneously three times weekly. Or 40,000 units subcutaneously once weekly. If hemoglobin level hasn't increased by at least 1 g/dl in the absence of RBC transfusion, increase dose to 60,000 units subcutaneously weekly. *Infants and children ages 6 months to 18 years‡:* 25 to 300 units/kg subcutaneously or I.V. three to seven times weekly.

🚫 **Adjust-a-dose:** Give the lowest dose that will gradually increase hemoglobin to a level where blood transfusion isn't necessary.

Withhold drug if hemoglobin level exceeds 13 g/dl. Reduce dosage by 25% and resume therapy when hemoglobin level is less than 12 g/dl. If hemoglobin level increases by more than 1 g/dl in any 2-week period, reduce dosage by 25%.

▶ **To reduce need for allogenic blood transfusion in anemic patients undergoing elective, noncardiac, nonvascular surgery.** *Adults:* 300 units/kg subcutaneously once daily for 10 days before surgery, on the day of surgery, and for 4 days after surgery. Or 600 units/kg subcutaneously in once-weekly doses (21, 14, and 7 days before surgery), plus a fourth dose on day of surgery.

▶ **Anemia related to rheumatoid arthritis and rheumatic disease‡.** *Adults:* 50 to 200 units/kg subcutaneously three times weekly.
▶ **Anemia related to prematurity‡.** *Neonates:* 25 to 100 units/kg subcutaneously three times weekly.

▼ I.V. administration

• Don't shake.
• Give drug by direct injection without dilution.
• If patient is having dialysis, drug may be given into venous return line after dialysis session. To keep drug from adhering to tubing, inject drug with blood still in the line; then flush with normal saline solution.
⊗ **Incompatibilities**
Other I.V. drugs.

Contraindications and cautions

• Contraindicated in patients with uncontrolled hypertension and in patients with hypersensitivity to mammal-cell–derived products or albumin.

⚠ **Lifespan:** In pregnant women, use cautiously. In breast-feeding women, use cautiously because it's unknown if the drug appears in breast milk. In children younger than age 1 month, safety and effectiveness haven't been established.

Adverse reactions

CNS: asthenia, dizziness, fatigue, fever, headache, paresthesia, *seizures.*
CV: *edema, hypertension,* increased clotting of arteriovenous grafts.
GI: abdominal pain and constipation in children, diarrhea, nausea, vomiting.
Hematologic: iron deficiency, thrombocytosis.
Metabolic: *hyperkalemia,* hyperphosphatemia, hyperuricemia.
Musculoskeletal: *arthralgia.*
Respiratory: cough, shortness of breath.
Skin: rash, urticaria.
Other: injection-site reaction.

Interactions

None significant.

Effects on lab test results

• May increase BUN, creatinine, uric acid, potassium, phosphate, and hemoglobin levels and hematocrit.
• May increase platelet count.

Pharmacokinetics

Absorption: After subcutaneous use, systemic absorption is delayed, incomplete, and variable compared with I.V. use.
Distribution: Unknown.
Metabolism: Unknown.
Excretion: Unknown. *Half-life:* 4 to 13 hours.

Route	Onset	Peak	Duration
I.V.	1 wk	Immediate	Unknown
SubQ	1–6 wk	5–24 hr	Unknown

Action

Chemical effect: Mimics effects of erythropoietin, a naturally occurring hormone produced by the kidneys. It functions as both growth and differentiating factors, enhancing the rate of RBC production.
Therapeutic effect: Corrects anemia.

Available forms

Injection: 2,000 units/ml, 3,000 units/ml, 4,000 units/ml, 10,000 units/ml, 20,000 units/ml, 40,000 units/ml

NURSING PROCESS

⏱ Assessment

• Assess patient's CBC and blood pressure before starting therapy.
• Assess effectiveness by monitoring CBC results. Suggested target hemoglobin range is 10 to 12 g/dl. Hematocrit may rise and cause excessive clotting. Watch for evidence of blood clot formation, such as shortness of breath and cold, swollen, or pulseless limb.
⚠ **ALERT:** May increase the risk for serious CV events, including death, when given to a target hemoglobin greater than 12 g/dl. Monitor hemoglobin level closely. Hemoglobin shouldn't exceed 12 g/dl and the rate of hemoglobin increase shouldn't exceed 1 g/dl in 2 weeks.
• Patient's response depends on amount of endogenous erythropoietin. Patients with 500 units/L or more usually have transfusion-dependent anemia and probably won't respond to drug. Those with levels below 500 units/L usually respond well.
• Before and during therapy, monitor patient's iron level. Most patients need supplemental iron to support erythropoiesis.
• Monitor blood pressure closely. Up to 80% of patients with chronic renal impairment have hy-

pertension. Blood pressure may rise, especially when hematocrit is increasing in early part of therapy.
• After injection (usually within 2 hours), some patients complain of pain or discomfort in their long bones and pelvis and of coldness and sweating. Symptoms may persist for up to 12 hours and then disappear.
• If adverse GI reaction occurs, monitor patient's hydration.
• Assess patient's and family's knowledge of drug therapy.

🔆 Nursing diagnoses

• Ineffective protection related to reduced production of endogenous erythropoietin
• Risk for deficient fluid volume related to drug-induced adverse GI reactions
• Deficient knowledge related to drug therapy

▷ Planning and implementation

⚠ **ALERT:** Hemoglobin levels of 12 g/dl or greater achieved with erythropoiesis-stimulating agents is associated with increased risk of tumor growth and shortened survival in cancer patients, and CV events in patients with chronic kidney failure.
• When used in an HIV-infected patient, individualize the dosage based on response. Dosage recommendations are for patients with endogenous erythropoietin levels of 500 units/L or less and cumulative zidovudine doses of 4.2 g per week or less.
• Patient may need additional heparin to prevent clotting during dialysis.
• Start diet restrictions or drug therapy to control blood pressure.
Patient teaching
• Advise patient that blood specimens will be drawn weekly for blood counts and that dosage adjustments may be made based on results.
• Warn patient to avoid hazardous activities, such as driving or operating heavy machinery, early in therapy; excessively rapid rise in hematocrit may increase the risk of seizures.
• Tell patient to notify prescriber if adverse reactions occur.

✓ Evaluation

• Patient's blood count is normal.
• Patient maintains adequate hydration throughout therapy.
• Patient and family state understanding of drug therapy.

eprosartan mesylate

(eh-proh-SAR-ten MEH-sih-layt)

Teveten

Pharmacologic class: angiotensin II receptor antagonist

Therapeutic class: antihypertensive

Pregnancy risk category: C (D in second and third trimesters)

Indications and dosages

▶ **Hypertension.** *Adults:* Initially 600 mg P.O. daily. Daily dosage ranges from 400 to 800 mg given as single daily dose or two divided doses. Drug can be given alone or with other antihypertensives.

Contraindications and cautions

• Contraindicated in patients hypersensitive to drug or any of its components.

• Use cautiously in patients with an activated renin-angiotensin system, such as volume- or salt-depleted patients, and in patients whose renal function may depend on the activity of the renin-angiotensin-aldosterone system, such as patients with severe heart failure.

• Use cautiously in patients with renal artery stenosis.

⚕ **Lifespan:** In pregnant and breast-feeding women, drug is contraindicated. In children, safety and effectiveness haven't been established. In elderly patients, use cautiously because of decreased response to drug.

Adverse reactions

CNS: depression, dizziness, fatigue, headache.

CV: chest pain, dependent edema, hypertriglyceridemia.

EENT: pharyngitis, rhinitis, sinusitis.

GI: abdominal pain, diarrhea, dyspepsia.

GU: UTI.

Hematologic: *neutropenia.*

Musculoskeletal: arthralgia, myalgia.

Respiratory: bronchitis, cough, upper respiratory tract infection.

Other: injury, viral infection.

Interactions

None significant.

Effects on lab test results

• May increase BUN and triglyceride levels. May decrease hemoglobin level and hematocrit.

• May decrease neutrophil count.

Pharmacokinetics

Absorption: Absolute bioavailability of single oral dose is about 13%.

Distribution: About 98% protein-bound.

Metabolism: No active metabolites.

Excretion: Eliminated by biliary and renal excretion. *Half-life:* 5 to 9 hours.

Route	Onset	Peak	Duration
P.O.	1–2 hr	1–3 hr	24 hr

Action

Chemical effect: Blocks vasoconstrictor and aldosterone-secreting effects of angiotensin II by selectively blocking binding of angiotensin II to its receptor sites in many tissues, such as vascular smooth muscle and the adrenal gland.

Therapeutic effect: Lowers blood pressure.

Available forms

Tablets: 400 mg, 600 mg

NURSING PROCESS

Assessment

• Monitor blood pressure closely at start of therapy. If hypotension occurs, place patient in supine position and give normal saline solution I.V.

• Determine patient's fluid balance and sodium level before starting drug therapy.

• In elderly patients, watch for a slightly decreased response to drug.

• Be alert for adverse reactions.

• Assess patient's and family's knowledge of drug therapy.

Nursing diagnoses

• Risk for injury related to presence of hypertension

• Risk for infection related to neutropenia

• Deficient knowledge related to drug therapy

Planning and implementation

• Correct hypovolemia and hyponatremia before starting therapy to reduce risk of symptomatic hypotension.

• A transient episode of hypotension isn't cause for stopping therapy altogether. Restart once patient's blood pressure is stabilized.

• Drug may be used alone or with other antihypertensives, such as diuretics and calcium channel blockers. Maximum blood pressure response may take 2 to 3 weeks.

• Monitor patient for facial or lip swelling because angioedema has occurred with other angiotensin II antagonists.

Patient teaching

• Advise woman of childbearing age to use reliable contraception and to notify prescriber immediately if pregnancy is suspected. Drug will need to be stopped under medical supervision.

• Advise patient to report facial or lip swelling and signs and symptoms of infection, such as fever or sore throat.

• Tell patient to notify prescriber before taking OTC product to treat a dry cough.

• Inform patient that drug may be taken without regard to meals.

• Tell patient to store drug at a controlled room temperature (68° to 77° F [20° to 25° C]).

☑ Evaluation

• Patient's blood pressure is well controlled, and patient remains free of injury.

• WBC count is normal.

• Patient and family state understanding of drug therapy.

eptifibatide
(ep-tih-FIH-beh-tide)
Integrilin

Pharmacologic class: glycoprotein IIb/IIIa inhibitor
Therapeutic class: antiplatelet
Pregnancy risk category: B

Indications and dosages

▶ **Acute coronary syndrome (unstable angina or non–ST segment elevation MI) in patients with creatinine level below 2 mg/dl, being managed medically and in those undergoing percutaneous coronary intervention (PCI).** *Adults:* 180 mcg/kg I.V. bolus as soon as possible after diagnosis, followed by a continuous I.V. infusion of 2 mcg/kg per minute until hospital discharge or start of coronary artery by-

pass graft surgery, up to 72 hours. If undergoing PCI, continue infusion until hospital discharge, or for up to 18 to 24 hours after the procedure, whichever comes first, up to 96 hours. Give patients weighing more than 121 kg (267 lb) a maximum bolus of 22.6 mg followed by a maximum infusion rate of 15 mg/hour.

◻ Adjust-a-dose: For adults with creatinine clearance less than 50 ml/minute or a creatinine level between 2 and 4 mg/dl, give 180 mcg/kg I.V. bolus as soon as possible after diagnosis, followed by an infusion rate of 1 mcg/kg per minute. For patients weighing more than 121 kg (267 lb), the maximum bolus dose is 22.6 mg and the maximum infusion rate is 7.5 mg/hour.

▶ **Patients with creatinine level below 2 mg/dl, undergoing PCI.** *Adults:* 180 mcg/kg I.V. bolus given immediately before the procedure, immediately followed by an infusion of 2 mcg/kg/minute and a second I.V. bolus of 180 mcg/kg given 10 minutes after the first bolus. Continue infusion until hospital discharge or for up to 18 to 24 hours, whichever comes first; infuse for a minimum of 12 hours. Give patients weighing more than 121 kg a maximum bolus of 22.6 mg followed by a maximum of 15 mg/hour.

◻ Adjust-a-dose: For adults with creatinine clearance less than 50 ml/minute or a creatinine level between 2 and 4 mg/dl, give 180 mcg/kg immediately before the procedure, immediately followed by an infusion of 1 mcg/kg per minute and a second bolus of 180 mcg/kg given 10 minutes after the first bolus. Give patients weighing more than 121 kg a maximum of 22.6 mg/bolus followed by a maximum rate of 7.5 mg/hour.

▼ I.V. administration

• Drug is intended for use with heparin and aspirin.

• Inspect solution for particulate matter before use. If particles are visible, sterility is suspect. Discard the solution.

• Drug may be given in same I.V. line with normal saline solution or normal saline and 5% dextrose; main infusion may also contain up to 60 mEq/L of potassium chloride.

• Drug may be given in same I.V. line as alteplase, atropine, dobutamine, heparin, lidocaine, meperidine, metoprolol, midazolam, morphine, nitroglycerin, or verapamil.

• When obtaining I.V. access, avoid use of noncompressible sites (such as subclavian or jugular veins).
• Withdraw bolus dose from 10-ml vial into a syringe and give by I.V. push over 1 to 2 minutes. Give I.V. infusion undiluted directly from 100-ml vial using an infusion pump.
• If patient needs thrombolytic therapy, stop infusion.
• Refrigerate vials at 36° to 46° F (2° to 8° C). Protect from light until use. Discard any unused solution left in vial.

⊗ **Incompatibilities**
Furosemide.

Contraindications and cautions

• Contraindicated in patients hypersensitive to drug or its components and in those with a history of bleeding diathesis, evidence of active abnormal bleeding within previous 30 days, severe hypertension (systolic blood pressure over 200 mm Hg or diastolic blood pressure over 110 mm Hg) not adequately controlled with antihypertensives, major surgery within previous 6 weeks, history of stroke within 30 days, history of hemorrhagic stroke, current or planned use of another parenteral glycoprotein IIb/IIIa inhibitor, or platelet count below 100,000/mm³. Also contraindicated in patients whose creatinine level is 2 mg/dl or higher (for the 180-mcg/kg bolus and 2-mcg/kg/minute infusion) or 4 mg/dl or higher (for the 135-mcg/kg bolus and 0.5-mcg/kg/minute infusion) and in patients dependent on dialysis.
🜲 **Lifespan:** In pregnant women, use cautiously. In breast-feeding women, use cautiously because it's unknown if the drug appears in breast milk. In children, safety and effectiveness haven't been established.

Adverse reactions

CV: hypotension.
GU: hematuria.
Hematologic: BLEEDING, *thrombocytopenia.*
Other: bleeding at femoral artery access site.

Interactions

Drug-drug. *Clopidogrel, dipyridamole, NSAIDs, thrombolytics, ticlopidine, warfarin:* May increase risk of bleeding. Monitor patient closely.
Glycoprotein IIb/IIIa inhibitors: May increase risk of serious bleeding. Don't give together.

Effect on lab test results

• May decrease platelet count.

Pharmacokinetics

Absorption: Given I.V.
Distribution: 25% protein-bound.
Metabolism: None reported. No major metabolites are detected.
Excretion: 50% of drug is excreted in urine.
Half-life: 2½ hours.

Route	Onset	Peak	Duration
I.V.	Immediate	Immediate	4–6 hr after therapy

Action

Chemical effect: Reversibly binds to the glycoprotein IIb/IIIa receptor on human platelets and inhibits platelet aggregation.
Therapeutic effect: Prevents clot formation.

Available forms

Injection: 10-ml (2 mg/ml), 100-ml (0.75 mg/ml, 2 mg/ml) vials

NURSING PROCESS

📝 **Assessment**
• Obtain history of patient's underlying medical conditions, especially conditions that increase risk of bleeding.
• Obtain accurate patient weight. Use drug cautiously in patients weighing more than 143 kg (315 lb).
• Determine creatinine and hemoglobin levels, hematocrit, platelet count, PT, INR, and PTT before start of therapy and regularly thereafter.
• Monitor patient for bleeding.
• Assess patient's and family's knowledge of drug therapy.

🔷 **Nursing diagnoses**
• Ineffective cardiopulmonary tissue perfusion related to presence of acute coronary syndrome
• Risk for injury related to increased bleeding tendencies
• Deficient knowledge related to drug therapy

▶ **Planning and implementation**
• Stop this drug and heparin, and achieve sheath hemostasis by standard compressive techniques at least 4 hours before hospital discharge.

Reactions may be *common*, uncommon, *life-threatening*, or COMMON AND LIFE-THREATENING.

• In patients undergoing coronary artery bypass graft surgery, stop infusion before surgery.
• Minimize use of arterial and venous punctures, I.M. injections, urinary catheters, and nasotracheal and nasogastric tubes.
• If platelet count is less than 100,000/mm³, notify prescriber and stop both this drug and heparin.

Patient teaching
• Explain that drug is a blood thinner used to prevent heart attack.
• Explain that the benefits of the drug far outweigh the risk of serious bleeding.
• Instruct patient to report chest discomfort or other adverse events immediately.

☑ Evaluation
• Patient maintains adequate cardiopulmonary tissue perfusion.
• Patient has no life-threatening bleeding episode.
• Patient and family state understanding of drug therapy.

HIGH ALERT!

erlotinib
(ur-LOE-tih-nib)
Tarceva

Pharmacologic class: human epidermal growth factor receptor 1 (HER1)/epidermal growth factor receptor (EGFR)–tyrosine kinase inhibitor
Therapeutic class: antineoplastic
Pregnancy risk category: D

Indications and dosages

▶ **Locally advanced or metastatic non–small-cell lung cancer after failure of at least one other chemotherapeutic agent.** *Adults:* 150 mg P.O. once daily taken at least 1 hour before or 2 hours after meals. Continue until disease progresses or intolerable toxicity occurs.
▶ **First-line treatment of locally advanced, unresectable, or metastatic pancreatic cancer in combination with gemcitabine.** *Adults:* 100 mg P.O. once daily taken at least 1 hour before or 2 hours after meals. Continue until disease progression or intolerable toxicity occurs.
⊟ Adjust-a-dose: In patients with severe skin reactions or severe diarrhea refractory to loperamide, reduce dosage in 50-mg decrements or stop therapy.

Contraindications and cautions

• Use cautiously in patients with pulmonary disease or liver impairment and in those who have received or are receiving chemotherapy because it may worsen adverse pulmonary effects.
☀ Lifespan: In pregnant women, use only if benefits outweigh risks to fetus. If patient becomes pregnant during therapy, drug may harm fetus and increase risk of miscarriage. Women shouldn't breast-feed while taking this drug. In children, safety and effectiveness haven't been established.

Adverse reactions

CNS: *fatigue.*
EENT: *conjunctivitis, keratoconjuctivitis sicca.*
GI: abdominal pain, *anorexia, diarrhea, nausea,* stomatitis, *vomiting.*
Respiratory: cough, dyspnea, ***pulmonary toxicity.***
Skin: *acne, dry skin,* pruritus, *rash.*
Other: *infection.*

Interactions

Drug-drug. *Anticoagulants, such as warfarin:* May increase risk of bleeding. Monitor PT and INR.
Atazanavir, clarithromycin, indinavir, itraconazole, ketoconazole, nefazodone, nelfinavir, ritonavir, saquinavir, telithromycin, troleandomycin, voriconazole: May decrease erlotinib metabolism. Use together cautiously, and consider reducing erlotinib dosage.
Carbamazepine, phenobarbital, phenytoin, rifabutin, rifampicin: May increase erlotinib metabolism. Erlotinib dosage may need to be increased.
Drug-herb. *St. John's wort:* May increase erlotinib metabolism. Erlotinib dosage may need to be increased. Discourage use together.

Effects on lab test results

• May increase ALT, AST, and bilirubin levels.
• May increase PT and INR.

Pharmacokinetics

Absorption: About 60%.
Distribution: About 93% protein-bound to albumin and alpha₁-acid glycoprotein.

Metabolism: Mainly by CYP3A4 and partly by CYP1A2 and CYP1A1.
Excretion: 83% in feces. *Half-life:* 36 hours.

Route	Onset	Peak	Duration
P.O.	Unknown	4 hr	Unknown

Action

Chemical effect: Probably inhibits tyrosine kinase activity in EGFR, which is expressed on the surface of normal and cancer cells, and is particularly selective for HER1.
Therapeutic effect: Increases survival of patients with locally advanced or metastatic non–small-cell lung cancer.

Available forms

Tablets: 25 mg, 100 mg, 150 mg

NURSING PROCESS

Assessment

• Assess patient's underlying condition before therapy.
• Monitor liver function tests periodically during therapy. If values change dramatically, consider reducing dosage or stopping drug.
• Monitor patient for severe diarrhea, and give loperamide if needed.
• Assess patient's and family's knowledge of drug therapy.

Nursing diagnoses

• Ineffective health maintenance related to presence of neoplastic disease
• Risk for deficient fluid volume related to drug-induced adverse GI reactions
• Deficient knowledge related to drug therapy

Planning and implementation

• Rarely, serious interstitial lung disease may occur. If patient develops dyspnea, cough, or fever, withhold therapy. Stop drug if interstitial lung disease develops.
• Overdose may cause diarrhea, rash, and liver transaminase elevations. If overdose occurs, withhold drug and treat symptoms.
Patient teaching
• Tell woman of childbearing age to use contraception while taking drug and for 2 weeks afterward.
• Tell patient to immediately report new or worsened cough, shortness of breath, eye irrita-

tion, or severe or persistent diarrhea, nausea, anorexia, or vomiting.
• Instruct patient to take drug 1 hour before or 2 hours after food.
• Explain the likelihood of serious interactions with other drugs and herbal supplements and the need to tell prescriber about any change in drugs and supplements taken.

Evaluation

• Patient responds to drug therapy.
• Patient maintains adequate hydration.
• Patient and family state understanding of drug therapy.

ertapenem sodium
(ur-tah-PEN-uhm SOH-dee-um)
Invanz

Pharmacologic class: carbapenem
Therapeutic class: antibiotic
Pregnancy risk category: B

Indications and dosages

▶ **Complicated intra-abdominal infections caused by** *Escherichia coli, Clostridium clostridioforme, Eubacterium lentum, Peptostreptococcus,* **or** *Bacteroides fragilis, distasonis, ovatus, thetaiotaomicron,* **or** *uniformis.*
Adults and children age 13 and older: 1 g I.V. or I.M. once daily for 5 to 14 days.
Infants and children age 3 months to 12 years: 15 mg/kg I.V. every 12 hours for 5 to 14 days. Don't exceed 1 g daily.
▶ **Complicated skin and skin-structure infections, including diabetic foot infection without osteomyelitis, caused by** *Staphylococcus aureus* **(methicillin-susceptible strains),** *Streptococcus agalactiae, Streptococcus pyogenes, E. coli, Klebsiella pneumoniae, Proteus mirabilis, B. fragilis, Peptostreptococcus* **species,** *Porphyromonas asaccharolytica,* **or** *Prevotella bivia. Adults and children age 13 and older:* 1 g I.M. or I.V. over 30 minutes once daily for 7 to 14 days. Diabetic foot infection may need up to 28 days of treatment.
Infants and children age 3 months to 12 years: 15 mg/kg I.M. or I.V. over 30 minutes Every 12 hours for 7 to 14 days. Don't exceed 1 g daily.
▶ **Community-acquired pneumonia caused by** *Streptococcus pneumoniae* **(penicillin-**

susceptible strains), *Haemophilus influenzae* (beta-lactamase–negative strains), or *Moraxella catarrhalis. Adults and children age 13 and older:* 1 g I.V. or I.M. once daily for 10 to 14 days. If improvement occurs after at least 3 days of therapy, appropriate oral therapy may be used to complete the full course of therapy.

Infants and children age 3 months to 12 years: 15 mg/kg I.V. every 12 hours for 10 to 14 days. Don't exceed 1 g daily. If patient improves after at least 3 days of treatment, use appropriate oral therapy to complete the full course of treatment.

▶ **Complicated UTI, including pyelonephritis, caused by *E. coli* or *K. pneumoniae*.** *Adults and children age 13 and older:* 1 g I.V. or I.M. once daily for 10 to 14 days. If improvement occurs after at least 3 days, appropriate oral therapy may be used to complete the full course of therapy.

Infants and children age 3 months to 12 years: 15 mg/kg I.V. every 12 hours for 10 to 14 days. Don't exceed 1 g daily. If patient improves after at least 3 days of treatment, use appropriate oral therapy to complete the full course of treatment.

▶ **Acute pelvic infections, including postpartum endomyometritis, septic abortion, and postsurgical gynecologic infections caused by *S. agalactiae*, *E. coli*, *B. fragilis*, *Peptostreptococcus* species, or *P. bivia*.** *Adults and children age 13 and older:* 1 g I.V. or I.M. once daily for 3 to 10 days.

Infants and children age 3 months to 12 years: 15 mg/kg I.V. every 12 hours for 3 to 10 days. Don't exceed 1 g daily.

Adjust-a-dose: In adults, if creatinine clearance is 30 ml/minute or less, give 500 mg daily. Give supplemental dose of 150 mg after a hemodialysis session only in patients who receive a daily dose of 500 mg within 6 hours before hemodialysis. If drug is given 6 hours or more before hemodialysis, no supplemental dose is needed.

▼ I.V. administration

● Reconstitute the contents of a 1-g drug vial with 10 ml of water for injection, normal saline injection, or bacteriostatic water for injection. Don't use diluents containing dextrose. Shake well to dissolve, and immediately transfer contents of the reconstituted vial to 50 ml of normal saline injection.

● Infuse over 30 minutes. Complete the infusion within 6 hours of reconstitution.

● Don't store lyophilized powder above 77° F (25° C).

● Reconstituted solution, immediately diluted in normal saline injection, may be stored at room temperature and used within 6 hours or stored for 24 hours under refrigeration (41° F [5° C]) and used within 4 hours after removal from refrigeration. Don't freeze solutions of ertapenem.

⊗ **Incompatibilities**

Diluents containing dextrose (alpha-D-glucose), other I.V. drugs.

Contraindications and cautions

● Contraindicated in patients hypersensitive to the drug or any of its components or to other drugs in the same class; also contraindicated in patients who have had anaphylactic reactions to beta-lactams. I.M. use is contraindicated in patients hypersensitive to local anesthetics of the amide type. (Lidocaine hydrochloride is used as the diluent.)

● Use cautiously in patients with CNS disorders or compromised renal function because seizures may occur. Ertapenem sodium may be removed by hemodialysis, if needed.

⚖ **Lifespan:** In pregnant women, use only if benefits outweigh risks to the fetus. In breastfeeding women, drug appears in breast milk. In elderly patients with renal impairment, select dose carefully and monitor renal function.

Adverse reactions

CNS: altered mental status, anxiety, asthenia, dizziness, fatigue, fever, headache, insomnia, pain, *seizures.*

CV: chest pain, edema, hypertension, hypotension, swelling, tachycardia.

EENT: pharyngitis.

GI: abdominal distention, abdominal pain, acid regurgitation, constipation, *diarrhea,* dyspepsia, oral candidiasis, nausea, *pseudomembranous colitis, vomiting.*

GU: hematuria, renal dysfunction, urine retention, vaginitis.

Hematologic: anemia, coagulation abnormalities, eosinophilia, *leukopenia, neutropenia, thrombocytopenia,* thrombocytosis.

Hepatic: jaundice.

Metabolic: hyperglycemia, *hyperkalemia,* hypernatremia.

Musculoskeletal: leg pain.

Respiratory: cough, crackles, dyspnea, *respiratory distress,* rhonchi.

Skin: erythema, extravasation, infused vein complication (infusion site pain and redness, phlebitis, thrombophlebitis), pruritus, rash.
Other: chills, hypersensitivity reactions, *septicemia.*

Interactions

Drug-drug. *Probenecid:* May reduce renal clearance and increase half-life. Avoid use together.

Effects on lab test results

• May increase ALT, AST, alkaline phosphatase, BUN, creatinine, glucose, potassium, sodium, and bilirubin levels. May decrease albumin, sodium bicarbonate, and hemoglobin levels and hematocrit.
• May increase PT, PTT, eosinophil count, and urinary RBC and WBC counts. May decrease segmented neutrophil and WBC counts. May increase or decrease platelet count.

Pharmacokinetics

Absorption: Almost completely absorbed after I.M. use. Mean bioavailability of 90%.
Distribution: Highly protein-bound, mainly to albumin.
Metabolism: Doesn't inhibit metabolism mediated by any cytochrome P-450 isoforms. Stable against hydrolysis by a variety of betalactamases, including penicillinase, cephalosporinase, and extended-spectrum beta-lactamase. Hydrolyzed by metallo-beta-lactamases.
Excretion: Mainly by the kidneys. *Half-life:* 4 hours.

Route	Onset	Peak	Duration
I.V.	Immediate	30 min	24 hr
I.M.	Unknown	2 hr	24 hr

Action

Chemical effect: Inhibition of cell wall synthesis is mediated through ertapenem binding to penicillin-binding proteins.
Therapeutic effect: Kills susceptible bacteria.

Available forms

Injection: 1 g

NURSING PROCESS

Assessment
• Check for previous penicillin, cephalosporin, or other beta-lactam hypersensitivity.

• If giving I.M., check for hypersensitivity to local, amide-type anesthetics.
• Obtain specimens for culture and sensitivity testing before giving first dose. Therapy may start before results are available.
• Monitor renal, hepatic, and hematopoietic function during prolonged therapy.
• Be alert for adverse reactions, particularly diarrhea, seizures, and superinfection.
• Assess patient's and family's knowledge of drug therapy.

Nursing diagnoses
• Diarrhea related to drug-induced adverse reaction
• Ineffective health maintenance related to underlying infectious disease process
• Deficient knowledge related to anti-infective therapy

Planning and implementation
ALERT: Don't mix or infuse with other drugs.
• When giving I.M., reconstitute contents of a 1-g vial of drug with 3.2 ml of 1% lidocaine hydrochloride injection (without epinephrine). See prescribing information for lidocaine hydrochloride. Shake vial thoroughly to form solution. Immediately withdraw contents of the vial and give by deep I.M. injection into a large muscle, such as gluteal muscles or lateral part of the thigh. Use reconstituted I.M. solution within 1 hour of preparing. Don't give reconstituted solution I.V.
• Avoid inadvertent injection into a blood vessel during I.M. delivery.
• If diarrhea persists during therapy, stop drug and collect stool specimen for culture to rule out pseudomembranous colitis.
• Vomiting is more common in children than in adults.
• If allergic reaction occurs, stop drug immediately and give immediate treatment with airway management, epinephrine, oxygen, and I.V. steroids.
• Continue anticonvulsants in patients with known seizure disorders. If focal tremors, myoclonus, or seizures occur, evaluate patient neurologically and give anticonvulsants if not given before. Decrease or stop drug after reexamining dosage.
• Overdose may cause nausea, diarrhea, and dizziness. If an overdose occurs, stop drug and

---

Reactions may be common, *uncommon,* **life-threatening,** *or* **COMMON AND LIFE-THREATENING.**

treat supportively until drug has been eliminated from the body.

⊛ ALERT: Don't confuse Avinza with Invanz.

Patient teaching
• Inform patient of potential adverse reactions and urge him to notify prescriber immediately if they occur.
• Tell patient to alert prescriber if he develops diarrhea.

✓ Evaluation
• Patient tolerates and responds well to drug therapy.
• Patient doesn't develop colitis or any other adverse reactions from drug therapy.
• Patient and family state understanding of drug therapy.

erythromycin base
(eh-rith-roh-MIGH-sin bays)
Apo-Erythro, Eryc✐, Ery-Tab, Erythromycin Delayed-Release, Erythromycin Filmtabs, PCE Dispertab

erythromycin estolate

erythromycin ethylsuccinate
Apo-Erythro-ES ♦, E.E.S., E.E.S. Granules, EryPed, EryPed 200, EryPed 400

erythromycin lactobionate
Erythrocin Lactobionate

erythromycin stearate
Apo-Erythro-S ♦, Erythrocin Stearate

Pharmacologic class: macrolide
Therapeutic class: antibiotic
Pregnancy risk category: B

Indications and dosages

▶ **Acute pelvic inflammatory disease caused by *Neisseria gonorrhoeae*.** *Adults:* 500 mg erythromycin lactobionate I.V. every 6 hours for 3 days; then 250 mg erythromycin base, estolate, or stearate P.O. every 6 hours or 333 mg every 8 hours for 7 days. Or 400 mg ethylsuccinate P.O. every 6 hours for 7 days.

▶ **Endocarditis prophylaxis for dental procedures in patients allergic to penicillin.** *Adults:* Initially 800 mg ethylsuccinate or 1 g stearate

P.O. 1 hour before procedure; then 400 mg ethylsuccinate or 500 mg stearate P.O. 6 hours later.
Children: Initially 20 mg/kg ethylsuccinate or stearate P.O. 1 hour before procedure; then 10 mg/kg 6 hours later.

▶ **Intestinal amebiasis.** *Adults:* 250 mg erythromycin base, estolate, or stearate, or 400 mg ethylsuccinate, P.O. every 6 hours, or 333 mg erythromycin base every 8 hours, or 500 mg every 12 hours for 10 to 14 days.
Children: 30 to 50 mg/kg erythromycin base, estolate, ethylsuccinate, or stearate P.O. daily in divided doses every 6 hours for 10 to 14 days.

▶ **Mild to moderately severe respiratory tract, skin, and soft-tissue infections caused by sensitive *Streptococcus pyogenes, Bordetella pertussis, Corynebacterium diphtheriae, Diplococcus pneumoniae, Listeria monocytogenes,* or *Mycoplasma pneumoniae*.** *Adults:* 250 to 500 mg erythromycin base, estolate, or stearate P.O. every 6 hours; or 400 to 800 mg erythromycin ethylsuccinate P.O. every 6 hours; or 15 to 20 mg/kg I.V. daily as continuous infusion or in divided doses every 6 hours for 10 to 21 days, depending on severity and source of infection, until oral dosage can be taken.
Children: 20 to 50 mg/kg oral erythromycin salts P.O. daily in divided doses every 6 hours; or 15 to 20 mg/kg I.V. daily in divided doses every 4 to 6 hours.

▶ **Syphilis.** *Adults:* 500 mg erythromycin base, estolate, or stearate P.O. q.i.d. for 15 days.

▶ **Legionnaire's disease.** *Adults:* 1 to 4 g P.O. or I.V. daily in divided doses for 10 to 14 days.

▶ **Uncomplicated urethral, endocervical, or rectal infections when tetracyclines are contraindicated.** *Adults:* 500 mg erythromycin base, estolate, or stearate or 800 mg ethylsuccinate P.O. q.i.d. or 666 mg erythromycin base P.O. every 8 hours for at least 7 days.

▶ **Urogenital *Chlamydia trachomatis* infections during pregnancy.** *Adults:* 500 mg erythromycin base, estolate, or stearate P.O. q.i.d. or 666 mg every 8 hours for at least 7 days; or 250 mg erythromycin base, estolate, or stearate, or 333 mg every 8 hours, or 500 mg every 12 hours, or 400 mg ethylsuccinate P.O. q.i.d. for at least 14 days.

▶ **Conjunctivitis caused by *C. trachomatis* in neonates.** *Neonates:* 50 mg/kg P.O. daily in four divided doses for 14 days or longer.

▶ **Pneumonia of infancy caused by *C. trachomatis.*** *Infants:* 50 mg/kg P.O. daily in four divided doses for at least 2 but usually 3 weeks; a second course may be needed.

▶ **Early form of Lyme disease in persons allergic to penicillins and cephalosporins and for whom tetracyclines are contraindicated‡.** *Adults and children age 8 and older:* 250 to 500 mg erythromycin base P.O. t.i.d. or q.i.d. Or 30 to 40 mg/kg P.O. daily in divided doses for 10 to 30 days.

Children younger than age 8: Give 30 to 40 mg/kg erythromycin base P.O. daily in divided doses (not to exceed adult dose) for 10 to 30 days.

▶ **Early Lyme disease manifested as erythema migrans‡.** *Adults:* 500 mg erythromycin base P.O. q.i.d. for 14 to 21 days.

Children: 12.5 mg/kg erythromycin base P.O. q.i.d. (maximum, 500 mg/dose) for 14 to 21 days.

▶ **Diarrhea caused by *Campylobacter jejuni‡.*** *Adults:* 500 mg erythromycin base P.O. q.i.d. for 7 days.

▶ **Genital, inguinal, or anorectal lymphogranuloma venereum‡.** *Adults:* 500 mg erythromycin base P.O. q.i.d. for 21 days.

▶ **Chancroid caused by *Haemophilus ducreyi‡.*** *Adults:* 500 mg P.O. t.i.d. or q.i.d. for 7 days, until ulcers or lymph nodes are healed.

▶ **Tetanus caused by *Clostridium tetani‡.*** *Adults:* 500 mg P.O. every 6 hours for 10 days.

▶ **Granuloma inguinale‡.** *Adults:* 500 mg P.O. q.i.d. for at least 21 days.

▼ I.V. administration

● Prepare the initial solution by adding 10 ml sterile water for injection to the 500-mg vial or 20 ml diluent to the 1-g vial. All other diluents may cause precipitation. Use only preservative-free sterile water for injection. Dilute each 250 mg in at least 100 ml of normal saline solution, lactated Ringer's injection, or Normosol-R.
● Don't give by I.V. bolus.
● Infuse over 1 hour or by continuous infusion.

⊗ **Incompatibilities**
Ascorbic acid injection, colistimethate, dextrose 2.5% in half-strength Ringer's lactate, dextrose 5% in lactated Ringer's solution, dextrose 5% in normal saline solution, D₅W, dextrose 10% in water, floxacillin, furosemide, heparin sodium, linezolid, metoclopramide, dextrose 5% in Normosol-M, Ringer's injection, vitamin B complex with C. Don't give with other I.V. drugs.

Contraindications and cautions

● Contraindicated in patients hypersensitive to drug, any of its components, or other macrolides. Also contraindicated in patients taking pimozide. Erythromycin estolate is contraindicated in patients with hepatic disease.
● Use other erythromycin salts cautiously in patients with impaired liver function.
⚕ **Lifespan:** In pregnant women, use cautiously. In breast-feeding women, use cautiously because the drug appears in breast milk. The American Academy of Pediatrics considers erythromycin compatible with breast-feeding. In neonates, avoid I.V. drug because it may contain benzyl alcohol.

Adverse reactions

CNS: dizziness, fever, headache.
CV: venous irritation or thrombophlebitis after I.V. injection, *ventricular arrhythmias.*
EENT: hearing loss.
GI: abdominal pain and cramping, diarrhea, nausea, *pseudomembranous colitis,* vomiting.
Hepatic: cholestatic hepatitis.
Skin: eczema, rash, urticaria.
Other: *anaphylaxis,* overgrowth of nonsusceptible bacteria or fungi.

Interactions

Drug-drug. *Carbamazepine:* May increase carbamazepine level and risk of toxicity. Avoid use together.
Clindamycin, lincomycin: May be antagonistic. Don't use together.
Cyclosporine: May increase cyclosporine level. Monitor patient closely for toxicity.
Digoxin: May increase digoxin level. Monitor patient for digoxin toxicity.
Disopyramide: May increase disopyramide level; may result, in some cases, in arrhythmias and prolonged QT intervals. Monitor ECG.
Ergot alkaloids: May cause acute ergot toxicity. Monitor carefully.
HMG-CoA reductase inhibitors: May increase risk of myopathy and rhabdomyolysis. Avoid use together.
Midazolam, triazolam: May increase effects of these drugs. Monitor patient closely.

Reactions may be *common*, uncommon, *life-threatening*, or COMMON AND LIFE-THREATENING.

Oral anticoagulants: May increase anticoagulant effects. Monitor PT and INR closely; monitor patient for bleeding.

Strong CYP3A inhibitors (such as diltiazem or verapamil): May increase risk of life-threatening cardiac condition. Don't use together.

Tacrolimus: May increase tacrolimus level and risk of adverse reactions, such as nephrotoxicity. Use together cautiously.

Theophylline: May decrease erythromycin level and increase risk of theophylline toxicity. Use together cautiously.

Vinblastine: May increase risk of vinblastine toxicity. Use together cautiously.

Drug-herb. *Pill-bearing spurge:* May inhibit CYP3A enzymes and alter drug metabolism. Discourage use together.

Effects on lab test results

- May increase CK, AST, ALT, alkaline phosphatase, and bilirubin levels. May decrease bicarbonate level.
- May increase eosinophil, neutrophil, and platelet counts.
- May falsely elevate urinary catecholamines, 17-hydroxycorticosterone, and 17-ketosteroids. May interfere with colorimetric assays, resulting in falsely elevated AST and ALT levels.

Pharmacokinetics

Absorption: Most erythromycin salts are absorbed in duodenum. Because erythromycin base is acid-sensitive, it must be buffered or have enteric coating to prevent destruction by gastric acid. Acid salts and esters (estolate, ethylsuccinate, and stearate) aren't affected by gastric acidity; they're unaffected or may even be enhanced by food. Give erythromycin base and stearate preparations on empty stomach.

Distribution: Widely distributed in most body tissues and fluids except CSF, where it appears at low levels. About 80% of erythromycin base and 96% of erythromycin estolate are protein-bound.

Metabolism: Partially metabolized in liver.

Excretion: Mainly unchanged in bile. *Half-life:* About 1½ hours.

Route	Onset	Peak	Duration
P.O.	Unknown	1–4 hr	Unknown
I.V.	Immediate	Immediate	Unknown

Action

Chemical effect: Inhibits bacterial protein synthesis by binding to 50S subunit of ribosome.

Therapeutic effect: Inhibits bacterial growth.

Available forms

erythromycin base

Capsules (delayed-release): 250 mg

Tablets (enteric-coated): 250 mg, 333 mg, 500 mg

Tablets (filmtabs): 250 mg, 500 mg

erythromycin estolate

Capsules: 250 mg

Oral suspension: 125 mg/5 ml, 250 mg/5 ml

erythromycin ethylsuccinate

Oral suspension: 100 mg/2.5 ml, 200 mg/5 ml, 400 mg/5 ml

Powder for oral suspension: 200 mg/5 ml, 400 mg/5 ml

Tablets: 400 mg

erythromycin lactobionate

Injection: 500-mg, 1-g vials

erythromycin stearate

Tablets (film-coated): 250 mg, 500 mg

NURSING PROCESS

Assessment

- Obtain history of patient's infection before starting therapy, and reassess regularly.
- Obtain appropriate specimen for culture and sensitivity tests before starting therapy. Begin therapy pending test results.
- Be alert for adverse reactions and drug interactions.
- If adverse GI reaction occurs, monitor patient's hydration.
- Monitor liver function. Drug may increase levels of alkaline phosphatase, ALT, AST, and bilirubin. Erythromycin estolate (most frequently used of all forms of erythromycin) may cause serious hepatotoxicity in adults (reversible cholestatic jaundice). A patient who develops hepatotoxicity may react similarly to other erythromycin forms.
- If high doses given I.V., monitor patient for hearing loss.
- Assess patient's and family's knowledge of drug therapy.

Nursing diagnoses

- Risk for infection related to presence of susceptible bacteria

• Risk for deficient fluid volume related to potential for drug-induced adverse GI reactions
• Deficient knowledge related to drug therapy

Planning and implementation
⑤ **ALERT:** The American Heart Association no longer recommends using erythromycin to prevent bacterial endocarditis. However, practitioners who have successfully used the drug as prophylaxis in individual patients may continue to do so.
• When giving suspension, note concentration.
• For best absorption, give oral form with full glass of water 1 hour before or 2 hours after meals. Coated tablets may be taken with meals. Tell patient not to drink fruit juice with drug.
• Coated tablets or encapsulated pellets cause less GI upset; they may be more tolerable in patients who can't tolerate drug.
Patient teaching
• Tell patient how to take oral drug.
• Tell patient to take entire amount of drug exactly as prescribed, even after he feels better.
• Instruct patient to notify prescriber if adverse reaction occurs, especially nausea, abdominal pain, and fever.

✓ Evaluation
• Patient is free from infection.
• Patient maintains adequate hydration with therapy.
• Patient and family state understanding of drug therapy.

escitalopram oxalate
(es-sigh-TAL-uh-pram OCKS-uh-layt)
Lexapro✐

Pharmacologic class: SSRI
Therapeutic class: anxiolytic, antidepressant
Pregnancy risk category: C

Indications and dosages

▶ **Major depressive disorder; generalized anxiety disorder.** *Adults:* Initially 10 mg P.O. daily, increasing to 20 mg, if needed, after at least 1 week.
▶ **Panic disorder‡.** *Adults:* 10 mg P.O. daily.
🔲 **Adjust-a-dose:** For elderly patients and those with hepatic impairment, 10 mg P.O. daily initially and as maintenance dosage.

Contraindications and cautions

• Contraindicated in patients hypersensitive to drug or its components or to citalopram. Also contraindicated within 14 days of MAO inhibitor therapy.
• Use cautiously in patients with suicidal ideation, a history of mania, seizure disorders, or renal or hepatic impairment. Also use cautiously in patients with diseases that produce altered metabolism or hemodynamic responses.
⚖ **Lifespan:** In pregnant women, use drug only if the benefits to the woman outweigh the risks to the fetus. Breast-feeding women should stop breast-feeding or stop drug. Drug appears in breast milk. In children, safety and effectiveness haven't been established. In elderly patients, use cautiously because they may have greater sensitivity to drug.

Adverse reactions

CNS: abnormal dreams, dizziness, fatigue, fever, *headache,* impaired concentration, *insomnia,* irritability, lethargy, light-headedness, migraine, paresthesia, *somnolence,* tremor, vertigo.
CV: chest pain, flushing, hypertension, palpitations.
EENT: blurred vision, earache, rhinitis, sinusitis, tinnitus.
GI: abdominal pain, constipation, cramps, diarrhea, dry mouth, flatulence, gastroesophageal reflux, heartburn, increased or decreased appetite, indigestion, *nausea,* vomiting.
GU: anorgasmia, *ejaculation disorder,* impotence, menstrual cramps, urinary frequency, UTI.
Metabolic: weight gain or loss.
Musculoskeletal: arthralgia, extremity pain, muscle cramps, myalgia.
Respiratory: bronchitis, cough.
Skin: increased sweating, rash.
Other: decreased libido, flulike symptoms, toothache, yawning.

Interactions

Drug-drug. *Carbamazepine:* May increase escitalopram clearance caused by cytochrome P-450 induction. Monitor patient for expected antidepressant effect, and adjust dose if needed. *Cimetidine:* May increase escitalopram level. Monitor patient for adverse reactions to escitalopram.
Citalopram: May cause additive effects. Avoid use together.

CNS drugs: May cause additive effects. Use together cautiously.

Desipramine, other drugs metabolized by CYP2D6: May increase levels of these drugs. Use together cautiously.

Lithium: May enhance serotonergic effect of escitalopram. Use together cautiously, and monitor lithium level.

MAO inhibitors: May cause serious, sometimes fatal, reactions. Avoid using drug within 14 days of MAO inhibitor.

SNRIs and triptans: May increase serotonergic effects, leading to weakness, enhanced reflex response, and incoordination. Use these drugs together cautiously.

Tricyclic antidepressants: May increase antidepressant level. Use together cautiously. Monitor antidepressant level. Reduce antidepressant dosage if needed.

Drug-lifestyle. *Alcohol use:* May increase CNS effects. Discourage using together.

Effects on lab test results

None reported.

Pharmacokinetics

Absorption: Absolute bioavailability is 80%.
Distribution: About 56% protein-bound.
Metabolism: Extensive, mainly by CYP3A4 and CYP2C19 to inactive metabolites.
Excretion: About 8% unchanged in urine. *Half-life:* 27 to 32 hours.

Route	Onset	Peak	Duration
P.O.	Unknown	5 hr	Unknown

Action

Chemical effect: May increase serotonergic activity in the CNS by inhibiting neuronal reuptake of serotonin.
Therapeutic effect: Relieves depression and anxiety.

Available forms

Oral solution: 5 mg/5 ml
Tablets: 5 mg, 10 mg, 20 mg

NURSING PROCESS

Assessment
- Obtain history of patient's medical condition before starting therapy.
- Closely monitor patients at high risk of suicide.
- Assess patient for history of drug abuse, and observe for signs of misuse or abuse.
- Assess patient's and family's knowledge of drug therapy.

Nursing diagnoses
- Ineffective coping related to underlying condition
- Interrupted family processes related to underlying condition
- Deficient knowledge related to drug therapy

Planning and implementation
- In case of overdose, establish and maintain an airway, induce vomiting, and give activated charcoal. Closely observe and monitor vital signs and cardiac health, and maintain supportive care. Dialysis isn't effective, and no known antidote exists.

ALERT: May increase the risk of suicidal thinking and behavior in young adults ages 18 to 24 during the first 2 months of treatment. Monitor patient closely.

ALERT: Don't confuse Lexapro with Celexa or Loxitane.

Patient teaching
- Inform patient that symptoms will improve gradually over several weeks rather than immediately.
- Tell patient to continue taking drug as prescribed even though improvement may not occur for 1 to 4 weeks.
- Tell patient to use caution while driving or operating hazardous machinery because of drug's potential to impair judgment, thinking, and motor skills.
- Advise the patient and his family to report suicidal thinking and behavior to prescriber immediately.
- Advise patient to consult prescriber before taking other prescription or OTC drugs.
- Tell patient that drug may be taken in the morning or evening with or without food.
- Encourage patient to avoid alcohol while taking drug.
- Tell patient to notify prescriber if she's pregnant or breast-feeding.

Evaluation
- Patient can carry out activities vital to usual role performance.
- Patient doesn't experience interrupted family processes.

• Patient and family state understanding of drug therapy.

esmolol hydrochloride

(EZ-moh-lohl high-droh-KLOR-ighd)
Brevibloc

Pharmacologic class: beta blocker
Therapeutic class: antiarrhythmic
Pregnancy risk category: C

Indications and dosages

▶ **Supraventricular tachycardia; control of ventricular rate in patients with atrial fibrillation or flutter in perioperative, postoperative, or other emergent circumstances; noncompensatory sinus tachycardia when heart rate requires specific interventions.** *Adults:* Loading dose is 500 mcg/kg/minute by I.V. infusion over 1 minute, followed by 4-minute maintenance infusion of 50 mcg/kg/minute. If adequate response doesn't occur within 5 minutes, repeat loading dose and infuse 100 mcg/kg/minute for 4 minutes. Repeat loading dose and increase maintenance infusion stepwise, as needed. Maximum maintenance infusion for tachycardia is 200 mcg/kg/minute.

▶ **Management of perioperative and postoperative tachycardia or hypertension.** *Adults:* For perioperative therapy, 80 mg (about 1 mg/kg) I.V. bolus over 30 seconds, followed by 150 mcg/kg/minute I.V., if needed. Adjust infusion rate, p.r.n., to maximum of 300 mcg/kg/minute. Postoperative therapy is the same as for supraventricular tachycardia, although dosages adequate for control may be as high as 300 mcg/kg/minute.

▼ I.V. administration

• Don't give by I.V. push; use infusion-control device. The 10-mg/ml single-dose vial may be used without diluting, but injection concentrate (250 mg/ml) must be diluted to no more than 10 mg/ml before infusion. Remove 20 ml from 500 ml of D₅W, lactated Ringer's solution, or half-normal or normal saline solution, and add two ampules of drug.
• Don't give more than 200 mcg/kg/minute.
• When patient's heart rate becomes stable, replace drug with a longer-acting antiarrhythmic, such as propranolol, digoxin, or verapamil;

30 minutes after giving the first dose of a replacement, reduce infusion rate by 50%. Monitor patient response, and if pulse is controlled for 1 hour after giving second dose of replacement, stop infusion.
• If local reaction develops at infusion site, change to another site. Avoid using butterfly needles.
• Don't abruptly stop giving the drug because withdrawal effects may occur. If immediate withdrawal is needed, use caution.
• Drug is intended for short-term use, no longer than 48 hours.
• Watch for irritation and infiltration because extravasation may cause tissue damage or necrosis.

⊗ **Incompatibilities**
Diazepam, furosemide, procainamide, thiopental sodium, warfarin sodium, 5% sodium bicarbonate injection.

Contraindications and cautions

• Contraindicated in patients with sinus bradycardia, heart block greater than first-degree, cardiogenic shock, or overt heart failure.
• Use cautiously in patients with impaired kidney function, diabetes, or bronchospasm.
☀ **Lifespan:** In pregnant women, use cautiously. In breast-feeding women, use cautiously because it's unknown if the drug appears in breast milk. In children, safety and effectiveness haven't been established.

Adverse reactions

CNS: agitation, confusion, dizziness, fatigue, headache, somnolence.
CV: HYPOTENSION, peripheral ischemia.
EENT: nasal congestion.
GI: *nausea,* vomiting.
Respiratory: *bronchospasm,* dyspnea, wheezing.
Other: induration at infusion site, inflammation.

Interactions

Drug-drug. *Digoxin:* May increase digoxin level by 10% to 20%. Monitor digoxin level.
Morphine: May increase esmolol level. Adjust esmolol carefully.
Prazosin: May increase the risk of orthostatic hypotension in the early phases of use together. Assist patient to stand slowly until effects are known.

Reserpine, other catecholamine-depleting drugs: May cause additive bradycardia and hypotension. Adjust esmolol carefully.
Succinylcholine: Esmolol may prolong neuromuscular blockade. Monitor patient.
Verapamil: May increase the effects of both drugs. Monitor cardiac function closely, and decrease dosages if needed.

Effects on lab test results

• May increase LDH level. May decrease hemoglobin level.

Pharmacokinetics

Absorption: Given I.V.
Distribution: Rapid. 55% protein-bound.
Metabolism: Rapid.
Excretion: By kidneys as metabolites. *Half-life:* About 9 minutes.

Route	Onset	Peak	Duration
I.V.	Immediate	30 min	< 30 min

Action

Chemical effect: Decreases heart rate, myocardial contractility, and blood pressure.
Therapeutic effect: Restores normal sinus rhythm.

Available forms

Injection: 10 mg/ml, 250 mg/ml

NURSING PROCESS

🔲 Assessment

• Obtain history of patient's arrhythmias before starting therapy.
• Monitor ECG and blood pressure continuously during infusion. Up to 50% of patients develop hypotension. Monitor patient closely, especially if blood pressure was low before therapy.
• Be alert for adverse reactions and drug interactions.
• Assess patient's and family's knowledge of drug therapy.

🔲 Nursing diagnoses

• Decreased cardiac output related to presence of arrhythmias
• Ineffective cerebral tissue perfusion related to drug-induced hypotension
• Deficient knowledge related to drug therapy

🔲 Planning and implementation

• If patient develops severe dose-related hypotension, decrease dose or stop infusion and immediately notify prescriber. Hypotension will reverse within 30 minutes.
• If patient develops symptoms of heart failure (shortness of breath, night cough, swelling of the limbs), notify prescriber.
Patient teaching
• Inform patient of need for continuous ECG, blood pressure, and heart rate monitoring to assess effectiveness of drug and detect adverse reactions.

🔲 Evaluation

• Patient regains normal cardiac output with correction of arrhythmias.
• Patient's blood pressure remains normal throughout therapy.
• Patient and family state understanding of drug therapy.

esomeprazole magnesium
(ee-soh-MEP-rah-zohl mag-NEEZ-ee-uhm)
Nexium

esomeprazole sodium
Nexium I.V.

Pharmacologic class: proton pump inhibitor
Therapeutic class: antisecretory
Pregnancy risk category: B

Indications and dosages

▶ **Gastroesophageal reflux disease (GERD), healing of erosive esophagitis.** *Adults:* 20 or 40 mg P.O. daily for 4 to 8 weeks. If symptoms persist, use for an additional 4 to 8 weeks.
Children and adolescents ages 12 to 17: Give 20 or 40 mg P.O. once daily for up to 8 weeks.
▶ **Long-term maintenance of healing in erosive esophagitis.** *Adults:* 20 mg P.O. daily for no longer than 6 months.
▶ **Long-term treatment of pathological hypersecretory conditions, including Zollinger-Ellison syndrome.** *Adults:* 40 mg P.O. b.i.d. Adjust dosage based on patient response.
▶ **Eradication of *Helicobacter pylori* to reduce duodenal ulcer recurrence.** *Adults:* Combination triple therapy with esomeprazole magnesium 40 mg P.O. daily plus amoxicillin

1,000 mg P.O. b.i.d. and clarithromycin 500 mg P.O. b.i.d., all for 10 days.

▶ **Short-term treatment of GERD in patients with a history of erosive esophagitis who are unable to take drug orally.** *Adults:* 20 or 40 mg I.V. once daily by direct injection over 3 minutes or by I.V. infusion over 10 to 30 minutes for up to 10 days. Switch patient to oral therapy as soon as possible.

▶ **Reduction of risk of gastric ulcers in patients on continuous NSAID therapy.** *Adults:* 20 to 40 mg P.O. once daily for up to 6 months.

◙ **Adjust-a-dose:** For patients with severe hepatic impairment, maximum dosage is 20 mg P.O. daily.

▼ I.V. administration

• Reconstitute 20- or 40-mg vial with 5 ml of D_5W, normal saline solution, or lactated Ringer's injection, and give by I.V. bolus over 3 minutes. Or further dilute to a total volume of 50 ml and give I.V. over 10 to 30 minutes.
• Flush I.V. line with D_5W, normal saline solution, or lactated Ringer's injection before and after administration.
• Store reconstituted solution and admixture at room temperature. Use reconstituted solution within 12 hours. For admixture diluted with D_5W, give within 6 hours. If diluted with normal saline solution or lactated Ringer's injection, use within 12 hours.
⊗ **Incompatibilities**
Don't infuse with other I.V. drugs.

Contraindications and cautions

• Contraindicated in patients hypersensitive to any component of esomeprazole or omeprazole. Combination triple therapy for the eradication of *H. pylori* is contraindicated in patients hypersensitive to clarithromycin, macrolide antibiotics, amoxicillin, or penicillin.
• Use cautiously in patients with severe hepatic insufficiency.
🎍 **Lifespan:** In pregnant women, use only if benefits outweigh risks to the fetus. In breastfeeding women, use cautiously because it's unknown whether drug appears in breast milk. In children, safety and effectiveness haven't been established.

Adverse reactions

CNS: headache.

GI: abdominal pain, constipation, diarrhea, dry mouth, flatulence, nausea, vomiting.

Interactions

Drug-drug. *Amoxicillin, clarithromycin:* May increase esomeprazole level. Monitor patient for toxicity.
Diazepam: May decrease diazepam clearance and increase level of diazepam. Monitor patient for diazepam toxicity.
Digoxin, iron salts, ketoconazole: May interfere with drug absorption. Monitor patient closely.
Other drugs metabolized by CYP2C19: May alter esomeprazole clearance. Monitor patient closely, especially elderly patient or patient with hepatic insufficiency.
Warfarin: May prolong PT and INR causing abnormal bleeding. Monitor the patient and PT and INR carefully.
Drug-food. *Any food:* May reduce bioavailability. Advise patient to take drug 1 hour before eating.

Effects on lab test results

• May increase creatinine, uric acid, bilirubin, alkaline phosphatase, ALT, AST, potassium, sodium, thyroxine, thyroid-stimulating hormone, and hemoglobin levels and hematocrit.
• May increase WBC and platelet counts.

Pharmacokinetics

Absorption: The level following a 40-mg dose is three times higher than after a 20-mg dose. Repeated daily 40-mg doses yield systemic bioavailability of 90%; a single 40-mg dose yields 64%. Giving drug with food reduces mean level by 33% to 53%.
Distribution: About 97% protein-bound.
Metabolism: Extensive in the liver by CYP2C19 to form hydroxy and desmethyl metabolites. CYP2C19 exhibits polymorphism. About 3% of whites and 15% to 20% of Asians who lack CYP2C19 may have decreased levels. CYP3A4 metabolizes the remaining amount.
Excretion: About 80% excreted as inactive metabolites in urine. Systemic clearance of esomeprazole decreases with multiple doses.
Half-life: 1 to 1½ hours.

Route	Onset	Peak	Duration
P.O.	Unknown	1½ hr	13–17 hr
I.V.	Unknown	Unknown	Unknown

Reactions may be *common*, uncommon, *life-threatening*, or COMMON AND LIFE-THREATENING.

Action

Chemical effect: Suppresses gastric secretion through proton pump inhibition. Inhibits the H^+-K^+-ATPase pump in gastric parietal cells, thereby reducing gastric acidity by blocking the final step in acid production.
Therapeutic effect: Decreases gastric acid.

Available forms

Capsules (delayed-release containing enteric-coated pellets): 20 mg, 40 mg
Powder for injection: 20 mg, 40 mg in single-use vials

NURSING PROCESS

☑ Assessment

• Assess patient's condition before and during drug therapy. Patients with a history of gastric ulcers or those age 60 and older on continuous NSAID therapy have increased risk of gastric ulcers.
• Monitor liver function test results because drug is extensively metabolized by CYP2C19. In patients with hepatic insufficiency, drug increases liver function test values.
• Long-term therapy with omeprazole has caused atrophic gastritis. Be alert for adverse reactions.
• Assess patient's and family's knowledge of drug therapy.

✥ Nursing diagnoses

• Impaired tissue integrity related to underlying gastroesophageal condition
• Imbalanced nutrition: less than body requirements related to decreased oral intake due to underlying gastroesophageal disorder
• Deficient knowledge related to drug therapy

▷ Planning and implementation

• Give esomeprazole at least 1 hour before meals because food decreases the extent of absorption.
• Overdose may result in confusion, drowsiness, blurred vision, tachycardia, nausea, diaphoresis, dry mouth, and headache. Provide supportive care. Dialysis is not effective.
• Urge patient to avoid alcohol and foods that increase gastric secretions.
Patient teaching
• Tell patient to take drug exactly as prescribed and at least 1 hour before meals.

• If patient has trouble swallowing capsule, suggest that he open it, sprinkle contents into applesauce, and swallow applesauce immediately. Warn against crushing or chewing the drug pellets.
• Tell patient to report continued or worsened symptoms or any adverse reaction.

☑ Evaluation

• Patient responds positively to drug therapy.
• Patient can tolerate liquids and foods orally without any nausea or vomiting.
• Patient and family state understanding of drug therapy.

HIGH ALERT!

estazolam
(eh-STAZ-uh-lam)

Pharmacologic class: benzodiazepine
Therapeutic class: hypnotic
Pregnancy risk category: X
Controlled substance schedule: IV

Indications and dosages

▶ **Insomnia.** *Adults:* 1 mg P.O. at bedtime. Some patients may need 2 mg.
▧ **Adjust-a-dose:** For elderly patients, give 1 mg P.O. at bedtime; use higher doses cautiously. Frail, elderly, or debilitated patients may take 0.5 mg, but this low dose may be only marginally effective.

Contraindications and cautions

• Contraindicated in patients hypersensitive to drug or any of its components.
• Use cautiously in patients with hepatic, renal, or pulmonary disease; depression; or suicidal tendencies.
⚘ **Lifespan:** In pregnant or breast-feeding women, drug is contraindicated. In children, safety and effectiveness haven't been established. In elderly or debilitated patients, use cautiously; monitor for excessive sedation.

Adverse reactions

CNS: abnormal thinking, asthenia, daytime drowsiness, dizziness, fatigue, headache, hypokinesia, somnolence.
GI: abdominal pain, dyspepsia.
Musculoskeletal: back pain, stiffness.
Respiratory: cold symptoms, pharyngitis.

Interactions

Drug-drug. *Cimetidine, disulfiram, hormonal contraceptives, isoniazid:* May impair metabolism and clearance of benzodiazepines and prolong their half-life. Monitor patient for CNS depression.

CNS depressants, including antihistamines, benzodiazepines, opioid analgesics: May increase CNS depression. Avoid use together.

Digoxin, phenytoin: May increase levels of these drugs, resulting in toxicity. Monitor levels closely.

Fluconazole, itraconazole, ketoconazole, miconazole: May increase and prolong drug level, CNS depression, and psychomotor impairment. Don't use together.

Rifampin: May increase metabolism and clearance and decrease half-life. Watch for decreased effectiveness.

Theophylline: May act as a drug antagonist. Watch for decreased effectiveness.

Drug-herb. *Catnip, kava, lady's slipper, lemon balm, passionflower, sassafras, skullcap, valerian:* May enhance sedative effects. Discourage use together.

Drug-lifestyle. *Alcohol use:* May increase CNS and respiratory depression. Strongly discourage use together.

Smoking: May increase drug metabolism and clearance and decrease half-life. Monitor patient for decreased effectiveness.

Effects on lab test results

• May increase ALT and AST levels.

Pharmacokinetics

Absorption: Rapid and complete.
Distribution: 93% protein-bound.
Metabolism: Extensive.
Excretion: Metabolites excreted mainly in urine. *Half-life:* 10 to 24 hours.

Route	Onset	Peak	Duration
P.O.	Unknown	1–3 hr	Unknown

Action

Chemical effect: May act on limbic system and thalamus of CNS by binding to specific benzodiazepine receptors.
Therapeutic effect: Promotes sleep.

Available forms

Tablets: 1 mg, 2 mg

NURSING PROCESS

⚕ Assessment
• Obtain history of patient's sleep pattern before starting therapy, and reassess regularly.
• Monitor liver and kidney function and CBC periodically during long-term therapy.
• Be alert for adverse reactions and drug interactions.
• Watch for withdrawal symptoms. If drug is stopped suddenly, patients who have received 6 weeks of continuous therapy may experience withdrawal.
• Assess patient's and family's knowledge of drug therapy.

⊞ Nursing diagnoses
• Sleep deprivation related to underlying condition
• Risk for trauma related to drug-induced adverse CNS reactions
• Deficient knowledge related to drug therapy

▶ Planning and implementation
• Before leaving bedside, make sure patient has swallowed drug.
• Take precautions to prevent hoarding by depressed, suicidal, or drug-dependent patient, or patient who has history of drug abuse.

Patient teaching
• Tell patient not to increase drug dose on his own, but to inform prescriber if he thinks that drug is no longer effective.
• Warn patient to avoid hazardous activities that require mental alertness or physical coordination. For inpatient (particularly elderly patient), supervise walking and raise side rails.
• Warn patient that additive depressant effects can occur if alcohol is consumed while taking drug or within 24 hours afterward.
• If patient uses a hormonal contraceptive, recommend another birth-control method during therapy because drug may enhance contraceptive hormone metabolism and decrease its effect.

✓ Evaluation
• Patient can sleep.
• Patient's safety is maintained.
• Patient and family state understanding of drug therapy.

Reactions may be *common*, uncommon, *life-threatening*, or COMMON AND LIFE-THREATENING.

estradiol (oestradiol)

(eh-stray-DYE-ol)

Alora, Climara, Esclim, Estrace🖉, Estrace Vaginal Cream, Estraderm, Estradot ♦, Estring, Evamist, FemPatch, Gynodiol, Menostar, Oesclim ♦, Vivelle, Vivelle-Dot

estradiol acetate

Femring Vaginal Ring

estradiol cypionate

Depo-Estradiol

estradiol gel

EstroGel, Divigel

estradiol hemihydrate

Estrasorb, Vagifem

estradiol valerate (oestradiol valerate)

Delestrogen

Pharmacologic class: hormone
Therapeutic class: estrogen replacement, antineoplastic
Pregnancy risk category: X

Indications and dosages

▶ **Vasomotor symptoms, vulvar and vaginal atrophy, hypoestrogenism from hypogonadism, castration, or primary ovarian failure.** *Adults:* 1 to 2 mg estradiol P.O. daily in cycles of 21 days on and 7 days off or cycles of 5 days on and 2 days off. Or 0.025-mg daily Esclim transdermal system applied to a clean, dry area of the trunk twice weekly. Adjust dosage, if needed, after the first 2 or 3 weeks of therapy, then at 3 to 6 months, p.r.n. Or 1 Estraderm transdermal system delivering 0.05 mg/24 hours applied twice weekly. Or, the Vivelle transdermal system delivering either 0.05 mg/24 hours or 0.0375 mg/24 hours applied twice weekly. Or, the Climara system delivering 0.05 mg/24 hours or 0.1 mg/24 hours applied transdermally once weekly in cycles of 3 weeks on and 1 week off. Or, 1 to 5 mg estradiol cypionate I.M. every 3 to 4 weeks. Or 10 to 20 mg estradiol valerate I.M. every 4 weeks, p.r.n. Or Estrasorb topical emulsion delivering 0.05 mg estradiol/day: Ap-

ply contents of two 1.74-g foil pouches daily, using one pouch for each thigh and calf.

▶ **Atrophic vaginitis, kraurosis vulvae.** *Women:* 2 to 4 g estradiol intravaginal applications of cream daily for 1 to 2 weeks. When vaginal mucosa is restored, maintenance dosage of 1 g one to three times weekly in a cycle. Or 0.05 mg/24 hours Climara applied weekly in a cycle. Or 0.05 mg/24 hours Estraderm applied twice weekly in a cycle. Or 10 to 20 mg estradiol valerate I.M. every 4 weeks, p.r.n.

▶ **Palliative therapy for advanced, inoperable breast cancer.** *Men and postmenopausal women:* 10 mg estradiol P.O. t.i.d. for 3 months.

▶ **Palliative therapy for advanced inoperable prostate cancer.** *Men:* 1 to 2 mg estradiol P.O. t.i.d. Or 30 mg estradiol valerate I.M. every 1 to 2 weeks.

▶ **To prevent postmenopausal osteoporosis in high-risk patients for whom non-estrogen therapy is inappropriate.** *Women:* 0.025 mg daily Vivelle-Dot, or Alora, or 0.5 mg daily Estraderm applied to a clean, dry area of the trunk twice weekly. Or 0.025 mg daily Climara patch applied once weekly, continuously. Or 0.014 mg daily Menostar patch applied to clean, dry area of the lower abdomen once weekly.

▶ **Vasomotor symptoms.** *Women:* 0.05 mg daily Climara patch applied once weekly, continuously. Or, 0.25 mg, 0.5 mg, or 1 g Divigel applied daily to the right or left thigh. Or, one spray daily to inner surface of forearm. May increase to 2 or 3 sprays daily based on patient response.

▶ **Moderate to severe vasomotor symptoms and vulvar and vaginal atrophy unresponsive to vaginal products.** *Women:* 1.25 EstroGel applied to skin in thin layer, wrist to shoulder, once daily.

Contraindications and cautions

● Contraindicated in patients with thrombophlebitis, thromboembolic disorders, estrogen-dependent neoplasia, breast or reproductive organ cancer (except as palliative therapy), or undiagnosed abnormal genital bleeding. Also contraindicated in patients with history of thrombophlebitis or thromboembolic disorders linked to estrogen use (except as palliative therapy of breast and prostate cancer) and in patients with liver dysfunction or disease.
● Use cautiously in patients with cerebrovascular or coronary artery disease, asthma, bone dis-

eases, migraine, seizures, or cardiac or renal dysfunction and in women with strong family history of breast cancer or who have breast nodules, fibrocystic disease, or abnormal mammogram findings. Use the lowest effective dose.

• This drug hasn't been approved for prevention of cognitive disorders or memory loss.

🎐 **Lifespan:** In pregnant and breast-feeding women, drug is contraindicated. In children, use is contraindicated except in some adolescents with pubertal delay because of risk of early epiphyseal closure, breast enlargement, vaginal cornification or bleeding, and male pubertal abnormalities.

Adverse reactions

CNS: chorea, depression, *dizziness, headache, seizures.*
CV: edema, hypertension, ***thromboembolism,*** thrombophlebitis.
EENT: abdominal cramps, bloating, diarrhea, intolerance of contact lenses, worsening of myopia or astigmatism.
GI: constipation, *nausea, **pancreatitis,*** vomiting.
GU: altered cervical secretions, altered menstrual flow, amenorrhea, breakthrough bleeding, cervical erosion, dysmenorrhea, ***endometrial cancer,*** enlargement of uterine fibromas, impotence, testicular atrophy, vaginal candidiasis.
Hepatic: cholestatic jaundice, gallbladder disease, ***hepatic adenoma.***
Metabolic: hypercalcemia, hyperglycemia, hyperthyroidism, hypothyroidism, increased appetite, weight changes.
Respiratory: *upper respiratory infection.*
Skin: dermatitis, erythema nodosum, hair loss, melasma, pruritus, urticaria.
Other: abnormal Pap smear, ***breast cancer,*** *breast changes* (tenderness, enlargement, secretion), flulike symptoms, gynecomastia.

Interactions

Drug-drug. *Bromocriptine:* May cause amenorrhea, interfering with bromocriptine effects. Avoid use together.
Carbamazepine, phenobarbital, rifampin: May decrease estrogen effectiveness. Monitor patient closely.
Corticosteroids: May enhance effects. Monitor patient closely.

Cyclosporine: May increase risk of toxicity. Monitor cyclosporine levels often.
Dantrolene, other hepatotoxic drugs: May increase risk of hepatotoxicity. Monitor patient closely.
Hydantoins: May cause loss of seizure control and increase risk of breakthrough bleeding, spotting, and pregnancy. Monitor patient closely.
Itraconazole, ketoconazole, macrolides, ritonavir: May increase estrogen level. Watch for increased adverse effects.
Oral anticoagulants: May decrease anticoagulant effects; may need to adjust dosage. Monitor PT and INR.
Tamoxifen: May interfere with tamoxifen effectiveness. Avoid use together.
Thyroid hormones: May alter thyroxine and thyrotropin levels. Increase thyroid hormone dosage as needed.
Topiramate: May increase estrogen metabolism and decrease effectiveness. Monitor patient closely.
Drug-herb. *St. John's wort:* May decrease estrogen level. Monitor patient for decreased effectiveness and changes in bleeding patterns.
Drug-food. *Caffeine:* May increase caffeine level. Monitor effects.
Drug-lifestyle. *Smoking:* May increase risk of CV effects. If smoking continues, may need alternative therapy. Urge patient to stop smoking.

Effects on lab test results

• May increase total T_4, thyroid-binding globulin, triglyceride, and clotting factor VII, VIII, IX, and X levels.
• May increase PT and norepinephrine-induced platelet aggregation.

Pharmacokinetics

Absorption: Well absorbed but substantially inactivated by liver after P.O. use. Absorbed rapidly and lasts days after I.M. use. Readily absorbed into systemic circulation after transdermal use.
Distribution: Highest levels in fat. About 50% to 80% protein-bound.
Metabolism: Mainly in liver.
Excretion: Mainly through kidneys. *Half-life:* Unknown.

Reactions may be *common,* uncommon, ***life-threatening***, or **COMMON AND LIFE-THREATENING**.

Route	Onset	Peak	Duration
P.O., I.M., vaginal	Unknown	Unknown	Unknown
Transdermal			
Esclim	Unknown	27–30 hr	Unknown
Estrasorb	Immediate	Unknown	Unknown
Gel	Immediate	1 hr	24–36 hr

Action

Chemical effect: Increases synthesis of DNA, RNA, and protein and reduces release of follicle-stimulating hormone and luteinizing hormone from pituitary gland.
Therapeutic effect: Replaces estrogen in women and treats some male prostate and breast cancers.

Available forms

estradiol
Gel (individual-use packets): 0.25 mg, 0.5 mg, 1 g
Spray: 1.53 mg
Tablets (micronized): 0.5 mg, 1 mg, 1.5 mg, 2 mg
Transdermal gel: 0.06%
Transdermal patch: 0.014 mg/day, 0.025 mg/24 hours, 0.0375 mg/24 hours, 0.05 mg/24 hours, 0.06 mg/day, 0.075 mg/24 hours, 0.1 mg/24 hours
Vaginal cream (in nonliquefying base): 0.01%
Vaginal ring: 0.0075 mg/24 hours
estradiol acetate
Vaginal ring: 0.05 mg/24 hours, 0.1 mg/24 hours
estradiol cypionate
Injection (in oil): 5 mg/ml
estradiol gel
Topical emulsion: 4.35 mg
estradiol hemihydrate
Topical emulsion: 4.35 mg hemihydrate/1.74 g; 3.48 g emulsion delivers 0.05 mg estradiol/day
Vaginal tablets: 25 mcg
estradiol valerate
Injection (in oil): 10 mg/ml, 20 mg/ml, 40 mg/ml

NURSING PROCESS

Assessment
• Obtain history of patient's underlying condition before starting therapy, and reassess regularly.

• Make sure patient has thorough physical examination before starting estrogen therapy.
• Ask patient about allergies, especially to foods or plants. Estradiol is available as aqueous solution or as solution in peanut oil; estradiol cypionate, as solution in cottonseed oil or vegetable oil; estradiol valerate, as solution in castor oil, sesame oil, or vegetable oil.
• Patient receiving long-term therapy should have yearly gynecologic and physical examinations. Periodically monitor lipid level, blood pressure, body weight, and liver function.
• Assess patient's and family's knowledge of drug therapy.

Nursing diagnoses
• Ineffective health maintenance related to underlying condition
• Ineffective tissue perfusion (cerebral, peripheral, pulmonary, or myocardial) related to drug-induced thromboembolism
• Deficient knowledge related to drug therapy

Planning and implementation
• Give oral drug at mealtimes or at bedtime (for once-daily dose) to minimize nausea.
• To give as I.M. injection, make sure drug is well-dispersed in solution by rolling vial between palms. Inject deep into large muscle. Rotate injection sites to prevent muscle atrophy. Never give drug I.V.
• Apply transdermal patch to clean, dry, hairless, intact skin on abdomen or buttocks. Don't apply to breasts, waistline, or other areas where clothing can loosen patch. When applying, ensure good contact with skin, especially around edges, and hold in place with palm for about 10 seconds. Rotate application sites.
• Begin transdermal patch 1 week after withdrawal of oral therapy, or sooner if menopausal symptoms appear before end of week.
⚕ ALERT: Risk of MI, deep vein thrombosis, invasive breast cancer, pulmonary embolism, and stroke is increased in postmenopausal women ages 50 to 79 who are being treated with estrogen and progestin. Risk of dementia is increased in postmenopausal women age 65 or older.
• Apply Divigel to 5″ by 7″ area of the thigh; alternate right and left thigh to avoid skin irritation.
⚕ ALERT: EstroGel dries in 2 to 5 minutes. Avoid fire, flame, or smoking until gel is dry because gel contains alcohol.

• Because of risk of thromboembolism, stop therapy at least 1 month before procedures that increase risk of prolonged immobilization or thromboembolism, such as knee or hip surgery. If you suspect thromboembolism, withhold drug and notify prescriber.

⊛ **ALERT:** Estrogen preparations aren't interchangeable.

Patient teaching

• Inform patient about adverse effects of estrogen.

• Emphasize importance of regular physical examinations. In postmenopausal women, estrogen replacement therapy for longer than 5 years may increase risk of endometrial cancer. Tell patient that risk is reduced by using cyclic rather than continuous therapy and lowest dosages of estrogen. Drug probably doesn't increase risk of breast cancer.

• Teach patient how to use vaginal cream. Tell her to wash vaginal area with soap and water before applying. Tell her to apply drug at bedtime or to lie flat for 30 minutes after application to minimize drug loss.

• Warn patient to immediately report abdominal pain; pain, numbness, or stiffness in legs or buttocks; pressure or pain in chest; shortness of breath; severe headaches; visual disturbances, such as blind spots, flashing lights, or blurriness; vaginal bleeding or discharge; breast lumps; swelling of hands or feet; yellow skin or sclera; dark urine; and light-colored stools.

• Explain to patient receiving cyclic therapy for postmenopausal symptoms that, although withdrawal bleeding may occur during week off drug, fertility hasn't been restored. Pregnancy can't occur because she hasn't ovulated.

• Teach patient using Estrasorb topical emulsion to rub into thigh and calf until thoroughly absorbed, rub excess on hands into buttocks, and let dry before covering with clothing. Tell patient to wash hands thoroughly.

• Teach patient using transdermal gel (Estro-Gel) to apply in a thin layer on one arm and let dry before smoking, nearing flames, dressing, or letting someone touch that arm. Recommend bathing before application to maintain full dosage.

• Teach patient using Divigel to use entire contents of package to cover 5″ by 7″ area of thigh and to alternate use of right and left thigh. Wait for gel to dry before dressing and for 1 hour before bathing. Wash hands after application.

• Instruct patient that spray should be applied in the morning, starting near the elbow of the inner forearm. Allow to dry for about 2 minutes before covering. Don't wash area for at least 30 minutes. Tell patient not to apply to any other area.

• Tell diabetic patient to report elevated glucose test results so antidiabetic dosage can be adjusted.

• Teach woman how to perform routine breast self-examination.

☑ **Evaluation**

• Patient shows improvement in underlying condition.

• Patient has no thromboembolic event during therapy.

• Patient and family state understanding of drug therapy.

estradiol and norgestimate
(eh-stray-DYE-ol and nor-JESS-tih-mayt)
Prefest

estrogens, conjugated, and medroxyprogesterone
(ESS-troh-jenz, KAHN-jih-gayt-ed, and med-roks-ee-proh-JESS-ter-ohn)
Premphase, Prempro

Pharmacologic class: hormones
Therapeutic class: combined estrogen and progestin
Pregnancy risk category: X

Indications and dosages

▶ **Moderate to severe vasomotor symptoms and vulvar and vaginal atrophy caused by menopause; prevention of osteoporosis in women with an intact uterus.** *Women:* 1 mg estradiol (pink tablet) P.O. daily for 3 days; then 1 mg estradiol/0.09 mg norgestimate (white tablet) P.O. daily for 3 days (Prefest). Repeat cycle until blister card is empty. Or 0.625 mg/2.5 mg (Prempro) P.O. once daily; can increase to 0.625 mg/5 mg tablet if needed. Or 0.625 mg conjugated estrogens (maroon tablet) P.O. once daily on days 1 through 14 and 0.625 mg conjugated estrogen/5 mg medroxyprogesterone (light blue tablet) P.O. once daily (Premphase) on days 15 through 28.

Contraindications and cautions

• Contraindicated in patients hypersensitive to any component of drugs and in patients with cancer of the breast, estrogen-dependent neoplasia, undiagnosed abnormal vaginal bleeding, or active or previous thrombophlebitis or thromboembolic disorders. Hormone replacement therapy is contraindicated for cardiac disease prevention.

• Use cautiously in women who have had a hysterectomy, are overweight, or have abnormal lipid profiles, gallbladder disease, or impaired liver function.

⊛ **ALERT:** Don't use estrogens and progestins to prevent CV disease. The Women's Health Initiative study reported increased risks of MI, stroke, invasive breast cancer, pulmonary embolism, and deep vein thrombosis in postmenopausal women during 5 years of combination therapy. Because of these risks, give estrogens and progestins at the lowest effective dose and for the shortest duration.

⚛ **Lifespan:** In women who are or may be pregnant, drug is contraindicated.

Adverse reactions

CNS: depression, dizziness, fatigue, *headache, pain, seizures, stroke.*

CV: edema, *pulmonary embolism, MI, thromboembolism.*

EENT: intolerance of contact lenses, pharyngitis, sinusitis, worsening of myopia or astigmatism.

GI: abdominal pain, flatulence, *nausea,* weight changes.

GU: decreased libido, dysmenorrhea, *endometrial cancer,* vaginal bleeding, vaginitis.

Hepatic: gallbladder disease, *hepatic adenoma.*

Musculoskeletal: arthralgia, back pain, myalgia.

Respiratory: cough, upper respiratory tract infection.

Other: *breast cancer,* breast pain, flulike symptoms, tooth disorder, viral infection.

Interactions

Drug-drug. *Bromocriptine:* May cause amenorrhea, interfering with bromocriptine effects. Avoid use together.

Carbamazepine, phenobarbital, rifampin: May decrease effectiveness of estrogen therapy. Monitor patient closely.

Corticosteroids: May enhance effects. Monitor patient closely.

Cyclosporine: May increase risk of toxicity. Monitor cyclosporine level often.

Dantrolene, other hepatotoxic drugs: May increase risk of hepatotoxicity. Monitor patient closely.

Hydantoins: May cause loss of seizure control and increased risk of breakthrough bleeding, spotting, and pregnancy. Monitor patient closely.

Itraconazole, ketoconazole, macrolides, ritonavir: May increase estrogen level. Monitor patient for increased adverse effects.

Oral anticoagulants: May decrease anticoagulant effects. Dosage adjustments may be needed. Monitor PT and INR.

Tamoxifen: May interfere with tamoxifen effectiveness. Avoid use together.

Thyroid hormones: May alter thyroxine and thyrotropin levels. Increase thyroid hormone dosage as needed.

Topiramate: May increase estrogen metabolism and decrease effectiveness. Monitor patient closely.

Drug-herb. *St. John's wort:* May decrease estrogen level. Watch for decreased effectiveness and changes in bleeding patterns.

Drug-food. *Caffeine:* May increase caffeine level. Monitor effects.

Drug-lifestyle. *Smoking:* May increase risk of CV effects. If smoking continues, patient may need alternative therapy. Urge patient to stop smoking.

Effects on lab test results

• May increase glucose, calcium, thyroxine-binding globulin, LDL, triglyceride, total circulating corticosteroid and sex steroid, total plasma cortisol, fibrinogen, plasminogen antigen, and blood clotting factor VII, VIII, IX, and X levels. May decrease folate, metyrapone, HDL, and antithrombin III levels.

• May increase PT, PTT, platelet aggregation time, and platelet count. May decrease T_3 resin uptake, glucose tolerance, and cortisol secretion rate.

Pharmacokinetics

Absorption: Unknown.

Distribution: Wide. Highly protein-bound.

Metabolism: Mainly metabolized in the liver.

Excretion: Mainly in urine. *Half-life:* About 16 hours for estrogens and 8 to 9 hours for progestins in postmenopausal women.

Route	Onset	Peak	Duration
P.O.			
estrogens	Unknown	Varies	Unknown
progestins	Rapid	1–2 hr	Several days

Action

Chemical effect: Circulating estrogens modulate pituitary secretion of gonadotropins, luteinizing hormone, and follicle-stimulating hormone. Estrogen-replacement therapy reduces elevated levels of these hormones in postmenopausal women. Estrogens also contribute to the reduction of the rate of bone turnover. Progestins counter estrogenic effects by decreasing the number of nuclear estradiol receptors and suppressing epithelial DNA synthesis in endometrial tissue.

Therapeutic effect: Relieves menopausal vasomotor symptoms and vaginal dryness; reduces the severity of osteoporosis.

Available forms

Prefest
Blister card of 15 pink and 15 white tablets. Pink tablets are 1 mg estradiol; white tablets are 1 mg estradiol and 0.09 mg norgestimate.

Premphase
Dial pack of 14 maroon and 14 light blue tablets. Maroon tablets are 0.625 mg estrogen; light blue tablets are 0.625 mg estrogen and 5 mg medroxyprogesterone.

Prempro
Dial pack of 28 tablets, available in these doses: 0.3 mg estrogen and 1.5 mg medroxyprogesterone, 0.45 mg and 1.5 mg, 0.625 mg and 2.5 mg, 0.625 mg and 5 mg.

NURSING PROCESS

🗒 Assessment

• Obtain history of patient's underlying condition before therapy, and reassess regularly thereafter.
• Make sure patient has a thorough physical examination before starting drug therapy.
• Assess patient's risk of venous thromboembolism.
• Assess patient's risk of cancer because hormone replacement therapy may increase the risk of breast cancer in postmenopausal women.

• Be alert for adverse reactions.
• Assess patient's and family's knowledge of drug therapy.

⊕ Nursing diagnoses

• Ineffective peripheral tissue perfusion related to drug-induced thromboembolism
• Ineffective health maintenance related to underlying condition
• Deficient knowledge related to drug therapy

⊠ Planning and implementation

⚛ ALERT: Combined product may increase risk of MI, stroke, invasive breast cancer, pulmonary embolism, and deep vein thrombosis in postmenopausal women ages 50 to 79. There's also an increased risk of probable dementia in postmenopausal women age 65 and older.

• Reassess patient at 6-month intervals to make sure treatment is still needed.
• Monitor patient for hypercalcemia if she has breast cancer and bone metastases. If severe hypercalcemia occurs, notify the prescriber and stop the drug; take the appropriate measures to reduce calcium level.

Patient teaching

• Explain the risks of estrogen therapy, including breast cancer, uterine cancer, abnormal blood clotting, gallbladder disease, heart disease, and stroke.
• Tell patient to immediately report any undiagnosed, persistent, or recurring abnormal vaginal bleeding.
• Instruct women to perform monthly breast examinations and have a yearly breast examination by a health care provider. Also recommend annual mammogram if patient is older than age 50.
• Tell patient to immediately report pain in the calves or chest, sudden shortness of breath, coughing blood, severe headache, vomiting, dizziness, faintness, changes in vision or speech, and weakness or numbness in arms or legs. These are warning signals of blood clots.
• Urge patient to report evidence of liver problems, such as yellowing of skin or eyes and upper right quadrant pain.
• Instruct patient to report pain, swelling, or tenderness in abdomen, which may indicate gallbladder problems.
• Tell patient to store drug at room temperature away from excessive heat and moisture. It remains stable for 18 months.

☑ Evaluation

- Patient has no thromboembolic event during therapy.
- Patient's underlying condition improves.
- Patient and family state understanding of drug therapy.

estrogens, conjugated (estrogenic substances, conjugated; oestrogens, conjugated)

(ESS-troh-jenz, KAHN-jih-gayt-ed)

C.E.S. ♦ , Cenestin, Enjuvia, Premarin, Premarin Intravenous

Pharmacologic class: hormone
Therapeutic class: estrogen, antineoplastic, antiosteoporotic
Pregnancy risk category: X

Indications and dosages

▶ **Abnormal uterine bleeding caused by hormonal imbalance.** *Women:* 25 mg I.V. or I.M. Repeat dose in 6 to 12 hours, if needed.

▶ **Vulvar or vaginal atrophy.** *Women:* 0.5 to 2 g cream intravaginally once daily in cycles of 3 weeks on, 1 week off. Or 0.3 mg P.O. daily.

▶ **Female castration, primary ovarian failure.** *Adults:* Initially 1.25 mg P.O. daily in cycles of 3 weeks on, 1 week off. Adjust dosage as needed.

▶ **Hypogonadism.** *Women:* 0.3 to 0.625 mg P.O. daily, given cyclically 3 weeks on, 1 week off.

▶ **Moderate to severe vasomotor symptoms with or without moderate to severe symptoms of vulvar and vaginal atrophy related to menopause.** *Women:* 0.3 mg P.O. daily, or cyclically 25 days on, 5 days off for atrophy; 0.45 mg P.O. daily for vasomotor symptoms.

▶ **Palliative therapy for inoperable prostate cancer.** *Men:* 1.25 to 2.5 mg P.O. t.i.d.

▶ **Palliative therapy for breast cancer.** *Adults:* 10 mg P.O. t.i.d. for 3 months or longer.

▶ **To prevent osteoporosis in women with an increased risk but for whom non-estrogen therapy is inappropriate.** *Adults:* 0.3 to 0.625 mg P.O. daily, or cyclically, 25 days on, 5 days off.

▽ I.V. administration

- Refrigerate before reconstituting.
- Withdraw 5 ml of air from vial before adding diluent.
- Reconstitute powder for injection with diluent provided (sterile water for injection with benzyl alcohol). Gently agitate to mix drug. Avoid shaking container.
- When giving by direct I.V. injection, give slowly to avoid flushing.

⊗ **Incompatibilities**
Acidic solutions, ascorbic acid.

Contraindications and cautions

- Contraindicated in patients with thrombophlebitis, thromboembolic disorders, estrogen-dependent neoplasia, breast or reproductive organ cancer (except for palliative therapy), or undiagnosed abnormal genital bleeding.
- Use cautiously in patients with cerebrovascular or coronary artery disease, asthma, bone disease, migraine, seizures, or cardiac, hepatic, or renal dysfunction and in women with a close family history of breast or genital tract cancer or who have breast nodules, fibrocystic disease, or abnormal mammogram findings.

⚘ **Lifespan:** In children and in pregnant or breast-feeding women, drug is contraindicated.

Adverse reactions

CNS: chorea, depression, dizziness, headache, lethargy, *seizures, stroke.*
CV: edema, hypertension, *MI, pulmonary embolism, thromboembolism,* thrombophlebitis.
EENT: intolerance of contact lenses, worsening of myopia or astigmatism.
GI: abdominal cramps, anorexia, bloating, constipation, diarrhea, *nausea, pancreatitis,* vomiting.
GU: altered cervical secretions, altered menstrual flow, amenorrhea, breakthrough bleeding, cervical erosion, dysmenorrhea, *endometrial cancer,* enlargement of uterine fibromas, impotence, testicular atrophy, vaginal candidiasis.
Hepatic: cholestatic jaundice, gallbladder disease, *hepatic adenoma.*
Metabolic: hypercalcemia, hyperglycemia, increased appetite, weight changes.
Skin: dermatitis, erythema nodosum, flushing (with rapid I.V. use), hair loss, hirsutism, melasma, urticaria.
Other: *breast cancer,* breast changes (tenderness, enlargement, secretion), gynecomastia.

Interactions

Drug-drug. *Bromocriptine:* May cause amenorrhea, interfering with bromocriptine effects. Avoid use together.

Carbamazepine, phenobarbital, rifampin: May decrease estrogen effectiveness. Monitor patient closely.

Corticosteroids: May enhance effects. Monitor patient closely.

Cyclosporine: May increase risk of toxicity. Monitor cyclosporine level often.

Dantrolene, other hepatotoxic drugs: May increase risk of hepatotoxicity. Monitor patient closely.

Hydantoins: May cause loss of seizure control and increased risk of breakthrough bleeding, spotting, and pregnancy. Monitor patient closely.

Itraconazole, ketoconazole, macrolides, ritonavir: May increase estrogen level. Monitor patient for increased adverse effects.

Oral anticoagulants: May decrease anticoagulant effects. Dosage adjustments may be needed. Monitor PT and INR.

Tamoxifen: May interfere with tamoxifen effectiveness. Avoid use together.

Thyroid hormones: May alter thyroxine and thyrotropin levels. Increase thyroid hormone dosage as needed.

Topiramate: May increase estrogen metabolism and decrease effectiveness. Monitor patient closely.

Drug-herb. *St. John's wort:* May decrease estrogen level. Watch for decreased effectiveness and changes in bleeding patterns.

Drug-food. *Caffeine:* May increase caffeine level. Monitor effects.

Drug-lifestyle. *Smoking:* May increase risk of CV effects. If smoking continues, consider alternative therapy. Urge patient to stop smoking.

Effects on lab test results

• May increase glucose, calcium, total T_4, thyroid-binding globulin, phospholipid, triglyceride, and clotting factor VII, VIII, IX, and X levels.

• May increase PT and norepinephrine-induced platelet aggregation.

Pharmacokinetics

Absorption: Rapid, continuing for days after I.M. use.

Distribution: Highest levels in fat. About 50% to 80% protein-bound.

Metabolism: Mainly in liver.

Excretion: Mostly through kidneys. *Half-life:* Unknown.

Route	Onset	Peak	Duration
P.O., I.V., I.M., vaginal	Unknown	Unknown	Unknown

Action

Chemical effect: Increases synthesis of DNA, RNA, and protein in responsive tissues; also reduces release of follicle-stimulating hormone and luteinizing hormone from pituitary gland.

Therapeutic effect: Provides estrogen replacement, relieves vasomotor menopausal symptoms and vaginal dryness, helps prevent severity of osteoporosis, and provides palliation for prostate and breast cancer.

Available forms

Injection: 25 mg/5 ml

Tablets: 0.3 mg, 0.45 mg, 0.625 mg, 0.9 mg, 1.25 mg

Vaginal cream: 0.625 mg/g

NURSING PROCESS

Assessment

• Obtain history of patient's underlying condition before starting therapy, and reassess regularly.

• Make sure patient has thorough physical examination before starting estrogen therapy.

• Patient receiving long-term therapy should have yearly examinations. Periodically monitor lipid levels, blood pressure, body weight, and liver function.

• Be alert for adverse reactions and drug interactions.

• Assess patient's and family's knowledge of drug therapy.

Nursing diagnoses

• Ineffective health maintenance related to underlying condition

• Ineffective tissue perfusion (cerebral, peripheral, pulmonary, or myocardial) related to drug-induced thromboembolism

• Deficient knowledge related to drug therapy

Planning and implementation

• Give oral forms at mealtimes or at bedtime (for once-daily dose) to minimize nausea.

- When giving I.M., inject deep into large muscle. Rotate injection sites to prevent muscle atrophy.
- Use I.M. or I.V. to rapidly treat dysfunctional uterine bleeding or to reduce surgical bleeding.
- Because of risk of thromboembolism, stop therapy at least 1 month before procedures that may prolong immobilization, such as knee or hip surgery. If thromboembolism is suspected, withhold drug, notify prescriber, and provide supportive care.

⊛ ALERT: Estrogens aren't interchangeable.

Patient teaching
- Inform patient about adverse effects.
- Emphasize importance of regular physical examinations. In postmenopausal women, using the drug for longer than 5 years may increase risk of endometrial carcinoma. This risk is reduced by using cyclic rather than continuous therapy and lowest dosages. Drug probably doesn't increase risk of breast cancer.
- Teach patient how to use vaginal cream. Tell her to wash vaginal area with soap and water before applying. Tell her to apply drug at bedtime or to lie flat for 30 minutes after application to minimize drug loss.
- Explain to patient on cyclic therapy for postmenopausal symptoms that, although withdrawal bleeding may occur during week off drug, fertility hasn't been restored. Pregnancy can't occur because she hasn't ovulated.
- Warn patient to immediately report abdominal pain; pain, numbness, or stiffness in legs or buttocks; pressure or pain in chest; shortness of breath; severe headaches; visual disturbances, such as blind spots, flashing lights, or blurriness; vaginal bleeding or discharge; breast lumps; swelling of hands or feet; yellow skin or sclera; dark urine; and light-colored stools.
- Tell diabetic patient to report elevated glucose test results so antidiabetic dosage can be adjusted.
- Teach woman how to perform routine breast self-examination.

☑ **Evaluation**
- Patient shows improvement in underlying condition.
- Patient has no thromboembolic event during therapy.
- Patient and family state understanding of drug therapy.

estrogens, esterified
(ESS-troh-jenz, ESS-tehr-eh-fighd)
Menest

Pharmacologic class: hormone
Therapeutic class: antineoplastic, estrogen
Pregnancy risk category: X

Indications and dosages

▶ **Inoperable prostate cancer.** *Men:* 1.25 to 2.5 mg P.O. t.i.d.
▶ **Breast cancer with metastasis.** *Men and postmenopausal women:* 10 mg P.O. t.i.d. for 3 or more months.
▶ **Hypogonadism.** *Women:* 2.5 to 7.5 mg P.O. daily in divided doses in cycles of 20 days on, 10 days off.
▶ **Female castration, primary ovarian failure.** *Women:* 2.5 mg P.O. daily to t.i.d. in cycles of 3 weeks on, 1 week off.
▶ **Vasomotor menopausal symptoms.** *Women:* Average dosage is 1.25 mg P.O. daily in cycles of 3 weeks on, 1 week off.
▶ **Atrophic vaginitis or urethritis.** *Women:* 0.3 to 1.25 mg P.O. daily in cycles of 3 weeks on, 1 week off.
▶ **Prevention of osteoporosis in women at significant risk for whom non-estrogen therapy is inappropriate.** *Women:* Initially 0.3 mg P.O. daily; may increase to maximum, 1.25 mg daily.

Contraindications and cautions

- Contraindicated in patients with breast cancer (except when metastatic disease is present), estrogen-dependent neoplasia, active thrombophlebitis or thromboembolic disorders, undiagnosed abnormal genital bleeding, hypersensitivity to drug, or history of thromboembolic disease.
- Use cautiously in patients with history of hypertension, depression, cardiac or renal dysfunction, liver impairment, bone diseases, migraine, seizures, or diabetes mellitus.

🜲 Lifespan: In children and in pregnant or breast-feeding women, drug is contraindicated.

Adverse reactions

CNS: headache, dizziness, chorea, depression, lethargy, *seizures, stroke.*
CV: edema, hypertension, *MI, pulmonary embolism,* thrombophlebitis, *thromboembolism.*

EENT: intolerance of contact lenses, worsening of myopia or astigmatism.
GI: abdominal cramps, anorexia, bloating, constipation, diarrhea, nausea, *pancreatitis,* vomiting.
GU: altered cervical secretions, altered menstrual flow, amenorrhea, breakthrough bleeding, *breast and endometrial cancers,* cervical erosion, dysmenorrhea, enlargement of uterine fibromas, impotence, testicular atrophy, vaginal candidiasis.
Hepatic: cholestatic jaundice, gallbladder disease, *hepatic adenoma.*
Metabolic: hypercalcemia, increased appetite, weight changes.
Skin: dermatitis, erythema nodosum, hair loss, hirsutism, melasma, rash.
Other: breast changes (tenderness, enlargement, secretion), gynecomastia.

Interactions

Drug-drug. *Bromocriptine:* May cause amenorrhea, interfering with bromocriptine effects. Avoid use together.
Carbamazepine, phenobarbital, rifampin: May decrease estrogen effectiveness. Monitor patient closely.
Corticosteroids: May enhance effects. Monitor patient closely.
Cyclosporine: May increase risk of toxicity. Monitor cyclosporine level often.
Dantrolene, other hepatotoxic drugs: May increase risk of hepatotoxicity. Monitor patient closely.
Hydantoins: May cause loss of seizure control and increased risk of breakthrough bleeding, spotting, and pregnancy. Monitor patient closely.
Itraconazole, ketoconazole, macrolides, ritonavir: May increase estrogen level. Watch for increased adverse effects.
Oral anticoagulants: May decrease anticoagulant effects. Dosage adjustments may be needed. Monitor PT and INR.
Tamoxifen: May interfere with tamoxifen effectiveness. Avoid use together.
Thyroid hormones: May alter thyroxine and thyrotropin levels. Increase thyroid hormone dose as needed.
Topiramate: May increase estrogen metabolism and decrease effectiveness. Monitor patient closely.
Drug-herb. *St. John's wort:* May decrease estrogen level. Watch for decreased effectiveness and changes in bleeding patterns.

Drug-food. *Caffeine:* May increase caffeine level. Monitor effects.
Drug-lifestyle. *Smoking:* May increase risk of CV effects. Urge patient to stop smoking. If smoking continues, patient may need alternative therapy.

Effects on lab test results

• May increase glucose, calcium, total T_4, thyroid-binding globulin, phospholipid, triglyceride, and clotting factor VII, VIII, IX, and X levels.
• May increase PT and norepinephrine-induced platelet aggregation.

Pharmacokinetics

Absorption: Well absorbed but substantially inactivated by liver.
Distribution: Highest levels in fat. About 50% to 80% protein-bound.
Metabolism: Mainly in liver.
Excretion: Mainly by kidneys. *Half-life:* Unknown.

Route	Onset	Peak	Duration
P.O.	Unknown	Unknown	Unknown

Action

Chemical effect: Increases synthesis of DNA, RNA, and protein and reduces release of follicle-stimulating hormone and luteinizing hormone from pituitary gland.
Therapeutic effect: Provides estrogen replacement, hinders prostate and breast cancer cell growth, and relieves menopausal vasomotor symptoms and vaginal dryness.

Available forms

Tablets: 0.3 mg, 0.625 mg, 1.25 mg, 2.5 mg
Tablets (film-coated): 0.3 mg, 0.625 mg, 1.25 mg, 2.5 mg

NURSING PROCESS

Assessment

• Obtain history of patient's underlying condition before starting therapy, and reassess regularly thereafter.
• Make sure patient has thorough physical examination before starting drug therapy.
• Patient receiving long-term therapy should have yearly examinations. Periodically monitor

---

lipid levels, blood pressure, body weight, and liver function.
- Be alert for adverse reactions and drug interactions.
- Assess patient's and family's knowledge of drug therapy.

🔢 Nursing diagnoses
- Ineffective health maintenance related to underlying condition
- Ineffective tissue perfusion (cerebral, peripheral, pulmonary, or myocardial) related to drug-induced thromboembolism
- Deficient knowledge related to drug therapy

▶ Planning and implementation
- Give oral forms at mealtimes or bedtime (for once-daily dose) to minimize nausea.
- Because of risk of thromboembolism, stop therapy at least 1 month before procedures that may cause prolonged immobilization or thromboembolism, such as knee or hip surgery. If thromboembolism is suspected, withhold drug, notify prescriber, and provide supportive care.
- **⚠ ALERT:** Estrogens aren't interchangeable.

Patient teaching
- Inform patient about adverse effects.
- Emphasize importance of regular physical examinations. Tell a postmenopausal woman who uses the drug for longer than 5 years that it may increase her risk for endometrial carcinoma, but that this risk is reduced by using cyclic rather than continuous therapy and the lowest dosages of estrogen. Also inform her that the drug probably doesn't increase risk of breast cancer.
- Explain to patient on cyclic therapy for postmenopausal symptoms that although withdrawal bleeding may occur during the week off, fertility hasn't been restored. Pregnancy can't occur because she hasn't ovulated.
- Warn patient to immediately report abdominal pain; pain, numbness, or stiffness in legs or buttocks; pressure or pain in chest; shortness of breath; severe headaches; visual disturbances, such as blind spots, flashing lights, or blurriness; vaginal bleeding or discharge; breast lumps; swelling of hands or feet; yellow skin or sclera; dark urine; and light-colored stools.
- Tell diabetic patient to report elevated glucose test results so antidiabetic dosage can be adjusted.
- Teach woman how to perform routine breast self-examination.

☑ Evaluation
- Patient shows improvement in underlying condition.
- Patient has no thromboembolic event during therapy.
- Patient and family state understanding of drug therapy.

estropipate (piperazine estrone sulfate)
(ess-troh-PIH-payt)
Ogen, Ortho-Est

Pharmacologic class: hormone
Therapeutic class: estrogen
Pregnancy risk category: X

Indications and dosages

▶ **Management of moderate-to-severe vasomotor symptoms, vulvar and vaginal atrophy.** *Women:* 0.75 to 6 mg P.O. daily 3 weeks on, 1 week off, or 2 to 4 g of vaginal cream daily. Typically dosage given on cyclic, short-term basis.

▶ **Primary ovarian failure, female castration, hypogonadism.** *Women:* Given cyclically with 1.5 to 9 mg P.O. daily for first 3 weeks and then 8 to 10 day rest period. If bleeding doesn't occur by end of rest period, repeat cycle.

▶ **To prevent osteoporosis.** *Women:* 0.75 mg P.O. daily for 25 days of 31-day cycle. Repeat cycle as needed.

Contraindications and cautions

- Contraindicated in patients with active thrombophlebitis, thromboembolic disorders, estrogen-dependent neoplasia, undiagnosed genital bleeding, or breast, reproductive organ, or genital cancer.
- Use cautiously in patients with cerebrovascular or coronary artery disease, asthma, depression, bone disease, migraine, seizures, or cardiac, hepatic, or renal dysfunction and in women with family history (mother, grandmother, sister) of breast or genital tract cancer or who have breast nodules, fibrocystic disease, or abnormal mammogram findings. Use the lowest effective dose for the shortest duration.
- This drug has not been approved for the prevention of cognitive disorders or memory loss.

⚖ **Lifespan:** In children and in pregnant or breast-feeding women, drug is contraindicated.

Adverse reactions

CNS: depression, dizziness, headache, migraine, *seizure, stroke.*
CV: edema, *MI, pulmonary embolism, thromboembolism,* thrombophlebitis.
GI: abdominal cramps, bloating, *nausea,* vomiting.
GU: breakthrough bleeding, candidiasis, cystitis-like syndrome, dysmenorrhea, *endometrial and breast cancers,* increased size of uterine fibromas, vaginal amenorrhea.
Hepatic: cholestatic jaundice.
Metabolic: hypercalcemia, weight changes.
Skin: *erythema multiforme,* erythema nodosum, hair loss, hemorrhagic eruption, hirsutism, melasma.
Other: aggravation of porphyria, breast engorgement or enlargement, libido changes.

Interactions

Drug-drug. *Bromocriptine:* May cause amenorrhea, interfering with bromocriptine effects. Avoid use together.
Carbamazepine, phenobarbital, rifampin: May decrease estrogen effectiveness. Monitor patient closely.
Corticosteroids: May enhance effects. Monitor patient closely.
Cyclosporine: May increase risk of toxicity. Monitor cyclosporine level often.
Dantrolene, other hepatotoxic drugs: May increase risk of hepatotoxicity. Monitor patient closely.
Hydantoins: May cause loss of seizure control and increased risk of breakthrough bleeding, spotting, and pregnancy. Monitor patient closely.
Itraconazole, ketoconazole, macrolides, ritonavir: May increase estrogen level. Watch for increased adverse effects.
Oral anticoagulants: May decrease anticoagulant effects. Dosage adjustments may be needed. Monitor PT and INR.
Tamoxifen: May interfere with tamoxifen effectiveness. Avoid use together.
Thyroid hormones: May alter thyroxine and thyrotropin levels. Increase thyroid hormone dosage as needed.
Topiramate: May increase estrogen metabolism and decrease effectiveness. Monitor patient closely.

Drug-herb. *St. John's wort:* May decrease estrogen level. Watch for decreased effectiveness and changes in bleeding patterns.
Drug-food. *Caffeine:* May increase caffeine level. Monitor effects.
Drug-lifestyle. *Smoking:* May increase risk of CV effects. Urge patient to stop smoking. If smoking continues, patient may need alternate therapy.

Effects on lab test results

• May increase calcium, total T_4, thyroid-binding globulin, phospholipid, triglyceride, and clotting factor VII, VIII, IX, and X levels.
• May increase PT and norepinephrine-induced platelet aggregation.

Pharmacokinetics

Absorption: Not well characterized after P.O. or intravaginal use.
Distribution: Highest levels in fat. About 50% to 80% protein-bound.
Metabolism: Mainly in liver.
Excretion: Mainly by kidneys. *Half-life:* Unknown.

Route	Onset	Peak	Duration
P.O., vaginal	Unknown	Unknown	Unknown

Action

Chemical effect: Increases synthesis of DNA, RNA, and protein and reduces release of follicle-stimulating hormone and luteinizing hormone from pituitary gland.
Therapeutic effect: Provides estrogen replacement, relieves menopausal vasomotor symptoms, and helps reduce severity of osteoporosis.

Available forms

Tablets: 0.625 mg, 1.25 mg, 2.5 mg, 5 mg as sodium estrone sulfate (equivalent to 0.75 mg, 1.5 mg, 3 mg, 6 mg as estropipate)
Vaginal cream: 1.5 mg/g (0.15%)

NURSING PROCESS

⚖ **Assessment**
• Obtain history of patient's underlying condition before starting therapy, and reassess regularly.
• Make sure patient has thorough physical examination before starting drug therapy.

• Patient receiving long-term therapy should have yearly examinations. Periodically monitor lipid level, blood pressure, body weight, and liver function.
• Be alert for adverse reactions and drug interactions.
• Assess patient's and family's knowledge of drug therapy.

Nursing diagnoses
• Ineffective health maintenance related to underlying condition
• Ineffective tissue perfusion (cerebral, peripheral, pulmonary, or myocardial) related to drug-induced thromboembolism
• Deficient knowledge related to drug therapy

▶ Planning and implementation
• Give oral forms with meals or at bedtime (for once-daily dose) to minimize nausea.
• Because of risk of thromboembolism, stop therapy at least 1 month before procedures that may cause prolonged immobilization or thromboembolism, such as knee or hip surgery. If thromboembolism is suspected, withhold drug, notify prescriber, and provide supportive care.
Ⓢ ALERT: Estrogens aren't interchangeable.
Patient teaching
• Inform patient about adverse effects.
• Emphasize importance of regular physical examinations. Tell a postmenopausal woman who uses the drug for longer than 5 years that it may increase her risk of endometrial carcinoma, but that the risk is reduced by using cyclic rather than continuous therapy and the lowest dosages of estrogen. Also inform her that the drug probably doesn't increase risk of breast cancer.
• Teach patient how to use vaginal cream. Tell her to wash vaginal area with soap and water before applying. Tell her to use drug at bedtime or to lie flat for 30 minutes after application to minimize drug loss.
• Explain to patient on cyclic therapy for postmenopausal symptoms that although withdrawal bleeding may occur during the week off, fertility hasn't been restored. Pregnancy can't occur because she hasn't ovulated.
• Explain to patient being treated for hypogonadism that therapy length depends on her endometrial response to drug. If satisfactory withdrawal bleeding doesn't occur, oral progestin may be added. Explain to patient that despite re-

turn of withdrawal bleeding, pregnancy can't occur because she isn't ovulating.
• Warn patient to immediately report abdominal pain; pain, numbness, or stiffness in legs or buttocks; pressure or pain in chest; shortness of breath; severe headaches; visual disturbances, such as blind spots, flashing lights, or blurriness; vaginal bleeding or discharge; breast lumps; swelling of hands or feet; yellow skin or sclera; dark urine; and light-colored stools.
• Tell diabetic patient to report elevated glucose test results so antidiabetic dosage can be adjusted.
• Teach women how to perform routine breast self-examination.

☑ Evaluation
• Patient shows improvement in underlying condition.
• Patient has no thromboembolic event during therapy.
• Patient and family state understanding of drug therapy.

HIGH ALERT!
---

eszopiclone
(ess-zoe-PICK-lone)
Lunesta✎

Pharmacologic class: pyrrolopyrazine derivative
Therapeutic class: hypnotic
Pregnancy risk category: C
Controlled substance schedule: IV

Indications and dosages
▶ **Insomnia.** *Adults:* 2 mg P.O. immediately before bedtime. Increase to 3 mg if needed.
Elderly patients having trouble falling asleep: 1 mg P.O. immediately before bedtime. Increase to 2 mg if needed.
Elderly patients having trouble staying asleep: 2 mg P.O. immediately before bedtime.
Ⓢ **Adjust-a-dose:** In patients with severe hepatic impairment, start with 1 mg P.O. In patients who also take a potent CYP3A4 inhibitor, start with 1 mg and increase to 2 mg if needed.

Contraindications and cautions
• Use cautiously in patients with diseases or conditions that could affect metabolism or hemodynamic responses. Also use cautiously in

patients with compromised respiratory function, severe hepatic impairment, or signs and symptoms of depression.

⚖ **Lifespan:** In pregnant women, use only if benefits outweigh risk to the fetus. In breastfeeding women, use cautiously because it isn't known if drug appears in breast milk. In children, safety and effectiveness haven't been established. Elderly patients may be more sensitive to drug effects.

Adverse reactions

CNS: abnormal dreams, anxiety, confusion, depression, dizziness, hallucinations, *headache,* nervousness, neuralgia, pain, *somnolence.*
EENT: unpleasant taste.
GI: diarrhea, dry mouth, dyspepsia, nausea, vomiting.
GU: UTI.
Respiratory: respiratory infection.
Skin: pruritus, rash.
Other: accidental injury, decreased libido, viral infection, ***anaphylaxis, angioedema.***

Interactions

Drug-drug. *CNS depressants:* May have additive CNS effects. Adjust dosage of either drug as needed.
CYP3A4 inhibitors (clarithromycin, itraconazole, ketoconazole, nefazodone, nelfinavir, ritonavir, troleandomycin): May decrease eszopiclone elimination, increasing the risk of toxicity. Use together cautiously.
Olanzapine: May impair cognitive function or memory. Use together cautiously.
Rifampicin: May decrease eszopiclone activity. Don't use together.
Drug-food. *High-fat meals:* May decrease eszopiclone absorption and decrease drug effects. Discourage high-fat meals with or just before taking drug.
Drug-lifestyle. *Alcohol:* May decrease psychomotor ability. Discourage use together.

Effects on lab test results

None reported.

Pharmacokinetics

Absorption: Rapid.
Distribution: In plasma. About 50% to 60% protein-bound.
Metabolism: By CYP3A4 in the liver, with two mainly inactive metabolites.

Excretion: In urine, mainly as metabolites.
Half-life: 6 hours.

Route	Onset	Peak	Duration
P.O.	Rapid	1 hr	Unknown

Action

Chemical effect: Drug probably interacts with gamma amino-butyric acid receptors at binding sites close to or connected to benzodiazepine receptors.
Therapeutic effect: Promotes sleep.

Available forms

Tablets: 1 mg, 2 mg, 3 mg

NURSING PROCESS

⚕ Assessment
• Evaluate patient for physical and psychiatric disorders before treatment.
• Be alert for drug interactions and adverse reactions. Anaphylaxis and angioedema may occur as early as the first dose.
• If patient is still having trouble sleeping after using drug for short-term therapy, check for other psychological disorders.
• Monitor patient for changes in behavior, including complex sleep disorders and those that suggest depression or suicidal thinking.
• Assess patient's and family's knowledge of drug therapy.

⊕ Nursing diagnoses
• Sleep deprivation related to insomnia
• Risk for injury related to drug-induced adverse CNS reactions
• Deficient knowledge related to drug therapy

▶ Planning and implementation
⊛ ALERT: Give drug immediately before patient goes to bed or after patient has gone to bed and has trouble falling asleep.
• Use the lowest effective dose.
• Use only for short periods (for example, 7 to 10 days).
• Overdose may cause impaired consciousness, hypotension, and CNS depression.
• Treat overdose symptomatically and supportively; flumazenil may be helpful. It isn't known if eszopiclone is removed by dialysis.

Reactions may be *common,* uncommon, *life-threatening*, or COMMON AND LIFE-THREATENING.

Patient teaching

• Urge patient to take drug immediately before going to bed because drug may cause dizziness or light-headedness.
• Caution patient not to take eszopiclone unless he can get a full night's sleep.
• Advise patient to avoid taking drug after a high-fat meal.
• Tell patient to avoid activities that require mental alertness until the drug's effects are known.
• Advise patient to avoid alcohol while taking drug.
• Urge patient to immediately report changes in behavior and thinking, including complex sleep-related behaviors.
• Warn patient not to stop drug abruptly or change dose without consulting the prescriber.
• Inform patient that tolerance or dependence may develop if drug is taken for a prolonged period.

☑ Evaluation

• Patient no longer experiences insomnia with drug therapy.
• Patient does not experience injury from adverse CNS reactions.
• Patient and family state understanding of drug therapy.

etanercept

(ee-TAN-er-sept)
Enbrel

Pharmacologic class: tumor necrosis factor (TNF) blocker
Therapeutic class: antirheumatic
Pregnancy risk category: B

Indications and dosages

▶ **Psoriatic arthritis, ankylosing spondylitis, moderately to severely active rheumatoid arthritis.** *Adults:* 25 mg subcutaneously twice weekly, on same day or 72 to 96 hours apart, or 50 mg subcutaneously from prefilled syringe once weekly. Continue methotrexate, glucocorticoids, salicylates, NSAIDs, or analgesics during therapy.
▶ **Moderate to severely active polyarticular-course juvenile rheumatoid arthritis in patients who have had an inadequate response to one or more disease-modifying anti-**

rheumatic drugs. *Children ages 4 to 17:* Give 0.4 mg/kg (maximum, 25 mg/dose) subcutaneously twice weekly, on same day or 72 to 96 hours apart.
▶ **Chronic moderate to severe plaque psoriasis in patients who are candidates for systemic therapy or phototherapy.** *Adults:* 50 mg subcutaneously twice weekly, 3 to 4 days apart for 3 months. Then, reduce dosage to 50 mg subcutaneously once weekly.

Contraindications and cautions

• Contraindicated in patients hypersensitive to drug or any of its components and in those with sepsis. Stop giving the drug to a patient who develops a serious infection or sepsis. Use of live vaccines during drug therapy is contraindicated.
• Use cautiously in patients with a history of recurring infections and in those with underlying diseases that predispose them to infection, such as diabetes or heart failure. Also use cautiously in patients with CNS demyelinating disorders and in those with a history of significant hematologic abnormalities.
⚠ **Lifespan:** In pregnant women, use cautiously. Breast-feeding women should stop drug or stop breast-feeding. In children younger than age 4, safety and effectiveness haven't been established.

Adverse reactions

CNS: asthenia, dizziness, *headache.*
EENT: pharyngitis, rhinitis, sinusitis.
GI: abdominal pain, dyspepsia.
Respiratory: cough, respiratory disorder, *upper respiratory tract infections.*
Skin: rash.
Other: infections, injection site reaction, *malignancies.*

Interactions

Drug-drug. *Live-virus vaccinations:* Transmission of infection remains unknown. Avoid use together.

Effects on lab test results

• May cause positive antinuclear antibody or positive anti–double-stranded DNA antibodies measured by radioimmunoassay and *Crithidia luciliae* assay.

Pharmacokinetics

Absorption: Level peaks in 72 hours.

Rapid onset   *Liquid form contains alcohol.*   ◆Canada   †OTC   ✐Photoguide   ‡Off-label use

Distribution: Unknown.
Metabolism: Unknown.
Excretion: Unknown. *Half-life:* 115 hours.

Route	Onset	Peak	Duration
SubQ	Unknown	3 days	Unknown

Action

Chemical effect: Binds specifically to TNF and blocks its action, reducing inflammatory and immune responses found in rheumatoid arthritis.
Therapeutic effect: Reduces signs and symptoms of rheumatoid arthritis.

Available forms

Injection: 25-mg single-use vial, 50-mg/ml prefilled syringe

NURSING PROCESS

℞ Assessment
• Obtain history of patient's underlying condition before starting therapy, and reassess regularly.
• Obtain accurate immunization history from parents or guardians of juvenile rheumatoid arthritis patients. Patient should be brought up-to-date with all immunizations before starting drug.
• Monitor patient for infection.
• Assess patient's and family's knowledge of drug therapy.

⊕ Nursing diagnoses
• Acute pain related to underlying condition
• Risk for infection related to drug-induced adverse reactions
• Deficient knowledge related to drug therapy

▷ Planning and implementation
• Drug is for subcutaneous injection only.
• Reconstitute aseptically with 1 ml of supplied sterile bacteriostatic water for injection, USP (0.9% benzyl alcohol). Don't filter reconstituted solution during preparation or administration. Inject diluent slowly into vial. Minimize foaming by gently swirling during dissolution rather than shaking. Dissolution takes less than 5 minutes.
• Inspect solution for particulates and discoloration before use. Reconstituted solution should be clear and colorless. Don't use solution if it's discolored or cloudy, or if particulates exist.
• Don't add other drugs or diluents to reconstituted solution.

• Use reconstituted solution as soon as possible. Solution may be refrigerated in vial for up to 6 hours at 36° to 46° F (2° to 8° C).
• Inject at least 1 inch from another injection site; don't use areas where skin is tender, bruised, red, or hard. Give in the thigh, abdomen, and upper arm. Rotate sites regularly.
• Don't give live vaccines during therapy.
• Drug may affect defenses against infection. If serious infection occurs, notify prescriber and stop therapy.
• Needle cover of diluent syringe contains dry natural rubber (latex). Don't allow those sensitive to latex to handle cover.
⚠ **ALERT:** Don't confuse Enbrel with Levbid.
Patient teaching
• If patient will be administering drug, teach mixing and injection techniques, including rotation of injection sites.
• Instruct patient to use puncture-resistant container to dispose of needles and syringes.
• Tell patient that injection site reactions typically occur within first month of therapy and decrease thereafter.
• Urge patient to avoid live vaccines during therapy. Stress importance of alerting other health care providers of etanercept use.
• Instruct patient to promptly report evidence of infection to prescriber.

✓ Evaluation
• Patient's pain decreases.
• Patient is free from infection.
• Patient and family state understanding of drug therapy.

ethacrynate sodium
(eth-uh-KRIH-nayt SOH-dee-um)
Sodium Edecrin

ethacrynic acid
Edecrin

Pharmacologic class: loop diuretic
Therapeutic class: diuretic
Pregnancy risk category: B

Indications and dosages

▶ **Acute pulmonary edema.** *Adults:* 50 mg or 0.5 to 1 mg/kg I.V. to maximum dose of

---

100 mg. Usually, only one dose is needed; occasionally, second dose may be required.

▶ **Edema.** *Adults:* 50 to 200 mg P.O. daily. Refractory cases may require up to 200 mg b.i.d. *Children age 1 and older:* Initial dose is 25 mg P.O.; increase cautiously in 25-mg increments daily until desired effect is achieved.

▶ **Hypertension‡.** *Adults:* Initially 25 mg P.O. daily. Adjust dosage as needed. Maximum maintenance dosage is 200 mg P.O. daily in two divided doses.

▼ I.V. administration

• Reconstitute vacuum vial with 50 ml of D_5W or normal saline solution.
• Give slowly through I.V. line of running infusion or by direct injection over several minutes.
• If more than one I.V. dose is needed, use new injection site to avoid thrombophlebitis.
• Discard unused solution after 24 hours. Don't use cloudy or opalescent solutions.

⊗ **Incompatibilities**
Hydralazine, Normosol-M, procainamide, ranitidine, reserpine, solutions or drugs with pH below 5, tolazoline, triflupromazine, whole blood and its derivatives.

Contraindications and cautions

• Contraindicated in patients hypersensitive to the drug or any of its components and in those with anuria.
• Use cautiously in patients with electrolyte abnormalities, advanced cirrhosis of the liver, hepatic encephalopathy, or renal impairment.
🜺 Lifespan: In pregnant women, use cautiously. In breast-feeding women, it's unknown if drug appears in breast milk. In infants, drug is contraindicated.

Adverse reactions

CNS: confusion, fatigue, fever, headache, malaise, nervousness, vertigo.
CV: orthostatic hypotension, volume depletion and dehydration.
EENT: blurred vision, hearing loss, tinnitus, transient deafness (with too-rapid I.V. injection).
GI: anorexia, cramping, diarrhea, GI bleeding, nausea, *pancreatitis,* vomiting.
GU: frequent urination, hematuria, nocturia, oliguria, polyuria.
Hematologic: *agranulocytosis, neutropenia, thrombocytopenia.*

Metabolic: dilutional hyponatremia, hyperglycemia, hyperuricemia, hypochloremic alkalosis, hypocalcemia, hypokalemia, *hypomagnesemia,* impaired glucose tolerance.
Skin: dermatitis, rash.
Other: chills.

Interactions

Drug-drug. *Aminoglycoside antibiotics:* May potentiate ototoxic adverse reactions of both drugs. Use together cautiously.
Antihypertensives: May increase risk of hypotension. Use together cautiously.
Chlorothiazide, chlorthalidone, hydrochlorothiazide, indapamide, metolazone: May cause excessive diuretic response, resulting in serious electrolyte abnormalities or dehydration. Adjust doses carefully while monitoring patient closely for excessive diuretic responses.
Cisplatin: May increase risk of ototoxicity. Avoid use together.
Digoxin: May increase risk of digoxin toxicity from ethacrynate-induced hypokalemia. Monitor potassium and digoxin levels.
Lithium: May decrease lithium clearance, increasing risk of lithium toxicity. Monitor lithium level.
Metolazone: May cause profound diuresis and enhance electrolyte loss. Use together cautiously.
NSAIDs: May decrease diuretic effectiveness. Use together cautiously.
Warfarin: May potentiate anticoagulant effect. Use together cautiously.
Drug-herb. *Licorice root:* May contribute to potassium depletion caused by diuretics. Discourage licorice root intake.
Drug-lifestyle. *Sun exposure:* Photosensitivity may occur. Discourage prolonged or unprotected exposure to sunlight.

Effects on lab test results

• May increase glucose, BUN, and uric acid levels. May decrease potassium, sodium, calcium, and magnesium levels.
• May decrease granulocyte, neutrophil, and platelet counts.

Pharmacokinetics

Absorption: Ethacrynic acid is absorbed rapidly from GI tract. Ethacrynate sodium is given I.V.
Distribution: Unknown.

Metabolism: Unknown.
Excretion: Unknown. *Half-life:* 1 hour.

Route	Onset	Peak	Duration
P.O.	30 min	2 hr	6–8 hr
I.V.	5 min	15–30 min	2 hr

Action

Chemical effect: Inhibits sodium and chloride reabsorption at renal tubules and ascending loop of Henle.
Therapeutic effect: Promotes sodium and water excretion.

Available forms

Injection: 50 mg (with 62.5 mg of mannitol and 0.1 mg of thimerosal)
Tablets: 25 mg, 50 mg

NURSING PROCESS

⚕ Assessment
• Obtain history of patient's underlying condition before starting therapy.
• Monitor effectiveness by regularly checking urine output, weight, peripheral edema, and breath sounds.
• Monitor fluid intake, blood pressure, and electrolyte levels.
• Monitor uric acid levels, especially in patients with history of gout.
• Be alert for adverse reactions and drug interactions.
• Assess patient's and family's knowledge of drug therapy.

⊕ Nursing diagnoses
• Excess fluid volume related to underlying condition
• Impaired urinary elimination related to diuretic therapy
• Deficient knowledge related to drug therapy

▷ Planning and implementation
• Give drug with food or milk because P.O. use may cause GI upset.
• To prevent nocturia, give P.O. doses in morning.
• Don't mix with whole blood or its derivatives.
• Don't give subcutaneously or I.M. because of local pain and irritation.
• Potassium chloride and sodium supplements may be needed.

• If diarrhea occurs, notify prescriber because severe diarrhea may warrant stopping drug.
Patient teaching
• Advise patient to avoid sudden posture changes and to rise slowly to avoid orthostatic hypotension.
• Advise diabetic patient to closely monitor glucose level.
• Teach patient and family to identify and report signs of hypersensitivity or fluid and electrolyte disturbances.
• Teach patient to monitor fluid volume by daily weight and intake and output.
• Tell patient to take oral drug early in day to avoid interruption of sleep by nocturia.

☑ Evaluation
• Patient is free from edema.
• Patient demonstrates adjustment of lifestyle to deal with altered patterns of urinary elimination.
• Patient and family state understanding of drug therapy.

ethambutol hydrochloride
(ee-THAM-byoo-tall high-droh-KLOR-ighd)
Etibi ◆ , Myambutol

Pharmacologic class: semisynthetic antituberculotic
Therapeutic class: antituberculotic
Pregnancy risk category: B

Indications and dosages

▶ **Adjunct therapy for pulmonary tuberculosis.** *Adults and children age 13 and older:* For patients who haven't received previous antitubercular therapy, 15 mg/kg P.O. daily. For patients who have received previous antitubercular therapy, 25 mg/kg P.O. daily for 60 days until cultures are negative; then decrease to 15 mg/kg P.O. daily.
▶ **Adjunct therapy for pulmonary *Mycobacterium avium* complex infections in patients without HIV‡.** *Adults:* 25 mg/kg P.O. daily for 2 months followed by 15 mg/kg P.O. daily until cultures are negative for 1 year.
▶ **Adjunct therapy for disseminated *Mycobacterium avium* complex infections‡.** *Adults:* 15 mg/kg P.O. daily for patient's lifetime.

Contraindications and cautions

• Contraindicated in patients hypersensitive to drug and in patients with optic neuritis.
• Use cautiously in patients with impaired kidney function, cataracts, recurrent eye inflammations, gout, or diabetic retinopathy.
⚞ **Lifespan:** In pregnant women, use cautiously. In breast-feeding women, use cautiously because it's unknown if the drug appears in breast milk. In children younger than age 13, drug is contraindicated.

Adverse reactions

CNS: confusion, dizziness, fever, hallucinations, headache, malaise, peripheral neuritis.
EENT: dose-related optic neuritis; loss of color discrimination, especially red and green; vision loss.
GI: abdominal pain, anorexia, nausea, vomiting.
Hematologic: *thrombocytopenia.*
Respiratory: bloody sputum.
Skin: dermatitis, pruritus, *toxic epidermal necrolysis.*
Other: *anaphylactoid reactions,* precipitation of gout.

Interactions

Drug-drug. *Aluminum salts:* May delay and reduce absorption of ethambutol. Separate doses by several hours.

Effects on lab test results

• May increase ALT, AST, bilirubin, and uric acid levels. May decrease glucose level.
• May decrease platelet count.

Pharmacokinetics

Absorption: Rapid.
Distribution: Wide. 8% to 22% protein-bound.
Metabolism: Undergoes partial hepatic metabolism.
Excretion: After 24 hours, about 50% of unchanged drug and 8% to 15% of its metabolites in urine; 20% to 25% in feces. *Half-life:* About 3½ hours.

Route	Onset	Peak	Duration
P.O.	Unknown	2–4 hr	Unknown

Action

Chemical effect: May interfere with synthesis of one or more metabolites of susceptible bacte-

ria, altering cellular metabolism during cell division.
Therapeutic effect: Hinders bacterial growth.

Available forms

Tablets: 100 mg, 400 mg

NURSING PROCESS

☑ Assessment

• Obtain history of patient's infection before starting therapy.
• Perform visual acuity and color discrimination tests before and during therapy (monthly when dose is 25 mg/kg or more).
• Monitor the drug's effectiveness by regularly assessing for improvement in patient's condition and evaluating culture and sensitivity test results.
• Obtain AST and ALT levels before starting therapy. Then monitor AST and ALT levels every 2 to 4 weeks.
• Monitor uric acid level; observe patient for symptoms of gout.
• Be alert for adverse reactions and drug interactions.
• Assess patient's and family's knowledge of drug therapy.

⊕ Nursing diagnoses

• Risk for infection related to presence of susceptible bacteria
• Disturbed sensory perception (visual) related to drug-induced adverse reactions
• Deficient knowledge related to drug therapy

▷ Planning and implementation

• Anticipate the need for a lower dose in a patient with impaired kidney function.
• Always give ethambutol with other antituberculotics to prevent development of resistant organisms.
⑤ **ALERT:** Don't confuse ethambutol with Ethmozine.
Patient teaching
• Reassure patient that visual disturbances will disappear several weeks to months after the therapy ends.
• Warn patient not to perform hazardous activities if visual disturbances or adverse CNS reactions occur.
• Emphasize need for regular follow-up care.

☑ **Evaluation**
- Patient is free from infection.
- Patient regains pretreatment vision.
- Patient and family state understanding of drug therapy.

ethinyl estradiol and desogestrel

(ETH-ih-nill es-truh-DIGH-ol and DAY-so-jest-rul)
monophasic: **Apri, Desogen, Ortho-Cept**
biphasic: **Kariva, Mircette**
triphasic: **Cyclessa, Velivet**

ethinyl estradiol and ethynodiol diacetate

monophasic: **Demulen 1/35, Demulen 1/50, Zovia 1/35E, Zovia 1/50E**

ethinyl estradiol and levonorgestrel

continuous use: **Lybrel**
emergency: **Preven**
extended cycle: **Seasonique**
monophasic: **Alesse, Aviane, Lessina, Levlen, Levlite, Levora, Nordette, Portia**
triphasic: **Enpresse, Tri-Levlen, Triphasil, Trivora**

ethinyl estradiol and norethindrone

monophasic: **Balziva, Brevicon, Genora 0.5/35, Genora 1/35, ModiCon, Norethin 1/35E, Norinyl 1+35, Ortho-Novum 1/35, Ovcon-35, Ovcon-50**
biphasic: **Necon 10/11, Nortrel, Ortho-Novum 10/11**
triphasic: **Necon 7/7/7, Nortrel 7/7/7, Ortho-Novum 7/7/7, Tri-Norinyl**

ethinyl estradiol and norethindrone acetate

monophasic: **Junel 1/20, Junel 1.5/30, Loestrin 21 1/20, Loestrin 21 1.5/30, Necon 1/35, Nortrel 1/35**
triphasic: **Estrostep**

ethinyl estradiol and norgestimate

monophasic: **MonoNessa, Ortho-Cyclen, Sprintec**
triphasic: **Ortho Tri-Cyclen, Ortho Tri-Cyclen Lo, Tri-Sprintec**

ethinyl estradiol and norgestrel

monophasic: **Cryselle, Lo/Ovral, Lo/Ovral 28, Low-Ogestrel, Ogestrel 0.5/50, Ovral**

ethinyl estradiol, norethindrone acetate, and ferrous fumarate

monophasic: **Femcon FE, Junel Fe 1/5/30, Junel Fe 1/20, Loestrin Fe 1/20, Loestrin 1.5/30, Loestrin 24 Fe, Microgestin Fe 1/20, Microgestin Fe 1.5/30**

mestranol and norethindrone

monophasic: **Necon 1/50, Norinyl 1+50, Ortho-Novum 1/50**
triphasic: **Estrostep Fe, Estrostep 21**

Pharmacologic class: hormonal contraceptive
Therapeutic class: estrogen with progestin
Pregnancy risk category: X

Indications and dosages

▶ **Contraception.** *Women:* One monophasic tablet P.O. daily, beginning on day 5 of menstrual cycle (first day of menstrual flow is day 1) or may start on first Sunday after menstruation ends. With 20- and 21-tablet packages, new cycle begins 7 days after last tablet taken. With 28-tablet packages, dosage is one tablet daily without interruption; extra tablets are placebos or contain iron. Or first-color biphasic tablet P.O. daily for 10 days; then next color tablet for 11 days. Or one triphasic tablet P.O. daily in sequence specified by brand. Or one transdermal patch, changed weekly. Or one extended-cycle (Seasonique) light blue–green tablet P.O. once daily for 84 consecutive days followed by one yellow tablet for consecutive 7 days; then repeat cycle. Or one tablet daily (Lybrel).
▶ **Moderate acne vulgaris in women and girls age 15 and older who have no known contraindications to hormonal contraceptive therapy, desire hormonal contraception, have achieved menarche, and are unresponsive to topical antiacne drugs.** *Women and girls age*

---

15 and older: One tablet Estrostep, Ortho Tri-Cyclen, or Tri-Sprintec P.O. daily. (21 tablets contain active ingredients, and seven are inert.)

Contraindications and cautions

• Contraindicated in patients with thromboembolic disorders, cerebrovascular or coronary artery disease, diplopia or ocular lesion arising from ophthalmic vascular disease, classic migraine, MI, known or suspected breast cancer, known or suspected estrogen-dependent neoplasia, benign or malignant liver tumors, active liver disease or history of cholestatic jaundice with pregnancy or prior use of hormonal contraceptives, or undiagnosed abnormal vaginal bleeding.

• Use cautiously in patients with cardiac, renal, or hepatic insufficiency; gallbladder disease; hyperlipidemia; hypertension; migraine; seizure disorders; or asthma.

☀ **Lifespan:** In adolescents, hormonal contraception isn't advised until after at least 2 years of well-established menstrual cycles and completion of physiologic maturation to avoid later fertility and menstrual problems. In women who are pregnant or suspect they may be pregnant and in breast-feeding women, drug is contraindicated.

Adverse reactions

CNS: depression, *dizziness, headache,* lethargy, migraine, **stroke.**
CV: edema, hypertension, **pulmonary embolism, thromboembolism.**
EENT: diplopia, exophthalmos, intolerance of contact lenses, worsening of myopia or astigmatism.
GI: abdominal cramps, anorexia, bloating, constipation, diarrhea, granulomatous colitis, nausea, **pancreatitis,** vomiting.
GU: amenorrhea, *breakthrough bleeding,* cervical erosion or abnormal secretions, dysmenorrhea, enlargement of uterine fibromas, vaginal candidiasis.
Hepatic: cholestatic jaundice, gallbladder disease, **liver tumors.**
Metabolic: changes in appetite, hypercalcemia, hyperglycemia, weight gain.
Skin: acne, **erythema multiforme,** rash.
Other: breast changes (tenderness, enlargement, secretion) hirsutism.

Interactions

Drug-drug. *Alprazolam, chlordiazepoxide, diazepam, temazepam:* May prolong the half-life of these drugs. Watch for adverse effects.
Antibiotic, such as penicillins and tetracycines: May interfere with effectiveness causing menstrual irregularities and pregnancy. Advise patient to use supplemental birth control while on antibiotics.
Atorvastatin: May increase estrogen level. Monitor patient closely.
Beta blockers, corticosteroids, theophyllines, tricyclic antidepressants: May enhance effects of these drugs. Monitor patient closely.
Bromocriptine: May cause amenorrhea, interfering with bromocriptine effects. Avoid use together.
Carbamazepine, phenobarbital, phenytoin, rifampin: May decrease effectiveness of estrogen therapy. Monitor patient closely.
Cyclosporine: May inhibit cyclosporine metabolism, increasing the risk of toxicity. Avoid use together, if possible. If given together, monitor cyclosporine level and renal and hepatic function. Adjust cyclosporine dosage as needed.
Dantrolene, other hepatotoxic drugs: May increase risk of hepatotoxicity. Monitor patient closely.
Griseofulvin, penicillins, sulfonamides, tetracyclines: May decrease effectiveness of hormonal contraceptives. Discourage use together, or suggest barrier contraception for the duration of therapy.
Lamotrigine, lorazepam, oxazepam, temazepam: May increase clearance of these drugs. Monitor patient for lack of effect.
Oral anticoagulants: May decrease anticoagulant effects. Dosage adjustments may be needed. Monitor PT and INR.
Selegiline: May increase selegiline levels. Monitor patient closely.
Tamoxifen: May interfere with tamoxifen effectiveness. Avoid use together.
Drug-herb. *St. John's wort:* May decrease estrogen level. Watch for decreased effectiveness and changes in bleeding patterns.
Drug-food. *Caffeine:* May increase caffeine level. Monitor effects.
Drug-lifestyle. *Smoking:* May increase risk of CV effects and thrombosis. Discourage patient from smoking. If smoking continues, patient may need a different form of contraception.

Effects on lab test results

• May increase glucose, calcium, fibrinogen, triglyceride, phospholipid, total T_4, thyroid-binding globulin, plasminogen, liver enzyme, and clotting factor II, VII, VIII, IX, X, and XII levels.

• May increase PT and norepinephrine-induced platelet aggregation.

Pharmacokinetics

Absorption: Mostly well absorbed.
Distribution: Wide. Extensively protein-bound.
Metabolism: Mainly in liver.
Excretion: In urine and feces. *Half-life:* 6 to 20 hours.

Route	Onset	Peak	Duration
P.O., transdermal	Unknown	Varies	Unknown

Action

Chemical effect: Inhibits ovulation through negative feedback mechanism directed at hypothalamus. Estrogen suppresses secretion of follicle-stimulating hormone, blocking follicle development and ovulation. Progestin suppresses secretion of luteinizing hormone so ovulation can't occur. Progestin thickens cervical mucus, which interferes with sperm migration and prevents implantation.

Therapeutic effect: Prevents pregnancy and relieves signs and symptoms of endometriosis.

Available forms

monophasic

ethinyl estradiol and desogestrel
Tablets: ethinyl estradiol 30 mcg and desogestrel 0.15 mg (Apri, Desogen, Ortho-Cept); ethinyl estradiol 25 mcg and desogestrel 0.1 mg

ethinyl estradiol and ethynodiol diacetate
Tablets: ethinyl estradiol 35 mcg and ethynodiol diacetate 1 mg (Demulen 1/35, Zovia 1/35E); ethinyl estradiol 50 mcg and ethynodiol diacetate 1 mg (Demulen 1/50, Zovia 1/50E)

ethinyl estradiol and levonorgestrel
Tablets: ethinyl estradiol 30 mcg and levonorgestrel 0.15 mg (Levlen, Levora, Nordette, Portia); ethinyl estradiol 20 mcg, levonorgestrel 0.1 mg (Alesse, Aviane, Lessina, Levlite); levonorgestrel/ethinyl estradiol tablets 0.15 mg/ 0.03 mg and ethinyl estradiol tablets 0.01 mg (Seasonique); ethinyl estradiol 20 mcg and levonorgesterel 90 mcg (Lybrel)

ethinyl estradiol and norethindrone
Tablets: ethinyl estradiol 35 mcg and norethindrone 0.4 mg (Balziva, Ovcon-35); ethinyl estradiol 35 mcg and norethindrone 0.5 mg (Brevicon, Necon, Nortrel, ModiCon); ethinyl estradiol 35 mcg and norethindrone 1 mg (Necon 1/35, Nortrel 1/35, Norinyl 1+35, Ortho-Novum 1/35); ethinyl estradiol 50 mcg and norethindrone 1 mg (Ovcon-50)

ethinyl estradiol, norethindrone, and ferrous fumarate
Tablets (chewable): ethinyl estradiol 35 mcg, norethindrone 0.4 mg and ferrous fumarate 75 mg (Femcon FE)

ethinyl estradiol and norethindrone acetate
Tablets: ethinyl estradiol 20 mcg and norethindrone acetate 1 mg (Loestrin 21 1/20); ethinyl estradiol 30 mcg and norethindrone acetate 1.5 mg (Loestrin 21 1.5/30)

ethinyl estradiol and norgestimate
Tablets: ethinyl estradiol 35 mcg and norgestimate 0.25 mg (Ortho-Cyclen)

ethinyl estradiol and norgestrel
Tablets: ethinyl estradiol 30 mcg and norgestrel 0.3 mg (Cryselle, Lo/Ovral, Lo/Ovral 28, Low-Ogestrel); ethinyl estradiol 50 mcg and norgestrel 0.5 mg (Ovral, Ovral 28, Ogestrel 0.5/50)

ethinyl estradiol, norethindrone acetate, and ferrous fumarate
Tablets: ethinyl estradiol 20 mcg, norethindrone acetate 1 mg, and ferrous fumarate 75 mg (Loestrin Fe 1/20, Microgestin Fe 1/20); ethinyl estradiol 30 mcg, norethindrone acetate 1.5 mg, and ferrous fumarate 75 mg (Loestrin Fe 1.5/30, Microgestin Fe 1.5/30)

mestranol and norethindrone
Tablets: mestranol 50 mcg and norethindrone 1 mg (Necon 1/50, Norinyl 1+50, Ortho-Novum 1/50)

biphasic

ethinyl estradiol and desogestrel
Tablets: ethinyl estradiol 20 mcg and desogestrel 0.15 mg (Kariva, Mircette)

ethinyl estradiol and norethindrone
Tablets: ethinyl estradiol 35 mcg and norethindrone 0.5 mg during phase 1 (10 days); ethinyl estradiol 35 mcg and norethindrone 1 mg during phase 2 (11 days) (Necon 10/11, Ortho-Novum 10/11)

triphasic

ethinyl estradiol and desogestrel
Tablets: desogestrel 0.1 mg and ethinyl estradiol 25 mcg (7 tablets); desogestrel 0.125 mg and

ethinyl estradiol 25 mcg (7 tablets); desogestrel 0.15 mg and ethinyl estradiol 25 mcg (7 tablets) (Cyclessa); 0.1 mg desogestrel and 0.025 mg ethinyl estradiol (7 tablets); 0.125 mg desogestrel and 0.025 mg ethinyl estradiol (7 tablets); and 0.15 mg desogestrel and 0.025 mg ethinyl estradiol (7 tablets) (Velivet)

ethinyl estradiol and levonorgestrel
Tablets: ethinyl estradiol 30 mcg and levonorgestrel 0.05 mg during phase 1 (6 days); ethinyl estradiol 40 mcg and levonorgestrel 0.075 mg during phase 2 (5 days); ethinyl estradiol 30 mcg and levonorgestrel 0.125 mg during phase 3 (10 days) (Tri-Levlen, Triphasil, Trivora-28, Enpresse)
Transdermal patch: ethinyl estradiol 0.045 mg and levonorgestrel 0.015 mg

ethinyl estradiol and norethindrone
Tablets: ethinyl estradiol 35 mcg and norethindrone 0.5 mg during phase 1 (7 days); ethinyl estradiol 35 mcg and norethindrone 1 mg during phase 2 (9 days); ethinyl estradiol 35 mcg and norethindrone 0.5 mg during phase 3 (5 days) (Tri-Norinyl); ethinyl estradiol 35 mcg and norethindrone 0.5 mg during phase 1 (7 days); ethinyl estradiol 35 mcg and norethindrone 0.75 mg during phase 2 (7 days); ethinyl estradiol 35 mcg and norethindrone 1 mg during phase 3 (7 days) (Necon 7/7/7, Nortrel 7/7/7, Ortho-Novum 7/7/7)

ethinyl estradiol and norethindrone acetate
Tablets: ethinyl estradiol 0.02 mg and norethindrone acetate 1 mg (5 tablets), ethinyl estradiol 0.03 mg and norethindrone acetate 1 mg (7 tablets), ethinyl estradiol 0.035 mg and norethindrone acetate 1 mg (9 tablets) (Estrostep Fe, Estrostep 21)

ethinyl estradiol and norgestimate
Tablets: ethinyl estradiol 35 mcg and norgestimate 0.18 mg during phase 1 (7 days); ethinyl estradiol 35 mcg and norgestimate 0.215 mg during phase 2 (7 days); ethinyl estradiol 35 mcg and norgestimate 0.25 mg during phase 3 (7 days) (Ortho Tri-Cyclen)

NURSING PROCESS

Assessment
• Obtain history of patient's fertility or underlying endometriosis before starting therapy.
• Monitor the drug's effectiveness by determining if pregnancy test is negative or if patient

with endometriosis has diminished signs and symptoms.
• Periodically monitor lipid levels, blood pressure, body weight, and liver function.
• Be alert for adverse reactions and drug interactions.
• Assess patient's and family's knowledge of drug therapy.

Nursing diagnoses
• Health-seeking behavior (prevention of pregnancy) related to family planning
• Acute pain related to drug-induced headache
• Deficient knowledge related to drug therapy

Planning and implementation
• Make sure patient has been properly instructed about prescribed hormonal contraceptive before she takes first dose.
ALERT: Make sure patient has negative pregnancy test before therapy starts.
• If patient develops granulomatous colitis, stop therapy and notify prescriber.
• Stop drug at least 1 week before surgery to decrease risk of thromboembolism. Tell patient to use other, nonhormonal birth control.
ALERT: Don't confuse Nortrel 7/7/7 with Nortrel 0.5/35 or Nortrel 1/35.
ALERT: Don't confuse Necon 7/7/7 with Nortrel 7/7/7.

Patient teaching
• Tell patient to take tablets at same time each day; nighttime doses may reduce nausea and headaches.
• Advise patient to use barrier birth control for first week of first cycle.
• Tell patient that missed doses in midcycle greatly increase likelihood of pregnancy.
• If one pill is missed, take pill as soon as possible; if remembered on the next day, take two pills, then continue regular dosage schedule. Use additional contraception for remainder of cycle.
• If two consecutive pills are missed, take two pills a day for next 2 days; then resume regular dosage schedule. Use additional contraception for the next 7 days or preferably for the remainder of cycle.
• If two consecutive pills are missed in the third week or if patient misses three consecutive pills, tell patient to contact prescriber for dosage instructions.

• Tell patient taking chewable tablets to chew tablet and follow with a full glass of water or to swallow whole.

• Warn patient that headache, nausea, dizziness, breast tenderness, spotting, and breakthrough bleeding are common at first. Effects will diminish after 3 to 6 months.

• If spotting or breakthrough bleeding with extended- or continuous-use pills lasts for longer than 7 consecutive days, tell patient to contact prescriber.

• Instruct patient to weigh herself at least twice weekly and to report sudden weight gain or edema to prescriber.

• Warn patient to avoid exposure to ultraviolet light or prolonged exposure to sunlight.

⚡ **ALERT:** Warn patient to immediately report abdominal pain; numbness, stiffness, or pain in legs or buttocks; pressure or pain in chest; shortness of breath; severe headache; visual disturbances, such as blind spots, blurriness, or flashing lights; undiagnosed vaginal bleeding or discharge; two consecutive missed menstrual periods; lumps in breast; swelling of hands or feet; or severe pain in abdomen.

• Advise patient that smoking while using hormonal contraceptives increases risks of thromboembolic events.

• Teach patient how to perform breast self-examination.

• If one menstrual period is missed and tablets have been taken on schedule, tell patient to continue taking them. If two consecutive menstrual periods are missed, tell patient to stop drug and have pregnancy test. Progestins may cause birth defects if taken early in pregnancy.

• Advise patient not to take same drug for longer than 12 months without consulting prescriber. Stress importance of Papanicolaou test and annual gynecologic examination.

• Advise patient to check with prescriber about how soon pregnancy may be attempted after hormonal therapy is stopped.

• Warn patient that she may not be able to become pregnant immediately after drug is stopped.

• Advise women on prolonged contraceptive therapy to stop drug and use other nonhormonal birth control. Periodically reassess patient while off hormone therapy.

☑ **Evaluation**
• Patient doesn't become pregnant.

• Patient obtains relief from drug-induced headache with administration of mild analgesic.

• Patient and family state understanding of drug therapy.

ethinyl estradiol and drospirenone
(ETH-ih-nill es-truh-DIGH-ol and droh-SPEER-ih-nohn)
Yasmin, YAZ

Pharmacologic class: hormonal contraceptive
Therapeutic class: estrogen and progestin
Pregnancy risk category: X

Indications and dosages

▶ **Contraception.** *Women and postpubertal girls:* 1 yellow tablet Yasmin P.O. for 21 consecutive days; then 1 white inert tablet on days 22 through 28 per menstrual cycle. Begin either on the first day of menstrual period (day 1 start) or on the first Sunday after menstruation starts (Sunday start).

◢ **NEW INDICATION: Premenstrual dysphoric disorder; contraception; moderate acne vulgaris.** *Women:* One light-pink tablet YAZ P.O. daily for 24 consecutive days followed by one white tablet P.O. for 4 consecutive days per menstrual cycle. Begin either on the first day of menstrual period (day 1 start) or on the first Sunday after menstruation starts (Sunday start).

Contraindications and cautions

• Contraindicated in women with hepatic dysfunction, tumor, or disease; renal or adrenal insufficiency; thrombophlebitis, thromboembolic disorders, or history of deep vein thrombosis or thromboembolic disorders; cerebrovascular or coronary artery disease; known or suspected breast cancer, endometrial cancer, or other estrogen-dependent neoplasia; unexplained vaginal bleeding; or cholestatic jaundice of pregnancy or jaundice with other contraceptive pill use. Also contraindicated in women older than age 35 who smoke 15 or more cigarettes daily.

• Use cautiously in patients with risk factors for CV disease, such as hypertension, hyperlipidemias, obesity, and diabetes.

☀ **Lifespan:** In women who are pregnant or suspect they may be pregnant, drug is contraindicated. In breast-feeding women, drug is con-

traindicated. In girls who haven't reached menarche, drug is contraindicated.

Adverse reactions

CNS: asthenia, depression, dizziness, emotional lability, headache, migraine, nervousness, **stroke.**
CV: edema, hypertension, **mesenteric thrombosis, MI, thromboembolism,** thrombophlebitis.
EENT: cataracts, intolerance to contact lenses, pharyngitis, retinal thrombosis, sinusitis, steepening of corneal curvature.
GI: abdominal cramping, abdominal pain, bloating, changes in appetite, colitis, diarrhea, gastroenteritis, nausea, vomiting.
GU: amenorrhea, breakthrough bleeding, change in cervical erosion and secretion, change in menstrual flow, cystitis, cystitis-like syndrome, dysmenorrhea, **hemolytic uremic syndrome,** leukorrhea, menstrual disorder, premenstrual syndrome, renal impairment, spotting, temporary infertility, UTI, vaginal candidiasis, vaginitis.
Hepatic: benign liver tumors, **Budd-Chiari syndrome,** cholestatic jaundice, gallbladder disease, **hepatic adenomas.**
Metabolic: porphyria, reduced tolerance to carbohydrates, weight gain.
Musculoskeletal: back pain.
Respiratory: bronchitis, **pulmonary embolism,** upper respiratory tract infection.
Skin: acne, **erythema multiforme,** erythema nodosum, hemorrhagic eruption, hirsutism, loss of scalp hair, melasma, pruritus, rash.
Other: breast changes, changes in libido, decreased lactation.

Interactions

Drug-drug. *ACE inhibitors, aldosterone antagonists, angiotensin II receptor antagonists, heparin, NSAIDs, potassium-sparing diuretics:* May increase risk of hyperkalemia. Monitor potassium level.
Acetaminophen: May decrease acetaminophen level. Adjust acetaminophen dosage as needed.
Ampicillin, griseofulvin, penicillins, tetracycline: May decrease contraceptive effect. Encourage use of additional birth control while taking the antibiotic.
Ascorbic acid, atorvastatin: May increase contraceptive level. Monitor patient for adverse effects.
Carbamazepine, phenobarbital, phenytoin: May increase metabolism of ethinyl estradiol and de-

crease contraceptive effectiveness. Encourage use of another form of birth control.
Clofibrate, morphine, salicylic acid, temazepam: May decrease levels and increase clearance of these drugs. Monitor effectiveness.
Cyclosporine, prednisolone, theophylline: May increase levels of these drugs. Monitor patient for adverse effects and toxicity.
Phenylbutazone, rifampin: May decrease contraceptive effectiveness and increase breakthrough bleeding. Encourage use of another form of birth control.
Drug-herb. *St. John's wort:* May decrease contraceptive effect and increase breakthrough bleeding. Encourage use of additional birth control, or discourage use together.
Drug-lifestyle. *Smoking:* May increase risk of CV adverse effects and thromboembolism. Warn patient to avoid smoking and tobacco products while taking hormonal contraceptives.

Effects on lab test results

• May increase circulating total thyroid hormone, triglyceride, other binding protein, sex hormone–binding globulin, total circulating endogenous sex steroid, corticoid, potassium, folate, liver enzyme, and clotting factors VII, VIII, IX, and X levels.
• May increase PT. May decrease glucose tolerance.

Pharmacokinetics

Absorption: Steady-state level occurs after 10 days for drospirenone and during second half of treatment cycle for ethinyl estradiol.
Distribution: Wide. Drospirenone is about 97% bound to nonspecific proteins. Ethinyl estradiol is about 98% bound to albumin and other nonspecific proteins.
Metabolism: Drospirenone is metabolized mainly by metabolites in plasma and to a minor extent in the liver by CYP3A4 to inactive metabolites. Ethinyl estradiol is mainly metabolized by hydroxylation and subject to presystemic conjugation in the small bowel and the liver.
Excretion: Small amounts of drospirenone unchanged in urine and feces. Ethinyl estradiol as metabolites in urine and feces. *Half-life:* drospirenone, 30 hours; ethinyl estradiol, 24 hours.

Route	Onset	Peak	Duration
P.O.	Unknown	1–3 hr	Unknown

Action

Chemical effect: Suppresses gonadotropins, follicle-stimulating hormone, and luteinizing hormone, thereby preventing ovulation, changing the cervical mucus to increase the difficulty of penetration by sperm and changing the endometrium to increase the difficulty of implantation.

Therapeutic effect: Reduces the opportunity for conception.

Available forms

Tablets: 21 yellow tablets containing 3 mg drospirenone and 30 mcg ethinyl estradiol, and 7 inert white tablets (Yasmin); 3 mg drospirenone and 20 mcg ethinyl estradiol (YAZ)

NURSING PROCESS

Assessment
- Determine if patient is pregnant before giving drug.
- Find out if the patient smokes, and investigate her medical history, CV health, and potassium level before starting therapy.
- Assess and be alert for adverse reactions. The use of contraceptives increases the risk of MI, thromboembolism, stroke, hepatic neoplasia, gallbladder disease, and hypertension, especially in patients with hypertension, diabetes, hyperlipidemia, and obesity.
- Monitor patient's laboratory results during drug therapy.
- Assess patient's and family's knowledge of contraception and drug therapy.

Nursing diagnoses
- Risk for injury related to drug-induced adverse reactions
- Health-seeking behavior for the prevention of pregnancy related to family planning
- Deficient knowledge of contraceptive drug therapy

Planning and implementation
- Because of the postpartum risk of thromboembolism, don't start drug earlier than 4 to 6 weeks after delivery.
- If patient misses two consecutive periods, tell her to obtain a negative pregnancy test result before continuing contraceptive. If pregnancy test is positive, tell her to immediately stop taking the drug.

- In patients scheduled to have elective surgery that may increase the risk of thromboembolism, stop contraceptive use from at least 4 weeks before until 2 weeks after surgery. Also avoid use during and after prolonged immobilization. Advise patient to use another form of birth control.
- Overdose may cause nausea and withdrawal bleeding. Monitor potassium and sodium levels, and watch for signs of metabolic acidosis.
- If loss of vision, proptosis, diplopia, papilledema, or retinal vascular lesions occur, stop use and evaluate patient. Recommend that contact lens wearers be evaluated by an ophthalmologist if they have changes in vision or lens intolerance.
- Evaluate patient who has unusual breakthrough bleeding for malignancy or pregnancy.
- If patient develops sharp or crushing chest pains, hemoptysis, sudden shortness of breath, calf pain, breast lumps, severe stomach pains, difficulty sleeping, weakness, fatigue, or jaundice, stop drug. Notify prescriber immediately and offer supportive treatment p.r.n.

Patient teaching
- Inform patient that pills are used to prevent pregnancy and don't protect against HIV and other sexually transmitted diseases.
- Advise patient of the dangers of smoking while taking hormonal contraceptives. Suggest that she choose a different form of birth control if she continues smoking.
- Tell patient to schedule yearly gynecologic examinations and perform monthly breast self-examinations.
- Inform patient that spotting, light bleeding, or stomach upset may occur during the first one to three packs of pills. Tell her to continue taking the pills and to notify prescriber if these symptoms persist.
- Tell patient to take the pill at the same time each day, preferably during the evening or at bedtime.
- Tell patient to immediately report sharp chest pain, coughing of blood, or sudden shortness of breath, pain in the calf, crushing chest pain or chest heaviness, sudden severe headache or vomiting, dizziness or fainting, visual or speech disturbances, weakness or numbness in an arm or leg, loss of vision, breast lumps, severe stomach pain or tenderness, difficulty sleeping, lack of energy, fatigue, change in mood, jaundice with fever, loss of appetite, dark urine, or light-colored bowel movements.

Reactions may be *common*, uncommon, *life-threatening*, or COMMON AND LIFE-THREATENING.

• Tell patient to notify prescriber if she wears contact lenses and notices a change in vision or has difficulty wearing the lenses.

• Advise patient to use additional birth control during the first 7 days of the first cycle of hormonal contraceptive.

• Tell patient that the risk of pregnancy increases with each active yellow tablet she forgets to take.

• If patient misses 1 tablet, tell her to take it as soon as she remembers and to take the next pill at the regular time.

• Tell patient to use additional birth control and notify prescriber if she isn't sure what to do about missed pills.

☑ Evaluation

• Patient doesn't suffer from any drug-induced adverse reactions.

• Patient doesn't become pregnant.

• Patient and family state understanding of drug therapy.

ethinyl estradiol and etonogestrel vaginal ring

(ETH-ih-nill es-truh-DIGH-ol and et-oh-noe-JESS-trel)
NuvaRing

Pharmacologic class: intravaginal hormonal contraceptive
Therapeutic class: progestin and estrogen
Pregnancy risk category: X

Indications and dosages

▶ **Contraception.** *Women:* Insert one ring vaginally, and leave in place for 3 weeks. Insert new ring exactly 1 week after the previous ring was removed, even if still menstruating.

Contraindications and cautions

• Contraindicated in patients hypersensitive to the drug or any of its components and in patients older than age 35 who smoke 15 or more cigarettes daily. Also contraindicated in patients with thrombophlebitis, thromboembolic disorder, history of deep vein thrombophlebitis, cerebral vascular or coronary artery disease (current or previous), valvular heart disease with complications, severe hypertension, diabetes with vascular complications, headache with focal neuro-

logic symptoms, major surgery with prolonged immobilization, known or suspected cancer of the endometrium or breast, estrogen-dependent neoplasia, abnormal undiagnosed vaginal bleeding, jaundice related to pregnancy or previous use of hormonal contraceptive, active liver disease, or benign or malignant hepatic tumors.

• Use cautiously in patients with hypertension, hyperlipidemias, obesity, diabetes, a condition that could be aggravated by fluid retention, a history of depression, or impaired liver function.

☀ **Lifespan:** In women who are or may be pregnant, drug is contraindicated. In breast-feeding women, drug isn't recommended; tell patient to use alternative forms of contraception until baby is weaned. In women who choose not to breast-feed, don't start drug earlier than 4 weeks after delivery. In girls who haven't reached menarche, drug is contraindicated. In postmenopausal women, don't use.

Adverse reactions

CNS: emotional lability, *headache.*
EENT: sinusitis.
GI: nausea.
GU: device-related events (such as foreign body sensation, coital difficulties, device expulsion), *leukorrhea,* vaginal discomfort, *vaginitis.*
Metabolic: weight gain.
Respiratory: upper respiratory tract infection.

Interactions

Drug-drug. *Acetaminophen, ascorbic acid, atorvastatin, itraconazole:* May increase ethinyl estradiol level. Monitor patient for adverse effects.
Ampicillin, barbiturates, carbamazepine, felbamate, griseofulvin, oxcarbazepine, phenylbutazone, phenytoin, rifampin, tetracyclines, topiramate: May decrease contraceptive effectiveness and increase risk of pregnancy, breakthrough bleeding, or both. Tell patient to use an additional form of contraception while taking these drugs.
Clofibric acid, morphine, salicylic acid, temazepam: May increase clearance of these drugs. Monitor patient for effectiveness.
Cyclosporine, prednisolone, theophylline: May increase levels of these drugs. Monitor cyclosporine and theophylline levels, and adjust dosages if needed.
Protease inhibitors: May increase or decrease the bioavailability of estrogen or progestin. Suggest other forms of birth control.

E

Drug-herb. *St. John's wort:* May reduce contraceptive effectiveness, increase risk of pregnancy, and increase risk of breakthrough bleeding. Discourage use together.

Drug-lifestyle. *Smoking:* May increase risk of serious CV side effects and thromboembolism, especially in women age 35 and older who smoke 15 or more cigarettes daily. Urge patient to quit smoking.

Effects on lab test results

• May increase prothrombin, thyroid-binding globulin (leading to increased circulating total thyroid hormone levels), other binding protein, sex hormone–binding globulin, triglyceride, lipoprotein, other lipid, and clotting factor VII, VIII, IX, and X levels. May decrease antithrombin III and folate levels.

• May increase norepinephrine-induced platelet aggregation. May decrease T_3 resin uptake and glucose tolerance.

Pharmacokinetics

Absorption: Rapid. Bioavailability of etonogestrel is 100% and ethinyl estradiol is 55.6%.
Distribution: Etonogestrel is 66% protein-bound and 32% bound to sex hormone–binding globulin. Ethinyl estradiol is about 98% nonspecific protein-bound and increases levels of sex hormone–binding globulin.
Metabolism: Both components of drug are metabolized in the liver by CYP3A4.
Excretion: Mainly in urine, bile, and feces. *Half-life:* ethinyl estradiol, 45 hours; etonogestrel, 29 hours.

Route	Onset	Peak	Duration
Vaginal	Immediate	Unknown	Unknown

Action

Chemical effect: Suppresses gonadotropins, which inhibits ovulation, increases the viscosity of cervical mucus (decreasing the ability of sperm to enter the uterus), and alters the endometrial lining (reducing potential for implantation).
Therapeutic effect: Decreases risk of pregnancy.

Available forms

Vaginal ring: Delivers 0.120 mg etonogestrel and 0.015 mg ethinyl estradiol daily

NURSING PROCESS

⚕ Assessment

• Assess patient for pregnancy before giving the drug.
• Find out if the patient smokes, and investigate her medical history, CV health, and risk factors before starting drug.
• Be alert for adverse reactions.
• Use of contraceptives increases the risk of MI, thromboembolism, stroke, hepatic neoplasia, gallbladder disease, and hypertension, especially in patients with hypertension, diabetes, hyperlipidemia, and obesity. Monitor patient for related signs and symptoms.
• Monitor patient's laboratory results during drug therapy.
• Assess patient's and family's knowledge of contraception and drug therapy.

⊕ Nursing diagnoses

• Risk for injury related to drug-induced adverse reactions
• Health-seeking behavior for the prevention of pregnancy related to family planning
• Deficient knowledge of contraceptive drug therapy

▷ Planning and implementation

• Stop drug at least 4 weeks before and for 2 weeks after procedures that may increase the risk of thromboembolism and during and after prolonged immobilization.
• If patient develops unexplained partial or complete loss of vision, proptosis, diplopia, papilledema, or retinal vascular lesions, stop drug.
• If patient has hypertension or renal disease, monitor blood pressure closely. If blood pressure rises, stop drug.
• If migraine begins or worsens or if patient has recurrent, persistent, or severe headaches, stop drug.
• If jaundice occurs, stop drug. The hormones may be poorly metabolized in patients with liver disease.
• If patient has persistent or severe abnormal menstrual bleeding, look for cause. If amenorrhea occurs, rule out pregnancy.
• If depression occurs, stop drug to determine whether depression is drug-related.
• If patient hasn't adhered to the prescribed regimen and a menstrual period is missed, if prescribed regimen is adhered to and two periods

are missed, or if the patient has retained the ring for longer than 4 weeks, rule out pregnancy.
• Overdose may cause nausea, vomiting, vaginal bleeding, or other menstrual irregularities. Offer supportive treatment.

Patient teaching
• Teach patient or provide patient with instructions for proper placement of vaginal ring. Also encourage proper handwashing before and after ring insertion to prevent vaginal infections.
• If the ring is removed or expelled (for example, while removing a tampon or moving the bowels), tell patient to wash with cool to lukewarm water and reinsert immediately. If the ring stays out for longer than 3 hours, contraceptive may not be effective. Recommend backup contraception until the reinserted ring is used continuously for 7 days.
• Emphasize the importance of having annual physical examinations to check for adverse effects or developing contraindications.
• Tell patient that drug doesn't protect against HIV and other sexually transmitted diseases.
• Advise patient not to smoke while using contraceptive.
• Tell patient not to use a diaphragm if backup birth control is needed.
• Tell patient who wears contact lenses to contact an ophthalmologist if vision or lens tolerance changes.

☑ Evaluation
• Patient doesn't suffer from any drug-induced adverse reactions or vaginal infections.
• Patient doesn't become pregnant.
• Patient and family state understanding of drug therapy.

ethinyl estradiol and norelgestromin transdermal system
(ETH-ih-nill es-truh-DIGH-ol and nor-el-GESS-troh-min)
Ortho Evra

Pharmacologic class: transdermal hormonal contraceptive
Therapeutic class: estrogen and progestin
Pregnancy risk category: X

Indications and dosages

▶ **Contraception.** *Women:* Apply one patch weekly for 3 weeks. Week 4 is patch-free. On the day after week 4 ends, apply a new patch to start a new 4-week cycle. Apply each new patch on the same day of the week.

Contraindications and cautions

• Contraindicated in patients hypersensitive to the drug or any of its components and in those with a history of deep vein thrombosis or related disorder; history of cerebrovascular or coronary artery disease; past or current known or suspected breast cancer, endometrial cancer, or other known or suspected estrogen-dependent neoplasia; hepatic adenoma or carcinoma; or known or suspected pregnancy. Also contraindicated in patients with thrombophlebitis, thromboembolic disorders, valvular heart disease with complications, severe hypertension, diabetes with vascular involvement, headaches with focal neurologic symptoms, major surgery with prolonged immobilization, undiagnosed abnormal genital bleeding, cholestatic jaundice of pregnancy or jaundice with previous hormonal contraceptive use, or acute or chronic hepatocellular disease with abnormal liver function.
• Use cautiously in patients with CV disease risk factors, with conditions that might be aggravated by fluid retention, or with a history of depression.
🜲 **Lifespan:** In breast-feeding women, safety and effectiveness haven't been established; advise another form of birth control. In girls who haven't reached menarche, safety and effectiveness haven't been evaluated; don't use.

Adverse reactions

CNS: cerebral hemorrhage, emotional lability, headache.
CV: edema, hypertension, *MI, thromboembolic events.*
EENT: contact lens intolerance.
GI: abdominal pain, nausea, vomiting.
GU: changes in menstrual flow, menstrual cramps, vaginal candidiasis.
Hepatic: benign liver tumors, gallbladder disease, *hepatic adenomas.*
Metabolic: weight changes.
Respiratory: upper respiratory tract infection.
Skin: application site reaction.
Other: breast tenderness, enlargement, or secretion.

E

Interactions

Drug-drug. *Acetaminophen, clofibric acid, morphine, salicylic acid, temazepam:* May decrease levels or increase clearance of these drugs. Monitor patient closely for lack of drug effect.
Ampicillin, barbiturates, carbamazepine, felbamate, griseofulvin, oxcarbazepine, phenylbutazone, phenytoin, rifampin, topiramate: May decrease contraceptive effectiveness, resulting in unintended pregnancy or breakthrough bleeding. If used together, encourage backup contraceptive.
Ascorbic acid, atorvastatin, itraconazole, ketoconazole: May increase hormone levels. Use together cautiously.
Cyclosporine, prednisolone, theophylline: May increase levels of these drugs. Monitor patient for adverse effects.
Protease inhibitors: May alter contraceptive effectiveness and safety. Use together cautiously.
Drug-herb. *St. John's wort:* May reduce contraceptive effectiveness and cause breakthrough bleeding. Discourage use together.
Drug-lifestyle. *Smoking:* May increase risk of serious CV side effects, especially in those older than age 35 who smoke 15 or more cigarettes daily. Urge patient to stop smoking.

Effects on lab test results

• May increase clotting factor VII, VIII, IX, and X; prothrombin; circulating total thyroid hormone; triglyceride; other binding protein; sex hormone–binding globulin; total circulating endogenous sex steroid; and corticoid levels. May decrease antithrombin III and folate levels.
• May decrease free T_3 resin uptake and glucose tolerance.

Pharmacokinetics

Absorption: Rapid. Maintained at a steady state while the patch is worn.
Distribution: Norelgestromin and norgestrel (a metabolite) are more than 97% protein-bound. Ethinyl estradiol is extensively bound to albumin.
Metabolism: In the liver.
Excretion: Norelgestromin and ethinyl estradiol are eliminated in 28 hours and 17 hours, respectively. The metabolites are eliminated in the

urine and feces. *Half-life:* 6 to 45 hours (ethinyl estradiol); 28 hours (norelgestromin).

Route	Onset	Peak	Duration
Transdermal	Rapid	2 days	Unknown

Action

Chemical effect: Suppresses gonadotropins and inhibits ovulation. Changes cervical mucus, complicating entry of sperm into the uterus, and changes endometrium, decreasing the likelihood of implantation.
Therapeutic effect: Reduces risk of pregnancy.

Available forms

Transdermal patch: norelgestromin 6 mg and ethinyl estradiol 0.75 mg (releases 150 mcg of norelgestromin and 20 mcg of ethinyl estradiol every 24 hours)

NURSING PROCESS

Assessment
• Rule out pregnancy before giving drug.
• Find out if the patient smokes, and investigate her medical history and CV health before starting drug.
• Be alert for any drug-induced adverse reactions.
• Monitor patient for adverse signs and symptoms related to contraceptive use: increased risk of MI, thromboembolism, stroke, hepatic neoplasia, gallbladder disease, and hypertension, especially in patients with hypertension, diabetes, hyperlipidemia, and obesity.
• Monitor patient's laboratory results during drug therapy.
• Assess patient's knowledge of contraception and drug therapy.

Nursing diagnoses
• Risk for injury related to drug-induced adverse reactions
• Health seeking behavior for the prevention of pregnancy related to family planning
• Deficient knowledge of contraceptive drug therapy

Planning and implementation
• Encourage women with a history of hypertension or renal disease to use a different contraceptive. If Ortho Evra is used, monitor blood

---

pressure closely; if hypertension occurs, stop use.
• Drug may be less effective in women weighing 90 kg (198 lb) or more.
• Cigarette smoking increases the risk of serious CV adverse effects. This risk increases especially in women age 35 and older who smoke 15 or more cigarettes per day.
• If used postpartum or postabortion, risk of thromboembolic disease increases.
• If breakthrough bleeding occurs for more than a few cycles, remove patch and assess cause.
• If no withdrawal bleeding occurs on patch-free week, resume on the next scheduled patch-change day. If withdrawal bleeding fails to occur for two consecutive cycles, rule out pregnancy.
• If skin becomes irritated, the patch may be removed and a new patch applied at a different site until the next patch-change day.
• Stop use at least 4 weeks before and for 2 weeks after elective surgery that increases risk of thromboembolism and during and after prolonged immobilization.
• If patient has vision loss, proptosis, diplopia, papilledema, retinal vascular lesions, or recurrent, persistent, or severe headaches, stop use.
• If jaundice occurs, stop use.
• If patient becomes severely depressed, stop use and evaluate whether the depression is drug related.

Patient teaching
• Emphasize the importance of having annual physical examinations to check for adverse effects or developing contraindications.
• Tell patient that the contraceptive patch doesn't protect against HIV and other sexually transmitted diseases.
• Advise patient to immediately apply a new patch once the used patch is removed, on the same day of the week, every 7 days for 3 weeks. Week 4 is patch-free. Tell patient to expect bleeding to occur during this time.
• Advise patient to start a new cycle, applying a new patch on the usual patch-change day, regardless of when the menstrual period starts or ends.
• Teach patient how to properly apply the patch.
• Tell patient to apply each patch to a new clean, dry area of the skin on the buttocks, abdomen, upper outer arm, or upper torso to avoid irritation. Tell patient not to apply to the breasts or to skin that's red, irritated, or cut. Instruct pa-

tient to avoid creams, oils, powder, or makeup on or near the skin where the patch will be placed because it may cause the patch to become loose.
• Tell patient what to do if a patch is partially or completely detached.
• Tell patient what to do if she forgets to change her patch.
• If patient wants to change her patch-change day, tell her to complete her current cycle and apply a new patch on the desired day during the patch-free week. There shouldn't be more than 7 consecutive patch-free days.
• Tell patient what to do if she misses a menstrual period.
• Tell patient to immediately stop drug if pregnancy is confirmed.
• Tell patient who wears contact lenses to contact an ophthalmologist if visual changes or changes in lens tolerance develop.
• Stress that if patient isn't sure what to do about mistakes with patch use, she should use backup birth control, such as a condom, spermicide, or diaphragm. She should contact her prescriber for further instructions.

☑ Evaluation
• Patient doesn't have any drug-induced adverse reactions.
• Patient doesn't become pregnant.
• Patient and family state understanding of drug therapy.

etodolac (ultradol)
(eh-toh-DOH-lak)
Lodine, Lodine XL

Pharmacologic class: NSAID
Therapeutic class: analgesic, antiarthritic
Pregnancy risk category: C (D in third trimester)

Indications and dosages

▶ **Acute pain.** *Adults:* 200 to 400 mg P.O. of film-coated tablets or capsules every 6 to 8 hours. Maximum dose is 1,200 mg daily.
▶ **Acute or long-term management of osteoarthritis or rheumatoid arthritis.** *Adults:* 600 to 1,000 mg P.O. daily of film-coated tablets or capsules in two divided doses. For extended-release tablets, usual dosage is 400 to

1,000 mg P.O. once daily. Maximum dose is 1,200 mg daily.

Contraindications and cautions

• Contraindicated in patients hypersensitive to the drug or any of its components and in those with history of aspirin- or NSAID-induced asthma, rhinitis, urticaria, or other allergic reactions.
• Use cautiously in patients with history of GI bleeding, ulceration, and perforation; in patients with renal or hepatic impairment, heart failure, hypertension, or cardiac function impairments; and in those predisposed to fluid retention.

⚕ **Lifespan:** In pregnant women during first and second trimesters, use cautiously. During third trimester, drug is contraindicated. In breast-feeding women, use cautiously because it's unknown if the drug appears in breast milk. In children younger than age 18, safety and effectiveness haven't been established.

Adverse reactions

CNS: *asthenia,* depression, *dizziness,* drowsiness, fever, headache, insomnia, *malaise,* nervousness, syncope.
CV: edema, fluid retention, flushing, ***heart failure,*** hypertension, palpitations.
EENT: blurred vision, dry mouth, photophobia, tinnitus.
GI: abdominal pain, anorexia, constipation, diarrhea, *dyspepsia,* flatulence, gastritis, ***GI bleeding,*** melena, nausea, peptic ulceration, ***perforation,*** thirst, ulcerative stomatitis, vomiting.
GU: dysuria, ***renal impairment,*** urinary frequency.
Hematologic: hemolytic anemia, ***leukopenia, thrombocytopenia, agranulocytosis.***
Hepatic: *hepatitis.*
Metabolic: weight gain.
Respiratory: *asthma.*
Skin: pruritus, rash, photosensitivity, ***Stevens-Johnson syndrome.***
Other: chills.

Interactions

Drug-drug. *ACE inhibitors, beta blockers, diuretics:* May blunt the effects of these drugs. Monitor patient closely.
Antacids: May decrease peak drug levels. Monitor patient for decreased etodolac effect.
Aspirin: May reduce protein-binding of etodolac without altering its clearance. Significance isn't known. Avoid use together.
Cyclosporine: May impair elimination and increase risk of nephrotoxicity. Avoid use together.
Digoxin, lithium, methotrexate: May impair elimination of these drugs, increasing levels and risk of toxicity. Monitor blood levels.
Phenytoin: May increase phenytoin level. Monitor patient and level for toxicity.
Warfarin: May decrease protein-binding of warfarin but doesn't alter clearance. Although no dosage adjustment is needed, monitor PT and INR closely, and watch for bleeding.
Drug-herb. *Dong quai, feverfew, garlic, ginger, horse chestnut, red clover:* May increase risk of bleeding. Discourage use together.
St. John's wort: May increase risk of photosensitivity. Discourage use together.
Drug-lifestyle. *Alcohol use:* May increase chance of adverse effects. Discourage use together.
Sun exposure: May cause photosensitivity reactions. Urge patient to avoid unprotected or prolonged exposure to sunlight.

Effects on lab test results

• May increase BUN and creatinine levels. May decrease uric acid and hemoglobin levels and hematocrit.
• May increase liver function test values. May decrease platelet, granulocyte, and WBC counts.
• May cause false-positive test for urinary bilirubin.

Pharmacokinetics

Absorption: Well absorbed from GI tract.
Distribution: To liver, lungs, heart, and kidneys.
Metabolism: Extensive.
Excretion: In urine, mainly as metabolites; 16% is excreted in feces. *Half-life:* 7¼ hours.

Route	Onset	Peak	Duration
P.O.	≤ 30 min	1–2 hr	4–12 hr

Action

Chemical effect: May inhibit prostaglandin synthesis.
Therapeutic effect: Relieves inflammation and pain.

Available forms

Capsules: 200 mg, 300 mg

Reactions may be *common,* uncommon, ***life-threatening,*** or COMMON AND LIFE-THREATENING.

Tablets (extended-release): 400 mg, 500 mg, 600 mg
Tablets (film-coated): 400 mg, 500 mg

NURSING PROCESS

🖅 Assessment
• Obtain history of patient's underlying condition before starting therapy.
• Be alert for adverse reactions and drug interactions.
• Assess patient's and family's knowledge of drug therapy.

🔅 Nursing diagnoses
• Acute pain related to underlying condition
• Risk for injury related to drug-induced adverse reactions
• Deficient knowledge related to drug therapy

▷ Planning and implementation
• Give drug with milk or meals to minimize GI discomfort.
• **ⓢ ALERT:** Don't confuse Lodine with codeine or iodine.
Patient teaching
• Advise patient that serious GI toxicity, including peptic ulceration and bleeding, can occur as a result of taking NSAIDs, despite absence of GI symptoms. Teach patient the signs and symptoms of GI bleeding, such as dark tarry stools, generalized weakness, and coffee-ground emesis, and tell him to contact prescriber immediately if they occur.
• Tell patient to take drug with milk or food.
• Instruct patient to notify prescriber if other adverse reactions occur or if drug doesn't relieve pain.
• Advise patient to use sunblock, wear protective clothing, and avoid prolonged exposure to sunlight to prevent photosensitivity reactions.
• Tell patient not to use drug during last trimester of pregnancy.
• Advise patients taking long-term NSAIDs to have periodic CBC and liver and renal function tests.

✓ Evaluation
• Patient is free from pain.
• Patient has no injury as result of drug-induced adverse reactions.
• Patient and family state understanding of drug therapy.

HIGH ALERT!

etoposide (VP-16)
(eh-toh-POH-sighd)
Etopophos, Toposar, VePesid

E

Pharmacologic class: podophyllotoxin
Therapeutic class: antineoplastic
Pregnancy risk category: D

Indications and dosages

▶ **Testicular cancer.** *Adults:* 50 to 100 mg/m^2 I.V. on 5 consecutive days every 3 to 4 weeks; or 100 mg/m^2 on days 1, 3, and 5 every 3 to 4 weeks for three to four courses of therapy.
▶ **Small-cell carcinoma of lung.** *Adults:* 35 mg/m^2/day I.V. for 4 days; or 50 mg/m^2/day I.V. for 5 days. P.O. dose is two times I.V. dose rounded to nearest 50 mg.
▶ **AIDS-related Kaposi sarcoma‡.** *Adults:* 150 mg/m^2 I.V. for 3 consecutive days every 4 weeks. Repeat cycles as needed.

▽ I.V. administration

• Keep diphenhydramine, hydrocortisone, epinephrine, and needed emergency equipment available to establish airway in case of anaphylaxis.
• Don't give drug through membrane-type in-line filter because diluent may dissolve filter.
• Dilute drug for infusion in either D$_5$W or normal saline solution to 0.2 or 0.4 mg/ml. Higher concentrations may crystallize.
• Give drug by slow I.V. infusion (over at least 30 minutes) to prevent severe hypotension.
• If systolic blood pressure falls below 90 mm Hg, stop infusion and notify prescriber.
• Solutions diluted to 0.2 mg/ml are stable 96 hours at room temperature in plastic or glass unprotected from light; solutions diluted to 0.4 mg/ml are stable 48 hours under same conditions.
⊗ **Incompatibilities**
Cefepime hydrochloride, filgrastim, gallium nitrate, idarubicin.

Contraindications and cautions

• Contraindicated in patients hypersensitive to the drug or any of its components.
• Use cautiously in patients who have had cytotoxic or radiation therapy.
⚕ **Lifespan:** In pregnant women, use cautiously and only when benefits outweigh risks to fe-

---

tus. In breast-feeding women, drug is contraindicated. In children, safety and effectiveness haven't been established.

Adverse reactions

CNS: peripheral neuropathy.
CV: hypotension.
GI: abdominal pain, anorexia, diarrhea, nausea, stomatitis, vomiting.
Hematologic: anemia, LEUKOPENIA, *myelosuppression* (dose-limiting), THROMBOCYTOPENIA.
Skin: reversible alopecia.
Other: *anaphylaxis,* rash.

Interactions

Drug-drug. *Warfarin:* May further prolong PT. Monitor patient for bleeding, and monitor PT and INR.

Effects on lab test results

• May decrease hemoglobin level and hematocrit.
• May decrease WBC, RBC, platelet, and neutrophil counts.

Pharmacokinetics

Absorption: Moderate across GI tract after P.O. use. Bioavailability ranges from 25% to 75%, with average of 50% of dose being absorbed.
Distribution: Wide in body tissues. Crosses blood–brain barrier to limited and variable extent. About 94% protein-bound.
Metabolism: Only small portion of dose is metabolized in liver.
Excretion: Mainly in urine as unchanged drug; smaller amount in feces. *Half-life:* Initial, 30 minutes to 2 hours; terminal, 5¼ to 11 hours.

Route	Onset	Peak	Duration
P.O., I.V.	Unknown	Unknown	Unknown

Action

Chemical effect: Unknown.
Therapeutic effect: Inhibits selected cancer cell growth.

Available forms

Capsules: 50 mg
Injection: 20 mg/ml
Powder for injection: 100 mg

NURSING PROCESS

✍ Assessment
• Obtain history of patient's underlying condition before starting therapy.
• Obtain baseline blood pressure before therapy, and monitor blood pressure at 30-minute intervals during infusion.
• Monitor effectiveness by noting results of follow-up diagnostic tests and overall physical health and by regularly checking tumor size and rate of growth through appropriate studies. Etoposide has produced complete remission in small-cell lung cancer and testicular cancer.
• Monitor CBC. Observe patient for signs of bone marrow suppression.
• Be alert for adverse reactions and drug interactions.
• Assess patient's and family's knowledge of drug therapy.

⊕ Nursing diagnoses
• Ineffective health maintenance related to presence of neoplastic disease
• Ineffective protection related to drug induced adverse hematologic reactions
• Deficient knowledge related to drug therapy

▶ Planning and implementation
• Follow facility policy to reduce risks. Preparation and administration of parenteral form creates carcinogenic, mutagenic, and teratogenic risks for staff.
• Store capsules in refrigerator.
Patient teaching
• Warn patient to watch for signs of infection and bleeding. Teach patient how to take infection-control and bleeding precautions.
• Tell patient that reversible hair loss may occur.
• Instruct patient to report discomfort, pain, or burning at I.V. insertion site.

✓ Evaluation
• Patient exhibits positive response to therapy.
• Patient's immune function returns to normal when therapy stops.
• Patient and family state understanding of drug therapy.

E

```
HIGH ALERT!
```

exemestane

(ecks-eh-MES-tayn)
Aromasin

Pharmacologic class: aromatase inhibitor
Therapeutic class: antineoplastic
Pregnancy risk category: D

Indications and dosages

▶ **Advanced breast cancer in postmenopausal women whose disease has progressed
after tamoxifen therapy.** *Women:* 25 mg P.O.
once daily after a meal.
▶ **Adjuvant treatment of postmenopausal
women with estrogen-receptor–positive early
breast cancer after 2 to 3 years of tamoxifen
therapy, to complete 5 consecutive years of
adjuvant hormonal therapy.** *Women:* 25 mg
P.O. once daily after a meal.
▶ **Prevention of prostate cancer.** *Men:* 25 mg
P.O. once daily after a meal.

Contraindications and cautions

• Contraindicated in patients hypersensitive to
drug or any of its components.
⚠ **Lifespan:** In premenopausal women, drug is
contraindicated.

Adverse reactions

CNS: *anxiety,* asthenia, confusion, *depression,*
dizziness, *fatigue, fever,* generalized weakness,
headache, hypoesthesia, *insomnia, pain,* pares-
thesia.
CV: chest pain, edema, *hot flashes,* hypertension.
EENT: pharyngitis, rhinitis, sinusitis.
GI: abdominal pain, anorexia, constipation, di-
arrhea, dyspepsia, nausea, vomiting.
GU: UTI.
Metabolic: increased appetite.
Musculoskeletal: *arthralgia,* back pain, patho-
logic fractures, skeletal pain.
Respiratory: bronchitis, coughing, *dyspnea,*
upper respiratory tract infection.
Skin: *alopecia,* dermatitis, *increased sweating,*
itching, rash.
Other: flulike symptoms, infection, lymph-
edema.

Interactions

Drug-drug. *CYP3A4 inducers, such as phenytoin and rifampicin:* May reduce therapeutic ef-

fects of exemestane; increase dose to 50 mg
once daily.
Drugs that contain estrogen: May interact.
Don't give together.
Drug-herb. *St. John's wort:* May decrease ef-
fectiveness of drug. Discourage use together.

Effects on lab test results

• May increase bilirubin, alkaline phosphatase,
and creatinine levels.

Pharmacokinetics

Absorption: Rapid, with about 42% of dose absorbed from the GI tract after P.O. use. Level increases by 40% after a high-fat meal.
Distribution: Extensive in tissues. 90% protein-
bound.
Metabolism: Extensive by the liver. Main liver
isoenzyme is CYP3A4.
Excretion: Equal in urine and feces. *Half-life:*
24 hours.

Route	Onset	Peak	Duration
P.O.	Unknown	1–2 hr	Unknown

Action

Chemical effect: Acts as a false substrate for
the aromatase enzyme, the principal enzyme
that converts androgens to estrogens in premenopausal and postmenopausal women. Results in lower levels of circulating estrogens.
Therapeutic effect: Hinders growth of
estrogen-dependent breast cancer cells.

Available forms

Tablets: 25 mg

```
NURSING PROCESS
```

⚕ Assessment
• Assess patient's breast cancer before starting
therapy and regularly thereafter.
• Monitor patient for adverse reactions.
• If adverse GI reactions occur, monitor pa-
tient's hydration.
• Assess patient's and family's knowledge of
drug therapy.

⊕ Nursing diagnoses
• Ineffective health maintenance related to presence of breast cancer

- Impaired physical mobility related to potential adverse musculoskeletal effects
- Deficient knowledge related to drug therapy

▶ Planning and implementation
- Give drug only to postmenopausal women.
- Don't give with drugs that contain estrogen because doing so could interfere with intended action.
- Continue treatment in patients with advanced breast cancer until tumor progression is evident.
- Patients with early breast cancer who have taken tamoxifen for 2 to 3 years should take exemestane to complete the 5-year course, unless cancer reoccurs or is found in the other breast.
- **⑤ ALERT:** Don't confuse exemestane with estramustine.

Patient teaching
- Tell patient to take drug after a meal.
- Inform patient that she may need to take drug for a long period.
- Advise patient to report adverse effects to prescriber.

☑ Evaluation
- Patient responds well to drug.
- Patient has no musculoskeletal adverse reactions.
- Patient and family state understanding of drug therapy.

HIGH ALERT!

exenatide
(ecks-EHN-uh-tighd)
Byetta

Pharmacologic class: incretin mimetic
Therapeutic class: antidiabetic
Pregnancy risk category: C

Indications and dosages

▶ **Adjunctive therapy to improve glycemic control in patients with type 2 diabetes who take metformin, a sulfonylurea, a thiazolidinedione, or a combination of metformin and a sulfonylurea or a thiazolidinedione, but haven't achieved adequate glycemic control.**
Adults: 5 mcg subcutaneously b.i.d. within 60 minutes before morning and evening meals (or before the two main meals of the day, about 6 hours or more apart). Increase to 10 mcg b.i.d. after 1 month, as needed.

Contraindications and cautions

- Contraindicated in patients hypersensitive to drug or its components. Don't give to patients with type 1 diabetes or diabetic ketoacidosis. Avoid in patients with end-stage renal disease, creatinine clearance less than 30 ml/minute, or severe GI disease.
- **⚠ Lifespan:** In pregnant women, use only if benefits justify risks to the fetus. In breast-feeding women, use cautiously because it isn't known if drug appears in breast milk. In children, safety and effectiveness haven't been established.

Adverse reactions

CNS: dizziness, headache, jittery feeling.
GI: diarrhea, dyspepsia, nausea, vomiting.
Metabolic: *hypoglycemia.*
Skin: excessive sweating.
Other: injection site reaction.

Interactions

Drug-drug. *Drugs that are rapidly absorbed:* May slow gastric emptying and reduce absorption of some oral drugs. Use cautiously together. *Oral drugs that need to maintain a threshold level to maintain effectiveness (antibiotics, hormonal contraceptives):* May reduce rate and extent of absorption of these drugs. Give these drugs at least 1 hour before giving exenatide. *Sulfonylureas:* May increase the risk of hypoglycemia. Reduce sulfonylurea dose, as needed, and monitor patient closely.

Effects on lab test results

None reported.

Pharmacokinetics

Absorption: Peaks in plasma in about 2 hours.
Distribution: Volume of about 28.3 L after a single dose.
Metabolism: Not metabolized.
Excretion: Mainly by glomerular filtration.
Half-life: About 2½ hours.

Route	Onset	Peak	Duration
SubQ	Unknown	2 hr	10 hr

Action

Chemical effect: Reduces fasting and postprandial glucose levels in type 2 diabetes by stimulating insulin production in response to elevated

glucose levels, inhibiting glucagon release after meals and slowing gastric emptying.
Therapeutic effect: Lowers glucose level.

Available forms

Injection: 5 mcg/dose in 1.2-ml prefilled pen, 10 mcg/dose in 2.4-ml prefilled pen (60 doses)

NURSING PROCESS

🜛 Assessment
• Assess GI function before treatment starts.
• Monitor blood glucose level regularly and glycosylated hemoglobin level periodically.
• Monitor patient for adverse reactions and drug interactions.
• Assess patient's and family's knowledge of drug therapy.

🜯 Nursing diagnoses
• Risk for injury related to drug-induced hypoglycemia
• Ineffective health maintenance related to hyperglycemia
• Deficient knowledge related to drug therapy

▶ Planning and implementation
• Drug comes in two strengths; check cartridge carefully before use.
• Overdose may cause rapid decline in blood glucose levels, leading to severe nausea and vomiting, tachycardia, restlessness, and dizziness.
• Provide symptomatic care for hypoglycemia. If patient is responsive, give fast-acting oral carbohydrate. If unresponsive, give I.V. glucose.
• ⚠ **ALERT:** Monitor patient for unexplained, persistent, severe abdominal pain, with or without vomiting. Stop drug if pancreatitis is suspected and don't restart if pancreatitis is confirmed or no other cause is found.
• Drug may be stored at room temperatures between 36° to 77° F (2° to 15° C) after first use.
• ⚠ **ALERT:** Don't confuse exenatide (Byetta) with ezetimibe (Zetia).

Patient teaching
• Explain the risks of exenatide.
• Review proper use and storage of dosage pen, particularly the one-time setup for each new pen.

• Inform patient that prefilled pen doesn't include a needle; explain which needle length and gauge is appropriate.
• Instruct patient to inject drug in the thigh, abdomen, or upper arm within 60 minutes before morning and evening meals. Caution against injecting drug after a meal.
• Advise patient that drug may decrease appetite, food intake, and body weight and that these changes don't warrant a change in dosage.
• Review steps for managing hypoglycemia, especially if patient takes a sulfonylurea.
• Advise patient to immediately seek medical care if they have persistent, severe abdominal pain, with or without vomiting.
• Stress importance of proper storage (refrigerated), infection prevention, and timing of exenatide dose in relation to other oral drugs.

✔ Evaluation
• Patient sustains no injury.
• Patient's glucose level is normal with drug therapy.
• Patient and family state understanding of drug therapy.

ezetimibe
(eh-ZET-eh-mighb)
Zetia⬩

Pharmacologic class: selective cholesterol absorption inhibitor
Therapeutic class: antilipemic
Pregnancy risk category: C

Indications and dosages

▶ **Primary hypercholesterolemia, alone or with HMG-CoA reductase inhibitors; adjunct to atorvastatin or simvastatin in patients with homozygous familial hypercholesterolemia; homozygous sitosterolemia to reduce sitosterol and campesterol levels.**
Adults: 10 mg P.O. daily.
▶ **Adjunct to fenofibrate and diet to reduce elevated total-C, LDL-C, Apo B and non-HDL-C in patients with mixed hyperlipidemia.** *Adults:* 10 mg P.O. once daily with or without food, taken at the same time as fenofibrate.

Contraindications and cautions

- Contraindicated in patients allergic to any component of the drug. Use with a HMG-CoA reductase inhibitor is contraindicated in patients with active hepatic disease or unexplained increase in transaminase levels.

☀ **Lifespan:** In pregnant women, use only if benefits outweigh risks to fetus. If used in pregnant women, don't give with an HMG-CoA reductase inhibitor. In breast-feeding women, use cautiously because it's unknown if drug appears in breast milk. In children, safety and effectiveness haven't been established. In elderly patients, use cautiously because they may have a greater sensitivity to drug.

Adverse reactions

CNS: dizziness, fatigue, headache.
CV: chest pain.
EENT: pharyngitis, sinusitis.
GI: abdominal pain, diarrhea.
Musculoskeletal: arthralgia, back pain, myalgia.
Respiratory: cough, upper respiratory tract infection.
Other: viral infection.

Interactions

Drug-drug. *Aluminum/magnesium antacids, bile acid sequestrant (cholestyramine):* May decrease ezetimibe level. Give ezetimibe at least 2 hours before or 4 hours after cholestyramine.
Cyclosporine, fenofibrate, gemfibrozil: May increase ezetimibe level. Monitor patient closely for adverse effects.
Fibrates: May increase excretion of cholesterol into gallbladder bile. Avoid use together.

Effects on lab test results

- May increase liver function test values.

Pharmacokinetics

Absorption: Absorbed and conjugated to an active metabolite.
Distribution: More than 90% protein-bound.
Metabolism: Mainly and rapidly in the small intestine and liver via glucuronide conjugation.
Excretion: Biliary and renal. *Half-life:* 22 hours.

Route	Onset	Peak	Duration
P.O.	Unknown	4–12 hr	Unknown

Action

Chemical effect: Inhibits absorption of cholesterol by the small intestine. Decreases hepatic cholesterol stores and increases cholesterol clearance.
Therapeutic effect: Lowers cholesterol levels.

Available forms

Tablets: 10 mg

NURSING PROCESS

▣ Assessment

- Obtain history of patient's underlying condition before starting therapy.
- Monitor total cholesterol, LDL, HDL, and triglyceride levels before and during therapy.
- Assess patient's and family's knowledge of drug therapy.

⊕ Nursing diagnoses

- Risk for injury related to elevated cholesterol levels
- Deficient knowledge related to drug therapy

▶ Planning and implementation

- Use drug only after diet and other nondrug therapy prove ineffective. Have patient follow a standard low-cholesterol diet before and during therapy.
- Before starting drug, evaluate patient for secondary causes of dyslipidemia.
- When drug is used with an HMG-CoA reductase inhibitor, check liver function test results at start of therapy and thereafter according to facility policy.
- Use with an HMG-CoA reductase inhibitor significantly reduces total cholesterol, LDL, apolipoprotein B, and triglyceride levels and (except with pravastatin) increases HDL level more than use of an HMG-CoA reductase inhibitor alone.

⊛ **ALERT:** Don't confuse Zetia with Zebeta, Zestril, or Zyrtec.

Patient teaching
- Emphasize importance of following a cholesterol-lowering diet.
- Tell patient he may take drug without regard to meals.
- Advise patient to notify prescriber of unexplained muscle pain, weakness, or tenderness.
- Urge patient to tell prescriber if he's taking herbal or dietary supplements.

Reactions may be *common*, uncommon, *life-threatening*, or COMMON AND LIFE-THREATENING.

- Advise patient to visit his prescriber for routine follow-up and blood tests.
- Tell patient to notify prescriber if she becomes pregnant.

☑ **Evaluation**
- Patient's cholesterol level is within normal limits.
- Patient and family state understanding of drug therapy.

famciclovir
(fam-SIGH-kloh-veer)
Famvir

Pharmacologic class: synthetic acyclic guanine derivative
Therapeutic class: antiviral
Pregnancy risk category: B

Indications and dosages

▶ **Acute herpes zoster.** *Adults:* 500 mg P.O. every 8 hours for 7 days.
▷ **Adjust-a-dose:** For patients with renal impairment, if creatinine clearance is 40 to 59 ml/minute, give 500 mg every 12 hours. If clearance is 20 to 39 ml/minute, give 500 mg every 24 hours. If clearance is less than 20 ml/minute, give 250 mg every 24 hours.
▶ **Recurrent genital herpes.** *Adults:* 1,000 mg P.O. b.i.d. for a single day. Start therapy at the first sign or symptom.
▷ **Adjust-a-dose:** If creatinine clearance is 40 to 59 ml/minute, give 500 mg every 12 hours for 1 day. If clearance is 20 to 39 ml/minute, give 500 mg P.O. as a single dose. If clearance is less than 20 ml/minute, give 250 mg as a single dose. If patient is undergoing hemodialysis, give 250 mg as a single dose after dialysis session.
▶ **Long-term suppressive therapy of recurrent episodes of genital herpes.** *Adults:* 250 mg P.O. b.i.d. for up to 1 year.
▷ **Adjust-a-dose:** If creatinine clearance is 20 to 39 ml/minute, give 125 mg every 12 hours. If clearance is less than 20 ml/minute, give 125 mg every 24 hours.

▶ **Recurrent herpes labialis (cold sores).**
Adults: 1,500 mg P.O. for one dose. Give at the first sign or symptom of cold sore.
▷ **Adjust-a-dose:** If creatinine clearance is 40 to 59 ml/minute, give 750 mg as a single dose. If clearance is 20 to 39 ml/minute, give 500 mg P.O. as a single dose. If clearance is less than 20 ml/minute, give 250 mg as a single dose. If patient is undergoing hemodialysis, give 250 mg as a single dose after dialysis session.
▶ **Recurrent herpes simplex virus infections in HIV-infected patients.** *Adults:* 500 mg P.O. b.i.d. for 7 days.
▷ **Adjust-a-dose:** If creatinine clearance is 20 to 39 ml/minute, give 500 mg every 24 hours. If clearance is less than 20 ml/minute, give 250 mg every 24 hours.

Contraindications and cautions

- Contraindicated in patients hypersensitive to drug or any of its components.
- Use cautiously in patients with renal or hepatic impairment. Dosage adjustment may be needed.
≉ **Lifespan:** In pregnant women, use only if benefits outweigh risks to fetus. In breast-feeding women, use cautiously because it's unknown if drug appears in breast milk. In men, use cautiously because of risk of decreased fertility. In children, safety and effectiveness haven't been established.

Adverse reactions

CNS: dizziness, fatigue, *headache,* paresthesia, somnolence.
EENT: pharyngitis, sinusitis.
GI: abdominal pain, anorexia, constipation, diarrhea, *nausea,* vomiting.
Musculoskeletal: arthralgia, back pain.
Skin: pruritus; zoster-related signs, symptoms, and complications.

Interactions

Drug-drug. *Probenecid:* May increase level of famciclovir. Monitor patient for increased adverse effects.

Effects on lab test results

- May increase AST, ALT, total bilirubin, creatinine, amylase, and lipase levels. May decrease hemoglobin level and hematocrit.
- May decrease WBC and neutrophil counts.

Pharmacokinetics

Absorption: Absolute bioavailability is 77%.
Distribution: Less than 20% protein-bound.
Metabolism: Extensive, in liver to active drug, penciclovir, and inactive metabolites.
Excretion: Mainly in urine. *Half-life:* 2 to 3 hours.

Route	Onset	Peak	Duration
P.O.	Unknown	≤ 1 hr	Unknown

Action

Chemical effect: Converted to penciclovir, which enters viral cells and inhibits DNA polymerase and viral DNA synthesis.
Therapeutic effect: Inhibits viral replication. Spectrum of activity includes herpes simplex types 1 and 2 and varicella zoster viruses.

Available forms

Tablets: 125 mg, 250 mg, 500 mg

NURSING PROCESS

℞ Assessment

• Assess patient's viral infection before starting therapy, and reassess regularly throughout therapy.
• Be alert for adverse reactions and drug interactions.
• If adverse GI reactions occur, monitor patient's hydration.
• Assess patient's and family's knowledge of drug therapy.

⊕ Nursing diagnoses

• Risk for infection related to presence of virus susceptible to famciclovir
• Risk for deficient fluid volume related to drug's adverse GI reactions
• Deficient knowledge related to drug therapy

▷ Planning and implementation

• Give a lower dose in patients with renal insufficiency.
• Drug may be taken with or without food.
Patient teaching
• Teach patient how to prevent spread of infection to others.
• Urge patient to recognize and report early symptoms of herpes infection, such as tingling, itching, or pain.

☑ Evaluation

• Patient is free from infection.
• Patient maintains adequate hydration.
• Patient and family state understanding of drug therapy.

famotidine

(fam-OH-tih-deen)
Acid Control Pepcid ♦ †, Pepcid†⊘, Pepcid AC†, Pepcid RPD, Ulcidine ♦

Pharmacologic class: H_2-receptor antagonist
Therapeutic class: antisecretory
Pregnancy risk category: B

Indications and dosages

▶ **Duodenal ulcer (short-term therapy).**
Adults: For acute therapy, 40 mg P.O. once daily at bedtime or 20 mg P.O. b.i.d. Maintenance, 20 mg P.O. once daily at bedtime.
▶ **Benign gastric ulcer (short-term therapy).**
Adults: 40 mg P.O. daily at bedtime for 8 weeks.
▶ **Pathologic hypersecretory conditions (such as Zollinger-Ellison syndrome).** *Adults:* 20 mg P.O. every 6 hours, up to 160 mg every 6 hours.
▶ **Gastroesophageal reflux disease (GERD).**
Adults: 20 mg P.O. b.i.d. for up to 6 weeks. For esophagitis caused by GERD, 20 to 40 mg b.i.d. for up to 12 weeks.
Children ages 1 to 16: Give 1 mg/kg/day P.O. in divided doses b.i.d. up to 80 mg daily.
▶ **Peptic ulcer in children.** *Children ages 1 to 16:* Give 0.5 mg/kg/day P.O. at bedtime or divided b.i.d. up to 40 mg daily.
▶ **Heartburn, prevention of heartburn.**
Adults: 10 mg Pepcid AC P.O. 15 to 60 minutes before meals (prevention) or 10 mg Pepcid AC P.O. with water when symptoms occur. Maximum, 20 mg daily. Drug shouldn't be taken daily for longer than 2 weeks without prescriber authorization.
▶ **Hospitalized patients with intractable ulcerations or hypersecretory conditions or patients who can't take oral drugs.** *Adults:* 20 mg I.V. every 12 hours.
Children ages 1 to 16: Give 0.25 mg/kg I.V. every 12 hours, up to 40 mg daily.
▧ **Adjust-a-dose:** If creatinine clearance is less than 50 ml/minute (moderate renal impairment)

---

or less than 10 ml/minute (severe renal impairment) dose may be reduced to half-strength or interval prolonged to 36 to 48 hours, if needed, to avoid excess drug accumulation.

▼I.V. administration

• For I.V. injection, dilute 2 ml (20 mg) with compatible I.V. solution to total volume of either 5 or 10 ml. Compatible solutions include sterile water for injection, normal saline injection, D₅W or dextrose 10% in water injection, 5% sodium bicarbonate injection, and lactated Ringer's injection. Inject over at least 2 minutes.
• For intermittent I.V. infusion, dilute 20 mg (2 ml) drug in 100 ml of compatible solution. Solution is stable for 48 hours at room temperature after dilution. Infuse over 15 to 30 minutes.
• If infiltration or phlebitis occurs, apply warm compresses and use different site for next dose.
• Store premixed injection at room temperature. Store unmixed injection in refrigerator at 36° to 46° F (2° to 8° C).
⊗ **Incompatibilities**
Amphotericin B cholesterol complex, azithromycin, cefepime, piperacillin with tazobactam.

Contraindications and cautions

• Contraindicated in patients hypersensitive to drug or any of its components. Injection may contain benzyl alcohol as a preservative; some preparations contain phenylalanine.
⚖ Lifespan: In pregnant women, use cautiously. In breast-feeding women, use cautiously because it isn't known if the drug appears in breast milk. In children younger than 1 year old, drug is contraindicated.

Adverse reactions

CNS: dizziness, fever, *headache,* malaise, paresthesia, vertigo.
CV: flushing, palpitations.
EENT: orbital edema, tinnitus.
GI: anorexia, constipation, diarrhea, dry mouth, taste disorder.
Musculoskeletal: musculoskeletal pain.
Skin: acne, dry skin.
Other: transient irritation at I.V. site.

Interactions

None significant.

Effects on lab test results

• May increase BUN, creatinine, and liver enzyme levels.

Pharmacokinetics

Absorption: 40% to 45%.
Distribution: Wide.
Metabolism: 30% to 35% by liver.
Excretion: Mostly unchanged in urine. *Half-life:* 2½ to 3½ hours.

Route	Onset	Peak	Duration
P.O.	≤1 hr	1–3 hr	10–12 hr
I.V.	≤1 hr	20 min	10–12 hr

Action

Chemical effect: Competitively inhibits action of H₂ at receptor sites of parietal cells, decreasing gastric acid secretion.
Therapeutic effect: Decreases gastric acid levels and prevents heartburn.

Available forms

Gelcaps: 10 mg
Injection: 10 mg/ml, 20 mg/50 ml (premixed)
Powder for oral suspension: 40 mg/5 ml after reconstitution
Tablets: 10 mg†, 20 mg, 40 mg
Tablets (chewable): 10 mg†
Tablets (orally-disintegrating): 20 mg, 40 mg

NURSING PROCESS

▣ Assessment
• Assess creatinine clearance before treatment.
• Assess patient's GI disorder before starting therapy and reassess regularly.
• Be alert for adverse reactions.
• Determine if patient has phenylalanine sensitivity.
• Assess patient's and family's knowledge of drug therapy.

⊕ Nursing diagnoses
• Impaired tissue integrity related to underlying GI disorder
• Deficient knowledge related to drug therapy

▶ Planning and implementation
• Give daily doses or last dose of the day at bedtime.
• Store reconstituted oral suspension below 86° F (30° C). Discard after 30 days.

Patient teaching
- Tell patient to take drug with food. Remind him that drug is most effective if taken at bedtime. Tell patient taking 20 mg b.i.d. to take one dose at bedtime.
- With prescriber's knowledge, allow patient to take antacids, especially at beginning of therapy when pain is severe.
- Urge patient not to smoke because it may increase gastric acid secretion and worsen disease.
- Advise patient not to take drug for longer than 8 weeks unless specifically ordered by prescriber. Tell patient not to self-medicate for heartburn longer than 2 weeks without prescriber's knowledge.

✅ Evaluation
- Patient reports decrease in or relief of GI pain with drug.
- Patient and family state understanding of drug therapy.

felodipine
(feh-LOH-dih-peen)
Plendil, Renedil ◆

Pharmacologic class: calcium channel blocker
Therapeutic class: antihypertensive
Pregnancy risk category: C

Indications and dosages

▶ **Hypertension.** *Adults:* Initially, 5 mg P.O. daily. Adjust dosage based on response, usually at no less than 2-week intervals. Usual dosage is 2.5 to 10 mg daily.
Elderly patients: 2.5 mg P.O. daily; adjust as for adults. Maximum, 10 mg daily.

Contraindications and cautions

- Contraindicated in patients hypersensitive to drug or any of its components.
- Use cautiously in patients with heart failure, particularly those receiving beta blockers, and in patients with impaired hepatic function.
- ⚠ **Lifespan:** In pregnant and breast-feeding women, use cautiously. In children, safety and effectiveness haven't been established.

Adverse reactions

CNS: asthenia, dizziness, *headache,* paresthesia.

CV: chest pain, *flushing,* palpitations, *peripheral edema.*
EENT: gingival hyperplasia, rhinorrhea, pharyngitis.
GI: abdominal pain, constipation, diarrhea, nausea.
Musculoskeletal: back pain, muscle cramps.
Respiratory: cough, upper respiratory infection.
Skin: rash.

Interactions

Drug-drug. *Anticonvulsants:* May decrease felodipine level. Avoid use together.
Cimetidine, erythromycin, itraconazole, ketoconazole: May decrease felodipine clearance. Give lower doses of felodipine.
Metoprolol: May alter pharmacokinetics of metoprolol. No dosage adjustment needed. Monitor patient for adverse effects.
Tacrolimus: May increase tacrolimus level. Monitor tacrolimus level and adjust dose as needed.
Theophylline: May slightly decrease theophylline level. Monitor patient's response carefully.
Drug-herb. *St. John's wort:* May increase felodipine metabolism. Discourage use together.
Drug-food. *Grapefruit, lime:* May increase level and adverse effects of drug. Discourage use together.

Effects on lab test results

None reported.

Pharmacokinetics

Absorption: Almost complete, but extensive first-pass metabolism reduces absolute bioavailability to about 20%.
Distribution: More than 99% protein-bound.
Metabolism: Possibly hepatic.
Excretion: More than 70% in urine and 10% in feces as metabolites. *Half-life:* 11 to 16 hours.

Route	Onset	Peak	Duration
P.O.	2–5 hr	2½–5 hr	24 hr

Action

Chemical effect: Prevents entry of calcium ions into vascular smooth muscle and cardiac cells.
Therapeutic effect: Lowers blood pressure.

Available forms

Tablets (extended-release): 2.5 mg, 5 mg, 10 mg

NURSING PROCESS

🏥 Assessment
• Assess patient's blood pressure before starting therapy, and reassess regularly.
• Be alert for adverse reactions and drug interactions.
• Assess patient's and family's knowledge of drug therapy.

🔷 Nursing diagnoses
• Risk for injury related to presence of hypertension
• Excess fluid volume related to drug-induced peripheral edema
• Deficient knowledge related to drug therapy

▶ Planning and implementation
• Drug may be given with or without food.
⚠ **ALERT:** Don't confuse Plendil with Isordil.
Patient teaching
• Instruct patient to swallow tablets whole and not to crush or chew them.
• Tell patient to take drug even when he feels better, to watch his diet, and to check with prescriber or pharmacist before taking other drugs, including OTC and herbal remedies.
• Advise patient to practice good oral hygiene and to see dentist regularly.

✅ Evaluation
• Patient's blood pressure is normal.
• Patient doesn't develop complications from peripheral edema.
• Patient and family state understanding of drug therapy.

fenofibrate
(feh-noh-FIGH-brayt)
Antara, Lipofen, Lofibra, TriCor, Triglide

Pharmacologic class: fibric acid derivative
Therapeutic class: antilipemic
Pregnancy risk category: C

Indications and dosages

▶ **Hypertriglyceridemia (Fredrickson types IV and V hyperlipidemia) in patients who don't respond adequately to diet alone.** For all forms, adjust dosage based on patient response and lipid determinations performed at 4- to 8-week intervals.
Antara
Adults: Initially, 43 to 130 mg P.O. daily. Maximum, 130 mg daily.
Lipofen
Adults: Initially, 50 to 150 mg daily. Maximum, 150 mg daily.
Lofibra
Adults: Initially, 67 to 200 mg (capsules) or 54 to 160 mg (tablets) daily. Maximum, 200 mg (capsules) or 160 mg (tablets) daily.
TriCor
Adults: Initially, 48 to 145 mg daily. Maximum, 145 mg daily.
Triglide
Adults: Initially, 50 to 160 mg daily. Maximum, 160 mg daily.
▶ **Primary hypercholesterolemia or mixed dyslipidemia (Fredrickson types IIa and IIb) in patients who don't respond adequately to diet alone.** If lipid levels fall significantly below target range, may reduce following dosages:
Antara
Adults: Initially, 130 mg P.O. daily.
Lipofen
Adults: Initially, 150 mg daily.
Lofibra
Adults: Initially, 200 mg (capsules) or 160 mg (tablets) daily.
TriCor
Adults: Initially, 145 mg daily.
Triglide
Adults: Initially, 160 mg daily.
📉 **Adjust-a-dose:** If creatinine clearance is less than 50 ml/minute or patient is elderly, start with 43 mg (Antara), 50 mg (Lipofen), 67 mg (Lofibra capsules), 54 mg (Lofibra tablets), 48 mg (TriCor), or 50 mg (Triglide) daily. Increase only after evaluating renal function and triglyceride level at this dose.

Contraindications and cautions

• Contraindicated in patients hypersensitive to drug or any of its components and in those with gallbladder disease, hepatic dysfunction, primary biliary cirrhosis, severe renal dysfunction, or unexplained persistent liver function abnormalities.
• Use cautiously in patients with history of pancreatitis.
⚠ **Lifespan:** In pregnant women, use only if benefits outweigh risks to fetus. Breast-feeding

F

women should stop the drug or stop breast-feeding. In children, safety and effectiveness haven't been established. In elderly patients, start with lower dosage.

Adverse reactions

CNS: asthenia, *dizziness,* fatigue, *headache,* insomnia, pain, paresthesia.
CV: *arrhythmias.*
EENT: blurred vision, conjunctivitis, earache, eye floaters, eye irritation, rhinitis, sinusitis.
GI: abdominal pain, constipation, diarrhea, dyspepsia, eructation, flatulence, increased appetite, nausea, *pancreatitis,* vomiting.
GU: polyuria, vaginitis.
Hepatic: cholelithiasis.
Musculoskeletal: arthralgia, myalgia, myositis, *rhabdomyolysis.*
Respiratory: cough.
Skin: pruritus, rash.
Other: decreased libido, flulike syndrome, hypersensitivity reaction, *infection.*

Interactions

Drug-drug. *Bile acid sequestrants:* May bind drug and inhibit absorption. Give drug 1 hour before or 4 to 6 hours after bile acid sequestrants.
Coumarin-type anticoagulants: May increase anticoagulant effect. Monitor PT and INR closely. Reduce anticoagulant dosage if needed.
Cyclosporine, immunosuppressants, nephrotoxic drugs: May cause renal dysfunction, which may compromise the elimination of drug. Use together cautiously.
HMG-CoA reductase inhibitors: May increase risk of myopathy, rhabdomyolysis, and acute renal impairment from use of HMG-CoA reductase inhibitors with gemfibrozil (another fibrate derivative). Don't use together.
Drug-food. *Any food:* May increase absorption. Give drug with meals.
Drug-lifestyle. *Alcohol use:* May elevate triglyceride level. Discourage use together.

Effects on lab test results

- May increase BUN, creatinine, ALT, and AST levels. May decrease uric acid and hemoglobin levels and hematocrit.
- May decrease WBC count.

Pharmacokinetics

Absorption: Good.

Distribution: 99% protein-bound.
Metabolism: Rapidly hydrolyzed by esterases to active metabolite, fenofibric acid.
Excretion: 60% in urine, mainly as metabolites, and 25% in feces. *Half-life:* 20 hours.

Route	Onset	Peak	Duration
P.O.	Unknown	6–8 hr	Unknown

Action

Chemical effect: May inhibit triglyceride synthesis, decreasing amount of very–low-density lipoproteins released into circulation. May stimulate breakdown of triglyceride-rich protein.
Therapeutic effect: Decreases triglyceride levels.

Available forms

Capsules: 50 mg, 100 mg, 150 mg
Capsules (micronized): 43 mg, 67 mg, 87 mg, 130 mg, 134 mg, 200 mg
Tablets: 40 mg, 48 mg, 50 mg, 54 mg, 107 mg, 120 mg, 145 mg, 160 mg

NURSING PROCESS

🔍 Assessment

- Assess baseline lipid levels and liver function test results before starting therapy and periodically thereafter.
- Be alert for adverse reactions and drug interactions.
- Assess patient's and family's knowledge of drug therapy.

🔄 Nursing diagnoses

- Impaired tissue integrity: muscular related to adverse drug reaction
- Risk for infection related to adverse drug reactions
- Deficient knowledge related to drug therapy

▶ Planning and implementation

- Stop giving the drug to a patient who doesn't have an adequate response after 2 months of therapy with maximum dose.
- Give tablets with meals to increase bioavailability.
- Evaluate renal function and triglyceride levels in patient with severe renal impairment before increasing dose.
- Counsel patient on importance of adhering to triglyceride-lowering diet.

Reactions may be *common,* uncommon, *life-threatening*, or COMMON AND LIFE-THREATENING.

⊛ **ALERT:** Don't confuse Tricor with Tracleer.

Patient teaching

• Advise patient to promptly report symptoms of unexplained muscle weakness, pain, or tenderness, especially if accompanied by malaise or fever.

• Urge patient to take drug with meals to optimize drug absorption.

• Advise patient to continue weight-control measures, including diet and exercise, and to reduce alcohol intake before starting therapy.

• Instruct patient who also takes bile acid resin to take fenofibrate 1 hour before or 4 to 6 hours after bile acid resin.

☑ Evaluation

• Patient remains free of myositis and rhabdomyolysis.

• Patient remains free from infection.

• Patient and family state understanding of drug therapy.

HIGH ALERT

fentanyl citrate
(FEN-tuh-nihl SIGH-trayt)
Sublimaze

fentanyl hydrochloride iontophoretic transdermal system
Ionsys

fentanyl transdermal system
Duragesic-12, Duragesic-25, Duragesic-50, Duragesic-75, Duragesic-100

fentanyl transmucosal
Actiq, Fentora

Pharmacologic class: opioid
Therapeutic class: analgesic, anesthetic
Pregnancy risk category: C
Controlled substance schedule: II

Indications and dosages

▶ **Adjunct to general anesthetic.** *Adults and children older than age 12:* For low-dose therapy, 2 mcg/kg I.V. For moderate-dose therapy, 2 to 20 mcg/kg I.V.; then 25 to 100 mcg I.V. or I.M., p.r.n. For high-dose therapy, 20 to 50 mcg/kg I.V.; then 25 mcg to one-half initial loading dose I.V., p.r.n.

Children ages 2 to 12: Give 2 to 3 mcg/kg I.V. or I.M. during induction and maintenance phases of general anesthesia.

▶ **Adjunct to regional anesthesia.** *Adults:* 50 to 100 mcg I.M. or slow I.V. over 1 to 2 minutes.

▶ **Postoperative pain.** *Adults:* 50 to 100 mcg I.M. every 1 to 2 hours, p.r.n.

▶ **Short-term management of acute postoperative pain in patients who need opioid analgesia during hospitalization.** *Adults:* First, give a different opioid until patient is comfortable. Then, apply Ionsys system to intact, nonirritated skin on the chest or upper outer arm. To activate a dose, instruct the patient to firmly press the dose-delivery button twice within 3 seconds. Each actuation of the system delivers 40 mcg of fentanyl. A beep indicates the start of delivery of each dose, and a red light remains on throughout the 10-minute delivery period. A maximum of six 40-mcg doses can be delivered each hour. Each system operates for 80 doses or up to 24 hours. A maximum of three systems can be used sequentially, applied to a different skin site, for a total of 72 hours of pain management.

▶ **To manage persistent, moderate to severe chronic pain in opioid-tolerant patients who require continuous, around-the-clock opioid analgesics for an extended period of time.** *Adults and children age 2 or older:* When converting to Duragesic, the initial dose is based on the daily dose, potency and characteristics of the current opioid therapy, the reliability of the relative potency estimates used to calculate the needed dose of fentanyl, the degree of opioid tolerance, and the condition of the patient. Each system may be worn for 72 hours, although some adult patients may need systems to be applied every 48 hours during the initial period. May increase dose 3 days after the first dose and then every 6 days thereafter.

▶ **Breakthrough cancer pain in opioid-tolerant patients.** *Adults:* Initially, 200 mcg Actiq P.O. (transmucosally); adjust dosage based on response. Have patient suck on each unit for 15 minutes. An additional unit may be given 30 minutes after start of the previous dose. Don't use more than 2 units per episode of breakthrough pain. Or, initially, 100 mcg Fentora between the upper cheek and gum. May repeat same dose once per breakthrough episode after at least 30 minutes. Adjust in 100-mcg in-

crements. Doses above 400 mcg can be increased by 200 mcg. Generally, dosage should be increased when patient needs more than one dose per breakthrough episode. Once a successful maintenance dose has been established, re-evaluate if patient has more than four breakthrough episodes per day.

▶ **Switching from Actiq to Fentora.** *Adults:* If current Actiq dose is 200 to 400 mcg, start with 100 mcg Fentora. If current Actiq dose is 600 to 800 mcg, use 200 mcg Fentora. If current Actiq dose is 1,200 to 1,600 mcg, use 400 mcg Fentora.

▽ I.V. administration

• Only staff trained in giving I.V. anesthetics and managing their adverse effects should give drug I.V.
• Keep naloxone and resuscitation equipment available when giving drug I.V.
• Drug is commonly used I.V. with droperidol to produce neuroleptanalgesia.
⊗ **Incompatibilities**
Azithromycin, fluorouracil, lidocaine, methohexital, pentobarbital sodium, phenytoin, thiopental.

Contraindications and cautions

• Contraindicated in patients intolerant of drug. Transdermal fentanyl is contraindicated in patients hypersensitive to adhesives; patients who need postoperative pain management; patients who have acute, mild, or intermittent pain that can be managed with nonopioid drugs; and patients who aren't opioid tolerant. Don't use in patients with increased intracranial pressure, impaired consciousness, or coma.
• Use cautiously in debilitated patients and in patients with brain tumors, increased CSF pressure, COPD, decreased respiratory reserve, potentially compromised respirations, hepatic or renal disease, or bradyarrhythmias.
⚘ Lifespan: In pregnant women, use cautiously. In breast-feeding women, use cautiously because it's unknown if the drug appears in breast milk. Actiq is contraindicated for use during labor and delivery. In children younger than age 2, safety and effectiveness of I.V. drug haven't been established. In children younger than age 16, safety and effectiveness of Actiq haven't been established. In children younger than age 12 and children younger than age 18 weighing less than 50 kg (110 lb), transdermal system is

contraindicated. In elderly patients, use all forms cautiously because dosages may have prolonged CNS and respiratory effects.

Adverse reactions

CNS: anxiety, *asthenia, clouded sensorium, confusion,* depression, dizziness, *euphoria,* hallucinations, headache, nervousness, *sedation, somnolence.*
CV: *arrhythmias, bradycardia,* chest pain, hypertension, hypotension.
EENT: dry mouth.
GI: abdominal pain, constipation, ileus, nausea, vomiting.
GU: urine retention.
Respiratory: *apnea,* dyspnea, hypoventilation, *respiratory depression.*
Skin: diaphoresis, pruritus.
Other: physical dependence, reaction at application site (edema, erythema, papules).

Interactions

Drug-drug. *CNS depressants, general anesthetics, hypnotics, MAO inhibitors, opioid analgesics, sedatives, tricyclic antidepressants:* May have additive effects. Use together cautiously. Reduce fentanyl dosage by one-fourth or one-third. Reduce dosages of other drugs.
Diazepam: May cause CV depression when given with high doses of fentanyl. Monitor patient closely.
Droperidol: May cause hypotension and decreased pulmonary arterial pressure. Monitor patient closely.
Potent CYP3A4 inhibitors (clarithromycin, erythromycin, itraconazole, ketoconazole, nefazodone, nelfinavir, ritonavir, troleandomycin): May increase analgesia, CNS depression, and hypotensive effects. Monitor patient's respiratory status and vital signs.
Protease inhibitors: May increase CNS and respiratory depression. Monitor patient closely.
Drug-lifestyle. *Alcohol use:* May have additive effects. Discourage use together.

Effects on lab test results

None reported.

Pharmacokinetics

Absorption: Varies with drug route.
Distribution: Accumulates in adipose tissue and skeletal muscle.
Metabolism: In liver.

Reactions may be *common,* uncommon, *life-threatening,* or COMMON AND LIFE-THREATENING.

Excretion: In urine. *Half-life:* 3½ hours (parenteral), 5 to 15 hours (transmucosal), 18 hours (transdermal).

Route	Onset	Peak	Duration
I.V.	1–2 min	3–5 min	30–60 min
I.M.	7–15 min	20–30 min	1–2 hr
Transmucosal	15 min	20–30 min	Unknown
Transdermal	12–24 hr	24–72 hr	72 hr

Action

Chemical effect: May bind with opiate receptors in CNS, altering both perception of and emotional response to pain.
Therapeutic effect: Relieves pain.

Available forms

Injection: 50 mcg/ml
Iontophoretic transdermal system: 40 mcg/dose
Transdermal system: patches designed to release 12.5, 25, 50, 75, or 100 mcg of fentanyl per hour
Transmucosal lozenge (Actiq): 200 mcg, 400 mcg, 600 mcg, 800 mcg, 1,200 mcg, 1,600 mcg
Transmucosal tablets (Fentora): 100 mcg, 200 mcg, 400 mcg, 600 mcg, 800 mcg

NURSING PROCESS

Assessment
• Assess patient's underlying condition before starting therapy.
• Evaluate degree of pain relief provided by each dose.
• Periodically monitor postoperative vital signs and bladder function. Because drug decreases both rate and depth of respirations, monitoring of arterial oxygen saturation (Sao_2) may help assess respiratory depression.
④ ALERT: Transdermal patch levels peak between 24 and 72 hours after initial application and dose increases. Monitor patients for life-threatening hypoventilation, especially during these times.
• Be alert for adverse reactions and drug interactions.
• Assess patient's and family's knowledge of drug therapy.

Nursing diagnoses
• Acute pain related to underlying condition

• Ineffective breathing pattern related to respiratory depression
• Deficient knowledge related to drug therapy

➤ Planning and implementation
• For better analgesic effect, give drug before patient has intense pain.
• When drug is used postoperatively, encourage patient to turn, cough, and breathe deeply to prevent atelectasis.
④ ALERT: Only the patient should activate the iontophoretic transdermal system.
④ ALERT: Fentora and Actiq aren't bioequivalent and can't be substituted on a mcg-per-mcg basis.
• To give transmucosal lozenge:
– Open childproof foil package with scissors immediately before use.
– Place lozenge or tablet in patient's mouth between the cheek and gum.
– Actiq should be actively sucked while Fentora should be allowed to dissolve.
– Make sure patient consumes the lozenge or tablet in about 15 minutes. Faster or slower consumption may reduce its effects.
– If signs of excess opioid effects appear before the entire lozenge or tablet dissolves, remove it from the patient's mouth and decrease future doses.
④ ALERT: Ask patient and caregivers about the presence of children in the home because lozenges and tablets may be fatal to a child. Explain how to dispose of lozenges properly.
• Don't use transdermal patch for postoperative pain.
• Use dosage equivalency charts to calculate transdermal dose based on daily morphine intake—for example, for every 90 mg of oral morphine or 15 mg of I.M. morphine daily, give 25 mcg/hour of transdermal drug.
• Adjust dosage gradually in patient using transdermal patch. Delay dosage adjustment until after at least two applications. Reaching steady-state levels of new dosage may take up to 6 days.
• High doses can produce muscle rigidity, which can be reversed with neuromuscular blockers; however, patient must be artificially ventilated.
• Immediately report respiratory rate below 12 breaths/minute or decreased respiratory volume or Sao_2.

• Most patients have good control of pain for 3 days while wearing transdermal patch, but a few may need a new application after 48 hours. Because drug level rises for first 24 hours after application, analgesic effect can't be evaluated on the first day. Make sure patient has adequate supplemental analgesic to prevent breakthrough pain.

• When reducing opioid therapy or switching to a different analgesic, withdraw transdermal patch gradually. Because drug level drops gradually after removal, give half of equianalgesic dose of new analgesic 12 to 18 hours after removal.

⊛ **ALERT:** Don't confuse fentanyl with sufentanil.

Patient teaching

• Teach patient proper application of transdermal patch. Instruct patient to clip hair at application site, but to avoid razors, which may irritate skin. Tell him to wash area with clear water if needed, but not with soaps, oils, lotions, alcohol, or other substances that may irritate skin or prevent adhesion. Urge him to dry area completely before application.

• Tell patient to remove transdermal system from package just before applying, to hold in place for 10 to 20 seconds, and to be sure edges of patch adhere to the skin.

• Teach patient to dispose of transdermal patch by folding so that adhesive side adheres to itself, and then flushing it down toilet.

• If patient needs another patch after 72 hours, tell him to apply it to new site and to be sure to remove old patch

• Inform patient that heat from fever or environment may increase transdermal delivery and cause toxicity, which requires dosage adjustment. Instruct patient to notify prescriber if fever occurs or if he will be spending time in hot climate.

⊛ **ALERT:** Strongly warn patient to keep drug safely secured, away from children.

• Advise parent or caregiver to place transdermal patch on the upper back for a child or a patient who's cognitively impaired, to reduce the chance the patch will be removed and placed in the mouth.

• Teach patient how to properly take transmucosal dose or how to apply transmucosal systems.

⊛ **ALERT:** Teach patient proper disposal of transmucosal Actiq units.

☑ **Evaluation**
• Patient is free from pain.
• Patient maintains adequate ventilation throughout drug therapy.
• Patient and family state understanding of drug therapy.

ferrous fumarate
(FEH-rus FYOO-muh-rayt)
Femiron†, **Feostat**†, **Feostat Drops**†, **Hemocyte**†, **Ircon**†, **Nephro-Fer**†, **Palafer**♦ †

ferrous gluconate
Fergon†, **Novo-ferrogluc** ♦

ferrous sulfate
Feosol*†, **Feratab**†, **Fer-Gen-Sol Drops**†, **Fer-In-Sol***†, **Fer-Iron Drops**†, **Fero-Gradumet**†, **FeroSul**†, **Irospan**†, **Mol-Iron**†

ferrous sulfate, dried
Feosol†, **Slow-Fe**†

Pharmacologic class: oral iron supplement
Therapeutic class: hematinic
Pregnancy risk category: A

Indications and dosages

▶ **Iron deficiency.** *Adults:* 150 to 300 mg elemental iron P.O. daily given in three divided doses.
Children: 3 to 6 mg/kg P.O. daily given in one to three divided doses.
Premature infants: 2 to 4 mg/kg P.O. daily given in one to two divided doses. Maximum, 15 mg/day.

Contraindications and cautions

• Contraindicated in patients hypersensitive to drug or its ingredients; patients with primary hemochromatosis, hemosiderosis, hemolytic anemia (unless iron deficiency anemia is also present), peptic ulcer disease, regional enteritis, or ulcerative colitis; and patients receiving repeated blood transfusions.

• Use cautiously on long-term basis.

⚘ **Lifespan:** In breast-feeding women, iron supplements usually are recommended. In children, use cautiously and don't give extended-

release forms. In elderly patients, may cause constipation.

Adverse reactions

GI: anorexia, *black stools, constipation,* diarrhea, epigastric pain, *nausea,* vomiting.
Other: temporary staining of teeth (drops, suspension).

Interactions

Drug-drug. *Antacids, cholestyramine resin, levodopa, tetracycline, vitamin E:* May decrease iron absorption. Separate doses by 2 to 4 hours.
Chloramphenicol: May increase iron response. Watch patient carefully.
Fluoroquinolones, penicillamine, tetracyclines: May decrease GI absorption of these drugs, possibly decreasing levels and effectiveness. Separate doses by 2 to 4 hours.
L-thyroxine: May decrease L-thyroxine absorption. Separate doses by at least 2 hours. Monitor thyroid function.
Levodopa, methyldopa: May decrease absorption and effectiveness of levodopa and methyldopa. Monitor patient for decreased effects of these drugs.
Vitamin C: May increase iron absorption. Suggest patient take vitamin C with drug.
Drug-food. *Cereals, cheese, coffee, eggs, milk, tea, whole-grain breads, yogurt:* May impair oral iron absorption. Advise against use together.

Effects on lab test results

None reported.

Pharmacokinetics

Absorption: Mainly at duodenum and proximal jejunum. For enteric-coated and some extended-release formulas, may be decreased. With food, may decrease by 33% to 50%.
Distribution: Binds immediately to carrier protein, transferrin, then to bone marrow for incorporation into hemoglobin.
Metabolism: Liberated by destruction of hemoglobin but is conserved and reused by body.
Excretion: Healthy people lose only small amounts of mineral each day. Men and postmenopausal women lose about 1 mg daily and premenopausal women about 1.5 mg daily. The loss usually occurs in nails, hair, feces, and urine. *Half-life:* Unknown.

Route	Onset	Peak	Duration
P.O.	≤ 4 days	7–10 days	2–4 mo

Action

Chemical effect: Provides elemental iron, an essential component in formation of hemoglobin.
Therapeutic effect: Relieves iron deficiency.

Available forms

ferrous fumarate
(Each 100 mg provides 33 mg of elemental iron.)
Tablets: 90 mg†, 324 mg†, 325 mg†, 350 mg†
Tablets (chewable): 100 mg†
Tablets (timed-release): 150 mg†
ferrous gluconate
(Each 100 mg provides 11.6 mg of elemental iron.)
Tablets: 225 mg†, 300 mg†, 324 mg† (contains 37 mg elemental iron), 325 mg†
ferrous sulfate
(About 20% elemental iron; dried and powdered, it's about 32% elemental iron.)
Drops: 75 mg/0.6 ml†
Elixir: 220 mg/5 ml*†
Tablets: 195 mg†, 300 mg†, 325 mg†, 187 mg (dried)†, 200 mg (dried)†
Tablets (extended-release): 160 mg (dried)†

NURSING PROCESS

Assessment
• Obtain baseline assessment of patient's iron deficiency before starting therapy.
• Evaluate hemoglobin level, hematocrit, and reticulocyte count during therapy.
• Be alert for adverse reactions and drug interactions.
• Assess patient's and family's knowledge of drug therapy.

Nursing diagnoses
• Fatigue related to iron deficiency
• Constipation related to adverse effect of drug therapy on GI tract
• Deficient knowledge related to drug therapy

Planning and implementation
• Give tablets with juice or water, but not with milk or antacids.
• Dilute liquid forms in juice or water, but not in milk or antacids.

- To avoid staining teeth, give suspension or elixir with straw and place drops at back of throat.
- Don't crush or allow patient to chew extended-release forms.
- GI upset may be related to dose. Preferably give drug between meals, but if GI upset continues, may give with food, except eggs, milk products, coffee, and tea, which may impair absorption. Enteric-coated or sustained-release forms reduce GI upset but also reduce amount absorbed.
- Oral iron may turn stools black. Although this unabsorbed iron is harmless, it could mask presence of melena. Have stools tested for presence of blood.

Patient teaching

Ⓢ **ALERT:** Inform parents that as few as three tablets can poison a child.
- If patient misses a dose, tell him to take it as soon as he remembers but not to double the dose.
- Advise patient to avoid taking drug with certain foods that may impair oral iron absorption, including yogurt, cheese, eggs, milk, whole-grain breads and cereals, tea, and coffee.
- Teach dietary measures for preventing constipation.
- Advise patient to report constipation and changes in stool color or consistency.

☑ Evaluation
- Patient reports fatigue is no longer a problem in daily life.
- Patient states appropriate measures to prevent or relieve constipation.
- Patient and family state understanding of drug therapy.

fexofenadine hydrochloride
(feks-oh-FEN-uh-deen high-droh-KLOR-ighd)
Allegra

Pharmacologic class: H_1-receptor antagonist
Therapeutic class: antihistamine
Pregnancy risk category: C

Indications and dosages

▶ **Seasonal allergic rhinitis.** *Adults and children age 12 and older:* 60 mg P.O. b.i.d. or 180 mg P.O. once daily.

Children ages 2 to 11: Give 30 mg P.O. b.i.d.
▶ **Chronic idiopathic urticaria.** *Children age 12 and older:* 60 mg P.O. b.i.d. or 180 mg P.O. once daily.
Children ages 2 to 11: Give 30 mg P.O. b.i.d.
Children ages 6 months to 2 years: 15 mg (2.5 ml) P.O. b.i.d.
Ⓢ **Adjust-a-dose:** For adults with renal impairment, increase dosage interval to every 24 hours. For children ages 2 to 11, give 30 mg daily. For children ages 6 months to 2 years, give 15 mg daily.

Contraindications and cautions

- Contraindicated in patients hypersensitive to the drug or any of its components.
- Use cautiously in patients with renal impairment.

⚕ **Lifespan:** In pregnant women, use only if benefits outweigh risks to the fetus, and avoid use in the third trimester. In breast-feeding women, use cautiously because it's unknown if drug appears in breast milk.

Adverse reactions

CNS: fatigue, drowsiness, *headache.*
GI: dyspepsia, nausea.
GU: dysmenorrhea.
Musculoskeletal: back pain.
Respiratory: cough, sinusitis.
Other: viral infection.

Interactions

Drug-drug. *Aluminum- or magnesium-containing antacids:* May interfere with absorption of fexofenadine. Separate doses.
Erythromycin, ketoconazole: May increase fexofenadine levels. Prolonged QT interval has occurred with other antihistamines. Monitor patient closely.
Drug-lifestyle. *Alcohol:* May increase sedative effects. Discourage use together.
Drug-food. *Apple, grapefruit, and orange juice:* May decrease GI absorption of drug, reducing effects. Discourage use together.

Effects on lab test results

None reported.

Pharmacokinetics

Absorption: Rapid.
Distribution: 60% to 70% protein-bound.
Metabolism: Unknown.

Reactions may be *common,* uncommon, *life-threatening,* or COMMON AND LIFE-THREATENING.

Excretion: Mainly in feces. *Half-life:* 14½ hours.

Route	Onset	Peak	Duration
P.O.	Unknown	3 hr	14 hr

Action

Chemical effect: Selectively inhibits peripheral H_1-receptors.
Therapeutic effect: Relieves symptoms of seasonal allergies.

Available forms

Capsules: 60 mg
Oral suspension: 30 mg/5 ml
Tablets: 30 mg, 60 mg, 180 mg
Tablets (orally-disintegrating): 30 mg

NURSING PROCESS

Assessment

• Assess patient's seasonal allergy symptoms before starting therapy and regularly thereafter.
• Monitor patient for adverse reactions.
• Assess patient's and family's knowledge of drug therapy.

Nursing diagnoses

• Risk for injury related to fatigue and drowsiness caused by drug
• Ineffective health maintenance related to underlying condition
• Deficient knowledge related to drug therapy

Planning and implementation

• Reduce daily dosage in patient with renal impairment or currently on dialysis.
• Avoid giving with apple, orange, or grapefruit juice.
• **ALERT:** Don't confuse Allegra with Viagra.
Patient teaching
• Instruct patient not to exceed prescribed dose and to take drug only when affected by seasonal allergy symptoms.
• Warn patient not to drink alcohol and to avoid hazardous activities that require alertness until the drug's CNS effects are known.
• Tell patient that coffee or tea may reduce drowsiness. Suggest sugarless gum, hard candy, or ice chips to relieve dry mouth.
• Tell patient to avoid taking drug with apple, orange, or grapefruit juice.

• Tell parents to keep oral solution tightly closed in a cool, dry place and to shake it well before using.

Evaluation

• Patient experiences limited fatigue and drowsiness caused by the drug.
• Patient responds well to the drug.
• Patient and family state understanding of drug therapy.

HIGH ALERT

filgrastim (granulocyte colony-stimulating factor; G-CSF)
(fil-GRAH-stem)
Neupogen

Pharmacologic class: biologic response modifier
Therapeutic class: colony-stimulating factor, hematopoietic
Pregnancy risk category: C

Indications and dosages

▶ **To decrease risk of infection in patients with nonmyeloid cancers receiving myelosuppressive antineoplastics followed by bone marrow transplant.** *Adults and children:*
10 mcg/kg I.V. or subcutaneously daily at least 24 hours after cytotoxic chemotherapy and bone marrow infusion. Adjust later doses according to neutrophil response.
▶ **Congenital neutropenia.** *Adults:* 6 mcg/kg subcutaneously b.i.d. Adjust dosage based on response.
▶ **Idiopathic or cyclic neutropenia.** *Adults:* 5 mcg/kg subcutaneously daily. Adjust dosage based on response.
▶ **Peripheral blood progenitor cell collection.** *Adults:* 10 mcg/kg subcutaneously daily for at least 4 days before first leukapheresis and continuing until the last leukapheresis is completed.
▶ **To decrease risk of infection in patients with nonmyeloid cancers receiving myelosuppressive antineoplastics, agranulocytosis‡, pancytopenia with colchicine overdose‡, acute leukemia‡, hematologic toxicity with zidovudine therapy‡.** *Adults and children:*
5 mcg/kg I.V. or subcutaneously daily as single dose. May increase in increments of 5 mcg/kg for each chemotherapy cycle, depending on du-

ration and severity of nadir of absolute neutrophil count (ANC).

▶ **Myelodysplasia‡.** *Adults:* 0.3 to 10 mcg/kg subcutaneously daily.

▶ **Neutropenia from HIV infection‡.** *Adults and adolescents:* 5 to 10 mcg/kg subcutaneously or I.V. daily for 2 to 4 weeks.

▼ I.V. administration

• Dilute in 50 to 100 ml of D_5W. If final concentration will be 2 to 15 mcg/ml, add albumin at 2 mg/ml (0.2%) to minimize binding of drug to plastic containers or tubing.
• Give by intermittent infusion over 15 to 60 minutes or continuous infusion over 24 hours.
• Refrigerate drug at 36° to 46° F (2° to 8° C). Don't freeze; avoid shaking. Store at room temperature for maximum of 6 hours; discard after 6 hours.

⊗ **Incompatibilities**
Amphotericin B, cefepime, cefonicid, cefotaxime, cefoxitin, ceftizoxime, ceftriaxone, cefuroxime, clindamycin, dactinomycin, etoposide, fluorouracil, furosemide, heparin sodium, mannitol, methylprednisolone sodium succinate, metronidazole, mitomycin, piperacillin, prochlorperazine edisylate, sodium solutions, thiotepa.

Contraindications and cautions

• Contraindicated in patients hypersensitive to proteins derived from *Escherichia coli* or to the drug or any of its components.
⚱ **Lifespan:** In pregnant women, use cautiously. In breast-feeding women, use cautiously because it's unknown if the drug appears in breast milk.

Adverse reactions

CNS: *fatigue, fever,* headache, weakness.
CV: *arrhythmias,* chest pain, *MI.*
GI: constipation, *diarrhea, mucositis, nausea,* stomatitis, *vomiting.*
GU: hematuria, proteinuria.
Hematologic: leukocytosis, *thrombocytopenia.*
Musculoskeletal: *skeletal pain.*
Respiratory: cough, dyspnea.
Skin: *alopecia,* cutaneous vasculitis, rash.
Other: hypersensitivity reactions.

Interactions

Drug-drug. *Chemotherapeutics:* May cause sensitivity in rapidly dividing myeloid cells.

Don't use filgrastim within 24 hours of chemotherapy.

Effects on lab test results

• May increase creatinine, uric acid, alkaline phosphatase, and LDH levels.
• May increase WBC count. May decrease platelet count.

Pharmacokinetics

Absorption: Rapid.
Distribution: Unknown.
Metabolism: Unknown.
Excretion: Unknown. *Half-life:* About 3½ hours.

Route	Onset	Peak	Duration
I.V.	5–60 min	24 hr	1–7 days
SubQ	5–60 min	2–8 hr	1–7 days

Action

Chemical effect: Stimulates proliferation and differentiation of hematopoietic cells. Drug is specific for neutrophils.
Therapeutic effect: Raises WBC count.

Available forms

Injection: 300 mcg/ml in 1-ml and 1.6-ml single-use vials; 300 mcg/0.5 ml, 480 mcg/ 0.8 ml in prefilled syringes

NURSING PROCESS

▨ **Assessment**
• Assess patient's underlying condition before starting therapy.
• Obtain baseline CBC and platelet count before and during therapy.
• Be alert for adverse reactions and drug interactions.
• Ask patient about skeletal pain.
• Assess patient's and family's knowledge of drug therapy.

⊞ **Nursing diagnoses**
• Ineffective protection related to underlying condition or treatment
• Acute pain related to adverse drug effects on skeletal muscle
• Deficient knowledge related to drug therapy

▶ Planning and implementation
• Don't give drug within 24 hours of cytotoxic chemotherapy.
• Once dose is withdrawn from vial, discard the unused portion. Vials are for single-dose use and contain no preservatives.
• Give daily for up to 2 weeks or until ANC has returned to 10,000/mm³ after the expected chemotherapy-induced neutrophil nadir.
⚠ ALERT: Rare cases of splenic rupture have occurred.
⚠ ALERT: Don't confuse Neupogen with Neumega or Neulasta.
Patient teaching
• Teach patient how to give drug and how to dispose of used needles, syringes, drug containers, and unused drug.
• Tell patient to report bruising or spontaneous bleeding, such as frequent nosebleeds.
• Teach patient how to manage skeletal pain.
• Tell patient to immediately report upper left abdominal or shoulder pain, because these may be signs of splenic rupture.

✓ Evaluation
• Patient's WBC count is normal.
• Patient reports skeletal pain is bearable or relieved with analgesic administration and comfort measures.
• Patient and family state understanding of drug therapy.

finasteride
(fin-ES-teh-righd)
Propecia, Proscar

Pharmacologic class: steroid derivative
Therapeutic class: androgen synthesis inhibitor
Pregnancy risk category: X

Indications and dosages
▶ **To reduce the progression of BPH symptoms.** *Men:* 5 mg Proscar P.O. daily with or without doxazosin.
▶ **To reduce risk of acute urine retention and need for surgery, including prostatectomy and transurethral resection of prostate; symptomatic BPH; adjunct therapy after radical prostatectomy‡, first-stage prostate cancer‡, acne‡, or hirsutism‡.** *Adults:* 5 mg Proscar P.O. daily.

▶ **Male pattern baldness.** *Men:* 1 mg Propecia P.O. daily.

Contraindications and cautions
• Contraindicated in patients hypersensitive to drug or any of its components or to other 5-alpha-reductase inhibitors, such as dutasteride. Use cautiously in patients with liver dysfunction.
⚠ **Lifespan:** In women and children, drug is contraindicated.

Adverse reactions
GU: decreased volume of ejaculate, impotence.
Other: decreased libido.

Interactions
None significant.

Effects on lab test results
• May decrease prostate-specific antigen (PSA) level.

Pharmacokinetics
Absorption: Not clearly defined, but average bioavailability may be as high as 63%.
Distribution: 90% protein-bound. Crosses blood–brain barrier.
Metabolism: Extensive.
Excretion: 39% in urine as metabolites; 57% in feces. *Half-life:* Unknown.

Route	Onset	Peak	Duration
P.O.	Unknown	1–2 hr	2 wk

Action
Chemical effect: Competitively inhibits steroid 5-reductase, an enzyme that forms potent androgen 5-dihydrotestosterone (DHT) from testosterone. Because DHT influences development of the prostate gland, lower levels will relieve symptoms of BPH. For male pattern baldness, a balding scalp contains higher amounts of DHT; drug lowers scalp and serum DHT levels.
Therapeutic effect: Relieves symptoms of BPH, reduces hair loss, and promotes hair growth.

Available forms
Tablets: 1 mg, 5 mg

NURSING PROCESS

🔧 Assessment
• Before starting therapy, assess patient's BPH and evaluate him for conditions that could mimic BPH, including hypotonic bladder; prostate cancer, infection, or stricture; and neurologic conditions. Carefully monitor patients with large residual urine volume or severely diminished urine flow. These patients may not be candidates for therapy.
• Assess patient for improvement in BPH symptoms.
• Perform periodic digital rectal examinations.
• Be alert for adverse reactions and drug interactions.
• Carefully evaluate sustained increases in PSA levels, which could indicate noncompliance or disease progression.
• Assess patient's and family's knowledge of drug therapy.

🔆 Nursing diagnoses
• Impaired urinary elimination related to BPH
• Ineffective sexuality pattern related to drug-induced impotence
• Deficient knowledge related to drug therapy

🔷 Planning and implementation
• Because it's impossible to identify which patients will respond to therapy, keep in mind that a minimum of 6 months of therapy may be needed.
Patient teaching
• Warn woman who is or may become pregnant not to handle crushed or broken tablets because of risk of adverse effects on fetus.
• Reassure patient that, although drug may decrease volume of ejaculate, it doesn't appear to impair normal sexual function. Impotence and decreased libido have occurred in less than 4% of patients.
• Tell patient taking drug for male pattern baldness that he may not notice any effects for 3 months or longer.
• Warn patient not to donate blood until at least 1 month after final dose.
• Tell patient that drug may be taken without regard to meals.

✅ Evaluation
• Patient's BPH symptoms diminish.

• Patient states appropriate ways to manage sexual dysfunction.
• Patient and family state understanding of drug therapy.

---

flecainide acetate
(FLEH-kay-nyd AS-ih-tayt)
Tambocor

Pharmacologic class: benzamide derivative
Therapeutic class: antiarrhythmic
Pregnancy risk category: C

Indications and dosages

▶ **Paroxysmal supraventricular tachycardia; paroxysmal atrial fibrillation or flutter in patients without structural heart disease.**
Adults: 50 mg P.O. every 12 hours. Increase in increments of 50 mg b.i.d. every 4 days until effectiveness is achieved. Maximum, 300 mg daily.

▶ **Life-threatening ventricular arrhythmias, such as sustained ventricular tachycardia.**
Adults: 100 mg P.O. every 12 hours. Increase in increments of 50 mg b.i.d. every 4 days until effectiveness is achieved. Maximum, 400 mg daily for most patients.

🔲 **Adjust-a-dose:** For patients with renal impairment, if creatinine clearance is more than 35 ml/minute, initial dose is 100 mg every 12 hours. If clearance is 35 ml/minute or less, initial dose is 100 mg once daily or 50 mg b.i.d. Adjust doses cautiously for all renally impaired patients. When flecainide is used with amiodarone, decrease flecainide dosage by 50%.

Contraindications and cautions

• Contraindicated in patients hypersensitive to the drug or any of its components and in those with cardiogenic shock, second- or third-degree AV block, recent MI, or right bundle branch block related to left hemiblock (in absence of artificial pacemaker or implantable cardioverter–defibrillator).
• Use cautiously in patients with heart failure, cardiomyopathy, severe renal or hepatic disease, prolonged QT interval, sick sinus syndrome, or blood dyscrasia.
☀ **Lifespan:** In pregnant women, use cautiously. Breast-feeding women should stop breast-

---

feeding or not use the drug. In children, safety and effectiveness haven't been established.

Adverse reactions

CNS: anxiety, asthenia, ataxia, depression, *dizziness,* fatigue, fever, *headache,* insomnia, *light-headedness,* malaise, paresthesia, *syncope,* tremor, vertigo.
CV: *arrhythmias, cardiac arrest,* chest pain, edema, flushing, *heart failure,* palpitations.
EENT: blurred vision, other visual disturbances.
GI: abdominal pain, anorexia, constipation, diarrhea, dyspepsia, nausea, vomiting.
Respiratory: *dyspnea.*
Skin: rash.

Interactions

Drug-drug. *Amiodarone, cimetidine:* May alter pharmacokinetics. Watch for toxicity. Decrease flecainide dose by 50%.
Digoxin: May increase digoxin level by 15% to 25%. Monitor digoxin level; watch for toxicity.
Disopyramide, verapamil: May have additive negative inotropic properties with flecainide. Avoid use together.
Propranolol, other beta blockers: May increase flecainide and propranolol levels by 20% to 30%. Monitor patient for propranolol and flecainide toxicity.
Urine acidifying and alkalinizing drugs: May substantially alter excretion of flecainide. Monitor patient for flecainide toxicity or decreased effectiveness.
Drug-lifestyle. *Smoking:* May lower drug level. Discourage smoking.

Effects on lab test results

None reported.

Pharmacokinetics

Absorption: Rapid and almost complete; bioavailability is 85% to 90%.
Distribution: Possibly wide. 40% protein-bound.
Metabolism: In liver to inactive metabolites; 30% escapes metabolism.
Excretion: In urine. *Half-life:* 12 to 27 hours.

Route	Onset	Peak	Duration
P.O.	Unknown	2–3 hr	Unknown

Action

Chemical effect: Decreases excitability, conduction velocity, and automaticity as result of slowed atrial, AV node, His-Purkinje system, and intraventricular conduction and causes slight but significant prolongation of refractory periods in these tissues.
Therapeutic effect: Restores normal sinus rhythm.

Available forms

Tablets: 50 mg, 100 mg, 150 mg

NURSING PROCESS

Assessment
• Assess patient's arrhythmia before starting therapy.
• Monitor effectiveness by continuous ECG monitoring initially; long-term oral administration requires regular ECG readings.
• Monitor level, especially in patient with renal impairment or heart failure. Therapeutic level ranges from 0.2 to 1 mcg/ml. Risk of adverse effects increases when trough level exceeds 1 mcg/ml.
• Monitor potassium level regularly.
• Be alert for adverse reactions and drug interactions.
• Assess patient's and family's knowledge of drug therapy.

Nursing diagnoses
• Decreased cardiac output related to underlying arrhythmia
• Ineffective protection related to drug-induced new arrhythmias
• Deficient knowledge related to drug therapy

Planning and implementation
• If used to prevent ventricular arrhythmias, give drug only to patient with documented life-threatening arrhythmias.
• If patient has pacemaker or implantable cardioverter–defibrillator, check that pacing threshold was determined 1 week before and after starting therapy because drug can alter endocardial pacing thresholds.
• Correct hypokalemia or hyperkalemia before giving drug because these electrolyte disturbances may alter effect.

• Twice-daily administration enhances patient compliance.
• Because of drug's long half-life, its full effect may take 3 to 5 days. Give I.V. lidocaine with drug for first several days.
• Keep emergency equipment nearby when giving drug.
• If ECG disturbances occur, withhold drug, obtain rhythm strip, and notify prescriber immediately.

Patient teaching
• Stress importance of taking oral drug exactly as prescribed.
• Warn patient to avoid hazardous activities that require alertness or good vision if adverse CNS or visual reaction occurs.
• Tell patient to limit fluid and sodium intake to minimize heart failure or fluid retention and to weigh himself daily on the same scale at around the same time. Urge him to report promptly sudden weight gain.

☑ Evaluation
• Patient regains normal cardiac output with abolishment of underlying arrhythmia after drug therapy.
• Patient doesn't develop new arrhythmias.
• Patient and family state understanding of drug therapy.

fluconazole
(floo-KON-uh-zohl)
Diflucan⬦

Pharmacologic class: bis-triazole derivative
Therapeutic class: antifungal
Pregnancy risk category: C

Indications and dosages

▶ **Oropharyngeal and esophageal candidiasis.** *Adults:* 200 mg P.O. or I.V. on first day, followed by 100 mg daily. Higher doses (up to 400 mg daily) may be used for esophageal disease. Continue for 2 weeks after symptoms resolve.
Children: 6 mg/kg P.O. or I.V. on first day, followed by 3 mg/kg daily for at least 2 weeks.
▶ **Systemic candidiasis.** *Adults:* 400 mg P.O. or I.V. on first day, followed by 200 mg daily. Continue at least 4 weeks or for 2 weeks after symptoms resolve.

Children: 6 to 12 mg/kg P.O. or I.V. daily.
▶ **Cryptococcal meningitis.** *Adults:* 400 mg P.O. or I.V. on first day, followed by 200 mg once daily. Higher doses (up to 400 mg daily) may be used. Continue for 10 to 12 weeks after CSF culture is negative.
Children: 12 mg/kg P.O. or I.V. on first day; follow with 6 mg/kg P.O. or I.V. daily for 10 to 12 weeks after CSF culture becomes negative.
▶ **To prevent candidiasis in bone marrow transplant.** *Adults:* 400 mg. P.O. or I.V. once daily. Start prophylaxis several days before anticipated granulocytopenia. Continue therapy for 7 days after neutrophil count rises above 1,000/mm³.
▶ **To suppress relapse of cryptococcal meningitis in patients with AIDS.** *Adults:* 200 mg P.O. or I.V. daily.
Children: 3 to 6 mg/kg P.O. daily.
▶ **Vulvovaginal candidiasis.** *Adults:* 150 mg P.O. as a single dose.
▶ **Candidal infection, long-term suppression in patients with HIV infection‡.** *Adults:* 100 to 200 mg P.O. or I.V. daily.
▶ **To prevent mucocutaneous candidiasis, cryptococcosis, coccidioidomycosis, or histoplasmosis in patients with HIV infection‡.**
Adults: 200 to 400 mg P.O. or I.V. daily.
Children and infants: 2 to 8 mg/kg P.O. daily.
⎍ Adjust-a-dose: For patients with renal impairment, give an initial loading dose of 50 to 400 mg. If creatinine clearance is 50 ml/minute or less, reduce dosage by 50% in patients not receiving dialysis. For patients on hemodialysis, give 100% of usual dose after each dialysis session.

▼I.V. administration

• Don't remove protective overwrap from I.V. bags until just before use to ensure product sterility. Plastic container may show some opacity from moisture absorbed during sterilization. This is normal; it won't affect the drug and will dissipate over time.
• Give by continuous infusion at no more than 200 mg/hour. Use infusion pump. To prevent air embolism, don't connect in series with other infusions.
⊗ **Incompatibilities**
Amphotericin B, amphotericin B cholesteryl sulfate complex, ampicillin sodium, calcium gluconate, cefotaxime sodium, ceftazidime, ceftriaxone, cefuroxime sodium, chloramphenicol

sodium succinate, clindamycin phosphate, diazepam, digoxin, erythromycin lactobionate, furosemide, haloperidol lactate, hydroxyzine hydrochloride, imipenem and cilastatin sodium, pentamidine, piperacillin sodium, ticarcillin disodium, trimethoprim-sulfamethoxazole. Don't add other drugs.

Contraindications and cautions

• Contraindicated in patients hypersensitive to drug or any of its components.
• Although no information exists regarding cross-sensitivity, use cautiously in patients hypersensitive to other antifungal azole compounds.

☀ **Lifespan:** In pregnant women, use cautiously. In breast-feeding women, don't give.

Adverse reactions

CNS: headache.
GI: abdominal pain, diarrhea, *nausea*, vomiting.
Hepatic: *hepatotoxicity.*
Skin: rash, *Stevens-Johnson syndrome.*
Other: *anaphylaxis.*

Interactions

Drug-drug. *Alprazolam, chlordiazepoxide, clonazepam, clorazepate, diazepam, estazolam, flurazepam, midazolam, quazepam, triazolam:* May increase and prolong levels of these drugs, CNS depression, and psychomotor impairment. Don't use together.
Amitriptyline: May increase amitriptyline levels. Avoid combining, if possible.
Atorvastatin, fluvastatin, lovastatin, pravastatin, simvastatin: May increase levels and adverse effects of these HMG-CoA reductase inhibitors. Avoid use together. If they must be given together, reduce dose of HMG-CoA reductase inhibitor.
Carbamazepine: May increase carbamazepine level. Monitor levels closely.
Cyclosporine, phenytoin, tacrolimus: May increase levels of these drugs. Monitor cyclosporine or phenytoin level, and watch for drug toxicity.
Isoniazid, oral sulfonylureas, phenytoin, rifampin, valproic acid: May increase risk of elevated hepatic transaminases. Monitor patient and level closely.
Oral antidiabetics (glipizide, glyburide, tolbutamide): May increase levels of these drugs.

Monitor patient for enhanced hypoglycemic effect.
Rifampin: May enhance fluconazole metabolism. Monitor patient for lack of response.
Theophylline: May decrease theophylline clearance. Monitor level.
Warfarin: May increase risk of bleeding. Monitor PT and INR.
Zidovudine: May increase zidovudine activity. Monitor patient closely.
Drug-lifestyle. *Alcohol use:* May increase risk of hepatotoxicity. Discourage use together.

Effects on lab test results

• May increase alkaline phosphatase, ALT, AST, bilirubin, and GGT levels.
• May decrease WBC and platelet counts.

Pharmacokinetics

Absorption: Rapid and complete.
Distribution: Wide. 12% protein-bound.
Metabolism: Partial.
Excretion: Mainly by kidneys; more than 80% unchanged in urine. *Half-life:* 20 to 50 hours.

Route	Onset	Peak	Duration
P.O.	Unknown	1–2 hr	Unknown
I.V.	Immediate	Immediate	Unknown

Action

Chemical effect: Inhibits fungal cytochrome P-450, an enzyme responsible for fungal sterol synthesis, and weakens fungal cell walls.
Therapeutic effect: Hinders fungal growth.

Available forms

Injection: 200 mg/100 ml, 400 mg/200 ml
Powder for oral suspension: 10 mg/ml, 40 mg/ml
Tablets: 50 mg, 100 mg, 150 mg, 200 mg

NURSING PROCESS

🔎 **Assessment**

• Assess patient's fungal infection before starting therapy, and reassess regularly.
• Periodically monitor liver function during prolonged therapy. Although adverse hepatic effects are rare, they can be serious.
• Be alert for adverse reactions and drug interactions.

- If adverse GI reactions occur, monitor patient's hydration.
- Assess patient's and family's knowledge of drug therapy.

✛ Nursing diagnoses
- Risk for infection related to presence of susceptible fungi
- Risk for deficient fluid volume related to adverse GI reactions
- Deficient knowledge related to drug therapy

▶ Planning and implementation
- If patient develops mild rash, monitor him closely. If lesions progress, stop drug and notify prescriber.

Patient teaching
- Urge patient to adhere to regimen and to return for follow-up.
- Tell patient to report adverse reactions to prescriber.

☑ Evaluation
- Patient is free from infection.
- Patient maintains adequate hydration.
- Patient and family state understanding of drug therapy.

flucytosine
(5-fluorocytosine, 5FC)
(floo-SIGH-toh-seen)
Ancobon

Pharmacologic class: fluorinated pyrimidine
Therapeutic class: antifungal
Pregnancy risk category: C

Indications and dosages

▶ **Severe fungal infections caused by susceptible strains of *Candida* (including septicemia, endocarditis, urinary tract and pulmonary infections) and *Cryptococcus* (meningitis, pulmonary infection, and possible UTI).** *Adults:* 50 to 150 mg/kg P.O. daily in divided doses given every 6 hours. Use the lower initial dose in patients with renal insufficiency.
▶ **Chromomycosis‡.** *Adults:* 150 mg/kg P.O. daily.

Contraindications and cautions

- Contraindicated in patients hypersensitive to the drug or any of its components.
- Use cautiously in those with hepatic or renal impairment or bone marrow suppression.
☀ **Lifespan:** In pregnant women, use cautiously. Breast-feeding women should stop breast-feeding or not use the drug. In children, safety and effectiveness haven't been established.

Adverse reactions

CNS: ataxia, confusion, dizziness, fatigue, hallucinations, headache, paresthesia, parkinsonism, peripheral neuropathy, psychosis, sedation, vertigo, weakness.
CV: *cardiac arrest,* chest pain.
EENT: hearing loss.
GI: abdominal pain, diarrhea, dry mouth, duodenal ulcer, *hemorrhage,* nausea, ulcerative colitis, vomiting.
GU: azotemia, crystalluria, *renal impairment.*
Hematologic: *agranulocytosis,* anemia, *aplastic anemia, bone marrow suppression,* eosinophilia, *leukopenia, thrombocytopenia.*
Hepatic: jaundice.
Metabolic: *hypoglycemia,* hypokalemia.
Respiratory: dyspnea, *respiratory arrest.*
Skin: occasional rash, photosensitivity, pruritus, urticaria.

Interactions

Drug-drug. *Amphotericin B:* May have synergistic effects and enhance toxicity when used together. Monitor patient.
Cytosine: May inactivate the antifungal activity of flucytosine. Monitor patient.

Effects on lab test results

- May increase urine urea, alkaline phosphatase, ALT, AST, bilirubin, creatinine, and BUN levels. May decrease glucose, potassium, and hemoglobin levels and hematocrit.
- May increase eosinophil count. May decrease WBC, platelet, and granulocyte counts.

Pharmacokinetics

Absorption: 75% to 90%; food decreases absorption rate.
Distribution: Wide. CSF levels vary from 60% to 100% of blood levels. 2% to 4% protein-bound.
Metabolism: Only small amounts.

Excretion: 75% to 95% unchanged in urine.
Half-life: 2½ to 6 hours.

Route	Onset	Peak	Duration
P.O.	Unknown	1–2 hr	Unknown

Action

Chemical effect: May penetrate fungal cells where it's converted to fluorouracil—a known metabolic antagonist—and causes defective protein synthesis.
Therapeutic effect: Hinders fungal growth, including some strains of *Cryptococcus* and *Candida*.

Available forms

Capsules: 250 mg, 500 mg

NURSING PROCESS

Assessment

• Assess patient's fungal infection before starting therapy, and reassess regularly.
• Before starting therapy, obtain hematologic tests and renal and liver function studies. Make sure susceptibility tests showing that organism is flucytosine-sensitive are on chart.
• Monitor blood, liver, and renal function studies frequently; obtain susceptibility tests weekly to monitor drug resistance.
• If possible, regularly perform blood level assays of drug to maintain flucytosine at therapeutic level (25 to 120 mcg/ml). Higher levels may be toxic.
• Be alert for adverse reactions and drug interactions.
• If adverse GI reaction occurs, monitor patient's hydration.
• Assess patient's and family's knowledge of drug therapy.

Nursing diagnoses

• Risk for infection related to presence of susceptible fungi
• Risk for deficient fluid volume related to adverse GI reactions
• Deficient knowledge related to drug therapy

Planning and implementation

• Give capsules over 15 minutes to reduce adverse GI reactions.

Patient teaching

• Inform patient that therapeutic response may take weeks or months.
• Tell patient how to take capsules.
• Warn patient to avoid activities requiring mental alertness if adverse CNS reactions occur.

Evaluation

• Patient is free from infection.
• Patient maintains adequate hydration throughout drug therapy.
• Patient and family state understanding of drug therapy.

HIGH ALERT

fludarabine phosphate
(floo-DAR-uh-been FOS-fayt)
Fludara

Pharmacologic class: antimetabolite, purine antagonist
Therapeutic class: antineoplastic
Pregnancy risk category: D

Indications and dosages

▶ **B-cell chronic lymphocytic leukemia in patients who either haven't responded or have responded inadequately to at least one standard alkylating drug regimen, mycosis fungoides‡, hairy cell leukemia‡, and Hodgkin and malignant lymphoma‡.** *Adults:* 25 mg/m² I.V. over 30 minutes for 5 consecutive days. Repeat cycle every 28 days.
Adjust-a-dose: For patients with renal impairment, if creatinine clearance is 30 to 70 ml/minute, decrease dose by 20%. If clearance is less than 30 ml/minute, don't give drug.
▶ **Chronic lymphocytic leukemia‡.** *Adults:* Usually, 18 to 30 mg/m² I.V. over 30 minutes for 5 consecutive days every 28 days. Therapy is based on patient's response and tolerance.

I.V. administration

• Preparing and giving the drug have mutagenic, teratogenic, and carcinogenic risks. Follow facility policy to reduce risks.
• To prepare solution from lyophilized powder, add 2 ml of sterile water for injection to solid cake of drug. Drug will dissolve within 15 seconds; each ml will contain 25 mg of drug. Di-

lute this solution or injection further in 100 or 125 ml of D_5W or normal saline injection.
● Check injection for particulate matter or discoloration; reconstituted solution should be clear.
● Use within 8 hours of reconstitution.
● Store drug in refrigerator at 36° to 46° F (2° to 8° C).

⊗ **Incompatibilities**
Acyclovir sodium, amphotericin B, chlorpromazine, daunorubicin, ganciclovir, hydroxyzine hydrochloride, prochlorperazine edisylate.

Contraindications and cautions

● Contraindicated in patients hypersensitive to the drug or any of its components.
● Use cautiously in patients with renal insufficiency.
⚜ **Lifespan:** In pregnant women, use only if benefits outweigh risks to fetus. In breastfeeding women and in children, safety and effectiveness haven't been established.

Adverse reactions

CNS: agitation, cerebellar syndrome, *coma, confusion,* depression, *fatigue, fever,* headache, *malaise,* pain, *paresthesia,* peripheral neuropathy, sleep disorder, *stroke,* transient ischemic attack, *weakness.*
CV: aneurysm, angina, *arrhythmias, deep vein thrombosis,* edema, *heart failure, hemorrhage, MI,* phlebitis, *supraventricular tachycardia.*
EENT: delayed blindness (with high doses), epistaxis, hearing loss, pharyngitis, sinusitis, *visual disturbances.*
GI: *anorexia,* constipation, *diarrhea,* esophagitis, GI BLEEDING, mucositis, *nausea,* stomatitis, *vomiting.*
GU: dysuria, hematuria, proteinuria, *renal impairment,* urinary hesitancy, *UTI.*
Hematologic: anemia, *myelosuppression, neutropenia, thrombocytopenia.*
Hepatic: cholelithiasis, *liver failure.*
Metabolic: dehydration, hyperglycemia, hyperphosphatemia, hyperuricemia.
Musculoskeletal: myalgia.
Respiratory: allergic pneumonitis, bronchitis, *cough, dyspnea,* hemoptysis, *hypoxia, pneumonia, pulmonary toxicity, upper respiratory infection.*
Skin: alopecia, diaphoresis, pruritus, *rash,* seborrhea.

Other: *anaphylaxis,* chills, INFECTION, tumor lysis syndrome.

Interactions

Drug-drug. *Anticoagulants:* May interfere with anticoagulant response. Monitor PT; adjust dosage as needed.
Estrogens: May decrease fludarabine metabolism. Monitor patient.
Other myelosuppressants: May increase toxicity. Avoid use together.
Pentostatin: May increase risk of pulmonary toxicity. Avoid use together.
Salicylates: May decrease effect of salicylates and increase ulcerogenic effects. Avoid use together.

Effects on lab test results

● May increase glucose, phosphate, potassium, and uric acid levels. May decrease hemoglobin level and hematocrit.
● May decrease platelet and neutrophil counts.

Pharmacokinetics

Absorption: Given I.V.
Distribution: Unknown.
Metabolism: Rapidly dephosphorylated and then phosphorylated intracellularly to its active metabolite.
Excretion: 23% in urine as unchanged active metabolite. *Half-life:* About 10 hours.

Route	Onset	Peak	Duration
I.V.	7–21 hr	Unknown	Unknown

Action

Chemical effect: Unknown; actions may be multifaceted. After conversion to its active metabolite, fludarabine interferes with DNA synthesis by inhibiting DNA polymerase alpha, ribonucleotide reductase, and DNA primase.
Therapeutic effect: Kills susceptible cancer cells.

Available forms

Injection: 50 mg/2 ml
Powder for injection: 50 mg

NURSING PROCESS

🔃 **Assessment**
● Assess patient's underlying condition before starting therapy, and reassess regularly.

Reactions may be *common,* uncommon, *life-threatening,* or COMMON AND LIFE-THREATENING.

• Careful hematologic monitoring is needed, especially of neutrophil and platelet counts, because bone marrow suppression can be severe.
• Be alert for adverse reactions and drug interactions.
• Assess patient's and family's knowledge of drug therapy.

🔱 Nursing diagnoses
• Ineffective health maintenance related to presence of leukemia
• Ineffective protection related to drug-induced immunosuppression
• Deficient knowledge related to drug therapy

⟩ Planning and implementation
• Optimum duration of therapy isn't known. Recommendations suggest three additional cycles after achieving maximum response.
Patient teaching
• Warn patient to watch for evidence of infection and bleeding.
• Tell patient to notify prescriber if adverse reactions occur.

☑ Evaluation
• Patient shows positive response to fludarabine therapy.
• Patient develops no serious infections or bleeding complications.
• Patient and family state understanding of drug therapy.

fludrocortisone acetate
(floo-droh-KOR-tuh-sohn AS-ih-tayt)

Pharmacologic class: mineralocorticoid
Therapeutic class: adrenocortical steroid
Pregnancy risk category: C

Indications and dosages
▶ **Adrenal insufficiency (partial replacement), adrenogenital syndrome.** *Adults:* 0.1 to 0.2 mg P.O. daily.
▶ **Orthostatic hypotension‡.** *Adults:* 0.1 to 0.4 mg P.O. daily.

Contraindications and cautions
• Contraindicated in patients hypersensitive to drug or any of its components and in those with systemic fungal infections.

• Use cautiously in patients with hypothyroidism, cirrhosis, ocular herpes simplex, emotional instability with psychotic tendencies, nonspecific ulcerative colitis, diverticulitis, fresh intestinal anastomoses, active or latent peptic ulcer, renal insufficiency, hypertension, osteoporosis, and myasthenia gravis.
⚖ **Lifespan:** In pregnant women, use only if benefits outweigh risks to fetus. In breast-feeding women, use cautiously because it's unclear if the drug appears in breast milk. In children, long-term use may delay growth and maturation.

Adverse reactions
CNS: dizziness, headache, *seizures.*
CV: cardiac hypertrophy, *edema,* **heart failure,** hypertension, *sodium and water retention.*
EENT: cataracts, glaucoma.
GI: peptic ulcer.
Metabolic: hyperglycemia, hypokalemia.
Musculoskeletal: weakness.
Skin: allergic rash, **anaphylaxis,** bruising, diaphoresis, urticaria.

Interactions
Drug-drug. *Amphotericin B, drugs that deplete potassium (such as thiazide diuretics):* May enhance potassium-wasting effects of fludrocortisone. Monitor potassium levels.
Barbiturates, phenytoin, rifampin: May increase clearance of fludrocortisone acetate. Monitor patient for effect.
Drug-food. *Food containing sodium:* May increase blood pressure. Advise patient to limit sodium intake.

Effects on lab test results
• May increase glucose level. May decrease potassium level.

Pharmacokinetics
Absorption: Good.
Distribution: To muscle, liver, skin, intestines, and kidneys. Extensively protein-bound. Only unbound portion is active.
Metabolism: In liver to inactive metabolites.
Excretion: In urine; insignificant amount in feces. *Half-life:* 18 to 36 hours.

Route	Onset	Peak	Duration
P.O.	Varies	Varies	1–2 days

Action

Chemical effect: Increases sodium reabsorption and potassium and hydrogen secretion at distal convoluted tubule of nephron.
Therapeutic effect: Increases sodium level and decreases potassium and hydrogen levels.

Available forms

Tablets: 0.1 mg

NURSING PROCESS

⚡ Assessment
• Assess patient's underlying condition before starting therapy, and reassess regularly.
• Monitor patient's blood pressure, weight, and electrolyte levels.
• Be alert for adverse reactions and drug interactions.
• Assess patient's and family's knowledge of drug therapy.

⊕ Nursing diagnoses
• Ineffective health maintenance related to underlying adrenal condition
• Excess fluid volume related to drug-induced adverse reactions
• Deficient knowledge related to drug therapy

⟩ Planning and implementation
• Drug is used with cortisone or hydrocortisone in patients with adrenal insufficiency.
• If hypertension occurs, notify prescriber, who may lower dosage by 50%.
• Potassium supplements may be needed for excessive potassium loss.
• Signs of overdose include excessive weight gain, edema, hypertension, hypokalemia, and enlarged heart. Stop therapy for a few days until symptoms subside, and then resume drug at a lower dose.
Patient teaching
• Tell patient to notify prescriber about worsened symptoms, such as hypotension, weakness, cramping, and palpitations.
• Warn patient that mild peripheral edema is common.

☑ Evaluation
• Patient's health is improved.
• Patient develops no sodium and water retention.

• Patient and family state understanding of drug therapy.

---

flumazenil
(floo-MAZ-ih-nil)
Romazicon

Pharmacologic class: benzodiazepine antagonist
Therapeutic class: antidote
Pregnancy risk category: C

Indications and dosages

▶ **Complete or partial reversal of sedative effects of benzodiazepines after anesthesia or short diagnostic procedures (conscious sedation).** *Adults:* Initially, 0.2 mg I.V. over 15 seconds. If patient doesn't reach desired level of consciousness (LOC) after 45 seconds, repeat dose. Repeat at 1-minute intervals until cumulative dose of 1 mg has been given (initial dose plus four more doses), if needed. Most patients respond after 0.6 to 1 mg of drug. In case of resedation, repeat dose after 20 minutes, but don't give more than 1 mg at any one time and no more than 3 mg/hour.
▶ **Suspected benzodiazepine overdose.**
Adults: Initially, 0.2 mg I.V. over 30 seconds. If patient doesn't reach desired LOC after 30 seconds, give 0.3 mg over 30 seconds. If patient still doesn't respond adequately, give 0.5 mg over 30 seconds; repeat 0.5-mg doses p.r.n. at 1-minute intervals up to a cumulative dose of 3 mg. Most patients with benzodiazepine overdose respond to cumulative doses between 1 and 3 mg; rarely, patients who respond partially after 3 mg may need additional doses. Don't give more than 5 mg over 5 minutes initially. Sedation that persists after this dosage is unlikely to be caused by benzodiazepines. In case of resedation, repeat dose after 20 minutes, but don't give more than 1 mg at any one time and no more than 3 mg/hour.

▼ I.V. administration

• Compatible solutions include D_5W, lactated Ringer's injection, and normal saline solution.
• Give drug into I.V. line in large vein with free-flowing I.V. solution to minimize pain at injection site.

F

• Discard within 24 hours any unused drug that has been drawn into syringe or diluted.
⊗ **Incompatibilities**
None reported.

Contraindications and cautions

• Contraindicated in patients hypersensitive to drug, any of its components, or benzodiazepines; patients who show evidence of serious cyclic antidepressant overdose; and those who received a benzodiazepine to treat a potentially life-threatening condition (such as status epilepticus).
• Use cautiously in patients at high risk for developing seizures; patients who recently have received multiple doses of parenteral benzodiazepine; patients displaying signs of seizure activity; patients who may be at risk for unrecognized benzodiazepine dependence, such as ICU patients; and patients with head injury, psychiatric, or alcohol-dependency problems.
⚠ **Lifespan:** In pregnant women, use cautiously. In breast-feeding women, use cautiously because it's unknown if the drug appears in breast milk. In children, safety and effectiveness haven't been established.

Adverse reactions

CNS: agitation, *dizziness,* emotional lability, *headache,* insomnia, **seizures,** tremor.
CV: *arrhythmias,* cutaneous vasodilation, palpitations.
EENT: abnormal or blurred vision.
GI: nausea, vomiting.
Respiratory: dyspnea, hyperventilation.
Skin: diaphoresis.
Other: pain at injection site.

Interactions

Drug-drug. *Antidepressants, drugs that can cause seizures or arrhythmias:* May cause seizures or arrhythmias after effect of benzodiazepine overdose is removed. Use with caution, if at all, in cases of mixed overdose.

Effects on lab test results

None reported.

Pharmacokinetics

Absorption: Given I.V.
Distribution: Rapid. 50% protein-bound.
Metabolism: By liver.

Excretion: 90% to 95% appears in urine as metabolites. *Half-life:* 54 minutes.

Route	Onset	Peak	Duration
I.V.	Unknown	Unknown	Unknown

Action

Chemical effect: Competitively inhibits actions of benzodiazepines on GABA-benzodiazepine receptor complex.
Therapeutic effect: Awakens patient from sedative effects of benzodiazepines.

Available forms

Injection: 0.1 mg/ml in 5- and 10-ml multiple-dose vials

NURSING PROCESS

📋 Assessment
• Assess patient's sedation before starting therapy.
• Assess patient's LOC often.
• Be alert for adverse reactions and drug interactions.
⊛ **ALERT:** Monitor patient closely for resedation that may occur after reversal of benzodiazepine effects because drug's duration of action is shorter than that of benzodiazepines. Monitor patient closely after long-acting benzodiazepines, such as diazepam, or high doses of short-acting benzodiazepines, such as 10 mg of midazolam. In most cases, severe resedation is unlikely in patient who shows no signs of resedation 2 hours after 1-mg dose of flumazenil.
• Monitor patient's ECG for evidence of arrhythmias.
• Assess patient's and family's knowledge of drug therapy.

🔷 Nursing diagnoses
• Ineffective protection related to sedated state
• Decreased cardiac output related to drug-induced seizures
• Deficient knowledge related to drug therapy

▶ Planning and implementation
• If arrhythmias or other adverse reactions occur, notify prescriber and treat accordingly.
Patient teaching
• Warn patient to avoid hazardous activities within 24 hours.

- Tell patient not to use alcohol, CNS depressants, or OTC drugs for 24 hours.
- Give family members important instructions or provide patient with written instructions.

☑ Evaluation
- Patient is awake and alert.
- Patient maintains adequate cardiac output.
- Patient and family state understanding of drug therapy.

HIGH ALERT

fluorouracil (5-fluorouracil, 5-FU)
(floo-roh-YOOR-uh-sil)
Carac, Efudex, Fluoroplex

Pharmacologic class: antimetabolite
Therapeutic class: antineoplastic
Pregnancy risk category: D (injection); X (topical)

Indications and dosages

▶ **Colon, rectal, breast, stomach, and pancreatic cancers.** *Adults:* 12 mg/kg I.V. daily for 4 days; if no toxicity, give 6 mg/kg on days 6, 8, 10, and 12; then begin single weekly maintenance dose of 10 to 15 mg/kg I.V. after toxicity (if any) from initial course subsides. Dosages based on lean body weight. Maximum single dose, 800 mg.

▶ **Palliative therapy of advanced colorectal cancer.** *Adults:* 425 mg/m² I.V. daily for 5 consecutive days. Give with 20 mg/m² of leucovorin I.V. Repeat at 4-week intervals for two additional courses; then repeat at intervals of 4 to 5 weeks, as tolerated.

▶ **Multiple actinic (solar) keratoses; superficial basal cell carcinoma.** *Adults:* Apply cream or topical solution b.i.d.

▶ **Multiple actinic (solar) keratosis of the face and anterior scalp.** *Adults:* Apply a thin layer of cream or topical solution to the washed and dried affected area daily for up to 4 weeks.

▽ I.V. administration

- Give antiemetic to reduce nausea before giving drug.
- Preparing and giving drug create carcinogenic, mutagenic, and teratogenic risks for staff. Follow facility policy to reduce risks.
- Drug may be given by direct injection without dilution.

- For I.V. infusion, drug may be diluted with D₅W, sterile water for injection, or normal saline injection.
- Infuse slowly over 2 to 8 hours. Don't use cloudy solution. If crystals form, dissolve by warming.
- Use plastic I.V. containers for giving continuous infusions. Solution is more stable in plastic I.V. bags than in glass bottles.

⊗ **Incompatibilities**
Aldesleukin, amphotericin B cholesterol complex, carboplatin, cisplatin, cytarabine, diazepam, doxorubicin, droperidol, epirubicin, fentanyl citrate, filgrastim, gallium nitrate, leucovorin calcium, metoclopramide, morphine sulfate, ondansetron, topotecan, vinorelbine tartrate.

Contraindications and cautions

- Contraindicated in patients hypersensitive to the drug or any of its components; in those with poor nutrition, bone marrow suppression (WBC count of 5,000/mm³ or less or platelet counts of 100,000/mm³ or less), or potentially serious infections; and in those who have had major surgery within the previous month.
- Use cautiously after high-dose pelvic radiation therapy and in patients who have received alkylating drugs. Also use cautiously in patients who have impaired hepatic or renal function or widespread neoplastic infiltration of bone marrow.

⚖ Lifespan: In pregnant and breast-feeding women, drug is contraindicated. In children, safety and effectiveness haven't been established.

Adverse reactions

CNS: acute cerebellar syndrome, ataxia, confusion, disorientation, euphoria, headache, *malaise*, nystagmus, *weakness.*
CV: angina, *myocardial ischemia,* thrombophlebitis.
EENT: epistaxis, lacrimal duct stenosis, lacrimation, photophobia, visual changes.
GI: anorexia, diarrhea, *GI bleeding,* GI ulcer, nausea, stomatitis, vomiting.
Hematologic: *agranulocytosis,* anemia, *leukopenia, thrombocytopenia.*
Skin: *burning, pain,* soreness, suppuration, and swelling with topical use; contact dermatitis; *dermatitis; erythema;* erythematous, desquamative rash of hands and feet; nail changes; photo-

---

Reactions may be *common,* uncommon, *life-threatening*, or **COMMON AND LIFE-THREATENING.**

sensitivity; pigmented palmar creases; *pruritus; reversible alopecia; scaling.*
Other: *anaphylaxis.*

Interactions

Drug-drug. *Leucovorin calcium, previous therapy with alkylating drugs:* May increase fluorouracil toxicity. Use cautiously.
Drug-lifestyle. *Sun exposure:* Photosensitivity reactions may occur. Urge patient to avoid unprotected or prolonged sun exposure.

Effects on lab test results

• May increase alkaline phosphatase, AST, ALT, bilirubin, LDH, and urine 5-hydroxyindoleacetic acid levels. May decrease hemoglobin level and hematocrit.
• May decrease WBC, RBC, platelet, and granulocyte counts.

Pharmacokinetics

Absorption: Unknown for topical forms.
Distribution: Wide; crosses blood–brain barrier.
Metabolism: Most of drug degraded in liver; small amount converted in tissues to active metabolite.
Excretion: Metabolites mainly through lungs as carbon dioxide. *Half-life:* 20 minutes.

Route	Onset	Peak	Duration
I.V., Topical	Unknown	Unknown	Unknown

Action

Chemical effect: Inhibits DNA synthesis.
Therapeutic effect: Inhibits cell growth of selected cancers.

Available forms

Cream: 0.5%, 1%, 5%
Injection: 50 mg/ml
Topical solution: 2%, 5%

NURSING PROCESS

☒ Assessment
• Assess patient's condition before starting therapy and reassess regularly.
• Monitor fluid intake and output, CBC, platelet count, and renal and hepatic function tests.
• Be alert for adverse reactions and interactions.
• Fluorouracil toxicity may be delayed for 1 to 3 weeks. Lowest WBC count is 9 to 14 days

after each dose; lowest platelet count is 7 to 14 days after each dose.
• Monitor patient receiving topical form for serious adverse reaction. Ingestion and systemic absorption may cause leukopenia, thrombocytopenia, stomatitis, diarrhea, or GI ulceration, bleeding, and hemorrhage. Application to large ulcerated areas may cause systemic toxicity.
• Watch for stomatitis or diarrhea (signs of toxicity).
• Assess patient's and family's knowledge of drug therapy.

⊕ Nursing diagnoses
• Ineffective health maintenance related to underlying neoplastic condition
• Ineffective protection related to adverse hematologic reactions
• Deficient knowledge related to drug therapy

▷ Planning and implementation
⑤ **ALERT:** Drug is sometimes ordered as 5≠fluorouracil or 5-FU. The numeral 5 is part of drug name and shouldn't be confused with dosage units.
• When giving topically, apply cautiously near eyes, nose, and mouth.
• Avoid occlusive dressings because they increase risk of inflammatory reactions in adjacent normal skin.
• Wash hands immediately after handling topical form.
• Wash and dry affected area; wait 10 minutes. Apply thin layer of cream to affected area.
• Use 1% topical form on face. Higher concentrations are used for thicker-skinned areas or resistant lesions.
• Use 5% topical form for superficial basal cell carcinoma confirmed by biopsy.
• May apply sunscreen and moisturizer 2 hours after application.
• Risk of local irritation isn't increased by extending therapy from 2 to 4 weeks; irritation typically resolves within 2 weeks of stopping drug.
• Don't refrigerate fluorouracil.
• If drug spills, use sodium hypochlorite 5% (household bleach) to inactivate it.
• If diarrhea occurs, stop giving the drug and notify prescriber.
• If WBC count is less than 2,000/mm³, consider protective isolation.

Patient teaching

• Warn patient that alopecia may occur, but it's reversible.

• Advise patient to avoid prolonged exposure to sunlight or ultraviolet light when topical form is used.

• Tell patient to use sunblock to avoid inflammatory erythematous dermatitis. Long-term use of drug may cause erythematous, desquamative rash of hands and feet, which may be treated with pyridoxine (50 to 150 mg P.O. daily) for 5 to 7 days.

• Warn patient that topically treated area may be unsightly during therapy and for several weeks after. Full healing may take 1 to 2 months. Local irritation typically resolves 2 weeks after drug is stopped.

• Inform patient that sunscreen and a moisturizer may be applied 2 hours after drug application.

☑ Evaluation

• Patient shows positive response to fluorouracil therapy.

• Patient develops no serious adverse hematologic reactions.

• Patient and family state understanding of drug therapy.

fluoxetine hydrochloride
(floo-OKS-eh-teen high-droh-KLOR-ighd)
Prozac◆, Prozac Weekly, Sarafem Pulvules

Pharmacologic class: SSRI
Therapeutic class: antidepressant
Pregnancy risk category: C

Indications and dosages

▶ **Depression, obsessive-compulsive disorder (OCD).** *Adults:* Initially, 20 mg P.O. in morning; increase by patient's response. May be given b.i.d. in morning and at noon. Maximum, 80 mg daily.
Children ages 7 to 17: For OCD, 10 mg P.O. daily. After 2 weeks, increase dosage to 20 mg daily to maximum of 60 mg daily. In lower-weight children, increase dosage to 20 to 30 mg daily after several weeks. Maximum, 60 mg daily.
Children ages 8 to 18: For depression, 10 to 20 mg P.O. daily. After 1 week, increase to

20 mg daily. Start lower-weight children at 10 mg daily and increase dosage to 20 mg daily after several weeks.

▶ **Maintenance therapy for depression in stabilized patients.** *Adults:* 90 mg Prozac Weekly P.O. once weekly. Start 7 days after the last daily dose of Prozac 20 mg.

▶ **Moderate to severe bulimia nervosa.** *Adults:* 60 mg daily P.O. in the morning.

▶ **Premenstrual dysphoric disorder (PMDD).** *Women:* 20 mg Sarafem P.O. daily every day of the menstrual cycle or starting 14 days before the anticipated onset of menstruation through the first full day of menses and repeating with each new cycle. Maximum, 80 mg daily.

▶ **Panic disorder with or without agoraphobia.** *Adults:* 10 mg P.O. daily. May increase in 10-mg increments at intervals of no less than 1 week to maximum dosage of 60 mg.

▶ **Anorexia nervosa‡.** *Adults:* 40 mg P.O. daily in weight-restored patients.

▶ **Depression linked to bipolar disorder‡.** *Adults:* 20 to 60 mg P.O. daily.

▶ **Cataplexy‡.** *Adults:* 20 mg P.O. daily or b.i.d. in conjunction with CNS stimulant therapy.

▶ **Alcohol dependence‡.** *Adults:* 60 mg P.O. daily.

▶ **To prevent migraine headaches‡.** *Adults:* 10 to 40 mg P.O. daily.

▶ **Posttraumatic stress disorder‡, Raynaud phenomenon‡.** *Adults:* 20 to 60 mg P.O. daily.

▶ **Generalized anxiety disorder‡, hot flashes‡.** *Adults:* 20 mg P.O. daily.

Contraindications and cautions

• Sarafem isn't approved for children.

• Contraindicated in patients hypersensitive to the drug or any of its components and in those taking MAO inhibitors within 14 days of starting therapy. Don't give MAO inhibitors or thioridazine within 5 weeks of discontinuing fluoxetine.

• Use cautiously in children and adolescents as drug may increase the risk of suicidal thinking.

• Use cautiously in patients at high risk for suicide and in those with history of mania, seizures, diabetes mellitus, or hepatic, renal, or CV disease.

≋ **Lifespan:** In pregnant women, use cautiously. In breast-feeding women, it's unknown if drug appears in breast milk. In children younger

than age 7, safety and effectiveness in OCD haven't been established. In children younger than age 8, safety and effectiveness in major depressive disorder haven't been established. In children, safety and effectiveness for panic disorder, PMDD, and bulimia nervosa haven't been established. In adults age 65 and older treated for depression, start with lower dosage.

Adverse reactions

CNS: anxiety, asthenia, dizziness, drowsiness, fatigue, fever, headache, insomnia, nervousness, somnolence, tremor.
CV: palpitations.
EENT: nasal congestion, pharyngitis, sinusitis.
GI: abdominal pain, *anorexia,* constipation, *diarrhea, dry mouth,* dyspepsia, flatulence, increased appetite, *nausea,* vomiting.
Metabolic: weight loss.
Musculoskeletal: muscle pain.
Respiratory: cough, *respiratory distress,* upper respiratory infection.
Skin: pruritus, rash, urticaria.
Other: flulike syndrome, hot flushes, sexual dysfunction.

Interactions

Drug-drug. *Amphetamines, dextromethorphan, dihydroergotamine, meperidine, SSRIs, sumatriptan, tramadol, trazodone:* May increase risk of serotonin syndrome. Avoid use together.
Benzodiazepines, tricyclic antidepressants: May increase CNS effects. Monitor patient and level closely; adjust dosages if needed.
Carbamazepine, clozapine, cyclosporine, flecainide, haloperidol, propafenone, ritonavir, vinblastine: May increase levels of these drugs. Monitor levels and patient for adverse effects.
Cyproheptadine: May reverse or decrease pharmacologic effect. Monitor patient closely.
Insulin, oral antidiabetics: May alter glucose levels and need for antidiabetic. Adjust dosage.
Lithium: May alter lithium level. Monitor lithium level closely.
Phenelzine, selegiline, tranylcypromine: May cause serotonin syndrome (CNS irritability, shivering, and altered consciousness). Don't give drug within 2 weeks of an SSRI.
Phenytoin: May increase phenytoin level and risk of toxicity. Monitor phenytoin level and adjust dosage.

Sumatriptan: May cause weakness, hyperreflexia, and incoordination. Monitor the patient closely.
Thioridazine: May raise level of thioridazine, leading to a higher risk of serious ventricular arrhythmias and sudden death. Don't give within 5 weeks of each other.
Tryptophan: May increase toxic reaction with agitation, GI distress, and restlessness. Don't use together.
Warfarin, other highly protein-bound drugs: May increase level of fluoxetine or other highly protein-bound drugs. Monitor level of these drugs closely.
Drug-herb. *St. John's wort:* May increase the risk of serotonin syndrome. Discourage use together.
Drug-lifestyle. *Alcohol use:* May increase CNS depression. Discourage use together.

Effects on lab test results

None reported.

Pharmacokinetics

Absorption: Good.
Distribution: 95% protein-bound.
Metabolism: Mainly in liver to active metabolites.
Excretion: By kidneys. *Half-life:* 2 to 3 days.

Route	Onset	Peak	Duration
P.O.	1–4 wk	6–8 hr	Unknown

Action

Chemical effect: May inhibit CNS neuronal uptake of serotonin.
Therapeutic effect: Relieves depression and obsessive-compulsive behaviors.

Available forms

Capsules: 10 mg, 20 mg, 40 mg
Capsules (delayed-release): 90 mg (Prozac Weekly)
Oral solution: 20 mg/5 ml
Tablets: 10 mg, 15 mg, 20 mg, 40 mg

NURSING PROCESS

☘ Assessment
• Assess patient's condition before starting therapy, and reassess regularly.
• Be alert for adverse reactions and drug interactions.

• Observe closely for evidence of suicidal thoughts or behaviors until depression is relieved.

• Assess patient's and family's knowledge of drug therapy.

⬡ Nursing diagnoses
• Ineffective coping related to patient's underlying condition
• Sleep deprivation related to drug-induced insomnia
• Deficient knowledge related to drug therapy

▶ Planning and implementation
• An elderly or debilitated patient, or a patient with renal or hepatic dysfunction, may need a lower dose or less frequent administration.

⚠ **ALERT:** Drug may increase the risk of suicidal thinking and behavior in young adults ages 18 to 24 during the first 2 months of treatment. Monitor patient closely.

• Give drug in morning to prevent insomnia.
• Give antihistamines or topical corticosteroids to treat rashes or pruritus.
• Low-weight children may need several weeks between dosage increases.

⚠ **ALERT:** Don't confuse Prozac with Prilosec.
⚠ **ALERT:** Don't confuse Sarafem with Serophene.

Patient teaching
• Tell patient not to take drug in afternoon or evening because fluoxetine commonly causes nervousness and insomnia.
• Instruct patient to take drug with or without food.
• Advise patient and his family to monitor for suicidal thinking and behavior, and to report to prescriber immediately.
• Warn patient to avoid hazardous activities that require alertness and psychomotor coordination until the drug's CNS effects are known.
• Advise patient to consult prescriber before taking any other prescription or OTC drugs.

✓ Evaluation
• Patient behavior and communication indicate an improvement of depression with drug therapy.
• Patient has no insomnia with drug use.
• Patient and family state understanding of drug therapy.

fluphenazine decanoate
(floo-FEN-uh-zeen deh-kuh-NOH-ayt)
Modecate Concentrate ◆

fluphenazine hydrochloride

Pharmacologic class: phenothiazine (piperazine derivative)
Therapeutic class: antipsychotic
Pregnancy risk category: C

Indications and dosages

▶ **Psychotic disorders.** *Adults:* Initially, 2.5 to 10 mg hydrochloride P.O. daily in divided doses every 6 to 8 hours; may increase cautiously to 20 mg. Maintenance, 1 to 5 mg P.O. daily. Or 1.25 mg hydrochloride I.M. initially; then 2.5 to 10 mg I.M. daily in divided doses every 6 to 8 hours. Or 12.5 to 25 mg decanoate I.M. or subcutaneously every 4 to 6 weeks. Maximum dose, 100 mg.
Elderly patients: Initially 1 to 2.5 mg P.O. daily. Adjust according to response. Maximum dose is 15 mg.

Contraindications and cautions

• Contraindicated in patients hypersensitive to drug or any of its components and in those with CNS depression, bone marrow suppression, other blood dyscrasia, subcortical damage, liver damage, or coma.
• Use cautiously in debilitated patients and those with pheochromocytoma, severe CV disease, peptic ulcer, fever, exposure to extreme heat or cold or phosphorous insecticides, respiratory disorder, hypocalcemia, seizure disorder, severe reactions to insulin or electroconvulsive therapy, mitral insufficiency, glaucoma, or prostatic hyperplasia. Use parenteral form cautiously in patients with asthma and patients allergic to sulfites.

☀ **Lifespan:** In pregnant women, use cautiously. In breast-feeding women, use cautiously because it's unknown if the drug appears in breast milk. In children, safety and effectiveness haven't been established. In elderly patients, use cautiously.

Adverse reactions

CNS: dizziness, drowsiness, EEG changes, extrapyramidal reactions, *neuroleptic malignant*

---

syndrome, pseudoparkinsonism, sedation, *seizures,* tardive dyskinesia.

CV: ECG changes, orthostatic hypotension, tachycardia.

EENT: *blurred vision, dry mouth,* nasal congestion, ocular changes.

GI: constipation.

GU: dark urine, inhibited ejaculation, menstrual irregularities, *urine retention.*

Hematologic: *agranulocytosis, aplastic anemia,* eosinophilia, hemolytic anemia, *leukopenia.*

Hepatic: cholestatic jaundice.

Metabolic: increased appetite, weight gain.

Skin: mild photosensitivity.

Other: allergic reactions, gynecomastia.

Interactions

Drug-drug. *Antacids:* May inhibit absorption of oral phenothiazines. Separate doses by at least 2 hours.

Anticholinergics: May increase anticholinergic effects. Avoid use together.

Barbiturates, lithium: May decrease phenothiazine effect. Observe patient.

Centrally-acting antihypertensives: May decrease antihypertensive effect. Monitor blood pressure.

CNS depressants: May increase CNS depression. Avoid use together.

Drug-lifestyle. *Alcohol use:* May increase CNS depression, particularly psychomotor skills. Strongly discourage use together.

Sun exposure: May increase risk of photosensitivity. Discourage prolonged or unprotected exposure to sun.

Effects on lab test results

• May decrease hemoglobin level and hematocrit.

• May increase eosinophil count. May decrease WBC, granulocyte, and platelet counts. May alter liver function test values.

Pharmacokinetics

Absorption: For tablet, erratic and variable.
Distribution: Wide. CNS levels are usually higher than those in blood. 91% to 99% protein-bound.
Metabolism: Extensive.
Excretion: Mostly in urine. *Half-life:* Hydrochloride, 15 hours; decanoate, 7 to 10 days.

Route	Onset	Peak	Duration
P.O.	≤1 hr	30 min	6–8 hr
I.M., SubQ	1–3 days	Unknown	1–6 wk

Action

Chemical effect: Unknown; may block dopamine receptors in brain.
Therapeutic effect: Relieves psychotic signs and symptoms.

Available forms

fluphenazine decanoate
Depot injection: 25 mg/ml, 100 mg/ml ♦
fluphenazine hydrochloride
Elixir: 2.5 mg/5 ml*
I.M. injection: 2.5 mg/ml
Oral concentrate: 5 mg/ml*
Tablets: 1 mg, 2.5 mg, 5 mg, 10 mg

NURSING PROCESS

⚕ Assessment

• Assess patient's condition before starting therapy and regularly thereafter.

• Monitor therapy with weekly bilirubin tests during first month, periodic blood tests (CBC and liver function), and periodic renal function and ophthalmic tests (long-term use).

• Be alert for adverse reactions and drug interactions.

• Monitor patient for tardive dyskinesia, which may occur after prolonged use. Reaction may not appear until months or years later and may disappear spontaneously or persist for life despite no longer taking the drug.

• Assess patient's and family's knowledge of drug therapy.

⊕ Nursing diagnoses

• Disturbed thought processes related to psychosis

• Impaired physical mobility related to extrapyramidal reactions

• Deficient knowledge related to drug therapy

▷ Planning and implementation

Ⓢ **ALERT:** Oral concentrates are up to 10 times more concentrated than elixir. Check dosage order carefully.

• Dilute liquid concentrate with water, fruit juice (except apple), milk, or semisolid food just before administration.

- When giving I.M. or subcutaneously, for long-acting oil preparation form (decanoate), use dry needle of at least 21G. Allow 24 to 96 hours for onset of action. Note and report adverse reactions in patient taking these drug forms.
- Oral liquid and parenteral forms can cause contact dermatitis. Wear gloves when preparing solutions, and avoid contact with skin and clothing.
- Protect drug from light. Slight yellowing of liquid or concentrate is common and doesn't affect potency. Discard markedly discolored solutions.
- If patient, especially a pregnant woman or a child, develops symptoms of blood dyscrasia (fever, sore throat, infection, cellulitis, weakness) or extrapyramidal reactions for longer than a few hours, don't give the next dose. Notify prescriber.
- Acute dystonic reactions may be treated with diphenhydramine.
- Don't abruptly stop the drug unless a severe adverse reaction occurs. After abruptly stopping long-term therapy, patient may experience gastritis, nausea, vomiting, dizziness, tremor, feeling of warmth or cold, diaphoresis, tachycardia, headache, and insomnia.

Patient teaching

- Warn patient to avoid activities that require alertness and psychomotor coordination until the drug's CNS effects are known.
- Tell patient not to mix concentrate with beverages containing caffeine, tannics (such as tea), or pectinates (such as apple juice).
- Tell patient not to drink alcohol during therapy.
- Advise patient to relieve dry mouth with sugarless gum or hard candy.
- Have patient report urine retention or constipation.
- Tell patient to use sun block and to wear protective clothing.
- Inform patient that drug may discolor urine.
- Stress importance of not stopping drug suddenly.

☑ **Evaluation**
- Patient demonstrates decrease in psychotic behavior.
- Patient maintains pretreatment physical mobility.
- Patient and family state understanding of drug therapy.

HIGH ALERT

flurazepam hydrochloride
(floo-RAH-zuh-pam high-droh-KLOR-ighd)
Dalmane, Novo-Flupam♦, Somnol♦, Som Pam♦

Pharmacologic class: benzodiazepine
Therapeutic class: sedative-hypnotic
Pregnancy risk category: X
Controlled substance schedule: IV

Indications and dosages

▶ **Insomnia.** *Adults:* 15 to 30 mg P.O. at bedtime. Dose repeated once, if needed.
◩ **Adjust-a-dose:** In elderly and debilitated patients, maximum dose is 15 mg.

Contraindications and cautions

- Contraindicated in patients hypersensitive to drug or any of its components and in pregnancy.
- Use cautiously in patients with impaired hepatic or renal function, chronic pulmonary insufficiency, mental depression, suicidal tendencies, or history of drug abuse.
- ❀ **Lifespan:** In pregnant women, drug is contraindicated. In breast-feeding women, drug is contraindicated because it isn't known if drug appears in breast milk. In children younger than age 15, safety and effectiveness haven't been established. In elderly patients, use cautiously and at a lower dose because they're more susceptible to CNS effects of drug.

Adverse reactions

CNS: ataxia, *coma,* confusion, *daytime sedation,* disorientation, *disturbed coordination, dizziness, drowsiness,* hallucinations, *headache,* lethargy, light-headedness, nervousness, staggering.
GI: abdominal pain, diarrhea, heartburn, nausea, vomiting.
Other: *anaphylaxis, angioedema,* physical or psychological dependence.

Interactions

Drug-drug. *Cimetidine:* May increase sedation from decreased hepatic metabolism of benzodiazepines. Monitor patient carefully.
CNS depressants, including opioid analgesics: May cause excessive CNS depression. Use together cautiously.

Digoxin: May increase digoxin level and risk of digoxin toxicity. Monitor patient and digoxin level closely.

Disulfiram, hormonal contraceptives, isoniazid: May decrease metabolism of benzodiazepines, leading to toxicity. Monitor patient closely.

Fluconazole, itraconazole, ketoconazole, miconazole: May increase and prolong level, CNS depression, and psychomotor impairment. Don't use together.

Phenytoin: May increase phenytoin level. Monitor patient for toxicity.

Rifampin: May increase benzodiazepine metabolism. Monitor patient for decreased effectiveness.

Theophylline: May antagonize flurazepam. Monitor patient for decreased effectiveness.

Drug-herb. *Catnip, kava, lady's slipper, lemon balm, passionflower, sassafras, skullcap, valerian:* May increase sedative effects. Discourage use together.

Drug-lifestyle. *Alcohol use:* May cause additive CNS and respiratory depression. Strongly discourage use together.

Smoking: May increase benzodiazepine metabolism. Discourage use together.

Effects on lab test results

● May increase AST, ALT, total and direct bilirubin, and alkaline phosphatase levels.

Pharmacokinetics

Absorption: Rapid.
Distribution: Wide. About 97% protein-bound.
Metabolism: In liver to active metabolite.
Excretion: In urine. *Half-life:* 2 to 4 days.

Route	Onset	Peak	Duration
P.O.	Unknown	30 min–1 hr	Unknown

Action

Chemical effect: Unknown; may act on limbic system, thalamus, and hypothalamus of CNS to produce hypnotic effects.
Therapeutic effect: Promotes sleep and calmness.

Available forms

Capsules: 15 mg, 30 mg
Tablets: 15 mg ◆, 30 mg ◆

⬛ Assessment

● Assess patient's sleep patterns and CNS before starting therapy.
● Be alert for adverse reactions and drug interactions. Anaphylaxis and angioedema may occur as early as first dose.
● Assess patient's and family's knowledge of drug therapy.

⬥ Nursing diagnoses

● Sleep deprivation related to underlying problem
● Risk for trauma related to drug-induced adverse CNS reactions
● Deficient knowledge related to drug therapy

▶ Planning and implementation

● Before leaving bedside, make sure patient has swallowed capsule.
Patient teaching
● Encourage patient to continue drug, even if it doesn't relieve insomnia on the first night.
● Warn patient to avoid activities that require alertness or physical coordination. For inpatient, particularly for elderly patient, supervise walking and raise bed rails.
● Advise patient that physical and psychological dependence is possible with long-term use.
● Warn patient about possible complex sleep-related behaviors.

✅ Evaluation

● Patient notes drug-induced sleep.
● Patient's safety is maintained.
● Patient and family state understanding of drug therapy.

flutamide
(FLOO-tuh-mighd)
Euflex ◆

Pharmacologic class: nonsteroidal antiandrogen
Therapeutic class: antineoplastic
Pregnancy risk category: D

Indications and dosages

▶ **Locally advanced (stage B2) or metastatic (stage D2) prostatic carcinoma.** *Adults:*

F

250 mg P.O. every 8 hours. Used with luteinizing hormone–releasing hormone analogues such as leuprolide acetate.

▶ **Hirsutism in women‡.** *Adults:* 250 mg P.O. daily.

Contraindications and cautions

• Contraindicated in patients hypersensitive to the drug or any of its components and in those with severe hepatic impairment.

⚠ **Lifespan:** In women and girls, drug is contraindicated. In boys, safety and effectiveness haven't been established. In elderly patients, use drug cautiously because its half-life is prolonged.

Adverse reactions

CNS: anxiety, confusion, depression, drowsiness, nervousness, paresthesia.
CV: hypertension, peripheral edema.
GI: anorexia, diarrhea, nausea, vomiting.
GU: impotence, urine discoloration.
Hematologic: anemia, hemolytic anemia, *leukopenia, thrombocytopenia.*
Hepatic: *hepatic encephalopathy, hepatitis, liver failure.*
Skin: photosensitivity, rash.
Other: gynecomastia, hot flashes, loss of libido.

Interactions

Drug-drug. *Warfarin:* May increase PT. Monitor patient's PT and INR.
Drug-lifestyle. *Sun exposure:* May cause sensitivity reactions. Warn patient to avoid unprotected or prolonged sun exposure.

Effects on lab test results

• May increase BUN, creatinine, and liver enzyme levels. May decrease hemoglobin level and hematocrit.
• May decrease WBC and platelet counts.

Pharmacokinetics

Absorption: Rapid and complete.
Distribution: Concentrates in prostate. 95% protein-bound.
Metabolism: More than 97% occurs rapidly, with at least six metabolites.
Excretion: More than 95% in urine. *Half-life:* 6 hours.

Route	Onset	Peak	Duration
P.O.	Unknown	2 hr	Unknown

Action

Chemical effect: Inhibits androgen uptake or prevents androgen binding in cell nuclei in target tissues.
Therapeutic effect: Hinders prostatic cancer cell activity.

Available forms

Capsules: 125 mg
Tablets: 250 mg ◆

NURSING PROCESS

Assessment
• Assess patient's prostatic cancer before starting therapy.
• Monitor liver function tests before starting treatment and periodically during therapy.
• Be alert for adverse reactions.
• If adverse GI reaction occurs, monitor hydration.
• Assess patient's and family's knowledge of drug therapy.

Nursing diagnoses
• Ineffective health maintenance related to presence of prostatic cancer
• Risk for deficient fluid volume related to adverse GI reactions
• Deficient knowledge related to drug therapy

Planning and implementation
• Drug may be given with or without meals.
• Give with luteinizing hormone–releasing antagonist (such as leuprolide acetate).
Patient teaching
• Make sure patient knows that flutamide must be taken continuously with drug used for medical castration (such as leuprolide acetate) to allow full benefit of therapy. Leuprolide suppresses testosterone production, and flutamide inhibits testosterone action at cellular level. Together they can impair growth of androgen-responsive tumors. Advise patient not to stop either drug.
• Tell patient to notify prescriber if adverse reactions occur.
• Instruct patient to avoid prolonged exposure to sun and other ultraviolet light. Use sunscreens and protective clothing until tolerance is determined.

Evaluation
• Patient responds well to drug.

• Patient maintains adequate hydration throughout drug therapy.
• Patient and family state understanding of drug therapy.

fluticasone propionate
(FLOO-tih-ka-sohn proh-PIGH-oh-nayt)
Flonase, Flovent Diskus,Flovent HFA

Pharmacologic class: corticosteroid
Therapeutic class: intranasal and inhalation anti-inflammatory
Pregnancy risk category: C

Indications and dosages

▶ **Asthma prevention and chronic asthma in patients who need oral corticosteroids.** *Adults and children age 12 and older previously taking bronchodilators alone:* Initially, 88 mcg Flovent HFA b.i.d. to maximum of 440 mcg b.i.d. Or 100 mcg Flovent Diskus b.i.d. to maximum of 500 mcg b.i.d.
Adults and children age 12 and older previously taking inhaled corticosteroids: Initially, 88 to 220 mcg Flovent HFA b.i.d. to maximum of 440 mcg b.i.d. In patients with poor asthma control, initial doses of Flovent HFA may be above 88 mcg b.i.d. Or 100 to 250 mcg Flovent Diskus b.i.d. to maximum of 500 mcg b.i.d. In patients with poor asthma control, initial doses of Flovent Diskus may be above 100 mcg b.i.d.
Adults and children age 12 and older previously taking oral corticosteroids: 440 mcg to a maximum of 880 mcg Flovent HFA b.i.d. Or 500 to 1,000 mcg Flovent Diskus b.i.d. to maximum of 1,000 mcg b.i.d.
Adults and children age 12 and older starting HFA or inhalation aerosol therapy who are receiving oral corticosteroid therapy: Reduce prednisone dosage to no more than 2.5 mg daily on a weekly basis, beginning after at least 1 week of therapy with fluticasone.
Children ages 4 to 11: Give 88 mcg Flovent Diskus b.i.d.
▶ **Management of nasal symptoms of seasonal and perennial allergic and nonallergic rhinitis.** *Adults:* 2 sprays (100 mcg) Flonase in each nostril once daily or 1 spray (50 mcg) b.i.d. Reduce dosage to 1 spray in each nostril daily for maintenance therapy. Or, for seasonal allergic rhinitis, 2 sprays (100 mcg) in each nostril once daily p.r.n. for symptom control, although greater symptom control may be achieved with regular use.
Children age 4 and older: Initially 1 spray (50 mcg) Flonase in each nostril once daily. If patient doesn't respond, increase to 2 sprays (100 mcg) in each nostril daily. Once adequate control is achieved, decrease dose to 1 spray in each nostril daily. Maximum dosage is 2 sprays in each nostril daily.

Contraindications and cautions

• Contraindicated in patients hypersensitive to any of the components of these preparations. Also contraindicated as primary therapy for patients with status asthmaticus or other acute episodes of asthma in whom intensive measures are needed.
• Use cautiously in patients with ocular herpes simplex or untreated systemic, bacterial, viral, fungal, or parasitic infection, and in those with active or quiescent pulmonary tuberculosis.
⚠ **Lifespan:** In pregnant women, use only if benefits outweigh risks to fetus. In breastfeeding women, use cautiously because it's unknown if the drug appears in breast milk. In children younger than age 12, safety and effectiveness of the HFA and inhalation aerosols haven't been studied. In children younger than age 4, safety and effectiveness of the nasal formulation hasn't been studied.

Adverse reactions

CNS: dizziness, fever, *headache,* migraine, nervousness.
EENT: acute nasopharyngitis, conjunctivitis, dysphonia, earache, epistaxis, eye irritation, hoarseness, laryngitis, mouth irritation, nasal congestion, nasal discharge, *oral candidiasis,* otitis media, *pharyngitis,* rhinitis, sinusitis, sneezing, tonsillitis.
GI: abdominal discomfort, abdominal pain, colitis, diarrhea, nausea, viral gastroenteritis, vomiting.
GU: candidiasis of vagina, dysmenorrhea, irregular menstrual cycle, pelvic inflammatory disease, vaginitis, vulvovaginitis.
Metabolic: cushingoid features, weight gain.
Musculoskeletal: aches and pains, disorder or symptoms of neck sprain or strain, growth retardation in children, pain in joints, sore muscles.
Respiratory: bronchitis, chest congestion, dyspnea, irritation from inhalant, *upper respiratory tract infection.*

Skin: dermatitis, urticaria.
Other: dental problems, influenza.

Interactions

Drug-drug. *Ketoconazole:* May increase mean fluticasone level. Use care when giving fluticasone with long-term ketoconazole and other CYP3A4 inhibitors.
Ritonavir: May reduce cortisol concentrations resulting in Cushing syndrome and adrenal suppression. Don't give together unless benefit outweighs risk.

Effects on lab test results

• May increase glucose level.
• May cause an abnormal response to the 6-hour cosyntropin (corticotropin) stimulation test with high doses.

Pharmacokinetics

Absorption: Mostly systemic, with 30% of the delivered dose reaching the lungs. Less than 2% from the nasal mucosa.
Distribution: 91% protein-bound.
Metabolism: Via CYP3A4.
Excretion: In feces, mainly as unchanged drug and metabolites. *Half-life:* 3 hours.

Route	Onset	Peak	Duration
Inhalation	24 hr	1–2 wk	Several days
Nasal	12 hr–3 days	4–7 days	Several days

Action

Chemical effect: Inhibits many cell types and mediator production or secretion involved in asthma.
Therapeutic effect: Improves breathing ability by reducing inflammation.

Available forms

Nasal suspension: 50-mcg/metered spray
Oral HFA: 44 mcg/actuation, 110 mcg/actuation, 220 mcg/actuation
Oral inhalation powder: 50 mcg/actuation, 100 mcg/actuation, 250 mcg/actuation

NURSING PROCESS

⚚ Assessment
• Obtain history of patient's underlying condition before starting therapy, and reassess regularly.

• Because of risk of systemic absorption of inhaled corticosteroids, observe patient carefully for evidence of systemic corticosteroid effects.
• Monitor patient, especially postoperatively or during periods of stress, for evidence of inadequate adrenal response.
• Monitor growth in children closely because growth suppression may occur.
• Assess patient's and family's knowledge of drug therapy.

⊕ Nursing diagnoses
• Ineffective breathing pattern related to respiratory condition
• Impaired oral mucous membrane related to potential adverse effect of oral candidiasis
• Deficient knowledge related to drug therapy

▶ Planning and implementation
• During withdrawal from oral corticosteroids, patient may have symptoms of systemically active corticosteroid withdrawal, such as joint or muscle pain, lethargy, and depression, despite maintenance or even improvement of respiratory function.
• Bronchospasm may occur with an immediate increase in wheezing after a dose. If bronchospasm occurs following inhalation, treat immediately with a fast-acting inhaled bronchodilator.
• If patient is using a bronchodilator regularly, administer it at least 5 minutes before corticosteroid.
⑤ ALERT: Use lowest effective dose in children to minimize growth suppression.
Patient teaching
• Tell patient that drug isn't intended to relieve acute bronchospasm.
• For proper use of drug and to attain maximum improvement, tell patient to use drug at regular intervals as directed.
• Instruct patient not to increase dosage but to contact prescriber if symptoms don't improve or if condition worsens.
• Instruct patient to contact prescriber immediately if episodes of asthma aren't responsive to bronchodilators. During such episodes, patients may need therapy with oral corticosteroids.
• Warn patient to avoid exposure to chickenpox or measles, and if exposed to immediately consult prescriber.
• Tell patient to carry or wear medical identification indicating that he may need supplemen-

---

tary corticosteroids during stress or a severe asthma attack.

• During periods of stress or a severe asthma attack, instruct patient who has been withdrawn from systemic corticosteroids to immediately resume oral corticosteroids (in large doses) and to contact prescriber for further instruction. Instruct him to rinse his mouth after inhalation.

• Instruct patient to shake canister well before using HFA, and to avoid spraying into the eyes.

☑ **Evaluation**
• Patient has normal breathing pattern.
• Patient doesn't develop oral candidiasis.
• Patient and family state understanding of drug therapy.

fluticasone propionate and salmeterol inhalation powder
(FLOO-tih-ka-sohn proh-PY-oh-nayt and sal-MEH-teh-rohl)
Advair Diskus 100/50, Advair Diskus 250/50, Advair Diskus 500/50, Advair HFA 45/21, Advair HFA 115/21, Advair HFA 230/21

Pharmacologic class: corticosteroid, long-acting beta$_2$ agonist
Therapeutic class: anti-inflammatory, bronchodilator
Pregnancy risk category: C

Indications and dosages

▶ **Chronic asthma.** *Adults and children age 12 and older:* 1 oral inhalation of Advair Diskus or 2 inhalations of Advair HFA b.i.d., morning and evening, at least 12 hours apart. Maximum oral inhalation of Advair Diskus is 500/50 b.i.d. Maximum oral inhalation of Advair HFA is 230/21 b.i.d.
Adults and children older than age 12 not taking an inhaled corticosteroid: 1 oral inhalation of Advair Diskus 100/50 b.i.d.
Adults and children older than age 12 taking beclomethasone dipropionate: If daily dose of beclomethasone dipropionate is 160 mcg or less, start with 1 oral inhalation of Advair Diskus 100/50 b.i.d. or 2 inhalations of Advair HFA 45/21 b.i.d. If beclomethasone dipropionate daily dose is 320 mcg, start with 1 oral inhalation

of Advair Diskus 250/50 b.i.d. or 2 inhalations of Advair HFA 115/21 b.i.d. If beclomethasone dipropionate daily dose is 340 mcg start with one inhalation of Advair Diskus 550/50 b.i.d. or 2 inhalations of Advair HFA 230/21 b.i.d.
Adults and children older than age 12 taking budesonide: If daily dose of budesonide is 400 mcg or less, start with 1 oral inhalation of Advair Diskus 100/50 b.i.d. or 2 oral inhalations of Advair HFA 45/21 b.i.d. If budesonide daily dose is 800 to 1,200 mcg, start with 1 oral inhalation of Advair Diskus 250/50 b.i.d. or 2 oral inhalations of Advair HFA 115/21 b.i.d. If budesonide daily dose is 1,600 mcg, start with 1 oral inhalation of Advair Diskus 500/50 b.i.d. or 2 oral inhalations of Advair HFA 230/21 b.i.d.
Adults and children older than age 12 taking flunisolide CFC: If daily dose of flunisolide is 1,000 mcg or less, start with 1 oral inhalation of Advair Diskus 100/50 b.i.d. or 2 oral inhalations of Advair HFA 45/21 b.i.d. If flunisolide daily dose is 1,250 to 2,000 mcg, start with 1 oral inhalation of Advair Diskus 250/50 b.i.d. or 2 oral inhalations of Advair HFA 115/21 b.i.d.
Adults and children older than age 12 taking fluticasone HFA inhalation aerosol: If daily dose of fluticasone HFA inhalation aerosol is 320 mcg or less, start with 1 oral inhalation of Advair Diskus 100/50 b.i.d. or 2 oral inhalations of Advair HFA 45/21 b.i.d. If daily dose of fluticasone HFA inhalation aerosol is 640 mcg, start with one oral inhalation of Advair Diskus 250/50 b.i.d. or 2 oral inhalations Advair HFA 115/21 b.i.d.
Adults and children older than age 12 taking fluticasone propionate inhalation aerosol: If daily dose of fluticasone propionate inhalation aerosol is 176 mcg or less, start with 1 oral inhalation of Advair Diskus 100/50 b.i.d. or 2 oral inhalations of Advair HFA 45/21 b.i.d. If fluticasone propionate inhalation aerosol daily dose is 440 mcg, start with 1 oral inhalation of Advair Diskus 250/50 b.i.d. or 2 oral inhalations of Advair HFA 115/21 b.i.d. If fluticasone propionate inhalation aerosol daily dose is 660 to 880 mcg, start with 1 oral inhalation of Advair Diskus 500/50 b.i.d. or 2 oral inhalations of Advair HFA 230/21 b.i.d.
Adults and children older than age 12 taking fluticasone propionate inhalation powder: If fluticasone propionate inhalation powder daily dose is 200 mcg or less, start with 1 oral inhala-

F

tion of Advair Diskus 100/50 b.i.d. or 2 oral inhalations of Advair HFA 45/21 b.i.d. If fluticasone propionate inhalation powder daily dose is 500 mcg, start with 1 oral inhalation of Advair Diskus 250/50 b.i.d. or 2 oral inhalations of Advair HFA 115/21 b.i.d. If fluticasone propionate inhalation powder daily dose is 1,000 mcg, start with 1 oral inhalation of Advair Diskus 500/50 b.i.d. or 2 oral inhalations of Advair HFA 230/21 b.i.d.

Adults and children older than age 12 taking mometasone furoate inhalation powder: If mometasone furoate inhalation powder daily dose is 220 mcg or less, start with 1 oral inhalation of Advair Diskus 100/50 b.i.d. or 2 oral inhalations of Advair HFA 45/21 b.i.d. If mometasone furoate inhalation powder daily dose is 440 mcg, start with 1 oral inhalation of Advair Diskus 250/50 b.i.d. or 2 oral inhalations of Advair HFA 115/21 b.i.d. If mometasone furoate inhalation powder daily dose is 880 mcg, start with 1 oral inhalation of Advair Diskus 500/50 b.i.d. or 2 oral inhalations of Advair HFA 230/21 b.i.d.

Adults and children older than age 12 taking triamcinolone acetonide: If triamcinolone acetonide daily dose is 1,000 mcg or less, start with 1 oral inhalation of Advair Diskus 100/50 b.i.d. or 2 oral inhalations of Advair HFA 45/21 b.i.d. If triamcinolone acetonide daily dose is 1,100 to 1,600 mcg, start with 1 oral inhalation of Advair Diskus 250/50 b.i.d. or 2 oral inhalations of Advair HFA 115/21 b.i.d.

Children ages 4 to 11: Give 1 oral inhalation of Advair Diskus 100/50 b.i.d., morning and evening, at least 12 hours apart. Advair HFA isn't approved for children under the age of 12.

Adjust-a dose: In all patients, after asthma has been controlled, adjust to lowest effective dosage.

▶ **Maintenance therapy for airflow obstruction in patients with COPD from chronic bronchitis.** *Adults:* 1 inhalation Advair Diskus 250/50 b.i.d., about 12 hours apart. Advair HFA is not approved for use in COPD.

Contraindications and cautions

• Contraindicated in patients hypersensitive to the drug or any of its components. Also contraindicated as primary therapy for status asthmaticus or other potentially life-threatening acute asthmatic episodes.

• Drug isn't indicated for exercise-induced bronchospasms.

• Use cautiously in patients with active or quiescent respiratory tuberculosis infection; untreated systemic fungal, bacterial, viral, or parasitic infection; or ocular herpes simplex. Also use cautiously in patients with CV disorders, especially coronary insufficiency, cardiac arrhythmias, and hypertension; in patients with seizure disorders or thyrotoxicosis; in patients unusually responsive to sympathomimetic amines; and in patients with hepatic impairment (because salmeterol is metabolized mainly in the liver).

• Salmeterol has been linked to asthma-related deaths; only use in patients not adequately controlled on other asthma drugs.

Lifespan: In pregnant women, use only if benefits outweigh risks to fetus. In breast-feeding women, use cautiously; it isn't known if drug is found in breast milk. In children younger than age 4, safety and effectiveness haven't been established. Closely monitor growth in children because growth suppression may occur. Maintain child on lowest effective dose to minimize potential for growth suppression.

Adverse reactions

CNS: agitation, compressed nerve syndromes, fever, *headache,* hypnagogic drowsiness, nervousness, pain, sleep disorder, tremor.
CV: *arrhythmias,* chest pains, fluid retention, palpitations, rapid heart rate.
EENT: blood in nasal mucosa, congestion, conjunctivitis, dysphonia, eye redness, hoarseness, keratitis, nasal irritation, oral candidiasis, *pharyngitis,* rhinitis, rhinorrhea, sinusitis, sneezing, viral eye infections.
GI: abdominal pain and discomfort, appendicitis, constipation, diarrhea, gastroenteritis, nausea, oral discomfort and pain, oral erythema and rashes, oral ulcerations, unusual taste, vomiting.
Musculoskeletal: arthralgia, articular rheumatism, back pain, bone and cartilage disorders, muscle pain, muscle stiffness, rigidity, tightness.
Respiratory: bronchitis, cough, lower viral respiratory infection, *paradoxical bronchospasms,* pneumonia, *severe asthma or asthma-related deaths,* upper respiratory tract infection.
Skin: disorders of sweat and sebum, skin flakiness, sweating, urticaria, viral skin infections.
Other: allergic reactions, allergies, bacterial infections, dental discomfort and pain, influenza.

Reactions may be *common*, uncommon, *life-threatening*, or COMMON AND LIFE-THREATENING.

Interactions

Drug-drug. *Beta blockers:* May block pulmonary effect of salmeterol, producing severe bronchospasm in patients with asthma. Avoid use together. If needed, use a cardioselective beta blocker cautiously.

Cytochrome P-450 inhibitors (such as ketoconazole): May increase fluticasone level and adverse effects. Use together cautiously.

Loop diuretics, thiazide diuretics: May cause or worsen ECG changes or hypokalemia. Use together cautiously.

MAO inhibitors, tricyclic antidepressants: May potentiate the action of salmeterol on the vascular system. Avoid use within 2 weeks of these drugs.

Effects on lab test results

• May increase or decrease liver function test values.

Pharmacokinetics

Absorption: *Fluticasone propionate:* systemic. *Salmeterol:* local. With long-term therapy, salmeterol appears in blood within 45 minutes.
Distribution: *Fluticasone:* 91% protein-bound and weakly and reversibly bound to erythrocytes. *Salmeterol:* 96% protein-bound.
Metabolism: Mainly by CYP3A4.
Excretion: *Fluticasone:* less than 5% of a dose in urine as metabolites, with remainder in feces as an unchanged drug and metabolite. *Salmeterol:* 25% and 60% in urine and feces, respectively, over 7 days. *Fluticasone half-life:* 8 hours; *salmeterol half-life:* 5½ hours.

Route	Onset	Peak	Duration
Inhalation			
salmeterol	20 min	Unknown	12 hr
fluticasone	Unknown	1–2 hr	Unknown

Action

Chemical effect: Fluticasone's action is unknown. Salmeterol xinafoate stimulates intracellular adenyl cyclase, the enzyme that catalyzes conversion of adenosine triphosphate (ATP) to cAMP. Increased cAMP levels relax bronchial smooth muscle and inhibit release of mediators of immediate hypersensitivity from cells, especially mast cells.
Therapeutic effect: Reduces inflammation in the lungs and opens airways to improve pulmonary function.

Available forms

Aerosol spray: 45 mcg fluticasone and 21 mcg salmeterol, 115 mcg fluticasone and 21 mcg salmeterol, 230 mcg fluticasone and 21 mcg salmeterol
Inhalation powder: 100 mcg fluticasone and 50 mcg salmeterol, 250 mcg fluticasone and 50 mcg salmeterol, 500 mcg fluticasone and 50 mcg salmeterol

NURSING PROCESS

Assessment
• Obtain patient's medical history, and assess patient before starting therapy.
ALERT: Chronic overdose of fluticasone may cause signs and symptoms of hypercorticism. Salmeterol overdose may cause seizures, angina, hypertension, hypotension, tachycardia, arrhythmias, nervousness, headache, tremor, muscle cramps, dry mouth, palpitations, nausea, prolonged QT interval, ventricular arrhythmia, hypokalemia, hyperglycemia, cardiac arrest, and death. Stop drug and give a cardioselective beta blocker. Monitor cardiac condition.
• Monitor patient for urticaria, angioedema, rash, bronchospasm, or other signs of hypersensitivity, which may occur immediately after a dose of Advair Diskus.
• Monitor patient for increased use of inhaled short-acting beta₂ agonist. The dose of Advair Diskus may need to be increased.
• Monitor patient for hypercorticism and adrenal suppression. If these occur, reduce dosage slowly.
• Monitor patient for eosinophilia, vasculitic rash, worsening pulmonary symptoms, cardiac complications, or neuropathy, which may be signs of a serious eosinophilic condition.
• Monitor patient for signs or symptoms of thrush.
• Assess patient's and family's knowledge of drug therapy.

Nursing diagnoses
• Ineffective airway clearance related to underlying asthmatic condition
• Activity intolerance related to underlying asthmatic condition
• Deficient knowledge related to proper inhalation with the device and drug therapy

❯ Planning and implementation

⑤ **ALERT:** Don't switch patient directly from systemic corticosteroids to Advair Diskus. Hypothalamic-pituitary-adrenal axis suppression from corticosteroid therapy requires gradual weaning of steroid before replacement with inhaled steroid to avoid risk of death from adrenal insufficiency.

● After asthma has been controlled, adjust to the lowest effective dosage.

⑤ **ALERT:** Don't start Advair Diskus therapy during rapidly deteriorating or potentially life-threatening episodes of asthma. Serious acute respiratory events, including death, can occur, especially in blacks.

⑤ **ALERT:** When a patient uses Advair Diskus, make sure the patient has an inhaled, short-acting beta$_2$ agonist (such as albuterol) for acute symptoms that occur between doses of Advair Diskus.

⑤ **ALERT:** Advair Diskus can produce paradoxical bronchospasm. If it does, treat immediately with a short-acting, inhaled bronchodilator (such as albuterol) and stop Advair Diskus therapy.

● If patient is exposed to chickenpox, give varicella zoster immune globulin as prophylaxis. If chickenpox develops, give an antiviral.

● If patient is exposed to measles, give pooled I.M. immunoglobulin as prophylaxis.

● Store at controlled room temperature (68° F to 77° F [20° to 25° C]) in a dry place away from direct heat or sunlight. Discard the device 1 month after removal from the moisture-protective overwrap pouch or after every foil-wrapped blister has been used, whichever comes first. Don't attempt to take the device apart.

Patient teaching

● Instruct patient on most effective use of the Advair Diskus.

● Instruct patient to keep the Advair Diskus in a dry place, to avoid washing the mouthpiece or other parts of the device, and to avoid taking the Diskus apart.

● Tell patient to stop taking an oral or inhaled long-acting beta$_2$ agonist simultaneously when beginning Advair Diskus.

⑤ **ALERT:** Explain that Advair Diskus is used only for long-term maintenance and not for acute symptoms of asthma or for prevention of exercise-induced bronchospasm. Urge patient to use a short-acting beta$_2$ agonist (such as albuterol) for relief of acute symptoms.

● Instruct patient to rinse mouth after each inhalation to prevent oral candidiasis.

● Inform patient that improvement may be seen within 30 minutes after an Advair dose; however, the full benefit may not occur for 1 week or more.

⑤ **ALERT:** Instruct patient not to exceed prescribed dose under any circumstances.

● Instruct patient to report decreasing effects or increasing use of the short-acting beta$_2$ agonist inhaler immediately to his prescriber.

● Instruct patient not to use Advair Diskus with a spacer device.

● Tell patient to report palpitations, chest pain, rapid heart rate, tremor, or nervousness immediately to prescriber. Also instruct patient to avoid stimulants, such as caffeine, while on Advair Diskus therapy because they may increase these adverse reactions.

● Instruct patient to contact prescriber immediately if exposed to chickenpox or measles.

✓ Evaluation

● Patient's activity tolerance increases.

● Patient has a normal breathing pattern and optimal air exchange.

● Patient and family state understanding of drug therapy.

fluvastatin sodium
(floo-vuh-STAH-tin SOH-dee-um)
Lescol, Lescol XL

Pharmacologic class: HMG-CoA reductase inhibitor
Therapeutic class: cholesterol inhibitor
Pregnancy risk category: X

Indications and dosages

▶ **To reduce LDL and total cholesterol levels in patients with primary hypercholesterolemia (types IIa and IIb) or to slow progression of coronary atherosclerosis in patients with coronary artery disease; elevated triglyceride and apolipoprotein B levels in patients with primary hypercholesterolemia and mixed dyslipidemia whose response to dietary restriction and other nonpharmacologic measures has been inadequate.** *Adults:* Initially, 20 to 40 mg P.O. at bedtime. Increase if needed to maximum of 80 mg daily (in divid-

ed doses). Or 80 mg extended-release tablet P.O. daily.

▶ **To reduce the risk of undergoing coronary revascularization procedures.** *Adults:* For patients who need LDL cholesterol reduction of 25% or more, initially 40 mg (regular-release) P.O. or 80 mg (extended-release) P.O. once daily in the evening. Or 40 mg (regular-release) P.O. b.i.d. For patients requiring LDL cholesterol reduction of less than 25%, initially 20 mg P.O. daily. The recommended range is 20 to 80 mg daily.

Adjust-a-dose: If levels of ALT or AST persist at least three times the upper limit of normal, stop giving the drug. Drug is primarily cleared hepatically, so dosage adjustments for mild to moderate renal impairment aren't needed. Exercise caution with severe renal impairment.

Contraindications and cautions

• Contraindicated in patients hypersensitive to drug or any of its components and in those with active liver disease or conditions that cause unexplained, persistent elevations of transaminase levels. Also contraindicated during pregnancy.
• Use cautiously in patients with severe renal impairment or with history of liver disease or heavy alcohol use.

⚠ **Lifespan:** In pregnant and breast-feeding women and women of childbearing age, drug is contraindicated. In children, safety and effectiveness haven't been established.

Adverse reactions

CNS: dizziness, fatigue, headache, insomnia.
EENT: pharyngitis, rhinitis, sinusitis.
GI: abdominal pain, constipation, diarrhea, dyspepsia, flatulence, nausea, vomiting.
Hematologic: hemolytic anemia, *leukopenia, thrombocytopenia.*
Musculoskeletal: arthralgia, arthropathy, myalgia, *rhabdomyolysis.*
Respiratory: bronchitis, cough, *upper respiratory infection.*
Skin: rash.
Other: hypersensitivity reactions, tooth disorder.

Interactions

Drug-drug. *Cholestyramine, colestipol:* May bind with fluvastatin in GI tract and decrease

absorption. Separate administration times by at least 4 hours.
Cimetidine, omeprazole, ranitidine: May decrease fluvastatin metabolism. Monitor patient for enhanced effects.
Cyclosporine and other immunosuppressants, erythromycin, gemfibrozil, niacin: May increase risk of polymyositis and rhabdomyolysis. Avoid use together.
Digoxin: May increase digoxin level. Monitor digoxin level carefully.
Fluconazole, itraconazole, ketoconazole: May increase fluvastatin level and adverse effects. Avoid use together. If they must be given together, reduce dosage of fluvastatin.
Rifampin: May increase rifampin metabolism and decrease level. Monitor patient for lack of effect.
Drug-herb. *Red yeast rice:* May increase the risk of adverse events or toxicity. Discourage use together.
Drug-lifestyle. *Alcohol use:* May increase risk of hepatotoxicity. Discourage use together.

Effects on lab test results

• May increase ALT, AST, bilirubin, and CK levels. May decrease hemoglobin level and hematocrit.
• May decrease platelet and WBC counts.

Pharmacokinetics

Absorption: Rapid and almost complete on empty stomach.
Distribution: More than 98% protein-bound.
Metabolism: Complete.
Excretion: About 5% in urine, 90% in feces as metabolites. *Half-life:* Less than 1 hour.

Route	Onset	Peak	Duration
P.O.	Unknown	30–45 min	Unknown

Action

Chemical effect: Inhibits HMG-CoA reductase, an early (and rate-limiting) step in synthetic pathway of cholesterol.
Therapeutic effect: Lowers blood LDL and cholesterol levels.

Available forms

Capsules: 20 mg, 40 mg
Tablets (extended-release): 80 mg

NURSING PROCESS

📝 Assessment
• Assess patient's LDL and total cholesterol levels before starting therapy, and evaluate regularly.
• Perform liver function tests periodically.
• Be alert for adverse reactions and drug interactions.
• Assess patient's and family's knowledge of drug therapy.

🔲 Nursing diagnoses
• Risk for injury related to elevated LDL and cholesterol blood levels
• Diarrhea related to adverse effect of drug on GI tract
• Deficient knowledge related to drug therapy

▶ Planning and implementation
• Start drug only after diet and other nondrug therapies have proven ineffective.
• Give drug at bedtime to enhance effectiveness.
• Maintain standard low-cholesterol diet during therapy.
Patient teaching
• Tell patient that drug may be taken with or without food; effectiveness is enhanced if taken in evening.
• Teach patient about proper dietary management, weight control, and exercise. Explain their importance in controlling lipid levels.
• Warn patient to restrict alcohol consumption.
• Tell patient to inform prescriber of any adverse reactions, particularly muscle aches, weakness and pains.
• Tell patient that blood for liver function tests will be drawn periodically.
• Tell patient to stop drug and notify prescriber about planned, suspected, or known pregnancy.

✓ Evaluation
• Patient's LDL and total cholesterol levels are within normal limits.
• Patient maintains normal bowel pattern.
• Patient and family state understanding of drug therapy.

fluvoxamine maleate
(floo-VOKS-uh-meen MAL-ee-ayt)
Luvox

Pharmacologic class: SSRI
Therapeutic class: antidepressant
Pregnancy risk category: C

Indications and dosages

▶ **Obsessive-compulsive disorder (OCD), depression‡.** *Adults:* Initially, 50 mg P.O. daily at bedtime. Increase in 50-mg increments every 4 to 7 days until maximum benefit occurs. Maximum, 300 mg daily. If total daily amount exceeds 100 mg, divide and give in two doses. *Children ages 8 to 17:* Give 25 mg P.O. at bedtime. Maximum daily dose for children ages 8 to 11 is 200 mg. Maximum daily dose for children ages 12 to 17 is 300 mg. Increase initial dosage every 4 to 7 days, as needed. Divide doses greater than 50 mg b.i.d.
⬛ **Adjust-a-dose:** For elderly patients and patients with hepatic impairment, initially 25 mg P.O. daily then increase gradually to a maximum daily dose of 200 mg.

Contraindications and cautions

• Contraindicated in patients hypersensitive to SSRIs or any of their ingredients and within 2 weeks of an MAO inhibitor. Use with thioridazine or pimozide is contraindicated because ventricular arrhythmias and death may occur.
• Use cautiously in patients with hepatic dysfunction, suicidal ideation, conditions that may affect hemodynamic responses or metabolism, or history of mania or seizures.
⚠ **Lifespan:** In pregnant women and in breast-feeding women, use cautiously. In adolescents and children, use cautiously because the drug can increase risk of suicidal thinking or behavior. In children younger than age 8, drug is contraindicated for OCD. In children, drug is contraindicated for major depressive disorder. In elderly patients, use cautiously and start at a lower dose.

Adverse reactions

CNS: agitation, anxiety, asthenia, CNS stimulation, depression, *dizziness,* headache, hypertonia, *insomnia, nervousness, somnolence,* tremor.
CV: palpitations, vasodilation.

Reactions may be *common,* uncommon, *life-threatening,* or COMMON AND LIFE-THREATENING.

EENT: amblyopia.

GI: anorexia, constipation, *diarrhea, dry mouth,* dyspepsia, dysphagia, flatulence, *nausea,* taste perversion, vomiting.

GU: abnormal ejaculation, anorgasmia, impotence, urinary frequency, urine retention.

Respiratory: dyspnea, upper respiratory tract infection, yawning.

Skin: sweating.

Other: chills, flulike syndrome, decreased libido, tooth disorder.

Interactions

Drug-drug. *Benzodiazepines, theophylline, warfarin:* May reduce clearance of these drugs. Use together cautiously (except for diazepam, which shouldn't be given with fluvoxamine). Adjust dosage as needed.

Carbamazepine, clozapine, haloperidol, methadone, metoprolol, propranolol, tricyclic antidepressants: May increase levels of these drugs. Use together cautiously. Monitor patient closely for adverse reactions. Adjust dosage if needed.

Diltiazem: May cause bradycardia. Monitor heart rate.

Lithium, tryptophan: May increase fluvoxamine effects. Use together cautiously.

Phenelzine, selegiline, tranylcypromine: May cause serotonin syndrome, which may include CNS irritability, shivering, and altered consciousness. Use together may also cause severe excitation, hyperpyrexia, myoclonus, delirium, and coma. Don't give an MAO inhibitor within 2 weeks of an SSRI.

Pimozide, thioridazine: May prolong QT interval. Avoid use together.

Triptans, sumatriptan: May cause serotonin syndrome, including weakness, hyperreflexia, and incoordination. Avoid use together. If combination is needed, monitor patient closely.

Drug-herb. *St. John's wort:* May cause serotonin syndrome. Discourage use together.

Drug-food. *Caffeine:* May decrease caffeine elimination and increase caffeine effects. Discourage use together.

Drug-lifestyle. *Alcohol use:* May increase CNS effects. Discourage use together.

Smoking: May decrease effectiveness of drug. Discourage patient from smoking.

Sun exposure: May cause photosensitivity. Discourage prolonged or unprotected exposure to sunlight.

Effects on lab test results

None reported.

Pharmacokinetics

Absorption: Good.
Distribution: 77% protein-bound.
Metabolism: In liver.
Excretion: In urine. *Half-life:* 17 hours.

Route	Onset	Peak	Duration
P.O.	3–10 wk	3–8 hr	Unknown

Action

Chemical effect: May selectively inhibit neuronal uptake of serotonin, which is thought to reduce obsessive-compulsive disorders.
Therapeutic effect: Decreases obsessive-compulsive behavior.

Available forms

Tablets: 25 mg, 50 mg, 100 mg

NURSING PROCESS

Assessment
• Assess patient's condition before starting therapy, and reassess regularly. Patient may need several weeks of therapy before having a positive response.
• Be alert for adverse reactions and drug interactions.
• Assess child with OCD for signs of depression, including suicidal thoughts and behaviors.
• Assess patient's and family's knowledge of drug therapy.

Nursing diagnoses
• Ineffective coping related to underlying condition
• Diarrhea related to adverse effect of drug on GI tract
• Deficient knowledge related to drug therapy

Planning and implementation
• Don't give drug within 14 days of MAO inhibitor therapy.
ALERT: Drug may increase the risk of suicidal thinking and behavior in young adults ages 18 to 24 during the first 2 months of treatment. Monitor patient closely.
• Give drug at bedtime, with or without food.
ALERT: Don't confuse Luvox with Lasix.

(§) **ALERT:** Don't confuse fluvoxamine with fluvoxate or fluoxetine.

Patient teaching
• Instruct patient not to stop drug abruptly but to first consult prescriber.
• Advise patient and his family to monitor for suicidal thinking and behavior and to contact the prescriber immediately.
• Warn patient to avoid hazardous activities until the drug's CNS effects are known.
• Advise patient not to drink alcoholic beverages during therapy.
• Inform patient that smoking may decrease effectiveness of drug.
• Tell patient that drug may be taken with or without food.
• Instruct woman to notify prescriber about planned, suspected, or known pregnancy.
• Tell patient who develops rash, hives, or related allergic reaction to notify prescriber.
• Inform patient that several weeks of therapy may be needed to obtain full antidepressant effect. Once improvement has occurred, advise patient not to stop drug unless directed by prescriber.
• Advise patient to check with prescriber before taking OTC drugs or herbal remedies because interactions can occur.

✓ **Evaluation**
• Patient's obsessive-compulsive behaviors are diminished.
• Patient maintains normal bowel patterns.
• Patient and family state understanding of drug therapy.

folic acid (vitamin B₉)
(FOH-lek AS-id)
Folvite, Novo-Folacid ◆

Pharmacologic class: folic acid derivative
Therapeutic class: vitamin
Pregnancy risk category: A

Indications and dosages

▶ **To maintain health.** *Adults and children age 4 and older:* 0.4 mg P.O. daily.
Pregnant or lactating women: 0.8 mg P.O. daily.
Children younger than age 4: Up to 0.3 mg P.O. daily.
Infants: Up to 0.1 mg P.O. daily.

▶ **Megaloblastic or macrocytic anemia caused by folic acid or other nutritional deficiency, hepatic disease, alcoholism, intestinal obstruction, excessive hemolysis.** *Adults and children age 4 and older:* 0.4 mg to 1 mg P.O., subcutaneously, or I.M. daily. After anemia caused by folic acid deficiency is corrected, proper diet and supplements are needed to prevent recurrence.
Pregnant and breast-feeding women: 0.8 mg P.O., subcutaneously, or I.M. daily.
Children younger than age 4: Up to 0.3 mg P.O., subcutaneously, or I.M. daily.
▶ **Prevention of megaloblastic anemia in pregnancy.** *Adults:* Up to 1 mg P.O., subcutaneously, or I.M. daily throughout pregnancy.
▶ **Nutritional supplement.** *Adults:* 0.1 mg P.O., subcutaneously, or I.M. daily.
Children: 0.05 mg P.O. daily.
▶ **To test folic acid deficiency in patients with megaloblastic anemia without masking pernicious anemia.** *Adults and children:* 0.1 to 0.2 mg P.O. or I.M. for 10 days with diet low in folate and vitamin B₁₂.
▶ **Tropical sprue.** *Adults:* 3 to 15 mg P.O. daily.

Contraindications and cautions

• Contraindicated in patients with undiagnosed vitamin B₁₂ deficiency or undiagnosed anemia as it may improve the hematologic symptoms while the neurologic complications progress.
⚠ **Lifespan:** In pregnant women, folic acid therapy is recommended to prevent fetal neural tube defects.

Adverse reactions

CNS: general malaise.
GI: anorexia, bitter taste, flatulence, nausea.
Respiratory: *bronchospasm.*
Other: allergic reactions (erythema, pruritus, rash).

Interactions

Drug-drug. *Aminosalicylic acid, chloramphenicol, methotrexate, sulfasalazine, trimethoprim:* May antagonize folic acid. Monitor patient for decreased folic acid effect. Use together cautiously.
Anticonvulsants (such as phenobarbital, phenytoin): May increase anticonvulsant metabolism and decrease anticonvulsant blood levels. Monitor patient closely.

Effects on lab test results
• May decrease RBC count.

Pharmacokinetics
Absorption: Rapid after P.O. use.
Distribution: Complete; liver contains about half of total body stores. Concentrated actively in CSF.
Metabolism: In liver.
Excretion: Excess is unchanged in urine; small amounts in feces. *Half-life:* Unknown.

Route	Onset	Peak	Duration
P.O., I.M., SubQ	Unknown	30–60 min	Unknown

Action
Chemical effect: Stimulates normal erythropoiesis and nucleoprotein synthesis.
Therapeutic effect: Nutritional supplement.

Available forms
Injection: 5 mg/ml with 1.5% benzyl alcohol
Tablets: 0.1 mg†, 0.4 mg†, 0.8 mg†, 1 mg

NURSING PROCESS

⚡ Assessment
• Assess patient's folic acid deficiency before starting therapy.
• Evaluate CBC and assess patient's physical status throughout therapy.
• Be alert for adverse reactions and drug interactions.
• Assess patient's and family's knowledge of drug therapy.

⊕ Nursing diagnoses
• Imbalanced nutrition: less than body requirements related to presence of folic acid deficiency
• Deficient knowledge related to drug therapy

▷ Planning and implementation
• Patient with small-bowel resection and intestinal malabsorption may need parenteral administration.
• Don't mix with other drugs in same syringe for I.M. injections.
• Protect from light and heat; store at room temperature.
• Give vitamin B$_{12}$ with this therapy, if needed.

• Make sure patient is getting properly balanced diet.
⚠ **ALERT:** Some preparations contain benzyl alcohol. Don't use in infants and children.
⚠ **ALERT:** Don't confuse folic acid with folinic acid.
Patient teaching
• Teach patient proper nutrition to prevent recurrence of anemia.
• Tell patient to report hypersensitivity reactions or breathing difficulty.
• Urge patient to avoid alcohol because it increases folic acid requirements.

☑ Evaluation
• Patient's CBC is normal.
• Patient and family state understanding of drug therapy.

HIGH ALERT

fondaparinux sodium
(fon-duh-PAIR-in-ux SOH-dee-uhm)
Arixtra

Pharmacologic class: inhibitor of activated factor X (Xa)
Therapeutic class: anticoagulant
Pregnancy risk category: B

Indications and dosages

▶ **To prevent deep vein thrombosis and pulmonary embolism in patients undergoing abdominal surgery or surgery for hip fracture, hip replacement, or knee replacement.** *Adults who weigh 50 kg (110 lb) or more:* 2.5 mg subcutaneously once daily for 5 to 9 days. Give initial dose after hemostasis is established, 6 to 8 hours after surgery. Giving the dose earlier than 6 hours after surgery increases the risk for major bleeding.
▶ **Acute deep vein thrombosis with warfarin; acute pulmonary embolism with warfarin when therapy is initiated in the hospital.**
Adults who weigh more than 100 kg (220 lb): 10 mg subcutaneously daily for 5 to 9 days.
Adults who weigh 50 to 100 kg: 7.5 mg subcutaneously daily for 5 to 9 days.
Adults who weigh less than 50 kg: 5 mg subcutaneously daily for 5 to 9 days.

For all patients, begin oral anticoagulant therapy as soon as possible, usually within 72 hours.

Contraindications and cautions

• Contraindicated in patients with creatinine clearance less than 30 ml/minute; in those who are hypersensitive to the drug or as prophylaxis for abdominal, hip, or knee surgery in patients who weigh less than 50 kg; and in those with active major bleeding, bacterial endocarditis, or thrombocytopenia with a positive test result for antiplatelet antibody during therapy.
• Use cautiously in patients also being treated with platelet inhibitors and in those at increased risk for bleeding, such as patients who have congenital or acquired bleeding disorders, a bleeding diathesis, active ulcerative and angiodysplastic GI disease, or hemorrhagic stroke; and patients who recently had brain, spinal, or ophthalmologic surgery. Also use cautiously in patients who have had epidural or spinal anesthesia or spinal puncture because they have an increased risk of epidural or spinal hematoma (which may cause permanent paralysis). Use cautiously in patients undergoing elective hip surgery with mild or moderate renal impairment. Also use caution in patients with a creatinine clearance of 30 to 50 ml/minute, a history of heparin-induced thrombocytopenia, uncontrolled arterial hypertension, or a history of recent GI ulceration, diabetic retinopathy, or hemorrhage.
⚖ **Lifespan:** In pregnant women, use only if benefits outweigh risks to fetus. In breastfeeding women, use cautiously because it's unknown if drug appears in breast milk. In children, safety and effectiveness haven't been established. In elderly patients, use cautiously because the risk of major bleeding increases with age.

Adverse reactions

CNS: confusion, dizziness, *fever,* headache, insomnia, pain, **spinal and epidural hematomas.**
CV: edema, hypotension.
GI: constipation, diarrhea, dyspepsia, *nausea,* vomiting.
GU: urine retention, UTI.
Hematologic: anemia, hematoma, **hemorrhage, postoperative hemorrhage, thrombocytopenia.**
Metabolic: hypokalemia.
Skin: bullous eruption, increased wound drainage, mild local irritation (injection site bleeding, pruritus, rash), purpura, rash.

Interactions

Drug-drug. *Drugs that increase risk of bleeding (anticoagulants, NSAIDs, platelet inhibitors, salicylates):* May increase risk of hemorrhage. If drugs must be used together, monitor patient closely.

Effects on lab test results

• May increase creatinine, AST, ALT, and bilirubin levels. May decrease potassium and hemoglobin levels and hematocrit.
• May decrease platelet count.

Pharmacokinetics

Absorption: Rapid and complete; 100% bioavailability.
Distribution: Mainly in blood. At least 94% bound to antithrombin III (AT-III).
Metabolism: Not studied.
Excretion: Up to 77% in urine unchanged in 72 hours. *Half-life:* 17 to 21 hours.

Route	Onset	Peak	Duration
SubQ	Unknown	2–3 hr	Unknown

Action

Chemical effect: Binds to AT-III and potentiates the natural neutralization of factor Xa by AT-III. Neutralization of factor Xa interrupts the coagulation cascade, thereby inhibiting formation of thrombin and thrombus development.
Therapeutic effect: Prevents the formation of blood clots.

Available forms

Injection (single-dose prefilled syringes): 2.5 mg/0.5 ml, 5 mg/0.4 ml, 7.5 mg/0.6 ml, 10 mg/0.8 ml

NURSING PROCESS

Assessment
• Assess patient's underlying condition before starting therapy.
• Be alert for adverse reactions and drug interactions.
• Patient who has received epidural or spinal anesthesia is at increased risk for epidural or spinal hematoma, which may result in long-term or permanent paralysis. Monitor patient closely for neurological impairment.

• Monitor renal function periodically, and stop drug in patient who develops unstable renal function or severe renal impairment.
• Routinely assess patient for signs and symptoms of bleeding, and regularly monitor CBC, platelet count, creatinine level, and stool occult blood test results. If platelet count is less than 100,000/mm³, stop drug.
• Effect may last for 2 to 4 days after stopping drug in patient with normal renal function.
• Don't use PT and PTT tests to measure effectiveness.
• Assess patient's and family's knowledge of drug therapy.

Nursing diagnoses
• Risk for injury related to potential for thrombosis or pulmonary emboli development from underlying condition
• Risk for trauma related to increased risk of bleeding and hemorrhaging due to drug therapy
• Deficient knowledge related to anticoagulant therapy

Planning and implementation
• Give by subcutaneous injection only, in fatty tissue only, rotating injection sites.
• Visually inspect the single-dose prefilled syringe for particulate matter and discoloration before administration.
• Don't mix with other injections.
🕭 ALERT: Don't use interchangeably with heparin, low–molecular-weight heparins, or heparinoids.
• To avoid loss of drug, don't expel air bubble from the syringe.
• If patient begins to overtly bleed while being given the drug, apply strong pressure to the injection area and immediately notify the prescriber.
• Overdose may lead to hemorrhagic complications. Stop giving the drug and treat bleeding appropriately.
🕭 ALERT: Don't confuse Arixtra with the lab test anti-factor Xa, sometimes written anti-Xa.
🕭 ALERT: Don't confuse Arixtra with Bextra.
Patient teaching
• Teach patient signs and symptoms of bleeding. If any occur, patient should immediately contact the prescriber.
• Instruct patient to avoid OTC products that contain aspirin, other salicylates, or NSAIDs and other non-prescribed anticoagulants.

• Teach patient the correct way to give drug to himself subcutaneously.
• Show patient the different sites for injection, and explain that he must alternate injection sites to prevent hardening of fatty tissues.
• Teach patient the proper disposal of the syringe.

✓ Evaluation
• Patient has no pulmonary embolus or thrombus during drug therapy.
• Patient is free from any injury or bleeding.
• Patient and family state understanding of drug therapy.

formoterol fumarate inhalation powder
(for-MOE-tur-all FYOO-muh-rayt)
Foradil Aerolizer, Perforomist

Pharmacologic class: selective long-acting beta₂ agonist
Therapeutic class: bronchodilator
Pregnancy risk category: C

Indications and dosages

▶ **Preventive and maintenance therapy for bronchospasm in patients with reversible obstructive airway disease or nocturnal asthma who usually need short-acting inhaled beta₂ agonists.** *Adults and children age 5 and older:* One 12-mcg capsule by inhalation via Aerolizer inhaler every 12 hours. Don't give more than one capsule b.i.d. (24 mcg daily). If symptoms are present between doses, use a short-acting beta₂ agonist for immediate relief.
▶ **To prevent exercise-induced bronchospasm.** *Adults and children age 12 and older:* One 12-mcg capsule by inhalation via Aerolizer inhaler at least 15 minutes before exercise, given occasionally, p.r.n. Avoid giving additional doses within 12 hours of first dose.
▶ **Maintenance therapy for COPD.** *Adults:* One 12-mcg capsule by inhalation via Aerolizer inhaler every 12 hours. Total daily dosage of greater than 24 mcg isn't recommended.
◼ **NEW INDICATION:** **Prevention of bronchoconstriction in patients with COPD (chronic bronchitis, emphysema).** *Adults:* One 20 mcg/2 ml vial by oral inhalation via a jet

nebulizer every 12 hours. Maximum dosage 40 mcg/day.

Contraindications and cautions

• Contraindicated in patients hypersensitive to drug or any of its components.
• Use cautiously in patients with CV disease, particularly coronary insufficiency, cardiac arrhythmias, and hypertension; in those who are unusually responsive to sympathomimetic amines; and in those with diabetes mellitus because hyperglycemia and ketoacidosis have occurred rarely with use of beta agonists. Also use cautiously in patients with lactose or milk allergy, seizure disorders, or thyrotoxicosis.
• Do not use to treat acute asthma attack or bronchospasm.
☀ **Lifespan:** In pregnant women, use cautiously because drug may interfere with uterine contractility. In breast-feeding women, use cautiously because it isn't known if drug appears in breast milk. In children younger than age 5, safety and effectiveness haven't been established for asthma. In children younger than age 12, safety and effectiveness haven't been established for exercise-induced bronchospasm.

Adverse reactions

CNS: dizziness, fatigue, headache, insomnia, malaise, nervousness, tremor.
CV: angina, *arrhythmias,* chest pain, hypertension, hypotension, palpitations, tachycardia.
EENT: dry mouth, dysphonia, tonsillitis.
GI: nausea.
Metabolic: hyperglycemia, hypokalemia, *metabolic acidosis.*
Musculoskeletal: muscle cramps.
Respiratory: bronchitis, chest infection, dyspnea.
Skin: rash.
Other: viral infection.

Interactions

Drug-drug. *Adrenergics:* May potentiate sympathetic effects of formoterol. Use together cautiously.
Beta blockers: May antagonize effects of beta agonists, causing bronchospasm in asthmatic patients. Avoid use except when benefits outweigh risks. Use cardioselective beta blockers cautiously to minimize risk of bronchospasm.

Corticosteroids, diuretics, xanthine derivatives: May potentiate hypokalemic effect of formoterol. Use together cautiously.
Loop or thiazide diuretics: May worsen ECG changes or hypokalemia with beta agonists. Use together cautiously, and monitor patient closely.
MAO inhibitors, tricyclic antidepressants, and other drugs that prolong the QT interval: May increase risk of ventricular arrhythmias. Use together cautiously.

Effects on lab test results

• May decrease potassium level. May increase glucose level.

Pharmacokinetics

Absorption: Rapid. Drug levels peak within 5 minutes after a 120-mcg dose.
Distribution: 61% to 64% protein-bound.
Metabolism: Mainly by CYP2D6, CYP2C19, CYP2C9, and CYP2A6. At therapeutic level, doesn't appear to inhibit cytochrome P-450 enzymes.
Excretion: 59% to 62% in urine and 32% to 34% in feces over 5 days. *Half-life:* Unknown.

Route	Onset	Peak	Duration
Inhalation	1–3 min	½–1½ hr	12 hr

Action

Chemical effect: Relaxes bronchial smooth muscle by acting on $beta_2$-adrenergic receptors; stimulates intracellular adenyl cyclase, the enzyme responsible for catalyzing the conversion of adenosine triphosphate (ATP) to cAMP. Increase in cAMP leads to relaxation of bronchial smooth muscle and inhibition of mediator release from mast cells.
Therapeutic effect: Prevents and controls bronchospasm.

Available forms

Capsules for inhalation: 12 mcg
Inhalation solution: 20 mcg/2 ml vial

NURSING PROCESS

▨ **Assessment**

• Assess patient's underlying condition before starting therapy, and reassess regularly.
• Evaluate patient's use of short-acting $beta_2$ agonists for immediate relief of bronchospasm. Drug may be used with short-acting $beta_2$ ago-

nists, inhaled corticosteroids, and theophylline therapy to manage asthma.

• Assess patient's and family's knowledge of drug therapy.

🔆 Nursing diagnoses

• Impaired gas exchange related to underlying pulmonary condition

• Risk for activity intolerance related to underlying pulmonary condition

• Deficient knowledge related to formoterol fumarate therapy

▷ Planning and implementation

• Before use, store drug in refrigerator. After use, drug may be stored at room temperature.

• Don't remove capsule from unopened blister until immediately before use.

• Give capsules only by oral inhalation and only with the Aerolizer inhaler.

• Don't use Foradil Aerolizer with a spacer device.

• For patient using drug twice daily, don't give additional doses to prevent exercise-induced bronchospasm.

• Don't use as a substitute for short-acting beta$_2$ agonists for immediate relief of bronchospasm, or as a substitute for inhaled or oral corticosteroids.

• Don't begin use in patients with rapidly deteriorating or significantly worsening asthma.

• If usual dose doesn't control symptoms of bronchoconstriction and the patient's short-acting beta$_2$ agonist becomes less effective, reevaluate patient and therapy.

• For patient who formerly used regularly scheduled short-acting beta$_2$ agonists, decrease use of these drugs to an as-needed basis when long-acting therapy starts.

• Don't let the patient exhale into the device.

• Pierce capsules only once. To minimize risk of shattering capsule, strictly follow storage and use instructions. The Aerolizer contains a screen that will catch any broken pieces of the capsule before they enter the patient's mouth or lungs.

• Drug may cause life-threatening paradoxical bronchospasm. If this occurs, immediately stop giving the drug and use a different drug.

• Monitor patient for tachycardia, hypertension, and other adverse CV effects. If they occur, stop drug.

• Watch for immediate hypersensitivity reactions, such as anaphylaxis, urticaria, angioedema, rash, and bronchospasm.

• Signs and symptoms of overdose include excessive beta blocker stimulation (tachycardia, tremor, hypotension) and exaggerated adverse effects, leading to cardiac arrest and death. To treat overdose, stop drug, monitor cardiac condition, give appropriate symptomatic relief or supportive therapy, and use cardioselective beta blockers cautiously. It's unknown whether dialysis is beneficial.

⚠ **ALERT:** Capsules shouldn't be swallowed.

⚠ **ALERT:** Don't confuse Foradil with Toradol.

Patient teaching

• Tell patient not to increase the dosage or frequency of use without medical advice.

• Warn patient not to stop or reduce other drugs taken for asthma.

• Advise patient that drug isn't for acute asthmatic episodes; instead, he should use short-acting beta$_2$ agonist.

• Advise patient to report worsening symptoms, decreasing effectiveness, or increasing use of short-acting beta$_2$ agonist.

• Tell patient to report nausea, vomiting, shakiness, headache, fast or irregular heartbeat, chest pain, or sleeplessness.

• Tell patient being treated for exercise-induced bronchospasm to take drug at least 15 minutes before exercise. Additional doses can't be taken for 12 hours.

• Tell patient not to use the Foradil Aerolizer with a spacer device or to exhale or blow into the inhaler.

• Advise patient to avoid washing the Aerolizer and to always keep it dry. Advise patient to use the new device that comes with each refill.

• Tell patient to avoid exposing capsules to moisture and to handle them only with dry hands.

☑ Evaluation

• Patient's pulmonary symptoms improve.

• Patient's activity intolerance improves.

• Patient and family state understanding of drug therapy.

fosamprenavir calcium
(foss-am-PREH-nuh-veer CAL-see-um)
Lexiva

Pharmacologic class: protease inhibitor
Therapeutic class: antiretroviral
Pregnancy risk category: C

Indications and dosages

▶ **HIV infection with other antiretrovirals.**
Adults: In patients previously untreated,
1,400 mg P.O. b.i.d. (without ritonavir). Or
1,400 mg P.O. once daily and ritonavir 200 mg
P.O. once daily. Or 1,400 mg P.O. once daily
and ritonavir 100 mg P.O. once daily. Or
700 mg P.O. b.i.d. and ritonavir 100 mg P.O.
b.i.d. In patients previously treated with a protease inhibitor, 700 mg P.O. b.i.d. plus ritonavir
100 mg P.O. b.i.d.

🔲 **Adjust-a-dose:** If patient takes efavirenz,
fosamprenavir, and ritonavir once daily, give an
additional 100 mg daily of ritonavir (300 mg total). If patient has mild or moderate hepatic impairment and takes fosamprenavir without ritonavir, reduce dosage to 700 mg P.O. b.i.d. Avoid
use in patients with severe hepatic impairment
because dose can't be reduced below 700 mg.

Contraindications and cautions

• Contraindicated in patients hypersensitive to
amprenavir or any of its components. Also contraindicated with dihydroergotamine, ergonovine, ergotamine, flecainide, methylergonovine,
midazolam, pimozide, propafenone, and triazolam.
• Use cautiously in patients allergic to sulfonamides and those with mild to moderate hepatic
impairment. Avoid use in patients with severe
hepatic impairment.
⚕ **Lifespan:** In pregnant women, breast-
feeding women, and children, safety and effectiveness haven't been established.

Adverse reactions

CNS: depression, fatigue, headache, oral pares-
thesia.
GI: abdominal pain, diarrhea, nausea, vomiting.
Skin: pruritus, *rash.*

Interactions

Drug-drug. *Amitriptyline, cyclosporine,
imipramine, tacrolimus:* May increase levels of
these drugs. Monitor drug levels.
*Antiarrhythmics (amiodarone, lidocaine, quini-
dine):* May increase antiarrhythmic level. Use
together cautiously, and monitor antiarrhythmic
levels.
Atorvastatin: May increase atorvastatin level.
Give 20 mg daily or less of atorvastatin and
monitor patient carefully. Or consider other
HMG-CoA reductase inhibitors, such as fluvastatin, pravastatin, or rosuvastatin.
*Benzodiazepines (alprazolam, clorazepate, di-
azepam, flurazepam):* May increase benzodiazepine level. Decrease benzodiazepine dosage
if needed.
*Calcium channel blockers (amlodipine, dilti-
azem, felodipine, isradipine, nicardipine,
nifedipine, nimodipine, nisoldipine, verapamil):*
May increase calcium channel blocker level.
Use together cautiously.
*Carbamazepine, dexamethasone, H_2-receptor
antagonists, phenobarbital, phenytoin, proton-
pump inhibitors:* May decrease amprenavir level. Use together cautiously.
Delavirdine: May cause loss of virologic response and resistance to delavirdine. Avoid use
together.
*Dihydroergotamine, ergonovine, ergotamine,
flecainide, methylergonovine, midazolam, pimozide, propafenone, triazolam:* May cause serious adverse reactions. Avoid use together.
Efavirenz, nevirapine, saquinavir: May decrease
amprenavir level. Appropriate combination doses haven't been established.
Efavirenz with ritonavir: May decrease amprenavir level. Increase ritonavir by 100 mg daily
(300 mg total) when giving efavirenz, fosamprenavir, and ritonavir once daily. No change needed in ritonavir when giving efavirenz, fosamprenavir, and ritonavir twice daily.
Ethinyl estradiol and norethindrone: May increase ethinyl estradiol and norethindrone levels. Recommend nonhormonal contraception.
Indinavir, nelfinavir: May increase amprenavir
level. Appropriate combination doses haven't
been established.
Itraconazole, ketoconazole: May increase ketoconazole and itraconazole levels. Reduce ketoconazole or itraconazole dosage as needed if
patient takes more than 400 mg daily of fosamprenavir. Don't give more than 200 mg daily.

Lopinavir with ritonavir: May decrease amprenavir and lopinavir levels. Appropriate combination doses haven't been established.

Lovastatin, simvastatin: May increase risk of myopathy, including rhabdomyolysis. Avoid use together.

Methadone: May decrease methadone level. Increase methadone dosage if needed.

Rifabutin: May increase rifabutin level. Obtain CBC weekly to watch for neutropenia and decrease rifabutin dosage by at least half. If patient takes ritonavir, decrease dosage by at least 75% from the usual 300 mg daily. Maximum, 150 mg every other day or three times weekly.

Rifampin: May decrease amprenavir level and drug effect. Avoid use together.

Sildenafil, tadalafil, vardenafil: May increase levels of these drugs. Recommend cautious use of sildenafil at 25 mg every 48 hours, tadalafil 10 mg every 72 hours, or vardenafil at no more than 2.5 mg every 24 hours. If patient takes ritonavir, recommend cautious use of vardenafil at no more than 2.5 mg every 72 hours. Tell patient to report adverse events.

Warfarin: May alter warfarin level. Monitor INR.

Drug-herb. *St. John's wort:* May cause loss of virologic response and resistance to fosamprenavir or its class of protease inhibitors. Discourage use together.

Effects on lab test results

• May increase lipase, triglyceride, AST, and ALT levels.
• May decrease neutrophil count.

Pharmacokinetics

Absorption: Food has no effect.
Distribution: 90% protein-bound.
Metabolism: Rapid and almost complete via CYP3A4.
Excretion: Unknown. *Half-life:* About 8 hours.

Route	Onset	Peak	Duration
P.O.	Unknown	1½–4 hr	Unknown

Action

Chemical effect: Converts rapidly to amprenavir, which binds to the active site of HIV-1 protease and causes formation of immature noninfectious viral particles.
Therapeutic effect: Hinders HIV activity.

Available forms

Tablets: 700 mg

NURSING PROCESS

Assessment
• Monitor patient with hemophilia for spontaneous bleeding.
• During initial therapy, monitor patient for such opportunistic infections as *Mycobacterium avium* complex, CMV, *Pneumocystis jiroveci (carinii)* pneumonia, and tuberculosis.
• Assess patient for redistribution or accumulation of body fat, as in central obesity, dorsocervical fat enlargement (buffalo hump), peripheral wasting, facial wasting, breast enlargement, and a cushingoid appearance.
• Assess patient's and family's knowledge of drug therapy.

Nursing diagnoses
• Risk for infection related to presence of HIV
• Risk for deficient fluid volume related to adverse GI reactions
• Deficient knowledge related to drug therapy

Planning and implementation
• Patient with hepatitis B or C, or noticeable increase in transaminase level before therapy, may have an increased risk of transaminase elevation. Monitor patient.
Patient teaching
• Tell patient that drug doesn't reduce the risk of transmitting HIV to others.
• Inform patient that the drug may reduce the risk of progression to AIDS and death.
• Explain that drug must be used with other antiretrovirals.
• Tell patient not to alter the dosage or stop taking drug without consulting the prescriber.
• Urge patient to inform the prescriber about sulfa allergy.
• Because this drug may interact with many drugs, urge patient to tell the prescriber about any prescription or OTC drugs and herbal products that he takes (especially St. John's wort).
• Explain that body fat may redistribute or accumulate.

Evaluation
• Patient responds well to therapy.
• Patient maintains adequate hydration.

• Patient and family state understanding of drug therapy.

---

foscarnet sodium (phosphonoformic acid)
(fos-KAR-net SOH-dee-um)
Foscavir

Pharmacologic class: pyrophosphate analogue
Therapeutic class: antiviral
Pregnancy risk category: C

Indications and dosages

▶ **CMV retinitis in patients with AIDS.**
Adults: Initially, 60 mg/kg I.V. over 1 hour every 8 hours, or 90 mg/kg I.V. over 1½ to 2 hours every 12 hours for 2 to 3 weeks, depending on response. Follow with maintenance infusion of 90 to 120 mg/kg I.V. daily over 2 hours.
▧ **Adjust-a-dose:** In patients with renal impairment, adjust dosage if creatinine clearance is less than 1.5 ml/kg/minute. If clearance is less than 0.4 ml/kg/minute, stop drug.
▶ **Mucocutaneous acyclovir-resistant herpes simplex virus infections.** *Adults:* 40 mg/kg I.V. infused over at least 1 hour, every 8 or 12 hours for 2 to 3 weeks or until healed.
▧ **Adjust-a-dose:** In patients with renal impairment, if creatinine clearance is less than 1.5 ml/kg/minute, adjust dosage. If clearance is less than 0.4 ml/kg/minute, stop drug.
▶ **Varicella zoster infection‡.** *Adults:* 40 mg/kg I.V. every 8 hours for 14 to 21 days.

▼ I.V. administration

• If infusing via central venous access, the standard 24-mg/ml solution may or may not be diluted. When using a peripheral venous catheter, dilute solution to 12 mg/ml with D_5W or normal saline solution.
• To reduce the risk of nephrotoxicity, give 750 to 1,000 ml of normal saline solution or D_5W before first dose and then with each subsequent dose.
• Don't exceed recommended dosage, infusion rate, or frequency of administration. All doses must be individualized based on patient's renal function.

• Use infusion pump to give drug over at least 1 hour.
• Use solution within 24 hours of first entry into sealed bottle.
⊗ **Incompatibilities**
Acyclovir, amphotericin B, co-trimoxazole, dextrose 30%, diazepam, digoxin, diphenhydramine, dobutamine, droperidol, ganciclovir, gentamicin, haloperidol, lactated Ringer's solution, leucovorin, lorazepam, midazolam, morphine, pentamidine, phenytoin, prochlorperazine, promethazine, solutions containing calcium (such as total parenteral nutrition), trimetrexate, vancomycin.

Contraindications and cautions

• Contraindicated in patients hypersensitive to drug or any of its components.
• Use cautiously and at a lower dose in a patient with abnormal renal function because drug will accumulate and toxicity will increase. Because drug is nephrotoxic, it may worsen renal impairment. Some nephrotoxicity occurs in most patients treated with drug.
❧ **Lifespan:** In pregnant women, use cautiously. In breast-feeding women, use cautiously because it's unknown if the drug appears in breast milk. In children, safety and effectiveness haven't been established. In elderly patients, use cautiously because they are more likely to have decreased renal function.

Adverse reactions

CNS: abnormal coordination, aggressive reaction, agitation, amnesia, anxiety, aphasia, *asthenia,* ataxia, cerebrovascular disorder, confusion, dementia, depression, *dizziness,* EEG abnormalities, *fatigue, fever,* generalized spasms, *headache, hypoesthesia,* insomnia, *malaise,* meningitis, nervousness, *neuropathy,* pain, *paresthesia,* **seizures,** sensory disturbances, somnolence, stupor, tremor.
CV: ECG abnormalities, edema, facial edema, first-degree AV block, flushing, hypertension, hypotension, palpitations, sinus tachycardia.
EENT: conjunctivitis, eye pain, pharyngitis, rhinitis, sinusitis, visual disturbances.
GI: *abdominal pain, anorexia,* constipation, *diarrhea,* dry mouth, dysphagia, flatulence, melena, *nausea, **pancreatitis, rectal hemorrhage,*** taste perversion, ulcerative stomatitis, *vomiting.*
GU: abnormal renal function, ***acute renal impairment,*** albuminuria, candidiasis, dysuria,

nephrotoxicity, polyuria, urethral disorder, urine retention, UTI.
Hematologic: anemia, ***bone marrow suppression, granulocytopenia, leukopenia,*** lymphadenopathy, ***thrombocytopenia, thrombosis.***
Hepatic: abnormal hepatic function.
Metabolic: hypocalcemia, hypokalemia, ***hypomagnesemia,*** hyponatremia, hypophosphatemia or hyperphosphatemia.
Musculoskeletal: arthralgia, leg cramps, myalgia.
Respiratory: ***bronchospasm,*** *cough, dyspnea,* hemoptysis, ***pneumonic respiratory insufficiency, pneumothorax,*** pulmonary infiltration, ***stridor.***
Skin: erythematous rash, *increased sweating,* pruritus, *rash,* seborrhea, skin discoloration, skin ulceration.
Other: abscess, back or chest pain, bacterial or fungal infections, flulike symptoms, inflammation, lymphoma-like disorder, pain at infusion site, rigors, sarcoma, ***sepsis.***

Interactions

Drug-drug. *Nephrotoxic drugs (such as aminoglycosides, amphotericin B):* May increase risk of nephrotoxicity. Avoid use together.
Pentamidine: May increase risk of nephrotoxicity and severe hypocalcemia. Don't use together.
Zidovudine: May increase risk or severity of anemia. Monitor blood counts.

Effects on lab test results

• May increase BUN, creatinine, phosphate, ALT, AST, alkaline phosphatase, and bilirubin levels. May decrease calcium, magnesium, phosphate, potassium, sodium, and hemoglobin levels and hematocrit.
• May decrease granulocyte and WBC counts. May increase or decrease platelet count.

Pharmacokinetics

Absorption: Given I.V.
Distribution: 14% to 17% protein-bound.
Metabolism: None.
Excretion: 80% to 90% unchanged in urine.
Half-life: 3 hours.

Route	Onset	Peak	Duration
I.V.	Immediate	Immediate	Unknown

Action

Chemical effect: Blocks pyrophosphate binding sites on DNA polymerases and reverse transcriptases.
Therapeutic effect: Kills virus.

Available forms

Injection: 24 mg/ml in 250- and 500-ml bottles

NURSING PROCESS

Assessment
• Assess patient's infection before therapy and regularly thereafter.
• Obtain electrolyte levels and creatinine clearance before therapy, two or three times weekly during induction and at least once every 1 or 2 weeks during maintenance.
• Drug may cause dose-related transient decrease in ionized calcium, which may not show up in laboratory values. Watch for tetany and seizures with abnormal electrolyte levels.
• Monitor patient's hemoglobin level and hematocrit. Patient may develop anemia severe enough that he needs transfusions.
• Be alert for adverse reactions and drug interactions.
• Assess patient's and family's knowledge of drug therapy.

Nursing diagnoses
• Risk for infection related to presence of herpes virus susceptible to drug
• Disturbed sensory perception (tactile) related to drug's adverse effect
• Deficient knowledge related to drug therapy

Planning and implementation
• Because drug is highly toxic and toxicity is probably dose-related, use lowest effective maintenance dosage.
Patient teaching
• Advise patient to report circumoral tingling, numbness in limbs, and paresthesia.

Evaluation
• Patient is free from infection.
• Patient has no adverse neurologic reactions.
• Patient and family state understanding of drug therapy.

fosinopril sodium
(foh-SIN-oh-pril SOH-dee-um)
Monopril✍

Pharmacologic class: ACE inhibitor
Therapeutic class: antihypertensive
Pregnancy risk category: C (D in second and third trimesters)

Indications and dosages

▶ **Hypertension.** *Adults:* Initially, 10 mg P.O. daily. Adjust dosage based on blood pressure at peak and trough levels. Usual dosage, 20 to 40 mg daily. Maximum, 80 mg daily. May divide dosage.
Children ages 6 to 16, weighing 50 kg (110 lb) or more: Give 5 to 10 mg P.O. daily.
▶ **Adjunct therapy for heart failure.** *Adults:* Initially, 10 mg P.O. once daily. Increase dosage over several weeks to maximum tolerable, but no more than 40 mg P.O. daily. If possible, stop diuretic therapy.
⊠ Adjust-a-dose: For patients who have heart failure with moderate to severe renal impairment or who are being vigorously diuresed, give initial dose of 5 mg P.O. daily.

Contraindications and cautions

• Contraindicated in patients hypersensitive to drug or any of its components or to other ACE inhibitors, including patients with a history of ACE inhibitor–induced angioedema and patients with hereditary or idiopathic angioedema. Avoid use in patients with renal artery stenosis.
• Use cautiously in patients with impaired renal or hepatic function.
⚘ Lifespan: In pregnant women, use only if benefits outweigh risks to fetus. In breast-feeding women, drug is contraindicated. In children younger than age 6 or those weighing less than 50 kg, safety and effectiveness haven't been established.

Adverse reactions

CNS: dizziness, fatigue, headache, paresthesia, sleep disturbance, *stroke,* syncope.
CV: angina, chest pain, hypotension, *MI,* orthostatic hypotension, palpitations, rhythm disturbances.
EENT: sinusitis, tinnitus.

GI: abdominal distention, abdominal pain, constipation, diarrhea, dry mouth, nausea, *pancreatitis,* vomiting.
GU: renal insufficiency.
Hepatic: *hepatitis.*
Metabolic: *hyperkalemia.*
Musculoskeletal: arthralgia, musculoskeletal pain, myalgia.
Respiratory: *bronchospasm;* dry, persistent, tickling, nonproductive cough.
Skin: photosensitivity, pruritus, rash, urticaria.
Other: *angioedema,* decreased libido, gout, sexual dysfunction.

Interactions

Drug-drug. *Antacids:* May impair absorption. Separate administration times by at least 2 hours.
Diuretics, other antihypertensives: May increase risk of excessive hypotension. Stop diuretic or lower fosinopril dosage.
Lithium: May increase lithium level and toxicity. Avoid use together.
Potassium-sparing diuretics, potassium supplements, sodium substitutes containing potassium: May increase risk of hyperkalemia. Monitor potassium level.
Drug-herb. *Licorice:* May cause sodium retention and increase blood pressure, interfering with ACE inhibitor effect. Discourage ingestion of licorice during drug therapy.
Drug-food. *Salt substitutes containing potassium:* May increase risk of hyperkalemia. Monitor potassium closely.
Drug-lifestyle. *Alcohol use:* May have additive hypotensive effects. Discourage use together.

Effects on lab test results

• May increase BUN, creatinine, and potassium levels. May decrease hemoglobin level and hematocrit.
• May increase liver function test values.

Pharmacokinetics

Absorption: Slow, mainly in proximal small intestine.
Distribution: More than 95% protein-bound.
Metabolism: Mainly in liver and gut.
Excretion: 50% in urine; remainder in feces.
Half-life: 11½ hours.

Route	Onset	Peak	Duration
P.O.	≤1 hr	2–6 hr	24 hr

Reactions may be *common,* uncommon, *life-threatening*, or COMMON AND LIFE-THREATENING.

Action

Chemical effect: Inhibits ACE, preventing conversion of angiotensin I to angiotensin II, a potent vasoconstrictor, which decreases peripheral arterial resistance, and aldosterone secretion.
Therapeutic effect: Lowers blood pressure.

Available forms

Tablets: 10 mg, 20 mg, 40 mg

NURSING PROCESS

🔲 Assessment

• Assess blood pressure before starting therapy and regularly thereafter.
• Assess renal and hepatic function before starting therapy and regularly thereafter.
• Monitor potassium intake and potassium level. Diabetic patients, those with renal impairment, and those receiving drugs that can increase potassium levels may develop hyperkalemia.
• Other ACE inhibitors have been linked to agranulocytosis and neutropenia. Monitor CBC with differential counts before therapy, every 2 weeks for first 3 months of therapy, and periodically thereafter.
• If adverse GI reaction occurs, monitor patient's hydration.
• Assess patient's and family's knowledge of drug therapy.

⊕ Nursing diagnoses

• Risk for injury related to presence of hypertension
• Risk for deficient fluid volume related to adverse GI reactions
• Deficient knowledge related to drug therapy

▷ Planning and implementation

• Drug may be taken with food, but it slows absorption.
Patient teaching
• Tell patient to avoid salt substitutes because they may contain potassium, which increases the risk of hyperkalemia.
• Urge patient to report signs of infection (such as fever and sore throat); easy bruising or bleeding; swelling of tongue, lips, face, eyes, mucous membranes, or limbs; difficulty swallowing or breathing; and hoarseness.
• Tell patient to use caution in hot weather and during exercise. Inadequate fluid intake, vomit-

ing, diarrhea, and excessive perspiration can lead to light-headedness and syncope.
• Tell woman to notify prescriber about planned, suspected, or known pregnancy. Drug will probably need to be stopped.

☑ Evaluation

• Patient's blood pressure is normal.
• Patient maintains adequate hydration throughout drug therapy.
• Patient and family state understanding of drug therapy.

fosphenytoin sodium

(fahs-FEN-eh-toyn SOH-dee-um)
Cerebyx

Pharmacologic class: hydantoin
Therapeutic class: anticonvulsant
Pregnancy risk category: D

Indications and dosages

▶ **Status epilepticus.** *Adults:* 15 to 20 mg phenytoin sodium equivalent (PE)/kg I.V. at 100 to 150 mg PE/minute as loading dose; then 4 to 6 mg PE/kg I.V. daily as maintenance dose. (Phenytoin may be used instead of fosphenytoin as maintenance, using the appropriate dose.)
▶ **To prevent and treat seizures during neurosurgery (nonemergent loading or maintenance doses).** *Adults:* Loading dose of 10 to 20 mg PE/kg I.M. or I.V. at infusion rate not exceeding 150 mg PE/minute. Maintenance dosage is 4 to 6 mg PE/kg I.V. or I.M. daily.
▶ **Short-term substitution for oral phenytoin therapy.** *Adults:* Same total daily dosage equivalent as oral phenytoin sodium therapy given as a single daily dose I.M. or I.V. at infusion rate not exceeding 150 mg PE/minute. Some patients may need more frequent doses.

▽ I.V. administration

• Dilute drug in D_5W or normal saline solution for injection to yield 1.5 to 25 mg PE/ml.
• Don't exceed 150 mg PE/minute.
• Monitor patient's ECG, blood pressure, and respirations throughout period of highest phenytoin levels—about 10 to 20 minutes after end of fosphenytoin infusion.

• Refrigerate at 36° to 46° F (2° C to 8° C). Don't keep at room temperature for longer than 48 hours.
⊗ **Incompatibilities**
Other I.V. drugs.

Contraindications and cautions

• Contraindicated in patients hypersensitive to drug or any of its components, phenytoin, or other hydantoins. Also contraindicated in patients with sinus bradycardia, SA block, second- or third-degree AV block, Adams-Stokes syndrome, or acute hepatotoxicity. Drug isn't indicated for absence seizures.
• Use cautiously in patients with renal and hepatic disease or in those with hypoalbuminemia.
⚖ **Lifespan:** In pregnant women, use drug only if nature, frequency, and severity of seizures pose a serious threat to the patient. In breast-feeding women, use cautiously. In children, safety and effectiveness haven't been established. In elderly patients, use a lower dose because of their decreased metabolism and decreased phenytoin clearance.

Adverse reactions

CNS: abnormal thinking, agitation, asthenia, *ataxia,* **brain edema,** decreased reflexes, *dizziness,* dysarthria, headache, extrapyramidal syndrome, fever, hypoesthesia, increased reflexes, incoordination, *intracranial hypertension,* nervousness, paresthesia, speech disorder, *somnolence,* stupor, vertigo.
CV: hypotension, hypertension, tachycardia, tremor, facial edema, vasodilation, *severe CV reactions, ventricular fibrillation.*
EENT: amblyopia, deafness, diplopia, *nystagmus,* tinnitus.
GI: constipation, dry mouth, nausea, taste perversion, tongue disorder, vomiting.
Hepatic: *hepatotoxicity.*
Metabolic: hypokalemia.
Musculoskeletal: back pain, myasthenia, pelvic pain.
Respiratory: pneumonia.
Skin: ecchymosis, *pruritus,* rash.
Other: accidental injury, chills, infection, injection-site reaction and pain.

Interactions

Drug-drug. *Amiodarone, chloramphenicol, chlordiazepoxide, cimetidine, diazepam, dicumarol, disulfiram, estrogens, ethosuximide,* *fluoxetine, H$_2$-receptor antagonists, halothane, isoniazid, methylphenidate, phenothiazines, phenylbutazone, salicylates, succinimides, sulfonamides, tolbutamide, trazodone:* May increase phenytoin level and therapeutic effects. Use together cautiously.
Carbamazepine, reserpine: May decrease phenytoin level. Monitor patient.
Coumarin, digitoxin, doxycycline, estrogens, furosemide, hormonal contraceptives, quinidine, rifampin, theophylline, vitamin D: May decrease effectiveness of these drugs because of increased hepatic metabolism. Monitor patient closely.
Phenobarbital, sodium valproate, valproic acid: May increase or decrease phenytoin level. Monitor patient.
Tricyclic antidepressants: May lower seizure threshold and require adjustments in phenytoin dosage. Use cautiously.
Drug-lifestyle. *Acute alcohol use:* May increase phenytoin level and toxic effects. Discourage alcohol use.
Chronic alcohol use: May decrease phenytoin level. Monitor patient; discourage alcohol use.

Effects on lab test results

• May increase alkaline phosphatase, GGT, and glucose levels. May decrease potassium and T$_4$ levels.
• May decrease platelet, WBC, granulocyte, leukocyte, and RBC counts.

Pharmacokinetics

Absorption: Complete.
Distribution: Wide. 95% to 99% protein-bound.
Metabolism: In the liver; undergoes rapid hydrolysis to phenytoin.
Excretion: In the urine as phenytoin metabolites. *Half-life:* 15 minutes.

Route	Onset	Peak	Duration
I.V.	Unknown	Immediate	Unknown
I.M.	Unknown	30 min	Unknown

Action

Chemical effect: Because fosphenytoin is a prodrug of phenytoin, their action is the same: stabilizing neuronal membranes.
Therapeutic effect: Prevents and controls seizures.

Reactions may be *common*, uncommon, *life-threatening*, or COMMON AND LIFE-THREATENING.

Available forms

Injection: 2 ml (150 mg fosphenytoin sodium equivalent to 100 mg phenytoin sodium), 10 ml (750 mg fosphenytoin sodium equivalent to 500 mg phenytoin sodium)

NURSING PROCESS

⚞ Assessment
• Don't give drug I.M. for status epilepticus because therapeutic phenytoin levels may not occur as rapidly as with I.V. use.
• Don't monitor phenytoin level until about 2 hours after the end of I.V. infusion or 4 hours after I.M. injection.
• Assess patient's and family's knowledge of drug therapy.

⊕ Nursing diagnoses
• Risk for trauma related to seizures
• Deficient knowledge related to drug therapy

▷ Planning and implementation
• Drug should always be prescribed and dispensed in PE units. Don't make any adjustments in recommended dose when substituting fosphenytoin for phenytoin, or vice versa.
• I.M. use generates systemic phenytoin levels similar to oral phenytoin sodium, allowing essentially interchangeable use.
⚕**ALERT:** Abruptly stopping the drug may cause status epilepticus. Substitute another drug, or reduce the dosage of this drug gradually.
⚕**ALERT:** Don't confuse Cerebyx with Celexa or Celebrex.
Patient teaching
• Warn patient that sensory disturbances may occur with I.V. use.
• Instruct patient to immediately report adverse reactions, especially rash.

☑ Evaluation
• Patient is free from seizures.
• Patient and family state understanding of drug therapy.

frovatriptan succinate
(froh-vah-TRIP-tan SUK-seh-nayt)
Frova⌀

Pharmacologic class: serotonin 5-HT$_1$ receptor agonist
Therapeutic class: antimigraine drug
Pregnancy risk category: C

Indications and dosages

▶ **Migraine attacks with or without aura.**
Adults: 2.5 mg P.O. taken at the first sign of migraine. If headache recurs after initial relief, a second tablet may be given after waiting at least 2 hours. Don't give more than 3 tablets daily.

Contraindications and cautions

• Contraindicated in patients hypersensitive to drug or any of the inactive ingredients. Also contraindicated in patients with history of or current ischemic heart disease, coronary artery vasospasm (including Prinzmetal variant angina), or other significant underlying CV conditions. Don't use in patients with cerebrovascular syndromes, such as stroke of any type or transient ischemic attacks, or in patients with peripheral vascular disease, including, but not limited to, ischemic bowel disease. Contraindicated in patients with uncontrolled hypertension and in patients with hemiplegic or basilar migraine.
⚖ Lifespan: In pregnant women, use drug only if benefits outweigh risks to fetus. In breastfeeding women, use cautiously because it's unknown if drug appears in breast milk. In children, safety and effectiveness haven't been established. In elderly patients, no special dosage has been suggested, but experience is limited.

Adverse reactions

CNS: anxiety, dizziness, dysesthesia, headache, hypoesthesia, insomnia, fatigue, pain, paresthesia, somnolence, *stroke.*
CV: *cardiac arrhythmias,* chest pain, flushing, hypertension, *MI,* palpitations.
EENT: abnormal vision, rhinitis, sinusitis, tinnitus.
GI: abdominal pain, diarrhea, dry mouth, dyspepsia, nausea, vomiting.
Musculoskeletal: skeletal pain.
Skin: increased sweating.
Other: hot or cold sensation.

F

Interactions

Drug-drug. *Ergotamine or ergot-type drugs (such as dihydroergotamine or methysergide):* May cause prolonged vasospastic reactions. Don't use within 24 hours of each other.

5-HT$_{1B/1D}$ agonists: May have additive effects. Use of other 5-HT$_1$ agonists within 24 hours of frovatriptan isn't recommended.

Hormonal contraceptives, propranolol: May increase bioavailability of frovatriptan. Monitor patient for adverse effects.

SSRIs (such as citalopram, fluoxetine, fluvoxamine, paroxetine, sertraline), SNRIs (duloxetine, venlafaxine): May cause serotonin syndrome. Monitor patient closely.

Effects on lab test results

None reported.

Pharmacokinetics

Absorption: Oral bioavailability 20% in men and 30% in women. Food delays the time to peak, but not bioavailability.
Distribution: 15% protein-bound.
Metabolism: In the liver, by CYP1A2. Drug doesn't appear to induce or inhibit cytochrome P-450.
Excretion: In urine and feces. *Half-life:* 26 hours.

Route	Onset	Peak	Duration
P.O.	Unknown	2–4 hr	Unknown

Action

Chemical effect: May inhibit excessive dilation of extracerebral intracranial arteries in migraine headaches.
Therapeutic effect: Relieves pain caused by migraines.

Available forms

Tablets: 2.5 mg

NURSING PROCESS

🔲 Assessment
• Assess underlying condition before starting therapy, and reassess regularly throughout therapy.
• Obtain complete medical history, paying particular attention to history of CV and cerebrovascular disease.

• Assess patient's and family's knowledge of drug therapy.

⊕ Nursing diagnoses
• Acute pain related to migraine headache
• Activity intolerance related to migraine headache
• Deficient knowledge related to frovatriptan succinate therapy

⟫ Planning and implementation
⑤ ALERT: Don't give within 24 hours of another 5-HT$_1$ agonist or an ergotamine or ergotlike drug.
⑤ ALERT: Serious cardiac events, including acute MI and life-threatening cardiac rhythm disturbances may occur within a few hours of giving 5-HT$_1$ agonists.
• Drug may bind to the melanin of the eye and cause ophthalmic effects. No specific ophthalmic monitoring is recommended.
• The safety of treating an average of more than four migraine attacks in a 30-day period hasn't been established.
• If used in a patient with risk factors for unrecognized coronary artery disease (such as hypertension, hypercholesterolemia, smoking, obesity, strong family history of coronary artery disease, woman with surgical or physiologic menopause, man older than age 40), give the first dose in a medically staffed and equipped facility. Obtain an ECG after the first dose. Periodically assess cardiac condition in intermittent, long-term users of 5-HT$_1$ agonists or those who have or acquire risk factors during therapy.

Patient teaching
• Instruct patient to take the dose at the first sign of a migraine headache. If the headache comes back after the first dose, a second dose may be taken after 2 hours. Tell patient not to take more than 3 tablets in a 24-hour period.
• Inform patient that, in rare cases, patients have experienced serious heart problems, stroke, or high blood pressure after taking the drug.
• Advise patient to take extra care or avoid driving and operating machinery if dizziness or fatigue develops.
• Emphasize importance of immediately reporting rash, itching, or pain, tightness, heaviness, or pressure in the chest, throat, neck, or jaw after taking the drug.

Reactions may be *common*, uncommon, *life-threatening*, or COMMON AND LIFE-THREATENING.

• Instruct patient not to take drug within 24 hours of taking another serotonin receptor agonist or ergotamine-type drugs.

✓ Evaluation

• Patient is relieved of pain.
• Patient's activity tolerance returns to baseline.
• Patient and family state understanding of drug therapy.

HIGH ALERT

fulvestrant
(full-VESS-trant)
Faslodex

Pharmacologic class: estrogen receptor antagonist
Therapeutic class: antineoplastic
Pregnancy risk category: D

Indications and dosages

▶ **Hormone-receptor–positive metastatic breast cancer in postmenopausal women with disease progression following antiestrogen therapy.** *Adults:* 250 mg by slow I.M. injection into buttock once monthly.

Contraindications and cautions

• Contraindicated in patients hypersensitive to drug or any of its components.
• Use cautiously in patients with moderate or severe hepatic impairment.
♨ **Lifespan:** In pregnant women, drug is contraindicated. Women of childbearing age should avoid getting pregnant while taking the drug. Breast-feeding women should stop breast-feeding or not take the drug. In children, safety and effectiveness haven't been established.

Adverse reactions

CNS: anxiety, *asthenia,* depression, dizziness, fever, *headache,* insomnia, *pain,* paresthesia.
CV: chest pain, peripheral edema, *vasodilation.*
EENT: *pharyngitis.*
GI: *abdominal pain,* anorexia, *constipation, diarrhea, nausea, vomiting.*
GU: UTI.
Hematologic: anemia.
Musculoskeletal: arthritis, *back pain, bone pain,* pelvic pain.
Respiratory: *cough, dyspnea.*
Skin: rash, sweating.

Other: accidental injury, flulike syndrome, *injection-site pain.*

Interactions

None reported.

Effects on lab test results

• May decrease hemoglobin level and hematocrit.

Pharmacokinetics

Absorption: Unknown.
Distribution: Extensive and rapid. 99% protein-bound.
Metabolism: Extensive, via several pathways.
Excretion: Hepatically cleared, 90% in feces.
Half-life: 29 to 51 days.

Route	Onset	Peak	Duration
I.M.	Unknown	7 days	1 mo

Action

Chemical effect: Competitively binds estrogen receptors and down-regulates estrogen-receptor protein in breast cancer cells.
Therapeutic effect: Fights cancer cells.

Available forms

Injection: 50 mg/ml in 2.5-ml and 5-ml pre-filled syringes

NURSING PROCESS

✏ Assessment

• Monitor hemoglobin level and hematocrit before starting therapy and during therapy.
• Confirm that patient isn't pregnant before starting therapy.
• Observe injection site for local reaction.
• Assess patient's and family's knowledge of drug therapy.

⊕ Nursing diagnoses

• Risk for imbalanced nutrition: less than body requirements, related to side effects of therapy
• Acute pain related to side effects of therapy
• Deficient knowledge related to drug therapy

▶ Planning and implementation

• Because drug is given I.M., don't use in patients with bleeding diatheses or thrombocytopenia or in those taking anticoagulants.

---

⑨ **ALERT:** The drug is packaged in one 5-ml prefilled syringe or two 2.5-ml prefilled syringes. If using the 2.5-ml syringes, both syringes must be given to achieve the full 250-mg recommended monthly dose.

• Expel the gas bubble from syringe before administration.

Patient teaching

• Tell patient the most common adverse reactions are GI symptoms, headache, back pain, hot flushes, and sore throat.

• Advise women of childbearing age to avoid pregnancy and to report suspected pregnancy immediately. Drug crosses the placenta after a single I.M. dose and harms the fetus.

☑ Evaluation

• Patient maintains adequate nutrition during therapy.

• Patient doesn't experience pain as an adverse effect.

• Patient and family state understanding of therapy.

furosemide (frusemide)
(fyoo-ROH-seh-mighd)
Lasix✐, Lasix Special ◆ , Novo-semide ◆

Pharmacologic class: loop diuretic
Therapeutic class: diuretic, antihypertensive
Pregnancy risk category: C

Indications and dosages

▶ **Acute pulmonary edema.** *Adults:* 40 mg I.V. injected slowly over 1 to 2 minutes; then 80 mg I.V. in 1 to 1½ hours, if needed.
Infants and children: 1 mg/kg I.M. or I.V. If desired results don't occur after 2 hours, may increase initial dose by 1 mg/kg. Separate doses by at least 2 hours.

▶ **Edema.** *Adults:* 20 to 80 mg P.O. daily in morning; second dose in 6 to 8 hours. Carefully adjust up to 600 mg daily, if needed. Or 20 to 40 mg I.M. or I.V.; increase by 20 mg every 2 hours until desired response occurs. Give I.V. dose slowly over 1 to 2 minutes.
Infants and children: 2 mg/kg P.O. daily; increase by 1 to 2 mg/kg in 6 to 8 hours, if needed. Carefully adjust up to 6 mg/kg daily, if needed. Or 1 mg/kg slow I.V.; increase by 1 mg/kg every 2 hours until desired response.

▶ **Heart failure and chronic renal impairment.** *Adults:* 2 to 2.5 g daily P.O. or I.V. Maximum I.V. injection, 1 g daily over 30 minutes.

▶ **Hypertension.** *Adults:* 40 mg P.O. b.i.d. Adjust dosage according to response.

▶ **Hypercalcemia‡.** *Adults:* 80 to 100 mg I.V. every 1 to 2 hours. Or 120 mg P.O. daily.

▽ I.V. administration

• Dilute with D_5W, normal saline solution, or lactated Ringer's solution.

• To avoid ototoxicity, infuse no more than 4 mg/minute.

• Give drug by direct injection over 1 to 2 minutes.

• Avoid exposing injection to light; it may discolor and become unusable.

• Use prepared infusion solution within 24 hours.

⊗ **Incompatibilities**
Acidic solutions, aminoglycosides, amiodarone, ascorbic acid, bleomycin, buprenorphine, chlorpromazine, diazepam, dobutamine, doxapram, doxorubicin, droperidol, epinephrine, erythromycin, esmolol, fluconazole, fructose 10% in water, gentamicin, hydralazine, idarubicin, invert sugar 10% in electrolyte #2, isoproterenol, meperidine, metoclopramide, milrinone, morphine, netilmicin, norepinephrine, ondansetron, prochlorperazine, promethazine, quinidine, vinblastine, vincristine.

Contraindications and cautions

• Contraindicated in patients hypersensitive to drug or any of its components and in those with anuria.

• Use cautiously in patients with hepatic cirrhosis.

• Patients with allergy to sulfonamides may also be allergic to furosemide.

⚘ **Lifespan:** In pregnant women, use only if benefits outweigh risks to fetus. In breastfeeding women, don't use drug.

Adverse reactions

CNS: dizziness, fever, headache, paresthesia, restlessness, vertigo, weakness.
CV: orthostatic hypotension, thrombophlebitis (with I.V. use), volume depletion, dehydration.
EENT: blurred or yellow vision, transient deafness.
GI: abdominal discomfort, anorexia, constipation, diarrhea, nausea, *pancreatitis,* vomiting.

Reactions may be *common,* uncommon, *life-threatening,* or COMMON AND LIFE-THREATENING.

GU: azotemia, frequent urination, nocturia, oliguria, polyuria.

Hematologic: *agranulocytosis,* anemia, *aplastic anemia, leukopenia, thrombocytopenia.*

Hepatic: hepatic dysfunction.

Metabolic: asymptomatic hyperuricemia; fluid and electrolyte imbalances, including dilutional hyponatremia, hypocalcemia, and hypomagnesemia; glucose intolerance; hyperglycemia; hypochloremic alkalosis; hypokalemia.

Musculoskeletal: muscle spasm.

Skin: dermatitis, photosensitivity, purpura.

Other: gout, transient pain at I.M. injection site.

Interactions

Drug-drug. *Aminoglycoside antibiotics, cisplatin:* May potentiate ototoxicity. Use together cautiously.

Amphotericin B, corticosteroids, corticotropin: May increase risk of hypokalemia. Monitor potassium level closely.

Antidiabetics: May decrease hypoglycemic effects. Monitor glucose level.

Antihypertensives: May increase risk of hypotension. Use together cautiously.

Chlorothiazide, chlorthalidone, hydrochlorothiazide, indapamide, metolazone: May cause excessive diuretic response, resulting in serious electrolyte abnormalities or dehydration. Adjust doses carefully while monitoring patient closely.

Digoxin, neuromuscular blockers: May increase toxicity from furosemide-induced hypokalemia. Monitor potassium level closely.

Ethacrynic acid: May increase risk of ototoxicity. Don't use together.

Lithium: May decrease lithium excretion, resulting in lithium toxicity. Monitor lithium level.

NSAIDs: May inhibit diuretic response. Use together cautiously.

Salicylates: May cause salicylate toxicity. Use together cautiously.

Drug-herb. *Aloe:* May increase drug effects. Monitor patient for dehydration.

Licorice: May cause rapid potassium loss. Monitor patient for hypokalemia; discourage licorice intake.

Drug-lifestyle. *Alcohol use:* May cause additive hypotensive and diuretic effect. Discourage use together.

Sun exposure: May cause photosensitivity reactions. Urge patient to avoid unprotected or prolonged sun exposure.

Effects on lab test results

● May increase glucose, cholesterol, and uric acid levels. May decrease potassium, sodium, calcium, magnesium, and hemoglobin levels and hematocrit.

● May decrease granulocyte, WBC, and platelet counts.

Pharmacokinetics

Absorption: 60% after P.O. use; unknown after I.M. use.

Distribution: 95% protein-bound.

Metabolism: Minimal.

Excretion: 50% to 80% in urine. *Half-life:* 30 minutes.

Route	Onset	Peak	Duration
P.O.	20–60 min	1–2 hr	6–8 hr
I.V.	5 min	30 min	2 hr
I.M.	Unknown	Unknown	Unknown

Action

Chemical effect: Inhibits sodium and chloride reabsorption at proximal and distal tubules and ascending loop of Henle.

Therapeutic effect: Promotes water and sodium excretion.

Available forms

Injection: 10 mg/ml

Oral solution: 40 mg/5 ml, 10 mg/ml

Tablets: 20 mg, 40 mg, 80 mg, 500 mg ◆

NURSING PROCESS

⚕ Assessment

● Assess patient's underlying condition before starting therapy. Monitor weight, peripheral edema, breath sounds, blood pressure, fluid intake and output, and electrolyte, glucose, BUN, and carbon dioxide levels.

● Monitor uric acid level, especially if patient has a history of gout.

● Be alert for adverse reactions and drug interactions.

● Assess patient's and family's knowledge of drug therapy.

⊕ Nursing diagnoses

● Excess fluid volume related to presence of edema

• Impaired urinary elimination related to diuretic therapy
• Deficient knowledge related to drug therapy

▶ **Planning and implementation**
• Give a P.O. or I.M. dose in the morning to prevent nocturia. Give a second dose in early afternoon.
• Store tablets in light-resistant container to prevent discoloration. Don't use yellowed injectable preparation.
• Refrigerate oral furosemide solution to ensure drug stability.
• If oliguria or azotemia develops or increases, notify prescriber.
Patient teaching
• Advise patient to stand slowly to prevent dizziness, not to drink alcohol, and to minimize strenuous exercise in hot weather.
• Instruct patient to report ringing in ears, severe abdominal pain, or sore throat and fever because they may indicate toxicity.
• **ALERT:** Discourage patient from storing different drugs in same container because this increases risk of errors. The most popular strengths of furosemide and digoxin are white tablets of similar size.
• Tell patient to check with prescriber before taking OTC drugs or herbal remedies.

✓ **Evaluation**
• Patient is free from edema.
• Patient demonstrates adjustment of lifestyle to cope with altered patterns of urinary elimination.
• Patient and family state understanding of drug therapy.

G

gabapentin
(geh-buh-PEN-tin)
Gabarone, Neurontin✐

Pharmacologic class: anticonvulsant
Therapeutic class: anticonvulsant
Pregnancy risk category: C

Indications and dosages

▶ **Adjunct therapy of partial seizures with and without secondary generalization in patients with epilepsy.** *Adults and children older than age 12:* Initially, 300 mg P.O. t.i.d. Increase dosage gradually based on response. Dosages of 900 to 1,800 mg daily in three divided doses are effective for most patients. Dosages up to 3,600 mg daily are well tolerated.
Children ages 3 to 12: Starting dosage, 10 to 15 mg/kg P.O. daily in three divided doses; adjust over 3 days to reach effective dosage.
Children ages 5 to 12: Effective dosage, 25 to 35 mg/kg P.O. daily in three divided doses.
Children ages 3 to 4: Effective dosage, 40 mg/kg P.O. daily in three divided doses.
⧅ Adjust-a-dose: For adults and children age 12 and older with renal impairment or undergoing hemodialysis, if creatinine clearance is 30 to 59 ml/minute, give 400 to 1,400 mg P.O. daily, divided b.i.d. If clearance is 15 to 29 ml/minute, give 200 to 700 mg P.O. daily. If clearance is less than 15 ml/minute, give 100 to 300 mg P.O. daily; reduce dosage in proportion to creatinine clearance (for example, for patients with a clearance of 7.5 ml/minute, give one-half the dose that a patient with 15 ml/minute would receive).
For dialysis patients, maintenance dosages are based on estimated creatinine clearance. Give supplemental postdialysis dose of 125 to 350 mg after each 4 hours of dialysis.
▶ **Postherpetic neuralgia.** *Adults:* 300 mg P.O. once daily on day 1, then 300 mg b.i.d. on day 2, and 300 mg t.i.d. on day 3. Adjust as needed for pain relief to maximum daily dosage, 1,800 mg, divided t.i.d.

Contraindications and cautions

• Contraindicated in patients hypersensitive to the drug or any of its components.
• ☀ **Lifespan:** In pregnant women, use cautiously. In breast-feeding women and in children younger than age 3, safety and effectiveness haven't been established. In children ages 3 to 12, use cautiously; drug may cause mild to moderate emotional lability, hostility, aggressive behavior, and hyperkinesias.

Adverse reactions

CNS: abnormal coordination, abnormal thinking, amnesia, *ataxia,* depression, *dizziness,* dysarthria, *fatigue,* nervousness, *nystagmus, somnolence, tremor,* twitching.

Reactions may be *common,* uncommon, *life-threatening,* or COMMON AND LIFE-THREATENING.

CV: peripheral edema, vasodilation.
EENT: *amblyopia, diplopia,* dry throat, pharyngitis, *rhinitis.*
GI: constipation, dry mouth, dyspepsia, nausea, vomiting.
GU: impotence.
Hematologic: *leukopenia.*
Metabolic: increased appetite, weight gain.
Musculoskeletal: back pain, fractures, myalgia.
Respiratory: cough.
Skin: abrasion, pruritus.
Other: dental abnormalities.

Interactions

Drug-drug. *Antacids:* May decrease gabapentin absorption. Separate administration times by at least 2 hours.
Morphine: May increase gabapentin level and risk of CNS depression. Decrease dose of either drug.
Drug-lifestyle. *Alcohol use:* May increase CNS depression. Discourage use together.

Effects on lab test results

• May decrease WBC count.
• May cause false-positive tests for urine protein when using Ames-N-Multistix SG dipstick test.

Pharmacokinetics

Absorption: Bioavailability isn't dose-proportional but averages 60%.
Distribution: Circulates largely unbound to protein.
Metabolism: Insignificant.
Excretion: By kidneys as unchanged drug.
Half-life: 5 to 7 hours.

Route	Onset	Peak	Duration
P.O.	Unknown	2–4 hr	Unknown

Action

Chemical effect: Unknown; although structurally related to GABA, drug doesn't interact with GABA receptors and isn't converted metabolically into GABA or a GABA agonist.
Therapeutic effect: Prevents and treats partial seizures and treats postherpetic neuralgia.

Available forms

Capsules: 100 mg, 300 mg, 400 mg
Solution: 250 mg/5 ml

Tablets (film-coated): 100 mg, 300 mg, 400 mg, 600 mg, 800 mg

NURSING PROCESS

Assessment

• Assess patient's disorder before starting therapy and regularly thereafter.
• Assess patient's renal function before starting therapy.
• Routine monitoring of level isn't needed. Drug doesn't appear to alter levels of other anticonvulsants.
• Be alert for adverse reactions and drug interactions.
• Assess patient's and family's knowledge of drug therapy.

Nursing diagnoses

• Risk for trauma related to seizures
• Risk for injury related to drug-induced adverse CNS reactions
• Deficient knowledge related to drug therapy

Planning and implementation

• Give first dose at bedtime to minimize drowsiness, dizziness, fatigue, and ataxia.
ALERT: If stopping drug or substituting another drug, do so gradually over at least 1 week to minimize risk of seizures. Don't abruptly stop other anticonvulsants when starting therapy.
• Take seizure precautions.
ALERT: Don't confuse Neurontin with Noroxin.
Patient teaching
• Tell patient drug can be taken with or without food.
• Warn patient to avoid hazardous activities until the drug's CNS effects are known.

Evaluation

• Patient is free from seizures.
• Patient has no injury from adverse CNS reactions.
• Patient and family state understanding of drug therapy.

galantamine hydrobromide

(gah-LAN-tah-meen high-droh-BROH-mighd)
Razadyne, Razadyne ER

Pharmacologic class: reversible, competitive acetylcholinesterase inhibitor
Therapeutic class: cholinomimetic
Pregnancy risk category: B

Indications and dosages

▶ **Mild to moderate dementia of Alzheimer type.** *Adults:* Initially, 4 mg P.O. b.i.d., preferably with morning and evening meals. If dose is well tolerated after minimum of 4 weeks of therapy, increase to 8 mg b.i.d. A further increase to 12 mg b.i.d. may be attempted only after at least 4 weeks of the previous dose. Recommended dosage range is 16 to 24 mg daily in two divided doses. Or if using the extended-release form, 8 mg P.O. once daily in the morning with food. Increase to 16 mg P.O. once daily after a minimum of 4 weeks. May further increase to 24 mg once daily after a minimum of 4 weeks, based on patient response and tolerability.

⚠ Adjust-a-dose: For patients with hepatic impairment (Child-Pugh score of 7 to 9), don't exceed 16 mg daily. For patients with a Child-Pugh score of 10 to 15, don't give drug. For patients with moderate renal impairment, don't exceed 16 mg daily. For patients with creatinine clearance less than 9 ml/minute, don't give drug. Adjusted dose is the same for regular and extended-release forms.

Contraindications and cautions

• Contraindicated in patients hypersensitive to the drug or any of its components.
• Use cautiously in patients with supraventricular cardiac conduction disorders and in those taking other drugs that significantly slow the heart rate. Use cautiously before or during procedures involving anesthesia with succinylcholine-type or other similar neuromuscular blockers. Use cautiously in patients with a history of peptic ulcer disease and in those taking NSAIDs. Because of the potential for cholinomimetic effects, use cautiously in patients with bladder outflow obstruction, seizures, asthma, or COPD.

♨ Lifespan: In pregnant women, use only if benefits outweigh risks to fetus. In breast-feeding women, use cautiously because it's unknown if drug appears in breast milk. In children, safety and effectiveness haven't been established.

Adverse reactions

CNS: depression, dizziness, fatigue, headache, insomnia, somnolence, syncope, tremor.
CV: *bradycardia,* heart block.
EENT: rhinitis.
GI: abdominal pain, anorexia, *diarrhea,* dyspepsia, *nausea, vomiting.*
GU: hematuria, UTI.
Hematologic: anemia.
Metabolic: weight loss.

Interactions

Drug-drug. *Amitriptyline, fluoxetine, fluvoxamine, quinidine:* May decrease galantamine clearance. Monitor patient closely.
Anticholinergics: May antagonize activity of anticholinergics. Monitor patient.
Cholinergics (such as bethanechol, succinylcholine): May have a synergistic effect. Monitor patient closely. May need to avoid use before procedures using general anesthesia with succinylcholine-type neuromuscular blockers.
Cimetidine, erythromycin, ketoconazole, paroxetine: May increase bioavailability of galantamine. Monitor patient closely.

Effects on lab test results

• May decrease hemoglobin level and hematocrit.

Pharmacokinetics

Absorption: Rapid and good, with an oral bioavailability of about 90%. Levels peak in 1 hour. In elderly patients, levels are 30% to 40% higher than in young, healthy people.
Distribution: Mainly to blood. Protein-binding isn't significant.
Metabolism: In liver by CYP2D6 and CYP3A4 and glucuronidated. Using with inhibitors of these enzyme systems may modestly increase bioavailability.
Excretion: In urine, unchanged, as glucuronide and metabolites. *Half-life:* About 7 hours.

Route	Onset	Peak	Duration
P.O.	Unknown	1 hr	Unknown

Action

Chemical effect: Unknown; may enhance cholinergic function by increasing acetylcholine level in the brain.
Therapeutic effect: Improves cognition in patients with Alzheimer disease.

Available forms

Capsules (extended-release): 8 mg, 16 mg, 24 mg
Oral solution: 4 mg/ml
Tablets: 4 mg, 8 mg, 12 mg

NURSING PROCESS

Assessment
• Assess underlying condition before starting therapy, and reassess regularly.
• Bradycardia and heart block have been reported in patients with and without underlying cardiac conduction abnormalities. Consider all patients at risk for adverse effects on cardiac conduction.
• Patients are at increased risk for gastric ulcers because of the potential for increased gastric acid secretion. Monitor patient closely for symptoms of active or occult GI bleeding.
• Assess patient's and family's knowledge of drug therapy.

Nursing diagnoses
• Risk for injury due to wandering related to Alzheimer disease
• Risk for imbalanced fluid volume related to drug-induced adverse GI reactions
• Deficient knowledge related to drug therapy

Planning and implementation
ALERT: Razadyne tablets should be given twice daily and Razadyne ER capsules once daily. To avoid errors, verify any prescription that suggests a different dosing schedule.
• Give drug with food and ensure adequate fluid intake to decrease the risk of nausea and vomiting.
• If drug is stopped for several days, restart at the lowest dose and increase, at a minimum of 4-week intervals, to the previous dose.
• Use proper technique when dispensing the oral solution with the pipette. Dispense measured amount in a liquid and give right away. Oral solution and tablets are bioequivalent.

• Don't give more than 16 mg daily in patients with moderate hepatic or renal impairment.
• In case of overdose, contact a poison control center. Treat symptoms and provide support. Atropine I.V. may be used as an antidote; give an initial dose of 0.5 to 1 mg and base subsequent doses on response. It's unknown if drug is removed by dialysis.

Patient teaching
• Advise patient or his caregiver that the conventional tablets should be taken with morning and evening meals and the extended-release capsules should be taken with the morning meal.
• Inform patient or caregiver that dosage increases should occur at no more than 4-week intervals.
• Explain that nausea and vomiting occur in less than 25% of patients.
• Advise patient or caregiver that following the recommended dosing and administration schedule can minimize common adverse effects.
• Tell patient or caregiver, if therapy is interrupted for several days or longer, to restart the drug at the lowest dose and increase based on the prescriber's dosing schedule.
• Advise patient or caregiver to report signs and symptoms of bradycardia immediately to the prescriber.
• Advise patient or caregiver that drug may enhance cognitive function, but may not alter the underlying disease process.

Evaluation
• Patient's cognition improves and tendency to wander decreases.
• Patient and family state that drug-induced adverse GI reactions haven't occurred.
• Patient and family state understanding of drug therapy.

ganciclovir (DHPG)
(gan-SIGH-kloh-veer)
Cytovene, Cytovene-IV

Pharmacologic class: synthetic nucleoside
Therapeutic class: antiviral
Pregnancy risk category: C

Indications and dosages

▶ **CMV retinitis in immunocompromised patients, including those with AIDS.** *Adults:* 5 mg/kg I.V. over 1 hour every 12 hours for

14 to 21 days, followed by 5 mg/kg I.V. daily for 7 days weekly, or 6 mg/kg I.V. daily for 5 of 7 days weekly. Or, following I.V. induction therapy, give 1,000 mg P.O. t.i.d. with food or 500 mg P.O. six times a day every 3 hours with food while awake.

▶ **To prevent CMV disease in transplant recipients at risk for CMV disease.** *Adults:* 5 mg/kg I.V. over 1 hour every 12 hours for 7 to 14 days, followed by 5 mg/kg I.V. once daily, or 6 mg/kg I.V. once daily for 5 of 7 days weekly. Alternatively, 1,000 mg P.O. t.i.d. with food. Length of therapy in transplant recipients depends on duration and degree of immunosuppression.

▶ **To prevent CMV disease in patients with advanced HIV infection at risk for development of CMV disease.** *Adults:* 1,000 mg P.O. t.i.d. with food.

▶ **Other CMV infections‡.** *Adults:* 5 mg/kg I.V. over 1 hour every 12 hours for 14 to 21 days. Or 2.5 mg/kg I.V. over 1 hour every 8 hours for 14 to 21 days.

⬛ Adjust-a-dose: For patients with renal impairment, adjust dosage according to the table at the top of page 603. For patients receiving hemodialysis, see dosages for creatinine clearance greater than 10 ml/minute.

▼ I.V. administration

• Reconstitute with 10 ml sterile water for injection. Shake vial to dissolve drug.
• Further dilute appropriate dose in normal saline solution, D₅W, Ringer's lactate, or Ringer's solution (typically 100 ml).
• Use caution when preparing alkaline solution.
• Infuse over 1 hour. Faster infusions will cause increased toxicity. Never exceed recommended infusion rate. Use infusion pump. Don't give as I.V. bolus or by rapid infusion.
• Infusion concentrations greater than 10 mg/ml aren't recommended.

⊗ **Incompatibilities**
Aldesleukin, amifostine, aztreonam, cefepime, cytarabine, doxorubicin hydrochloride, fludarabine, foscarnet, ondansetron, paraben (bacteriostatic agent), piperacillin sodium with tazobactam, sargramostim, vinorelbine. Manufacturer recommends not giving with other I.V. drugs.

Contraindications and cautions

• Contraindicated in patients hypersensitive to ganciclovir or acyclovir. Patients with allergies

to acyclovir may also react to ganciclovir. Also contraindicated in those with absolute neutrophil count below 500/mm³ or platelet count below 25,000/mm³.
• Use cautiously and at a lower dosage in patients with renal impairment.

⚕ Lifespan: In pregnant women, use only if benefits outweigh risks to the fetus. In breast-feeding women, use cautiously because it isn't known if drug appears in breast milk. In children, safety and effectiveness haven't been established.

Adverse reactions

CNS: altered dreams, ataxia, behavioral changes, *coma,* confusion, dizziness, headache, pain, *seizures.*
CV: *arrhythmias,* hypertension, hypotension.
EENT: retinal detachment in CMV retinitis.
GI: anorexia, diarrhea, nausea, vomiting.
GU: hematuria.
Hematologic: *agranulocytosis,* anemia, *granulocytopenia, leukopenia, thrombocytopenia.*
Other: inflammation, phlebitis at injection site.

Interactions

Drug-drug. *Cytotoxic drugs:* May increase toxic effects, especially hematologic effects and stomatitis. Monitor patient closely.
Imipenem and cilastatin: May heighten seizure activity. Monitor patient closely.
Immunosuppressants (such as azathioprine, corticosteroids, cyclosporine): May enhance immune and bone marrow suppression. Use together cautiously.
Probenecid: May increase ganciclovir level. Monitor patient closely.
Zidovudine: May increase risk of granulocytopenia. Monitor patient closely.

Effects on lab test results

• May increase creatinine, ALT, AST, GGT, and alkaline phosphatase levels. May decrease hemoglobin level and hematocrit.
• May decrease granulocyte, platelet, neutrophil, and WBC counts.

Pharmacokinetics

Absorption: Poor. Bioavailability is about 5% under fasting conditions.
Distribution: Concentrates in CMV-infected cells.
Metabolism: Less than 10%.

Excretion: Mostly unchanged. *Half-life:* About 3 hours.

Route	Onset	Peak	Duration
P.O.	Unknown	3 hr	Unknown
I.V.	Immediate	Immediate	Unknown

Action

Chemical effect: Unknown, may inhibit viral DNA synthesis of CMV.
Therapeutic effect: Inhibits CMV.

Available forms

Capsules: 250 mg, 500 mg
Injection: 500 mg/vial

NURSING PROCESS

⚗ Assessment
• Assess patient's condition before starting therapy and regularly thereafter.
• Obtain CBC, neutrophil, and platelet counts every 2 days during twice-daily ganciclovir use and at least weekly thereafter.
• Monitor hydration if adverse GI reaction occurs with oral drug.
• Be alert for adverse reactions and drug interactions.
• Assess patient's and family's knowledge of drug therapy.

🔬 Nursing diagnoses
• Risk for infection related to CMV retinitis
• Ineffective protection related to adverse hematologic reactions
• Deficient knowledge related to drug therapy

▶ Planning and implementation
• Give oral form of drug with food.
• ⑤ **ALERT:** Don't give drug subcutaneously or I.M. because severe tissue irritation could result.
• ⑤ **ALERT:** Encourage fluid intake; ensure adequate hydration during drug infusion.
• Alert prescriber to signs of renal impairment because the dosage will need adjustment.
• Capsules are linked to a risk of rapid progression of CMV retinitis. Don't use capsules for induction therapy; use only as maintenance therapy in patients who benefit from not taking drug I.V.
Patient teaching
• Tell patient to take oral form of drug with food.

• Stress importance of drinking adequate fluids throughout therapy.
• Advise patient to report pain or discomfort at I.V. site.
• Instruct patient about infection-control and bleeding precautions.

✓ Evaluation
• Patient is free from infection.
• Patient has no serious adverse hematologic reactions.
• Patient and family state understanding of drug therapy.

gatifloxacin ophthalmic solution
(gah-ti-FLOCKS-ah-sin off-THAL-mick suh-LOO-shun)
Zymar

Pharmacologic class: fluoroquinolone
Therapeutic class: antibiotic
Pregnancy risk category: C

Indications and dosages

▶ **Bacterial conjunctivitis.** *Adults and children age 1 and older:* While patient is awake, instill 1 drop into affected eyes every 2 hours up to eight times daily for 2 days. Then, instill 1 drop up to q.i.d. for 5 more days.

Contraindications and cautions

• Contraindicated in patients hypersensitive to the drug or any of its components or to quinolones or any of their components.
• ⚖ **Lifespan:** In pregnant women, use cautiously. In breast-feeding women, use cautiously because it's unknown if the drug appears in breast milk. In children younger than age 1 year, drug is contraindicated.

Adverse reactions

CNS: headache.
EENT: chemosis, conjunctival hemorrhage, *conjunctival irritation,* discharge, dry eyes, eye irritation, eyelid edema, *increased lacrimation, keratitis,* pain, *papillary conjunctivitis,* red eyes, reduced visual acuity.
GI: taste disturbance.

Interactions

None reported.

Effects on lab test results

None reported.

Pharmacokinetics

Absorption: Unknown.
Distribution: Unknown.
Metabolism: Unknown.
Excretion: Unknown. *Half-life:* Unknown.

Route	Onset	Peak	Duration
Ophthalmic	Unknown	Unknown	Unknown

Action

Chemical effect: Inhibits DNA gyrase and topoisomerase, preventing cell replication and division.
Therapeutic effect: Kills susceptible bacteria.

Available forms

Solution: 0.3% in 2.5- and 5-ml bottles

NURSING PROCESS

Assessment
• Monitor therapy for effectiveness.
• Monitor patient for adverse reactions.
• Assess patient's and family's knowledge of drug therapy.

Nursing diagnoses
• Disturbed sensory perception (visual) related to eye infection
• Deficient knowledge related to drug therapy

Planning and implementation
• Don't inject solution subconjunctivally or into the anterior chamber of the eye.
• Systemic drug causes serious hypersensitivity reactions. If allergic reaction occurs, stop giving the drug and treat symptoms.
• Monitor patient for superinfection.
Patient teaching
• Tell patient to immediately stop taking the drug and seek medical treatment if evidence of a serious allergic reaction develops, such as itching, rash, swelling of the face or throat, or difficulty breathing.
• Tell patient not to wear contact lenses.
• Warn patient to avoid touching the applicator tip to anything, including eyes and fingers.
• Teach patient that prolonged use may encourage infections with nonsusceptible bacteria.

Evaluation
• Patient recovers from infection.
• Patient and family state understanding of drug therapy.

gemfibrozil
(jem-FIGH-broh-zil)
Gen-Fibro ◆ , Lopid

Pharmacologic class: fibric acid derivative
Therapeutic class: antilipemic
Pregnancy risk category: C

Indications and dosages

▶ **Type IV and V hyperlipidemia unresponsive to diet and other drugs; reduction of risk of coronary heart disease in patients with type IIb hyperlipidemia who can't tolerate or who are refractory to therapy with bile acid sequestrants or niacin.** *Adults:* 1,200 mg P.O. daily in two divided doses, 30 minutes before morning and evening meals. If no benefit occurs after 3 months, stop drug.

Contraindications and cautions

• Contraindicated in patients hypersensitive to the drug or any of its components and in those with hepatic or severe renal dysfunction (including primary biliary cirrhosis) or gallbladder disease.
 Lifespan: In pregnant women, use cautiously. In breast-feeding women and in children, safety and effectiveness haven't been established.

Adverse reactions

CNS: blurred vision, dizziness, fatigue, headache.
GI: *abdominal and epigastric pain,* diarrhea, *dyspepsia,* flatulence, nausea, taste perversion, vomiting.
Hematologic: *bone marrow hypoplasia, leukopenia, severe anemia, thrombocytopenia.*
Hepatic: bile duct obstruction, gallstones.
Musculoskeletal: painful limbs, *rhabdomyolysis.*
Skin: dermatitis, pruritus, rash.

Interactions

Drug-drug. *Cyclosporine:* May decrease cyclosporine effects. Monitor cyclosporine level.

Reactions may be *common,* uncommon, *life-threatening,* or COMMON AND LIFE-THREATENING.

HMG-CoA reductase inhibitors: May lead to myopathy with rhabdomyolysis. Don't use together.
Oral anticoagulants: May increase effects of oral anticoagulants. Monitor patient.
Repaglinide: May increase repaglinide level. Avoid use together.

Effects on lab test results

• May increase ALT, AST, and CK levels. May decrease potassium and hemoglobin levels and hematocrit.
• May decrease eosinophil, WBC, and platelet counts.

Pharmacokinetics

Absorption: Good.
Distribution: 95% protein-bound.
Metabolism: By liver.
Excretion: Mainly in urine. *Half-life:* 1¼ hours.

Route	Onset	Peak	Duration
P.O.	2–5 days	> 4 wk	Unknown

Action

Chemical effect: Inhibits peripheral lipolysis and also reduces triglyceride synthesis in liver.
Therapeutic effect: Lowers triglyceride levels and raises HDL levels.

Available forms

Tablets: 600 mg

NURSING PROCESS

Assessment

• Obtain patient's triglyceride and HDL levels before starting therapy and regularly thereafter.
• Obtain CBC and liver function tests periodically during first 12 months of therapy.
• Be alert for adverse reactions and drug interactions.
• Assess patient's and family's knowledge of drug therapy.

Nursing diagnoses

• Risk for injury related to elevated blood lipids and cholesterol levels
• Diarrhea related to drug's adverse effect on GI tract
• Deficient knowledge related to drug therapy

Planning and implementation

• Give drug 30 minutes before breakfast and dinner.
• Make sure patient is following standard low-cholesterol diet.

Patient teaching

• Instruct patient to take drug 30 minutes before breakfast and dinner.
• Teach patient dietary management of lipids (restricting total fat and cholesterol intake) and measures to control other cardiac disease risk factors. If appropriate, suggest weight control, exercise, and smoking cessation programs.
• Advise patient to avoid driving or other potentially hazardous activities until drug's CNS effects are known.
• Tell patient to observe bowel movements and to report signs of steatorrhea or bile duct obstruction (nausea, vomiting, abdominal or epigastric pain, and diarrhea).

Evaluation

• Patient's triglyceride and cholesterol levels are normal.
• Patient regains normal bowel patterns.
• Patient and family state understanding of drug therapy.

gemifloxacin mesylate

(geh-mih-FLOCKS-a-sin MESS-ih-late)
Factive

Pharmacologic class: fluoroquinolone
Therapeutic class: antibacterial
Pregnancy risk category: C

Indications and dosages

▶ **Acute bacterial exacerbation of chronic bronchitis caused by** *Streptococcus pneumoniae, Haemophilus influenzae, Haemophilus parainfluenzae, Moraxella catarrhalis.* *Adults:* 320 mg P.O. once daily for 5 days.

▶ **Mild to moderate community-acquired pneumonia caused by** *S. pneumoniae* **(including penicillin-resistant strains),** *H. influenzae, M. catarrhalis, Mycoplasma pneumoniae, Chlamydia pneumoniae, Klebsiella pneumoniae.* *Adults:* 320 mg P.O. once daily for 7 days.

Adjust-a-dose: For patients with renal impairment, if creatinine clearance is 40 ml/minute or less or if patient receives routine hemodialysis

or continuous ambulatory peritoneal dialysis, reduce dosage to 160 mg P.O. once daily.

Contraindications and cautions

• Contraindicated in patients hypersensitive to fluoroquinolones or any of their components, those with a history of prolonged QT interval, those with uncorrected electrolyte disorders, and those taking a class IA or III antiarrhythmic.

• Use cautiously in patients with epilepsy, predisposition to seizures, or renal impairment.

⚖ **Lifespan:** In pregnant women, use only if benefits outweigh risks to fetus. In breast-feeding women, use cautiously because it isn't known if drug appears in breast milk. In children, safety and effectiveness of drug haven't been established.

Adverse reactions

CNS: dizziness, fatigue, headache.
GI: abdominal pain, diarrhea, nausea, *pseudomembranous colitis,* vomiting.
Musculoskeletal: ruptured tendons.
Skin: rash.
Other: hypersensitivity reactions.

Interactions

Drug-drug. *Antacids (magnesium or aluminum), didanosine, iron, multivitamins containing metal cations (such as zinc), sucralfate:* May decrease gemifloxacin level. Give gemifloxacin at least 3 hours before or 2 hours after these drugs.
Antiarrhythmics (amiodarone, procainamide, quinidine, sotalol): May increase risk of prolonged QT interval. Avoid use together.
Drugs that affect QT interval (such as antidepressants, antipsychotics, erythromycin): May increase risk of prolonged QT interval. Use together cautiously.
Probenecid: May increase gemifloxacin level. Use together cautiously.
Warfarin: May increase anticoagulation effects. Monitor patient's PT and INR.
Drug-lifestyle. *Sun exposure:* May increase risk of photosensitivity. Discourage excessive or unprotected exposure to ultraviolet light or sunlight.

Effects on lab test results

• May increase ALT and AST levels.

Pharmacokinetics

Absorption: Rapid and unaffected by food.
Distribution: Wide, especially to lung tissue and fluids. 60% to 70% protein-bound.
Metabolism: Limited, mainly hepatic; some minor metabolites formed.
Excretion: In feces and urine as unchanged drug and metabolites. *Half-life:* 4 to 12 hours.

Route	Onset	Peak	Duration
P.O.	Unknown	½–2 hr	Unknown

Action

Chemical effect: Prevents cell growth by inhibiting DNA gyrase and topoisomerase IV, which interferes with DNA synthesis.
Therapeutic effect: Kills susceptible bacteria.

Available forms

Tablets: 320 mg

NURSING PROCESS

⚡ Assessment

• Serious and occasionally fatal hypersensitivity reaction may occur. Monitor patient carefully.
• Drug may cause CNS effects, such as tremors and anxiety. Monitor patient carefully.
• Carefully monitor patient's liver enzyme levels. Liver enzyme levels may rise during therapy but will resolve afterward.
• Assess patient's and family's knowledge of drug therapy.

⊕ Nursing diagnoses

• Risk for infection related to presence of bacteria susceptible to drug
• Risk for injury related to adverse effects of drug therapy
• Deficient knowledge related to drug therapy

▷ Planning and implementation

• Rash is more likely to appear in a patient younger than age 40, especially women and those taking hormone therapy. Stop giving drug if rash appears.
• Drug may cause tendon rupture, arthropathy, or osteochondrosis. Stop drug if patient reports pain, inflammation, or signs of muscle rupture.
• If patient has a photosensitivity reaction, stop giving drug.
• Serious diarrhea may indicate pseudomembranous colitis. Stop drug if needed.

• Keep patient adequately hydrated to avoid concentration of urine.

• In acute overdose, empty patient's stomach by inducing vomiting or performing gastric lavage. Hydrate patient if needed, and continue treating symptoms. Hemodialysis removes 20% to 30% of a dose.

Patient teaching

• Instruct patient to finish full course of therapy, even if symptoms improve.

• Tell patient to stop drug and seek medical care if evidence of hypersensitivity reaction develops.

• Tell patient to report serious diarrhea.

• Instruct patient to drink fluids liberally.

• Warn patient against taking OTC drugs or dietary supplements with this drug without consulting prescriber.

• Tell patient to avoid excessive exposure to sunlight or ultraviolet light.

• Urge patient to report pain, inflammation, or rupture of tendons.

• Warn patient to avoid driving or other hazardous activities until effects of drug are known.

✓ Evaluation

• Patient is free from infection after drug treatment.

• Patient remains free from injury from adverse reactions.

• Patient and family state understanding of drug therapy.

HIGH ALERT

gemtuzumab ozogamicin
(gem-TOO-zuh-mab oh-zoh-GAM-ih-sin)
Mylotarg

Pharmacologic class: monoclonal antibody
Therapeutic class: chemotherapeutic drug
Pregnancy risk category: D

Indications and dosages

▶ **Patients with CD33-positive acute myeloid leukemia in first relapse who are not considered candidates for cytotoxic chemotherapy.**
Adults age 60 and older: 9 mg/m² I.V. infusion over 2 hours every 14 days for a total of two doses. One hour before the infusion, give 50 mg of diphenhydramine P.O. and 650 to 1,000 mg of acetaminophen P.O. Additional doses of acetaminophen 650 to 1,000 mg P.O. can be given every 4 hours, p.r.n.

▽ I.V. administration

• During preparation and administration, protect from direct and indirect sunlight and unshielded fluorescent light.

• Administer in 100 ml of normal saline injection. Don't dilute in any other electrolyte solutions. Place the 100-ml I.V. bag into an ultraviolet light protectant bag. Use immediately.

• Use a separate I.V. line equipped with a low–protein-binding 1.2-micron terminal filter for administration of drug. May be infused by central or peripheral line.

• Don't give I.V. push or bolus.

• Monitor vital signs during infusion and for 4 hours after infusion.

⊗ **Incompatibilities**

• Other drugs, electrolyte solutions, or D₅W.

Contraindications and cautions

• Contraindicated in patients hypersensitive to drug or any of its components.

• Use cautiously in patients with hepatic impairment.

≋ **Lifespan:** Drug is indicated only for adults age 60 and older. In pregnant women, avoid using drug. Advise women of childbearing age not to become pregnant. Breast-feeding women should stop nursing or stop taking drug. It's unknown whether drug appears in breast milk. In children, safety and effectiveness haven't been established.

Adverse reactions

CNS: *asthenia, depression, dizziness, fever, headache, insomnia, pain.*
CV: hypertension, hypotension, tachycardia.
EENT: *epistaxis, pharyngitis, rhinitis.*
GI: *abdominal pain, anorexia, constipation, diarrhea, dyspepsia, enlarged abdomen, nausea, stomatitis, vomiting.*
GU: *hematuria,* VAGINAL HEMORRHAGE.
Hematologic: *anemia,* BLEEDING, LEUKOPENIA, NEUTROPENIA, NEUTROPENIC FEVER, SEVERE MYELOSUPPRESSION, THROMBOCYTOPENIA.
Hepatic: *hepatotoxicity, hyperbilirubinemia, veno-occlusive disease.*
Metabolic: hyperglycemia, hypokalemia, *hypomagnesemia.*
Musculoskeletal: arthralgia, back pain.
Respiratory: *acute respiratory distress syndrome,* dyspnea, *hypoxia, increased cough,* pneumonia, *pulmonary edema.*
Skin: *rash.*

Other: chills, herpes simplex, SEPSIS, *severe hypersensitivity reactions.*

Interactions

None reported.

Effects on lab test results

● May increase liver enzyme, LDH, and glucose levels. May decrease potassium, magnesium, and hemoglobin levels and hematocrit.
● May decrease leukocyte, neutrophil, and platelet counts.

Pharmacokinetics

Absorption: Given I.V.
Distribution: Unknown.
Metabolism: Unknown. Liver microsomal enzymes may be involved.
Excretion: Unknown. *Half-life:* Total and unconjugated calicheamicin, 45 and 100 hours, respectively, after the first dose. After the second dose, total calicheamicin, 60 hours.

Route	Onset	Peak	Duration
I.V.	Unknown	Unknown	Unknown

Action

Chemical effect: May bind to CD33 antigen on the surface of leukemic blasts in patients with acute myeloid leukemia, resulting in formation of a complex that's internalized by the cell. The calicheamicin derivative is then released inside the cell, causing DNA double-strand breaks and cell death.
Therapeutic effect: Kills cancer cells.

Available forms

Powder for injection: 5 mg

NURSING PROCESS

Assessment

● Monitor CBC and platelets before starting and during therapy.
● Monitor liver enzymes before and during therapy.
● Monitor patient for postinfusion reactions and tumor lysis syndrome.
● Monitor I.V. site for local reactions.
● Assess patient's and family's knowledge of drug therapy.

Nursing diagnoses

● Risk for injury related to adverse effects of drug
● Risk for infection related to drug-induced adverse hematologic reactions
● Deficient knowledge related to drug therapy

Planning and implementation

● Use only under the supervision of a prescriber experienced in the use of cancer drugs.
● Drug may produce a postinfusion symptom complex in the 24 hours immediately after the infusion; symptoms include chills, fever, hypotension, hypertension, hyperglycemia, hypoxia, or dyspnea.
● Tumor lysis syndrome may occur. Provide adequate hydration, and treat with allopurinol to prevent hyperuricemia.
● Drug isn't dialyzable.
● Severe myelosuppression will occur in all patients given the recommended dose. Careful hematologic monitoring is required.
● Monitor electrolytes, hepatic function, CBC, and platelets during therapy.
Patient teaching
● Inform patient about postinfusion symptoms, and instruct him to continue to take acetaminophen 650 to 1,000 mg every 4 hours p.r.n.
● Tell patient to watch for signs of infection (fever, sore throat, and fatigue) and bleeding (easy bruising, nosebleeds, bleeding gums, and melena). Tell patient to take temperature daily, before acetaminophen dose.

Evaluation

● Patient remains free from infection.
● Patient's laboratory values remain above critical levels throughout course of therapy.
● Patient and family state understanding of drug therapy.

gentamicin sulfate
(jen-tuh-MIGH-sin SUL-fayt)

Pharmacologic class: aminoglycoside
Therapeutic class: antibiotic
Pregnancy risk category: D

Indications and dosages

▶ **Serious infections caused by sensitive strains of** *Pseudomonas aeruginosa, Esche-*

---

richia coli, Proteus, Klebsiella, Serratia, Enterobacter, Citrobacter, Staphylococcus. Adults: 3 mg/kg daily in divided doses I.M. or I.V. every 8 hours. For life-threatening infections, up to 5 mg/kg daily in three to four divided doses. Reduce to 3 mg/kg daily as soon as indicated. *Children:* 2 to 2.5 mg/kg I.M. or I.V. every 8 hours.

Neonates older than age 1 week and infants: 2.5 mg/kg I.M. or I.V. every 8 hours.

Preterm infants and neonates age 1 week and younger: 2.5 mg/kg I.V. every 12 hours.

▶ **Meningitis.** *Adults:* 3 mg/kg daily in divided doses I.M. or I.V. every 8 hours. For life-threatening infections, up to 5 mg/kg daily in three to four divided doses. Reduce to 3 mg/kg daily as soon as indicated. Or 4 to 8 mg intrathecally daily.

Children and infants older than age 3 months: 2 to 2.5 mg/kg I.M. or I.V. every 8 hours. Or 1 to 2 mg intrathecally daily.

▶ **Endocarditis prophylaxis for GI or GU procedure or surgery.** *Adults:* 1.5 mg/kg to maximum dose, 80 mg, I.M. or I.V. 30 to 60 minutes before procedure or surgery. Give separately with ampicillin I.M. or I.V. followed in 6 hours by ampicillin or amoxicillin alone.

Children: 2 mg/kg I.M. or I.V. 30 to 60 minutes before procedure or surgery. Give separately with ampicillin I.M. or I.V. followed in 6 hours by ampicillin or amoxicillin alone.

▶ **Posthemodialysis to maintain therapeutic level.** *Adults:* 1 to 1.7 mg/kg I.M. or I.V. after each dialysis session. *Children:* 2 to 2.5 mg/kg I.M. or by I.V. infusion after each dialysis session.

⬛ **Adjust-a-dose:** In impaired renal function, dosage adjustment is needed. Serum concentrations of gentamicin should be monitored and dosing adjusted accordingly.

▼ I.V. administration

• When giving drug by intermittent I.V. infusion, dilute with 50 to 200 ml of D_5W or normal saline injection.

• Infuse over 30 minutes to 2 hours.

• After infusion, flush line with normal saline solution or D_5W.

⊗ Incompatibilities

Allopurinol, amphotericin B, ampicillin, azithromycin, cefazolin, cefepime, cefotaxime, ceftazidime, ceftriaxone sodium, cefuroxime, certain parenteral nutrition formulations, cytara-

bine, dopamine, fat emulsions, furosemide, heparin, hetastarch, idarubicin, indomethacin sodium trihydrate, nafcillin, propofol, ticarcillin, warfarin.

Contraindications and cautions

• Contraindicated in patients hypersensitive to drug or other aminoglycosides.

• Use cautiously in patients with renal impairment or neuromuscular disorders.

⚖ **Lifespan:** In pregnant women, don't use because drug is teratogenic. Beast-feeding women should stop the drug or stop breast-feeding. In neonates, infants, and the elderly, use drug cautiously.

Adverse reactions

CNS: headache, lethargy, numbness, paresthesias, peripheral neuropathy, *neurotoxicity, seizures,* twitching.

EENT: *ototoxicity.*

GU: NEPHROTOXICITY.

Hematologic: *agranulocytosis, leukopenia, thrombocytopenia.*

Other: hypersensitivity reactions.

Interactions

Drug-drug. *Acyclovir, amphotericin B, cisplatin, methoxyflurane, other aminoglycosides, vancomycin:* May increase ototoxicity and nephrotoxicity. Use together cautiously.

Atracurium, pancuronium, rocuronium, vecuronium: May increase neuromuscular blockade. Monitor patient closely.

Cephalothin: May increase nephrotoxicity. Use together cautiously; monitor renal function.

Dimenhydrinate: May mask symptoms of ototoxicity. Use with caution.

Diuretics: May increase ototoxicity. Avoid use together.

General anesthetics: May increase effects of nondepolarizing muscle relaxant, including prolonged respiratory depression. Use together only when necessary.

Indomethacin: May decrease renal clearance of gentamicin, leading to increased risk of toxicity.

I.V. loop diuretics (such as furosemide): May increase ototoxicity. Use cautiously.

Neurotoxic drugs: May increase neurotoxicity. Avoid use together.

Parenteral penicillins (such as ampicillin, ticarcillin): May inactivate gentamicin in vitro. Don't mix together.

G

Effects on lab test results

• May increase BUN, creatinine, nonprotein nitrogen, ALT, AST, bilirubin, and LDH levels. May decrease hemoglobin level and hematocrit.
• May increase eosinophil count. May decrease WBC, platelet, and granulocyte counts.

Pharmacokinetics

Absorption: Rapid and complete after I.M. use.
Distribution: Wide. CSF penetration is low even in adults with inflamed meninges. CSF levels are higher in neonates than adults. Protein-binding is minimal.
Metabolism: None.
Excretion: Mainly in urine. *Half-life:* 2 to 3 hours.

Route	Onset	Peak	Duration
I.V.	Immediate	15–30 min	Unknown
I.M.	Unknown	30–90 min	Unknown
Intrathecal	Unknown	Unknown	Unknown

Action

Chemical effect: Inhibits protein synthesis by binding to ribosomes.
Therapeutic effect: Kills susceptible bacteria (many aerobic gram-negative organisms and some aerobic gram-positive organisms). Drug may act against some aminoglycoside-resistant bacteria.

Available forms

Injection: 40 mg/ml (adult), 10 mg/ml (pediatric), 2 mg/ml (intrathecal)
I.V. infusion (premixed): 40 mg, 60 mg, 70 mg, 80 mg, 90 mg, 100 mg, 120 mg, 160 mg, 180 mg available in normal saline solution

NURSING PROCESS

🔍 Assessment

• Assess patient's infection and hearing before starting therapy and regularly thereafter.
• Obtain specimen for culture and sensitivity tests before giving the first dose. Begin therapy pending test results.
• Weigh patient and review baseline renal function studies before therapy and regularly during therapy. Notify prescriber of any changes; adjust dosage.
• Obtain blood for peak drug level 1 hour after I.M. injection and 30 minutes to 1 hour after I.V. infusion; for trough levels, draw blood just

before next dose. Don't collect blood in heparinized tube because heparin is incompatible with aminoglycosides.
• Peak level above 12 mcg/ml and trough level above 2 mcg/ml may increase risk of toxicity.
• Be alert for adverse reactions and drug interactions.
• Assess patient's and family's knowledge of drug therapy.

⊕ Nursing diagnoses

• Risk for infection related to presence of susceptible bacteria
• Impaired urinary elimination related to nephrotoxicity
• Deficient knowledge related to drug therapy

▶ Planning and implementation

• Give I.M. injection deep into large muscle mass (gluteal or midlateral thigh); rotate injection sites. Don't inject more than 2 g of drug per site.
• **⚠ ALERT:** Use preservative-free forms of gentamicin for intrathecal route.
• Hemodialysis (8 hours) removes up to 50% of drug.
• Notify prescriber about signs of decreasing renal function or changes in hearing.
• Therapy usually continues for 7 to 10 days. If no response occurs in 3 to 5 days, therapy may be stopped and new specimens obtained for culture and sensitivity testing.
• Therapeutic peak and trough levels are 4 to 12 mcg/ml and less than 2 mcg/ml, respectively.
• Make sure patient is well hydrated to minimize chemical irritation of renal tubules.
Patient teaching
• Instruct patient to notify prescriber about adverse reactions, such as changes in hearing.
• Emphasize importance of drinking at least 2 L of fluids daily, if not contraindicated.

✓ Evaluation

• Patient is free from infection.
• Patient maintains normal renal function throughout drug therapy.
• Patient and family state understanding of drug therapy.

Reactions may be *common,* uncommon, *life-threatening,* or COMMON AND LIFE-THREATENING.

glimepiride
(gligh-MEH-peh-righd)
Amaryl

Pharmacologic class: sulfonylurea
Therapeutic class: antidiabetic
Pregnancy risk category: C

Indications and dosages

▶ **Type 2 diabetes mellitus when hyperglycemia can't be managed by diet and exercise alone.** *Adults:* Initially, 1 to 2 mg P.O. once daily with first main meal of day. Usual maintenance dosage is 1 to 4 mg P.O. once daily. After reaching 2 mg, increase dosage in increments not exceeding 2 mg every 1 to 2 weeks, based on patient's response. Maximum, 8 mg daily.

▶ **Adjunct to insulin therapy in patients with type 2 diabetes mellitus whose hyperglycemia can't be managed by diet and exercise with oral antidiabetics.** *Adults:* 8 mg P.O. once daily with first main meal of day with low-dose insulin. Adjust insulin upward weekly based on patient's response.

▶ **Adjunct to metformin therapy in patients with type 2 diabetes mellitus whose hyperglycemia can't be managed by diet, exercise, and glimepiride or metformin alone.** *Adults:* 8 mg P.O. once daily with first main meal of the day with metformin. Adjust dosages based on patient's blood glucose response to determine minimum effective dosage of each drug.

⛌ Adjust-a-dose: For patients with renal or hepatic impairment, initial dose is 1 mg P.O. daily with breakfast; then adjust based on the patient's fasting glucose levels.

Contraindications and cautions

• Contraindicated in patients hypersensitive to the drug or any of its components, in those with diabetic ketoacidosis, and in those with allergies to sulfonamides or thiazide diuretics.
• Use cautiously in debilitated or malnourished patients and in those with adrenal, pituitary, hepatic, or renal insufficiency.
※ **Lifespan:** In pregnant and breast-feeding women, drug is contraindicated. In children, safety and effectiveness haven't been established. In elderly patients, use cautiously because they might be more sensitive to the drug.

Adverse reactions

CNS: asthenia, dizziness, headache.
EENT: changes in accommodation.
GI: nausea.
Hematologic: *agranulocytosis, aplastic anemia,* hemolytic anemia, *leukopenia, pancytopenia, thrombocytopenia.*
Hepatic: cholestatic jaundice.
Metabolic: *hypoglycemia.*
Skin: allergic skin reactions.

Interactions

Drug-drug. *Beta blockers:* May mask symptoms of hypoglycemia. Monitor glucose level carefully.
Drugs that produce hyperglycemia, thiazides and other diuretics: May lead to loss of glucose control. May require dosage adjustment.
Insulin: May increase risk of hypoglycemia. Monitor glucose level closely.
NSAIDs, other highly protein-bound drugs: May increase hypoglycemic action of sulfonylureas, such as glimepiride. Monitor patient carefully.
Drug-herb. *Aloe, bilberry leaf, bitter melon, burdock, dandelion, fenugreek, garlic, ginseng:* May improve glucose control, which may allow reduction of oral hypoglycemic. Tell patient to discuss herbs with prescriber before use.
Drug-lifestyle. *Alcohol use:* May alter glycemic control, most commonly toward hypoglycemia. May cause disulfiram-like reaction. Discourage use together.
Sun exposure: May cause photosensitivity. Discourage prolonged or unprotected exposure to the sun.

Effects on lab test results

• May increase BUN, creatinine, alkaline phosphatase, ALT, and AST levels. May decrease glucose, sodium, and hemoglobin levels and hematocrit.
• May decrease WBC, RBC, platelet, and granulocyte counts.

Pharmacokinetics

Absorption: Complete.
Distribution: Almost completely protein-bound.
Metabolism: Complete.
Excretion: In urine and feces. *Half-life:* 9 hours.

Route	Onset	Peak	Duration
P.O.	≤1 hr	2–3 hr	24 hr

Action

Chemical effect: Stimulates release of insulin from pancreatic beta cells; increases sensitivity of peripheral tissues to insulin.
Therapeutic effect: Lowers glucose levels.

Available forms

Tablets: 1 mg, 2 mg, 4 mg

NURSING PROCESS

🔖 Assessment
• Monitor fasting glucose periodically to determine therapeutic response. Also monitor glycosylated hemoglobin level, usually every 3 to 6 months, to more precisely assess long-term glycemic control.
• Assess patient's and family's knowledge of drug therapy.

✚ Nursing diagnoses
• Ineffective health maintenance related to hyperglycemia
• Risk for injury related to drug-induced hypoglycemia
• Deficient knowledge related to drug therapy

▶ Planning and implementation
• Oral hypoglycemic drugs have been linked to an increased risk of CV mortality compared with diet alone or with diet and insulin therapy.
• Give drug with the first meal of the day.
Patient teaching
• Tell patient to take drug with first meal of day.
• Stress importance of adhering to diet, weight-reduction, exercise, and personal hygiene programs.
• Explain to patient and family how to monitor glucose levels, identify signs and symptoms, and treat hyperglycemia and hypoglycemia.
• Advise patient to wear or carry medical identification that describes his condition.
• Instruct patient to avoid alcohol consumption during therapy.

☑ Evaluation
• Patient's glucose level is normal.
• Patient recognizes hypoglycemia early and treats it before injury occurs.
• Patient and family state understanding of drug therapy.

HIGH ALERT

glipizide
(GLIH-pih-zighd)
Glucotrol◊, Glucotrol XL◊

Pharmacologic class: sulfonylurea
Therapeutic class: antidiabetic
Pregnancy risk category: C

Indications and dosages

▶ **Adjunct to diet to lower glucose level in patients with type 2 diabetes mellitus.** *Adults:* Initially 5 mg immediate-release P.O. daily 30 minutes before breakfast. Maximum recommended total daily dose, 40 mg. Or 5 mg extended-release tablets P.O. daily. Adjust in 5-mg increments every 3 months depending on level of glycemic control. Maximum daily dose for extended-release tablets, 20 mg.
▣ **Adjust-a-dose:** In elderly patients with liver disease, 2.5 mg immediate-release or 5 mg extended-release. Maximum once-daily dose is 15 mg.
▶ **To replace insulin therapy.** *Adults:* If insulin dosage is more than 20 units daily, patient is started at usual dosage in addition to 50% of insulin. If insulin dosage is less than 20 units, stop insulin.

Contraindications and cautions

• Contraindicated in patients hypersensitive to the drug or any of its components, in those with diabetic ketoacidosis, and in those with allergies to sulfonamides or thiazide diuretics.
• Use cautiously in patients with renal and hepatic disease and in debilitated or malnourished patients.
⚖ **Lifespan:** In pregnant and breast-feeding women, drug is contraindicated. In children, safety and effectiveness haven't been established because of the rarity of type 2 diabetes mellitus in this population. In elderly patients, use cautiously.

Adverse reactions

CNS: dizziness, drowsiness, headache.
CV: facial flushing.
GI: constipation, nausea, vomiting.
Hematologic: *agranulocytosis, aplastic anemia, thrombocytopenia.*
Hepatic: cholestatic jaundice.

Reactions may be *common*, uncommon, *life-threatening*, or COMMON AND LIFE-THREATENING.

Metabolic: *hypoglycemia.*
Skin: rash, pruritus.

Interactions

Drug-drug. *Anabolic steroids, antifungal antibiotics, chloramphenicol, cimetidine, clofibrate, guanethidine, MAO inhibitors, phenylbutazone, probenecid, salicylates, sulfonamides:* May increase hypoglycemic activity. Monitor glucose level.
Beta blockers: May prolong hypoglycemic effect and mask symptoms of hypoglycemia. Use together cautiously.
Corticosteroids, glucagon, rifampin, thiazide diuretics: May decrease hypoglycemic response. Monitor glucose level.
Hydantoins: May increase hydantoin level. Monitor level.
Oral anticoagulants: May increase hypoglycemic activity or enhance anticoagulant effect. Monitor glucose level, PT, and INR.
Drug-herb. *Aloe, bilberry leaf, bitter melon, burdock, dandelion, fenugreek, garlic, ginseng:* May improve glucose control, which may allow reduction of oral hypoglycemic. Tell patient to discuss herbs with prescriber before use.
Drug-lifestyle. *Alcohol use:* May alter glycemic control, most commonly toward hypoglycemia. May also cause disulfiram-like reaction. Discourage use together.
Sun exposure: May cause photosensitivity. Discourage prolonged or unprotected sun exposure.

Effects on lab test results
• May increase BUN, creatinine, alkaline phosphatase, AST, and LDH levels. May decrease glucose and hemoglobin levels and hematocrit.
• May decrease granulocyte and platelet counts.

Pharmacokinetics
Absorption: Rapid and complete.
Distribution: In extracellular fluid. 98% to 99% protein-bound.
Metabolism: By liver to inactive metabolites.
Excretion: Mainly in urine. *Half-life:* 2 to 4 hours.

Route	Onset	Peak	Duration
P.O.	15–30 min	1–3 hr	10–24 hr

Action
Chemical effect: May stimulate insulin release from pancreas, reduce glucose output by liver, and increase peripheral sensitivity to insulin.
Therapeutic effect: Lowers glucose level.

Available forms
Tablets: 5 mg, 10 mg
Tablets (extended-release): 2.5 mg, 5 mg, 10 mg

NURSING PROCESS

Assessment
• Assess glucose level before starting therapy and regularly thereafter.
• Patient transferring from insulin therapy to oral antidiabetic needs glucose monitoring at least three times daily before meals.
• During periods of increased stress, such as from infection, fever, surgery, or trauma, patient may need insulin therapy. Monitor patient closely for hyperglycemia in these situations.
• Be alert for adverse reactions and drug interactions.
• Assess patient's and family's knowledge of drug therapy.

Nursing diagnoses
• Ineffective health maintenance related to hyperglycemia
• Risk for injury related to drug-induced hypoglycemia
• Deficient knowledge related to drug therapy

Planning and implementation
• Give drug about 30 minutes before meals.
• Some patients may attain effective control with once-daily dose; others show better response with divided doses.
• For a hypoglycemic reaction, give oral form of fast-acting carbohydrates or glucagon or I.V. glucose (if patient can't swallow or is comatose). Then give patient a complex carbohydrate snack when he awakens, and determine cause of the reaction.
• Make sure adjunct therapies, such as diet and exercise, are being used appropriately.
ALERT: Don't confuse glipizide with glyburide.
Patient teaching
• Teach patient about diabetes and the importance of following a therapeutic regimen: adher-

ing to specific diet, weight reduction, exercise and personal hygiene programs, and avoiding infection.
• Explain how to monitor glucose level and how to recognize and treat hypoglycemia and hyperglycemia.
• Tell patient not to change dosage without prescriber's consent and to report any adverse reactions.
• Advise patient not to take other drugs, including OTC drugs or herbal remedies, without first checking with prescriber.
• Instruct patient not to drink alcohol during drug therapy.
• Advise patient to carry medical identification at all times.

✓ Evaluation
• Patient's glucose level is normal with drug therapy.
• Patient doesn't experience hypoglycemia or hyperglycemia.
• Patient and family state understanding of drug therapy.

glucagon
(GLOO-kuh-gon)

Pharmacologic class: pancreatic hormone
Therapeutic class: antihypoglycemic
Pregnancy risk category: B

Indications and dosages

▶ **Hypoglycemia.** *Adults and children who weigh more than 20 kg (44 lb):* 1 mg I.V., I.M., or subcutaneously.
Children who weigh 20 kg or less: 0.5 mg I.V., I.M., or subcutaneously.
▶ **Diagnostic aid for radiologic examination.** *Adults:* 0.25 to 2 mg I.V. or 1 to 2 mg I.M. before start of radiologic procedure.

▼ I.V. administration

• Reconstitute drug in 1-unit vial with 1 ml of diluent. Use only diluent supplied by manufacturer.
• Don't exceed concentration of 1 mg/ml (1 unit/ml).
• For I.V. drip infusion, use dextrose solution, which is compatible with glucagon. Drug forms precipitate in chloride solutions.

• Inject directly into vein or into I.V. tubing of free-flowing compatible solution over 2 to 5 minutes. Interrupt primary infusion during glucagon injection (if using same I.V. line). Repeat in 15 minutes if needed.
• If patient fails to respond, give I.V. glucose. When patient responds, give supplemental carbohydrate promptly.
⊗ **Incompatibilities**
Sodium chloride solution, solutions with pH of 3 to 9.5.

Contraindications and cautions

• Contraindicated in patients hypersensitive to the drug or any or its components and in those with pheochromocytoma.
• Use cautiously in patients with history of insulinoma or pheochromocytoma.
☀ **Lifespan:** In pregnant women, use only if benefits outweigh risks to the fetus. In breastfeeding women, use cautiously because it's unknown if the drug appears in breast milk. In children, safety and effectiveness as a diagnostic aid haven't been established.

Adverse reactions

CV: hypotension.
GI: nausea, vomiting.
Respiratory: *respiratory distress.*
Skin: urticaria.
Other: allergic reactions.

Interactions

Drug-drug. *Oral anticoagulants:* May increase anticoagulant effect. Monitor PT and INR closely; monitor patient for bleeding.

Effects on lab test results

• May decrease potassium level.

Pharmacokinetics

Absorption: Unknown.
Distribution: Unknown.
Metabolism: Extensive by liver, in kidneys and plasma, and at its tissue receptor sites in plasma membranes.
Excretion: By kidneys. *Half-life:* 8 to 18 minutes.

Route	Onset	Peak	Duration
I.V., I.M., SubQ	Immediate	≤ 30 min	1–2 hr

Reactions may be *common*, uncommon, *life-threatening*, or COMMON AND LIFE-THREATENING.

Action

Chemical effect: Promotes catalytic depolymerization of hepatic glycogen to glucose.
Therapeutic effect: Raises glucose level.

Available forms

Powder for injection: 1 mg (1 unit)/vial

NURSING PROCESS

⚕ Assessment

• Assess patient's glucose level before starting therapy and after giving the drug.
• Be alert for adverse reactions and drug interactions.
• If patient vomits, monitor his hydration.
• Assess patient's and family's knowledge of drug therapy.

⊞ Nursing diagnoses

• Risk for injury related to hypoglycemia
• Risk for deficient fluid volume related to drug-induced vomiting
• Deficient knowledge related to drug therapy

▷ Planning and implementation

• For I.M use, reconstitute drug in 1-unit vial with 1 ml of diluent; reconstitute drug in 10-unit vial with 10 ml of diluent. Use only diluent supplied by manufacturer when preparing doses of 2 mg or less. For larger doses, dilute with sterile water for injection.
• Arouse lethargic patient as quickly as possible and give additional carbohydrates orally to prevent secondary hypoglycemic reactions. Notify prescriber that patient's hypoglycemic episode required glucagon use. If patient doesn't respond to drug, provide emergency intervention. Unstable hypoglycemic diabetic patient may not respond to drug. Give glucose I.V. instead.
• If patient can't retain some form of sugar for 1 hour because of nausea or vomiting, notify prescriber.
Patient teaching
• Instruct patient and family in proper drug administration.
• Teach them to recognize signs and symptoms of hypoglycemia, and tell them to notify prescriber immediately in emergencies.

☑ Evaluation

• Patient's glucose level returns to normal.

• Patient remains well hydrated.
• Patient and family state understanding of drug therapy.

HIGH ALERT

glyburide (glibenclamide)

(GLIGH-byoo-righd)
DiaBeta✐, Euglucon ◆, Gen-Glybe ◆,
Glynase PresTab, Micronase✐

Pharmacologic class: sulfonylurea
Therapeutic class: antidiabetic
Pregnancy risk category: B (for Micronase, Glynase); C (for DiaBeta)

Indications and dosages

▶ **Adjunct to diet to lower glucose level in patients with type 2 diabetes mellitus.** *Adults:* Initially, 1.25- to 5-mg regular tablets P.O. once daily with breakfast. For maintenance, 1.25 to 20 mg daily as single dose or in divided doses. Or, initially, 0.75- to 3-mg micronized formulation P.O. daily. For maintenance, 0.75 to 12 mg P.O. daily in single or divided doses.
▶ **To replace insulin therapy.** *Adults:* Initially, if insulin dosage is more than 40 units daily, 5-mg regular tablets or 3-mg micronized form P.O. once daily in addition to 50% of insulin dosage. If insulin dosage is 20 to 40 units daily, 5-mg regular tablets or 3-mg micronized form P.O. once daily while abruptly stopping insulin. If insulin dosage is less than 20 units daily, 2.5- to 5-mg regular tablets or 1.5- to 3-mg micronized form P.O. once daily while abruptly stopping insulin.

Contraindications and cautions

• Contraindicated in patients hypersensitive to the drug or any of its components, in those with diabetic ketoacidosis, and in those with allergies to sulfonamides or thiazide diuretics.
• Use cautiously in patients with hepatic or renal impairment and in debilitated or malnourished patients.
⚕ **Lifespan:** In pregnant women, breastfeeding women, and children, drug is contraindicated. In elderly patients, use cautiously.

Adverse reactions

CV: facial flushing.
GI: epigastric fullness, heartburn, nausea.

Hematologic: *agranulocytosis, aplastic anemia, thrombocytopenia.*
Hepatic: cholestatic jaundice.
Metabolic: *hypoglycemia.*
Skin: pruritus, rash.

Interactions

Drug-drug. *Anabolic steroids, chloramphenicol, clofibrate, guanethidine, MAO inhibitors, phenylbutazone, salicylates, sulfonamides:* May increase hypoglycemic activity. Monitor glucose level.
Beta blockers: May prolong hypoglycemic effect and mask symptoms of hypoglycemia. Use together cautiously.
Corticosteroids, glucagon, rifampin, thiazide diuretics: May decrease hypoglycemic response. Monitor glucose level.
Hydantoins: May increase hydantoin level. Monitor level.
Oral anticoagulants: May increase hypoglycemic activity or enhance anticoagulant effect. Monitor glucose level, PT, and INR.
Drug-herb. *Aloe, bilberry leaf, bitter melon, burdock, dandelion, fenugreek, garlic, ginseng:* May improve glucose control and allow reduction of oral hypoglycemic. Tell patient to discuss herbs with prescriber before use.
Drug-lifestyle. *Alcohol use:* May alter glycemic control, most commonly hypoglycemia. May also cause disulfiram-like reaction. Discourage use together.
Sun exposure: May cause photosensitivity. Discourage prolonged or unprotected exposure to sunlight.

Effects on lab test results

• May increase BUN, alkaline phosphatase, bilirubin, AST, ALT, and LDH levels. May decrease glucose and hemoglobin levels and hematocrit.
• May decrease WBC, platelet, and granulocyte counts.

Pharmacokinetics

Absorption: Almost complete.
Distribution: 99% protein-bound.
Metabolism: Complete.
Excretion: As metabolites in urine and feces in equal proportions. *Half-life:* 10 hours.

Route	Onset	Peak	Duration
P.O.	45–60 min	2–4 hr	24 hr

Action

Chemical effect: May stimulate insulin release from pancreas, reduce glucose output by liver, increase peripheral sensitivity to insulin, and cause mild diuresis.
Therapeutic effect: Lowers glucose levels.

Available forms

Tablets: 1.25 mg, 2.5 mg, 5 mg
Tablets (micronized): 1.5 mg, 3 mg, 4.5 mg, 6 mg

NURSING PROCESS

Assessment
• Assess glucose level before starting therapy and regularly thereafter.
• Patient transferring from insulin therapy to oral antidiabetic needs glucose monitoring at least three times daily before meals.
• During periods of increased stress, such as from infection, fever, surgery, or trauma, patient may need insulin therapy. Monitor patient closely for hyperglycemia in these situations.
• Be alert for adverse reactions and drug interactions.
• Assess patient's and family's knowledge of drug therapy.

Nursing diagnoses
• Ineffective health maintenance related to hyperglycemia
• Risk for injury related to drug-induced hypoglycemia
• Deficient knowledge related to drug therapy

Planning and implementation
• Micronized glyburide (Glynase PresTab) contains drug in smaller particle size and isn't bioequivalent to regular tablets. Adjust dose in a patient who has been taking Micronase or DiaBeta.
• Although most patients take drug once daily, patient taking more than 10 mg daily may achieve better results with twice-daily dosage.
• For hypoglycemic reaction, give oral form of fast-acting carbohydrates or, if patient can't swallow or is comatose, glucagon or I.V. glucose. Then give patient a complex carbohydrate snack when patient is conscious, and determine cause of reaction.
• Make sure that adjunct therapy, such as diet and exercise, is appropriate.
ALERT: Don't confuse glyburide with glipizide.

Patient teaching
• Teach patient about diabetes and the importance of following therapeutic regimen by adhering to specific diet, weight reduction, exercise, and personal hygiene programs and by avoiding infection.
• Explain how to monitor glucose level and recognize and treat hypoglycemia and hyperglycemia.
• Tell patient not to change dosage without prescriber's consent and to report any adverse reactions.
• Advise patient not to take OTC drugs or herbal remedies without first checking with prescriber.
• Instruct patient not to drink alcohol during drug therapy.
• Advise patient to wear or carry medical identification at all times.

✓ Evaluation
• Patient's glucose level is normal with drug therapy.
• Patient doesn't experience hypoglycemia.
• Patient and family state understanding of drug therapy.

HIGH ALERT

goserelin acetate
(GOH-seh-reh-lin AS-ih-tayt)
Zoladex, Zoladex 3-Month, Zoladex LA ◆

Pharmacologic class: luteinizing hormone–releasing hormone (LH-RH) analogue
Therapeutic class: antineoplastic
Pregnancy risk category: X (for endometriosis); D (for advanced breast cancer)

Indications and dosages
▶ **Endometriosis, advanced breast cancer.**
Women: One 3.6-mg implant subcutaneously every 28 days into upper abdominal wall for 6 months in endometriosis, longer in breast cancer. For endometriosis, maximum duration of therapy is 6 months.
▶ **Palliative therapy of advanced carcinoma of the prostate.** *Men:* One 10.8-mg implant subcutaneously every 12 weeks or 3.6 mg implant subcutaneously every 4 weeks into upper abdominal wall, given with radiotherapy and Flutamide.
▶ **Endometrial thinning before endometrial ablation for dysfunctional uterine bleeding.**

Women: One or two 3.6-mg implants subcutaneously into upper abdominal wall. Give each implant 4 weeks apart.

Contraindications and cautions
• Contraindicated in patients hypersensitive to LH-RH, LH-RH agonist analogues, goserelin acetate, or any of its components.
• The 10.8-mg implant is contraindicated for use in women.
• Use cautiously in patients with risk factors for osteoporosis, such as family history of osteoporosis, chronic alcohol or tobacco abuse, or use of drugs that affect bone density.
⚠ **Lifespan:** In pregnant women, breast-feeding women, and children, drug is contraindicated.

Adverse reactions
CNS: anxiety, depression, dizziness, emotional lability, fever, headache, insomnia, lethargy, pain, *stroke.*
CV: *arrhythmias,* chest pain, edema, *heart failure,* hypertension, *MI,* peripheral vascular disorder.
GI: constipation, diarrhea, nausea, ulcer, vomiting.
GU: amenorrhea, *impotence, lower urinary tract symptoms,* renal insufficiency, urinary obstruction, UTI, vaginal dryness.
Hematologic: anemia.
Metabolic: hyperglycemia, weight increase.
Musculoskeletal: loss of bone mineral density.
Respiratory: COPD, upper respiratory tract infection.
Skin: diaphoresis, rash.
Other: breast swelling and tenderness, changes in breast size, chills, gout, *hot flushes, sexual dysfunction.*

Interactions
None reported.

Effects on lab test results
• May increase ALT, AST, LDL, HDL, cholesterol, triglyceride, calcium, and glucose levels. May decrease hemoglobin level and hematocrit.
• May alter diagnostic tests of pituitary-gonadotropic and gonadal function.

Pharmacokinetics
Absorption: Slow.
Distribution: Minimally protein-bound.

G

Metabolism: Hydrolysis of C-terminal amino acids.
Excretion: Mostly via kidneys, 20% unchanged. *Half-life:* About 4 hours.

Route	Onset	Peak	Duration
SubQ	2–4 wk	12–15 days	Throughout therapy

Action

Chemical effect: Acts on pituitary to decrease release of follicle-stimulating hormone and LH, resulting in dramatically lowered levels of sex hormones.
Therapeutic effect: Decreases effects of sex hormones on tumor growth in prostate gland and tissue growth in uterus.

Available forms

Implants: 3.6 mg, 10.8 mg

NURSING PROCESS

☑ Assessment
• Assess patient's condition before starting therapy and regularly thereafter.
• When used for prostate cancer, drug may initially worsen symptoms because it initially increases testosterone levels. Patient may have increased bone pain. Rarely, disease (spinal cord compression or ureteral obstruction) may worsen.
• Be alert for adverse reactions.
• Assess patient's and family's knowledge of drug therapy.

⊞ Nursing diagnoses
• Ineffective health maintenance related to underlying condition
• Acute pain related to drug's adverse effect
• Deficient knowledge related to drug therapy

⊳ Planning and implementation
• Give under supervision of prescriber.
• Give drug into upper abdominal wall. After cleaning area with alcohol swab (and injecting local anesthetic), stretch patient's skin with one hand while grasping barrel of syringe with the other. Insert needle into subcutaneous fat; then change direction of needle so that it parallels abdominal wall. Push in needle until hub touches patient's skin, and then withdraw about 1 cm (this creates a gap for drug to be injected) before depressing plunger completely.

• To avoid need for new syringe and injection site, don't aspirate after inserting needle.
• Implant comes in preloaded syringe. If package is damaged, don't use syringe. Make sure drug is visible in translucent chamber.
• After implantation, area requires bandage after needle is withdrawn.
• If implants require removal, schedule patient for ultrasound to locate them.
• Notify prescriber of adverse reactions, and provide supportive care.

Patient teaching
• Advise patient to report every 28 days for new implant. A delay of a couple of days is permissible.
• Tell patient to call prescriber if menstruation persists or breakthrough bleeding occurs. Menstruation should stop during therapy.
• After therapy ends, inform patient that she may experience delayed return of menses. Persistent amenorrhea is rare.
• Warn patient that pain may occur.

☑ Evaluation
• Patient responds well to drug.
• Patient has no pain.
• Patient and family state understanding of drug therapy.

granisetron hydrochloride
(grah-NEEZ-eh-trohn high-droh-KLOR-ighd)
Kytril

Pharmacologic class: selective 5-hydroxytryptamine (5-HT$_3$) receptor antagonist
Therapeutic class: antiemetic, antinauseant
Pregnancy risk category: B

Indications and dosages

▶ **Prevention of nausea and vomiting caused by emetogenic chemotherapy.** *Adults and children age 2 and older:* 10 mcg/kg undiluted and given by direct injection over 30 seconds, or diluted and infused over 5 minutes. Begin infusion within 30 minutes before chemotherapy starts. Or, for adults, 1 mg P.O. up to 1 hour before chemotherapy and repeated 12 hours later. Or, for adults, 2 mg P.O. daily within 1 hour before chemotherapy.
▶ **Prevention of nausea and vomiting from radiation, including total body irradiation**

Reactions may be *common*, uncommon, *life-threatening*, or COMMON AND LIFE-THREATENING.

and fractionated abdominal radiation.
Adults: 2 mg P.O. once daily within 1 hour of
radiation.

▶ **Postoperative nausea and vomiting.** *Adults:*
1 mg I.V. undiluted and given over 30 seconds.
For prevention, give before anesthesia induction
or immediately before reversal.

▼ I.V. administration

• Dilute drug with normal saline injection or
D_5W to make 20 to 50 ml.
• Infuse over 5 minutes, beginning within
30 minutes before chemotherapy starts and only
on days chemotherapy is given.
• Diluted solutions are stable for 24 hours at
room temperature.
⊗ **Incompatibilities**
Other I.V. drugs.

Contraindications and cautions

• Contraindicated in patients hypersensitive to
the drug or any of its components.
⚠ **Lifespan:** In pregnant women, use cautiously. In breast-feeding women, use cautiously because it's unknown if the drug appears in breast
milk. In children, safety and effectiveness
haven't been established for postoperative nausea and vomiting. In children younger than age
2, safety and effectiveness haven't been established for nausea and vomiting from chemotherapy. Safety and effectiveness of oral drug
haven't been established in children of any age.

Adverse reactions

CNS: agitation, anxiety, *asthenia,* CNS stimulation, *dizziness, fever, headache,* insomnia, *pain,*
somnolence.
CV: *bradycardia,* hypertension, hypotension.
GI: abdominal pain, *constipation,* decreased appetite, diarrhea, dyspepsia, flatulence, *nausea,*
taste disorder, *vomiting.*
GU: *oliguria,* UTI.
Hematologic: anemia, *leukopenia, leukocytosis, thrombocytopenia.*
Respiratory: cough, dyspnea, increased sputum.
Skin: alopecia, dermatitis, rash, urticaria.
Other: *anaphylaxis,* hypersensitivity reactions,
infection.

Interactions

Drug-herb. *Horehound:* May enhance serotonergic effects. Discourage use together.

Effects on lab test results

• May increase ALT and AST levels. May decrease hemoglobin level and hematocrit.
• May decrease WBC and platelet counts.

Pharmacokinetics

Absorption: Unknown.
Distribution: Distributed freely between plasma and RBCs. About 65% protein-bound.
Metabolism: By liver.
Excretion: In urine and feces. *Half-life:* 5 to
9 hours.

Route	Onset	Peak	Duration
P.O., I.V.	Unknown	Unknown	Unknown

Action

Chemical effect: Located in the CNS at the
area postrema (chemoreceptor trigger zone) and
in the peripheral nervous system on nerve terminals of the vagus nerve. Drug's blocking action
may occur at both sites.
Therapeutic effect: Prevents nausea and vomiting from chemotherapy and anesthesia.

Available forms

Injection: 0.1 mg/ml, 1 mg/ml
Oral solution: 1 mg/5 ml
Tablets: 1 mg

NURSING PROCESS

🔖 Assessment
• Assess patient's chemotherapy and GI reactions before starting therapy.
• Monitor patient for nausea and vomiting.
• Be alert for adverse reactions.
• If drug is ineffective or diarrhea occurs, monitor hydration.
• Assess patient's and family's knowledge of
drug therapy.

⊕ Nursing diagnoses
• Risk for deficient fluid volume related to nausea and vomiting
• Acute pain related to drug-induced headache
• Deficient knowledge related to drug therapy

▶ Planning and implementation
• Give oral form of drug 1 hour before chemotherapy; repeat in 12 hours.
⚠ **ALERT:** Don't mix with other drugs. Compatibility data are limited.

- If patient has nausea or vomits, alert prescriber.

Patient teaching
- Tell patient to notify prescriber if adverse drug reactions occur.

☑ Evaluation
- Patient has no nausea or vomiting with chemotherapy.
- Patient's headache is relieved with mild analgesic.
- Patient and family state understanding of drug therapy.

guaifenesin (glyceryl guaiacolate)
(gwah-FEH-nih-sin)
Allfen Jr., Diabetic Tussin EX†, Guiatuss*†, Humibid Maximum Strength†, Humibid Pediatric, Hytuss†, Hytuss-2X†, Liquibid, Mucinex†, Mucinex ER, Mucinex Mini-Melts†, Naldecon Senior EX†, Organidin NR, Robitussin*†, Scot-tussin Expectorant†, Siltussin SA†, X-Peet

Pharmacologic class: propanediol derivative
Therapeutic class: expectorant
Pregnancy risk category: C

Indications and dosages

▶ **Expectorant.** *Adults and children age 12 and older:* Give 200 to 400 mg P.O. every 4 hours, or 600 to 1,200 mg extended-release capsules every 12 hours. Maximum, 2,400 mg daily.
Children ages 6 to 11: Give 100 to 200 mg P.O. every 4 hours. Maximum, 1,200 mg daily.
Children ages 2 to 5: Give 50 to 100 mg P.O. every 4 hours. Maximum, 600 mg daily.

Contraindications and cautions
- Contraindicated in patients hypersensitive to the drug or any of its components.
- ⚠ **Lifespan:** In pregnant women, use cautiously. In breast-feeding women, safety and effectiveness haven't been established. In children younger than age 2 years, safety and effectiveness haven't been established. For children younger than age 12, don't give extended-release form.

Adverse reactions
CNS: drowsiness.
GI: diarrhea, stomach pain, nausea (with large doses), vomiting.
Skin: rash.

Interactions
None significant.

Effects on lab test results
- May decrease serum uric acid level.
- May falsify results of 5-hydroxyindoleacetic acid and vanillylmandelic acid tests.

Pharmacokinetics
Absorption: Good.
Distribution: Unknown.
Metabolism: Unknown.
Excretion: Renal, as inactive metabolites. *Half-life:* 1 hour.

Route	Onset	Peak	Duration
P.O.	Unknown	Unknown	Unknown

Action
Chemical effect: Increases production of respiratory tract fluids to help liquefy and reduce viscosity of tenacious secretions.
Therapeutic effect: Thins respiratory secretions for easier removal.

Available forms
Capsules: 200 mg†
Capsules (extended-release): 300 mg
Granules: 50 mg†, 100 mg†
Liquid: 100 mg/5 ml†, 200 mg/5 ml†
Syrup: 100 mg/5 ml†
Tablets: 100 mg†, 200 mg, 400 mg
Tablets (extended-release): 600 mg†, 1,200 mg†

NURSING PROCESS

⧩ Assessment
- Assess patient's sputum production before and after giving drug.
- Be alert for adverse reactions.
- If adverse GI reactions occur, monitor patient's hydration.
- Assess patient's and family's knowledge of drug therapy.

Reactions may be *common*, uncommon, *life-threatening*, or COMMON AND LIFE-THREATENING.

Nursing diagnoses
- Ineffective airway clearance related to underlying condition
- Risk for deficient fluid volume related to adverse GI reactions
- Deficient knowledge related to drug therapy

Planning and implementation
- Give drug with a full glass of water.

Patient teaching
- Inform patient that persistent cough may indicate a serious condition. Tell him to contact prescriber if cough lasts longer than 1 week, recurs frequently, or accompanies a high fever, rash, or severe headache.
- Advise patient to take each dose with a full glass of water before and after dose. Increasing fluid intake may prove beneficial.
- For granules, tell patient to empty entire packet onto tongue and swallow and not to chew.
- **ALERT:** Advise patient not to break, crush, or chew extended-release tablets.
- Encourage patient to perform deep-breathing exercises.

Evaluation
- Patient's lungs are clear and respiratory secretions are normal.
- Patient maintains adequate hydration.
- Patient and family state understanding of drug therapy.

haloperidol
(hal-oh-PER-uh-dol)
Haldol, Novo-Peridol ♦

haloperidol decanoate
Haldol Decanoate, Haldol LA ♦

haloperidol lactate
Haldol

Pharmacologic class: butyrophenone derivative
Therapeutic class: antipsychotic
Pregnancy risk category: C

Indications and dosages
▶ **Psychotic disorders.** *Adults and children age 12 and older:* Initial range is 0.5 to 5 mg P.O. b.i.d. or t.i.d. Or 2 to 5 mg I.M. every 4 to 8 hours, although hourly administration may be needed until control is obtained. Maximum, 100 mg P.O. daily.
Children ages 3 to 11: Give 0.05 to 0.15 mg/kg P.O. given b.i.d. or t.i.d. Severely disturbed children may need higher doses.
▶ **Chronically psychotic patients who need prolonged therapy.** *Adults:* Initially, 10 to 20 times previous daily dosage of oral haloperidol equivalent up to a maximum of 100 mg decanoate given I.M. every 4 weeks. Usual maintenance dosage, 10 to 15 times previous daily dosage in oral haloperidol equivalents.
▶ **Nonpsychotic behavior disorders, hyperactivity.** *Children ages 3 to 12:* Give 0.05 to 0.075 mg/kg P.O. b.i.d. or t.i.d. Maximum, 6 mg P.O. daily.
▶ **Tourette syndrome.** *Adults:* 0.5 to 1.5 mg P.O. t.i.d. Some patients may require up to 10 mg/day in two or three divided doses.
Children ages 3 to 12: Give 0.05 to 0.075 mg/ kg P.O. b.i.d. or t.i.d.
▶ **Delirium‡.** *Adults:* 1 to 2 mg I.V. every 2 to 4 hours.

I.V. administration
- I.V. form not recommended; best I.V. dosage hasn't been established.
- ⊗ **Incompatibilities**
Allopurinol, amphotericin B, benztropine, cefepime, diphenhydramine, fluconazole, foscarnet, heparin, hydromorphone, hydroxyzine, ketorolac, morphine, nitroprusside, piperacillin, and tazobactam.

Contraindications and cautions
- Contraindicated in patients hypersensitive to the drug or any of its components and in those with parkinsonism, coma, or CNS depression.
- Use cautiously in debilitated patients; in patients who take anticonvulsants, anticoagulants, antiparkinsonians, or lithium; and in patients with a history of seizures or EEG abnormalities, severe CV disorders, allergies, glaucoma, or urine retention.
- **Lifespan:** In pregnant women, use only if benefits outweigh risks to fetus. In breastfeeding women, drug is contraindicated. In children younger than age 3 or those who weigh

less than 15 kg (33 lb), use is contraindicated. In elderly patients, use cautiously. Elderly patients need a lower initial dose and a more gradual dosage adjustment.

Adverse reactions

CNS: *neuroleptic malignant syndrome,* sedation, *seizures,* severe extrapyramidal reactions, tardive dyskinesia.
CV: *bradycardia,* ECG changes, hypertension, hypotension, tachycardia, *torsades de pointes.*
EENT: blurred vision.
GU: menstrual irregularities, urine retention.
Hematologic: leukocytosis, *leukopenia.*
Hepatic: jaundice.
Skin: rash.
Other: gynecomastia.

Interactions

Drug-drug. *Carbamazepine:* May decrease haloperidol level. Monitor patient.
CNS depressants: May increase CNS depression. Avoid use together.
Fluoxetine: May cause severe extrapyramidal reaction. Don't use together.
Lithium: May cause lethargy and confusion with high doses. Monitor patient.
Methyldopa: May cause symptoms of dementia or psychosis. Monitor patient.
Phenytoin, rifampin: May decrease haloperidol level. Monitor patient.
Drug-herb. *Nutmeg:* May cause loss of symptom control or interference with therapy for psychiatric illness. Discourage use together.
Drug-lifestyle. *Alcohol use:* May increase CNS depression. Discourage use together.

Effects on lab test results

• May increase liver function test values. May increase or decrease WBC count.

Pharmacokinetics

Absorption: 60% after P.O. use; 70% of I.M. dose within 30 minutes. I.M. route provides 4 to 10 times more active drug than oral route.
Distribution: Wide, with high levels in adipose tissue. 91% to 99% protein-bound.
Metabolism: Extensive.
Excretion: 40% in urine within 5 days; 15% in feces by way of biliary tract. *Half-life:* P.O., 24 hours; I.M., 21 hours.

Route	Onset	Peak	Duration
P.O.	Unknown	3–6 hr	Unknown
I.M.			
lactate	Unknown	10–20 min	Unknown
decanoate	Unknown	3–9 days	Unknown

Action

Chemical effect: May block postsynaptic dopamine receptors in brain.
Therapeutic effect: Decreases psychotic behaviors.

Available forms

haloperidol
Tablets: 0.5 mg, 1 mg, 2 mg, 5 mg, 10 mg, 20 mg
haloperidol decanoate
Injection: 50 mg/ml, 100 mg/ml
haloperidol lactate
Injection: 5 mg/ml
Oral concentrate: 2 mg/ml

NURSING PROCESS

Assessment
• Assess patient's disorder before starting therapy and regularly thereafter.
• Be alert for adverse reactions and drug interactions.
• Monitor patient for tardive dyskinesia, which may not appear until months or years later and may disappear spontaneously or persist for life despite stopping use of the drug.
• Assess patient's and family's knowledge of drug therapy.

Nursing diagnoses
• Disturbed thought processes related to underlying condition
• Impaired physical mobility related to extrapyramidal effects
• Deficient knowledge related to drug therapy

Planning and implementation
⚠ ALERT: Give long-acting form of the drug by deep I.M. injection in gluteal region, using a 21G needle. Don't exceed 3 ml for each injection.
⚠ ALERT: I.V. form not recommended; optimum I.V. dosage has not been established.

Reactions may be *common*, uncommon, *life-threatening*, or COMMON AND LIFE-THREATENING.

(S) **ALERT:** Sudden death, QT prolongation, and torsades de pointes may occur when administered I.V. or at higher than recommended doses.
• When changing from oral to injection form, give patient 10 to 15 times oral dose once monthly (maximum, 100 mg).
• Protect drug from light. Slight yellowing of liquid or concentrate is common and doesn't affect potency. Discard markedly discolored solutions.
• Don't abruptly stop giving the drug unless severe adverse reaction occurs.
• Acute dystonic reactions may be treated with diphenhydramine.
Patient teaching
• Warn patient to avoid activities that require alertness and psychomotor coordination until the drug's CNS effects are known.
• Tell patient not to drink alcohol while taking drug.
• Tell patient to relieve dry mouth with sugarless gum or hard candy.
• Instruct patient to take drug exactly as prescribed and not to double doses to compensate for missed ones.

☑ Evaluation
• Patient has decreased psychotic behavior and agitation.
• Patient maintains physical mobility.
• Patient and family state understanding of drug therapy.

HIGH ALERT

heparin sodium
(HEH-prin SOH-dee-um)
Hepalean ♦, Heparin Leo ♦, Heparin Lock Flush Solution (with Tubex), Hep-Lock

Pharmacologic class: anticoagulant
Therapeutic class: heparin
Pregnancy risk category: C

Indications and dosages
Heparin dosage is highly individualized depending on patient's disease state, age, and renal and hepatic health.
▶ **Deep vein thrombosis, pulmonary embolism.** *Adults:* Initially, 10,000 units as I.V. bolus; then adjust according to PTT and give I.V. every 4 to 6 hours (5,000 to 10,000 units). Or 5,000 units as I.V. bolus; then 20,000 to

40,000 units in 24 hours by I.V. infusion pump. Adjust hourly rate 4 to 6 hours after bolus dose according to PTT.
Children: Initially, 50 units/kg I.V. drip. Maintenance dosage is 100 units/kg I.V. drip over 4 hours. For constant infusion, 20,000 units/m² daily. Adjust dosages according to PTT.
▶ **Embolism prevention.** *Adults:* 5,000 units subcutaneously every 8 to 12 hours. In surgical patients, give first dose 2 hours before procedure; follow with 5,000 units subcutaneously every 8 to 12 hours for 5 to 7 days or until patient is fully ambulatory.
▶ **Open-heart surgery.** *Adults:* (total body perfusion) 150 to 400 units/kg continuous I.V. infusion.
▶ **DIC.** *Adults:* 50 to 100 units/kg I.V. every 4 hours as a single injection or constant infusion. If no improvement in 4 to 8 hours, stop drug.
Children: 25 to 50 units/kg I.V. every 4 hours as a single injection or constant infusion. If no improvement in 4 to 8 hours, stop drug.
▶ **Maintaining patency of I.V. indwelling catheters.** *Adults:* 10 to 100 units I.V. flush. Use sufficient volume to fill device. Not intended for therapeutic use.
▶ **Unstable angina‡.** *Adults:* 70 to 80 units/kg I.V. loading dose; follow by infusion maintaining PTT at 1.5 to 2 times control level during first week of anginal pain.
▶ **Post MI, cerebral thrombosis in evolving stroke, left ventricular thrombi, heart failure, history of embolism, and atrial fibrillation‡.**
Adults: 5,000 units subcutaneously every 12 hours empirically. Or 75 units/kg continuous infusion to maintain PTT at 1.5 to 2 times control value; follow by warfarin sodium.

▼ I.V. administration
• Check order and vial carefully. Heparin comes in various concentrations.
• Give drug I.V. using infusion pump to provide maximum safety because of long-term effects and irregular absorption when given subcutaneously.
• Check constant I.V. infusions regularly, even when pumps are in good working order, to prevent giving too much or too little.
• Never piggyback other drugs into infusion line while heparin infusion is running. Many antibiotics and other drugs deactivate heparin. Never mix any drug with heparin in syringe when bolus therapy is used.

• If I.V. bag is empty, restart it as soon as possible and reschedule bolus dose immediately. Don't skip dose or increase rate to catch up.

⊗ **Incompatibilities**
Alteplase, amikacin, amiodarone, ampicillin sodium, atracurium, chlorpromazine, ciprofloxacin, codeine phosphate, cytarabine, dacarbazine, daunorubicin, dextrose 4.3% in sodium chloride solution 0.18%, diazepam, diltiazem, dobutamine, doxorubicin, doxycycline hyclate, droperidol, ergotamine, erythromycin gluceptate or lactobionate, filgrastim, gentamicin, haloperidol lactate, hydrocortisone sodium succinate, hydroxyzine hydrochloride, idarubicin, kanamycin, labetalol, levorphanol, meperidine, methadone, methotrimeprazine, methylprednisone sodium succinate, morphine sulfate, netilmicin, nicardipine, penicillin G potassium, penicillin G sodium, pentazocine lactate, phenytoin sodium, polymyxin B sulfate, prochlorperazine edisylate, promethazine hydrochloride, quinidine gluconate, 1/6 M sodium lactate, streptomycin, tobramycin sulfate, trifluoperazine, triflupromazine, vancomycin, vinblastine, warfarin; solutions containing a phosphate buffer, sodium carbonate, or sodium oxalate.

Contraindications and cautions

• Contraindicated in patients hypersensitive to the drug or any of its components.
• Use very cautiously in patients with active bleeding; blood dyscrasia; bleeding tendencies, such as hemophilia, thrombocytopenia, or hepatic disease with hypoprothrombinemia; suspected intracranial hemorrhage; suppurative thrombophlebitis; inaccessible ulcerative lesions (especially of GI tract) and open ulcerative wounds; extensive denudation of skin; ascorbic acid deficiency and other conditions causing increased capillary permeability; subacute bacterial endocarditis; shock; advanced renal disease; threatened abortion; and severe hypertension. Also use very cautiously during or after brain, eye, or spinal cord surgery; during spinal tap or spinal anesthesia; and during continuous tube drainage of stomach or small intestine. Although heparin is clearly hazardous in these conditions, risk versus benefits must be evaluated. Use cautiously in patients with mild hepatic or renal disease, alcoholism, an occupation with a risk of physical injury, or a history of allergies, asthma, or GI ulcerations.

• Be aware of the possibility of delayed onset of heparin-induced thrombocytopenia (HIT), a serious antibody-mediated reaction resulting from irreversible aggregation of platelets. HIT may progress to development of venous and arterial thromboses, referred to as heparin-induced thrombocytopenia and thrombosis (HITT). Thrombotic events may be the initial presentation for HITT, which can occur several weeks after stopping heparin therapy. Patients who have thrombocytopenia or thrombosis after stopping heparin should be evaluated for HIT and HITT.
⚠ **Lifespan:** In pregnant women who need anticoagulation, most clinicians use heparin. Use it cautiously, especially during the last trimester and immediately postpartum, because of the increased risk of maternal hemorrhage. Heparin doesn't appear in breast milk. In neonates, safety and effectiveness haven't been established. In elderly patients, use cautiously and at a lower dosage.

Adverse reactions

CNS: fever.
EENT: conjunctivitis, lacrimation, rhinitis.
Hematologic: *hemorrhage, overly prolonged clotting time, thrombocytopenia, white clot syndrome.*
Skin: cutaneous or subcutaneous necrosis, hematoma, irritation, mild pain, pruritus, ulceration, urticaria.
Other: *anaphylaxis,* burning feet, chills, *hypersensitivity reactions.*

Interactions

Drug-drug. *Antiplatelet drugs, aspirin, salicylates:* May increase the risk of bleeding. Monitor coagulation tests and patient closely for bleeding.
Oral anticoagulants: May cause additive anticoagulation. Monitor PT, INR, and PTT; monitor patient for bleeding.
Thrombolytics: May increase risk of hemorrhage. Monitor patient closely for bleeding.
Drug-herb. *Dong quai, feverfew, garlic, ginger, horse chestnut, motherwort, red clover:* May increase risk of bleeding. Monitor patient closely for bleeding.

Effects on lab test results

• May increase ALT and AST levels.
• May increase INR, PT, and PTT. May decrease platelet count.

Pharmacokinetics

Absorption: Peak level varies.
Distribution: Extensively bound to lipoprotein, globulins, and fibrinogen.
Metabolism: Thought to be removed by reticuloendothelial system, with some metabolism occurring in liver.
Excretion: Small amount in urine as unchanged drug. *Half-life:* 1 to 2 hours. Dose-dependent and nonlinear and may be disproportionately prolonged at higher doses.

Route	Onset	Peak	Duration
I.V.	Immediate	Unknown	Unknown
SubQ	20–60 min	2–4 hr	Unknown

Action

Chemical effect: Accelerates formation of antithrombin III–thrombin complex and deactivates thrombin, preventing conversion of fibrinogen to fibrin.
Therapeutic effect: Decreases ability of blood to clot.

Available forms

Products are derived from beef lung or porcine intestinal mucosa.
heparin sodium
Carpuject: 5,000 units/ml
Disposable syringes: 1,000 units/ml; 2,500 units/ml; 5,000 units/ml; 7,500 units/ml; 10,000 units/ml; 15,000 units/ml; 20,000 units/ml; 40,000 units/ml
Premixed I.V. solutions: 1,000 units in 500 ml of normal saline solution; 2,000 units in 1,000 ml of normal saline solution; 12,500 units in 250 ml of half-normal saline solution; 25,000 units in 250 ml of half-normal saline solution; 25,000 units in 500 ml of half-normal saline solution; 10,000 units in 100 ml of D_5W; 12,500 units in 250 ml of D_5W; 25,000 units in 250 ml of D_5W; 25,000 units in 500 ml of D_5W; 20,000 units in 500 ml of D_5W
Unit-dose ampules: 1,000 units/ml; 5,000 units/ml; 10,000 units/ml
Vials: 1,000 units/ml; 2,500 units/ml; 5,000 units/ml; 7,500 units/ml; 10,000 units/ml; 15,000 units/ml; 20,000 units/ml; 40,000 units/ml
heparin sodium flush
Disposable syringes: 10 units/ml, 100 units/ml
Vials: 10 units/ml, 100 units/ml

Assessment
• Assess patient's underlying condition before starting therapy.
• Draw blood to establish baseline coagulation values before starting therapy.
• Monitor the drug's effectiveness by measuring PTT carefully and regularly. Anticoagulation is present when PTT values are 1½ to 2 times control values.
• To avoid falsely elevated PTT, always draw blood 30 minutes before next dose. Draw blood for PTT 8 hours after start of continuous I.V. heparin therapy. Don't draw blood for PTT from I.V. tubing of heparin infusion; draw blood from opposite arm.
• Be alert for adverse reactions and drug interactions.
• Monitor platelet counts regularly. Thrombocytopenia caused by heparin may be linked to a type of arterial thrombosis known as white clot syndrome.
• Solutions more concentrated than 100 units/ml can irritate blood vessels.
• Assess patient's and family's knowledge of drug therapy.

Nursing diagnoses
• Risk for injury related to potential for thrombosis or emboli development from underlying condition
• Ineffective protection related to increased bleeding risks
• Deficient knowledge related to drug therapy

Planning and implementation
• Give low-dose injections sequentially between iliac crests in lower abdomen deep into subcutaneous fat. Inject drug slowly. Leave needle in place for 10 seconds after injection, then withdraw. Don't massage after subcutaneous injection. Watch for bleeding at injection site. Alternate sites every 12 hours.
• Drug requirements are higher in early phases of thrombogenic diseases and febrile states, lower when patient's condition stabilizes.
• Place notice above patient's bed to inform I.V. team or laboratory staff to apply pressure dressings after taking blood.
• Take precautions to reduce bleeding.

• To minimize the risk of hematoma, avoid excessive I.M. injection of other drugs. If possible, don't give I.M. injections at all.

⚠ ALERT: To treat severe overdose, use protamine sulfate, a heparin antagonist. Base dosage on heparin dose, the route used, and time elapsed since it was given. As a general rule, 1 to 1.5 units of protamine/100 units of heparin are given if only a few minutes have elapsed; 0.5 to 0.75 mg protamine/100 units heparin if 30 to 60 minutes have elapsed; and 0.25 to 0.375 mg protamine/100 units heparin if 2 or more hours have elapsed.

• Abruptly stopping the drug may increase coagulability, and heparin therapy is usually followed by oral anticoagulants for prophylaxis.

⚠ ALERT: Don't give heparin I.M.

⚠ ALERT: Don't give heparin with low–molecular-weight heparins.

⚠ ALERT: Spell out "units" to reduce the risk of misreading "U" as a zero.

⚠ ALERT: Don't confuse heparin with Hespan.

⚠ ALERT: Don't confuse heparin sodium injection 10,000 units/ml and Hep-Lock 10 units/ml.

Patient teaching

• Instruct patient and family to watch for signs of bleeding and to immediately notify the prescriber.

• Tell patient to avoid OTC drugs containing aspirin, other salicylates, some herbal remedies, and other drugs that may interact with heparin.

☑ **Evaluation**

• Patient's PTT reflects goal of heparin therapy.
• Patient has no injury from bleeding.
• Patient and family state understanding of drug therapy.

hepatitis B immune globulin, human

(hep-uh-TIGH-tus bee ih-MYOON GLOH-byoo-lin, HYOO-mun)

BayHep B, HBIG, HepaGam B, HyperHEP B S/D, Nabi-HB

Pharmacologic class: immunoglobulin
Therapeutic class: hepatitis B prophylaxis
Pregnancy risk category: C

Indications and dosages

▶ **Hepatitis B exposure in high-risk patients.**
Adults and children: 0.06 ml/kg I.M. within 7 days after exposure (preferably within first 24 hours). If patient refuses hepatitis B vaccine, repeat dosage 28 days after exposure.
Neonates born to patients who test positive for hepatitis B surface antigen (HBsAg): 0.5 ml I.M. within 12 hours of birth.

◾ **NEW INDICATION:** **To prevent hepatitis B recurrence following liver transplantation in HBsAg-positive liver transplant patients.**
Adults: 20,000 international units I.V. at rate of 2 ml/min. Give the first dose simultaneously with the grafting of the transplanted liver (anhepatic phase); then daily on days 1 through 7, every 2 weeks from day 14 through 12 weeks, and then monthly from month 4 onward.

◻ **Adjust-a-dose:** Adjust dosage to maintain serum anti-HB levels of 500 international units/L within first week after transplantation.

Contraindications and cautions

• Contraindicated in patients with a history of anaphylactic reactions to immune serum.
• Use cautiously in patients with severe thrombocytopenia or any coagulation disorder that would contraindicate I.M. injections.

🔹 **Lifespan:** In pregnant women, use cautiously. In breast-feeding women, use cautiously because it isn't known if drug appears in breast milk.

Adverse reactions

CNS: *headache.*
Musculoskeletal: *myalgia.*
Skin: urticaria.
Other: *anaphylaxis, angioedema,* injection-site reactions.

Interactions

Drug-drug. *Live-virus vaccines:* May interfere with response to live-virus vaccines. Defer routine immunization for 3 months.

Effects on lab test results

None reported.

Pharmacokinetics

Absorption: Slow.
Distribution: Unknown.
Metabolism: Unknown.

Excretion: Unknown. *Half-life:* Antibodies to HBsAg, 21 days.

Route	Onset	Peak	Duration
I.M.	1–6 days	3–11 days	≥ 2 mo

Action

Chemical effect: Provides passive immunity to hepatitis B.
Therapeutic effect: Prevents hepatitis B.

Available forms

Injection: 1-ml, 5-ml vials; 0.5 ml and 1.0 ml prefilled syringes

NURSING PROCESS

☒ Assessment
• Assess patient's allergies and reaction to immunizations before starting therapy.
• Monitor effectiveness by checking patient's antibody titers.
• Be alert for anaphylaxis.
• Assess patient's and family's knowledge of drug therapy.

⊕ Nursing diagnoses
• Ineffective protection related to lack of immunity to hepatitis B
• Deficient knowledge related to drug therapy

▷ Planning and implementation
• Do not give I.V.
• Inject drug into anterolateral aspect of thigh or deltoid muscle in older children and adults; inject into anterolateral aspect of thigh for neonates and children younger than age 3.
• Make sure epinephrine 1:1,000 is available in case anaphylaxis occurs.
• To prevent neutralization, do not give Hep B immune globulin and Hep B vaccine in same site or same syringe.
• For postexposure prophylaxis (for example, needle stick, direct contact), drug is usually given with hepatitis B vaccine.
Patient teaching
• Instruct patient to immediately report respiratory difficulty.

☑ Evaluation
• Patient exhibits passive immunity to hepatitis B.

• Patient and family state understanding of drug therapy.

high–molecular-weight hyaluronan
(HI–mow-LECK-yuh-lerr-wayt high-al-your-RON-ann)
Euflexxa, Hyalgan, Orthovisc, Supartz, Synvisc

Pharmacologic class: hyaluronic acid derivative
Therapeutic class: viscosupplement; analgesic
Pregnancy risk category: NR

Indications and dosages

▶ **To reduce pain caused by osteoarthritis of the knee in patients who haven't responded to nondrug therapy or simple analgesics.**
Adults: Intra-articular injection (one syringe) into affected knee once weekly for a total of three to five injections.

Contraindications and cautions

• Contraindicated (except Euflexxa) in patients allergic to hyaluronate preparations, birds, eggs, feathers, and poultry.
• Contraindicated in patients with infection or skin disease in area of injection site or joint.
🌣 Lifespan: In pregnant women, use only if benefits outweigh risks to fetus. In breast-feeding women and in children, safety and effectiveness haven't been established.

Adverse reactions

CNS: dizziness, *headache,* pain.
CV: *hypotensive crisis.*
Musculoskeletal: *arthralgia,* back pain, bursitis.
Other: anaphylactoid reaction, injection-site pain.

Interactions

Drug-drug. *Skin preparation disinfectants that contain quaternary ammonium salts:* May cause hyaluronan to precipitate. Don't use together.

Effects on lab test results

None reported.

Pharmacokinetics

Absorption: None.

Distribution: None.
Metabolism: None.
Excretion: None. *Half-life:* Unknown.

Route	Onset	Peak	Duration
Intra-articular	Unknown	Unknown	Unknown

Action

Chemical effect: Supplements body's natural supply of hyaluronan, which acts as a shock absorber and lubricant in the joints.
Therapeutic effect: Relief of pain in knee joints in osteoarthritis patients.

Available forms

Injection: 16 mg/2 ml (Synvisc), 20 mg/2 ml (Euflexxa, Hyalgan), 25 mg/2.5 ml (Supartz), 30 mg/2 ml (Orthovisc)

NURSING PROCESS

⚗ Assessment
• Assess patient for joint effusion before giving the drug. Remove joint effusion before injecting drug.
• Evaluate patient's degree of pain relief. Pain may not be relieved until after the third injection.
• Assess patient for injection-site reactions. Inflammation may increase briefly in affected knee in a patient with inflammatory osteoarthritis.
• Assess patient's and family's knowledge of drug therapy.

⊕ Nursing diagnoses
• Acute pain related to underlying medical condition
• Impaired physical mobility related to underlying medical condition
• Deficient knowledge related to drug therapy

▷ Planning and implementation
• Drug should be given by staff trained in intra-articular administration.
• Use an 18G to 21G needle. Inject contents of one syringe into one knee. If needed, use a second syringe for the second knee.
• Don't give less than three injections in a treatment cycle.
• Safety and effectiveness of drug use for more than one treatment cycle or in joints other than the knee aren't known.

• Give drug immediately after opening. Store in original package at room temperature (lower than 77° F [25° C]); don't freeze. Discard unused drug.

Patient teaching
• Tell patient that pain and inflammation may increase briefly after the injection.
• Urge patient to avoid strenuous or weight-bearing activity, such as running or tennis, for longer than an hour within 48 hours of an injection.
• Tell patient to report injection-site reactions, such as pain, swelling, itching, heat, rash, bruising, or redness.
• Inform patient that a treatment cycle includes at least three injections and that pain may not be relieved until after the third injection.
• Caution patient to report planned or suspected pregnancy.

☑ Evaluation
• Patient is free from pain.
• Patient has full physical mobility.
• Patient and family state understanding of drug therapy.

---

hydralazine hydrochloride
(high-DRAL-uh-zeen high-droh-KLOR-ighd)
Apresoline, Novo-Hylazin ◆

Pharmacologic class: peripheral vasodilator
Therapeutic class: antihypertensive
Pregnancy risk category: C

Indications and dosages

▶ **Essential hypertension (orally, alone or with other antihypertensives); severe essential hypertension (parenterally, to lower blood pressure quickly).** *Adults:* Initially, 10 mg P.O. q.i.d.; gradually increase to 50 mg q.i.d. if needed. Maximum recommended dosage is 200 mg daily, but some patients may need 300 to 400 mg daily. Or give 10 to 20 mg I.V. slowly and repeat if needed. Switch to P.O. antihypertensives as soon as possible. Or 10 to 50 mg I.M.; repeat if needed. Switch to P.O. form as soon as possible.

▶ **To manage hypertensive emergencies related to pregnancy (preeclampsia, eclampsia).** *Adults:* 5 to 10 mg I.V.; repeat every 20 to 30 minutes if needed to achieve adequate

---

blood pressure control. Or, infuse at 0.5 to 10 mg/hour.

► **To manage severe heart failure‡.** *Adults:* Initially 50 to 75 mg P.O.; then adjust according to patient's response. Most patients respond to 200 to 600 mg daily, divided every 6 to 12 hours, but daily dosages as high as 3 g have been given.

▼ I.V. administration

• Drug is compatible with normal saline solution, Ringer's and lactated Ringer's solutions, and several other common I.V. solutions. Manufacturer doesn't recommend mixing drug in infusion solutions.
• Drug changes color in most infusion solutions, but the change doesn't indicate loss of potency.
• Give drug slowly and repeat if needed, usually every 4 to 6 hours.
• Monitor blood pressure closely.
⊗ **Incompatibilities**
Aminophylline, ampicillin sodium, chlorothiazide, dextrose 10% in lactated Ringer's solution, dextrose 10% in normal saline solution, D_5W, diazoxide, doxapram, edetate calcium disodium, ethacrynate, fructose 10% in normal saline solution, fructose 10% in water, furosemide, hydrocortisone sodium succinate, mephentermine, metaraminol bitartrate, methohexital, nitroglycerin, phenobarbital sodium, verapamil.

Contraindications and cautions

• Contraindicated in patients hypersensitive to the drug or any of its components and in those with coronary artery disease or mitral valvular rheumatic heart disease.
• Use cautiously in patients with suspected cardiac disease, stroke, or severe renal impairment, and in those taking other antihypertensives.
⚘ **Lifespan:** In pregnant women, use cautiously. In breast-feeding women and in children, safety and effectiveness haven't been established.

Adverse reactions

CNS: dizziness, *headache,* peripheral neuritis.
CV: angina, **arrhythmias,** orthostatic hypotension, palpitations, tachycardia.
GI: anorexia, diarrhea, nausea, vomiting.
Hematologic: *agranulocytopenia, leukopenia, neutropenia.*

Metabolic: sodium retention, *weight gain.*
Skin: rash.
Other: *lupuslike syndrome.*

Interactions

Drug-drug. *Diazoxide, MAO inhibitors:* May cause severe hypotension. Use together cautiously.
Epinephrine: May decrease pressor effects of epinephrine. Monitor patient's response.
Indomethacin: May decrease hydralazine effects. Monitor patient.
Metoprolol, propranolol: May increase levels and effects of these drugs. Monitor patient closely; adjust dosage of either drug if needed.

Effects on lab test results

• May decrease hemoglobin level and hematocrit.
• May decrease neutrophil, WBC, RBC, granulocyte, and platelet counts.

Pharmacokinetics

Absorption: Rapid after P.O. use; food enhances absorption. Unknown after I.M. use.
Distribution: Wide. 88% to 90% protein-bound.
Metabolism: Extensive, in GI mucosa and liver.
Excretion: Mainly in urine. *Half-life:* 3 to 7 hours.

Route	Onset	Peak	Duration
P.O.	20–30 min	1–2 hr	2–4 hr
I.V.	≤ 5 min	15–30 min	2–6 hr
I.M.	10–30 min	1 hr	2–6 hr

Action

Chemical effect: Unknown. As a direct-acting vasodilator, it relaxes arteriolar smooth muscle.
Therapeutic effect: Lowers blood pressure.

Available forms

Injection: 20 mg/ml
Tablets: 10 mg, 25 mg, 50 mg, 100 mg

NURSING PROCESS

☞ **Assessment**
• Assess blood pressure before starting therapy and regularly thereafter.
• Monitor CBC, lupus erythematosus cell preparation, and antinuclear antibody titer determination during long-term therapy.

• Be alert for adverse reactions and drug interactions, especially lupuslike reactions at high drug dosages.
• Assess patient's and family's knowledge of drug therapy.

⬚ Nursing diagnoses
• Risk for injury related to presence of hypertension
• Excess fluid volume related to sodium retention
• Deficient knowledge related to drug therapy

⬚ Planning and implementation
• Give oral form of drug with meals to increase absorption.
• Some clinicians combine hydralazine therapy with diuretics and beta blockers to decrease sodium retention and tachycardia and to prevent angina.
• Compliance may be improved by giving drug twice daily. Check with prescriber.
⬚ **ALERT:** Don't confuse hydralazine with hydroxyzine.
Patient teaching
• Instruct patient to take oral form with meals.
• Inform patient that orthostatic hypotension can be minimized by rising slowly and not changing position suddenly.
• Tell patient not to abruptly stop taking the drug, but to call prescriber if adverse reactions occur.
• Tell patient to limit sodium intake.

⬚ Evaluation
• Patient's blood pressure is normal.
• Fluid retention doesn't develop.
• Patient and family state understanding of drug therapy.

hydrochlorothiazide
(high-droh-klor-oh-THIGH-uh-zighd)
**Apo-Hydro ♦, Aquazide-H, Diuchlor HI,
Esidrix, Ezide, Hydro-Par, Microzide,
Novo-Hydrazide ♦, Nu-Hydro ♦, Oretic,
Urozide ♦**

Pharmacologic class: thiazide diuretic
Therapeutic class: diuretic, antihypertensive
Pregnancy risk category: B

Indications and dosages
▶ **Edema.** *Adults:* 25 to 100 mg P.O. daily or intermittently.
▶ **Hypertension.** *Adults:* 12.5 to 50 mg P.O. once daily. May increase or decrease daily dosage based on blood pressure.
Children ages 2 to 12: Give 2.2 mg/kg or 60 mg/m² P.O. daily in two divided doses. Usual dosage range is 37.5 to 100 mg P.O. daily.
Infants and children ages 6 months to younger than 2 years: 2.2 mg/kg or 60 mg/m² P.O. daily in two divided doses. Usual dosage range is 12.5 to 37.5 mg P.O. daily.
Infants younger than age 6 months: Up to 3.3 mg/kg daily in two divided doses.

Contraindications and cautions
• Contraindicated in patients with anuria and in patients hypersensitive to other thiazides or sulfonamide derivatives.
• Use cautiously in patients with severe renal disease, impaired hepatic function, and progressive hepatic disease.
⬚ **Lifespan:** In pregnant women, drug isn't recommended. In breast-feeding women, safety and effectiveness haven't been established. In elderly patients, use lower initial dose.

Adverse reactions
CV: orthostatic hypotension, volume depletion and dehydration.
GI: anorexia, nausea, *pancreatitis.*
GU: frequent urination, nocturia, polyuria, *renal impairment.*
Hematologic: *agranulocytosis, aplastic anemia, leukopenia, thrombocytopenia.*
Hepatic: *hepatic encephalopathy.*
Metabolic: asymptomatic hyperuricemia, dilutional hyponatremia, fluid and electrolyte imbalances, hypercalcemia, hyperglycemia, hypochloremia, hypokalemia, impaired glucose tolerance, *metabolic alkalosis.*
Skin: dermatitis, photosensitivity, rash.
Other: *anaphylactic reactions;* gout; hypersensitivity reactions, such as pneumonitis and vasculitis.

Interactions
Drug-drug. *Antidiabetics:* May decrease hypoglycemic effectiveness. Monitor glucose level, and adjust dosage if needed.

Antihypertensives: May have additive antihypertensive effect. Use together cautiously; monitor blood pressure closely.

Barbiturates, opioids: May increase orthostatic hypotensive effect. Monitor patient closely.

Bumetanide, ethacrynic acid, furosemide, torsemide: May cause excessive diuretic response, resulting in serious electrolyte abnormalities or dehydration. Adjust doses while monitoring patient for excessive diuretic responses.

Cholestyramine, colestipol: May decrease intestinal absorption of thiazides. Give drugs separately.

Diazoxide: May increase antihypertensive, hyperglycemic, and hyperuricemic effects. Use together cautiously.

Digoxin: May increase risk of digoxin toxicity from hydrochlorothiazide-induced hypokalemia. Monitor potassium and digoxin levels.

Lithium: May decrease lithium excretion, increasing risk of toxicity. Monitor level.

NSAIDs: May increase risk of NSAID-induced renal impairment. Monitor patient closely.

Drug-herb. *Dandelion:* May interfere with diuretic activity. Discourage use together.

Licorice root: May contribute to the potassium depletion caused by thiazides. Discourage use together.

Drug-lifestyle. *Alcohol use:* May increase orthostatic hypotensive effect. Discourage use together.

Sun exposure: May increase photosensitivity. Urge patient to avoid unprotected or prolonged sun exposure.

Effects on lab test results

• May increase glucose, cholesterol, triglyceride, calcium, and uric acid levels. May decrease potassium, sodium, chloride, and hemoglobin levels and hematocrit.

• May decrease granulocyte, WBC, and platelet counts.

Pharmacokinetics

Absorption: Varies with drug forms.
Distribution: 40% to 68% protein-bound.
Metabolism: None.
Excretion: Unchanged in urine. *Half-life:* 5½ to 15 hours.

Route	Onset	Peak	Duration
P.O.	2 hr	4–6 hr	6–12 hr

Action

Chemical effect: Increases sodium and water excretion by inhibiting sodium and chloride reabsorption in the distal segment of the nephron.
Therapeutic effect: Promotes sodium and water excretion, thereby lowering blood pressure.

Available forms

Capsules: 12.5 mg
Oral solution: 50 mg/5 ml
Tablets: 25 mg, 50 mg, 100 mg

NURSING PROCESS

📝 Assessment

• Assess patient's edema or blood pressure before starting therapy.
• Monitor the drug's effectiveness by regularly checking blood pressure, urine output, and weight. In a patient with hypertension, therapeutic response may be delayed several days.
• Monitor electrolyte levels.
• Monitor creatinine and BUN levels regularly. If these levels are more than twice normal, monitor patient for decreased effectiveness.
• Monitor uric acid level, especially in patient with history of gout.
• Be alert for adverse reactions and drug interactions.
• Assess patient's and family's knowledge of drug therapy.

🔅 Nursing diagnoses

• Ineffective health maintenance related to presence of edema or hypertension
• Impaired urinary elimination related to diuretic effect of drug
• Deficient knowledge related to drug therapy

▶ Planning and implementation

• Give drug in morning to prevent nocturia.
• If nausea occurs, give drug with food.
• Drug may be used with potassium-sparing diuretic to prevent potassium loss.

Patient teaching
• Advise patient to take drug with food to minimize GI upset.
• Warn patient not to change position suddenly and to rise slowly to avoid orthostatic hypotension.
• Instruct patient not to drink alcohol during drug therapy.

H

- Advise patient to use sunblock to prevent photosensitivity reactions.
- Tell patient to check with prescriber before taking OTC drugs or herbal remedies.

☑ **Evaluation**

- Patient's blood pressure is normal, and no edema is present.
- Patient demonstrates adjustment of lifestyle to accommodate altered patterns of urinary elimination.
- Patient and family state understanding of drug therapy.

hydrocortisone
(high-droh-KOR-tuh-sohn)
Cortef, Cortenema, Hydrocortone

hydrocortisone acetate
Cortifoam, Hydrocortone Acetate

hydrocortisone cypionate
Cortef

hydrocortisone sodium phosphate
Hydrocortone Phosphate

hydrocortisone sodium succinate
A-hydroCort, Solu-Cortef

Pharmacologic class: adrenocortical steroid
Therapeutic class: glucocorticoid
Pregnancy risk category: NR

Indications and dosages

▶ **Severe inflammation, adrenal insufficiency.** *Adults:* 20 to 240 mg hydrocortisone or cypionate P.O. daily. Or 5 to 75 mg acetate injected into joints or soft tissue. Give once every 2 to 3 weeks, although some conditions may require weekly injections. Dosage varies with degree of inflammation and size and location of the joint or soft tissues. Or 15 to 240 mg phosphate I.V., I.M., or subcutaneously daily, divided into 12-hour intervals. Or, initially, 100 to 500 mg succinate I.V. or I.M.; may repeat every 2 to 6 hours if needed.

▶ **Adjunct for ulcerative colitis and proctitis.** *Adults:* 1 enema (100 mg) hydrocortisone or acetate P.R. nightly for 21 days.
▶ **Shock.** *Adults:* Initially, 50 mg/kg succinate I.V. repeated in 4 hours or every 24 hours, as needed. Or 0.5 mg to 2 g I.V. every 2 to 6 hours, as needed.
Children: 0.16 to 1 mg/kg or 6 to 30 mg/m^2 phosphate I.M. or succinate I.M. or I.V. daily or b.i.d.

▼ I.V. administration

- Don't use acetate or suspension form I.V.
- Hydrocortisone sodium phosphate may be added directly to D_5W or normal saline solution for I.V. administration.
- Reconstitute hydrocortisone sodium succinate with bacteriostatic water or bacteriostatic sodium chloride solution before adding to I.V. solutions. When giving by direct I.V. injection, inject over at least 30 seconds. For infusion, dilute with D_5W, normal saline solution, or D_5W in normal saline solution to 1 mg/ml or less.
- When giving as direct injection, inject directly into vein or I.V. line containing free-flowing compatible solution over 30 seconds to several minutes.
- When giving as intermittent or continuous infusion, dilute solution per manufacturer's instructions and give over prescribed duration. If used for continuous infusion, change solution every 24 hours.

⊗ **Incompatibilities**
Hydrocortisone sodium phosphate: doxapram, mitoxantrone, sargramostim.
Hydrocortisone sodium succinate: amobarbital, ampicillin sodium, bleomycin, ciprofloxacin, colistimethate, cytarabine, dacarbazine, diazepam, dimenhydrinate, ephedrine, ergotamine, furosemide, heparin sodium, hydralazine, idarubicin, Ionosol B with invert sugar 10%, kanamycin, methylprednisolone sodium succinate, midazolam, nafcillin, pentobarbital sodium, phenobarbital sodium, phenytoin, prochlorperazine edisylate, promethazine hydrochloride, sargramostim, vancomycin, vitamin B complex with C.

Contraindications and cautions

- Contraindicated in patients hypersensitive to drug or any of its components, and in those with systemic fungal infections. Hydrocortisone

sodium succinate is contraindicated in premature infants.

• Use cautiously in patients with GI ulcer, renal disease, hypertension, osteoporosis, diabetes mellitus, hypothyroidism, cirrhosis, diverticulitis, nonspecific ulcerative colitis, recent intestinal anastomoses, thromboembolic disorders, seizures, myasthenia gravis, heart failure, tuberculosis, ocular herpes simplex, emotional instability, psychotic tendencies, and recent MI.

⚘ **Lifespan:** In pregnant women, use cautiously. In breast-feeding women, use cautiously. Drug isn't recommended in high doses. In children, use cautiously because long-term use may delay growth and maturation.

Adverse reactions

Most adverse reactions are dose- or duration-dependent.

CNS: *euphoria, insomnia,* pseudotumor cerebri, psychotic behavior, *seizures.*

CV: *arrhythmias,* edema, *heart failure,* hypertension, *thromboembolism.*

EENT: cataracts, glaucoma.

GI: GI irritation, increased appetite, *pancreatitis,* peptic ulceration.

Metabolic: carbohydrate intolerance, hyperglycemia, hypokalemia.

Musculoskeletal: growth suppression in children, muscle weakness, osteoporosis.

Skin: acne, delayed wound healing, easy bruising, hirsutism, various skin eruptions.

Other: *acute adrenal insufficiency with increased stress (infection, surgery, or trauma) or abrupt withdrawal after long-term therapy,* susceptibility to infections.

Interactions

Drug-drug. *Aspirin, indomethacin, NSAIDs:* May increase risk of GI distress and bleeding. Give together cautiously.

Barbiturates, phenytoin, rifampin: May decrease corticosteroid effect; may require increased dosage.

Live-attenuated virus vaccines, other toxoids and vaccines: May decrease antibody response and increase risk of neurologic complications. Avoid use together.

Oral anticoagulants: May alter dosage requirements. Monitor PT and INR closely.

Potassium-depleting drugs (such as thiazide diuretics): May enhance potassium-wasting

effects of hydrocortisone. Monitor potassium level.

Skin-test antigens: May decrease skin response. Defer skin testing until therapy is completed.

Drug-lifestyle. *Alcohol use:* May increase risk of GI effects. Discourage use together.

Effects on lab test results

• May increase glucose and cholesterol levels. May decrease potassium and calcium levels.

Pharmacokinetics

Absorption: Rapid after P.O. use. Variable after I.M. or intra-articular injection. Unknown after rectal use.

Distribution: To muscle, liver, skin, intestines, and kidneys. Extensively protein-bound. Only unbound portion is active.

Metabolism: Metabolized in liver.

Excretion: Inactive metabolites and small amounts of unmetabolized drug excreted in urine; insignificant amount in feces. *Half-life:* 8 to 12 hours.

Route	Onset	Peak	Duration
P.O., I.V., I.M., P.R.	Varies	Varies	Varies

Action

Chemical effect: Not clearly defined; may stabilize leukocyte lysosomal membranes, suppress immune response, stimulate bone marrow, and influence nutrient metabolism.

Therapeutic effect: Reduces inflammation, suppresses immune function, and raises adrenocorticoid hormonal levels.

Available forms

hydrocortisone
Enema: 100 mg/60 ml
Tablets: 5 mg, 10 mg, 20 mg
hydrocortisone acetate
Enema: 10% aerosol foam (provides 90 mg/application)
Injection: 25-mg/ml*, 50-mg/ml* suspension
Suppositories: 25 mg
hydrocortisone cypionate
Oral suspension: 10 mg/5 ml
hydrocortisone sodium phosphate
Injection: 50-mg/ml solution
hydrocortisone sodium succinate
Injection: 100 mg/vial*, 250 mg/vial*, 500 mg/vial*, 1,000 mg/vial*

H

NURSING PROCESS

⌨ Assessment
• Assess patient's condition before starting therapy and regularly thereafter.
• Monitor patient's weight, blood pressure, and electrolyte levels.
• Monitor patient for stress. Fever, trauma, surgery, and emotional problems may increase adrenal insufficiency.
• Periodically measure growth and development during high-dose or prolonged therapy in infants and children.
• Be alert for adverse reactions and drug interactions.
• Assess patient's and family's knowledge of drug therapy.

🔁 Nursing diagnoses
• Ineffective health maintenance related to underlying condition
• Ineffective protection related to immunosuppression
• Deficient knowledge related to drug therapy

▷ Planning and implementation
• For better results and less toxicity, give once-daily dose in morning.
• Give oral dose with food.
• Give I.M. injection deep into gluteal muscle. Rotate injection sites to prevent muscle atrophy.
• Rectal suppositories may produce the same systemic effects as other forms of hydrocortisone. If therapy must exceed 21 days, stop gradually by giving every other night for 2 or 3 weeks.
⚠ ALERT: Avoid subcutaneous injection because atrophy and sterile abscesses may occur.
• Injectable forms aren't used for alternate-day therapy.
• High-dose therapy usually doesn't continue beyond 48 hours.
• Always adjust to lowest effective dose, and gradually reduce dosage after long-term therapy.
• Give potassium supplements.
• If evidence of adrenal insufficiency appears, notify prescriber and increase dosage.
• Notify prescriber about adverse reactions. Provide supportive care.
⚠ ALERT: Avoid abbreviating drug as HCT, which can be misread as HCTZ (hydrochlorothiazide).

⚠ ALERT: Don't confuse Solu-Cortef with Solu-Medrol.

Patient teaching
• Teach patient signs of early adrenal insufficiency (fatigue, muscle weakness, joint pain, fever, anorexia, nausea, dyspnea, dizziness, and fainting).
• Instruct patient to carry or wear medical identification that identifies need for supplemental systemic glucocorticoids during stress.
⚠ ALERT: Tell patient not to abruptly stop taking the drug without prescriber's consent. Abruptly stopping therapy may lead to rebound inflammation, fatigue, weakness, arthralgia, fever, dizziness, lethargy, depression, fainting, orthostatic hypotension, dyspnea, anorexia, and hypoglycemia. After prolonged use, sudden withdrawal may be fatal.
• Warn patient receiving long-term therapy about cushingoid symptoms, and tell him to report sudden weight gain or swelling to prescriber.
• Advise him to consider exercise or physical therapy, to ask his prescriber about vitamin D or calcium supplements, and to have periodic ophthalmic examinations.
• Warn patient about easy bruising.

✅ Evaluation
• Patient's condition improves.
• Serious complications related to drug-induced immunosuppression don't develop.
• Patient and family state understanding of drug therapy.

HIGH ALERT

hydromorphone hydrochloride (dihydromorphinone hydrochloride)
(high-droh-MOR-fohn high-droh-KLOR-ighd)
Dilaudid, Dilaudid-HP

Pharmacologic class: opioid
Therapeutic class: analgesic, antitussive
Pregnancy risk category: C
Controlled substance schedule: II

Indications and dosages

▶ **Moderate to severe pain.** *Adults:* 2 to 4 mg P.O. every 4 to 6 hours p.r.n. Or 1 to 2 mg I.M., subcutaneously, or I.V. (slowly over at least 2 to

---

3 minutes) every 4 to 6 hours p.r.n. Or 3-mg rectal suppository every 6 to 8 hours p.r.n.
▶ **Cough.** *Adults:* 1 mg P.O. every 3 to 4 hours p.r.n.
Children ages 6 to 12: Give 0.5 mg P.O. every 3 to 4 hours p.r.n.

▽▼ I.V. administration

• For infusion, drug may be mixed in D₅W, normal saline solution, D₅W in normal saline solution, D₅W in half-normal saline solution, or Ringer's or lactated Ringer's solutions.
• For direct injection, give over at least 2 minutes.
• Respiratory depression and hypotension may occur. Monitor respiration and circulation often.
⊗ **Incompatibilities**
Alkalines, amphotericin B cholesterol complex, ampicillin sodium, bromides, cefazolin, dexamethasone, diazepam, gallium nitrate, haloperidol, heparin sodium, iodides, minocycline, phenobarbital sodium, phenytoin sodium, prochlorperazine edisylate, sargramostim, sodium bicarbonate, sodium phosphate, thiopental.

Contraindications and cautions

• Contraindicated in patients hypersensitive to drug or any of its components, patients with intracranial lesions from increased intracranial pressure, patients with status asthmaticus, and whenever ventilatory function is depressed in the absence of resuscitative equipment. Also contraindicated as obstetric analgesia.
• Use with extreme caution in patients with COPD, cor pulmonale, a substantially decreased respiratory reserve, hypoxia, hypercapnia, or respiratory depression. Use cautiously in debilitated patients and in patients with hepatic or renal disease, hypothyroidism, Addison disease, prostatic hypertrophy, urethral stricture, CNS depression or coma, toxic psychosis, gallbladder disease, acute alcoholism, alcohol withdrawal, kyphoscoliosis, or sulfite sensitivity (because drug contains sodium metabisulfite and may cause allergic-type reactions, including anaphylactic symptoms or asthmatic episodes, especially in people with asthma). Also use cautiously after GI surgery.
※ **Lifespan:** In pregnant women, use only if potential benefits to mother outweigh risks to fetus. During labor and delivery, don't use drug. Women shouldn't breast-feed while receiving drug. In children, safety and effectiveness

haven't been established except as listed for cough. In elderly patients, use cautiously.

Adverse reactions

CNS: *clouded sensorium, dizziness, euphoria, sedation, seizures, somnolence.*
CV: *bradycardia,* hypotension.
EENT: blurred vision, diplopia, nystagmus.
GI: constipation, ileus, nausea, vomiting.
GU: urine retention.
Respiratory: *bronchospasm, respiratory depression.*
Other: induration with repeated subcutaneous injections, physical dependence.

Interactions

Drug-drug. *CNS depressants, general anesthetics, hypnotics, MAO inhibitors, other opioid analgesics, sedatives, tranquilizers, tricyclic antidepressants:* May have additive effects. Use together cautiously. Reduce hydromorphone dose, and monitor patient response.
Drug-lifestyle. *Alcohol use:* May have additive effects. Discourage use together.

Effects on lab test results

• May increase amylase and lipase levels.

Pharmacokinetics

Absorption: Good.
Distribution: Unknown.
Metabolism: Mainly in liver.
Excretion: Mainly in urine. *Half-life:* 2½ to 4 hours.

Route	Onset	Peak	Duration
P.O.	30 min	30 min–2 hr	4–5 hr
I.V.	10–15 min	15–30 min	2–3 hr
I.M.	15 min	30–60 min	4–5 hr
SubQ	15 min	30–90 min	4 hr
P.R.	Unknown	Unknown	4 hr

Action

Chemical effect: Binds with opiate receptors in CNS, altering perception of and emotional response to pain. Suppresses cough reflex by direct action on cough center in medulla.
Therapeutic effect: Relieves pain and cough.

Available forms

Injection: 1 mg/ml, 2 mg/ml, 4 mg/ml, 10 mg/ml

Injection (lyophilized powder): 250 mg/vial
Liquid: 5 mg/5 ml
Suppositories: 3 mg
Tablets: 2 mg, 4 mg, 8 mg

NURSING PROCESS

Assessment
• Assess patient's pain or cough before and after giving drug.
• Drug may worsen or mask gallbladder pain.
• Drug is a commonly abused opioid. Be alert for addictive behavior or drug abuse.
• Be alert for adverse reactions and drug interactions.
• Assess patient's and family's knowledge of drug therapy.

Nursing diagnoses
• Acute pain related to underlying condition
• Ineffective breathing pattern related to respiratory depression
• Deficient knowledge related to drug therapy

Planning and implementation
• For better analgesic effect, give drug before patient's pain becomes intense.
• Dilaudid-HP, a highly concentrated form (10 mg/ml), may be given in smaller volumes to prevent discomfort caused by large-volume I.M. or subcutaneous injections. Check dosage carefully.
• To avoid induration with subcutaneous injection, rotate injection sites.
• Keep resuscitation equipment and opioid antagonist (naloxone) available.
• Postoperatively, encourage patient to turn, cough, and deep-breathe to avoid atelectasis.
• Recommend increased intake of fiber and fluids and a stool softener to prevent constipation during maintenance therapy.
• Signs and symptoms of overdose include respiratory depression, CNS depression progressing to stupor or coma, flaccid muscles, cold and clammy skin, bradycardia, hypotension, and constricted pupils. Severe overdose may include apnea, circulatory collapse, cardiac arrest, and death.
• To treat overdose, ensure a patent airway and provide ventilation as needed. If patient is conscious and received the oral form of drug, gastric lavage or induced emesis may be useful in removing unabsorbed drug. If patient is unconscious and has a secure airway, activated charcoal may be given by NG tube; a saline cathartic or sorbitol may be added to the first dose. If patient has significant respiratory or circulatory depression, give naloxone; use caution if patient may be physically dependent on hydromorphone. Provide symptomatic and supportive treatment, including I.V. fluids, vasopressors, and other measures as needed.

Patient teaching
• Advise ambulatory patient to be careful when getting out of bed or walking. Warn patient to avoid activities that require mental alertness until the drug's CNS effects are known.
• Encourage patient to ask for drug before pain becomes severe.
• If patient's respiratory rate decreases, tell patient or caregiver to notify prescriber.
• Instruct patient to avoid alcohol consumption during drug therapy.

Evaluation
• Patient is free from pain.
• Patient maintains adequate breathing patterns.
• Patient and family state understanding of drug therapy.

✳ New Drug

hydroxocobalamin
(high-DROX-oh-koh-ball-ah-min)
Cyanokit

Pharmacologic class: hydroxylated form of vitamin B_{12}
Therapeutic class: antidote
Pregnancy risk category: C

Indications and dosages

▶ **Cyanide poisoning.** *Adults:* Initially, 5 g I.V. over 15 minutes. May give another 5-g dose over 15 minutes to 2 hours based on severity of poisoning and patient's condition.

▽ I.V. administration
• Add 100 ml normal saline solution to each vial. If normal saline solution isn't available, use lactated Ringer's or 5% dextrose solution.
• With vial in upright position, fill to the line. Then rotate vial for 30 seconds to mix solution. Don't shake.

Reactions may be *common,* uncommon, *life-threatening,* or COMMON AND LIFE-THREATENING.

• Inspect the solution. It should be dark red and contain no particulate matter. If it looks otherwise, don't use.
• Infuse the solution over 7½ minutes.
• Repeat this process for the second vial.
• Store dry vials at room temperature. Reconstituted solution is stable for 6 hours at temperatures below 104° F (40° C).

⊗ **Incompatibilities**
Don't give through same I.V. line with diazepam, dobutamine, dopamine, fentanyl, nitroglycerin, pentobarbital, propofol, or thiopental because particles may form. Don't give through same I.V. line with sodium thiosulfate, sodium nitrite, or ascorbic acid because these drugs are chemically incompatible.

Give blood products through separate lines; don't administer simultaneously.

Contraindications and cautions

• Use cautiously in patients with history of hypersensitivity to hydroxocobalamin or cyanocobalamin and in patients with hypertension.
✷ **Lifespan:** In pregnant women, use only if potential benefit to mother outweighs risk to fetus. In breast-feeding women, use cautiously; it isn't known if drug appears in breast milk. In children, safety and effectiveness haven't been established.

Adverse reactions

CNS: dizziness, headache, memory impairment, restlessness.
CV: chest discomfort, *ECG abnormalities,* edema, flushing, *hypertension,* increased heart rate, ventricular extrasystoles.
EENT: dry throat, eye irritation and redness, swelling, throat tightness.
GI: abdominal discomfort, diarrhea, dyspepsia, dysphagia, hematochezia, nausea, vomiting.
GU: *chromaturia* (red urine).
Respiratory: dyspnea, pleural effusion.
Skin: *erythema,* infusion site reaction, pruritus, *rash.*

Interactions

Drug-drug. *Cyanide antidotes:* Effect of giving more than one cyanide antidote isn't known. Give through separate lines.
Drug-lifestyle. *Sun exposure:* May lead to photosensitivity reaction. Tell patient to avoid direct sunlight while skin is discolored.

Effects on lab test results

• May increase blood creatinine, triglyceride, cholesterol, total protein, glucose, albumin, alkaline phosphatase, and bilirubin levels; urine glucose, protein, ketones, bilirubin, urobilinogen, and nitrite levels; and hemoglobin level. May decrease ALT and amylase levels.
• May increase urine pH and RBC, WBC, and basophil counts.
• May increase or decrease aPTT, PT, and phospate, uric acid, AST, CK, CK-MB, and LDH levels.

Pharmacokinetics

Absorption: Given I.V.
Distribution: Binds to plasma proteins.
Metabolism: Unknown.
Excretion: Renal, mainly in the first 24 hours, although red color may last up to 35 days after infusion. *Half life:* 26 to 31 hr.

Route	Onset	Peak	Duration
I.V.	Rapid	Unknown	Unknown

Action

Chemical effect: Binds cyanide ions. Each hydroxocobalamin molecule can bind one cyanide ion, forming cyanocobalamin, which is then excreted in urine.
Therapeutic effect: Elimination of cyanide from the body.

Available forms

Injection: 2.5 g vial, two vials per kit

NURSING PROCESS

🔖 **Assessment**
• Assess if patient is hypersensitive to hydroxocobalamin or cyanocobalamin.
• Assess baseline vital signs.
• Assess kidney and liver studies. Safety and efficacy haven't been established in patients with renal or hepatic impairment.
• Assess patient's and family's knowledge of drug therapy.

🔅 **Nursing diagnoses**
• Ineffective health maintenance related to cyanide ingestion
• Risk for injury related to drug-induced adverse reactions
• Deficient knowledge related to drug therapy

≫ Planning and implementation

- Hydroxocobalamin's deep red color may affect the results of some laboratory tests, including those involving urine, blood chemistry, hematology, and coagulation.
- Obtaining a serum sample to test for cyanide poisoning before treatment isn't required but may be helpful for documentation.
- Monitor patient's blood pressure during and after infusion.
- Photosensitivity reactions are possible.
- Because the drug is cleared unchanged in the kidney, oxalate crystals may occur.

Patient teaching
- Explain that skin may turn red for up to 2 weeks after infusion and may increase the risk of photosensitivity. Urge patient to avoid direct sun while skin is discolored.
- Inform patient that urine may be red for up to 5 weeks after infusion.
- Tell patient that an acne-like rash appears in some people 7 to 28 days after infusion and usually resolves without treatment in a few weeks.
- If patient was breast-feeding, instruct her to consult prescriber about whether to resume after the infusion.
- Urge patient to disclose a history of hypertension because blood pressure may increase during infusion.
- Tell patient that the result of some blood and urine tests may be altered for several days after infusion.

☑ Evaluation

- Patient responds positively to drug therapy.
- Patient sustains no injury from adverse reactions.
- Patient and family state understanding of drug therapy.

hydroxychloroquine sulfate
(high-droks-ee-KLOR-oh-kwin SUL-fayt)
Plaquenil

Pharmacologic class: 4-aminoquinoline
Therapeutic class: antimalarial, anti-inflammatory
Pregnancy risk category: C

Indications and dosages

▶ **Suppressive prophylaxis of malaria attacks caused by *Plasmodium vivax*, *P. malariae*, *P. ovale*, and susceptible strains of *P. falciparum*.** *Adults:* 310 mg base P.O. weekly on same day of week. Begin 1 to 2 weeks before exposure and continue for 4 weeks after leaving endemic areas.
Children: 5 mg base/kg P.O. weekly, not to exceed 310 mg.
Patients untreated before exposure: Initial loading dose is doubled (620 mg for adults, 10 mg/kg for children) P.O. in two divided doses 6 hours apart.
▶ **Acute malarial attacks.** *Adults:* Initially, 620 mg base P.O.; then 310 mg base after 6 hours; then 310 mg base daily for 2 days.
Children: Initial dose, 10 mg base/kg (up to 620 mg base); second dose, 5 mg base/kg (up to 310 mg base) 6 hours after first dose; third dose, 5 mg base/kg 18 hours after second dose; fourth dose, 5 mg base/kg 24 hours after third dose.
▶ **Lupus erythematosus (chronic discoid and systemic).** *Adults:* 400 mg (sulfate) P.O. daily or b.i.d., continued for several weeks or months, depending on response. Prolonged maintenance dosage: 200 to 400 mg (sulfate) daily.
▶ **Rheumatoid arthritis.** *Adults:* Initially, 400 to 600 mg (sulfate) P.O. daily. When good response occurs (usually in 4 to 12 weeks), reduce dosage by 50% and continue at 200 to 400 mg daily.

Contraindications and cautions

- Contraindicated in patients hypersensitive to the drug or any of its components and in patients with retinal or visual field changes or porphyria.
- Use cautiously in patients with severe GI, neurologic, or blood disorders, and in patients with hepatic disease or alcoholism because drug concentrates in liver. Also use cautiously in those with G6PD deficiency or psoriasis because drug may worsen these conditions.
- ☀ **Lifespan:** In pregnant women, use cautiously. In breast-feeding women, safety and effectiveness haven't been established. In children who need long-term therapy, drug is contraindicated.

Adverse reactions

CNS: ataxia, dizziness, fatigue, hypoactive deep tendon reflexes, irritability, lassitude, night-

---

hydroxychloroquine sulfate   649

H

mares, nystagmus, psychic stimulation, *seizures,* toxic psychosis, vertigo.
EENT: ototoxicity, retinopathy, serious visual disturbances.
GI: abdominal cramps, anorexia, diarrhea, nausea, vomiting.
Hematologic: *agranulocytosis, aplastic anemia, hemolysis in patients with G6PD deficiency, leukopenia, thrombocytopenia.*
Metabolic: weight loss.
Musculoskeletal: skeletal muscle weakness.
Skin: alopecia, bleaching of hair, lichen planus eruptions, pleomorphic skin eruptions, pruritus, skin and mucosal pigment changes.

Interactions

Drug-drug. *Aluminum and magnesium salts, kaolin:* May decrease GI absorption. Separate administration times.
Cimetidine: May decrease hepatic metabolism of hydroxychloroquine. Monitor patient for toxicity.
Cyclosporines: May increase levels of these drugs. Monitor drug levels and adjust dosage of cyclosporine accordingly.
Digoxin: May increase levels of digoxin. Monitor patient and drug levels for digoxin toxicity.
Epinephrine: Vasopressor effects are inhibited by hydroxyzine. Use a different vasopressor, if needed.
Mefloquine: May increase risk of seizures. Avoid use together.
Metoprolol: May increase CV effects. Consider use of alternate beta-blocker.

Effects on lab test results

• May decrease hemoglobin level and hematocrit.
• May decrease granulocyte, WBC, and platelet counts.

Pharmacokinetics

Absorption: Good and almost complete.
Distribution: Concentrates in liver, spleen, kidneys, heart, and brain and is strongly bound in melanin-containing cells. Drug is protein-bound.
Metabolism: By liver.
Excretion: Mostly unchanged in urine. *Half-life:* 32 to 50 days.

Route	Onset	Peak	Duration
P.O.	Unknown	2–4½ hr	Unknown

Action

Chemical effect: May bind to and alter properties of DNA in susceptible organisms.
Therapeutic effect: Prevents or hinders growth of *P. malariae, P. ovale, P. vivax,* and *P. falciparum.* Relieves inflammation.

Available forms

Tablets: 200 mg (equivalent to 155-mg base)

NURSING PROCESS

Assessment
• Assess patient's condition before starting therapy and regularly thereafter.
• Make sure baseline and periodic ophthalmic examinations are performed because blindness can occur. Check periodically for ocular muscle weakness after long-term use.
• Obtain audiometric tests before, during, and after therapy, especially long-term therapy.
• Monitor CBC and liver function studies periodically during long-term therapy.
• Assess patient for overdose, which can quickly lead to headache, drowsiness, visual disturbances, CV collapse, and seizures, followed by cardiopulmonary arrest. Children are extremely susceptible to toxicity, so don't give them long-term therapy.
• Be alert for adverse reactions and drug interactions.
• Assess patient's and family's knowledge of drug therapy.

Nursing diagnoses
• Risk for infection related to susceptible organisms
• Disturbed sensory perception (visual and auditory) related to adverse reactions to drug
• Deficient knowledge related to drug therapy

Planning and implementation
• Give drug right before or after meals on same day of each week.
• Notify prescriber immediately about severe blood disorder that can't be attributed to disease. Blood reaction may require stopping the drug.

Patient teaching
- Advise patient to take drug immediately before or after meals on same day each week to enhance compliance for prophylaxis.
- If adverse CNS or visual disturbances occur, warn patient to avoid hazardous activities.
- Tell patient to promptly report visual or auditory changes.

✓ Evaluation
- Patient is free from infection.
- Patient maintains normal visual and auditory function.
- Patient and family state understanding of drug therapy.

HIGH ALERT

hydroxyurea
(high-droks-ee-yoo-REE-uh)
Droxia, Hydrea

Pharmacologic class: antimetabolite
Therapeutic class: antineoplastic; antisickling drug
Pregnancy risk category: D

Indications and dosages
Dosage and indications for hydroxyurea may vary. Check current literature for recommended protocol.
▶ **Solid tumors.** *Adults:* 80 mg/kg Hydrea P.O. as a single dose every 3 days; or 20 to 30 mg/kg Hydrea P.O. as a single daily dose.
▶ **Head and neck cancers, excluding the lip.** *Adults:* 80 mg/kg Hydrea P.O. as a single dose every 3 days.
▶ **Resistant chronic myelocytic leukemia.** *Adults:* 20 to 30 mg/kg Hydrea P.O. as a single daily dose.
▶ **To reduce the frequency of painful crises and to reduce the need for blood transfusions in patients with sickle cell anemia with recurrent moderate-to-severe painful crises (typically at least 3 during the preceding 12 months).** *Adults:* Base dosage on the patient's actual or ideal weight, whichever is less. The initial dose is 15 mg/kg Droxia P.O. as a single daily dose. The patient's blood count must be monitored every 2 weeks; see package insert for dosage adjustment.

Contraindications and cautions
- Contraindicated in patients hypersensitive to the drug or any of its components and in those with marked bone marrow depression and severe anemia.
- Use cautiously in patients with renal dysfunction and in the elderly.
☀ **Lifespan:** In pregnant women, use only if benefits outweigh risks to fetus. In breast-feeding women, drug is contraindicated. In children, safety and effectiveness haven't been established. Elderly patients may be more sensitive to the drug and require a lower dosage.

Adverse reactions
CNS: disorientation, dizziness, drowsiness, fever, hallucinations, headache, malaise, *seizures.*
GI: anorexia, diarrhea, nausea, stomatitis, vomiting.
GU: *renal toxicity.*
Hematologic: anemia, *bone marrow suppression, leukopenia, megaloblastosis, thrombocytopenia.*
Metabolic: hyperuricemia.
Skin: mucositis, pruritus, rash.
Other: chills.

Interactions
Drug-drug. *Cytotoxic drugs, radiation therapy:* May enhance toxicity of hydroxyurea. Use together cautiously.

Effects on lab test results
- May increase liver enzyme, BUN, creatinine, and uric acid levels. May decrease hemoglobin level and hematocrit.
- May decrease WBC, RBC, and platelet counts.

Pharmacokinetics
Absorption: Good. Level is higher with a large, single dose than with divided doses.
Distribution: Crosses blood-brain barrier.
Metabolism: 50% of dose degraded in liver.
Excretion: 50% of drug in urine as unchanged drug; metabolites excreted through lungs as carbon dioxide and in urine as urea. *Half-life:* 3 to 4 hours.

Route	Onset	Peak	Duration
P.O.	Unknown	2 hr	Unknown

Reactions may be *common*, uncommon, *life-threatening*, or COMMON AND LIFE-THREATENING.

Action

Chemical effect: Unknown; thought to inhibit DNA synthesis.
Therapeutic effect: Hinders growth of certain cancer cells.

Available forms

Capsules: 200 mg, 300 mg, 400 mg, 500 mg

NURSING PROCESS

Assessment
• Assess patient's condition before therapy and regularly thereafter.
• Measure CBC, BUN, uric acid, and creatinine levels.
• Auditory and visual hallucinations and hematologic toxicity increase with decreased renal function.
• Radiation therapy may increase risk or severity of GI distress or stomatitis.
• Be alert for adverse reactions and drug interactions.
• Assess patient's and family's knowledge of drug therapy.

Nursing diagnoses
• Ineffective health maintenance related to presence of neoplastic disease
• Ineffective protection related to adverse hematologic reactions
• Deficient knowledge related to drug therapy

Planning and implementation
⚡ **ALERT:** Patients who have received or are currently receiving interferon may be at a greater risk of cutaneous vasculitic toxicities. Monitor them closely.
• Keep patient hydrated.
• Dosage modification may be needed after chemotherapy or radiation therapy.
• Bone marrow suppression is dose-limited and dose-related, with rapid recovery.
Patient teaching
• If patient can't swallow capsules, tell him to empty contents of capsules into water and drink immediately.
• Warn patient to watch for signs of infection (fever, sore throat, fatigue) and bleeding (easy bruising, nosebleed, bleeding gums, melena). Instruct patient to take infection-control and bleeding precautions. Tell patient to take temperature daily.

• Tell patient or caregiver to wear gloves when handling drug or its container and to wash their hands before and after contact with the bottle or capsule. If powder from capsule is spilled, wipe it up immediately with a damp towel and dispose of the towel in a closed container, such as a plastic bag.
• Advise woman of childbearing age not to become pregnant during therapy and to consult with prescriber before becoming pregnant.

Evaluation
• Patient responds well to drug therapy.
• Serious infections or bleeding complications don't develop.
• Patient and family state understanding of drug therapy.

hydroxyzine hydrochloride
(high-DROKS-ihzeen high-droh -KLOR-ighd)
hydroxyzine pamoate
Vistaril

Pharmacologic class: piperazine derivative
Therapeutic class: anxiolytic, sedative, antihistamine, antipruritic, antiemetic, antispasmodic
Pregnancy risk category: C

Indications and dosages

▸ **Anxiety.** *Adults:* 50 to 100 mg P.O. q.i.d.
Children age 6 and older: 50 to 100 mg P.O. daily in divided doses.
Children younger than age 6: Give 50 mg P.O. daily in divided doses.
▸ **Adjunct preoperative and postoperative sedation.** *Adults:* 25 to 100 mg P.O. or I.M. every 4 to 8 hours.
Children: 0.6 mg/kg P.O or I.M. every 4 to 6 hours.
▸ **Pruritus from allergies.** *Adults:* 25 mg P.O. t.i.d. or q.i.d.
Children age 6 and older: 50 to 100 mg P.O. daily in divided doses.
Children younger than age 6: Give 50 mg P.O. daily in divided doses.
▸ **Psychiatric and emotional emergencies, including acute alcoholism.** *Adults:* 50 to 100 mg I.M. every 4 to 6 hours p.r.n.
▸ **Nausea and vomiting (excluding nausea and vomiting of pregnancy).‡** *Adults:* 25 to 100 mg I.M. every 4 to 8 hours.

Contraindications and cautions

• Contraindicated in patients hypersensitive to hydroxyzine or cetirizine.

⚠ **Lifespan:** In pregnancy, safety has not been established. In breast-feeding women, safety and effectiveness haven't been established. In elderly patients, use cautiously and at lower doses.

Adverse reactions

CNS: *drowsiness,* involuntary motor activity.
GI: *dry mouth.*
Other: hypersensitivity reactions, marked discomfort at I.M. injection site.

Interactions

Drug-drug. *CNS depressants:* May increase CNS depression. Use cautiously at lower doses.
Epinephrine: Inhibits and reverses vasopressor effect of epinephrine. If vasopressor is required, don't use epinephrine.
MAO inhibitors: May enhance anticholinergic effects. Use together cautiously.
Drug-lifestyle. *Alcohol use:* May increase CNS depression. Discourage use together.
Sun exposure: Photosensitivity may occur. Urge patient to avoid unprotected or prolonged sun exposure.

Effects on lab test results

• May cause false elevations of urine 17-hydroxycorticosteroids, depending on test method used.

Pharmacokinetics

Absorption: Rapid and complete after P.O. use. Unknown for I.M. use.
Distribution: Unknown.
Metabolism: Almost complete.
Excretion: Mainly in urine. *Half-life:* 3 hours.

Route	Onset	Peak	Duration
P.O.	15–30 min	2 hr	4–6 hr
I.M.	Unknown	Unknown	4–6 hr

Action

Chemical effect: Unknown; may suppress activity in key regions of subcortical area of CNS.
Therapeutic effect: Relieves anxiety and itching, promotes calmness, and alleviates nausea and vomiting.

Available forms

hydroxyzine embonate
Capsules: 25 mg, 50 mg
hydroxyzine hydrochloride
Injection: 25 mg/ml*, 50 mg/ml*
Syrup: 10 mg/5 ml*
Tablets: 10 mg, 25 mg, 50 mg, 100 mg
hydroxyzine pamoate
Capsules: 25 mg, 50 mg, 100 mg
Oral suspension: 25 mg/5 ml

NURSING PROCESS

Assessment
• Assess patient's condition before therapy and regularly thereafter.
• Be alert for adverse reactions and drug interactions.
• Assess patient's and family's knowledge of drug therapy.

Nursing diagnoses
• Ineffective health maintenance related to underlying condition
• Risk for injury related to adverse CNS reactions
• Deficient knowledge related to drug therapy

Planning and implementation
• Give a lower dose to an elderly or debilitated patient.
• Parenteral form (hydroxyzine hydrochloride) for I.M. use only; Z-track injection method is preferred. Aspirate I.M. injection carefully to prevent inadvertent intravascular injection. Inject deep into large muscle mass.
ALERT: Never give drug I.V.
ALERT: Don't confuse hydroxyzine with hydralazine.
Patient teaching
• Warn patient to avoid hazardous activities until CNS effects of drug are known.
• Tell patient to avoid alcohol during drug therapy.
• Suggest sugarless hard candy or gum to relieve dry mouth.

Evaluation
• Patient has improved health.
• Patient doesn't experience injury.
• Patient and family state understanding of drug therapy.

Reactions may be *common,* uncommon, *life-threatening,* or COMMON AND LIFE-THREATENING.

ibandronate sodium
(ih-BAN-druh-nayt SOH-dee-um)
Boniva

Pharmacologic class: bisphosphonate
Therapeutic class: bone resorption inhibitor
Pregnancy risk category: C

Indications and dosages

▶ **Postmenopausal osteoporosis.** *Adults:* For treatment or prevention, 2.5 mg P.O. daily or 150 mg P.O. once monthly. Drug should be taken first thing in the morning with a large glass of plain water, 1 hour before food or other drugs, and patient must remain standing or seated upright for 60 minutes. Or, for treatment only, 3 mg I.V. bolus over 15 to 30 seconds once every 3 months.

▼ I.V. administration

• Injection is for I.V. use only. Don't give I.M. or subcutaneously.
• Give the 3-mg/3-ml dose using the ¾-inch safety needle provided with the prefilled 5-ml syringe.
• Syringes are for single use only.
• Inspect prefilled syringe for particles and discoloration before giving. Don't use if particles are visible or product is discolored.
⊗ **Incompatibilities**
Calcium-containing solutions and other I.V. drugs.

Contraindications and cautions

• Contraindicated in patients hypersensitive to ibandronate and patients with uncorrected hypocalcemia. Oral form contraindicated in patients who are unable to stand or sit upright for 60 minutes. Not recommended for patients with severe renal impairment (creatinine clearance less than 30 ml/minute).
• Use cautiously in patients with a history of GI disorders.
⚖ Lifespan: In pregnant women, use only if benefits outweigh risks to fetus. In breast-feeding women, use cautiously because it isn't

known if drug appears in breast milk. In children, safety and effectiveness haven't been established.

Adverse reactions

CNS: asthenia, dizziness, headache, insomnia, nerve root lesion, vertigo.
CV: hypertension.
EENT: nasopharyngitis, pharyngitis.
GI: abdominal pain, constipation, diarrhea, *dyspepsia,* gastritis, nausea, vomiting.
GU: UTI.
Musculoskeletal: arthralgia, arthritis, *back pain,* joint disorder, limb pain, localized osteoarthritis, muscle cramps, myalgia, osteonecrosis.
Respiratory: bronchitis, pneumonia, upper respiratory tract infection.
Skin: rash.
Other: allergic reaction, infection, influenza, tooth disorder.

Interactions

Drug-drug. *Aspirin, NSAIDs:* May increase GI irritation. Use together cautiously.
Aluminum-, calcium-, magnesium-, or iron-containing products: May decrease ibandronate absorption. Give ibandronate 60 minutes before vitamins, minerals, or antacids.
Drug-food. *Food, milk, and beverages other than water:* May decrease ibandronate absorption. Give drug on an empty stomach with plain water.
Drug-lifestyle. *Alcohol use:* May decrease ibandronate absorption and increase risk of esophageal irritation. Discourage use together.

Effects on lab test results

• May increase cholesterol level. May decrease total alkaline phosphatase level.
• May interfere with bone-imaging agents.

Pharmacokinetics

Absorption: Absorbed in the upper GI tract; bioavailability is low and significantly impaired by food or non-water beverages.
Distribution: Rapidly binds to bone or is eliminated.
Metabolism: Not metabolized.

Excretion: Unchanged in urine and feces; 50% to 60% excreted by kidneys. *Half-life:* 37 to 157 hours in patients taking the 150-mg dose.

Route	Onset	Peak	Duration
P.O.	Unknown	½–2 hr	Unknown
I.V.	Rapid	Unknown	Unknown

Action

Chemical effect: Inhibits the osteoclast activity of bone breakdown and removal to reduce bone loss.
Therapeutic effect: Increases bone mass.

Available forms

Injection: 3-mg/3-ml prefilled syringe
Tablets: 2.5 mg, 150 mg

NURSING PROCESS

🕮 Assessment
• Assess patient for adequate intake of calcium and vitamin D.
• Monitor patient for signs or symptoms of esophageal irritation, including dysphagia, painful swallowing, retrosternal pain, and heartburn.
• Monitor patient for bone, joint, and muscle pain, which may be severe or incapacitating.
• Watch for signs and symptoms of uveitis and scleritis.
• Assess patient's and family's knowledge of drug therapy.

⊕ Nursing diagnoses
• Risk for injury related to decreased bone mass
• Risk for deficient fluid volume related to drug-induced GI upset
• Deficient knowledge related to drug therapy

➤ Planning and implementation
• Correct hypocalcemia or other disturbances of bone and mineral metabolism before therapy.
• Give drug in the morning 60 minutes before the first meal or fluid and before any other drugs.
• ⑤ **ALERT:** Bisphosphonates may lead to osteonecrosis, mainly in the jaw. Dental surgery may worsen the condition. If the patient needs dental procedures, assess the risk of stopping ibandronate.

• Signs of possible overdose include hypocalcemia, hypophosphatemia, upset stomach, dyspepsia, esophagitis, gastritis, or ulcer.
• Treatment of overdose includes giving milk or antacids to enhance binding of ibandronate. Avoid emesis to minimize gastric irritation. Keep patient upright during management of overdose. Dialysis isn't helpful.

Patient teaching
• Tell patient receiving I.V. form, if she misses a dose, reschedule the missed dose as soon as possible. Subsequent injections should be rescheduled once every 3 months from that dose. She shouldn't receive more than one dose in a 3-month timeframe.
• Tell patient taking the monthly dose to take it on the same date each month and to wait at least 7 days between doses if she misses a scheduled dose.
• Instruct patient to take drug 60 minutes before eating or drinking in the morning and before any other drugs, including OTC products, such as calcium, antacids, and vitamins.
• Advise patient to swallow drug whole with a full glass of plain water while standing or sitting and to remain upright for at least 60 minutes after taking drug.
• Caution patient to take only with plain water and no other beverage.
• Instruct patient not to chew or suck on the tablet.
• Advise patient to take calcium and vitamin D supplements as directed by prescriber.
• Tell patient to report any bone, joint, or muscle pain.
• Advise patient to stop drug and immediately report signs and symptoms of esophageal irritation, such as dysphagia, painful swallowing, retrosternal pain, or heartburn.

✓ Evaluation
• Patient does not suffer any injury related to decreased bone mass.
• Patient maintains adequate hydration.
• Patient and family state understanding of drug therapy.

---

ibuprofen

(igh-byoo-PROH-fen)

Advil†, Advil Children's†, Advil Infants' Drops†, Advil Junior Strength†, Advil Liqui-Gels†, Advil Migraine†, Genpril Caplets†, Genpril Tablets†, IBU†, Ibu-Tab†, Menadol†, Midol Cramp†, Midol IB†, Motrin†, Motrin Children's†, Motrin Drops†, Motrin IB Caplets†, Motrin IB Gelcaps†, Motrin IB Tablets†, Motrin Infants' Drops†, Motrin Junior Strength†, Motrin Migraine Pain Caplets†, Novo-Profen ◆, PediaCare Fever†

Pharmacologic class: NSAID
Therapeutic class: analgesic, antipyretic, anti-inflammatory
Pregnancy risk category: C

Indications and dosages

▶ **Rheumatoid arthritis, osteoarthritis.**
Adults: 300 to 800 mg P.O. t.i.d. or q.i.d., not to exceed 3.2 g P.O. daily.
Children: 20 to 40 mg/kg P.O. daily, divided into three to four doses.
▶ **Mild to moderate pain, dysmenorrhea.**
Adults: 400 mg P.O every 4 to 6 hours p.r.n.
Children ages 6 months to 12 years: 10 mg/kg per dose P.O. every 6 to 8 hours. Maximum, 40 mg/kg daily.
▶ **Fever, minor aches and pains.** *Adults and children older than age 12:* Give 200 to 400 mg P.O. every 4 to 6 hours p.r.n. Don't exceed 1.2 g P.O. daily or give for longer than 3 days for fever or 10 days for pain unless directed by pre-scriber.
Children ages 6 months to 12 years: If tempera-ture is below 102.5° F (39° C), recommended dosage is 5 mg/kg P.O. every 6 to 8 hours p.r.n. Treat higher temperatures with 10 mg/kg P.O. every 6 to 8 hours p.r.n. to maximum dosage of 40 mg/kg daily.

Contraindications and cautions

• Contraindicated in patients hypersensitive to the drug or any of its components and in those with nasal polyps, angioedema, and broncho-spastic reaction to aspirin or other NSAIDs.
• Use cautiously in patients with GI disorders, history of peptic ulcer disease, hepatic or renal

disease, cardiac decompensation, hypertension, or intrinsic coagulation defects.

♨ Lifespan: In pregnant and breast-feeding women, drug isn't recommended. In infants younger than age 6 months, safety and effective-ness haven't been established. In elderly pa-tients, use cautiously at a lower dose because they are at greater risk for adverse GI effects.

Adverse reactions

CNS: aseptic meningitis, cognitive dysfunction, *dizziness, drowsiness, headache.*
CV: edema, *heart failure,* hypertension, *periph-eral edema.*
EENT: *tinnitus,* visual disturbances.
GI: epigastric distress, nausea, occult blood loss, peptic ulceration.
GU: reversible renal failure.
Hematologic: *agranulocytosis,* anemia, *aplas-tic anemia, leukopenia, neutropenia, pancy-topenia,* prolonged bleeding time, *thrombocy-topenia.*
Respiratory: *bronchospasm.*
Skin: photosensitivity reactions, pruritus, rash, *Stevens-Johnson syndrome,* urticaria.

Interactions

Drug-drug. *Antihypertensives, furosemide, thi-azide diuretics:* May decrease effectiveness of diuretics or antihypertensives. Monitor patient.
Aspirin: May decrease drug level and increase risk of adverse GI reactions. Monitor patient.
Corticosteroids: May increase risk of adverse GI reactions. Avoid use together.
Cyclosporine: May increase nephrotoxicity of both drugs. Avoid use together.
Digoxin: May increase digoxin level. Monitor level closely for digoxin toxicity.
Lithium, oral anticoagulants: May increase lev-els or effects of these drugs. Monitor patient for toxicity.
Methotrexate: May increase risk of methotrex-ate toxicity. Monitor patient closely.
Probenecid: May increase level and toxicity of NSAIDs. Monitor patient for signs of toxicity.
Drug-herb. *Dong quai, feverfew, garlic, ginger, horse chestnut, red clover:* May increase risk of bleeding. Monitor patient closely for bleeding.
St. John's wort: May increase risk of photosen-sitivity reactions. Advise patient to avoid unpro-tected or prolonged exposure to sunlight.

Drug-lifestyle. *Alcohol use:* May increase risk of adverse GI reactions. Discourage use together.

Smoking: May increase risk for gastric ulceration. Discourage use together.

Sun exposure: May cause photosensitivity reactions. Advise patient to avoid unprotected or prolonged exposure to sunlight.

Effects on lab test results

● May increase BUN, creatinine, ALT, AST, potassium levels. May decrease glucose and hemoglobin levels and hematocrit.

● May decrease neutrophil, WBC, RBC, platelet, and granulocyte counts.

Pharmacokinetics

Absorption: Rapid and complete from GI tract.
Distribution: Highly protein-bound.
Metabolism: Undergoes biotransformation in liver.
Excretion: Mainly in urine, with some biliary excretion. *Half-life:* 2 to 4 hours.

Route	Onset	Peak	Duration
P.O.	≤ 30 min	2–4 hr	≥ 4 hr

Action

Chemical effect: May inhibit prostaglandin synthesis.
Therapeutic effect: Relieves pain, fever, and inflammation.

Available forms

Caplets: 200 mg†
Capsules (liquid-filled): 200 mg†
Oral drops: 40 mg/ml†
Oral suspension: 100 mg/5 ml†
Tablets: 100 mg†, 200 mg†, 400 mg, 600 mg, 800 mg
Tablets (chewable): 50 mg†, 100 mg†
Tablets (film-coated): 100 mg†, 200 mg†, 400 mg, 600 mg, 800 mg

NURSING PROCESS

🔲 Assessment

● Assess patient's underlying condition before starting therapy.

● Evaluate patient for relief from pain, fever, or inflammation. Full effects on arthritis may take 2 to 4 weeks.

● Check renal and hepatic function periodically in long-term therapy.

● Be alert for adverse reactions and drug interactions.

● Assess patient's and family's knowledge of drug therapy.

🔲 Nursing diagnoses

● Chronic pain related to underlying condition
● Risk for injury related to drug-induced adverse reactions
● Deficient knowledge related to drug therapy

▷ Planning and implementation

● Give with meals or milk to reduce adverse GI reactions.

● If drug is ineffective, notify prescriber.

● If renal or hepatic abnormalities occur, stop drug and notify prescriber.

Patient teaching

● Tell patient to take drug with meals or milk to reduce adverse GI reactions.

● Tell adult patient using OTC drug not to exceed 1.2 g daily, not to give drug to children younger than age 12, and not to take drug for extended periods without consulting prescriber.

● Ibuprofen can negate the antiplatelet effect of low-dose aspirin therapy. Tell patient how to safely use ibuprofen along with aspirin therapy.

● Warn patient that using drug with aspirin, alcohol, or corticosteroids may increase the risk of adverse GI reactions.

● Serious GI toxicity, including peptic ulceration and bleeding, can occur in patients taking NSAIDs, despite absence of GI symptoms.

● Teach patient to recognize and report signs and symptoms of GI bleeding.

● Instruct patient not to drink alcohol during therapy.

● Instruct patient to use sunblock, wear protective clothing, and avoid prolonged exposure to sunlight.

● Inform patient that ankle swelling may occur, but tell him to call prescriber promptly if weight increases by 3 to 5 pounds/week, or if he develops shortness of breath, cough, or palpitations.

🔲 Evaluation

● Patient is free from pain.
● Patient doesn't experience injury from adverse reactions.
● Patient and family state understanding of drug therapy.

Reactions may be *common*, uncommon, *life-threatening*, or COMMON AND LIFE-THREATENING.

ibutilide fumarate
(igh-BYOO-tih-lighd FYOO-muh-rayt)
Corvert

Pharmacologic class: ibutilide derivative
Therapeutic class: class III antiarrhythmic
Pregnancy risk category: C

Indications and dosages

▶ **Rapid conversion of recent atrial fibrillation or atrial flutter to sinus rhythm.** *Adults who weigh 60 kg (132 lb) or more:* 1 mg I.V. over 10 minutes.
Adults who weigh less than 60 kg (132 lb): 0.01 mg/kg I.V. over 10 minutes.

▼ I.V. administration

• Give undiluted or diluted in 50 ml of diluent. Add to normal saline solution for injection or D_5W injection before infusion. Add contents of one 10-ml vial (0.1 mg/ml) to a 50-ml infusion bag to form admixture of about 0.017 mg/ml ibutilide fumarate. Drug is compatible with polyvinyl chloride plastic bags and polyolefin bags.
• Admixtures with approved diluents are chemically and physically stable for 24 hours at room temperature or 48 hours if refrigerated.
• Inspect parenteral drugs for particles and discoloration before giving.
• Stop infusion if arrhythmia stops or if patient develops sustained or nonsustained ventricular tachycardia or significantly prolonged QT interval. If arrhythmia doesn't stop within 10 minutes after infusion ends, give a second 10-minute infusion of equal strength.
⊗ **Incompatibilities**
None reported.

Contraindications and cautions

• Contraindicated in patients hypersensitive to the drug or any of its components.
• Contraindicated for use in patients with history of polymorphic ventricular tachycardia, such as torsades de pointes.
• Use cautiously in patients with hepatic or renal dysfunction; usually, no dosage adjustments are needed.
☀ **Lifespan:** In pregnant women, use cautiously. In breast-feeding women and in children,

safety and effectiveness haven't been established.

Adverse reactions

CNS: headache, syncope.
CV: *AV block, bradycardia,* bundle branch block, *heart failure,* hypertension, hypotension, *nonsustained ventricular tachycardia,* palpitations, *QT interval prolongation, sustained polymorphic ventricular tachycardia,* tachycardia, ventricular extrasystoles.
GI: nausea.
GU: *renal failure.*

Interactions

Drug-drug. *Class IA antiarrhythmics (such as disopyramide, procainamide, quinidine), other class III drugs (such as amiodarone, sotalol):* May increase risk of prolonged refractory state. Avoid use together.
Digoxin: Supraventricular arrhythmias may mask cardiotoxicity from excessive digoxin levels. Use cautiously.
H_1-receptor antagonist antihistamines, phenothiazines, tetracyclic antidepressants, tricyclic antidepressants, other drugs that prolong QT interval: May increase risk of proarrhythmias. Monitor patient closely.

Effects on lab test results

None reported.

Pharmacokinetics

Absorption: Given I.V.
Distribution: Highly distributed. About 40% protein-bound.
Metabolism: Not clearly defined.
Excretion: In urine and feces. *Half-life:* Averages about 6 hours.

Route	Onset	Peak	Duration
I.V.	Unknown	Unknown	Unknown

Action

Chemical effect: Prolongs action potential in isolated cardiac myocyte and increases atrial and ventricular refractoriness; has mainly class III properties.
Therapeutic effect: Restores normal sinus rhythm.

Available forms

Injection: 0.1 mg/ml in 10-ml vials

NURSING PROCESS

⚖ Assessment

• Assess patient's arrhythmia before starting therapy.

• ⚠ **ALERT:** Monitor ECG continuously during therapy and for at least 4 hours afterward (or until QT interval returns to baseline) because drug can induce or worsen ventricular arrhythmias. If ECG shows arrhythmias, monitor it longer.

• Be alert for adverse reactions and drug interactions.

• Assess patient's and family's knowledge of drug therapy.

✚ Nursing diagnoses

• Decreased cardiac output related to arrhythmias

• Risk for injury related to life-threatening arrhythmias

• Deficient knowledge related to drug therapy

⟩ Planning and implementation

• Drug should be given only by skilled personnel. During and after administration, have available proper equipment and facilities for a cardiac emergency, such as cardiac monitor, intracardiac pacer, cardioverter or defibrillator, and drugs for sustained ventricular tachycardia.

• Correct hypokalemia and hypomagnesemia before therapy to reduce risk of proarrhythmia.

Patient teaching

• Tell patient to promptly report adverse reactions, especially headaches, dizziness, weakness, palpitations, or chest pains.

• Instruct patient to report any discomfort at injection site.

✔ Evaluation

• Patient regains normal sinus rhythm.

• Life-threatening arrhythmia doesn't develop.

• Patient and family state understanding of drug therapy.

HIGH ALERT

idarubicin hydrochloride

(igh-duh-ROO-bih-sin high-droh-KLOR-ighd)
Idamycin PFS

Pharmacologic class: anthracycline antibiotic
Therapeutic class: antineoplastic
Pregnancy risk category: D

Indications and dosages

▶ **Acute myeloid leukemia, including French-American-British classifications M1 through M7, with other approved antileukemic drugs.** *Adults:* 12 mg/m² by slow I.V. injection (over 10 to 15 minutes) daily for 3 days with 100 mg/m² of cytarabine by continuous I.V. infusion daily for 7 days or cytarabine as 25-mg/m² bolus followed by 200 mg/m² by continuous infusion daily for 5 days. Give second course, if needed. If patient develops severe mucositis, don't give until recovery is complete, and reduce dosage by 25%.

✂ Adjust-a-dose: For patients with hepatic or renal impairment, reduce dosage. If bilirubin level is above 5 mg/dl, withhold drug.

▽ I.V. administration

• Preparation and administration of drug have carcinogenic, mutagenic, and teratogenic risks. Follow facility policy to reduce risks.

• Reconstitute to final concentration of 1 mg/ml using normal saline solution for injection. Add 5 ml to 5-mg vial or 10 ml to 10-mg vial. Don't use bacteriostatic saline solution. Vial is under negative pressure.

• Give over 10 to 15 minutes into free-flowing I.V. infusion of normal saline solution or D₅W running into large vein. If extravasation occurs, stop infusion immediately, elevate limb, and notify prescriber. Apply intermittent ice packs for 30 minutes immediately and then 30 minutes q.i.d. for 4 days. Consult plastic surgery promptly if pain, erythema, edema, vesication, or ulceration occurs.

• Reconstituted solutions are stable for 72 hours at 59° to 86° F (15° to 30° C), 7 days if refrigerated. Label unused solutions with chemotherapy hazard label.

⊗ Incompatibilities

Acyclovir sodium, alkaline solutions, allopurinol, ampicillin sodium with sulbactam, cefazolin, cefepime, ceftazidime, clindamycin

phosphate, dexamethasone sodium phosphate, etoposide, furosemide, gentamicin, heparin, hydrocortisone sodium succinate, lorazepam, meperidine, methotrexate sodium, piperacillin sodium with tazobactam, sodium bicarbonate, teniposide, vancomycin, vincristine.

Contraindications and cautions

• Use cautiously in patients with bone marrow suppression induced by previous drug therapy or radiotherapy and in patients with impaired hepatic or renal function, heart disease, or previous therapy with anthracyclines at high cumulative doses or other potentially cardiotoxic drugs.

⚕ Lifespan: In pregnant and breast-feeding women, use cautiously. In children, safety and effectiveness haven't been established.

Adverse reactions

CNS: *altered mental status, fever, headache,* peripheral neuropathy, *seizures.*
CV: *arrhythmias,* atrial fibrillation, *cardiomyopathy,* chest pain, *heart failure, MI,* myocardial insufficiency, *myocardial toxicity.*
GI: *cramps, diarrhea, mucositis, nausea, severe enterocolitis with perforation,* vomiting.
Hematologic: HEMORRHAGE, MYELOSUPPRESSION.
Skin: *alopecia,* bullous erythrodermatous rash on palms and soles, erythema at previously irradiated sites, rash, tissue necrosis at injection site if extravasation occurs, urticaria, urticaria at injection site.
Other: INFECTION.

Interactions

None reported.

Effects on lab test results

• May increase BUN, creatinine, and uric acid and levels. May decrease hemoglobin level and hematocrit.
• May increase liver function test values. May decrease RBC, WBC, and platelet counts.

Pharmacokinetics

Absorption: Given I.V.
Distribution: 97% lipophilic and tissue-bound, with highest levels in nucleated blood and bone marrow cells.
Metabolism: Extensively outside of liver. Metabolite is cytotoxic.

Excretion: Mainly biliary. *Half-life:* 20 to 22 hours.

Route	Onset	Peak	Duration
I.V.	Unknown	≤ 3 min	Unknown

Action

Chemical effect: May inhibit nucleic acid synthesis by intercalation; interacts with enzyme topoisomerase II.
Therapeutic effect: Hinders growth of susceptible leukemic cells.

Available forms

Powder for injection: 1 mg/ml available in 5-, 10-, and 20-mg vials

NURSING PROCESS

✍ Assessment

• Assess patient's condition before starting therapy and regularly thereafter.
• Assess patient for systemic infection, and control infection before therapy begins.
• Monitor CBC and hepatic and renal function test results frequently.
• Be alert for adverse reactions and drug interactions, especially signs of heart failure, infection, and hemorrhage.
• Assess patient's and family's knowledge of drug therapy.

⊞ Nursing diagnoses

• Ineffective health maintenance related to presence of underlying condition
• Ineffective protection related to adverse hematologic reactions
• Deficient knowledge related to drug therapy

▶ Planning and implementation

• Take appropriate preventive measures (including adequate hydration) before starting treatment.
⚠ ALERT: Never give drug I.M. or subcutaneously.
• Hyperuricemia may result from rapid destruction of leukemic cells. Give allopurinol.
⚠ ALERT: Don't confuse idarubicin with daunorubicin, doxorubicin, or epirubicin.
Patient teaching
• Teach patient to recognize and report signs of extravasation, infection, bleeding, and heart failure, such as shortness of breath and leg swelling.

• Advise patient that red urine for several days is normal and doesn't indicate blood in urine.
• Advise women of childbearing age to use a reliable contraceptive during therapy and to consult with prescriber before becoming pregnant.

✓ Evaluation
• Patient responds well to drug.
• Serious adverse hematologic reactions don't develop.
• Patient and family state understanding of drug therapy.

HIGH ALERT

ifosfamide
(igh-FOHS-fuh-mighd)
IFEX

Pharmacologic class: alkylating drug
Therapeutic class: antineoplastic
Pregnancy risk category: D

Indications and dosages

▶ **Testicular cancer.** *Adults:* 1.2 g/m^2 I.V. daily for 5 consecutive days. Repeat every 3 weeks or after patient recovers from hematologic toxicity.
▶ **Lung cancer, Hodgkin and malignant lymphoma, breast cancer, acute lymphocytic leukemia, ovarian cancer, gastric cancer, pancreatic cancer, sarcomas, cervical cancer, and uterine cancer‡.** *Adults:* 1.2 to 2.5 g/m^2 I.V. daily for 3 to 5 days, with cycles of therapy repeated as needed.

▼ I.V. administration

• Follow facility policy to reduce risks. Preparation and administration are linked to carcinogenic, mutagenic, and teratogenic risks.
• Reconstitute each gram of drug with 20 ml of diluent to yield 50 mg/ml. Use sterile water for injection or bacteriostatic water for injection. Solutions may be further diluted with sterile water, dextrose 2.5% or 5% in water, half-normal or normal saline solution for injection, D$_5$W and normal saline solution for injection, or lactated Ringer's injection.
• Infuse each dose over at least 30 minutes.
• Ifosfamide and mesna are physically compatible and may be mixed in same I.V. solution.
• Reconstituted solution is stable for 1 week at room temperature or 6 weeks if refrigerated. If

drug was reconstituted with sterile water, however, use solution within 6 hours.
⊗ **Incompatibilities**
Cefepime, methotrexate sodium.

Contraindications and cautions

• Contraindicated in patients hypersensitive to the drug or any of its components and in those with severely depressed bone marrow function.
• Use cautiously in patients with renal impairment or compromised bone marrow from leukopenia, granulocytopenia, extensive bone marrow metastases, previous radiation therapy, or previous therapy with cytotoxic drugs.
🜲 **Lifespan:** In pregnant and breast-feeding women, drug is contraindicated. In children, safety and effectiveness haven't been established.

Adverse reactions

CNS: ataxia, *coma, confusion, depressive psychosis,* lethargy, *seizures, somnolence.*
GI: *nausea, vomiting.*
GU: *hematuria, hemorrhagic cystitis, nephrotoxicity.*
Hematologic: *leukopenia, myelosuppression, thrombocytopenia.*
Metabolic: *metabolic acidosis.*
Skin: *alopecia.*
Other: infection.

Interactions

Drug-drug. *Anticoagulants, aspirin:* May increase risk of bleeding. Avoid use together.
Barbiturates, chloral hydrate, phenytoin: May increase ifosfamide toxicity by inducing hepatic enzymes that hasten formation of toxic metabolites. Monitor patient closely.
Mesna: May decrease ifosfamide-induced bladder toxicity. May be given together.
Myelosuppressants: May enhance hematologic toxicity. Dosage adjustment may be needed.

Effects on lab test results

• May increase BUN, creatinine, bilirubin, and liver enzyme levels. May decrease hemoglobin level and hematocrit.
• May decrease WBC, RBC, and platelet counts.

Pharmacokinetics

Absorption: Given I.V.
Distribution: Crosses blood-brain barrier, but its metabolites don't, so alkylation doesn't occur in CSF.

Reactions may be *common,* uncommon, *life-threatening,* or COMMON AND LIFE-THREATENING.

Metabolism: About 50% of dose is metabolized in liver.
Excretion: Mainly in urine. *Half-life:* About 14 hours.

Route	Onset	Peak	Duration
I.V.	Unknown	Unknown	Unknown

Action

Chemical effect: Cross-links strands of cellular DNA and interferes with RNA transcription, which causes growth imbalance that leads to cell death.
Therapeutic effect: Kills cancer cells.

Available forms

Injection: 1 g (supplied with 200-mg ampule of mesna), 3 g (supplied with 400-mg ampule of mesna)

NURSING PROCESS

Assessment
• Assess patient's condition before starting therapy and regularly thereafter.
• Obtain urinalysis before each dose. If microscopic hematuria is present, evaluate patient for hemorrhagic cystitis. Adjust dosage of mesna, a protecting agent given with drug, if needed.
• Monitor CBC and renal and liver function test results.
• Be alert for adverse reactions and drug interactions.
• Assess patient for mental status changes. Dosage may need to be decreased or therapy stopped.
• Assess patient's and family's knowledge of drug therapy.

Nursing diagnoses
• Ineffective health maintenance related to presence of cancer
• Ineffective protection related to adverse CNS and hematologic reactions
• Deficient knowledge related to drug therapy

Planning and implementation
• Give antiemetic before giving drug to decrease nausea.
• Give drug with mesna to prevent hemorrhagic cystitis. Give mesna with or before drug to prevent cystitis. Give at least 2 L of fluids daily, either P.O. or I.V.

• Don't give drug at bedtime; infrequent voiding at night may increase risk of cystitis. If cystitis develops, stop giving drug and notify prescriber.
• Bladder irrigation with normal saline solution may decrease possibility of cystitis.
• Institute infection control and bleeding precautions.
⑤ **ALERT:** Don't confuse ifosfamide with cyclophosphamide.

Patient teaching
• Tell patient to void frequently to minimize contact of drug and its metabolites with bladder mucosa.
• Warn patient to watch for evidence of infection (fever, sore throat, fatigue), CNS effects (somnolence and dizziness), and bleeding (easy bruising, nosebleed, bleeding gums, melena). Teach patient about infection-control and bleeding precautions, and tell him to report adverse effects. Tell him to take his temperature daily.
• Instruct patient to avoid OTC drugs that contain aspirin.
• Stress importance of adequate fluid intake. Explain that it may help prevent hemorrhagic cystitis.
• Warn patient that hyperpigmentation may occur.

Evaluation
• Patient responds well to drug.
• Serious infections and CNS and bleeding complications don't develop.
• Patient and family state understanding of drug therapy.

iloprost
(IGH-loe-prost)
Ventavis

Pharmacologic class: prostacyclin analogue
Therapeutic class: vasodilator
Pregnancy risk category: C

Indications and dosages

▶ **Pulmonary arterial hypertension in patients with New York Heart Association Class III or IV symptoms.** *Adults:* Initially, 2.5 mcg inhaled using the I-neb or Prodose adaptive aerosol delivery (AAD) system. As tolerated, increase to 5 mcg inhaled 6 to 9 times daily while

awake, p.r.n., but no more than every 2 hours. Maximum, 5 mcg nine times daily.

Route	Onset	Peak	Duration
Inhalation	Unknown	Unknown	30–60 min

Contraindications and cautions

• No known contraindications. Don't use in patients whose systolic blood pressure is less than 85 mm Hg.

• Use drug cautiously in patients who have hepatic or renal impairment and in patients with COPD, severe asthma, or acute pulmonary infection.

⚖ **Lifespan:** In pregnant women, use only if benefits outweigh risk to fetus. In breast-feeding women, breast-feeding should be stopped because it isn't known if drug appears in breast milk. In children, safety and effectiveness haven't been established. In elderly patients, use cautiously and start with a low dosage.

Adverse reactions

CNS: *headache,* insomnia, *syncope.*
CV: chest pain, **heart failure, hypotension,** palpitations, peripheral edema, **supraventricular tachycardia,** *vasodilation.*
EENT: tongue pain.
GI: *nausea,* vomiting.
GU: renal failure.
Musculoskeletal: back pain, muscle cramps, *trismus.*
Respiratory: *cough,* dyspnea, hemoptysis, pneumonia, **pulmonary edema.**
Other: *flulike syndrome.*

Interactions

Drug-drug. *Anticoagulants:* May increase the risk of bleeding. Monitor patient closely.
Antihypertensive drugs, vasodilators: May increase effects of these drugs. Monitor patient's blood pressure.

Effects on lab test results

• May increase alkaline phosphatase and GGT levels.

Pharmacokinetics

Absorption: No GI absorption.
Distribution: 60% protein-bound, mainly to albumin.
Metabolism: To inactive metabolites.
Excretion: Mainly in urine; some in feces.
Half-life: 20 to 30 minutes.

Action

Chemical effect: Lowers pulmonary arterial pressure by dilating systemic and pulmonary arterial beds. Drug also affects platelet aggregation, although effect in pulmonary hypertension treatment isn't known.
Therapeutic effect: Improved exercise tolerance, fewer symptoms, and lack of deterioration.

Available forms

Inhalation solution: 10 mcg/ml (given only using the I-neb delivery system); 20 mcg/2-ml single-use ampule (should be given using the Prodose AAD system, but can be done with the I-neb)

NURSING PROCESS

🔍 Assessment

• Assess patient's underlying condition, and assess regularly thereafter.
• Monitor patient's vital signs carefully at start of treatment.
• Monitor patient for syncope.
• Monitor patient for evidence of pulmonary edema; stop treatment immediately.
• Assess patient's and family's knowledge of drug therapy.

⊕ Nursing diagnoses

• Ineffective tissue perfusion (cardiopulmonary) related to underlying condition
• Risk for injury related to drug-induced syncope
• Deficient knowledge related to drug therapy

▶ Planning and implementation

• Keep drug away from skin and eyes.
• Administer drug only through Prodose AAD device.
• Take care not to inhale drug while providing treatment.
• Overdose may cause hypotension, headache, flushing, nausea, vomiting, and diarrhea.
• To treat overdose, stop the inhalation session as needed. Monitor patient closely, and provide symptomatic treatment.

Patient teaching

• Advise patient to take drug exactly as prescribed using Prodose AAD.

Reactions may be *common,* uncommon, ***life-threatening***, or COMMON AND LIFE-THREATENING.

- Urge patient to follow manufacturer's instructions for preparing and inhaling drug.
- Advise patient to keep a backup Prodose AAD device in case the original malfunctions.
- Tell patient to keep drug away from skin and eyes and to rinse the area immediately if contact occurs.
- Caution patient not to ingest the drug solution.
- Inform patient that drug may cause dizziness and fainting. Urge him to stand up slowly from a sitting or lying position and to report worsening of symptoms.
- Tell patient to take drug before physical exertion but no more than every 2 hours.
- Discourage exposing other people—especially pregnant women and babies—to drug.
- Teach patient how to clean equipment and safely dispose of used ampules after each treatment. Caution patient not to save or use leftover solution.

☑ Evaluation
- Patient's pulmonary artery pressure decreases and patient reaches pulmonary hemodynamic stability.
- Patient maintains a stable blood pressure and doesn't experience syncope.
- Patient and family state understanding of drug therapy.

HIGH ALERT

imatinib mesylate
(ih-MAH-tin-nib MEH-suh-layt)
Gleevec

Pharmacologic class: protein-tyrosine kinase inhibitor
Therapeutic class: antineoplastic
Pregnancy risk category: D

Indications and dosages

▪ **NEW INDICATION: Aggressive systemic mastocytosis (ASM) without the D816V c-Kit mutation or with c-Kit mutatational status unknown, hypereosinophilic syndrome, chronic eosinophilic leukemia.** *Adults:* 400 mg P.O. daily. For ASM associated with eosinophilia, starting dose is 100 mg daily.
▶ **Chronic myeloid leukemia (CML) in blast crisis, in accelerated phase, or in chronic phase after failure of interferon-alpha therapy; newly diagnosed Philadelphia chromosome–positive (Ph+) chronic-phase CML.**
Adults: For chronic-phase CML, 400 mg. daily as single dose with a meal and large glass of water. For accelerated-phase CML or blast crisis, 600 mg P.O. daily as single dose with a meal and large glass of water. Continue treatment as long as patient continues to benefit. May increase daily dose to 600 mg P.O. in chronic phase or to 800 mg P.O. (400 mg P.O. b.i.d.) in accelerated phase or blast crisis. Increase dosage only if no severe adverse reactions and no severe non–leukemia-related neutropenia or thrombocytopenia occur in the following circumstances: disease progression (at any time), failure to achieve a satisfactory hematologic response after at least 3 months of treatment, or loss of a previously achieved hematologic response.
Children age 2 and older: For newly diagnosed Ph+ chronic-phase CML only, give 340 mg/m²/ day P.O. Don't exceed 600 mg.
▪ **NEW INDICATION: Dermatofibrosarcoma protuberans.** *Adults:* 800 mg P.O. daily.
▪ **NEW INDICATION: Myelodysplastic or myeloproliferative disease.** *Adults:* 400 mg P.O. daily.
▶ **Patients with kit (CD117)-positive unresectable or metastatic malignant GI stromal tumors (GIST).** *Adults:* 400 or 600 mg P.O. daily.
▪ **NEW INDICATION: Ph+ acute lymphoblastic leukemia.** *Adults:* 600 mg P.O. daily.
▶ **Ph+ chronic-phase CML in patients whose disease has recurred after stem cell transplant or who are resistant to interferon-alpha therapy.** *Children age 3 and older:* 260 mg/m² P.O. as single daily dose or divided into two doses, taken with a meal and large glass of water. May increase dosage to 340 mg/m² daily.
� Adjust-a-dose: Withhold treatment or reduce dosage based on bilirubin or liver transaminase levels, severity of fluid retention, or hematologic toxicities.

Contraindications and cautions

- Contraindicated in patients hypersensitive to the drug or any of its components.
- Use cautiously in hepatically impaired patients.
- **☠ Lifespan:** In pregnant and breast-feeding women, drug is contraindicated. In children younger than age 3, safety and effectiveness haven't been established. In elderly patients, use

cautiously because they may have an increased risk of edema when taking drug.

Adverse reactions

CNS: CEREBRAL HEMORRHAGE, *dizziness, fatigue, fever, headache, insomnia,* weakness.
CV: *edema,* **heart failure.**
EENT: *epistaxis,* nasopharyngitis.
GI: *abdominal pain, anorexia,* constipation, *diarrhea, dyspepsia,* GI HEMORRHAGE, *nausea, vomiting.*
GU: *renal failure.*
Hematologic: *anemia,* HEMORRHAGE, **neutropenia, thrombocytopenia.**
Hepatic: *liver toxicity.*
Metabolic: *hypokalemia, weight increase.*
Musculoskeletal: arthralgia, *muscle cramps, musculoskeletal pain, myalgia.*
Respiratory: *cough,* dyspnea, *nasopharyngitis, pleural effusion,* pneumonia, **pulmonary edema,** *upper respiratory tract infection.*
Skin: petechiae, pruritus, *rash.*
Other: night sweats.

Interactions

Drug-drug. *Acetaminophen:* May increase risk of liver toxicity. Monitor patient.
Cyclosporine, dihydropyridine calcium channel blockers, certain HMG-CoA reductase inhibitors, pimozide, triazolobenzodiazepines: May increase levels of these drugs. Monitor drug levels and patient for toxicity.
CYP3A4 inducers (carbamazepine, dexamethasone, phenobarbital, phenytoin, rifampin): May increase metabolism and decrease imatinib level. Use cautiously.
CYP3A4 inhibitors (clarithromycin, erythromycin, itraconazole, ketoconazole): May decrease metabolism and increase imatinib level. Monitor patient for toxicity.
Warfarin: May alter warfarin metabolism. Avoid use together; instead, use standard heparin or a low–molecular-weight heparin.
Drug-herb. *St. John's wort:* May decrease drug effects. Warn patient not to use together.

Effects on lab test results

- May increase creatinine, bilirubin, alkaline phosphatase, AST, and ALT levels. May decrease potassium and hemoglobin levels and hematocrit.
- May decrease neutrophil and platelet counts.

Pharmacokinetics

Absorption: Well absorbed.
Distribution: 98% protein-bound.
Metabolism: Mainly by CYP3A4.
Excretion: Mainly in feces as metabolites.
Half-life: 18 to 40 hours.

Route	Onset	Peak	Duration
P.O.	Unknown	2–4 hr	Unknown

Action

Chemical effect: Inhibits Bcr-Abl tyrosine kinase, the abnormal tyrosine kinase created in CML. Inhibits tumor growth of Bcr-Abl–transfected murine myeloid cells and Bcr-Abl–positive leukemia lines derived from CML patients in blast crisis.
Therapeutic effect: Stops tumor growth.

Available forms

Tablets: 100 mg, 400 mg

NURSING PROCESS

⚚ Assessment

- Assess neoplastic disease before starting therapy, and reassess regularly.
- Obtain baseline weight before starting therapy, and then weigh patient daily. Evaluate and treat unexpected and rapid weight gain.
- Assess patient's and family's knowledge of drug therapy.
- Monitor patient closely for fluid retention, which can be severe.
- Monitor CBC weekly for first month, biweekly for second month, and periodically thereafter.
- Monitor liver function test results carefully because severe hepatotoxicity may occur. Decrease dosage as needed.
- Because the long-term safety of this drug isn't known, carefully monitor renal toxicity, liver toxicity, and immunosuppression.

⊕ Nursing diagnoses

- Ineffective health maintenance related to neoplastic disease
- Risk for falls related to drug-induced adverse reactions
- Deficient knowledge related to drug therapy

▶ Planning and implementation

- For CML, increase dosage only if no severe adverse reactions and no severe non–leukemia-

---

related neutropenia or thrombocytopenia has occurred under the following circumstances: disease progression (at any time), failure to achieve a satisfactory hematologic response after at least 3 months of treatment, or loss of a previously achieved hematologic response.
• Because GI irritation is common, give drug with food.
• For patients unable to swallow tablets, dissolve tablets in water or apple juice (50 ml for 100-mg tablet or 200 ml for 400-mg tablet). Stir and have patient drink immediately.

Patient teaching
• Instruct patient to take drug with food and a large glass of water.
• Urge patient to report to the prescriber any adverse effects, such as fluid retention, signs of bleeding, or infection.
• Advise patient to have periodic liver and kidney function tests and tests to determine blood counts.
• Tell patient to avoid OTC products with acetaminophen.

✔ Evaluation
• Patient shows positive response to drug therapy on follow-up studies.
• Patient doesn't experience falls.
• Patient and family state understanding of drug therapy.

imipenem and cilastatin sodium
(im-ih-PEN-em and sigh-luh-STAT-in SO-dee-um)
Primaxin IM, Primaxin IV

Pharmacologic class: carbapenem (thienamycin class); beta-lactam antibiotic
Therapeutic class: antibiotic
Pregnancy risk category: C

Indications and dosages

▶ **Mild to moderate lower respiratory tract, skin, skin structure, intra-abdominal, and gynecologic infections; serious lower respiratory and urinary tract, intra-abdominal, and gynecologic infections; bacterial septicemia; bone and joint infections; serious soft-tissue infections; endocarditis; polymicrobic infections.** *Adults who weigh at least 70 kg (154 lb):* 500 to 750 mg I.M. every 12 hours. Or 250 mg to 1 g I.V. every 6 to 8 hours. Maximum I.V.

dosage is 50 mg/kg or 4 g daily, whichever is less.
Children age 3 months and older: 15 to 25 mg/kg I.V. every 6 hours. Maximum dosage for fully susceptible organisms is 2 g daily and for moderately susceptible organisms, 4 g daily (based on adult studies).
Infants ages 4 weeks to 3 months and weighing at least 1.5 kg (3.3 lb): 25 mg/kg I.V. every 6 hours.
Neonates ages 1 to 4 weeks and weighing at least 1.5 kg: 25 mg/kg I.V. every 8 hours.
Neonates younger than 1 week and weighing at least 1.5 kg: 25 mg/kg I.V. every 12 hours.
▨ **Adjust-a-dose:** For patients who weigh less than 70 kg (154 lb), use lower dose or longer intervals between doses if needed.
For patients with renal impairment, if creatinine clearance is 6 to 20 ml/minute, give 125 to 250 mg I.V. every 12 hours. If clearance is less then 5 ml/minute, withhold drug unless hemodialysis starts within 48 hours.

▽ I.V. administration
• When reconstituting powder, shake until solution is clear. Solutions may range from colorless to yellow; variations of color within this range don't affect drug's potency. After reconstitution, solution is stable for 10 hours at room temperature and for 48 hours when refrigerated.
• Don't give drug by direct I.V. bolus injection. Give 250- or 500-mg dose by I.V. infusion over 20 to 30 minutes. Infuse each 1-g dose over 40 to 60 minutes. If nausea occurs, slow infusion.
⊗ **Incompatibilities**
Antibiotics, dextrose 5% in lactated Ringer's injection, other I.V. drugs including allopurinol, amiodarone, amphotericin B cholesterol complex, azithromycin, etoposide, fluconazole, gemcitabine, lorazepam, meperidine, midazolam, milrinone, sargramostim, sodium bicarbonate.

Contraindications and cautions
• Contraindicated in patients hypersensitive to drug or any of its components.
• Use cautiously in patients allergic to penicillins or cephalosporins and in those with history of seizure disorders, especially if they also have compromised renal function.
▲ **Lifespan:** In pregnant women, use cautiously. In breast-feeding women, use cautiously because it's unknown if drug appears in breast

milk. In children younger than age 12, I.M. safety and effectiveness haven't been established. In children with CNS infections, I.V. use isn't recommended because of risk of seizures. In children who weigh less than 30 kg (66 lb) with renal impairment, use is contraindicated. In elderly patients, use cautiously because they may have decreased renal function.

Adverse reactions

CNS: dizziness, fever, *seizures,* somnolence.
CV: hypotension, thrombophlebitis.
GI: diarrhea, nausea, *pseudomembranous colitis,* vomiting.
Skin: pruritus, rash, urticaria.
Other: hypersensitivity reactions *(anaphylaxis),* pain at injection site.

Interactions

Drug-drug. *Beta-lactam antibiotics:* May cause in vitro antagonism. Avoid use together.
Cyclosporine: May increase adverse CNS effects of both drugs, possibly because of additive or synergistic toxicity. Avoid use together.
Ganciclovir: May cause seizures. Avoid use together.
Probenecid: May increase cilastatin levels. Avoid use together.

Effects on lab test results

● May increase BUN, creatinine, ALT, AST, alkaline phosphatase, bilirubin, and LDH levels. May decrease hemoglobin level and hematocrit.
● May increase eosinophil count. May decrease WBC and platelet counts.

Pharmacokinetics

Absorption: Imipenem is about 75% bioavailable; cilastatin is about 95% bioavailable.
Distribution: Rapid and wide. About 20% of imipenem is protein-bound; 40% of cilastatin is protein-bound.
Metabolism: Imipenem is metabolized by kidney dehydropeptidase I, resulting in low urine levels. Cilastatin inhibits this enzyme, reducing imipenem metabolism.
Excretion: About 70% excreted unchanged by kidneys. *Half-life:* 1 hour after I.V. dose; 2 to 3 hours after I.M. dose.

Route	Onset	Peak	Duration
I.V.	Unknown	Immediate	Unknown
I.M.	Unknown	1–2 hr	Unknown

Action

Chemical effect: Imipenem is bactericidal and inhibits bacterial cell wall synthesis. Cilastatin inhibits enzymatic breakdown of imipenem in kidneys, making it effective in urinary tract.
Therapeutic effect: Kills susceptible organisms, including many gram-positive, gram-negative, and anaerobic bacteria.

Available forms

Powder for I.M. injection: 500- and 750-mg vials
Powder for I.V. injection: 250- and 500-mg vials

NURSING PROCESS

⚁ Assessment
● Assess patient's infection before starting therapy and regularly thereafter.
● Obtain urine specimen for culture and sensitivity tests before starting therapy. Start therapy pending test results.
● Be alert for adverse reactions and drug interactions.
● If adverse GI reaction occurs, monitor patient's hydration status.
● Assess patient's and family's knowledge of drug therapy.

⚁ Nursing diagnoses
● Risk for infection related to presence of susceptible organisms
● Risk for deficient fluid volume related to adverse GI reactions
● Deficient knowledge related to drug therapy

▶ Planning and implementation
● Reconstitute drug for I.M. injection with 1% lidocaine hydrochloride (without epinephrine) as directed.
⚠ **ALERT:** If seizures develop and persist despite anticonvulsants, notify prescriber, stop giving the drug, and institute seizure precautions and protocols.
Patient teaching
● Instruct patient to report adverse reactions because supportive therapy may be needed.
● Warn patient about pain at injection site.

☑ Evaluation
● Patient is free from infection.

Reactions may be *common,* uncommon, *life-threatening*, or COMMON AND LIFE-THREATENING.

• Patient maintains adequate hydration throughout therapy.
• Patient and family state understanding of drug therapy.

imipramine hydrochloride
(ih-MIP-ruh-meen high-droh-KLOR-ighd)
Impril ◆ , Novo-pramine ◆ , Tofranil

imipramine pamoate
Tofranil-PM

Pharmacologic class: dibenzazepine-derivative tricyclic antidepressant
Therapeutic class: antidepressant
Pregnancy risk category: D

Indications and dosages

▶ **Depression.** *Adults:* 75 to 100 mg P.O. daily in divided doses; increase in 25- to 50-mg increments to maximum dosage. Or 25 mg P.O. daily; increase in 25-mg increments every other day. Or entire dosage may be given at bedtime. Maximum dosage is 200 mg P.O. daily for outpatients, 300 mg P.O. daily for inpatients, and 100 mg P.O. daily for elderly patients.
▶ **Enuresis.** *Children age 6 and older:* 25 mg P.O. 1 hour before bedtime. If no response within 1 week, increase dosage 50 mg nightly for children younger than age 12 or 75 mg nightly for children age 12 and older. Maximum, 2.5 mg/kg P.O. daily.
▶ **Attention-deficit/hyperactivity disorder‡.** *Children age 6 and older:* 2 to 5 mg/kg P.O. given in two to three divided daily doses.

Contraindications and cautions

• Contraindicated in patients hypersensitive to the drug or any of its components, patients receiving MAO inhibitors, and patients in acute recovery phase of MI.
• Use cautiously in patients at risk for suicide, those receiving thyroid drugs, and those with a history of urine retention or angle-closure glaucoma, increased intraocular pressure, CV disease, impaired hepatic function, hyperthyroidism, seizure disorder, or renal impairment.
⚥ **Lifespan:** In pregnant and breast-feeding women, don't use. In children, safety and effectiveness haven't been established for treating depression. In elderly patients, use lower dose

and more gradual dose increases to avoid toxicity.

Adverse reactions

CNS: confusion, *dizziness, drowsiness,* EEG changes, excitation, extrapyramidal reactions, headache, nervousness, **seizures, stroke,** tremor, weakness.
CV: *arrhythmias,* ECG changes, *heart block,* hypertension, *MI, orthostatic hypotension,* tachycardia.
EENT: *blurred vision,* mydriasis, tinnitus.
GI: anorexia, *constipation, dry mouth,* nausea, paralytic ileus, vomiting.
GU: impotence, testicular swelling, *urine retention.*
Metabolic: hyperglycemia, **hypoglycemia.**
Skin: *diaphoresis,* photosensitivity reactions, rash, urticaria.
Other: altered libido, galactorrhea and breast enlargement, gynecomastia, hypersensitivity reactions, SIADH.

Interactions

Drug-drug. *Barbiturates, CNS depressants:* May increase CNS depression. Avoid use together.
Cimetidine, methylphenidate: May increase imipramine level. Monitor patient for adverse reactions.
Clonidine: May cause loss of blood pressure control with potentially life-threatening elevations in blood pressure. Don't use together.
Epinephrine, norepinephrine: May cause life-threatening hypertensive effect. Use cautiously; monitor patient's blood pressure.
MAO inhibitors: May cause hyperpyretic crisis, severe seizures, and death. Don't use together.
SSRIs: May increase effects of tricyclic antidepressants; symptoms may persist several weeks after fluoxetine therapy stops. Monitor symptoms closely.
Drug-herb. *SAMe, St. John's wort:* May increase serotonin level. Discourage use together.
Yohimbe: May increase blood pressure effects. Avoid use together.
Drug-lifestyle. *Alcohol use:* May increase CNS depression. Discourage use together.
Smoking: May decrease imipramine level. Monitor patient for lack of effect; discourage patient from smoking.
Sun exposure: May increase risk of photosensitivity reactions. Advise patient to avoid unprotected or prolonged exposure to sunlight.

Effects on lab test results

- May increase or decrease glucose level.
- May increase liver function test values.

Pharmacokinetics

Absorption: Rapid and complete.
Distribution: Wide. 90% protein-bound.
Metabolism: By liver. A significant first-pass effect may explain variable level in different patients taking same dose.
Excretion: Mostly in urine. *Half-life:* 11 to 25 hours.

Route	Onset	Peak	Duration
P.O.	Unknown	1–2 hr	Unknown

Action

Chemical effect: Increases amount of norepinephrine, serotonin, or both in CNS by blocking their reuptake by presynaptic neurons.
Therapeutic effect: Relieves depression and childhood enuresis (hydrochloride form).

Available forms

imipramine hydrochloride
Tablets: 10 mg, 25 mg, 50 mg
imipramine pamoate
Capsules: 75 mg, 100 mg, 125 mg, 150 mg

NURSING PROCESS

⏱ Assessment

- Assess patient's condition before starting therapy and regularly thereafter.
- Observe patient closely for evidence of suicidal thoughts or behaviors until depression is relieved.
- Be alert for adverse reactions and drug interactions.
- Assess patient's and family's knowledge of drug therapy.

⊕ Nursing diagnoses

- Ineffective coping related to depression
- Deficient knowledge related to drug therapy

▷ Planning and implementation

- Give a lower dose to an elderly or a debilitated patient, an adolescent, or a patient with aggravated psychotic symptoms.
- Ⓢ **ALERT:** Drug may increase the risk of suicidal thinking and behavior in young adults ages 18

to 24 during the first 2 months of treatment. Monitor patient closely.
- Although doses can be given up to four times daily, patients also may receive entire daily dose at one time because of drug's long action.
- Don't abruptly stop giving the drug. After abruptly stopping long-term therapy, the patient may experience nausea, headache, and malaise. These symptoms don't indicate addiction. Provide supportive treatment.
- Drug causes high risk of orthostatic hypotension. Check sitting and standing blood pressures after initial dose.
- Because of hypertensive episodes during surgery in patients receiving tricyclic antidepressants, gradually stop giving the drug over several days before surgery.
- If signs of psychosis occur or increase, notify prescriber, lower the dose, and institute safety precautions.
- Ⓢ **ALERT:** Don't confuse imipramine with desipramine or amitriptyline.

Patient teaching
- Advise patient to take full dose at bedtime, but warn about possible morning orthostatic hypotension.
- Suggest taking drug with food or milk if it causes stomach upset.
- Suggest relieving dry mouth with sugarless chewing gum or hard candy. Encourage good dental prophylaxis because persistent dry mouth may increase the risk of dental caries.
- Tell patient not to drink alcohol or smoke during therapy.
- Warn patient to avoid hazardous activities until the drug's CNS effects are known.
- Warn the patient not to abruptly stop taking the drug.
- Ⓢ **ALERT:** Advise patient and his family to monitor for mood changes, especially suicidal thinking and behavior, and to report to prescriber immediately.
- Advise patient to consult prescriber before taking other prescription drugs, OTC drugs, or herbal remedies.
- Advise patient to use sunblock, wear protective clothing, and avoid prolonged exposure to sunlight to prevent photosensitivity reactions.

☑ Evaluation

- Patient behavior and communication show diminished depression.

Reactions may be *common*, uncommon, *life-threatening*, or COMMON AND LIFE-THREATENING.

• Patient and family state understanding of drug therapy.

---

immune globulin intramuscular (gamma globulin, IG, IGIM)

(ih-MYOON GLOB-yoo-lin in-truh-MUS-kyoo-ler)
GamaSTAN S/D

immune globulin intravenous (IGIV)

Carimune NF, Flebogamma, Gammagard Liquid, Gammagard S/D, Gamunex, Iveegam EN, Octagam, Polygam S/D

Pharmacologic class: immunologic drug
Therapeutic class: immune serum
Pregnancy risk category: C

Indications and dosages

▶ **Primary humoral immunodeficiency (IGIV); primary defective antibody synthesis, such as agammaglobulinemia or hypogammaglobulinemia, in patients who are at increased risk of infection.**
BayGam
Adults and children: Initially, 1.3 ml/kg I.M. Maintenance, 0.66 ml/kg (at least 100 mg/kg) every 3 to 4 weeks. Maximum single dose of IGIM is 30 to 50 ml in adults and 20 to 30 ml in infants and small children.
Carimune, Panglobulin
Adults and children: 200 mg/kg I.V. monthly. Start with 0.5 to 1 ml/minute of 3% solution; gradually increase to 2.5 ml/minute after 15 to 30 minutes.
Gammagard S/D
Adults and children: 200 to 400 mg/kg I.V.; then monthly doses of 100 mg/kg. Start infusion at 0.5 ml/kg/hour and increase to maximum of 4 ml/kg/hour. Dosage is related to patient response.
Gammar-P IV
Adults: 200 to 400 mg/kg I.V. every 3 to 4 weeks, infused at 0.01 ml/kg/minute; if no problems develop, increase to 0.02 ml/kg/minute after 15 to 30 minutes. Maximum infusion rate is 0.06 ml/kg/minute.
Adolescents and children: 200 to 400 mg/kg I.V. every 3 to 4 weeks.

Iveegam EN
Adults and children: 200 mg/kg I.V. monthly, infused at 1 to 2 ml/minute for 5% solution. May increase to maximum of 800 mg/kg or give more often to produce desired effect.
Octagam
Adults and children: 100 to 200 mg/kg I.V. monthly at 0.01 to 0.02 ml/kg/minute for 30 minutes. If no discomfort, rate can slowly be increased to a maximum of 0.08 ml/kg/minute.
Polygam S/D
Adults and children: 200 to 400 mg/kg I.V. at 0.5 ml/kg/hour, increasing to a maximum of 4 ml/kg/hour. Subsequent dose is 100 mg/kg I.V. monthly.
Venoglobulin-S
Adults and children: 200 mg/kg I.V. monthly, infused at 0.01 to 0.02 ml/kg/minute for 30 minutes; if tolerated, increase 5% solution to 0.08 ml/kg/minute and 10% solution to 0.05 ml/kg/minute. If immune globulin G levels aren't adequate, increase to 300 to 400 mg/kg and give more than once monthly.
▶ **Idiopathic thrombocytopenic purpura (IGIV).**
Carimune, Panglobulin
Adults and children: 400 mg/kg I.V. for 2 to 5 consecutive days, depending on platelet count and immune response.
Gammagard S/D, Polygam S/D
Adults and children: 1,000 mg/kg I.V. as a single dose. Give up to three doses on alternate days, if needed.
Octagam
Adults and children: 400 mg/kg of 5% solution I.V. for 5 days, or 1,000 mg/kg of 10% solution I.V. for 1 to 2 days with maintenance dosage of 10% solution at 400 to 1,000 mg/kg I.V. single infusion to maintain 30,000/mm^3 platelet count.
Venoglobulin-S
Adults and children: Maximum of 2,000 mg/kg I.V. over 5 days or less. Maintenance, 1,000 mg/kg, if needed.
▶ **Bone marrow transplant (IGIV).** *Adults older than age 20:* Give 500 mg/kg of 5% or 10% solution I.V. Octagam on days 7 and 2 before transplantation, and then weekly until 90 days after transplantation.
▶ **B-cell chronic lymphocytic leukemia (IGIV).** *Adults:* 400 mg/kg I.V. Gammagard S/D or Polygam S/D every 3 to 4 weeks.
▶ **Pediatric HIV infection (IGIV).** *Children:* 400 mg/kg I.V. once every 2 to 4 weeks.

▶ **Kawasaki syndrome (IGIV).**
Iveegam EN
Adults: 400 mg/kg I.V. daily over 2 hours for 4 consecutive days, or a single dose of 2,000 mg/kg I.V. over 10 to 12 hours. Start within 10 days of disease onset. Give with aspirin (80 to 100 mg/kg P.O. daily through day 14; then 3 to 10 mg/kg P.O. daily for 5 weeks).
Gammagard S/D, Polygam S/D
Adults: Either a single dose of 1 g/kg or 400 mg/kg I.V. daily for 4 days starting within 7 days of fever onset. Give with aspirin (80 to 100 mg/kg in four divided daily doses).

▶ **Hepatitis A exposure (IGIM).** *Adults and children:* 0.02 ml/kg I.M. as soon as possible after exposure. Up to 0.06 ml/kg may be given for prolonged or intense exposure.

▶ **Measles exposure (IGIM).** *Adults and children:* 0.02 ml/kg I.M. within 6 days after exposure.

▶ **Measles postexposure prophylaxis (IGIM).** *Immunocompromised children:* 0.5 ml/kg I.M. (maximum, 15 ml) within 6 days after exposure.

▶ **Chickenpox exposure (IGIM).** *Adults and children:* 0.6 to 1.2 ml/kg I.M. as soon as possible after exposure.

▶ **Rubella exposure in first trimester of pregnancy (IGIM).** *Women:* 0.55 ml/kg I.M. as soon as possible after exposure (within 72 hours).

▼ **I.V. administration**

● I.V. products aren't interchangeable. Gammagard requires a filter, which is supplied by the manufacturer.
● Most adverse effects are related to rapid infusion rate. Infuse slowly.
● In patients with a risk of a thrombotic event, avoid infusion solutions more concentrated than 5%, start infusion at no more than 0.5 ml/kg/hour, and speed up slowly and only if well tolerated to a maximum rate of 4 ml/kg/hour.
⊗ **Incompatibilities**
Don't mix with other I.V. drugs.

Contraindications and cautions

● Contraindicated in patients hypersensitive to the drug or any of its components, in patients with a history of an allergic response to thimerosal, and in patients with selective immune globulin A deficiencies.

● I.M. administration contraindicated in patients with severe thrombocytopenia or other coagulation-bleeding disorders.
● Use Gammagard S/D cautiously in patients with renal impairment. Renal dysfunction may occur more often with preparations stabilized in glucose (Carimune NF).
● Use caution when giving drug to patients with a history of CV disease or thrombotic episodes because I.V. drug may cause thrombotic events. The exact cause of this is unknown.
⚖ **Lifespan:** In pregnant women, use cautiously. In breast-feeding women, use cautiously because it's unknown if the drug appears in breast milk.

Adverse reactions

CNS: faintness, fever, malaise, severe headache requiring hospitalization.
CV: chest pain, *heart failure*, *MI*.
GI: nausea, vomiting.
GU: *acute renal impairment, acute tubular necrosis, nephrotic syndrome,* osmotic nephrosis.
Musculoskeletal: muscle stiffness at injection site.
Respiratory: *pulmonary embolism,* transfusion-related acute lung injury.
Skin: erythema, urticaria.
Other: *anaphylaxis.*

Interactions

Drug-drug. *Live-virus vaccines:* Antibodies in the vaccine may interfere with drug therapy. Don't give within 6 months after giving immune globulin.

Effects on lab test results

● May increase BUN and creatinine levels.

Pharmacokinetics

Absorption: Slow.
Distribution: Evenly between intravascular and extravascular spaces.
Metabolism: Unknown.
Excretion: Unknown. *Half-life:* 21 to 24 days in immunocompromised patients.

Route	Onset	Peak	Duration
I.V.	Immediate	Immediate	Unknown
I.M.	Unknown	2–5 days	Unknown

Action

Chemical effect: Provides passive immunity by increasing antibody titer. The primary component is immune globulin G.
Therapeutic effect: Helps prevent infections.

Available forms

IGIM
Injection: 150 to 180 mg of protein/ml, 2-ml and 10-ml vials
IGIV
Injection: 5% and 10% in 50-ml, 100-ml, and 200-ml vials; 5% in 1-g, 2.5-g, 5-g, and 10-g single-use bottles
Powder for injection: 50 mg protein/ml in 2.5-g, 5-g, and 10-g vials; 5-g vials (Iveegam); 1-g, 3-g, 6-g, and 12-g vials (Carimune NF)

NURSING PROCESS

Assessment
• Obtain history of allergies and reactions to immunizations.
• Observe patient for signs of anaphylaxis or other adverse reactions immediately after injection.
• Inspect injection site for local reactions.
• Monitor effectiveness by checking antibody titers after administration.
• Assess patient's and family's knowledge of drug therapy.

Nursing diagnoses
• Ineffective protection related to lack of or decreased immunity
• Ineffective breathing pattern related to anaphylaxis
• Deficient knowledge related to drug therapy

Planning and implementation
• Give I.M. injection in gluteal region. Divide any dose larger than 10 ml, and inject into several muscle sites to reduce local discomfort.
• If 6 weeks or more have passed since exposure or since symptoms have begun, don't give immune globulin to help prevent hepatitis A.
• Make sure epinephrine 1:1,000 is available in case of anaphylaxis.
ⓢ **ALERT:** I.V. and I.M. products aren't interchangeable.
Patient teaching
• Instruct patient to immediately report respiratory difficulty.

• Tell patient that local reactions may occur at injection site.
• Instruct patient to promptly notify prescriber if adverse reaction persists or becomes severe.

Evaluation
• Patient exhibits increased passive immunity.
• Patient shows no signs of anaphylaxis.
• Patient and family state understanding of drug therapy.

indapamide
(in-DAP-uh-mighd)
Lozide ◆ , Lozol

Pharmacologic class: thiazide-like diuretic
Therapeutic class: diuretic, antihypertensive
Pregnancy risk category: B

Indications and dosages

▶ **Edema.** *Adults:* Initially, 2.5 mg P.O. daily in morning. Increase to 5 mg daily after 1 week, if needed.
▶ **Hypertension.** *Adults:* Initially, 1.25 mg P.O. daily in morning. Increase to 2.5 mg daily after 4 weeks. Increase to 5 mg daily after 4 more weeks.

Contraindications and cautions

• Contraindicated in patients hypersensitive to the drug, any of its components, or other sulfonamide-derived drugs. Also contraindicated in patients with anuria.
• Use cautiously in patients with severe renal disease, impaired hepatic function, and progressive hepatic disease.
⚠ **Lifespan:** In pregnant women, use cautiously. In breast-feeding women and children, safety and effectiveness haven't been established.

Adverse reactions

CNS: *dizziness, headache,* irritability, *lightheadedness,* nervousness, weakness.
CV: orthostatic hypotension, volume depletion and dehydration.
GI: nausea, *pancreatitis.*
GU: frequent urination, nocturia, polyuria.
Metabolic: anorexia, hyperuricemia, hypochloremia, hypokalemia, hyponatremia, *metabolic alkalosis.*
Musculoskeletal: muscle cramps and spasms.

Skin: dermatitis, photosensitivity reactions, rash.
Other: gout.

Interactions

Drug-drug. *Antihypertensives:* May cause severe hypotension. Use together cautiously.
Bumetanide, ethacrynic acid, furosemide, torsemide: May cause excessive diuretic response, resulting in serious electrolyte abnormalities or dehydration. Adjust dosages carefully while monitoring the patient for excessive diuretic responses.
Diazoxide: May increase antihypertensive, hyperglycemic, and hyperuricemic effects. Use together cautiously.
Digoxin: May increase risk of digoxin toxicity from indapamide-induced hypokalemia. Monitor potassium and digoxin levels.
Lithium: May decrease lithium clearance and increase risk of toxicity. Use together cautiously.
NSAIDs: May reduce the diuretic, natriuretic, and antihypertensive effects. Monitor patient.
Drug-lifestyle. *Sun exposure:* May cause photosensitivity reactions. Avoid prolonged and unprotected exposure to sunlight.

Effects on lab test results

• May increase glucose, cholesterol, triglyceride, and uric acid levels. May decrease potassium, sodium, and chloride levels.

Pharmacokinetics

Absorption: Complete.
Distribution: Wide because of its lipophilicity. 71% to 79% protein-bound.
Metabolism: Undergoes significant hepatic metabolism.
Excretion: Mainly in urine; smaller amounts in feces. *Half-life:* About 14 hours.

Route	Onset	Peak	Duration
P.O.	1–2 hr	≤ 2 hr	≤ 36 hr

Action

Chemical effect: Unknown; probably inhibits sodium reabsorption in distal segment of nephron. Also has direct vasodilating effect, possibly from calcium channel-blocking action.
Therapeutic effect: Promotes water and sodium excretion and lowers blood pressure.

Available forms

Tablets: 1.25 mg, 2.5 mg

NURSING PROCESS

⚖ Assessment
• Assess patient's underlying condition before starting therapy.
• Monitor effectiveness by assessing fluid intake and output, weight, and blood pressure. In hypertensive patient, therapeutic response may be delayed several days.
• Monitor electrolytes and glucose levels.
• Monitor creatinine and BUN levels regularly. If these levels are more than twice normal, drug is less effective.
• Monitor uric acid level, especially if patient has history of gout.
• Be alert for adverse reactions and drug interactions.
• Assess patient's and family's knowledge of drug therapy.

⊕ Nursing diagnoses
• Risk for injury related to presence of hypertension
• Excessive fluid volume related to presence of edema
• Deficient knowledge related to drug therapy

▷ Planning and implementation
• To prevent nocturia, give drug in the morning.
• Drug may be used with potassium-sparing diuretic to prevent potassium loss.
Patient teaching
• Advise patient not to suddenly change position, and to rise slowly to avoid orthostatic hypotension.
• Advise patient to use sunblock and avoid prolonged exposure to sunlight to prevent photosensitivity reactions.
• Teach patient to monitor fluid volume by recording daily weight and intake and output.
• Tell patient to avoid high-sodium foods and to choose high-potassium foods.
• Advise patient to take drug early in day to avoid nocturia.

☑ Evaluation
• Patient's blood pressure is normal.
• Patient is free from edema.
• Patient and family state understanding of drug therapy.

Reactions may be *common*, uncommon, *life-threatening*, or COMMON AND LIFE-THREATENING.

indinavir sulfate

(in-DIH-nuh-veer SUL-fayt)

Crixivan

Pharmacologic class: protease inhibitor
Therapeutic class: antiretroviral
Pregnancy risk category: C

Indications and dosages

▶ **HIV infection.** *Adults:* 800 mg P.O. every 8 hours, 1 hour before or 2 hours after a meal.

Adjust-a-dose: For patients with mild to moderate hepatic insufficiency resulting in cirrhosis, reduce dosage to 600 mg P.O. every 8 hours.

Contraindications and cautions

• Contraindicated in patients hypersensitive to the drug or any of its components.
• Contraindicated in patients also taking amiodarone, ergot derivatives, midazolam, triazolam, cisapride, or pimozide.
• Use cautiously and at a reduced dosage in patients with hepatic insufficiency.

Lifespan: In pregnant women, use only if benefits outweigh risks to fetus. In breastfeeding women, use cautiously because it isn't known if drug appears in breast milk. In children, safety and effectiveness haven't been established.

Adverse reactions

CNS: asthenia, dizziness, fatigue, headache, insomnia, malaise, somnolence.
GI: *abdominal pain,* acid regurgitation, anorexia, diarrhea, dry mouth, *nausea,* taste perversion, vomiting.
GU: *acute renal failure, nephrolithiasis.*
Hematologic: *hemolytic anemia, neutropenia.*
Hepatic: *hepatic failure,* hyperbilirubinemia.
Metabolic: *hyperglycemia, new onset diabetes mellitus.*
Musculoskeletal: back pain, flank pain.
Other: redistribution and accumulation of body fat.

Interactions

Drug-drug. *Amiodarone, cisapride, ergot derivatives, pimozide:* May be fatal. Don't give together.

Amprenavir, saquinavir: May increase levels of these drugs. Dosage adjustments probably aren't needed.
Carbamazepine: May decrease indinavir level. Avoid use together.
Clarithromycin: May alter clarithromycin level. Monitor patient.
Delavirdine, itraconazole, ketoconazole: May increase indinavir level. Consider reducing indinavir dosage to 600 mg every 8 hours.
Didanosine: May need normal gastric pH for optimal absorption of indinavir. Give these drugs and indinavir at least 1 hour apart on an empty stomach.
Efavirenz, nevirapine: May decrease indinavir level. Increase indinavir to 1,000 mg every 8 hours.
HMG-CoA reductase inhibitors: May increase levels of these drugs and increase risk of myopathy and rhabdomyolysis. Avoid use together.
Midazolam, triazolam: May inhibit metabolism of these drugs (because of competition for CYP3A4 by indinavir) and increase risk of serious or life-threatening events, such as arrhythmias or prolonged sedation. Don't give together.
Nelfinavir: May increase levels of indinavir by 50% and nelfinavir by 80%. Monitor patient closely.
Rifabutin: May increase rifabutin level and decrease indinavir level. Give indinavir 1,000 mg every 8 hours and decrease rifabutin to either 150 mg daily or 300 mg two to three times weekly.
Rifampin: May significantly decrease indinavir level because rifampin is a potent inducer of CYP3A4. Avoid use together.
Ritonavir: May increase indinavir level by two to five times. Adjust dosage to indinavir 400 mg b.i.d. and ritonavir 400 mg b.i.d., or indinavir 800 mg b.i.d. and ritonavir 100 to 200 mg b.i.d.
Sildenafil, tadalafil, vardenafil: May increase levels of these drugs and the risk of adverse effects (hypotension, visual changes, priapism). Tell patient not to exceed 25 mg of sildenafil in a 48-hour period, 10 mg of tadalafil in a 72-hour period, or 2.5 mg vardenafil in a 24-hour period.
Drug-herb. *St. John's wort:* May reduce indinavir level by more than 50%. Discourage use together.
Drug-food. *Any food:* May substantially decrease absorption of oral indinavir. Give drug on an empty stomach.

Grapefruit juice: May decrease level and therapeutic effect of indinavir. Advise patient to take drug with liquid other than grapefruit juice.

Effects on lab test results

• May increase ALT, AST, bilirubin, amylase, triglyceride, cholesterol, and glucose levels. May decrease hemoglobin level and hematocrit.
• May decrease neutrophil and platelet counts.

Pharmacokinetics

Absorption: Rapid.
Distribution: 60% protein-bound.
Metabolism: By liver and kidneys.
Excretion: In urine. *Half-life:* 2 hours.

Route	Onset	Peak	Duration
P.O.	Unknown	< 1 hr	1–8 hr

Action

Chemical effect: Binds to and inhibits protease active sites. Prevents cleavage of viral polyproteins, resulting in formation of immature, noninfectious viral particles.
Therapeutic effect: Reduces symptoms of HIV.

Available forms

Capsules: 100 mg, 200 mg, 333 mg, 400 mg

NURSING PROCESS

Assessment
• Monitor adverse reactions and drug interactions.
• Assess patient's and family's knowledge of drug therapy.

Nursing diagnoses
• Risk for infection related to presence of virus
• Risk for deficient fluid volume related to effect on kidneys
• Deficient knowledge related to drug therapy

Planning and implementation
• Give at least 48 oz (1.5 L) of fluids every 24 hours to maintain adequate hydration.
• Give drug on an empty stomach, 1 hour before or 2 hours after a meal.
Patient teaching
• Instruct patient to use barrier contraception.
• If patient misses a dose, advise him to take the next dose at regularly scheduled time and not to double the dose.

• Instruct patient to take drug on an empty stomach with water 1 hour before or 2 hours after a meal.
• Instruct patient to store capsules in the original container and to keep the desiccant in the bottle.
• Instruct patient to drink at least 48 oz (1.5 L) of fluid daily.
• Advise HIV-positive women to prevent transmitting virus to infant by not breast-feeding.
• Instruct patient to promptly report evidence of nephrolithiasis (flank pain, hematuria) or diabetes (increased thirst, polyuria).
• Advise patient taking sildenafil, tadalafil, or vardenafil that he may be at increased risk for adverse reactions, such as hypotension, visual changes, and priapism, and that he should promptly report any symptoms to prescriber. Patient shouldn't take more than 25 mg of sildenafil in a 48-hour period, 10 mg of tadalafil in a 72-hour period, or 2.5 mg of vardenafil in a 24-hour period.

Evaluation
• Patient's health improves, and signs and symptoms of underlying condition diminish with use of drug.
• Patient maintains adequate hydration.
• Patient and family state understanding of drug therapy.

indomethacin
(in-doh-METH-uh-sin)
Indocid ♦ , Indocin*, Indocin SR, Novo-Methacin ♦ , Nu-Indo, Pro-Indo, Rhodacine

indomethacin sodium trihydrate
Indocid PDA ♦ , Indocin I.V.

Pharmacologic class: NSAID
Therapeutic class: analgesic, antipyretic, anti-inflammatory
Pregnancy risk category: C (D in third trimester)

Indications and dosages

▶ **Moderate to severe rheumatoid arthritis or osteoarthritis, ankylosing spondylitis.**
Adults: 25 mg P.O. b.i.d. or t.i.d. with food or antacids. Increase by 25 mg or 50 mg daily every 7 days up to 200 mg daily. Or 50 mg P.R.

q.i.d. Or 75-mg sustained-release capsule P.O. to start, in morning or at bedtime, followed, if needed, by another 75 mg b.i.d.

▶ **Acute gouty arthritis.** *Adults:* 50 mg P.O. t.i.d. Reduce dose as soon as possible; then stop. Don't use sustained-release capsules.

▶ **Acute painful shoulders (bursitis or tendinitis).** *Adults:* 75 to 150 mg P.O. daily t.i.d. or q.i.d. with food or antacids for 7 to 14 days.

▶ **To close hemodynamically significant patent ductus arteriosus in premature infants.** *Neonates less than 48 hours old:* 0.2 mg/kg I.V. followed by two doses of 0.1 mg/kg at 12- to 24-hour intervals.
Neonates ages 2 to 7 days: 0.2 mg/kg I.V. followed by two doses of 0.2 mg/kg at 12- to 24-hour intervals.
Neonates more than 7 days old: 0.2 mg/kg I.V. followed by two doses of 0.25 mg/kg at 12- to 24-hour intervals.

▶ **Pericarditis‡.** *Adults:* 75 to 200 mg P.O. daily in three to four divided doses.

▶ **Dysmenorrhea‡.** *Adults:* 25 mg P.O. t.i.d. with food or antacids.

▶ **Bartter syndrome‡.** *Adults:* 150 mg P.O. daily with food or antacids.
Children: 0.5 to 2 mg/kg P.O. in divided doses.

▼ I.V. administration

• Reconstitute powder for injection with sterile water for injection or normal saline solution. For each 1-mg vial, add 1 ml of diluent to yield 1 mg/ml; add 2 ml of diluent to yield 0.5 mg/ml.
• Use only preservative-free diluents to prepare I.V. injection. Never use diluents containing benzyl alcohol because it has been linked to fatal gasping syndrome in neonates. Because injection contains no preservatives, reconstitute immediately before administration and discard unused solution.
• Give by direct injection over 20 to 30 minutes per published literature although the optimum rate has not been established by the manufacturer.
• If patient has anuria or marked oliguria, don't give second or third scheduled I.V. dose; instead, notify prescriber.

⊗ **Incompatibilities**
Amino acid injection, calcium gluconate, cimetidine, dextrose injection, dobutamine, dopa-

mine, gentamicin, levofloxacin, solutions with pH less than 6, tobramycin sulfate, tolazoline.

Contraindications and cautions

• Contraindicated in patients hypersensitive to the drug or any of its components and in those with a history of aspirin- or NSAID-induced asthma, rhinitis, or urticaria. Suppositories contraindicated in patients with a history of proctitis or recent rectal bleeding.
• Because of its high risk of adverse effects during prolonged use, don't use drug routinely as analgesic or antipyretic.
• Use cautiously in patients with epilepsy, parkinsonism, hepatic or renal disease, CV disease, infection, mental illness or depression, or history of GI disease.
⚕ **Lifespan:** In pregnant and breast-feeding women, drug is contraindicated. In children younger than age 14, safety and effectiveness haven't been established by manufacturer. In infants with untreated infection, active bleeding, coagulation defects, thrombocytopenia, congenital heart disease (in whom patency of ductus arteriosus is needed for satisfactory pulmonary or systemic blood flow), necrotizing enterocolitis, or renal impairment, drug is contraindicated. In elderly patients, use cautiously.

Adverse reactions

P.O. and P.R.
CNS: confusion, drowsiness, depression, *dizziness, headache,* peripheral neuropathy, psychic disturbances, *seizures,* syncope, vertigo.
CV: edema, *heart failure,* hypertension.
EENT: blurred vision, corneal and retinal damage, hearing loss, tinnitus.
GI: anorexia, diarrhea, *GI bleeding,* nausea, peptic ulceration, vomiting.
GU: *acute renal failure,* hematuria.
Hematologic: *aplastic anemia, agranulocytosis,* hemolytic anemia, iron-deficiency anemia, *leukopenia, thrombocytopenic purpura.*
Metabolic: *hyperkalemia.*
Respiratory: respiratory distress.
Skin: pruritus, rash, *Stevens-Johnson syndrome,* urticaria.
Other: *anaphylaxis, angioedema,* hypersensitivity reactions.
I.V.
GI: *GI bleeding,* vomiting.
GU: azotemia, renal dysfunction.

Metabolic: *hyperkalemia, hypoglycemia,* hyponatremia.
Respiratory: *respiratory distress.*
Other: *anaphylaxis, angioedema,* hypersensitivity reactions, rash.

Interactions

Drug-drug. *Aminoglycosides, cyclosporine, methotrexate:* May increase toxicity of these drugs. Avoid use together.
Antihypertensives: May decrease antihypertensive effect. Monitor blood pressure closely.
Aspirin: May decrease indomethacin level and increase the risk of GI toxicity. Avoid use together.
Corticosteroids: May increase risk of GI toxicity. Don't use together.
Diflunisal, probenecid: May decrease indomethacin excretion. Monitor patient for increased adverse reactions to indomethacin.
Digoxin: May prolong digoxin half-life. Use together cautiously; monitor digoxin level.
Dipyridamole: May enhance fluid retention. Avoid use together.
Furosemide, thiazide diuretics: May impair response to both drugs. Avoid using together, if possible.
Lithium: May increase lithium level. Monitor patient for lithium toxicity.
Triamterene: May cause nephrotoxicity. Monitor patient closely.
Drug-herb. *Dong quai, feverfew, garlic, ginger, horse chestnut, red clover:* May increase risk of bleeding. Monitor patient closely for bleeding.
Senna: May block laxative effects. Discourage use together.
St. John's wort: May increase risk of photosensitivity. Advise patient to avoid unprotected or prolonged exposure to sunlight.
Drug-lifestyle. *Alcohol use:* May increase risk of GI toxicity. Discourage use together.

Effects on lab test results

• May increase AST, ALT, BUN, creatinine, and potassium levels. May decrease glucose, sodium, and hemoglobin levels and hematocrit.
• May decrease WBC, granulocyte, and platelet counts.

Pharmacokinetics

Absorption: Rapid and complete.
Distribution: Highly protein-bound.
Metabolism: In liver.

Excretion: Mainly in urine, with some biliary excretion. *Half-life:* 4¼ hours.

Route	Onset	Peak	Duration
P.O.	30 min	1–4 hr	4–6 hr
I.V.	Immediate	Immediate	Unknown
P.R.	2–4 hr	Unknown	4–6 hr

Action

Chemical effect: Unknown; produces anti-inflammatory, analgesic, and antipyretic effects, possibly by inhibiting prostaglandin synthesis.
Therapeutic effect: Relieves pain, fever, and inflammation.

Available forms

indomethacin
Capsules: 25 mg, 50 mg
Capsules (sustained-release): 75 mg
Oral suspension: 25 mg/5 ml
Suppositories: 50 mg
indomethacin sodium trihydrate
Injection: 1-mg vials

NURSING PROCESS

Assessment
• Assess patient's condition before starting therapy and regularly thereafter.
• Monitor patient carefully for bleeding and for reduced urine output during I.V. use.
• Be alert for adverse reactions and drug interactions.
• Assess patient's and family's knowledge of drug therapy.

Nursing diagnoses
• Chronic pain related to underlying condition
• Risk for injury related to adverse reactions
• Deficient knowledge related to drug therapy

Planning and implementation
• If GI upset occurs, give oral form of drug with food, milk, or antacid.
• If ductus arteriosus reopens, give second course of one to three doses. If ineffective, surgery may be needed.
• If patient has bleeding or reduced urine output, stop giving the drug and notify prescriber.
• Drug may enhance hypothalamic-pituitary-adrenal axis response to dexamethasone suppression test.
• Notify prescriber if drug is ineffective.

Patient teaching

• Tell patient to take oral form of drug with food, milk, or antacid if GI upset occurs.
• Inform patient that use of oral form with aspirin, alcohol, or corticosteroids may increase risk of adverse GI reactions.
• Teach patient signs and symptoms of GI bleeding, and tell him to report them to prescriber. Serious GI toxicity, including peptic ulceration and bleeding despite absence of GI symptoms, can occur in patients taking oral NSAIDs.
• Instruct patient not to drink alcohol during therapy.
• Tell patient to notify prescriber immediately about visual or hearing changes. Patient receiving long-term oral therapy should have regular eye and hearing examinations, CBC, and renal function tests to detect toxicity.
• Advise patient to avoid hazardous activities if adverse CNS reactions occur.

☑ Evaluation

• Patient is free from pain.
• Patient doesn't experience injury from adverse reactions.
• Patient and family state understanding of drug therapy.

infliximab
(in-FLICKS-ih-mab)
Remicade

Pharmacologic class: monoclonal antibody
Therapeutic class: anti-inflammatory
Pregnancy risk category: B

Indications and dosages

▶ **Moderate to severe active Crohn disease; to reduce the number of draining fistulas and maintain fistula closure in patients with Crohn disease.** *Adults:* 5 mg/kg by I.V. infusion over at least 2 hours, given as an induction regimen at 0, 2, and 6 weeks, followed by a maintenance regimen of 5 mg/kg every 8 weeks thereafter. For adults who respond and then stop responding, consider giving 10 mg/kg. Patients who don't respond by week 14 are unlikely to respond to continued therapy; consider stopping drug.

▶ **Moderate to severe active Crohn disease.** *Children:* 5 mg/kg given as I.V. induction regimen at 0, 2, and 6 weeks, followed by a maintenance regimen of 5 mg/kg every 8 weeks.
▶ **Moderate to severe active rheumatoid arthritis, with methotrexate.** *Adults:* 3 mg/kg by I.V. infusion over at least 2 hours. Give additional doses of 3 mg/kg at 2 and 6 weeks after initial infusion and every 8 weeks thereafter. If response is inadequate, increase to 10 mg/kg or give every 4 weeks.
▶ **Ankylosing spondylitis.** *Adults:* 5 mg/kg by I.V. infusion over at least 2 hours. Give additional doses of 5 mg/kg at 2 and 6 weeks after first infusion and then every 6 weeks thereafter.
▶ **Psoriatic arthritis, with or without methotrexate.** *Adults:* 5 mg/kg by I.V. infusion over at least 2 hours. Give additional doses of 5 mg/kg at 2 and 6 weeks after first infusion and then every 8 weeks thereafter.
▶ **Moderate to severe ulcerative colitis.** *Adults:* Induction dose, 5 mg/kg I.V. over 2 hours given at 0, 2, and 6 weeks, followed by a maintenance dose of 5 mg/kg every 8 weeks thereafter.
▶ **Chronic severe plaque psoriasis.** *Adults:* 5 mg/kg by I.V. infusion over at least 2 hours. Repeat dosage in 2 and 6 weeks; then give 5 mg/kg every 8 weeks thereafter.

▽ I.V. administration

• Drug is incompatible with plasticized polyvinyl chloride equipment or devices; prepare only in glass infusion bottles or polypropylene or polyolefin infusion bags.
• Give through polyethylene-lined administration sets with an in-line, sterile, nonpyrogenic, low–protein-binding filter (pore size of 1.2 mm or less).
• Reconstitute with 10 ml sterile solution for injection using syringe with 21G or smaller needle. Don't shake; gently swirl to dissolve powder. Solution should be colorless to light yellow and opalescent; it may contain a few translucent particles. If you see other particles or discoloration, don't use.
• Vials don't contain antibacterial preservatives; use reconstituted drug immediately.
• Dilute total volume of reconstituted drug to 250 ml with normal saline solution for injection. Infusion concentration range is 0.4 to 4 mg/ml.
• Infuse within 3 hours of preparation and for at least 2 hours after starting.

• If an infusion reaction occurs, stop the infusion, notify prescriber, and give acetaminophen, antihistamines, corticosteroids, and epinephrine.
⊗ **Incompatibilities**
Other I.V. drugs.

Contraindications and cautions

• Contraindicated in patients hypersensitive to murine proteins or any other of the drug's components.
• In patients with mild heart failure (New York Heart Association [NYHA] Class I or II), use cautiously. Doses greater than 5 mg/kg are contraindicated in patients with moderate to severe heart failure (NYHA Class III or IV).
• Use cautiously in patients with a history of hematologic abnormalities or those with CNS demyelinating or seizure disorders.
⚖ **Lifespan:** In pregnant women, give only if benefits outweigh risks to fetus. In breast-feeding women, stop breast-feeding or don't use the drug. In elderly patients, use cautiously.

Adverse reactions

CNS: depression, dizziness, *fatigue, fever, headache,* insomnia, malaise, pain, systemic and cutaneous vasculitis.
CV: chest pain, flushing, *hypertension,* hypotension, *pericardial effusion,* peripheral edema, tachycardia.
EENT: conjunctivitis, *pharyngitis,* rhinitis, *sinusitis.*
GI: *abdominal pain,* constipation, *diarrhea, dyspepsia,* flatulence, intestinal obstruction, mouth pain, *nausea,* ulcerative stomatitis, vomiting.
GU: dysuria, increased urinary frequency, *UTI.*
Hematologic: anemia, hematoma, *leukopenia, neutropenia, pancytopenia.*
Musculoskeletal: *arthralgia,* arthritis, *back pain,* myalgia.
Respiratory: *bronchitis, coughing,* dyspnea, *upper respiratory tract infection.*
Skin: acne, alopecia, candidiasis, dry skin, ecchymosis, eczema, erythema, erythematous rash, increased sweating, maculopapular rash, papular rash, pruritus, *rash,* urticaria.
Other: abscess, chills, flulike syndrome, hot flushes, hypersensitivity reaction, *severe opportunistic infections,* toothache, tuberculosis.

Interactions

Drug-drug. *Anakinra:* May increase the risk of serious infection and neutropenia. Avoid use together.
Live-virus vaccines: No data are available on response to vaccines or on the secondary transmission of infection by live-virus vaccines. Don't use together.

Effects on lab test results

• May increase liver enzyme levels. May decrease hemoglobin level and hematocrit.

Pharmacokinetics

Absorption: Given I.V.
Distribution: Mainly in the vascular compartment.
Metabolism: Unknown.
Excretion: Unknown. *Half-life:* 9½ days.

Route	Onset	Peak	Duration
I.V.	Unknown	Unknown	Unknown

Action

Chemical effect: Binds to tumor necrosis factor (TNF)-alpha to neutralize it and inhibit its binding with receptors, reducing the infiltration of inflammatory cells and production of TNF-alpha in inflamed areas of the intestine.
Therapeutic effect: Relieves inflammation.

Available forms

Injection: 100-mg vials

NURSING PROCESS

↗ Assessment
• Obtain history of patient's underlying condition before starting therapy, and reassess regularly.
• Use in Crohn disease and ulcerative colitis only after patient has had an inadequate response to conventional therapy.
• Observe patient for infusion-related reactions, including fever, chills, pruritus, urticaria, dyspnea, hypotension, hypertension, and chest pain, within 2 hours of infusion.
• Monitor liver function test results.
• Observe patient for development of lymphomas and infection. Patients with chronic Crohn disease and long-term exposure to immunosuppressants are more likely to develop lymphomas and infections.

• Consider stopping treatment in patient who develops significant hematologic abnormalities or CNS adverse reactions.
• Drug may affect normal immune responses. Monitor patient for development of autoimmune antibodies and lupus-like syndrome; stop giving the drug if symptoms develop. Symptoms should resolve.
• Tuberculosis, invasive fungal infections, and other fatal opportunistic infections may occur.
• In patient with heart failure, monitor patient's cardiac status.
• Assess patient's and family's knowledge of drug therapy.

Nursing diagnoses
• Chronic pain related to inflammation of the GI tract
• Imbalanced nutrition: less than body requirements related to underlying medical condition
• Deficient knowledge related to drug therapy

Planning and implementation
• If patient develops new or worsening symptoms of heart failure, notify the prescriber.
ALERT: Don't confuse infliximab with rituximab.
• Patient may develop tuberculosis, invasive fungal infections, or other opportunistic infection. Test patient for latent tuberculosis infection with a tuberculin skin test. Start treatment of latent tuberculosis infection before therapy.
• Patient may develop histoplasmosis, listeriosis, and pneumocystosis. For patients who have lived in regions where histoplasmosis is endemic, carefully consider the benefits and risks before starting therapy.
Patient teaching
• Tell patient about infusion reaction symptoms and the need to report them to prescriber.
• Inform patient of postinfusion adverse effects, and tell him to promptly report them.
• Advise patient to seek immediate medical attention for signs and symptoms of infection or strange or unusual bleeding or bruising.
• Advise parent to have child up-to-date for all vaccines before therapy starts.

Evaluation
• Patient is free from pain.
• Patient maintains adequate nutrition.
• Patient and family state understanding of drug therapy.

influenza virus vaccine live, intranasal
(inn-floo-EHN-zah VY-russ vack-SEEN LYV inn-truh-NAZ-ul)
FluMist

Pharmacologic class: neuraminidase inhibitor
Therapeutic class: antiviral
Pregnancy risk category: C

Indications and dosages
▶ **Active immunization for influenza A and B viruses.** *Adults and children ages 9 to 49:* Give 0.2 ml per season (0.1 ml per nostril).
Children ages 2 to 8 (not previously vaccinated with FluMist): Two doses of 0.2 ml each (0.1 ml per nostril), at least 1 month apart.
Children ages 2 to 8 (previously vaccinated with FluMist): 0.2 ml per season (0.1 ml per nostril).

Contraindications and cautions
• Contraindicated in patients hypersensitive to the drug or any of its components, including eggs or egg products. Also contraindicated in patients who may be immunosuppressed or have altered or compromised immune status as a consequence of treatment with systemic corticosteroids, alkylating drugs, antimetabolites, radiation, or other immunosuppressive therapies. Contraindicated in patients with known or suspected immune deficiency diseases, such as combined immunodeficiency, agammaglobulinemia, or thymic abnormalities; conditions such as HIV infection, malignancy, leukemia, or lymphoma; or a history of Guillain-Barré syndrome or asthma or reactive airway disease.
Lifespan: In pregnant women, drug is contraindicated. In breast-feeding women, use cautiously because it's unknown if drug appears in breast milk. In children ages 2 to 17 receiving aspirin or drugs that contain aspirin, drug is contraindicated because of the link with Reye syndrome. Contraindicated in children younger than 5 years with recurrent wheezing, unless benefits outweigh the risk. In children younger than age 2 and adults age 50 and older, safety and effectiveness haven't been established.

Adverse reactions
CNS: fever, headache, irritability.
EENT: nasal congestion, runny nose, sore throat.

GI: vomiting.
Musculoskeletal: muscle aches.
Respiratory: cough.
Other: chills, decreased activity.

Interactions

Drug-drug. *Antivirals active against influenza A or B viruses:* May cause synergistic or decreased effect. Wait 48 hours after stopping antiviral therapy before giving vaccine. Don't give antivirals within 2 weeks of vaccine.
Aspirin: May cause Reye syndrome. Avoid use together.

Effects on lab test results

None reported.

Pharmacokinetics

Absorption: Unknown.
Distribution: Unknown.
Metabolism: Unknown.
Excretion: Unknown. *Half-life:* Unknown.

Route	Onset	Peak	Duration
Intranasal	Unknown	Unknown	Unknown

Action

Chemical effect: May play a role in prevention and recovery from infection. Induces influenza strain-specific serum antibodies.
Therapeutic effect: Protects against influenza.

Available forms

Intranasal spray: 0.2 ml pre-filled, single use

NURSING PROCESS

Assessment
● Assess patient's health and immune status.
● To prevent allergic or other adverse reaction, review patient's history for possible sensitivity to influenza vaccine components, including eggs and egg products.
● Be alert for adverse reactions.
● Assess patient's and family's knowledge of therapy.

Nursing diagnoses
● Risk for infection related to influenza A and B virus
● Deficient knowledge related to vaccine therapy

Planning and implementation
ALERT: Keep epinephrine injection (1:1,000) or compatible treatment readily available in case of an acute anaphylactic reaction.
● Don't give drug until at least 72 hours after a patient's fever has started.
● Advise vaccine recipient and the parents of immunized child to avoid close contact within the same household with immunocompromised people for at least 21 days.
● Report adverse reactions. The U.S. Department of Health and Human Services has established a Vaccine Adverse Event Reporting System to manage reports of suspected adverse reactions for any vaccine (1-800-822-7967). Reporting forms may also be obtained at the FDA Web site (http://vaers.hhs.gov).
● Give drug before exposure to influenza. The peak of influenza varies from year to year, but typically occurs between late December and early March. Because the duration of protection from drug isn't known and yearly variation in the influenza strains is possible, revaccinate annually to increase the likelihood of protection.
● Don't give with other vaccines.
● Drug may not protect 100% of patients.
● Thaw drug before giving. To thaw, hold the sprayer in the palm of the hand and support the plunger rod with the thumb. Give the vaccine immediately. Or thaw drug in a refrigerator, and store at 36° to 46° F (2° to 8° C) for no more than 24 hours before use. When thawed, drug is a colorless to pale yellow liquid that's clear to slightly cloudy. Some particulates may be present, but they don't affect use.
● Give half contents of sprayer into each nostril while the recipient is in an upright position. Insert the tip of the sprayer just inside the nose, and depress the plunger to spray. The dose-divider clip is removed from the sprayer to give the second half of the dose into the other nostril.
● Formulation changes seasonally. Check package insert for dosage changes.

Patient teaching
● Inform parents of children ages 2 to 8 that two doses of the drug are required the first time it's used.
● Tell patient to avoid close contact within the same household with immunocompromised people for at least 21 days.
● Instruct patient to report any suspected adverse reaction to the prescriber or clinic where the vaccine was given.

Reactions may be *common*, uncommon, *life-threatening*, or COMMON AND LIFE-THREATENING.

- Inform patient that annual revaccination may increase the likelihood of protection and that not every person who receives the vaccine will be protected.

✔ Evaluation
- Patient remains free from adverse effects of the therapy.
- Patient does not contract influenza A or B virus.
- Patient and family state understanding of vaccine therapy.

---

insulin aspart (rDNA origin) injection
(IN-suh-lin AS-part)
NovoLog

insulin aspart (rDNA origin) protamine suspension and insulin aspart (rDNA origin) injection
NovoLog 70/30

Pharmacologic class: human insulin analogue
Therapeutic class: antidiabetic
Pregnancy risk category: B

Indications and dosages

▶ **Control of hyperglycemia in diabetes mellitus.** *Adults and children age 6 and older:* 0.5 to 1 unit/kg NovoLog subcutaneously daily within 5 to 10 minutes of start of meal. About 50% to 70% of the daily insulin requirement may be provided by this drug and the remainder by intermediate-acting or long-acting insulin. Initially, dosage for NovoLog external insulin infusion pumps is based on the total daily insulin dosage of the previous regimen. Give 50% of the total dosage as a bolus at mealtime and the remainder as basal infusion. Adjust dosage as needed. Or give NovoLog 70/30 b.i.d. within 15 minutes of meals.

Contraindications and cautions

- Contraindicated during episodes of hypoglycemia and in patients hypersensitive to Novo-Log or its excipients.
- Use cautiously in patients prone to hypoglycemia and hypokalemia, such as patients who are fasting, have autonomic neuropathy, or are us-

ing potassium-lowering drugs or drugs sensitive to potassium levels.

⚖ **Lifespan:** In breast-feeding women, use cautiously because it's unknown if drug appears in breast milk. In children younger than age 6, safety and effectiveness haven't been established.

Adverse reactions
Metabolic: *hyperkalemia, hypoglycemia.*
Skin: lipodystrophy, pruritus, rash.
Other: allergic reactions, injection site reactions.

Interactions
Drug-drug. *ACE inhibitors, disopyramide, fibrates, fluoxetine, MAO inhibitors, oral antidiabetics, propoxyphene, salicylates, somatostatin analogue (octreotide), sulfonamide antibiotics:* May enhance the blood glucose–lowering effects of insulin and increase risk of hypoglycemia. Monitor glucose level and signs of hypoglycemia. May require insulin dosage adjustment.
Beta blockers, clonidine, guanethidine, reserpine: May mask symptoms of hypoglycemia. Use cautiously in patients with diabetes.
Corticosteroids, danazol, diuretics, estrogens, isoniazid, niacin, phenothiazine derivatives, progestogens (hormonal contraceptives), somatropin, sympathomimetics (such as epinephrine, salbutamol, terbutaline), thyroid hormones: May reduce the blood glucose–lowering effect of insulin and may cause hyperglycemia. Monitor glucose level. May require insulin dosage adjustment.
Lithium salts, pentamidine: May enhance or weaken blood glucose–lowering effect of insulin, causing hypoglycemia or hyperglycemia. Pentamidine may cause hypoglycemia, which may sometimes be followed by hyperglycemia. Monitor glucose level.
Drug-lifestyle. *Alcohol use:* May increase the blood glucose–lowering effects of insulin. Discourage use together.
Marijuana use: May increase glucose level. Tell patient about this interaction.
Smoking: May increase glucose level and decrease response to insulin. Discourage patient from smoking; have patient monitor glucose level closely.

Effects on lab test results
- May decrease glucose and potassium levels.

Pharmacokinetics

Absorption: Bioavailable as regular human insulin. Faster absorption and onset and shorter duration of action compared to regular human insulin.
Distribution: 0% to 9% protein-bound, similar to regular insulin.
Metabolism: Unknown.
Excretion: Unknown. *Half-life:* 81 minutes.

Route	Onset	Peak	Duration
SubQ			
NovoLog	15–30 min	1–3 hr	3–5 hr
NovoLog 70/30	Rapid	1–4 hr	24 hr

Action

Chemical effect: Binds to insulin receptors on muscle and fat cells, lowers glucose level, facilitates the cellular uptake of glucose, and inhibits the output of glucose from the liver.
Therapeutic effect: Lowers glucose level.

Available forms

10-ml vial for injection: 100 units/ml
3-ml PenFill cartridges: 100 units/ml
3-ml FlexPen prefilled syringe: 100 units/ml

NURSING PROCESS

� Assessment

• Assess underlying condition before starting therapy, and reassess regularly.
• Monitor glucose level before starting therapy and regularly throughout therapy.
• Monitor patient's glycosylated hemoglobin level regularly.
• Monitor urine ketones when glucose level is elevated.
• Monitor patient for injection-site reactions.
• Monitor patient with an external insulin pump for erythematous, pruritic, or thickened skin at injection site.
• Assess patient's and family's knowledge of drug therapy.

� Nursing diagnoses

• Risk for impaired skin integrity related to adverse drug effects
• Risk for injury related to drug-induced hypoglycemia
• Deficient knowledge related to insulin aspart therapy

� Planning and implementation

• Give NovoLog 5 to 10 minutes before the start of a meal. Give NovoLog 70/30 up to 15 minutes before the start of a meal. Because of drug's rapid onset and short duration of action, patients may need the addition of longer-acting insulins to prevent before-meal hyperglycemia.
• Give subcutaneously into the abdominal wall, thigh, or upper arm. Rotate sites to minimize lipodystrophies.
• Monitor patient for hypoglycemia, which may occur as a result of an excess of insulin relative to food intake, energy expenditure, or both. The warning signs and symptoms of hypoglycemia include shaking, sweating, dizziness, fatigue, hunger, irritability, confusion, blurred vision, headaches, or nausea and vomiting. Treat mild episodes of hypoglycemia with oral glucose. Adjust drug dosage, meal patterns, or exercise, if needed. Treat more severe episodes involving coma, seizure, or neurologic impairment with I.M. or subcutaneous glucagon or concentrated I.V. glucose. Sustain carbohydrate intake and observe because hypoglycemia may recur.
• Look at insulin vial before use. NovoLog should appear as a clear, colorless solution. It should never contain particulate matter, appear cloudy or viscous, or be discolored. NovoLog 70/30 should appear uniformly white and cloudy and should never contain particulate matter or be discolored.
• Don't use drug after its expiration date. Discard after expiration date.
• Store drug between 36° and 46° F (2° and 8° C). Don't freeze. Don't expose vials to excessive heat or sunlight. Open vials are stable at room temperature for 28 days.
• ⑤ ALERT: Pump or infusion-set malfunctions or insulin degradation can lead to hyperglycemia and ketosis in a short time because of a subcutaneous depot of fast-acting insulin.
• Don't dilute or mix insulin aspart with any other insulin when using an external insulin pump.
• Insulin aspart is recommended for use with Disetronic H-TRON plus V100 with Disetronic 3.15 plastic cartridges and Classic or Tender infusion sets, and MiniMed Models 505, 506, and 507 with MiniMed 3-ml syringes and Polyfin or Sof-set infusion sets. The use of insulin aspart in quick-release infusion sets and cartridge adapters has not been assessed.
• Replace infusion sets and insulin aspart in the reservoir and choose a new infusion site every

---

Reactions may be *common*, uncommon, *life-threatening*, or COMMON AND LIFE-THREATENING.

48 hours or less to avoid insulin degradation and infusion set malfunction.

• Discard drug exposed to temperatures higher than 98.6° F (37° C). The temperature may exceed room temperature when the pump housing, cover, tubing, or sport case is exposed to sunlight or radiant heat.

⚠ **ALERT:** Spell out "units" to reduce the risk of error of misreading "U" as a zero.

⚠ **ALERT:** Don't confuse NovoLog 70/30 with Novolin 70/30.

⚠ **ALERT:** Don't confuse NovoLog with Novolin or Humalog.

Patient teaching
• Inform patient of the drug's risks and benefits.
• Teach patient to recognize symptoms of hypoglycemia and hyperglycemia and how to treat them.
• Instruct patient on injection techniques, timing of dose to meals, adherence to meal planning, importance of regular glucose monitoring and periodic glycosylated hemoglobin testing, and proper storage of insulin.
• Tell woman to notify prescriber if she plans to become or becomes pregnant. Information on drug in pregnancy or lactation isn't available.
• Instruct patient to report changes at injection site, including redness, itchiness, or thickened skin.
• Tell patient not to dilute or mix insulin aspart with any other insulin when using an external insulin pump.
• Teach patient how to properly use the external insulin pump.

☑ **Evaluation**
• Patient doesn't experience adverse reactions from drug.
• Patient's glucose level is within the normal range.
• Patient and family state understanding of drug therapy.

HIGH ALERT

insulin detemir
(IN-suh-lin DEH-teh-meer)
Levemir

Pharmacologic class: insulin analogue
Therapeutic class: antidiabetic
Pregnancy risk category: C

Indications and dosages

▶ **Hyperglycemia in patients with diabetes mellitus who need basal (long-acting) insulin.**
Adults and children age 6 and older: Base dosage on patient response and glucose level. In insulin-naive patients with type 2 diabetes, start with 0.1 to 0.2 units/kg subcutaneously once daily in the evening or 10 units once or b.i.d. based on glucose level. Patients with type 1 or 2 diabetes receiving basal-bolus treatment or basal insulin only may switch to insulin detemir on a unit-to-unit basis adjusted to glycemic target.

Contraindications and cautions

• Contraindicated in patients hypersensitive to insulin detemir or its excipients. Don't give drug with an insulin infusion pump.
• Use cautiously in patients with hepatic or renal impairment; they may need dosage adjustment.
☀ **Lifespan:** In pregnant women, use only if benefits outweigh risks to the fetus. In breast-feeding women, use cautiously; it isn't known whether drug appears in breast milk. In children, safety and efficacy haven't been established. In elderly patients, starting dosage, increments of change, and maintenance dosage should be conservative; hypoglycemia may be harder to recognize in these patients.

Adverse reactions

CV: edema.
Metabolic: HYPOGLYCEMIA, sodium retention, *weight gain.*
Skin: injection site reactions, lipodystrophy, pruritus, rash.
Other: allergic reactions.

Interactions

Drug-drug. *ACE inhibitors, antidiabetic drugs, disopyramide, fibrates, fluoxetine, MAO inhibitors, octreotide, propoxyphene, salicylates, sulfonamides:* May increase blood glucose–lowering effect of insulin and risk of hypoglycemia. Monitor blood glucose carefully.
Beta blockers, clonidine, guanethidine, reserpine: May decrease or conceal signs of hypoglycemia. Avoid use together if possible.
Beta blockers, clonidine, lithium salts: May increase or decrease blood glucose–lowering effect of insulin. Monitor blood glucose level carefully.
Corticosteroids, danazol, diuretics, estrogens, isoniazid, phenothiazines, progestogens (hormonal contraceptives), somatropin, sympath-

omimetics, thyroid hormones: May decrease blood glucose–lowering effect of insulin. Monitor blood glucose level carefully.

Insulin other than insulin detemir: May alter the action of one or both insulins if mixed together. Don't mix or dilute insulin detemir with other insulins.

Pentamidine: May cause initial hypoglycemia followed by hyperglycemia. Use together cautiously.

Drug-lifestyle. *Alcohol use:* May increase or decrease blood glucose–lowering effect of insulin. Discourage use together.

Marijuana use: May increase glucose level. Tell patient about this interaction.

Smoking: May increase glucose level and decrease response to insulin. Discourage patient from smoking; have patient monitor glucose level closely.

Effects on lab test results

● May decrease glucose level.

Pharmacokinetics

Absorption: Slow and prolonged.
Distribution: 98% bound to albumin.
Metabolism: Unknown.
Excretion: Unknown. *Half life:* 5 to 7 hours.

Route	Onset	Peak	Duration
SubQ	Unknown	6–8 hr	6–23 hr

Action

Chemical effect: Regulates glucose metabolism by binding to insulin receptors, facilitating cellular uptake of glucose into muscle and fat, and inhibiting release of glucose from liver.
Therapeutic effect: Lowers glucose level.

Available forms

Injection: 100 units/ml in 10-ml vials, 3-ml cartridges (PenFill), 3-ml prefilled syringes (InnoLet, FlexPen)

NURSING PROCESS

⏱ Assessment
● Monitor blood glucose level routinely in all patients receiving insulin.
● Measure patient's glycosylated hemoglobin level periodically.
● Watch for hyperglycemia, especially if patient's diet or exercise patterns change.

● Assess patient for signs and symptoms of hypoglycemia. Insulin dosages may need adjustment.
● Assess patient's and family's knowledge of drug therapy.

⚅ Nursing diagnoses
● Risk for injury related to drug-induced hypoglycemia
● Ineffective health maintenance related to hyperglycemia
● Deficient knowledge related to drug therapy

❯ Planning and implementation
Ⓢ **ALERT:** Don't give this drug by I.V. or I.M. route.
Ⓢ **ALERT:** Don't mix or dilute insulin detemir with other insulins.
Ⓢ **ALERT:** Spell out "units" to reduce the risk of misreading "U" as a zero.
● Early warning symptoms of hypoglycemia may be less pronounced in patients who take beta blockers and patients with long-standing diabetes, diabetic nerve disease, or intensified diabetes control. Monitor glucose level closely in these patients because severe hypoglycemia could develop before symptoms do.
● Insulin dosages may need adjustment if patient experiences illness, emotional disturbance, or other stresses or if patient changes his usual meal plan or exercise level.

Patient teaching
● Teach diabetes management, including glucose monitoring, injection techniques, and continuous rotation of injection sites.
Ⓢ **ALERT:** Teach patient not to mix insulin detemir with any other insulin or solution.
● Instruct patient to use only solution that's clear and colorless, with no visible particles.
● Tell patient to recognize and report signs and symptoms of hyperglycemia, such as nausea, vomiting, drowsiness, flushed dry skin, dry mouth, increased urination, thirst, and loss of appetite.
● Urge patient to check blood glucose level often to achieve control and to avoid hyperglycemia and hypoglycemia.
● Teach patient to recognize and report signs and symptoms of hypoglycemia, such as sweating, dizziness, light-headedness, headache, drowsiness, and irritability.

Reactions may be *common,* uncommon, *life-threatening,* or COMMON AND LIFE-THREATENING.

• Advise patient to carry a quick source of simple sugar, such as hard candy or glucose tablets, in case of hypoglycemia.
• Caution patient not to stop insulin abruptly or change the amount or type of insulin used without consulting prescriber.
• Advise patient to avoid alcohol because it lowers the glucose level.
• Caution woman to consult prescriber before trying to become pregnant.
• Tell patient to store unused vials, cartridges, and prefilled syringes in the refrigerator at 36° to 46° F (2° to 8° C).
• After initial use, vials may be refrigerated or stored at room temperature, below 86° F (30° C), away from direct heat and light, for up to 42 days. Cartridges or prefilled syringes may be stored at room temperature, below 86° F (30° C). Tell patient not to store or refrigerate insulin with a needle in place.
• Caution against freezing insulin detemir and against using insulin detemir that has been frozen.

☑ **Evaluation**
• Patient does not experience drug-induced hypoglycemia.
• Patient's glucose level remains within normal limits with drug therapy.
• Deficient knowledge related to drug therapy.

HIGH ALERT

insulin glargine (rDNA)
(IN-suh-lin GLAR-gene)
Lantus

Pharmacologic class: insulin analogue
Therapeutic class: antidiabetic
Pregnancy risk category: C

Indications and dosages

▶ **Management of type 1 or type 2 diabetes mellitus in patients who need basal (long-acting) insulin for the control of hyperglycemia.** *Adults and children age 6 and older:* Individualize dosage. Start drug subcutaneously at the same dose as the current insulin dose at the same time each day.

▶ **Management of type 2 diabetes mellitus in patients previously treated with oral antidiabetics.** *Adults:* 10 units subcutaneously once daily at bedtime. Adjust p.r.n. to total daily dosage of 2 units to 100 units subcutaneously at the same time each day.

Contraindications and cautions
• Contraindicated in patients hypersensitive to insulin glargine or its excipients. Don't use drug during episodes of hypoglycemia.
• Use cautiously in patients with renal or hepatic impairment, and adjust dosage as directed.
❦ **Lifespan:** In breast-feeding women, use cautiously because it's unknown if the drug appears in breast milk. In children younger than age 6, safety and effectiveness haven't been established. In elderly patients, use cautiously to avoid hypoglycemia.

Adverse reactions
EENT: retinopathy.
Metabolic: *hypoglycemia.*
Skin: lipodystrophy, pruritus, rash.
Other: allergic reactions, pain at injection site.

Interactions
Drug-drug. *ACE inhibitors, disopyramide, fibrates, fluoxetine, MAO inhibitors, octreotide, oral antidiabetics, propoxyphene, salicylates, sulfonamide antibiotics:* May cause hypoglycemia and increased insulin effect. Monitor glucose level. Insulin glargine dosage may need adjustment.
Beta blockers, clonidine, guanethidine, reserpine: May decrease or conceal signs of hypoglycemia. Use cautiously.
Beta blockers, clonidine, lithium salts: May increase or decrease blood glucose–lowering effect of insulin. Monitor blood glucose level carefully.
Corticosteroids, danazol, diuretics, estrogens, isoniazid, phenothiazines (prochlorperazine, promethazine), progestins (hormonal contraceptives), sympathomimetics (albuterol, epinephrine, terbutaline), thyroid hormones: May reduce the blood glucose–lowering effect of insulin. Monitor glucose level. Insulin glargine dosage may need adjustment.
Guanethidine, reserpine: May mask signs of hypoglycemia. Avoid using together, if possible. Monitor glucose level carefully.
Lithium: May increase or decrease blood glucose–lowering effect of insulin. Monitor glucose level. Insulin glargine dosage may need adjustment.

I

Pentamidine: May cause hypoglycemia, which may be followed by hyperglycemia. Avoid using together, if possible.

Drug-herb. *Aloe, bilberry leaf, bitter melon, burdock, dandelion, fenugreek, garlic, ginseng:* May improve glucose control and allow a reduced antidiabetic dosage. Tell patient to discuss the use of herbal remedies with prescriber before use.

Licorice root: May increase dosage requirements of insulin. Discourage use together.

Drug-lifestyle. *Alcohol use:* May increase glucose-lowering effects of insulin. Discourage use together.

Emotional stress, exercise: May increase or decrease glucose-lowering effect of insulin. Monitor glucose level. Insulin glargine dosage may need adjustment.

Marijuana use: May increase glucose level. Tell patient about this interaction.

Smoking: May increase glucose level and decrease response to insulin. Discourage patient from smoking; have patient monitor glucose level closely.

Effects on lab test results
• May decrease glucose level.

Pharmacokinetics
Absorption: Slower, more prolonged absorption than NPH and a relatively constant level over 24 hours with no pronounced peak when compared with NPH insulin. After injection into subcutaneous tissue, the acidic solution is neutralized, leading to formation of microprecipitates. From these microprecipitates, small amounts of insulin glargine are slowly released.
Distribution: Unknown.
Metabolism: Partly metabolized to form two active metabolites similar to insulin.
Excretion: Unknown. *Half-life:* Unknown.

Route	Onset	Peak	Duration
SubQ	Slow	None	10¾–24 hr

Action
Chemical effect: Increases glucose transport across muscle and fat cell membranes to reduce glucose level. Promotes conversion of glucose to its storage form, glycogen.
Therapeutic effect: Lowers glucose level.

Available forms
Injection: 100 units per ml in 10-ml vials, 3-ml cartridges (OptiClik) or 3-ml disposable insulin device (SoloStar)

NURSING PROCESS

Assessment
• Obtain history of patient's underlying condition before starting therapy, and reassess regularly. As with any insulin, the desired glucose level and the doses and timing of antidiabetic drug must be determined individually.
• Monitor glucose level closely.
• Monitor patient for hypoglycemia. Early symptoms may be different or less pronounced in patients with long-standing diabetes, diabetic nerve disease, or intensified diabetes control.
• Assess patient's and family's knowledge of drug therapy.

Nursing diagnoses
• Ineffective health maintenance related to hyperglycemia
• Risk for injury related to drug-induced hypoglycemia
• Deficient knowledge related to drug therapy

Planning and implementation
• Drug isn't intended for I.V. use. Its prolonged action depends on injection into the subcutaneous space.
• Because of its prolonged duration, insulin glargine isn't the insulin of choice for diabetic ketoacidosis.
• The rate of absorption and onset and the duration of action may be affected by exercise and other circumstances, such as illness and emotional stress.
• Don't dilute drug or mix it with any other insulin or solution.
• As with any insulin therapy, lipodystrophy may occur at injection site and delay insulin absorption. Rotate injection sites to reduce lipodystrophy.
⚠ ALERT: Spell out "units" to reduce the risk of misreading "U" as a zero.
• Store unopened vials at 36° F to 46° F (2° to 8° C). Don't freeze. Discard opened vials, whether refrigerated or not, after 28 days. May store opened vials at room temperature away from direct heat and light.
⚠ ALERT: Don't confuse Lantus with Lente.

Patient teaching

• Teach patient proper glucose-monitoring techniques and proper diabetes management.
• Teach diabetic patient signs and symptoms of hypoglycemia, such as fatigue, weakness, confusion, headache, and pale skin.
• Advise patient to treat mild episodes of hypoglycemia with oral glucose tablets. Encourage patient to always carry glucose tablets in case of a hypoglycemic episode.
• Teach patient the importance of maintaining a diabetic diet. Explain that adjustments in drug dosage, meal patterns, and exercise may be needed to regulate blood glucose.
• Tell patient that any change of insulin should be made cautiously and only under medical supervision. Changes in insulin strength, manufacturer, type (regular, NPH, insulin analogues), species (animal, human), or method of manufacture (ribosomal DNA versus animal source) may warrant a dosage change. Oral antidiabetic treatment may need to be adjusted.
• Tell patient to consult prescriber before using OTC drugs.
• Advise patient not to dilute or mix any other insulin or solution with insulin glargine. Tell patient to discard the vial if the solution is cloudy.
• Instruct patient to store insulin glargine vials in the refrigerator, if possible.

✓ Evaluation

• Patient's blood glucose level is normal.
• Patient doesn't experience hypoglycemic reactions.
• Patient and family state understanding of drug therapy.

insulin glulisine (rDNA origin)
(IN-suh-lin GLOO-lih-seen)
Apidra

Pharmacologic class: human insulin analogue
Therapeutic class: antidiabetic
Pregnancy risk category: C

Indications and dosages

▶ **Diabetes mellitus.** *Adults:* Individualize dosage. Give subcutaneous injection within 15 minutes before a meal or within 20 minutes after meal starts if regimen also includes a longer-acting insulin or basal insulin analogue.

Or give subcutaneous infusion using an external infusion pump. Or give I.V. as ordered.

▼ I.V. administration

• Mix in normal saline solution to a concentration of 1 unit/ml.
• Use only polyvinyl chloride I.V. infusion bags and tubing.
• Monitor blood glucose and potassium levels closely.
• Insulin glulisine is equally potent to regular human insulin by I.V. route.
⊗ **Incompatibilities**
Other I.V. drugs, including other insulins; solutions other than normal saline.

Contraindications and cautions

• Contraindicated during periods of hypoglycemia and in patients hypersensitive to insulin glulisine or one of its excipients.
• Use cautiously in patients with moderate to severe renal or hepatic dysfunction.
🐾 **Lifespan:** In pregnant women, safety and effectiveness haven't been established. In breastfeeding women, use cautiously because it's unknown if the drug appears in breast milk. In children, safety and effectiveness haven't been established.

Adverse reactions

Metabolic: *hypoglycemia.*
Skin: *injection-site reactions,* lipodystrophy, pruritus, rash.
Other: allergic reactions, ***anaphylaxis,*** insulin antibody production.

Interactions

Drug-drug. *ACE inhibitors, disopyramide, fibrates, fluoxetine, MAO inhibitors, oral antidiabetics, pentoxifylline, propoxyphene, salicylates, sulfonamide antibiotics:* May increase blood glucose–lowering effects. Monitor glucose level, and watch for evidence of hypoglycemia.
Beta blockers, clonidine, guanethidine, reserpine: May decrease or conceal signs of hypoglycemia. Avoid use together if possible.
Beta blockers, clonidine, lithium, pentamidine: May cause unpredictable response to insulin. Use together cautiously; monitor patient closely.
Clozapine, corticosteroids, danazol, diazoxide, diuretics, estrogens, glucagons, isoniazid, olanzapine, phenothiazines, progestogens, protease inhibitors, somatropin, sympathomimetics (such

as albuterol, epinephrine, and terbutaline), thyroid hormones: May decrease blood glucose–lowering effects. Monitor glucose level carefully.

Drug-lifestyle. *Alcohol:* May increase or decrease drug effects, resulting in either hypoglycemia or hyperglycemia. Discourage alcohol use.
Marijuana use: May increase glucose level. Tell patient about this interaction.
Smoking: May increase glucose level and decrease response to insulin. Discourage patient from smoking; have patient monitor glucose level closely.

Effects on lab test results

• May decrease glucose level.

Pharmacokinetics

Absorption: Absorbed rapidly, faster than regular insulin.
Distribution: Wide.
Metabolism: Bound and inactivated in peripheral tissues plus primary metabolism in the liver.
Excretion: Renal filtration. *Half-life:* 13 minutes (I.V.); 42 minutes (subQ).

Route	Onset	Peak	Duration
I.V.	Rapid	Unknown	Unknown
SubQ	15 min	34–91 min	105–210 min

Action

Chemical effect: Increases peripheral glucose uptake by skeletal muscle and fat and decreases hepatic glucose production.
Therapeutic effect: Lowers glucose level.

Available forms

Injection: 10-ml vials (3-ml cartridges for Opti-Clik) of 100 units/ml

NURSING PROCESS

🕮 Assessment
• Monitor patient for signs and symptoms of hyperglycemia, including drowsiness, fruity breath, frequent urination, and thirst.
• Monitor patient for signs and symptoms of hypoglycemia, including cool, diaphoretic skin; shaking; trembling; confusion; headache; irritability; hunger; tachycardia; and nausea.
• Look for early warning signs of hypoglycemia. They may be different or less pronounced in patients who take beta blockers, who have

had an oral antidiabetic added to the regimen, or who have long-term diabetes or diabetic nerve disease.
• Assess injection site for redness, swelling, or itching.
• Monitor injection site for lipodystrophy. Lipodystrophy may delay insulin absorption.
• Assess patient's and family's knowledge of drug therapy.

✥ Nursing diagnoses
• Ineffective health maintenance related to presence of underlying disease
• Risk for injury related to drug-induced hypoglycemia
• Deficient knowledge related to drug therapy

▶ Planning and implementation
• Use with a longer-acting or basal insulin analogue.
🕔 **ALERT:** Drug has a more rapid onset and shorter duration of action than regular human insulin. Give within 15 minutes before or immediately after a meal.
🕔 **ALERT:** Spell out "units" to reduce the risk of misreading "U" as a zero.
• Don't mix drug in a syringe with other insulins except NPH.
• When drug is used in an external subcutaneous infusion pump, don't mix with other insulins or with a diluent.
• Adjust dosage for changes in insulin strength, manufacturer, or type and in physical activity or usual meal plan and during illness, emotional disturbances, or stress.
Patient teaching
• Tell patient to take drug within 20 minutes of eating.
• Teach patient how to give subcutaneous insulin injections.
• Tell patient to use drug only if clear and colorless, without visible particles.
• Tell patient not to mix drug in a syringe with any insulin other than NPH.
• If patient is mixing drug with NPH, tell patient to use U-100 syringes, to draw insulin glulisine into the syringe before NPH insulin, and to inject the mixture immediately.
• Instruct patient to rotate injection sites to avoid injection-site reactions.
• If patient is using an external infusion pump, teach proper use of the device. Tell patient not to mix drug with other insulin or diluents. In-

struct patient to change the infusion set, reservoir with insulin, and infusion site every 48 hours.

• Teach patient the signs and symptoms of hypoglycemia (sweating, rapid pulse, trembling, confusion, headache, irritability, and nausea). Advise the patient to treat these symptoms by eating or drinking something containing sugar.

• Tell the patient to contact his prescriber for dosage adjustments if hypoglycemia occurs frequently.

• Show patient how to monitor and log his glucose levels to assess diabetes control.

• Explain the possible long-term complications of diabetes and the importance of regular preventive therapy. Urge patient to follow prescribed diet and exercise regimen. To further reduce the increased risk of heart disease, encourage patient to stop smoking and lose weight.

• Instruct patient to wear or carry identification showing that he has diabetes.

• Tell patient to store unopened vials in the refrigerator. Opened vials must be stored below 77° F (25° C) and should be used within 28 days. Drug should be protected from direct heat and light.

☑ **Evaluation**
• Patient's glucose level is normal.
• Patient doesn't experience hypoglycemia.
• Patient and family state understanding of drug therapy.

HIGH ALERT

insulin (regular)
(IN-suh-lin)
Humulin R, Humulin R Regular U-500 (concentrated), Novolin R, Novolin R PenFill, Novolin R Prefilled

insulin (lispro)
Humalog

insulin lispro protamine and insulin lispro
Humalog Mix 75/25

isophane insulin suspension (NPH)
Humulin N, Novolin N, Novolin N PenFill, Novolin N Prefilled

isophane insulin suspension and insulin injection combinations
Humulin 50/50, Humulin 70/30, Novolin 70/30, Novolin 70/30 PenFill, Novolin 70/30 Prefilled

---

Pharmacologic class: pancreatic hormone
Therapeutic class: antidiabetic
Pregnancy risk category: B (C; oral inhalation)

Indications and dosages

▶ **Moderate to severe diabetic ketoacidosis or hyperosmolar hyperglycemia (regular insulin).** *Adults older than age 20:* Give loading dose of 0.15 units/kg I.V. by direct injection, followed by 0.1 unit/kg/hour as a continuous infusion. When glucose level reaches 250 to 300 mg/dl, decrease insulin infusion to 0.05 to 0.1 unit/kg/hour. When glucose level is 150 to 200 mg/dl in patients with diabetic ketoacidosis or 250 to 300 mg/dl in those with hyperosmolar hyperglycemia, start infusion of D₅W in half-normal saline solution separately from the insulin infusion. Give insulin dose (intermediate-acting insulin is recommended) subcutaneously 1 to 2 hours before stopping insulin infusion.
Adults and children age 20 or younger: Loading dose isn't recommended. Start with 0.1 unit/kg/hour by I.V. infusion. Once condition improves, decrease insulin infusion to 0.05 unit/kg/hour. When glucose level is 250 mg/dl, start infusion of D₅W in half-normal saline solution separately from the insulin infusion.

▶ **Mild diabetic ketoacidosis (regular insulin).** *Adults older than age 20:* Give loading dose of 0.4 to 0.6 unit/kg divided in two equal parts, with half the dose given by direct I.V. injection and half given I.M. or subcutaneously. Subsequent doses can be based on 0.1 unit/kg/hour I.M. or subcutaneously.

▶ **Newly diagnosed diabetes mellitus (regular insulin).** *Adults older than age 20:* Individualize therapy. Initially, 0.5 to 1 unit/kg/day subcutaneously as part of a regimen with short-acting and long-acting insulin therapy.
Adults and children age 20 or younger: Individualize therapy. Initially, 0.1 to 0.25 unit/kg subcutaneously every 6 to 8 hours for 24 hours; then adjust accordingly.

▶ **Control of hyperglycemia with Humalog and longer-acting insulin in patients with**

---

type 1 diabetes mellitus. *Adults:* Dosage varies among patients and must be determined by prescriber familiar with patient's metabolic needs, eating habits, and other lifestyle variables. Inject subcutaneously within 15 minutes before or after a meal.

▶ **Control of hyperglycemia with Humalog and sulfonylureas in patients with type 2 diabetes mellitus.** *Adults and children older than age 3:* Dosage varies among patients and must be determined by prescriber familiar with patient's metabolic needs, eating habits, and other lifestyle variables. Inject subcutaneously within 15 minutes before or after a meal.

▶ **Hyperkalemia‡.** *Adults:* 50 ml of dextrose 50% given over 5 minutes, followed by 5 to 10 units of regular insulin by I.V. push.

▼ I.V. administration

• Give only regular insulin I.V. Inject directly into vein or into a port close to I.V. access site. Intermittent infusion isn't recommended. If given by continuous infusion, infuse drug diluted in normal saline solution at prescribed rate.
• Regular insulin is used in patients with circulatory collapse, diabetic ketoacidosis, or hyperkalemia.
• Don't use Humulin R (concentrated) U-500 I.V.
• Don't use intermediate- or long-acting insulins for coma or other emergency requiring rapid drug action.
• Ketosis-prone type 1, severely ill, and newly diagnosed diabetic patients with very high glucose levels may need hospitalization and I.V. treatment with regular fast-acting insulin.
⊗ **Incompatibilities**
Aminophylline, amobarbital, chlorothiazide, cytarabine, digoxin, diltiazem, dobutamine, dopamine, levofloxacin, methylprednisolone sodium succinate, nafcillin, norepinephrine, pentobarbital sodium, phenobarbital sodium, phenytoin sodium, ranitidine, sodium bicarbonate, thiopental.

Contraindications and cautions

• Contraindicated in hypoglycemia and in patients hypersensitive to insulin or any of its ingredients.
⚖ **Lifespan:** In pregnant and breast-feeding women, insulin is drug of choice to treat diabetes.

Adverse reactions

Metabolic: hyperglycemia (rebound or Somogyi effect), *hypoglycemia.*
Respiratory: dyspnea, *increased cough,* reduced pulmonary function, *respiratory tract infection.*
Skin: itching, rash, redness, stinging, swelling, urticaria, warmth at injection site.
Other: *anaphylaxis,* hypersensitivity reactions, lipoatrophy, lipohypertrophy, rash.

Interactions

Drug-drug. *AIDS antiretrovirals, corticosteroids, dextrothyroxine, epinephrine, thiazide diuretics:* May decrease insulin response. Monitor patient for hyperglycemia.
Anabolic steroids, clofibrate, guanethidine, MAO inhibitors, salicylates, tetracyclines: May prolong hypoglycemic effect. Monitor glucose level carefully.
Beta blockers, clonidine: May decrease or conceal signs of hypoglycemia. Use together cautiously.
Hormonal contraceptives: May decrease glucose tolerance in diabetic patients. Monitor glucose level, and adjust insulin dosage carefully.
Drug-herb. *Basil, bay, bee pollen, burdock, ginseng, glucomannan, horehound, marshmallow, myrrh, sage:* May affect glycemic control. Monitor glucose level carefully.
Drug-lifestyle. *Alcohol use:* May increase the blood glucose–lowering effects of insulin. Discourage use together.
Marijuana use: May increase glucose level. Tell patient about this interaction.
Smoking: May increase glucose level and decrease response to insulin. Discourage smoking; have patient monitor glucose level closely.

Effects on lab test results

• May decrease glucose, magnesium, and potassium levels.

Pharmacokinetics

Absorption: Highly variable after subcutaneous use depending on insulin type and injection site.
Distribution: Wide.
Metabolism: Some is bound and inactivated by peripheral tissues, but most appears to be degraded in liver and kidneys.

Excretion: Filtered by renal glomeruli; undergoes some tubular reabsorption. *Half-life:* About 9 minutes after I.V. use.

Route	Onset	Peak	Duration
I.V.	≤ 30 min	15–30 min	30 min–1 hr
SubQ	15 min–8 hr	2–30 hr	5–36 hr

Action

Chemical effect: Increases glucose transport across muscle and fat cell membranes to reduce glucose level. Promotes conversion of glucose to its storage form, glycogen.
Therapeutic effect: Lowers blood glucose level.

Available forms

Available without a prescription
insulin (regular)
Injection (human): 100 units/ml (Humulin R, Novolin R, Novolin R PenFill, Novolin R Prefilled)
isophane insulin suspension (NPH)
Injection (human): 100 units/ml (Humulin N, Novolin N, Novolin N PenFill, Novolin N Prefilled)
insulin zinc suspension (lente)
Injection (human): 100 units/ml (Novolin L)
isophane insulin suspension and insulin injection combinations
Injection (human): 100 units/ml (Humulin 50/50, Humulin 70/30, Novolin 70/30, Novolin 70/30 PenFill, Novolin 70/30 Prefilled)
Available by prescription only
insulin (regular)
Injection (human): 500 units/ml (Humulin R Regular U-500 [concentrated])
insulin (lispro)
Injection (human): 100 units/ml (Humalog)
insulin lispro protamine and insulin lispro
Injection (human): 100 units/ml (Humalog Mix 75/25)

NURSING PROCESS

🔬 Assessment

• Assess patient's glucose level before starting therapy and regularly thereafter. If patient is under stress, unstable, pregnant, recently diagnosed, or taking drugs that can interact with insulin, monitor level more frequently.
• Monitor patient's glycosylated hemoglobin level regularly.

• Monitor urine ketone level when glucose level is elevated.
• Be alert for adverse reactions and drug interactions.
• Monitor injection sites for local reactions.
• Assess patient's and family's knowledge of drug therapy.

⊕ Nursing diagnoses

• Ineffective health maintenance related to hyperglycemia
• Risk for injury related to drug-induced hypoglycemia
• Deficient knowledge related to drug therapy

⊠ Planning and implementation

⊕ **ALERT:** Dose is always expressed in USP units. Use only syringes calibrated for particular concentration of insulin given (such as U-100 for 100 units/ml insulin).
⊕ **ALERT:** Spell out "units" to reduce the risk of misreading the "U" as a zero.
• Insulin resistance may develop; large insulin doses are needed to control symptoms of diabetes in these patients. U-500 insulin is available as Regular (Concentrated) for such patients. Although not normally stocked in every pharmacy, it's readily available. Give hospital pharmacy sufficient notice before the need to refill in-house prescription. Never store U-500 insulin in same area with other insulin preparations because of danger of severe overdose if given accidentally to other patients.
• To mix insulin suspension, swirl vial gently or rotate between palms or between palm and thigh. Don't shake vigorously because doing so causes bubbling and air in syringe.
• Humalog insulin has a rapid onset of action. Give 15 minutes before meals.
• Regular insulin may be mixed with NPH insulins in any proportion.
• Switching from separate injections to prepared mixture may alter patient response. Whenever NPH is mixed with regular insulin in same syringe, give immediately to avoid loss of potency.
• Don't use insulin that has changed color or become clumped or granular.
• Check expiration date on vial before using.
• Usual route is subcutaneous. Pinch fold of skin with fingers starting at least 3 inches apart, and insert needle at 45- to 90-degree angle.

• Press but don't rub site after injection. Rotate and chart injection sites to avoid overuse of one area. Rotate injection sites within same anatomic region to help diabetic patients achieve better control.
• Ketosis-prone type 1, severely ill, and newly diagnosed diabetic patients with very high glucose levels may require hospitalization and I.V. treatment with regular fast-acting insulin.
• Store drug in cool area. Refrigeration is desirable but not essential except for concentrated regular insulin.
• Notify prescriber of sudden changes in glucose levels, dangerously high or low levels, or ketosis.
• If patient develops diabetic ketoacidosis or hyperglycemic hyperosmolar nonketotic coma, provide supportive treatment.
• Treat hypoglycemic reaction with oral form of rapid-acting glucose if patient can swallow, or with glucagon or I.V. glucose if patient can't be roused. Follow with complex carbohydrate snack when patient is awake, and determine cause of reaction.
• Make sure patient is following appropriate diet and exercise programs. Adjust insulin dosage when other aspects of regimen are changed.
• Discuss with prescriber how to deal with noncompliance.
• Treat lipoatrophy or lipohypertrophy according to prescribed protocol.
Patient teaching
• Tell patient that insulin relieves symptoms but doesn't cure disease.
• Inform patient about nature of disease; importance of following therapeutic regimen; adherence to specific diet, weight reduction, exercise, and personal hygiene programs; and ways of avoiding infection. Review timing of injections and eating, and explain that meals must not be skipped.
• Stress that accuracy of measurement is very important, especially with concentrated regular insulin. Aids, such as a magnifying sleeve or dose magnifier, may improve accuracy. Instruct patient and family how to measure and give insulin.
• Advise patient not to alter order of mixing insulins or change model or brand of syringe or needle.
• Tell patient that glucose monitoring and urine ketone tests are essential guides to dosage and

success of therapy. Stress the importance of recognizing hypoglycemic symptoms because insulin-induced hypoglycemia is hazardous and may cause brain damage if prolonged. Most adverse effects are self-limiting and temporary.
• Teach patient about proper use of equipment for monitoring glucose level.
• Instruct patient not to drink alcohol during therapy.
• Advise patient not to smoke within 30 minutes after insulin injection. Smoking decreases absorption.
• Tell patient that marijuana use may increase insulin requirements.
• Advise patient to wear or carry medical identification at all times, to carry ample insulin supply and syringes on trips, to have carbohydrates (lump of sugar or candy) on hand for emergencies, and to note time-zone changes for dose scheduling when traveling.

☑ **Evaluation**
• Patient's glucose level is normal.
• Patient sustains no injury from drug-induced hypoglycemia.
• Patient and family state understanding of drug therapy.

HIGH ALERT

interferon alfa-2b, recombinant (IFN-alpha 2)
Intron-A

Pharmacologic class: biological response modifier
Therapeutic class: antineoplastic, immunomodulator
Pregnancy risk category: C

Indications and dosages

▶ **Hairy cell leukemia.** *Adults:* 2 million international units/m^2 alfa-2b I.M. or subcutaneously three times weekly for induction and maintenance.
▶ **Condylomata acuminata.** *Adults:* 1 million international units alfa-2b per lesion, intralesionally, three times weekly for 3 weeks. May repeat after 12 to 16 weeks if results are not satisfactory.
▶ **Kaposi sarcoma.** *Adults:* 30 million international units/m^2 alfa-2b subcutaneously or I.M.

three times weekly. Maintain dose unless disease progresses. Maximal response achieved after 16 weeks. May decrease dosage for severe adverse affects.

▶ **Chronic hepatitis C.** *Adults:* 3 million international units alfa-2b subcutaneously or I.M. three times weekly. In patients tolerating therapy with normalization of ALT at 16 weeks of treatment, extend therapy to 18 to 24 months. If no normalization of ALT at 16 weeks of treatment, consider stopping therapy.

▶ **Chronic hepatitis B.** *Adults:* 30 to 35 million international units alfa-2b subcutaneously or I.M. weekly either as 5 million international units daily or 10 million international units three times weekly for 16 weeks.

Children ages 1 to 17: Give 3 million international units/m² alfa-2b subcutaneously three times weekly for 1 week; then escalate dosage to 6 million international units/m² subcutaneously three times weekly (up to 10 million international units/m² subcutaneously three times weekly) for 16 to 24 weeks.

▶ **Malignant melanoma.** *Adults:* 20 million international units/m² alfa-2b daily given as I.V. infusion 5 days in a row for 4 weeks. For maintenance therapy, 10 million international units/m² subcutaneously three times weekly for 48 weeks. If adverse effects occur, stop therapy until they subside, and then resume therapy at 50% of the previous dose. If intolerance persists, stop therapy.

▶ **Initial treatment of aggressive follicular malignant lymphoma with combination chemotherapy containing anthracycline.** *Adults:* 5 million international units alfa-2b subcutaneously three times weekly for up to 18 months.

▶ **Metastatic renal cell carcinoma‡.** *Adults:* 5 to 20 million international units alfa-2b subcutaneously daily or three times weekly.

Contraindications and cautions

• Contraindicated in patients hypersensitive to the drug, its components, or mouse protein.
• Use cautiously in patients with severe hepatic or renal function impairment, seizure disorders, compromised CNS function, cardiac disease, or myelosuppression.
• Alpha interferons cause or aggravate fatal or life-threatening neuropsychiatric, autoimmune, ischemic, and infectious disorders. Monitor patient closely. Stop drug in patients with persist-

ently severe or worsening signs or symptoms of these conditions.

⚖ **Lifespan:** In pregnant women, use cautiously. In breast-feeding women, stop drug or stop breast-feeding. In children, safety and effectiveness haven't been established.

Adverse reactions

CNS: anxiety, apathy, confusion, *depression,* difficulty in thinking or concentrating, *dizziness,* fatigue, gait disturbances, *headache, insomnia, irritability,* lethargy, nervousness, numbness, paresthesia, poor coordination, sedation, syncope, vertigo.

CV: *arrhythmias,* chest pain, *cyanosis,* edema, flushing, *heart failure, hypertension,* hypotension, *MI,* palpitations.

EENT: conjunctivitis, dry or inflamed oropharynx, earache, excessive salivation, eye irritation, pharyngitis, rhinitis, rhinorrhea, sinusitis, visual disturbances.

GI: abdominal fullness, *abdominal pain, anorexia,* constipation, *diarrhea,* dysgeusia, esophagitis, flatulence, gastric distress, gingivitis, hypermotility, *nausea,* stomatitis, vomiting.

GU: transient impotence.

Hematologic: anemia, *leukopenia, mild thrombocytopenia, neutropenia.*

Hepatic: *hepatitis.*

Respiratory: *coughing, dyspnea,* tachypnea.

Skin: *diaphoresis,* dryness, partial alopecia, *pruritus, rash,* urticaria.

Other: *flulike syndrome,* hot flushes, *injection site reaction.*

Interactions

Drug-drug. *Aminophylline, theophylline:* May reduce theophylline clearance. Monitor level.

Cardiotoxic, hematotoxic, or neurotoxic drugs: May increase effects of these drugs. Monitor patient closely.

CNS depressants: May increase CNS effects. Avoid use together.

Interleukin-2: May increase risk of renal impairment from interleukin-2. Monitor patient closely.

Live-virus vaccines: May increase risk of adverse reactions and decreased antibody response. Don't use together.

Zidovudine: May have synergistic adverse effects between alfa-2b and zidovudine. Carefully monitor WBC count.

Drug-lifestyle. *Alcohol use:* May increase risk of GI bleeding. Discourage use together.
Sun exposure: May cause photosensitivity reactions. Discourage prolonged or unprotected sun exposure.

Effects on lab test results

• May increase calcium, potassium, AST, ALT, alkaline phosphatase, LDH, triglyceride, and fasting glucose levels. May decrease hemoglobin level and hematocrit.
• May increase PT, INR, and PTT. May decrease WBC, neutrophil, and platelet counts.

Pharmacokinetics

Absorption: More than 80% absorbed after I.M. or subcutaneous injection.
Distribution: Wide and rapid.
Metabolism: Drug appears to be metabolized in liver and kidneys.
Excretion: Reabsorbed from glomerular filtrate with minor biliary elimination. *Half-life:* 3½ to 8½ hours.

Route	Onset	Peak	Duration
I.M.	Unknown	3¾ hr	Unknown
SubQ	Unknown	7¼ hr	Unknown
Intralesional	Unknown	Unknown	Unknown

Action

Chemical effect: May involve direct antiproliferative action against tumor cells or viral cells to inhibit replication and change immune response by enhancing phagocytic macrophages and by augmenting specific cytotoxicity of lymphocytes for target cells.
Therapeutic effect: Inhibits growth of certain tumor cells and viral cells.

Available forms

alfa-2b (Intron A)
Multidose pens: 18 million international units (3 million international units per dose); 30 million international units (5 million international units per dose); 60 million international units (10 million international units per dose)
Powder for injection with diluent: 5 million international units/vial; 10 million international units/vial; 18 million international units/multidose vial; 25 million international units/vial; 50 million international units/vial
Solution for injection: 3 million international units/vial or syringe; 5 million international

units/vial or syringe; 10 million international units/vial; 18 million international units/multidose vial; 25 million international units/vial

Assessment

• Assess patient's condition before starting therapy and regularly thereafter.
• Obtain allergy history. Drug contains phenol as preservative and albumin as stabilizer.
• Assess patient for flulike symptoms before starting therapy; these tend to diminish with continued therapy.
• Alpha interferons may cause or aggravate fatal or life-threatening neuropsychiatric, autoimmune, ischemic, and infectious disorders. Monitor patients closely. Stop drug in patients with persistently severe or worsening signs or symptoms of these conditions. In many, but not all, cases, these disorders resolve after stopping therapy.
• Monitor blood studies. Tests include CBC with differential, platelet count, blood chemistry and electrolyte studies, liver function, and, if patient has cardiac disorder or advanced stages of cancer, ECGs. Any effects are dose-related and reversible. Recovery occurs within several days or weeks after withdrawal.
• Be alert for adverse reactions and drug interactions.
• Assess patient's and family's knowledge of drug therapy.

Nursing diagnoses

• Ineffective health maintenance related to underlying condition
• Risk for injury related to drug-induced adverse CNS reactions
• Deficient knowledge related to drug therapy

Planning and implementation

• Premedicate patient with acetaminophen to minimize flulike symptoms.
• Give drug at bedtime to minimize daytime drowsiness.
• Make sure patient is well hydrated, especially during initial stages of treatment.
ALERT: Different brands of interferon may not be equivalent and may require different dosages.
• Give subcutaneously if patient's platelet count is below 50,000/mm³.

• When giving interferon alfa-2b for condylomata acuminata, use only 10 million– international units vial because dilution of other strengths for intralesional use results in hypertonic solution. Don't reconstitute 10 million–international units vial with more than 1 ml of diluent. Use tuberculin or similar syringe and 25G to 30G needle. Don't inject too deeply beneath lesion or too superficially. As many as five lesions can be treated at one time. To ease discomfort, give drug in evening with acetaminophen.

• Refrigerate drug.

• Notify prescriber of severe adverse reactions, which may require a lower dose or stopping the drug.

• Using drug with blood dyscrasia–causing drugs, bone marrow suppressants, or radiation therapy may increase bone marrow suppression. A lower dose may be needed.

Patient teaching

• Advise patient that laboratory tests will be performed before starting therapy and periodically thereafter.

• Instruct patient in proper oral hygiene because bone marrow–suppressant effects may lead to microbial infection, delayed healing, and gingival bleeding. Drug may decrease salivary flow.

• Emphasize need to follow prescriber's instructions about taking and recording temperature. Explain how and when to take acetaminophen.

• Advise patient to check with prescriber for instructions after missing dose.

• Tell patient that drug may cause temporary hair loss; explain that it will grow back when therapy ends.

• Teach patient how to prepare and give drug and how to dispose of used needles, syringes, containers, and unused drug. Give him a copy of information for patients included with product, and make sure he understands it. Also provide information on drug stability.

• Warn patient not to receive any immunization without prescriber's approval and to avoid contact with people who have taken polio vaccine. Use with live-virus vaccine may increase adverse reactions and decrease patient's antibody response. Patient is at increased risk for infection.

• Instruct patient to avoid alcohol during drug therapy.

• Advise patient to report signs of depression.

☑ **Evaluation**

• Patient shows improved health.

• Patient sustains no injury from adverse CNS reactions.

• Patient and family state understanding of drug therapy.

HIGH ALERT

interferon beta-1b, recombinant
(in-ter-FEER-on BAY-tuh wun bee ree-CAHM-bih-nehnt)
Betaseron

Pharmacologic class: biological response modifier
Therapeutic class: antiviral, immunoregulator
Pregnancy risk category: C

Indications and dosages

▶ **To reduce frequency of exacerbations in patients with relapsing multiple sclerosis.**
Adults: 0.0625 mg subcutaneously every other day for weeks 1 and 2; then 0.125 mg subcutaneously every other day for weeks 3 and 4; then 0.1875 mg subcutaneously every other day for weeks 5 and 6; then 0.25 mg subcutaneously every other day thereafter.

Contraindications and cautions

• Contraindicated in patients hypersensitive to interferon beta or human albumin.

⚠ **Lifespan:** In pregnant and breast-feeding women, use only if benefits outweigh risks to the fetus or infant. In children, safety and effectiveness haven't been established.

Adverse reactions

CNS: anxiety, confusion, depersonalization, depression, dizziness, emotional lability, headache, *malaise, seizures,* somnolence, *suicidal tendencies.*
CV: *hemorrhage,* peripheral edema.
EENT: laryngitis.
GI: abdominal pain, constipation, diarrhea, nausea, vomiting.
GU: impotence, menstrual disorders, urinary urgency.
Hematologic: *leukopenia, neutropenia.*
Hepatic: *liver failure.*
Respiratory: bronchitis, dyspnea, sinusitis, upper respiratory tract infection.
Skin: alopecia, skin disorders, sweating.

Other: breast pain, flulike symptoms, hypersensitivity reaction, inflammation, lymphadenopathy, necrosis at injection site, pain, pelvic pain, thyroid disorders.

Interactions

Drug-lifestyle. *Sun exposure:* May cause photosensitivity reactions. Discourage prolonged or unprotected sun exposure.

Effects on lab test results

• May increase ALT and bilirubin levels.
• May decrease WBC and neutrophil counts.

Pharmacokinetics

Absorption: Bioavailability is 50% after subcutaneous injection.
Distribution: Unknown.
Metabolism: Unknown.
Excretion: Unknown. *Half-life:* 8 minutes to 4¼ hours.

Route	Onset	Peak	Duration
SubQ	Unknown	1–8 hr	Unknown

Action

Chemical effect: Attaches to membrane receptors and causes cellular changes, including increased protein synthesis.
Therapeutic effect: Decreases neurologic disturbances seen during exacerbations of multiple sclerosis.

Available forms

Powder for injection: 0.3 mg with separate 1.2-ml prefilled syringe of sodium chloride, 0.54% diluent

NURSING PROCESS

⚖ Assessment

• Assess patient's underlying condition before starting therapy.
• Monitor frequency of exacerbations after drug therapy begins.
• Monitor WBC counts, platelet counts, and blood chemistries, including liver function test results.
⚠ **ALERT:** Serious liver damage can occur with therapy, including hepatic failure and need for liver transplant. Monitor liver function 1, 3, and 6 months after treatment starts, then periodically thereafter.

• Be alert for adverse reactions.
• Monitor patient for depression and suicidal ideation.
• Assess patient's and family's knowledge of drug therapy.

✛ Nursing diagnoses

• Ineffective health maintenance related to exacerbations of multiple sclerosis
• Risk for injury related to drug-induced adverse CNS reactions
• Deficient knowledge related to drug therapy

▶ Planning and implementation

• Premedicate patient with acetaminophen to minimize flulike symptoms.
• To reconstitute, inject 1.2 ml of supplied diluent (0.54% saline solution for injection) into vial and gently swirl to dissolve drug. Don't shake. Reconstituted solution will contain 8 million units (0.25 mg)/ml. Discard vials that contain particles or discolored solution.
• Inject preparation immediately.
• Store at room temperature. Once reconstituted, may refrigerate for up to 3 hours before use.
• Rotate injection sites to minimize local reactions.
Patient teaching
• Warn woman of childbearing age about dangers to fetus. Tell her to notify prescriber promptly if she becomes pregnant.
• Teach patient how to give subcutaneous injections, including solution preparation, use of aseptic technique, rotation of injection sites, and equipment disposal. Periodically reevaluate patient's technique.
• Advise patient to take drug at bedtime to minimize mild flulike symptoms.
• Advise patient of need for blood testing to check liver status and need to report anorexia, fatigue, malaise, dark urine, light feces, or jaundice to prescriber promptly.
• Advise patient to report thoughts of depression or suicidal ideation.

✓ Evaluation

• Patient exhibits decreased frequency of exacerbations.
• Patient sustains no injury from adverse CNS reactions.
• Patient and family state understanding of drug therapy.

interferon gamma-1b
(in-ter-FEER-on GAH-muh WUN BEE)
Actimmune

Pharmacologic class: biological response modifier
Therapeutic class: immunomodulator; antineoplastic
Pregnancy risk category: C

Indications and dosages

▶ **To delay disease progression in patients with severe, malignant osteopetrosis; chronic granulomatous disease.** *Patients with body surface area greater than 0.5 m²:* 50 mcg/m² (1 million international units/m²) subcutaneously three times weekly in the deltoid or anterior thigh.
Patients with body surface area 0.5 m² or less: 1.5 mcg/kg/dose subcutaneously three times weekly in the deltoid or anterior thigh.

Contraindications and cautions

• Contraindicated in patients hypersensitive to the drug or any of its components or to genetically engineered products derived from *Escherichia coli*.
• Use cautiously in patients with cardiac disease, compromised CNS function, or seizure disorders.
• Drug metabolized by cytochrome P-450. Use cautiously with other drugs using same system of metabolism.
⚠ Lifespan: In pregnant women, use cautiously. In breast-feeding women, use cautiously because it's unknown if drug appears in breast milk. In children younger than age 1, safety and effectiveness haven't been established.

Adverse reactions

CNS: decreased mental status, depression, fatigue, gait disturbance.
GI: diarrhea, nausea, vomiting.
Hematologic: *neutropenia, thrombocytopenia.*
Skin: rash.
Other: flulike syndrome, erythema and tenderness at injection site.

Interactions

Drug-drug. *Myelosuppressive drugs:* May have additive myelosuppression. Monitor patient closely.
Zidovudine: May have additive bone marrow suppression. Consider reducing dosage.

Effects on lab test results

• May increase liver enzyme levels.
• May decrease neutrophil and platelet counts.

Pharmacokinetics

Absorption: About 90% absorbed after subcutaneous or I.M. use.
Distribution: Unknown.
Metabolism: Unknown.
Excretion: Unknown. *Half-life:* 6 hours.

Route	Onset	Peak	Duration
SubQ	Unknown	≤ 7 hr	Unknown

Action

Chemical effect: Acts as interleukin-type lymphokine. Drug has potent phagocyte-activating properties and enhances oxidative metabolism of tissue macrophages.
Therapeutic effect: Promotes phagocytes.

Available forms

Injection: 100 mcg (2 million international units)/0.5-ml vial

⚗ Assessment
• Assess patient's condition before starting therapy and regularly thereafter.
• Be alert for adverse reactions and drug interactions. Flulike symptoms include headache, fever, chills, myalgia, and arthralgia.
• If adverse GI reactions occur, monitor patient's hydration status.
• Assess patient's and family's knowledge of drug therapy.

⊕ Nursing diagnoses
• Ineffective health maintenance related to underlying condition
• Risk for deficient fluid volume related to adverse GI reactions
• Deficient knowledge related to drug therapy

⯈ Planning and implementation
• Premedicate with acetaminophen to minimize symptoms at beginning of therapy. Flulike symptoms tend to diminish with continued therapy.
• Discard unused portion. Each vial is for single-dose use and doesn't contain preservative.
• Give drug at bedtime to reduce discomfort from flulike symptoms.
• Refrigerate drug immediately. Vials must be stored at 36° to 46° F (2° to 8° C). Don't freeze. Don't shake vial; avoid excessive agitation. Discard vials that have been left at room temperature for longer than 12 hours.
Patient teaching
• Teach patient and family how to give drug and how to dispose of used needles, syringes, containers, and unused drug. Give him a copy of patient information included with product, and make sure he understands it.
• Instruct patient to notify prescriber if adverse reaction occurs.

☑ Evaluation
• Patient responds well to drug.
• Patient maintains adequate hydration.
• Patient and family state understanding of drug therapy.

ipratropium bromide
(ip-ruh-TROH-pee-um BROH-mighd)
Atrovent, Atrovent HFA

Pharmacologic class: anticholinergic
Therapeutic class: bronchodilator
Pregnancy risk category: B

Indications and dosages
⯈ **Bronchospasm caused by COPD.** *Adults and children age 12 and older:* 2 inhalations q.i.d. Additional inhalations may be needed to maximum of 12 total inhalations in 24 hours. Or use inhalation solution, 500 mcg every 6 to 8 hours via oral nebulizer.
⯈ **Rhinorrhea linked to allergic and nonallergic perennial rhinitis.** *Adults and children age 6 and older:* 2 sprays of 0.03% nasal spray in each nostril b.i.d. or t.i.d.

⯈ **Rhinorrhea caused by the common cold.**
Adults and children age 12 and older: 2 sprays of 0.06% nasal spray per nostril t.i.d. or q.i.d. *Children ages 5 to 11:* Give 2 sprays of 0.06% nasal spray per nostril t.i.d.
⯈ **Rhinorrhea linked to seasonal allergic rhinitis.** *Adults and children age 5 and older:* 2 sprays of 0.06% nasal spray per nostril q.i.d.

Contraindications and cautions
• Contraindicated in patients hypersensitive to the drug, its components, or atropine or its derivatives and in those hypersensitive to soya lecithin or related food products, such as soybeans and peanuts.
• Use cautiously in patients with angle-closure glaucoma, prostatic hyperplasia, or bladder-neck obstruction.
• Safety and effectiveness of use beyond 4 days for rhinorrhea from the common cold or 3 weeks for seasonal allergic rhinitis haven't been established.
⚖ **Lifespan:** In pregnant women, use cautiously. In breast-feeding women, use cautiously because it's unknown if the drug appears in breast milk. In children younger than age 12, safety of oral inhaler or nebulizer hasn't been established.

Adverse reactions
CNS: dizziness, headache, nervousness.
CV: chest pain, palpitations.
EENT: blurred vision, burning eyes, epistaxis.
GI: constipation, dry mouth, GI distress, nausea.
Respiratory: bronchitis, *bronchospasm,* cough, upper respiratory tract infection.
Skin: rash.

Interactions
Drug-drug. *Anticholinergics:* May increase anticholinergic effects. Avoid use together.
Cromolyn sodium: Will precipitate if mixed in same nebulizer. Don't use together.
Drug-herb. *Jaborandi tree, pill-bearing spurge:* May decrease drug effects. Use cautiously.

Effects on lab test results
None reported.

Pharmacokinetics
Absorption: Not readily absorbed into systemic circulation.
Distribution: Not distributed.

Reactions may be *common,* uncommon, *life-threatening,* or COMMON AND LIFE-THREATENING.

Metabolism: Small amount that's absorbed is metabolized in liver.
Excretion: Absorbed drug excreted in urine and bile; remainder excreted unchanged in feces.
Half-life: About 2 hours.

Route	Onset	Peak	Duration
Inhalation	5–15 min	1–2 hr	3–6 hr

Action

Chemical effect: Inhibits vagally mediated reflexes by antagonizing acetylcholine.
Therapeutic effect: Relieves bronchospasms and symptoms of seasonal allergic rhinitis.

Available forms

Inhaler: 17 mcg/metered dose (HFA), 18 mcg/metered dose
Nasal spray: 0.03% (21 mcg/spray), 0.06% (42 mcg/spray)
Solution for inhalation: 0.02% (500-mcg vial)

NURSING PROCESS

Assessment
• Assess patient's condition before and after drug therapy; monitor peak expiratory flow.
• Be alert for adverse reactions and drug interactions.
• Assess patient's and family's knowledge of drug therapy.

Nursing diagnoses
• Ineffective breathing pattern related to patient's underlying condition
• Acute pain related to drug-induced headache
• Deficient knowledge related to drug therapy

Planning and implementation
 ALERT: Drug isn't effective for treating acute episodes of bronchospasm when rapid response is needed.
• Don't exceed 12 total inhalations in 24 hours; total nasal sprays shouldn't exceed 8 in each nostril in 24 hours.
• If giving more than one inhalation, let 2 minutes elapse between inhalations. If giving more than one type of inhalant, always give bronchodilator first and wait 5 minutes before giving the other.
• Give drug on time to ensure maximal effect.
• If drug fails to relieve bronchospasms, notify prescriber.

 ALERT: Don't confuse Atrovent with Alupent.
Patient teaching
• Warn patient that drug isn't effective for treating acute episodes of bronchospasm where rapid response is needed.
• Give patient these instructions for using metered-dose inhaler: clear nasal passages and throat. Breathe out, expelling as much air from lungs as possible. Place mouthpiece well into mouth, and inhale deeply as you release dose from inhaler. Hold breath for several seconds, remove mouthpiece, and exhale slowly.
• Tell patient to avoid accidentally spraying into eyes. Temporary blurring of vision may result.
• Tell patient to wait at least 2 minutes before repeating when using more than one inhalation.
• If patient also uses a corticosteroid inhaler, tell him to use ipratropium first and then wait about 5 minutes before using the corticosteroid. This process allows bronchodilator to open air passages for maximum effectiveness of the corticosteroid.
• Tell patient to take a missed dose as soon as remembered, unless it's almost time for next dose. In that case, tell him to skip the missed dose and not to double the dose.
• Tell patient to rinse mouth after using oral inhaler.

Evaluation
• Patient's bronchospasms are relieved.
• Patient doesn't suffer from any drug-induced headaches.
• Patient and family state understanding of drug therapy.

irbesartan
(ir-buh-SAR-tun)
Avapro

Pharmacologic class: angiotensin II receptor antagonist
Therapeutic class: antihypertensive
Pregnancy risk category: C (D in second and third trimesters)

Indications and dosages

▶ **Hypertension.** *Adults and children age 13 and older:* Initially 150 mg P.O. daily; increase to a maximum of 300 mg daily, if needed.

Children ages 6 to 12 years: Initially, 75 mg P.O. daily; increase to a maximum of 150 mg daily, if needed.

▶ **Nephropathy in type 2 diabetic patients.**
Adults: 300 mg P.O. daily.

▧ **Adjust-a-dose:** In patients who are volume- or salt-depleted, give lower initial dose of 75 mg P.O. daily.

Contraindications and cautions

• Contraindicated in patients hypersensitive to the drug or any of its components.
• Use cautiously in volume- or salt-depleted patients and in patients with renal impairment or renal artery stenosis.

✾ **Lifespan:** In pregnant women, drug should be stopped as soon as possible; use in the second and third trimesters can cause fetal death. Breast-feeding women should stop the drug or stop breast-feeding. In children younger than age 6, safety and effectiveness haven't been established.

Adverse reactions

CNS: anxiety, dizziness, fatigue, headache.
CV: chest pain, edema, tachycardia.
EENT: pharyngitis, rhinitis, sinus abnormality.
GI: abdominal pain, diarrhea, dyspepsia, nausea, vomiting.
GU: UTI.
Metabolic: *hyperkalemia.*
Musculoskeletal: musculoskeletal trauma or pain.
Respiratory: *upper respiratory tract infection.*
Skin: rash.

Interactions

Drug-drug. *Potassium-sparing drugs, potassium supplements:* Use cautiously because of risk of hyperkalemia.

Effects on lab test results

• May increase potassium level.

Pharmacokinetics

Absorption: Rapid and complete, with an average absolute bioavailability of 60% to 80%.
Distribution: Wide. 90% protein-bound.
Metabolism: Mainly by conjugation and oxidation.
Excretion: Biliary and renal. About 20% is recovered in urine and the rest in feces. *Half-life:* 11 to 15 hours.

Route	Onset	Peak	Duration
P.O.	Unknown	1½–2 hr	24 hr

Action

Chemical effect: Inhibits the vasoconstricting and aldosterone-secreting effects of angiotensin II by selectively blocking binding of angiotensin II to receptor sites in many tissues.
Therapeutic effect: Lowers blood pressure.

Available forms

Tablets: 75 mg, 150 mg, 300 mg

NURSING PROCESS

⚕ Assessment

• Monitor patient's blood pressure regularly. Dizziness and orthostatic hypotension may occur more frequently in patients with type 2 diabetes mellitus and renal disease.
• Monitor patient's electrolytes, particularly potassium, and assess patient for volume or salt depletion before starting drug therapy.
• Make sure a woman of childbearing age uses effective birth control before starting this drug because of danger to fetus in second and third trimesters.
• Assess patient's and family's knowledge of drug therapy.

⊕ Nursing diagnoses

• Risk for deficient fluid volume in volume- or sodium-depleted patients
• Risk of injury related to the presence of hypertension
• Deficient knowledge related to drug therapy

▶ Planning and implementation

• If drug is needed to control blood pressure, give with a diuretic or other antihypertensive.
• If patient becomes hypotensive, place in a supine position and give an I.V. infusion of normal saline solution.

Patient teaching
• Warn woman of childbearing age about consequences of exposing fetus to drug. Tell her to call prescriber immediately if she suspects she is pregnant.
• Tell patient that drug may be taken once daily with or without food.
• Instruct patient to avoid driving and hazardous activities until CNS effects of drug are known.

Reactions may be *common,* uncommon, *life-threatening*, or COMMON AND LIFE-THREATENING.

✓ Evaluation

• Patient doesn't experience hypotension as a result of volume or salt depletion.
• Patient's blood pressure remains within normal limits, and drug therapy doesn't cause injury.
• Patient and family state understanding of drug therapy.

iron dextran
(IGH-ern DEKS-tran)
DexFerrum, Dexiron ♦, InFeD, Infufer ♦

Pharmacologic class: parenteral iron supplement
Therapeutic class: hematinic
Pregnancy risk category: C

Indications and dosages

▶ **Iron deficiency anemia.** Total dose (in ml) is based on patient's weight and hemoglobin (Hgb) level using the following formula:

$$\text{Dose (ml)} = 0.0442 \text{ (desired Hgb} - \text{observed Hgb)} \times \text{weight**} + (0.26 \times \text{weight})$$

**Ideal body weight (IBW) or actual body weight if less than IBW, in kilograms

For children 5 to 15 kg, use actual weight in kg.

One ml iron dextran provides 50 mg elemental iron.
Adults and children: For I.M. use, 0.5-ml test dose injected by Z-track method. If no reactions occur, maximum daily doses are 0.5 ml (25 mg) for infants weighing less than 5 kg (11 lb), 1 ml (50 mg) for children weighing less than 10 kg (22 lb), and 2 ml (100 mg) for heavier children and adults. For I.V. use, 0.5-ml test dose injected over 30 seconds for InFeD, but for DexFerrum, inject over at least 5 minutes. If no reactions occur in 1 hour, remainder of therapeutic dose is given I.V. Therapeutic dose repeated I.V. daily. Maximum single dose is 100 mg of undiluted iron. Give slowly (1 ml/minute).

▽ I.V. administration

• Check facility policy before giving drug I.V.
• Use I.V. when patient has insufficient muscle mass for deep I.M. injection, impaired absorption from muscle as a result of stasis or edema, possibility of uncontrolled I.M. bleeding from trauma (as may occur in hemophilia), or massive and prolonged parenteral therapy (as may be needed in chronic substantial blood loss).
• When I.V. dose is complete, flush vein with 10 ml of normal saline solution. Have patient rest for 15 to 30 minutes after I.V. administration.

⊗ **Incompatibilities**
Other I.V. drugs, parenteral nutrition solutions for I.V. infusion.

Contraindications and cautions

• Contraindicated in patients hypersensitive to drug or any of its components and in those with acute infectious renal disease or anemia disorders (except iron deficiency anemia).
• Use cautiously in patients who have serious hepatic impairment, rheumatoid arthritis, or other inflammatory diseases, and in patients with history of significant allergies or asthma.

⚖ **Lifespan:** In pregnant women, use only when benefits outweigh risks to the fetus. In breast-feeding women, use cautiously because it's unknown if the drug appears in breast milk. In children younger than age 4 months, safety and effectiveness haven't been studied.

Adverse reactions

CNS: arthralgia, dizziness, headache, malaise, myalgia, syncope, transitory paresthesia, weakness.
CV: *arrhythmias,* bradycardia, chest pain, chest tightness, hypertension, hypotensive reaction, peripheral vascular flushing with overly rapid I.V. administration, *shock,* tachycardia.
GI: abdominal pain, diarrhea, metallic taste, nausea, transient loss of taste, vomiting.
Respiratory: *bronchospasm.*
Skin: *brown discoloration* at I.M. injection site, rash, urticaria.
Other: *anaphylaxis;* atrophy; delayed sensitivity reactions; fibrosis; necrosis; *soreness, inflammation, and local phlebitis* at I.V. injection site; sterile abscess.

Interactions

Drug-drug. *Chloramphenicol:* May increase iron level because of decreased iron clearance and erythropoiesis. Consult prescriber about using together.

Effects on lab test results

• May increase bilirubin and hemoglobin levels and hematocrit. May decrease calcium level.
• May falsely increase bilirubin level. May falsely decrease calcium level.
• May interfere with bone scans involving 99m Tc-diphosphonate.

Pharmacokinetics

Absorption: In two stages: 60% after 3 days and up to 90% by 3 weeks. Remainder is absorbed over several months or longer.
Distribution: During first 3 days, local inflammation facilitates passage of drug into lymphatic system; drug is then ingested by macrophages, which enter lymph and blood.
Metabolism: Cleared from plasma by reticuloendothelial cells of liver, spleen, and bone marrow.
Excretion: Trace amounts in urine, bile, and feces. *Half-life:* 6 hours.

Route	Onset	Peak	Duration
I.V., I.M.	72 hr	Unknown	3–4 wk

Action

Chemical effect: Provides elemental iron, a component of hemoglobin.
Therapeutic effect: Increases level of iron, an essential component of hemoglobin.

Available forms

Injection: 50 mg elemental iron/ml

NURSING PROCESS

Assessment

• Assess patient's iron deficiency before starting therapy.
• Monitor the drug's effectiveness by evaluating hemoglobin level, hematocrit, and reticulocyte count, and monitor patient's health status.
• Be alert for adverse reactions and drug interactions.
• Observe patient for delayed reactions (1 to 2 days), which may include arthralgia, backache, chills, dizziness, headache, malaise, fever, myalgia, nausea, and vomiting.
• Assess patient's and family's knowledge of drug therapy.

Nursing diagnoses

• Ineffective health maintenance related to iron deficiency
• Risk for injury related to potential drug-induced anaphylaxis
• Deficient knowledge related to drug therapy

Planning and implementation

• Don't give iron dextran with oral iron preparations.
• I.M. or I.V. injections of iron are recommended only for patients for whom oral administration is impossible or ineffective.
⊛ **ALERT:** I.M. or I.V. test dose is required.
• When giving I.M., use a 19G or 20G needle that is 2 to 3 inches long. Inject drug deep into upper outer quadrant of buttock—never into arm or other exposed area. Use Z-track method to avoid leakage into subcutaneous tissue and staining of skin.
• Minimize skin staining by using separate needle to withdraw drug from its container.
• Keep epinephrine and resuscitation equipment readily available to treat anaphylaxis.
Patient teaching
• Warn patient to avoid OTC vitamins that contain iron.
• Teach patient to recognize and report symptoms of reaction or toxicity.

Evaluation

• Patient's hemoglobin level, hematocrit, and reticulocyte count are normal.
• Patient doesn't experience anaphylaxis.
• Patient and family state understanding of drug therapy.

iron sucrose
(IGH-ern SOO-krohs)
Venofer

Pharmacologic class: polynuclear iron (III)-hydroxide in sucrose
Therapeutic class: hematinic
Pregnancy risk category: B

Indications and dosages

▶ **Iron deficiency anemia in patients undergoing long-term hemodialysis who are receiving supplemental erythropoietin therapy.**
Adults: 100 mg (5 ml) of elemental iron I.V.

directly in the dialysis line either by slow injection over 2 to 5 minutes or by infusion over 15 minutes during the dialysis session, one to three times weekly for a total of 1,000 mg in 10 doses. Repeat, if needed.

▶ **Iron deficiency anemia in chronic kidney disease patients not on dialysis.** *Adults:* 200 mg by slow I.V. injection undiluted over 2 to 5 minutes on five separate occasions during a 14-day period to a total cumulative dose of 1,000 mg.

▼ I.V. administration

• Inspect drug for particulates and discoloration before giving it.
• For slow injection, give 1 ml (20 mg elemental iron) undiluted solution per minute, not exceeding one vial (100 mg elemental iron) per injection.
• For infusion, dilute to a maximum of 100 ml in normal saline solution immediately before infusion, and infuse 100 mg elemental iron over at least 15 minutes.
• Giving by infusion may reduce the risk of hypotension.
• Transferrin saturation values increase rapidly after I.V. delivery of iron sucrose. Measure iron level 48 hours after an I.V. dose.

⊗ **Incompatibilities**
Other I.V. drugs, parenteral nutrition infusions.

Contraindications and cautions

• Contraindicated in patients with evidence of iron overload, patients hypersensitive to drug or its components, and patients with anemia not caused by iron deficiency.
✺ **Lifespan:** In pregnant women, use cautiously. In breast-feeding women, use cautiously because it's not known whether drug appears in breast milk. In children, safety and effectiveness of drug haven't been established. In elderly patients, make dose selection conservatively; these patients may have decreased hepatic, renal, and cardiac function and other diseases and drug therapies.

Adverse reactions

CNS: asthenia, dizziness, fever, headache, malaise, pain.
CV: chest pain, fluid retention, *heart failure,* hypertension, *hypotension.*
GI: abdominal pain, diarrhea, nausea, taste perversion, vomiting.

Musculoskeletal: bone and muscle pain, *leg cramps.*
Respiratory: cough, dyspnea, pneumonia.
Skin: pruritus.
Other: accidental injury, *anaphylaxis,* hypersensitivity reaction, injection-site reaction, *sepsis.*

Interactions

Drug-drug. *Oral iron preparations:* May reduce absorption of these compounds. Avoid use together.

Effects on lab test results

• May increase liver enzyme levels.

Pharmacokinetics

Absorption: Given I.V.
Distribution: Mainly in blood and somewhat in extravascular fluid. A significant amount of iron is also distributed in the liver, spleen, and bone marrow.
Metabolism: Dissociated by reticuloendothelial system into iron and sucrose.
Excretion: About 75% of sucrose and 5% of the iron component are eliminated by urinary excretion in 24 hours. *Half-life:* 6 hours.

Route	Onset	Peak	Duration
I.V.	Unknown	Unknown	Variable

Action

Chemical effect: Iron component of dissociated drug eventually replenishes depleted body iron stores, significantly increasing iron and ferritin levels and decreasing total iron-binding capacity.
Therapeutic effect: Increases iron level.

Available forms

Injection: 20 mg/ml of elemental iron in 5-ml vial

NURSING PROCESS

🔍 Assessment

• Assess underlying condition before starting therapy, and reassess regularly.
• Monitor ferritin and hemoglobin levels, hematocrit, and transferrin saturation.
• Monitor patient for adverse reactions or hypersensitivity reactions to the drug.
• Assess patient's and family's knowledge of drug therapy.

🔲 Nursing diagnoses
- Acute pain related to adverse drug effects
- Ineffective health maintenance related to iron deficiency
- Deficient knowledge related to iron sucrose therapy

▶ Planning and implementation
- Monitor patient for symptoms of overdose or too-rapid infusion, which include hypotension, headache, nausea, dizziness, joint aches, paresthesia, abdominal and muscle pain, edema, and CV collapse.
- Observe patient for rare but fatal hypersensitivity reactions characterized by anaphylaxis, loss of consciousness, collapse, hypotension, dyspnea, or seizures.
- Withhold dose in patient with evidence of iron overload.

Patient teaching
- Instruct patient to notify prescriber if symptoms of overdose occur, such as headache, nausea, dizziness, joint aches, paresthesia, or abdominal and muscle pain.
- Warn patient not to take OTC vitamins containing iron.

☑ Evaluation
- Patient doesn't experience pain.
- Patient's hemoglobin level and hematocrit are normal.
- Patient and family state understanding of iron sucrose therapy.

isoniazid (isonicotinic acid hydride INH)
(igh-soh-NIGH-uh-sid)
Isotamine ◆ , Nydrazid

Pharmacologic class: isonicotinic acid hydrazine
Therapeutic class: antituberculotic
Pregnancy risk category: C

Indications and dosages

▶ **Actively growing tubercle bacilli with other antituberculotics.** *Adults and children age 15 and older:* 5 mg/kg P.O. or I.M. daily in single dose, maximum 300 mg P.O. or I.M. daily, continued for 6 months to 2 years. Or

15 mg/kg (maximum dosage 900 mg/daily) two to three times weekly.
Infants and children: 10 to 15 mg/kg P.O. or I.M. daily in single dose, maximum 300 mg P.O. or I.M. daily, continued for 18 months to 2 years. Or 20 to 40 mg/kg (maximum dose 900 mg/daily) two to three times weekly.

▶ **Prevention of tubercle bacilli in those closely exposed to tuberculosis or those with positive skin tests whose chest X-rays and bacteriologic studies are consistent with non-progressive tuberculosis.** *Adults:* 300 mg P.O. daily in single dose, for 6 months to 1 year.
Infants and children: 10 mg/kg P.O. daily in single dose. Maximum, 300 mg P.O. daily for 1 year.

Contraindications and cautions
- Contraindicated in patients with acute hepatic disease or isoniazid-related liver damage.
- Use cautiously in patients with chronic non–isoniazid-related liver disease, seizure disorders (especially in those taking phenytoin), severe renal impairment, chronic alcoholism, or I.V. drug abuse.

❧ **Lifespan:** In pregnant women, use cautiously. In breast-feeding women, small amounts of drug appear in breast milk but aren't sufficient to cause harm or therapeutic benefit to the infant. In elderly patients, use cautiously.

Adverse reactions
CNS: paresthesias, *peripheral neuropathy,* psychosis, *seizures.*
GI: constipation, dry mouth, epigastric distress, nausea, vomiting.
Hematologic: *agranulocytosis, aplastic anemia,* eosinophilia, hemolytic anemia, *leukopenia, methemoglobinemia, neutropenia, thrombocytopenia.*
Hepatic: *hepatitis.*
Metabolic: hyperglycemia, *metabolic acidosis.*
Other: hypersensitivity reactions, irritation at I.M. injection site, rheumatic syndrome and lupuslike syndrome.

Interactions
Drug-drug. *Acetaminophen:* May increase hepatotoxic effects of acetaminophen. Don't give together.
Antacids and laxatives containing aluminum: May decrease rate and amount of isoniazid ab-

sorbed. Give isoniazid at least 1 hour before antacid or laxative.

Carbamazepine: May increase risk of isoniazid hepatotoxicity. Use together cautiously.

Carbamazepine, phenytoin: May increase levels of these anticonvulsants. Monitor patient closely.

Corticosteroids: May decrease therapeutic effect of isoniazid. Monitor patient's need for larger isoniazid dose.

Cyclosporine: May increase adverse CNS effects of cyclosporine. Monitor patient closely.

Disulfiram: May cause neurologic symptoms, including changes in behavior and coordination. Avoid use together.

Ketoconazole: May decrease ketoconazole level. Monitor patient closely.

Oral anticoagulants: May increase anticoagulation. Monitor patient for signs of bleeding.

Rifampin: May increase risk of hepatotoxicity. Monitor patient closely.

SSRIs: May cause serotonin syndrome. Use with caution.

Theophylline: May increase theophylline level. Monitor level closely, and adjust theophylline dosage.

Drug-food. *Foods containing tyramine:* May cause hypertensive crisis. Tell patients to avoid such foods altogether.

Drug-lifestyle. *Alcohol use:* May increase risk of isoniazid-related hepatitis. Discourage use together.

Effects on lab test results

• May increase transaminase, glucose, and bilirubin levels. May decrease calcium, phosphate, and hemoglobin levels and hematocrit.

• May increase eosinophil count. May decrease WBC, granulocyte, neutrophil, and platelet counts.

Pharmacokinetics

Absorption: Complete and rapid after P.O. use. Also absorbed readily after I.M. injection.

Distribution: Wide.

Metabolism: Mainly in liver. Rate of metabolism varies individually; fast acetylators metabolize drug five times faster than others. About 50% of blacks and whites are slow acetylators; more than 80% of Chinese, Japanese, and Eskimos are fast acetylators.

Excretion: Mainly in urine; some in saliva, sputum, feces, and breast milk. *Half-life:* 1 to 4 hours.

Route	Onset	Peak	Duration
P.O., I.M.	Unknown	1–2 hr	Unknown

Action

Chemical effect: May inhibit cell wall biosynthesis by interfering with lipid and DNA synthesis.

Therapeutic effect: Kills susceptible bacteria, such as *Mycobacterium tuberculosis, M. bovis,* and some strains of *M. kansasii.*

Available forms

Injection: 100 mg/ml
Oral solution: 50 mg/5 ml
Tablets: 100 mg, 300 mg

NURSING PROCESS

Assessment
• Assess patient's infection before starting therapy by physical examination and culture and sensitivity testing.
• Monitor patient for improvement, and evaluate culture and sensitivity tests.
• Be alert for adverse reactions and drug interactions.
• Monitor hepatic function closely for changes.
• Monitor patient for paresthesia of hands and feet, which usually precedes peripheral neuropathy, especially in patients who are malnourished, alcoholic, diabetic, or slow acetylators.
• Assess patient's and family's knowledge of drug therapy.

Nursing diagnoses
• Risk for infection related to presence of susceptible bacteria
• Disturbed sensory perception (tactile) related to drug-induced peripheral neuropathy
• Deficient knowledge related to drug therapy

Planning and implementation
• Give oral form of drug 1 hour before or 2 hours after meals to avoid decreased absorption.
• Switch from I.M. to P.O. form as soon as possible.
• **ALERT:** Always give isoniazid with other antituberculotics to prevent development of resistant organisms.
• Give pyridoxine to prevent peripheral neuropathy, especially in malnourished patients.

Patient teaching

• Tell patient to take drug as prescribed; warn against stopping drug without prescriber's consent.
• Advise patient to take with food if GI irritation occurs.
• Instruct patient not to drink alcohol during therapy.
• Instruct patient to avoid certain foods (fish, such as skip jack and tuna, and foods containing tyramine, such as aged cheese, beer, and chocolate) because drug acts like an MAO inhibitor.
• Tell patient to notify prescriber immediately if symptoms of liver impairment occur (loss of appetite, fatigue, malaise, jaundice, dark urine).
• Urge patient to comply with treatment, which may last for months or years.

☑ Evaluation

• Patient is free from infection.
• Patient maintains normal peripheral nervous system function.
• Patient and family state understanding of drug therapy.

HIGH ALERT

isoproterenol hydrochloride
(igh-soh-proh-TEER-uh-nol)
Isuprel

Pharmacologic class: adrenergic
Therapeutic class: bronchodilator, cardiac stimulant
Pregnancy risk category: C

Indications and dosages

▶ **Bronchospasm during anesthesia.** *Adults:* Dilute 1 ml of a 1:5,000 solution with 10 ml of normal saline of D_5W. Give 0.01 to 0.02 mg I.V. (0.5 ml to 1 ml). Repeat as needed. Or, 0.01 to 0.02 mg of 1:50,000 solution undiluted I.V. (0.5 ml to 1 ml). Repeat as needed.
▶ **Heart block and ventricular arrhythmias.** *Adults:* Initially, 0.02 to 0.06 mg hydrochloride I.V. Subsequent doses 0.01 to 0.2 mg I.V. or 5 mcg/minute I.V. Or 0.2 mg I.M. initially; then 0.02 to 1 mg, as needed.
Children: Give half of initial adult dosage of hydrochloride.
▶ **Shock.** *Adults and children:* 0.5 to 5 mcg/minute hydrochloride by continuous I.V. infusion. Usual concentration is 1 mg (5 ml) in

500 ml D_5W. Infusion rate adjusted according to heart rate, central venous pressure, blood pressure, and urine flow.
▶ **Postoperative cardiac patients with bradycardia‡.** *Children:* I.V. infusion of 0.029 mcg/kg/minute.
▶ **As an aid in diagnosing the cause of mitral regurgitation‡.** *Adults:* 4 mcg/minute I.V. infusion.
▶ **As an aid in diagnosing coronary artery disease or lesions‡.** *Adults:* 1 to 3 mcg/minute I.V. infusion.

▼ I.V. administration

• If injection solution is discolored or contains precipitate, don't use.
• Give drug by direct injection or I.V. infusion. For infusion, drug may be diluted with most common I.V. solutions.
• If heart rate exceeds 110 beats/minute with I.V. infusion, notify prescriber. Doses sufficient to increase heart rate to more than 130 beats/minute may induce ventricular arrhythmias.
• When giving I.V. isoproterenol to treat shock, closely monitor blood pressure, central venous pressure, ECG, arterial blood gas measurements, and urine output. Carefully adjust infusion rate according to these measurements. Use continuous infusion pump to regulate flow rate.
⊗ **Incompatibilities**
Alkalies, aminophylline, furosemide, metals, sodium bicarbonate.

Contraindications and cautions

• Contraindicated in patients with tachycardia caused by digitalis intoxication, in those with arrhythmias (other than those that may respond to treatment with isoproterenol), and in those with angina pectoris.
• Use cautiously in patients with renal or CV disease, coronary insufficiency, diabetes, hyperthyroidism, or history of sensitivity to sympathomimetic amines.
⚕ **Lifespan:** In pregnant and breast-feeding women, use cautiously. In children and elderly patients, use cautiously.

Adverse reactions

CNS: *Adams-Stokes syndrome,* dizziness, *headache,* insomnia, mild tremor, nervousness, weakness.

Reactions may be *common,* uncommon, *life-threatening*, or COMMON AND LIFE-THREATENING.

CV: angina, *arrhythmias, cardiac arrest,* flushing of face, labile blood pressure, palpitations, tachycardia.
GI: nausea, vomiting.
Metabolic: hyperglycemia.
Respiratory: *bronchospasm.*
Skin: diaphoresis.

Interactions

Drug-drug. *Beta blockers, such as propranolol:* May block bronchodilating effect of isoproterenol. If used together, monitor patient carefully.
Sympathomimetics, such as epinephrine: May increase risk of arrhythmias. Avoid use together.

Effects on lab test results

• May increase glucose level.

Pharmacokinetics

Absorption: Rapid
Distribution: Wide.
Metabolism: By conjugation in GI tract and by enzymatic reduction in liver, lungs, and other tissues.
Excretion: Mainly in urine. *Half-life:* Unknown.

Route	Onset	Peak	Duration
I.V.	Immediate	Unknown	< 1 hr

Action

Chemical effect: Relaxes bronchial smooth muscle by acting on $beta_2$-adrenergic receptors. As cardiac stimulant, acts on $beta_1$-adrenergic receptors in heart.
Therapeutic effect: Relieves bronchospasms and heart block and restores normal sinus rhythm after ventricular arrhythmia.

Available forms

Injection: 20 mcg/ml (1:50,000 solution), 200 mcg/ml (1:5,000 solution)

NURSING PROCESS

🔲 Assessment

• Assess patient's underlying condition before starting therapy.
• Monitor blood pressure, heart rate, urine flow and electrocardiogram for arrhythmias and ischemia.

• Be alert for adverse reactions and drug interactions.
• This drug may aggravate ventilation and perfusion abnormalities. Even when ease of breathing is improved, arterial oxygen tension may fall paradoxically.
• Assess patient's and family's knowledge of drug therapy.

🔲 Nursing diagnoses

• Ineffective health maintenance related to underlying condition
• Risk for injury related to drug-induced adverse reactions
• Deficient knowledge related to drug therapy

▶ Planning and implementation

• Drug doesn't treat blood or fluid volume deficit. Correct volume deficit before giving vasopressors.
• If adverse reactions occur, notify prescriber; adjust dosage or stop drug if needed.
• If precordial distress or angina occurs, stop drug immediately.
• ⑤ **ALERT:** Don't confuse Isuprel with Ismelin or Isordil.
• Use only in surgical or acute care settings.
Patient teaching
• Tell patient to report chest pain or shortness of breath.

☑ Evaluation

• Patient has improved health.
• Patient sustains no injury from adverse reactions.
• Patient and family state understanding of drug therapy.

isosorbide dinitrate
(igh-soh-SOR-bighd digh-NIGH-trayt)
Apo-ISDN ◆, Cedocard SR ◆, Dilatrate-SR, Isochron, Isordil Titradose, Novo-Sorbide ◆

isosorbide mononitrate
IMDUR, ISMO, Monoket

Pharmacologic class: nitrate
Therapeutic class: antianginal, vasodilator
Pregnancy risk category: C

Indications and dosages

▶ **Acute angina (S.L. form only), prophylaxis in situations likely to cause angina.** *Adults:* 2.5 to 5 mg S.L. tablets for prompt relief of angina, repeated every 5 to 10 minutes (maximum of three doses for each 30-minute period). For prevention, 2.5 to 10 mg every 2 to 3 hours. Or, 5 to 40 mg isosorbide dinitrate P.O. b.i.d. or t.i.d. for prevention only (use smallest effective dose). Or, 30 to 60 mg isosorbide mononitrate using Imdur P.O. once daily on arising; increased to 120 mg once daily after several days, if needed. Or, 20 mg isosorbide mononitrate using ISMO or Monoket b.i.d. with the two doses given 7 hours apart.

▶ **Adjunctive treatment of heart failure‡.** *Adults:* 20 mg isosorbide dinitrate with 37.5 mg hydralazine P.O. t.i.d. Maximum dose is 40 mg isosorbide dinitrate and 75 mg hydralazine P.O. t.i.d.

▶ **Diffuse esophageal spasm without gastroesophageal reflux‡.** *Adults:* 10 to 30 mg isosorbide dinitrate P.O. q.i.d.

Contraindications and cautions

• Contraindicated in patients hypersensitive to nitrates, in those with idiosyncratic reactions to nitrates, and in those with severe hypotension, shock, or acute MI with low left ventricular filling pressure.

• Use cautiously in patients with blood volume depletion (such as that resulting from diuretic therapy) or mild hypotension.

⚘ **Lifespan:** In pregnant women, use cautiously. In breast-feeding women, use cautiously because it's unknown if drug appears in breast milk. In children, safety and effectiveness haven't been established.

Adverse reactions

CNS: dizziness, *headache,* weakness.
CV: ankle edema, fainting, *flushing,* orthostatic hypotension, palpitations, tachycardia.
GI: nausea, vomiting.
Skin: cutaneous vasodilation.
Other: hypersensitivity reactions, sublingual burning.

Interactions

Drug-drug. *Antihypertensives:* May increase hypotensive effects. Monitor patient closely during initial therapy.

Sildenafil, tadalafil, vardenafil: May increase hypotensive effects. Avoid use together.
Drug-lifestyle. *Alcohol use:* May increase hypotension. Discourage use together.

Effects on lab test results

None reported.

Pharmacokinetics

Absorption: Dinitrate is well absorbed from GI tract but undergoes first-pass metabolism, resulting in bioavailability of about 50% (depending on dosage form used). Mononitrate is also absorbed well, with almost 100% bioavailability.
Distribution: Widely throughout body.
Metabolism: In liver to active metabolites.
Excretion: In urine. *Half-life:* Dinitrate P.O., 5 to 6 hours; S.L., 2 hours; mononitrate, about 5 hours.

Route	Onset	Peak	Duration
P.O.	2–60 min	2–60 min	1–12 hr
S.L.	2–5 min	2–5 min	1–2 hr

Action

Chemical effect: May reduce cardiac oxygen demand by decreasing left ventricular end diastolic pressure (preload) and, to a lesser extent, systemic vascular resistance (afterload). May increase blood flow through collateral coronary vessels.
Therapeutic effect: Relieves angina.

Available forms

isosorbide dinitrate
Capsules (extended-release): 40 mg
Tablets: 5 mg, 10 mg, 20 mg, 30 mg, 40 mg
Tablets (S.L.): 2.5 mg, 5 mg
Tablets (sustained-release): 40 mg
isosorbide mononitrate
Tablets: 10 mg, 20 mg
Tablets (extended-release): 30 mg, 60 mg, 120 mg

NURSING PROCESS

▨ **Assessment**
• Assess patient's angina before and regularly during therapy.
• Monitor blood pressure, heart rate and rhythm, and intensity and duration of drug response.
• Be alert for adverse reactions and drug interactions.

- Assess patient's and family's knowledge of drug therapy.

Nursing diagnoses
- Acute pain related to angina
- Risk for injury related to drug-induced adverse reactions
- Deficient knowledge related to drug therapy

Planning and implementation
- To prevent tolerance, don't give drug during an 8- to 12-hour period daily. The dosage regimen for isosorbide mononitrate (one tablet on awakening with second dose in 7 hours, or one extended-release tablet daily) is intended to offer a nitrate-free period during the day to minimize nitrate tolerance.
- Give drug on empty stomach, either 30 minutes before or 1 to 2 hours after meals, and have patient swallow tablets whole.
- Give S.L. form of drug at first sign of angina. Have patient wet tablet with saliva, place it under his tongue until completely absorbed, and sit down and rest. Dose may be repeated every 5 to 10 minutes for maximum of three doses.
- ⚡ ALERT: Don't stop therapy abruptly because coronary vasospasm may occur.
- If patient's pain doesn't subside, notify prescriber immediately.
- ⚡ ALERT: Don't confuse Isordil with Isuprel or Inderal.
- ⚡ ALERT: Don't confuse Coronex (isosorbide dinitrate) with Coronex (the herbal supplement for male virility and vitality).

Patient teaching
- Advise patient to take drug regularly, as prescribed, and to keep it accessible at all times.
- ⚡ ALERT: Advise patient that stopping drug abruptly causes coronary vasospasm.
- Tell patient to take S.L. tablet at first sign of attack. Explain that tablet should be wet with saliva and placed under tongue until completely absorbed, and that patient should sit down and rest until pain subsides. Tell patient that dose may be repeated every 5 to 10 minutes for up to three doses. If pain doesn't subside, tell patient to get medical help promptly.
- If patient complains of tingling sensation with S.L. use, suggest holding tablet in buccal pouch.
- ⚡ ALERT: Warn patient not to confuse S.L. form with P.O. form.
- Instruct patient taking P.O. form to take tablet on empty stomach, either 30 minutes before or

1 to 2 hours after meals, and to swallow tablet whole.
- Tell patient to minimize orthostatic hypotension by changing to upright position slowly. Tell him to go up and down stairs carefully and to lie down at first sign of dizziness.
- Instruct patient to avoid alcohol during therapy.
- Tell patient to store drug in cool place, in tightly closed container, away from light.

Evaluation
- Patient is free from pain.
- Patient sustains no injury from adverse reactions.
- Patient and family state understanding of drug therapy.

isotretinoin
(igh-soh-TREH-tih-noyn)
Accutane, Accutane Roche ♦ , Amnesteem, Claravis, Clarus ♦ , Sotret

Pharmacologic class: retinoic acid derivative
Therapeutic class: antiacne drug
Pregnancy risk category: X

Indications and dosages
▶ **Severe recalcitrant nodular acne unresponsive to conventional therapy.** *Adults and children ages 12 to 17:* Give 0.5 to 1 mg/kg P.O. daily in two divided doses for 15 to 20 weeks. Maximum daily dosage, 2 mg/kg.
▶ **Keratinization disorders resistant to conventional therapy, prevention of skin cancer‡.** *Adults:* Dosage varies with specific disease and severity of the disorder. Dosages up to 2 to 4 mg/kg P.O. daily have been used. Consult literature for specific recommendations.
▶ **Squamous cell cancer of the head and neck‡.** *Adults:* 50 to 100 mg/m² P.O.

Contraindications and cautions
- Contraindicated in patients hypersensitive to parabens, which are used as preservatives.
- Use cautiously in patients with genetic predisposition or history of osteoporosis, osteomalacia, or other disorders of bone metabolism. Also use cautiously in patients with a history of mental illness or family history of psychiatric disorders, asthma, liver disease, diabetes, heart disease, osteoporosis, weak bones, or anorexia nervosa.

⚖ **Lifespan:** In women of childbearing age, drug is contraindicated unless patient has had negative serum pregnancy test within 2 weeks of beginning therapy, will begin drug therapy on second or third day of next menstrual period, and will comply with stringent contraceptive measures for 1 month before therapy, during therapy, and at least 1 month after therapy. In pregnant women, drug is contraindicated. In breast-feeding women, use cautiously. In children younger than age 12, safety and effectiveness haven't been established. In children ages 12 to 17, use cautiously.

Adverse reactions

CNS: *aggressive and violent behavior,* depression, emotional instability, *fatigue, headache,* pseudotumor cerebri (benign intracranial hypertension), psychosis, *seizure, stroke, suicide.*
CV: hypertriglyceridemia.
EENT: *conjunctivitis,* corneal deposits, decreased night vision, dry eyes, hearing impairment, intolerance to contact lenses, visual disturbances.
GI: *acute pancreatitis,* gum bleeding and inflammation, inflammatory bowel disease, nausea, nonspecific GI symptoms, vomiting.
Hematologic: anemia.
Hepatic: *hepatitis,* increased liver enzymes.
Metabolic: hyperglycemia.
Musculoskeletal: *arthralgia,* arthritis, back pain, bone abnormalities, calcification of tendons and ligaments, decreases in bone mineral density, musculoskeletal symptoms, premature epiphyseal closure, *rhabdomyolysis,* skeletal hyperostosis, tendonitis.
Skin: *cheilosis, dry skin,* peeling of palms and toes, photosensitivity, *rash,* skin infection, thinning of hair.

Interactions

Drug-drug. *Corticosteroids:* May increase risk of osteoporosis. Use together cautiously.
Medicated soaps and cleansers, medicated cover-ups, topical resorcinol peeling agents (benzoyl peroxide), and preparations containing alcohol: May have cumulative drying effect. Use cautiously.
Microdosed progesterone birth control pills that don't contain estrogen: May decrease contraceptive effectiveness. Advise using alternative contraceptive methods.

Phenytoin: May increase risk of osteomalacia. Use together cautiously.
Tetracyclines: May increase risk of pseudotumor cerebri. Avoid use together.
Vitamin A products: May have additive toxic effect. Avoid use together.
Drug-food. *Any food:* May increase absorption of drug. Have patient take drug with food.
Drug-lifestyle. *Alcohol use:* May increase risk of hypertriglyceridemia. Discourage use together.
Sun exposure: May increase photosensitivity reactions. Advise patient to use sunscreen and wear protective clothing.

Effects on lab test results

• May increase CK, ALT, AST, alkaline phosphatase, uric acid, glucose, and triglyceride levels. May decrease hemoglobin level and hematocrit.
• May increase platelet count.

Pharmacokinetics

Absorption: Rapid.
Distribution: Wide. 99.9% protein-bound, mainly to albumin.
Metabolism: In liver and possibly in gut wall.
Excretion: Unknown. *Half-life:* 30 minutes to 39 hours.

Route	Onset	Peak	Duration
P.O.	Unknown	3 hr	Unknown

Action

Chemical effect: May normalize keratinization, reversibly decrease size of sebaceous glands, and alter composition of sebum to less viscous form that is less likely to plug follicles.
Therapeutic effect: Improves skin integrity.

Available forms

Capsules: 10 mg, 20 mg, 30 mg, 40 mg
Softgel capsules: 10 mg, 20 mg, 30 mg, 40 mg

NURSING PROCESS

🗒 **Assessment**
• Assess patient's skin before starting therapy and regularly thereafter.
• Obtain baseline lipid studies, liver function test results, and pregnancy test before therapy. Monitor these values at regular intervals until response to drug is established (usually about 4 weeks).

- Monitor glucose and CK levels in patients who engage in vigorous physical activity.
- Be alert for adverse reactions and drug interactions.
- Osteoporosis, osteopenia, bone fractures, and delayed healing of bone fractures have been seen in patients taking isotretinoin. While a causal relationship hasn't been established, an effect can't be ruled out. Long-term effects haven't been studied. It's important not to exceed the recommended dose or duration.
- Most adverse reactions appear to be dose-related, occurring at dosages greater than 1 mg/kg daily. They're usually reversible when therapy is stopped or dosage reduced.
- To minimize the risk of fetal exposure, drug is only available through restricted distribution program approved by the FDA called iPLEDGE.
- Actively monitor mood and behavioral changes because of risk of significant psychological changes including suicidal thoughts and behavior.
- Assess patient's and family's knowledge of drug therapy.

Nursing diagnoses
- Impaired skin integrity related to underlying skin condition
- Impaired tissue integrity related to adverse reactions
- Deficient knowledge related to drug therapy

Planning and implementation
- Start second course of therapy at least 8 weeks after completion of first course because improvement may continue after stopping drug.
- Any suspected fetal exposure to drug must be immediately reported to the FDA's MedWatch program at 1-800-FDA-1088 and the iPLEDGE pregnancy registry at 1-866-495-0654 or www.ipledgeprogram.com.
- Give drug with meals or shortly thereafter to enhance absorption.
- **ALERT:** Screen patient with headache, nausea and vomiting, or visual disturbances for papilledema. Signs and symptoms of pseudotumor cerebri require an immediate stop to therapy and prompt neurologic intervention.

Patient teaching
- Advise patient to take drug with milk, meals, or shortly after meals to ensure adequate absorption.

- Tell patient to immediately report visual disturbances and bone, muscle, or joint pain.
- Warn patient that contact lenses may feel uncomfortable during therapy.
- Warn patient against using abrasives, medicated soaps and cleansers, acne preparations containing peeling agents, and topical alcohol preparations (including cosmetics, aftershave, cologne) because these agents cause cumulative irritation or excessive drying of skin.
- Instruct patient not to drink alcohol during therapy.
- Urge patient to report mood changes, such as increased hostility or depression, and suicidal thinking immediately; these may be drug related.
- Tell patient to avoid prolonged exposure to sunlight, to use sunblock, and to wear protective clothing.
- **ALERT:** Advise patient not to donate blood during or for 30 days after therapy; severe fetal abnormalities may occur if a pregnant woman receives blood containing isotretinoin.
- Advise women of childbearing age to use two reliable forms of contraception simultaneously within 1 month of treatment, during treatment and for 1 month after treatment as prescribed under the iPLEDGE program, and to report suspected pregnancy immediately.

Evaluation
- Patient has improved skin condition.
- Patient is free from conjunctivitis, corneal deposits, and dry eyes.
- Patient and family state understanding of drug therapy.

itraconazole
(ih-truh-KAHN-uh-zohl)
Sporanox

Pharmacologic class: synthetic triazole
Therapeutic class: antifungal
Pregnancy risk category: C

Indications and dosages
▶ **Pulmonary and extrapulmonary blastomycosis, histoplasmosis.** *Adults:* 200 mg P.O. (capsules) daily. Dosage may be increased as needed and tolerated in 100-mg increments to maximum of 400 mg daily. Divide doses larger than 200 mg daily into two doses. Continue treatment

for at least 3 months. In life-threatening illness, loading dose of 200 mg t.i.d. is given for 3 days. Or give 200 mg by I.V. infusion over 1 hour b.i.d. for four doses; then 200 mg I.V. once daily.

▶ **Aspergillosis.** *Adults:* 200 to 400 mg P.O. (capsules) daily. Or give 200 mg by I.V. infusion over 1 hour b.i.d. for four doses; then decrease to 200 mg I.V. once daily for up to 14 days.

▶ **Onychomycosis for toenails with or without fingernail involvement.** *Adults:* 200 mg P.O. (capsules) once daily for 12 weeks.

▶ **Onychomycosis for fingernails.** *Adults:* Two treatment phases, each consisting of 200 mg P.O. (capsules) b.i.d. for 1 week. Phases are separated by a 3-week period without drug.

▶ **Esophageal candidiasis.** *Adults:* 100 to 200 mg P.O. (oral solution) swished in mouth vigorously and swallowed daily for a minimum of 3 weeks.

▶ **Oropharyngeal candidiasis.** *Adults:* 200 mg P.O. (oral solution) swished in mouth vigorously and swallowed daily for 1 to 2 weeks. For patients unresponsive to fluconazole tablets, give 100 mg swished in mouth vigorously and swallowed b.i.d. for 2 to 4 weeks.

▄▀ **NEW INDICATION: Empiric coverage for febrile neutropenia.** *Adults*: 200 mg I.V. b.i.d. for four doses; then 200 mg daily for up to 14 days.

▶ **Prevention of fungal infections in HIV-infected individuals with severe and frequent recurrences.**‡ *Adults*: 200 mg P.O. daily.

▼ I.V. administration

● Injection form shouldn't be used in patients with creatinine clearance below 30 ml/minute.
● Distributed in a kit that includes a 50-ml bag of normal saline solution for injection and filtered infusion set.
● Administer through a designated line.
● Don't give drug by I.V. bolus injection.
● Infuse over 60 minutes, using an infusion set with a filter.
● Flush I.V. line with 15 to 20 ml of normal saline solution (not bacteriostatic) after each infusion.
⊗ Incompatibilities
● Dextrose solution, lactated Ringer's solution.

Contraindications and cautions

● Contraindicated in patients hypersensitive to the drug or any of its components. Also contraindicated in patients with ventricular dysfunc-

tion, heart failure, or a history of heart failure. Also contraindicated in patients receiving cisapride, oral midazolam, triazolam, pimozide, dofetilide, or quinidine; HMG-CoA reductase inhibitors metabolized by CYP3A4 (lovastatin, simvastatin); ergot alkaloids (dihydroergotamine, ergonovine, methylergonovine).

● Use cautiously in patients with hypochlorhydria (they may not absorb drug as readily as patients with normal gastric acidity), in HIV-infected patients (hypochlorhydria can accompany HIV infection), and in those with liver disease.

🔊 **Lifespan:** In pregnant women, use cautiously. In breast-feeding women, drug is contraindicated because it appears in breast milk. In children, safety and effectiveness haven't been established.

Adverse reactions

CNS: abnormal dreaming, anxiety, asthenia, depression, dizziness, fatigue, fever, *headache,* malaise, pain, somnolence, tremor.
CV: edema, **heart failure,** hypertension, hypertriglyceridemia, orthostatic hypotension.
EENT: pharyngitis, rhinitis, sinusitis.
GI: abdominal pain, anorexia, constipation, diarrhea, dyspepsia, flatulence, increased appetite, gastritis, gastroenteritis, gingivitis, *nausea,* ulcerative stomatitis, vomiting.
GU: albuminuria, cystitis, impotence, UTI.
Hematologic: *neutropenia.*
Hepatic: *hepatotoxicity, impaired hepatic function, liver failure.*
Metabolic: hypokalemia.
Musculoskeletal: myalgia.
Respiratory: *pulmonary edema,* upper respiratory tract infection.
Skin: pruritus, rash.
Other: *angioedema,* decreased libido, herpes zoster, hypersensitivity reactions, injury, *Stevens-Johnson syndrome,* urticaria.

Interactions

Drug-drug. *Alprazolam, chlordiazepoxide, clonazepam, clorazepate, diazepam, estazolam, flurazepam, midazolam, quazepam, triazolam:* May increase and prolong levels of these drugs, CNS depression, and psychomotor impairment. Don't use together.
Antacids, H₂-receptor antagonists, phenytoin, rifampin: May decrease itraconazole level. Avoid use together.

Reactions may be *common,* uncommon, **life-threatening**, or COMMON AND LIFE-THREATENING.

Antineoplastics (busulfan, docetaxel, vinca alkaloids): May inhibit metabolism of these drugs, resulting in toxicity. Avoid use together.
Aripiprazole: May increase levels of this drug. Decrease aripiprazole dosage by 50%.
Atorvastatin, fluvastatin, lovastatin, pravastatin, simvastatin: May increase levels and adverse effects of these HMG-CoA reductase inhibitors. Don't use together.
Buspirone, carbamazepine, corticosteroids, cyclosporine, digoxin: May increase levels of these drugs. Monitor level closely.
Calcium channel blockers: May increase negative inotropic effect, causing edema. Use together with caution, and adjust dosages as necessary.
Didanosine: May decrease therapeutic effect of itraconazole. Give itraconazole at least 2 hours before didanosine.
Dofetilide, pimozide, quinidine: May increase levels of these drugs by CYP3A4 metabolism, causing serious CV events, including torsades de pointes, prolonged QT interval, ventricular tachycardia, cardiac arrest, or sudden death. Use together is contraindicated.
Isoniazid: May decrease itraconazole level. Monitor patient closely.
Macrolide antibiotics (clarithromycin, erythromycin): May increase concentrations of itraconazole. Adjust dosage accordingly.
Oral anticoagulants: May enhance anticoagulant effects. Monitor PT and INR closely.
Oral antidiabetics: May cause hypoglycemia. Monitor glucose level.
Protease inhibitors: May increase concentrations of protease inhibitors, resulting in toxicity. Use together with caution.
Rifabutin, rifampin, rifamycin: May reduce the effectiveness of itraconazole. Avoid use together.
Drug-food. *Cola:* May increase drug level and adverse effects. Advise patient to take drug with water.
Grapefruit: May delay absorption of drug. Advise patient to avoid grapefruit products.
Orange juice: May decrease level and therapeutic effects of drug. Advise patient to avoid taking drug with orange juice.

Effects on lab test results
• May increase alkaline phosphatase, ALT, AST, bilirubin, and GGT levels. May decrease potassium level.

Pharmacokinetics
Absorption: For oral solution, bioavailability is maximal when taken without food; for capsules, it's with a full meal.
Distribution: 99.8% protein-bound. Extensively distributed in tissues susceptible to infection.
Metabolism: Extensively by liver.
Excretion: In feces and urine. *Half-life:* 1 to 8¼ hours.

Route	Onset	Peak	Duration
P.O.			
Fasting	Unknown	2 hr	Unknown
Non-fasting	Unknown	5 hr	Unknown
I.V.	Unknown	Unknown	Unknown

Action
Chemical effect: Interferes with fungal cell wall synthesis by inhibiting formation of ergosterol and increasing cell wall permeability.
Therapeutic effect: Hinders fungi, including *Aspergillus* sp. and *Blastomyces dermatitidis.*

Available forms
Capsules: 100 mg
Injection: 10 mg/ml in a kit with 25-ml ampule, 50-ml bag of normal saline solution for injection, and a filtered infusion set
Oral solution: 10 mg/ml

NURSING PROCESS

Assessment
• Assess patient's infection before starting therapy and regularly thereafter.
• Before starting treatment, obtain nail specimens for potassium hydroxide preparation, fungal culture, or nail biopsy to confirm diagnosis of onychomycosis.
• Monitor liver and renal function test results.
• Be alert for adverse reactions and drug interactions.
• Assess patient's and family's knowledge of drug therapy.

Nursing diagnoses
• Risk for infection related to presence of susceptible fungi
• Risk for deficient fluid volume related to adverse reactions
• Deficient knowledge related to drug therapy

▶ Planning and implementation

• Don't use in patient with baseline liver impairment, unless in a life-threatening situation where benefit exceeds risk. If signs of liver dysfunction occur, monitor liver function closely and stop therapy; don't restart unless the benefit exceeds the risk.
• Give capsules with food. Don't give oral solution with food.
🚫 **ALERT:** Oral solution and capsules aren't interchangeable.
• If signs and symptoms of heart failure occur, stop drug.
• Report signs and symptoms of liver disease and abnormal liver test results.

Patient teaching
• Teach patient to recognize and report signs and symptoms of liver disease (anorexia, dark urine, pale feces, unusual fatigue, or jaundice) and heart failure (weight gain more than 3 to 5 lb in 1 week, ankle or leg swelling, new shortness of breath).
• Tell patient to take capsules with food to ensure maximum absorption.
• Instruct patient to swish oral solution vigorously in the mouth (10 ml at a time) for several seconds and then swallow. Oral solution should be taken without food, if possible.

☑ Evaluation

• Patient is free from infection.
• Patient maintains adequate fluid balance.
• Patient and family state understanding of drug therapy.

kaolin and pectin mixtures
(KAY-oh-lin and PEK-tin MIX-cherz)
Kaodene Non-Narcotic†, Kaolin w/Pectin†, Kao-Spen†, Kapectolin†

Pharmacologic class: absorbent
Therapeutic class: antidiarrheal
Pregnancy risk category: NR

Indications and dosages

▶ **Mild, nonspecific diarrhea.** *Adults:* With regular-strength suspension, 60 to 120 ml P.O. after each bowel movement. With liquid, 45 ml P.O. one to three times daily or after each loose bowel movement.
Children ages 6 to 12: With regular-strength suspension, 30 to 60 ml P.O. after each bowel movement. With liquid, 22.5 ml P.O. one to three times daily or after each loose bowel movement.
Children ages 3 to 6: With regular-strength suspension, 15 to 30 ml P.O. after each bowel movement. With liquid, 15 ml P.O. one to three times daily or after each loose bowel movement.

Contraindications and cautions

• Don't use in patients with diarrhea linked to pseudomembranous colitis or caused by toxigenic bacteria.
• Use cautiously in patients with bleeding disorders or salicylate sensitivity.
⚖ **Lifespan:** In pregnant women and in children, use cautiously.

Adverse reactions

GI: constipation; fecal impaction or ulceration (in infants and elderly or debilitated patients after long-term use).

Interactions

Drug-drug. *Oral drugs:* May decrease drug absorption. Separate administration times by at least 2 or 3 hours.

Effects on lab test results

None reported.

Pharmacokinetics

Absorption: None.
Distribution: None.
Metabolism: None.
Excretion: In stool. *Half-life:* Unknown.

Route	Onset	Peak	Duration
P.O.	Unknown	Unknown	Unknown

Action

Chemical effect: Decreases fluid content of feces, although total water loss seems to remain the same.
Therapeutic effect: Alleviates diarrhea.

Reactions may be *common*, uncommon, *life-threatening*, or COMMON AND LIFE-THREATENING.

Available forms

Liquid: 3.9 g kaolin and 194.4 mg pectin per 30 ml with bismuth subsalicylate (Kaodene)
Oral suspension: 5.2 g kaolin and 260 mg pectin per 30 ml† (Kao-Spen), 90 g kaolin and 2 g pectin per 30 ml† (Kapectolin†, Kaolin w/Pectin†)

NURSING PROCESS

🗲 Assessment
• Assess patient's bowel patterns before and after therapy.
• Be alert for adverse GI reactions and drug interactions.
• Assess patient's and family's knowledge of drug therapy.

🔁 Nursing diagnoses
• Diarrhea related to underlying condition
• Constipation related to long-term use of drug
• Deficient knowledge related to drug therapy

▶ Planning and implementation
• Read label carefully. Check dosage and strength.
• Give dose after each loose bowel movement.
• Don't use in place of specific therapy for underlying cause of diarrhea.
Patient teaching
• Warn patient not to use drug to replace therapy for underlying cause of the disease.
• Advise patient not to use drug for longer than 2 days.

☑ Evaluation
• Patient reports decrease in or absence of loose stools.
• Patient doesn't have constipation.
• Patient and family state understanding of drug therapy.

ketoconazole
(kee-toh-KAHN-uh-zohl)
Nizoral, Nizoral A-D

Pharmacologic class: imidazole derivative
Therapeutic class: antifungal
Pregnancy risk category: C

Indications and dosages

▶ **Systemic candidiasis, chronic mucocandidiasis, oral thrush,** *candiduria, coccidioidomycosis, histoplasmosis, chromomycosis, paracoccidioidomycosis,* **severe cutaneous dermatophyte infection resistant to therapy with topical or oral griseofulvin.** *Adults and children who weigh more than 40 kg (88 lb):* Initially, 200 mg P.O. daily in single dose. Increase to 400 mg once daily in patients who don't respond to lower dosage.
Children age 2 and older: 3.3 to 6.6 mg/kg P.O. daily as single dose.
Note: Minimum treatment for candidiasis is 7 to 14 days; for other systemic fungal infections, 6 months; for resistant dermatophyte infections, at least 4 weeks.

▶ **Cutaneous candidiasis, tinea corporis, tinea pedis, tinea cruris, and tinea versicolor.** *Adults:* Apply cream once daily to cover the affected area and area immediately surrounding it. Treat candidal infection, tinea cruris, tinea corporis, and tinea versicolor for 2 weeks. Patients with tinea pedis require 6 weeks of treatment.

▶ **Seborrheic dermatitis.** *Adults:* Apply cream or foam to affected area b.i.d. for 4 weeks or until resolved. Apply gel to affected area once daily for 2 weeks.

▶ **Dandruff.** *Adults:* Moisten hair and scalp with water. Gently massage shampoo over the entire scalp area for about 1 minute. Rinse thoroughly with warm water. Repeat, leaving shampoo on scalp for an additional 3 minutes. After second thorough rinse, dry hair with towel or warm airflow. Use shampoo twice weekly for 4 weeks with at least 3 days between each shampooing. Then use as needed.

Contraindications and cautions

• Contraindicated in patients hypersensitive to the drug or any of its components.
• Use cautiously in patients with hepatic disease and in those taking other hepatotoxic drugs.
⚜ **Lifespan:** In pregnant women, use cautiously. Breast-feeding women should stop breast-feeding or use another drug. In children younger than age 2, safety hasn't been established.

Adverse reactions

CNS: dizziness, headache, nervousness, *suicidal tendencies.*
GI: abdominal pain, constipation, diarrhea, *nausea, vomiting.*

K

Hematologic: *thrombocytopenia.*
Hepatic: *hepatotoxicity.*
Skin: itching, stinging (cream).
Other: gynecomastia with tenderness.

Interactions

Drug-drug. *Alprazolam, chlordiazepoxide, clonazepam, clorazepate, diazepam, estazolam, flurazepam, quazepam:* May increase and prolong levels, CNS depression, and psychomotor impairment. Don't use together.
Antacids, anticholinergics, H_2-receptor antagonists, proton pump inhibitors, sucralfate: May decrease ketoconazole absorption. Wait at least 2 hours after ketoconazole dose before giving these drugs.
Astemizole, cisapride, and terfenadine: May cause increased levels of drug resulting in QT interval prolongation and arrhythmias. Don't use together.
Atorvastatin, fluvastatin, lovastatin, pravastatin, simvastatin: May increase level and adverse effects of these HMG-CoA reductase inhibitors. Avoid this combination. If they must be given together, reduce dosage of HMG-CoA reductase inhibitor.
Corticosteroids: May increase corticosteroid bioavailability and may decrease clearance, possibly resulting in toxicity. Monitor patient closely.
Cyclosporine, methylprednisolone, tacrolimus: May increase levels of these drugs. Adjust their dosages, and monitor their levels closely.
Didanosine: Therapeutic effects of ketoconazole may be decreased by the buffers in the chewable tablets.
Isoniazid, rifampin: May increase ketoconazole metabolism. Monitor patient for decreased antifungal effect.
Oral anticoagulants: May enhance anticoagulant response may be enhanced. Monitor PT and INR.
Oral midazolam, triazolam: May increase levels of these drugs, which may increase or prolong sedative or hypnotic effects. Avoid using together.

Effects on lab test results

• May increase lipid, alkaline phosphatase, ALT, and AST levels. May decrease hemoglobin level and hematocrit.
• May decrease platelet and WBC counts.

Pharmacokinetics

Absorption: Decreased by raised gastric pH and may be increased in extent and consistency by food.
Distribution: Into bile, saliva, cerumen, synovial fluid, and sebum. Penetration into CSF is erratic and probably minimal. About 84% to 99% protein-bound.
Metabolism: In liver.
Excretion: Mainly in feces, with smaller amount in urine. *Half-life:* 8 hours.

Route	Onset	Peak	Duration
P.O.	Unknown	1–2 hr	Unknown

Action

Chemical effect: Inhibits purine transport and DNA, RNA, and protein synthesis; increases cell wall permeability, making fungus more susceptible to osmotic pressure.
Therapeutic effect: Kills or hinders growth of susceptible fungi, including most pathogenic fungi.

Available forms

Cream: 2%
Shampoo: 1%†, 2%
Tablets: 200 mg

NURSING PROCESS

✍ Assessment

• Assess patient's infection before starting therapy and regularly thereafter.
• Evaluate laboratory studies for eradication of fungi.
• Be alert for adverse reactions and drug interactions.
• If adverse GI reactions occur, monitor patient's hydration.
• Obtain liver function test results before the start of therapy and at frequent intervals during therapy.
• Assess patient's and family's knowledge of drug therapy.

Nursing diagnoses

• Risk for infection related to presence of susceptible fungi
• Risk for deficient fluid volume related to adverse GI reactions
• Deficient knowledge related to drug therapy

Planning and implementation

• Because of risk of serious hepatotoxicity, don't use for less serious conditions, such as fungus infections of skin or nails.
• Monitor for signs of hepatic dysfunction such as jaundice, fatigue, nausea, vomiting, dark urine or pale stool.
• To minimize nausea, divide daily amount into two doses. Also, give drug with meals to help decrease nausea.
• Have patient dissolve each tablet in 4 ml aqueous solution of 0.2N hydrochloric acid and sip mixture through straw to avoid contact with teeth. Have patient drink full glass (8 oz) of water afterward.

⑤ ALERT: Cream contains sulfites, which can cause allergic reactions in susceptible individuals.

Patient teaching
• Instruct patient with achlorhydria to dissolve each tablet in 4 ml aqueous solution of 0.2N hydrochloric acid, sip mixture through a straw (to avoid contact with teeth), and drink a glass of water after the dose because drug requires gastric acidity to dissolve and absorb completely.
• Make sure patient understands that therapy will continue until all tests indicate that active fungal infection has subsided. If drug is stopped too soon, infection will recur.
• Reassure patient that nausea will subside.
• Tell patient that shampoo and cream are for external use only and to avoid contact with eyes.
• Instruct patient to separate doses of H_2-receptor antagonists, antacids, anticholinergics, proton pump inhibitors, and sucralfate at least 2 hours from drug, as drug requires stomach acidity to work properly.

☑ Evaluation

• Patient is free from infection.
• Patient maintains adequate hydration.
• Patient and family state understanding of drug therapy.

ketoprofen
(kee-toh-PROH-fen)
Actron†, Apo-Keto ♦, Apo-Keto-E ♦, Apo-Keto SR ♦, Novo-Keto ♦, Rhodis ♦, Rhodis-EC ♦

Pharmacologic class: NSAID

Therapeutic class: analgesic, antipyretic, anti-inflammatory
Pregnancy risk category: B (D in third trimester)

Indications and dosages

▶ **Rheumatoid arthritis and osteoarthritis.**
Adults: 75 mg t.i.d., 50 mg q.i.d., or 200 mg as sustained-release tablet once daily. Maximum, 300 mg daily. Or, where suppository is available, 100 mg P.R. b.i.d. or one suppository at bedtime (with P.O. form during day).
▶ **Mild to moderate pain; dysmenorrhea.**
Adults: 25 to 50 mg P.O. every 6 to 8 hours, p.r.n. Maximum, 300 mg daily.
▶ **Minor aches and pain or fever†.** *Adults:* 12.5 mg with full glass of water every 4 to 6 hours. Don't exceed 25 mg in 4 hours or 75 mg in 24 hours.

🕗 **Adjust-a-dose:** In patients with mildly impaired renal function, the maximum total daily dosage is 150 mg. In more severe renal impairment (GFR less than 25 ml/minute or end-stage renal impairment), the maximum total daily dose is 100 mg. In patients with impaired liver function and serum albumin level less than 3.5 g/dl, the maximum initial total daily dosage is 100 mg. Reduce initial dosage in patients age 75 and older.

Contraindications and cautions

• Contraindicated in patients hypersensitive to the drug or any of its components, and in those with a history of aspirin- or NSAID-induced asthma, urticaria, or other allergic reactions.
• Use cautiously in patients with a history of peptic ulcer disease, renal or liver dysfunction, hypertension, heart failure, or fluid retention.

☀ **Lifespan:** In pregnant women, don't use drug during the third trimester. In breast-feeding women, don't use because drug appears in breast milk. In children, safety and effectiveness haven't been established. In children younger than age 16, safety and effectiveness of OTC use haven't been established.

Adverse reactions

CNS: *depression,* dizziness, *excitation, headache, malaise, nervousness.*
EENT: *laryngeal edema,* tinnitus, visual disturbances.

GI: *abdominal pain,* anorexia, *constipation, diarrhea, flatulence, nausea,* peptic ulceration, stomatitis, vomiting.
GU: *nephrotoxicity.*
Hematologic: *agranulocytosis,* prolonged bleeding time, *thrombocytopenia.*
Metabolic: *edema.*
Respiratory: *bronchospasm,* dyspnea.
Skin: exfoliative dermatitis, photosensitivity, rash.

Interactions

Drug-drug. *Anticoagulants:* May increase anticoagulant effect. Monitor patient for signs and symptoms of bleeding.
Aspirin: May increase risk of adverse GI reactions and increase ketoprofen levels. Avoid use together.
Corticosteroids: May increase risk of adverse GI reactions. Avoid use together.
Hydrochlorothiazide, other diuretics: May decrease diuretic effectiveness. Monitor patient for lack of effect.
Lithium, methotrexate: May increase levels of these drugs, leading to toxicity. Monitor levels closely.
Other NSAIDs: May increase risk of bleeding. Monitor patient.
Probenecid: May increase ketoprofen level. Avoid use together.
Drug-herb. *Dong quai, feverfew, garlic, ginger, horse chestnut, red clover:* May increase risk of bleeding. Monitor patient closely.
St. John's wort: May increase risk of photosensitivity reactions. Advise patient to avoid unprotected or prolonged exposure to sunlight.
Drug-lifestyle. *Alcohol use:* May increase risk of GI toxicity. Discourage use together.
Sun exposure: May cause photosensitivity reactions. Advise patient to avoid unprotected or prolonged exposure to sunlight.

Effects on lab test results

- May increase BUN level.
- May increase bleeding time and liver function test values. May decrease WBC and platelet counts.

Pharmacokinetics

Absorption: Rapid and complete.
Distribution: Highly protein-bound.
Metabolism: Extensive, in liver.

Excretion: In urine. *Half-life:* 2 to 5½ hours for extended-release forms.

Route	Onset	Peak	Duration
P.O., P.R.	1–2 hr	½–2 hr	3–4 hr
P.O. Extended-release	2–3 hr	6–9 hr	24–48 hr

Action

Chemical effect: May inhibit prostaglandin synthesis.
Therapeutic effect: Relieves pain, fever, and inflammation.

Available forms

Capsules: 25 mg, 50 mg, 75 mg
Capsules (extended-release): 100 mg, 150 mg, 200 mg
Suppositories: 100 mg ♦
Tablets: 12.5 mg†
Tablets (enteric-coated): 50 mg ♦, 100 mg ♦
Tablets (sustained-release): 200 mg ♦

NURSING PROCESS

Assessment
- Assess patient's pain before and after giving the drug. Full effect may not occur for 2 to 4 weeks.
- Check renal and hepatic function every 6 months during long-term therapy.
- Be alert for adverse reactions and drug interactions.
- If adverse GI reactions occur, monitor patient's hydration.
- Assess patient's and family's knowledge of drug therapy.

Nursing diagnoses
- Chronic pain related to underlying condition
- Risk for deficient fluid volume related to adverse GI reactions
- Deficient knowledge related to drug therapy

Planning and implementation
- Sustained-release form isn't recommended for patients in acute pain.
- May give drug with antacids, food, or milk to minimize adverse GI effects.
- Inform lab technician that patient is taking drug; it may interfere with tests for glucose and iron levels, depending on testing method used.

Patient teaching

- Patient may take drug with milk or meals if he experiences adverse GI effects.
- Tell patient that full therapeutic effect may be delayed for 2 to 4 weeks.
- Instruct patient to report adverse visual or auditory reactions immediately.
- Teach patient to recognize and immediately report evidence of GI bleeding. Explain that serious GI toxicity, including peptic ulceration and bleeding, can occur in patients taking NSAIDs even without GI symptoms.
- Inform patient that use with aspirin, alcohol, or corticosteroids may increase risk of adverse GI reactions.
- Advise patient to use sun block, wear protective clothing, and avoid prolonged exposure to sunlight. Explain that drug may cause photosensitivity reactions.

☑ Evaluation

- Patient is free from pain.
- Patient maintains normal hydration.
- Patient and family state understanding of drug therapy.

---

ketorolac tromethamine
(KEE-toh-roh-lak troh-METH-uh-meen)
Acular, Acular LS, Acular PF

Pharmacologic class: NSAID
Therapeutic class: analgesic, anti-inflammatory
Pregnancy risk category: C (D in third trimester)

Indications and dosages

▶ **Short-term management of pain.** *Adults younger than age 65:* Base dosage on patient response. Initially, 60 mg I.M. or 30 mg I.V. as single dose or doses of 30 mg I.M. or I.V. every 6 hours. Maximum, 120 mg daily. To switch to P.O. route, initially give 20 mg P.O., and then 10 mg P.O. every 4 to 6 hours, p.r.n., up to 40 mg daily. Maximum combined use of drug not to exceed 5 days.
Adults age 65 and older, patients with renal impairment, and those weighing less than 50 kg (110 lb): Initially, 30 mg I.M. or 15 mg I.V. as single dose or doses of 15 mg I.M. or I.V. every 6 hours. Maximum, 60 mg daily. To switch to P.O. route, 10 mg P.O. every 4 to 6 hours, if

needed, up to 40 mg daily. Maximum combined use of drug not to exceed 5 days.
▶ **Ocular itching caused by seasonal allergic rhinitis.** *Adults:* 1 drop (0.25 mg) q.i.d.
▶ **Postoperative inflammation following cataract surgery.** *Adults:* 1 drop to affected eye q.i.d. starting 24 hours after surgery and continuing for the first 2 postoperative weeks.
▶ **Pain and burning or stinging following corneal refractive surgery.** *Adults:* 1 drop in the operated eye q.i.d., p.r.n., for up to 4 days.

▽ I.V. administration

- Injection solution contains alcohol.
- Give I.V. bolus over at least 15 seconds.
⊗ **Incompatibilities**
Haloperidol lactate; nalbuphine; solutions that result in a relatively low pH, such as hydroxyzine, meperidine, morphine sulfate, and prochlorperazine; thiethylperazine.

Contraindications and cautions

- Contraindicated in patients hypersensitive to the drug or any of its components; in those with a history of nasal polyps, angioedema, bronchospastic reactivity, or allergic reactions to aspirin or other NSAIDs; in patients receiving aspirin or other NSAIDs; in those with advanced renal impairment; and in those at risk for renal impairment as a result of volume depletion. Also contraindicated in patients with a high risk of bleeding and in those with suspected or confirmed cerebrovascular bleeding, hemorrhagic diathesis, and incomplete hemostasis.
- Contraindicated for perioperative pain in patients requiring coronary artery bypass graft surgery.
- Not recommended for intrathecal or epidural administration because of its alcohol content.
- Use cautiously in patients in the perioperative period, and in patients with hepatic or renal impairment, history of serious GI events or peptic ulcer disease, cardiac decompensation, hypertension, or coagulation disorders.
≋ **Lifespan:** In pregnant women, safety during first two trimesters hasn't been established; drug is contraindicated in third trimester. In breastfeeding women, use cautiously because trace amounts have been detected in breast milk. In children, safety of oral form hasn't been established; I.M. and I.V. use are safe in children age 2 and older; ophthalmic solutions are safe for children age 3 and older.

K

Adverse reactions

CNS: dizziness, drowsiness, *headache,* insomnia, syncope,
CV: edema, hypertension, palpitations.
EENT: corneal edema, keratitis (ocular form), ocular irritation, *transient stinging and burning.*
GI: diarrhea, *dyspepsia, GI pain, nausea.*
GU: hematuria, polyuria, **renal failure.**
Hematologic: anemia, eosinophilia, purpura.
Skin: sweating.
Other: pain at injection site.

Interactions

Drug-drug. *Antihypertensives, diuretics:* May decrease effectiveness of these drugs. Monitor reactions closely.
Cyclosporine: May increase risk of nephrotoxicity. Use together cautiously.
Lithium: May increase lithium level. Monitor level closely.
Low–molecular-weight heparin, salicylates, warfarin: May increase levels of free (unbound) salicylates or warfarin in blood. Significance is unknown.
Methotrexate: May decrease methotrexate clearance and increase toxicity. Don't use together.
Drug-herb. *Dong quai, feverfew, garlic, ginger, horse chestnut, red clover:* May increase risk of bleeding. Monitor patient closely.
St. John's wort: May increase risk of photosensitivity reactions. Advise patient to avoid unprotected or prolonged exposure to sunlight.

Effects on lab test results

• May increase BUN and creatinine levels. May decrease hemoglobin level and hematocrit.
• May increase eosinophil count and liver function test values.

Pharmacokinetics

Absorption: Complete after I.M. use. After P.O. use, food delays absorption but doesn't decrease amount absorbed.
Distribution: More than 99.9% protein-bound.
Metabolism: Mainly in liver.
Excretion: More than 90% in urine, with the remainder in feces. *Half-life:* 4 to 6 hours.

Route	Onset	Peak	Duration
P.O.	30–60 min	30–60 min	6–8 hr
I.V.	Immediate	Immediate	8 hr
I.M.	≤ 30 min	1–2 hr	6–8 hr

Action

Chemical effect: May inhibit prostaglandin synthesis.
Therapeutic effect: Relieves pain and inflammation.

Available forms

Injection: 15 mg/ml, 30 mg/ml
Ophthalmic solution: 0.4%, 0.5%
Tablets: 10 mg

NURSING PROCESS

⚗ Assessment

• Assess patient's pain before and after drug therapy.
• Be alert for adverse reactions and drug interactions.
• Assess patient's and family's knowledge of drug therapy.

⊕ Nursing diagnoses

• Acute pain related to underlying condition
• Risk for injury related to drug-induced adverse CNS reactions
• Deficient knowledge related to drug therapy

▶ Planning and implementation

⚠ **ALERT:** Drug may cause peptic ulcers, GI bleeding, or perforation of the stomach or intestines, which may be fatal. These events may occur without warning.
⚠ **ALERT:** Drug may increase risk of serious CV thrombotic events, MI, and stroke, which may be fatal.
• When switching from I.M. to P.O., don't exceed 120 mg (including maximum of 40 mg P.O.) on day of transition.
• I.M. use may cause pain at injection site. Apply pressure to site for 15 to 30 seconds after injection to minimize local effects.
• If pain persists or worsens, notify prescriber.
⚠ **ALERT:** Don't confuse Toradol with Foradil.
⚠ **ALERT:** Duration of therapy should not exceed 5 days.
Patient teaching
• Teach patient to recognize and immediately report signs and symptoms of GI bleeding. Explain that serious GI toxicity, even without any symptoms, can occur.
• Instruct patient not to administer eye drops while wearing contact lenses.

- Advise patient to report persistent or worsening pain.
- Explain that drug is intended only for short-term use.

✓ **Evaluation**
- Patient is free from pain.
- Patient sustains no injury from adverse reactions.
- Patient and family state understanding of drug therapy.

ketotifen fumarate
(kee-toe-TYE-fen FOO-muh-rayt)
Alaway, Zaditor

Pharmacologic class: histamine antagonist and mast cell stabilizer
Therapeutic class: ophthalmic antihistamine
Pregnancy risk category: C

Indications and dosages

▶ **To temporarily prevent itching of eye caused by allergic conjunctivitis.** *Adults and children age 3 and older:* Instill 1 drop in affected eye every 8 to 12 hours.

Contraindications and cautions

- Contraindicated in patients hypersensitive to the drug or any of its components.
- **Lifespan:** In pregnant women, use cautiously. In breast-feeding women, use cautiously; it's unknown if topical ocular drug appears in breast milk. In children younger than age 3, safety and effectiveness haven't been established.

Adverse reactions

CNS: *headaches.*
EENT: burning or stinging of eyes, *conjunctival infection,* conjunctivitis, dry eyes, eye discharge, eye pain, eyelid disorder, itching of eyes, keratitis, lacrimation disorder, mydriasis, ocular allergic reactions, ocular rash, pharyngitis, photophobia, *rhinitis.*
Other: flulike syndrome.

Interactions

None reported.

Effects on lab test results

None reported.

Pharmacokinetics

Absorption: Unknown.
Distribution: Unknown.
Metabolism: Unknown.
Excretion: Unknown. *Half-life:* Unknown.

Route	Onset	Peak	Duration
Ophthalmic	Within min	Unknown	Unknown

Action

Chemical effect: Inhibits release of mediators from cells involved in hypersensitivity reactions.
Therapeutic effect: Temporary prevention of eye itching.

Available forms

Ophthalmic solution: 0.025% solution in 5-ml and 7.5-ml bottles

NURSING PROCESS

Assessment
- Assess underlying condition before starting therapy, and reassess regularly during therapy.
- Monitor patient for sensitivity reactions.
- Monitor patient for signs of infection.
- Assess patient's and family's knowledge of drug therapy.

Nursing diagnoses
- Impaired tissue integrity related to drug-induced adverse EENT reactions
- Deficient knowledge related to ketotifen fumarate therapy

Planning and implementation
- Drug is for ophthalmic use only and not for injection or oral use.
- Drug isn't indicated for use with irritation related to contact lenses.
- Preservative in drug may be absorbed by soft contact lenses. Have patient remove contact lenses before giving drops, and tell him not to reinsert them for at least 10 minutes.
Patient teaching
- Teach patient proper instillation technique. Tell him to avoid contaminating dropper tip and solution and not to touch eyelids or surrounding areas with dropper tip of bottle.
- Tell patient not to wear contact lenses if eyes are red. Warn patient not to use drug to treat irritation related to contact lenses.

• Instruct patient who wears soft contact lenses and whose eyes aren't red to wait at least 10 minutes after instilling drug before inserting contact lenses.
• Advise patient to report adverse reactions to prescriber.
• Instruct patient to keep bottle tightly closed when not in use.

✔ Evaluation
• Patient demonstrates appropriate management of any adverse EENT reactions.
• Patient and family state understanding of therapy.

HIGH ALERT

labetalol hydrochloride
(lah-BAY-tuh-lol high-droh-KLOR-ighd)
Normodyne, Trandate

Pharmacologic class: alpha and beta blocker
Therapeutic class: antihypertensive
Pregnancy risk category: C

Indications and dosages
▶ **Hypertension.** *Adults:* 100 mg P.O. b.i.d. with or without diuretic. Adjust dosage in increments of 100 mg b.i.d. every 2 or 3 days. Maintenance dosage, 200 to 400 mg b.i.d. Some patients may need 1.2 to 2.4 g/day.
▶ **Severe hypertension, hypertensive emergency.** *Adults:* 200 mg I.V. diluted for infusion at 2 mg/minute until obtaining satisfactory response; then stop infusion. Or give by repeated I.V. injection; initially, 20 mg I.V. slowly over 2 minutes. Then repeat injections of 40 to 80 mg every 10 minutes, as needed to maximum dose, 300 mg.

▽ I.V. administration
• Dilute 200 mg in 160 ml for 1 mg/ml solution for infusion. May use 200 mg/250 ml solution.
• Dilute with D$_5$W, normal saline solutions, Ringer's solution, or lactated Ringer's solution.
• Give diluted infusion with infusion-control device.

• Give direct I.V. injection over 2 minutes at 10-minute intervals.
• Monitor blood pressure every 5 minutes for 30 minutes, then every 30 minutes for 2 hours, then every hour for 6 hours.
• When given I.V. for hypertensive emergency, drug produces rapid, predictable fall in blood pressure within 5 to 10 minutes.
• Have patient lie down for 3 hours after infusion.
• Store drug at 36° to 86° F (2° to 30° C) and protect from light.
⊗ **Incompatibilities**
Alkali solutions, cefoperazone, ceftriaxone, furosemide, heparin, nafcillin, sodium bicarbonate, thiopental, warfarin.

Contraindications and cautions
• Contraindicated in patients hypersensitive to the drug or any of its components and in those with bronchial asthma, overt cardiac failure, greater than first-degree heart block, cardiogenic shock, severe bradycardia, and other conditions linked to severe and prolonged hypotension.
• Use cautiously in patients with heart failure, hepatic impairment, chronic bronchitis, emphysema, peripheral vascular disease, or pheochromocytoma.
⚖ **Lifespan:** In pregnant and breast-feeding women, use cautiously. In children, safety and effectiveness haven't been established. Elderly patients typically need a lower maintenance dosage.

Adverse reactions
CNS: *dizziness,* fatigue, headache, transient scalp tingling, vivid dreams.
CV: *bradycardia, orthostatic hypotension,* peripheral vascular disease, *ventricular arrhythmias.*
EENT: nasal stuffiness.
GI: diarrhea, nausea, vomiting.
GU: sexual dysfunction, urine retention.
Respiratory: increased airway resistance.
Skin: rash.

Interactions
Drug-drug. *Beta agonists:* May lessen the bronchodilator effect of these drugs in patients with bronchospasm. Increase dosage of these bronchodilators.
Cimetidine: May enhance labetalol's effect. Give together cautiously; monitor patient for adverse reactions.

Reactions may be *common,* uncommon, *life-threatening,* or **COMMON AND LIFE-THREATENING.**

Diuretics and other antihypertensives: May increase hypotension. Monitor patient and adjust dosage.

Glutethimide: May decrease effects of labetalol. Adjust labetalol dosage carefully to reach optimal blood pressure control.

Halothane: May increase hypotension. Monitor blood pressure.

Insulin, oral antidiabetics: May change required dosage in previously stabilized diabetic patients. Observe patient carefully.

Tricyclic antidepressants: May increase risk of tremor. Monitor patient.

Effects on lab test results

• May increase glucose, transaminase, and blood urea levels.
• May cause false-positive result for amphetamines in urine drug screen.

Pharmacokinetics

Absorption: 90% to 100%, but drug undergoes extensive first-pass metabolism in liver and only about 25% reaches circulation unchanged.
Distribution: Wide. About 50% protein-bound.
Metabolism: Extensive, in liver and possibly GI mucosa.
Excretion: About 5% unchanged in urine; remainder as metabolites in urine and feces.
Half-life: About 5½ hours after I.V. use; 6 to 8 hours after P.O. use.

Route	Onset	Peak	Duration
P.O.	≤ 20 min	2–4 hr	8–12 hr
I.V.	2–5 min	5 min	2–4 hr

Action

Chemical effect: May be related to reduced peripheral vascular resistance as a result of alpha-adrenergic blockade.
Therapeutic effect: Lowers blood pressure.

Available forms

Injection: 5 mg/ml
Tablets: 100 mg, 200 mg, 300 mg

NURSING PROCESS

☝ Assessment

• Obtain history of patient's hypertension before starting therapy.
• Check blood pressure often. Drug masks common signs of shock.

• Be alert for adverse reactions and drug interactions.
• With oral form, full antihypertensive effect is usually seen within the first 1 to 3 hours of initial dose or dose change.
• Assess patient's and family's knowledge of drug therapy.

🔲 Nursing diagnoses

• Ineffective health maintenance related to presence of hypertension
• Risk for trauma related to drug-induced hypotension
• Deficient knowledge related to drug therapy

▶ Planning and implementation

• If dizziness occurs, give at bedtime or give smaller doses t.i.d. to help minimize it.
🔵 **ALERT:** Don't confuse Trandate with Tridrate or Trental.
Patient teaching
• Tell patient that abruptly stopping therapy can worsen angina and cause MI.
• Inform patient that rising slowly and avoiding sudden position changes can minimize dizziness.

☑ Evaluation

• Patient's blood pressure is normal.
• Patient doesn't experience trauma caused by drug-induced hypotension.
• Patient and family state understanding of drug therapy.

lactulose

(LAK-tyoo-lohs)
Cephulac, Cholac, Constilac, Constulose, Enulose, Generlac, Hepotalac, Kristalose

Pharmacologic class: disaccharide
Therapeutic class: laxative
Pregnancy risk category: B

Indications and dosages

▶ **Constipation.** *Adults:* 10 to 20 g (15 to 30 ml) P.O. daily, increase to 60 ml/day, if needed.

▶ **To prevent and treat hepatic encephalopathy, including hepatic precoma and coma in patients with severe hepatic disease.** *Adults:* Initially, 20 to 30 g (30 to 45 ml) P.O. t.i.d. or

q.i.d. until two to three soft stools are produced daily. Usual dosage, 60 to 100 g total daily. Or 200 g (300 ml) diluted with 700 ml of water or normal saline solution and given as retention enema every 4 to 6 hours, p.r.n.
Adolescents and older children: 27 to 60 g (40 to 90 ml) daily in divided doses.
Infants: 1.67 to 6.67 g (2.5 to 10 ml) daily in divided doses.

For all patients, the desired effect is two to three stools daily. If diarrhea occurs with first dose, reduce dosage immediately. If diarrhea persists, stop drug.

▶ **To induce bowel evacuation in geriatric patients with colonic retention of barium and severe constipation after a barium meal examination‡.** *Adults:* 3.3 to 6.7 g P.O. b.i.d. for 1 to 4 weeks.

▶ **To restore bowel movements after hemorrhoidectomy‡.** *Adults:* 10 g P.O. twice during day before surgery and 5 days afterward.

Contraindications and cautions

● Contraindicated in patients on low-galactose diet.
● Use cautiously in patients with diabetes mellitus because drug contains lactose, galactose, and other sugars.
≉ **Lifespan:** In pregnant women, use only when clearly needed. In breast-feeding women, use cautiously; it's unknown if the drug appears in breast milk. In children, use for chronic constipation is contraindicated. In elderly patients, use cautiously because they may be more susceptible to hyponatremia.

Adverse reactions

GI: *abdominal cramps and distention, belching, diarrhea, flatulence,* nausea, vomiting.

Interactions

Drug-drug. *Antacids, antibiotics, oral neomycin:* May decrease effectiveness of lactulose. Avoid use together.

Effects on lab test results

● May increase glucose level. May decrease ammonia, chloride, potassium, and sodium levels.

Pharmacokinetics

Absorption: Minimal.
Distribution: Local, mainly in colon.
Metabolism: By colonic bacteria.

Excretion: Mostly in feces; absorbed portion in urine.

Route	Onset	Peak	Duration
P.O.	24–48 hr	Varies	Varies
P.R.	Unknown	Unknown	Unknown

Action

Chemical effect: Produces osmotic effect in colon. Resulting distention promotes peristalsis. Decreases blood ammonia build-up that causes hepatic encephalopathy, probably as result of bacterial degradation, which lowers pH of colon contents.
Therapeutic effect: Relieves constipation, decreases blood ammonia concentration.

Available forms

Crystals for reconstitution: 10 g/packet, 20 g/packet
Solution: 10 g/15 ml, 3.33 g/5 ml

NURSING PROCESS

⚕ Assessment
● Assess patient's condition before starting therapy and regularly thereafter to monitor drug effectiveness. If patient has hepatic encephalopathy, assess mental condition.
● Monitor patient's electrolyte levels during long-term use.
● In a patient with hepatic disease, monitor ammonia level.
● Be alert for adverse reactions and drug interactions.
● Assess patient's and family's knowledge of drug therapy.

⊕ Nursing diagnoses
● Constipation related to underlying condition
● Deficient knowledge related to drug therapy

▶ Planning and implementation
③ **ALERT:** Don't confuse lactulose with lactose.
● Replace fluid loss.
● Diarrhea may indicate overdose.
● To minimize sweet taste, dilute with water or fruit juice or give with food.
● If enema isn't retained for at least 30 minutes, repeat dose.
③ **ALERT:** For a patient undergoing electrocautery procedures during proctoscopy or colonoscopy, the accumulation of hydrogen gas,

---

combined with an electrical spark may cause an explosion. For a patient undergoing electro-cautery procedures, give an enema with a non-fermentable solution.
• Store drug at room temperature, preferably below 86° F (30° C); don't freeze.
Patient teaching
• Advise patient to dilute drug with juice or water, or to take with food to improve taste.
• Inform patient of adverse reactions and tell him to notify prescriber if reactions become bothersome or if more than two or three soft stools daily are passed.

☑ **Evaluation**
• Patient's constipation is relieved.
• Patient and family state understanding of drug therapy.

lamivudine (3TC)
(la-MIH-vyoo-deen)
Epivir, Epivir-HBV

Pharmacologic class: nucleoside reverse transcriptase inhibitor
Therapeutic class: antiretroviral
Pregnancy risk category: C

Indications and dosages
▶ **HIV infection (with other antiretrovirals).**
Adults and children age 16 and older: 300 mg Epivir P.O. once daily or 150 mg P.O. b.i.d.
Children ages 3 months to 16 years: 4 mg/kg Epivir P.O. b.i.d. Maximum, 150 mg b.i.d.
Neonates age 30 days and younger‡: 2 mg/kg Epivir P.O. b.i.d.
◩ **Adjust-a-dose:** For adults and adolescents with renal impairment, if creatinine clearance is 30 to 49 ml/minute, give 150 mg Epivir P.O. daily; if clearance is 15 to 29 ml/minute, give 150 mg P.O. on day 1, then 100 mg daily; if clearance is 5 to 14 ml/minute, give 150 mg on day 1, then 50 mg daily; if clearance is less than 5 ml/minute, give 50 mg on day 1, then 25 mg daily.
▶ **Chronic hepatitis B with evidence of hepatitis B virus (HBV) replication and active liver inflammation.** *Adults:* 100 mg Epivir-HBV P.O. once daily.
Children ages 2 to 17: Give 3 mg/kg Epivir-HBV once daily. Maximum daily, 100 mg.

◩ **Adjust-a-dose:** For adult patients with renal impairment, if creatinine clearance is 30 to 49 ml/minute, give 100 mg Epivir-HBV as first dose, then 50 mg P.O. daily; if clearance is 15 to 29 ml/minute, give 100 mg first dose, then 25 mg P.O. daily; if clearance is 5 to 14 ml/minute, give 35 mg first dose, then 15 mg P.O. daily; if clearance is less than 5 ml/minute, give 35 mg first dose, then 10 mg P.O. daily.

Contraindications and cautions
• Contraindicated in patients hypersensitive to the drug or any of its components, as well as in combination antiretroviral therapy with abacavir, lamivudine, and tenofovir, and with didanosine, lamivudine, and tenofovir because of early drug resistance in HIV-infected patients.
• Epivir-HBV is contraindicated for patients coinfected with HBV and HIV.
• Safety and effectiveness of Epivir-HBV in all patients for longer than 1 year haven't been established; ideal length of therapy isn't known.
• Use cautiously in patients with decompensated liver disease or organ transplant. Use cautiously and at a reduced dosage in patients with renal impairment.
⚘ **Lifespan:** In pregnant women, use only if benefits outweigh risks to the fetus. Breast-feeding women should stop breast-feeding or take another drug. In children younger than age 2, safety and effectiveness in chronic hepatitis B haven't been established. In children with history of pancreatitis or other significant risk factors for pancreatitis, use cautiously, if at all.

Adverse reactions
For HIV-infected patients
CNS: depressive disorders, *dizziness, fatigue, fever, headache, insomnia, malaise, neuropathy, sleep disorders.*
EENT: *nasal symptoms.*
GI: abdominal cramps, abdominal pain, *anorexia, diarrhea,* dyspepsia, *hepatomegaly* (in children), *nausea,* **pancreatitis,** vomiting.
Hematologic: anemia, lymphadenopathy (in children), **neutropenia, thrombocytopenia.**
Musculoskeletal: arthralgia, *musculoskeletal pain,* myalgia.
Respiratory: *cough.*
Skin: rash (*rashes* in children).
Other: chills, **lactic acidosis.**
For hepatitis B patients
CNS: *fatigue, fever, headache, malaise.*

EENT: ear, nose, and throat infections; sore throat.
GI: abdominal pain and discomfort, *diarrhea, nausea, vomiting.*
Musculoskeletal: arthralgia, *myalgia.*
Skin: rash.
Other: *lactic acidosis.*

Interactions

Drug-drug. *Co-trimoxazole:* May increase lamivudine bioavailability. Dosage adjustment isn't needed. Avoid giving lamivudine with high doses of co-trimoxazole for *Pneumocystis jiroveci (carinii)* pneumonia and toxoplasmosis.
Zalcitabine: May inhibit activation of both drugs. Avoid use together.

Effects on lab test results

• May increase ALT and bilirubin levels. May decrease hemoglobin level and hematocrit.
• May decrease neutrophil and platelet counts.

Pharmacokinetics

Absorption: Rapid for HIV-infected patients.
Distribution: Possibly into extravascular spaces. Volume is independent of dose and doesn't correlate with body weight. Less than 36% protein-bound.
Metabolism: To trans-sulfoxide.
Excretion: Mainly unchanged in urine. *Half-life:* 5 to 7 hours.

Route	Onset	Peak	Duration
P.O.	Unknown	1–3 hr	Unknown

Action

Chemical effect: Inhibits HIV reverse transcription by viral DNA chain termination and RNA- and DNA-dependent DNA polymerase activities.
Therapeutic effect: Reduces the symptoms of HIV infection, reduces liver inflammation of chronic hepatitis B and may seroconvert some patients.

Available forms

Epivir
Oral solution: 10 mg/ml
Tablets: 150 mg, 300 mg
Epivir-HBV
Oral solution: 5 mg/ml
Tablets: 100 mg

NURSING PROCESS

⚕ Assessment

• Obtain history of patient's underlying condition before starting therapy, and reassess regularly thereafter to monitor drug effectiveness.
• Test patient with HBV for HIV before and throughout therapy because drug isn't appropriate for those dually infected.
⊛ ALERT: Some patients with chronic HBV infection may have recurrent hepatitis after stopping the drug. Patients with liver disease may have more severe effects; monitor liver function tests, markers of HBV replication, and clinical signs regularly after stopping therapy.
• Monitor renal function before and during therapy.
• Monitor patient's CBC, platelet count, and liver function. Report any abnormalities to prescriber.
• Assess patient's and family's knowledge of drug therapy.

⊕ Nursing diagnoses

• Risk for infection related to the presence of HIV
• Risk for injury related to drug-induced CNS adverse reactions
• Deficient knowledge related to drug therapy

▶ Planning and implementation

• Safety and effectiveness of drug haven't been established for chronic hepatitis B in a patient infected with both HIV and HBV. Drug-resistant HBV variations may occur in such a patient; HIV drug resistance often occurs also.
⊛ ALERT: Lactic acidosis and severe hepatomegaly, including fatal cases, have been reported.
• If signs, symptoms, or laboratory abnormalities suggest pancreatitis, stop therapy immediately and notify prescriber.
• An Antiretroviral Pregnancy Registry has been established to monitor maternal-fetal outcomes of pregnant women exposed to drug. To register a pregnant woman, call 1-800-258-4263, or register online at www.apregistry.com.
⊛ ALERT: Don't confuse lamivudine with lamotrigine.
Patient teaching
• Inform patient that long-term effects of drug are unknown.
• Stress importance of taking drug exactly as prescribed.

Reactions may be *common*, uncommon, *life-threatening*, or COMMON AND LIFE-THREATENING.

• Teach patient the signs and symptoms of pancreatitis. Advise him to report signs and symptoms immediately.

✓ Evaluation
• Patient responds well to drug therapy.
• Patient sustains no injury as a result of drug-induced CNS adverse reactions.
• Patient and family state understanding of drug therapy.

lamivudine and zidovudine
(la-MIH-vyoo-deen and zy-DOH-vyoo-deen)
Combivir

Pharmacologic class: nucleoside reverse transcriptase inhibitor
Therapeutic class: antiretroviral
Pregnancy risk category: C

Indications and dosages
▶ **HIV infection.** *Adults and children age 12 and older who weigh more than 50 kg (110 lb):* One tablet P.O. b.i.d.

Contraindications and cautions
• Contraindicated in patients hypersensitive to the drug or any of its components, those who need dosage adjustments (such as those who weigh less than 50 kg), those with creatinine clearance less than 50 ml/minute, and those with impaired hepatic function. Also contraindicated in patients with dose-limiting adverse effects.
• For patients infected with HIV and hepatitis B virus (HBV), safety and effectiveness of lamivudine haven't been established. Drug-resistant HBV variations may occur in these patients after receiving combination drug.
※ Lifespan: In pregnant women, use only if benefits outweigh risks to the fetus. Breast-feeding women should stop breast-feeding or use another drug. In children younger than age 12, drug is contraindicated.

Adverse reactions
CNS: depression, *dizziness, fatigue, fever, headache, insomnia, malaise, neuropathy.*
EENT: *nasal signs and symptoms.*
GI: abdominal cramps, abdominal pain, *anorexia, diarrhea,* dyspepsia, *nausea, vomiting.*

Hematologic: *neutropenia,* severe anemia.
Hepatic: *severe hepatomegaly with steatosis.*
Musculoskeletal: arthralgia, *musculoskeletal pain,* myalgia.
Respiratory: *cough.*
Skin: rash.
Other: *chills, lactic acidosis.*

Interactions
Drug-drug. *Atovaquone, fluconazole, methadone, probenecid, valproic acid given with zidovudine:* May increase bioavailability of zidovudine. Dosage adjustment isn't needed.
Co-trimoxazole, nelfinavir: May increase bioavailability of lamivudine. Dosage adjustment isn't needed. Avoid giving lamivudine with high doses of co-trimoxazole for *Pneumocystis jiroveci (carinii)* pneumonia and toxoplasmosis.
Ganciclovir, interferon-alfa, and other bone marrow suppressive or cytotoxic drugs: May increase hematologic toxicity of zidovudine. Use cautiously as with other reverse transcriptase inhibitors.
Nelfinavir, ritonavir: May decrease bioavailability of zidovudine. Dosage modification isn't needed.
Zalcitabine: May inhibit intracellular phosphorylation of one another. Avoid using these drugs together.

Effects on lab test results
• May increase ALT, AST, and amylase levels. May decrease hemoglobin level and hematocrit.
• May decrease neutrophil count.

Pharmacokinetics
Absorption: Rapid for both drugs, with bioavailability of 86% and 64%, respectively.
Distribution: Extensive for both drugs; minimally protein-bound.
Metabolism: About 5% for lamivudine; 74% for zidovudine.
Excretion: Mainly in urine. *Half-lives of lamivudine and zidovudine:* 5 to 7 hours and ½ to 3 hours, respectively.

Route	Onset	Peak	Duration
P.O.	Unknown	Unknown	Unknown

Action
Chemical effect: Inhibits reverse transcriptase by DNA chain termination. Both drugs are also weak inhibitors of DNA polymerase. Together,

L

they act synergistically by suppressing or delaying the emergence of resistant strains that can occur with retroviral monotherapy, because dual resistance requires multiple mutations.
Therapeutic effect: Reduces the symptoms of HIV infection.

Available forms

Tablets: 150 mg lamivudine and 300 mg zidovudine

NURSING PROCESS

⚕ Assessment
● Obtain history of patient's underlying condition before starting therapy, and reassess regularly thereafter to monitor the drug's effectiveness.
● Watch for hematologic toxicity by taking frequent blood counts, especially in patients with advanced HIV infection.
● Assess patient's fine motor skills and peripheral sensation for evidence of peripheral neuropathies.
⚠ ALERT: In a patient with chronic HBV infection, hepatitis may recur when drug is stopped. Patients with pre-existing liver disease may have more severe consequences. In patient with liver disease and HBV, periodically monitor liver function test results and markers of HBV replication.
● Assess patient's and family's knowledge of drug therapy.

⚕ Nursing diagnoses
● Risk for infection related to the presence of HIV
● Disturbed sensory perception (tactile) related to drug-induced peripheral neuropathy
● Deficient knowledge related to drug therapy

▷ Planning and implementation
⚠ ALERT: Fatal lactic acidosis and severe hepatomegaly with steatosis may occur. If patient develops signs or symptoms of lactic acidosis or severe hepatotoxicity, stop drug.
● Use drug cautiously in patients with bone marrow suppression (granulocyte count below 1,000/mm³ or hemoglobin level below 9.5 g/dl).
● An Antiretroviral Pregnancy Registry has been established to monitor maternal-fetal outcomes of pregnant women exposed to drug. To register a pregnant patient call 1-800-258-4263 or register online at www.apregistry.com.

Patient teaching
● Explain to patient that therapy won't cure HIV infection and that he may continue to have illness.
● Warn patient that HIV transmission can still occur with drug therapy. Educate patient about using barrier contraception when engaging in sexual activities to prevent disease transmission.
● Teach patient signs and symptoms of neutropenia and anemia (fever, chills, infection, fatigue), and instruct him to immediately report them to the prescriber.
● Tell patient to have blood counts followed closely while taking drug, especially if he has advanced disease.
● Advise patient to consult prescriber or pharmacist before taking other drugs.
● Warn patient to report abdominal pain immediately.
● Instruct patient to report evidence of myopathy or myositis, such as muscle inflammation, pain, weakness, and a decrease in muscle size.
● Stress importance of taking combination drug therapy exactly as prescribed to reduce the development of drug resistance.
● Tell patient he may take combination with or without food.
● Inform woman that breast-feeding is contraindicated with an HIV infection, whether or not she is taking drug.

✓ Evaluation
● Patient responds well to drug.
● Patient doesn't develop peripheral neuropathy.
● Patient and family state understanding of drug therapy.

lamotrigine
(lah-MOH-trih-jeen)
Lamictal

Pharmacologic class: phenyltriazine
Therapeutic class: anticonvulsant, mood stabilizer
Pregnancy risk category: C

Indications and dosages

▶ **Adjunct therapy for partial seizures caused by epilepsy or generalized seizures of Lennox-Gastaut syndrome.** *Adults and children older than age 12:* For patients taking

valproic acid with other enzyme-inducing anti-convulsants, 25 mg P.O. every other day for 2 weeks; then 25 mg P.O. daily for 2 weeks. Continue to increase, as appropriate, by 25 to 50 mg/day every 1 to 2 weeks until effective maintenance dosage of 100 to 400 mg daily, given in one or two divided doses, is reached. When added to valproic acid alone, mainte-nance dosage is 100 to 200 mg P.O. daily. For patients receiving enzyme-inducing anticonvul-sants and not valproic acid, 50 mg P.O. daily for 2 weeks; then 100 mg P.O. daily in two divided doses for 2 weeks. Increase, as needed, by 100 mg daily every 1 to 2 weeks. Maintenance dosage, 300 to 500 mg P.O. daily in two divided doses.

Children ages 2 to 12 who weigh 6.7 to 40 kg (15 to 88 lb): For patients taking valproic acid with other enzyme-inducing anticonvulsants, 0.15 mg/kg P.O. daily in one or two divided doses (round down to nearest whole tablet) for 2 weeks, followed by 0.3 mg/kg daily in one or two divided doses for another 2 weeks. Then maintenance dosage, 1 to 5 mg/kg daily (maxi-mum, 200 mg daily in one to two divided dos-es). For patients receiving enzyme-inducing an-ticonvulsants and not valproic acid, 0.6 mg/kg P.O. daily in two divided doses (round down to nearest whole tablet) for 2 weeks, followed by 1.2 mg/kg daily in two divided doses for anoth-er 2 weeks. Maintenance dosage, 5 to 15 mg/kg daily (maximum, 400 mg daily in two divided doses).

▶ **Adjunctive therapy for primary general-ized tonic-clonic seizures.** *Adults and children age 12 and older:* Dosage is based on other antiepileptics taken. For patients also taking valproate: for weeks 1 and 2, give 25 mg P.O. every other day; for weeks 3 and 4, give 25 mg daily; then increase by 25 to 50 mg/day every 1 to 2 weeks to maintenance dosage of 100 to 400 mg daily in one or two divided doses or, 100 to 200 mg daily with valproate alone. For patients taking antiepileptics other than carba-mazepine, phenobarbital, phenytoin, primidone, or valproate: for weeks 1 and 2, give 25 mg P.O. daily; for weeks 3 and 4, give 50 mg P.O. daily; then increase by 50 mg/day every 1 to 2 weeks to maintenance dosage of 225 to 375 mg daily in two divided doses. For patients taking carba-mazepine, phenobarbital, phenytoin, or primi-done, and not valproate: for weeks 1 and 2, give 50 mg P.O. daily; for weeks 3 and 4, give

100 mg daily in two divided doses; then in-crease by 100 mg daily every 1 to 2 weeks to maintenance dosage of 300 to 500 mg daily in 2 divided dosages.

Children ages 2 to 12: Dosage is based on other antiepileptics taken. For patients also taking val-proate: for weeks 1 and 2, give 0.15 mg/kg P.O. daily in one or two divided doses; for weeks 3 and 4, give 0.3 mg/kg daily in one or two di-vided doses; then increase to maintenance dos-age of 1 to 5 mg/kg daily; maximum dosage, 200 mg daily, or 1 to 3 mg/kg daily with val-proate alone. For patients taking antiepileptics other than carbamazepine, phenobarbital, phenytoin, primidone, or valproate: for weeks 1 and 2, give 0.3 mg/kg P.O. daily in one or two divided doses; for weeks 3 and 4, give 0.6 mg/ kg daily in two divided doses; then increase to maintenance dosage of 4.5 to 7.5 mg/kg daily; maximum dosage, 300 mg daily. For patients taking carbamazepine, phenobarbital, pheny-toin, or primidone, and not valproate: for weeks 1 and 2, give 0.6 mg/kg P.O. daily in two divid-ed doses; for weeks 3 and 4, give 1.2 mg/kg dai-ly in two divided doses; increase to maintenance dosage of 5 to 15 mg/kg daily in two divided doses; maximum dosage, 400 mg daily.

▶ **To convert patients from monotherapy with a hepatic enzyme-inducing anticonvul-sant to lamotrigine.** *Adults and children age 16 and older:* Add 50 mg P.O. once daily to current therapy for 2 weeks, followed by 100 mg P.O. daily in two divided doses for 2 weeks. Then in-crease daily dosage by 100 mg every 1 to 2 weeks until maintenance dosage of 500 mg daily in two divided doses is reached. Gradually withdraw hepatic enzyme-inducing anticonvul-sant in 20% decrements weekly for 4 weeks.

◤ **Adjust-a-dose:** For patients with severe renal impairment or moderate to severe hepatic im-pairment, use lower maintenance dosage.

▶ **Bipolar disorder.** *Adults not taking carba-mazepine (or other enzyme-inducing drugs) or valproic acid:* Target dose, 200 mg daily. Initial-ly, 25 mg daily for weeks 1 and 2; then 50 mg daily for weeks 3 and 4; then 100 mg daily for week 5; then 200 mg daily for weeks 6 and 7. *Adults taking carbamazepine (or other enzyme-inducing drugs) and not taking valproic acid:* Target dose, 400 mg/day. Initially, 50 mg daily for weeks 1 and 2; then 100 mg daily in divided doses for weeks 3 and 4; then 200 mg daily in divided doses for week 5; then 300 mg daily in

divided doses for week 6; and up to 400 mg daily in divided doses for week 7.

Adults taking valproic acid: Target dosage is 100 mg/day. Initially, 25 mg every other day for weeks 1 and 2; then 25 mg daily for weeks 3 and 4; then 50 mg daily for week 5; then 100 mg daily for weeks 6 and 7.

☒ **Adjust-a-dose:** If other psychotropic drugs are withdrawn following stabilization, adjust dosage.

Contraindications and cautions

• Contraindicated in patients hypersensitive to the drug or any of its components.
• Use cautiously in patients with renal, hepatic, or cardiac impairment.

⚖ **Lifespan:** In pregnant women, use only when benefits outweigh risks to the fetus. In breast-feeding women, use cautiously, it isn't known if drug appears in breast milk. In children, drug is only indicated as adjunctive therapy for the generalized seizures of Lennox-Gastaut syndrome. For other uses, safety and effectiveness haven't been established in children younger than age 16.

Adverse reactions

CNS: aggravated reaction, anxiety, *ataxia,* concentration disturbance, decreased memory, depression, *dizziness,* emotional lability, fever, *headache,* incoordination, insomnia, irritability, malaise, mind racing, *seizures,* sleep disorder, *somnolence,* speech disorder, *suicide attempts,* tremor, vertigo.
CV: palpitations.
EENT: *blurred vision, diplopia,* nystagmus, pharyngitis, rhinitis, vision abnormality.
GI: abdominal pain, anorexia, constipation, diarrhea, dry mouth, dyspepsia, *nausea, vomiting.*
GU: amenorrhea, dysmenorrhea, vaginitis.
Musculoskeletal: dysarthria, muscle spasm, neck pain.
Respiratory: cough, dyspnea.
Skin: acne, alopecia, pruritus, rash, *Stevens-Johnson syndrome, toxic epidermal necrolysis.*
Other: chills, flulike syndrome, hot flushes, infection, tooth disorder.

Interactions

Drug-drug. *Acetaminophen:* May reduce lamotrigine level, decreasing therapeutic effects. Monitor patient.

Carbamazepine, oxcarbazepine, phenobarbital, phenytoin, primidone, rifamycins: May decrease lamotrigine steady-state level. Monitor patient closely for decreased effect.
Folate inhibitors (such as co-trimoxazole, methotrexate): May have additive effect because lamotrigine inhibits dihydrofolate reductase, an enzyme involved in folic acid synthesis. Monitor patient closely for adverse effects and toxicities.
Hormonal contraceptives, progestins: May reduce lamotrigine level. Adjust lamotrigine dosage if needed.
Valproic acid: May decrease lamotrigine clearance, which increases steady-state levels. Monitor patient closely for toxicity.
Drug-herb. *Evening primrose oil:* May lower the seizure threshold. Discourage use together.
Drug-lifestyle. *Sun exposure:* May cause photosensitivity reactions. Urge patient to avoid unprotected or prolonged exposure to sunlight.

Effects on lab test results

None reported.

Pharmacokinetics

Absorption: Rapid and complete with negligible first-pass metabolism.
Distribution: 55% protein-bound.
Metabolism: Mainly by glucuronic acid conjugation.
Excretion: Mainly in urine. *Half-life:* 14½ to 70¼ hours, depending on dosage schedule and use of other anticonvulsants.

Route	Onset	Peak	Duration
P.O.	Unknown	1½–4½ hr	Unknown

Action

Chemical effect: May inhibit release of glutamate and aspartate, excitatory neurotransmitters in the brain, through action at sodium channels.
Therapeutic effect: Prevents partial seizures, stabilizes mood.

Available forms

Tablets: 25 mg, 100 mg, 150 mg, 200 mg
Tablets (chewable dispersible): 2 mg, 5 mg, 25 mg

Reactions may be *common,* uncommon, *life-threatening,* or **COMMON AND LIFE-THREATENING.**

NURSING PROCESS

☑ Assessment
• Obtain history of patient's disorder before starting therapy.
• Evaluate patient for reduction in frequency and duration of seizures after therapy begins. Check adjunct anticonvulsant level periodically.
• Monitor signs and symptoms of bipolar disorder and suicidal thoughts.
• Assess patient's and family's knowledge of drug therapy.

🔄 Nursing diagnoses
• Risk for trauma related to seizures
• Risk for impaired skin integrity related to dermatologic reactions
• Deficient knowledge related to drug therapy

▷ Planning and implementation
• If drug is added to therapy that includes valproic acid, lower dosage.
⚠ **ALERT:** Don't abruptly stop giving the drug because doing so increases the risk of seizures and unstable mood. Taper drug over at least 2 weeks.
⚠ **ALERT:** Rash may be life-threatening. If one develops, stop giving the drug and immediately notify prescriber. Don't restart.
⚠ **ALERT:** Don't confuse Lamictal with Lamisil, levothyroxine, or Lomotil.
Patient teaching
• Inform patient that drug may cause rash. Combination therapy with valproic acid and lamotrigine is more likely to cause a serious rash. Tell patient to immediately report rash or signs or symptoms of hypersensitivity because they could be life threatening.
• Instruct patient to avoid prolonged exposure to sunlight, use sun block, and wear protective clothing to avoid photosensitivity.
• Warn patient not to engage in hazardous activity until the drug's CNS effects are known.

☑ Evaluation
• Patient is seizure-free.
• Patient doesn't develop drug-induced skin reactions.
• Patient and family state understanding of drug therapy.

lansoprazole
(lan-SOH-pray-zohl)
Prevacid✐, **Prevacid I.V.**, **Prevacid SoluTab**

Pharmacologic class: proton-pump inhibitor
Therapeutic class: gastric antisecretory
Pregnancy risk category: B

Indications and dosages

▶ **Short-term therapy for active duodenal ulcer.** *Adults:* 15 mg P.O. daily for 4 weeks.
▶ **Maintenance of healed duodenal ulcers; maintenance of healing erosive esophagitis.** *Adults:* 15 mg P.O. daily.
▶ **Short-term therapy for erosive esophagitis.** *Adults:* 30 mg P.O. daily for up to 8 weeks. If healing doesn't occur, give additional 8 weeks of therapy. Maintenance dosage for healing is 15 mg P.O. daily.
Children ages 12 to 17: Give 30 mg P.O. once daily for up to 8 weeks.
Children ages 1 to 11 who weigh 30 kg (66 lb) or less: 15 mg P.O. daily for up to 12 weeks.
Children ages 1 to 11 who weigh more than 30 kg: 30 mg P.O. daily for up to 12 weeks.
▶ **Short-term therapy for erosive esophagitis when the patient isn't able to take oral drug.** *Adults:* 30 mg I.V. daily, over 30 minutes, for up to 7 days. As soon as the patient can take oral drug, switch to P.O. and continue for 6 to 8 weeks.
▶ **Short-term therapy for active benign gastric ulcer.** *Adults:* 30 mg P.O. daily for up to 8 weeks.
▶ ***Helicobacter pylori* eradication to reduce risk of duodenal ulcer recurrence.** *Adults:* For triple therapy, 30 mg P.O. lansoprazole with 500 mg P.O. clarithromycin and 1 g P.O. amoxicillin, each given every 12 hours for 14 days. For dual therapy, 30 mg P.O. lansoprazole with 1 g P.O. amoxicillin, each given every 8 hours for 14 days.
▶ **Long-term therapy for pathologic hypersecretory conditions, including Zollinger-Ellison syndrome.** *Adults:* Initially, 60 mg P.O. daily. Increase dosage as needed. If more than 120 mg daily, give in divided doses.
▶ **Short-term therapy for symptomatic gastroesophageal reflux disease.** *Adults:* 15 mg P.O. daily for up to 8 weeks.

L

Children ages 12 to 17: Give 15 mg P.O. daily for up to 8 weeks.

Children ages 1 to 11 who weigh 30 kg (66 lb) or less: 15 mg P.O. daily for up to 12 weeks.

Children ages 1 to 11 who weigh more than 30 kg: 30 mg P.O. daily for up to 12 weeks.

▶ **NSAID-related ulcer in patients who are continuing NSAIDs.** *Adults:* 30 mg P.O. daily for 8 weeks.

▶ **To reduce risk of NSAID-related ulcer in a patient who has a history of gastric ulcer and needs NSAIDs.** *Adults:* 15 mg P.O. daily for up to 12 weeks.

▼ I.V. administration

• Reconstitute with 5 ml sterile water for injection only.

• Mix gently until the powder is dissolved.

• Infuse over 30 minutes using the provided 1.2 micron in-line filter, which will remove any precipitate that forms when reconstituted solution comes in contact with I.V. solutions.

⊗ **Incompatibilities**
Other I.V. drugs.

Contraindications and cautions

• Contraindicated in patients hypersensitive to the drug or any of its components.

• Drug isn't recommended as maintenance therapy for patients with active duodenal ulcers or erosive esophagitis.

⚠ **Lifespan:** In pregnant women, use only when benefits outweigh risks to the fetus. In breast-feeding women, don't use; it isn't known if drug appears in breast milk. In children younger than age 1, safety and effectiveness haven't been established.

Adverse reactions

GI: abdominal pain, diarrhea, nausea.

Interactions

Drug-drug. *Ampicillin esters, digoxin, iron salts, ketoconazole:* May interfere with absorption of these drugs. Monitor patient closely.

Sucralfate: May delay lansoprazole absorption. Give lansoprazole at least 30 minutes before sucralfate.

Theophylline: May slightly increase theophylline clearance. Use together cautiously. Adjust dosage, if needed, when lansoprazole is started or stopped.

Drug-herb. *Male fern:* May inactivate drug in alkaline environments. Discourage use together. *St. John's wort:* May increase risk of photosensitivity reactions. Advise patient to avoid unprotected or prolonged exposure to sunlight.

Drug-food. *Food:* May decrease absorption of drug when taken with meals. Take drug on an empty stomach, before meals.

Effects on lab test results

None reported.

Pharmacokinetics

Absorption: Rapid.
Distribution: 97% protein-bound.
Metabolism: Extensive, in liver.
Excretion: Mainly in feces, minimally in urine.
Half-life: Less than 2 hours.

Route	Onset	Peak	Duration
P.O.	Unknown	2 hr	> 24 hr

Action

Chemical effect: Inhibits proton pump and binds to hydrogen or potassium adenosine triphosphatase, located at secretory surface of gastric parietal cells.
Therapeutic effect: Decreases gastric acid formation.

Available forms

Capsules (delayed-release): 15 mg, 30 mg
Injection: 30-mg single-use vial
Oral suspension (delayed-release): 15 mg/packet, 30 mg/packet
Tablets (delayed-release, orally-disintegrating): 15 mg (contains 2.5 mg phenylalanine), 30 mg (contains 5.1 mg phenylalanine)

NURSING PROCESS

📝 **Assessment**
• Assess patient's condition before starting therapy and regularly thereafter to monitor drug's effectiveness.
• Be alert for adverse reactions and drug interactions.
• Assess patient's and family's knowledge of drug therapy.

🔢 **Nursing diagnoses**
• Impaired tissue integrity related to underlying condition

Reactions may be *common*, uncommon, *life-threatening*, or COMMON AND LIFE-THREATENING.

• Ineffective health maintenance related to drug-induced adverse reactions
• Deficient knowledge related to drug therapy

▶ **Planning and implementation**

⚠ **ALERT:** Orally-disintegrating tablets contain phenylalanine. Assess patient for sensitivity before starting therapy.
• Give drug on an empty stomach.
• If giving by NG tube, mix contents of capsule with 40 ml of apple juice in a syringe and give within 3 to 5 minutes. Flush with additional apple juice to ensure entire dose is given and to maintain patency of the tube.
• If giving capsule to a patient who has difficulty swallowing, empty contents of capsule into about 2 oz (60 ml) of apple, cranberry, grape, orange, pineapple, prune, tomato, or vegetable juice, mix briefly, and use within 30 minutes. To ensure complete dose, rinse glass with two or more servings of juice and have patient drink immediately. Or mix contents of capsule with 1 tbs of applesauce, pudding, cottage cheese, yogurt, or strained pears and have patient swallow immediately. Tell him not to chew or crush granules.
• For the oral suspension, empty packet contents into 30 ml of water. Stir well and have patient drink immediately. Tell patient not to chew or crush the contents of the capsules or the suspension. Don't use with other liquids or food. If any material remains after drinking, add more water, stir, and have patient drink immediately.
• Place orally-disintegrating tablets on the patient's tongue and allow to dissolve completely. Water isn't needed. If using NG tube or oral syringe, dissolve 15-mg tablet in 4 ml water or 30-mg tablet in 10 ml water.

⚠ **ALERT:** Don't crush drug or allow patient to chew it.
• If adverse reaction occurs, notify prescriber and provide supportive care.
• Adjust dosage in patients with severe liver disease.

Patient teaching
• Tell patient not to crush or chew drug and to take it before a meal.
• Explain how to mix drug with other liquids if patient has difficulty swallowing.
• Tell patient to allow orally-disintegrating tablets to dissolve on tongue until the particles can be swallowed.

• Instruct patient to notify prescriber if any adverse reactions occur.

☑ **Evaluation**
• Patient regains normal GI tissue integrity.
• Patient doesn't experience serious adverse reactions.
• Patient and family state understanding of drug therapy.

✴ **New Drug**

HIGH ALERT

lapatinib
(lah-PAH-tih-nihb)
Tykerb

Pharmacologic class: kinase inhibitor
Therapeutic class: antineoplastic
Pregnancy risk category: D

Indications and dosages

▶ **With capecitabine, advanced or metastatic breast cancer when tumors overexpress HER2 in patient who has received prior therapy including an anthracycline, a taxane, and trastuzumab.** *Adults:* 1,250 mg (5 tablets of 250 mg each) P.O. once daily as a single dose on days 1 through 21, with 2,000 mg/m²/day capecitabine. Capecitabine is given P.O. in 2 doses, about 12 hours apart, on days 1 to 14, in a repeating 21-day cycle.

▣ **Adjust-a-dose:** If left ventricular function (LVEF) decreases due to treatment, stop the drug. After 2 weeks, if LVEF returns to normal and patient is asymptomatic, resume at reduced dosage of 1,000 mg/day and monitor LVEF.

For severe hepatic impairment (Child-Pugh Class C), reduce dosage to 750 mg/day.

In patients with grade 2 or higher toxicity by NCI Common Terminology Criteria for Adverse Events (known as NCI CTCAE), if initial episode of toxicity improves to grade 1 or lower, resume normal dose of 1,250 mg/day. If toxicity recurs, resume at a lower dose of 1,000 mg/day.

Contraindications and cautions

• Use cautiously in patients with left ventricular dysfunction, conditions that may decrease LVEF, severe hepatic impairment, hypokalemia, hypomagnesemia, or diarrhea.

L

Lifespan: In pregnant women, drug may harm fetus; inform patient of risk. It's unknown if drug is found in breast milk; tell patient to stop nursing or stop drug, depending on importance of the drug to the mother. In children, safety and effectiveness haven't been established. Elderly patients may experience greater sensitivity to the drug.

Adverse reactions

CV: *decreased left ventricular cardiac function or ejection fraction, prolonged QT interval.*
EENT: *mucosal inflammation.*
GI: *diarrhea, nausea, vomiting, stomatitis, dyspepsia.*
Hematologic: *anemia,* **neutropenia.**
Musculoskeletal: *arm or leg pain, back pain.*
Respiratory: *dyspnea.*
Skin: *palmar-plantar erythrodysesthesia, rash, dry skin.*
Other: *insomnia.*

Interactions

Drug-drug. *Antiarrhythmics, other drugs that lead to prolonged QT interval, cumulative high-dose anthracycline:* May prolong QTc interval. Avoid using together.
CYP2C8 inhibitors, P-glycoprotein substrates: May increase lapatinib level. Avoid using together.
Strong CYP3A4 inducers (dexamethasone, phenytoin, carbamazepine, rifampin, rifabutin, rifapentine, phenobarbital): May significantly decrease lapatinib level. Avoid using together or gradually increase lapatinib dosage as tolerated, to 4,500 mg/day.
Strong CYP3A4 inhibitors (ketoconazole, itraconazole, clarithromycin, atazanavir, indinavir, nefazodone, nelfinavir, ritonavir, saquinavir, telithromycin, voriconazole): May significantly increase lapatinib level. Avoid using together or reduce lapatinib dosage to 500 mg/day.
Drug-herb. *St. John's wort:* May significantly decrease drug level. Avoid using together or gradually increase lapatinib dosage as tolerated, to 4,500 mg/day.
Drug-food. *All food:* May increase exposure to drug. Give at least one hour before or one hour after a meal.
Grapefruit: May increase drug level. Avoid using together.

Effects on lab test results

• May increase total bilirubin, AST, and ALT levels. May decrease hemoglobin level.
• May decrease platelet and neutrophil counts.

Pharmacokinetics

Absorption: Incomplete and variable; increased by eating.
Distribution: Highly bound to albumin and alpha-1 glycoprotein.
Metabolism: CYP450 metabolized (primarily 3A4, 3A5, 2C19, 2C8) to oxidized metabolites.
Excretion: Mostly through metabolism; 27% via feces; negligible via kidneys. *Half-life:* 14¼ hours; after repeated dosing, 24 hours.

Route	Onset	Peak	Duration
P.O.	Up to 1½ hr	4 hr	Unknown

Action

Chemical effect: Inhibits tumor cell growth with additive effects when given with capecitabine.
Therapeutic effect: Slows tumor growth.

Available forms

Tablets: 250 mg

NURSING PROCESS

Assessment
• Evaluate LVEF before using and monitor during treatment.
• Correct hypokalemia and hypomagnesemia before using.
• Assess patient's and family's knowledge of drug therapy.

Nursing diagnoses
• Ineffective health maintenance related to presence of neoplastic disease
• Risk for deficient fluid volume related to drug-induced adverse GI reactions
• Deficient knowledge related to drug therapy

Planning and implementation
• Monitor for excessive diarrhea, give prophylactic antidiarrheals, and correct electrolytes as needed.
• Monitor for anemia and neutropenia.
• No antidote exists for overdose. Administer supportive treatment based on symptoms.

Reactions may be *common*, uncommon, *life-threatening*, or COMMON AND LIFE-THREATENING.

Patient teaching
- Instruct patient to store drug at room temperature.
- Tell patient to report the following immediately to his health care provider: shortness of breath, palpitations, fatigue, diarrhea, changes in medications or OTC preparations.
- Tell patient not to divide doses but to take drug once daily, regardless of number of tablets per dose, one hour before or after a meal.
- Remind patient to take capecitabine as prescribed.
- Instruct patient that if a dose is missed, it should be taken as soon as they remember. If the dose is late by several hours, tell him to call his health care provider for guidance as to whether he should take or skip the drug.
- Tell patient not to eat grapefruit or drink grapefruit juice during therapy.

☑ Evaluation
- Patient responds well to therapy.
- Patient doesn't develop serious side effects.
- Patient and family state understanding of drug therapy.

HIGH ALERT

leflunomide
(leh-FLOO-noh-mighd)
Arava

Pharmacologic class: dihydro-orotate dehydrogenase inhibitor
Therapeutic class: immunomodulator
Pregnancy risk category: X

Indications and dosages
▶ **Active rheumatoid arthritis (RA), to reduce signs and symptoms, to retard structural damage based on X-ray evidence of erosions and joint space narrowing, to improve physical function.** *Adults:* Initially, 100 mg P.O. every 24 hours for 3 days followed by a daily dose of 20 mg. If this dosage isn't tolerated, decrease to 10 mg daily.

Contraindications and cautions
- Contraindicated in patients hypersensitive to the drug or any of its components.
- Use cautiously in patients with hepatic insufficiency, hepatitis B or C, severe immunodeficiency, bone marrow dysplasia, or severe uncontrolled infections.
- Use cautiously in patients with renal insufficiency.

☀ **Lifespan:** In pregnant and breast-feeding women, drug is contraindicated. In children, safety and effectiveness haven't been established. In men attempting to father children, drug isn't recommended.

Adverse reactions
CNS: anxiety, asthenia, depression, dizziness, fever, headache, insomnia, malaise, migraine, neuralgia, neuritis, paresthesia, sleep disorder, vertigo.
CV: angina pectoris, chest pain, *hypertension,* palpitations, peripheral edema, tachycardia, varicose veins, vasculitis, vasodilation.
EENT: blurred vision, cataracts, conjunctivitis, enlarged salivary gland, epistaxis, eye disorders, pharyngitis, rhinitis, sinusitis.
GI: abdominal pain, anorexia, cholelithiasis, colitis, constipation, *diarrhea,* dry mouth, dyspepsia, esophagitis, flatulence, gastritis, gastroenteritis, gingivitis, melena, mouth ulcer, nausea, oral candidiasis, stomatitis, taste perversion, vomiting.
GU: albuminuria, cystitis, dysuria, hematuria, menstrual disorder, pelvic pain, prostate disorder, urinary frequency, UTI, vaginal candidiasis.
Hematologic: anemia, hyperlipidemia.
Metabolic: *diabetes mellitus,* hyperglycemia, hyperthyroidism, hypokalemia, weight loss.
Musculoskeletal: arthralgia, arthrosis, back pain, bone necrosis, bone pain, bursitis, joint disorder, leg cramps, muscle cramps, myalgia, neck pain, synovitis, tendon rupture, tenosynovitis.
Respiratory: *asthma,* bronchitis, dyspnea, increased cough, lung disorders, pneumonia, *respiratory infection.*
Skin: acne, *alopecia,* contact dermatitis, dry skin, ecchymosis, eczema, fungal dermatitis, hair discoloration, hematoma, increased sweating, maculopapular rash, nail disorder, pruritus, *rash,* skin nodule, skin discoloration, skin disorder, subcutaneous nodule, skin ulcer.
Other: abscess, allergic reaction, cyst, flulike syndrome, hernia, herpes simplex, herpes zoster, injury or accident, pain, tooth disorder.

Interactions

Drug-drug. *Charcoal, cholestyramine:* May decrease leflunomide level. Sometimes used for this effect in overdose.
Live vaccines: May alter immune response. Avoid live vaccines during therapy, and remember leflunomide's long half-life when considering a live vaccine after therapy stops.
Methotrexate, other hepatotoxic drugs: May increase risk of hepatotoxicity. Monitor liver enzyme levels.
NSAIDs (diclofenac, ibuprofen): May increase NSAID level. Significance is unknown; monitor patient.
Rifampin: May increase active leflunomide metabolite level. Use together cautiously.
Tolbutamide: May increase tolbutamide levels. Significance is unknown; monitor patient.

Effects on lab test results

• May increase AST, ALT, glucose, lipid, T_4, and CK levels. May decrease potassium, TSH, and hemoglobin levels and hematocrit.

Pharmacokinetics

Absorption: 80%.
Distribution: Low. Extensively bound to albumin.
Metabolism: Main route unknown.
Excretion: Renal and biliary; 43% in urine, 48% in feces. *Half-life:* 15 to 18 days.

Route	Onset	Peak	Duration
P.O.	Unknown	6–12 hr	Unknown

Action

Chemical effect: Inhibits dihydroorotate dehydrogenase, an enzyme involved in pyrimidine synthesis, and is antiproliferative and anti-inflammatory.
Therapeutic effect: Reduces pain and inflammation related to RA.

Available forms

Tablets: 10 mg, 20 mg

NURSING PROCESS

Assessment

• Assess patient's condition before starting therapy, and regularly thereafter to monitor drug effectiveness.

• Be alert for adverse reactions and drug interactions.
• Monitor platelet and WBC counts and ALT and hemoglobin levels and hematocrit, at baseline and at monthly intervals during the first 6 months; if stable, continue monitoring every 6 to 8 weeks. If used with methotrexate (MTX) or other immunosuppressant, monitor patient's AST, ALT, and albumin levels monthly.
ALERT: Severe liver damage, sometimes fatal, may rarely occur. Most cases of severe liver damage occur within 6 months of therapy in a patient with multiple risk factors for hepatotoxicity (liver disease, other hepatotoxins).
• Monitor for overlapping hematologic toxicity when switching to another antirheumatic.
• Because of drug's long half-life, carefully observe patient after reducing dosage because level may take several weeks to decline.
• Assess patient's and family's knowledge of drug therapy.

Nursing diagnoses

• Ineffective health maintenance related to underlying disease
• Deficient knowledge related to drug therapy

Planning and implementation

• If ALT level increases to between two and three times the upper limit of normal (ULN), lower the dose to 10 mg daily. This may allow you to continue use under close monitoring. If ALT level stays between two and three times ULN despite the lower dose, or if ALT level increases to more than three times ULN, stop giving the drug, give cholestyramine or charcoal, and monitor the patient closely. Give additional doses of cholestyramine or charcoal if needed.
ALERT: Drug can cause fetal harm when given during pregnancy. Stop giving the drug to a woman planning to become pregnant, and notify prescriber.
• Stop drug in a man who plans to father a child. Tell him to take 8 g cholestyramine P.O. t.i.d. for 11 days to remove drug. Check levels.
• If bone marrow suppression occurs, stop the drug and start cholestyramine or charcoal therapy.
• Some immunosuppressants, possibly including leflunomide, increase the risk of cancer, particularly lymphoproliferative disorders. Use drug only when benefits exceed risks.

Patient teaching

• Explain the need for frequent blood test monitoring.

• Instruct patient to use contraceptive measures during drug therapy and until drug is no longer active.

• If a woman suspects she is pregnant, advise her to immediately notify the prescriber.

• Advise breast-feeding woman not to breast-feed during therapy.

• Tell patient that live-virus vaccines should be avoided during therapy.

• Tell patient that he may continue taking aspirin, other NSAIDs, and low-dose corticosteroids, but that combined use of drug with antimalarials, I.M. or P.O. gold, penicillamine, azathioprine, or MTX hasn't been adequately studied. Instruct patient to review all drugs with prescriber before use.

☑ Evaluation

• Patient's symptoms of RA improve.

• Patient and family state understanding of drug therapy.

leucovorin calcium
(citrovorum factor, folinic acid)
(loo-koh-VOR-in KAL-see-um)

Pharmacologic class: formyl derivative (active reduced form of folic acid)
Therapeutic class: vitamin, antidote
Pregnancy risk category: C

Indications and dosages

▶ **Overdose of folic acid antagonist.** *Adults and children:* P.O., I.M., or I.V. dose equivalent to weight of antagonist given.

▶ **Rescue after high methotrexate dose given as cancer therapy.** *Adults and children:* 10 mg/m^2 P.O., I.M., or I.V. every 6 hours until methotrexate level falls below 5×10^{-8} M.

▶ **Megaloblastic anemia caused by congenital enzyme deficiency.** *Adults and children:* 3 to 6 mg I.M. daily; then 1 mg P.O. or I.M. daily for life.

▶ **Folate-deficient megaloblastic anemia.**
Adults and children: Up to 1 mg P.O. or I.M. daily. Duration of therapy depends on hematologic response.

▶ **Hematologic toxicity caused by pyrimethamine or trimethoprim therapy.** *Adults and children:* 5 to 15 mg P.O. or I.M. daily.

▶ **Palliative treatment of advanced colorectal carcinoma.** *Adults:* 20 mg/m^2 I.V., followed by fluorouracil, for 5 consecutive days. Repeat every 4 weeks for two more courses; then every 4 to 5 weeks, if tolerated.

▼ I.V. administration

• Give leucovorin I.V. to patients with GI toxicity (diarrhea, stomatitis, vomiting) when doses exceed 25 mg.

• When using powder for injection, reconstitute drug in 50-mg vial with 5 ml, 100 mg vial with 10 ml, or 350-mg vial with 17 ml of sterile water or bacteriostatic water for injection. When doses are greater than 10 mg/m^2 don't use diluents containing benzyl alcohol, especially in neonates.

• Don't give faster than 160 mg/minute because of the calcium concentration.

• Protect drug from light and heat, especially reconstituted parenteral forms.

⊗ Incompatibilities
Droperidol, fluorouracil, foscarnet, sodium bicarbonate.

Contraindications and cautions

• Contraindicated in patients with pernicious anemia and other megaloblastic anemias caused by lack of vitamin B$_{12}$.

⚘ Lifespan: In breast-feeding women, use cautiously; it's unknown if drug appears in breast milk. In neonates, injection form is contraindicated because it contains benzyl alcohol. In children, use cautiously because drug may increase risk of seizures.

Adverse reactions

Respiratory: *bronchospasm.*
Skin: hypersensitivity reactions (erythema, pruritus, rash).

Interactions

Drug-drug. *Anticonvulsants:* May decrease anticonvulsant effectiveness. Monitor patient closely.
Fluorouracil: May enhance fluorouracil toxicity. Adjust fluorouracil dosage if needed.
Methotrexate: May decrease intrathecal methotrexate effectiveness. Avoid use together.

L

Effects on lab test results
None reported.

Pharmacokinetics
Absorption: Rapid after P.O. use.
Distribution: Throughout body; liver contains about one-half of total body folate stores.
Metabolism: In liver.
Excretion: By kidneys. *Half-life:* 6¼ hours.

Route	Onset	Peak	Duration
P.O.	20–30 min	2–3 hr	3–6 hr
I.V.	5 min	10 min	3–6 hr
I.M.	10–20 min	< 1 hr	3–6 hr

Action
Chemical effect: Readily converts to other folic acid derivatives.
Therapeutic effect: Raises folic acid level.

Available forms
Injection: 3 mg/ml in 1-ml ampule; 10 mg/ml in 5-ml vial
Powder for injection: 50-mg, 100-mg, and 350-mg vials for reconstitution
Tablets: 5 mg, 15 mg, 25 mg

NURSING PROCESS

Assessment
• Assess patient's condition before starting therapy and regularly thereafter to monitor drug effectiveness.
• Monitor creatinine level daily to detect renal dysfunction.
• Be alert for adverse reactions and drug interactions.
• Monitor patient for rash, wheezing, pruritus, and urticaria, which can signal drug allergy.
• Assess patient's and family's knowledge of drug therapy.

Nursing diagnoses
• Ineffective health maintenance related to underlying condition
• Deficient knowledge related to drug therapy

Planning and implementation
• Drug may mask diagnosis of pernicious anemia.
• Follow leucovorin rescue schedule and protocol closely to maximize therapeutic response.

• Don't give simultaneously with systemic methotrexate.
ALERT: Don't confuse leucovorin (folinic acid) with folic acid. To avoid confusion, don't refer to leucovorin as folinic acid.
Patient teaching
• Explain to patient reasons for drug therapy.

Evaluation
• Patient's condition improves.
• Patient and family state understanding of drug therapy.

HIGH ALERT

leuprolide acetate
(loo-PROH-lighd AS-ih-tayt)
Eligard, Lupron, Lupron Depot, Lupron Depot-Ped, Lupron Depot-3 Month, Lupron Depot-4 Month, Lupron for Pediatric Use

Pharmacologic class: synthetic analogue of gonadotropin-releasing hormone
Therapeutic class: antineoplastic, luteinizing hormone-releasing hormone agonist
Pregnancy risk category: X

Indications and dosages
▶ **Advanced prostate cancer.** *Men:* 1 mg subcutaneously daily. Or 7.5 mg I.M. depot injection monthly. Or 7.5 mg Eligard subcutaneously once monthly. Or 22.5 mg I.M. every 3 months (84 days). Or 22.5 mg Eligard subcutaneously every 3 months. Or 30 mg I.M. depot injection every 4 months (16 weeks). Or 30 mg Eligard subcutaneously every 4 months. Or 45 mg Eligard subcutaneously every 6 months.
▶ **Endometriosis.** *Women:* 3.75 mg I.M. as single injection once monthly. Or 11.25 mg I.M. every 3 months (depot injection only). Recommended duration of treatment is 6 months.
▶ **Central precocious puberty.** *Children:* Initially, 0.3 mg/kg (minimum, 7.5 mg) I.M. depot injection as a single injection every 4 weeks. Increase dosage in increments of 3.75 mg every 4 weeks, if needed. This will be considered the maintenance dosage. Or 50 mcg/kg subcutaneously (injection form) daily. If total downregulation isn't achieved, increase dosage by 10 mcg/kg daily. This becomes the maintenance dosage. Stop drug before girls reach age 11 and before boys reach age 12.

▶ **Uterine leiomyomata (depot only).** *Women:*
3.75 mg I.M. monthly or one dose of 11.25 mg
I.M. with iron therapy. Recommended duration
of therapy is 3 months or less.

Contraindications and cautions

• Contraindicated in patients hypersensitive to
drug, its components, or other gonadotropin-
releasing hormone analogues and in women
with undiagnosed vaginal bleeding.
• Use cautiously in patients hypersensitive to
benzyl alcohol.
❋ **Lifespan:** In women, the 30-mg depot form
is contraindicated. In pregnant and breast-
feeding women, drug is contraindicated. In
neonates, drug is contraindicated because it contains benzyl alcohol.

Adverse reactions

CNS: depression, dizziness, headache, pain.
CV: angina, *arrhythmias, MI,* peripheral edema.
GI: nausea, vomiting.
GU: impotence.
Musculoskeletal: *decreased bone density,* tran-
sient bone pain (during first week of therapy).
Respiratory: *pulmonary embolism.*
Skin: skin reactions at injection site.
Other: decreased libido, gynecomastia, *hot
flushes.*

Interactions

None significant.

Effects on lab test results

• May increase BUN, creatinine, bilirubin, alkaline phosphatase, LDH, glucose, uric acid, albumin, calcium, phosphorus, total cholesterol,
LDL, and triglyceride levels. May decrease
potassium, HDL, and hemoglobin levels and
hematocrit.
• May increase WBC count. May decrease PT,
PTT, RBC, and platelet counts.
• May give inaccurate reading of pituitary go-
nadotropic and gonadal functions during therapy and for up to 12 weeks afterwards.

Pharmacokinetics

Absorption: Rapid and complete after subcuta-
neous use; unknown for I.M. use.
Distribution: Unknown. About 7% to 15%
protein-bound at therapeutic level.
Metabolism: Unknown.
Excretion: Unknown. *Half-life:* 3 hours.

Route	Onset	Peak	Duration
I.M., SubQ	Unknown	4 hr	1–3 mo

Action

Chemical effect: Initially stimulates but then
inhibits release of gonadotropin-releasing hormone, resulting in testosterone and estrogen
suppression.
Therapeutic effect: Hinders prostatic cancer
cell growth, eases signs and symptoms of endometriosis, and inhibits progression of puberty
in children. Also decreases uterine and fibroid
volume.

Available forms

Injection: 5 mg/ml in 2.8-ml multiple-dose vial
Microspheres for injection, lyophilized:
3.75 mg, 7.5 mg, 11.25 mg, 15 mg, 22.5 mg,
30 mg
Suspension for depot injection: 7.5 mg,
22.5 mg, 30 mg, 45 mg (single-use kit)

NURSING PROCESS

🔖 **Assessment**
• Assess patient's condition before starting therapy and regularly thereafter to monitor drug effectiveness.
• Be alert for adverse reactions.
• Assess patient's and family's knowledge of
drug therapy.

🔄 **Nursing diagnoses**
• Ineffective health maintenance related to un-
derlying condition
• Disturbed thought processes related to drug-
induced depression
• Deficient knowledge related to drug therapy

▶ **Planning and implementation**
🔔 **ALERT:** Never give drug by I.V. injection.
🔔 **ALERT:** Different products have specific mixing and administration instructions. Read the
manufacturer's directions closely. When using
the two-syringe mixing system, after connecting
the syringes, inject the liquid contents from syringe A into the powder in syringe B. Mix product by pushing contents back and forth between
syringes for about 45 seconds. (Shaking syringes won't provide adequate mixing.) The suspension will be colorless to pale yellow. The
7.5-mg suspension should be light tan to tan.

L

Use immediately after mixing. Attach the needle provided in the kit and inject subcutaneously.
• Give once-monthly depot injection under medical supervision. Use supplied diluent to reconstitute. (Discard extra diluent.) Draw 1 ml into syringe with 22G needle. (When preparing Lupron Depot-3 Month 22.5 mg, use a 23G or larger needle.) Withdraw 1.5 ml from ampule for the 3-month formulation. Inject into vial and shake well. Suspension will appear milky. Although suspension is stable for 24 hours after reconstitution, it doesn't contain a bacteriostatic agent. Use immediately.
• When using prefilled dual-chamber syringes, screw white plunger into end stopper until stopper begins to turn. Remove and discard tab around base of needle. Hold syringe upright and release diluent by slowly pushing plunger until first stopper is at blue line in middle of barrel. Gently shake syringe to form a uniform milky suspension. If particles adhere to stopper, tap syringe. Remove needle guard and advance plunger to expel air from syringe. Inject entire contents I.M. as for a normal injection.
• Drug is a nonsurgical alternative to orchiectomy or estrogen therapy for advanced prostate cancer.
(🚫) ALERT: A fractional dose of drug formulated to be given every 3 months isn't equivalent to same dose of once-monthly formulation.

Patient teaching
• Before starting therapy in a child with central precocious puberty, make sure parents understand importance of continuous therapy.
• Carefully instruct patient who will give subcutaneous injection about proper administration technique, and advise him to use only syringes provided by manufacturer.
• Advise patient that if another syringe must be substituted, a low-dose insulin syringe (U-100, 0.5 ml) is acceptable.
• Advise patient to store drug at room temperature, protected from light and heat.
• Reassure patient with a history of undesirable effects from other endocrine therapies that this drug is much easier to tolerate. Tell patient that adverse effects are transient and will disappear after about 1 week.
• Warn patient that worsening of prostate cancer symptoms may occur when therapy starts.
• Instruct woman to have a bone-density evaluation before and after therapy. Recommend supplemental calcium to minimize bone loss.

✔ Evaluation
• Patient exhibits improvement in underlying condition.
• Patient demonstrates pretherapy thought processes.
• Patient and family state understanding of drug therapy.

levalbuterol hydrochloride
(leev-al-BYOO-teh-rohl high-droh-KLOR-ighd)
Xopenex, Xopenex HFA

Pharmacologic class: beta$_2$ agonist
Therapeutic class: bronchodilator
Pregnancy risk category: C

Indications and dosages

▶ **To prevent or treat bronchospasm in patients with reversible obstructive airway disease.** *Adults and children age 12 and older:* 0.63 mg (3 ml) solution for inhalation by nebulizer t.i.d. every 6 to 8 hours. Patients with more severe asthma who don't respond adequately to 0.63-mg doses may benefit from 1.25 mg t.i.d. *Children ages 6 to 11:* Give 0.31 mg given t.i.d. by nebulizer. Maximum dosage 0.63 mg t.i.d.
▶ **Treatment of acute episode of bronchospasm or prevention of asthmatic symptoms.** *Adults and children age 4 and older:* 2 inhalations (90 mcg) every 4 to 6 hours. In some patients, 1 inhalation every 4 hours is sufficient.

Contraindications and cautions

• Contraindicated in patients hypersensitive to the drug or any of its components, or racemic albuterol.
• Use cautiously in patients with CV disorders, especially coronary insufficiency, hypertension, and arrhythmias. Also use cautiously in patients with seizure disorders, hyperthyroidism, or diabetes mellitus and in patients who are unusually responsive to sympathomimetic amines.
⚘ Lifespan: In pregnant women, use only when benefits outweigh risks to fetus. In breast-feeding women, use cautiously. In children younger than age 6 and patients age 65 and older, safety and effectiveness are unknown.

Adverse reactions

CNS: anxiety, dizziness, *headache,* migraine, nervousness, pain, tremor.

Reactions may be *common,* uncommon, *life-threatening,* or COMMON AND LIFE-THREATENING.

CV: tachycardia.
EENT: *rhinitis,* sinusitis, turbinate edema.
GI: dyspepsia.
Musculoskeletal: leg cramps.
Respiratory: *asthma exacerbation, bronchospasm,* increased cough.
Other: accidental injury, flulike syndrome, *viral infection.*

Interactions

Drug-drug. *Beta blockers:* May block pulmonary effect of drug and may cause severe bronchospasm. Don't use together. If drug is needed, a cardioselective beta blocker may be considered, but give it with caution.
Digoxin: May decrease digoxin level up to 22%. Monitor digoxin level, and monitor patient for loss of therapeutic effect.
Epinephrine, short-acting sympathomimetic aerosol bronchodilators: May increase adverse adrenergic effects. To avoid serious CV effects, use additional adrenergics with caution.
Loop and thiazide diuretics: May increase risk of ECG changes and hypokalemia. Use together cautiously; monitor cardiac condition and potassium level.
MAO inhibitors, tricyclic antidepressants: May increase levalbuterol action on the vascular system. Use caution when giving these drugs within 2 weeks of each other.

Effects on lab test results

None reported.

Pharmacokinetics

Absorption: Some.
Distribution: Unknown.
Metabolism: Unknown.
Excretion: Unknown. *Half-life:* 3¼ to 4 hours.

Route	Onset	Peak	Duration
Inhalation			
Solution	10–17 min	90 min	5–8 hr
Aerosol	Unknown	< 1 hr	Unknown

Action

Chemical effect: Activates beta$_2$ receptors on airway smooth muscle, which causes smooth muscle from trachea to terminal bronchioles to relax, relieving bronchospasm and reducing airway resistance. Inhibits the release of mediators from mast cells in the airway.
Therapeutic effect: Improves ventilation.

Available forms

Inhalation aerosol: 15 g containing 200 actuations
Solution for inhalation: 0.31 mg, 0.63 mg, or 1.25 mg in 3-ml vials

NURSING PROCESS

Assessment
• Obtain history of patient's underlying condition before starting therapy, and reassess regularly to monitor drug effectiveness.
• Make sure that patient has a thorough physical examination before starting drug therapy.
• Be alert for adverse reactions and drug interactions.
• Assess patient's and family's knowledge of drug therapy.

Nursing diagnoses
• Impaired gas exchange related to underlying respiratory condition
• Risk for injury related to drug-induced adverse reactions
• Deficient knowledge related to drug therapy

Planning and implementation
ALERT: Drug may produce life-threatening paradoxical bronchospasm. If this reaction occurs, immediately stop giving the drug and start alternative therapy.
• Rarely, drug may produce significant CV effects. If they occur, stop the drug.
• Compatibility, effectiveness, and safety of levalbuterol when mixed with other drugs in a nebulizer haven't been established.
Patient teaching
• Warn patient to stop taking the drug and notify prescriber if drug worsens breathing.
• Tell patient to call prescriber immediately if drug becomes less effective, if signs and symptoms worsen, or if drug is needed more often than usual.
• Urge patient not to increase the dose or frequency without consulting prescriber.
• Tell patient to prime the inhaler before first use or if it has not been used for more than 3 days. To prime inhaler, release 4 test sprays into the air away from the face.
• Tell patient to breathe as calmly, deeply, and evenly as possible until no more mist is formed in the nebulizer reservoir (5 to 15 minutes).

- Teach patient to correctly use and clean nebulizer unit.
- Tell patient that the drug's effects may last up to 8 hours.
- Urge patient to use other inhalations and anti-asthma drugs only as directed while taking this drug.
- Tell woman to notify prescriber if she becomes pregnant or intends to breast-feed.
- Tell patient to keep unopened vials in foil pouch. Once the foil pouch is opened, use vials within 2 weeks. Inform patient that vials removed from the pouch should be protected from light and heat and used within 1 week.

☑ Evaluation

- Patient's respiration improves.
- Patient doesn't experience injury from adverse reactions caused by drug.
- Patient and family state understanding of drug therapy.

levetiracetam
(lee-veh-tih-RACE-ah-tam)
Keppra

Pharmacologic class: pyrrolidine derivative
Therapeutic class: anticonvulsant
Pregnancy risk category: C

Indications and dosages

▶ **Adjunctive treatment of partial-onset seizures in epilepsy.** *Adults and adolescents age 16 and older:* Initially, 500 mg P.O. or I.V. b.i.d. Increase dosage by 500 mg b.i.d., if needed, for seizure control at 2-week intervals to maximum, 1,500 mg b.i.d.
Children ages 4 to 16: Give 10 mg/kg P.O. b.i.d. Increase dosage by 10 mg/kg b.i.d. at 2-week intervals to recommended dose of 30 mg/kg b.i.d. If patient can't tolerate this dose, it may be reduced. Patients who weigh 20 kg or less should use the oral solution.
▪ **NEW INDICATION:** Adjunctive therapy in the treatment of primary generalized tonic-clonic seizures in patients with idiopathic generalized epilepsy. *Adults and adolescents age 16 and older:* Initially 500 mg P.O. b.i.d. Increase dosage by 500 mg b.i.d. every 2 weeks to recommended dosage of 1,500 mg b.i.d.

Children ages 6 to 16: Initially, 10 mg/kg P.O. b.i.d. Increase dosage by 10 mg/kg b.i.d. at 2-week intervals to recommended dosage of 30 mg/kg b.i.d. For children weighing more than 20 kg (44 lb) use either tablets or oral solution. For children who weigh 20 kg (44 lb) or less, use the oral solution.
▶ **Adjunctive treatment of myoclonic seizures in juvenile myoclonic epilepsy.**
Adults and adolescents age 12 and older: Initially, 500 mg P.O. b.i.d. Increase by 1,000 mg/day every 2 weeks to 3,000 mg daily.
▩ **Adjust-a-dose:** For adults with renal impairment, if creatinine clearance is greater than 80 ml/minute, give 500 to 1,500 mg every 12 hours; if clearance is 50 to 80 ml/minute, give 500 to 1,000 mg every 12 hours; if clearance is 30 to 50 ml/minute, give 250 to 750 mg every 12 hours; if clearance is less than 30 ml/minute, give 250 to 500 mg every 12 hours. For dialysis patients, give 500 to 1,000 mg every 24 hours. Give one dose of 250 to 500 mg after dialysis.

▼ I.V. administration

- Dilute drug before giving it.
- Dilute 500-mg, 1,000-mg, or 1,500-mg dose in 100 ml normal saline, D_5W, or lactated Ringer's injection, and infuse over 15 minutes.
- Drug is compatible with diazepam, lorazepam, and valproate sodium for 24 hours at a controlled room temperature.
⊗ **Incompatibilities**
None reported.

Contraindications and cautions

- Contraindicated in patients hypersensitive to the drug or any of its components.
- Use cautiously in immunocompromised patients and in those with poor renal function.
⚘ **Lifespan:** In breast-feeding women, use cautiously; it isn't known if the drug appears in breast milk. In children younger than age 4, drug isn't indicated. I.V. form should not be used for children. In elderly patients, use cautiously because of their greater risk of falls.

Adverse reactions

CNS: amnesia, anxiety, *asthenia*, ataxia, depression, dizziness, emotional lability, *headache,* hostility, nervousness, paresthesia, *somnolence,* vertigo.
EENT: diplopia, pharyngitis, rhinitis, sinusitis.
GI: anorexia.

Reactions may be *common,* uncommon, ***life-threatening***, or COMMON AND LIFE-THREATENING.

Hematologic: *leukopenia, neutropenia.*
Musculoskeletal: pain.
Respiratory: cough.
Other: infection.

Interactions

Drug-drug. *Antihistamines, benzodiazepines, opioids, tricyclic antidepressants, other drugs that cause drowsiness:* May lead to severe sedation. Avoid use together.
Carbamazepine, clozapine, and other drugs known to cause leukopenia or neutropenia: May increase the risk of infection. Monitor patient closely; monitor hematologic studies.
Drug-lifestyle. *Alcohol use:* Increases risk of severe sedation. Discourage use together.

Effects on lab test results

• May decrease WBC and neutrophil counts.

Pharmacokinetics

Absorption: Rapid. Level peaks in about 1 hour. When given with food, peak level is delayed by about 1½ hours and level will be slightly lower. Level reaches steady-state in about 2 days.
Distribution: Minimally protein-bound.
Metabolism: No active metabolites.
Excretion: About 66% of drug is unchanged by glomerular filtration and tubular reabsorption.
Half-life: About 7 hours in patients with normal renal function.

Route	Onset	Peak	Duration
P.O., I.V.	1 hr	1 hr	12 hr

Action

Chemical effect: May inhibit kindling in hippocampus, preventing simultaneous neuronal firing that leads to seizures.
Therapeutic effect: Prevents seizures.

Available forms

Injection: 100 mg/ml in 5-ml single-use vials
Oral solution: 100 mg/ml
Tablets: 250 mg, 500 mg, 750 mg, 1,000 mg

NURSING PROCESS

Assessment
• Obtain history of patient's underlying condition before starting therapy, and reassess regularly to monitor drug effectiveness.

• Assess renal function before starting therapy.
• Monitor patient closely for dizziness, which may lead to falls.
• Assess patient's and family's knowledge of drug therapy.

Nursing diagnoses
• Risk for trauma related to seizures
• Risk for infection related to drug-induced leukopenia and neutropenia
• Deficient knowledge related to drug therapy

Planning and implementation
• Drug can be taken with or without food.
• Use drug only with other anticonvulsants. It isn't recommended for monotherapy.
• Taper drug to reduce the risk of seizures.
ALERT: Don't confuse Keppra with Kaletra.
Patient teaching
• Tell patient to use a calibrated device for measuring a dose of oral solution; a household spoon is inadequate.
• Warn patient that drug may cause dizziness and somnolence and to use extra care when rising to a sitting or standing position to avoid becoming dizzy or falling; also to avoid driving, bike riding or other activities that may be hazardous until drugs effects are known.
• Advise patient to call prescriber, but not to abruptly stop taking drug, if an adverse reaction occurs.
• Tell patient to take drug with other prescribed seizure drugs.
• Inform patient that drug can be taken with or without food.

Evaluation
• Patient is free from seizures.
• Patient doesn't develop infection.
• Patient and family state understanding of drug therapy.

✳ New Drug

levocetirizine dihydrochloride
(LEH-voh-see-TEER-ah-zeen)
Xyzal

Pharmacologic class: H_1-receptor antagonist
Therapeutic class: antihistamine
Pregnancy risk category: B

Indications and dosages

▶ **Seasonal and perennial allergic rhinitis.**
Adults and children ages 12 and older: 5 mg
P.O. once daily in the evening.
Children ages 6 to 11: Give 2.5 mg P.O. once
daily in the evening.

▶ **Uncomplicated skin manifestations of
chronic idiopathic urticaria.** *Adults and children ages 12 and older:* 5 mg P.O. once daily in
the evening.
Children ages 6 to 11 years: 2.5 mg P.O. once
daily in the evening.

Adjust-a-dose: For adults and children ages
12 and older with creatinine clearance 50 to
80 ml/minute, give 2.5 mg P.O. once daily; creatinine clearance 30 to 50 ml/minute, 2.5 mg P.O.
every other day; and creatinine clearance 10 to
30 ml/minute, 2.5 mg P.O. twice weekly (once
every 3 to 4 days). Avoid use in patients with
end-stage renal disease or those undergoing hemodialysis. No adjustment is needed for patients with only hepatic impairment. Avoid use
in children ages 6 to 11 with impaired renal
function.

Contraindications and cautions

• Contraindicated in patients hypersensitive to
drug or to cetirizine.
• Contraindicated in patients with creatinine
clearance less than 10 ml/minute or those undergoing hemodialysis.
• Contraindicated in patients ages 6 to 11 with
impaired renal function.

Lifespan: In pregnant women, use drug only
if clearly needed. In breast-feeding women,
drug isn't recommended because it's likely to be
found in breast milk.

In children younger than age 6, safety and effectiveness haven't been established. In children, drug levels may be increased and clearance may be slower than in adults. In elderly
patients, since renal function is usually reduced,
adjust dosage if appropriate and monitor patient
for side effects.

Adverse reactions

CNS: fatigue, somnolence, pyrexia.
EENT: dry mouth, epistaxis (ages 6 to 12
years), nasopharyngitis, pharyngitis.
Respiratory: cough.

Interactions

Drug-drug. *CNS depressants:* May have additive effects when taken with this drug. Avoid using together.
Ritonavir: May increase the serum concentration and decrease the half-life of levocetirizine.
Use together cautiously.
Theophylline: May decrease the clearance of levocetirizine. Use together cautiously.
Drug-lifestyle. *Alcohol use:* May have additive
effects while taking drug. Avoid use together.

Effects on lab test results

None reported.

Pharmacokinetics

Absorption: Rapid and extensive absorption.
Distribution: 91% to 92% bound by plasma
proteins.
Metabolism: Less than 14% of the dose. Meta-
bolic pathways include CYP3A4.
Excretion: 85% in urine and 13% in feces.
Half-life: 8 hours.

Route	Onset	Peak	Duration
P.O.	Unknown	1 hr	24 hr

Action

Chemical effect: Effects mediated through H_1
receptor inhibition.
Therapeutic effect: Relieves symptoms of seasonal and year-round allergies and treats hives.

Available forms

Tablets: 5 mg, scored

NURSING PROCESS

Assessment
• Assess renal function before and during use.
• Monitor patient for adverse reactions.

Nursing diagnoses
• Risk for injury related to sedation
• Impaired oral mucous membrane related to
dry mouth

Planning and implementation
• Overdose may cause drowsiness in adults. In
children, overdose initially causes agitation and
restlessness, followed by drowsiness. No specific antidote is available. Symptomatic and supportive treatment is recommended.

Reactions may be *common,* uncommon, *life-threatening*, or COMMON AND LIFE-THREATENING.

- Drug isn't effectively removed by dialysis.
- Increase fluid intake or humidify air to prevent dry mucous membranes.

Patient teaching

- Warn patients not to perform hazardous tasks or those requiring alertness and coordination until CNS effects are known.
- Advise patient to avoid use of alcohol and other CNS depressants while taking this drug.
- Tell patient to avoid hazardous activities or those that require mental alertness until he knows how his body responds.
- Inform woman that this drug shouldn't be used if she's pregnant or breast-feeding.
- Tell patient if a dose is missed, to take the dose as soon as possible, but if it's almost time for the next dose or if he gets drowsy from the drug, to skip the missed dose and take the next dose on schedule; he shouldn't double the dose.
- Advise patient to use warm water rinses, ice chips, or sugarless gum or candy to relieve dry mouth.
- Advise patient to avoid use of mouthwashes that may worsen dry mouth.

☑ **Evaluation**

- Patient sustains no injury from sedation.
- Patient maintains normal mucous membranes.
- Patient and family state understanding of drug.

levodopa

(lee-voh-DOH-puh)
Larodopa

Pharmacologic class: precursor of dopamine
Therapeutic class: antiparkinsonian
Pregnancy risk category: C

Indications and dosages

▶ **Idiopathic parkinsonism, postencephalitic parkinsonism, and symptomatic parkinsonism after carbon monoxide or manganese intoxication or with cerebral arteriosclerosis.**
Adults and children older than age 12: Initially, 0.5 to 1 g P.O. daily divided into two or more doses with food; increase by no more than 0.75 g daily every 3 to 7 days until daily dosage of 3 to 6 g is reached. Maximum, 8 g daily. Adjust dosage carefully to patient requirements,

tolerance, and response. Closely supervise higher dosages.

Contraindications and cautions

- Contraindicated in patients hypersensitive to the drug or any of its components, in those who have taken an MAO inhibitor within 14 days, and in those with acute angle-closure glaucoma, melanoma, or undiagnosed skin lesions.
- Use cautiously in patients with severe CV, renal, hepatic, or pulmonary disorders; peptic ulcer; psychiatric illness; MI with residual arrhythmias; bronchial asthma; emphysema; or endocrine disease.

⚱ **Lifespan:** In pregnant women, use cautiously; safety hasn't been established. In breast-feeding women, drug is contraindicated. In children age 12 and younger, safety and effectiveness haven't been established.

Adverse reactions

CNS: *abnormal movements (choreiform, dyskinetic, dystonic), aggressive behavior, anxiety, ataxia, bradykinetic episodes, delirium, dementia, disturbing dreams, euphoria, fatigue, hallucinations, involuntary grimacing and head movements, malaise, memory loss, mood changes, muscle twitching, myoclonic body jerks, nervousness, psychiatric disturbance,* **seizures,** *severe depression,* **suicidal tendencies,** *tremor.*
CV: **cardiac irregularities,** flushing, hypertension, *orthostatic hypotension,* phlebitis.
EENT: activation of latent Horner syndrome, *blepharospasm,* blurred vision, diplopia, mydriasis or miosis, nasal discharge, oculogyric crises, widening of palpebral fissures.
GI: *anorexia,* bitter taste, constipation, diarrhea, dry mouth, epigastric pain, excessive salivation, flatulence, *nausea, vomiting.*
GU: darkened urine, incontinence, priapism, urinary frequency, urine retention.
Hematologic: **agranulocytosis,** hemolytic anemia, **leukopenia.**
Hepatic: **hepatotoxicity.**
Metabolic: weight loss.
Respiratory: hiccups, hyperventilation.
Other: dark perspiration, excessive and inappropriate sexual behavior.

Interactions

Drug-drug. *Antacids:* May increase levodopa absorption. Give antacids 1 hour after levodopa.

Anticholinergics: May increase gastric deactivation and decrease intestinal absorption of levodopa. Avoid use together.

Benzodiazepines: May decrease levodopa's therapeutic value. Monitor patient closely.

Furazolidone, procarbazine: May increase risk of severe hypertension. Avoid use together.

Inhaled halogen anesthetics, sympathomimetics: May increase risk of arrhythmias. Monitor ECG and vital signs closely.

MAO inhibitors (phenelzine, tranylcypromine): May cause a hypertensive reaction. Don't use together.

Metoclopramide: May accelerate gastric emptying of levodopa. Give metoclopramide 1 hour after levodopa.

Papaverine, phenothiazines and other antipsychotics, phenytoin, rauwolfia alkaloids: May decrease levodopa effect. Use together cautiously.

Pyridoxine (vitamin B_6): May decrease the effectiveness of levodopa. Avoid use together. (Pyridoxine has little to no effect on the combination drug levodopa and carbidopa.)

Tricyclic antidepressants: May delay absorption and decrease bioavailability of levodopa. Hypertensive episodes have occurred. Monitor patient closely.

Drug-herb. *Kava:* May interfere with drug and with natural dopamine, worsening symptoms of Parkinson disease. Discourage use together.

Rauwolfia: May decrease effectiveness of levodopa. Discourage use together.

Drug-food. *Foods high in protein:* May decrease levodopa absorption. Don't give with high-protein foods.

Drug-lifestyle. *Cocaine:* May increase risk of arrhythmias. Inform patient of this interaction.

Effects on lab test results

• May increase BUN, ALT, AST, alkaline phosphatase, LDH, bilirubin, and uric acid levels. May decrease hemoglobin level and hematocrit.
• May decrease WBC and granulocyte counts.
• May falsely increase urine catecholamine level. May falsely decrease urine vanillylmandelic acid level. May cause false-positive Coombs test or tests for urine glucose with reagents that use copper sulfate. May cause false-negative results with tests that use glucose enzymatic methods. May cause false-positive or false-negative tests for urine ketones and urine phenylketonuria.

Pharmacokinetics

Absorption: Rapid, by active amino acid transport system, with 30% to 50% reaching general circulation.

Distribution: Wide to most body tissues but not CNS, which receives less than 1% of dose because of extensive metabolism in periphery.

Metabolism: 95% of levodopa is converted to dopamine.

Excretion: Mainly in urine. *Half-life:* 1 to 3 hours.

Route	Onset	Peak	Duration
P.O.	Unknown but varies greatly	1–3 hr	About 5 hr

Action

Chemical effect: May be decarboxylated to dopamine, countering dopamine depletion in extrapyramidal centers.

Therapeutic effect: Improves voluntary movement.

Available forms

Capsules: 100 mg, 250 mg, 500 mg
Tablets: 100 mg, 250 mg, 500 mg

NURSING PROCESS

Assessment

• Assess patient's condition before starting therapy and regularly thereafter to monitor drug effectiveness.
• Observe and monitor vital signs, especially during dosage adjustments.
• Test patient receiving long-term therapy regularly for diabetes and acromegaly; periodically monitor kidney, liver, and hematopoietic function.
• Assess mental status before initiation of treatment and periodically thereafter.
• Be alert for adverse reactions and drug interactions.
• Assess patient's and family's knowledge of drug therapy.

Nursing diagnoses

• Impaired physical mobility related to presence of parkinsonism
• Disturbed thought processes related to drug-induced adverse reactions
• Deficient knowledge related to drug therapy

Planning and implementation

• To minimize GI upset, give drug with food but not a high-protein meal, which can impair absorption and reduce effectiveness.

• In a patient undergoing surgery, continue drug as long as oral intake is permitted, usually until 6 to 24 hours before surgery. Resume drug as soon as patient can take oral drug.

• Protect drug from heat, light, and moisture. If preparation darkens, discard because it has lost potency.

🛈 **ALERT:** Muscle twitching and eyelid twitching may be early signs of drug overdose. Report signs immediately.

• Reestablish effectiveness of lower dose by not giving the drug for a period of time (called a drug holiday). Because the drug holiday may cause symptoms that resemble neuroleptic malignant syndrome, observe patient when drug is abruptly stopped or the dose is abruptly lowered.

Patient teaching

• Advise patient to take drug with food, but not with high-protein meals. If patient has trouble swallowing pills, tell him or family member to crush tablets and mix with applesauce or baby food.

• Teach patient and family that behavioral or thought changes may occur and to report symptoms promptly for evaluation.

• Warn patient and family not to increase dosage without prescriber's orders.

• Warn patient about dizziness and light-headedness, especially at start of therapy. Tell patient to change positions slowly and dangle legs before getting out of bed. Elastic stockings may help control this reaction.

• Advise patient and family that multivitamin preparations, fortified cereals, and certain OTC drugs may contain pyridoxine (vitamin B_6), which can block effects of levodopa.

• Warn patient about risk of arrhythmias if he uses cocaine while taking drug.

✓ Evaluation

• Patient has improved physical mobility.
• Patient maintains normal thought process.
• Patient and family state understanding of drug therapy.

levodopa and carbidopa
(lee-vuh-DOH-puh and kar-bih-DOH-puh)
Parcopa, Sinemet, Sinemet CR

Pharmacologic class: dopamine precursor and decarboxylase inhibitor combination
Therapeutic class: antiparkinsonian
Pregnancy risk category: C

Indications and dosages

▶ **Idiopathic Parkinson disease, postencephalitic parkinsonism, and symptomatic parkinsonism resulting from carbon monoxide or manganese intoxication.** *Adults:* 1 tablet of 100 mg levodopa and 25 mg carbidopa or 1 tablet of 100 mg levodopa and 10 mg carbidopa P.O. t.i.d. followed by increase of 1 tablet daily or every other day if needed; maximum daily, 8 tablets. Substitute 250 mg levodopa and 25 mg carbidopa or 100 mg levodopa and 10 mg carbidopa tablets as required. Determine optimum daily dosage by carefully adjusting dosage for each patient. Patients taking conventional tablets may receive extended-release tablets; dosage is calculated on current levodopa intake. Initially, give extended-release tablets equal to 10% more levodopa per day, increase as needed and tolerated to 30% more levodopa per day. Give in divided doses at intervals of 4 to 8 hours.

Contraindications and cautions

• Contraindicated in patients hypersensitive to drugs or any of its components; in patients with acute angle-closure glaucoma, melanoma, or undiagnosed skin lesions; and within 14 days of MAO inhibitor therapy.

• Use cautiously in patients with severe CV, renal, hepatic, endocrine, or pulmonary disorders; history of peptic ulcer; psychiatric illness; MI with residual arrhythmias; bronchial asthma; emphysema; or well-controlled, chronic, open-angle glaucoma.

☀ **Lifespan:** In pregnant women, use cautiously. In breast-feeding women, drug combination is contraindicated. In children, safety and effectiveness haven't been established.

Adverse reactions

CNS: *abnormal movements (choreiform, dyskinetic, dystonic),* anxiety, *ataxia,* bradykinetic

L

episodes, delirium, dementia, disturbing dreams, euphoria, fatigue, hallucinations, *head movements, involuntary grimacing,* malaise, memory loss, muscle twitching, *myoclonic body jerks,* nervousness, psychiatric disturbances, *severe depression, suicidal tendencies,* tremors.
CV: *cardiac irregularities,* flushing, hypertension.
EENT: activation of latent Horner syndrome, *blepharospasm,* blurred vision, diplopia, excessive salivation, mydriasis or miosis, nasal discharge, oculogyric crises, widening of palpebral fissures.
GI: anorexia, bitter taste, dry mouth, nausea, vomiting, and weight loss at start of therapy; constipation; diarrhea; epigastric pain; flatulence.
GU: darkened urine, priapism, urinary frequency, urinary incontinence, urine retention.
Hematologic: hemolytic anemia.
Hepatic: *hepatotoxicity.*
Respiratory: hiccups, hyperventilation.
Skin: dark perspiration, phlebitis.
Other: excessive and inappropriate sexual behavior.

Interactions

Drug-drug. *Antacids:* May increase absorption of levodopa components. Monitor patient closely.
Antihypertensives: May have additive hypotensive effects. Use together cautiously; monitor blood pressure.
Iron salts: May decrease bioavailability of levodopa and carbidopa. Give iron 1 hour before or 2 hours after giving levodopa and carbidopa.
MAO inhibitors: May increase risk of severe hypertension. Don't use together.
Papaverine, phenytoin: May antagonize antiparkinsonian. Avoid use together.
Phenothiazines, other antipsychotics: May antagonize antiparkinsonian. Use together cautiously; monitor for decreased effect.
Drug-herb. *Kava:* May interfere with action of levodopa and natural dopamine, worsening Parkinson symptoms. Discourage use together.
Octacosanol: May worsen dyskinesia. Discourage use together.
Drug-food. *Foods high in protein:* May decrease absorption of levodopa. Warn against taking drug with high-protein foods.

Effects on lab test results

• May decrease hemoglobin level and hematocrit.
• May decrease platelet, granulocyte, and WBC counts.
• May falsely increase levels of uric acid, urine ketones, urine catecholamines, and urine vanillylmandelic acid, depending on reagent and test method used.

Pharmacokinetics

Absorption: 40% to 70%.
Distribution: Wide to most body tissues, except CNS.
Metabolism: For carbidopa, not extensive. It inhibits levodopa, increasing its own absorption.
Excretion: 30% unchanged in urine within 24 hours. When given with carbidopa, amount of levodopa unchanged in urine is increased by about 6%. *Half-life:* 1 to 2 hours.

Route	Onset	Peak	Duration
P.O.			
Regular-release	Unknown	40 min	Unknown
Extended-release	Unknown	2½ hr	Unknown

Action

Chemical effect: Unknown for levodopa. May be decarboxylated to dopamine, countering depletion of striatal dopamine in extrapyramidal centers. Carbidopa inhibits peripheral decarboxylation of levodopa without affecting levodopa's metabolism within CNS, making more levodopa available to be decarboxylated to dopamine in brain.
Therapeutic effect: Improves voluntary movement.

Available forms

Tablets: carbidopa 10 mg with levodopa 100 mg (Sinemet 10-100), carbidopa 25 mg with levodopa 100 mg (Sinemet 25-100), carbidopa 25 mg with levodopa 250 mg (Sinemet 25-250)
Tablets (extended-release): carbidopa 25 mg with levodopa 100 mg, carbidopa 50 mg with levodopa 200 mg (Sinemet CR)
Tablets (orally-disintegrating): carbidopa 10 mg with levodopa 100 mg, carbidopa 25 mg with levodopa 100 mg, carbidopa 25 mg with levodopa 250 mg

---

Reactions may be *common*, uncommon, *life-threatening*, or COMMON AND LIFE-THREATENING.

NURSING PROCESS

◈ Assessment
• Assess patient's underlying condition before therapy and regularly thereafter. Therapeutic response usually follows each dose, disappears within 5 hours, and may vary considerably.
• Be alert for adverse reactions and drug interactions.
• ⊛ ALERT: Immediately report muscle twitching and blepharospasm, which may be early signs of drug overdose.
• Test patients receiving long-term therapy regularly for diabetes and acromegaly, and perform periodic tests of liver, renal, and hematopoietic function.
• Assess patient's and family's knowledge of drug therapy.

⊞ Nursing diagnoses
• Impaired physical mobility related to underlying parkinsonian syndrome
• Disturbed thought processes related to drug-induced CNS adverse reactions
• Deficient knowledge related to drug therapy

▷ Planning and implementation
• If patient is being treated with levodopa only, stop that drug at least 8 hours before starting levodopa and carbidopa combination.
• Give drug with food to minimize adverse GI reactions.
• Adjust dosage according to patient's response and tolerance.
• If vital signs or mental condition change significantly, don't give drug. Notify the prescriber, and then lower the dose or stop giving the drug.
• Treat patient with open-angle glaucoma with caution. Monitor patient closely. Watch for change in intraocular pressure and arrange for periodic eye exams.
Patient teaching
• Caution patient and family not to increase dosage without consulting the prescriber.
• Warn patient of dizziness and orthostatic hypotension, especially at start of therapy. Tell patient to change positions slowly and to dangle legs before getting out of bed. Elastic stockings may control this adverse reaction.
• Teach patient and family that behavioral or thought changes may occur and to report symptoms promptly for evaluation.

• Instruct patient to report adverse reactions and therapeutic effects.
• Inform patient that pyridoxine (vitamin B₆) doesn't reverse beneficial effects of levodopa and carbidopa. Multivitamins can be taken without decreased drug effectiveness.

☑ Evaluation
• Patient exhibits improved mobility with reduction of muscular rigidity and tremor.
• Patient remains mentally alert.
• Patient and family state understanding of drug therapy.

levodopa, carbidopa, and entacapone
(lee-vuh-DOH-puh, kar-bih-DOH-puh, and en-TAH-kah-pohn)
Stalevo 50, Stalevo 100, Stalevo 150

Pharmacologic class: dopamine precursor, decarboxylase inhibitor, and catechol-*O*-methyltransferase (COMT) inhibitor
Therapeutic class: antiparkinsonian
Pregnancy risk category: C

Indications and dosages
▷ **Idiopathic parkinsonism.** *Adults:* Individualize and carefully adjust the optimum daily dosage according to response. For maintenance therapy, reduce the total daily dosage by either decreasing the strength of this drug or by decreasing the frequency by extending the time between doses. When more levodopa is needed, give the next higher strength of this drug or increase the frequency to maximum, eight doses daily without exceeding the maximum daily dosage.

Contraindications and cautions
• Contraindicated in patients hypersensitive to drug or any of its components and in patients with angle-closure glaucoma, suspicious undiagnosed skin lesions, or a history of melanoma. Also contraindicated within 14 days of MAO inhibitor therapy. If the intraocular pressure is well controlled, patients with chronic open-angle glaucoma may use drug.
• Use cautiously in patients with liver, renal, or endocrine disease or biliary obstruction. Also

use cautiously in patients with past or current psychosis, severe CV or pulmonary disease, bronchial asthma, or history of MI with residual arrhythmias.

⚖ **Lifespan:** In pregnant women, use only if benefits outweigh risks to the fetus. In breast-feeding women, use cautiously. In children, safety and effectiveness haven't been established.

Adverse reactions

CNS: agitation, anxiety, asthenia, dizziness, *dyskinesia*, fatigue, hallucinations, *hyperkinesia*, hypokinesia, **neuroleptic malignant syndrome**, somnolence, syncope.
CV: chest pain, hypotension.
GI: abdominal pain, constipation, *diarrhea*, dry mouth, dyspepsia, flatulence, gastritis, gastrointestinal disorder, *nausea*, taste disorder, vomiting.
GU: *nephrotoxicity*, urine discoloration.
Hematologic: *agranulocytosis*, anemia, *leukopenia*, *thrombocytopenia*.
Musculoskeletal: back pain.
Respiratory: dyspnea.
Skin: sweating.
Other: bacterial infection.

Interactions

Drug-drug. *Antihypertensives:* May cause postural hypotension. Adjust antihypertensive dosage, if needed.
Dopamine D$_2$-receptor antagonists (such as butyrophenones, isoniazid, metoclopramide, phenothiazines, and risperidone): May reduce levodopa effects. Avoid use together.
Drugs metabolized by COMT, such as alpha-methyldopa, apomorphine, bitolterol, dobutamine, dopamine, epinephrine, isoetharine, isoproterenol, and norepinephrine: May increase heart rate, arrhythmias, and excessive changes in blood pressure. Use together cautiously.
Drugs that interfere with biliary excretion, glucuronidation, and intestinal beta-glucuronidase, including cholestyramine, probenecid, and some antibiotics (ampicillin, chloramphenicol, erythromycin, rifampicin): May interfere with entacapone excretion. Use together cautiously.
Hydantoin, papaverine: May reduce levodopa effects. Avoid use together.
Iron salts: May reduce the bioavailability of drug. Adjust dosage if needed.
Metoclopramide: May increase bioavailability of carbidopa and levodopa by increasing gastric emptying. Adjust dosage if needed.

Nonselective MAO inhibitors: May cause a hypertensive reaction. Don't use within 14 days of each other.
Selegiline: May cause severe hypotension. Avoid use together.
Tricyclic antidepressants: May cause hypertension and dyskinesia. Use together cautiously.
Drug-food. *Foods high in protein, such as legumes, liquid protein shakes, and red meat:* May delay and reduce the absorption of levodopa. Give drug on an empty stomach.

Effects on lab test results

• May increase growth hormone level. May decrease prolactin level. May increase or decrease BUN and bilirubin levels.
• May increase liver function test values.
• May cause a false-positive Coombs test. May cause a false-positive reaction for urinary ketone bodies when using a test tape.

Pharmacokinetics

Absorption: Varies. Carbidopa level peaks within 2½ to 3½ hours. Levodopa level peaks in 1 to 1½ hours. Entacapone level peaks within 1½ hours.
Distribution: Levodopa and carbidopa are minimally protein-bound. Entacapone is 98% bound to albumin.
Metabolism: Carbidopa is metabolized to two main metabolites. Levodopa is extensively metabolized to various metabolites. Entacapone is almost completely metabolized.
Excretion: Carbidopa, primarily in urine unchanged; entacapone, 10% in urine, 90% in feces; levodopa, unknown. *Half-life:* 1½ to 2 hours for carbidopa, 1 to 5 hours for levodopa, and 1 to 4 hours for entacapone.

Route	Onset	Peak	Duration
P.O.	< 1 hr	1–1½ hr	Unknown

Action

Chemical effect: Levodopa, a dopamine precursor, converts to dopamine in the brain. Carbidopa inhibits the decarboxylation of peripheral levodopa. When given with levodopa, carbidopa permits more intact levodopa to be transported into the brain. Entacapone is a selective and reversible inhibitor of COMT.
Therapeutic effect: Decreases symptoms of Parkinson disease.

Available forms

Tablets: 12.5 mg carbidopa, 50 mg levodopa, and 200 mg entacapone (Stalevo 50); 25 mg carbidopa, 100 mg levodopa, and 200 mg entacapone (Stalevo 100); 37.5 mg carbidopa, 150 mg levodopa, and 200 mg entacapone (Stalevo 150)

NURSING PROCESS

⏱ Assessment
• Periodically evaluate hepatic, hematopoietic, CV, and renal function.
• Monitor patient for mental disturbances such as hallucinations or depression with suicidal tendencies.
• Be alert for adverse reactions and interactions.
• Assess patient's and family's knowledge of drug therapy.

⊕ Nursing diagnoses
• Impaired physical mobility related to underlying parkinsonism
• Risk for injury related to drug-induced adverse reactions
• Deficient knowledge related to drug therapy

▷ Planning and implementation
• Patients taking 200-mg entacapone tablet with each dose of standard-release levodopa and carbidopa can be switched to the corresponding strength of this drug containing the same amount of levodopa and carbidopa.
• Patients who experience signs and symptoms of end-of-dose "wearing off" on standard-release levodopa and carbidopa and have a history of moderate or severe dyskinesia, or take more than 600 mg of levodopa per day are likely to require a reduction in daily levodopa dose when entacapone is added. Adjust dosage with levodopa and carbidopa (1:4 ratio) and entacapone, then transfer to a corresponding dose of this drug once the patient is stabilized.
• Don't cut or break tablets.
• If dyskinesia occurs, reduce dosage.
⚠ ALERT: If abruptly reducing or stopping drug, especially in a patient also taking an antipsychotic, observe him carefully for a syndrome resembling neuroleptic malignant syndrome: elevated temperature, muscle rigidity, involuntary movements, altered consciousness, confusion, tachycardia, tachypnea, sweating, hypertension or hypotension, leukocytosis, myoglobinuria, and increased myoglobin level.

⚠ ALERT: Check for overdose by monitoring respiratory, renal, and CV functions. Use supportive measures along with repeated doses of charcoal over time. Also give I.V. fluids and ensure adequate airway.

Patient teaching
• Advise patient to take drug on an empty stomach preferably, or at least not with high-protein meals or drinks.
• Tell patient to take drug exactly as prescribed.
• Tell patient not to cut or break tablets.
• Warn patient of adverse reactions, such as hallucinations, diarrhea, nausea, and discolored urine, and instruct him to notify prescriber if they occur.
• Instruct patient to notify prescriber of any and all drugs taken to prevent any drug interactions.

☑ Evaluation
• Patient has improved physical mobility.
• Patient doesn't suffer any injury from adverse reactions.
• Patient and family state understanding of drug therapy.

levofloxacin
(lee-voh-FLOCKS-uh-sihn)
Levaquin♦

Pharmacologic class: fluorinated carboxyquinolone
Therapeutic class: broad-spectrum antibiotic
Pregnancy risk category: C

Indications and dosages

▶ **Acute bacterial sinusitis caused by susceptible strains of *Streptococcus pneumoniae, Moraxella catarrhalis,* or *Haemophilus influenzae.*** *Adults:* 500 mg P.O. or I.V. daily for 10 to 14 days; or, 750 mg P.O. or I.V. daily for 5 days.
▶ **Acute bacterial exacerbation of chronic bronchitis caused by *Staphylococcus aureus, S. pneumoniae, M. catarrhalis,* or *H. influenzae* or *parainfluenzae.*** *Adults:* 500 mg P.O. or I.V. daily for 7 days.
▶ **Community-acquired pneumonia caused by *S. pneumoniae* resistant to two or more of the following antibiotics: penicillin, second-generation cephalosporins, macrolides, tetracyclines, trimethoprim, and sulfamethoxa-**

zole; or by *S. aureus, M. catarrhalis, H. influenzae, H. parainfluenzae, Klebsiella pneumoniae, Chlamydia pneumoniae, Legionella pneumophila, Mycoplasma pneumoniae,* or *S. pneumoniae. Adults:* 500 mg P.O. or I.V. daily for 7 to 14 days. Or, 750 mg P.O. or I.V. once daily for 5 days (not for multidrug-resistant *S. pneumoniae*).

▪ NEW INDICATION: Complicated UTI caused by *Escherichia coli, K. pneumoniae,* or *Proteus mirabilis* and acute pyelonephritis caused by *E. coli. Adults:* 750 mg P.O. or I.V. for 5 days.

▧ Adjust-a-dose: For patients with renal impairment, if creatinine clearance is 20 to 49 ml/minute, give 750 mg P.O. or I.V. every 48 hours. If creatinine clearance is 10 to 19 ml/minute or patient is on hemodialysis, give 750 mg initially and then 500 mg every 48 hours.

▪ NEW INDICATION: Nosocomial pneumonia caused by methicillin-susceptible *S. aureus, Pseudomonas aeruginosa, Serratia marcescens, E. coli, K. pneumoniae, H. influenzae,* or *S. pneumoniae. Adults:* 750 mg P.O. or I.V. daily for 10 to 14 days.

Use adjunctive therapy as indicated. Where *P. aeruginosa* is documented or presumed, combination therapy with an antipseudomonal beta-lactam is recommended.

▧ Adjust-a-dose: For patients with renal impairment, if creatinine clearance is 20 to 49 ml/minute, give initial dose of 750 mg every 48 hours. If creatinine clearance is 10 to 19 ml/minute, give 750 mg initially and then 500 mg every 48 hours. For patients on hemodialysis or chronic ambulatory peritoneal dialysis, give initial dose of 750 mg and then 500 mg every 48 hours.

▶ Mild to moderate skin and skin-structure infections caused by *S. aureus* or *Streptococcus pyogenes. Adults:* 500 mg P.O. or I.V. daily for 7 to 10 days.

▶ Chronic bacterial prostatitis caused by *E. coli, E. faecalis,* or *Staphylococcus epidermidis. Adults:* 500 mg P.O. or I.V. daily for 28 days.

**▶ Prevention of inhalation anthrax following confirmed or suspected exposure to *Bacillus anthracis. Adults:* 500 mg I.V. or P.O. every 24 hours for 60 days.

▧ Adjust-a-dose: For patients with renal impairment, if creatinine clearance is 20 to 49 ml/minute, give initial dose of 500 mg and then 250 mg once daily; or (if not treating multidrug-resistant *S. pneumoniae*), give 750 mg initially and then 750 mg every 48 hours. If clearance is 10 to 19 ml/minute, initial dose is 500 mg and then 250 mg every 48 hours; or give 750 mg initially and then 500 mg every 48 hours. For patients on hemodialysis or chronic ambulatory peritoneal dialysis, give initial dose of 500 mg and then 250 mg every 48 hours; or give 750 mg initially and then 500 mg every 48 hours.

▶ Complicated skin and skin structure infections caused by methicillin-sensitive *S. aureus, E. faecalis, S. pyogenes, P. mirabilis;* nosocomial pneumonia caused by methicillin-susceptible *S. aureus, P. aeruginosa, Serratia marcescens, E. coli, K. pneumoniae, H. influenzae,* or *S. pneumoniae. Adults:* 750 mg P.O. or I.V. daily for 7 to 14 days.

▧ Adjust-a-dose: For patients with renal impairment, if creatinine clearance is 20 to 49 ml/minute, give 750 mg initially and then 750 mg every 48 hours. If clearance is 10 to 19 ml/minute or patient is on hemodialysis or chronic ambulatory peritoneal dialysis, give 750 mg initially and then 500 mg every 48 hours.

▶ Mild to moderate UTI caused by *Enterococcus faecalis, Enterobacter cloacae, E. coli, K. pneumoniae, Proteus mirabilis,* or *Pseudomonas aeruginosa. Adults:* 250 mg P.O. or I.V. daily for 10 days.

▶ Mild to moderate acute pyelonephritis caused by *E. coli. Adults:* 250 mg P.O. or I.V. daily for 10 days.

▧ Adjust-a-dose: For patients with renal impairment, if creatinine clearance is 10 to 19 ml/minute, give 250 mg initially and then 250 mg every 48 hours.

▶ Mild to moderate uncomplicated UTI caused by *Escherichia coli, K. pneumoniae,* or *Staphylococcus saprophyticus. Adults:* 250 mg P.O. daily for 3 days.

▶ Traveler's diarrhea‡. *Adults:* 500 mg P.O. as a single dose with loperamide hydrochloride.

▶ To prevent traveler's diarrhea‡. *Adults:* 500 mg P.O. daily during period of risk, for up to 3 weeks.

▶ Uncomplicated cervical, urethral, or rectal gonorrhea‡. *Adults and adolescents:* 250 mg P.O. as a single dose.

▶ Disseminated gonococcal infection‡. *Adults and adolescents:* 250 mg I.V. daily and continue for 24 to 48 hours after improvement begins. Switch to 500 mg P.O. daily to complete at least 1 week of therapy.

Reactions may be *common,* uncommon, *life-threatening,* or COMMON AND LIFE-THREATENING.

▶ **Nongonococcal urethritis; urogenital chlamydial infections‡.** *Adults and adolescents:* 500 mg P.O. daily for 7 days.

▶ **Acute pelvic inflammatory disease‡.** *Adults and adolescents:* 500 mg I.V. daily with or without metronidazole 500 mg every 8 hours. Stop parenteral drug 24 hours after improvement; then begin 100 mg P.O. b.i.d. of doxycycline to complete 14 days of therapy. Or give 500 mg P.O. levofloxacin daily for 14 days with or without metronidazole 500 mg b.i.d. for 14 days.

▽ I.V. administration

• Dilute in single-use vials with D_5W or normal saline solution for injection to yield 5 mg/ml.
• Make sure reconstituted solution is clear, slightly yellow, and free of particulates.
• Give only by I.V. infusion over 60 minutes for 500 mg or 90 minutes for 750 mg.
• Diluted solution is stable for 72 hours at room temperature, 14 days when refrigerated in plastic containers, and 6 months when frozen. Thaw at room temperature or in refrigerator.
⊗ Incompatibilities
Mannitol 20%, multivalent cations (such as magnesium), sodium bicarbonate 5%. Don't mix drug with other drugs.

Contraindications and cautions

• Contraindicated in patients hypersensitive to the drug, any of its components, or other fluoroquinolones.
⚞ Lifespan: In pregnant women, use only when benefits outweigh risks to fetus. Breast-feeding women should either stop breast-feeding or use another drug. In children, safety and effectiveness haven't been established. In elderly patients with renal impairment, adjust dosage.

Adverse reactions

CNS: dizziness, *encephalopathy,* headache, insomnia, pain, paresthesia, *seizures.*
CV: abnormal ECG, chest pain, palpitations, vasodilation.
GI: abdominal pain, constipation, diarrhea, dyspepsia, flatulence, nausea, *pseudomembranous colitis,* vomiting.
GU: vaginitis.
Hematologic: eosinophilia, hemolytic anemia, *lymphocytopenia.*
Metabolic: *hypoglycemia.*
Musculoskeletal: back pain, tendon rupture.
Respiratory: allergic pneumonitis.

Skin: *erythema multiforme,* photosensitivity reactions, pruritus, rash, *Stevens-Johnson syndrome.*
Other: *anaphylaxis,* hypersensitivity reactions, *multisystem organ failure.*

Interactions

Drug-drug. *Aluminum hydroxide, aluminum-magnesium hydroxide, calcium carbonate, magnesium hydroxide:* May decrease levofloxacin effects. Give antacid at least 6 hours before or 2 hours after levofloxacin.
Antidiabetics: May alter glucose level. Monitor it closely.
Iron salts: May decrease levofloxacin absorption, reducing anti-infective response. Give at least 2 hours apart.
NSAIDs: May increase CNS stimulation. Monitor patient for seizures.
Sucralfate, zinc-containing products: May interfere with GI absorption of levofloxacin. Give at least 2 hours apart.
Theophylline: May decrease theophylline clearance with some fluoroquinolones. Monitor theophylline levels.
Warfarin: May increase anticoagulant effects. Monitor PT and INR closely.
Drug-lifestyle. *Sun exposure:* May cause photosensitivity reactions. Urge patient to avoid unprotected or prolonged exposure to sunlight.

Effects on lab test results

• May decrease glucose and hemoglobin levels and hematocrit.
• May increase eosinophil count. May decrease WBC and lymphocyte counts.
• May cause false-positive opiate assay results.

Pharmacokinetics

Absorption: Rapid and complete.
Distribution: Wide.
Metabolism: Limited.
Excretion: Mainly unchanged in urine. *Half-life:* About 6 to 8 hours.

Route	Onset	Peak	Duration
P.O.	Unknown	1–2 hr	30–36 hr
I.V.	Immediate	1–1½ hr	30–36 hr

Action

Chemical effect: Inhibits bacterial DNA gyrase and prevents DNA replication, transcription,

repair, and recombination in susceptible bacteria.
Therapeutic effect: Kills susceptible bacteria.

Available forms

Infusion (premixed): 250 mg in 50 ml D_5W, 500 mg in 100 ml D_5W, 750 mg in 150 ml D_5W (5 mg/ml)
Oral solution: 25 mg/ml
Single-use vials: 500 mg, 750 mg (25 mg/ml)
Tablets: 250 mg, 500 mg, 750 mg

NURSING PROCESS

Assessment
• Obtain specimen for culture and sensitivity tests before starting therapy and as needed to detect bacterial resistance. Therapy may begin pending results.
• Obtain history of seizure disorders or other CNS diseases, such as cerebral arteriosclerosis, before starting therapy.
• Monitor glucose level and renal, hepatic, and hematopoietic blood studies.
• Assess patient's and family's knowledge of drug therapy.

Nursing diagnoses
• Risk for infection related to presence of bacteria susceptible to drug
• Risk for deficient fluid volume related to drug-induced adverse GI reactions
• Deficient knowledge related to drug therapy

Planning and implementation
• Give oral drugs with plenty of fluids.
• Oral solution should be taken 1 hour before or 2 hours after eating.
• P.O. and I.V. dosages are interchangeable.
• Oral solution is as effective as tablet form and is flexible, which is helpful for patients with renal impairment.
⑤ ALERT: If *P. aeruginosa* is or is suspected to be the cause, give combination therapy with an antipseudomonal beta-lactam.
• Treat acute hypersensitivity reactions with epinephrine, oxygen, I.V. fluids, antihistamines, corticosteroids, pressor amines, and airway management.
• If patient has symptoms of excessive CNS stimulation (restlessness, tremor, confusion, hallucinations), stop drug and notify prescriber. Take seizure precautions.

• Most antibacterials can cause pseudomembranous colitis. If diarrhea occurs, notify prescriber. If symptoms are severe or unrelieved by appropriate treatment, stop giving the drug.
Patient teaching
• Tell patient to take drug as prescribed, even if symptoms resolve.
• Advise patient to take drug with plenty of fluids and to avoid antacids, sucralfate, and products containing iron or zinc for at least 2 hours before and after each dose.
• Warn patient to avoid hazardous tasks until the drug's CNS effects are known.
• Advise patient to avoid excessive sunlight, use sunblock, and wear protective clothing when outdoors.
• Instruct patient to stop taking the drug and notify prescriber if rash or other signs or symptoms of hypersensitivity develop.
• Tell patient to notify prescriber if he experiences pain or inflammation; tendon rupture can occur with drug.
• Instruct diabetic patient to monitor glucose level and notify prescriber if a hypoglycemic reaction occurs; may need to stop drug.
• Instruct patient to notify prescriber about loose stools or diarrhea.

Evaluation
• Patient is free from infection after drug therapy.
• Patient maintains adequate hydration throughout drug therapy.
• Patient and family state understanding of drug therapy.

levothyroxine sodium (T4, L-thyroxine sodium)
(lee-voh-thigh-ROKS-een SOH-dee-um)
Eltroxin ♦, Levothroid, Levoxyl✎, Synthroid, Thyro-Tabs, Unithroid

Pharmacologic class: thyroid hormone
Therapeutic class: thyroid hormone replacement
Pregnancy risk category: A

Indications and dosages

▶ **Myxedema coma.** *Adults:* 300 to 500 mcg I.V., followed by parenteral maintenance dosage

of 75 to 100 mcg I.V. daily. Switch patient to oral maintenance as soon as possible.

▶ **Thyroid hormone replacement.** *Adults:* Initially, 25 to 50 mcg P.O. daily; increase by 25 mcg P.O. every 4 to 8 weeks until desired response occurs. Maintenance dosage is 75 to 200 mcg P.O. daily.

Children older than age 12: More than 150 mcg or 2 to 3 mcg/kg P.O. daily.

Children ages 6 to 12: Give 100 to 150 mcg or 4 to 5 mcg/kg P.O. daily.

Children ages 1 to 5: Give 75 to 100 mcg or 5 to 6 mcg/kg P.O. daily.

Children ages 6 months to 1 year: Give 50 to 75 mcg or 6 to 8 mcg/kg P.O. daily.

Children younger than age 6 months: Give 25 to 50 mcg or 8 to 10 mcg/kg P.O. daily.

Patients older than age 65: Give 2.5 to 50 mcg P.O. daily; increase by 12.5 to 25 mcg every 6 to 8 weeks, depending on response.

▼ I.V. administration

• Don't confuse mg with mcg dosage (1 mg = 1,000 mcg).

• Initial I.V. dose is about half the previously established oral dose of tablets when used for maintenance of euthyroid state.

• Prepare dose immediately before injection. Dilute powder for injection with 5 ml of normal saline solution for injection or bacteriostatic saline solution injection with benzyl alcohol to 200- or 500-mcg vial; don't use other diluents. Resulting solutions contain 40 or 100 mcg/ml, respectively.

• Inject into vein over 1 to 2 minutes.

• Monitor blood pressure and heart rate closely. High initial dosage is usually tolerated by patients in myxedema coma. Normal levels of T_4 occur within 24 hours, followed by a threefold increase in T_3 in 3 days.

⊗ **Incompatibilities**
Other I.V. solutions.

Contraindications and cautions

• Contraindicated in patients hypersensitive to the drug or any of its components, and in patients with acute MI uncomplicated by hypothyroidism, untreated thyrotoxicosis, or uncorrected adrenal insufficiency.

• Use cautiously in patients with angina pectoris, hypertension, other CV disorders, renal insufficiency, or ischemia. Also use cautiously in

patients with diabetes mellitus, diabetes insipidus, myxedema, or dysphagia.

• Use cautiously in patients with arteriosclerosis. Rapid replacement in these patients may precipitate angina, coronary occlusion, or stroke.

≋ **Lifespan:** In breast-feeding women, use cautiously; it's unknown if the drug appears in breast milk. Children typically need a higher dose than adults. Adults older than age 60 typically need a lower dose than younger adults.

Adverse reactions

CNS: fever, headache, *insomnia, nervousness, tremor.*

CV: angina pectoris, ***arrhythmias, cardiac arrest,*** hypertension, palpitations, tachycardia.

GI: appetite change; choking, gagging, or dysphagia, particularly when not taken with fluids; diarrhea; nausea.

GU: menstrual irregularities.

Metabolic: weight loss.

Musculoskeletal: leg cramps.

Skin: diaphoresis.

Other: heat intolerance.

Interactions

Drug-drug. *Cholestyramine, colestipol:* May impair levothyroxine absorption. Separate doses by 4 to 5 hours.

Insulin, oral antidiabetics: May increase glucose level. Monitor glucose level when starting or changing dosage, and adjust dosage if needed.

I.V. phenytoin: May release free thyroid. Monitor patient for tachycardia.

Oral anticoagulants: May increase PT. Decrease anticoagulants by about one-third when initiating thyroid replacement therapy, monitor PT and INR, and adjust dosage to desired range, if needed.

Sympathomimetics (such as epinephrine): May increase risk of coronary insufficiency. Monitor patient closely.

Effects on lab test results

• May alter results of radioactive iodine uptake studies.

Pharmacokinetics

Absorption: Good.
Distribution: Wide. 99% protein-bound.

Metabolism: Mainly in liver, kidneys, and intestines.
Excretion: 20% to 40% in feces. *Half-life:* 3 to 4 days in hyperthyroidism, 9 to 10 days in hypothyroidism.

Route	Onset	Peak	Duration
P.O. I.V., I.M.	24 hr	Unknown	Unknown

Action

Chemical effect: Not fully defined; stimulates metabolism by accelerating cellular oxidation.
Therapeutic effect: Raises thyroid hormone levels in body.

Available forms

Powder for injection: 200 mcg/vial, 500 mcg/vial
Tablets: 0.025 mg, 0.05 mg, 0.075 mg, 0.088 mg, 0.1 mg, 0.112 mg, 0.125 mg, 0.137 mg, 0.15 mg, 0.175 mg, 0.2 mg, 0.3 mg

NURSING PROCESS

Assessment

• Assess patient's condition before starting therapy and regularly thereafter to monitor drug effectiveness. Monitor TSH monthly until stable, then yearly if asymptomatic.
• Be alert for adverse reactions and drug interactions.
• In patient with coronary artery disease who must receive thyroid hormone, monitor carefully for coronary insufficiency.
• Assess patient for swallowing difficulties before giving the drug. Advise all patients to take tablet with water.
• Assess patient's and family's knowledge of drug therapy.

Nursing diagnoses

• Ineffective health maintenance related to presence of hypothyroidism
• Risk for injury related to drug-induced adverse reactions
• Deficient knowledge related to drug therapy

Planning and implementation

⑤ ALERT: Doses of alternative brands of thyroid replacement drugs may not be equivalent, particularly between levothyroxine sodium (synthetic T_4), liothyronine (synthetic T_3), and thyroid hormone from animals (Armour thyroid, desiccated thyroid).
• Thyroid hormone replacement requirements are about 25% lower in patients older than age 60 than in younger adults.
• I.M. use typically isn't recommended because of variable absorption and difficulty regulating dose.
• Patients with adult hypothyroidism are unusually sensitive to thyroid hormone. Start patient at lowest dose and adjust to higher dose until reaching a euthyroid state based on symptoms and laboratory data.
• When changing from levothyroxine to liothyronine, stop levothyroxine then begin liothyronine at a low dose. Increase liothyronine dosage in small increments after residual effects of levothyroxine disappear. When changing from liothyronine to levothyroxine, to avoid relapse start levothyroxine several days before stopping liothyronine.
• Thyroid hormones alter thyroid non-serum test results. Stop drug 4 weeks before test.
• In patient taking a prescribed anticoagulant with thyroid hormones, lower the dosage of anticoagulant if needed.
⑤ ALERT: Don't confuse levothyroxine sodium with liothyronine sodium, liotrix, or Lamictal.
Patient teaching
• Stress importance of compliance. Tell patient to take thyroid hormones at same time each day, preferably 30 to 60 minutes before breakfast, to maintain constant hormone levels, prevent insomnia, and increase absorption.
• Instruct patient (especially an elderly patient) to immediately notify prescriber about chest pain, palpitations, sweating, nervousness, shortness of breath, or other signs of overdose or aggravated CV disease.
• Advise patient who has achieved stable response not to change brands without physician advice.
• Advise female patient to alert prescriber if she becomes pregnant.
• Tell patient to report unusual bleeding and bruising.

Evaluation

• Patient's thyroid hormone levels are normal.
• Patient doesn't experience any adverse reactions.
• Patient and family state understanding of drug therapy.

Reactions may be *common*, uncommon, *life-threatening*, or COMMON AND LIFE-THREATENING.

HIGH ALERT

lidocaine hydrochloride (lignocaine hydrochloride)

(LIGH-doh-kayn high-droh-KLOR-ighd)
LidoPen Auto-Injector, Xylocaine, Xylocard ◆

Pharmacologic class: amide derivative
Therapeutic class: ventricular antiarrhythmic
Pregnancy risk category: B

Indications and dosages

▶ **Ventricular arrhythmias resulting from MI, cardiac manipulation, or digoxin toxicity.** *Adults:* 50 to 100 mg (1 to 1.5 mg/kg) by I.V. bolus at 25 to 50 mg/minute. Repeat bolus dose every 3 to 5 minutes until arrhythmias subside or adverse reactions develop. Don't exceed 300-mg total bolus during 1-hour period. Simultaneously, start a constant infusion of 20 to 50 mcg/kg/minute (or 1 to 4 mg/minute). If single bolus has been given, smaller bolus dose may be repeated 5 to 10 minutes after start of infusion to maintain therapeutic level. After 24 hours of continuous infusion, decrease rate by half. Or 200 to 300 mg I.M., followed by second I.M. dose 60 to 90 minutes later, if needed. Change to I.V. form as soon as possible. *Children:* 1 mg/kg by I.V. bolus, followed by infusion of 20 to 50 mcg/kg/minute.
⧄ **Adjust-a-dose:** For elderly patients, patients who weigh less than 50 kg (110 lb) and patients with heart failure or hepatic disease, give half the normal adult dose.
▶ **Status epilepticus‡.** *Adults:* 1 mg/kg I.V. bolus; then, if seizures continue, give 0.5 mg/kg 2 minutes after first dose. May use an infusion of 30 mcg/kg/minute.

▼ I.V. administration

• Use drug without preservatives. Read label carefully.
• Injections (additive syringes and single-use vials) containing 40, 100, or 200 mg/ml are for preparing I.V. infusion solutions and must be diluted before use.
• Add 1 g of drug (using 25 ml of 4% or 5 ml of 20% injection) to 1 L of D_5W injection to provide a solution containing 1 mg/ml.
• If patient is fluid restricted, use a more concentrated solution of up to 8 mg/ml.

• Patients receiving infusion must be on a cardiac monitor and must be attended at all times. Use infusion-control device to give infusion precisely. Don't exceed 4 mg/minute because doing so greatly increases the risk of toxicity.
⊗ **Incompatibilities**
Fentanyl citrate (higher pH formulations), methohexital sodium, phenytoin sodium.

Contraindications and cautions

• Contraindicated in patients hypersensitive to amide-type local anesthetics and in those with Adams-Stokes syndrome, Wolff-Parkinson-White syndrome, or severe degrees of SA, AV, or intraventricular block in absence of artificial pacemaker.
• Use cautiously and reduce dosage in patients with complete or second-degree heart block or sinus bradycardia, in those with heart failure or renal or hepatic disease, and in those who weigh less than 50 kg.
☀ **Lifespan:** In pregnant women, use only when benefits outweigh risks to the fetus. In breast-feeding women and in children, safety and effectiveness haven't been established. In elderly patients, use cautiously.

Adverse reactions

CNS: *confusion,* depression, euphoria, lethargy, *light-headedness,* muscle twitching, paresthesia, *restlessness, seizures,* slurred speech, somnolence, *stupor, tremor.*
CV: *bradycardia, cardiac arrest,* hypotension, *new or worsened arrhythmias.*
EENT: *blurred or double vision, tinnitus.*
Respiratory: *respiratory arrest, status asthmaticus.*
Skin: diaphoresis.
Other: *anaphylaxis,* cold sensation, soreness at injection site.

Interactions

Drug-drug. *Atenolol, metoprolol, nadolol, pindolol, propranolol:* May reduce hepatic metabolism of lidocaine, increasing risk of lidocaine toxicity. Give bolus doses of lidocaine at a slower rate, and monitor lidocaine level closely.
Cimetidine: May decrease lidocaine clearance, increasing the risk of lidocaine toxicity. Use a different H_2-antagonist. Monitor lidocaine level closely.

L

Phenytoin, procainamide, propranolol, quinidine: May have additive cardiac depressant effects. Monitor patient.

Succinylcholine: May prolong neuromuscular blockage. Monitor patient for increased effects.

Tocainide: May increase risk of adverse reactions. Avoid use together.

Drug-herb. *Pareira:* May increase neuromuscular blockade. Avoid use together.

Drug-lifestyle. *Smoking:* May increase lidocaine metabolism. Monitor patient closely; discourage patient from smoking.

Effects on lab test results

• May increase CK level.

Pharmacokinetics

Absorption: Nearly complete.
Distribution: Wide, especially to adipose tissue.
Metabolism: Most of drug in liver to two active metabolites.
Excretion: 90% as metabolites; less than 10% in urine unchanged. *Half-life:* 1½ to 2 hours (may be prolonged in patients with heart failure or hepatic disease).

Route	Onset	Peak	Duration
I.V.	Immediate	30–60 min	10–20 min
I.M.	5–15 min	10 min	2 hr

Action

Chemical effect: Decreases depolarization, automaticity, and excitability in ventricles during diastolic phase by direct action on tissues.
Therapeutic effect: Abolishes ventricular arrhythmias.

Available forms

Infusion (premixed): 0.2% (2 mg/ml), 0.4% (4 mg/ml), 0.8% (8 mg/ml)
Injection for direct I.V. use: 1% (10 mg/ml), 2% (20 mg/ml)
Injection for I.M. use: 300 mg/3 ml automatic injection device
Injection for I.V. admixtures: 4% (40 mg/ml), 10% (100 mg/ml), 20% (200 mg/ml)

NURSING PROCESS

⏣ Assessment

• Assess patient's condition before starting therapy and regularly thereafter to monitor drug effectiveness.

⊛ **ALERT:** Patient receiving infusion must be on cardiac monitor and attended to at all times.

• Monitor patient's response, especially ECG, blood pressure, and electrolytes, BUN, and creatinine levels.
• Check for therapeutic level (2 to 5 mcg/ml).
• Be alert for adverse reactions and drug interactions.

⊛ **ALERT:** Monitor patient for toxicity. Seizures may be the first sign. Severe reactions usually are preceded by somnolence, confusion, and paresthesia.

• Assess patient's and family's knowledge of drug therapy.

⊕ Nursing diagnoses

• Decreased cardiac output related to presence of ventricular arrhythmia
• Disturbed thought processes related to adverse CNS reactions
• Deficient knowledge related to drug therapy

⊳ Planning and implementation

⊛ **ALERT:** If using I.M. drug in patient with suspected MI, test isoenzymes before starting therapy because patients receiving I.M. drug show sevenfold increase in CK level. Such an increase originates in skeletal muscle, not cardiac muscle.

⊛ **ALERT:** Give I.M. injections only in deltoid muscle.

• Use only the 10% solution for I.M. injection. Read label carefully.
• If signs of toxicity (such as dizziness) occur, immediately stop giving the drug and notify prescriber. Continued infusion could lead to seizures and coma. Give oxygen by way of nasal cannula. Keep oxygen and cardiopulmonary resuscitation equipment available.
• If arrhythmias worsen or if ECG changes, such as with a widening QRS complex or substantially prolonged PR interval, stop drug and notify prescriber.

Patient teaching
• Explain purpose of drug to patient.
• Tell patient or caregiver to report any adverse reactions.
• Instruct patient to avoid smoking during drug therapy.

☑ Evaluation

• Patient's cardiac output returns to normal with abolishment of ventricular arrhythmia.

Reactions may be *common*, uncommon, *life-threatening*, or COMMON AND LIFE-THREATENING.

- Patient maintains normal thought processes throughout therapy.
- Patient and family state understanding of drug therapy.

linezolid
(lih-NEH-zoe-lid)
Zyvox

Pharmacologic class: oxazolidinone
Therapeutic class: antibiotic
Pregnancy risk category: C

Indications and dosages

▶ **Vancomycin-resistant** *Enterococcus faecium* **infections, including those with bacteremia.** *Adults and children age 12 and older:* 600 mg I.V. or P.O. every 12 hours for 14 to 28 days.
Neonates 7 days or older, infants, and children age 11 and younger: 10 mg/kg I.V. or P.O. every 8 hours for 14 to 28 days.
Neonates younger than 7 days old: 10 mg/kg I.V. or P.O. every 12 hours for 14 to 28 days. If neonate doesn't respond or when he is 7 days old, increase to 10 mg/kg every 8 hours.
▶ **Nosocomial pneumonia caused by** *Staphylococcus aureus* **(methicillin-susceptible [MSSA] and methicillin-resistant [MRSA] strains) or** *Streptococcus pneumonia* **(multidrug-resistant strains [MDRSP] only); complicated skin and skin-structure infections, including diabetic foot infections without osteomyelitis, caused by** *S. aureus* **(MSSA and MRSA),** *Streptococcus pyogenes,* **or** *Streptococcus agalactiae;* **community-acquired pneumonia caused by** *S. pneumoniae* **(including MDRSP), including those with bacteremia, or** *S. aureus* **(MSSA only).** *Adults and children age 12 and older:* 600 mg I.V. or P.O. every 12 hours for 10 to 14 days.
Neonates 7 days or older, infants, and children age 11 and younger: 10 mg/kg I.V. or P.O. every 8 hours for 10 to 14 days.
Preterm neonates younger than 7 days old: 10 mg/kg I.V. or P.O. every 12 hours for 10 to 14 days. Increase to 10 mg/kg every 8 hours if neonate doesn't respond or when he is 7 days old.
▶ **Uncomplicated skin and skin-structure infections caused by** *S. aureus* **(MSSA only)**

or *S. pyogenes.* *Adults:* 400 mg P.O. every 12 hours for 10 to 14 days.
Children ages 12 to 18: Give 600 mg P.O. every 12 hours for 10 to 14 days.
Children ages 5 to 11: Give 10 mg/kg P.O. every 12 hours for 10 to 14 days.
Neonates 7 days or older, infants, and children younger than age 5: Give 10 mg/kg P.O. every 8 hours for 10 to 14 days.
Neonates younger than 7 days old: 10 mg/kg I.V. or P.O. every 12 hours for 10 to 14 days. Increase to 10 mg/kg every 8 hours if neonate doesn't respond or when he is 7 days old.

▽ I.V. administration

- Drug is compatible with D_5W, normal saline solution for injection, and lactated Ringer's injection.
- Infuse over 30 to 120 minutes. Don't infuse in a series connection.
- Store drug at room temperature in its protective overwrap. The solution may turn yellow over time, but potency isn't affected. Use within 21 days.
⊗ **Incompatibilities**
Amphotericin B, ceftriaxone sodium, chlorpromazine hydrochloride, diazepam, erythromycin lactobionate, pentamidine isethionate, phenytoin sodium, trimethoprim-sulfamethoxazole. Don't mix with other I.V. drugs.

Contraindications and cautions

- Contraindicated in patients hypersensitive to the drug or any of its components.
- Safety and effectiveness of therapy for longer than 28 days haven't been studied.
☀ **Lifespan:** In pregnant women, use only if benefits outweigh risks to the fetus. In breast-feeding women, use cautiously.

Adverse reactions

CNS: dizziness, fever, *headache,* insomnia.
GI: altered taste, constipation, *diarrhea, nausea,* oral candidiasis, ***pseudomembranous colitis,*** tongue discoloration, vomiting.
GU: vaginal candidiasis.
Hematologic: anemia, *leukopenia, neutropenia, thrombocytopenia.*
Skin: rash.
Other: fungal infection.

Interactions

Drug-drug. *Adrenergics (such as dopamine, epinephrine, pseudoephedrine):* Increases risk of hypertension. Monitor blood pressure and heart rate. Start continuous infusions of dopamine and epinephrine at lower doses, and adjust to response.
Serotoninergics: Increases risk of serotonin syndrome (confusion, delirium, restlessness, tremor, blushing, diaphoresis, hyperpyrexia). If these symptoms occur, stop serotoninergic.
Drug-food. *Foods and beverages high in tyramine (such as aged cheese, air-dried meat, draft beer, red wine, sauerkraut, soy sauce):* May increase blood pressure. Advise patient to avoid these foods; explain that tyramine content of meals shouldn't exceed 100 mg.

Effects on lab test results

• May increase ALT, AST, bilirubin, alkaline phosphatase, creatinine, BUN, amylase, and lipase levels. May decrease hemoglobin level and hematocrit.
• May decrease WBC, neutrophil, and platelet counts.

Pharmacokinetics

Absorption: Rapid and complete. Bioavailability is about 100%.
Distribution: Good. About 31% protein-bound.
Metabolism: Undergoes oxidative metabolism to two inactive metabolites.
Excretion: At steady-state, about 30% unchanged in urine and about 50% as metabolites.
Half-life: 6¼ hours.

Route	Onset	Peak	Duration
P.O.			
Tablet	Unknown	1 hr	4¾–5½ hr
Suspension	Unknown	1 hr	4½ hr
I.V.	Unknown	½ hr	4¾ hr

Action

Chemical effect: Bacteriostatic against enterococci and staphylococci. Bactericidal against most strains of streptococci. Interferes with bacterial protein synthesis.
Therapeutic effect: Hinders or kills susceptible bacteria.

Available forms

Injection: 2 mg/ml

Powder for oral suspension: 100 mg/5 ml when reconstituted
Tablets: 400 mg, 600 mg

NURSING PROCESS

Assessment

• Obtain history of patient's underlying condition before starting therapy, and reassess regularly to monitor drug effectiveness.
• Obtain specimen for culture and sensitivity tests before starting therapy. Use sensitivity results to guide subsequent therapy.
• Monitor platelet count in patient with increased risk of bleeding, patient with thrombocytopenia, patient taking drugs that may cause thrombocytopenia, or patient taking linezolid for longer than 14 days.
• Monitor patient for persistent diarrhea; if it occurs, consider the possibility of pseudomembranous colitis.
• Assess patient's and family's knowledge of drug therapy.

Nursing diagnoses

• Risk for infection related to presence of susceptible bacteria
• Risk for injury related to drug-induced adverse reactions
• Deficient knowledge related to drug therapy

Planning and implementation

• Because inappropriate use of antibiotics may lead to resistant organisms, carefully consider other drugs before starting therapy, especially in an outpatient setting.
• No dosage adjustment is needed when switching from I.V. to P.O. dosage forms.
ALERT: Don't confuse Zyvox with Zovirax. They both come in a 400-mg tablet.
Patient teaching
• Inform patient that tablets and oral suspension may be taken with or without meals.
• Stress to patient the importance of completing the entire course of therapy, even if he feels better.
• Tell patient to alert prescriber if he has hypertension, is taking cough or cold preparations, or is taking a selective serotonin reuptake inhibitor or another antidepressant.
• Inform patient with phenylketonuria that each 5 ml of oral suspension contains 20 mg of

---

phenylalanine. Tablets and injection don't contain phenylalanine.

☑ Evaluation

• Patient is free from infection.
• Patient sustains no injury as a result of drug-induced adverse reactions.
• Patient and family state understanding of drug therapy.

※ **New Drug**

lisdexamfetamine dimesylate
(lihs-deks-am-FETT-ah-meen dy-MEHS-eh-layt)
Vyvanse

Pharmacologic class: amphetamine
Therapeutic class: CNS stimulant
Pregnancy risk category: C
Controlled substance schedule: II

Indications and dosages

▶ **Attention deficit hyperactivity disorder (ADHD).** *Children ages 6 to 12:* Initially, 30 mg P.O. once daily in the morning. Increase by 20 mg at weekly intervals to a maximum of 70 mg daily.

Contraindications and cautions

• Contraindicated in patients hypersensitive to sympathomimetic amines or in those with idiosyncratic reactions to them, in agitated patients, in those with advanced arteriosclerosis, hyperthyroidism, symptomatic CV disease, structural cardiac abnormalities, glaucoma, or moderate to severe hypertension, or in those with a history of drug abuse.
• Contraindicated within 14 days of MAO inhibitor therapy.
• Use cautiously in patients with a history of arrhythmias, MI, stroke, or seizures; in those with pre-existing psychosis, bipolar disorder, or aggressive behavior; or in those with Tourette syndrome.
※ **Lifespan:** In pregnant women, safety and effectiveness haven't been established. Use during pregnancy only if the potential benefit outweighs the risk to the fetus. Breast-feeding isn't recommended because of the potential for serious adverse effects in breast-fed infants. In children younger than age 6, don't use. In elderly patients, safety and effectiveness haven't been established.

Adverse reactions

CNS: fever, dizziness, *headache,* somnolence, labile affect, initial insomnia, *insomnia, irritability,* tic, hallucinations, delusional thinking, aggressive or hostile behavior.
CV: *ventricular hypertrophy.*
EENT: abnormal vision, blurred vision.
GI: *abdominal pain,* dry mouth, nausea, vomiting, *decreased appetite.*
Metabolic: slow growth, weight loss.
Skin: rash.

Interactions

Drug-drug. *Adrenergic blockers:* May inhibit adrenergic-blocking effects. Avoid using together.
Antihistamines: May inhibit sedative effects of these drugs. Monitor patient.
Antihypertensives, veratrum alkaloids: May inhibit antihypertensive effects of these drugs. Avoid using together.
Chlorpromazine, haloperidol: May decrease effectiveness of amphetamines. Monitor patient closely.
Ethosuximide: May delay absorption of this drug. Monitor patient closely.
Lithium: May inhibit anorectic and CNS stimulation effects of amphetamine. Monitor patient closely.
MAO inhibitors: May cause severe hypertension or hypertensive crisis. Avoid using within 14 days of MAO inhibitor therapy.
Meperidine: May increase the analgesic effect of this drug. Use together cautiously.
Norepinephrine: May increase adrenergic effects of the drug. Monitor patient closely.
Phenobarbital, phenytoin: May delay intestinal absorption of these drugs and enhance their anticonvulsant effects. Monitor patient.
Propoxyphene: Fatal seizures can occur with overdose of the drug. Don't use together.
Tricyclic antidepressants: May cause adverse CV effects. Avoid using together.
Urine acidifiers (ammonium chloride, sodium acid phosphate), methenamine: May decrease level and increase renal excretion of amphetamine. Monitor patient for decreased drug effects.
Drug-food. *Caffeine:* May increase CNS stimulation. Discourage using together.

Effects on lab test results

• May increase corticosteroid level.
• May interfere with urinary steroid test.

Pharmacokinetics

Absorption: Rapid. Food delays peak concentration by 1 hour.
Distribution: No information available.
Metabolism: Undergoes first-pass metabolism in intestine, liver, or both. Isn't metabolized through cytochrome P-450 system.
Excretion: Primarily in urine. *Half-life:* Less than 1 hour.

Route	Onset	Peak	Duration
P.O.	Rapid	1 hr	Unknown

Action

Chemical effect: Thought to increase the release of norepinephrine and dopamine into extraneuronal spaces by blocking their reuptake into the presynaptic neuron.
Therapeutic effect: Increases attention and decreases impulsivity and hyperactivity.

Available forms

Capsules: 30 mg, 50 mg, 70 mg

NURSING PROCESS

Assessment
• Monitor the patient for signs of drug dependence or abuse.
• Monitor patient closely for CV adverse effects, new or worsening behavior (aggression, mania), vision problems, or seizures.
• Monitor blood pressure and pulse routinely.
• Growth may be suppressed with long-term stimulant use. Monitor child for growth and weight gain. If growth is suppressed or if weight gain is lower than expected, stop treatment.

Nursing diagnoses
• Ineffective health maintenance related to underlying condition
• Disturbed sleep pattern related to drug-induced insomnia
• Deficient knowledge related to drug therapy

Planning and implementation
• Overdose may cause restlessness, tremor, hyperreflexia, tachypnea, confusion, combativeness, hallucinations, panic states, hyperpyrexia, rhabdomyolysis, nausea, vomiting diarrhea, abdominal cramps, arrhythmias, and hypertension or hypotension; followed by fatigue and depression. Coma or seizures usually precede death.

• Treat overdose symptomatically and supportively. Activated charcoal, catharsis, and gastric lavage may be considered after securing the patient's airway and controlling agitation with sedation. If acute severe hypertension occurs, administer phentolamine I.V. However, a gradual drop in blood pressure usually results when patient is adequately sedated. Chlorpromazine may be used to reverse central stimulant effects of the amphetamine.
• Give the lowest effective dose in the morning. Afternoon doses may cause insomnia.
• Effectiveness of this drug when taken longer than 4 weeks isn't known. Periodically interrupt therapy to determine whether continued therapy is necessary.

The drug may trigger Tourette syndrome. Monitor the child, especially at start of therapy.

Patient teaching
• Diagnosis of ADHD must be based on complete history and evaluation of the child with consultation of psychological, educational, and social resources.
• Tell your child's health care provider about any other prescription medications, nonprescription medications, herbs, and supplements your child may be taking.
• Tell the patient or caregiver that the drug should be taken in the morning to prevent insomnia.
• Advise patient or caregiver not to stop the drug abruptly, as this may cause severe fatigue and depression.
• Capsules may be swallowed whole, or the contents may be dissolved in a glass of water and taken immediately.
• Caution the patient to avoid activities that require alertness or good psychomotor coordination until the CNS effects of the drug are known.
• Warn the patient with seizure disorder that drug may decrease seizure threshold. Urge him to notify his prescriber if a seizure occurs.
• Tell the patient or caregiver to report worsening aggression, hallucinations, delusions, or mania. Instruct the patient or caregiver to report palpitations or visual disturbances.
• Advise the patient to avoid beverages containing caffeine while taking the drug.
• If a dose is missed, give the dose in the morning as soon as possible. Don't give the missed dose in the afternoon because it may prevent the child from going to sleep at night. Give the next dose the following morning.

Reactions may be *common*, uncommon, *life-threatening*, or COMMON AND LIFE-THREATENING.

☑ Evaluation

- Patient responds positively to drug therapy.
- Patient doesn't experience insomnia related to drug therapy.
- Patient and family state understanding of drug therapy.

lisinopril
(ly-SIN-uh-pril)
Prinivil◆, Zestril

Pharmacologic class: ACE inhibitor
Therapeutic class: antihypertensive
Pregnancy risk category: C (D in second and third trimesters)

Indications and dosages

▶ **Hypertension.** *Adults:* Initially, 10 mg P.O. daily. If patient also takes a diuretic, reduce initial dosage to 5 mg P.O. daily. Usual effective dosage is 20 to 40 mg daily. Maximum dosage, 80 mg daily.
Children ages 6 to 16: Initially, 0.07 mg/kg P.O. once daily (up to 5 mg total). Adjust dosage by blood pressure response. Doses above 0.61 mg/kg (or in excess of 40 mg) haven't been tested in children.
▶ **Adjunct therapy in heart failure (with diuretics and digoxin).** *Adults:* Initially, 5 mg P.O. daily. Usual effective dosage range is 5 to 20 mg daily. In patients with hyponatremia (sodium level below 130 mEq/L) or creatinine above 3 mg/dl, start with 2.5 mg P.O. once daily.
▶ **Hemodynamically stable patients within 24 hours of acute MI to improve survival.** *Adults:* Initially, 5 mg P.O. Then 5 mg P.O. after 24 hours, 10 mg P.O. after 48 hours, and 10 mg P.O. once daily for 6 weeks. In patients with systolic blood pressure of 120 mm Hg or less at start of therapy or during first 3 days after an MI, reduce dosage to 2.5 mg.

Contraindications and cautions

- Contraindicated in patients hypersensitive to ACE inhibitors and in those with a history of angioedema from previous therapy with an ACE inhibitor.
- Use cautiously in patients with impaired kidney function; adjust dosage as directed. Also use cautiously in patients at risk for hyperkalemia (those with renal insufficiency or diabetes or who use drugs that raise potassium level).
🔥 **Lifespan:** In pregnant women, use in first trimester when benefits to woman exceed risks to fetus. In last two trimesters, drug is contraindicated. In breast-feeding women, use cautiously. In children younger than age 6 and in children with GFR of less than 30 ml/minute, safety and effectiveness haven't been established.

Adverse reactions

CNS: depression, *dizziness, fatigue, headache,* paresthesia, somnolence.
CV: chest pain, hypotension, *orthostatic hypotension.*
EENT: nasal congestion.
GI: *diarrhea,* dysgeusia, dyspepsia, nausea.
GU: impotence.
Metabolic: *hyperkalemia.*
Musculoskeletal: *muscle cramps.*
Respiratory: *dry, persistent, tickling, nonproductive cough.*
Skin: rash.
Other: *angioedema, anaphylaxis,* decreased libido.

Interactions

Drug-drug. *Capsaicin:* May cause or worsen coughing caused by ACE inhibitors. Monitor patient closely.
Digoxin: May increase digoxin level. Monitor level.
Diuretics: May cause excessive hypotension. Stop diuretics for 2 to 3 days or increase salt intake before lisinopril therapy or reduce lisinopril dosage to 5 mg P.O. once daily. Monitor blood pressure closely until stabilized.
Indomethacin: May lessen hypotensive effect. Monitor blood pressure.
Insulin, oral antidiabetics: May increase risk of hypoglycemia, especially when starting lisinopril. Monitor glucose closely.
Lithium: May increase lithium level. Monitor patient for toxicity.
Phenothiazines: May increase effects of drug. Monitor blood pressure.
Potassium-sparing diuretics, potassium supplements: May increase risk of hyperkalemia. Monitor potassium level.
Thiazide diuretics: May lessen potassium loss caused by thiazide diuretics. Monitor potassium level.

L

Tizanidine: May cause severe hypotension. Monitor patient closely.

Drug-herb. *Licorice:* May cause sodium retention and increase blood pressure, interfering with ACE inhibitor effects. Discourage use together.

Drug-food. *Salt substitutes with potassium:* May increase risk of hyperkalemia. Monitor patient closely; discourage patient from using unless directed by prescriber.

Effects on lab test results

• May increase BUN, creatinine, potassium, and bilirubin levels.
• May increase liver function test values.

Pharmacokinetics

Absorption: Variable.
Distribution: Wide, although minimally to brain. Insignificantly protein-bound.
Metabolism: None.
Excretion: Unchanged in urine. *Half-life:* 12 hours.

Route	Onset	Peak	Duration
P.O.	1 hr	7 hr	24 hr

Action

Chemical effect: Unknown; may result primarily from suppression of renin-angiotensin-aldosterone system.
Therapeutic effect: Lowers blood pressure.

Available forms

Tablets: 2.5 mg, 5 mg, 10 mg, 20 mg, 40 mg

NURSING PROCESS

Assessment

• Assess patient's condition before starting therapy and regularly thereafter to monitor drug effectiveness. Beneficial effects may take several weeks to appear.
• Monitor WBC with differential counts before therapy, every 2 weeks for first 3 months, and periodically thereafter.
• Be alert for adverse reactions and drug interactions.
• Assess patient's and family's knowledge of drug therapy.

Nursing diagnoses

• Risk for injury related to presence of hypertension

• Decreased cardiac output related to drug-induced hypotension
• Deficient knowledge related to drug therapy

Planning and implementation

• If drug doesn't control blood pressure, add diuretics.
ALERT: Don't confuse lisinopril with fosinopril or Lioresal.
ALERT: Don't confuse Prinivil with Proventil or Prilosec.
ALERT: Don't confuse Zestril with Zostrix, Zetia, Zebeta, or Zyrtec.
Patient teaching
• Advise patient to report signs or symptoms of angioedema (including laryngeal edema), such as breathing difficulty or swelling of face, eyes, lips, or tongue.
• Tell patient that light-headedness may occur, especially during first few days of therapy. Tell him to rise slowly to avoid this effect and to report symptoms to prescriber. If syncope occurs, tell patient to stop taking drug and call prescriber immediately.
• Tell patient not to abruptly stop taking the drug but to call the prescriber if an adverse reaction occurs.
• Advise patient to report signs of infection, such as fever and sore throat.
• Tell patient to notify prescriber and stop taking the drug if she becomes pregnant.

Evaluation

• Patient's blood pressure is within normal limits.
• Patient maintains adequate cardiac output throughout therapy.
• Patient and family state understanding of drug therapy.

lithium carbonate
(LITH-ee-um KAR-buh-nayt)
Carbolith ♦ , Duralith ♦ , Lithane ♦ , Lithobid

lithium citrate
Lithium Citrate Syrup

Pharmacologic class: alkali metal
Therapeutic class: antipsychotic
Pregnancy risk category: D

Indications and dosages

▶ **To prevent or control acute manic or mixed episodes in patients with bipolar disorder.** *Adults:* 300 to 600 mg P.O. up to q.i.d., increasing on basis of drug level to achieve therapeutic dosage, usually 1,800 mg P.O. daily. Therapeutic drug level is 1 to 1.5 mEq/L for acute mania; 0.6 to 1.2 mEq/L for maintenance therapy; and 2 mEq/L as maximum level.

▶ **Major depression, schizoaffective disorder, schizophrenic disorder, alcohol dependence‡.** *Adults:* 300 mg lithium carbonate P.O. t.i.d. or q.i.d.

▶ **Apparent mixed bipolar disorder in children‡.** *Children:* Initially, 15 to 60 mg/kg or 0.5 to 1.5 g/m² lithium carbonate P.O. daily in three divided doses. Don't exceed usual adult dosage. Adjust dosage based on patient's response and lithium level. Usual range, 150 to 300 mg daily in divided doses to maintain lithium level of 0.5 to 1.2 mEq/L.

▶ **Chemotherapy-induced neutropenia in children and patients with AIDS receiving zidovudine‡.** *Adults and children:* 300 to 1,000 mg P.O. daily.

Contraindications and cautions

• Contraindicated if therapy can't be closely monitored.

• Use cautiously in patients receiving neuroleptics, neuromuscular blockers, or diuretics; in debilitated patients; and in patients with thyroid disease, seizure disorder, renal or CV disease, severe debilitation or dehydration, or sodium depletion.

⚠ Lifespan: In pregnant and breast-feeding women, drug is contraindicated. In children younger than age 12, safety and effectiveness haven't been established. In elderly patients, use cautiously because of possible decreased rate of excretion.

Adverse reactions

CNS: ataxia, *coma*, confusion, dizziness, drowsiness, EEG changes, *epileptiform seizures*, headache, impaired speech, incoordination, lethargy, psychomotor retardation, restlessness, stupor, syncope, tremor, worsened organic mental syndrome, weakness.
CV: ankle and wrist edema, *arrhythmias*, hypotension, *reversible ECG changes*.
EENT: blurred vision, tinnitus.

GI: abdominal pain, anorexia, diarrhea, dry mouth, flatulence, indigestion, metallic taste, nausea, thirst, vomiting.
GU: albuminuria, glycosuria, polyuria, *renal toxicity*.
Hematologic: *reversible leukocytosis*.
Metabolic: goiter, hyponatremia, hypothyroidism, transient hyperglycemia.
Skin: acne, alopecia, diminished or absent sensation, drying and thinning of hair, pruritus, psoriasis, rash.

Interactions

Drug-drug. *Acetazolamide, aminophylline, sodium bicarbonate, urine alkalinizers:* May increase lithium excretion. Avoid salt loads; monitor lithium levels for increase.
Carbamazepine, indomethacin, methyldopa, NSAIDs, piroxicam, probenecid: May increase lithium effects. Monitor patient for lithium toxicity.
Diuretics: May increase reabsorption of lithium by kidneys with a toxic effect. Use cautiously, and monitor lithium and electrolyte levels (especially sodium).
Fluoxetine: May increase lithium level. Monitor patient for toxicity.
Neuroleptics: May cause encephalopathy. Watch for signs and symptoms (lethargy, tremor, extrapyramidal symptoms), and stop drug if they occur.
Neuromuscular blockers: May cause prolonged paralysis or weakness. Monitor patient closely.
Thyroid hormones: May induce hypothyroidism. Monitor thyroid function, and treat with thyroid hormones as needed.

Effects on lab test results

• May increase glucose level. May decrease sodium, T_3, T_4, and protein-bound iodine levels.
• May increase ^{131}I uptake and WBC and neutrophil counts.

Pharmacokinetics

Absorption: Complete within 8 hours.
Distribution: Wide. Levels in thyroid gland, bone, and brain exceed serum levels.
Metabolism: Not metabolized.
Excretion: 95% unchanged in urine. *Half-life:* 18 hours (adolescents) to 36 hours (elderly).

Route	Onset	Peak	Duration
P.O.	Unknown	½–3 hr	Unknown

Action

Chemical effect: Unknown; probably alters chemical transmitters in CNS, possibly by interfering with ionic pump mechanisms in brain cells, and may compete with sodium ions.
Therapeutic effect: Stabilizes mood.

Available forms

lithium carbonate
Capsules: 150 mg, 300 mg, 600 mg
Tablets: 300 mg (300 mg = 8.12 mEq lithium)
Tablets (controlled-release): 300 mg, 450 mg
lithium citrate
Syrup (sugarless): 8 mEq of lithium per 5 ml (8 mEq lithium = 300 mg of lithium carbonate)

NURSING PROCESS

Assessment

• Assess patient's condition before starting therapy and regularly thereafter to monitor drug effectiveness. Expect delay of 1 to 3 weeks before drug's beneficial effects occur.
• Monitor baseline ECG, thyroid and kidney studies, and electrolyte levels.
• Monitor lithium blood level 8 to 12 hours after first dose, usually before morning dose, two or three times weekly in first month, and then weekly to monthly during maintenance therapy. With blood levels below 1.5 mEq/L, adverse reactions usually remain mild, although toxicity may occur even at therapeutic levels.
• Check urine-specific gravity, and report level below 1.005, which may indicate diabetes insipidus.
• Monitor glucose level closely. Lithium may alter glucose tolerance in diabetic patient.
• Be alert for adverse reactions and drug interactions.
• Assess patient's and family's knowledge of drug therapy.

Nursing diagnoses

• Disturbed thought processes related to presence of bipolar disorder
• Ineffective health maintenance related to drug-induced endocrine dysfunction
• Deficient knowledge related to drug therapy

Planning and implementation

ALERT: Don't confuse Lithobid with Levbid, Lithonate with Lithostat, or Lithotabs with Lithobid or Lithostat.
• Monitoring lithium level is crucial to safe use of drug. Don't use in patient who can't have level checked regularly.
• Give with plenty of water and after meals to minimize GI reactions.
• Before leaving bedside, make sure patient has swallowed drug.
• Notify prescriber if patient's behavior hasn't improved in 3 weeks or if it worsens.
• Perform outpatient follow-up of thyroid and kidney function every 6 to 12 months. Palpate thyroid to check for enlargement.
Patient teaching
• Tell patient to take drug with plenty of water and after meals to minimize GI upset.
• Explain that lithium has narrow therapeutic margin of safety. A blood level that's even slightly high can be dangerous.
• Warn patient and family to watch for signs of toxicity (diarrhea, vomiting, tremor, drowsiness, muscle weakness, ataxia) and to expect transient nausea, polyuria, thirst, and discomfort during the first few days. Tell patient not to stop taking the drug abruptly unless he has symptoms of toxicity. If he does, he should call his prescriber and not take the next dose.
• Warn patient to avoid activities that require alertness and good psychomotor coordination until the drug's CNS effects are known.
• Tell patient not to switch brands or take other prescription or OTC drugs without prescriber's approval.
• Advise patient to wear or carry medical identification.

Evaluation

• Patient exhibits improved behavior and thought processes.
• Patient maintains normal endocrine function throughout therapy.
• Patient and family state understanding of drug therapy.

HIGH ALERT

lomustine (CCNU)
(loh-MUH-steen)
CeeNU

Pharmacologic class: alkylating drug, nitrosourea
Therapeutic class: antineoplastic
Pregnancy risk category: D

Indications and dosages

▶ **Brain tumor, Hodgkin and other lymphomas.** *Adults and children:* 100 to 130 mg/m²
P.O. as single dose every 6 weeks. Reduce dosage according to degree of bone marrow suppression. Don't repeat doses until WBC count is more than 4,000/mm³ and platelet count is more than 100,000/mm³.

Contraindications and cautions

• Contraindicated in patients hypersensitive to the drug or any of its components.
• Use cautiously in patients with lowered platelet, WBC, or RBC count and in those receiving other myelosuppressant drugs.
✲ **Lifespan:** In pregnant and breast-feeding women, drug is contraindicated.

Adverse reactions

GI: *nausea*, stomatitis, *vomiting.*
GU: *nephrotoxicity,* progressive azotemia, *renal impairment.*
Hematologic: anemia, *bone marrow suppression, leukopenia, thrombocytopenia.*
Hepatic: *hepatotoxicity.*
Respiratory: *pulmonary fibrosis.*
Other: *secondary malignant disease.*

Interactions

Drug-drug. *Anticoagulants, aspirin:* Increases bleeding risk. Avoid use together.

Effects on lab test results

• May increase urine urea, liver enzyme, BUN, and creatinine levels. May decrease hemoglobin level and hematocrit.
• May decrease WBC, RBC, and platelet counts.

Pharmacokinetics

Absorption: Rapid and good.

Distribution: Wide. Crosses blood–brain barrier to significant extent.
Metabolism: Rapid and extensive in liver.
Excretion: Metabolites mainly in urine. *Half-life:* 1 to 2 days.

Route	Onset	Peak	Duration
P.O.	Unknown	Unknown	Unknown

Action

Chemical effect: Cross-links strands of cellular DNA and interferes with RNA transcription.
Therapeutic effect: Kills selected cancer cells.

Available forms

Capsules: 10 mg, 40 mg, 100 mg, dose pack (two 10-mg, two 40-mg, two 100-mg capsules)

NURSING PROCESS

 Assessment
• Assess patient's condition before starting therapy and regularly thereafter to monitor drug effectiveness.
• Monitor CBC weekly because bone marrow toxicity is delayed by 4 to 6 weeks after treatment.
• Periodically monitor liver function test results.
• Be alert for adverse reactions and drug interactions.
• Assess patient's and family's knowledge of drug therapy.

 Nursing diagnoses
• Ineffective health maintenance related to presence of neoplastic disease
• Ineffective protection related to adverse hematologic reactions
• Deficient knowledge related to drug therapy

 Planning and implementation
• Give antiemetic before giving drug to help patient avoid nausea.
• Give 2 to 4 hours after meals because drug is better absorbed on an empty stomach.
• Repeat dose only when CBC results reveal safe blood counts.
• Institute infection control and bleeding precautions.
Patient teaching
• Warn patient to watch for signs of infection (fever, sore throat, fatigue) and bleeding (easy

bruising, nosebleeds, bleeding gums, melena) and to take temperature daily.
• Instruct patient to avoid OTC products containing aspirin.
• Advise woman of childbearing age to avoid pregnancy during therapy and to consult with prescriber before becoming pregnant.

☑ Evaluation
• Patient responds well to therapy.
• Patient regains normal hematologic function.
• Patient and family state understanding of drug therapy.

loperamide
(loh-PEH-ruh-mighd)
Imodium, Imodium A-D†, Kaopectate II Caplets†, Maalox Anti-Diarrheal Caplets†, Neo-Diaral†, Pepto Diarrhea Control†

Pharmacologic class: piperidine derivative
Therapeutic class: antidiarrheal
Pregnancy risk category: B

Indications and dosages

▶ **Acute diarrhea.** *Adults and children age 12 and older:* Initially, 4 mg P.O.; then 2 mg after each unformed stool. Maximum dosage, 16 mg daily.
Children ages 8 to 12 who weigh more than 30 kg (66 lb): 2 mg P.O. t.i.d. on first day. On subsequent days, doses of 1 mg/10 kg of body weight may be given after each unformed stool. Maximum dosage, 6 mg daily.
Children ages 6 to 8 who weigh 20 to 30 kg (44 to 66 lb): 2 mg P.O. b.i.d. on first day. On subsequent days, doses of 1 mg/10 kg of body weight may be given after each unformed stool. Maximum dosage, 4 mg daily.
Children ages 2 to 5 who weigh 13 to 20 kg (29 to 44 lb): 1 mg P.O. t.i.d. on first day. On subsequent days, give doses of 1 mg/10 kg of body weight after each unformed stool. Maximum dosage, 3 mg daily.
▶ **Chronic diarrhea.** *Adults:* Initially, 4 mg P.O.; then 2 mg after each unformed stool until diarrhea subsides. Adjust dosage to individual response. Maximum dosage, 16 mg daily. If patient doesn't improve in 10 days, consider different therapy.

Children‡: 0.08 to 0.24 mg/kg P.O. daily in two to three divided doses. Report persistent diarrhea to prescriber.
▶ **Self-medication of acute diarrhea including traveler's diarrhea.** *Adults:* 4 mg† after first loose bowel movement followed by 2 mg† after each subsequent loose bowel movement; maximum, 8 mg P.O. daily for 2 days.

Contraindications and cautions

• Contraindicated in patients hypersensitive to the drug or any of its components; in patients for whom constipation must be avoided; in patients with pseudomembranous colitis from antibiotic use; and patients with *Shigella, Salmonella,* or enteroinvasive *Escherichia coli* infection. OTC form is contraindicated in patients with bloody diarrhea and those with temperature over 101° F (38° C).
• Use cautiously in patients with hepatic disease because of risk of encephalopathy.
☀ **Lifespan:** In pregnant women, use cautiously. In breast-feeding women, use cautiously; it's unknown if the drug appears in breast milk. In children younger than age 2, drug is contraindicated.

Adverse reactions

CNS: dizziness, drowsiness, fatigue.
GI: abdominal pain, distention, or discomfort; *constipation;* dry mouth; nausea; vomiting.
Skin: rash.
Other: hypersensitivity reactions.

Interactions

Drug-drug. *Saquinavir:* May increase loperamide level and decrease saquinavir level. Avoid use together.

Effects on lab test results

None reported.

Pharmacokinetics

Absorption: Poor.
Distribution: Unknown.
Metabolism: In liver.
Excretion: Mainly in feces; less than 2% in urine. *Half-life:* 9 to 14½ hours.

Route	Onset	Peak	Duration
P.O.	Unknown	2½–5 hr	24 hr

Reactions may be *common*, uncommon, *life-threatening*, or COMMON AND LIFE-THREATENING.

Action
Chemical effect: Inhibits peristalsis, prolonging passage of intestinal contents.
Therapeutic effect: Relieves diarrhea.

Available forms
Capsules: 2 mg†
Oral liquid*: 1 mg/5 ml†, 1 mg/ml†
Tablets: 2 mg†

NURSING PROCESS

⚡ Assessment
• Assess patient's diarrhea before starting therapy and regularly thereafter to monitor drug effectiveness.
• Be alert for adverse reactions.
⚠ **ALERT:** Monitor children closely for CNS effects because they may be more sensitive than adults.
• Monitor patient's hydration.
• Assess patient's and family's knowledge of drug therapy.

⊞ Nursing diagnoses
• Diarrhea related to underlying condition
• Risk for deficient fluid volume related to drug-induced adverse GI reactions
• Deficient knowledge related to drug therapy

▷ Planning and implementation
• If patient doesn't improve in 48 hours, stop therapy.
• If patient has severe abdominal pain, bloating, or firmness or if drug is ineffective, notify prescriber.
• If drug is given by NG tube, flush tube to clear it and ensure drug's passage to stomach.
⚠ **ALERT:** Oral liquids are available in different concentrations. Check dose carefully. For children, consider an oral liquid product that doesn't contain alcohol.
⚠ **ALERT:** Don't confuse Imodium with Ionamin.
Patient teaching
• Advise patient not to exceed recommended dosage.
• Tell patient with acute diarrhea to contact prescriber if patient doesn't improve within 48 hours. For chronic diarrhea, tell patient to notify prescriber and stop taking the drug if no improvement occurs after taking 16 mg daily for at least 10 days.

• Advise patient to stop taking drug and to notify prescriber immediately if abdominal pain, bloating, or firmness develop because of risk of toxic megacolon.

✓ Evaluation
• Patient's diarrhea is relieved.
• Patient is adequately hydrated throughout therapy.
• Patient and family state understanding of drug therapy.

lopinavir and ritonavir
(loe-PIN-a-veer and rih-TOH-nuh-veer)
Kaletra✐

Pharmacologic class: protease inhibitor
Therapeutic class: antiretroviral
Pregnancy risk category: C

Indications and dosages
▶ **HIV infection, with other antiretrovirals in treatment-naive adults.** *Adults:* 800 mg lopinavir and 200 mg ritonavir (4 tablets or 10 ml) P.O. with food once daily or 400 mg lopinavir and 100 mg ritonavir with food b.i.d.
▶ **HIV infection, with other antiretrovirals in treatment-experienced patients.** *Adults and children older than age 12:* Give 400 mg lopinavir and 100 mg ritonavir (2 tablets or 5 ml) P.O. b.i.d.
Children ages 6 months to 12 years who weigh 15 to 40 kg (33 to 88 lb): 10 mg/kg (lopinavir content) P.O. b.i.d. with food up to a maximum of 400 mg lopinavir and 100 mg ritonavir in children weighing more than 40 kg.
Children ages 6 months to 12 years who weigh 7 to 15 kg (15 to 33 lb): 12 mg/kg (lopinavir content) P.O. b.i.d. with food.
⧄ **Adjust-a-dose:** In treatment-experienced patients older than age 12 also taking efavirenz, nevirapine, fosamprenavir without ritonavir, or nelfinavir, consider dosage of 600 mg lopinavir and 150 mg ritonavir (3 tablets) P.O. b.i.d. For patients using oral solution and also taking efavirenz, nevirapine, amprenavir, or nelfinavir, 533 mg lopinavir and 133 mg ritonavir (6.5 ml) b.i.d. with food is recommended.
    In treatment-experienced patients ages 6 months to 12 years also taking amprenavir, efavirenz, or nevirapine and weighing 7 to

15 kg, give 13 mg/kg (lopinavir content) P.O. b.i.d. with food. For patients weighing 15 to 45 kg, give 11 mg/kg (lopinavir content) P.O. b.i.d. with food up to a maximum dose of 533 mg lopinavir and 133 mg ritonavir b.i.d. In children weighing more than 45 kg, use adult dosage.

Contraindications and cautions

• Contraindicated in patients hypersensitive to the drug or any of its components.

• Use cautiously in patients with a history of pancreatitis or with hepatic impairment, hepatitis B or C, marked elevations in liver enzyme levels, or hemophilia.

⚘ **Lifespan:** In breast-feeding women, either stop breast-feeding or use another drug. In infants younger than age 6 months, safety and effectiveness haven't been established. In elderly patients, use cautiously because of possible decreased rate of excretion.

Adverse reactions

CNS: abnormal dreams, abnormal thinking, agitation, amnesia, anxiety, asthenia, ataxia, confusion, depression, dizziness, dyskinesia, emotional lability, *encephalopathy,* fever, headache, hypertonia, insomnia, malaise, nervousness, neuropathy, pain, paresthesia, peripheral neuritis, somnolence, tremor.

CV: chest pain, *deep vein thrombosis,* edema, facial edema, hypertension, palpitations, peripheral edema, thrombophlebitis, vasculitis.

EENT: abnormal vision, eye disorder, otitis media, sialadenitis, sinusitis, stomatitis, taste perversion, tinnitus, ulcerative stomatitis.

GI: abdominal pain, abnormal stools, anorexia, cholecystitis, constipation, *diarrhea,* dry mouth, dyspepsia, dysphagia, enterocolitis, eructation, esophagitis, fecal incontinence, flatulence, gastritis, gastroenteritis, GI disorder, *hemorrhagic colitis,* increased appetite, *nausea, pancreatitis,* vomiting.

GU: abnormal ejaculation, decreased libido, gynecomastia, hypogonadism, renal calculus, urine abnormality.

Hematologic: anemia, *leukopenia,* lymphadenopathy, *neutropenia, thrombocytopenia* in children.

Hepatic: hyperbilirubinemia in children.

Metabolic: Cushing syndrome, dehydration, decreased glucose tolerance, *hypercholesterolemia,* hyperglycemia, hyperuricemia, hypona-

tremia in children, hypothyroidism, *lactic acidosis,* weight loss.

Musculoskeletal: arthralgia, arthrosis, back pain, myalgia.

Respiratory: bronchitis, dyspnea, *lung edema.*

Skin: acne, alopecia, benign skin neoplasm, dry skin, exfoliative dermatitis, furunculosis, nail disorder, pruritus, rash, skin discoloration, sweating.

Other: chills, flulike syndrome, viral infection.

Interactions

Drug-drug. *Amiodarone, bepridil, lidocaine, quinidine:* May increase antiarrhythmic levels. Use cautiously. Monitor levels of these drugs; adjust dosage, if needed.

Amprenavir, efavirenz, nelfinavir, nevirapine: May decrease lopinavir level. Consider increasing lopinavir and ritonavir dose. Don't use a once-daily Kaletra regimen with these drugs.

Antiarrhythmics (flecainide, propafenone), pimozide: May increase risk of cardiac arrhythmias. Don't use together.

Atovaquone, methadone: May decrease levels of these drugs. Consider increasing doses of these drugs.

Carbamazepine, corticosteroids, phenobarbital, phenytoin: May decrease lopinavir level. Use cautiously.

Clarithromycin: May increase clarithromycin levels in patients with renal impairment. Adjust clarithromycin dosage.

Cyclosporine, rapamycin, tacrolimus: May increase levels of these drugs. Monitor therapeutic levels.

Delavirdine: May increase lopinavir level. May be prescribed together for this effect.

Didanosine: May decrease absorption of didanosine because lopinavir and ritonavir dose is taken with food. Give didanosine 1 hour before or 2 hours after lopinavir and ritonavir.

Dihydroergotamine, ergonovine, ergotamine, methylergonovine: May increase risk of ergot toxicity characterized by peripheral vasospasm and ischemia. Don't use together.

Disulfiram, metronidazole: May increase risk of disulfiram-like reaction. Avoid use together.

Felodipine, nicardipine, nifedipine: May increase levels of these drugs. Use cautiously. Monitor patient.

Fluticasone: May significantly increase fluticasone exposure and significantly decreased cortisol level, which may lead to systemic corticoste-

roid effects (including Cushing syndrome). Don't use together, if possible.

HMG-CoA reductase inhibitors: May increase risk of adverse reactions, such as myopathy and rhabdomyolysis. Atorvastatin, fluvastatin, and pravastatin may be used with careful monitoring. Avoid using lovastatin or simvastatin.

Hormonal contraceptives (ethinyl estradiol): May decrease effectiveness of contraceptives. Recommend nonhormonal contraception.

Indinavir, saquinavir: May increase level of these drugs. May be prescribed together for this effect.

Itraconazole, ketoconazole: May increase levels of these drugs. Don't give more than 200 mg/day of these drugs.

Methadone: May decrease methadone absorption. May need to increase dosage. Monitor patient closely.

Midazolam, triazolam: May prolong or increase sedation or respiratory depression. Don't use together.

Phosphodiesterase type 5 inhibitors (sildenafil, tadalafil, vardenafil): May increase levels and risk of adverse effects of these drugs, such as hypotension and prolonged erection. Don't exceed 25 mg of sildenafil in 48 hours, 10 mg of tadalafil in 72 hours, or 2.5 mg of vardenafil in 72 hours. Use cautiously, and monitor patient for adverse reactions.

Rifabutin: May increase rifabutin level. Decrease rifabutin dosage by 75%; monitor patient for adverse effects.

Rifampin: May decrease effectiveness of lopinavir and ritonavir. Avoid use together.

Trazodone: May increase trazodone level, causing nausea, dizziness, hypotension, and syncope. Avoid use together. If unavoidable, use cautiously with a lower dose of trazodone.

Warfarin: May affect warfarin level. Monitor PT and INR.

Drug-herb. *St. John's wort:* May cause loss of virologic response and resistance to drug. Discourage use together.

Drug-food. *Any food:* May increase absorption of oral solution. Give drug with food.

Effects on lab test results

● May increase amylase, liver enzyme, glucose, uric acid, cholesterol, and triglyceride levels. May decrease hemoglobin level and hematocrit. In children, may increase bilirubin level and decrease sodium level.

● May decrease WBC, neutrophil, and platelet counts.

Pharmacokinetics

Absorption: Levels peak in 4 hours. Drug is better absorbed when taken with food.
Distribution: Lopinavir is 98% or 99% protein-bound.
Metabolism: Lopinavir is extensively metabolized by the CYP3A isoenzyme. Ritonavir is a potent inhibitor of CYP3A, which inhibits lopinavir metabolism and increases lopinavir level.
Excretion: In urine and feces. Less than 3% of drug is excreted unchanged. *Half-life:* About 6 hours.

Route	Onset	Peak	Duration
P.O.	Unknown	4 hr	6 hr

Action

Chemical effects: Inhibits HIV protease. Ritonavir inhibits lopinavir metabolism, increasing lopinavir level.
Therapeutic effect: Prevents cleavage of the Gag-Pol polyprotein, resulting in the production of immature, noninfectious viral particles.

Available forms

Capsule: 133.3 mg lopinavir and 33.3 mg ritonavir
Solution: lopinavir 400 mg and ritonavir 100 mg per 5 ml (80 mg and 20 mg per ml)
Tablets: 100 mg lopinavir and 25 mg ritonavir, 200 mg lopinavir and 50 mg ritonavir

NURSING PROCESS

Assessment
● Assess underlying condition before starting therapy, and reassess regularly to monitor drugs' effectiveness.
● Monitor total cholesterol and triglycerides before starting therapy and periodically thereafter.
● To monitor maternal-fetal outcomes of pregnant women exposed to lopinavir and ritonavir, an Antiretroviral Pregnancy Registry has been established. Enroll patients by calling 1-800-258-4263, or register online at www.apregistry.com.
ALERT: This drug interacts with many other drugs. Review all drugs that patient is currently taking.

• Assess patient's and family's knowledge of drug therapy.

Nursing diagnoses
• Risk for falls related to drug-induced adverse CNS effects
• Risk for powerlessness related to chronic disease and need for aggressive medical management
• Deficient knowledge related to drug therapy

Planning and implementation
• Tablets may be taken without regard to meals. Oral solution must be taken with food.
• **ALERT:** Tablets must be swallowed whole. Don't crush, divide, or let patient chew.
• Refrigerated drug remains stable until expiration date on package. If stored at room temperature, use drug within 2 months.
• Monitor patient for signs of fat redistribution, including central obesity, buffalo hump, peripheral wasting, breast enlargement, and cushingoid appearance.
• Watch for evidence of pancreatitis: nausea, vomiting, abdominal pain, and increased lipase and amylase values.
• Monitor patient for signs of bleeding.
• For an overdose, induce emesis or perform gastric lavage. Activated charcoal may be used to aid in removing unabsorbed drug. Dialysis is unlikely to help remove drug.
• **ALERT:** Don't confuse Kaletra with Keppra.
Patient teaching
• Tell patient to take oral solution with food.
• Tell patient also taking didanosine to take it 1 hour before or 2 hours after lopinavir and ritonavir.
• Advise patient to report side effects to prescriber.
• Tell patient to immediately report severe nausea, vomiting, or abdominal pain.
• Warn patient to tell prescriber about any other prescription or nonprescription drug he is taking, including herbal supplements.
• Tell patient that drug doesn't cure HIV.
• If patient takes a drug for erectile dysfunction, caution about an increased risk of adverse events, including hypotension, visual changes, and priapism, and the need to promptly report any symptoms. Tell him not to take more than directed.

• Advise HIV-infected mothers not to breast-feed because breast-feeding may transmit HIV to their infants.

✓ Evaluation
• Patient doesn't experience falls.
• Patient has adequate support, personal and professional, to deal with emotional aspects of having HIV disease.
• Patient and family state understanding of drug therapy.

loratadine
(loo-RAH-tuh-deen)
Alavert†, Claritin†, Claritin Reditabs†, Claritin Syrup†, Claritin-D 12 Hour†, Claritin-D 24 Hour†, Clear-Atadine†, Dimetapp Children's ND Non-Drowsy Allergy†, Tavist ND Allergy†, Triaminic Allerchews†

Pharmacologic class: peripherally selective piperidine
Therapeutic class: antihistamine
Pregnancy risk category: B

Indications and dosages
▶ **Allergic rhinitis, chronic idiopathic urticaria.** *Adults and children age 6 and older:* 10 mg P.O. daily.
Children ages 2 to 5: Give 5 mg P.O. daily.
Adjust-a-dose: For patients with renal or hepatic impairment, adjust dosage as follows: in adults and children age 6 and older with liver impairment or creatinine clearance less than 30 ml/minute, give 10 mg every other day. In children ages 2 to 5 with liver impairment or renal insufficiency, give 5 mg every other day.

Contraindications and cautions
• Contraindicated in patients hypersensitive to the drug or any of its components.
• Use cautiously in patients with hepatic impairment.
⚠ **Lifespan:** In pregnant women, use only when benefits outweigh risks to the fetus. In breast-feeding women, use cautiously because it isn't known if drug appears in breast milk. In children younger than age 2, safety and effectiveness haven't been established.

Adverse reactions

CNS: drowsiness, fatigue, *headache,* insomnia, nervousness.
EENT: *dry mouth.*

Interactions

Drug-drug. *Erythromycin, ketoconazole:* May increase loratadine level. Monitor patient closely.
Drug-lifestyle. *Alcohol use:* May increase CNS depression. Discourage use together.

Effects on lab test results

None reported.

Pharmacokinetics

Absorption: Good. Food may delay peak levels by 1 hour.
Distribution: Doesn't readily cross blood-brain barrier. About 97% protein-bound.
Metabolism: Extensive, although specific enzyme system hasn't been identified.
Excretion: About 80%, distributed equally between urine and feces. *Half-life:* 8½ hours.

Route	Onset	Peak	Duration
P.O.	1 hr	4–6 hr	24 hr

Action

Chemical effect: Blocks effects of histamine at H1-receptor sites. Drug's chemical structure prevents entry into CNS, preventing sedation.
Therapeutic effect: Relieves allergy symptoms.

Available forms

Syrup: 5 mg/5 ml†
Tablets: 10 mg†
Tablets (chewable): 5 mg†
Tablets (orally-disintegrating): 5 mg†, 10 mg†

NURSING PROCESS

Assessment
• Assess patient's condition before starting therapy and regularly thereafter to monitor drug effectiveness.
• Be alert for adverse reactions and drug interactions.
• Assess patient's and family's knowledge of drug therapy.

Nursing diagnoses
• Ineffective health maintenance related to underlying allergy condition
• Fatigue related to drug's adverse effect
• Deficient knowledge related to drug therapy

Planning and implementation
• Give drug on an empty stomach.
• If drug is ineffective, notify prescriber.
Patient teaching
• Tell patient to take drug at least 2 hours after a meal, to avoid eating for at least 1 hour after taking drug, and to take drug only once daily.
• Advise patient taking rapidly-disintegrating tablets to place tablet on the tongue, where it disintegrates within a few seconds. It can be swallowed with or without water.
• Tell patient to contact prescriber if symptoms persist or worsen.
• Advise patient to stop taking drug 4 days before allergy skin tests to preserve accuracy of tests.
• Tell patient not to drink alcohol and not to drive or engage in other activities that require alertness until the drug's CNS effects are known.

Evaluation
• Patient states that allergy symptoms are relieved.
• Patient describes coping strategies for fatigue.
• Patient and family state understanding of drug therapy.

HIGH ALERT

lorazepam
(loo-RAZ-eh-pam)
Ativan, Lorazepam Intensol, Novo-Lorazem ♦

Pharmacologic class: benzodiazepine
Therapeutic class: anxiolytic, sedative-hypnotic
Pregnancy risk category: D
Controlled substance schedule: IV

Indications and dosages

▶ **Anxiety.** *Adults:* 2 to 6 mg P.O. daily in divided doses. Maximum, 10 mg daily.
▶ **Insomnia caused by anxiety.** *Adults:* 2 to 4 mg P.O. at bedtime.

⚓ **Adjust-a-dose:** For elderly patients, initially, 1 to 2 mg P.O. daily in divided doses. Adjust as needed and as tolerated.

▶ **Status epilepticus.** *Adults:* 4 mg I.V. If seizures continue or recur after 10 to 15 minutes, another 4 mg may be given. Drug may be given I.M. if I.V. access is not available. *Children‡:* 0.05 to 0.1 mg/kg I.V.

▶ **Premedication before operative procedure.** *Adults:* 0.05 mg/kg I.M. 2 hours before procedure. Maximum dosage, 4 mg. Or 2 mg total or 0.044 mg/kg I.V., whichever is smaller.

▶ **Nausea and vomiting caused by emetogenic cancer chemotherapy‡.** *Adults:* 2.5 mg P.O. the evening before chemotherapy; repeat just after the initiation of chemotherapy. Or 1.5 mg/m² (maximum, 3 mg) I.V. over 5 minutes, 45 minutes before chemotherapy.

▼ I.V. administration

• Have emergency resuscitation equipment and oxygen available.
• Dilute with equal volume of sterile water for injection, normal saline solution for injection, or D_5W injection.
• Don't exceed 2-mg dose preoperatively in patients older than age 50.
• Check respirations before each dose and every 5 to 15 minutes thereafter until respiratory condition is stable.
• Give drug slowly, at no more than 2 mg/minute.
⊗ **Incompatibilities**
Aldesleukin, aztreonam, buprenorphine, foscarnet, idarubicin, imipenem-cilastatin sodium, ondansetron hydrochloride, sargramostim, sufentanil citrate, thiopental.

Contraindications and cautions

• Contraindicated in patients hypersensitive to the drug, any of its components, or other benzodiazepines. Contraindicated in patients with acute angle-closure glaucoma or acute alcohol intoxication. I.M. and I.V. forms contraindicated in patients with renal or hepatic impairment.
• Use cautiously in patients with pulmonary impairment. Use oral forms cautiously in patients with renal or hepatic impairment. Also use cautiously and at a reduced dosage in acutely ill or debilitated patients.
⚖ **Lifespan:** In pregnant and breast-feeding women, drug is contraindicated. In elderly patients, use cautiously and at a lower dosage.

Adverse reactions

CNS: anterograde amnesia, *drowsiness,* fainting, *hangover, lethargy,* psychosis, restlessness.
CV: transient hypotension.
EENT: visual disturbances.
GI: abdominal discomfort, dry mouth.
GU: incontinence, urine retention.
Other: *acute withdrawal syndrome.*

Interactions

Drug-drug. *CNS depressants:* May increase CNS depression. Avoid use together.
Digoxin: May increase digoxin level, increasing toxicity. Monitor level.
Levodopa: May decrease antiparkinson effect. Monitor patient.
Scopolamine: May increase the risk of sedation, hallucinations, and irrational behavior. Monitor patient.
Drug-herb. Catnip, kava, lady's slipper, lemon balm, passion flower, sassafras, skullcap, valerian: May enhance sedative effects. Discourage use together.
Drug-lifestyle. *Alcohol use:* May cause additive CNS effects. Strongly discourage use together.
Smoking: May decrease drug effectiveness. Monitor patient closely; discourage patient from smoking.

Effects on lab test results

• May increase liver function test values.

Pharmacokinetics

Absorption: Good with P.O. use; unknown with I.M. use.
Distribution: Wide. 85% protein-bound.
Metabolism: In liver.
Excretion: In urine. *Half-life:* 10 to 20 hours.

Route	Onset	Peak	Duration
P.O.	1 hr	2 hr	12–24 hr
I.V.	1–5 min	1–1½ hr	6–8 hr
I.M.	15–30 min	1–1½ hr	6–8 hr

Action

Chemical effect: May stimulate gamma-aminobutyric receptors in ascending reticular activating system.
Therapeutic effect: Relieves anxiety and promotes calmness and sleep.

Available forms

Injection: 2 mg/ml, 4 mg/ml

Reactions may be *common,* uncommon, *life-threatening*, or COMMON AND LIFE-THREATENING.

Oral solution (concentrated): 2 mg/ml
Tablets: 0.5 mg, 1 mg, 2 mg
Tablets (S.L.): 0.5 mg ♦, 1 mg ♦, 2 mg ♦

NURSING PROCESS

⚄ Assessment
• Assess patient's condition before starting therapy and regularly thereafter to monitor drug effectiveness.
• Monitor liver, kidney, and hematopoietic function studies periodically in patient receiving repeated or prolonged therapy.
• Be alert for adverse reactions and drug interactions.
• Assess patient's and family's knowledge of drug therapy.

⚄ Nursing diagnoses
• Anxiety related to underlying condition
• Risk for injury related to drug-induced adverse CNS effects
• Deficient knowledge related to drug therapy

▷ Planning and implementation
• For I.M. injection, inject drug deep into muscle mass. Don't dilute.
• Refrigerate parenteral form to prolong shelf life.
⊛ **ALERT:** Possibility of abuse and addiction exists. Don't abruptly stop giving the drug after long-term use. Withdrawal symptoms may occur.
⊛ **ALERT:** Don't confuse lorazepam with alprazolam or Lovaza.
Patient teaching
• Warn patient to avoid hazardous activities until the drug's CNS effects are known.
• Tell patient not to drink alcohol or smoke during therapy.
• Explain the risks of dependence and addiction with prolonged use of drug.
• Teach patient not to stop drug abruptly after prolonged use because of risk of seizures or other withdrawal symptoms.

☑ Evaluation
• Patient is less anxious.
• Patient doesn't experience injury as result of adverse CNS reactions.
• Patient and family state understanding of drug therapy.

losartan potassium
(loh-SAR-tan poh-TAH-see-um)
Cozaar◈

Pharmacologic class: angiotensin II receptor antagonist
Therapeutic class: antihypertensive
Pregnancy risk category: C (D in second and third trimesters)

Indications and dosages
▶ **Nephropathy in type 2 diabetes mellitus.**
Adults: 50 mg P.O. daily. Increase dose to 100 mg daily based on blood pressure response.
▶ **Hypertension.** *Adults:* Initially, 25 to 50 mg P.O. daily. Maximum, 100 mg daily in one or two divided doses.
▶ **To reduce risk of stroke in patients with hypertension and left ventricular hypertrophy.** *Adults:* Initially, 50 mg P.O. once daily. Adjust dosage based on blood pressure response, adding hydrochlorothiazide 12.5 mg once daily, increasing losartan to 100 mg daily, or both. If further adjustments are needed, may increase the daily dose of hydrochlorothiazide to 25 mg.
⧄ **Adjust-a-dose:** In patient with impaired liver function or volume depletion (such as patient taking diuretic), use initial dose of 25 mg.

Contraindications and cautions
• Contraindicated in patients hypersensitive to the drug or any of its components.
• Use cautiously in patients with impaired kidney or liver function and in volume-depleted, hypotensive patients.
⚘ **Lifespan:** In pregnant women, drug is contraindicated in second and third trimesters; use very cautiously in first trimester. If pregnancy occurs, stop drug as soon as possible. Breast-feeding women should stop breast-feeding or use another drug. In children, safety and effectiveness haven't been established.

Adverse reactions
For hypertension and left ventricular hypertrophy
CNS: asthenia, dizziness, fatigue, headache, insomnia.
CV: chest pain, edema.
EENT: nasal congestion, pharyngitis, sinus disorder, sinusitis.

GI: abdominal pain, diarrhea, dyspepsia, nausea.
Musculoskeletal: back or leg pain, muscle cramps, myalgia.
Respiratory: cough, upper respiratory tract infection.
Other: *anaphylaxis, angioedema.*
For nephropathy
CNS: *asthenia,* diabetic neuropathy, *fatigue,* fever, hypoesthesia.
CV: *chest pain, diabetic vascular disease,* hypotension, orthostatic hypotension.
EENT: cataract, sinusitis.
GI: *diarrhea,* dyspepsia, gastritis.
GU: UTI.
Hematologic: *anemia.*
Metabolic: *hyperkalemia,* HYPOGLYCEMIA, weight gain.
Musculoskeletal: *back pain,* leg or knee pain, muscle weakness.
Respiratory: *bronchitis,* cough.
Skin: cellulitis.
Other: *anaphylaxis, angioedema,* infection, *flulike syndrome,* trauma.

Interactions

Drug-drug. *Fluconazole:* May increase antihypertensive effects and adverse reactions. Monitor patient.
Indomethacin: May decrease hypotensive effect. Monitor blood pressure.
Phenobarbital: May decrease losartan absorption. Monitor patient.
Potassium-sparing diuretics, potassium supplements: May cause hyperkalemia. Monitor potassium level.
Rifamycins: May decrease antihypertensive effects. Monitor blood pressure.
Drug-herb. *Red yeast rice:* May increase the risk of adverse events or toxicity because herb contains components similar to those of statin drugs. Discourage use together.
Drug-food. *Salt substitutes containing potassium:* May increase risk of hyperkalemia. Monitor patient closely; advise patient to use only under prescriber's guidance.

Effects on lab test results

None reported.

Pharmacokinetics

Absorption: Good with extensive first-pass metabolism; systemic bioavailability of drug is 33%.
Distribution: Highly protein-bound.

Metabolism: Involves CYP2C9 and CYP3A4.
Excretion: Mainly in feces with smaller amount in urine. *Half-life:* 2 hours.

Route	Onset	Peak	Duration
P.O.	Unknown	1–4 hr	Unknown

Action

Chemical effect: Inhibits vasoconstricting and aldosterone-secreting effects of angiotensin II by selectively blocking binding of angiotensin II to receptor sites in many tissues, including vascular smooth muscle and adrenal glands.
Therapeutic effect: Lowers blood pressure.

Available forms

Tablets: 25 mg, 50 mg, 100 mg

NURSING PROCESS

Assessment
• Assess patient's blood pressure before starting therapy and regularly thereafter to monitor drug's effectiveness. When drug is used alone, its effect on blood pressure is notably less in black patients than in patients of other races.
• Regularly assess creatinine and BUN levels to check kidney function. Patients with severe heart failure whose kidney function depends on angiotensin-aldosterone system may develop acute renal impairment during therapy. Monitor patient closely, especially during first few weeks of therapy.
• Be alert for adverse reactions.
• If patient is taking a diuretic, watch for symptomatic hypotension.
• Assess patient's and family's knowledge of drug therapy.

Nursing diagnoses
• Risk for injury related to presence of hypertension
• Sleep deprivation related to drug-induced insomnia
• Deficient knowledge related to drug therapy

Planning and implementation
• Black patients with hypertension and left ventricular hypertrophy have a lower risk of stroke with atenolol than with this drug, but the cause is unknown.
• Drug can be used alone or with other antihypertensives.

• Determine trough level to measure effect. If giving once daily isn't effective, divide same total daily into two daily doses or increase dose.
• Give once-daily dose in the morning to prevent insomnia.
• If pregnancy is suspected, stop giving the drug and immediately notify prescriber.
⚠ **ALERT:** Don't confuse Cozaar with Zocor.

Patient teaching
• Tell patient to avoid sodium substitutes because they may contain potassium, which can cause hyperkalemia in patients taking drug.
• Tell woman of childbearing age to notify prescriber immediately if she suspects she is pregnant.

☑ **Evaluation**
• Patient's blood pressure is normal.
• Patient states that insomnia hasn't occurred.
• Patient and family state understanding of drug therapy.

lovastatin (mevinolin)
(loh-vuh-STAH-tin)
Altoprev, Mevacor✐

Pharmacologic class: HMG-CoA reductase inhibitor
Therapeutic class: cholesterol-lowering drug
Pregnancy risk category: X

Indications and dosages

▶ **Primary prevention of coronary artery disease; coronary artery disease; hyperlipidemia.** *Adults:* Initially, 20 mg immediate-release tablets P.O. once daily with evening meal. Recommended range is 10 to 80 mg in single or two divided doses; maximum dosage, 80 mg daily. Or 20 to 60 mg extended-release P.O. at bedtime. Starting dose of 10 mg can be used for patients requiring smaller reductions. Usual dosage range is 10 to 60 mg daily for the extended-release tablets.
▶ **Heterozygous familial hypercholesterolemia.** *Children ages 10 to 17:* Give 10 to 40 mg P.O. (immediate-release) daily with evening meal. In patients requiring reductions in LDL level of 20% or more, start with 20 mg daily.
▧ **Adjust-a-dose:** For patients also taking cyclosporine, give 10 mg P.O. daily, not to exceed 20 mg daily. Avoid use of drug with fibrates or

niacin; if used with either, don't give more than 20 mg of lovastatin daily. If using with amiodarone or verapamil (immediate-release), don't exceed 40 mg/day.
For patients with renal impairment, if creatinine clearance is less than 30 ml/minute, take care when considering dosage increase above 20 mg daily.

Contraindications and cautions

• Contraindicated in patients hypersensitive to the drug or any of its components, and in those with active liver disease or conditions linked to unexplained persistent elevations of transaminase levels.
• Use cautiously in patients who consume substantial quantities of alcohol or have history of liver disease.
⚘ **Lifespan:** In pregnant and breast-feeding women, drug is contraindicated. In women of childbearing age, drug is contraindicated unless they have no risk of pregnancy. In children younger than age 10, safety and effectiveness haven't been established.

Adverse reactions

CNS: dizziness, headache, peripheral neuropathy.
EENT: blurred vision.
GI: abdominal pain or cramps, constipation, diarrhea, dysgeusia, dyspepsia, flatulence, heartburn, nausea.
Musculoskeletal: muscle cramps, myalgia, myositis, *rhabdomyolysis.*
Skin: pruritus, rash.

Interactions

Drug-drug. *Bile acid sequestrants:* May decrease lovastatin bioavailability. Give separately.
Cyclosporine or other immunosuppressants, erythromycin, gemfibrozil, niacin: May increase risk of polymyositis and rhabdomyolysis. Monitor patient closely.
Digoxin: May slightly elevate digoxin level. Monitor patient.
Fluconazole, itraconazole, ketoconazole: May increase lovastatin level and adverse effects. Avoid this combination. If drugs must be given together, reduce lovastatin dosage.
Isradipine: May increase lovastatin clearance and its metabolites by increasing hepatic blood

flow. Monitor patient for loss of therapeutic effect.

Nicotinic acid: May increase risk of severe myopathy or rhabdomyolysis. Monitor patient closely.

Oral anticoagulants: May enhance oral anticoagulant effects. Monitor PT and INR.

Drug-herb. *Red yeast rice:* May increase risk of adverse events or toxicity because herb contains components similar to those of drug. Discourage use together.

Drug-lifestyle. *Alcohol use:* May increase risk of hepatotoxicity. Discourage use together.

Sun exposure: May cause photosensitivity reactions. Tell patient to avoid unprotected or prolonged exposure to sunlight.

Effects on lab test results

• May increase ALT, AST, and CK levels. May decrease lipid level.

Pharmacokinetics

Absorption: About 30%. Giving with food improves levels of total inhibitors by about 30%. Extended-release tablets have greater bioavailability than immediate-release tablets.

Distribution: Less than 5% because of extensive first-pass hepatic extraction. More than 95% protein-bound.

Metabolism: In liver.

Excretion: About 80% in feces, about 10% in urine. *Half-life:* 3 hours.

Route	Onset	Peak	Duration
P.O.	Unknown	2–6 hr	4–6 wk
P.O. Extended-release	Unknown	14 hr	Unknown

Action

Chemical effect: Inhibits HMG-CoA reductase. This enzyme is an early and rate-limiting step in synthetic pathway of cholesterol.

Therapeutic effect: Lowers LDL and total cholesterol levels.

Available forms

Tablets: 10 mg, 20 mg, 40 mg
Tablets (extended-release): 10 mg, 20 mg, 40 mg, 60 mg

NURSING PROCESS

⚖ Assessment

• Obtain history of patient's lipoprotein and cholesterol levels before starting therapy, and reassess regularly to monitor drug effectiveness.

• Use for heterozygous familial hypercholesterolemia in girls who are at least 1 year postmenarche and boys (ages 10 to 17) who have the following findings after an adequate trial of diet therapy: LDL level higher than 189 mg/dl or LDL level higher than 160 mg/dl with a family history of premature CV disease or two or more other CV disease risk factors.

• Perform liver function tests before starting therapy and periodically thereafter.

• Be alert for adverse reactions and drug interactions.

• Assess patient's and family's knowledge of drug therapy.

⚕ Nursing diagnoses

• Risk for injury related to underlying condition
• Acute pain related to drug-induced adverse musculoskeletal reactions
• Deficient knowledge related to drug therapy

▷ Planning and implementation

• Begin drug therapy only after diet and other nondrug therapies have proven ineffective. Make sure patient follows a low-cholesterol diet.

• Give drug with evening meal; absorption is enhanced and cholesterol biosynthesis is greater in evening.

⚠ ALERT: Don't confuse lovastatin with Lotensin, Leustatin, or Livostin. Don't confuse Mevacor with Mivacron.

Patient teaching

• Instruct patient to take drug with evening meal.

• Advise patient not to crush or chew extended-release tablets.

• Teach patient to manage lipid level by restricting total fat and cholesterol intake. If appropriate, recommend weight control, exercise, and smoking cessation programs to control other cardiac disease risk factors.

• Advise patient to have periodic eye examinations.

• Tell patient to store drug at room temperature in light-resistant container.

• Instruct patient to avoid alcohol consumption during drug therapy.

Reactions may be *common*, uncommon, *life-threatening*, or COMMON AND LIFE-THREATENING.

⊛ **ALERT:** Inform patient that drug is contraindicated during pregnancy. Tell her to notify prescriber immediately if she becomes pregnant.

☑ **Evaluation**
• Patient's LDL and cholesterol levels are within normal limits.
• Patient doesn't experience musculoskeletal pain.
• Patient and family state understanding of drug therapy.

lubiprostone
(loo-bee-PROSS-tohn)
Amitiza⌀

Pharmacologic class: chloride channel activator
Therapeutic class: laxative
Pregnancy risk category: C

Indications and dosages

▶ **Chronic idiopathic constipation.** *Adults:* 24 mcg P.O. b.i.d. with food.

Contraindications and cautions

• Contraindicated in patients hypersensitive to drug or its components and in those with a history of mechanical GI obstruction.
• Use cautiously in women who are or may become pregnant.
⚕ **Lifespan:** In pregnant patients, use only if benefits outweigh risks to fetus. In breast-feeding patients, mother should stop breast-feeding or stop drug therapy. In children, safety and effectiveness haven't been established. In elderly patients, use cautiously due to increased likelihood of hepatic or renal insufficiency.

Adverse reactions

CNS: anxiety, depression, dizziness, fatigue, *headache,* insomnia, pyrexia.
CV: chest pain, peripheral edema.
EENT: nasopharyngitis, pharyngolaryngeal pain, sinusitis.
GI: abdominal distention, abdominal pain or discomfort, constipation*, diarrhea,* dry mouth, dyspepsia, flatulence, gastroesophageal reflux disease, loose stools, *nausea,* stomach discomfort, viral gastroenteritis, vomiting.
GU: UTI.
Metabolic: weight gain.

Musculoskeletal: arthralgia, back pain, limb pain, muscle cramps.
Respiratory: bronchitis, cough, dyspnea, upper respiratory tract infection.
Other: influenza.

Interactions

None reported.

Effects on lab test results

None reported.

Pharmacokinetics

Absorption: Low systemic availability.
Distribution: 94% bound to plasma proteins.
Metabolism: Rapid and extensive in stomach and jejunum.
Excretion: Trace amount in feces. *Half-life:* Unknown.

Route	Onset	Peak	Duration
P.O.	Unknown	1 hr	Unknown

Action

Chemical effect: Increases intestinal fluid secretion by activating chloride channels, and increases intestinal motility.
Therapeutic effect: Relieves constipation.

Available forms

Capsules: 24 mcg

NURSING PROCESS

▦ **Assessment**
• Obtain history of bowel disorder, GI status, fluid intake, nutritional status, exercise habits, and normal patterns of elimination.
• Monitor effectiveness by checking frequency and characteristics of stools. Relief is defined as three or more spontaneous bowel movements weekly.
• Be alert for adverse reactions. Nausea, diarrhea, and headache are the most common.
• Assess patient's and family's understanding of drug therapy.

⊞ **Nursing diagnoses**
• Constipation related to interruption of normal pattern of elimination
• Risk for deficient fluid volume due to drug-induced diarrhea
• Deficient knowledge related to drug therapy

⬧ Planning and implementation
• Auscultate bowel sounds at least once per shift. Check for pain and cramping.
• Don't give drug to a patient with severe diarrhea.
Patient teaching
• Tell patient to take drug with food.
• Explain that patient may have diarrhea during treatment; advise against taking the drug if he develops severe diarrhea.
• Advise patient about a proper diet and the need to drink plenty of fluids.

☑ Evaluation
• Patient reports return of normal bowel pattern of elimination.
• Patient is free from deficient fluid volume.
• Patient and family state understanding of drug therapy.

lymphocyte immune globulin (LIG) (antithymocyte globulin [equine], ATG)
(LIM-foh-sight ih-MYOON GLOH-byoo-lin)
Atgam

Pharmacologic class: immunoglobulin
Therapeutic class: immunosuppressant
Pregnancy risk category: C

Indications and dosages
▶ **To prevent acute renal allograft rejection.**
Adults and children: 15 mg/kg I.V. daily for 14 days, followed by alternate-day doses for 14 days. Give first dose within 24 hours of transplantation.
▶ **Acute renal allograft rejection.** *Adults and children:* 10 to 15 mg/kg I.V. daily for 14 days, followed by alternate-day doses for 14 days. Start therapy when rejection is diagnosed.
▶ **Aplastic anemia.** *Adults:* 10 to 20 mg/kg I.V. daily for 8 to 14 days. Additional alternate-day therapy up to total of 21 doses can be given.
▶ **Skin allotransplantation** ‡. *Adults:* 10 mg/ kg I.V. 24 hours before allograft; then 10 to 15 mg/kg every other day. Maintenance dosage ranges from 5 to 40 mg/kg daily based on response. Therapy usually continues until allograft covers less than 20% of total body surface area, usually 40 to 60 days.

▼ I.V. administration
• Dilute dose in 250 to 1,000 ml of half-normal or normal saline solution for injection. Don't exceed final concentration of 4 mg/ml. When adding drug to solution, make sure container is inverted so drug doesn't contact air inside container. The proteins in drug can be denatured by air. Gently rotate or swirl container to mix contents; don't shake because this may cause excessive foaming and may alter drug.
• Allow diluted drug to reach room temperature before infusion.
• Infuse with in-line filter with pore size of 0.2 to 1 micron over no less than 4 hours (most facilities specify 4 to 8 hours) into a vascular shunt, arterial venous fistula, or high-flow central vein.
• Don't use solutions that are more than 12 hours old, including actual infusion time.
• Refrigerate drug at 35° to 47° F (2° to 8° C). Don't freeze. Drug is heat sensitive.
⊗ **Incompatibilities**
Acidic solutions, dextrose solutions, solutions with low salt concentration.

Contraindications and cautions
• Contraindicated in patients hypersensitive to the drug or any of its components.
• Use cautiously in patients receiving additional immunosuppressive therapy (such as corticosteroids and azathioprine) because of increased risk of infection.
⚖ Lifespan: In pregnant women, use cautiously. In breast-feeding women, drug isn't recommended because it's unknown if drug is excreted in breast milk.

Adverse reactions
CNS: headache, malaise, *seizures.*
CV: *chest pain,* edema, *hypotension, iliac vein obstruction,* renal artery stenosis, tachycardia, thrombophlebitis.
EENT: laryngospasm.
GI: abdominal distention, diarrhea, epigastric pain, *nausea,* stomatitis, *vomiting.*
Hematologic: *aplastic anemia,* hemolysis, *leukopenia,* lymphadenopathy, *thrombocytopenia.*
Metabolic: hyperglycemia.
Musculoskeletal: arthralgia.
Respiratory: *dyspnea,* hiccups, *pulmonary edema.*
Skin: rash.

Reactions may be *common,* uncommon, *life-threatening,* or COMMON AND LIFE-THREATENING.

Other: *anaphylaxis,* febrile reactions, infection, night sweats, serum sickness.

Interactions

Drug-drug. *Immunosuppressants, muromonab-CD3:* May increase risk of infection. Monitor patient closely.

Effects on lab test results

• May increase liver enzyme and glucose levels. May decrease hemoglobin level and hematocrit.
• May decrease WBC and platelet counts.

Pharmacokinetics

Absorption: Given I.V.
Distribution: Unknown.
Metabolism: Unknown.
Excretion: About 1% in urine, mainly as unchanged drug. *Half-life:* About 6 days.

Route	Onset	Peak	Duration
I.V.	Unknown	5 days	Unknown

Action

Chemical effect: Inhibits cell-mediated immune responses by either altering T-cell function or eliminating antigen-reactive T cells.
Therapeutic effect: Prevents or relieves evidence of renal allograft rejection; also relieves signs and symptoms of aplastic anemia.

Available forms

Injection: 50 mg of equine immunoglobulin/ml

NURSING PROCESS

Assessment

• Assess patient's condition before starting therapy and regularly thereafter to monitor drug effectiveness.
• Be alert for adverse reactions and drug interactions.
• Assess patient's and family's knowledge of drug therapy.

Nursing diagnoses

• Ineffective health maintenance related to underlying condition
• Ineffective immune protection related to adverse hematologic reactions
• Deficient knowledge related to drug therapy

Planning and implementation

• Perform an intradermal skin test at least 1 hour before giving the first dose. Marked local swelling or erythema larger than 10 mm indicates increased risk of severe systemic reaction, such as anaphylaxis. Severe reactions to skin test, such as hypotension, tachycardia, dyspnea, generalized rash, or anaphylaxis, rule out further use.
⚠ ALERT: Keep airway adjuncts and anaphylaxis drugs at bedside while giving the drug.
Patient teaching
• Warn patient that he'll likely develop a fever. Instruct him to report adverse drug effects.
• Instruct patient to take infection-control and bleeding precautions.

Evaluation

• Patient responds well to therapy.
• Patient doesn't experience serious adverse hematologic reactions.
• Patient and family state understanding of drug therapy.

HIGH ALERT

magnesium chloride
(mag-NEE-see-um KLOR-ighd)
Chloromag, Slow-Mag†

magnesium sulfate

Pharmacologic class: magnesium salts
Therapeutic class: anticonvulsant, mineral, antiarrhythmic
Pregnancy risk category: A

Indications and dosages

▶ **Mild hypomagnesemia.** *Adults:* 1 g I.M. every 6 hours for four doses, depending on magnesium level.
▶ **Severe hypomagnesemia (magnesium level 0.8 mEq/L or less with symptoms).** *Adults:* Up to 2 mEq (0.5 ml of 50% solution)/kg I.M. within a 4-hour period may be given, or 5 g (about 40 mEq) I.V. in 1 L of solution over 3 hours. Subsequent doses depend on magnesium level.

▶ **Magnesium supplementation.** *Adults:* 54 to 483 mg P.O. daily in divided doses (chloride form only).

▶ **Magnesium supplementation in total parenteral nutrition (TPN).** *Adults:* 8 to 24 mEq I.V. daily added to TPN solution. *Infants:* 2 to 10 mEq I.V. daily added to TPN solution. Each 2 ml of 50% solution contains 1 g, or 8.12 mEq, magnesium sulfate.

▶ **Hypomagnesemic seizures.** *Adults:* 1 to 2 g of 10% solution I.V. over 15 minutes; then 1 g I.M. every 4 to 6 hours, based on patient's response and magnesium level.

▶ **Seizures caused by hypomagnesemia in acute nephritis.** *Children:* 20 to 40 mg/kg I.M. p.r.n. to control seizures. Dilute the 50% concentration to a 20% solution and give 0.1 to 0.2 ml/kg of the 20% solution. Or, 100 to 200 mg/kg as a 1% to 3% solution I.V. slowly over one hour with 50% of dose given in first 15 to 20 minutes. Adjust dosage according to magnesium level and seizure response.

▶ **Paroxysmal atrial tachycardia in patients unresponsive to other therapies‡.** *Adults:* 3 to 4 g I.V. of 10% solution over 30 seconds with close monitoring of ECG.

▶ **To reduce CV morbidity and mortality from acute MI‡.** *Adults:* 2 g I.V. over 5 to 15 minutes, followed by infusion of 18 g over 24 hours (12.5 mg/minute). Start as soon as possible, and no longer than 6 hours after MI.

▶ **To manage preterm labor‡.** *Adults:* 4 to 6 g I.V. over 20 minutes as a loading dose, followed by maintenance infusions of 2 to 4 g/hour for 12 to 24 hours, as tolerated, after contractions subside.

▶ **Severe acute asthma unresponsive to conventional therapy‡.** *Children:* 25 to 50 mg/kg (up to 2 g) I.V. over 10 to 20 minutes.

▼ I.V. administration

• Solutions must be diluted to 20% (200 mg/ml) or less before administration.

• Inject I.V. bolus dose slowly. Use infusion pump for continuous infusion to avoid respiratory or cardiac arrest. Don't exceed 150 mg/minute (1.5 ml of a 10% solution). Rapid drip causes heat sensation.

• When giving I.V. for severe hypomagnesemia, watch for respiratory depression and evidence of heart block. Give dose only when respirations are more than 16 breaths/minute.

• Monitor vital signs every 15 minutes when giving drug I.V.

• For preterm labor, monitor I.V. fluids and rates carefully to avoid circulatory overload. Monitor patient for pulmonary edema.

⊗ **Incompatibilities**
Alcohol in high concentrations, alkali carbonates and bicarbonates, amiodarone, amphotericin B, arsenates, barium, calcium gluconate, cefepime, ciprofloxacin, clindamycin, cyclosporine, dobutamine, ethanol, heavy metals, hydrocortisone sodium succinate, I.V. fat emulsion 10%, polymyxin B, procaine, salicylates, sodium bicarbonate, soluble phosphates, tartrates.

Contraindications and cautions

• Contraindicated in patients with myocardial damage, marked myocardial disease, or heart block. I.V. form is contraindicated in patients with preeclampsia during the 2 hours preceding delivery. Magnesium chloride is contraindicated in patients with renal impairment.

• Use magnesium sulfate cautiously in patients with impaired kidney function.

⚖ **Lifespan:** Use during all trimesters of pregnancy if clearly needed except during active labor when drug is contraindicated. Continuous I.V. infusion longer than 24 hours in toxemic mothers may cause neonatal magnesium toxicity. In breast-feeding women small amount of drug is excreted in breast milk but use if clearly needed. Elderly patients may need a lower dose because of renal insufficiency. If patient is severely renally impaired, don't exceed 20 g in 48 hours.

Adverse reactions

CNS: *depressed deep tendon reflexes,* drowsiness, flaccid paralysis, hypothermia, perioral paresthesia, *seizures,* tetany, twitching carpopedal spasm.
CV: *arrhythmias; circulatory collapse; depressed cardiac function; heart block;* hypotension; *slow, weak pulse.*
Metabolic: hypocalcemia.
Respiratory: *respiratory paralysis.*
Other: diaphoresis, flushing.

Interactions

Drug-drug. *Anesthetics, CNS depressants:* May cause additive CNS depression. Use together cautiously.

Reactions may be *common,* uncommon, *life-threatening,* or COMMON AND LIFE-THREATENING.

Digoxin: May cause serious cardiac conduction changes. Give cautiously.

Neuromuscular blockers: May increase neuromuscular blockage. Use cautiously; monitor patient for increased effects.

Nitrofurantoin, penicillamine, tetracyclines: May decrease bioavailability with oral magnesium supplements. Separate doses by 2 to 3 hours.

Effects on lab test results

• May increase magnesium level. May decrease calcium and potassium levels.

Pharmacokinetics

Absorption: 35% to 40% of P.O. dose. High-fat diets may interfere.

Distribution: About 30% is bound intracellularly to proteins and energy-rich phosphates.

Metabolism: None.

Excretion: Parenteral dose mainly in urine, P.O. dose in urine and feces. *Half-life:* Unknown.

Route	Onset	Peak	Duration
P.O.	Unknown	4 hr	4–6 hr
I.V.	Immediate	Unknown	30 min
I.M.	1 hr	Unknown	3–4 hr

Action

Chemical effect: Replaces and maintains magnesium levels; as anticonvulsant, reduces muscle contractions by interfering with release of acetylcholine at myoneural junction.

Therapeutic effect: Raises magnesium levels, alleviates seizures, and restores normal sinus rhythm.

Available forms

magnesium chloride

Injectable solutions: 20% (1.97 mEq/ml)

Tablets (delayed-release): 64 mg elemental magnesium

magnesium sulfate

Injectable solutions: 10% (0.8 mEq/ml), 12.5% (1 mEq/ml), 50% (4 mEq/ml)

NURSING PROCESS

📝 Assessment

• Assess patient's condition before therapy and regularly thereafter to monitor drug effectiveness.

• Check magnesium level after repeated doses.

🛑 **ALERT:** Watch for respiratory depression and signs of heart block. Make sure respirations are 16 breaths/minute before each dose.

• Monitor patient's fluid intake and output. Make sure output is 100 ml or more during the 4 hours before giving.

• Be alert for adverse reactions and drug interactions.

• Assess patient's and family's knowledge of drug therapy.

🔋 Nursing diagnoses

• Ineffective health maintenance related to underlying condition

• Risk for injury related to drug-induced adverse reactions

• Deficient knowledge related to drug therapy

➤ Planning and implementation

• Keep I.V. calcium gluconate available at bedside to reverse magnesium intoxication.

• For cases of severe hypermagnesemia, peritoneal dialysis or hemodialysis may be needed.

• Undiluted 50% solutions may be given to adults by deep I.M. injection. When giving to children, dilute solutions to 20% or less.

🛑 **ALERT:** Test knee-jerk (patellar) reflexes before each additional dose. If no reflex, notify prescriber and withhold magnesium until reflexes return. Check magnesium level because it may be toxic. Signs of hypermagnesemia begin to appear at a level of 4 mEq/L.

• If used to treat seizures, take appropriate seizure precautions.

Patient teaching

• Instruct patient taking parenteral drug to immediately report any adverse reactions.

• Review oral administration schedule with patient. Tell him not to take more than prescribed.

✓ Evaluation

• Patient has positive response to drug administration.

• Patient sustains no injury from adverse reactions.

• Patient and family state understanding of drug therapy.

magnesium citrate (citrate of magnesia)
(mag-NEE-see-um SIH-trayt)

magnesium hydroxide
Dulcolax†, Milk of Magnesia†, Milk of Magnesia Concentrated†, Phillips' Chewable†, Phillips' Milk of Magnesia†, Phillips' Milk of Magnesia Concentrated†

magnesium sulfate
Epsom salts†

Pharmacologic class: magnesium salts
Therapeutic class: saline laxatives
Pregnancy risk category: NR

Indications and dosages

▶ **Constipation, to evacuate bowel before surgery.** *Adults and children age 12 and older:* 11 to 25 g magnesium citrate P.O. daily as single dose or divided. Or 2 to 4 tbs magnesium hydroxide at bedtime or on rising, followed by 240 ml (8 oz) of liquid. Or 10 to 30 g magnesium sulfate P.O. daily as single dose or divided.
Children ages 6 to 11: Give 5.5 to 12.5 g magnesium citrate P.O. daily as single dose or divided. Or 1 to 2 tbs magnesium hydroxide followed by 240 ml (8 oz) of liquid. Don't use dosage cup. Or 5 to 10 g magnesium sulfate P.O. daily as single dose or divided.
Children ages 2 to 5: Give 2.7 to 6.25 g magnesium citrate P.O. daily as single dose or divided. Or 1 to 3 tsp magnesium hydroxide followed by 240 ml (8 oz) of liquid. Don't use dosage cup. Or 2.5 to 5 g magnesium sulfate P.O. daily as single dose or divided.

▶ **Acid indigestion, gastroesophageal reflux disease, peptic ulcer disease, heartburn.**
Adults and children age 12 and older: Don't use dosage cup. 1 to 3 tsp magnesium hydroxide with a little water, up to q.i.d., or as directed by prescriber. Or, for adults, 5 to 15 ml magnesium citrate P.O. t.i.d. or q.i.d.

Contraindications and cautions

• Contraindicated in patients with abdominal pain, nausea, vomiting, other symptoms of appendicitis or acute surgical abdomen, myocardial damage, heart block, fecal impaction, rectal fissures, intestinal obstruction or perforation, or renal disease.
• Use cautiously in patients with rectal bleeding.
☀ **Lifespan:** In pregnant women, use cautiously. During labor and delivery, drug is contraindicated. In breast-feeding women, use cautiously; small amounts of the drug appears in breast milk. In children, use cautiously.

Adverse reactions

GI: *abdominal cramping, diarrhea,* laxative dependence with long-term or excessive use, *nausea.*
Metabolic: fluid and electrolyte disturbances.

Interactions

Drug-drug. *Benzodiazepines, chloroquine, corticosteroids, digoxin, H_2 antagonists, hydantoins, iron, nitrofurantoin, penicillamine, phenothiazines, tetracyclines:* May decrease pharmacologic effects of these drugs. Monitor patient.
Ciprofloxacin, levofloxacin, lomefloxacin, moxifloxacin, norfloxacin, ofloxacin: May decrease effects of quinolones. Give drug at least 6 hours before or 2 hours after quinolones.
Dicumarol, quinidine, sulfonylureas: May increase effects of these drugs. Monitor patient.
Oral drugs: May impair absorption. Separate doses.

Effects on lab test results

• May increase or decrease fluid and electrolyte levels with prolonged use.

Pharmacokinetics

Absorption: About 15% to 30% may be systemic (posing risk to patients with renal impairment).
Distribution: Unknown.
Metabolism: Unknown.
Excretion: Unabsorbed drug in feces; absorbed drug rapidly in urine. *Half-life:* Unknown.

Route	Onset	Peak	Duration
P.O.	30 min–3 hr	Varies	Varies

Action

Chemical effect: Reduces total acid load in GI tract, elevates gastric pH to inhibit pepsin, strengthens gastric mucosal barrier, and increases esophageal sphincter tone.

Therapeutic effect: Soothes stomach upset, relieves constipation, and raises magnesium level.

Available forms

magnesium citrate
Oral solution: about 3.85 to 4.71 mEq magnesium/5 ml†
magnesium hydroxide
Liquid: 400 mg/5 ml†, 800 mg/5 ml†
Tablets (chewable): 311 mg†
magnesium sulfate
Granules: about 40 mEq magnesium/5 g†

NURSING PROCESS

Assessment
• Assess patient's condition before therapy and regularly thereafter to monitor drug effectiveness.
• Before giving drug for constipation, determine whether patient has adequate fluid intake, exercise, and diet.
ALERT: Monitor electrolyte levels during prolonged use. Magnesium may accumulate in patients with renal insufficiency.
• Be alert for adverse reactions and drug interactions.
• Assess patient's and family's knowledge of drug therapy.

Nursing diagnoses
• Constipation related to underlying condition
• Diarrhea related to therapy
• Deficient knowledge related to drug therapy

Planning and implementation
• Give the drug at a time that doesn't interfere with scheduled activities or sleep.
• Chill magnesium citrate before use to improve its palatability.
• Shake suspension well. Give with large amount of water when used as laxative. When giving through NG tube, make sure tube is placed properly and is patent. After instilling drug, flush tube with water to ensure passage to stomach and to maintain tube patency.
ALERT: Drug is for short-term therapy only.
• Magnesium sulfate is more potent than other saline laxatives.
Patient teaching
• Teach patient about dietary sources of bulk, such as bran, other high-fiber cereals, and fresh fruit and vegetables.

• Warn patient that frequent or prolonged use may cause dependence.

Evaluation
• Patient's constipation is relieved.
• Diarrhea doesn't develop.
• Patient and family state understanding of drug therapy.

magnesium oxide
(mag-NEE-see-um OKS-ighd)
Mag-Caps†, Mag-Ox 400†, Maox 420†, Uro-Mag†

Pharmacologic class: magnesium salt
Therapeutic class: antacid, mineral
Pregnancy risk category: NR

Indications and dosages
▶ **Antacid.** *Adults:* 140 mg (capsules) P.O. 3 to 4 times daily, or 400 to 800 mg (tablets) daily.
▶ **Mild hypomagnesemia.** *Adults:* 400 to 840 mg P.O. daily based on magnesium level.

Contraindications and cautions
• In patients with renal disease, use cautiously and under the supervision of a physician.
Lifespan: In pregnant women, use cautiously. In breast-feeding women, use cautiously; it's unknown if the drug appears in breast milk.

Adverse reactions
GI: abdominal pain, *diarrhea,* nausea.
Metabolic: hypermagnesemia.

Interactions
Drug-drug. *Allopurinol, antibiotics (including fluoroquinolones and tetracyclines), diflunisal, digoxin, iron, isoniazid, penicillamine, phenothiazines, quinidine:* May decrease pharmacologic effect, possibly because of impaired absorption. Separate doses.
Enteric-coated drugs: May release prematurely in stomach. Separate doses by at least 1 hour.

Effects on lab test results
• May increase magnesium level.

Pharmacokinetics
Absorption: Small.
Distribution: Unknown.

Metabolism: None.
Excretion: Unabsorbed drug in feces; absorbed drug in urine. *Half-life:* Unknown.

Route	Onset	Peak	Duration
P.O.			
Fasting	20 min	Unknown	20–60 min
Nonfasting	20 min	Unknown	20–60 min

Action

Chemical effect: Reduces total acid load in GI tract, elevates gastric pH to inhibit pepsin, strengthens gastric mucosal barrier, and increases esophageal sphincter tone.
Therapeutic effect: Soothes stomach upset, relieves constipation, and raises magnesium level.

Available forms

Capsules: 140 mg (84.5 mg elemental magnesium)†
Tablets: 400 mg (241.3 mg elemental magnesium)†, 420 mg†, 500 mg†

NURSING PROCESS

🔹 Assessment
• Assess patient's condition before therapy and regularly thereafter to monitor drug effectiveness.
🔹 **ALERT:** Monitor magnesium level. In a patient with renal impairment on long-term therapy, watch for signs and symptoms of hypermagnesemia (hypotension, nausea, vomiting, depressed reflexes, respiratory depression, and coma).
• Be alert for adverse reactions and drug interactions.
• Assess patient's and family's knowledge of drug therapy.

🔹 Nursing diagnoses
• Ineffective health maintenance related to underlying condition
• Risk for injury related to potential for hypermagnesemia
• Deficient knowledge related to drug therapy

🔹 Planning and implementation
• Don't give other oral drugs 1 to 2 hours before or after therapy.
• If patient has diarrhea, use a different drug.

Patient teaching
• Advise patient not to take drug indiscriminately or to switch antacids without prescriber's advice.

☑ Evaluation
• Patient responds well to therapy.
• Patient maintains normal magnesium level throughout therapy.
• Patient and family state understanding of drug therapy.

mannitol
(MAN-ih-tol)
Osmitrol, Resectisol

Pharmacologic class: osmotic diuretic
Therapeutic class: diuretic
Pregnancy risk category: C

Indications and dosages

▶ **Test dose for marked oliguria or suspected inadequate kidney function.** *Adults and children older than age 12:* Give 200 mg/kg or 12.5 g as 15% or 20% I.V. solution over 3 to 5 minutes. Response is adequate if 30 to 50 ml of urine/hour is excreted over 2 to 3 hours. If response is inadequate, give second test dose. If still no response after second dose, stop drug. *Children age 12 and younger‡:* 200 mg/kg or 6 g/m² I.V. as a 15% or 20% solution over 3 to 5 minutes. Measure response adequacy as above.
▶ **Oliguria.** *Adults and children older than age 12:* Give 50 to 100 g I.V. of a 15% to 25% solution.
Children age 12 and younger‡: 2 g/kg or 60 g/m² I.V. as a 15% or 20% solution.
▶ **To prevent oliguria or acute renal impairment.** *Adults and children older than age 12:* Give 50 to 100 g I.V. of concentrated solution, followed by 5% to 10% solution. Exact concentration determined by fluid requirements.
▶ **Edema; ascites caused by renal, hepatic, or cardiac failure.** *Adults and children older than age 12:* Give 100 g I.V. as 10% to 20% solution over 2 to 6 hours.
Children age 12 and younger‡: 2 g/kg or 60 g/m² I.V. as a 15% or 20% solution over 2 to 6 hours.

Reactions may be *common*, uncommon, *life-threatening*, or **COMMON AND LIFE-THREATENING**.

▶ **To reduce intraocular or intracranial pressure.** *Adults and children older than age 12:* Give 1.5 to 2 g/kg as 15% to 25% I.V. solution over 30 to 60 minutes.
Children age 12 and younger‡: 2 g/kg or 60 g/m² I.V. as a 15% or 20% solution over 30 to 60 minutes.
▶ **Diuresis in drug intoxication.** *Adults and children older than age 12:* Concentration depends on fluid requirement and urine output. If benefit not seen after 200 mg, discontinue infusion.
Children age 12 and younger‡: 2 g/kg or 60 g/m² I.V. as a 5% or 10% solution, p.r.n.
▶ **Irrigating solution during transurethral resection of prostate.** *Adults:* 2.5% solution, p.r.n.

▼ I.V. administration

• Crystals may form in solution at low temperatures or in concentrations greater than 15%. To dissolve, warm bottle in hot water bath and shake vigorously. Cool to body temperature before giving. Don't use solution with undissolved crystals.
• Give as intermittent or continuous infusion, using in-line filter and infusion pump. Direct injection isn't recommended. Check I.V. line patency at infusion site before and during administration.
• Watch for signs of infiltration, including inflammation, edema, and necrosis.
⊗ **Incompatibilities**
Blood products, cefepime, doxorubicin liposomal, filgrastim, imipenem-cilastatin, meropenem, potassium chloride, sodium chloride, strongly acidic or alkaline solutions.

Contraindications and cautions

• Contraindicated in patients hypersensitive to the drug or any of its components, and in those with anuria, severe pulmonary congestion, frank pulmonary edema, severe heart failure, severe dehydration, metabolic edema, progressive renal disease or dysfunction, or active intracranial bleeding except during craniotomy.
⚱ **Lifespan:** In pregnant women, use cautiously. In breast-feeding women, use cautiously; it's unknown if drug appears in breast milk.

Adverse reactions

CNS: headache, confusion, *seizures.*
CV: *circulatory overload, heart failure,* tachycardia; chest pain.

EENT: blurred vision, rhinitis.
GI: thirst, nausea, vomiting, *diarrhea.*
GU: urine retention.
Metabolic: *water intoxication,* cellular dehydration, electrolyte imbalances.

Interactions

Drug-drug. *Lithium:* Increases urinary excretion of lithium. Monitor patient closely; monitor lithium level.

Effects on lab test results

• May cause electrolyte imbalance.

Pharmacokinetics

Absorption: Given I.V.
Distribution: Remains in extracellular compartment; doesn't cross blood-brain barrier.
Metabolism: Minimal.
Excretion: In urine. *Half-life:* About 1½ hours.

Route	Onset	Peak	Duration
I.V.	30–60 min	≤ 1 hr	6–8 hr

Action

Chemical effect: Increases osmotic pressure of glomerular filtrate, inhibiting tubular reabsorption of water and electrolytes. This elevates blood osmolality, enhancing water and sodium flow into extracellular fluid.
Therapeutic effect: Increases water excretion, decreases intracranial or intraocular pressure, prevents or treats kidney dysfunction, and promotes excretion of drug overdosage.

Available forms

Injection: 5%, 10%, 15%, 20%, 25%
Irrigation solution: 5 g/100 ml

NURSING PROCESS

Assessment
• Assess patient's condition before therapy and regularly thereafter to monitor the drug's effectiveness.
• Monitor vital signs, central venous pressure, and fluid intake and output hourly. Insert urethral catheter in comatose or incontinent patient because therapy is based on strict evaluation of fluid intake and output. In patient with urethral catheter, use hourly urometer collection bag for accurate evaluation.

• Monitor weight and kidney function, as well as serum and urine sodium and potassium levels, daily.
• Be alert for adverse reactions and drug interactions.
• Assess patient's and family's knowledge of drug therapy.

🔯 Nursing diagnoses
• Ineffective health maintenance related to underlying condition
• Risk for deficient fluid volume related to drug-induced adverse GI reactions
• Deficient knowledge related to drug therapy

▷ Planning and implementation
• For maximum intraocular pressure reduction before surgery, give 1 to 1¼ hours before surgery.
• When used as irrigating solution for prostate surgery, a concentration of 3.5% or greater is needed to avoid hemolysis.
• If patient's oliguria increases or he has adverse reactions, notify prescriber immediately.
Patient teaching
• Tell patient he may feel thirsty or have a dry mouth, and emphasize the importance of drinking only the amount of fluid provided.
• Instruct patient to immediately report pain in chest, back, or legs, or shortness of breath.

☑ Evaluation
• Patient responds well to mannitol.
• Patient maintains adequate hydration throughout therapy.
• Patient and family state understanding of drug therapy.

✳ New Drug

maraviroc
(MAHR-ay-vih-rowk)
Selzentry

Pharmacologic class: CCR5 coreceptor antagonist
Therapeutic class: antiretroviral
Pregnancy risk category: B

Indications and dosages

▶ **Combination treatment of CCR5-tropic HIV-1 with evidence of viral replication and resistant to multiple agents with CYP3A4 in-** hibitors or strong CYP3A inhibitors. *Adults:* 150 mg P.O. b.i.d.
▶ **Combination treatment of CCR5-tropic HIV-1 with evidence of viral replication and resistant to multiple agents with nucleoside reverse transcriptase inhibitors, or other drugs that are not strong CYP3A inhibitors or CYP3A inducers.** *Adults:* 300 mg P.O. b.i.d.
▶ **Combination treatment of CCR5-tropic HIV-1 with evidence of viral replication and resistant to multiple agents with CYP3A inducers, without a strong CYP3A inhibitor.** *Adults:* 600 mg P.O. b.i.d.

Contraindications and cautions
• Contraindicated in patients with dual, mixed, or CXCR4-tropic HIV-1.
• Contraindicated in treatment-naïve patients.
• Use cautiously in patients with preexisting liver dysfunction, those patients who are coinfected with viral hepatitis B or C, those at risk for CV events, those with a history of postural hypotension, and those also taking a drug known to lower blood pressure.
🜍 **Lifespan:** In pregnant women, use only if the potential benefit justifies the risk to the fetus. To avoid risk of postnatal transmission of HIV infection and serious adverse reactions, an HIV-infected mother shouldn't breast-feed her infant. In children younger than age 16, safety hasn't been established. In elderly patients with diminished hepatic and renal function, use with caution.

Adverse reactions

CNS: dizziness, paresthesias, sensory abnormalities, peripheral neuropathy.
CV: unstable angina, *acute cardiac failure,* coronary artery disease, *myocardial infarction,* myocardial ischemia.
GI: abdominal pain, constipation, dyspepsia, stomatitis, appetite disorders.
Hepatic: *cirrhosis*, *hepatic failure,* cholestatic jaundice.
Metabolic: lipodystrophies.
Musculoskeletal: muscle pains, myositis, osteonecrosis, *rhabdomyolysis.*
Respiratory: *upper respiratory tract infection,* bronchitis, sinusitis, *cough.*
Skin: rash, pruritus, dermatitis, eczema.
Other: *pyrexia,* herpes infection.

Reactions may be *common,* uncommon, *life-threatening,* or COMMON AND LIFE-THREATENING.

Interactions

Drug-drug. *Clarithromycin; CYP3A inhibitors; delavirdine; itraconazole; ketoconazole; nefazodone; protease inhibitors, except tipranavir and ritonavir; telithromycin:* May increase levels of maraviroc. Maraviroc dose should be decreased.
CYP3A inducers including efavirenz: May decrease the levels of maraviroc. Maraviroc dose should be increased.
Drug-herb. *St. John's wort:* May decrease maraviroc levels and lead to a loss of virologic response and possible resistance to maraviroc. Using together isn't recommended.

Effects on lab test results

• May increase AST, ALT, total bilirubin, amylase and lipase levels.
• May decrease absolute neutrophil count.

Pharmacokinetics

Absorption: Bioavailability is 23% to 33%.
Distribution: 76% protein-bound.
Metabolism: By CYP3A to inactive metabolites.
Excretion: 20% excreted in the urine, and 76% excreted in the feces. *Half-life:* 14 to 18 hours.

Route	Onset	Peak	Duration
P.O.	Unknown	½ to 4 hr	Unknown

Action

Chemical effect: Blocks viral entry into cells by binding to CCR5 receptor, preventing the initiation of HIV replication.
Therapeutic effect: To treat HIV infection.

Available forms

Tablets: 150 mg, 300 mg

NURSING PROCESS

Assessment
• Monitor cardiac status during therapy.
• Test women for pregnancy before therapy.
• Monitor liver function tests periodically during therapy.
• Assess patient's and family's knowledge of drug therapy.

Nursing diagnoses
• Ineffective protection related to underlying HIV infection

• Risk for injury related to adverse reactions
• Deficient knowledge related to drug therapy

Planning and implementation
• Patients should be monitored closely for signs and symptoms of infection during therapy.
• In a patient with signs or symptoms of hepatitis or with increased liver enzymes combined with rash or other systemic symptoms, consider stopping drug.
• Treatment of overdose should include general supportive measures and careful assessment of patient vital signs, blood pressure and ECG. Drug may be removed by hemodialysis.
• To monitor maternal-fetal outcomes of pregnant women, register patients in the Antiretroviral Pregnancy Registry by calling 1-800-258-4263.

Patient teaching
• Instruct patient to promptly report signs or symptoms of hepatitis or allergic reaction (rash, yellow eyes or skin, dark urine, vomiting, abdominal pain).
• Caution patient that drug isn't a cure for HIV infection and that he may still develop illness associated with HIV infection, including opportunistic infections.
• Caution patient that drug hasn't been shown to reduce the risk of transmission of HIV to others through sexual contact, sharing needles, or blood contamination.
• Advise patient that he should avoid driving or operating machinery if he experiences dizziness during therapy.
• Instruct woman to inform her physician if she is pregnant or plans to become pregnant during therapy.
• Instruct patient to take daily as prescribed. He shouldn't stop, change dose, or change schedule without consulting prescriber.

Evaluation
• Patient remains free from infection.
• Patient sustains no injury from adverse reactions.
• Patient and family state understanding of drug therapy.

mebendazole
(meh-BEN-duh-zohl)
Vermox

Pharmacologic class: benzimidazole
Therapeutic class: anthelmintic
Pregnancy risk category: C

Indications and dosages

▶ **Pinworm.** *Adults and children older than age 2:* Give 100 mg P.O. as single dose. If infection persists for 3 weeks, repeat therapy.
▶ **Roundworm, whipworm, hookworm.** *Adults and children older than age 2:* Give 100 mg P.O. b.i.d. for 3 days. If infection persists for 3 weeks, repeat therapy.
▶ **Trichinosis‡.** *Adults and children older than age 2:* Give 200 to 400 mg P.O. t.i.d. for 3 days, then 400 to 500 mg t.i.d. for 10 days.
▶ **Capillariasis‡.** *Adults and children older than age 2:* Give 200 mg P.O. b.i.d. for 20 days.
▶ **Toxocariasis‡.** *Adults and children:* 100 to 200 mg P.O. b.i.d. for 5 days.
▶ **Dracunculiasis‡.** *Adults and children older than age 2:* Give 400 to 800 mg P.O. daily for 6 days.

Contraindications and cautions

• Contraindicated in patients hypersensitive to the drug or any of its components.
⚠ Lifespan: In pregnant women, use cautiously. In breast-feeding women, safety and effectiveness haven't been established. In children younger than 2 years, safety and effectiveness haven't been established.

Adverse reactions

GI: diarrhea, transient abdominal pain.

Interactions

Drug-drug. *Carbamazepine, hydantoins:* May reduce level of mebendazole, possibly decreasing its therapeutic effect. Monitor patient for effect.
Cimetidine: Increases mebendazole level. Monitor patient for toxicity.

Effects on lab test results

None reported.

Pharmacokinetics

Absorption: About 5% to 10%; varies widely among patients.
Distribution: Highly protein-bound.
Metabolism: To inactive metabolites.
Excretion: Mostly in feces; 2% to 10% in urine. *Half-life:* 3 to 9 hours.

Route	Onset	Peak	Duration
P.O.	Unknown	2–5 hr	Varies

Action

Chemical effect: Selectively and irreversibly inhibits uptake of glucose and other nutrients in susceptible helminths.
Therapeutic effect: Kills helminth infestation.

Available forms

Tablets (chewable): 100 mg

NURSING PROCESS

Assessment
• Assess patient's condition before therapy and regularly thereafter to monitor the drug's effectiveness.
• Be alert for adverse reactions and drug interactions.
• Assess patient's and family's knowledge of drug therapy.

Nursing diagnoses
• Risk for infection related to presence of helminths
• Diarrhea related to drug-induced adverse GI reactions
• Deficient knowledge related to drug therapy

Planning and implementation
• Tablets may be chewed, swallowed whole, or crushed and mixed with food.
• Give drug to all family members to decrease risk of spreading infection.
• No dietary restrictions, laxatives, or enemas are needed.
Patient teaching
• Teach patient about personal hygiene, especially good hand-washing technique. To avoid reinfection, teach patient to wash perianal area daily, to change undergarments and bedclothes daily, and to wash hands and clean fingernails before meals and after bowel movements.
• Advise patient not to prepare food for others.

☑ Evaluation

• Patient is free from infestation.
• Patient's bowel pattern returns to normal after therapy is stopped.
• Patient and family state understanding of drug therapy.

mecasermin rinfabate
(meh-KAH-sur-men RIHN-fah-bayt)
Iplex

Pharmacologic class: human insulin growth factor
Therapeutic class: growth factor
Pregnancy risk category: C

Indications and dosages

▶ **Growth failure in children with severe primary insulin growth factor-1 (IGF-1) deficiency or children with growth hormone gene deletion who have developed neutralizing antibodies to growth hormone.** *Children age 3 and older:* Initially, 0.5 mg/kg subcutaneously. Adjust to therapeutic range (1 to 2 mg/kg once daily) based on glucose and IGF-1 levels. Give at about the same time each day, before the morning or evening meal, as long as the child maintains a balanced diet.

Contraindications and cautions

• Contraindicated in patients with closed epiphyses, active or suspected cancer, or allergy to mecasermin rinfabate or any component of the drug. I.V. use is also contraindicated. Don't use in place of growth hormone or for other causes of growth failure.
⚘ **Lifespan:** In pregnant or breast-feeding women, use cautiously. In children younger than age 3, safety and effectiveness haven't been established.

Adverse reactions

CNS: dizziness, *headache,* intracranial hypertension.
EENT: otitis media, papilledema, *tonsillar hypertrophy.*
GI: vomiting.
GU: hematuria, ovarian cysts.
Hematologic: *iron deficiency anemia.*
Metabolic: hyperglycemia, *hypoglycemia.*

Musculoskeletal: arthralgia, bone pain, *muscle atrophy,* scoliosis.
Other: *enlarged thyroid, pain,* injection site reaction, lymphadenopathy, snoring.

Interactions

None known.

Effects on lab test results

• May increase AST, LDH, and transaminase levels. May increase or decrease glucose level.

Pharmacokinetics

Absorption: Rapid.
Distribution: Less than 2% of total IGF-1 exists as free form.
Metabolism: None.
Excretion: *IGF-1 half-life:* More than 12 hours.

Route	Onset	Peak	Duration
SubQ			
IGF-1	1 hr	5–17½ hr	Unknown
IGFBP-3	1 hr	10½–28½ hr	Unknown

Action

Chemical effect: Promotes growth because synthetic drug is identical to endogenous insulin-like growth factor-binding protein-3 (IGFBP-3) and IGF-1.
Therapeutic effect: Promotes growth.

Available forms

Injection: 36 mg/0.6-ml vial

NURSING PROCESS

☑ Assessment

• Make sure child has had a fundoscopic eye exam before therapy starts.
• Monitor blood glucose level carefully, especially in small children, whose oral intake can be inconsistent.
• Check patient regularly for adenotonsillar enlargement. Ask parent or caregiver if the child has developed snoring, sleep apnea, or reduced hearing.
• Monitor patient for changes typical of acromegaly.

⊕ Nursing diagnoses

• Delayed growth and development related to primary IGF-1 deficiency

• Ineffective health maintenance related to adverse metabolic reactions
• Deficient knowledge related to drug therapy

▶ Planning and implementation

• Give drug at the same time each day. Because of its insulin-like effects, withhold dose if patient can't or won't eat.
• If drug produces rapid growth, patient may be at risk for slipped capital femoral epiphysis or progression of scoliosis. Monitor patient closely.
• Acute overdose may produce hypoglycemia (dizziness, tiredness, hunger, irritability, sweating, nausea, fast or irregular heartbeat). If mild, treat with oral glucose. If severe, give parenteral glucagon or I.V. glucose.
• Long-term overdose may cause acromegaly (enlarged hands and feet; increased sweating; oily skin; acne; thickening of facial features, especially the nose; increased prominence of jaw or forehead). Notify prescriber, and monitor patient.

Patient teaching
• Explain that drug must be kept frozen until ready to use. Tell parent or caregiver to discard unused drug after 2 months, even if it has been frozen.
• Instruct parent to thaw drug at room temperature for about 45 minutes before giving it and to give it within 1 hour of thawing. Explain that drug must be discarded if not used within 2 hours of thawing because it may not work.
• Warn parent not to use drug if it's cloudy.
• Tell parent to give drug before the same meal daily and to withhold dose if the child is unable or unwilling to eat.
• Teach parent how to inject drug and dispose of syringes properly.
• Tell parent to inject drug into child's upper arm, upper thigh, stomach area, or buttocks. Caution against injecting it into a muscle or vein.
• To decrease injection site reactions, advise parent to rotate injection sites.
• Tell parent to regularly monitor the child's blood glucose level. Review signs and symptoms of hypoglycemia, including dizziness, tiredness, hunger, irritability, sweating, nausea, and a fast or irregular heartbeat.
• Advise parent and child to keep a quick source of sugar (such as orange juice, glucose gel, or candy) readily available in case of hypoglycemia.
• Explain that child should avoid hazardous activities while the dosage is being adjusted.

Hypoglycemia can cause unconsciousness, seizures, or death.
• Advise parent to have the child's tonsils checked regularly and to monitor child for enlarged tonsils and snoring or sleep apnea.
• Tell parent to notify prescriber if child develops nausea and vomiting with headache, hypoglycemic episodes, a limp, hip or knee pain, snoring, trouble swallowing, earaches, or breathing problems.

☑ Evaluation
• Patient exhibits growth.
• Patient's thyroid function studies and glucose level are normal.
• Patient and family state understanding of drug therapy.

HIGH ALERT

mechlorethamine hydrochloride (nitrogen mustard)
(meh-klor-ETH-uh-meen high-droh-KLOR-ighd)
Mustargen

Pharmacologic class: alkylating drug
Therapeutic class: antineoplastic
Pregnancy risk category: D

Indications and dosages

▶ **Hodgkin lymphoma.** *Adults and children:* 6 mg/m^2 I.V. daily on days 1 and 8 of 28-day cycle given with other antineoplastics, such as mechlorethamine-vincristine-procarbazine-prednisone (MOPP). Repeat dosage for six cycles.
Adjust-a-dose: Reduce subsequent doses by 50% during MOPP therapy when WBC count is between 3,000 and 3,999/mm^3, and by 75% when WBC count is between 1,000 and 2,999/mm^3; or when platelet count is between 50,000 and 100,000/mm^3.
▶ **Polycythemia vera, chronic lymphocytic leukemia, chronic myelocytic leukemia, bronchogenic cancer, lymphosarcoma, mycosis fungoides.** *Adults and children:* 0.4 mg/kg I.V. daily as a single dose or divided into 2 doses of 0.2 mg/kg or 4 doses of 0.1 mg/kg. Base dosage on ideal dry body weight without edema or ascites. Subsequent courses can't be given until patient has recovered hematologically, usually within 3 weeks.

Reactions may be *common*, uncommon, *life-threatening*, or COMMON AND LIFE-THREATENING.

▼ I.V. administration

• Preparation and administration of parenteral form are linked to carcinogenic, mutagenic, and teratogenic risks. Follow facility protection policy to reduce risks.
• Prepare solution immediately before infusion because it's unstable. Use within 15 minutes, and discard unused solution.
• Reconstitute drug using 10 ml of sterile water for injection. Resulting solution contains 1 mg/ml of drug. Give by direct injection into I.V. line containing free-flowing compatible solution.
• Don't use solutions that are discolored or contain particulates. Don't use vials that appear to contain droplets of water.
• Make sure I.V. solution doesn't extravasate because drug is a potent vesicant. If it does, infiltrate area with sterile (1/6 molar) isotonic sodium thiosulfate and apply cold compresses for 6 to 12 hours.
• Dispose of used equipment properly and according to facility policy. Neutralize unused solution with equal volume of 5% sodium bicarbonate and 5% sodium thiosulfate for 45 minutes.

⊗ **Incompatibilities**
Allopurinol, cefepime, methohexital.

Contraindications and cautions

• Contraindicated in patients with infectious disease or previous anaphylactic reactions to the drug.
• Use cautiously in patients with chronic lymphatic lymphoma caused by increased drug toxicity.
• Use cautiously in patients with widely disseminated neoplasms. In patients with inoperable neoplasms or in the terminal stage of the disease, weigh risks and discomfort from use against limited potential gain.
⚖ **Lifespan:** Women of childbearing age shouldn't become pregnant while taking drug. In pregnant women, use cautiously because of risks to the fetus. Breast-feeding women should stop breast-feeding or not take the drug. In children, safety and effectiveness of drug haven't been established.

Adverse reactions

CNS: drowsiness, headache, vertigo, weakness.
CV: thrombophlebitis.
EENT: hearing loss, tinnitus.
GI: anorexia, metallic taste, nausea, vomiting.

Hematologic: *agranulocytosis,* anemia, *lymphocytopenia, myelosuppression, thrombocytopenia.*
Skin: *alopecia,* rash, severe irritation if drug extravasates or touches skin, sloughing.
Other: *anaphylaxis,* herpes zoster, *secondary malignant disease.*

Interactions

Drug-drug. *Anticoagulants, aspirin:* May increase risk of bleeding. Monitor PT and INR and monitor patient for bleeding; adjust dosage, if needed.

Effects on lab test results

• May increase urine urea level. May decrease hemoglobin level and hematocrit.
• May increase PT and INR. May decrease platelet, granulocyte, lymphocyte, WBC, and RBC counts.

Pharmacokinetics

Absorption: Incomplete, probably from deactivation by body fluids in cavity.
Distribution: Doesn't cross blood–brain barrier.
Metabolism: Converted rapidly to its active form, which reacts quickly with various cellular components before being deactivated.
Excretion: Metabolites in urine. *Half-life:* Unknown.

Route	Onset	Peak	Duration
I.V., intra-cavitary	Rapid	Unknown	Unknown

Action

Chemical effect: Cross-links strands of cellular DNA and interferes with RNA transcription, causing imbalance of growth that leads to cell death.
Therapeutic effect: Kills certain cancer cells.

Available forms

Injection: 10-mg vials

NURSING PROCESS

▣ **Assessment**
• Assess patient's condition before therapy and regularly thereafter to monitor drug effectiveness.
• Monitor CBC and platelet counts regularly. Mild anemia begins in 2 to 3 weeks.

M

- Monitor uric acid level.
- Be alert for adverse reactions and drug interactions.
- Monitor patient for signs and symptoms of infection caused by immunosuppression. Myelosuppression peaks in 4 to 10 days and lasts 10 to 21 days per cycle.
- Neurotoxicity and ototoxicity increases with dose and patient age.
- Assess patient's and family's knowledge of drug therapy.

⊕ Nursing diagnoses
- Ineffective health maintenance related to presence of neoplastic disease
- Risk for infection related to adverse hematologic reactions
- Deficient knowledge related to drug therapy

▷ Planning and implementation
⊛ **ALERT:** Drug is highly toxic. Avoid inhaling dust or vapors. Also avoid contact with skin or mucous membranes. Use personal protection equipment, clean drug equipment, and neutralize unused drug according to manufacturer's instructions.
- Give under the supervision of a physician experienced in the use of chemotherapy drugs.
- To prevent hyperuricemia with resulting uric acid nephropathy, make sure patient is adequately hydrated.
- If patient develops the acute phase of herpes zoster, stop giving the drug to avoid progression to generalized herpes zoster.

Patient teaching
- Warn patient to watch for signs of infection (fever, sore throat, fatigue) and bleeding (easy bruising, nosebleeds, bleeding gums, melena). Have patient take temperature daily.
- Instruct patient to avoid OTC products that contain aspirin.
- Advise woman of childbearing age to avoid becoming pregnant during therapy and to consult with prescriber before attempting to become pregnant.

☑ Evaluation
- Patient responds positively to drug.
- Patient regains normal hematologic parameters.
- Patient and family state understanding of drug therapy.

meclizine hydrochloride (meclozine hydrochloride)
(MEK-lih-zeen high-droh-KLOR-ighd)
Antivert†, Antivert/25, Antivert/50, Antrizine, Bonamine ♦, Bonine†, Dramamine Less Drowsy Formula†, Meni-D

Pharmacologic class: piperazine-derivative antihistamine; anticholinergic
Therapeutic class: antiemetic, antivertigo drug
Pregnancy risk category: B

Indications and dosages
▶ **Vertigo, dizziness.** *Adults:* 25 to 100 mg P.O. daily in divided doses. Dosage varies with patient response.
▶ **Motion sickness.** *Adults:* 25 to 50 mg P.O. 1 hour before travel, repeat daily for duration of journey.

Contraindications and cautions
- Contraindicated in patients hypersensitive to the drug or any of its components.
- Use cautiously in patients with asthma, glaucoma, or prostatic hyperplasia.
⚕ **Lifespan:** In pregnant women, safety and effectiveness haven't been established. In breastfeeding women, use cautiously; it's unknown if drug appears in breast milk. In children, safety and effectiveness haven't been established.

Adverse reactions
CNS: *drowsiness,* excitation, fatigue, nervousness.
CV: hypotension, palpitations, tachycardia.
EENT: blurred vision.
GI: anorexia, diarrhea, dry mouth, nausea, vomiting.
GU: urinary frequency.
Skin: rash, urticaria.

Interactions
Drug-drug. *CNS depressants:* May increase drowsiness. Use together cautiously; monitor patient for safety.

Effects on lab test results
None reported.

Pharmacokinetics
Absorption: Unknown.

Reactions may be *common,* uncommon, *life-threatening*, or COMMON AND LIFE-THREATENING.

Distribution: Good.
Metabolism: May be in liver.
Excretion: Unchanged in feces; metabolites in urine. *Half-life:* About 6 hours.

Route	Onset	Peak	Duration
P.O.	30–60 min	Unknown	4–24 hr

Action

Chemical effect: May affect neural pathways originating in labyrinth to inhibit nausea and vomiting.
Therapeutic effect: Relieves vertigo and nausea.

Available forms

Capsules: 25 mg, 30 mg†
Tablets: 12.5 mg, 25 mg†, 50 mg
Tablets (chewable): 25 mg†

NURSING PROCESS

⚚ Assessment

• Assess patient's condition before therapy and regularly thereafter to monitor drug effectiveness.
• Be alert for adverse reactions and drug interactions.
• Assess patient's and family's knowledge of drug therapy.

🔵 Nursing diagnoses

• Risk for injury related to vertigo
• Risk for deficient fluid volume related to motion sickness
• Deficient knowledge related to drug therapy

▷ Planning and implementation

• Don't abruptly stop giving the drug after long-term therapy. Paradoxical reactions or sudden reversal of improved state may occur.
🔵 **ALERT:** Don't confuse Antivert with Axert.
Patient teaching
• Advise patient to refrain from driving and performing other hazardous activities that require alertness until the drug's CNS effects are known.
• If drug is to be used long-term, stress the importance of not abruptly stopping it.
• Advise patient not to use alcohol while taking this drug and to consult prescriber before taking this drug if he's already taking sedatives or tranquilizers.

✓ Evaluation

• Patient states that vertigo is relieved.
• Patient states that motion sickness doesn't occur.
• Patient and family state understanding of drug therapy.

medroxyprogesterone acetate

(med-roks-ee-proh-JES-ter-ohn AS-ih-tayt)
Amen, Cycrin, Depo-Provera, Provera℘

Pharmacologic class: synthetic hormone
Therapeutic class: progestin, antineoplastic
Pregnancy risk category: X

Indications and dosages

▶ **Abnormal uterine bleeding caused by hormonal imbalance.** *Women:* 5 or 10 mg P.O. daily for 5 to 10 days beginning on day 16 or 21 of menstrual cycle. If patient also has received estrogen, 10 mg P.O. daily for 10 days beginning on day 16 of cycle.
▶ **Secondary amenorrhea.** *Women:* 5 or 10 mg P.O. daily for 5 to 10 days.
▶ **Endometrial or renal carcinoma.** *Adults:* 400 to 1,000 mg I.M. weekly. If disease improves within a few weeks to months and seems stable, it may be possible to maintain response with 400 mg monthly.
▶ **Endometrial hyperplasia.** *Postmenopausal women who haven't had a hysterectomy and are taking 0.625 mg conjugated estrogens:* 5 or 10 mg P.O. daily for 12 to 14 consecutive days per month, starting on day 1 or day 16 of the cycle.
▶ **Contraception.** *Women:* 150 mg I.M. once every 3 months.
▶ **Paraphilia‡.** *Men:* Initially, 200 mg I.M. b.i.d. or t.i.d. or 500 mg I.M. weekly. Base dosage on response.

Contraindications and cautions

• Contraindicated in patients hypersensitive to the drug or any of its components and in those with active thromboembolic disorders, breast cancer, undiagnosed abnormal vaginal bleeding, missed abortion, hepatic dysfunction, or a history of thromboembolic disorders, cerebrovascular disease, or stroke. Tablets are contraindicated in patients with liver dysfunction or known or suspected genital cancer.

M

• Use cautiously in patients with diabetes mellitus, seizure disorder, migraine, cardiac or renal disease, asthma, or depression.

⚖ **Lifespan:** In pregnant women, drug is contraindicated. In breast-feeding women, drug has no adverse effects on infants; it may increase milk production and duration of lactation.

Adverse reactions

CNS: asthenia, depression, dizziness, lethargy, migraine, nervousness, *stroke.*
CV: edema, hypertension, *thromboembolism,* thrombophlebitis.
EENT: intolerance of contact lenses.
GI: abdominal cramps, nausea, vomiting.
GU: abnormal secretions, amenorrhea, breakthrough bleeding, cervical erosion, dysmenorrhea, uterine fibromas, vaginal candidiasis.
Hepatic: *cholestatic jaundice,* gallbladder disease, *tumors.*
Metabolic: hyperglycemia, *weight gain.*
Respiratory: *pulmonary embolism.*
Skin: acne, alopecia, induration, melasma, pain, rash, sterile abscesses.
Other: breast tenderness, enlargement, or secretion; decreased libido; hypersensitivity reactions.

Interactions

Drug-drug. *Aminoglutethimide, rifampin:* May decrease progestin effects. Monitor patient for diminished therapeutic response. Tell patient to use nonhormonal contraceptive during therapy with these drugs.
Bromocriptine: May cause amenorrhea, interfering with bromocriptine's effects. Avoid use together.
Drug-food. *Caffeine:* May increase caffeine levels. Monitor patient for effect.
Drug-lifestyle. *Smoking:* May increase risk of adverse CV effects. If smoking continues, may need alternative therapy. Discourage patient from smoking.

Effects on lab test results

• May increase thyroxin-binding globulin and T4 levels.
• May increase liver function test values.

Pharmacokinetics

Absorption: Rapid.
Distribution: Extensively protein-bound, mainly to albumin and corticosteroid-binding globulin.

Metabolism: Rapid, mainly in the liver.
Excretion: Mainly in urine. *Half-life:* 2¼ to 9 hours P.O., 10 weeks I.M.

Route	Onset	Peak	Duration
P.O.	Rapid	1–2 hr	3–5 days
I.M.	Rapid	24 hr	3–4 mo

Action

Chemical effect: Acts as progestin: suppresses ovulation, possibly by inhibiting pituitary gonadotropin secretion.
Therapeutic effect: Regulates menses or acts as a contraceptive depending on dose; promotes anti-androgenic effects in men; and slows growth of some cancer cells.

Available forms

Injection (suspension): 150 mg/ml, 400 mg/ml
Tablets: 2.5 mg, 5 mg, 10 mg

NURSING PROCESS

Assessment
• Assess patient's condition before therapy and regularly thereafter to monitor drug effectiveness.
• Be alert for adverse reactions and drug interactions.
• Monitor injection sites for evidence of sterile abscess.
• Assess patient's and family's knowledge of drug therapy.

Nursing diagnoses
• Ineffective health maintenance related to underlying condition
• Excessive fluid volume related to drug-induced edema
• Deficient knowledge related to drug therapy

Planning and implementation
• Rotate injection sites to prevent muscle atrophy.
Patient teaching
• Explain to patient adverse effects of progestins before giving the first dose.
• Instruct patient not to smoke or use caffeine during therapy.
ALERT: Tell patient to immediately report unusual symptoms and to stop taking drug and notify prescriber about disturbed vision or migraine.

Reactions may be *common,* uncommon, *life-threatening*, or COMMON AND LIFE-THREATENING.

- Teach woman how to perform routine monthly breast self-examination.
- Warn patient that I.M. injection may be painful.

☑ Evaluation
- Patient responds well to drug therapy.
- Patient doesn't develop fluid excess throughout drug therapy.
- Patient and family state understanding of drug therapy.

mefloquine hydrochloride
(MEF-loh-kwin high-droh-KLOR-ighd)
Lariam

Pharmacologic class: quinine derivative
Therapeutic class: antimalarial
Pregnancy risk category: C

Indications and dosages

▶ **Acute malaria infections caused by mefloquine-sensitive strains of *Plasmodium falciparum* and *P. vivax*.** *Adults age 17 and older:* 1,250 mg P.O. as single dose, with 240 ml (8 oz) water. Give patients with *P. vivax* infections primaquine or other 8-aminoquinoline to avoid relapse of initial infection after therapy.
Children age 6 months to 16 years: 20 to 25 mg/kg in 2 divided doses given 6 to 8 hours apart, with ample water.

▶ **To prevent malaria.** *Adults:* 250 mg P.O. once weekly. Give 1 week before patient enters endemic area and continue for 4 weeks after return. Can begin prophylaxis 2 to 3 weeks before departure when taken with other drugs.
Children: The recommended prophylactic dose is 5 mg/kg body weight once weekly.

One 250-mg tablet should be taken once weekly in children weighing more than 45 kg. In children weighing less than 45 kg, the weekly dose decreases in proportion to body weight: 31 to 45 kg, ¾ tablet; 21 to 30 kg, ½ tablet; 11 to 20 kg, ¼ tablet; 5 to 10 kg, ⅛ tablet (approximate tablet fraction based on a dosage of 5 mg/kg body weight).

Contraindications and cautions
- Contraindicated in patients hypersensitive to the drug or related compounds. Don't give as prevention to patients with active depression, a recent history of depression, generalized anxiety disorder, psychosis, schizophrenia, other major psychiatric disorder, or a history of seizures.
- Use cautiously in patients with a history of depression and in patients with cardiac disease or seizure disorders.

☀ **Lifespan:** In pregnant women, use cautiously. In breast-feeding women, use cautiously; it's unknown if the drug appears in breast milk. In infants less than 6 months, safety and effectiveness haven't been established.

Adverse reactions

CNS: ataxia, dizziness, fatigue, fever, headache, mood changes, panic attacks, *seizures, suicide,* syncope, tremor.
CV: chest pain, edema, extrasystoles.
EENT: tinnitus.
GI: diarrhea, dyspepsia, GI discomfort, loose stools, loss of appetite, *nausea,* vomiting.
Skin: rash.
Other: chills.

Interactions

Drug-drug. *Beta blockers, quinidine, quinine:* May cause ECG abnormalities and cardiac arrest. Avoid use together.
Chloroquine, quinine: May increase risk of seizures. Do not use together.
Halofantrine: May increase risk of fatal prolongation of QTc interval. Don't use together.
Oral live typhoid vaccine: May reduce effectiveness of immunization. Complete immunization at least 3 days before giving drug.
Valproic acid, other anticonvulsants: May cause loss of seizure control by lowering drug levels. Check anticonvulsant level.

Effects on lab test results
- May increase transaminase levels. May decrease hemoglobin level and hematocrit.
- May decrease WBC and platelet counts.

Pharmacokinetics

Absorption: Good, enhanced with food.
Distribution: Concentrated in RBCs. About 98% protein-bound.
Metabolism: By liver.
Excretion: Primarily by liver; small amounts in urine. *Half-life:* About 21 days.

Route	Onset	Peak	Duration
P.O.	Unknown	7–24 hr	Unknown

M

Action
Chemical effect: May be related to its ability to form complexes with hemin.
Therapeutic effect: Inhibits or kills malaria-causing organisms.

Available forms
Tablets: 250 mg

NURSING PROCESS

🔢 Assessment
• Assess patient's condition before therapy and regularly thereafter to monitor drug effectiveness.
• Periodically monitor liver function.
• Be alert for adverse reactions and drug interactions.
• If patient has an adverse GI reaction, monitor his hydration.
• Assess patient's and family's knowledge of drug therapy.

🔢 Nursing diagnoses
• Risk for infection related to presence of malaria organisms
• Risk for deficient fluid volume related to drug-induced adverse reactions
• Deficient knowledge related to drug therapy

🔢 Planning and implementation
🔅 **ALERT:** During preventive use, psychiatric symptoms may precede a more serious reaction. Stop giving the drug, and use an alternative.
• If *P. falciparum* infection is life-threatening or overwhelming, start with an I.V. antimalarial drug, and complete therapy with mefloquine.
• Because health risks from simultaneous administration of quinine and mefloquine are great, don't begin therapy within 12 hours of last dose of quinine or quinidine.
• Patients with infections caused by *P. vivax* are at high risk for relapse because drug doesn't eliminate hepatic phase (exoerythrocytic parasites). Follow-up therapy with primaquine or an 8-aminoquinoline is advisable.
• Give drug with food and full glass of water to minimize adverse GI reactions.
• If a pediatric patient vomits and a significant loss of drug product is observed or suspected because of vomiting, a second full dose of mefloquine HCl should be administered to patients who vomit less than 30 minutes after

receiving the drug. If vomiting occurs 30 to 60 minutes after a dose, an additional half-dose should be given. If vomiting recurs, the patient should be monitored closely and alternative malaria treatment considered if improvement is not observed within a reasonable period of time.

Patient teaching
• Advise patient to take drug on the same day each week when using it for prevention and to take with food and a full 8-ounce glass of water.
• Advise caregiver to contact prescriber if child vomits following drug administration.
• Advise patient to use caution when performing hazardous activities that require alertness and coordination because dizziness, disturbed sense of balance, and neuropsychiatric reactions may occur.
• Instruct patient taking drug as prevention to stop taking the drug and notify prescriber if he notices signs or symptoms of impending toxicity, such as unexplained anxiety, depression, confusion, or restlessness.
• For patient undergoing long-term therapy, recommend that he have periodic ophthalmologic examinations.

🔢 Evaluation
• Patient is free from infection.
• Patient maintains adequate hydration throughout therapy.
• Patient and family state understanding of drug therapy.

HIGH ALERT

megestrol acetate
(meh-JES-trol AS-ih-tayt)
Megace, Megace ES

Pharmacologic class: synthetic progestin
Therapeutic class: antineoplastic
Pregnancy risk category: D (tablets); X (oral suspension)

Indications and dosages
▶ **Breast cancer.** *Adults:* 40 mg P.O. q.i.d.
▶ **Endometrial cancer.** *Women:* 40 to 320 mg P.O. daily in divided doses.
▶ **Anorexia, cachexia, or unexplained significant weight loss in patients with AIDS.**
Adults: 800 mg P.O. (20 ml regular oral suspension) or 625 mg P.O. (5 ml concentrated ES oral suspension) once daily.

▶ **Anorexia or cachexia in patients with neoplastic disease‡.** *Adults:* 480 to 600 mg P.O. daily.

Contraindications and cautions

• Contraindicated in patients hypersensitive to the drug or any of its components.
• Use cautiously in patients with history of thrombophlebitis.
☀ **Lifespan:** In pregnant women, drug is contraindicated in the first 4 months of pregnancy. In breast-feeding women, use cautiously; it's unknown if drug appears in breast milk. In children, safety and effectiveness haven't been established.

Adverse reactions

CV: *heart failure,* hypertension, *thromboembolism,* thrombophlebitis.
GI: abdominal pain, nausea, vomiting.
GU: breakthrough menstrual bleeding.
Metabolic: increased appetite, weight gain.
Musculoskeletal: back pain, carpal tunnel syndrome.
Respiratory: *pulmonary embolism.*
Skin: alopecia, hirsutism.
Other: breast tenderness.

Interactions

Drug-drug. *Dofetilide:* May increase risk of cardiotoxicity. Monitor QT interval.

Effects on lab test results

• May increase glucose level.

Pharmacokinetics

Absorption: Good.
Distribution: May be stored in fatty tissue. Highly protein-bound.
Metabolism: Complete.
Excretion: In urine. *Half-life:* 2¼ to 9 hours.

Route	Onset	Peak	Duration
P.O.	Rapid	1–2 hr	3–5 days

Action

Chemical effect: Changes tumor's hormonal environment and alters neoplastic process. Mechanism of appetite stimulation is unknown.
Therapeutic effect: Hinders cancer cell growth and increases appetite.

Available forms

Oral suspension: 40 mg/ml
Oral suspension (concentrated): 125 mg/ml
Tablets: 20 mg, 40 mg

NURSING PROCESS

▨ Assessment

• Assess patient's condition before therapy and regularly thereafter to monitor drug effectiveness.
• Be alert for adverse reactions.
• If patient has an adverse GI reaction, monitor his hydration.
• Assess patient's and family's knowledge of drug therapy.

⊕ Nursing diagnoses

• Ineffective health maintenance related to underlying condition
• Risk for deficient fluid volume related to drug-induced adverse GI reactions
• Deficient knowledge related to drug therapy

▷ Planning and implementation

• Two months is adequate trial when treating cancer.
• If patient develops pronounced back pain, abdominal pain, headache, or nausea and vomiting, notify prescriber.
Patient teaching
• Inform patient that therapeutic response isn't immediate.
ⓈALERT: Tell patient the ES oral suspension is more concentrated than the regular oral suspension so a smaller amount is needed for the proper dose.
• Advise breast-feeding woman to stop breast-feeding during therapy because of infant toxicity.
• Encourage women to use nonhormonal contraceptives during therapy.

☑ Evaluation

• Patient responds well to therapy.
• Patient maintains adequate hydration throughout therapy.
• Patient and family state understanding of drug therapy.

meloxicam
(mell-OX-ih-kam)
Mobic

Pharmacologic class: NSAID
Therapeutic class: anti-inflammatory, analgesic
Pregnancy risk category: C

Indications and dosages

▶ **Osteoarthritis or rheumatoid arthritis.**
Adults: 7.5 mg P.O. once daily. May increase to maximum of 15 mg P.O. once daily.
▶ **Pauciarticular or polyarticular course juvenile rheumatoid arthritis.** *Children ages 2 to 17:* Give 0.125 mg/kg P.O. once daily, up to a maximum of 7.5 mg daily.

Contraindications and cautions

• Contraindicated in patients hypersensitive to the drug or any of its components and in those who have had asthma, urticaria, or allergic-type reactions after taking aspirin or other NSAIDs. Contraindicated in patients with severe renal impairment and for treating perioperative pain after coronary artery bypass surgery.
• Use cautiously in patients with a history of ulcers or GI bleeding and in patients with dehydration, anemia, hepatic disease, renal disease, hypertension, fluid retention, heart failure, or asthma.
⚜ Lifespan: In pregnant women, avoid use especially during the third trimester. In breast-feeding women, don't use drug. In children younger that age 2, safety and effectiveness haven't been established. In elderly and debilitated patients, use cautiously because of greater risk of fatal GI bleeding.

Adverse reactions

CNS: anxiety, confusion, depression, dizziness, fatigue, fever, headache, insomnia, malaise, nervousness, paresthesia, *seizures,* somnolence, syncope, tremor, vertigo.
CV: angina, *arrhythmias,* edema, *heart failure,* hypertension, hypotension, *MI,* palpitations, *shock,* tachycardia.
EENT: abnormal vision, conjunctivitis, pharyngitis, tinnitus.
GI: abdominal pain, colitis, constipation, diarrhea, dry mouth, duodenal ulcer, dyspepsia, esophagitis, flatulence, gastric ulcer, gastritis, GI reflux, *hemorrhage,* increased appetite, nausea, *pancreatitis,* taste perversion, vomiting.
GU: albuminuria, hematuria, *renal impairment,* urinary frequency, UTI.
Hematologic: *agranulocytosis,* anemia, *leukopenia,* purpura, *thrombocytopenia.*
Hepatic: bilirubinemia, *hepatitis,* jaundice, *liver failure.*
Metabolic: dehydration, weight changes.
Musculoskeletal: arthralgia, back pain.
Respiratory: *asthma, bronchospasm,* cough, dyspnea, upper respiratory tract infection.
Skin: alopecia, bullous eruption, *erythema multiforme, exfoliative dermatitis,* photosensitivity reactions, pruritus, rash, *Stevens-Johnson syndrome,* sweating, *toxic epidermal necrolysis,* urticaria.
Other: accidental injury, allergic reaction, *anaphylactoid reactions, angioedema,* flulike symptoms.

Interactions

Drug-drug. *ACE inhibitors:* May decrease antihypertensive effects. Monitor patient's blood pressure.
Aspirin: May increase risk of adverse effects. Avoid use together.
Bile acid sequestrants: May increase clearance of meloxicam. Monitor patient's pain level.
Cyclosporine: May increase risk of nephrotoxicity. Monitor patient.
Lithium: May increase lithium level. Monitor lithium level closely for toxicity.
Methotrexate: May increase the toxicity of methotrexate. Use cautiously together.
Thiazide and loop diuretics: May reduce sodium excretion linked to diuretics, leading to sodium retention. Monitor patient for edema and increased blood pressure.
Warfarin: May increase PT or INR. Monitor PT and INR, and check for signs and symptoms of bleeding.
Drug-herb. *Dong quai, feverfew, garlic, ginger, horse chestnut, ma huang, meadowsweet, red clover:* May increase risk of bleeding. Discourage use together.
St. John's wort: May increase risk of photosensitivity reactions. Advise patient to avoid unprotected or prolonged exposure to sunlight.
Drug-lifestyle. *Alcohol use:* May increase risk of GI irritation and bleeding. Monitor patient for bleeding; discourage use together.

Reactions may be *common,* uncommon, *life-threatening,* or COMMON AND LIFE-THREATENING.

Smoking: May increase risk of GI irritation and bleeding. Monitor patient for bleeding; discourage patient from smoking.

Effects on lab test results

• May increase BUN, creatinine, ALT, AST, and bilirubin levels. May decrease hemoglobin level and hematocrit.
• May decrease WBC and platelet counts.

Pharmacokinetics

Absorption: Bioavailability is 89% and doesn't appear to be affected by food or antacids. Steady-state conditions are reached after 5 days of daily administration.
Distribution: 99.4% protein-bound.
Metabolism: Almost complete, to pharmacologically inactive metabolites.
Excretion: In both urine and feces, mainly as metabolites. *Half-life:* 15 to 20 hours.

Route	Onset	Peak	Duration
P.O.	Unknown	Unknown	Unknown

Action

Chemical effect: May be related to prostaglandin (cyclooxygenase) synthetase inhibition.
Therapeutic effect: Relief of signs and symptoms of osteoarthritis.

Available forms

Oral suspension: 7.5 mg/5 ml
Tablets: 7.5 mg, 15 mg

NURSING PROCESS

⚕ Assessment

• Obtain accurate history of drug allergies. Drug can produce allergic-like reactions in patients hypersensitive to aspirin and other NSAIDs.
• Assess patient for increased risk of GI bleeding. Risk factors include history of ulcers or GI bleeding, therapy with corticosteroids or anticoagulants, long duration of NSAID therapy, smoking, alcoholism, old age, and poor overall health.
• Monitor patient for signs and symptoms of overt and occult bleeding.
⚠ ALERT: NSAIDs may increase the risk of serious thrombotic events, MI, or stroke. The risk may increase with duration of use and be higher in patients with CV disease or risk factors for CV disease.

• Monitor children for abdominal pain, vomiting, diarrhea, headache, and pyrexia, which may occur more commonly than in adults.
• Monitor patient for fluid retention; closely monitor patient who has hypertension, edema, or heart failure.
• Monitor liver function.
• Assess patient's and family's knowledge of drug therapy.

⊕ Nursing diagnoses

• Chronic pain related to underlying condition
• Risk for injury related to drug-induced adverse reactions
• Deficient knowledge related to drug therapy

▶ Planning and implementation

• Drug may be taken with food to prevent GI upset.
• Rehydrate dehydrated patient before therapy.
• If patient develops evidence of liver disease (eosinophilia, rash), stop giving the drug.
• Use oral suspension to improve accuracy of doses in lighter-weight children.
Patient teaching
• Tell patient to notify prescriber about history of allergic reactions to aspirin or other NSAIDs before therapy.
• Oral solution may be substituted on a milligram-per-milligram basis for tablets. Shake suspension gently before use.
• Tell patient to report signs and symptoms of GI ulcerations and bleeding, such as vomiting blood, blood in stool, and black, tarry stools.
• Instruct patient to report skin rash, weight gain, or edema.
• Advise patient to report warning signs of hepatotoxicity (nausea, fatigue, lethargy, pruritus, jaundice, right upper quadrant tenderness, and flulike symptoms).
• Warn patient with a history of asthma that it may recur during therapy and that he should stop taking the drug and notify prescriber if it does.
• Tell woman to notify prescriber if she becomes pregnant or is planning to become pregnant during therapy.
• Inform patient that it may take several days before consistent pain relief is achieved.

✓ Evaluation

• Patient is free from pain.
• Patient sustains no injury as a result of drug-induced adverse reactions.

M

• Patient and family state understanding of drug therapy.

melphalan (L-phenylalanine mustard)
(MEL-feh-len)
Alkeran

Pharmacologic class: nitrogen mustard; alkylating drug
Therapeutic class: antineoplastic
Pregnancy risk category: D

Indications and dosages

▶ **Multiple myeloma.** *Adults:* 6 mg P.O. daily for 2 to 3 weeks; then stop drug for up to 4 weeks or until WBC and platelet counts begin to rise again; then give maintenance dosage of 2 mg daily.

▶ **Alternative therapy for multiple myeloma.** *Adults:* 0.15 mg/kg P.O. daily for 7 days at 2- to 6-week intervals, then begin maintenance therapy at or less than 0.05 mg/kg/day when WBC and platelet counts increase. Or 0.25 mg/kg P.O. daily for 4 days, repeat every 4 to 6 weeks. Or 10 mg/day for 7 to 10 days, maintenance therapy at 2 mg/day, adjust dosage within 1- to 3-mg range daily based on hematological response. Or for patients who can't tolerate oral therapy, give 16 mg/m² by I.V. infusion over 15 to 20 minutes every 2 weeks for four doses. After patient has recovered from toxicity, give drug every 4 weeks.

Adjust-a-dose: For patients with renal impairment, reduce I.V. dosage by 50% to reduce risk of severe leukopenia and drug-related death.

▶ **Nonresectable advanced ovarian cancer.** *Women:* 0.2 mg/kg P.O. daily for 5 days. Repeat every 4 to 6 weeks, depending on bone marrow recovery.

I.V. administration

• Follow facility policy to reduce risks. Preparation and administration of parenteral form are linked to carcinogenic, mutagenic, and teratogenic risks for personnel.
• Because drug isn't stable in solution, reconstitute immediately before giving, using 10 ml of sterile diluent supplied by manufacturer. Shake vigorously until solution is clear. Resulting so-

lution contains 5 mg/ml. Immediately dilute required dose in normal saline solution for injection. Don't exceed a final concentration of 0.45 mg/ml.
• Give promptly after diluting because reconstituted product begins to degrade within 30 minutes. After final dilution, nearly 1% of drug degrades every 10 minutes. Administration must be completed within 60 minutes of reconstitution.
• Give by I.V. infusion over 15 to 20 minutes.
• Don't refrigerate reconstituted product because precipitate will form.

⊗ **Incompatibilities**
Amphotericin B, chlorpromazine, D₅W, lactated Ringer's injection. Compatibility with normal saline injection depends on concentration.

Contraindications and cautions

• Contraindicated in patients hypersensitive to the drug or any of its components and in those whose disease is resistant to drug. Patients hypersensitive to chlorambucil may have cross-sensitivity to drug.
• Drug isn't recommended for patients with severe leukopenia, thrombocytopenia, anemia, or chronic lymphocytic leukemia.
Lifespan: In pregnant and breast-feeding women, drug isn't recommended. In children, safety and effectiveness haven't been established.

Adverse reactions

Hematologic: *bone marrow suppression, leukopenia, thrombocytopenia.*
Hepatic: *hepatotoxicity.*
Respiratory: pneumonitis, *pulmonary fibrosis.*
Skin: alopecia, dermatitis, pruritus, rash.
Other: *anaphylaxis,* hypersensitivity reactions.

Interactions

Drug-drug. *Anticoagulants, aspirin:* May increase risk of bleeding. Use cautiously together.
Antigout drugs: May decrease effectiveness. Dosage adjustments may be needed.
Bone marrow suppressants: May have additive toxicity. Monitor patient closely.
Carmustine: May reduce carmustine lung toxicity threshold. Monitor patient closely for signs of toxicity.
Cisplatin: May affect melphalan's pharmacokinetics by inducing renal dysfunction and altering melphalan clearance. Monitor patient for toxicity.

Cyclosporine: May increase toxicity of cyclosporine, particularly nephrotoxicity. Monitor cyclosporine level and renal function tests.
Interferon alfa: May decrease melphalan level. Monitor level closely.
Nalidixic acid: May increase risk of severe hemorrhagic necrotic enterocolitis in children. Monitor patient closely.
Vaccines: May decrease effectiveness of killed-virus vaccines and increase risk of toxicity from live-virus vaccines. Postpone routine immunization for at least 3 months after last dose of melphalan.
Drug-food. *Any food:* May decrease absorption of oral drug. Separate administration times; give drug on an empty stomach.

Effects on lab test results

• May increase urine urea level. May decrease hemoglobin level and hematocrit.
• May decrease RBC, WBC, and platelet counts.

Pharmacokinetics

Absorption: Incomplete and variable.
Distribution: Rapid and wide in total body water. Initially 50% to 60% protein-bound, increasing to 80% to 90%.
Metabolism: Extensively deactivated by hydrolysis.
Excretion: Mainly in urine. *Half-life:* 2 hours.

Route	Onset	Peak	Duration
P.O., I.V.	Unknown	Unknown	Unknown

Action

Chemical effect: Cross-links strands of cellular DNA and interferes with RNA transcription.
Therapeutic effect: Kills certain cancer cells.

Available forms

Injection: 50 mg
Tablets (scored): 2 mg

NURSING PROCESS

🗣 Assessment
• Assess patient's condition before therapy and regularly thereafter to monitor drug effectiveness.
• Monitor uric acid level and CBC.
• Be alert for adverse reactions and drug interactions.
• Assess patient's and family's knowledge of drug therapy.

🖳 Nursing diagnoses
• Ineffective health maintenance related to presence of neoplastic disease
• Risk for infection related to adverse hematologic reactions
• Deficient knowledge related to drug therapy

▷ Planning and implementation
• Give under the supervision of a physician experienced in using chemotherapy drugs.
⚛ ALERT: Drug may cause leukemia. Use proper precautions.
• Dosage may need to be reduced in patient with renal impairment.
• Melphalan is drug of choice with prednisone in patients with multiple myeloma.
• Give drug on empty stomach.
• Anaphylaxis may occur. Keep antihistamines and steroids readily available.
⚛ ALERT: Don't confuse melphalan with Mephyton.
Patient teaching
• Tell patient to take oral drug on empty stomach.
• Warn patient to watch for signs of infection (fever, sore throat, fatigue) and bleeding (easy bruising, nosebleed, bleeding gums, melena). Have patient take temperature daily.
• Instruct patient to avoid OTC products that contain aspirin.
• Advise woman of childbearing age not to become pregnant during therapy and to consult with prescriber before becoming pregnant.

☑ Evaluation
• Patient responds well to therapy.
• Patient regains normal hematologic function when therapy is completed.
• Patient and family state understanding of drug therapy.

M

memantine hydrochloride
(MEHM-en-teen high-droh-KLOR-ighd)
Namenda

Pharmacologic class: N-methyl-D-aspartate (NMDA) receptor antagonist
Therapeutic class: Alzheimer disease drug
Pregnancy risk category: B

Indications and dosages

▶ **Moderate to severe Alzheimer-type dementia.** *Adults:* Initially, 5 mg P.O. once daily. Increase by 5 mg/day each week up to the target dosage. Maximum, 10 mg P.O. b.i.d. Divide doses larger than 5 mg b.i.d.

§ **Adjust-a-dose:** If the patient has moderate renal impairment, reduce dosage.

Contraindications and cautions

• Contraindicated in patients allergic to the drug or any of its components. In patients with severe renal impairment, drug isn't recommended.

• Use cautiously in patients with seizures, hepatic impairment, or moderate renal impairment. Also use cautiously in patients who may have an increased urine pH (from drugs, diet, renal tubular acidosis, or severe UTI).

⚖ **Lifespan:** In pregnant women, use only if benefits outweigh risks to the fetus. In breast-feeding women, use cautiously; it's unknown if the drug appears in breast milk. In children, safety and effectiveness haven't been established. In elderly patients, use cautiously.

Adverse reactions

CNS: abnormal gait, aggressiveness, agitation, anxiety, ataxia, confusion, depression, dizziness, fatigue, hallucinations, headache, hypokinesia, insomnia, pain, somnolence, *stroke,* syncope, transient ischemic attack, vertigo.
CV: edema, *heart failure,* hypertension.
EENT: cataracts, conjunctivitis.
GI: anorexia, constipation, diarrhea, nausea, vomiting.
GU: incontinence, urinary frequency, UTI.
Hematologic: anemia.
Metabolic: weight loss.
Musculoskeletal: arthralgia, back pain.
Respiratory: bronchitis, coughing, dyspnea, pneumonia, upper respiratory tract infection.
Skin: rash.
Other: falls, flulike symptoms, inflicted injury.

Interactions

Drug-drug. *Cimetidine, hydrochlorothiazide, quinidine, ranitidine, triamterene:* May alter drug levels. Monitor patient.
NMDA antagonists (amantadine, dextromethorphan, ketamine): May interact. Use together cautiously.
Urine alkalinizers (carbonic anhydrase inhibitors, sodium bicarbonate): May decrease

memantine clearance. Monitor patient for adverse effects.
Drug-herb. *Herbs that alkalinize urine:* May increase drug level and adverse effects. Discourage use together.
Drug-food. *Foods that alkalinize urine:* May increase drug level and adverse effects. Discourage use together.
Drug-lifestyle. *Alcohol use:* May decrease drug's effectiveness or increase adverse effects. Discourage use together.
Smoking: May alter levels of drug and nicotine. Discourage use together.

Effects on lab test results

• May increase alkaline phosphatase level. May decrease hemoglobin level and hematocrit.

Pharmacokinetics

Absorption: Good.
Distribution: About 45% protein-bound.
Metabolism: Little.
Excretion: Unchanged, mainly in urine. *Half-life:* 60 to 80 hours.

Route	Onset	Peak	Duration
P.O.	Unknown	3–7 hr	Unknown

Action

Chemical effect: Antagonizes NMDA receptors, the persistent activation of which seems to increase Alzheimer symptoms.
Therapeutic effect: Decreases dementia.

Available forms

Oral solution: 2 mg/ml
Tablets: 5 mg, 10 mg

NURSING PROCESS

📝 **Assessment**
• Assess patient's condition before therapy and regularly thereafter to monitor drug effectiveness.
• Assess patient's and family's knowledge of drug therapy.

🔷 **Nursing diagnoses**
• Acute or chronic confusion related to underlying disease
• Risk for imbalanced fluid volume related to drug-induced GI effects
• Deficient knowledge related to drug therapy

> **Planning and implementation**
- Drug isn't indicated for mild Alzheimer disease or other types of dementia.
- Give drug with or without food.

Patient teaching
- Explain that drug doesn't cure Alzheimer disease but may improve the symptoms.
- Tell patient to report adverse effects.
- Urge patient not to drink alcohol during therapy.
- Advise patient not to take herbal or OTC cold and cough or GI products without consulting the prescriber.

☑ **Evaluation**
- Patient's cognition improves, and he experiences less confusion.
- Patient and family state that adverse GI effects haven't occurred or have been managed effectively.
- Patient and family state understanding of drug therapy.

menotropins
(meh-noh-TROH-pins)
Menopur, Repronex

Pharmacologic class: gonadotropin
Therapeutic class: ovulation stimulant
Pregnancy risk category: X

Indications and dosages

▶ **Stimulation of ovulation in patients who have received gonadotropin-releasing hormone agonist pituitary suppression.** *Adults:* Initially, 225 units subcutaneously. Repronex may also be given I.M. Adjust subsequent dosages based on serum estradiol level, vaginal ultrasound, and patient response. Don't adjust more than once every 2 days, and don't exceed 75 to 150 units per adjustment for Repronex, or 150 units per adjustment for Menopur. Maximum daily dose is 450 units. Use beyond 12 days for Repronex, or 20 days for Menopur, isn't recommended.

Once follicular development is adequate, give 5,000 to 10,000 units of human chorionic gonadotropin (hCG) to induce final follicular maturation in preparation for oocyte retrieval. If the ovaries are abnormally enlarged on the last day of therapy, withhold hCG to reduce the chance of developing ovarian hyperstimulation syndrome.

Contraindications and cautions

- Contraindicated in patients hypersensitive to the drug or any of its components and in women with primary ovarian failure, uncontrolled thyroid or adrenal dysfunction, pituitary tumor, abnormal uterine bleeding, uterine fibromas, or ovarian cysts or enlargement.
≋ **Lifespan:** In pregnant women, breastfeeding women, and children, drug is contraindicated.

Adverse reactions

CNS: *headache, stroke.*
CV: *arterial occlusion,* fever, tachycardia.
GI: diarrhea, nausea, vomiting.
GU: multiple births, *ovarian enlargement,* ovarian hyperstimulation syndrome.
Hematologic: hemoconcentration with fluid loss into abdomen.
Respiratory: *acute respiratory distress syndrome,* atelectasis, *pulmonary embolism, pulmonary infarction.*
Other: *anaphylaxis, gynecomastia,* hypersensitivity reactions.

Interactions

None significant.

Effects on lab test results

None reported.

Pharmacokinetics

Absorption: Unknown.
Distribution: Unknown.
Metabolism: Unknown.
Excretion: In urine. *Half-life:* I.M., 60 hours.

Route	Onset	Peak	Duration
SubQ, I.M.	9–12 days	Unknown	Unknown

Action

Chemical effect: When given to women who haven't had primary ovarian failure, mimics follicle-stimulating hormone (FSH) in inducing follicular growth and luteinizing hormone (LH) in aiding follicular maturation.
Therapeutic effect: Stimulates ovulation.

M

Available forms

Injection: 75 units of LH and 75 units of FSH activity per ampule; 150 units of LH and 150 units of FSH activity per ampule

NURSING PROCESS

⏀ Assessment
• Assess patient's condition before therapy and regularly thereafter to monitor drug effectiveness.
• Be alert for adverse reactions.
⊛ **ALERT:** Monitor women for rare ovarian hyperstimulation syndrome (ovarian enlargement with possible pain and abdominal distention, ascites, and possible pleural effusion with hemoconcentration). Stop drug immediately and hospitalize patient for symptomatic treatment.
• Assess patient's and family's knowledge of drug therapy.

⊕ Nursing diagnoses
• Sexual dysfunction related to underlying disorder
• Risk for deficient fluid volume related to drug-induced adverse reactions
• Deficient knowledge related to drug therapy

▷ Planning and implementation
• Monitor patient closely to ensure adequate hormonal stimulation.
• Reconstitute with 1 ml (Menopur) or 1 to 2 ml (Repronex) of sterile normal saline solution. Use immediately.
• Rotate injection sites.
Patient teaching
• Teach patient correct administration technique.
• Discuss risk of multiple births.
• Encourage patient to have intercourse daily from the day before hCG is given until ovulation occurs.
• Tell patient that pregnancy usually occurs 4 to 6 weeks after therapy.
• Instruct patient to immediately report severe abdominal pain, bloating, swelling of hands or feet, nausea, vomiting, diarrhea, substantial weight gain, or shortness of breath.

☑ Evaluation
• Patient or partner becomes pregnant.
• Patient maintains adequate hydration throughout therapy.

• Patient and family state understanding of drug therapy.

HIGH ALERT

meperidine hydrochloride (pethidine hydrochloride)
(meh-PER-uh-deen high-droh-KLOR-ighd)
Demerol

Pharmacologic class: opioid
Therapeutic class: analgesic, adjunct to anesthesia
Pregnancy risk category: B; D (injection, for prolonged periods or high doses at term)
Controlled substance schedule: II

Indications and dosages

▶ **Moderate to severe pain.** *Adults:* 50 to 150 mg P.O., I.M., or subcutaneously every 3 to 4 hours, p.r.n. Or 15 to 35 mg/hour by continuous I.V. infusion.
Children: 1.1 to 1.75 mg/kg P.O., I.M., or subcutaneously, up to the adult dose, every 3 to 4 hours, p.r.n.
▶ **Preoperatively.** *Adults:* 50 to 100 mg I.M., I.V., or subcutaneously 30 to 90 minutes before surgery.
Children: 1 to 2.2 mg/kg I.M., I.V., or subcutaneously up to adult dose 30 to 90 minutes before surgery.
▶ **Adjunct to anesthesia.** *Adults:* Repeat slow I.V. injections of fractional doses (such as 10 mg/ml). Or continuous I.V. infusion of more dilute solution (1 mg/ml); adjust to needs of patient.
▶ **Obstetric analgesia.** *Adults:* 50 to 100 mg I.M. or subcutaneously when pain becomes regular; repeat at 1- to 3-hour intervals.

▽ I.V. administration
• Drug is compatible with most I.V. solutions, including D_5W, normal saline solution, and Ringer's or lactated Ringer's solutions.
• Keep resuscitation equipment and naloxone available.
• Give slowly by direct I.V. injection or slow continuous I.V. infusion.
⊗ Incompatibilities
Acyclovir, allopurinol, aminophylline, amobarbital, amphotericin B, cefepime, cefoperazone, doxorubicin liposomal, ephedrine, furosemide,

heparin, hydrocortisone sodium succinate, idarubicin, imipenem-cilastatin sodium, methyl-prednisolone sodium succinate, morphine, pentobarbital, phenobarbital sodium, phenytoin, sodium bicarbonate, sodium iodide, sulfonamides, thiopental.

Contraindications and cautions

• Contraindicated in patients hypersensitive to the drug or any of its components and in those who have received MAO inhibitors within 14 days.
• Use cautiously in debilitated patients and in patients with increased intracranial pressure, head injury, asthma, other respiratory conditions, supraventricular tachycardias, seizures, acute abdominal conditions, hepatic or renal disease, hypothyroidism, Addison disease, urethral stricture, or prostatic hyperplasia.
❈ **Lifespan:** In pregnant women, use cautiously. In breast-feeding women, use cautiously because it's unknown if drug appears in breast milk. In the elderly, use cautiously because of increased risk of renal insufficiency.

Adverse reactions

CNS: *clouded sensorium,* dizziness, euphoria, paradoxical excitement, sedation, *seizures,* somnolence, tremors.
CV: *bradycardia, cardiac arrest,* hypotension, *shock,* tachycardia.
GI: constipation, ileus, nausea, vomiting.
GU: urine retention.
Musculoskeletal: muscle twitching.
Respiratory: *respiratory arrest, respiratory depression.*
Skin: local tissue irritation and induration, phlebitis.
Other: pain at injection site, physical dependence.

Interactions

Drug-drug. *Chlorpromazine:* May cause excessive sedation and hypotension. Don't use together.
CNS depressants, general anesthetics, hypnotics, other opioid analgesics, phenothiazines, sedatives, tricyclic antidepressants: May cause respiratory depression, hypotension, profound sedation, or coma. Use together cautiously. Reduce meperidine dosage as directed.

MAO inhibitors: May increase CNS excitation or depression that can be severe or fatal. Don't use together.
Phenytoin: May decrease meperidine level. Monitor patient for decreased analgesia.
Drug-lifestyle. *Alcohol use:* May have additive CNS effects. Discourage use together.

Effects on lab test results

• May increase amylase and lipase levels.

Pharmacokinetics

Absorption: Unknown.
Distribution: Wide.
Metabolism: Mainly by hydrolysis in liver.
Excretion: Mainly in urine, enhanced by acidifying urine. *Half-life:* 2½ to 4 hours.

Route	Onset	Peak	Duration
P.O.	15 min	60–90 min	2–4 hr
I.V.	1 min	5–7 min	2–4 hr
I.M., SubQ	10–15 min	30–50 min	2–4 hr

Action

Chemical effect: Binds with opioid receptors in CNS, altering both perception of and emotional response to pain through unknown mechanism.
Therapeutic effect: Relieves pain.

Available forms

Injection: 25 mg/ml, 50 mg/ml, 75 mg/ml, 100 mg/ml
Injection (for infusion only): 10 mg/ml
Syrup: 50 mg/5 ml
Tablets: 50 mg, 100 mg

NURSING PROCESS

▨ **Assessment**
• Assess patient's pain before therapy and regularly thereafter to monitor drug effectiveness.
• Be alert for adverse reactions and drug interactions.
• Meperidine and its active metabolite normeperidine accumulate in the body. Monitor patient for increased toxic effect, especially in patient with renal impairment.
• Monitor respirations of neonate exposed to drug during labor.
• Don't stop drug abruptly after long-term use; doing so may cause withdrawal symptoms.
• Assess patient's and family's knowledge of drug therapy.

✦ Nursing diagnoses

• Acute pain related to underlying condition
• Risk for injury related to drug-induced adverse reactions
• Deficient knowledge related to drug therapy

▶ Planning and implementation

• Drug may be used in patients with pain who are allergic to morphine.
• Because drug toxicity often appears after several days of therapy, it isn't recommended for chronic pain.
• **ALERT:** If respiratory rate is less than 12 breaths/minute, if respiratory depth decreases, or if pupil size decreases, don't give drug.
• **ALERT:** Oral dose is less than half as effective as parenteral dose. Give I.M., if possible. When changing from parenteral to oral route, increase dose.
• Syrup has local anesthetic effect. Give with full glass of water.
• Subcutaneous injection is painful; avoid if possible.
• **ALERT:** Don't confuse Demerol with Demulen, Dymelor, or Temaril.

Patient teaching
• Warn outpatient to avoid hazardous activities until the drug's CNS effects are known.
• Instruct patient not to use alcohol during therapy.
• Teach patient to manage adverse reactions, such as constipation.
• Tell family members not to give the drug and to notify the prescriber if patient's respiratory rate decreases.

☑ Evaluation

• Patient is free from pain.
• Patient doesn't experience injury.
• Patient and family state understanding of drug therapy.

HIGH ALERT

mercaptopurine
(6-mercaptopurine, 6-MP)
(mer-cap-toh-PYOO-reen)
Purinethol

Pharmacologic class: antimetabolite
Therapeutic class: antineoplastic
Pregnancy risk category: D

Indications and dosages

▶ **Acute lymphatic leukemia (lymphocytic, lymphoblastic), acute myelogenous and acute myelomonocytic leukemia.** *Adults:* 2.5 mg/kg P.O. daily as single dose, up to 5 mg/kg P.O. daily. Maintenance dosage is 1.5 to 2.5 mg/kg P.O. daily.
Children age 5 and older: 2.5 mg/kg P.O. daily. Maintenance dosage is 1.5 to 2.5 mg/kg P.O. daily.
▶ **Intractable Crohn disease‡.** *Adults:* 1 to 1.5 mg/kg P.O. daily (maximum 125 mg/day) with other therapies.
Children: 1 to 1.5 mg/kg P.O. daily (maximum 75 mg/day) with other therapies.

Contraindications and cautions

• Contraindicated in patients whose disease has resisted drug.
• **Lifespan:** In pregnant and breast-feeding women, drug is contraindicated.

Adverse reactions

GI: anorexia, nausea, *pancreatitis,* stomatitis, vomiting.
Hematologic: anemia, *leukopenia, thrombocytopenia.*
Hepatic: biliary stasis, *hepatotoxicity,* jaundice.
Metabolic: hyperuricemia.
Skin: hyperpigmentation, rash.

Interactions

Drug-drug. *Allopurinol:* May slow inactivation of mercaptopurine. Decrease mercaptopurine to one-fourth or one-third normal dose.
Hepatotoxic drugs: May enhance hepatotoxicity of mercaptopurine. Monitor patient closely; monitor liver function test results.
Warfarin: May antagonize anticoagulant effect. Monitor PT and INR.

Effects on lab test results

• May increase alkaline phosphatase, bilirubin, and liver enzyme levels. May decrease hemoglobin level and hematocrit.
• May decrease WBC, RBC, and platelet counts.
• May falsely increase glucose and uric acid levels.

Pharmacokinetics

Absorption: Incomplete and variable; about 50%.

Reactions may be *common,* uncommon, *life-threatening,* or COMMON AND LIFE-THREATENING.

Distribution: Wide in total body water.
Metabolism: Extensive.
Excretion: In urine. *Half-life:* Unknown.

Route	Onset	Peak	Duration
P.O.	Unknown	Unknown	Unknown

Action

Chemical effect: Inhibits RNA and DNA synthesis. Strongly inhibits primary immune response by suppressing humoral immunity.
Therapeutic effect: Inhibits growth of certain cancer cells.

Available forms

Tablets (scored): 50 mg

NURSING PROCESS

🔬 Assessment
• Assess patient's condition before therapy and regularly thereafter to monitor drug effectiveness.
• Monitor blood count and transaminase, alkaline phosphatase, and bilirubin levels weekly during initiation of treatment until remission is achieved and monthly during maintenance.
• Observe patient for signs of bleeding and infection.
• Monitor fluid intake and output and uric acid level.
• Be alert for adverse reactions and drug interactions. Adverse GI reactions are less common in children.
⑤ **ALERT:** Watch for jaundice, clay-colored stools, and frothy, dark urine. Hepatic dysfunction is reversible when drug is stopped. If hepatic tenderness occurs, stop giving the drug and notify prescriber.
• Assess patient's and family's knowledge of drug therapy.

🔆 Nursing diagnoses
• Ineffective health maintenance related to presence of leukemia
• Risk for infection related to drug-induced adverse hematologic reactions
• Deficient knowledge related to drug therapy

▶ Planning and implementation
• Calculate dosage to the closest multiple of 25 mg.

• Adjust dosage after chemotherapy or radiation therapy and in a patient with depressed neutrophil or platelet count, or impaired liver or kidney function.
• Be aware that drug is usually used with other antineoplastics because response to monotherapy is poor.
⑤ **ALERT:** Sometimes drug is ordered as 6-mercaptopurine or 6-MP. The numeral 6 is part of drug name and doesn't signify number of dosage units. To prevent confusion, avoid these designations.
• Therapy must continue despite nausea and vomiting. If patient has an adverse GI reaction, notify prescriber and give an antiemetic.
• Encourage adequate fluid intake (3 L daily).
• Give allopurinol cautiously.
• If hepatic tenderness occurs, stop giving the drug and notify prescriber.
⑤ **ALERT:** Don't confuse Purinethol with propylthiouracil.
Patient teaching
• Tell patient to notify prescriber if vomiting occurs shortly after taking dose because antiemetic will be needed so drug therapy can continue.
• Instruct patient to watch for signs of infection (fever, sore throat, fatigue) and bleeding (easy bruising, nosebleed, bleeding gums, melena). Have patient take his temperature daily.
• Advise woman of childbearing age not to become pregnant during therapy and to consult with prescriber before becoming pregnant after therapy.

☑ Evaluation
• Patient responds well to therapy.
• Patient doesn't develop serious ill effects when hematologic studies are abnormal.
• Patient and family state understanding of drug therapy.

meropenem
(mer-oh-PEN-em)
Merrem I.V.

Pharmacologic class: synthetic broad-spectrum carbapenem
Therapeutic class: antibiotic
Pregnancy risk category: B

Indications and dosages

▶ **Complicated skin and skin structure infections caused by** *Staphylococcus aureus* **(beta-lactamase and non–beta-lactamase producing, methicillin-susceptible isolates only),** *Streptococcus pyogenes, Streptococcus agalactiae, viridans group streptococci, Enterococcus faecalis* **(excluding vancomycin-resistant isolates),** *Pseudomonas aeruginosa, Escherichia coli, Proteus mirabilis, Bacteroides fragilis,* **and** *Peptostreptococcus* **species.** *Adults and children weighing more than 50 kg (110 lb):* 500 mg I.V. every 8 hours over 15 to 30 minutes as I.V. infusion.

Children ages 3 months and older weighing 50 kg or less: 10 mg/kg I.V. every 8 hours over 15 to 30 minutes as I.V. infusion or over 3 to 5 minutes as I.V. bolus injection (5 to 20 ml); maximum dose is 500 mg I.V. every 8 hours.

▶ **Complicated appendicitis and peritonitis caused by viridans group streptococci,** *E. coli, Klebsiella pneumoniae, P. aeruginosa, Bacteroides fragilis, Bacteroides thetaiotaomicron,* **and** *Peptostreptococcus* **species.** *Adults and children weighing more than 50 kg:* 1 g I.V. every 8 hours over 15 to 30 minutes as I.V. infusion or over 3 to 5 minutes as I.V. bolus injection (5 to 20 ml).

Children ages 3 months and older, weighing 50 kg or less: 20 mg/kg I.V. every 8 hours over 15 to 30 minutes as I.V. infusion or over 3 to 5 minutes as I.V. bolus injection (5 to 20 ml); maximum dosage is 1 g I.V. every 8 hours.

📎 **Adjust-a-dose:** For adults with creatinine clearance of 26 to 50 ml/minute, give usual dose every 12 hours. If clearance is 10 to 25 ml/minute, give half usual dose every 12 hours; if clearance is less than 10 ml/minute, give half usual dose every 24 hours.

▶ **Bacterial meningitis caused by** *Streptococcus pneumoniae, Haemophilus influenzae,* **and** *Neisseria meningitides. Children weighing more than 50 kg:* 2 g I.V. every 8 hours.

Children ages 3 months and older weighing 50 kg or less: 40 mg/kg I.V. every 8 hours; maximum dose, 2 g I.V. every 8 hours.

▼ I.V. administration

• For I.V. bolus, add 10 ml of sterile water for injection to 500-mg/20-ml vial or add 20 ml to 1-g/30-ml vial. Shake to dissolve, and let stand until clear.

• For I.V. infusion, infusion vials (500 mg/100 ml and 1 g/100 ml) may be directly reconstituted with compatible infusion fluid. Or an injection vial may be reconstituted, then the resulting solution added to an I.V. container, and further diluted with appropriate infusion fluid. Don't use ADD-Vantage vials for this purpose.

• Follow manufacturer's guidelines closely when using ADD-Vantage vials.

• Use freshly prepared solutions of drug immediately.

• Stability of drug varies with form of drug used (injection vial, infusion vial, or ADD-Vantage container).

⊗ **Incompatibilities**
Other I.V. drugs.

Contraindications and cautions

• Contraindicated in patients hypersensitive to the drug, its components, or other drugs in the class. Also contraindicated in those who have had anaphylactic reactions to beta-lactams.

• Use cautiously and at a reduced dosage in patients with renal impairment.

⚜ **Lifespan:** In pregnant women, use only when benefits outweigh risks to the fetus. In breast-feeding women, use cautiously because it's unknown if the drug appears in breast milk. In infants younger than age 3 months, safety and effectiveness haven't been established.

Adverse reactions

CNS: agitation, confusion, headache, insomnia, nervousness, somnolence.

CV: *bradycardia, cardiac arrest, heart failure,* hypertension, hypotension, *MI, pulmonary embolism,* tachycardia, thrombophlebitis at injection site.

GI: anorexia, cholestatic jaundice, constipation, diarrhea, glossitis, nausea, oral candidiasis, *pseudomembranous colitis,* vomiting.

GU: dysuria, *renal failure.*

Hematologic: *agranulocytosis,* anemia, eosinophilia, *leukopenia, neutropenia.*

Respiratory: *apnea.*

Skin: *erythema multiforme,* pruritus, *Stevens-Johnson syndrome,* rash, *toxic epidermal necrolysis,* urticaria.

Other: *anaphylaxis, angioedema,* hypersensitivity reactions, inflammation at injection site, pain.

Reactions may be *common,* uncommon, *life-threatening,* or COMMON AND LIFE-THREATENING.

Interactions
Drug-drug. *Probenecid:* May inhibit renal meropenem excretion. Don't give together.

Effects on lab test results
• May increase ALT, AST, bilirubin, alkaline phosphatase, LDH, creatinine, and BUN levels. May decrease hemoglobin level and hematocrit.
• May increase eosinophil count. May decrease WBC count. May increase or decrease platelet count and PT.

Pharmacokinetics
Absorption: Given I.V.
Distribution: 2% protein-bound. Penetrates into most body fluids and tissues, including CSF.
Metabolism: In kidneys.
Excretion: In urine. *Half-life:* 1 hour.

Route	Onset	Peak	Duration
I.V.	Unknown	< 1 hr	Unknown

Action
Chemical effect: Readily penetrates the cell wall of most gram-positive and gram-negative bacteria to reach penicillin-binding protein targets, where it inhibits cell wall synthesis.
Therapeutic effect: Bactericidal.

Available forms
Powder for injection: 500 mg/20 ml, 500 mg/30 ml, 1 g/20 ml, 1 g/30 ml

NURSING PROCESS

Assessment
• Obtain specimen for culture and sensitivity tests before giving first dose. Therapy may begin pending test results.
⚠ ALERT: Serious and occasionally fatal hypersensitivity reactions may occur. Before therapy, determine whether patient has ever had a hypersensitivity reaction to penicillins, cephalosporins, other beta-lactams, or other allergens.
• Monitor patient for signs and symptoms of superinfection.
• Periodically assess organ-system functions during prolonged therapy.
• Assess patient's and family's knowledge of drug therapy.

Nursing diagnoses
• Risk for infection related to bacteria
• Risk for deficient fluid volume related to effect on kidneys
• Deficient knowledge related to drug therapy

Planning and implementation
• Drug isn't used to treat methicillin-resistant staphylococci.
• If patient develops diarrhea, suspect pseudomembranous colitis. If confirmed, stop giving the drug, begin fluid and electrolyte management, and give an antibacterial effective against *Clostridium difficile.*
• If overdose occurs (usually in patients with renal impairment), stop giving the drug and provide general supportive therapy until renal elimination occurs. Drug is removable by hemodialysis, if needed.
Patient teaching
• Instruct patient to report adverse reactions.

Evaluation
• Patient is free from infection.
• Patient maintains adequate hydration.
• Patient and family state understanding of drug therapy.

mesalamine
(5-aminosalicylic acid)
(mez-AL-uh-meen)
Asacol, Canasa, Lialda, Mesasal ♦, Novo-5 ASA ♦, Pentasa, Rowasa, Salofalk ♦

Pharmacologic class: salicylate
Therapeutic class: anti-inflammatory
Pregnancy risk category: B

Indications and dosages
▶ **Active mild to moderate distal ulcerative colitis, proctitis, proctosigmoiditis.** *Adults:* 800 mg P.O. (tablets) t.i.d. for total dose of 2.4 g daily for 6 weeks, or 1 g P.O. (capsules) q.i.d. for total dose of 4 g daily up to 8 weeks. Or, 1,000 mg suppository retained in the rectum for 1 to 3 hours or longer, if possible, once daily at bedtime. Or 4 g as retention enema once daily (preferably at bedtime) retained for about 8 hours. Usual course of therapy for P.R. form is 3 to 6 weeks.

► **Induction of remission of active, mild to moderate ulcerative colitis.** *Adults:* Two to four 1.2-g tablets P.O. once daily with a meal for a total daily dose of 2.4 to 4.8 g, for maximum of 8 weeks.

► **Maintenance of remission of ulcerative colitis.** *Adults:* 1.6 g P.O. daily in divided doses for 6 months. Or, 60 ml (4 g) rectal suspension every 2 to 3 nights or 1 to 3 g rectal suspension daily; retain for about 8 hours.

Contraindications and cautions

• Contraindicated in patients hypersensitive to the drug, any of its components, or salicylates.
• Use cautiously in patients with renal impairment; absorbed drug may cause nephrotoxicity.
⚘ **Lifespan:** In pregnant women, use cautiously. In breast-feeding women, rectal form of drug is contraindicated. Oral form may be used with caution. It's unknown if the drug appears in breast milk. In children, drug is contraindicated. In the elderly, use cautiously.

Adverse reactions

CNS: dizziness, fatigue, fever, headache, malaise.
GI: abdominal cramps, discomfort, or pain; *belching;* bloating; diarrhea; flatulence; *nausea; pancolitis; pancreatitis;* rectal pain; vomiting.
Respiratory: upper respiratory tract infection, wheezing.
Skin: acne, hair loss, pruritus, rash, urticaria.
Other: *anaphylaxis,* pain.

Interactions

None significant.

Effects on lab test results

• May increase BUN, creatinine, AST, ALT, alkaline phosphatase, LDH, amylase, and lipase levels.

Pharmacokinetics

Absorption: Poor with P.R. use.
Distribution: Not clearly defined.
Metabolism: Undergoes acetylation, but whether this takes place at colonic or systemic sites is unknown.
Excretion: P.O. form mainly in urine; most of P.R. form in feces. *Half-life:* About 5 to 10 hours.

Route	Onset	Peak	Duration
P.O., P.R.	Unknown	3–12 hr	Unknown

Action

Chemical effect: May act topically by inhibiting prostaglandin production in colon.
Therapeutic effect: Relieves inflammation in lower GI tract.

Available forms

Capsules (controlled-release): 250 mg, 500 mg
Rectal suspension: 4 g/60 ml
Suppositories: 500 mg, 1,000 mg
Tablets (delayed-release): 400 mg, 1.2 g

NURSING PROCESS

Assessment

• Assess patient's condition before therapy and regularly thereafter to monitor drug effectiveness.
• In patient on long-term therapy, periodically monitor kidney function.
• In patient sensitive to sulfites, drug may cause hypersensitivity reactions because it contains potassium metabisulfite.
• Be alert for adverse reactions.
• Assess patient's and family's knowledge of drug therapy.

Nursing diagnoses

• Impaired tissue integrity related to underlying condition
• Acute pain related to drug-induced adverse GI reactions
• Deficient knowledge related to drug therapy

Planning and implementation

• Have patient swallow tablets and capsules whole; don't crush or let him chew them.
• For maximum effectiveness, have patient retain suppository as long as possible. When giving rectal suspension, shake bottle before application.
⚠ **ALERT:** Don't confuse Asacol with Os-Cal or mesalamine with mecamylamine.

Patient teaching
• Teach patient how to take oral and rectal form, and instruct him to carefully follow instructions supplied with drug.
• Instruct patient to stop taking drug if he experiences fever or rash. Patient intolerant of sulfasalazine or aminosalicylic acid may also be hypersensitive to this drug.

Reactions may be *common*, uncommon, *life-threatening*, or COMMON AND LIFE-THREATENING.

☑ Evaluation
• Patient reports relief from GI symptoms.
• Patient states that no new pain is experienced during therapy.
• Patient and family state understanding of drug therapy.

mesna
(MEZ-nah)
Mesnex, Uromitexan ♦

Pharmacologic class: thiol derivative
Therapeutic class: uroprotectant
Pregnancy risk category: B

Indications and dosages

▶ **To prevent hemorrhagic cystitis in patients taking ifosfamide.** *Adults:* Dosage varies with amount of ifosfamide given. If using 1.2-g/m^2 ifosfamide, give 240 mg/m^2 as I.V. bolus with ifosfamide. Repeat dose at 4 hours and 8 hours to a total of 60% of the ifosfamide dose. Or, give 20% as a single bolus injection followed by two oral doses (40% each). If using 1.2-g/m^2 ifosfamide, give 240 mg/m^2 I.V. mesna with ifosfamide, then 480 mg/m^2 P.O. at 2 and 6 hours.
▶ **To prevent hemorrhagic cystitis in bone marrow recipients taking cyclophosphamide ‡.** *Adults:* Give 60% to 160% of the cyclophosphamide daily dose I.V. in three to five divided doses or by continuous infusion. Or, in patients receiving 50 to 60 mg/kg cyclophosphamide I.V. daily for 2 to 4 days, give 10 mg/kg I.V. loading dose followed by 60 mg/kg by continuous infusion over 24 hours. Give with each cyclophosphamide dose and continue for 24 hours after last dose of cyclophosphamide.

▽ I.V. administration
• Dilute drug in D$_5$W, dextrose 5% combined with normal saline solution for injection, normal saline solution for injection, or lactated Ringer's solution to obtain final solution of 20 mg/ml.
• After mixing, inspect drug for particulate matter and discoloration before administering.
• Drug and ifosfamide are compatible in same I.V. infusion.
• Although diluted solution is stable for 24 hours at room temperature, refrigerate after preparation and use within 6 hours. After open-

ing ampule, discard any unused drug because it decomposes quickly into inactive compound.
⊗ **Incompatibilities**
Amphotericin B, carboplatin, cisplatin.

Contraindications and cautions
• Contraindicated in patients hypersensitive to the drug or other compounds containing thiol.
☀ **Lifespan:** In pregnant women, use cautiously. In breast-feeding women and in children, safety and effectiveness haven't been established.

Adverse reactions
CNS: anxiety, *asthenia,* confusion, dizziness, *fatigue, fever,* headache, insomnia, pain, somnolence.
CV: chest pain, edema, flushing, hypotension, tachycardia.
GI: abdominal pain, anorexia, constipation, diarrhea, dyspepsia, nausea, vomiting.
GU: hematuria.
Hematologic: *anemia, granulocytopenia, leukopenia, thrombocytopenia.*
Metabolic: dehydration, hypokalemia.
Musculoskeletal: back pain.
Respiratory: dyspnea, coughing, pneumonia.
Skin: alopecia, increased sweating, pallor.
Other: *allergy,* injection site reaction.

Interactions
None significant.

Effects on lab test results
• May interfere with diagnostic tests for urine ketones.

Pharmacokinetics
Absorption: Unaffected by food.
Distribution: Remains in vascular compartment.
Metabolism: Rapid, to one metabolite.
Excretion: In urine. *Half-life:* 4 to 8 hours.

Route	Onset	Peak	Duration
P.O., I.V.	Unknown	Unknown	Unknown

Action
Chemical effect: Detoxifies urotoxic ifosfamide metabolites.
Therapeutic effect: Prevents ifosfamide from adversely affecting bladder tissue.

M

Available forms

Injection: 100 mg/ml in 10-ml vials (contains benzyl alcohol)
Tablets: 400 mg

NURSING PROCESS

⚕ Assessment
• Assess patient's condition before therapy and regularly thereafter to monitor drug effectiveness.
• Up to 6% of patients may not respond to drug's protective effects.
• Monitor urine samples for hematuria daily in patient taking mesna.
• Be alert for adverse reactions.
• If patient has an adverse GI reaction, monitor his hydration.
• Assess patient's and family's knowledge of drug therapy.

⊞ Nursing diagnoses
• Risk for deficient fluid volume related to drug-induced adverse GI reactions
• Deficient knowledge related to drug therapy

▷ Planning and implementation
• If patient vomits within 2 hours of taking drug P.O., repeat the dose or give I.V.
• Because drug is used with ifosfamide and other chemotherapeutics, it's difficult to determine adverse reactions attributable solely to this drug.
• Drug isn't effective in preventing hematuria from other causes (such as thrombocytopenia).
• Although formulated to prevent hemorrhagic cystitis from ifosfamide, drug won't protect against other toxicities linked to ifosfamide.
Patient teaching
• Instruct patient to report hematuria immediately and to notify prescriber about adverse GI reactions.

☑ Evaluation
• Patient maintains adequate hydration throughout therapy.
• Patient and family state understanding of drug therapy.

metaproterenol sulfate
(met-uh-proh-TER-eh-nul SUL-fayt)
Alupent

Pharmacologic class: beta agonist
Therapeutic class: bronchodilator
Pregnancy risk category: C

Indications and dosages

▶ **Asthma; bronchospasm.**
Oral
Adults and children age 9 and older or weighing more than 27.3 kg (60 lb): 20 mg P.O. t.i.d. to q.i.d.
Adults and children younger than age 9 or weighing less 27.3 kg (60 lb): 10 mg P.O. t.i.d. to q.i.d.
Children younger than age 6: Give 1.3 to 2.6 mg/kg/day P.O. in divided doses.
Aerosol inhalation
Adults and children older than age 12: Give 2 to 3 inhalations with at least 2 minutes between inhalations. Don't repeat inhalations more often than every 3 to 4 hours. Maximum, 12 inhalations daily.
Intermittent positive-pressure breathing (IPPB) or nebulizer
Adults and children age 12 and older: 0.2 to 0.3 ml of 5% solution diluted in 2.5 ml of normal saline solution or 2.5 ml of commercially available 0.4% or 0.6% solution every 4 hours, p.r.n.
Hand-bulb nebulizer
Adults and children age 12 and older: 10 inhalations of an undiluted 5% solution.
▶ **Acute asthma attacks.** *Children age 6 and older:* Use 5% solution for inhalation only. Give 0.1 to 0.2 ml in saline to a total volume of 3 ml given by nebulizer at time of attack.

Contraindications and cautions

• Contraindicated in patients hypersensitive to the drug or any of its components, in those receiving cyclopropane or halogenated hydrocarbon general anesthetics, and in those with tachycardia or arrhythmias caused by tachycardia, peripheral or mesenteric vascular thrombosis, or profound hypoxia or hypercapnia.
• Use cautiously in patients with hypertension, hyperthyroidism, heart disease, diabetes, or

cirrhosis and in patients who are receiving digoxin.

⚘ **Lifespan:** In pregnant women, use cautiously. In breast-feeding women, use cautiously. It's unknown if the drug appears in breast milk.

Adverse reactions

CNS: drowsiness, *nervousness,* tremors, *weakness.*
CV: *cardiac arrest,* ECG changes, hypertension, palpitations, tachycardia.
GI: heartburn, nausea, taste perversion, vomiting.
Respiratory: *paradoxical bronchoconstriction.*

Interactions

Drug-drug. *Aminophylline, theophylline:* May increase risk of cardiotoxicity. Monitor ECG and vital signs closely.
Other sympathomimetics: May have additive effects and toxicity. Separate administration times.
Propranolol, other beta blockers: May block bronchodilating effect of metaproterenol. Monitor patient.

Effects on lab test results

None reported.

Pharmacokinetics

Absorption: Good in GI tract. Minimally through the lungs.
Distribution: Wide.
Metabolism: Extensive on first pass through liver.
Excretion: In urine. *Half-life:* Unknown.

Route	Onset	Peak	Duration
P.O.	15 min	1 hr	1–4 hr
Inhalation	1 min	1 hr	2–6 hr
Nebulization	5–30 min	1 hr	2–6 hr

Action

Chemical effect: Relaxes bronchial smooth muscle by acting on beta$_2$-adrenergic receptors.
Therapeutic effect: Improves breathing.

Available forms

Aerosol inhaler: 0.65 mg/metered spray
Solution for nebulizer inhalation: 0.4%, 0.6%
Syrup: 10 mg/5 ml
Tablets: 10 mg, 20 mg

NURSING PROCESS

⚗ Assessment
• Assess patient's condition before therapy and regularly thereafter to monitor drug effectiveness.
• Be alert for adverse reactions and drug interactions.
• If patient has an adverse GI reaction, monitor his hydration.
• Assess patient's and family's knowledge of drug therapy.

⊕ Nursing diagnoses
• Impaired gas exchange related to underlying respiratory condition
• Risk for deficient fluid volume related to drug-induced adverse GI reactions
• Deficient knowledge related to drug therapy

▷ Planning and implementation
• Aerosol nebulization solution can be given by IPPB with drug diluted in normal saline solution or by hand-bulb nebulizer at full strength.
⚛ **ALERT:** Don't use solution if discolored or precipitated.
⚛ **ALERT:** Don't confuse metaproterenol with metoprolol or metipranolol.
⚛ **ALERT:** Don't confuse Alupent with Atrovent.
Patient teaching
• Give patient the following instructions for using metered-dose inhaler: clear nasal passages and throat. Breathe out, expelling as much air from lungs as possible. Place mouthpiece well into mouth and inhale deeply as you release a dose from inhaler. Hold breath for several seconds, remove mouthpiece, and exhale slowly. Allow 2 minutes between inhalations.
• Instruct patient to store drug in light-resistant container.
• Tell patient using corticosteroid inhaler to use bronchodilator first and then to wait 5 to 15 minutes before using corticosteroid. This allows bronchodilator to open air passages for maximum effectiveness of corticosteroid.
• Warn patient to immediately stop taking the drug and notify the prescriber if he has paradoxical bronchospasm.
• Tell patient that if dose doesn't work, he should notify his prescriber for an increase.

⚑ Evaluation
• Patient's respiratory status improves.

M

- Patient maintains adequate hydration.
- Patient and family state understanding of drug therapy.

metformin hydrochloride
(met-FOR-min high-droh-KLOR-ighd)
Fortamet, Glucophage◆, Glucophage XR◆, Glumetza, Riomet

Pharmacologic class: biguanide
Therapeutic class: antidiabetic
Pregnancy risk category: B

Indications and dosages

▶ **Adjunct to diet and exercise to lower glucose level in patients with type 2 diabetes mellitus.** *Adults (immediate-release form):* 500 mg P.O. b.i.d. or 850 mg P.O. daily, given with meals. Increase doses in increments of 500 mg weekly or 850 mg every 2 weeks to 2,000 mg daily, in divided doses. May also increase from 500 mg b.i.d. to 850 mg b.i.d. after 2 weeks. Maximum daily dose is 2,550 mg daily. Doses above 2,000 mg may be better tolerated given t.i.d. with meals.
Adults (extended-release form): 500 mg P.O. daily with the evening meal. Increase in increments of 500 mg weekly to a maximum of 2,000 mg once daily (2,500 mg for Fortamet) with the evening meal. If glycemic control isn't achieved with 2,000 mg once daily, consider a trial of 1,000 mg b.i.d. If higher doses are required, use immediate-release form.
Children ages 10 to 16: Give 500 mg P.O. b.i.d. (regular-release form). Increase dosage in increments of 500 mg weekly to a maximum of 2,000 mg daily in divided doses. Don't use extended-release form in children.
▶ **Adjunct to diet and exercise in type 2 diabetes, as monotherapy or with a sulfonylurea or insulin.** *Adults and adolescents age 17 and older:* Initially, 500 to 1,000 mg of Fortamet P.O. with evening meal. Increase dosage based on glucose level in increments of 500 mg/week to a maximum of 2,500 mg daily. When used with a sulfonylurea or insulin, base dosage on blood glucose level, and adjust slowly until desired therapeutic effect occurs. Decrease insulin dosage by 10% to 25% when fasting blood glucose level is less than 120 mg/dl.

▶ **Adjunct to diet and exercise in type 2 diabetes as monotherapy or with a sulfonylurea or insulin (Glumetza).** *Adults:* Initially, 1,000 mg P.O. once daily in the evening with food. Increase, as needed, by 500 mg in weekly increments up to a maximum of 2,000 mg daily. If glycemic control not attained at this dose, give 1,000 mg b.i.d.
When used with a sulfonylurea or insulin, base dosage on glucose level and adjust slowly until desired therapeutic effect occurs. Decrease insulin dosage by 10% to 25% when fasting blood glucose level is less than 120 mg/dl.
⬛ Adjust-a-dose: In malnourished or debilitated patients, don't adjust to maximum dosage.

Contraindications and cautions

- Contraindicated in patients hypersensitive to the drug or any of its components; those with hepatic disease, renal disease or dysfunction, or acute or chronic metabolic acidosis; and in heart failure patients who need other drugs. Temporarily withhold drug in patients undergoing radiologic studies involving parenteral administration of iodinated contrast materials; using such products may result in acute renal dysfunction. If patient enters hypoxic state, stop drug.
- Use cautiously in debilitated or malnourished patients and in those with adrenal or pituitary insufficiency because of increased risk of hypoglycemia.
⬛ Lifespan: In pregnant women, safety and effectiveness haven't been established. In breastfeeding women, use cautiously; it's unknown if drug appears in breast milk. In children younger than age 10, safety and effectiveness of regular form haven't been established. In children younger than age 17, safety and effectiveness of extended-release form haven't been established. In elderly patients, use cautiously.

Adverse reactions

CNS: asthenia, dizziness, headache.
GI: abdominal discomfort, *diarrhea, flatulence,* indigestion, *nausea,* unpleasant or metallic taste, *vomiting.*
Hematologic: megaloblastic anemia.
Metabolic: *lactic acidosis.*

Interactions

Drug-drug. *Calcium channel blockers, corticosteroids, estrogens, hormonal contraceptives, isoniazid, nicotinic acid, phenothiazines, pheny-*

toin, sympathomimetics, thiazide and other diuretics, thyroid drugs: May cause hyperglycemia. Monitor patient's glycemic control. Increase metformin dosage.

Cationic drugs (such as amiloride, cimetidine, digoxin, morphine, procainamide, quinidine, quinine, ranitidine, triamterene, trimethoprim, vancomycin): May reduce metformin clearance and increase metformin level. Monitor patient's glucose level. Adjust dosages, if needed.

Furosemide, nifedipine: May increase metformin level. Monitor patient and decrease dosage.

Iodinated contrast material: May cause lactic acidosis, leading to acute renal impairment. Withhold metformin on or before the day of the study, and resume after 48 hours, if renal function is normal.

Drug-herb. *Aloe, bilberry leaf, bitter melon, burdock, dandelion, fenugreek, garlic, ginseng:* May improve glucose control and allow reduction of antidiabetic. Tell patient to discuss use of herbal remedies with prescriber before therapy.

Drug-lifestyle. *Alcohol use:* May increase drug effects. Discourage use together.

Effects on lab test results

• May decrease pH, bicarbonate, triglyceride, total cholesterol, LDL, glucose, hemoglobin, and glycosylated hemoglobin levels and hematocrit.
• May decrease RBC count.

Pharmacokinetics

Absorption: Food decreases rate and extent for tablets, but increases extent for oral solution.
Distribution: Negligible.
Metabolism: None.
Excretion: Unchanged in urine. *Half-life:* About 6 hours.

Route	Onset	Peak	Duration
P.O.			
Regular	Unknown	2–4 hr	Unknown
Solution	Unknown	2½ hr	Unknown
Extended-release	Unknown	4–8 hr	24–48 hr

Action

Chemical effect: Decreases hepatic glucose production and intestinal absorption of glucose and improves insulin sensitivity (increases peripheral glucose uptake and utilization).

Therapeutic effect: Lowers blood glucose level.

Available forms

Oral solution: 500 mg/5 ml
Tablets: 500 mg, 850 mg, 1,000 mg
Tablets (extended-release): 500 mg, 750 mg, 1,000 mg

NURSING PROCESS

Assessment
• Assess patient's glucose level before therapy and regularly thereafter to monitor drug effectiveness.
• Assess patient's kidney function before therapy and reassess at least annually. If renal impairment is detected, expect prescriber to switch to different antidiabetic.
• Monitor patient's hematologic lab test results for megaloblastic anemia. Patients with low vitamin B12 or calcium intake or absorption may be more likely to develop a below-normal vitamin B12 level. Check their vitamin B12 level every 2 to 3 years.
• Be alert for adverse reactions and drug interactions.
• Monitor patient closely during times of stress, such as infection, fever, surgery, or trauma. Insulin therapy may be needed.
• The risk of drug-induced lactic acidosis is very low but may occur in diabetics with significant renal or hepatic insufficiency, other medical or surgical problems, and multiple drug therapies. The risk of lactic acidosis increases with the degree of renal impairment and patient's age. Don't give drug to patient age 80 or older unless measurement of creatinine clearance shows renal function is normal.
• Assess patient's and family's knowledge of drug therapy.

Nursing diagnoses
• Ineffective health maintenance related to presence of hyperglycemia
• Risk for deficient fluid volume related to drug-induced adverse GI reactions
• Deficient knowledge related to drug therapy

Planning and implementation
• When switching from standard oral antidiabetic (except chlorpropamide) to metformin, usually no transition period is needed. When

switching from chlorpropamide to metformin, use care during first 2 weeks of metformin therapy because prolonged retention of chlorpropamide increases risk of hypoglycemia during this time.

⊛ **ALERT:** Don't use extended-release formulation in children.

⊛ **ALERT:** Don't cut, crush, or chew extended-release tablets; swallow whole.

• If glucose level rises despite therapy, notify prescriber.

• If patient hasn't responded to 4 weeks of therapy using maximum dosage, add oral sulfonylurea while continuing metformin at maximum dosage. If patient still doesn't respond after several months, stop both drugs and start insulin therapy.

⊛ **ALERT:** If patient develops conditions linked to hypoxemia or dehydration, stop giving the drug immediately and notify prescriber because of risk of lactic acidosis.

• Stop therapy temporarily for a surgical procedure (except minor procedures not related to restricted intake of food and fluids), and don't restart until patient's oral intake and kidney function are normal.

Patient teaching

• Tell patient to take once-daily dose with breakfast (except Fortamet or Glumetza, which is to be taken with dinner) and twice-daily dose with breakfast and dinner.

• Tell patient not to crush or chew extended-release tablets.

• Instruct patient to stop drug and tell prescriber about unexplained hyperventilation, myalgia, malaise, unusual somnolence, or other symptoms of early lactic acidosis.

• Warn patient to avoid alcohol consumption while taking drug.

⊛ **ALERT:** Teach patient about diabetes and the importance of complying with therapy; adhering to diet, weight reduction, exercise, and hygiene programs; and avoiding infection. Explain how and when to monitor glucose level and how to differentiate between hypoglycemia and hyperglycemia.

• Tell patient not to change dose without prescriber's consent. Encourage patient to report abnormal glucose test results.

• Advise patient not to take other drugs, including OTC drugs, without checking with prescriber.

• Instruct patient to wear or carry medical identification.

☑ **Evaluation**

• Patient's glucose level is normal.

• Patient maintains adequate hydration throughout therapy.

• Patient and family state understanding of drug therapy.

HIGH ALERT

methadone hydrochloride
(METH-eh-dohn high-droh-KLOR-ighd)
Diskets, Dolophine, Methadose

Pharmacologic class: opioid
Therapeutic class: analgesic, opioid detoxification adjunct
Pregnancy risk category: C
Controlled substance schedule: II

Indications and dosages

▶ **Severe pain.** *Adults:* 2.5 to 10 mg P.O., I.M., or subcutaneously every 3 to 4 hours, p.r.n. If patient is opioid-naive, give every 8 to 12 hours. *Children‡:* 0.7 mg/kg P.O. every 4 to 6 hours.
▶ **Opioid withdrawal syndrome.** *Adults:* 15 to 40 mg P.O. daily initially based on previous opioid exposure (highly individualized). Maintenance dosage is 20 to 120 mg P.O. daily. Adjust dosage as needed. Daily doses greater than 120 mg require state and federal approval.

Contraindications and cautions

• Contraindicated in patients hypersensitive to the drug or any of its components.

• Use cautiously in debilitated patients and in patients with acute abdominal conditions, severe hepatic or renal impairment, hypothyroidism, Addison disease, prostatic hyperplasia, urethral stricture, head injury, increased intracranial pressure, asthma, or other respiratory conditions.

⚖ **Lifespan:** In pregnant women, use cautiously. In breast-feeding women, don't use. It's unknown if the drug appears in breast milk. In children, safety and effectiveness haven't been established. In elderly patients, use cautiously.

Adverse reactions

CNS: agitation, chorea, *clouded sensorium,* dizziness, *euphoria,* hallucinations, headache,

---

insomnia, light-headedness, *sedation, seizures, somnolence,* syncope.

CV: *arrhythmias, bradycardia, cardiac arrest, cardiomyopathy,* flushing, hypotension, phlebitis, *prolonged QT interval, shock.*

EENT: visual disturbances.

GI: abdominal pain, anorexia, constipation, glossitis, ileus, nausea, vomiting.

GU: urine retention.

Metabolic: hypokalemia, *hypomagnesia,* weight gain.

Respiratory: *pulmonary edema, respiratory arrest, respiratory depression.*

Skin: diaphoresis.

Other: decreased libido, induration after subcutaneous injection, pain at injection site, *physical dependence,* tissue irritation.

Interactions

Drug-drug. *Ammonium chloride and other urine acidifiers, phenytoin:* May reduce methadone effect. Monitor patient for decreased pain control.

Cimetidine: May increase methadone level. Monitor patient for increased CNS and respiratory depression.

CNS depressants, general anesthetics, hypnotics, MAO inhibitors, sedatives, tranquilizers, tricyclic antidepressants: May cause respiratory depression, hypotension, profound sedation, or coma. Use together cautiously and monitor patient.

Rifampin: May cause withdrawal symptoms; reduces blood levels of methadone. Use together cautiously.

Drug-lifestyle. *Alcohol use:* May have additive effects. Discourage patient from use together.

Effects on lab test results

● May increase amylase or lipase levels.

Pharmacokinetics

Absorption: Good in P.O. use; unknown in I.M. use.

Distribution: Highly bound to tissue protein.

Metabolism: Mainly in liver.

Excretion: Mainly in urine; metabolites in feces. *Half-life:* 15 to 25 hours.

Route	Onset	Peak	Duration
P.O.	30–60 min	1–2 hr	4–7 hr
I.M.	10–30 min	½–1 hr	4–7 hr
SubQ	Unknown	1–1½ hr	4–7 hr

Action

Chemical effect: Binds to opioid receptors at many sites in CNS, altering both perception of and emotional response to pain through unknown mechanism.

Therapeutic effect: Relieves pain and symptoms of opioid withdrawal.

Available forms

Dispersible tablets (for maintenance therapy): 40 mg
Injection: 10 mg/ml
Oral solution (contains 8% alcohol): 5 mg/ 5 ml, 10 mg/5 ml, 10 mg/ml (concentrate)
Tablets: 5 mg, 10 mg

NURSING PROCESS

Assessment
● Assess patient's pain or opioid dependence before and during therapy.
● Monitor patient closely because drug has cumulative effect. Marked sedation can occur after repeated doses.
⊛ ALERT: Respiratory depressant effect may last longer than analgesic effect. Monitor patient's respiratory status closely.
● Be alert for adverse reactions and drug interactions.
● Assess patient's and family's knowledge of drug therapy.

Nursing diagnoses
● Chronic pain related to underlying condition
● Ineffective coping related to opioid dependence
● Deficient knowledge related to drug therapy

Planning and implementation
● Liquid form is legally required in maintenance programs. Dissolve tablets in 120 ml of orange juice or powdered citrus drink.
● P.O. dose is one-half as potent as injected dose.
● Dispersible tablets are only available in 40 mg doses so they may not be appropriate for initial dosing in many patients.
● For parenteral use, I.M. injection is preferred. Rotate injection sites.
● Around-the-clock therapy is needed to manage severe, chronic pain.
● Duration of action is prolonged to 22 to 48 hours with repeated doses of drug. Depres-

M

sant effects from overdosage can also last 36 to 48 hours.

⊛ **ALERT:** Very high doses of methadone may cause QT interval prolongation and torsades de pointes.

⊛ **ALERT:** Don't confuse methadone with Metadate.

Patient teaching
• Warn patient about getting out of bed or walking. Warn outpatient to avoid hazardous activities until drug's CNS effects are known.
• Instruct patient to avoid alcohol consumption during drug therapy.

☑ Evaluation
• Patient is free from pain.
• Patient doesn't exhibit opioid withdrawal symptoms.
• Patient and family state understanding of drug therapy.

methamphetamine hydrochloride
(meth-am-FET-uh-meen high-droh-KLOR-ighd)
Desoxyn

Pharmacologic class: amphetamine
Therapeutic class: CNS stimulant, short-term adjunct anorexigenic, sympathomimetic amine
Pregnancy risk category: C
Controlled substance schedule: II

Indications and dosages

▶ **Attention deficit hyperactivity disorder.**
Children age 6 and older: Initially, 5 mg P.O. once daily or b.i.d., increase by 5-mg increments weekly p.r.n. Usual effective dosage is 20 to 25 mg daily.
▶ **Short-term adjunct in exogenous obesity.**
Adults and children older than age 12: Give 5 mg P.O. 30 minutes before each meal. Treatment should not exceed a few weeks.

Contraindications and cautions

• Contraindicated in patients hypersensitive to sympathomimetic amines; patients with idiosyncratic reactions to sympathomimetic amines; patients with moderate to severe hypertension, hyperthyroidism, symptomatic CV disease, advanced arteriosclerosis, glaucoma, or history of drug abuse; patients who have taken an MAO inhibitor within 14 days; and agitated patients.

• Use cautiously in patients who are debilitated, asthenic, psychopathic, or patients who have a history of suicidal or homicidal tendencies.

⚖ **Lifespan:** In pregnant and breast-feeding women, drug is contraindicated. In children younger than age 6, safety and effectiveness haven't been established. In elderly patients, use cautiously.

Adverse reactions

CNS: dizziness, euphoria, headache, hyperexcitability, *insomnia,* irritability, *nervousness,* psychotic episodes, *talkativeness,* tics, tremors, worsening of Tourette syndrome.
CV: *arrhythmias, cardiomyopathy,* hypertension, *palpitations, reflex bradycardia,* tachycardia.
EENT: blurred vision, mydriasis.
GI: abdominal cramps, *anorexia,* constipation, diarrhea, dry mouth, metallic taste, nausea, vomiting.
GU: impotence.
Skin: urticaria.
Other: altered libido, growth suppression in children.

Interactions

Drug-drug. *Acetazolamide, antacids, sodium bicarbonate:* May increase renal reabsorption. Monitor patient for enhanced effects.
Ammonium chloride, ascorbic acid: May decrease level and increase renal excretion of methamphetamine. Monitor patient for decreased methamphetamine effects.
Furazolidone: May increase sensitivity to amphetamines. Monitor patient for toxicity and adjust dosage as needed.
Guanethidine: May decrease the antihypertensive effectiveness of guanethidine. Monitor blood pressure.
Haloperidol, phenothiazines, tricyclic antidepressants: May increase CNS effects. Avoid use together.
Insulin, oral antidiabetics: May decrease antidiabetic requirement. Monitor glucose level.
MAO inhibitors: May cause severe hypertension; possible hypertensive crisis. Don't use within 14 days of MAO inhibitor therapy.
SSRIs: May increase sensitivity to sympathomimetics and increase risk of serotonin syndrome. Monitor and adjust dosage as needed.

Reactions may be *common,* uncommon, *life-threatening,* or COMMON AND LIFE-THREATENING.

Photoguide to tablets and capsules

This photoguide provides full-color photographs of some of the most commonly prescribed tablets and capsules. These drugs, organized by generic name, are shown in actual size and color with page references to corresponding drug information. Each drug is labeled with its trade name and its strength.

Adapted from Facts & Comparisons, St. Louis, Mo.

For the list of companies permitting the use of these photographs, see pages 1403-1404.

ACAMPROSATE CALCIUM

Campral
(page 96)

333 mg

ALENDRONATE SODIUM

Fosamax
(page 120)

10 mg　　　　　　40 mg　　　　　　70 mg

ALPRAZOLAM

Xanax
(page 130)

0.25 mg　　　　　0.5 mg　　　　　1 mg

2 mg

AMLODIPINE BESYLATE

Norvasc
(page 145)

2.5 mg　　　　　5 mg　　　　　10 mg

ANASTROZOLE

Arimidex
(page 162)

1 mg

ARIPIPRAZOLE

Abilify
(page 170)

10 mg   15 mg   30 mg

ATENOLOL

Tenormin
(page 180)

25 mg   50 mg   100 mg

ATOMOXETINE HYDROCHLORIDE

Strattera
(page 182)

10 mg   18 mg   25 mg

40 mg   60 mg

ATORVASTATIN CALCIUM

Lipitor
(page 183)

10 mg   20 mg   40 mg

80 mg

AZITHROMYCIN

Zithromax
(page 194)

250 mg   500 mg   600 mg

CAPTOPRIL

Capoten
(page 252)

12.5 mg   25 mg

CELECOXIB

Celebrex
(page 289)

100 mg   200 mg

CIPROFLOXACIN HYDROCHLORIDE

Cipro
(page 316)

250 mg   500 mg   750 mg

CITALOPRAM HYDROBROMIDE

Celexa
(page 321)

20 mg   40 mg

DARIFENACIN HYDROBROMIDE

Enablex
(page 376)

7.5 mg   15 mg

DESLORATADINE

Clarinex
(page 388)

5 mg

DIAZEPAM
Valium
(page 403)

2 mg

5 mg

10 mg

DILTIAZEM HYDROCHLORIDE
Cardizem
(page 417)

30 mg

90 mg

Cardizem CD
(page 417)

180 mg

360 mg

Cardizem LA
(page 417)

180 mg

240 mg

360 mg

DIVALPROEX SODIUM
Depakote
(page 1281)

125 mg

250 mg

500 mg

DULOXETINE HYDROCHLORIDE
Cymbalta
(page 459)

20 mg

30 mg

60 mg

ENALAPRIL MALEATE

Vasotec
(page 473)

2.5 mg   5 mg   10 mg

20 mg

ERYTHROMYCIN BASE

Eryc
(page 499)

250 mg

ESCITALOPRAM OXALATE

Lexapro
(page 502)

10 mg   20 mg

ESTRADIOL

Estrace
(page 509)

0.5 mg   1 mg   2 mg

ESZOPICLONE

Lunesta
(page 521)

1 mg   2 mg   3 mg

EZETIMBE

Zetia
(page 545)

10 mg

FAMOTIDINE

Pepcid

(page 548)

20 mg   40 mg

FLUCONAZOLE

Diflucan

(page 564)

100 mg   150 mg   200 mg

FLUOXETINE HYDROCHLORIDE

Prozac

(page 574)

10 mg   20 mg   40 mg

90 mg

FOSINOPRIL SODIUM

Monopril

(page 600)

10 mg   20 mg   40 mg

FROVATRIPTAN SUCCINATE

Frova

(page 603)

2.5 mg

FUROSEMIDE

Lasix

(page 606)

20 mg   40 mg   80 mg

GABAPENTIN

Neurontin
(page 608)

100 mg   300 mg   400 mg

GLIPIZIDE

Glucotrol
(page 622)

5 mg   10 mg

Glucotrol XL
(page 622)

5 mg   10 mg

GLYBURIDE

DiaBeta
(page 625)

1.25 mg   2.5 mg   5 mg

Micronase
(page 625)

1.25 mg   2.5 mg   5 mg

LANSOPRAZOLE

Prevacid
(page 731)

15 mg   30 mg

LEVOFLOXACIN

Levaquin
(page 751)

250 mg

500 mg

LEVOTHYROXINE SODIUM

Levoxyl
(page 754)

25 mcg

50 mcg

75 mcg

88 mcg

100 mcg

112 mcg

125 mcg

137 mcg

150 mcg

175 mcg

200 mcg

300 mcg

LISINOPRIL

Prinivil
(page 763)

5 mg

10 mg

20 mg

40 mg

LOPINAVIR AND RITONAVIR

Kaletra
(page 769)

200mg/50 mg

LOSARTAN POTASSIUM

Cozaar
(page 775)

25 mg

50 mg

LOVASTATIN

Mevacor
(page 777)

10 mg

20 mg

40 mg

LUBIPROSTONE

Amitiza
(page 779)

24 mcg

MEDROXYPROGESTERONE ACETATE

Provera
(page 795)

2.5 mg

5 mg

10 mg

METFORMIN HYDROCHLORIDE

Glucophage
(page 816)

500 mg

850 mg

1,000 mg

Glucophage XR
(page 816)

500 mg

METHYLPHENIDATE HYDROCHLORIDE

Ritalin
(page 828)

| 5 mg | 10 mg | 20 mg |

METOPROLOL SUCCINATE

Toprol-XL
(page 837)

| 50 mg | 100 mg | 200 mg |

MONTELUKAST SODIUM

Singulair
(page 863)

| 4 mg | 5 mg | 10 mg |

NIFEDIPINE

Procardia XL
(page 904)

| 30 mg | 60 mg | 90 mg |

NORTRIPTYLINE HYDROCHLORIDE

Pamelor
(page 919)

| 10 mg | 25 mg | 50 mg |

OMEPRAZOLE

Prilosec
(page 934)

| 10 mg | 20 mg | 40 mg |

OXYCODONE HYDROCHLORIDE

OxyContin
(page 947)

10 mg

20 mg

40 mg

80 mg

PHENYTOIN SODIUM

Dilantin Kapseals
(page 1000)

30 mg

100 mg

POTASSIUM CHLORIDE

K-Dur 20
(page 1017)

20 mEq

PRAVASTATIN SODIUM

Pravachol
(page 1027)

10 mg

20 mg

40 mg

QUINAPRIL HYDROCHLORIDE

Accupril
(page 1065)

5 mg

10 mg

20 mg

40 mg

RANOLAZINE

Ranexa
(page 1082)

500 mg

RASAGILINE

Azilect
(page 1083)

0.5 mg

1 mg

RISEDRONATE SODIUM

Actonel
(page 1099)

5 mg

35 mg

RISPERIDONE

Risperdal
(page 1101)

0.25 mg

0.5 mg

1 mg

2 mg

3 mg

4 mg

Risperdal M-Tab
(page 1101)

0.5 mg

ROSIGLITAZONE MALEATE

Avandia
(page 1111)

2 mg

4 mg

8 mg

ROSUVASTATIN CALCIUM

Crestor
(page 1113)

5 mg

10 mg

20 mg

40 mg

SERTRALINE HYDROCHLORIDE

Zoloft
(page 1129)

50 mg

100 mg

SILDENAFIL CITRATE

Viagra
(page 1135)

25 mg

50 mg

100 mg

SIMVASTATIN

Zocor
(page 1137)

5 mg

10 mg

20 mg

40 mg

SITAGLIPTIN PHOSPHATE

Januvia
(page 1142)

100 mg

SORAFENIB
Nexavar
(page 1156)

200 mg

SUNITINIB MALATE
Sutent
(page 1180)

12.5 mg   25 mg   50 mg

TERAZOSIN HYDROCHLORIDE
Hytrin
(page 1202)

1 mg   5 mg   10 mg

VARDENAFIL HYDROCHLORIDE
Levitra
(page 1286)

5 mg   10 mg   20 mg

VARENICLINE TARTRATE
Chantix
(page 1288)

0.5 mg   1mg

VENLAFAXINE HYDROCHLORIDE
Effexor XR
(page 1292)

75 mg   150 mg

VERAPAMIL HYDROCHLORIDE

Calan
(page 1294)

40 mg

80 mg

120 mg

WARFARIN SODIUM

Coumadin
(page 1311)

1 mg

2 mg

2.5 mg

3 mg

4 mg

5 mg

6 mg

7.5 mg

10 mg

ZOLPIDEM TARTRATE

Ambien
(page 1326)

5 mg

10 mg

Drug-herb. *Melatonin*: May enhance mono-aminergic effects of drug; may worsen insomnia. Discourage use together.
Drug-food. *Caffeinated beverages:* May increase drug effects. Discourage use together.

Effects on lab test results

• May increase corticosteroid level.

Pharmacokinetics

Absorption: Rapid.
Distribution: Wide.
Metabolism: In liver to at least seven metabolites.
Excretion: In urine. *Half-life:* 4 to 5 hours.

Route	Onset	Peak	Duration
P.O.	Unknown	Unknown	≤ 24 hr

Action

Chemical effect: Probably promotes nerve impulse transmission by releasing stored norepinephrine from nerve terminals in brain. Main sites appear to be cerebral cortex and reticular activating system. In hyperkinetic children, drug has paradoxical calming effect.
Therapeutic effect: Promotes calmness in children with attention deficit disorder and causes weight loss.

Available forms

Tablets: 5 mg

NURSING PROCESS

Assessment
• Assess patient's condition before therapy, and regularly thereafter to monitor drug effectiveness.
• Be alert for adverse reactions and drug interactions particularly growth suppression in children and cardiomyopathy with prolonged use.
• Assess patient's and family's knowledge of drug therapy.

Nursing diagnoses
• Ineffective health maintenance related to underlying condition
• Sleep deprivation related to drug-induced insomnia
• Deficient knowledge related to drug therapy

Planning and implementation
ⓢ **ALERT:** Don't confuse Desoxyn with digitoxin or digoxin.
• Store drug below 30° C (86° F).
• Drug isn't the first-line therapy for obesity. Use as anorexigenic is prohibited in some states.
• When used for obesity, make sure patient is on weight-reduction program.
• If tolerance to anorexigenic effect develops, notify prescriber and stop giving the drug.
Patient teaching
• Warn patient of high risk of abuse. Advise him that drug shouldn't be used to prevent fatigue.
• Advise patient to take last dose of drug at least 6 hours before bedtime.
• Warn patient to avoid activities that require alertness or good coordination until the drug's CNS effects are known.
• Tell patient not to use caffeine during therapy.
• Instruct patient to report signs of excessive stimulation.
• Instruct patient not to crush long-acting tablets.

Evaluation
• Patient has positive response to drug therapy.
• Patient doesn't experience insomnia.
• Patient and family state understanding of drug therapy.

methimazole
(meth-IH-muh-zohl)
Tapazole

Pharmacologic class: thyroid hormone antagonist
Therapeutic class: antithyroid drug
Pregnancy risk category: D

Indications and dosages

▶ **Hyperthyroidism.** *Adults:* If mild, 15 mg P.O. daily. If moderately severe, 30 to 40 mg daily. If severe, 60 mg daily. Daily dosage divided into three doses at 8-hour intervals. Maintenance dosage is 5 to 15 mg daily.
Children: 0.4 mg/kg P.O. daily in divided doses every 8 hours. Maintenance dosage is 0.2 mg/kg P.O. daily in divided doses every 8 hours. Or 0.5 to 0.7 mg/kg P.O. daily in three divided doses. Maintenance dosage is one-third to two-thirds of initial dose. Maximum dosage 30 mg/24 hours.

Contraindications and cautions

• Contraindicated in patients hypersensitive to the drug or any of its components.

⚖ **Lifespan:** In pregnant women, use cautiously. In breast-feeding women, use cautiously; it's unknown if drug appears in breast milk.

Adverse reactions

CNS: CNS stimulation, depression, drowsiness, headache, neuritis, neuropathies, paresthesias, vertigo.
GI: diarrhea, epigastric distress, loss of taste, nausea, salivary gland enlargement, vomiting.
Hematologic: *agranulocytosis, aplastic anemia, leukopenia,* lymphadenopathy, *thrombocytopenia.*
Hepatic: jaundice.
Metabolic: hypothyroidism.
Musculoskeletal: arthralgia, myalgia.
Skin: alopecia, rash, skin discoloration, urticaria.
Other: drug-induced fever.

Interactions

Drug-drug. *Anticoagulants:* May enhance anti–vitamin K effects. Monitor PT and INR.
Beta blockers, digoxin, theophylline: May increase levels of these drugs when a hyperthyroid patient becomes euthyroid. Reduce dosage of these drugs, if needed.

Effects on lab test results

• May decrease hemoglobin level and hematocrit.
• May decrease granulocyte, WBC, RBC, and platelet counts.

Pharmacokinetics

Absorption: Rapid.
Distribution: Concentrated in thyroid and isn't protein-bound.
Metabolism: Hepatic.
Excretion: Mainly in urine. *Half-life:* 5 to 13 hours.

Route	Onset	Peak	Duration
P.O.	Unknown	30 min–1 hr	Unknown

Action

Chemical effect: Inhibits oxidation of iodine in thyroid gland, blocking iodine's ability to combine with tyrosine to form T4. Also may prevent coupling of monoiodotyrosine and diiodotyrosine to form T4 and T3.
Therapeutic effect: Reduces thyroid hormone level.

Available forms

Tablets: 5 mg, 10 mg

NURSING PROCESS

📋 Assessment

• Assess patient's thyroid condition before therapy and regularly thereafter to monitor the drug's effectiveness.
• Monitor thyroid function studies.
• Monitor CBC and liver function periodically.
🔔 **ALERT:** Dosages higher than 30 mg daily increase risk of agranulocytosis, especially in patients older than age 40.
• Be alert for adverse reactions.
• Assess patient's and family's knowledge of drug therapy.

🔀 Nursing diagnoses

• Ineffective health maintenance related to presence of hyperthyroidism
• Risk for infection related to drug-induced adverse hematologic reactions
• Deficient knowledge related to drug therapy

➤ Planning and implementation

• Pregnant women may need a lower dosage as pregnancy progresses. Thyroid hormone may be added. Drug may be stopped during last weeks of pregnancy.
• Notify prescriber about signs and symptoms of hypothyroidism and adjust dosage.
🔔 **ALERT:** If severe rash occurs or cervical lymph nodes become enlarged, stop giving the drug and notify prescriber.
🔔 **ALERT:** Don't confuse methimazole with mebendazole, methazolamide, or rabeprazole.
Patient teaching
• Tell patient to take drug with meals.
• Warn patient to immediately report fever, sore throat, or mouth sores (signs of agranulocytosis); skin eruptions (sign of hypersensitivity); or anorexia, pruritus, right upper quadrant pain, and yellow skin or sclera (signs of hepatic dysfunction).
• Tell patient to ask prescriber about using iodized salt and eating shellfish.

Reactions may be *common*, uncommon, *life-threatening*, or COMMON AND LIFE-THREATENING.

- Warn patient against taking OTC cough products, because many contain iodine.
- Instruct patient to store drug in light-resistant container.

✓ Evaluation
- Patient has normal thyroid hormone level.
- Patient maintains normal hematologic parameters and remains free from infection throughout therapy.
- Patient and family state understanding of drug therapy.

HIGH ALERT

methotrexate
(amethopterin, MTX)
(meth-oh-TRECKS-ayt)
Trexall

methotrexate sodium
Methotrexate LPF, Rheumatrex Dose Pack

Pharmacologic class: antimetabolite
Therapeutic class: antineoplastic, immunosuppressant, antirheumatic
Pregnancy risk category: X

Indications and dosages

▶ **Trophoblastic tumors (choriocarcinoma, hydatidiform mole).** *Adults:* 15 to 30 mg P.O. or I.M. daily for 5 days. May repeat course after 1 or more weeks, based on response or toxicity. Three to five courses usually are used.

▶ **Acute lymphoblastic and lymphatic leukemia.** *Adults and children:* 3.3 mg/m² P.O. or I.M. daily for 4 to 6 weeks or until remission occurs; then 20 to 30 mg/m² P.O. or I.M. twice weekly. Or, 2.5 mg/kg I.V. every 14 days.

▶ **Meningeal leukemia.** *Adults and children:* 12 mg/m² intrathecally (maximum of 15 mg) every 2 to 5 days and repeat until cell count of CSF returns to normal, then give one additional dose. Or, 12 mg/m² once weekly for 2 weeks, then once monthly thereafter. Or intrathecal dose based on age in years: younger than 1 year, 6 mg; 1 year, 8 mg; 2 years, 10 mg; 3 years or older, 12 mg.

▶ **Burkitt lymphoma (stage I or stage II).** *Adults:* 10 to 25 mg P.O. daily for 4 to 8 days with 7- to 10-day rest intervals.

▶ **Lymphosarcoma (stage III).** *Adults:* 0.625 to 2.5 mg/kg P.O., I.M., or I.V. daily.

▶ **Osteosarcoma.** *Adults:* 12 g/m² I.V. as a 4-hour infusion. May increase to 15 g/m² in subsequent treatments if peak serum concentration at the end of infusion doesn't reach 1,000 micromolar (10–3 mol/L).

▶ **Mycosis fungoides.** *Adults:* 5 to 50 mg P.O. or I.M. once weekly. Or, 15 to 37.5 mg P.O. or I.M. twice weekly.

▶ **Psoriasis.** *Adults:* 10 to 25 mg P.O., I.M., or I.V. as single weekly dose. Do not exceed 30 mg/week. Or, 2.5 mg every 12 hours for 3 doses each week. Don't exceed 30 mg/week. A 5- to 10-mg test dose should be tried the week before therapy starts.

▶ **Rheumatoid arthritis.** *Adults:* Initially, 7.5 mg P.O. once weekly, or divided as 2.5 mg P.O. every 12 hours for three doses once a week. Gradually increase dosage to maximum, 20 mg weekly.
Adults‡: 7.5 to 15 mg I.M. once weekly.

▶ **Head and neck carcinoma‡.** *Adults:* 40 to 60 mg/m² I.V. once weekly. Response to therapy is limited to 4 months.

▼ I.V. administration

- Follow facility policy to reduce risks. Preparation and administration of parenteral forms are linked to carcinogenic, mutagenic, and teratogenic risks.
- Liquid methotrexate sodium injection with preservatives may be given undiluted except intrathecally or in high I.V. doses.
- Preservative-free liquid methotrexate sodium injection may be given undiluted or may be further diluted with normal saline solution.
- For reconstitution of lyophilized powders, reconstitute immediately before use, and discard unused drug. Dilute with D_5W or normal saline solution. Dilute the 20-mg vial to a concentration no greater than 25 mg/ml. Reconstitute 1-g vial with 19.4 ml of diluent for a maximum concentration of 50 mg/ml.
- For intrathecal use, only use 20-mg vials of powder with no preservatives. Reconstitute immediately before using, with preservative-free normal saline solution injection. Dilute to maximum of 1 mg/ml. Use only new vials of drug and diluent.
- Drug may be given daily or weekly, depending on the disease.

M

• Storage for 24 hours at 70° to 77° F (21° to 25° C) results in a product that is within 90% of label potency. Protect from light.

⊗ **Incompatibilities**

Bleomycin, chlorpromazine, dexamethasone sodium phosphate, droperidol, fluorouracil, gemcitabine, idarubicin, ifosfamide, metoclopramide, midazolam, nalbuphine, prednisolone, promethazine, propofol, sodium phosphate, vancomycin.

Contraindications and cautions

• Contraindicated in patients hypersensitive to the drug or any of its components and in those with psoriasis or rheumatoid arthritis who also have alcoholism, alcoholic liver, chronic liver disease, immunodeficiency syndromes, or blood dyscrasias.
• Use cautiously and at modified dosage in patients with impaired liver or kidney function, bone marrow suppression, aplasia, leukopenia, thrombocytopenia, or anemia. Also use cautiously in patients with infection, peptic ulceration, or ulcerative colitis and in debilitated patients.

☀ **Lifespan:** In pregnant and breast-feeding women, drug is contraindicated. In children younger than age 2, safety and effectiveness haven't been established for uses other than cancer. In elderly patients, use cautiously.

Adverse reactions

CNS: arachnoiditis, dizziness, headache, *leukoencephalopathy,* malaise, neurotoxicity, *seizures,* subacute demyelination.
EENT: blurred vision, gingivitis, pharyngitis.
GI: diarrhea, enteritis, *intestinal perforation,* nausea, stomatitis, vomiting.
GU: nephropathy, *renal impairment, renal failure,* TUBULAR NECROSIS.
Hematologic: *anemia, leukopenia, thrombocytopenia.*
Hepatic: *acute toxicity, chronic toxicity, cirrhosis, hepatic fibrosis.*
Metabolic: hyperuricemia.
Musculoskeletal: osteoporosis in children with long-term use.
Respiratory: pneumonitis, *pulmonary fibrosis, pulmonary interstitial infiltrates.*
Skin: alopecia, hyperpigmentation, photosensitivity reactions, pruritus, psoriatic lesions, rash, *urticaria.*
Other: *severe infections, sudden death.*

Interactions

Drug-drug. *Digoxin:* May decrease digoxin level. Monitor digoxin level.
Folic acid derivatives: May antagonize methotrexate effect. Monitor patient.
NSAIDs, phenylbutazone, salicylates, sulfonamides: May increase methotrexate toxicity. Use together cautiously; monitor methotrexate levels.
Phenytoin: May decrease phenytoin level. Monitor phenytoin level.
Probenecid: May impair excretion of methotrexate, causing increased levels, effects, and toxicity. Monitor level closely, and decrease dosage accordingly.
Procarbazine: May increase nephrotoxicity of methotrexate. Monitor renal function closely.
Vaccines: May inactivate vaccine; may increase risk of disseminated infection with live-virus vaccines. Consult with prescriber about safe time to give vaccine.
Drug-food. *Food:* May delay drug absorption and reduce peak levels of methotrexate. Take on empty stomach.
Drug-lifestyle. *Alcohol use:* May increase hepatotoxicity. Discourage use together.
Sun exposure: May cause photosensitivity reactions. Urge patient to avoid unprotected or prolonged exposure to sunlight.

Effects on lab test results

• May increase uric acid, BUN, creatinine, and liver enzyme levels. May decrease hemoglobin level and hematocrit.
• May decrease WBC, RBC, and platelet counts.

Pharmacokinetics

Absorption: For small P.O. doses, almost complete, but for large doses, incomplete and variable. For I.M. use, complete.
Distribution: Wide, with highest levels in kidneys, gallbladder, spleen, liver, and skin. About 50% protein-bound.
Metabolism: Only slight.
Excretion: Primarily in urine. *Half-life for doses below 30 mg/m^2:* About 3 to 10 hours. *Half-life for doses of 30 mg/m^2 and above:* 8 to 15 hours.

Route	Onset	Peak	Duration
P.O.	Unknown	1–2 hr	Unknown
I.V., intrathecal	Unknown	Immediate	24 hr
I.M.	Unknown	30 min–1 hr	Unknown

Reactions may be *common*, uncommon, *life-threatening*, or COMMON AND LIFE-THREATENING.

Action

Chemical effect: Prevents reduction of folic acid to tetrahydrofolate by binding to dihydrofolate reductase.
Therapeutic effect: Kills certain cancer cells and reduces inflammation.

Available forms

methotrexate
Tablets: 2.5 mg, 5 mg, 7.5 mg, 10 mg, 15 mg
methotrexate sodium
Injection (lyophilized powder, preservative free): 20 mg (as base); 1-g (as base) vials
Injection (preservative-free): 25 mg/ml in 2-, 4-, 8-, 10-, 20-, and 40-ml vials
Injection (with preservatives): 25 mg/ml in 2- and 10-ml vials
Tablets: 2.5 mg

NURSING PROCESS

🏷 Assessment
• Assess patient's condition before therapy and regularly thereafter to monitor drug effectiveness.
• Perform baseline pulmonary function tests before therapy, and repeat periodically.
• Monitor fluid intake and output daily.
• Monitor uric acid level.
• Watch for increases in AST, ALT, and alkaline phosphatase levels, which are signs of hepatic dysfunction.
• Regularly monitor CBC.
• Be alert for adverse reactions and drug interactions.
• Assess patient's and family's knowledge of drug therapy.

🔷 Nursing diagnoses
• Ineffective health maintenance related to underlying condition
• Risk for infection related to drug-induced adverse hematologic reactions
• Deficient knowledge related to drug therapy

▶ Planning and implementation
• CSF volume depends on age, not body surface area (BSA). Basing dose on BSA for meningeal leukemia may cause low CSF methotrexate level in children and high level and neurotoxicity in adults. Instead, base dose on patient's age. Elderly patients may need a reduced dosage because CSF volume and turnover may decrease with age.
• Arachnoiditis can develop within hours of intrathecal use but subacute neurotoxicity may begin a few weeks later.
• Have patient drink 2 to 3 L of fluids daily.
• **⑤ ALERT:** Alkalinize urine by giving sodium bicarbonate tablets to prevent precipitation of drug, especially with high doses. Maintain urine pH at more than 6.5. If BUN level reaches 20 to 30 mg/dl or creatinine level reaches 1.2 to 2 mg/dl, reduce dosage. Report BUN level over 30 mg/dl or creatinine level over 2 mg/dl, and stop drug.
• Rash, redness, ulcerations in the mouth, or adverse pulmonary reactions may signal serious complications. If patient develops ulcerative stomatitis, other severe adverse GI reaction, or pulmonary toxicity, stop giving the drug.
• Leucovorin rescue is used with high-dose (greater than 100 mg) protocols. This technique works against systemic toxicity but doesn't interfere with tumor cells' absorption of methotrexate.
Patient teaching
• Teach and encourage diligent mouth care to reduce risk of superinfection in mouth.
• Tell patient to take oral form on empty stomach.
• Advise patient to avoid prolonged exposure to sunlight, wear protective clothing, and use highly protective sunblock.
• Tell patient to continue leucovorin rescue despite severe nausea and vomiting and to tell prescriber. Parenteral leucovorin therapy may be needed.
• Warn patient not to become pregnant during or immediately after therapy, because of risk of spontaneous abortion or congenital anomalies.
• Instruct patient not to use alcohol during therapy.

☑ Evaluation
• Patient exhibits positive response to drug therapy.
• Patient has no serious complications when hematologic parameters are depressed during therapy.
• Patient and family state understanding of drug therapy.

M

methyldopa
(meth-il-DOH-puh)
Aldomet

methyldopate hydrochloride
Aldomet

Pharmacologic class: centrally acting anti-adrenergic
Therapeutic class: antihypertensive
Pregnancy risk category: B (P.O.), C (I.V.)

Indications and dosages

▶ **Hypertension, hypertensive crisis.** *Adults:* Initially, 250 mg P.O. b.i.d. to t.i.d. in first 48 hours. Then increase as needed every 2 days. Entire daily dosage may be given in evening or at bedtime. If other antihypertensives are added to or removed from therapy, adjust dosages as needed. Maintenance dosage, 500 mg to 2 g daily divided b.i.d. or q.i.d. Maximum daily dosage, 3 g. Or, 250 to 500 mg I.V. every 6 hours. Maximum dosage, 1 g every 6 hours. Switch to P.O. antihypertensives as soon as possible.
Children: Initially, 10 mg/kg P.O. daily in two to four divided doses. Or, 20 to 40 mg/kg I.V. daily in four divided doses. Increase dosage at least every 2 days until desired response occurs. Maximum, 65 mg/kg, 2 g/m^2, or 3 g daily, whichever is least.

▼I.V. administration

• Drug may contain sulfites.
• Dilute appropriate dose in 100 ml D$_5$W. Or, the required dose may be given in 5% dextrose injection at 10 mg/ml.
• Infuse slowly over 30 to 60 minutes.
• When control has been obtained, substitute oral therapy starting with the same parenteral dosage schedule.
⊗ **Incompatibilities**
Amphotericin B; drugs with poor solubility in acidic media, such as barbiturates and sulfonamides; methohexital; some total parenteral nutrition solutions.

Contraindications and cautions

• Contraindicated in patients hypersensitive to drug or any of its components (including sulfites), those with active hepatic disease (such as acute hepatitis) or active cirrhosis, and those taking MAO inhibitors. Also contraindicated if previous methyldopa therapy has been linked to liver disorders.
• Use cautiously in patients with renal impairment or a history of impaired liver function.
⚖ **Lifespan:** Drug has been used effectively in pregnant women without apparent harm to the fetus. In breast-feeding women, use cautiously; it's unknown if the drug appears in breast milk. In elderly patients, use cautiously because they may experience syncope from increased sensitivity.

Adverse reactions

CNS: asthenia, *decreased mental acuity,* depression, dizziness, headache, involuntary choreoathetoid movements, nightmares, psychic disturbances, *sedation,* weakness.
CV: aggravated angina, **bradycardia,** edema, **heart failure, myocarditis,** orthostatic hypotension.
EENT: nasal congestion.
GI: constipation, diarrhea, *dry mouth,* nausea, **pancreatitis,** vomiting.
GU: decreased libido, impotence.
Hematologic: hemolytic anemia, **thrombocytopenia.**
Hepatic: *hepatic necrosis.*
Metabolic: weight gain.
Skin: rash.
Other: *drug-induced fever,* galactorrhea, gynecomastia.

Interactions

Drug-drug. *Amphetamines, norepinephrine, phenothiazines, tricyclic antidepressants:* May decrease hypotensive effects. Monitor blood pressure carefully.
Antihypertensives, diuretics: May increase hypotensive effects. Decrease the methyldopa dosage.
Barbiturates: May increase likelihood of orthostatic hypotension. Monitor patient and blood pressure.
Haloperidol: May produce dementia and sedation. Use together cautiously.
Levodopa: May have additive hypotensive effects and may increase adverse CNS reactions. Monitor patient closely.
Lithium: May increase lithium level. Monitor lithium level and toxicity.

Reactions may be *common,* uncommon, *life-threatening*, or COMMON AND LIFE-THREATENING.

MAO inhibitors: May increase sympathetic stimulation, which may result in hypertensive crisis. Don't use together.
Oral iron therapy: May increase hypotensive effects. Use together cautiously; monitor blood pressure.
Drug-herb. *Capsicum:* May reduce antihypertensive effectiveness. Discourage use together.
Yohimbe: May interfere with blood pressure. Discourage use together.

Effects on lab test results

• May increase creatinine level. May decrease hemoglobin level and hematocrit.
• May decrease liver function test values and granulocyte, platelet, RBC, and WBC counts.
• May cause positive direct Coombs test.

Pharmacokinetics

Absorption: Partial.
Distribution: Wide. Weakly protein-bound.
Metabolism: Extensive in liver and intestinal cells.
Excretion: Absorbed drug in urine; unabsorbed drug in feces. *Half-life:* About 2 hours.

Route	Onset	Peak	Duration
P.O.	Unknown	4–6 hr	12–48 hr
I.V.	Unknown	4–6 hr	10–16 hr

Action

Chemical effect: May involve inhibition of central vasomotor centers, decreasing sympathetic outflow to heart, kidneys, and peripheral vasculature.
Therapeutic effect: Lowers blood pressure.

Available forms

methyldopa
Tablets: 250 mg, 500 mg
methyldopate hydrochloride
Injection: 50 mg/ml in 5- and 10-mg vials

NURSING PROCESS

Assessment
• Assess patient's blood pressure before therapy and regularly thereafter to monitor drug effectiveness.
• Monitor CBC with differential counts before therapy, every 2 weeks for first 3 months, and periodically thereafter.

• In patient who has received this drug for several months, positive reaction to direct Coombs test indicates hemolytic anemia. Monitor patient's Coombs test results.
• Be alert for adverse reactions and drug interactions.
• Assess patient's and family's knowledge of drug therapy.

Nursing diagnoses
• Ineffective health maintenance related to presence of hypertension
• Risk for injury related to drug-induced adverse CNS reactions
• Deficient knowledge related to drug therapy

Planning and implementation
• Report involuntary choreoathetoid movements. Drug may be stopped.
• Tolerance may occur, usually between the second and third months of therapy, and addition of a diuretic or a dosage adjustment may be needed. If patient's response changes significantly, notify prescriber.
• If hypertension occurs after dialysis, notify prescriber. Patient may need extra dose of drug.
• In a patient who needs blood transfusions, perform direct and indirect Coombs tests to prevent crossmatching problems.
ALERT: Don't confuse Aldomet with Aldoril or Anzemet.
Patient teaching
• Advise patient to report signs of infection, such as fever and sore throat.
• Tell patient to report adverse reactions but not to stop taking drug.
• Tell patient to check his weight daily and to report weight gain of more than 5 lb (2.27 kg). Diuretics can relieve sodium and water retention.
• Warn patient that drug may impair mental alertness, particularly at start of therapy. Once-daily dose at bedtime minimizes daytime drowsiness.
• Tell patient to rise slowly and avoid sudden position changes.
• Tell patient that dry mouth can be relieved with ice chips, sugarless gum, or hard candy.
• Advise patient that urine may turn dark in bleached toilet bowls.

Evaluation
• Patient's blood pressure is normal.

• Patient doesn't experience injury as result of drug-induced adverse CNS reactions.
• Patient and family state understanding of drug therapy.

methylphenidate hydrochloride
(meth-il-FEN-ih-dayt high-droh-KLOR-ighd)
Concerta, Metadate CD, Metadate ER, Methylin, Methylin ER, Ritalin◊, Ritalin LA, Ritalin SR

methylphenidate transdermal system
Daytrana

Pharmacologic class: piperidine derivative
Therapeutic class: CNS stimulant
Pregnancy risk category: NR (Metadate ER, Methylin, Methylin ER, Ritalin, Ritalin SR); C (Concerta, Daytrana, Metadate CD, Ritalin LA)
Controlled substance schedule: II

Indications and dosages

▶ **Attention deficit hyperactivity disorder (ADHD).** *Children age 6 and older:* Initially 5 mg, Methylin or Ritalin P.O. b.i.d. before breakfast and lunch. Increase in 5- to 10-mg increments weekly, as needed until an optimum daily dosage of 2 mg/kg is reached, not to exceed 60 mg/day. Ritalin SR, Metadate ER, Methylin ER, Metadate CD, or Ritalin LA may be used in place of above tablets by calculating the dose of methylphenidate in 8 hours, and giving the total dosage P.O. once daily before breakfast. Or, initially, 20 mg Metadate CD or Ritalin LA P.O. daily before breakfast; increase in 10-mg increments weekly to maximum, 60 mg daily. Or, for children age 6 to 12, initially, apply one 10-mg patch (Daytrana) to clean, dry, nonirritated skin on the hip, alternating sites daily. Avoid the waistline or where tight clothing may rub off the patch. Apply 2 hours before desired effect, and remove 9 hours later. Increase dosage weekly, as needed, to a maximum of 30 mg daily. Base final dose and wear time on patient response.
Adolescents ages 13 to 17 not on methylphenidate, or for patients on other stimulants: 18 mg P.O. extended-release Concerta once daily in the morning. Adjust dosage by 18 mg at weekly in-

tervals to a maximum of 72 mg P.O. (not to exceed 2 mg/kg) once daily in the morning.
Children ages 6 to 12 not on methylphenidate, or for patients on other stimulants: 18 mg P.O. extended-release Concerta once daily in the morning. Adjust dosage by 18 mg at weekly intervals to a maximum of 54 mg P.O. once daily in the morning.
Children age 6 and older on methylphenidate: If the previous methylphenidate daily dosage is 5 mg b.i.d. or t.i.d. or 20 mg of sustained-release, the recommended dose of Concerta is 18 mg P.O. every morning. If the previous methylphenidate daily dose is 10 mg b.i.d. or t.i.d. or 40 mg sustained-release, the recommended dosage of Concerta is 36 mg P.O. every morning. If the previous methylphenidate daily dosage is 15 mg b.i.d. or t.i.d. or 60 mg of sustained-release, the recommended dose of Concerta is 54 mg P.O. every morning. Maximum conversion daily dose is 54 mg. After conversion is complete, adjust adolescents ages 13 to 17 to maximum, 72 mg once daily (not to exceed 2 mg/kg).
▶ **Narcolepsy.** *Adults:* 10 mg Methylin or Ritalin P.O. b.i.d. or t.i.d. 30 to 45 minutes before meals. Dosage varies with patient needs; average dose is 40 to 60 mg P.O. daily. Ritalin SR, Metadate ER, and Methylin ER tablets may be used in place of methylphenidate tablets by calculating the dosage of methylphenidate in 8 hours and administering the total dosage P.O. once daily before breakfast.

Contraindications and cautions

• Contraindicated in patients hypersensitive to the drug or any of its components and in those with glaucoma, motor tics, family history or diagnosis of Tourette syndrome, or history of marked anxiety, tension, or agitation. Also contraindicated within 14 days of taking an MAO inhibitor. Avoid use in patients with structural cardiac abnormalities.
• Use cautiously in patients with hypertension, history of drug abuse, GI stricture or narrowing, seizures, or EEG abnormalities.
 Lifespan: In pregnant women, use cautiously. In breast-feeding women, use cautiously. It's unknown if the drug appears in breast milk. In children younger than age 6, safety and effectiveness haven't been established.

Reactions may be *common*, uncommon, *life-threatening*, or COMMON AND LIFE-THREATENING.

Adverse reactions

CNS: akathisia, dizziness, dyskinesia, headache, *insomnia*, mood swings, *nervousness, seizures*, Tourette syndrome.
CV: angina, changes in blood pressure and pulse rate, *palpitations, tachycardia.*
EENT: dry throat, pharyngitis, sinusitis.
GI: *abdominal pain, anorexia, decreased appetite, nausea, vomiting.*
Hematologic: *leukopenia, thrombocytopenia, thrombocytopenic purpura.*
Metabolic: delayed growth, weight loss.
Respiratory: cough, upper respiratory tract infection.
Skin: application site reaction (redness, swelling, papules), *erythema multiforme*, exfoliative dermatitis, rash, urticaria.
Other: viral infection.

Interactions

Drug-drug. *Anticonvulsants (such as phenobarbital, phenytoin, primidone), SSRIs, tricyclic antidepressants (clomipramine, desipramine, imipramine), warfarin:* May increase levels of these drugs. Monitor patient for adverse reactions, and decrease dosage of these drugs as needed. Monitor drug levels (or coagulation times if patient is also taking warfarin).
Centrally-acting antihypertensives: Decreases antihypertensive effect. Monitor blood pressure.
Clonidine: May cause serious adverse events. Avoid use together.
Coumadin: May increase levels. Monitor PT and INR and monitor patient for bleeding.
Drugs that increase gastric pH (antacids, H_2-receptor antagonists, proton pump inhibitors): May alter the release of Ritalin LA extended-release capsules. Separate administration times.
MAO inhibitors: May cause severe hypertension or hypertensive crisis. Don't use together or within 14 days of each other.
Drug-food. *Caffeine:* May increase amphetamine and related amine effects. Discourage use together.

Effects on lab test results

- May decrease hemoglobin level and hematocrit.
- May decrease WBC and platelet counts.

Pharmacokinetics

Absorption: Rapid and complete. Ritalin LA and Metadate CD have two distinct peaks.

Distribution: Unknown. Ritalin LA is 10% to 33% protein-bound.
Metabolism: By the liver.
Excretion: In urine. *Half-life:* 12 hours.

Route	Onset	Peak	Duration
P.O.			
Methylin, Ritalin	Unknown	2 hr	3–6 hr
Concerta	Unknown	6–8 hr	8–12 hr
Methylin ER, Ritalin SR	Unknown	4¾ hr	3–8 hr
Metadate CD	Unknown	1st peak, 1½ hr 2nd peak, 4½ hr	8–12 hr
Ritalin LA	Unknown	1st peak, 1–3 hr 2nd peak, 4–7 hr	8–12 hr
Transdermal	2 hr	Variable	12 hr

Action

Chemical effect: Probably promotes nerve impulse transmission by releasing stored norepinephrine from nerve terminals in brain. Main site appears to be cerebral cortex and reticular activating system.
Therapeutic effect: Promotes calmness in hyperkinesis, and prevents sleep.

Available forms

Capsules (extended-release) (Metadate CD, Ritalin LA): 10 mg, 20 mg, 30 mg, 40 mg
Oral solution: 5 mg/5 ml, 10 mg/5 ml
Tablets (chewable) (Methylin): 2.5 mg, 5 mg, 10 mg
Tablets (extended-release) (Metadate ER, Methylin ER, Ritalin SR): 10 mg, 20 mg
Tablets (extended-release core) (Concerta): 18 mg, 27 mg, 36 mg, 54 mg
Tablets (immediate-release) (Methylin, methylphenidate, Ritalin): 5 mg, 10 mg, 20 mg
Transdermal patch: 10 mg, 15 mg, 20 mg, 30 mg

NURSING PROCESS

Assessment

- Assess patient's condition before therapy and regularly thereafter to monitor drug effectiveness.
- Drug may precipitate Tourette syndrome in children. Monitor effects, especially at start of therapy.

M

• Observe patient for signs of excessive stimulation. Monitor blood pressure.
• Check CBC, differential, and platelet counts with long-term use, particularly if patient shows signs or symptoms of hematologic toxicity (fever, sore throat, easy bruising).
• Monitor height and weight in child receiving long-term therapy. Drug may delay growth, but child will attain normal height when drug is stopped.
⚐ **ALERT:** Chronic abuse can lead to marked tolerance and psychological dependence. Careful supervision is needed. Monitor patient for tolerance or psychological dependence.
• Be alert for adverse reactions and drug interactions.
• Assess patient's and family's knowledge of drug therapy.

⊕ Nursing diagnoses
• Ineffective health maintenance related to underlying condition
• Sleep deprivation related to drug induced insomnia
• Deficient knowledge related to drug therapy

▶ Planning and implementation
⚐ **ALERT:** This is drug of choice for ADHD and is usually stopped after puberty.
• Don't use to prevent fatigue.
• Metadate CD and Ritalin-LA may be swallowed whole, or the contents of the capsule may be sprinkled onto a small amount of cool applesauce and given immediately with a full glass of water.
• Give at least 6 hours before bedtime to prevent insomnia. Give after meals to reduce appetite suppression.
• Methylin ER and Ritalin SR tablets have a duration of about 8 hours and may be used in place of regular tablets when 8-hour dosage of sustained release tablets corresponds to the adjusted dosage of the regular tablets.
⚐ **ALERT:** Don't confuse Ritalin with Rifadin or Metadate with methadone.
Patient teaching
• Tell patient to swallow Ritalin SR and Concerta tablets whole and not to chew or crush them. Metadate CD or Ritalin LA may be swallowed whole, or the contents of the capsule may be sprinkled onto a small amount of cool applesauce and given immediately.

• Warn patient to avoid activities that require alertness until the drug's CNS effects are known.
• Tell patient to avoid caffeine.
• Advise patient with seizure disorder to notify prescriber.
• Inform patient that he will need more rest as drug effects wear off.
• Warn patient that the shell of the Concerta tablet may appear in the stool.
• Tell parent to apply patch immediately after opening; don't use if pouch seal is broken. Press firmly in place for about 30 seconds using the palm of your hand, being sure there is good contact with the skin—especially around the edges. Once applied correctly, the child may shower, bathe, or swim as usual.
• Inform parent if patch comes off, a new one may be applied on a different site, but the total wear time for that day should be 9 hours. Upon removal, fold patch in half so the sticky sides adhere to itself, and then flush down toilet or dispose of in a lidded container.
• Tell parent if the applied patch is missing, to ask the child when or how the patch came off.
• Encourage parent to use the application chart provided with the patch carton to keep track of application and removal.
• Tell parent to remove patch sooner than 9 hours if the child has decreased evening appetite or has difficulty sleeping.
• Tell parent the effects of the patch lasts for several hours after its removal.
• Warn parent and patient to avoid exposing patch to direct external heat sources such as heating pads, electric blankets, and heated water beds.
• Tell parent to notify prescriber if the child develops bumps, swelling, or blistering at the application site or is experiencing blurred vision or other serious side effects.

☑ Evaluation
• Patient responds positively to drug therapy.
• Patient doesn't experience insomnia during therapy.
• Patient and family state understanding of drug therapy.

Reactions may be *common*, uncommon, *life-threatening*, or COMMON AND LIFE-THREATENING.

methylprednisolone
(meth-il-pred-NIS-uh-lohn)
Medrol, Meprolone

methylprednisolone acetate
depMedalone 40, depMedalone 80, Depo-Medrol, Depopred-40, Depopred-80

methylprednisolone sodium succinate
A-MethaPred, Solu-Medrol

Pharmacologic class: glucocorticoid
Therapeutic class: anti-inflammatory, immunosuppressant
Pregnancy risk category: C (oral); NR (parenteral)

Indications and dosages

▶ **Severe inflammation or immunosuppression.** *Adults:* 2 to 60 mg methylprednisolone P.O. daily in four divided doses. Or 10 to 80 mg methylprednisolone acetate I.M. daily, or 4 to 80 mg into joint or soft tissue, as needed. May repeat every 1 to 5 weeks as needed. Or 10 to 250 mg methylprednisolone succinate I.M. or I.V. every 4 hours.
Children: 0.03 to 0.2 mg/kg or 1 to 6.25 mg/m^2 methylprednisolone succinate I.M. once or twice daily. Although dosage may be reduced in infants and children, give dose based more on severity of condition and response than by age or size. Don't give less than 0.5 mg/kg daily.
▶ **Shock.** *Adults:* 100 to 250 mg methylprednisolone succinate I.V. at 2- to 6-hour intervals. Or 30 mg/kg I.V. initially, repeat every 4 to 6 hours, as needed. Continue therapy for 2 to 3 days or until patient is stable.
▶ **Acute exacerbations of multiple sclerosis.** *Adults:* Give 200 mg I.M. prednisolone daily for 1 week, followed by 80 mg I.M. every other day for 1 month. (Note that 5 mg of prednisolone is equivalent to 4 mg of methylprednisolone.)
▶ **Severe lupus nephritis**‡. *Adults:* 1 g methylprednisolone succinate I.V. over 1 hour for 3 days. Continue orally at 0.5 mg/kg daily using prednisone or prednisolone.
Children: 30 mg/kg methylprednisolone succinate I.V. every other day for 6 doses.
▶ **To minimize motor and sensory defects caused by acute spinal cord injury**‡. *Adults:*
Initially, 30 mg/kg I.V. over 15 minutes, followed in 45 minutes by 5.4 mg/kg/hour I.V. infusion for 23 hours.
▶ **Adjunct treatment for moderate to severe** *Pneumocystis jiroveci (carinii)* **pneumonia**‡. *Adults and children older than age 13:* Give 30 mg I.V. b.i.d. for 5 days; then 30 mg I.V. daily for 5 days; then 15 mg I.V. daily for 11 days (or until completion of anti-infective therapy).

▼ I.V. administration

• Compatible solutions include D$_5$W, normal saline solution, and D$_5$W in normal saline solution.
• Use within 48 hours after mixing.
• Give only methylprednisolone sodium succinate I.V., never the acetate form. Reconstitute according to manufacturer's directions using supplied diluent or bacteriostatic water for injection with benzyl alcohol.
• For direct injection, inject diluted drug into vein or I.V. line containing free-flowing compatible solution over at least 1 minute. For shock, give massive doses over at least 10 minutes to prevent arrhythmias and circulatory collapse.
• For intermittent or continuous infusion, dilute solution according to manufacturer's instructions and give over prescribed duration. In continuous infusion, change solution every 24 hours.
• Rapid administration of large I.V. doses (0.5 to 1 g in less than 10 to 120 minutes) may result in circulatory collapse, cardiac arrhythmias, or fatal cardiac arrest.
⊗ **Incompatibilities**
Allopurinol, aminophylline, calcium gluconate, cephalothin, ciprofloxacin, cytarabine, diltiazem, docetaxel, doxapram, etoposide, filgrastim, gemcitabine, glycopyrrolate, metaraminol, nafcillin, ondansetron, paclitaxel, penicillin G sodium, potassium chloride, propofol, sargramostim, vinorelbine, vitamin B complex with C.

Contraindications and cautions

• Contraindicated in patients hypersensitive to drug or any of its components, and in those with systemic fungal infections.
• Use cautiously in patients with GI ulceration or renal disease, hypertension, osteoporosis, diabetes mellitus, hypothyroidism, cirrhosis, diverticulitis, nonspecific ulcerative colitis, recent intestinal anastomoses, thromboembolic disorders, seizures, myasthenia gravis, heart failure,

tuberculosis, ocular herpes simplex, emotional instability, or psychotic tendencies.

⚕ **Lifespan:** In pregnant women, use cautiously. In breast-feeding women, don't use because it's unknown if drug appears in breast milk. In premature infants, methylprednisolone acetate and methylprednisolone succinate are contraindicated because they contain benzyl alcohol.

Adverse reactions

CNS: *euphoria, insomnia,* pseudotumor cerebri, psychotic behavior.
CV: *arrhythmias, circulatory collapse,* edema, *fatal arrest, heart failure,* hypertension, *thromboembolism.*
EENT: cataracts, glaucoma.
GI: GI irritation, increased appetite, *pancreatitis,* peptic ulceration.
Metabolic: carbohydrate intolerance, growth suppression in children, hyperglycemia, hypokalemia.
Musculoskeletal: muscle weakness, osteoporosis.
Skin: acne, delayed wound healing, hirsutism, various skin eruptions.
Other: *acute adrenal insufficiency,* susceptibility to infections.

Interactions

Drug-drug. *Anticholinesterases:* May cause profound weakness. Use together cautiously.
Aspirin, indomethacin, other NSAIDs: May increase risk of GI distress and bleeding. Give together cautiously.
Cyclosporins: May increase risk of adverse events and convulsions. May need to increase methylprednisolone dose.
CYP3A4 inducers (barbiturates, ephedrine, phenytoin, rifampin): May decrease corticosteroid effect. Increase corticosteroid dosage.
CYP3A4 inhibitors (ketoconazole, macrolides): May decrease glucocorticoid clearance. Adjust dosage, if needed.
Hormonal contraceptives: May decrease corticosteroid metabolism. Dosage of steroid may need to be reduced.
Oral anticoagulants: May alter dosage requirements. Monitor PT and INR closely.
Potassium-depleting drugs (such as thiazide and loop diuretics): May increase potassium-wasting effects. Monitor potassium level.
Skin-test antigens: May decrease response. Defer skin testing until therapy is completed.

Toxoids, live-virus vaccines: May decrease antibody response and increase risk of neurologic complications. Avoid use together.

Effects on lab test results

• May increase glucose and cholesterol levels. May decrease potassium and calcium levels.

Pharmacokinetics

Absorption: Good after P.O. use; sodium succinate is rapid while acetate is much slower.
Distribution: Rapid to muscle, liver, skin, intestines, and kidneys.
Metabolism: In liver.
Excretion: Primarily in urine. *Half-life:* 18 to 36 hours.

Route	Onset	Peak	Duration
P.O.	Rapid	1–2 hr	30–36 hr
I.V.	Immediate	Immediate	Unknown
I.M.	6–48 hr	Unknown	4–8 days

Action

Chemical effect: Not clear; decreases inflammation, mainly by stabilizing leukocyte lysosomal membranes. Drug also suppresses immune response, stimulates bone marrow, and influences protein, fat, and carbohydrate metabolism.
Therapeutic effect: Relieves inflammation and suppresses immune system function.

Available forms

methylprednisolone
Tablets: 2 mg, 4 mg, 8 mg, 16 mg, 24 mg, 32 mg
methylprednisolone acetate
Injection (suspension): 20 mg/ml, 40 mg/ml, 80 mg/ml
methylprednisolone sodium succinate (contains benzyl alcohol)
Injection: 40-, 125-, 500-, 1,000-, and 2,000-mg vials

NURSING PROCESS

Assessment
• Assess patient's condition before therapy and regularly thereafter to monitor drug effectiveness.
• Watch for enhanced response in patient with hypothyroidism or cirrhosis.
• Monitor patient's weight, blood pressure, electrolyte levels (especially glucose), and sleep

patterns. Euphoria may initially interfere with sleep, but patient typically adjusts to drug after 1 to 3 weeks.
• Be alert for adverse reactions and drug interactions.
• Assess patient's and family's knowledge of drug therapy.

Nursing diagnoses
• Ineffective health maintenance related to underlying condition
• Risk for injury related to drug-induced adverse reactions
• Deficient knowledge related to drug therapy

Planning and implementation
⚠ **ALERT:** Salt formulations are not interchangeable.
• Drug may be used for alternate-day therapy.
• For better results and less risk of toxicity, give once-daily dose in morning.
• Don't inject subcutaneously. Atrophy and sterile abscesses may occur.
• Give with food whenever possible. Critically ill patients may also need antacid or H_2-receptor antagonist therapy.
• Give I.M. injection deep into gluteal muscle.
• Dermal atrophy may occur with large dose of acetate salt. Use multiple small injections rather than single large dose, and rotate injection sites.
⚠ **ALERT:** Don't give intrathecally because severe adverse reactions may occur.
• Don't use acetate salt when immediate onset of action is needed.
⚠ **ALERT:** Acute adrenal insufficiency may occur in patients on long term therapy who are under stress (infection, surgery, or trauma).
• Always adjust to lowest effective dosage.
• Give potassium supplements as appropriate.
• Gradually stop giving the drug after long-term therapy. Abruptly stopping drug may be fatal or cause inflammation, fatigue, weakness, arthralgia, fever, dizziness, lethargy, depression, fainting, orthostatic hypotension, dyspnea, anorexia, or hypoglycemia.
⚠ **ALERT:** Don't confuse Solu-Medrol with Solu-Cortef.
⚠ **ALERT:** Don't confuse methylprednisolone with medroxyprogesterone.
Patient teaching
• Tell patient most adverse reactions are dose or duration dependent.

• Tell patient not to abruptly stop taking the drug without prescriber's consent.
• Teach patient signs of early adrenal insufficiency: fatigue, muscle weakness, joint pain, fever, anorexia, nausea, dyspnea, dizziness, and fainting.
• Instruct patient to wear or carry medical identification.
• Warn patient receiving long-term therapy about cushingoid symptoms, and tell him to report sudden weight gain or swelling. Suggest exercise or physical therapy, and advise him to ask prescriber about vitamin D or calcium supplements.

✓ Evaluation
• Patient responds positively to drug therapy.
• Patient sustains no injury from adverse reactions.
• Patient and family state understanding of drug therapy.

metoclopramide hydrochloride
(met-oh-KLOH-preh-mighd high-droh-KLOR-ighd)
Apo-Metoclop ♦ , Maxolon, Octamide, Octamide PFS, Reglan

M

Pharmacologic class: para-aminobenzoic acid derivative; dopamine-receptor agonist
Therapeutic class: antiemetic, GI stimulant
Pregnancy risk category: B

Indications and dosages

▶ **To prevent or reduce nausea and vomiting induced by cisplatin alone or with other chemotherapeutics.** *Adults:* 1 to 2 mg/kg I.V. 30 minutes before chemotherapy; then repeat every 2 hours for two doses; then every 3 hours for three doses.

▶ **To prevent or reduce postoperative nausea and vomiting.** *Adults:* 10 to 20 mg I.M. near end of surgical procedure, repeat every 4 to 6 hours, p.r.n.

▶ **To facilitate small-bowel or upper G.I. intubation and aid in radiologic examinations.**
Adults and children older than age 14: Give 10 mg (2 ml) I.V. as single dose over 1 to 2 minutes.
Children ages 6 to 14: Give 2.5 to 5 mg I.V. (0.5 to 1 ml).
Children younger than age 6: Give 0.1 mg/kg I.V.

▶ **Delayed gastric emptying caused by diabetic gastroparesis.** *Adults:* 10 mg P.O. for mild symptoms; slow I.V. infusion for severe symptoms 30 minutes before meals and at bedtime for 2 to 8 weeks, depending on response.

▶ **Gastroesophageal reflux disease.** *Adults:* 10 to 15 mg P.O. q.i.d., p.r.n., 30 minutes before meals and at bedtime.

⃠ **Adjust-a-dose:** For patients with renal impairment, if creatinine clearance is less than 40 ml/minute, reduce initial dose by 50% and adjust dosage, as tolerated.

▼ I.V. administration

• Drug is compatible with D_5W, normal saline solution for injection, dextrose 5% in half-normal saline solution, Ringer's solution, and lactated Ringer's solution. Normal saline is the preferred diluent because drug is most stable in this solution.

• Dilute doses larger than 10 mg in 50 ml of compatible diluent, and infuse over at least 15 minutes.

• Give doses of 10 mg or less by direct injection over 1 to 2 minutes.

• Closely monitor blood pressure.

• If giving infusion mixture within 24 hours, protection from light is unnecessary. If protected from light and refrigerated, it's stable for 48 hours.

⊗ **Incompatibilities**

Allopurinol, amphotericin B, ampicillin, calcium gluconate, cefepime, chloramphenicol sodium succinate, cisplatin, doxorubicin liposomal, erythromycin lactobionate, fluorouracil, furosemide, methotrexate sodium, penicillin G potassium, propofol, sodium bicarbonate.

Contraindications and cautions

• Contraindicated in patients hypersensitive to the drug or any of its components; patients allergic to procainamide may also be allergic to metoclopramide. Also contraindicated in patients taking drugs that are likely to cause extrapyramidal reactions (butyrophenones, phenothiazines), in those for whom stimulation of GI motility might be dangerous (such as those with hemorrhage), and in those with pheochromocytoma or seizure disorder.

• Use cautiously in patients with a history of depression, Parkinson disease, hypertension, or renal impairment.

• Safety and effectiveness haven't been established for therapy that lasts longer than 12 weeks.

❧ **Lifespan:** In pregnant women, use cautiously. In breast-feeding women, use cautiously; it's unknown if the drug appears in breast milk. In elderly patients, use cautiously and at a reduced dosage.

Adverse reactions

CNS: *anxiety,* dizziness, *drowsiness,* dystonic reactions, extrapyramidal symptoms, fatigue, fever, headache, insomnia, *lassitude, restlessness,* sedation, *seizures, suicidal ideation,* tardive dyskinesia.

CV: *arrhythmias, AV block, bradycardia, heart failure,* hypotension, transient hypertension.

GI: bowel disturbances, diarrhea, nausea.

Hematologic: *agranulocytosis, leukopenia, neonatal methemoglobinemia, neutropenia.*

Skin: rash.

Other: loss of libido, prolactin secretion.

Interactions

Drug-drug. *Acetaminophen, aspirin, cyclosporine, diazepam, levodopa, lithium, tetracycline:* May increase absorption of these drugs. Monitor patient for adverse effects.

Anticholinergics, opioid analgesics: May antagonize GI motility effects of metoclopramide. Use together cautiously.

Cimetidine: May decrease bioavailability of cimetidine. Avoid use together.

CNS depressants: May cause additive CNS depression. Avoid use together.

Digoxin: May decrease absorption of digoxin. Monitor digoxin levels.

Insulin: May influence the rate of food absorption. Adjust insulin dosage, if needed.

Drug-lifestyle. *Alcohol use:* May cause additive CNS depression. Discourage use together.

Effects on lab test results

• May increase aldosterone and prolactin levels.

• May decrease neutrophil and granulocyte counts.

Pharmacokinetics

Absorption: After P.O. use, rapid and complete. After I.M. use, about 74% to 96% bioavailable.

Distribution: To most body tissues and fluids, including brain.

Reactions may be *common*, uncommon, *life-threatening*, or COMMON AND LIFE-THREATENING.

Metabolism: Not extensive.
Excretion: In urine and feces. *Half-life:* 4 to 6 hours.

Route	Onset	Peak	Duration
P.O.	30–60 min	1–2 hr	1–2 hr
I.V.	1–3 min	Unknown	1–2 hr
I.M.	10–15 min	Unknown	1–2 hr

Action

Chemical effect: Stimulates motility of upper GI tract by increasing lower esophageal sphincter tone. Blocks dopamine receptors at chemoreceptor trigger zone.
Therapeutic effect: Prevents or minimizes nausea and vomiting. Also reduces gag reflex, improves gastric emptying, and reduces gastric reflux.

Available forms

Injection: 5 mg/ml
Syrup: 5 mg/5 ml (sugar-free), 10 mg/ml
Tablets: 5 mg, 10 mg

NURSING PROCESS

📖 Assessment
• Assess patient's condition before therapy and regularly thereafter to monitor drug effectiveness.
• Monitor blood pressure often in patient taking I.V. form of drug.
• Be alert for adverse reactions and drug interactions.
• Assess patient's and family's knowledge of drug therapy.

⊕ Nursing diagnoses
• Risk for deficient fluid volume related to nausea and vomiting
• Risk for injury related to drug-induced adverse CNS reactions
• Deficient knowledge related to drug therapy

▷ Planning and implementation
• Dilute oral concentrate with water, juice, or carbonated beverage just before administration. Semisolid food, such as applesauce or pudding, also may be used.
• Commercially available I.M. preparations may be used without further dilution.

🔵 **ALERT:** Extrapyramidal effects caused by high drug doses are counteracted by 25 mg diphenhydramine I.V.
🔵 **ALERT:** Don't confuse Reglan with Relafen.
Patient teaching
• Instruct patient not to drink alcohol during therapy.
• Advise patient to avoid activities requiring alertness for 2 hours after taking each dose.

✓ Evaluation
• Patient responds positively to drug and doesn't develop fluid volume deficit.
• Patient doesn't experience injury from adverse reactions.
• Patient and family state understanding of drug therapy.

metolazone
(meh-TOH-luh-zohn)
Zaroxolyn

Pharmacologic class: quinazoline derivative
Therapeutic class: diuretic, antihypertensive
Pregnancy risk category: B

Indications and dosages

▶ **Edema in heart failure or renal disease.**
Adults: 5 to 20 mg P.O. daily.
▶ **Mild to moderate essential hypertension.**
Adults: Initially, 2.5 mg to 5 mg P.O. daily. Maintenance dosage determined by patient's blood pressure. If response is inadequate, add another antihypertensive.

Contraindications and cautions

• Contraindicated in patients hypersensitive to thiazides or other sulfonamide-derived drugs and in patients with anuria, hepatic coma, or precoma.
• Use cautiously in patients with impaired kidney or liver function.
⚖ **Lifespan:** In pregnant women, use only when benefits outweigh risks to the fetus. In breast-feeding women and in children, safety and effectiveness haven't been established.

Adverse reactions

CNS: *dizziness,* fatigue, headache.
CV: chest pain, orthostatic hypotension, palpitations, volume depletion.

M

GI: anorexia, nausea, *pancreatitis.*
GU: frequent urination, nocturia, polyuria.
Hematologic: *agranulocytosis, aplastic anemia, leukopenia, thrombocytopenia.*
Hepatic: *hepatic encephalopathy.*
Metabolic: dehydration, dilutional hyponatremia, glucose tolerance impairment, hypercalcemia, hypochloremia, hyperglycemia, hyperlipidemia, hyperuricemia, hypokalemia, *metabolic alkalosis.*
Musculoskeletal: acute gouty attacks, muscle cramps, swelling.
Skin: dermatitis, photosensitivity reactions, rash.
Other: hypersensitivity reactions.

Interactions

Drug-drug. *Amphotericin B, corticosteroids:* May cause hypokalemia. Monitor potassium level.
Barbiturates, opioids: May increase orthostatic hypotensive effect. Monitor blood pressure closely.
Bumetanide, ethacrynic acid, furosemide, torsemide: May cause excessive diuretic response resulting in serious electrolyte abnormalities or dehydration. Adjust dosages carefully while monitoring patient closely.
Cholestyramine, colestipol: May decrease intestinal absorption of thiazides. Separate doses by 1 hour.
Diazoxide: May increase antihypertensive, hyperglycemic, and hyperuricemic effects. Use together cautiously.
Digoxin: May increase risk of digoxin toxicity from metolazone-induced hypokalemia. Monitor potassium and digitalis levels.
Insulin, sulfonylureas: May increase requirements in diabetic patients. Adjust dosages.
Lithium: May decrease lithium clearance, increasing risk of lithium toxicity. Avoid giving together.
NSAIDs: May increase risk of NSAID-induced renal impairment. Monitor patient for signs of renal impairment.
Drug-lifestyle. *Alcohol use:* May increase orthostatic hypotensive effect. Discourage use together.
Sun exposure: May cause photosensitivity reactions. Urge patient to avoid unprotected or prolonged exposure to sunlight.

Effects on lab test results

• May increase glucose, calcium, cholesterol, pH, bicarbonate, uric acid, and triglyceride levels. May decrease potassium, sodium, magnesium, chloride, and hemoglobin levels and hematocrit.
• May decrease granulocyte, platelet, and WBC counts.

Pharmacokinetics

Absorption: About 65% in healthy adults; in cardiac patients, falls to 40%.
Distribution: 50% to 70% erythrocyte-bound. 33% protein-bound.
Metabolism: Insignificant.
Excretion: 70% to 95% unchanged in urine.
Half-life: About 14 hours.

Route	Onset	Peak	Duration
P.O.	≤ 1 hr	2–8 hr	12–24 hr

Action

Chemical effect: Increases sodium and water excretion by inhibiting sodium reabsorption in cortical diluting site of ascending loop of Henle.
Therapeutic effect: Promotes water and sodium elimination and lowers blood pressure.

Available forms

Tablets: 2.5 mg, 5 mg, 10 mg

NURSING PROCESS

Assessment
• Assess patient's condition before therapy and regularly thereafter to monitor the drug's effectiveness. In hypertensive patients, therapeutic response may be delayed several days.
• Unlike thiazide diuretics, drug is effective in patients with decreased kidney function.
• Monitor fluid intake and output, weight, blood pressure, and electrolyte level.
• Monitor uric acid level, especially in patient with a history of gout.
• Be alert for adverse reactions and drug interactions.
• Assess patient's and family's knowledge of drug therapy.

Nursing diagnoses
• Excess fluid volume related to presence of edema

- Risk for injury related to presence of hypertension
- Deficient knowledge related to drug therapy

▶ Planning and implementation

- Drug may be used with potassium-sparing diuretic to prevent potassium loss.
- Give drug in morning to prevent nocturia.
- Drug is used as adjunct in furosemide-resistant edema.

⚠ **ALERT:** Don't confuse Zaroxolyn with Zarontin or metolazone with metoprolol.

Patient teaching

- Advise patient to not change position suddenly and to rise slowly, to avoid orthostatic hypotension.
- Advise patient to wear protective clothing, avoid prolonged exposure to sunlight, and use sunblock to prevent photosensitivity reactions.
- Instruct patient to avoid alcohol consumption during drug therapy.

☑ Evaluation

- Patient doesn't have edema.
- Patient's blood pressure is normal.
- Patient and family state understanding of drug therapy.

---

metoprolol succinate
(meh-TOH-pruh-lol SUHK-seh-nayt)
Toprol-XL✎

metoprolol tartrate
(meh-TOH-pruh-lol TAR-trayt)
Betaloc ♦ , Betaloc Durules ♦ , Lopressor, Novo-metoprol ♦ , Nu-Metop ♦

Pharmacologic class: selective beta$_1$ blocker
Therapeutic class: antihypertensive, adjunct therapy of acute MI
Pregnancy risk category: C

Indications and dosages

▶ **Hypertension.** *Adults:* Initially, 50 to 100 mg succinate P.O. once daily. Adjust dosage as needed and tolerated at intervals of no less than 1 week to maximum, 400 mg daily. For metoprolol tartrate, initially, 100 mg P.O. daily in single or divided doses; usual maintenance dosage is 100 to 450 mg daily.

▶ **Early intervention in acute MI.** *Adults:* 5 mg tartrate I.V. push every 2 to 5 minutes up to a total of 15 mg based on hemodynamic status. Then, 15 minutes after last dose, 25 to 50 mg P.O. every 6 hours for 48 hours. Maintenance dosage is 100 mg P.O. b.i.d. In patients who do not tolerate full 15 mg dose in 10 to 15 minutes, may decrease oral dose to 25 mg initially. If severe intolerance, discontinue drug.

▶ **Angina pectoris.** *Adults:* Initially, 100 mg succinate P.O. daily as single dose. Increase at weekly intervals until adequate response or pronounced decrease in heart rate is seen. Safety and effectiveness of daily dose higher than 400 mg aren't known. Or, 100 mg metoprolol tartrate P.O. in two divided doses. Increase at weekly intervals until adequate response or pronounced decrease in heart rate is seen. Maintenance dosage, 100 to 400 mg P.O. daily.

▶ **Stable, symptomatic heart failure (New York Heart Association class II) resulting from ischemia, hypertension, or cardiomyopathy.** *Adults:* 25 mg succinate P.O. once daily for 2 weeks. In patients with more severe heart failure, start with 12.5 mg P.O. once daily for 2 weeks. Double the dose every 2 weeks as tolerated to a maximum of 200 mg daily.

▶ **Atrial tachyarrhythmias after acute MI‡.** *Adults:* 2.5 to 5 mg I.V. every 2 to 5 minutes to control rate up to 15 mg over a 10- to 15-minute period. Once heart rate is controlled or normal sinus rhythm is restored, therapy may continue with 50 mg P.O. b.i.d. for 24 hours starting 15 minutes after the last I.V. dose. Increase dosage to 100 mg P.O. b.i.d. as tolerated. When therapeutic response is achieved or if systolic blood pressure is less than 100 mm Hg or heart rate is less than 50 beats/minute, stop drug.

▶ **Unstable angina or non–ST-segment elevation MI at high risk for ischemic events‡.** *Adults:* 5 mg I.V. bolus every 5 minutes for 3 doses. May continue therapy with P.O. drug.

▽ I.V. administration

- Give drug undiluted and by direct injection.
- Drug is only compatible with meperidine hydrochloride or morphine sulfate, or with alteplase infusions at Y-site connection.
- Store drug at room temperature and protect from light. If solution is discolored or contains particulates, discard. Don't freeze.

⊗ **Incompatibilities**
Amphotericin B, other I.V. drugs.

M

Contraindications and cautions

• Contraindicated in patients hypersensitive to the drug or other beta blockers, and in those with sinus bradycardia, heart block greater than first-degree, cardiogenic shock, or overt cardiac failure when used to treat hypertension or angina. When used to treat MI, drug is also contraindicated in patients with heart rate below 45 beats/minute, second- or third-degree heart block, PR interval of 0.24 second or more with first-degree heart block, systolic blood pressure lower than 100 mm Hg, or moderate to severe cardiac failure.
• Use cautiously in patients with heart failure, diabetes, or respiratory or hepatic disease.
⚖ **Lifespan:** In pregnant women, use cautiously. In breast-feeding women, don't use; it's unknown if drug appears in breast milk. In children, safety and effectiveness haven't been established.

Adverse reactions

CNS: dizziness, fatigue, fever, lethargy.
CV: *AV block, bradycardia, heart failure,* hypotension, peripheral vascular disease.
GI: diarrhea, nausea, vomiting.
GU: decreased libido.
Musculoskeletal: arthralgia.
Respiratory: *bronchospasm,* dyspnea.
Skin: rash.

Interactions

Drug-drug. *Amobarbital, aprobarbital, butabarbital, butalbital, mephobarbital, pentobarbital, phenobarbital, primidone, secobarbital:* May reduce the effects of metoprolol. Increase beta blocker dose.
Antihypertensives: May produce additive effects. Monitor blood pressure.
Chlorpromazine: May decrease hepatic clearance. Monitor patient for increased beta blockade.
Cimetidine: May increase the pharmacologic effects of beta blocker. Consider another H_2 agonist or decrease the dose of beta blocker.
CYP2D6 inhibitors, such as amiodarone, fluoxetine, paroxetine, propafenone, quinidine: May increase metoprolol level. Monitor patient for increased adverse effects.
Digoxin, diltiazem: May cause excessive bradycardia and increase depressant effect on myocardium. Use together cautiously.

Hydralazine: May increase levels and effects of both drugs. Monitor patient closely. Adjust dosage of either drug, if needed.
Indomethacin: May decrease antihypertensive effect. Monitor blood pressure and adjust dosage.
Insulin, oral antidiabetics: May alter dosage requirements in previously stabilized diabetic patient. Observe patient carefully.
I.V. lidocaine: May reduce metabolism of lidocaine, increasing the risk of toxicity. Give bolus doses of lidocaine at a slower rate, and monitor lidocaine levels closely.
MAO inhibitors: May cause bradycardia during use with MAO inhibitors. Monitor ECG and patient closely.
Prazosin: May increase the risk of orthostatic hypotension in the early phases of use together. Assist patient to stand slowly until effects are known.
Rifampin: May increase metabolism of metoprolol. Monitor patient for decreased effect.
Thioamine: May alter pharmacokinetics of metoprolol, increasing the effects of metoprolol. Monitor patient.
Thyroid hormones: May impair actions of metoprolol when patient is converted to euthyroid state. Monitor patient.
Verapamil: May increase the effects of both drugs. Monitor cardiac function closely, and decrease dosages if needed.
Drug-food. *Any food:* May increase absorption. Give together.

Effects on lab test results

• May increase transaminase, alkaline phosphatase, LDH, and uric acid levels.

Pharmacokinetics

Absorption: Rapid and almost complete; food enhances absorption of metoprolol tartrate.
Distribution: Wide. About 12% protein-bound.
Metabolism: In liver.
Excretion: About 95% in urine. *Half-life:* 3 to 7 hours.

Route	Onset	Peak	Duration
P.O.	≤ 15 min	1–12 hr	6–24 hr
I.V.	≤ 5 min	20 min	5–8 hr

Action

Chemical effect: Unknown. Known to depress renin secretion.

Therapeutic effect: Reduces blood pressure; decreases myocardial contractility, heart rate, and cardiac output; reduces myocardial oxygen consumption; and helps to prevent myocardial tissue damage.

Available forms

metoprolol succinate
Tablets (extended-release): 25 mg, 50 mg, 100 mg, 200 mg
metoprolol tartrate
Injection: 1 mg/ml in 5-ml ampules and carpuject cartridge
Tablets: 50 mg, 100 mg
Tablets (extended-release): 100 mg ♦, 200 mg ♦

NURSING PROCESS

⚡ Assessment
• Assess patient's condition before therapy and regularly thereafter to monitor drug effectiveness.
• Monitor blood pressure often. Drug masks common signs of shock.
• Be alert for adverse reactions and drug interactions.
• Assess patient's and family's knowledge of drug therapy.

✦ Nursing diagnoses
• Ineffective health maintenance related to underlying disorder
• Risk for injury related to drug-induced adverse CNS reactions
• Deficient knowledge related to drug therapy

▶ Planning and implementation
⊙ **ALERT:** Always check patient's apical pulse rate before giving drug. If it's slower than 60 beats/minute, don't give the drug and immediately call the prescriber.
• Give drug with meals because food may increase absorption.
⊙ **ALERT:** Don't confuse metoprolol with metaproterenol or metolazone or Toprol XL with Topamax, Tegretol, or Tegretol-XR.
Patient teaching
• Tell patient that abruptly stopping therapy can worsen angina and precipitate MI. He should stop taking the drug gradually over 1 to 2 weeks.
• Instruct patient to take oral form with meals to enhance absorption.

• Advise patient to report adverse reactions to prescriber.
• Warn patient to avoid performing hazardous activities until the drug's CNS effects are known.

☑ Evaluation
• Patient responds well to therapy.
• Patient doesn't experience injury from adverse CNS reactions.
• Patient and family state understanding of drug therapy.

metronidazole
(met-roh-NIGH-duh-zohl)
Flagyl, Flagyl ER, Flagyl 375, Metric 21, MetroCream, MetroGel, MetroGel-vaginal, MetroLotion, NidaGel ♦, Noritate, Protostat

metronidazole hydrochloride
Flagyl I.V. RTU, Metro I.V., Novonidazol ♦

Pharmacologic class: nitroimidazole
Therapeutic class: antibacterial, antiprotozoal, amebicide
Pregnancy risk category: B

Indications and dosages
▶ **Amebic hepatic abscess.** *Adults:* 500 to 750 mg P.O. t.i.d. for 5 to 10 days.
Children: 35 to 50 mg/kg P.O. daily (in three doses) for 10 days.
▶ **Intestinal amebiasis.** *Adults:* 750 mg P.O. t.i.d. for 5 to 10 days.
Children: 35 to 50 mg/kg P.O. daily (in three doses) for 10 days; maximum of 750 mg/dose. Therapy is followed by P.O. iodoquinol.
▶ **Trichomoniasis.** *Adults:* 250 mg P.O. t.i.d. for 7 days, or 500 mg b.i.d. for 7 days or 2 g P.O. in single dose (may give 2-g dose as two 1-g doses on same day); allow 4 to 6 weeks between courses of therapy. Both partners should be treated.
Children: 5 mg/kg dose P.O. t.i.d. for 7 days. Maximum dosage, 2 g daily.
▶ **Refractory trichomoniasis.** *Adults:* 500 mg P.O. b.i.d. for 7 days. For repeated failures, 2 g P.O. daily for 3 to 5 days.
▶ **Bacterial infections caused by anaerobic microorganisms.** *Adults:* Loading dose, 15 mg/kg I.V. infused over 1 hour (about 1 g for 70-kg

M

[154-lb] adult). Maintenance dosage, 7.5 mg/kg I.V. or P.O. every 6 hours (about 500 mg for 70 kg adult). Give first maintenance dose 6 hours after loading dose. Maximum, 4 g daily. Manufacturer recommends a maximum of 7 to 10 days of therapy, but serious infections may require 2 to 3 weeks of therapy.

▶ **To prevent postoperative infection in contaminated or potentially contaminated colorectal surgery.** *Adults:* 15 mg/kg I.V. over 30 to 60 minutes and completed about 1 hour before surgery. Then, 7.5 mg/kg I.V. over 30 to 60 minutes at 6 and 12 hours after initial dose.

▶ **Inflammatory papules and pustules of acne rosacea.** *Adults:* If using a 0.75% preparation, apply thin film to affected area b.i.d., morning and evening. If using a 1% preparation, apply thin film to affected area once daily. Frequency and duration of therapy are adjusted after response is seen. Results are usually noticed within 3 weeks.

▶ **Pelvic inflammatory disease‡.** *Adults:* 500 mg I.V. every 8 hours with other drugs. Or, 500 mg P.O. b.i.d. for 14 days given with ofloxacin, 400 mg P.O. b.i.d.

▶ **Bacterial vaginosis‡.** *Adults:* 500 mg P.O. b.i.d. for 7 days. Or, 2 g P.O. as a single dose. Or, 250 mg P.O. t.i.d. for 7 days.

▶ **Active Crohn disease‡.** *Adults:* 400 mg P.O. b.i.d. For refractory perineal disease, 20 mg/kg (1 to 1.5 g) P.O. daily in three to five divided doses.

▶ **To prevent sexually transmitted diseases in sexual assault victims‡.** *Adults:* 2 g P.O. given with other drugs.

▶ **Helicobacter pylori with peptic ulcer disease‡.** *Adults:* 250 to 500 mg P.O. t.i.d. to q.i.d. given with other drugs. Continue for 7 to 14 days depending on the regimen used.
Children: 15 to 20 mg/kg P.O. daily, divided in two doses for 4 weeks given with other drugs.

▶ **Giardiasis‡.** *Adults:* 250 mg P.O. t.i.d. for 7 days.

❑ **Adjust-a-dose:** In patients with hepatic impairment, adjust dosage or frequency.

▼ I.V. administration

● No preparation is needed for Flagyl I.V. RTU form.
● Add 4.4 ml of sterile water for injection, bacteriostatic water for injection, sterile normal saline solution injection, or bacteriostatic nor-

mal saline solution injection. Reconstituted drug contains 100 mg/ml.
● Add contents of vial to 100 ml of D_5W, lactated Ringer's injection, or normal saline solution for final concentration of 5 mg/ml. Don't exceed a concentration of 8 mg/ml.
● The resulting highly acidic solution must be neutralized before giving. Carefully add 5 mEq of sodium bicarbonate for each 500 mg of metronidazole. Carbon dioxide will form and may need to be vented.
● Don't use equipment (needles, hubs) containing aluminum to reconstitute the drug or to transfer reconstituted drug. Equipment that contains aluminum will turn the solution orange; the potency isn't affected.
● Infuse drug over at least 1 hour. Don't give I.V. push.
● Don't refrigerate neutralized diluted solution. Precipitation may occur. If Flagyl I.V. RTU is refrigerated, crystals may form. These will disappear after solution is gently warmed to room temperature.

⊗ **Incompatibilities**
Aluminum, amino acid 10%, amphotericin B, aztreonam, ceftriaxone, dopamine, filgrastim, meropenem, warfarin; other I.V. drugs.

Contraindications and cautions

● Contraindicated in patients hypersensitive to the drug or other nitroimidazole derivatives.
● Use cautiously in patients receiving hepatotoxic drugs and in patients with history of blood dyscrasia or CNS disorder, retinal or visual field changes, hepatic disease, or alcoholism.
⚱ **Lifespan:** In pregnant women, don't use during first trimester unless benefits outweigh risks to the fetus. In breast-feeding women, use cautiously. It isn't known if drug appears in breast milk.

Adverse reactions

CNS: ataxia, confusion, depression, drowsiness, fatigue, fever, headache, incoordination, insomnia, irritability, neuropathy, paresthesia of limbs, psychic stimulation, restlessness, *seizures,* sensory neuropathy, vertigo, weakness.
CV: edema, flattened T wave, flushing, thrombophlebitis.
EENT: eye tearing.
GI: abdominal cramping, *anorexia,* constipation, diarrhea, dry mouth, metallic taste, *nausea,* proctitis, stomatitis, *vomiting.*

Reactions may be *common*, uncommon, *life-threatening*, or COMMON AND LIFE-THREATENING.

GU: cystitis, darkened urine, dry vagina and vulva, dyspareunia, dysuria, incontinence, polyuria, pyuria, sense of pelvic pressure.
Hematologic: *neutropenia, thrombocytopenia, transient leukopenia.*
Skin: burning and stinging, contact dermatitis, dry skin, local allergic reaction or irritation, pruritus, rash, worsening of rosacea.
Other: decreased libido, glossitis, gynecomastia, overgrowth of nonsusceptible organisms.

Interactions

Drug-drug. *Azathioprine, fluorouracil:* May increase risk of transient neutropenia. Use cautiously.
Barbiturates, phenobarbital, phenytoin: May decrease metronidazole effectiveness because of increased hepatic clearance. Monitor patient closely for effect.
Cimetidine: May increase risk of metronidazole toxicity because of inhibited hepatic metabolism. Monitor patient.
Disulfiram: May cause acute psychoses and confusional states. Don't use together.
Lithium: May increase lithium level, resulting in toxicity. Monitor lithium level closely.
Oral anticoagulants: May increase anticoagulant effects. Monitor patient for bleeding; monitor PT and INR.
Drug-lifestyle. *Alcohol use:* May cause disulfiram-like reaction (nausea, vomiting, headache, cramps, flushing). Discourage use together.

Effects on lab test results

• May decrease WBC and neutrophil counts.
• May falsely decrease AST, ALT, LDH and triglyceride levels.

Pharmacokinetics

Absorption: About 80%; food delays peak levels to about 2 hours.
Distribution: To most body tissues and fluids. Less than 20% protein-bound.
Metabolism: To active metabolite and to other metabolites.
Excretion: Primarily in urine; 6% to 15% in feces. *Half-life:* 6 to 8 hours.

Route	Onset	Peak	Duration
P.O.	Unknown	1–2 hr	Unknown
I.V.	Immediate	Immediate	Unknown
Topical	Unknown	6–10 hr	Unknown

Action

Chemical effect: Direct-acting trichomonacide and amebicide that works at both intestinal and extraintestinal sites.
Therapeutic effect: Hinders growth of selected organisms, including most anaerobic bacteria and protozoa.

Available forms

Capsules: 375 mg
Injection: 5 mg/ml
Tablets: 250 mg, 500 mg
Tablets (extended-release): 750 mg
Topical cream or gel: 0.75%; 1%
Topical lotion: 0.75%

NURSING PROCESS

Assessment
• Assess patient's infection before therapy and regularly thereafter to monitor drug effectiveness.
• Watch carefully for edema, especially in patients also receiving corticosteroids, because Flagyl I.V. RTU may cause sodium retention.
• Record number and character of stools when used in amebiasis.
• Be alert for adverse reactions and drug interactions.
• I.V. infusion may cause thrombophlebitis at site; observe closely.
• Assess skin for severity, areas of rosacea before and after therapy, and any local adverse reactions.
• Assess patient's and family's knowledge of drug therapy.

Nursing diagnoses
• Risk for infection related to presence of susceptible organisms
• Risk for deficient fluid volume related to drug-induced adverse GI reactions
• Deficient knowledge related to drug therapy

Planning and implementation
• Give drug (except Flagyl ER) with meals to minimize GI distress. Give Flagyl ER at least 1 hour before or 2 hours after meals.
• Use only after *T. vaginalis* has been confirmed by wet smear or culture or *E. histolytica* has been identified; simultaneously treat asymptomatic sexual partners to avoid reinfection.

M

- To treat trichomoniasis during pregnancy, give drug for 7 days instead of 2-g single dose.

Patient teaching
- Tell patient not to use alcohol or drugs that contain alcohol during therapy and for at least 48 hours after therapy is completed.
- Tell patient that metallic taste and dark or red-brown urine may occur.
- Instruct patient to take oral form with meals to minimize reactions.
- Urge patient to complete full course of therapy even if he feels better.
- Instruct patient in proper hygiene.
- Teach patient to cleanse affected skin areas twice daily before applying MetroLotion.
- Instruct users of topical drug to report worsening of rosacea promptly to prescriber.

☑ **Evaluation**
- Patient is free from infection.
- Patient maintains adequate hydration throughout therapy.
- Patient and family state understanding of drug therapy.

HIGH ALERT

mexiletine hydrochloride
(MEKS-il-eh-teen high-droh-KLOR-ighd)
Mexitil

Pharmacologic class: lidocaine analogue, sodium channel antagonist
Therapeutic class: class IB ventricular antiarrhythmic
Pregnancy risk category: C

Indications and dosages

▶ **Refractory life-threatening ventricular arrhythmias, including ventricular tachycardia and PVCs.** *Adults:* 200 mg (if rapid control of arrhythmia is not necessary) to 400 mg (for rapid arrhythmia control) P.O., followed by 200 mg every 8 hours. If satisfactory control isn't obtained, increase dosage in 2 to 3 days to 400 mg every 8 hours. Patients who respond well to a 12-hour schedule may be given up to 450 mg every 12 hours. Maximum daily dose is 1,200 mg.

▶ **Diabetic neuropathy** ‡. *Adults:* 200 mg P.O. daily for 2 days; then give 200 mg P.O. b.i.d. for 2 days followed by 200 mg P.O. t.i.d.

Contraindications and cautions

- Contraindicated in patients with cardiogenic shock or second- or third-degree AV block in absence of artificial pacemaker.
- Use cautiously in patients with first-degree heart block, ventricular pacemaker, sinus node dysfunction, intraventricular conduction disturbances, hypotension, severe heart failure, or seizure disorder.

⚠ **Lifespan:** In pregnant women, use cautiously. In breast-feeding women, use cautiously; it isn't known if drug appears in breast milk. In children, safety and effectiveness haven't been established.

Adverse reactions

CNS: ataxia, blurred vision, confusion, diplopia, *dizziness,* headache, nervousness, nystagmus, *tremor.*
CV: *arrhythmias, bradycardia,* chest pain, hypotension, palpitations, **widened QRS complex.**
GI: constipation, diarrhea, *heartburn,* nausea, vomiting.
Skin: rash.

Interactions

Drug-drug. *Antacids, atropine, opioids:* May slow mexiletine absorption. Monitor patient; separate doses.
Cimetidine: May increase or decrease mexiletine level. Monitor patient for effect or toxicities.
Methylxanthines (such as theophylline): May reduce clearance of methylxanthines, possibly resulting in toxicity. Monitor levels.
Metoclopramide: May accelerate absorption. Monitor patient for toxicity.
Phenobarbital, phenytoin, rifampin, urine acidifiers: May decrease mexiletine level. Monitor patient.
Urine alkalinizers: May increase mexiletine level. Monitor patient.
Drug-food. *Caffeine:* May reduce clearance of methylxanthines, resulting in toxicity. Monitor patient.

Effects on lab test results
- May increase AST level.

Pharmacokinetics

Absorption: About 90%.
Distribution: Wide. Volume declines in patients with liver disease, resulting in toxic levels with usual doses. About 50% to 60% of circulating drug is protein-bound.

Metabolism: Almost complete, in liver.
Excretion: In urine. *Half-life:* 10 to 12 hours.

Route	Onset	Peak	Duration
P.O.	½–2 hr	2–3 hr	Unknown

Action

Chemical effect: Blocks fast sodium channel in cardiac tissues without involvement of autonomic nervous system. Reduces acceleration and amplitude of action potential and decreases automaticity in Purkinje fibers. It also shortens action potential and, to a lesser extent, decreases the effective refractory period in Purkinje fibers.
Therapeutic effect: Abolishes ventricular arrhythmias.

Available forms

Capsules: 100 mg ♦ , 150 mg, 200 mg, 250 mg

NURSING PROCESS

⚎ Assessment
• Assess patient's condition until arrhythmia is abolished.
• Monitor drug levels. Therapeutic levels are 0.5 to 2 mcg/ml.
• Be alert for adverse reactions and drug interactions.
• Monitor patient for toxicity. Early signs include tremors—usually fine tremor of hands. As drug level increases, additional signs of toxicity such as dizziness, ataxia, and nystagmus may develop. Ask patient about these symptoms.
• If patient has an adverse GI reaction, monitor his hydration.
• Assess patient's and family's knowledge of drug therapy.

⊕ Nursing diagnoses
• Decreased cardiac output related to presence of ventricular arrhythmia
• Risk for deficient fluid volume related to drug-induced adverse GI reactions
• Deficient knowledge related to drug therapy

▷ Planning and implementation
• Give with meals or antacids to lessen GI distress.
• If patient appears to be good candidate for twice-a-day therapy, notify prescriber. This dose enhances compliance.

• Notify prescriber of any significant changes in blood pressure, heart rate, and heart rhythm.
Patient teaching
• Instruct patient taking oral form of drug to take it with food.
• Instruct patient to report adverse reactions.

☑ Evaluation
• Patient regains normal cardiac output.
• Patient maintains adequate hydration throughout therapy.
• Patient and family state understanding of drug therapy.

micafungin sodium
(my-kah-FUN-jin SOE-dee-um)
Mycamine

Pharmacologic class: echinocandin antifungal
Therapeutic class: antifungal
Pregnancy risk category: C

Indications and dosages

▶ **Esophageal candidiasis.** *Adults:* 150 mg I.V. daily for 10 to 30 days.
▶ **Prevention of candidal infection in hematopoietic stem cell transplant recipients.** *Adults:* 50 mg I.V. daily for 6 to 51 days.

▽ I.V. administration

• Use aseptic technique when preparing micafungin.
• Reconstitute each 50-mg vial with 5 ml of normal saline solution for injection or D_5W.
• To minimize foaming, dissolve powder by swirling the vial; don't shake it.
• Dilute dose in 100 ml of normal saline solution for injection.
• Flush I.V. line with normal saline solution for injection before infusing drug.
• Infuse drug over 1 hour.
• Reconstituted product and diluted infusion may be stored for up to 24 hours at room temperature.
• Protect diluted solution from light.
⊗ **Incompatibilities**
Other I.V. drugs.

Contraindications and cautions

• Contraindicated in patients hypersensitive to drug.

• Use cautiously in patients with severe hepatic disease.

≛ **Lifespan:** In pregnant women, only use if clearly needed. Use cautiously in breast-feeding women; it isn't known whether micafungin appears in breast milk. In children, safety hasn't been established.

Adverse reactions

CNS: delirium, headache, pyrexia, rigors.
CV: *shock.*
GI: abdominal pain, diarrhea, nausea, vomiting.
Hematologic: anemia, *leukopenia, neutropenia, thrombocytopenia.*
Hepatic: hepatocellular damage, hyperbilirubinemia.
Metabolic: hemolytic anemia, hypocalcemia, hypokalemia, *hypomagnesemia,* hypophosphatemia.
Skin: infusion site inflammation, phlebitis, pruritus, rash.

Interactions

Drug-drug. *Nifedipine:* May increase nifedipine level. Monitor blood pressure, and decrease nifedipine dosage if needed.
Sirolimus: May increase sirolimus level. Monitor patient for evidence of toxicity, and decrease the sirolimus dosage if needed.

Effects on lab test results

• May increase alkaline phosphatase, ALT, AST, bilirubin, BUN, creatinine, and LDH levels. May decrease calcium, magnesium, phosphorus, potassium, and hemoglobin levels and hematocrit.
• May decrease neutrophil and platelet counts.

Pharmacokinetics

Absorption: Given I.V.
Distribution: More than 99% protein-bound, mainly to albumin.
Metabolism: By several pathways in the liver.
Excretion: Mainly fecal.

Route	Onset	Peak	Duration
I.V.	Unknown	Unknown	Unknown

Action

Chemical effect: Inhibits synthesis of 1,3-b-D-glucan, which is an essential component of fungal cell walls that isn't found in mammal cells.

Therapeutic effect: Hinders fungal growth, including *Candida albicans, C. glabrata, C. krusei, C. parapsilosis,* and *C. tropicalis.*

Available forms

Lyophilized powder for injection: 50-mg single-use vial

NURSING PROCESS

⚗ Assessment

• Assess patient's fungal infection before treatment and regularly thereafter.
• Be alert for adverse reactions and drug interactions.
• Monitor hepatic and renal function during therapy.
• Monitor patient for hemolysis and hemolytic anemia.
• Assess patient's and family's knowledge of drug therapy.

⊕ Nursing diagnoses

• Infection related to presence of susceptible fungi
• Risk for injury related to potential for drug-induced hypersensitivity reaction
• Deficient knowledge related to drug therapy

▷ Planning and implementation

• Injection site reactions occur more often in patients receiving drug by peripheral I.V. route.
• Histamine-mediated reactions may occur more often if drug is infused over less than 1 hour.
• Stop infusion if patient develops signs of serious hypersensitivity reaction, including shock.
• Micafungin isn't removed by dialysis.
Patient teaching
• Advise patient to report pain or redness at infusion site.
• Tell patient to expect to undergo laboratory tests during treatment to monitor hematologic, renal, and hepatic function.

✓ Evaluation

• Patient responds to drug therapy and is free from infection.
• Patient has no hypersensitivity reaction.
• Patient and family state understanding of drug therapy.

HIGH ALERT

midazolam hydrochloride
(mid-AYZ-oh-lam high-droh-KLOR-ighd)

Pharmacologic class: benzodiazepine
Therapeutic class: sedative
Pregnancy risk category: D
Controlled substance schedule: IV

Indications and dosages

▶ **Preoperative sedation (to induce sleepiness or drowsiness and relieve apprehension).**
Adults younger than age 60: Give 0.07 mg to 0.08 mg/kg I.M. about 1 hour before surgery.
▶ **Moderate sedation before short diagnostic or endoscopic procedures.** *Adults younger than age 60:* Initially, up to 2.5 mg slow I.V.; repeat in 2 minutes if needed, in small increments of initial dose over at least 2 minutes. Total dose that exceeds 5 mg usually isn't needed.
Adults age 60 and older: 1.5 mg or less over at least 2 minutes. If additional adjustment is needed, give at no more than 1 mg over 2 minutes. Total doses exceeding 3.5 mg aren't usually needed.
▶ **Induction of general anesthesia.** *Adults younger than age 55:* If patient hasn't received preanesthesia drug, 0.3 to 0.35 mg/kg I.V. over 20 to 30 seconds. If patient has received preanesthesia drug, 0.15 to 0.35 mg/kg I.V. over 20 to 30 seconds. To complete induction, give additional increments of 25% of initial dose p.r.n. Total dose that exceeds 0.6 mg/kg usually isn't needed.
Adults age 55 and older: If patient hasn't been premedicated, 0.3 mg/kg I.V. over 20 to 30 seconds. If patient has received sedation or opioid, 0.2 mg/kg I.V. over 20 to 30 seconds. To complete induction, give additional increments of 25% of initial dose p.r.n.
▶ **To induce sleepiness and amnesia and to relieve apprehension before anesthesia or before or during procedures in children.**
Children: 0.1 to 0.15 mg/kg I.M. Doses up to 0.5 mg/kg can be used for more anxious patients. Total dose usually doesn't exceed 10 mg. I.M. depending on age of child.
Children ages 12 to 16: Initially, give dose of 2.5 mg or less I.V. slowly; repeat in 2 minutes, if needed, in small increments of initial dose over at least 2 minutes to achieve desired effect. Slowly titrate additional doses to maintain de-

sired level of sedation in increments of 25% of dose used to first reach the sedative endpoint. Total dose that exceeds 5 mg usually isn't needed.
Children ages 6 to 12: Give 0.025 to 0.05 mg/kg I.V. over 2 to 3 minutes. Additional doses may be given in small increments after 2 to 3 minutes. Total dose that exceeds 0.4 mg/kg usually isn't needed.
Children ages 6 months to 5 years: Initially, 0.05 to 0.1 mg/kg I.V. over 2 to 3 minutes. Additional doses may be given in small increments after 2 to 3 minutes. Total dose that exceeds 0.6 mg/kg usually isn't needed.
▶ **Continuous infusion for sedation of intubated patients in the critical care setting.**
Adults: Initially, 0.01 to 0.05 mg/kg I.V. over several minutes, repeat at 10- to 15-minute intervals, until adequate sedation is achieved. To maintain sedation, infuse initially at 0.02 to 0.1 mg/kg/hour. Some patients may need higher loading doses or infusion rates. Use the lowest effective rate.
Children: Initially, 0.05 to 0.2 mg/kg I.V. over at least 2 to 3 minutes; then continuous infusion at 0.06 to 0.12 mg/kg/hour. Increase or decrease infusion to maintain desired effect.
Neonates born at 32 weeks' gestation or later: Initially 0.06 mg/kg/hour. Adjust rate, as needed, using lowest possible rate.
Neonates born earlier than 32 weeks' gestation: Initially 0.03 mg/kg/hour. Adjust rate, as needed, using lowest possible rate.

▼ I.V. administration

• When mixing infusion, use 5-mg/ml vial, dilute to 0.5 mg/ml with D₅W or normal saline solution.
• Give slowly over at least 2 minutes, and wait at least 2 minutes when adjusting doses to desired effect.
• Watch for irritation and infiltration. Extravasation can cause tissue damage and necrosis.
⊗ **Incompatibilities**
Albumin, amphotericin B, ampicillin sodium, bumetanide, butorphanol, ceftazidime, cefuroxime, clonidine, dexamethasone sodium phosphate, dimenhydrinate, dobutamine, foscarnet, fosphenytoin, furosemide, hydrocortisone, imipenem-cilastatin sodium, methotrexate sodium, nafcillin, pentobarbital sodium, perphenazine, prochlorperazine edisylate, ranitidine hydrochloride, sodium bicarbonate, thiopental,

some total parenteral nutrition formulations, trimethoprim-sulfamethoxazole.

Contraindications and cautions

• Contraindicated in patients hypersensitive to the drug or any of its components and in those with acute angle-closure glaucoma, shock, coma, or acute alcohol intoxication.
• Use cautiously in patients with uncompensated acute illness and in debilitated patients.
☀ **Lifespan:** In pregnant women, drug is contraindicated. In breast-feeding women, use cautiously; it's unknown if the drug appears in breast milk. Use with caution in neonates and avoid rapid injection. In elderly patients, use drug cautiously.

Adverse reactions

CNS: amnesia, combativeness, headache, involuntary movements, oversedation.
CV: *cardiac arrest, hypotension,* variations in blood pressure and pulse rate.
GI: hiccups, nausea, vomiting.
Respiratory: APNEA, decreased respiratory rate.
Other: pain, tenderness at injection site.

Interactions

Drug-drug. *Cimetidine, verapamil:* May increase effects of benzodiazepine. Monitor patient closely.
CNS depressants: May increase risk of apnea. Monitor vital signs and respiratory condition closely.
CYP3A4 inducers (carbamazepine, phenobarbital, phenytoin, rifampin): May decrease midazolam level. Monitor patient for effect; adjust dosage if needed.
Diltiazem: May increase CNS depression and prolong midazolam effects. Use lower dose of midazolam.
Fluconazole, itraconazole, ketoconazole, miconazole: May increase and prolong levels, and may increase CNS depression and psychomotor impairment. Don't use together.
Hormonal contraceptives: May prolong benzodiazepine half-life. Monitor patient closely.
Indinavir, ritonavir: May cause prolonged or severe sedation and respiratory depression. Monitor patient closely.
Opioid analgesics: May increase midazolam's hypnotic effect and increase risk of hypotension. Monitor patient closely; adjust dosage as needed.

Rifamycin: May decrease midazolam levels. Monitor patient for effect.
Drug-food. *Grapefruit juice:* May increase bioavailability of oral midazolam. Discourage use together.
Drug-lifestyle. *Alcohol use:* May cause additive CNS effects. Strongly discourage use together.

Effects on lab test results

None reported.

Pharmacokinetics

Absorption: 80% to 100%.
Distribution: Large volume. About 97% protein-bound.
Metabolism: In liver by CYP3A4 isoenzyme.
Excretion: In urine. *Half-life:* 2 to 6 hours.

Route	Onset	Peak	Duration
P.O.	10–20 min	45–60 min	2–6 hr
I.V.	1½–5 min	Rapid	2–6 hr
I.M.	≤ 15 min	15–60 min	2–6 hr

Action

Chemical effect: May depress CNS at limbic and subcortical levels of brain by potentiating effects of GABA.
Therapeutic effect: Promotes calmness and sleep.

Available forms

Injection: 1 mg/ml, 5 mg/ml
Syrup: 2 mg/ml

NURSING PROCESS

📱 Assessment

• Assess patient's condition before therapy and regularly thereafter to monitor drug effectiveness.
• Monitor blood pressure, heart rate and rhythm, respirations, airway integrity, and arterial oxygen saturation during procedure, especially in patients premedicated with opioids.
• Assess patient's and family's knowledge of drug therapy.

📋 Nursing diagnoses

• Anxiety related to surgery
• Ineffective breathing pattern related to drug's effect on respiratory system
• Deficient knowledge related to drug therapy

Reactions may be *common*, uncommon, *life-threatening*, or COMMON AND LIFE-THREATENING.

> **Planning and implementation**

⚕ **ALERT:** Have oxygen and resuscitation equipment available in case of severe respiratory depression. Excessive dose or too rapid infusion may cause respiratory arrest, particularly in an elderly or debilitated patient.
• Abrupt withdrawal of drug can cause seizures.
• For I.M. dose, give deep into large muscle mass.
⚕ **ALERT:** Don't give by rapid injection to neonates.
• Drug contains benzyl alcohol preservative. Don't give by intrathecal or epidural route. May cause gasping syndrome in premature infants.
Patient teaching
• Use extra caution when teaching patient because drug will diminish predrug memory. Provide written information, family member instruction, and follow-up contact to ensure that patient has adequate information.
• Instruct patient not to use alcohol during therapy.

☑ **Evaluation**
• Patient exhibits calmness.
• Patient maintains adequate breathing pattern throughout therapy.
• Patient and family state understanding of drug therapy.

HIGH ALERT

miglitol
(MIG-lih-tall)
Glyset

Pharmacologic class: alpha-glucosidase inhibitor
Therapeutic class: antidiabetic
Pregnancy risk category: B

Indications and dosages

▶ **Type 2 diabetes mellitus where hyperglycemia can't be managed with diet alone; with a sulfonylurea when diet plus either miglitol or sulfonylurea alone yield inadequate glycemic control.** *Adults:* 25 mg P.O. t.i.d. with the first bite of each main meal; some patients may start at 25 mg P.O. daily to minimize GI side effects. Increase dosage after 4 to 8 weeks to maintenance dosage of 50 mg P.O. t.i.d. Further increase dosage after 3 months, based on glycosylated hemoglobin level, to maximum of 100 mg P.O. t.i.d.

Contraindications and cautions

• Contraindicated in patients hypersensitive to the drug or any of its components. Also contraindicated in patients with diabetic ketoacidosis, inflammatory bowel disease, colonic ulceration, or partial intestinal obstruction; patients predisposed to intestinal obstruction or those with chronic intestinal diseases related to disorders of digestion or absorption; and patients with conditions that may deteriorate as a result of increased gas formation in the intestine.
• Use cautiously in patients with serum creatinine more than 2 mg/dl.
• Use cautiously in patients also receiving insulin or oral sulfonylureas.
🜚 **Lifespan:** In pregnant women, use cautiously when benefits outweigh risks to the fetus. In breast-feeding women, don't use. In children, safety and effectiveness haven't been established.

Adverse reactions

GI: *abdominal pain, diarrhea, flatulence.*
Skin: rash.

Interactions

Drug-drug. *Digestive enzyme preparations (such as amylase, pancreatin), intestinal absorbents (such as charcoal):* May reduce the effectiveness of miglitol. Avoid use together.
Digoxin, propranolol, ranitidine: May decrease the bioavailability of these drugs. Monitor patient for loss of effectiveness and adjust dosages.
Insulin, oral sulfonylureas: May increase the effect of these drugs. Adjust dosage of these drugs if needed. Monitor these patients for hypoglycemia.
Drug-herb. *Aloe, bilberry leaf, bitter melon, burdock, dandelion, fenugreek, garlic, ginseng, stinging nettle:* May improve glucose level control, allowing for a reduced antidiabetic dosage. Advise patient to discuss the use of herbal remedies with prescriber before therapy.

Effects on lab test results

• May decrease iron and glucose levels.

Pharmacokinetics

Absorption: A 25-mg dose is completely absorbed, whereas a 100-mg dose is only 50% to 70% absorbed.

Distribution: Mainly into the extracellular fluid. Less than 4% protein-bound.
Metabolism: None.
Excretion: Mainly renal. More than 95% of a dose in urine as unchanged drug. *Half-life:* About 2 hours.

Route	Onset	Peak	Duration
P.O.	Unknown	2–3 hr	Unknown

Action

Chemical effect: Lowers glucose level through reversible inhibition of alpha glucosidases in the small intestine; they convert oligosaccharides and disaccharides to glucose. Inhibiting these enzymes delays glucose absorption. Drug has no effect on insulin secretion.
Therapeutic effect: Lowers glucose level.

Available forms

Tablets: 25 mg, 50 mg, 100 mg

NURSING PROCESS

Assessment

• Obtain history of patient's condition before therapy, and reassess regularly to monitor drug effectiveness.
• Regularly monitor glucose level, especially during increased stress, such as infection, fever, surgery, and trauma.
• Check glycosylated hemoglobin level every 3 months to monitor long-term glycemic control.
• Assess patient's and family's knowledge of drug therapy.

Nursing diagnoses

• Ineffective health maintenance related to hyperglycemia
• Risk for injury related to drug-induced hypoglycemia
• Deficient knowledge related to drug therapy

Planning and implementation

• Give with the first bite of each main meal.
• Manage type 2 diabetes with diet control, exercise program, and regular testing of urine and glucose levels.
• Treat mild to moderate hypoglycemia with dextrose, such as glucose tablets or gel, or orange juice with sugar packets. Severe hypoglycemia may require I.V. glucose or glucagon.

• GI adverse effects decrease with continued treatment.

Patient teaching

• Tell patient about the importance of adhering to prescriber's diet, weight reduction, and exercise instructions and to have glucose and glycosylated hemoglobin level tested regularly.
• Inform patient that drug therapy relieves symptoms but doesn't cure diabetes.
• Teach patient the signs and symptoms of hyperglycemia and hypoglycemia.
• Instruct patient to treat hypoglycemia with glucose tablets and to have a source of glucose readily available when miglitol is taken with a sulfonylurea or insulin.
• Advise patient to promptly seek medical advice during periods of stress such as fever, trauma, infection, or surgery, because drug requirements may change.
• Instruct patient to take drug three times a day with the first bite of each main meal.
• Show patient how and when to monitor glucose level.
• Advise patient that adverse GI effects are most common during the first few weeks of therapy and should improve over time.
• Urge patient to always carry medical identification.

Evaluation

• Patient's glucose level is normal.
• Patient sustains no injury from drug-induced hypoglycemia.
• Patient and family state understanding of drug therapy.

HIGH ALERT

milrinone lactate
(MIL-rih-nohn LAK-tayt)
Primacor

Pharmacologic class: bipyridine phosphodiesterase inhibitor
Therapeutic class: inotropic vasodilator
Pregnancy risk category: C

Indications and dosages

▶ **Short-term therapy for acute decompensated heart failure.** *Adults:* Loading dose is 50 mcg/kg I.V., given slowly over 10 minutes, followed by continuous I.V. infusion of 0.375 to 0.75 mcg/kg/minute. Adjust infusion dose based

on response. Maximum dosage is 1.13 mg/kg daily.

Adjust-a-dose: For patients with renal impairment, if creatinine clearance is 50 ml/minute or less, decrease dosage to achieve maximum effect, not to exceed 1.13 mg/kg I.V. daily.

▼ I.V. administration

• Dilute with half-normal or normal saline solution or D_5W. Prepare 100-mcg/ml solution by adding 180 ml of diluent per 20-mg (20-ml) vial, 150-mcg/ml solution by adding 113 ml of diluent per 20-mg (20-ml) vial, and 200-mcg/ml solution by adding 80 ml of diluent per 20-mg (20-ml) vial.
• Decreased blood pressure requires stopping or slowing infusion.
• Drug hasn't been shown to be safe or effective for more than 48 hours. Avoid using longer.
⊗ **Incompatibilities**
Bumetanide, furosemide, procainamide.

Contraindications and cautions

• Contraindicated in patients hypersensitive to the drug, or any of its components.
• Use cautiously in patients with severe aortic or pulmonic valvular disease in place of surgical correction of obstruction, or for patients in acute phase of MI.
• Use cautiously in patients with atrial flutter or fibrillation because drug slightly shortens AV node conduction time and may increase ventricular response rate.
Lifespan: In pregnant women, use cautiously. In breast-feeding women, use cautiously; it's unknown if the drug appears in breast milk. In children, safety and effectiveness haven't been established.

Adverse reactions

CNS: headache.
CV: chest pain, hypotension, VENTRICULAR ARRHYTHMIAS, *ventricular ectopic activity, ventricular fibrillation, ventricular tachycardia.*

Interactions

Drug-drug. *Nesiritide:* May increase hypotensive effect. Avoid use together.

Effects on lab test results

None reported.

Pharmacokinetics

Absorption: Given I.V.
Distribution: About 70% protein-bound.
Metabolism: About 12% to glucuronide metabolite.
Excretion: About 83% unchanged in urine.
Half-life: 2½ to 2¾ hours.

Route	Onset	Peak	Duration
I.V.	5–15 min	1–2 hr	3–6 hr

Action

Chemical effect: Produces inotropic action by increasing cellular levels of cAMP; produces vasodilation by relaxing vascular smooth muscle.
Therapeutic effect: Relieves acute signs and symptoms of heart failure.

Available forms

Injection: 1 mg/ml
Premixed injection: 200 mcg/ml in 100 ml D_5W injection; 200 mcg/ml in 200 ml D_5W injection

NURSING PROCESS

M

Assessment

• Assess patient's heart failure before therapy and regularly thereafter to monitor drug effectiveness.
• Monitor fluid and electrolyte levels, blood pressure, heart rate, and kidney function during therapy.
• Continuously monitor patient's ECG.
• Be alert for adverse reactions.
• Assess patient's and family's knowledge of drug therapy.

Nursing diagnoses

• Impaired gas exchange related to presence of heart failure
• Decreased cardiac output related to drug-induced cardiac arrhythmias
• Deficient knowledge related to drug therapy

Planning and implementation

• Drug is typically given with digoxin and diuretics.
• Inotropics may aggravate outflow tract obstruction in hypertrophic subaortic stenosis.
ALERT: Improvement of cardiac output may result in enhanced urine output. Reduce diuretic

dosage as heart failure improves. Potassium loss may predispose patient to digitalis toxicity.

⑤ **ALERT:** Don't confuse milrinone with inamrinone.

⑤ **ALERT:** Don't confuse Primacor with Primaxin.

Patient teaching
• Tell patient to report headache. Mild analgesic can be given for relief.

☑ Evaluation
• Patient exhibits adequate gas exchange as heart failure is resolved.
• Drug-induced arrhythmias don't develop during therapy.
• Patient and family state understanding of drug therapy.

minocycline hydrochloride
(migh-noh-SIGH-kleen high-droh-KLOR-ighd)
Dynacin, Minocin, Myrac, Solodyn

Pharmacologic class: tetracycline
Therapeutic class: antibiotic
Pregnancy risk category: D

Indications and dosages

▶ **Infections caused by sensitive gram-negative and gram-positive organisms, trachoma, amebiasis.** *Adults:* 200 mg I.V.; then 100 mg I.V. every 12 hours. Maximum 400 mg I.V. daily. Or 200 mg P.O. initially; then 100 mg P.O. every 12 hours. Some clinicians use 100 or 200 mg P.O. initially, followed by 50 mg q.i.d. *Children older than age 8:* Initially, 4 mg/kg P.O. or I.V., then 2 mg/kg P.O. every 12 hours. Give I.V. in 500- to 1,000-ml solution without calcium over 6 hours.

▶ **Gonorrhea in patients sensitive to penicillin.** *Adults:* Initially, 200 mg P.O.; then 100 mg every 12 hours for at least 4 days.

▶ **Syphilis in patients sensitive to penicillin.** *Adults:* Initially, 200 mg P.O.; then 100 mg every 12 hours for 10 to 15 days.

▶ **Meningococcal carrier state.** *Adults:* 100 mg P.O. every 12 hours for 5 days.

▶ **Uncomplicated urethral, endocervical, or rectal infection caused by** *Chlamydia trachomatis* **or** *Ureaplasma urealyticum. Adults:* 100 mg P.O. b.i.d. for at least 7 days.

▶ **Uncomplicated gonococcal urethritis in men.** *Adults:* 100 mg P.O. b.i.d. for 5 days.

▶ **Cholera.** *Adults:* Initially, 200 mg P.O., then 100 mg P.O. every 12 hours for 2 to 3 days.

▶ **Multibacillary leprosy‡.** *Adults:* 100 mg P.O. daily with clofazimine and ofloxacin for 6 months, followed by 100 mg P.O. daily for an additional 18 months in conjunction with clofazimine.

▶ **Nongonococcal urethritis caused by** *C. trachomatis* **or** *mycoplasma‡. Adults:* 100 mg P.O. daily in one or two divided doses for 1 to 3 weeks.

⑤ **Adjust-a-dose:** Decrease dosage or extend dosing intervals in patients with renal impairment to a maximum of 200 mg Minocin in 24 hours.

▼ I.V. administration

• Reconstitute 100 mg of powder with 5 ml of sterile water for injection, with further dilution of 500 to 1,000 ml of sodium chloride, 5% dextrose, D_5W, or Ringer's lactate for I.V. infusion.
• Infusions are usually given over 6 hours.
• Thrombophlebitis may develop. Watch for irritation and infiltration; extravasation can cause tissue damage and necrosis.
• Switch to P.O. form as soon as possible.
• Solution is stable for 24 hours at room temperature.

⊗ **Incompatibilities**
Adrenocorticotropic hormone, allopurinol, amifostine, aminophylline, amobarbital sodium, amphotericin B, bicarbonate infusion mixtures, calcium gluconate or calcium chloride, carbenicillin, cefazolin sodium, cephalothin sodium, chloramphenicol succinate, colistin sulfate, doxapram, heparin sodium, hydrocortisone sodium succinate, hydromorphone, iodine sodium, meperidine, morphine, penicillin, pentobarbital, phenytoin sodium, piperacillin sodium-tazobactam sodium, polymyxin, prochlorperazine, propofol, rifampin, sodium ascorbate, sulfadiazine, sulfisoxazole, thiopental sodium, thiotepa, vitamin K (sodium bisulfate or sodium salt), whole blood.

Contraindications and cautions

• Contraindicated in patients hypersensitive to the drug or other tetracyclines.
• Use cautiously in patients with impaired kidney or liver function.

⚓ **Lifespan:** In breast-feeding women, don't use because it's unknown if drug appears in breast milk. In children younger than age 8, don't use. Drug may cause permanent discoloration of teeth, enamel defects, and bone growth retardation. In pregnant women, don't use in the last trimester because of these same effects on the fetus.

Adverse reactions

CNS: *intracranial hypertension* (pseudotumor cerebri), light-headedness or dizziness from vestibular toxicity.
CV: pericarditis, *thrombophlebitis.*
EENT: dysphagia, glossitis.
GI: *anorexia, diarrhea,* enterocolitis, epigastric distress, inflammatory anogenital lesions, oral candidiasis, nausea, vomiting.
Hematologic: eosinophilia, *neutropenia, thrombocytopenia.*
Musculoskeletal: bone growth retardation.
Skin: increased pigmentation, maculopapular and erythematous rashes, photosensitivity reactions, urticaria.
Other: *anaphylaxis,* enamel defects, *hypersensitivity reactions,* permanent discoloration of teeth, superinfection.

Interactions

Drug-drug. *Antacids (including sodium bicarbonate) and laxatives containing aluminum, magnesium, or calcium; antidiarrheals:* May decrease antibiotic absorption. Give antibiotic 1 hour before or 2 hours after these drugs.
Cimetidine: May decrease absorption of minocycline. Monitor patient.
Digoxin: May increase digoxin level. Decrease digoxin dose, if needed.
Ferrous sulfate, other iron products, zinc: May decrease antibiotic absorption. Administer drug 3 hours after or 2 hours before iron.
Hormonal contraceptives: May decrease contraceptive effectiveness and increase risk of breakthrough bleeding. Recommend a nonhormonal contraceptive.
Methoxyflurane: May cause nephrotoxicity with tetracyclines. Avoid use together; monitor patient carefully.
Oral anticoagulants: May increase anticoagulant effect. Monitor PT and INR. Adjust dosage if needed.
Penicillins: May interfere with bactericidal action of penicillins. Avoid use together.

Drug-herb. *St. John's wort:* May increase photosensitivity reactions. Urge patient to avoid unprotected or prolonged exposure to sunlight.
Drug-lifestyle. *Sun exposure:* May cause photosensitivity reaction. Urge patient to avoid unprotected or prolonged exposure to sunlight.

Effects on lab test results

• May increase BUN and liver enzyme levels. May decrease hemoglobin level and hematocrit.
• May increase eosinophil count. May decrease platelet and neutrophil counts.
• May cause false-positive reading of copper sulfate tests, such as Clinitest (parenteral form). May cause false-negative reading of glucose enzymatic tests, such as Diastix (all forms).

Pharmacokinetics

Absorption: 90% to 100%.
Distribution: Wide, including into synovial, pleural, prostatic, and seminal fluids; bronchial secretions; saliva; and aqueous humor. CSF penetration is poor. 70% to 80% protein-bound.
Metabolism: Partial.
Excretion: In bile salts, urine, and feces. *Half-life:* 11 to 26 hours.

Route	Onset	Peak	Duration
P.O.	Unknown	1–4 hr	Unknown
I.V.	Immediate	Immediate	Unknown

Action

Chemical effect: May exert bacteriostatic effect by binding to ribosomal subunit of microorganisms, inhibiting protein synthesis.
Therapeutic effect: Hinders bacterial cell growth.

Available forms

Capsules: 50 mg, 75 mg, 100 mg
Capsules (pellet-filled): 50 mg, 100 mg
Injection: 100 mg/vial
Suspension: 50 mg/5 ml*
Tablets: 50 mg, 75 mg, 100 mg

NURSING PROCESS

☞ Assessment

• Assess patient's infection before therapy and regularly thereafter to monitor drug effectiveness.
• Obtain specimen for culture and sensitivity tests before giving first dose. Begin therapy pending results.

M

- Be alert for adverse reactions and drug interactions.
- If patient has an adverse GI reaction, monitor patient's hydration.
- Assess patient's and family's knowledge of drug therapy.

⊕ Nursing diagnoses
- Risk for infection related to presence of susceptible bacteria
- Risk for deficient fluid volume related to drug-induced adverse reactions
- Deficient knowledge related to drug therapy

▷ Planning and implementation
⊛ ALERT: Check expiration date. Outdated or degraded tetracyclines have been linked to reversible nephrotoxicity (Fanconi syndrome).
- Don't expose these drugs to light or heat. Keep cap tightly closed.
- Drug may cause tooth discoloration in children and young adults. If it occurs, inform prescriber.
⊛ ALERT: Don't confuse Minocin with niacin and Mithracin.
⊛ ALERT: Don't confuse Dynacin with DynaCirc.
Patient teaching
- Inform patient that drug may be taken with food, and instruct him to take drug exactly as prescribed.
- Instruct patient to take oral form with full glass of water and to avoid taking it within 1 hour of bedtime to avoid esophagitis.
- Warn patient to avoid hazardous tasks until the drug's CNS effects are known.
- Instruct patient to avoid direct sunlight and ultraviolet light, to use sunblock, and to wear protective clothing in order to avoid photosensitivity reaction.
- Advise patient who uses hormonal contraceptives that barrier method of contraception should also be used. Also inform her that she may experience breakthrough bleeding.

☑ Evaluation
- Patient is free from infection.
- Patient maintains adequate hydration throughout therapy.
- Patient and family state understanding of drug therapy.

mirtazapine
(mir-TAH-zuh-peen)
Remeron, Remeron SolTab

Pharmacologic class: piperazinoazepine
Therapeutic class: antidepressant
Pregnancy risk category: C

Indications and dosages

▶ **Depression.** *Adults:* Initially, 15 mg P.O. at bedtime. Maintenance dosage is 15 to 45 mg daily. Adjust dosage at intervals of at least 1 to 2 weeks.

Contraindications and cautions

- Contraindicated in patients hypersensitive to the drug or any of its components and in those taking MAO inhibitors.
- Use cautiously in patients with CV or cerebrovascular disease, seizure disorders, suicidal ideation, impaired hepatic or renal function, or history of mania or hypomania.
≋ Lifespan: In pregnant women, use only if benefits outweigh risks to the fetus. In breast-feeding women, use cautiously; it's unknown if the drug appears in breast milk. In children, safety and effectiveness haven't been established, and drug shouldn't be used to treat major depressive disorder. Increased risk of suicidal behavior has been noted in this population, although not proven to be attributable to drug.

Adverse reactions

CNS: abnormal dreams, abnormal thinking, asthenia, confusion, dizziness, neuropathy, neurosis, *somnolence,* tremor.
CV: edema, peripheral edema.
GI: constipation, dry mouth, increased appetite, nausea.
GU: urinary frequency.
Hematologic: *agranulocytosis, neutropenia.*
Metabolic: *weight gain.*
Musculoskeletal: back pain, myalgia.
Respiratory: dyspnea.
Other: flulike syndrome.

Interactions

Drug-drug. *Diazepam, other CNS depressants:* May have additive CNS effects. Avoid use together.

MAO inhibitors: May cause serious and sometimes fatal reactions. Don't use drug within 14 days of an MAO inhibitor.

Drug-lifestyle. *Alcohol use:* May have additive CNS effects. Discourage use together.

Effects on lab test results

• May increase ALT level.
• May decrease neutrophil and granulocyte counts.

Pharmacokinetics

Absorption: Rapid.
Distribution: 85% protein-bound.
Metabolism: Extensive.
Excretion: Mainly in urine; some in feces.
Half-life: About 20 to 40 hours.

Route	Onset	Peak	Duration
P.O.	Unknown	< 2 hr	Unknown

Action

Chemical effect: Enhances central noradrenergic and serotonergic action; potent antagonist of histamine receptors.
Therapeutic effect: Relieves depression.

Available forms

Tablets: 15 mg, 30 mg, 45 mg
Tablets (orally-disintegrating): 15 mg, 30 mg, 45 mg

NURSING PROCESS

Assessment

• Assess mental status before and regularly during treatment.
• Monitor for signs of infection and other adverse reactions.
• Assess patient's and family's knowledge of drug therapy.

Nursing diagnoses

• Disturbed thought processes related to adverse effects
• Risk for injury related to sedation and orthostatic hypotension
• Deficient knowledge related to drug therapy

Planning and implementation

• If patient develops a sore throat, fever, stomatitis, or other signs of infection with a low

WBC count, stop giving the drug and monitor him closely.

⑤ ALERT: Don't stop drug therapy abruptly because doing so increases the patient's risk of suicide. Monitor patient and take suicide precautions.

Patient teaching
• Instruct patient to remove orally-disintegrating tablet from blister pack and immediately place on the tongue. Tell him he won't need water to swallow the tablet because drug dissolves rapidly.
• Tell patient not to break or split tablet.
• Warn patient to avoid hazardous activities if somnolence occurs.
• Tell patient to report signs and symptoms of infection or flulike symptoms.
• Advise patient not to use alcohol or take other CNS depressants.
• Stress importance of compliance with therapy.
• Instruct patient not to take other drugs without prescriber's approval.
• Tell woman to notify prescriber if she suspects pregnancy or if she is breast-feeding.

☑ Evaluation

• Patient regains normal thought processes.
• Patient sustains no injury from adverse reactions.
• Patient and family state understanding of drug therapy.

misoprostol
(migh-soe-PROST-ole)
Cytotec

Pharmacologic class: prostaglandin E1 analogue
Therapeutic class: gastric mucosal protectant
Pregnancy risk category: X

Indications and dosages

▶ **Prevention of NSAID-induced gastric ulcer in elderly or debilitated patients at high risk for complications from gastric ulcer and in patients with history of NSAID-induced ulcer.** *Adults:* 200 mcg P.O. q.i.d. with food. If dosage isn't tolerated, decrease to 100 mcg P.O. q.i.d.

▶ **Duodenal or gastric ulcer‡.** *Adults:* 100 to 200 mcg P.O. q.i.d. with meals and at bedtime for 4 to 8 weeks.

Contraindications and cautions

• Contraindicated in patients with a known allergy to prostaglandins.

⚘ **Lifespan:** In pregnant women, don't use because of risk of uterine rupture and fetal death. In breast-feeding women, don't use because significant diarrhea in infants has been reported. In children, safety and effectiveness haven't been established.

Adverse reactions

CNS: headache, lethargy, vertigo.
GI: *abdominal pain,* constipation, *diarrhea,* dyspepsia, flatulence, nausea, *pancreatitis,* vomiting.
GU: cramps, dysmenorrhea, hematuria, hypermenorrhea, menstrual disorders, spotting, UTI.
Other: *anaphylaxis.*

Interactions

Drug-drug. *Antacids:* May reduce misoprostol level insignificantly. Monitor patient.

Effects on lab test results

• May increase alkaline phosphatase, aminotransferase, and cardiac enzyme levels. May decrease hemoglobin level and hematocrit.
• May increase erythrocyte sedimentation rate. May decrease platelet count.

Pharmacokinetics

Absorption: Rapid.
Distribution: Highly protein-bound.
Metabolism: Rapidly de-esterified to misoprostol acid, the biologically active metabolite.
Excretion: About 15% in feces; rest in urine.
Half-life: 20 to 40 minutes.

Route	Onset	Peak	Duration
P.O.	30 min	60–90 min	3 hr

Action

Chemical effect: Replaces gastric prostaglandins depleted by NSAID therapy. Decreases basal and stimulated gastric acid secretion and may increase gastric mucus and bicarbonate production.
Therapeutic effect: Protects gastric mucosa from ulcerating.

Available forms

Tablets: 100 mcg, 200 mcg

NURSING PROCESS

Assessment
• Obtain history of patient's GI condition before therapy.
• In woman of childbearing age, make sure that negative pregnancy test is obtained within 2 weeks before therapy begins.
• Be alert for adverse reactions and drug interactions.
• Assess patient's and family's knowledge of drug therapy.

Nursing diagnoses
• Risk for injury related to potential for gastric ulceration
• Acute pain related to headache
• Deficient knowledge related to drug therapy

Planning and implementation
⚕ **ALERT:** Take special precautions not to use drug in a pregnant woman. Make sure she is fully aware of dangers to fetus and that she receives both verbal and written warnings of these dangers. Also, make sure she can comply with effective contraceptive use.
• Uterine rupture is linked to certain risk factors, including later trimester pregnancies, higher doses of the drug, previous cesarean delivery or uterine surgery, and five or more previous pregnancies.
⚕ **ALERT:** Don't confuse misoprostol with mifepristone.
Patient teaching
• Instruct patient to report to prescriber headache, diarrhea that doesn't resolve within three weeks or is severe, and severe abdominal pain.
• Instruct patient not to share drug because it may cause miscarriage, usually with life-threatening bleeding, in women of childbearing age.
• Advise patient not to start therapy until the second or third day of the next normal menstrual period.

Evaluation
• Patient remains free from signs and symptoms of gastric ulceration.
• Patient states that drug-induced headache doesn't occur.
• Patient and family state understanding of drug therapy.

Reactions may be *common,* uncommon, *life-threatening*, or COMMON AND LIFE-THREATENING.

HIGH ALERT

mitomycin (mitomycin-C)
(myt-oh-MY-sin)
Mutamycin

Pharmacologic class: antibiotic
Therapeutic class: antineoplastic
Pregnancy risk category: NR

Indications and dosages

▶ **Disseminated adenocarcinomas of the pancreas and stomach.** *Adults:* 20 mg/m^2 I.V. as single dose. Repeat cycle after 6 to 8 weeks when WBC and platelet counts have returned to normal.

⑤ Adjust-a-dose: If WBC count at nadir after last dose is 2,000 to 2,999 mm^3 and platelet count is 25,000 to 74,999 mm^3, give 70% of regular dose. If WBC count is less than 2,000 mm^3 and platelet count is less than 25,000 mm^3, give 50% of regular dose.

▶ **Bladder cancer‡.** *Adults:* 20 to 60 mg intravesically once per week for 8 weeks.

▽ I.V. administration

● Preparation and administration are related to mutagenic, teratogenic, and carcinogenic risks to personnel. Follow facility policy to reduce risks.
● To reconstitute 5-mg vial use 10 ml sterile water for injection; to reconstitute 20-mg vial, use 40 ml of sterile water for injection; to reconstitute a 40-mg vial, use 80 ml sterile water for injection, to give a concentration of 0.5 mg/ml. Let stand at room temperature until complete dissolution occurs.
● Give drug into the Y-connector of a free-flowing I.V. line.
● Watch for irritation and infiltration. Extravasation can cause tissue damage, severe ulceration, and necrosis. If it occurs, stop infusion immediately and notify prescriber.
● When reconstituted with sterile water for injection to 0.5 mg/ml, drug is stable for 14 days refrigerated or 7 days at room temperature. When diluted to 20 to 40 mcg/ml, it's stable in D$_5$W for 3 hours, in normal saline solution for 12 hours, and in sodium lactate for 24 hours.
● The combination of 5 to 15 mg mitomycin and 1,000 to 10,000 units heparin in 30 ml of normal saline solution for injection is stable at room temperature for 48 hours.

⊗ Incompatibilities
Aztreonam, bleomycin, cefepime, etoposide, filgrastim, gemcitabine, piperacillin sodium-tazobactam sodium, sargramostim, vinorelbine.

Contraindications and cautions

● Contraindicated in patients hypersensitive to the drug or any of its components and in those with thrombocytopenia, coagulation disorder, or increased bleeding tendency from other causes.
⚘ **Lifespan:** In pregnant and breast-feeding women, use only when benefits outweigh risks to the fetus and infant. In children, safety and effectiveness haven't been established.

Adverse reactions

CNS: confusion, drowsiness, fatigue, *fever,* headache, neurologic abnormalities.
GI: anorexia, *nausea,* stomatitis, *vomiting.*
GU: *hemolytic uremic syndrome, renal toxicity.*
Hematologic: LEUKOPENIA, *microangiopathic hemolytic anemia,* THROMBOCYTOPENIA.
Respiratory: *acute respiratory distress syndrome,* dyspnea, *interstitial pneumonitis,* nonproductive cough, *pulmonary edema.*
Skin: cellulitis, ulceration, and sloughing with extravasation; desquamation, induration, pruritus, and *pain* at injection site; purple coloration of nail beds; *reversible alopecia.*
Other: *septicemia.*

Interactions

Drug-drug. *Vinca alkaloids:* May cause acute respiratory distress. Avoid use together.

Effects on lab test results

● May decrease hemoglobin level and hematocrit.
● May decrease platelet and WBC counts.

Pharmacokinetics

Absorption: Given I.V.
Distribution: Wide. Doesn't cross blood-brain barrier.
Metabolism: By hepatic microsomal enzymes and rapidly deactivated in kidneys, spleen, brain, and heart.
Excretion: Mainly in urine; small portion in bile and feces. Only 10% of dose as active drug. *Half-life:* About 50 minutes.

Route	Onset	Peak	Duration
I.V.	Unknown	Unknown	Unknown

M

Action

Chemical effect: Acts like alkylating drug, cross-linking strands of DNA. This causes imbalance of cell growth, leading to cell death.
Therapeutic effect: Kills certain cancer cells.

Available forms

Injection: 5-, 20-, and 40-mg vials

NURSING PROCESS

Assessment

• Assess patient's condition before therapy and regularly thereafter to monitor drug effectiveness.
• Obtain CBC and blood studies.
• Monitor kidney function tests.
• Be alert for adverse reactions and drug interactions.
• Assess patient's and family's knowledge of drug therapy.

Nursing diagnoses

• Ineffective health maintenance related to presence of neoplastic disease
• Ineffective protection related to adverse hematologic reactions
• Deficient knowledge related to drug therapy

Planning and implementation

• Never give drug I.M. or subcutaneously.
• Base dosage adjustments on nadir of leukocyte and platelet counts after previous dose.
• Hemolytic uremic syndrome is characterized by microangiopathic hemolytic anemia, thrombocytopenia, and renal impairment.
• Watch for leukopenia up to 8 weeks post infusion; also can be cumulative with successive doses.
⚠ ALERT: Don't confuse mitomycin with mithramycin.
Patient teaching
• Instruct patient to watch for signs of infection and bleeding and to take temperature daily.
• Warn patient that alopecia may occur, but assure him that it's reversible.
• Tell patient to promptly report to prescriber any adverse reaction.

Evaluation

• Patient responds well to therapy.
• Patient doesn't develop serious complications.

• Patient and family state understanding of drug therapy.

HIGH ALERT

mitoxantrone hydrochloride

(my-toh-ZAN-trohn hy-droh-KLOR-ighd)
Novantrone

Pharmacologic class: anthracinedione antibiotic
Therapeutic class: antineoplastic
Pregnancy risk category: D

Indications and dosages

▶ **Combination initial therapy for acute non-lymphocytic leukemia.** *Adults:* Induction begins with 12 mg/m^2 I.V. daily on days 1 through 3, given with 100 mg/m^2 daily of cytarabine on days 1 through 7. If response isn't adequate, give second induction. Maintenance therapy includes 12 mg/m^2 on days 1 and 2, given with cytarabine on days 1 through 5.
▶ **To reduce neurologic disability and frequency of relapse in chronic progressive, progressive relapsing, or worsening relapsing-remitting multiple sclerosis.** *Adults:* 12 mg/m^2 I.V. infusion over 5 to 15 minutes every 3 months.
▶ **Pain from advanced hormone-refractory prostate cancer.** *Adults:* 12 to 14 mg/m^2 I.V. infusion over 15 to 30 minutes every 21 days with corticosteroids.

I.V. administration

• Preparation and administration of parenteral form carries mutagenic, teratogenic, and carcinogenic risks. Check facility policy.
• Dilute dose (available as aqueous solution of 2 mg/ml in volumes of 10, 12.5, and 15 ml) in at least 50 ml of normal saline solution injection or D$_5$W injection. Give drug by direct injection into free-flowing I.V. line of normal saline solution or D$_5$W injection over at least 3 minutes, usually 15 to 30 minutes.
• Although drug isn't a vesicant, if dose extravasates, stop infusion immediately and notify prescriber. Apply ice packs over area of suspected extravasation and elevate extremity.
• Never give by subcutaneous, I.M., intra-arterial, or intrathecal route.
• Store undiluted solution at room temperature. Once vial is penetrated, undiluted solution may

be stored at room temperature for 7 days, or 14 days in refrigerator. Don't freeze.

⊗ **Incompatibilities**
Amphotericin B, aztreonam, cefepime, doxorubicin liposomal, heparin sodium, hydrocortisone, other I.V. drugs, paclitaxel, piperacillin sodium and tazobactam sodium, propofol, sargramostim.

Contraindications and cautions

• Contraindicated in patients hypersensitive to the drug or any of its components.
• Use cautiously in patients previously exposed to anthracyclines or other cardiotoxic drugs.
⚘ Lifespan: In pregnant and breast-feeding women, drug is contraindicated. In children, safety and effectiveness haven't been established.

Adverse reactions

CNS: headache, *seizures.*
CV: *arrhythmias, fatal myocardial toxicity, heart failure,* tachycardia.
EENT: conjunctivitis.
GI: abdominal pain, BLEEDING, diarrhea, mucositis, nausea, stomatitis, vomiting.
GU: *renal impairment,* uric acid nephropathy.
Hematologic: *myelosuppression, secondary acute myelogenous leukemia.*
Hepatic: *jaundice.*
Metabolic: hyperuricemia.
Respiratory: cough, dyspnea.
Skin: alopecia, ecchymoses, petechiae.

Interactions

None significant.

Effects on lab test results

• May increase ALT, AST, bilirubin, BUN, creatinine, and uric acid levels. May decrease hemoglobin level and hematocrit.
• May decrease WBC, RBC, and platelet counts.

Pharmacokinetics

Absorption: Given I.V.
Distribution: 78% protein-bound.
Metabolism: In liver.
Excretion: By renal and hepatobiliary systems.
Half-life: 5¼ days.

Route	Onset	Peak	Duration
I.V.	Unknown	Unknown	Unknown

Action

Chemical effect: Not fully understood; may be cell cycle–nonspecific. Drug reacts with DNA, producing cytotoxic effect.
Therapeutic effect: Hinders susceptible cancer cell growth.

Available forms

Injection: 2 mg/ml in 10-, 12.5-, and 15-ml vials

NURSING PROCESS

✎ Assessment
• Assess patient's condition before therapy and regularly thereafter to monitor drug effectiveness.
• Monitor CBC and other lab test results regularly.
• Monitor left ventricular ejection fraction and signs of heart failure or cardiac toxicity with each dose.
• Be alert for adverse reactions and drug interactions.
• Assess patient's and family's knowledge of drug therapy.

⊕ Nursing diagnoses
• Ineffective health maintenance related to presence of leukemia
• Risk for infection related to drug-induced myelosuppression
• Deficient knowledge related to drug therapy

▷ Planning and implementation
• Give under the supervision of a physician experienced in the use of cytotoxic chemotherapeutics.
• Don't give drug to a patient with neutrophil count below 1,500 cells/mm³ or left ventricular ejection fraction less than 50% unless benefits outweigh risks.
• Cardiotoxicity is linked to a cumulative dose greater than 140 mg/m².
• Myocardial toxicity may occur during treatment or months to years after therapy ends.
• Give allopurinol, if needed. Uric acid nephropathy can be avoided by adequately hydrating patient before and during therapy.
• If severe nonhematologic toxicity occurs during first course of therapy, delay second course until patient recovers.

M

Patient teaching
- Inform patient that urine may appear blue-green within 24 hours after administration, and that some bluish discoloration of sclera may occur. These effects aren't harmful.
- Teach patient infection control and bleeding precautions. Tell him to watch for and report signs of bleeding and infection.
- Tell patient to report sudden weight gain, peripheral edema, shortness of breath, or chest discomfort to prescriber immediately.
- Advise woman of childbearing age not to become pregnant during therapy and to consult prescriber before becoming pregnant.

☑ **Evaluation**
- Patient responds well to therapy.
- Patient develops no serious complications from drug-induced myelosuppression.
- Patient and family state understanding of drug therapy.

modafinil
(moh-DAFF-ih-nil)
Provigil

Pharmacologic class: CNS stimulant
Therapeutic class: analeptic
Pregnancy risk category: C
Controlled substance schedule: IV

Indications and dosages

▶ **Narcolepsy, obstructive sleep apnea/hypopnea syndrome.** *Adults:* 200 mg P.O. daily, given as a single dose in the morning.
▶ **Shift-work sleep disorder.** *Adults:* 200 mg P.O. once daily 1 hour before start of shift work.
▧ **Adjust-a-dose:** For patients with severe hepatic impairment, reduce dosage by 50%.

Contraindications and cautions

- Contraindicated in patients hypersensitive to the drug or any of its components. Don't use in patients with a history of left ventricular hypertrophy or ischemic ECG changes, chest pain, arrhythmias, or other signs or symptoms of mitral valve prolapse caused by CNS stimulant use.
- Use cautiously in patients with recent MI or unstable angina, in those with history of psychosis, and in those receiving therapy with MAO inhibitors.

- Use cautiously and at reduced dosage in patients with severe hepatic impairment, with or without cirrhosis.
- Safety and effectiveness of drug in patients with severe renal impairment hasn't been established.
▱ **Lifespan:** In pregnant women, use only when benefits outweigh risks to the fetus. In breast-feeding women, use cautiously because it's unknown if the drug appears in breast milk. In children younger than age 16, safety and effectiveness haven't been established. In elderly patients with renal or hepatic impairment, use cautiously and at a low dose.

Adverse reactions

CNS: amnesia, anxiety, ataxia, cataplexy, confusion, depression, dizziness, dyskinesia, emotional lability, fever, hallucination, *headache,* hypertonia, insomnia, nervousness, paresthesia, *suicidal ideation,* syncope, tremor.
CV: *arrhythmias,* chest pain, hypertension, hypotension, vasodilation.
EENT: abnormal vision, amblyopia, epistaxis, *rhinitis,* pharyngitis.
GI: anorexia, diarrhea, dry mouth, gingivitis, mouth ulcer, *nausea,* thirst, vomiting.
GU: abnormal ejaculation, abnormal urine, urine retention.
Hematologic: eosinophilia.
Metabolic: hyperglycemia.
Musculoskeletal: joint disorder, neck pain, rigid neck.
Respiratory: *asthma,* dyspnea, lung disorders.
Skin: dry skin, herpes simplex, rash, *Stevens-Johnson syndrome, toxic epidermal necrolysis.*
Other: chills, infection.

Interactions

Drug-drug. *Cyclosporine, theophylline:* May reduce levels of these drugs. Use together cautiously.
Drugs that induce CYP3A4 (carbamazepine, phenobarbital, rifampin), drugs that inhibit CYP3A4 (itraconazole, ketoconazole): May alter modafinil level. Monitor patient closely.
Drugs metabolized by CYP2C9 (diazepam, phenytoin, propranolol): May increase levels of these drugs. Use together cautiously, and adjust dosage as needed.
Hormonal contraceptives: May reduce levels of these drugs, resulting in reduced contraceptive effectiveness. Recommend additional or alterna-

tive contraceptive method during modafinil therapy and for 1 month afterward.

Methylphenidate: May delay modafinil absorption. Separate doses.

Phenytoin, warfarin: May inhibit CYP2C9 and increase levels of phenytoin and warfarin. Monitor patient closely for signs of toxicity.

Tricyclic antidepressants (clomipramine, desipramine): May increase tricyclic antidepressant levels. Reduce dosage of these drugs.

Drug-food. *Food:* May delay absorption by about 1 hour.

Effects on lab test results

• May increase glucose, GGT, and AST levels.
• May increase eosinophil count.

Pharmacokinetics

Absorption: Rapid, with levels peaking in 2 to 4 hours.
Distribution: Good. About 60% protein-bound, mainly to albumin.
Metabolism: About 90% in the liver.
Excretion: Less than 10% from the kidneys as unchanged drug. *Half-life:* 15 hours.

Route	Onset	Peak	Duration
P.O.	Unknown	2–4 hr	Unknown

Action

Chemical effect: Unknown. It provides wake-promoting actions similar to those of sympathomimetics, including amphetamines, but it's structurally distinct from amphetamines and doesn't appear to alter the release of either dopamine or norepinephrine to produce CNS stimulation.
Therapeutic effect: Improves daytime wakefulness.

Available forms

Tablets: 100 mg, 200 mg

NURSING PROCESS

Assessment

• Obtain history of patient's condition before therapy, and reassess regularly thereafter to monitor drug effectiveness.
• Assess patient's renal function before therapy.
• Closely monitor hypertensive patient.
• Assess patient's and family's knowledge of drug therapy.

Nursing diagnoses

• Sleep deprivation related to drug-induced insomnia
• Risk for injury related to drug-induced CNS adverse effects
• Deficient knowledge related to drug therapy

Planning and implementation

• Food has no effect on overall bioavailability, but it may delay modafinil absorption by 1 hour.
• Although single, daily, 400-mg dose is usually well tolerated, no consistent evidence exists that this dosage provides additional benefit beyond daily 200-mg doses.
Patient teaching
• Drug may impair judgment. Advise patient to be careful while driving or performing other activities that require alertness until the drug's CNS effects are known.
• Instruct patient not to take other prescription or OTC drugs without consulting prescriber because of possible drug interactions.
⊛ **ALERT:** Instruct patient to stop drug and contact prescriber immediately if he experiences psychiatric symptoms such as anxiety, mania, hallucination, and suicidal ideation.
• Advise patient not to drink alcohol during therapy.
⊛ **ALERT:** Tell patient to stop drug and notify prescriber immediately if he develops a rash, hives, or a related allergic reaction.
• Caution woman that use of hormonal contraceptives (including depot or implantable contraceptives) with modafinil tablets may increase the risk of pregnancy. Recommend barrier method as alternative or additional contraception during therapy and for 1 month after therapy ends.
• Advise woman to notify prescriber if she becomes pregnant or intends to become pregnant during therapy.
• Tell woman to notify prescriber if she's breast-feeding.

Evaluation

• Patient develops and maintains normal sleep-wake patterns.
• Patient has no adverse CNS effects.
• Patient and family state understanding of drug therapy.

M

moexipril hydrochloride
(moh-EKS-eh-pril high-droh-KLOR-ighd)
Univasc

Pharmacologic class: ACE inhibitor
Therapeutic class: antihypertensive
Pregnancy risk category: C (D in second and third trimesters)

Indications and dosages

▶ **Hypertension.** *Adults:* Initially, 7.5 mg P.O. daily in patients not receiving a diuretic, given 1 hour before meals. If inadequate response, increase or divide dose. Maintenance dosage, 7.5 to 30 mg daily in one or two divided doses 1 hour before meals.

Ⓢ **Adjust-a-dose:** For patients with renal impairment, if creatinine clearance is 40 ml/minute or less, start dosage at 3.75 mg P.O. daily. Maximum, 15 mg P.O. daily. For patients taking diuretics, if diuretic can't be discontinued, start dosage at 3.75 mg P.O. daily.

Contraindications and cautions

• Contraindicated in patients hypersensitive to the drug or any of its components, and in those with history of angioedema with previous ACE inhibitor therapy.
• Use cautiously in patients with impaired kidney function, heart failure, or renal artery stenosis.
⚖ Lifespan: In pregnant women, use cautiously during first trimester; contraindicated in second and third trimesters. In breast-feeding women, use cautiously; it's unknown if the drug appears in breast milk. In children, safety and effectiveness haven't been established.

Adverse reactions

CNS: *dizziness,* fatigue, headache, pain.
CV: chest pain, flushing, hypotension, orthostatic hypotension, peripheral edema.
EENT: pharyngitis, rhinitis, sinusitis.
GI: diarrhea, dyspepsia, nausea.
GU: urinary frequency.
Hematologic: *neutropenia.*
Metabolic: *hyperkalemia.*
Musculoskeletal: myalgia.
Respiratory: *persistent, nonproductive cough;* upper respiratory tract infection.
Skin: rash.

Other: *anaphylaxis, angioedema,* flulike syndrome.

Interactions

Drug-drug. *Antacids:* May decrease bioavailability of ACE inhibitors. Give drug on an empty stomach.
Digoxin: May increase or decrease digoxin level. Monitor digoxin level and patient closely.
Diuretics: May increase risk of excessive hypotension. Monitor blood pressure closely.
Indomethacin: May reduce hypotensive effects of ACE inhibitors. Avoid use together; monitor blood pressure.
Lithium: May increase lithium level and toxicity. Use together cautiously. Monitor lithium level often.
Potassium-sparing diuretics, potassium supplements: May increase risk of hyperkalemia. Monitor potassium level closely.
Drug-herb. *Capsaicin:* May cause or worsen coughing from ACE inhibitor therapy. Discourage use together.
Drug-food. *Salt substitutes that contain potassium:* May increase risk of hyperkalemia. Monitor potassium level closely; urge patient to avoid salt substitutes containing potassium.

Effects on lab test results

• May increase potassium level.
• May decrease neutrophil and granulocyte counts.

Pharmacokinetics

Absorption: Incomplete, with bioavailability of about 13%. Food significantly decreases bioavailability.
Distribution: About 50% protein-bound.
Metabolism: Extensive, to the active metabolite moexiprilat.
Excretion: Mainly in feces, with small amount in urine. *Half-life:* 2 to 9 hours.

Route	Onset	Peak	Duration
P.O.	1 hr	3–6 hr	24 hr

Action

Chemical effect: May suppress renin-angiotensin-aldosterone system. Inhibits ACE, inhibiting production of angiotensin II (a potent vasoconstrictor and stimulator of aldosterone secretion).
Therapeutic effect: Lowers blood pressure.

Available forms

Tablets: 7.5 mg, 15 mg

NURSING PROCESS

⚕ Assessment
• Assess patient's blood pressure before therapy begins.
• Measure blood pressure at lowest point just before dose to verify adequate control. Drug is less effective in reducing trough blood pressure in blacks than in others.
• Monitor patient for hypotension.
• Assess kidney function before therapy and periodically thereafter. Monitor potassium level.
• Monitor CBC with differential counts before therapy, especially in patient who has collagen-vascular disease with impaired kidney function.
• Be alert for adverse reactions and interactions.
• Assess patient's and family's knowledge of drug therapy.

⚙ Nursing diagnoses
• Risk for injury related to presence of hypertension
• Sleep deprivation related to cough
• Deficient knowledge related to drug therapy

▷ Planning and implementation
⚠ **ALERT:** Excessive hypotension can occur when drug is given with diuretics. If possible, stop giving diuretics 2 to 3 days before giving this drug to decrease risk of reaction. If drug doesn't adequately control blood pressure, restart diuretic with care.
⚠ **ALERT:** Angioedema involving tongue, glottis, or larynx may be fatal because of airway obstruction. Give epinephrine and ensure a patent airway.
• If cough interferes with patient's ability to sleep, notify prescriber.
Patient teaching
• Instruct patient to take drug on an empty stomach; high-fat meals can impair absorption.
• Tell patient to avoid salt substitutes. These products may contain potassium, which can cause hyperkalemia.
• Advise patient to rise slowly to minimize light-headedness. If syncope occurs, tell him to stop taking the drug and immediately call the prescriber.
• Urge patient to use caution in hot weather and during exercise. Inadequate fluid intake, vomit-

ing, diarrhea, and excessive perspiration can lead to light-headedness and syncope.
• Advise patient to report signs of infection, such as fever and sore throat; easy bruising or bleeding; swelling of tongue, lips, face, eyes, mucous membranes, or limbs; difficulty swallowing or breathing; and hoarseness.
• Tell woman to notify prescriber if she becomes pregnant.

☑ Evaluation
• Patient's blood pressure is normal.
• Patient states that sleep disturbance doesn't occur.
• Patient and family state understanding of drug therapy.

mometasone furoate
(moe-MEH-tah-zone FUHR-oh-ayt)
Asmanex Twisthaler

Pharmacologic class: corticosteroid
Therapeutic class: anti-inflammatory, antiasthmatic
Pregnancy risk category: C

Indications and dosages

▶ **Maintenance therapy for asthma; asthma in patients who need oral corticosteroids.**
Adults and children age 12 and older who use a bronchodilator or inhaled corticosteroids: Initially, 220 mcg by oral inhalation every day in the evening. Maximum, 440 mcg/day.
Adults and children age 12 and older who take oral corticosteroids: 440 mcg b.i.d. by oral inhalation. Maximum, 880 mcg/day. Reduce oral corticosteroid dosage by no more than 2.5 mg/day at weekly intervals starting at least 1 week after starting mometasone. After stopping oral corticosteroids, reduce mometasone dosage to the lowest effective amount.

Contraindications and cautions

• Contraindicated in patients hypersensitive to drug or its ingredients and as primary treatment of status asthmaticus or other acute episodes of asthma or bronchospasm.
• Use cautiously in patients at high risk for decreased bone mineral content (those with a family history of osteoporosis, prolonged immobilization, long-term use of drugs that reduce

bone mass), patients switching from systemic to inhaled corticosteroids, and patients with active or quiescent tuberculosis, untreated systemic infections, ocular herpes simplex, or immunosuppression.

⚜ **Lifespan:** In pregnant women, use only if benefits outweigh risks to the fetus. In breastfeeding women; use cautiously; it isn't known if drug appears in breast milk. In children younger than age 12, safety hasn't been established.

Adverse reactions

CNS: depression, fatigue, *headache,* insomnia.
EENT: *allergic rhinitis,* dry throat, dysphonia, earache, epistaxis, nasal irritation, *pharyngitis,* sinus congestion, sinusitis.
GI: abdominal pain, anorexia, dyspepsia, flatulence, gastroenteritis, nausea, oral candidiasis, vomiting.
GU: dysmenorrhea, menstrual disorder, UTI.
Musculoskeletal: arthralgia, back pain, myalgia, pain.
Respiratory: respiratory disorder, *upper respiratory tract infection.*
Other: accidental injury, flulike symptoms, infection.

Interactions

Drug-drug. *Ketoconazole:* May increase mometasone level. Use together cautiously.

Effects on lab test results

None reported.

Pharmacokinetics

Absorption: Low in plasma.
Distribution: None in RBCs.
Metabolism: Extensive in the liver by CYP3A4 to multiple metabolites.
Excretion: Mainly in feces; some in urine.
Half-life: 5 hours after I.V. use, not known for inhalation.

Route	Onset	Peak	Duration
Inhalation	Unknown	1–2.5 hr	Unknown

Action

Chemical effect: Unknown, although corticosteroids inhibit many cells and mediators involved in inflammation and the asthmatic response.

Therapeutic effect: Reduces inflammation in the lungs and airways to improve pulmonary function.

Available forms

Inhalation powder: 220 mcg per inhalation

NURSING PROCESS

▨ Assessment

• Obtain patient's medical history, including current treatments for asthma, before starting drug therapy.
⑧ **ALERT:** If patient is switching from an oral corticosteroid to an inhaled form, watch closely for evidence of adrenal insufficiency, such as fatigue, lethargy, weakness, nausea, vomiting, and hypotension.
• Because inhaled corticosteroids can be systemically absorbed, watch for cushingoid effects.
• If a woman takes corticosteroids during pregnancy, monitor newborn for hypoadrenalism.
• Assess patient for bone loss during long-term use.
• Watch for evidence of localized mouth infections, glaucoma, and immunosuppression.
• Monitor elderly patients for increased sensitivity to drug effects.
• Assess patient's and family's knowledge of drug therapy.

⊕ Nursing diagnoses

• Impaired gas exchange related to underlying condition and poor pulmonary function
• Activity intolerance related to underlying asthmatic condition
• Deficient knowledge related to drug therapy

▷ Planning and implementation

⑧ **ALERT:** Don't use this drug to treat acute bronchospasm.
• Wean patient slowly from systemic corticosteroids once he switches to mometasone. Monitor lung function tests, beta-agonist use, and asthma symptoms.
• After oral corticosteroids are withdrawn, it may take months for hypothalamic-pituitary-adrenal (HPA) function to recover. Patients are particularly vulnerable to adrenal insufficiency or adrenal crisis during this period of HPA recovery if they experience trauma, stress, infection, or surgery.

- Maximum benefits may not occur for 1 to 2 weeks or longer after mometasone therapy is initiated.

Patient teaching
- Tell patient to use the mometasone inhaler regularly and at the same time each day. If he uses it only once daily, tell him to do so in the evening.
- Caution patient not to use drug for immediate relief of an asthmatic attack or bronchospasm.
- Inform patient that maximum benefits may not occur for 1 to 2 weeks or longer after mometasone therapy starts; instruct him to notify the prescriber if his condition fails to improve or if it worsens.
- Explain that, if bronchospasm develops after taking mometasone, he should immediately use a fast-acting bronchodilator. Urge him to contact the prescriber immediately if bronchospasm doesn't respond to the fast-acting bronchodilator.
- ⊛ ALERT: If patient has been weaned from oral corticosteroids, urge him to resume them during severe asthmatic attack or periods of stress and to contact the prescriber for instructions.
- Warn patient to avoid exposure to chickenpox or measles and to notify the prescriber if such exposure occurs.
- Tell patient to report vision changes; long-term use of an inhaled corticosteroid may increase the risk of cataracts or glaucoma.
- Advise patient to write the date on a new inhaler on the day he opens it and to discard the unit after 45 days or when the dose counter reads "00".
- Instruct patient on the proper use and routine care of the inhaler.

☑ Evaluation
- Patient has normal respiratory rate and optimal air exchange.
- Patient experiences improved exercise and activity tolerance.
- Patient and family state understanding of drug therapy.

montelukast sodium
(mon-tih-LOO-kist SOH-dee-um)
Singulair◆

Pharmacologic class: leukotriene receptor antagonist
Therapeutic class: antiasthmatic
Pregnancy risk category: B

Indications and dosages

▶ **Asthma, seasonal allergic rhinitis.** *Adults and children age 15 and older:* One 10-mg tablet P.O. daily in the evening.
Children ages 6 to 14: Give 5-mg chewable tablet P.O. daily in the evening.
Children ages 2 to 5: Give 4-mg chewable tablet P.O. or one packet (4-mg) oral granules daily in the evening.
▶ **Asthma.** *Children ages 12 to 23 months:* One packet (4-mg) granules P.O. daily in the evening.
▶ **Perennial allergic rhinitis in children.** *Children 6 to 23 months:* One packet (4-mg) granules P.O. daily in the evening.
▶ **Prevention of exercise-induced bronchospasm‡.** *Adults and children age 15 and older:* 10 mg P.O. at least 2 hours before exercise. Additional dose shouldn't be taken if already taking a daily dose.
Children ages 6 to 14: Give 5 mg P.O. daily.

Contraindications and cautions

- Contraindicated in patients hypersensitive to the drug or any of its components and in patients with acute asthmatic attacks or status asthmaticus.
- Use cautiously and with appropriate monitoring when systemic corticosteroid dosages are reduced.
- ⚘ Lifespan: In children younger than age 6 months, safety and effectiveness haven't been established.

Adverse reactions

CNS: asthenia, dizziness, fatigue, fever, *headache.*
EENT: nasal congestion.
GI: abdominal pain, dyspepsia, infectious gastroenteritis.
GU: pyuria.
Respiratory: cough.

M

Skin: rash.
Other: dental pain, influenza, trauma.

Interactions

Drug-drug. *Phenobarbital, rifampin:* May decrease bioavailability of montelukast by inducing hepatic metabolism. Monitor patient closely for decreased effects.

Effects on lab test results

• May increase ALT and AST levels.

Pharmacokinetics

Absorption: Rapid with an oral bioavailability of 64% in adults without regard to meals.
Distribution: More than 99% bound to plasma proteins.
Metabolism: Extensive, by cytochrome P-450 isoenzymes in GI tract.
Excretion: About 86% in the feces. *Half-life:* 2¾ to 5½ hours.

Route	Onset	Peak	Duration
P.O.			
Chewable	Unknown	2–2½ hr	24 hr
Coated	Unknown	3–4 hr	24 hr
Granules	Unknown	2 hr	24 hr

Action

Chemical effect: Inhibits action of cysteinyl leukotriene1 (CysLT1) receptor by binding with CysLT1. This reduces early- and late-phase bronchoconstriction caused by antigen challenge.
Therapeutic effect: Improves breathing.

Available forms

Granules: 4-mg packet
Tablets (chewable): 4 mg, 5 mg
Tablets (film-coated): 10 mg

NURSING PROCESS

⚅ Assessment

• Assess patient's underlying condition before therapy and regularly thereafter to monitor drug effectiveness.
• Monitor patient for adverse reactions and drug interactions.
• Assess patient's and family's knowledge of drug therapy.

⚅ Nursing diagnoses

• Impaired gas exchange related to asthma

• Activity intolerance related to asthma
• Deficient knowledge related to drug therapy

▷ Planning and implementation

• Don't abruptly substitute drug for inhaled or oral corticosteroids.
• Drug isn't indicated for patients with acute asthmatic attacks or status asthmaticus. It's also not indicated as monotherapy for managing exercise-induced bronchospasm. Continue rescue drug for acute exacerbations.
• Give oral granules directly in mouth or mixed with a teaspoonful of cold or room-temperature applesauce, carrots, rice, or ice cream. After opening packet, give within 15 minutes. If mixed with food, don't store excess for future use; discard any unused portion.
• Granules aren't intended to be dissolved in liquid other than formula or breast milk. Other liquids may be given afterwards.
• Don't give oral granules with high-fat meals.
• Give drug daily in the evening for asthma or asthma with allergic rhinitis; in the morning, give only for allergic rhinitis.

Patient teaching

• Advise patient not to use drug on an as-needed basis but to take drug daily, even if asymptomatic, and to contact prescriber if asthma isn't well controlled.
• Warn patient not to reduce or stop taking any other prescribed antiasthma drugs without the prescriber's approval.
• Tell parent the oral granules may be given directly into the child's mouth, dissolved in 1 tsp of cold or room temperature baby formula or breast milk, or mixed in a spoonful of applesauce, carrots, rice, or ice cream.
• Warn patient that drug isn't beneficial in acute asthma attacks or in exercise-induced bronchospasm, and advise him to keep appropriate rescue drugs available.
• Advise patient with known aspirin sensitivity to continue not to use aspirin or other NSAIDs.
• Advise patient with phenylketonuria that chewable tablet contains phenylalanine.

☑ Evaluation

• Patient's respiratory signs and symptoms improve.
• Patient can perform normal activities of daily living.
• Patient and family state understanding of drug therapy.

Reactions may be *common,* uncommon, *life-threatening,* or COMMON AND LIFE-THREATENING.

HIGH ALERT

morphine hydrochloride
(MOR-feen high-droh-KLOR-ighd)
Doloral ◆, M.O.S. ◆, M.O.S.-SR ◆

morphine sulfate
Astramorph PF, Avinza, DepoDur, DMS
Concentrate, Duramorph PF, Infumorph 200,
Infumorph 500, Kadian, Morphine H.P. ◆,
M.O.S.-Sulfate ◆, MS Contin, MSIR, MS/L,
MS/L Concentrate, OMS Concentrate,
Oramorph SR, RMS Uniserts, Roxanol,
Roxanol 100, Roxanol T

Pharmacologic class: opioid agonist
Therapeutic class: analgesic
Pregnancy risk category: C
Controlled substance schedule: II

Indications and dosages

▶ **Severe pain.** *Adults:* 5 to 20 mg/70 kg subcutaneously or I.M. every 4 hours, p.r.n. Or 2 to 10 mg/70 kg I.V. every 4 hours, p.r.n. Or 10 to 30 mg P.O. every 4 hours, p.r.n. Or, 10 to 20 mg P.R. every 4 hours, p.r.n. Or 15 to 30 mg of controlled-release tablets P.O. every 8 to 12 hours. Or 5 mg of epidural injection by epidural catheter. Maximum total epidural dose, 10 mg. If adequate pain relief not obtained within 1 hour, give additional doses of 1 to 2 mg at intervals sufficient to assess effectiveness.
Children: 0.1 to 0.2 mg/kg I.M. or subcutaneously every 4 hours, p.r.n. Maximum single dose is 15 mg. Or, 0.05 to 0.1 mg/kg by slow I.V. injection.

▶ **Moderate to severe pain requiring continuous, around-the-clock opioid therapy.**
Adults: Give loading dose of 15 mg or more by continuous I.V. infusion; then continuous infusion (concentration of 1 mg/ml) of 0.8 to 80 mg/hour. Or individualize dosage of Avinza according to patient's previous drug schedule.
Children: Give 0.025 to 2.6 mg/kg/hour by I.V. infusion.

▶ **Pain following major surgery.** *Adults:* Inject 10 to 15 mg DepoDur (maximum 20 mg) by lumbar epidural administration into lumbar epidural space before surgery or after clamping of umbilical cord during cesarean delivery. Inject undiluted or dilute up to 5 ml total volume with preservative-free normal saline solution.

Don't mix with other drugs. Don't give other drugs into epidural space for at least 48 hours.

▽ I.V. administration

• Drug is compatible with most common I.V. solutions.
• For direct injection, dilute 2.5 to 15 mg in 4 or 5 ml of sterile water for injection and give over 4 to 5 minutes.
• For continuous infusion, mix with D_5W to yield 0.1 to 1 mg/ml.
⊗ **Incompatibilities**
Aminophylline, amobarbital, cefepime, chlorothiazide, fluorouracil, haloperidol, heparin sodium, meperidine, pentobarbital, phenobarbital sodium, phenytoin sodium, prochlorperazine, promethazine hydrochloride, sodium bicarbonate, thiopental.

Contraindications and cautions

• Contraindicated in patients hypersensitive to the drug or any of its components and in those with conditions that preclude I.V. administration of opioids (acute bronchial asthma or upper airway obstruction).
• Use cautiously in debilitated patients and in patients with head injury, increased intracranial pressure, seizures, chronic pulmonary disease, prostatic hyperplasia, severe hepatic or renal disease, acute abdominal conditions, hypothyroidism, Addison disease, or urethral stricture.
⚘ **Lifespan:** In pregnant women, use cautiously. In breast-feeding women, wait 2 to 3 hours after last dose before breast-feeding to avoid sedation in infant. In elderly patients, use cautiously.

Adverse reactions

CNS: *clouded sensorium,* dizziness, *euphoria,* nightmares, *sedation, seizures, somnolence.*
CV: *bradycardia, cardiac arrest,* flushing, *hypotension, shock.*
GI: constipation, ileus, nausea, vomiting.
GU: urine retention.
Hematologic: *thrombocytopenia.*
Respiratory: *respiratory arrest, respiratory depression.*
Skin: pruritus.
Other: *physical dependence.*

Interactions

Drug-drug. *Antihistamines, chloral hydrate, CNS depressants, general anesthetics, glu-*

M

tethimide, hypnotics, MAO inhibitors, methocarbamol, opioid analgesics, sedatives, tranquilizers, tricyclic antidepressants: May cause respiratory depression, hypotension, profound sedation, or coma. Use cautiously. Reduce morphine dosage, and monitor patient.

Drug-lifestyle. *Alcohol use:* May have additive CNS effects. Also, use with Avinza and Kadian may compromise the extended-release capsule characteristics and cause a life-threatening dose of morphine to be released. Urge patient to avoid using alcohol during drug therapy.

Effects on lab test results

• May increase amylase level.
• May decrease platelet count.

Pharmacokinetics

Absorption: Variable when given P.O.; unknown for other routes.
Distribution: Wide.
Metabolism: Mainly in liver.
Excretion: In urine and bile. *Half-life:* 2 to 3 hours.

Route	Onset	Peak	Duration
P.O.	1 hr	1–2 hr	4–12 hr
I.V.	< 5 min	20 min	4–5 hr
I.M.	10–30 min	30–60 min	4–5 hr
SubQ	10–30 min	50–90 min	4–5 hr
P.R.	20–60 min	20–60 min	4–5 hr
Epidural	15–60 min	15–60 min	24 hr
Intrathecal	15–60 min	Unknown	24 hr

Action

Chemical effect: Binds with opioid receptors in CNS, altering both perception of and emotional response to pain through unknown mechanism.
Therapeutic effect: Relieves pain.

Available forms

morphine hydrochloride ◆
Oral solution ◆ : 1 mg/ml, 5 mg/ml, 10 mg/ml, 20 mg/ml, 50 mg/ml
Suppositories ◆ : 10 mg, 20 mg, 30 mg
Syrup ◆ : 1 mg/ml, 5 mg/ml, 10 mg/ml, 20 mg/ml, 50 mg/ml
Tablets ◆ : 10 mg, 20 mg, 40 mg, 60 mg
Tablets (extended-release) ◆ : 30 mg, 60 mg
morphine sulfate
Capsules: 15 mg, 30 mg

Capsules (extended-release beads) (Avinza): 30 mg, 60 mg, 90 mg, 120 mg
Capsules (extended-release pellets) (Kadian): 10 mg, 20 mg, 30 mg, 50 mg, 60 mg, 80 mg, 100 mg, 200 mg
Injection (with preservative): 1 mg/ml, 2 mg/ml, 4 mg/ml, 5 mg/ml, 8 mg/ml, 10 mg/ml, 15 mg/ml, 25 mg/ml, 50 mg/ml
Injection (without preservative): 0.5 mg/ml, 1 mg/ml, 10 mg/ml, 15 mg/ml, 25 mg/ml, 50 mg/ml
Liposomal injection (preservative-free): 10 mg/ml, 15 mg/1.5 ml, 20 mg/2 ml
Oral solution: 10 mg/5 ml, 20 mg/5 ml
Oral solution (concentrated): 20 mg/ml, 100 mg/5 ml
Soluble tablets: 10 mg, 15 mg, 30 mg
Suppositories: 5 mg, 10 mg, 20 mg, 30 mg
Tablets: 15 mg, 30 mg
Tablets (extended-release): 15 mg, 30 mg, 60 mg, 100 mg, 200 mg
Tablets (sustained-release): 15 mg, 30 mg, 60 mg, 100 mg, 200 mg

NURSING PROCESS

Assessment
• Assess patient's pain before therapy and regularly thereafter to monitor drug effectiveness.
• Drug may worsen or mask gallbladder pain.
• Monitor patient for respiratory depression after administration. When given epidurally, monitor patient for up to 24 hours after injection. Check respiratory rate and depth every 30 to 60 minutes for 24 hours.
• Assess patient for constipation often; adjust GI drugs as needed when increasing morphine dose.
• Be alert for adverse reactions and drug interactions.
• Assess patient's and family's knowledge of drug therapy.

Nursing diagnoses
• Acute pain related to underlying condition
• Ineffective breathing pattern related to drug's depressive effect on respiratory system
• Deficient knowledge related to drug therapy

Planning and implementation
• Preservative-free preparations are available for giving by epidural or intrathecal route.

ⓢ **ALERT:** Highly concentrated injections containing 10 or 25 mg/ml are meant for continuous, controlled microinfusion devices. Don't use for I.M., subcutaneous, I.V epidural, or intrathecal individual doses because of the risk of substantial overdose.

• Solutions of various strengths are available as well as concentrated P.O. solutions (20 mg/ml, 100 mg/5 ml). Double-check the orders written against the strength you are giving carefully. Serious events and fatalities may occur from dispensing and using wrong concentrations.

• Don't crush or break extended- or sustained-release tablets.

• For use with gastrostomy tube, immediately give opened Kadian capsule pellets in 10 ml water, swirling them into prewetted gastrostomy tube. Flush with additional water to clear all pellets; don't use in NG tube and don't crush pellets.

• May open controlled-release capsules and sprinkle beads or pellets onto small amount of applesauce for immediate use P.O. Follow with 4 to 8 oz water.

• Store DepoDur in refrigerator. Unopened vials can be stored at room temperature for up to 7 days. After withdrawn from vial, drug can be stored at room temperature for up to 4 hours before use.

• No need to refrigerate rectal suppositories.

• If using S.L., measure solution with tuberculin syringe. Give dose a few drops at a time to maximize S.L. absorption and minimize swallowing.

• In some patients, P.R. and P.O. absorption may not be equivalent.

• Morphine is drug of choice in relieving pain of MI. It may cause transient decrease in blood pressure.

• Keep opioid antagonist and resuscitation equipment available.

• Around-the-clock therapy best manages severe, chronic pain.

ⓢ **ALERT:** If respiratory rate is below 12 breaths/ minute except in terminal conditions, don't give the dose. Notify prescriber.

• Because constipation is often severe with maintenance dosage, give stool softener or other laxative.

ⓢ **ALERT:** Don't confuse morphine with hydromorphone. Don't confuse Avinza with Invanz.

ⓢ **ALERT:** Dose of Kadian is not bioequivalent to other controlled-release formulations. Therefore, observe patient carefully for oversedation

or inadequate analgesia, and adjust dosage or time interval accordingly.

Patient teaching

• Teach patient use of standardized pain-rating scale to facilitate communication about analgesic effectiveness.

ⓢ **ALERT:** Consuming alcoholic beverages or drugs containing alcohol while taking Avinza may cause extended-release coating to fail, releasing a potentially fatal dose of morphine. Warn patient against the use of alcohol in any form, and stress need to read labels on OTC products carefully.

• Warn patient about getting out of bed or walking without assistance. Warn outpatient not to drive or perform other hazardous activities until the drug's CNS effects are known.

• Tell patient to report continued pain and not to increase dose independently.

• Tell patient that stool softeners or laxatives may be needed to avoid constipation.

• Instruct patient to keep opioids locked safely out of reach of children or cognitively impaired individuals.

• Instruct patient not to consume alcohol during therapy.

☑ **Evaluation**

• Patient states that pain is relieved.

• Patient maintains adequate breathing patterns throughout therapy.

• Patient and family state understanding of drug therapy.

moxifloxacin hydrochloride
(mox-ih-FLOX-uh-sin high-droh-CLOR-ighd)
Avelox, Avelox I.V.

Pharmacologic class: fluoroquinolone
Therapeutic class: antibiotic
Pregnancy risk category: C

Indications and dosages

▶ **Acute bacterial sinusitis caused by *Streptococcus pneumoniae, Haemophilus influenzae,* or *Moraxella catarrhalis*.** *Adults:* 400 mg P.O. or I.V. once daily for 10 days.

▶ **Acute bacterial exacerbation of chronic bronchitis caused by *S. pneumoniae, H. influenzae, H. parainfluenzae, Klebsiella pneumoniae, Staphylococcus aureus,* or *M. ca-***

tarrhalis. Adults: 400 mg P.O. or I.V. once daily for 5 days.

▶ **Community-acquired pneumonia caused by multidrug-resistant S. pneumoniae (resistance to two or more of the following antibiotics: penicillin, second-generation cephalosporins, macrolides, tetracyclines, trimethoprim and sulfamethoxazole),** *Chlamydia pneumoniae, H. influenzae, K. pneumoniae, Mycoplasma pneumoniae, M. catarrhalis,* **or** *S. aureus. Adults:* 400 mg P.O. or I.V. once daily for 7 to 14 days.

▶ **Uncomplicated skin and skin-structure infections caused by** *S. aureus* **and** *Streptococcus pyogenes. Adults:* 400 mg P.O daily for 7 days.

▶ **Complicated skin and skin structure infections caused by methicillin-susceptible** *S. aureus, Escherichia coli, K. pneumoniae,* **or** *Enterobacter cloacae. Adults:* 400 mg P.O. or I.V. every 24 hours for 7 to 21 days.

▶ **Complicated intra-abdominal infections caused by** *E. coli, Bacteroides fragilis, Streptococcus anginosus, Streptococcus constellatus, Enterococcus faecalis, Proteus mirabilis, Clostridium perfringens, Bacteroides thetaiotaomicron,* **or** *Peptostreptococcus species. Adults:* 400 mg P.O. or I.V. every 24 hours for 5 to 14 days. Therapy usually begins with the I.V. formulation.

▼ I.V. administration

• If particulate matter is visible, don't use.
• Flush I.V. line with a compatible solution such as D₅W, normal saline solution, or Ringer's lactate solution before and after use.
• Infuse over 60 minutes by direct infusion or through a Y-type I.V. infusion set. Avoid rapid infusion or bolus injection.
• Switch from I.V. to P.O. form when warranted.

⊗ **Incompatibilities**
Other I.V. drugs or additives.

Contraindications and cautions

• Contraindicated in patients hypersensitive to drug, any of its components, or other fluoroquinolones.
• Use cautiously in patients with known or suspected CNS disorders and in patients with risk factors that may predispose them to seizures or lower the seizure threshold. Use cautiously in

patients with prolonged QT interval or uncorrected hypokalemia.

☀ **Lifespan:** In pregnant women, breastfeeding women, and children, safety and effectiveness haven't been established. In elderly patients, monitor cardiac function carefully, especially with I.V. form.

Adverse reactions

CNS: anxiety, asthenia, confusion, dizziness, headache, insomnia, malaise, nervousness, pain, paresthesia, somnolence, tremor, vertigo.
CV: chest pain, hypertension, palpitations, peripheral edema, *prolonged QT interval,* tachycardia.
GI: abdominal pain, anorexia, constipation, diarrhea, dry mouth, dyspepsia, flatulence, GI disorder, glossitis, nausea, oral candidiasis, *pseudomembranous colitis,* stomatitis, taste perversion, vomiting.
GU: vaginal candidiasis, vaginitis.
Hematologic: eosinophilia, *leukopenia, thrombocytopenia, thrombocytosis.*
Hepatic: cholestatic jaundice, liver dysfunction.
Musculoskeletal: arthralgia, back pain, leg pain, myalgia, tendon rupture.
Respiratory: dyspnea.
Skin: phototoxicity, pruritus, rash (maculopapular, purpuric, pustular), sweating.
Other: *allergic reaction,* candidiasis, injection site reaction.

Interactions

Drug-drug. *Aluminum hydroxide, aluminummagnesium hydroxide, calcium carbonate, magnesium hydroxide:* May decrease moxifloxacin effects. Give antacid at least 4 hours before or 8 hours after.
Class IA (procainamide, quinidine) or Class III (amiodarone, sotalol) antiarrhythmics: May enhance adverse CV effects. Avoid use together.
Didanosine, metal cations (such as aluminum, iron, magnesium, zinc), multivitamins: May decrease absorption and lower levels. Give moxifloxacin at least 4 hours before or 8 hours after these drugs.
Drugs known to prolong the QT interval, such as antipsychotics, erythromycin, tricyclic antidepressants: May have an additive effect when combined with these drugs. Avoid use together.
NSAIDs: May increase risk of CNS stimulation and seizures. Don't use together.

Sucralfate: May decrease absorption of moxifloxacin, reducing anti-infective effect. If use together can't be avoided, give at least 6 hours apart.

Warfarin: May enhance anticoagulant effects. Monitor PT and INR closely.

Drug-lifestyle. *Sun exposure:* May cause photosensitivity reactions. Discourage prolonged or unprotected exposure to sunlight or tanning bed use.

Effects on lab test results

• May increase GGT, glucose, amylase, lipid, and LDH levels.
• May increase eosinophil count. May decrease WBC count. May increase or decrease platelet count, PT, and INR.

Pharmacokinetics

Absorption: Good.
Distribution: Wide. About 50% protein-bound.
Metabolism: About 50% to inactive conjugates.
Excretion: About 45% of dose unchanged in urine and feces. *Half-life:* About 12 hours.

Route	Onset	Peak	Duration
P.O., I.V.	Unknown	1–3 hr	24 hr

Action

Chemical effect: Inhibits the enzymes needed for bacterial DNA replication, transcription, repair, and recombination.
Therapeutic effect: Kills susceptible bacteria.

Available forms

Injection (premixed solution): 400 mg
Tablets (film-coated): 400 mg

NURSING PROCESS

Assessment

• Obtain history of patient's condition before therapy, and reassess regularly to monitor drug effectiveness.
• Obtain specimen for culture and sensitivity tests before first dose. Begin therapy pending culture results.
• Monitor patient for hypersensitivity reactions and symptoms of CNS toxicity, including seizures, prolonged QT interval, pseudomembranous colitis, phototoxicity, and tendon rupture.
• Assess patient's and family's knowledge of drug therapy.

Nursing diagnoses

• Risk for infection related to presence of bacteria susceptible to drug
• Risk for injury related to drug-induced adverse reactions
• Deficient knowledge related to drug therapy

Planning and implementation

• Correct hypokalemia before therapy.
• Give with or without food. Give at same time each day to provide consistent absorption.
• Provide plenty of fluids.
• The most common adverse reactions are nausea, vomiting, stomach pain, diarrhea, dizziness, and headache.
• Store drug at controlled room temperature.

Patient teaching
• Instruct patient to take drug once daily, at the same time each day.
• Tell patient to finish the entire course of therapy, even if symptoms resolve.
• Advise the patient to drink plenty of fluids and to take moxifloxacin 4 hours before or 8 hours after antacids, sucralfate, or products containing iron and zinc.
• Tell patient to avoid hazardous activities, such as driving or operating machinery, until the drug's CNS effects are known.
• Instruct patient to contact prescriber if he experiences adverse effects.

Evaluation

• Patient is free from infection after drug therapy.
• Patient sustains no injury as a result of drug-induced adverse reactions.
• Patient and family state understanding of drug therapy.

moxifloxacin hydrochloride ophthalmic solution

(mocks-ih-FLOCKS-ah-sin high-droe-KLOR-ighd off-THAL-mick suh-LOO-shun)
Vigamox

Pharmacologic class: fluoroquinolone
Therapeutic class: antibiotic
Pregnancy risk category: C

Indications and dosages

▶ **Bacterial conjunctivitis.** *Adults and children age 1 and older:* 1 drop into affected eye t.i.d. for 7 days.

Contraindications and cautions

• Contraindicated in patients hypersensitive to the drug, any of its components, or other fluoroquinolones. Contraindicated in patients with epithelial herpes simplex keratitis, vaccinia, varicella, mycobacterial infections of the eye, fungal diseases of the ocular structure, or use of steroid combinations after uncomplicated removal of a corneal foreign body.

⚠ **Lifespan:** In pregnant women, use only when benefits of therapy outweigh risks to the fetus. In breast-feeding women, use cautiously because it's unknown if the drug appears in breast milk. In children younger than age 1, don't use drug.

Adverse reactions

EENT: conjunctivitis; dry eyes; increased lacrimation; keratitis; ocular hyperemia; ocular discomfort, pain, and pruritus; otitis media; pharyngitis; reduced visual acuity; rhinitis; subconjunctival hemorrhage.
Respiratory: increased cough.
Skin: rash.
Other: fever, infection.

Interactions

None reported.

Effects on lab test results

None reported.

Pharmacokinetics

Absorption: Local.
Distribution: Local tissues and plasma 1,000 to 1,600 times less than oral doses.
Metabolism: Unknown.
Excretion: In urine and bile. *Half-life:* 13 hours.

Route	Onset	Peak	Duration
Ocular	Immediate	Unknown	Unknown

Action

Chemical effect: Inhibits DNA gyrase and topoisomerase IV, preventing cell replication, transcription, repair of bacterial DNA, and cell division.

Therapeutic effect: Kills susceptible bacteria causing infection.

Available forms

Solution: 0.5%

NURSING PROCESS

🗄 Assessment
• Assess patient's allergy history before therapy.
• Monitor patient for superinfection, particularly with repeated use.
• Monitor patient for adverse reactions.
• Assess patient's and family's knowledge of drug therapy.

🔁 Nursing diagnoses
• Risk for infection related to presence of bacteria susceptible to drug
• Disturbed visual sensory perception related to adverse effects of the drug
• Deficient knowledge related to drug therapy

▶ Planning and implementation
• Don't inject solution subconjunctivally, or into the eye's anterior chamber.
• Drug has caused serious hypersensitivity reactions; if patient has an allergic reaction, stop giving the drug and treat symptoms.

Patient teaching
• Tell patient to stop taking the drug and immediately seek medical treatment if he develops an allergic reaction (itching, rash, swelling of the face or throat, or difficulty breathing).
• Tell patient not to wear contact lenses during therapy.
• Instruct patient not to touch dropper tip to anything, including eyes and fingers.

✅ Evaluation
• Patient is free from infection after drug therapy.
• Patient doesn't experience adverse drug effects.
• Patient and family state understanding of drug therapy.

muromonab-CD3
(myoo-roh-MOH-nab see dee three)
Orthoclone OKT3

Pharmacologic class: monoclonal antibody
Therapeutic class: immunosuppressive
Pregnancy risk category: C

Indications and dosages

▶ **Acute allograft rejection in heart, liver, or kidney transplant.** *Adults:* 5 mg I.V. daily for 10 to 14 days.
Children: Initially, 2.5 mg/day (if 30 kg or less) or 5 mg/day (if more than 30 kg) I.V. as a single bolus over less than 1 minute for 10 to 14 days. Increase daily dosage in 2.5-mg increments to decrease CD3-positive cells.

▼ I.V. administration

• Don't give by infusion.
• Draw solution into syringe through low–protein-binding 0.2- or 0.22-micron filter. Discard filter and attach needle for bolus injection.
• Give bolus over less than 1 minute.
• Store drug in the refrigerator at 2° to 8° C (36° to 46° F). Do not freeze.
⊗ **Incompatibilities**
Other I.V. drugs.

Contraindications and cautions

• Contraindicated in patients hypersensitive to the drug or to other products of murine origin. Also contraindicated in patients who have anti-mouse antibody titers of 1:1,000 or more; who have fluid overload, as evidenced by chest X-ray or weight gain greater than 3% in the week before therapy; and who have history of or predisposition to seizures.
⚖ **Lifespan:** In pregnant and breast-feeding women, drug is contraindicated. In children, safety and effectiveness haven't been established.

Adverse reactions

CNS: *asthenia,* confusion, depression, dizziness, fatigue, *fever, headache,* lethargy, malaise, *meningitis,* nervousness, *seizures,* somnolence, tremor.
CV: *arrhythmia, bradycardia,* chest pain, edema, hypertension, hypotension, tachycardia, *vascular occlusion,* vasodilation.

EENT: photophobia, tinnitus.
GI: abdominal pain, anorexia, *diarrhea,* GI pain, *nausea, vomiting.*
GU: *renal dysfunction.*
Hematologic: anemia, *leukocytosis, leukopenia, thrombocytopenia.*
Musculoskeletal: arthralgia, myalgia.
Respiratory: *acute respiratory distress syndrome,* dyspnea, hyperventilation, *hypoxia,* pneumonia, *pulmonary edema,* respiratory congestion, wheezing.
Skin: diaphoresis, pruritus, *rash.*
Other: chills, *cytokine release syndrome,* hypersensitivity reactions, pain in trunk area.

Interactions

Drug-drug. *Immunosuppressants:* May increase risk of infection. Monitor patient closely.
Indomethacin: May increase muromonab-CD3 levels with CNS effects, including encephalopathy. Monitor patient closely.
Live-virus vaccines: May increase replication and effects of vaccine. Postpone vaccination when possible, and consult prescriber.

Effects on lab test results

• May increase BUN and creatinine levels. May decrease hemoglobin level and hematocrit.
• May decrease platelet count. May increase or decrease WBC count.

Pharmacokinetics

Absorption: Given I.V.
Distribution: Unknown.
Metabolism: Unknown.
Excretion: Unknown. *Half-life:* Unknown.

Route	Onset	Peak	Duration
I.V.	Immediately	Unknown	1 wk after therapy

Action

Chemical effect: Reacts in T-lymphocyte membrane with CD3 needed for antigen recognition and depletes blood of CD3-positive T cells.
Therapeutic effect: Halts acute allograft rejection in kidney transplantation.

Available forms

Injection: 1 mg/ml in 5-ml ampules

NURSING PROCESS

✒ Assessment
• Assess patient's condition before therapy and regularly thereafter to monitor drug effectiveness.
• Obtain chest X-ray within 24 hours before drug therapy.
• Assess patient for signs of fluid overload before therapy.
• Be alert for adverse reactions and drug interactions.
• If patient has an adverse GI reaction, monitor his hydration.
• Assess patient's and family's knowledge of drug therapy.

⊕ Nursing diagnoses
• Risk for injury related to presence of acute allograft rejection
• Risk for deficient fluid volume related to drug-induced adverse GI reactions
• Deficient knowledge related to drug therapy

⊵ Planning and implementation
• Begin therapy in facility equipped and staffed for cardiopulmonary resuscitation where patient can be closely monitored.
• Most adverse reactions develop within 30 minutes to 6 hours after first dose.
⚛ ALERT: Give antipyretic before giving drug to lower risk of expected pyrexia and chills. It is recommended that methylprednisolone sodium succinate 8 mg/kg be administered I.V. 1 to 4 hours before initial dose of muromonab-CD3 to reduce the risk for and severity of cytokine release syndrome.
• If second course of therapy is attempted, patient may develop antibodies to drug that can lead to loss of effectiveness and more severe adverse reactions; use for one course of therapy only.
Patient teaching
• Inform patient of expected adverse reactions, and reassure him that they will lessen as therapy progresses.

✓ Evaluation
• Patient shows no signs of organ rejection.
• Patient maintains adequate hydration.
• Patient and family state understanding of drug therapy.

mycophenolate mofetil
(migh-koh-FEN-oh-layt MOH-feh-til)
CellCept

mycophenolate mofetil hydrochloride
CellCept Intravenous

mycophenolate sodium
Myfortic

Pharmacologic class: mycophenolic acid derivative
Therapeutic class: immunosuppressant
Pregnancy risk category: D

Indications and dosages

▶ **Prevention of organ rejection in patients receiving allogenic renal transplant.** *Adults:* 1 g I.V. infused over 2 hours b.i.d. with cyclosporine and corticosteroids. Begin I.V. infusion within 24 hours after transplantation. For oral use, give 1 g P.O. b.i.d. as soon as possible after surgery. Or 720 mg delayed-release P.O. b.i.d. on an empty stomach.
Children age 1 and older: 600 mg/m² oral suspension P.O. b.i.d. up to a maximum daily dosage of 2 g/10 ml. Or give child with 1.25 m² to 1.5 m² body surface area 750 mg capsules P.O. b.i.d. Give child with a greater than 1.5 m² body surface area 1 g P.O. tablets or capsules b.i.d. For oral use, give as soon as possible after surgery.
⊠ Adjust-a-dose: For patients with renal impairment, if GFR is less than 25 ml/minute outside the immediate post-transplant period, avoid doses above 1 g b.i.d. If neutropenia develops, interrupt or reduce dose.
▶ **Prevention of organ rejection in patients receiving allogenic cardiac transplant.** *Adults:* 1.5 g P.O. or I.V. b.i.d. over no less than 2 hours, with cyclosporine and corticosteroids.
▶ **Prevention of organ rejection in patients receiving allogenic hepatic transplants.** *Adults:* 1 g I.V. b.i.d. over no less than 2 hours or 1.5 g P.O. b.i.d., with cyclosporine and corticosteroids.
⊠ Adjust-a-dose: If neutropenia develops, interrupt or reduce dose.

▼ I.V. administration

- Avoid direct contact with solution.
- Reconstitute under aseptic conditions.
- Reconstitute the contents of each CellCept Intravenous vial with 14 ml of D_5W. Use two vials to prepare a 1-g dose and 3 vials for a 1.5-g dose. Gently shake the vial to dissolve drug.
- For a 1-g dose, dilute 2 vials further into 140 ml of D_5W; for a 1.5-g dose, dilute three vials further into 210 ml of 5% dextrose injection. The final concentration of both solutions is 6 mg/ml.
- Never give drug by rapid or bolus I.V. injection. Give infusion over at least 2 hours.
- Use within 4 hours of reconstitution and dilution.
- ⊗ Incompatibilities
- Other I.V. solutions.

Contraindications and cautions

- Contraindicated in patients hypersensitive to the drug or any of its components.
- Use cautiously in patients with GI disorders.
- ≛ Lifespan: In pregnant and breast-feeding women, use only when benefits outweigh risks to fetus and infant. In children, safety and effectiveness for cardiac and hepatic transplantation haven't been established.

Adverse reactions

CNS: asthenia, dizziness, fever, headache, insomnia, pain, tremor.
CV: *chest pain, edema, hypertension,* peripheral edema, tachycardia.
EENT: pharyngitis.
GI: abdominal pain, constipation, diarrhea, dyspepsia, HEMORRHAGE, nausea, oral candidiasis, vomiting.
GU: hematuria, *kidney tubular necrosis,* UTI.
Hematologic: anemia, hypochromic anemia, leukocytosis, *leukopenia,* THROMBOCYTOPENIA.
Metabolic: *hypercholesteremia, hyperglycemia, hyperkalemia, hypokalemia, hypophosphatemia.*
Musculoskeletal: *back pain.*
Respiratory: bronchitis, *cough, dyspnea*, infection, pneumonia.
Skin: *acne,* rash.
Other: infection, *sepsis.*

Interactions

Drug-drug. *Acyclovir, ganciclovir, other drugs known to undergo tubular secretion:* May in-

crease risk of toxicity for both drugs. Monitor patient closely.
Antacids with magnesium and aluminum hydroxides: May decrease mycophenolate mofetil absorption. Separate doses.
Azathioprine: Hasn't been studied. Avoid use together.
Cholestyramine: May interfere with enterohepatic recirculation, reducing mycophenolate bioavailability. Don't give together.
Hormonal contraceptives: May reduce effectiveness of hormonal contraceptives. Advise patient to use barrier birth control methods.

Effects on lab test results

- May increase cholesterol and glucose levels. May decrease phosphorus and hemoglobin levels and hematocrit. May increase or decrease potassium level.
- May decrease platelet count. May increase or decrease WBC count.

Pharmacokinetics

Absorption: Good.
Distribution: 97% protein-bound.
Metabolism: Complete, to mycophenolic acid.
Excretion: Mainly in urine, with small amount in feces. *Half-life:* About 18 hours.

Route	Onset	Peak	Duration
P.O.	Unknown	Unknown	Unknown
I.V.	Unknown	Unknown	10–17 hr

Action

Chemical effect: Inhibits proliferative responses of T- and B-lymphocytes, suppresses antibody formation by B-lymphocytes, and may inhibit recruitment of leukocytes into sites of inflammation and graft rejection.
Therapeutic effect: Prevents organ rejection.

Available forms

mycophenolate mofetil
Capsules: 250 mg
Powder for oral suspension (contains aspartame): 200 mg/ml
Tablets: 500 mg
mycophenolate mofetil hydrochloride
Injection: 500 mg/vial
mycophenolate sodium
Tablets (delayed-release): 180 mg, 360 mg

NURSING PROCESS

⚕ Assessment
- Obtain a serum or urine pregnancy test within one week of beginning therapy and provide contraception counseling.
- Obtain history of patient's kidney transplant.
- Monitor CBC regularly.
- Be alert for adverse reactions and drug interactions.
- Assess patient's and family's knowledge of drug therapy.

⚕ Nursing diagnoses
- Ineffective health maintenance related to need for kidney transplant
- Risk for infection related to drug-induced immunosuppression
- Deficient knowledge related to drug therapy

⚕ Planning and implementation
- Administer drug under the supervision of a physician experienced in immunosuppressive therapy and management of renal, hepatic, or cardiac transplant patients.
- Give drug on an empty stomach.
- ⚠ ALERT: Because of risk of teratogenic effects, don't open or crush capsules. Avoid inhaling powder in capsules or letting it contact skin or mucous membranes. If it does, wash skin thoroughly with soap and water and rinse eyes with plain water.
- If patient develops neutropenia, notify prescriber.
- Women planning pregnancy should not use mycophenolate therapy unless other immunosuppressant drugs have not been successful. Risks, benefits, and alternative therapy should be discussed with patient.

Patient teaching
- Warn patient not to open or crush capsule but to swallow it whole on an empty stomach.
- Stress importance of not interrupting therapy without consulting prescriber.
- Tell woman to do a pregnancy test 1 week before therapy. Tell her to use two forms of contraception simultaneously unless abstinent and to use effective contraception until at least 6 weeks after therapy ends, even if she has a history of infertility (unless she has had a hysterectomy). If patient becomes pregnant, tell her to immediately contact her prescriber.

☑ Evaluation
- Patient shows no signs and symptoms of organ rejection.
- Neutropenia doesn't develop.
- Patient and family state understanding of drug therapy.

nabilone
(NAH-bi-lohn)
Cesamet

Pharmacologic class: cannabinoid
Therapeutic class: antiemetic
Pregnancy risk category: C
Controlled substance schedule: II

Indications and dosages

▶ **Chemotherapy-induced nausea and vomiting unresponsive to other antiemetic therapy.**
Adults: Usually 1 or 2 mg P.O. b.i.d. Give first dose 1 to 3 hours before chemotherapy starts and then b.i.d. to t.i.d. throughout the cycle. If needed, start with 1- or 2-mg dose the night before chemotherapy starts and continue 48 hours after the cycle ends. Maximum dosage is 6 mg daily, divided and given t.i.d.

Contraindications and cautions

- Contraindicated in patients hypersensitive to cannabinoids.
- Use cautiously in patients taking highly protein-bound drugs; patients taking sedatives, hypnotics, or other psychoactive drugs; and patients with hypertension, heart disease, hepatic or renal impairment, or current or previous mental illness or substance abuse.
- ⚕ Lifespan: In pregnant patients, use only if potential benefit justifies risk to fetus. Breast-feeding isn't recommended during treatment with nabilone. In children, safety and efficacy aren't known; use cautiously because of drug's psychoactive effects. In elderly patients, use cautiously because of drug's effects on heart rate and blood pressure.

Adverse reactions

CNS: anorexia, asthenia, *ataxia,* depersonalization, *depression, difficulty concentrating,* disorientation, *drowsiness,* dysphoria, *euphoria,* headache, *sleep disturbance, vertigo.*
CV: hypotension, orthostatic hypotension, tachycardia.
EENT: *visual disturbance.*
GI: *dry mouth,* nausea, thirst.
Metabolic: increased appetite.

Interactions

Drug-drug. *Anticholinergics, sympathomimetics, tricyclic antidepressants:* May increase hypertension, tachycardia, and drowsiness. Avoid use together if possible.
CNS depressants: May increase CNS depression. Use with extreme caution, and monitor patient carefully.
Highly protein-bound drugs: May be displaced by nabilone. Monitor patient and drug levels, as needed. Dosages may need adjustment.
Drug-lifestyle. *Alcohol use:* May increase CNS depression. Tell patient to avoid alcohol.
Marijuana: May cause additive effects. Discourage use.

Effects on lab test results

None reported.

Pharmacokinetics

Absorption: Complete in the GI tract.
Distribution: Rapid. Highly protein-bound.
Metabolism: Extensive in the liver through multiple cytochrome P-450 pathways. Several metabolites are formed.
Excretion: Mainly in feces via the biliary tract, less by the kidneys. *Half-life:* 2 hours for drug; 35 hours for metabolites.

Route	Onset	Peak	Duration
P.O.	Rapid	2 hr	Unknown

Action

Chemical effect: Drug probably exerts antiemetic effects by interacting with cannabinoid receptors in the CNS.
Therapeutic effect: Relieves chemotherapy-induced nausea and vomiting.

Available forms

Capsules: 1 mg

Assessment

• Obtain a detailed health history before treatment starts to rule out mental illness and substance abuse.
• Monitor drug's effectiveness by assessing patient for nausea and vomiting. Drug effects may persist for days after therapy ends.
• Be alert for adverse reactions and drug interactions.
• Monitor patient for physical or psychological dependence. Drug has high potential for abuse.
• Check supine and standing pulse and blood pressure before and periodically during treatment.
• Monitor patient's hydration, weight, and nutrition regularly.
• Assess patient's and family's knowledge of drug therapy.

Nursing diagnoses

• Risk for deficient fluid volume related to nausea and vomiting from chemotherapy
• Disturbed thought processes related to drug-induced adverse CNS reactions
• Deficient knowledge related to drug therapy

Planning and implementation

• Give drug only to patients who haven't responded satisfactorily to other antiemetics.
• Give drug 1 to 3 hours before chemotherapy starts and then 2 to 3 times daily throughout the cycle. Continue for up to 48 hours posttreatment.
• Make sure patient will remain under the supervision of a responsible adult during treatment.
• Then stopping drug, monitor patient for evidence of withdrawal, including mental distress, insomnia, and autonomic hyperactivity (sweating, rhinorrhea, loose stools, hiccups). Psychiatric reactions may persist up to 72 hours after treatment stops.
• In case of overdose, if patient is psychotic, keep the environment quiet and offer reassurance as needed. Monitor vital signs closely; watch especially for hypotension, orthostatic hypotension, hypertension, and tachycardia. Activated charcoal may decrease systemic absorption. Protect patient's airway, and maintain ven-

N

tilation, perfusion, and circulation. Treatment is symptomatic and supportive.

Patient teaching

• Tell patient that drug commonly causes dizziness, euphoria, disorientation, and drowsiness. Explain that depression, hallucinations, and psychosis are also possible.

• Stress that patient should remain under the supervision of a responsible adult, especially when treatment starts or dosage changes, because of drug's psychoactive effects.

• Advise patient to rise slowly from a reclining position and to sit with his feet on the floor before standing until drug's effects are known.

• Urge patient to avoid alcohol, sedatives, and hypnotics because of the increased risk of adverse effects.

• Caution patient to avoid driving and other hazardous activities during treatment.

• Explain that drug has a high abuse potential and should be used only as prescribed.

☑ **Evaluation**

• Patient maintains adequate hydration.

• Patient regains normal thought processes after effects of drug therapy have dissipated.

• Patient and family state understanding of drug therapy.

nabumetone
(nuh-BYOO-meh-tohn)

Pharmacologic class: NSAID
Therapeutic class: anti-inflammatory, analgesic, antipyretic
Pregnancy risk category: C; D (third trimester)

Indications and dosages

▶ **Rheumatoid arthritis, osteoarthritis.**
Adults: Initially, 1,000 mg P.O. daily as single dose or in divided doses b.i.d. Maximum, 2,000 mg daily.

Contraindications and cautions

• Contraindicated in patients hypersensitive to the drug or any of its components and in patients with history of aspirin- or NSAID-induced asthma, urticaria, or other allergic reactions.

• Use cautiously in patients with renal or hepatic impairment, peptic ulcer disease, heart failure, hypertension, or other conditions that may predispose patient to fluid retention.

⚖ **Lifespan:** In pregnant and breast-feeding women, only use when benefits outweigh risks to fetus and infant. In children, safety and effectiveness haven't been established. In the elderly, use cautiously because of possible impaired excretion.

Adverse reactions

CNS: *dizziness,* fatigue, *headache,* insomnia, nervousness, somnolence.
CV: *edema,* vasculitis.
EENT: tinnitus.
GI: abdominal pain, **bleeding,** constipation, diarrhea, dry mouth, dyspepsia, flatulence, gastritis, nausea, stomatitis, ulceration, vomiting.
Respiratory: dyspnea, pneumonitis.
Skin: increased sweating, *pruritus, rash.*

Interactions

Drug-drug. *Diuretics:* May decrease diuretic effectiveness. Monitor patient for effect.
Drugs highly bound to proteins (such as warfarin): May increase risk of adverse effects from displacement of drug by nabumetone. Use together cautiously; monitor patient for adverse effects.
Drug-herb. *Dong quai, feverfew, garlic, ginger, horse chestnut, red clover:* May increase risk of bleeding. Discourage use together.
St. John's wort: May increase risk of photosensitivity. Advise patient to avoid unprotected or prolonged exposure to sunlight.
Drug-food. *Any food:* May increase absorption rate. Give together.
Drug-lifestyle. *Alcohol use:* May increase risk of additive GI toxicity. Discourage use together.

Effects on lab test results

None reported.

Pharmacokinetics

Absorption: Good. Taking with food increases absorption rate and peak levels of principal metabolite but doesn't change total amount absorbed.
Distribution: More than 99% of metabolite is protein-bound.
Metabolism: To inactive metabolites in liver.

Excretion: Metabolites mainly in urine; about 9% in feces. *Half-life:* About 24 hours.

Route	Onset	Peak	Duration
P.O.	Unknown	2–4 hr	Unknown

Action

Chemical effect: Unknown; may inhibit prostaglandin synthesis.
Therapeutic effect: Relieves pain.

Available forms

Tablets: 500 mg, 750 mg

NURSING PROCESS

✎ Assessment

• Assess patient's arthritis before starting therapy and regularly thereafter to monitor drug effectiveness.
• During long-term therapy, periodically monitor renal and liver function, CBC, and hematocrit; assess patient for evidence of GI bleeding.
• Watch for fluid retention, especially in a patient with heart failure and hypertension.
• Be alert for adverse reactions and drug interactions.
• Assess patient's and family's knowledge of drug therapy.

✣ Nursing diagnoses

• Chronic pain related to arthritic condition
• Impaired tissue integrity related to adverse drug effect on GI mucosa
• Deficient knowledge related to drug therapy

▷ Planning and implementation

• Give drug with food to increase absorption rate.
• Notify prescriber about adverse reactions.
• ⊛ **ALERT:** Don't confuse Relafen with Rifadin.
Patient teaching
• Instruct patient to take drug with food, milk, or antacids for best absorption.
• Advise patient to limit alcohol intake because of additive GI toxicity.
• Teach patient to recognize and report signs and symptoms of GI bleeding.

✓ Evaluation

• Patient is free from pain.
• Patient's GI tissue integrity is maintained throughout drug therapy.

• Patient and family state understanding of drug therapy.

nadolol
(nay-DOH-lol)
Corgard

Pharmacologic class: nonselective beta blocker
Therapeutic class: antihypertensive, antianginal
Pregnancy risk category: C

Indications and dosages

▶ **Angina pectoris.** *Adults:* Initially, 40 mg P.O. once daily. Increase in 40- to 80-mg increments every 3 to 7 days until optimum response occurs. Usual maintenance dosage is 40 or 80 mg daily; a maximum dose of 160 or 240 mg may be needed.
▶ **Hypertension.** *Adults:* Initially, 20 to 40 mg P.O. once daily. Increase by 40- to 80-mg increments every 2 to 14 days until optimum response occurs. Usual maintenance dosage is 40 or 80 mg daily; doses up to 240 or 320 mg may be needed.
◫ **Adjust-a-dose:** In patients with renal impairment, if creatinine clearance is 31 to 50 ml/minute, give every 24 to 36 hours; if 10 to 30 ml/minute, give every 24 to 48 hours; if less than 10 ml/minute, give every 40 to 60 hours.
▶ **Arrhythmias‡.** *Adults:* 60 to 160 mg P.O. daily or in divided doses.
▶ **To prevent vascular headaches‡.** *Adults:* 20 to 40 mg P.O. daily; gradually increase to 120 mg daily, if needed.

Contraindications and cautions

• Contraindicated in patients with bronchial asthma, sinus bradycardia, greater than first-degree heart block, and cardiogenic shock.
• Use cautiously in patients undergoing major surgery involving general anesthesia and in those with heart failure, chronic bronchitis, emphysema, renal or hepatic impairment, or diabetes.
⚜ **Lifespan:** In pregnant women, use only if benefits outweigh risks to the fetus. In breast-feeding women, don't use because it's unknown if drug appears in breast milk. In children, safety and effectiveness haven't been established.

N

Adverse reactions

CNS: dizziness, fatigue, fever, lethargy.
CV: *bradycardia, heart failure, hypotension,*
peripheral vascular disease.
GI: constipation, diarrhea, nausea, vomiting.
Respiratory: *increased airway resistance.*

Interactions

Drug-drug. *Antihypertensives:* May enhance
antihypertensive effect. Monitor patient's blood
pressure closely.
Digoxin, diltiazem: May cause excessive bradycardia and affect AV conduction. Use together
cautiously; monitor ECG.
Epinephrine: May cause an initial hypertensive
episode followed by bradycardia. Stop beta
blocker 3 days before anticipated epinephrine
use. Monitor patient closely.
Insulin: May mask symptoms of hypoglycemia
as a result of beta blockade (such as tachycardia). Use cautiously in patients with diabetes.
I.V. lidocaine: May reduce hepatic metabolism
of lidocaine, increasing the risk of toxicity. Give
bolus doses of lidocaine at a slower rate, and
monitor lidocaine level closely.
NSAIDs: May decrease antihypertensive effect.
Monitor blood pressure and adjust dosage.
Oral antidiabetics: May alter dosage requirements in diabetic patients. Monitor glucose
level.
Prazosin: May increase the risk of orthostatic
hypotension early in use together. Teach patient
to stand slowly until effects are known.
Verapamil: May increase the effects of both
drugs. Monitor cardiac function closely for excessive bradycardia and decrease dosage.

Effects on lab test results

None reported.

Pharmacokinetics

Absorption: 30% to 40% without regard to
meals.
Distribution: Distributed throughout body.
About 30% protein-bound.
Metabolism: None.
Excretion: Most excreted unchanged in urine;
remainder in feces. *Half-life:* About 10 to
24 hours.

Route	Onset	Peak	Duration
P.O.	Unknown	2–4 hr	24 hr

Action

Chemical effect: Reduces cardiac oxygen demand by blocking catecholamine-induced increases in heart rate, blood pressure, and myocardial contraction. Depresses renin secretion.
Therapeutic effect: Lowers blood pressure, relieves and prevents recurrence of angina.

Available forms

Tablets: 20 mg, 40 mg, 80 mg, 120 mg, 160 mg

NURSING PROCESS

⏻ Assessment
• Assess patient's condition before starting therapy and regularly thereafter to monitor drug effectiveness.
• Drug masks common signs of shock, hyperthyroidism, and hypoglycemia.
• Be alert for adverse reactions and drug interactions.
• Assess patient's and family's knowledge of
drug therapy.

⊕ Nursing diagnoses
• Risk for injury related to presence of hyper-
tension
• Acute pain related to angina
• Deficient knowledge related to drug therapy

⊳ Planning and implementation
⚅ **ALERT:** Always check apical pulse before giving drug. If slower than 60 beats/minute, don't
give the dose. Notify prescriber.
• If patient develops severe hypotension, give
vasopressor.
⚅ **ALERT:** Reduce dosage gradually over 1 to
2 weeks. Abruptly stopping the drug can worsen
angina and MI.
⚅ **ALERT:** Don't confuse Corgard with Coreg.
Patient teaching
• Explain importance of taking drug as prescribed, even when feeling well.
• Warn patient not to abruptly stop taking the
drug.

☑ Evaluation
• Patient's blood pressure is normal.
• Patient reports reduced angina.
• Patient and family state understanding of drug
therapy.

Reactions may be *common*, uncommon, *life-threatening*, or **COMMON AND LIFE-THREATENING.**

nafcillin sodium
(naf-SIL-in SOH-dee-um)

Pharmacologic class: penicillinase-resistant penicillin
Therapeutic class: antibiotic
Pregnancy risk category: B

Indications and dosages

▶ **Systemic infections caused by susceptible organisms (including methicillin-sensitive *Staphylococcus aureus*).** *Adults and children who weigh 40 kg (88 lb) or more:* 500 mg to 1 g I.V. every 4 hours depending on severity of the infection.
Infants and children older than age 1 month: 50 to 200 mg/kg I.V. or I.M. daily in equally divided doses every 4 to 6 hours depending severity of the infection.
Neonates younger than age 7 days who weigh less than 2 kg (4.4 lb): 25 mg/kg I.V. or I.M. every 12 hours.
Neonates younger than age 7 days who weigh more than 2 kg: 25 mg/kg I.V. or I.M. every 8 hours.
Neonates ages 1 to 4 weeks who weigh less than 2 kg: 25 mg/kg I.V. or I.M. every 8 hours. Or 25 mg/kg every 12 hours for those who weigh less than 1.2 kg (2.6 lb).
Neonates ages 1 to 4 weeks who weigh more than 2 kg: 25 to 35 mg/kg I.V. or I.M. every 6 hours.
▶ **Meningitis.** *Adults and children who weigh 40 kg or more:* 100 to 200 mg/kg I.V. daily in divided doses every 4 to 6 hours.
Neonates younger than age 7 days who weigh more than 2 kg: 25 mg/kg I.V. or I.M. every 8 hours.
Neonates ages 1 to 4 weeks who weigh more than 2 kg: 35 mg/kg I.V. or I.M. every 6 hours.
▶ **Acute or chronic osteomyelitis caused by susceptible organism.** *Adults:* 1 to 2 g I.V. every 4 hours.
▶ **Native valve endocarditis caused by susceptible organisms.** *Adults and children who weigh 40 kg or more:* 2 g I.V. every 4 hours for 4 to 6 weeks, with gentamicin for the first 3 to 5 days.
Children: 200 mg/kg I.V. daily in equally divided doses every 4 to 6 hours for 6 weeks, with gentamicin for the first 3 to 5 days.

▼ I.V. administration

• After thawing at room temperature or under refrigeration, check and discard container with leaks, cloudiness, or precipitate.
• 10-40 mg/ml reconstituted vials are stable for 24 hours at room temperature.
• Give by intermittent I.V. infusion over at least 30 to 60 minutes.
• Give by intermittent I.V. injection, slowly giving the properly diluted nafcillin sodium over 5 to 10 minutes.
• Change I.V. site every 48 hours to reduce the risk of vein irritation.
⊗ **Incompatibilities**
Aminoglycosides, aminophylline, ascorbic acid, aztreonam, bleomycin, cytarabine, diltiazem, droperidol, gentamicin, hydrocortisone sodium succinate, insulin, labetalol, meperidine, methylprednisolone sodium succinate, midazolam, nalbuphine, pentazocine lactate, promazine, vancomycin, verapamil hydrochloride, vitamin B complex with C.

Contraindications and cautions

• Contraindicated in patients hypersensitive to the drug or other penicillins.
• Use cautiously in patients with GI distress and those with other drug allergies, especially to cephalosporins.
⚜ **Lifespan:** In pregnant women, use cautiously. In breast-feeding women, use cautiously because penicillins appear in breast milk.

Adverse reactions

CV: thrombophlebitis.
GI: *nausea,* vomiting, diarrhea.
Hematologic: *transient leukopenia, neutropenia, granulocytopenia, thrombocytopenia.*
Other: *anaphylaxis,* hypersensitivity reactions, vein irritation.

Interactions

Drug-drug. *Aminoglycosides:* May have synergistic effect; may use together for this effect. Monitor patient closely.
Cyclosporine: May cause subtherapeutic cyclosporine level. Monitor level.
Probenecid: May increase level of nafcillin. Probenecid may be used for this purpose.
Rifampin: May cause dose-dependent antagonism. Monitor patient closely.

N

Warfarin: May increase risk of bleeding when used with I.V. nafcillin. Monitor patient for bleeding.

Effects on lab test results

• May decrease neutrophil, granulocyte, WBC, and platelet counts.
• May falsely increase urine or serum proteins or cause false-positive results in certain tests for them.

Pharmacokinetics

Absorption: Administered I.V. or I.M.
Distribution: Wide. CSF penetration is poor but enhanced by meningeal inflammation. 70% to 90% protein-bound.
Metabolism: Metabolized primarily in liver; undergoes enterohepatic circulation.
Excretion: Excreted primarily in bile; 25% to 30% is excreted in urine unchanged. *Half-life:* 30 to 90 minutes.

Route	Onset	Peak	Duration
I.V.	Immediate	Immediate	Unknown
I.M.	Unknown	30–60 min	Unknown

Action

Chemical effect: Inhibits cell wall synthesis during microorganism multiplication; resists bacteria-produced penicillinases.
Therapeutic effect: Kills susceptible bacteria, such as penicillinase-producing staphylococci, and some gram-positive aerobic and anaerobic bacilli.

Available forms

Injection: 1 g, 2 g in premixed frozen container or as powder in Add-Vantage vials

NURSING PROCESS

Assessment

• Assess patient's infection before starting therapy and regularly thereafter to monitor the drug's effectiveness.
• Before giving drug, ask patient about allergic reactions to penicillins and cephalosporins. Remember that allergic reactions may occur even in patients with no history of penicillin allergy.
• Obtain specimen for culture and sensitivity tests before giving first dose. Begin therapy pending results.

ALERT: Monitor WBC counts twice weekly in patients receiving nafcillin for longer than 2 weeks. Neutropenia commonly occurs in the third week.
• Be alert for adverse reactions and drug interactions.
• If patient has an adverse GI reaction, monitor his hydration.
• Assess patient's and family's knowledge of drug therapy.

Nursing diagnoses

• Risk for infection related to susceptible bacteria
• Risk for deficient fluid volume related to drug-induced adverse GI reactions
• Deficient knowledge related to drug therapy

Planning and implementation

• Give drug at least 1 hour before bacteriostatic antibiotics.
• If urinalysis is abnormal, notify prescriber because this may indicate drug-induced interstitial nephritis.
Patient teaching
• Tell patient to notify prescriber if rash, fever, or chills develop.
• Instruct patient to report pain, burning, edema, or redness at I.V. site.

Evaluation

• Patient is free from infection.
• Patient maintains adequate hydration throughout drug therapy.
• Patient and family state understanding of drug therapy.

HIGH ALERT

nalbuphine hydrochloride
(NAL-byoo-feen hy-droh-KLOR-iyd)
Nubain

Pharmacologic class: synthetic opioid partial agonist/antagonist
Therapeutic class: analgesic, adjunct to anesthesia
Pregnancy risk category: B, D (with prolonged use or high dosage at term)

Indications and dosages

▶ **Moderate to severe pain.** *Adults:* For patient who weighs about 70 kg (154 lb), give 10 to

20 mg I.V., I.M., or subcutaneously every 3 to 6 hours, as appropriate. Maximum daily dosage is 160 mg.

▶ **Adjunct in balanced anesthesia.** *Adults:* 0.3 mg/kg to 3 mg/kg I.V. over 10 to 15 minutes, followed by maintenance doses of 0.25 to 0.5 mg/kg in single I.V. doses, p.r.n.

▼ I.V. administration

• Keep resuscitation equipment available.
• Inject slowly over at least 2 minutes into vein or into line containing compatible, free-flowing solution, such as D_5W, normal saline solution, or lactated Ringer's solution.
• Respiratory depression can be reversed with naloxone.
⊗ **Incompatibilities**
Allopurinol, amphotericin B, cefepime, diazepam, docetaxel, ketorolac, methotrexate sodium, nafcillin, pentobarbital sodium, piperacillin and tazobactam sodium, promethazine, sargramostim, sodium bicarbonate, thiethylperazine.

Contraindications and cautions

• Contraindicated in patients hypersensitive to the drug or sulfites present in some preparations of drug.
• Use cautiously in substance abusers and in those with emotional instability, head injury, increased intracranial pressure, impaired ventilation, MI accompanied by nausea and vomiting, upcoming biliary surgery, and hepatic or renal disease.
❄ **Lifespan:** In pregnant women, use cautiously. In breast-feeding women, use cautiously because it's unknown if drug appears in breast milk. In children, safety and effectiveness haven't been established.

Adverse reactions

CNS: confusion, crying, delusions, depression, dizziness, euphoria, hallucinations, headache, hostility, nervousness, restlessness, *sedation,* speech difficulty, unusual dreams, vertigo.
CV: *bradycardia,* hypertension, hypotension, tachycardia.
EENT: blurred vision.
GI: bitter taste, constipation, cramps, dry mouth, dyspepsia, nausea, vomiting.
GU: urinary urgency.
Respiratory: *pulmonary edema, respiratory depression.*

Skin: burning; itching; sweaty, clammy feeling; urticaria.

Interactions

Drug-drug. *CNS depressants, hypnotics, MAO inhibitors, sedatives, tranquilizers, tricyclic antidepressants:* May cause respiratory depression, hypertension, profound sedation, or coma. Dose of one or both drugs may need to be decreased.
General anesthetics: May increase respiratory depression, sedation, and coma; may cause hypertension or hypotension.
Opioid analgesics: May decrease analgesic effect and increase withdrawal symptoms. Avoid use together.
Drug-lifestyle. *Alcohol use:* May cause respiratory depression, hypertension, profound sedation, or coma. Discourage use together.

Effects on lab test results

• May interfere with enzymatic methods for detection of opioids.

Pharmacokinetics

Absorption: Unknown.
Distribution: Not measurably protein-bound.
Metabolism: In liver.
Excretion: In urine and bile. *Half-life:* 5 hours.

Route	Onset	Peak	Duration
I.V.	2–3 min	≤ 30 min	3–4 hr
I.M.	≤ 15 min	≤ 60 min	3–6 hr
SubQ	≤ 15 min	30–60 min	3–6 hr

Action

Chemical effect: Binds with opioid receptors in CNS, altering pain perception and response to pain by unknown mechanism.
Therapeutic effect: Relieves pain and enhances anesthesia.

Available forms

Injection: 10 mg/ml, 20 mg/ml

NURSING PROCESS

📝 **Assessment**
• Assess patient's pain or anesthetic requirement before starting therapy and regularly thereafter to monitor drug effectiveness.
• Observe for signs of withdrawal in patient receiving long-term opioid therapy.

• Monitor patient closely for respiratory depression.
• Monitor patient for signs and symptoms of constipation.
• Be alert for adverse reactions and drug interactions.
• Assess patient's and family's knowledge of drug therapy.

Nursing diagnoses
• Acute pain related to underlying condition
• Disturbed thought processes related to drug's effect on CNS
• Deficient knowledge related to drug therapy

Planning and implementation
• Psychological and physical dependence may occur with prolonged use.
• Drug acts as an opioid antagonist and may precipitate withdrawal syndrome. For patients receiving long-term opioid therapy, start with 25% of usual dose.
• Give stool softener or other laxative to prevent constipation. Encourage patient to drink fluids and eat fiber.
ALERT: If patient's respirations are shallow or rate is below 12 breaths/minute, withhold dose and notify prescriber.
ALERT: Don't confuse Nubain with Navane.
Patient teaching
• Warn ambulatory patient about getting out of bed or walking.
• Instruct outpatient to avoid hazardous activities until the drug's CNS effects are known.

Evaluation
• Patient is free from pain.
• Patient maintains normal thought processes throughout therapy.
• Patient and family state understanding of drug therapy.

naloxone hydrochloride
(nal-OKS-ohn high-droh-KLOR-ighd)
Narcan

Pharmacologic class: opioid antagonist
Therapeutic class: antidote
Pregnancy risk category: B

Indications and dosages

▶ **Known or suspected opioid-induced respiratory depression, including that caused by pentazocine and propoxyphene.** *Adults:* 0.4 to 2 mg I.V. May be given I.M. or subcutaneously if I.V. route unavailable. Repeat every 2 to 3 minutes, if needed. If no response is observed after 10 mg has been given, reevaluate diagnosis.
▶ **Postoperative reversal of opioid effects.**
Adults: 0.1 to 0.2 mg I.V. every 2 to 3 minutes, if needed.
Children: 0.005 to 0.01 mg/kg dose I.V. Repeat every 2 to 3 minutes, if needed.
Neonates (asphyxia neonatorum): 0.01 mg/kg I.V. into umbilical vein. May repeat every 2 to 3 minutes until response is obtained.
▶ **Naloxone challenge for diagnosing opiate dependence‡.** *Adults:* 0.16 mg I.M. naloxone; if no signs of withdrawal after 20 to 30 minutes, give second dose of 0.24 mg. Test is negative if no withdrawal symptoms within 30 minutes.

I.V. administration

• If 0.02 mg/ml isn't available for neonatal concentration, adult concentration (0.4 mg) may be diluted by mixing 0.5 ml with 9.5 ml of sterile water or saline solution for injection.
• Give continuous I.V. infusion to control adverse effects of epidural morphine.
⊗ **Incompatibilities**
All other I.V. drugs, especially preparations containing bisulfite, sulfite, long-chain or high–molecular-weight anions, or alkaline solutions.

Contraindications and cautions

• Contraindicated in patients hypersensitive to drug or any of its components.
• Use cautiously in patients with cardiac irritability and opioid addiction. Abrupt reversal of opioid-induced CNS depression may cause nausea, vomiting, diaphoresis, tachycardia, CNS excitement, and increased blood pressure.
Lifespan: In pregnant women, use cautiously. In breast-feeding women, safety and effectiveness haven't been established.

Adverse reactions

CNS: *seizures,* tremors.
CV: tachycardia and hypertension with high doses, *ventricular fibrillation.*
GI: nausea and vomiting with high doses.
Respiratory: *pulmonary edema.*
Other: *withdrawal symptoms.*

Reactions may be *common,* uncommon, *life-threatening*, or COMMON AND LIFE-THREATENING.

Interactions

None significant.

Effects on lab test results

None reported.

Pharmacokinetics

Absorption: Unknown.
Distribution: Rapid.
Metabolism: Rapid.
Excretion: In urine. *Half-life:* 60 to 90 minutes in adults, 3 hours in neonates.

Route	Onset	Peak	Duration
I.V.	1–2 min	Unknown	Varies
I.M., SubQ	2–5 min	Unknown	Varies

Action

Chemical effect: Unknown; may displace opioid analgesics from their receptors (competitive antagonism). Has no pharmacologic activity.
Therapeutic effect: Reverses opioid effects.

Available forms

Injection: 0.02 mg/ml, 0.4 mg/ml, 1 mg/ml

NURSING PROCESS

⏀ Assessment

• Assess patient's opioid use before starting therapy, and reassess regularly to monitor drug effectiveness.
• Duration of opioid action may exceed that of naloxone, causing relapse into respiratory depression. Monitor patient's respiratory depth and rate.
• Patients who receive naloxone to reverse opioid-induced respiratory depression may develop tachypnea.
• If patient has an adverse GI reaction, monitor his hydration.
• Assess patient's and family's knowledge of drug therapy.

⏀ Nursing diagnoses

• Ineffective health maintenance related to opioid use
• Risk for deficient fluid volume related to drug-induced adverse GI reactions
• Deficient knowledge related to drug therapy

⏀ Planning and implementation

• High doses of drug may cause withdrawal symptoms in opioid-dependent patients.
⏀ **ALERT:** Drug is effective only in reversing respiratory depression caused by opioids. Use flumazenil to treat respiratory depression caused by diazepam or other benzodiazepines.
⏀ **ALERT:** Provide oxygen, ventilation, and other resuscitation measures to patient with severe respiratory depression from acute opioid overdose.
⏀ **ALERT:** Don't confuse naloxone with naltrexone.

Patient teaching
• Instruct patient and family to report adverse reactions.

☑ Evaluation

• Patient responds well to drug.
• Patient maintains adequate hydration.
• Patient and family state understanding of drug therapy.

naltrexone hydrochloride

(nal-TREKS-ohn high-droh-KLOR-ighd)
Depade, ReVia, Vivitrol

N

Pharmacologic class: opioid antagonist
Therapeutic class: adjunct in opioid detoxification/cessation
Pregnancy risk category: C

Indications and dosages

▶ **Adjunct in maintaining opioid-free state in detoxified patients.** *Adults:* Initially, 25 mg P.O. If no withdrawal signs occur within 1 hour, additional 25 mg is given. Once patient takes 50 mg every 24 hours, flexible maintenance schedule may be used.
▶ **Alcohol dependence in combination with a treatment program.** *Adults:* 50 mg P.O. once daily for up to 12 weeks. Or, 380 mg I.M. every 4 weeks or once each month.

Contraindications and cautions

• Contraindicated in patients hypersensitive to the drug or any of its components; those who are receiving opioid analgesics, have a positive urine screen for opioids, or are opioid dependent; those who have acute opioid withdrawal; and those with acute hepatitis or liver failure.

• Use cautiously in patients with mild hepatic disease or history of recent hepatic disease.

⚠ **Lifespan:** In pregnant women, use cautiously. In breast-feeding women and in children, safety and effectiveness haven't been established.

Adverse reactions

CNS: *anxiety,* depression, *headache, insomnia, nervousness,* **suicidal ideation.**
GI: *abdominal pain,* anorexia, nausea, vomiting
Hematologic: lymphocytosis.
Hepatic: *hepatotoxicity.*
Musculoskeletal: *muscle and joint pain.*
Other: *injection site reaction* (I.M. form).

Interactions

Drug-drug. *Products containing opioids (such as cough and cold and antidiarrheal products):* May decrease response to these products. Recommend a nonopioid product.
Thioridazine: May increase somnolence and lethargy. Monitor patient closely.

Effects on lab test results

• May increase AST, ALT, and LDH levels.
• May increase lymphocyte count. May decrease platelet count (I.M. form).

Pharmacokinetics

Absorption: Good.
Distribution: Wide but variable. About 21% to 28% protein-bound.
Metabolism: Extensive. Its major metabolite may be pure antagonist and contribute to its effectiveness. Drug and metabolites may undergo enterohepatic recirculation.
Excretion: Mainly by kidneys. *Half-life:* About 4 hours; 5 to 10 days with I.M. form.

Route	Onset	Peak	Duration
P.O.	15–30 min	1–2 hr	24 hr
I.M.	Unknown	2 hr; then again in 2–3 days	> 1 month

Action

Chemical effect: May reversibly block subjective effects of I.V. opioids by occupying opiate receptors in brain.
Therapeutic effect: Helps prevent opioid dependence and treats alcohol dependence.

Available forms

Injectable suspension: 380 mg vial in single-use kit
Tablets: 25 mg, 50 mg, 100 mg

NURSING PROCESS

🗒 Assessment

• Assess patient's opioid or alcohol dependence before starting therapy and regularly thereafter to monitor drug effectiveness.
• Assess patient's and family's knowledge of drug therapy.

⊕ Nursing diagnoses

• Health-seeking behavior related to desire to remain free from opioid dependence
• Sleep deprivation related to drug-induced insomnia
• Deficient knowledge related to drug therapy

▷ Planning and implementation

🅢 **ALERT:** Begin therapy for opioid dependence after giving naloxone challenge, a provocative test of opioid dependence. If signs of opioid withdrawal persist after challenge, don't give the drug.
🅢 **ALERT:** Patient must be completely free from opioids before taking the drug, or severe withdrawal symptoms may occur. Wait at least 7 days in patient addicted to short-acting opioids, such as heroin and meperidine. Wait at least 10 days in patient addicted to longer-acting opioids, such as methadone.
• Use a nonopioid analgesic for analgesia. If an opioid analgesic is needed in an emergency, give an opioid analgesic in a higher dose than usual to surmount naltrexone's effect. Respiratory depression caused by opioid analgesic may be longer and deeper.
• For patient with opioid dependence who isn't expected to comply, use flexible maintenance regimen: 100 mg on Monday and Wednesday, 150 mg on Friday.
• I.M. injection should be given in gluteal muscle, alternating buttocks, using the kit components provided.
• Store Vivitrol in the refrigerator. Unrefrigerated, it can be stored at temperatures not exceeding 25° C (77° F) for no longer than 7 days before use. Vivitrol shouldn't be frozen.
• Use naltrexone only as part of comprehensive rehabilitation program.

Reactions may be *common,* uncommon, *life-threatening*, or COMMON AND LIFE-THREATENING.

(§) **ALERT:** Don't confuse naltrexone with naloxone.

Patient teaching
● Advise patient to wear or carry medical identification. Warn him to tell medical personnel that he takes naltrexone.
● Give patient names of nonopioid drugs he can take for pain, diarrhea, or cough.

☑ **Evaluation**
● Patient maintains opioid-free state.
● Patient reports no insomnia.
● Patient and family state understanding of drug therapy.

naproxen
(nuh-PROK-sin)
**EC-Naprosyn, Naprosyn, Novo-Naprox ♦,
Nu-Naprox ♦**

naproxen sodium
**Aleve†, Anaprox, Anaprox DS,
Apo-Napro-Na ♦, Apo-Napro-Na DS ♦,
Midol Extended Relief†, Naprelan, Novo-
Naprox Sodium ♦**

Pharmacologic class: NSAID
Therapeutic class: analgesic, antipyretic, anti-inflammatory
Pregnancy risk category: B; D (third trimester)

Indications and dosages

▶ **Rheumatoid arthritis, osteoarthritis, ankylosing spondylitis.** *Adults:* 250 to 500 mg naproxen P.O. b.i.d. Or, 375 mg to 500 mg EC-Naprosyn P.O. b.i.d. Or, 275 to 550 mg naproxen sodium P.O. b.i.d. Or, 750 mg or 1,000 mg Naprelan P.O. daily; may use 1,500 mg daily for limited periods. Or, where suppository is available, 500 mg P.R. at bedtime with naproxen P.O. during day.
▶ **Juvenile arthritis.** *Children age 2 and older:* 10 mg/kg naproxen P.O. in two divided doses.
▶ **Acute gout.** *Adults:* 750 mg naproxen P.O., followed by 250 mg every 8 hours until attack subsides. Or 825 mg naproxen sodium initially; then 275 mg every 8 hours until attack subsides. Or 1,000 mg to 1,500 mg Naprelan P.O. on the first day; then 1,000 mg daily until attack subsides.

▶ **Mild to moderate pain, primary dysmenorrhea, acute tendinitis and bursitis.** *Adults:* 500 mg naproxen P.O., followed by 250 mg every 6 to 8 hours p.r.n. Or 550 mg naproxen sodium P.O. initially; then 275 mg P.O. every 6 to 8 hours p.r.n. Or 1,000 mg Naprelan P.O. daily; use 1,500 mg P.O. daily for limited period.

Contraindications and cautions

● Contraindicated in patients hypersensitive to the drug or any of its components and in patients with asthma, rhinitis, or nasal polyps.
● Use cautiously in those with renal disease, CV disease, GI disorders, hepatic disease, or peptic ulcer disease.
☀ **Lifespan:** In women in the last trimester of pregnancy and in breast-feeding women, drug is contraindicated. In children younger than age 2, safety and effectiveness haven't been established. In elderly patients, use cautiously because of possible delayed excretion.

Adverse reactions

CNS: aseptic meningitis, cognitive dysfunction, *dizziness, drowsiness, headache.*
CV: digital vasculitis, palpitations, peripheral edema.
EENT: *tinnitus,* visual disturbances.
GI: *epigastric distress,* nausea, *occult blood loss,* peptic ulceration.
GU: *nephrotoxicity.*
Hematologic: *agranulocytosis, neutropenia, thrombocytopenia.*
Metabolic: *hyperkalemia.*
Respiratory: dyspnea.
Skin: *pruritus, rash,* urticaria.

Interactions

Drug-drug. *ACE inhibitors:* May increase risk of renal disease. Don't use together.
Aspirin, corticosteroids: May increase risk of adverse GI reactions. Use cautiously, and monitor patient for abdominal pain and bleeding.
Cyclosporine: May increase nephrotoxicity of both drugs. Monitor renal function tests.
Diuretics: May decrease effect of these drugs. Monitor patient.
Drugs that are highly protein-bound, oral anticoagulants, sulfonylureas: May increase risk of toxicity. Monitor patient closely.
Methotrexate: May increase risk of toxicity. Monitor levels.

N

Probenecid: May decrease naproxen elimination. Monitor patient for toxicity.
Drug-herb. *Dong quai, feverfew, garlic, ginger, horse chestnut, red clover:* May increase risk of bleeding. Discourage use together.
St. John's wort: May increase risk of photosensitivity. Advise patient to avoid unprotected or prolonged exposure to sunlight.
Drug-lifestyle. *Alcohol use:* May increase risk of adverse GI reactions. Discourage use together.

Effects on lab test results
• May increase BUN, creatinine, ALT, AST, and potassium levels.
• May increase bleeding time. May decrease granulocyte, platelet, and neutrophil counts.
• May interfere with urinary assays of 5-hydroxyindoleacetic acid and may falsely elevate urine 17-ketosteroid concentrations.

Pharmacokinetics
Absorption: Rapid and complete.
Distribution: Highly protein-bound.
Metabolism: In liver.
Excretion: In urine. *Half-life:* 10 to 20 hours.

Route	Onset	Peak	Duration
P.O.	≤1 hr	1–6 hr	7–12 hr
P.R.	Unknown	Unknown	Unknown

Action
Chemical effect: Unknown; produces anti-inflammatory, analgesic, and antipyretic effects, possibly by inhibiting prostaglandin synthesis.
Therapeutic effect: Relieves pain, fever, and inflammation.

Available forms
naproxen
Oral suspension: 125 mg/5 ml
Tablets: 250 mg, 375 mg, 500 mg
Tablets (delayed-release, enteric-coated): 375 mg, 500 mg
Tablets (extended-release) ◆ : 750 mg, 1,000 mg
naproxen sodium
275 mg naproxen sodium equals 250 mg naproxen
Tablets: 220 mg†, 275 mg, 550 mg
Tablets (controlled-release): 375 mg, 500 mg

NURSING PROCESS

Assessment
• Assess patient's condition before starting therapy and regularly thereafter to monitor drug effectiveness.
• Monitor CBC, electrolytes, and renal and hepatic function every 4 to 6 months during long-term therapy.
• NSAIDs may mask signs and symptoms of infection.
• If patient has an adverse GI reaction, monitor his hydration.
• Assess patient's and family's knowledge of drug therapy.

Nursing diagnoses
• Acute pain related to underlying condition
• Risk for deficient fluid volume related to drug-induced adverse GI reactions
• Deficient knowledge related to drug therapy

Planning and implementation
ALERT: Don't exceed 1.25 g of naproxen or 1.375 g of naproxen sodium daily.
• Give drug with food or milk to minimize GI upset.
• Suppository form isn't available in the United States.
• Don't use in patients with inflammatory lesion of the rectum or anus.
Patient teaching
• Tell patient taking prescription doses of naproxen for arthritis that full therapeutic effect may take 2 to 4 weeks.
• Tell patient to take a full glass of water or other liquid with each dose.
• Tell patient not to break, crush, or chew delayed-release tablets.
ALERT: Warn patient against taking naproxen and naproxen sodium at the same time.
• Teach patient to recognize and report evidence of GI bleeding. Serious GI toxicity, including peptic ulceration and bleeding, can occur in patients taking NSAIDs, despite absence of GI symptoms.
• Warn patient that use with aspirin, alcohol, or corticosteroids may increase risk of adverse GI reactions.
• Advise patient to have periodic eye examinations.

☑ **Evaluation**
• Patient is free from pain.
• Patient maintains adequate hydration.
• Patient and family state understanding of drug therapy.

naratriptan hydrochloride
(nah-rah-TRIP-tin high-droh-KLOR-ighd)
Amerge

Pharmacologic class: selective agonist of serotonin
Therapeutic class: antimigraine drug
Pregnancy risk category: C

Indications and dosages

▶ **Acute migraine headaches with or without aura.** *Adults:* 1 or 2.5 mg P.O. as a single dose. If headache returns or responds only partially, dose may be repeated after 4 hours, for maximum dosage of 5 mg in 24 hours.
▨ **Adjust-a-dose:** For patients with mild or moderate renal or hepatic impairment, don't use more than 2.5 mg P.O. in 24 hours. If creatinine clearance is less than 15 ml/minute or if patient has severe hepatic impairment, don't use drug.

Contraindications and cautions

• Contraindicated in patients hypersensitive to the drug or any of its components and in those who have received ergot-containing, ergot-type, or other 5-HT$_1$ agonists in the previous 24 hours. Also contraindicated in patients with a history or evidence of cardiac ischemia, cerebrovascular disease, peripheral vascular disease, significant underlying CV disease, uncontrolled hypertension, creatinine clearance below 15 ml/minute, or severe hepatic impairment (Child-Pugh grade C).
• Unless a CV evaluation deems patient free from cardiac disease, use cautiously in patient with risk factors for coronary artery disease, such as hypertension, hypercholesterolemia, obesity, diabetes, a strong family history of coronary artery disease, surgical or physiologic menopause (women), age older than 40 (men), and smoking. For patients with cardiac risk factors but a satisfactory CV evaluation, give first dose in a medical facility and consider ECG monitoring.

• Safety and effectiveness haven't been established for cluster headaches or for treating more than four migraine headaches in a 30-day period.
⚖ **Lifespan:** In pregnant women, drug is contraindicated. In breast-feeding women, small amounts of drug may appear in breast milk. In children, safety and effectiveness haven't been established. In elderly patients, drug is contraindicated.

Adverse reactions

CNS: dizziness, drowsiness, fatigue, malaise, paresthesias, syncope, vertigo.
CV: *atrial fibrillation, atrial flutter, coronary artery vasospasm,* increased blood pressure, *MI,* palpitations, PR- and *QT-interval prolongation,* PVCs, ST/T wave abnormalities, *tachyarrhythmias,* transient myocardial ischemia, *ventricular fibrillation, ventricular tachycardia.*
EENT: ear, nose, and throat infections; photophobia.
GI: hyposalivation, nausea, vomiting.
Other: pressure, tightness, and heaviness sensations; warm or cold temperature sensations.

Interactions

Drug-drug. *Ergot-containing or ergot-type drugs (dihydroergotamine, methysergide), other 5-HT$_1$ agonists:* May prolong vasospastic reactions. Don't give within 24 hours of naratriptan. *Hormonal contraceptives:* May slightly increase naratriptan levels. Monitor patient.
Sibutramine: May cause signs of serotonin syndrome, including CNS irritability, motor weakness, shivering, myoclonus may occur. Use together cautiously.
SSRIs, such as fluoxetine, fluvoxamine, paroxetine, sertraline: May cause weakness, hyperreflexia, and incoordination. Monitor patient.
Drug-lifestyle. *Smoking:* May increase naratriptan clearance. Discourage use together; urge patient to stop smoking.

Effects on lab test results

None reported.

Pharmacokinetics

Absorption: Good. Bioavailability of 70%.
Distribution: About 28% to 31% protein-bound.
Metabolism: To a number of inactive metabolites by wide range of cytochrome P-450 isoenzymes.

N

Excretion: Mainly in urine with 50% of dose recovered unchanged and 30% as metabolites. *Half-life:* 6 hours.

Route	Onset	Peak	Duration
P.O.	Unknown	2–3 hr	Unknown

Action

Chemical effect: May activate receptors in intracranial blood vessels, leading to vasoconstriction and relief from migraine headache; activation of receptors on sensory nerve endings in trigeminal system may inhibit proinflammatory neuropeptide release.
Therapeutic effect: Relieves migraine pain.

Available forms

Tablets: 1 mg, 2.5 mg

NURSING PROCESS

Assessment
• Assess baseline cardiac function before starting therapy. Perform periodic cardiac evaluation in patients who develop risk factors for coronary artery disease.
• Assess renal and liver function test results before starting drug therapy, and report abnormalities.
• Assess patient's and family's knowledge of drug therapy.

Nursing diagnoses
• Acute pain related to presence of migraine headache
• Risk for injury related to drug-induced adverse CV reactions
• Deficient knowledge related to drug therapy

Planning and implementation
• Give drug only for a definite diagnosis of migraine. Drug isn't intended to prevent migraine headaches or treat hemiplegic headaches, basilar migraines, or cluster headaches.
• If patient has pain or tightness in chest or throat, arrhythmias, or increased blood pressure, withhold the drug and notify prescriber.
• Don't give drug to a patient with history of coronary artery disease, hypertension, arrhythmias, or risk factors for coronary artery disease because drug may cause coronary vasospasm and hypertension.

• For patients with cardiac risk factors who have had a satisfactory cardiac evaluation, give first dose while monitoring ECG. Keep emergency equipment readily available.

Patient teaching
• Instruct patient to take drug only as prescribed.
• Tell patient that drug is intended to relieve migraine headaches, not to prevent them.
• Instruct patient to take dose soon after headache starts. If no response occurs to first tablet, tell patient to seek prescriber approval before taking second tablet. If prescriber approves a second dose, patient may take a second tablet, but no sooner than 4 hours after first tablet. Advise patient not to exceed two tablets in 24 hours.
• Teach patient to alert prescriber about risk factors for coronary artery disease or bothersome adverse effects.

Evaluation
• Patient has relief from migraine headache.
• Patient has no pain or tightness in chest or throat, arrhythmias, or increase in blood pressure.
• Patient and family state understanding of drug therapy.

✳ New Drug

natalizumab
(nah-tah-LIZ-yoo-mab)
Tysabri

Pharmacologic class: monoclonal antibody
Therapeutic class: immune response modifier
Pregnancy risk category: C

Indications and dosages

▶ **To slow the accumulation of physical disabilities and reduce the frequency of flare-ups in relapsing forms of multiple sclerosis for patients who failed to respond or were unable to tolerate other therapies.** *Adults:* 300 mg in 100 ml normal saline solution infused I.V. over 1 hour every 4 weeks.

▼ I.V. administration
• Dilute 300 mg in 100 ml normal saline solution.
• Invert I.V. bag gently to mix solution; don't shake.

Reactions may be *common*, uncommon, *life-threatening*, or COMMON AND LIFE-THREATENING.

- Infuse over 1 hour; don't give by I.V. push or bolus.
- Flush I.V. line with normal saline solution after infusion is complete.
- Refrigerate solution and use within 8 hours if not used immediately.

⊗ **Incompatibilities**

Any diluent other than normal saline solution. Don't mix or infuse with other drugs.

Contraindications and cautions

- Contraindicated in patients hypersensitive to drug or its components and in those with current or previous progressive multifocal leukoencephalopathy. Use with other immunosuppressants isn't recommended.

⚕ **Lifespan:** In pregnant patients, use only if clearly needed. In breast-feeding women, don't use drug. In children, safety and effectiveness haven't been established. In elderly patients, use caution; it isn't known whether they respond differently than younger adults.

Adverse reactions

CNS: *depression, fatigue, headache, **progressive multifocal leukoencephalopathy**, somnolence, vertigo.*
CV: chest discomfort.
EENT: tonsillitis.
GI: *abdominal discomfort, diarrhea, gastroenteritis.*
GU: amenorrhea, dysmenorrhea, irregular menstruation, urinary frequency, urinary urgency, *UTI, vaginitis.*
Metabolism: weight increase or decrease.
Musculoskeletal: *arthralgia, extremity pain,* muscle cramps, swollen joints.
Respiratory: *lower respiratory tract infection.*
Skin: dermatitis, pruritus, *rash.*
Other: herpes, hypersensitivity reaction, infection, *infusion-related reaction,* rigors, seasonal allergy, *tooth infections.*

Interactions

Drug-drug. *Corticosteroids, other immunosuppressants:* May increase risk of infection. Don't use together.

Effects on lab test results

- May increase liver function test values and lymphocyte, monocyte, eosinophil, basophil, and nucleated RBC counts.

Pharmacokinetics

Absorption: Unknown.
Distribution: Unknown.
Metabolism: Unknown.
Excretion: Unknown. *Half-life:* 7 to 15 days.

Route	Onset	Peak	Duration
I.V.	Unknown	Unknown	Unknown

Action

Chemical effect: Not fully defined. May block interaction between adhesion molecules on inflammatory cells and receptors on endothelial cells of vessel walls.
Therapeutic effect: Slows progression of multiple sclerosis.

Available forms

Injection: 300 mg/15 ml single-use vials

NURSING PROCESS

🔍 **Assessment**
- Make sure patient has had a brain MRI before therapy starts.
- Assess patient's condition before therapy and regularly thereafter to monitor drug effectiveness.
- Be alert for adverse reactions and drug interactions.
- Assess patient's and family's knowledge of drug therapy.

⊕ **Nursing diagnoses**
- Ineffective health maintenance related to underlying condition
- Risk for injury related to drug-induced adverse reactions
- Deficient knowledge related to drug therapy

▶ **Planning and implementation**
- Watch for evidence of hypersensitivity reaction during and for 1 hour after infusion. Evidence may include dizziness, urticaria, fever, rash, rigors, pruritus, nausea, flushing, hypotension, dyspnea, and chest pain.
- Patients who develop antibodies to drug have an increased risk of infusion-related reaction.
⚠ **ALERT:** Drug may cause progressive multifocal leukoencephalopathy. Withhold drug and notify prescriber at the first evidence that suggests progressive multifocal leukoencephalopathy.

N

Patient teaching
- Tell patient to read the Medication Guide before each infusion.
- Urge patient to immediately report progressively worsening symptoms persisting over several days, including changes in thinking, eyesight, balance, or strength.
- Advise patient to inform all the healthcare providers caring for him that he is receiving this drug.
- Tell patient to schedule follow-up appointments with prescriber at 3 and 6 months after the first infusion, then at least every 6 months thereafter.
- Urge patient to immediately report rash, hives, dizziness, fever, shaking chills, or itching while drug is infusing or up to 1 hour afterward.

☑ Evaluation
- Patient responds positively to drug therapy.
- Patient sustains no injury from adverse reactions.
- Patient and family state understanding of drug therapy.

HIGH ALERT

nateglinide
(na-TEG-lih-nighd)
Starlix

Pharmacologic class: amino acid derivative
Therapeutic class: antidiabetic
Pregnancy risk category: C

Indications and dosages

▶ **Alone or with metformin or a thiazolidinedione to lower glucose levels in patients with type 2 diabetes whose hyperglycemia isn't adequately controlled by diet and exercise and who haven't received long-term therapy with other antidiabetics.** *Adults:* 120 mg P.O. t.i.d., taken 1 to 30 minutes before meals. If patient's glycosylated hemoglobin level is near normal when therapy starts, he may receive 60 mg P.O. t.i.d.

Contraindications and cautions

- Contraindicated in patients hypersensitive to the drug or any of its components and in patients with type 1 diabetes or diabetic ketoacidosis.
- Use cautiously in malnourished patients and patients with moderate to severe liver dysfunction or adrenal or pituitary insufficiency.

☀ Lifespan: In pregnant women, don't use. In breast-feeding women, use cautiously; it's unknown if the drug appears in breast milk. In children, safety and effectiveness haven't been established. In elderly patients, use cautiously because some of these patients have greater sensitivity to the glucose-lowering effects than others.

Adverse reactions

CNS: dizziness.
GI: diarrhea.
Metabolic: *hypoglycemia.*
Musculoskeletal: arthropathy, back pain.
Respiratory: bronchitis, coughing, upper respiratory tract infection.
Other: accidental trauma, flulike symptoms.

Interactions

Drug-drug. *Corticosteroids, sympathomimetics, thiazides, thyroid drugs:* May reduce hypoglycemic action of nateglinide. Monitor patient for hyperglycemia, and monitor glucose levels closely.
MAO inhibitors, nonselective beta blockers, NSAIDs, salicylates: May increase hypoglycemic action of nateglinide. Monitor patient for hypoglycemia and monitor glucose levels closely.

Effects on lab test results

- May decrease glucose level.

Pharmacokinetics

Absorption: Rapid when taken immediately before a meal.
Distribution: 98% protein-bound, mainly to albumin.
Metabolism: In the liver.
Excretion: Rapid and complete. *Half-life:* About 1½ hours.

Route	Onset	Peak	Duration
P.O.	20 min	1 hr	4 hr

Action

Chemical effect: Stimulates insulin secretion from the pancreas.
Therapeutic effect: Lowers glucose level.

Available forms

Tablets: 60 mg, 120 mg

Reactions may be *common*, uncommon, *life-threatening*, or COMMON AND LIFE-THREATENING.

NURSING PROCESS

⊞ Assessment
• Assess underlying condition before starting therapy, and reassess regularly to monitor drug effectiveness.
• Monitor glucose level regularly to evaluate drug effectiveness.
• When other drugs are started or stopped, monitor glucose level closely to detect interactions.
• Periodically monitor glycosylated hemoglobin level.
• Assess patient's and family's knowledge of drug therapy.

⊞ Nursing diagnoses
• Ineffective health maintenance related to hyperglycemia
• Risk for injury related to adverse drug effect of hypoglycemia
• Deficient knowledge related to nateglinide therapy

▷ Planning and implementation
• Don't use with or instead of glyburide or other oral antidiabetics. Drug may be used with metformin or a thiazolidinedione.
• Give drug 1 to 30 minutes before a meal. If patient misses a meal, skip the scheduled dose.
ⓢ ALERT: Risk of hypoglycemia rises with strenuous exercise, alcohol ingestion, insufficient caloric intake, and use with other oral antidiabetics.
• Symptoms of hypoglycemia may be masked in patients with autonomic neuropathy and in those who use beta blockers.
• Insulin may be needed for glycemic control in patients with fever, infection, trauma, or impending surgery.
• Effectiveness may decline over time.
ⓢ ALERT: Observe patient for evidence of hypoglycemia, including sweating, rapid pulse, trembling, confusion, headache, irritability, and nausea. To minimize the risk of hypoglycemia, follow dose immediately with a meal. If hypoglycemia occurs and the patient remains conscious, give an oral form of glucose. If unconscious, give I.V. glucose.
Patient teaching
• Tell patient to take drug 1 to 30 minutes before a meal.

• To reduce the risk of hypoglycemia, advise patient to skip the scheduled dose if he misses a meal.
• Educate patient about the risk of hypoglycemia and its signs and symptoms (sweating, rapid pulse, trembling, confusion, headache, irritability, and nausea). Advise patient to treat these symptoms by eating or drinking something containing sugar.
• Teach patient how to monitor and log glucose levels to evaluate diabetes control.
• Instruct patient to adhere to the prescribed diet and exercise regimen.
• Explain the long-term complications of diabetes and the importance of regular preventive therapy.
• Encourage patient to wear or carry medical identification that shows he has diabetes.

☑ Evaluation
• Patient's glucose level is normal.
• Patient doesn't become hypoglycemic and sustains no injury.
• Patient and family state understanding of drug therapy.

nefazodone hydrochloride
(nef-AZ-oh-dohn high-droh-KLOR-ighd)

Pharmacologic class: serotonin modulator
Therapeutic class: antidepressant
Pregnancy risk category: C

Indications and dosages

▶ **Depression.** *Adults:* Initially, 200 mg P.O. daily in two divided doses. Increase dosage in increments of 100 to 200 mg daily at intervals of no less than 1 week. Usual daily dosage range, 300 to 600 mg. Maximum dosage is 600 mg.

Contraindications and cautions

• Contraindicated in patients hypersensitive to the drug or any of its components, other phenylpiperazine antidepressants, or in patients who are withdrawn from drug because of liver injury. Also contraindicated within 14 days of MAO inhibitor therapy.
• Use cautiously in patients with CV or cerebrovascular disease that could be worsened by hypotension (such as history of MI, angina, or

N

stroke) and conditions that predispose to hypotension (such as dehydration, hypovolemia, and therapy with antihypertensives).

• Also use cautiously in patients with history of mania.

⚖ **Lifespan:** In pregnant women, use cautiously. In breast-feeding women, use cautiously; it's unknown if drug appears in breast milk. In children, drug isn't approved for use because children may have an increased risk of suicidal behavior.

Adverse reactions

CNS: abnormal dreams, *asthenia,* ataxia, *confusion,* decreased concentration, *dizziness,* fever, headache, hypertonia, incoordination, insomnia, *light-headedness,* memory impairment, paresthesia, psychomotor retardation, *somnolence, suicidal ideation,* tremor.

CV: hypotension, orthostatic hypotension, peripheral edema, vasodilation.

EENT: *abnormal vision, blurred vision,* pharyngitis, tinnitus, visual field defect.

GI: *constipation,* diarrhea, *dry mouth,* dyspepsia, increased appetite, nausea, taste perversion, vomiting.

GU: urinary frequency, urine retention, UTI, vaginitis.

Hepatic: *liver failure.*

Metabolic: hyponatremia.

Musculoskeletal: arthralgia, neck rigidity.

Respiratory: cough.

Skin: pruritus, rash.

Other: breast pain, chills, flulike syndrome, infection, thirst.

Interactions

Drug-drug. *Alprazolam, triazolam:* May increase effects of these drugs. Avoid using together or substantially reduce dosage of alprazolam and triazolam.

Calcium channel blockers, HMG-CoA reductase inhibitors: May increase levels of these drugs. Adjust dosage if needed.

CNS-active drugs: May alter CNS activity. Use together cautiously.

Digoxin: May increase digoxin level. Use together cautiously and monitor digoxin levels.

MAO inhibitors (phenelzine, selegiline, tranylcypromine): May cause serotonin syndrome (CNS irritability, shivering, and altered consciousness). Don't give together. Wait at least

2 weeks after stopping an MAO inhibitor before giving any selective serotonin reuptake inhibitors. *Other drugs highly bound to proteins:* May increase adverse reactions. Monitor patient closely.

Sibutramine, sumatriptan: May cause severe excitation, hyperpyrexia, seizures, delirium, coma, or a fatal reaction. Avoid using together.

Drug-herb. *St. John's wort:* May cause additive effects and serotonin syndrome (CNS irritability, shivering, and altered consciousness). Discourage using together.

Drug-lifestyle. *Alcohol use:* Enhances CNS depression. Discourage using together.

Effects on lab test results

• May decrease sodium level.

Pharmacokinetics

Absorption: Rapid and complete.
Distribution: Wide. Extensively protein-bound.
Metabolism: Extensive.
Excretion: In urine. *Half-life:* 2 to 4 hours.

Route	Onset	Peak	Duration
P.O.	Unknown	1 hr	Unknown

Action

Chemical effect: Not precisely defined. Drug inhibits neuronal uptake of serotonin (5-HT$_2$) and norepinephrine; it also occupies serotonin and alpha$_1$-adrenergic receptors in CNS.
Therapeutic effect: Relieves depression.

Available forms

Tablets: 50 mg, 100 mg, 150 mg, 200 mg, 250 mg

NURSING PROCESS

🏵 **Assessment**
• Assess patient's depression before starting therapy and regularly thereafter to monitor the drug's effectiveness.

🏵 **ALERT:** Calculate a risk-benefit ratio before using drug for depression because of the risk for hepatic failure and emergence of suicidal ideation and attempts.

• Record mood changes. Monitor patient for suicidal tendencies.

• Be alert for adverse reactions and drug interactions.

- Assess patient's and family's knowledge of drug therapy.

🔷 Nursing diagnoses
- Disturbed thought processes related to depression
- Risk for injury related to drug-induced adverse CNS reactions
- Deficient knowledge related to drug therapy

▶ Planning and implementation
⚡ **ALERT:** Allow at least 7 days after stopping drug before starting patient on an MAO inhibitor. Allow at least 14 days after stopping an MAO inhibitor before starting patient on the drug.

⚡ **ALERT:** Drug may increase the risk of suicidal thinking and behavior in young adults ages 18 to 24 during the first 2 months of treatment. Monitor patient closely.

⚡ **ALERT:** Don't initiate therapy in patients with active liver disease or with elevated baseline transaminase levels. Preexisting liver disease doesn't appear to increase the likelihood of developing liver failure, but baseline abnormalities can complicate patient monitoring.

⚡ **ALERT:** If patient has signs and symptoms of liver dysfunction, such as AST or ALT levels greater than or equal to 3 times upper limit of normal, stop giving the drug and don't restart.

Patient teaching
- Warn patient not to engage in hazardous activity until the drug's CNS effects of drug are known.

⚡ **ALERT:** Instruct man with prolonged or inappropriate erections to stop drug at once and call prescriber.

- Instruct woman to call prescriber if she becomes pregnant or intends to become pregnant during therapy.
- Teach patient the signs and symptoms of liver dysfunction (jaundice, anorexia, GI complaints, and malaise), and tell him to immediately report them to prescriber.
- Instruct patient not to drink alcohol during therapy.
- Tell patient who develops rash, hives, or related allergic reaction to notify prescriber.
- Inform patient that several weeks of therapy may be needed to obtain full antidepressant effect. Once improvement occurs, tell patient not to stop drug until directed by prescriber.

⚡ **ALERT:** Inform family members to be particularly vigilant for suicidal tendencies during therapy with nefazodone. Report to prescriber immediately.
- Urge patient to notify prescriber before taking any OTC drugs.

☑ Evaluation
- Patient exhibits improved thought processes.
- Patient sustains no injuries from drug-induced adverse CNS reactions.
- Patient and family state understanding of drug therapy.

nelfinavir mesylate
(nel-FIN-uh-veer MES-ih-layt)
Viracept

Pharmacologic class: protease inhibitor
Therapeutic class: antiretroviral
Pregnancy risk category: B

Indications and dosages
▶ **HIV infection when antiretroviral therapy is warranted.** *Adults and children older than age 13:* Give 750 mg P.O. t.i.d., or 1,250 mg P.O. b.i.d. with meal.
Children ages 2 to 13: Give 45 to 55 mg/kg b.i.d. or 25 to 35 mg/kg t.i.d. with meal. Maximum dosage, 2,500 mg daily.
▶ **Prophylaxis after occupational exposure to HIV‡.** *Adults:* 750 mg P.O. t.i.d. with two other antiretrovirals for 4 weeks.

Contraindications and cautions
- Contraindicated in patients hypersensitive to the drug or any of its components and in patients receiving amiodarone, ergot derivatives, lovastatin, midazolam, pimozide, quinidine, simvastatin, or triazolam.
- Contraindicated in children and pregnant women not currently on Viracept therapy due to the presence of EMS, a known carcinogen. Children stable on a Viracept-containing regimen may stay on it. Pregnant women should be taken off Viracept.
- Use cautiously in patients with hepatic dysfunction or hemophilia type A and B.
☀ **Lifespan:** In pregnant women, use only when clearly needed. Women shouldn't breastfeed to avoid transmitting HIV to infant.

Adverse reactions

CNS: anxiety, asthenia, depression, dizziness, emotional lability, headache, malaise, paresthesia, *seizures,* sleep disorders, *suicidal ideation.*
EENT: conjunctivitis, iritis, pharyngitis, rhinitis, sinusitis.
GI: *diarrhea,* flatulence, mouth ulceration, nausea, *pancreatitis.*
GU: renal calculus, sexual dysfunction.
Hematologic: anemia, *leukopenia, thrombocytopenia.*
Hepatic: *hepatitis.*
Metabolic: dehydration, hyperlipidemia, hyperuricemia, *hypoglycemia.*
Musculoskeletal: arthralgia, myalgia, myasthenia, myopathy.
Respiratory: diaphoresis, dyspnea.
Skin: dermatitis, pruritus, rash, urticaria.
Other: allergic reactions, fever, redistribution or accumulation of body fat.

Interactions

Drug-drug. *Amiodarone, ergot derivatives, lovastatin, midazolam, pimozide, quinidine, simvastatin, triazolam:* May increase levels of these drugs, causing increased risk of serious or life-threatening adverse reactions. Avoid use together.
Atorvastatin, lovastatin, simvastatin: May increase level of these drugs. Use lowest dose, or consider using pravastatin or fluvastatin instead.
Azithromycin: May increase azithromycin level. Monitor patient for liver impairment.
Carbamazepine, phenobarbital: May reduce the nelfinavir effectiveness. Use together cautiously; monitor drug level and virologic response.
Cyclosporine, sirolimus, tacrolimus: May increase levels of these immunosuppressants. Use together cautiously.
Delavirdine, HIV protease inhibitors (indinavir or saquinavir), nevirapine: May increase protease inhibitor level. Use together cautiously.
Didanosine: May decrease didanosine absorption. Give nelfinavir with food at least 2 hours before or 1 hour after didanosine.
Ethinyl estradiol: May decrease level of contraceptive. Advise patient to use alternative contraceptive measures during therapy.
Methadone, phenytoin: May decrease levels of these drugs. Adjust dosage of these drugs accordingly.
Phosphodiesterase type 5 inhibitors (sildenafil, tadalafil, vardenafil): May increase adverse effects of these drugs. Use together cautiously. Don't exceed 25 mg of sildenafil in a 48-hour period, 10 mg of tadalafil in a 72-hour period, or 2.5 mg of vardenafil in a 72-hour period.
Rifabutin: May increase rifabutin level and decrease nelfinavir level. Reduce rifabutin dosage to half the usual amount, and increase nelfinavir to 1,250 mg b.i.d.
Drug-herb. *St. John's wort:* May decrease nelfinavir level. Discourage use together.

Effects on lab test results

- May increase ALT, AST, alkaline phosphatase, bilirubin, GGT, amylase, CK, and uric acid levels. May decrease hemoglobin level and hematocrit. May increase or decrease glucose level.
- May decrease WBC and platelet counts.

Pharmacokinetics

Absorption: Level peaks higher when drug is taken with food.
Distribution: More than 98% protein-bound.
Metabolism: Mainly by CYP3A and CYP2C19.
Excretion: Mainly in feces. *Half-life:* 3½ to 5 hours.

Route	Onset	Peak	Duration
P.O.	Unknown	2–4 hr	Unknown

Action

Chemical effect: Inhibits protease enzyme and prevents splitting of the viral polyprotein.
Therapeutic effect: Produces immature, noninfectious virus; prevention of AIDS progression.

Available forms

Powder (for suspension): 50 mg/g (as base) powder
Tablets (film-coated): 250 mg (as base), 625 mg (as base)

NURSING PROCESS

☼ Assessment

- Obtain baseline assessment of patient's condition before starting therapy, and reassess regularly to monitor drug's effectiveness.
- Monitor liver function test results.
- Assess patient for increased bleeding tendencies, especially if he has hemophilia type A or B.

- Monitor patient for excessive diarrhea, and treat as directed.
- Assess patient's and family's knowledge of drug therapy.

⊕ Nursing diagnoses
- Risk for injury related to adverse GI effects of drug
- Risk for impaired skin integrity secondary to drug-induced adverse effects
- Deficient knowledge related to drug therapy

⟫ Planning and implementation
- Give oral powder to children unable to take tablets. Mix powder with small amount of water, milk, formula, soy formula, soy milk, or dietary supplements. Tell patient to consume entire contents.
- Don't reconstitute drug with water in its original container.
- Use reconstituted powder within 6 hours.
- Mixing with acidic foods or juice isn't recommended because of the bitter taste.
- ⊛ ALERT: Children and pregnant women should avoid exposure to Viracept. See package insert for full prescribing details.
- Enroll pregnant women with the Antiretroviral Pregnancy Registry by calling 1-800-258-4263 or visiting www.apregistry.com.
- ⊛ ALERT: Don't confuse nelfinavir with nevirapine.

Patient teaching
- Advise patient to take drug with food.
- Explain that drug doesn't cure HIV infection or reduce the risk of transmitting HIV to others.
- Tell patient that the drug's long-term effects are unknown.
- Instruct patient to take drug daily as prescribed and not to alter dose or stop drug without medical approval.
- Tell patient that diarrhea is the most common adverse effect and that it can be controlled with loperamide.
- If patient misses a dose, tell him to take it immediately and then return to his normal schedule, but do not double the dose.
- ⊛ ALERT: Warn patient with phenylketonuria that powder contains 11.2 mg phenylalanine per gram.

- Instruct patient to report use of other prescribed or OTC drugs because of interactions.
- Advise patient taking sildenafil, tadalafil, or vardenafil of an increased risk of adverse events, including hypotension, visual changes, and priapism; tell him to promptly report any symptoms to prescriber. Tell him not to exceed 25 mg of sildenafil in a 48-hour period, 10 mg of tadalafil in a 72-hour period, or 2.5 mg of vardenafil in a 72-hour period.

☑ Evaluation
- Patient has no adverse GI reactions.
- Patient and family state understanding of drug therapy.
- Skin integrity remains intact.

neomycin sulfate
(nee-oh-MIGH-sin SUL-fayt)
Mycifradin, Neo-Fradin, Neo-Tabs

Pharmacologic class: aminoglycoside
Therapeutic class: antibiotic
Pregnancy risk category: D

Indications and dosages

▶ **Preoperative suppression of intestinal bacteria.** *Adults:* 1 g P.O. every hour for four doses; then 1 g every 4 hours for balance of 24 hours. For the 2- to 3-day regimen, 88 mg/kg/day in 6 equally divided doses at 4-hour intervals. Give a saline cathartic before first dose.
Children: 40 to 100 mg/kg daily P.O. divided every 4 to 6 hours. Give a saline cathartic before first dose.
▶ **Adjunct in hepatic coma.** *Adults:* 1 to 3 g P.O. q.i.d. for 5 to 6 days. Or 200 ml of 1% solution or 100 ml of 2% solution as enema retained for 20 to 60 minutes every 6 hours.
▶ **Hypercholesterolemia‡.** *Adults:* 500 mg to 2 g P.O. daily in 2 to 3 divided doses with or immediately after meals.

Contraindications and cautions

- Contraindicated in patients hypersensitive to other aminoglycosides and in those with intestinal obstruction.
- Use cautiously in patients with renal impairment, neuromuscular disorders, or ulcerative bowel lesions.

⚖ **Lifespan:** In pregnant women, only use drug when clearly needed because of the potential for harm. In breast-feeding women, safety and effectiveness haven't been established. In elderly patients, use cautiously.

Adverse reactions

CNS: headache, lethargy.
EENT: *ototoxicity.*
GI: nausea, vomiting.
GU: *nephrotoxicity.*
Skin: rash, urticaria.
Other: *hypersensitivity reactions.*

Interactions

Drug-drug. *Acyclovir, amphotericin B, cisplatin, methoxyflurane, other aminoglycosides, vancomycin:* May increase risk of nephrotoxicity. Use together cautiously.
Atracurium, pancuronium, rocuronium, vecuronium: May increase effects of nondepolarizing muscle relaxant, such as prolonged respiratory depression. Use together only when needed, and reduce dosage.
Cephalothin: May increase risk of nephrotoxicity. Use together cautiously; monitor renal function.
Digoxin: May decrease digoxin absorption. Monitor patient for loss of therapeutic effect.
Dimenhydrinate: May mask symptoms of ototoxicity. Use cautiously.
I.V. loop diuretics (such as furosemide): May increase risk of ototoxicity. Use cautiously; monitor hearing function.
Methotrexate: May decrease methotrexate effects. Monitor patient for decreased effect.
Oral anticoagulants: May inhibit vitamin K–producing bacteria; may increase anticoagulant effect. Monitor patient for bleeding; monitor PT and INR.

Effects on lab test results

• May increase BUN, creatinine, and nonprotein nitrogen levels.

Pharmacokinetics

Absorption: About 3%. Enhanced in patients with impaired GI motility or mucosal intestinal ulcerations.
Distribution: Local.
Metabolism: None.
Excretion: Mainly unchanged in feces. *Half-life:* 2 to 3 hours.

Route	Onset	Peak	Duration
P.O.	Unknown	1–4 hr	8 hr

Action

Chemical effect: Inhibits protein synthesis by binding directly to 30S ribosomal subunit.
Therapeutic effect: Kills susceptible bacteria, such as many aerobic gram-negative organisms and some aerobic gram-positive organisms. Inhibits ammonia-forming bacteria in GI tract, reducing ammonia and improving neurologic status of patients with hepatic encephalopathy.

Available forms

Oral solution: 125 mg/5 ml
Tablets: 500 mg

NURSING PROCESS

Assessment
• Assess patient's condition before starting therapy and regularly thereafter to monitor drug effectiveness.
• Evaluate patient's hearing before starting therapy and regularly thereafter.
• Monitor renal function (output, specific gravity, urinalysis, BUN and creatinine levels, and creatinine clearance).
• Be alert for adverse reactions and drug interactions.
• If patient has adverse GI reactions, monitor his hydration.
• Assess patient's and family's knowledge of drug therapy.

Nursing diagnoses
• Risk for infection related to organisms
• Risk for deficient fluid volume related to drug-induced adverse GI reactions
• Deficient knowledge related to drug therapy

Planning and implementation
ALERT: Never give drug parenterally.
• Drug is nonabsorbable at recommended dosage. More than 4 g daily may be systemically absorbed and lead to nephrotoxicity.
• Make sure patient is well hydrated while taking drug to minimize chemical irritation of renal tubules.
• For preoperative disinfection, provide low-residue diet and cathartic immediately before giving the drug orally.

• In adjunct therapy of hepatic coma, decrease patient's dietary protein and assess neurologic status frequently during therapy.

• The ototoxic and nephrotoxic properties of neomycin limit its usefulness.

• Drug is available with polymyxin B as urinary bladder irrigant.

• Notify prescriber about signs of decreasing renal function or complaints of tinnitus, vertigo, or hearing loss. Deafness may begin several weeks after drug is stopped.

Patient teaching

• Instruct patient to report adverse reactions, especially hearing loss or change in urinary elimination.

• Emphasize the need to drink 2 L of fluid each day.

• Tell patient to alert prescriber if infection worsens or doesn't improve.

☑ **Evaluation**

• Patient is free from infection.

• Patient maintains adequate hydration throughout drug therapy.

• Patient and family state understanding of drug therapy.

neostigmine bromide
(nee-oh-STIG-meen BROH-mighd)
Prostigmin

neostigmine methylsulfate
Prostigmin

Pharmacologic class: cholinesterase inhibitor
Therapeutic class: muscle stimulant
Pregnancy risk category: C

Indications and dosages

▶ **Myasthenia gravis.** *Adults:* 15 to 30 mg P.O. t.i.d. (range, 15 to 375 mg daily). Or, 0.5 mg (1:2,000 solution) subcutaneously, I.M., or I.V., p.r.n.
Children: 7.5 to 15 mg P.O. t.i.d. or q.i.d. or 2 mg/kg/day P.O. divided every 3 to 4 hours. Or, 0.01 to 0.04 mg/kg/dose I.M., I.V., or subcutaneously every 2 to 3 hours, p.r.n. Later doses must be highly individualized, depending on response and tolerance of adverse effects. Therapy may be required day and night.

▶ **To diagnose myasthenia gravis.** *Adults:* 0.022 mg/kg I.M. 30 minutes after 0.011 mg/kg I.M. of atropine sulfate.
Children: 0.025 to 0.04 mg/kg I.M. after 0.011 mg/kg atropine sulfate subcutaneously.

▶ **Postoperative abdominal distention and bladder atony.** *Adults:* 0.25 to 0.5 mg (1:4,000 solution) I.M. or subcutaneously every 4 to 6 hours for 2 to 3 days.

▶ **Antidote for nondepolarizing neuromuscular blockers.** *Adults:* 0.5 to 2.5 mg I.V. slowly. Repeat, p.r.n., to total of 5 mg. Before antidote dose, give 0.6 to 1.2 mg I.V. atropine sulfate.
Children age 12 months and older: 0.025 to 0.08 mg/kg/dose I.V. given with atropine or glycopyrrolate.
Infants up to age 12 months: 0.025 to 0.1 mg/kg/dose I.V. given with atropine or glycopyrrolate.

▶ **Supraventricular tachycardia from tricyclic antidepressant overdose‡.** *Children:* 0.5 to 1 mg I.V. slowly, followed by 0.25 to 0.5 mg I.V. every 1 to 3 hours, if needed.

▶ **Decrease small bowel transit time during radiography‡.** *Adults:* 0.5 to 0.75 mg subcutaneously.

▽ **I.V. administration**

• A 1:1,000 solution of injectable solution contains 1 mg/ml; a 1:2,000 solution contains 0.5 mg/ml.

• Give drug at slow, controlled rate of no more than 1 mg/minute in adults and 0.5 mg/minute in children.

⊗ **Incompatibilities**
None reported.

Contraindications and cautions

• Contraindicated in patients hypersensitive to cholinergics or bromide and in those with peritonitis or mechanical obstruction of intestine or urinary tract.

• Use cautiously in patients with bronchial asthma, bradycardia, seizure disorders, recent coronary occlusion, vagotonia, hyperthyroidism, arrhythmias, or peptic ulcer.

⚜ **Lifespan:** In pregnant women, safety and effectiveness haven't been established.

Adverse reactions

CNS: dizziness, headache, jitters, mental confusion.
CV: *bradycardia, cardiac arrest,* hypotension.

EENT: blurred vision, lacrimation, miosis.
GI: *abdominal cramps, diarrhea,* excessive salivation, *nausea, vomiting.*
GU: urinary frequency.
Musculoskeletal: *muscle cramps,* muscle fasciculations, muscle weakness.
Respiratory: *bronchoconstriction, bronchospasm, depressed respiratory drive, respiratory arrest.*
Skin: diaphoresis, rash (with bromide).
Other: *anaphylaxis,* hypersensitivity reactions.

Interactions

Drug-drug. *Aminoglycosides, anticholinergics, atropine, corticosteroids, magnesium sulfate, procainamide, quinidine:* May reverse cholinergic effects. Observe patient for lack of drug effect.

Effects on lab test results

None reported.

Pharmacokinetics

Absorption: 1% to 2% after P.O. use. Unknown after subcutaneous or I.M. use.
Distribution: About 15% to 25% of dose binds to serum albumin.
Metabolism: Hydrolyzed by cholinesterases and metabolized by microsomal liver enzymes.
Excretion: About 80% of drug in urine. *Half-life:* 52 to 53 minutes.

Route	Onset	Peak	Duration
P.O.	45–75 min	1–2 hr	2–4 hr
I.V.	4–8 min	1–2 hr	2–4 hr
I.M.	20–30 min	1–2 hr	2–4 hr
SubQ	Unknown	1–2 hr	2–4 hr

Action

Chemical effect: Inhibits destruction of acetylcholine released from parasympathetic and somatic efferent nerves. Acetylcholine accumulates, increasing stimulation of receptor.
Therapeutic effect: Stimulates muscle contraction.

Available forms

neostigmine bromide
Tablets: 15 mg
neostigmine methylsulfate
Injection: 0.25 mg/ml, 0.5 mg/ml, 1 mg/ml

NURSING PROCESS

Assessment
• Assess patient's condition before beginning therapy.
• Monitor patient's response after each dose. Watch closely for improvement in strength, vision, and ptosis 45 to 60 minutes after each dose. Show patient how to record variations in muscle strength.
• Monitor vital signs often.
• Assess patient's and family's knowledge of drug therapy.

Nursing diagnoses
• Impaired physical mobility related to condition
• Diarrhea related to drug's adverse effect on GI tract
• Deficient knowledge related to drug therapy

Planning and implementation
⊛ ALERT: For diagnosis of myasthenia gravis, stop any anticholinesterases for at least 8 hours before giving drug.
• For myasthenia gravis, schedule doses before fatigue. For example, if patient has dysphagia, schedule dose 30 minutes before each meal.
• Give atropine injection and provide respiratory support as needed.
• When drug is used to prevent abdominal distention and GI distress, use a rectal tube to help passage of gas.
⊛ ALERT: Although drug is commonly used to reverse effects of nondepolarizing neuromuscular blockers in patients who have undergone surgery, it may worsen blockade produced by succinylcholine.
• Patient may develop resistance to drug.
• Give oral drug with food or milk.
⊛ ALERT: Use I.M. drug instead of edrophonium to diagnose myasthenia gravis when lengthy procedures involving testing of limb strength are used.
⊛ ALERT: Don't confuse neostigmine with etomidate (Amidate) vials. They may look alike.
Patient teaching
• Tell patient to take drug with food or milk to reduce GI distress.
• When using for myasthenia gravis, explain that drug will relieve ptosis, double vision, difficulty chewing and swallowing, and trunk and limb weakness. Stress need to take drug exactly

---

Reactions may be *common,* uncommon, *life-threatening*, or COMMON AND LIFE-THREATENING.

as ordered. Explain that it may have to be taken for life.
• Advise patient to wear or carry medical identification indicating that he has myasthenia gravis.

☑ **Evaluation**
• Patient performs activities of daily living without assistance.
• Patient has normal bowel patterns.
• Patient and family state understanding of drug therapy.

HIGH ALERT

nesiritide
(neh-SIR-ih-tighd)
Natrecor

Pharmacologic class: human B-type natriuretic peptide
Therapeutic class: inotropic vasodilator
Pregnancy risk category: C

Indications and dosages

▶ **Acutely decompensated heart failure in patients with dyspnea at rest or with minimal activity.** *Adults:* 2 mcg/kg by I.V. bolus over 60 seconds followed by continuous infusion of 0.01 mcg/kg/minute.

▼ I.V. administration

• Use these formulas to calculate bolus volume (2 mcg/kg) and infusion flow rate (0.01 mcg/kg/minute):

$$\frac{\text{Bolus volume}}{(\text{ml})} = 0.33 \times \frac{\text{patient weight}}{(\text{kg})}$$

$$\frac{\text{Infusion flow rate}}{(\text{ml/hr})} = 0.1 \times \frac{\text{patient weight}}{(\text{kg})}$$

• Reconstitute one 1.5-mg vial with 5 ml of diluent (such as D_5W, normal saline solution, 5% dextrose and 0.2% saline solution injection, or 5% dextrose and half-normal saline solution) from a prefilled 250-ml I.V. bag.
• Don't shake vial. Gently rock until solution is clear and colorless.
• Withdraw contents of vial and add back to the 250-ml bag to yield 6 mcg/ml. Invert the bag several times to ensure complete mixing, and use the solution within 24 hours.

• Drug binds heparin and could bind the heparin lining of a heparin-coated catheter, decreasing the amount of drug delivered. Don't give drug through a central heparin-coated catheter.
• Before starting bolus dose, prime the tubing. Give the bolus over 60 seconds through a port in the tubing.
• Immediately after giving bolus, infuse drug at 0.1 ml/kg/hour to deliver 0.01 mcg/kg/minute.
• Store drug at a controlled room temperature or refrigerate. Stable for about 24 hours.
⊗ **Incompatibilities**
Bumetanide, enalaprilat, ethacrynate sodium, furosemide, heparin, hydralazine, insulin, sodium metabisulfite preservative.

Contraindications and cautions

• Contraindicated in patients hypersensitive to the drug or any of its components.
• Avoid using drug as primary therapy in patients with cardiogenic shock, systolic blood pressure below 90 mm Hg, low cardiac filling pressures, conditions in which cardiac output depends on venous return, or conditions that make vasodilators inappropriate, such as valvular stenosis, restrictive or obstructive cardiomyopathy, constrictive pericarditis, or pericardial tamponade.
⚹ **Lifespan:** In pregnant women, use cautiously. In breast-feeding women, use cautiously; it's unknown if the drug appears in breast milk. In children, safety and effectiveness haven't been established. Some older patients are more sensitive to drug effects than younger patients, but no overall difference in effectiveness has been noted.

Adverse reactions

CNS: anxiety, confusion, dizziness, fever, headache, insomnia, paresthesia, somnolence, tremor.
CV: angina, atrial fibrillation, AV node conduction abnormalities, *bradycardia, hypotension,* ventricular extrasystoles, *ventricular tachycardia.*
GI: abdominal pain, nausea, vomiting.
Hematologic: anemia.
Musculoskeletal: back pain, leg cramps.
Respiratory: *apnea,* cough.
Skin: pruritus, rash, sweating.
Other: injection-site reactions, pain at the site.

Interactions

Drug-drug. *ACE inhibitors:* May increase hypotension symptoms. Monitor blood pressure closely.

Effects on lab test results

• May increase creatinine level more than 0.5 mg/dl above baseline. May decrease hemoglobin level and hematocrit.

Pharmacokinetics

Absorption: Given I.V.
Distribution: Unknown.
Metabolism: Unknown.
Excretion: Three independent paths: lysosomal proteolysis after drug binds to cell surface receptors, proteolytic cleavage by endopeptidases in the vascular lumen, and renal filtration. *Half-life:* 18 minutes.

Route	Onset	Peak	Duration
I.V.	15 min	1 hr	3 hr

Action

Chemical effect: Binds to receptors on vascular smooth muscle and endothelial cells, which leads to relaxation of smooth muscles and dilation of veins and arteries.
Therapeutic effect: Produces a dose-dependent reduction in pulmonary capillary wedge pressure and systemic arterial pressure in patients with heart failure.

Available forms

Injection: Single-dose vials of 1.5-mg sterile, lyophilized powder

NURSING PROCESS

⬚ Assessment

• Assess underlying condition before starting therapy, and reassess regularly to monitor drug effectiveness.
⬚ **ALERT:** Drug may cause hypotension. Monitor patient's blood pressure closely, particularly if patient also takes an ACE inhibitor.
• Evaluate patient's renal function because drug affects renal function in some people. In patients with severe heart failure whose renal function depends on the renin-angiotensin-aldosterone system, therapy may lead to azotemia.

• Monitor patient's cardiac status before, during, and after giving drug.
• Assess patient's and family's knowledge of drug therapy.

⬚ Nursing diagnoses

• Ineffective tissue perfusion (cardiopulmonary) related to drug-induced hypotension
• Excess fluid volume related to heart failure
• Deficient knowledge related to drug therapy

⬚ Planning and implementation

• Because of hypotension, don't start drug at dose higher than recommended. If hypotension develops during administration, reduce dose or stop giving drug; then restart at a lower dose.
• Limited data exist about giving this drug for longer than 48 hours.
Patient teaching
• Tell patient to report discomfort at I.V. site.
• Urge patient to report symptoms of hypotension, such as dizziness, light-headedness, blurred vision, or sweating.
• Tell patient to report other adverse effects promptly.

⬚ Evaluation

• Patient's blood pressure remains normal during therapy.
• Patient's volume status improves.
• Patient and family state understanding of drug therapy.

nevirapine
(neh-VEER-uh-peen)
Viramune

Pharmacologic class: nonnucleoside reverse transcriptase inhibitor
Therapeutic class: antiretroviral
Pregnancy risk category: C

Indications and dosages

▶ **Adjunct for deteriorating patients with HIV-1 infection.** *Adults:* 200 mg P.O. daily for first 14 days, followed by 200 mg P.O. b.i.d. with nucleoside analogue antiretroviral drugs.
▶ **Adjunct therapy in children infected with HIV-1.** *Children age 8 and older:* 4 mg/kg P.O. once daily for first 14 days, followed by 4 mg/kg P.O. b.i.d. thereafter. Maximum, 400 mg daily.

Children ages 2 months to 7 years: 4 mg/kg
P.O. once daily for first 14 days, followed by
7 mg/kg P.O. b.i.d. thereafter. Maximum dosage
is 400 mg daily.

▶ *Prevention of maternal-fetal transmission of
HIV‡.* Mother: Give 200 mg P.O. as a single
dose at the onset of labor.
Neonate: Give 2 mg/kg P.O. as a single dose
48 to 72 hours after birth. Usually given with a
three-part zidovudine regimen.

Contraindications and cautions

• Contraindicated in patients hypersensitive to
the drug or any of its components and in those
with severe hepatic impairment.
• Use cautiously in patients with impaired
renal and hepatic function or coinfection with
hepatitis B or C. Use extreme caution in women
and patients with CD4 counts greater than
250 cells/mm³.
⚠ Lifespan: In pregnant women, use only if
benefits outweigh risks to the fetus. Women
shouldn't breast-feed to reduce risk of giving
HIV to infant. In the elderly, choose dose cautiously.

Adverse reactions

CNS: *fever, headache,* paresthesia.
GI: abdominal pain, diarrhea, *nausea,* ulcera-
tive stomatitis.
Hepatic: *hepatitis, hepatotoxicity.*
Musculoskeletal: myalgia.
Skin: blistering, rash, *Stevens-Johnson syn-
drome, toxic epidermal necrolysis.*
Other: fat redistribution, *severe hypersensitivi-
ty reactions.*

Interactions

Drug-drug. *CYP3A4 inhibitors (cimetidine,
macrolides):* May increase nevirapine level.
Monitor patient for adverse effects.
*Drugs extensively metabolized by CYP3A4
(rifabutin, rifampin):* May decrease plasma concentrations of these drugs. Adjust dosages of
these drugs if needed.
Hormonal contraceptives, protease inhibitors:
May decrease levels of these drugs. Monitor
patient for effect; advise patient to use nonhormonal contraception.
Ketoconazole: May decrease ketoconazole level
and increase nevirapine level. Avoid use together.

Drug-herb. *St. John's wort:* May decrease nevirapine level. Discourage use together.

Effects on lab test results

• May increase ALT, AST, GGT, and bilirubin
levels. May decrease hemoglobin level and
hematocrit.
• May decrease neutrophil count.

Pharmacokinetics

Absorption: Greater than 90%.
Distribution: Wide.
Metabolism: By liver.
Excretion: In urine and feces. *Terminal-phase
half-life:* 45 hours (single dose); 25 to 30 hours
(multiple doses).

Route	Onset	Peak	Duration
P.O.	Unknown	4 hr	Unknown

Action

Chemical effect: Binds to reverse transcriptase
and blocks RNA-dependent and DNA-dependent DNA polymerase activities.
Therapeutic effect: May inhibit replication of
HIV-1.

Available forms

Oral suspension: 50 mg/5 ml
Tablets: 200 mg

NURSING PROCESS

Assessment
• Obtain lab tests, including liver and renal
function tests, before and during therapy.
• Monitor patient for blistering, oral lesions,
conjunctivitis, muscle or joint aches, or general
malaise. Be especially alert for severe rash, rash
with fever, or rash with elevated AST and ALT
levels, which require stopping therapy. Report
such signs and symptoms immediately to prescriber.

Nursing diagnoses
• Risk for infection related to presence of virus
• Deficient knowledge related to drug therapy

Planning and implementation
• If clinical hepatitis occurs, stop therapy per-
manently.
• Use drug with at least one other antiretroviral.

• Notify the Antiretroviral Pregnancy Registry if woman is or becomes pregnant while taking drug by calling 1-800-258-4263 or visiting www.apregistry.com.

⚡ **ALERT:** Don't confuse nelfinavir with nevirapine.

Patient teaching

• Inform patient that drug doesn't cure HIV infection and that he can still develop illnesses in advanced HIV infection and can still transmit HIV to others.

• Instruct patient to report rash at once and to stop taking the drug if rash develops.

• Instruct women to use at least two barrier methods of contraception because hormonal contraceptive effectiveness is reduced.

• Tell patient not to take other drugs unless approved by prescriber.

• If therapy is interrupted for longer than 7 days, instruct patient to resume it as if for the first time.

• Tell patient with evidence of hepatitis (fatigue, malaise, anorexia, nausea, jaundice, liver tenderness or hepatomegaly, with or without initially abnormal transaminase levels) to stop taking the drug and immediately seek medical evaluation.

☑ **Evaluation**

• Patient shows no signs of worsening condition.

• Patient and family state understanding of drug therapy.

niacin (nicotinic acid, vitamin B₃)
(NIGH-uh-sin)
Niacor, Niaspan, Slo Niacin†

niacinamide (nicotinamide)†

Pharmacologic class: B-complex vitamin
Therapeutic class: vitamin B₃, antilipemic, peripheral vasodilator
Pregnancy risk category: A (C in dosages that exceed the RDA)

Indications and dosages

▶ **RDA.** *Neonates and infants younger than 6 months:* Give 2 mg.
Infants ages 7 months to 1 year: Give 4 mg.
Children ages 1 to 3: Give 6 mg.

Children ages 4 to 8: Give 8 mg.
Children ages 9 to 13: Give 12 mg.
Males age 14 and older: Give 16 mg.
Females age 14 and older: Give 14 mg.
Pregnant women: Give 18 mg.
Breast-feeding women: Give 17 mg.

▶ **Pellagra.** *Adults:* 300 to 500 mg P.O. daily in divided doses, depending on severity of niacin deficiency.
Children: Up to 300 mg P.O. daily, depending on severity of niacin deficiency. After symptoms subside, advise adequate nutrition and RDA supplements to prevent recurrence.

▶ **Hartnup disease.** *Adults:* 50 to 200 mg P.O. daily.

▶ **Niacin deficiency.** *Adults:* Up to 100 mg P.O. daily.

▶ **Hyperlipidemias, especially with hypercholesterolemia.** *Adults:* Initially, 250 mg P.O. as a single dose following evening meal. Then increase every 4 to 7 days to 1 to 2 g P.O. b.i.d. or t.i.d. with meals until desired LDL level is achieved. Maximum, 6 g daily. Alternatively, for extended-release tablets, start at 500 mg P.O. daily at bedtime for 1 to 4 weeks; then increase to 1,000 mg at bedtime during weeks 5 to 8. After week 8, increase by 500 mg every 4 weeks. Maximum, 2 g daily.

Contraindications and cautions

• Contraindicated in patients hypersensitive to the drug or any of its components and in those with hepatic dysfunction, active peptic ulcers, severe hypotension, or arterial hemorrhage.

• Use cautiously in patients with gallbladder disease, diabetes mellitus, or coronary artery disease and in patients with history of liver disease, peptic ulcer, allergy, or gout.

☼ **Lifespan:** In pregnant women, use above the RDA hasn't been studied. In breast-feeding women, use above the RDA isn't recommended. In children, safety of doses that exceed the RDA hasn't been established.

Adverse reactions

CNS: dizziness, transient headache.
CV: *arrhythmias, excessive peripheral vasodilation, flushing.*
GI: activation of peptic ulceration, *diarrhea,* epigastric or substernal pain, *nausea, vomiting.*
Hepatic: *hepatic dysfunction.*
Metabolic: hyperglycemia, hyperuricemia.
Skin: dryness, pruritus, tingling.

Reactions may be *common,* uncommon, *life-threatening*, or COMMON AND LIFE-THREATENING.

Interactions

Drug-drug. *Antihypertensives:* May increase risk of orthostatic hypotension. Use together cautiously; also warn patient about orthostatic hypotension.
HMG-CoA reductase inhibitors, such as lovastatin: May result in myopathy and rhabdomyolysis. Avoid use together.

Effects on lab test results

• May increase glucose, AST, ALT, and uric acid levels.

Pharmacokinetics

Absorption: Rapid after P.O. use. Unknown after subcutaneous or I.M. use.
Distribution: Wide.
Metabolism: By liver to active metabolites.
Excretion: In urine. *Half-life:* About 45 minutes.

Route	Onset	Peak	Duration
P.O.	Unknown	45 min	Unknown

Action

Chemical effect: Niacin and niacinamide stimulate lipid metabolism, tissue respiration, and glycogenolysis; niacin decreases synthesis of low-density lipoproteins and inhibits lipolysis in adipose tissue.
Therapeutic effect: Restores normal level of vitamin B_3, lowers triglyceride and cholesterol levels, and dilates peripheral blood vessels.

Available forms

niacin
Capsules (timed-release): 125 mg†, 250 mg†, 400 mg†, 500 mg†
Tablets: 50 mg†, 100 mg†, 250 mg†, 500 mg†
Tablets (extended-release): 500 mg, 750 mg, 1,000 mg
Tablets (timed-release): 250 mg†, 500 mg†, 750 mg†
niacinamide
Tablets: 50 mg†, 100 mg†, 500 mg†

NURSING PROCESS

Assessment

• Assess patient's condition before starting therapy and regularly thereafter to monitor drug effectiveness.
• Monitor hepatic function and glucose levels.

• Be alert for adverse reactions and drug interactions.
• If patient has an adverse GI reaction, monitor his hydration.
• Assess patient's and family's knowledge of drug therapy.

Nursing diagnoses

• Imbalanced nutrition: less than body requirements related to decreased intake of vitamin B_3
• Risk for deficient fluid volume related to drug-induced adverse GI reactions
• Deficient knowledge related to drug therapy

Planning and implementation

ALERT: Give aspirin (325 mg P.O. 30 minutes before niacin dose) to help reduce persistent or distressing flushing.
• Timed-release niacin or niacinamide may prevent excessive flushing that occurs with large doses, but this drug form also has been linked to hepatic dysfunction, even at doses as low as 1 g daily.
• Give drug with meals to minimize GI adverse effects.
ALERT: Don't confuse Nicobid and Nicotinex with Nicoderm, Nicotrol, or Nicorette.
Patient teaching
• Explain that skin flushing or warm sensation is usually harmless and will usually subside with continued use.
• Advise patient to decrease flushing by taking drug with a low-fat snack and not taking it after alcohol, hot beverages, hot or spicy foods, a hot shower, or exercise.
• Stress that drug is a potent drug that may cause serious adverse effects. Explain importance of adhering to therapy.
• Advise patient against self-medicating for hyperlipidemia.

Evaluation

• Patient's vitamin B_3 levels are normal.
• Patient maintains adequate hydration throughout drug therapy.
• Patient and family state understanding of drug therapy.

N

nifedipine

(nigh-FEH-duh-peen)

Adalat CC, Apo-Nifed ♦, Nifedical XL, Procardia XL⊘

Pharmacologic class: calcium channel blocker
Therapeutic class: antianginal
Pregnancy risk category: C

Indications and dosages

▶ **Vasospastic angina (Prinzmetal or variant angina), classic chronic stable angina pectoris.** *Adults:* Initially, 10 mg (short-acting capsules) P.O. t.i.d. Usual effective dosage range is 10 to 20 mg t.i.d. Some patients may require up to 30 mg q.i.d. Maximum daily dose is 180 mg. Adjust dosage over 7 to 14 days to evaluate response. Or, 30 to 60 mg (extended-release tablets, except Adalat CC) P.O. once daily. Maximum daily dose is 120 mg. Adjust dosage over 7 to 14 days to evaluate response.

▶ **Hypertension.** *Adults:* 30 or 60 mg P.O. (extended-release) once daily. Adjusted over 7 to 14 days. Doses larger than 90 mg (Adalat CC) and 120 mg (Procardia XL) aren't recommended.

Contraindications and cautions

• Contraindicated in patients hypersensitive to the drug or any of its components.
• Use cautiously in those with heart failure or hypotension. Use extended-release tablets cautiously in patients with severe GI narrowing because obstructive symptoms may occur.
⚖ **Lifespan:** In pregnant and breast-feeding women, drug is contraindicated. In children, safety and effectiveness haven't been established. In geriatric patients, use cautiously.

Adverse reactions

CNS: *dizziness, headache, light-headedness,* nervousness, somnolence, syncope, weakness.
CV: *flushing, **heart failure,** hypotension, MI,* palpitations, *peripheral edema.*
EENT: nasal congestion.
GI: abdominal discomfort, constipation, diarrhea, *nausea.*
Metabolic: hypokalemia.
Musculoskeletal: muscle cramps.

Respiratory: cough, dyspnea, ***pulmonary edema.***
Skin: pruritus, rash.

Interactions

Drug-drug. *Antiretrovirals, cimetidine, verapamil:* May decrease nifedipine metabolism. Monitor blood pressure closely, and adjust nifedipine dosage as needed.
Azole antifungals, dalfopristin, erythromycin, quinupristin: May increase nifedipine effects. Monitor blood pressure closely, and decrease nifedipine dosage as needed.
Digoxin: May increase digoxin level. Monitor digoxin level.
Diltiazem: May increase nifedipine effects. Monitor patient closely.
Fentanyl: May cause severe hypotension. Monitor blood pressure.
Phenytoin: May reduce phenytoin metabolism. Monitor phenytoin level.
Propranolol, other beta blockers: May cause hypotension and heart failure. Use together cautiously.
Quinidine: May decrease quinidine levels and effects and increase nifedipine effects. Monitor heart rate, and adjust nifedipine dosage as needed.
Rifamycins: May decrease nifedipine level. Monitor patient.
Tacrolimus: May increase tacrolimus level and risk for toxicity. Decrease tacrolimus dosage as needed.
Drug-herb. *Ginkgo:* May increase nifedipine effects. Discourage use together.
Ginseng: May increase nifedipine level and possibly cause toxicity. Discourage use together.
Melatonin, St. John's wort: May interfere with antihypertensive effect. Discourage use together.
Drug-food. *Grapefruit juice:* May increase nifedipine bioavailability. Discourage use together.

Effects on lab test results

• May increase ALT, AST, alkaline phosphatase, and LDH levels.

Pharmacokinetics

Absorption: Rapid and about 90%, but only about 45% to 75% reaches circulation because of significant first-pass effect in liver.
Distribution: About 92% to 98% protein-bound.

Reactions may be *common*, uncommon, ***life-threatening***, or **COMMON AND LIFE-THREATENING**.

Metabolism: In liver.
Excretion: In urine and feces as inactive metabolites. *Half-life:* 2 to 5 hours.

Route	Onset	Peak	Duration
P.O.	20 min	30–60 min	4–8 hr
P.O.			
Extended-release	20 min	6 hr	24 hr

Action

Chemical effect: Unknown; may inhibit calcium ion influx across cardiac and smooth-muscle cells, decreasing myocardial contractility and oxygen demand. Also may dilate coronary arteries and arterioles.
Therapeutic effect: Reduces blood pressure and prevents angina.

Available forms

Capsules: 10 mg, 20 mg
Tablets (extended-release): 30 mg, 60 mg, 90 mg

NURSING PROCESS

🔎 Assessment
• Assess patient's condition before starting therapy and regularly thereafter to monitor drug effectiveness.
• Monitor blood pressure regularly, especially in patients who take beta blockers or antihypertensives.
• Monitor potassium level regularly.
• Be alert for adverse reactions and drug interactions.
• Assess patient's and family's knowledge of drug therapy.

🔅 Nursing diagnoses
• Risk for injury related to presence of hypertension
• Chronic pain related to angina
• Deficient knowledge related to drug therapy

▶ Planning and implementation
• Don't give immediate-release form within 1 week of acute MI or in acute coronary syndrome.
• **ALERT:** Don't use nifedipine capsules sublingually to rapidly reduce severely high blood pressure. Excessive hypotension, MI, and death may result.

• Watch for symptoms of heart failure.
• **ALERT:** Don't confuse nifedipine with nimodipine or nicardipine.

Patient teaching
• If patient is kept on nitrate therapy while nifedipine dosage is adjusted, urge continued compliance. Patient may take S.L. nitroglycerin, as needed, for acute chest pain.
• Tell patient that chest pain may worsen briefly when therapy starts or dosage increases.
• Instruct patient to swallow extended-release tablets without breaking, crushing, or chewing them.
• Advise patient to avoid taking drug with grapefruit juice.
• Reassure patient taking the extended-release form that a wax-matrix "ghost" from the tablet may be passed in the stool. Drug is completely absorbed before this occurs.
• Tell patient to protect capsules from direct light and moisture and to store at room temperature.

☑ Evaluation
• Patient's blood pressure is normal.
• Patient's angina is less frequent and severe.
• Patient and family state understanding of drug therapy.

nisoldipine
(nigh-SOHL-dih-peen)
Sular

Pharmacologic class: calcium channel blocker
Therapeutic class: antihypertensive
Pregnancy risk category: C

Indications and dosages

▶ **Hypertension.** *Adults:* Initially, 20 mg P.O. once daily; then increase by 10 mg weekly or at longer intervals, as indicated. Usual maintenance dosage is 20 to 40 mg once daily. Dosages above 60 mg daily aren't recommended.
◻ **Adjust-a-dose:** For patients older than age 65 and those who have liver dysfunction, initial dosage is 10 mg P.O. daily.

Contraindications and cautions

• Contraindicated in patients hypersensitive to dihydropyridine calcium channel blockers.

• Use cautiously in patients with severe hepatic impairment, heart failure, or compromised ventricular function, and particularly in those taking beta blockers.

⚘ **Lifespan:** In pregnant women, use cautiously. In breast-feeding women, don't use drug. In children, safety and effectiveness haven't been established.

Adverse reactions

CNS: dizziness, *headache.*
CV: chest pain, palpitations, *peripheral edema,* vasodilation.
EENT: pharyngitis, sinusitis.
GI: nausea.
Skin: rash.

Interactions

Drug-drug. *Cimetidine:* May increase nisoldipine bioavailability and peak level. Monitor patient for increased adverse effects.
Quinidine: May decrease nisoldipine bioavailability but not peak level. Monitor patient.
Drug-food. *Grapefruit juice:* May increase peak drug level, increasing therapeutic and adverse effects. Give drug 1 hour before or after patient eats or drinks grapefruit.
High-fat meal: May increase peak drug level. Don't give drug with a high-fat meal.

Effects on lab test results

None reported.

Pharmacokinetics

Absorption: Good; high-fat foods significantly affect rate of release of drug.
Distribution: About 99% protein-bound.
Metabolism: Extensive.
Excretion: In urine. *Half-life:* 7 to 12 hours.

Route	Onset	Peak	Duration
P.O.	Unknown	6–12 hr	24 hr

Action

Chemical effect: Prevents entry of calcium ions into vascular smooth-muscle cells, causing dilation of arterioles, which decreases peripheral vascular resistance.
Therapeutic effect: Lowers blood pressure.

Available forms

Tablets (extended-release): 10 mg, 20 mg, 30 mg, 40 mg

NURSING PROCESS

🖎 Assessment
• Assess patient's blood pressure before starting therapy, and monitor regularly, especially during dosage adjustment.
• Monitor patient carefully. Some patients, especially those with severe obstructive coronary artery disease, may develop increased frequency, duration, or severity of angina or acute MI when starting calcium channel blocker therapy or increasing dose.
• Be alert for adverse reactions and interactions.
• Assess patient's and family's knowledge of drug therapy.

🖎 Nursing diagnoses
• Risk for injury related to hypertension
• Excess fluid volume related to edema
• Deficient knowledge related to drug therapy

▷ Planning and implementation
• Don't give drug with a high-fat meal or grapefruit products.
⚠ **ALERT:** Don't confuse nisoldipine with nifedipine or nicardipine.
Patient teaching
• Tell patient to take drug as prescribed.
• Instruct patient to swallow tablet whole and not to chew, divide, or crush it.

✓ Evaluation
• Patient's blood pressure is normal.
• Patient doesn't exhibit signs of edema.
• Patient and family state understanding of drug therapy.

nitrofurantoin macrocrystals
(nigh-troh-fyoo-RAN-toyn MAH-kroh-kris-tuls)
Macrobid, Macrodantin

nitrofurantoin microcrystals
Furadantin, Furalan, Macrodantin

Pharmacologic class: nitrofuran
Therapeutic class: urinary tract anti-infective
Pregnancy risk category: B

Indications and dosages

▶ **UTI caused by susceptible** *Escherichia coli, Staphylococcus aureus,* **enterococci, and**

certain strains of *Klebsiella* and *Enterobacter.*
Adults and children older than age 12: Give
50 to 100 mg P.O. q.i.d. with milk or meals. Or
100 mg Macrobid P.O. every 12 hours for 7
days.
Children ages 1 month to 12 years: 5 to 7 mg/
kg P.O. daily, divided q.i.d.

▶ **Long-term suppression therapy.** *Adults:*
50 to 100 mg P.O. at bedtime.
Children age 1 month and older: 1 to 2 mg/kg
P.O. at bedtime.

Contraindications and cautions

● Contraindicated in patients who are hypersensitive to the drug or any of its components. Contraindicated in patients with moderate to severe
renal impairment (creatinine clearance less than
60 ml/minute), anuria, or oliguria.
● Use cautiously in patients with renal impairment, anemia, diabetes mellitus, electrolyte abnormalities, vitamin B deficiency, debilitating
disease, or G6PD deficiency.
⚖ **Lifespan:** In pregnant women, use cautiously. In breast-feeding women, use cautiously; it's
unknown if the drug appears in breast milk. In
infants age 1 month and younger, drug is contraindicated.

Adverse reactions

CNS: *ascending polyneuropathy,* dizziness,
drowsiness, headache, *peripheral neuropathy.*
GI: abdominal pain, anorexia, diarrhea, nausea,
vomiting.
Hematologic: *agranulocytosis, hemolysis in*
patients with G6PD deficiency, leukopenia,
thrombocytopenia.
Hepatic: *hepatic necrosis, hepatitis.*
Respiratory: *asthma,* pulmonary sensitivity.
Skin: eczematous, erythematous, or maculopapular eruption; exfoliative dermatitis; pruritus; *Stevens-Johnson syndrome,* urticaria.
Other: *anaphylaxis,* drug fever, hypersensitivity reactions, overgrowth of nonsusceptible organisms in urinary tract, transient alopecia.

Interactions

Drug-drug. *Magnesium-containing antacids:*
May decrease nitrofurantoin absorption. Separate ingestion by 1 hour.
Probenecid, sulfinpyrazone: May increase blood
level and decrease urine level. May result in increased toxicity and lack of therapeutic effect.
Don't use together.

Quinolones (such as nalidixic acid, nor-
floxacin): May decrease effectiveness of
quinolone derivatives. Avoid use together.
Drug-food. *Any food:* May increase drug absorption. Give drug with food.

Effects on lab test results

● May increase phosphorus, bilirubin, and alkaline phosphatase levels. May decrease glucose
and hemoglobin levels and hematocrit.
● May decrease granulocyte and platelet counts.
● May cause false-positive results with urine
glucose test using copper sulfate reduction
method (Clinitest), Benedict's solution, or
Fehling's solution, but not with glucose enzymatic test.

Pharmacokinetics

Absorption: Good. Food aids drug's dissolution
and speeds absorption. Macrocrystal form has
slower dissolution and absorption.
Distribution: Into bile. 60% protein-bound.
Metabolism: Partially in liver.
Excretion: About 30% to 50% in urine. *Half-*
life: 15 minutes to 1 hour.

Route	Onset	Peak	Duration
P.O.	Unknown	Unknown	Unknown

Action

Chemical effect: Unknown; may interfere with
bacterial enzyme systems and cell wall formation.
Therapeutic effect: Hinders growth of many
common gram-positive and gram-negative urinary pathogens.

Available forms

nitrofurantoin macrocrystals
Capsules: 25 mg, 50 mg, 100 mg
Capsules (dual-release): 100 mg
nitrofurantoin microcrystals
Capsules: 50 mg, 100 mg
Oral suspension: 25 mg/5 ml
Tablets: 50 mg, 100 mg

NURSING PROCESS

▣ **Assessment**
● Assess patient's infection before starting therapy and regularly thereafter to monitor drug effectiveness.

- Obtain urine specimen for culture and sensitivity tests before starting therapy, and repeat as needed. Start therapy pending results.
- Monitor fluid intake and output. May turn urine darker or even brown.
- Monitor CBC and pulmonary status regularly.
- Assess patient for renal impairment before and during therapy, especially with high doses, and increased risk of ascending polyneuropathy.
- Be alert for adverse reactions and drug interactions.
- If patient has adverse GI reactions, monitor his hydration.
- Assess patient's and family's knowledge of drug therapy.

⊕ **Nursing diagnoses**
- Risk for infection related to susceptible bacteria
- Risk for deficient fluid volume related to drug-induced adverse GI reactions
- Deficient knowledge related to drug therapy

▷ **Planning and implementation**
- Drug has no effect on blood or tissue outside urinary tract.
- Notify prescriber if patient develops cough, chest pains, fever, chills, and dyspnea (signs of pulmonary sensitivity).
- Be aware that patients with G6PD deficiency who develop hemolysis during therapy will recover when drug is stopped.
- ⑤ **ALERT:** Hypersensitivity may develop during long-term therapy.
- Dual-release capsules (25-mg nitrofurantoin macrocrystals combined with 75-mg nitrofurantoin monohydrate) enable twice-daily dosing.
- Continue therapy for 3 days after urine specimens become sterile.
- Patient may experience fewer adverse GI effects with nitrofurantoin macrocrystals.
- Store drug in amber container. Avoid metals other than stainless steel or aluminum to avoid precipitate formation.

Patient teaching
- Tell patient to take drug with food or milk to minimize GI distress.
- Teach patient how to measure intake and output. Warn him that drug will turn urine darker or even brown.
- Instruct patient how to store drug.

☑ **Evaluation**
- Patient is free from infection.
- Patient maintains adequate hydration throughout drug therapy.
- Patient and family state understanding of drug therapy.

HIGH ALERT
---

nitroglycerin (glyceryl trinitrate)
(nigh-troh-GLIH-suh-rin)
Minitran, Nitrek, Nitro-Dur, Nitrogard, Nitroglyn, Nitrolingual, NitroMist, NitroQuick, Nitrostat, Nitro-Time

Pharmacologic class: nitrate
Therapeutic class: antianginal, vasodilator
Pregnancy risk category: C

Indications and dosages

▶ **Prevention of chronic anginal attacks.**
Adults: 2.5 mg or 2.6 mg sustained-release capsule every 8 to 12 hours. Or 2% ointment: Start with ½ inch of ointment and increase by ½-inch increments until headache occurs; then decrease to previous dose. Range of dosage with ointment is ¼ to 5 inches. Usual dose is 1 to 2 inches. Or Nitrodisc, Nitro-Dur, or Transderm-Nitro transdermal disk or pad, 0.2 to 0.4 mg/hour once daily.

▶ **Acute angina pectoris; to prevent or minimize anginal attacks when taken immediately before stressful events.** *Adults:* 1 S.L. tablet (grain [gr] ½₀₀, ⅟₁₅₀, ⅟₁₀₀) dissolved under tongue or in buccal pouch as soon as angina begins. Repeat every 5 minutes for up to 15 minutes if symptoms persist. Or, using Nitrolingual spray, 1 or 2 sprays into mouth, preferably onto or under tongue. Repeat every 3 to 5 minutes if symptoms persist, to maximum of three doses in 15-minute period. Or, 1 to 3 mg extended-release tablet buccally every 3 to 5 hours during waking hours.

▶ **Hypertension related to surgery; heart failure linked to MI; angina pectoris in acute situations; to produce controlled hypotension during surgery.** *Adults:* Initial infusion rate is 5 mcg/minute. Increase as needed by 5 mcg/minute every 3 to 5 minutes until response occurs. If 20-mcg/minute rate doesn't produce response, increase dosage by 10 to 20 mcg/minute every 3 to 5 minutes. Up to 100 mcg/minute I.V. may be needed.

► **Hypertensive crisis‡.** *Adults:* Infuse at 5 to 100 mcg/minute I.V.

▽ I.V. administration

• Mix in glass bottles, and avoid I.V. filters because drug binds to plastic. Regular polyvinyl chloride tubing can bind up to 80% of drug, requiring higher doses. Special nonabsorbent, nonpolyvinyl chloride tubing is available from manufacturer.
• Dilute drug with D_5W or normal saline solution for injection to no more than 400 mcg/ml.
• Always use same type of infusion set when changing I.V. lines.
• When changing concentration of nitroglycerin infusion, flush I.V. administration set with 15 to 20 ml of new concentration before use. This will clear line of old drug solution.
• Give with infusion control device and titrate to desired response.
⊗ **Incompatibilities**
Alteplase, bretylium, hydralazine, levofloxacin, phenytoin sodium, other I.V. drugs.

Contraindications and cautions

• Contraindicated in patients hypersensitive to nitrates and in those with early MI (S.L. form), severe anemia, increased intracranial pressure, angle-closure glaucoma, orthostatic hypotension, and allergy to adhesives (transdermal form). I.V. nitroglycerin is contraindicated in patients with hypovolemia, hypotension, cardiac tamponade, restrictive cardiomyopathy, constrictive pericarditis, or hypersensitivity to I.V. form.
• Use cautiously in patients with hypotension or volume depletion.
☀ **Lifespan:** In pregnant women, use cautiously. In breast-feeding women, use cautiously; it's unknown if the drug appears in breast milk. In children, safety and effectiveness haven't been established.

Adverse reactions

CNS: *dizziness, headache, throbbing,* weakness.
CV: fainting, *flushing, orthostatic hypotension,* palpitations, *tachycardia.*
EENT: S.L. burning.
GI: nausea, vomiting.
Skin: contact dermatitis (patch), cutaneous vasodilation, rash.
Other: hypersensitivity reactions.

Interactions

Drug-drug. *Alteplase:* May decrease t-PA antigen level. Avoid use together. If use together is unavoidable, use the lowest effective dose of nitroglycerin.
Antihypertensives: May increase hypotensive effect. Monitor patient closely.
Dihydroergotamine: May decrease antianginal effect or increase mean standing systolic blood pressure. Avoid use together.
Phosphodiesterase type 5 inhibitors (sildenafil, tadalafil, vardenafil): May cause severe hypotension. Use of nitrates in any form with erectile dysfunction drugs is contraindicated.
Drug-lifestyle. *Alcohol use:* May increase hypotension. Urge patient to avoid alcohol during therapy.

Effects on lab test results

• May interfere with Zlatkis-Zak color reaction, causing false report of decreased cholesterol level.

Pharmacokinetics

Absorption: For P.O. use, good but incomplete. For S.L. use, relatively complete. For topical or transdermal use, good.
Distribution: Wide. About 60% protein-bound.
Metabolism: In liver.
Excretion: Metabolites in urine. *Half-life:* About 1 to 4 minutes.

Route	Onset	Peak	Duration
P.O.	20–45 min	Unknown	3–8 hr
I.V.	Immediate	Immediate	3–5 min
Topical	30 min	Unknown	2–12 hr
Transdermal	30 min	Unknown	≤ 24 hr
S.L.	1–3 min	Unknown	30–60 min
Buccal	3 min	Unknown	5 hr
Translingual	2–4 min	Unknown	30–60 min

Action

Chemical effect: Reduces cardiac oxygen demand by decreasing left ventricular end-diastolic pressure (preload) and, to a lesser extent, systemic vascular resistance (afterload). Also increases blood flow through collateral coronary vessels.
Therapeutic effect: Prevents or relieves acute angina, lowers blood pressure, and helps minimize heart failure caused by MI.

N

Available forms

Aerosol (translingual): 0.4 mg metered spray
Capsules (sustained-release): 2.5 mg, 6.5 mg, 9 mg
I.V.: 5 mg/ml
I.V. premixed solutions in dextrose: 100 mcg/ml, 200 mcg/ml, 400 mcg/ml
Tablets (buccal extended-release): 2 mg, 3 mg
Tablets (S.L.): 0.3 mg (gr $\frac{1}{200}$), 0.4 mg (gr $\frac{1}{50}$), 0.6 mg (gr $\frac{1}{100}$)
Topical: 2% ointment
Transdermal: 0.1 mg/hr, 0.2 mg/hr, 0.3 mg/hr, 0.4 mg/hr, 0.6 mg/hr, 0.8 mg/hr

NURSING PROCESS

Assessment

• Assess patient's condition before starting therapy and regularly thereafter to monitor drug effectiveness.
• Monitor vital signs and drug response. Be particularly aware of blood pressure. Excessive hypotension may worsen MI.
• Be alert for adverse reactions and drug interactions.
• Assess patient's and family's knowledge of drug therapy.

Nursing diagnoses

• Acute or chronic pain related to angina
• Risk for injury related to drug-induced adverse reactions
• Deficient knowledge related to drug therapy

Planning and implementation

• Give P.O. tablets on empty stomach, either 30 minutes before or 1 to 2 hours after meals.
• Don't allow patient to swallow or chew S.L. tablets.
• Give S.L. tablet at first sign of attack. Wet tablet with patient's saliva, then place under patient's tongue until completely absorbed. Have patient sit and rest until pain subsides.
• Repeat dose every 5 minutes for up to three doses. If drug doesn't provide relief, immediately notify prescriber.
• If patient complains of tingling sensation with S.L. form, place tablet in buccal pouch.
• When giving translingual aerosol form, make sure patient doesn't inhale spray. Release it onto or under tongue, and have patient wait about 10 seconds or so before swallowing.

• To apply ointment, measure prescribed amount on application paper, and then place paper on any nonhairy area. Don't rub in. Cover with plastic film to aid absorption and protect clothing.
• If using Tape-Surrounded Appli-Ruler (TSAR) system, keep TSAR on skin to protect patient's clothing and to make sure that ointment remains in place.
• Remove excess ointment from previous site before applying next dose. Avoid getting ointment on fingers.
• Apply transdermal forms to any nonhairy area, except lower parts of arms or legs, to promote maximum absorption.
⊛ **ALERT:** Remove transdermal patch before defibrillation. Electric current may cause patch to arc, causing burn to patient or damage to paddles.
• When stopping transdermal therapy for angina, gradually reduce dosage and frequency of application over 4 to 6 weeks.
• If drug is ineffective, immediately notify prescriber and keep patient at rest.
• Drug may cause headache, especially at start of therapy. Lower the dose temporarily. Tolerance to drug without headache response may develop. Treat headache with aspirin or acetaminophen.
• Minimize drug tolerance with 10- to 12-hour daily nitrate-free interval. For example, remove transdermal system in early evening and apply a new system the next morning. Or omit the last daily dose of buccal, sustained-release, or ointment form. If tolerance is suspected, alter dosage.
⊛ **ALERT:** Don't confuse Nitro-Bid with Nicobid.
⊛ **ALERT:** Don't confuse nitroglycerin with nitroprusside.

Patient teaching
• Teach patient how to use prescribed form of drug.
• Tell patient to place transmucosal tablet between lip and gum above incisors, or between cheek and gum. Tablet should be allowed to dissolve slowly over 3 to 5 hours. If tablet is inadvertently swallowed, tell patient to replace it.
• Tell patient to swallow oral tablets whole and not to chew them.
• Instruct patient to take drug regularly, as prescribed, and to have it accessible at all times.
• Tell patient that abruptly stopping the drug causes coronary vasospasm.

Reactions may be *common*, uncommon, *life-threatening*, or COMMON AND LIFE-THREATENING.

• Inform patient that an additional dose may be taken before anticipated stress or at bedtime if angina is nocturnal.
• Instruct patient to use caution when wearing transdermal patch near microwave oven. Leaking radiation may heat metallic backing of patch and cause burns.
• Advise patient not to drink alcohol during therapy.
• Tell patient to change to upright position slowly. Advise him to go up and down stairs carefully and to lie down at first sign of dizziness.
• Urge patient to store drug in cool, dark place in tightly closed container. To ensure potency, tell him to replace S.L. tablets 6 months after opening (mark bottle with date opened), and to remove cotton because it absorbs drug.
• Tell patient to store S.L. tablets in original container or other container specifically approved for this use and to carry container in jacket pocket or purse, not in a pocket close to body.

☑ **Evaluation**
• Patient reports pain relief.
• Patient sustains no injury from adverse reactions.
• Patient and family state understanding of drug therapy.

HIGH ALERT

nitroprusside sodium
(nigh-troh-PRUHS-ighd SOH-dee-um)
Nipride ♦ , Nitropress

Pharmacologic class: vasodilator
Therapeutic class: antihypertensive
Pregnancy risk category: C

Indications and dosages

▶ **To lower blood pressure quickly in hypertensive emergencies; to produce controlled hypotension during anesthesia; to reduce preload and afterload in cardiac pump failure or cardiogenic shock (may be used with or without dopamine).** *Adults:* Begin infusion at 0.25 to 0.3 mcg/kg/minute I.V. and gradually titrate every few minutes to a maximum infusion rate of 10 mcg/kg/minute. Average dose is 3 mcg/kg/minute. Patients taking other antihypertensives are extremely sensitive to nitroprusside. Adjust dosage.

▼ **I.V. administration**

• Dissolve 50 mg in 2 to 3 ml of D_5W injection. Further dilute in 250, 500, or 1,000 ml of D_5W to provide solutions of 200, 100, or 50 mcg/ml, respectively. Reconstitute ADD-Vantage vials labeled as containing 50 mg of drug according to manufacturer's directions.
• Because drug is sensitive to light, wrap infusion bag in foil; wrapping the tubing isn't needed.
• Infuse with infusion pump. Drug is best given by piggyback through peripheral line with no other drug. Don't adjust rate of main line while drug is being infused. Even small bolus of nitroprusside can cause severe hypotension.
• Check blood pressure every 5 minutes at start of infusion and every 15 minutes thereafter.
• If severe hypotension occurs, stop infusion. Effects of drug reverse quickly. Notify prescriber.
• Start arterial pressure line. Adjust flow to specified level.
• If cyanide toxicity occurs, stop drug immediately and notify prescriber.
• Fresh solution will have faint brownish tint. Discard drug after 24 hours.
⊗ **Incompatibilities**
Bacteriostatic water for injection, other I.V. drug, or preservative.

Contraindications and cautions

• Contraindicated in patients hypersensitive to the drug or any of its components, and in those with compensatory hypertension (as in arteriovenous shunt or coarctation of aorta), inadequate cerebral circulation, congenital optic atrophy, or tobacco-induced amblyopia.
• Use cautiously in patients with increased intracranial pressure and in those with hypothyroidism, hepatic or renal disease, hyponatremia, or low vitamin B_{12} level.
⚖ **Lifespan:** In pregnant women, use cautiously. In breast-feeding women and in children, safety and effectiveness haven't been established.

Adverse reactions

CNS: absent reflexes, ataxia, ***coma***, dilated pupils, *dizziness, headache, **increased intracranial pressure,*** loss of consciousness, *muscle twitching, restlessness.*
CV: *bradycardia,* distant heart sounds, *hypotension,* palpitations, tachycardia, weak pulse.

N

GI: abdominal pain, nausea, vomiting.
Hematologic: *methemoglobinemia.*
Metabolic: *acidosis.*
Respiratory: dyspnea, shallow breathing.
Skin: *diaphoresis,* pink color.
Other: *cyanide toxicity, thiocyanate toxicity.*

Interactions

Drug-drug. *Antihypertensives:* May cause sensitivity to nitroprusside. Adjust dosage.
Ganglionic blockers, general anesthetics, negative inotropics, other antihypertensives: May have additive effects. Monitor blood pressure closely.
Sildenafil, tadalafil, vardenafil: May increase hypotensive effects. Don't use together.
Tricyclic antidepressants: May increase the pressor response and cause arrhythmias. Use with caution.

Effects on lab test results

• May increase creatinine, thiocyanide, and methemoglobin levels.

Pharmacokinetics

Absorption: Given I.V.
Distribution: Unknown.
Metabolism: Rapid in erythrocytes and tissues to cyanide radical and then converted to thiocyanate in liver.
Excretion: Mainly as metabolites in urine.
Half-life: 2 minutes.

Route	Onset	Peak	Duration
I.V.	Immediate	1–2 min	10 min

Action

Chemical effect: Relaxes arteriolar and venous smooth muscle.
Therapeutic effect: Lowers blood pressure and reduces preload and afterload.

Available forms

Injection: 50 mg/vial in 2-ml, 5-ml vials

NURSING PROCESS

⚖ Assessment
• Assess patient's condition before starting therapy.
• Obtain baseline vital signs before giving drug, and find out what parameters prescriber wants to achieve.

⑤ **ALERT:** Excessive doses or rapid infusion (greater than 15 mcg/kg/minute) can cause cyanide toxicity; check thiocyanate levels every 72 hours. Levels above 100 mcg/ml may cause toxicity. Watch for profound hypotension, metabolic acidosis, dyspnea, headache, loss of consciousness, ataxia, and vomiting.
• Be alert for adverse reactions and drug interactions.
• Assess patient's (if appropriate) and family's knowledge of drug therapy.

⊕ Nursing diagnoses
• Risk for injury related to hypertension
• Decreased cardiac output related to heart failure
• Deficient knowledge related to drug therapy

▷ Planning and implementation
• Keep patient in supine position when starting therapy or adjusting dose.
⑤ **ALERT:** Don't confuse nitroprusside with nitroglycerin.
Patient teaching
• Advise patient, if alert, to report adverse reactions or discomfort at the I.V. site immediately.

☑ Evaluation
• Patient's blood pressure is normal.
• Patient has normal cardiac output.
• Patient and family state understanding of drug therapy.

nizatidine
(ny-ZAT-ih-deen)
Axid, Axid AR†

Pharmacologic class: histamine$_2$ (H$_2$)-receptor antagonist
Therapeutic class: gastric antisecretory
Pregnancy risk category: B

Indications and dosages

▶ **Active duodenal ulcer.** *Adults:* 300 mg P.O. daily at bedtime. Or, 150 mg P.O. b.i.d.
▶ **Maintenance therapy for duodenal ulcer.** *Adults:* 150 mg P.O. daily at bedtime.
▶ **Benign gastric ulcer.** *Adults:* 150 mg P.O. b.i.d. or 300 mg P.O. at bedtime for 8 weeks.
▶ **Gastroesophageal reflux disease.** *Adults:* 150 mg P.O. b.i.d.

Reactions may be *common,* uncommon, *life-threatening*, or COMMON AND LIFE-THREATENING.

▶ **Relief or prevention of heartburn†.** *Adults:* 75-mg tablet 1 to 2 times daily.

⩔ **Adjust-a-dose:** For patients with renal impairment, if creatinine clearance is 20 to 50 ml/minute, give 150 mg P.O. daily for active duodenal ulcer or 150 mg every other day for maintenance therapy. If creatinine clearance is less than 20 ml/minute, give 150 mg P.O. every other day for active ulcer or 150 mg every third day for maintenance.

Contraindications and cautions

• Contraindicated in patients hypersensitive to H_2-receptor antagonists.
• Use cautiously in patients with renal impairment.
⚖ **Lifespan:** In pregnant women, use cautiously. In breast-feeding women, use cautiously; it's unknown if the drug appears in breast milk. In children, safety and effectiveness haven't been established.

Adverse reactions

CNS: fever, *somnolence.*
CV: *arrhythmias.*
Hematologic: *thrombocytopenia.*
Hepatic: *liver damage.*
Metabolic: hyperuricemia.
Skin: *diaphoresis,* exfoliative dermatitis, rash, urticaria.

Interactions

Drug-drug. *Aspirin:* May increase salicylate level (with high doses). Monitor patient for salicylate toxicity.
Drug-lifestyle. *Alcohol use:* May increase alcohol level. Discourage use together.

Effects on lab test results

• May increase liver enzyme and uric acid levels.
• May decrease platelet count.
• May cause false-positive test results for urobilinogen.

Pharmacokinetics

Absorption: Greater than 90%. May be slightly enhanced by food and slightly impaired by antacids.
Distribution: About 35% protein-bound.
Metabolism: Unknown, but may undergo hepatic metabolism.

Excretion: More than 90% excreted in urine; less than 6% in feces. *Half-life:* 1 to 2 hours.

Route	Onset	Peak	Duration
P.O.	≤ 30 min	30 min–3 hr	≤ 12 hr

Action

Chemical effect: Competitively inhibits action of H_2 at receptor sites of parietal cells.
Therapeutic effect: Decreases gastric acid secretion.

Available forms

Capsules: 75 mg†, 150 mg, 300 mg
Oral solution: 15 mg/ml
Tablets: 75 mg

NURSING PROCESS

🕮 **Assessment**
• Assess patient's condition before starting therapy and regularly thereafter to monitor drug effectiveness.
• Be alert for adverse reactions and drug interactions.
• Assess patient for abdominal pain. Note presence of blood in emesis, stool, or gastric aspirate.
• Assess patient's and family's knowledge of drug therapy.

✛ **Nursing diagnoses**
• Impaired tissue integrity related to ulceration of GI mucosa
• Decreased cardiac output related to drug-induced arrhythmias
• Deficient knowledge related to drug therapy

▶ **Planning and implementation**
• If needed, open capsules and mix contents with apple juice.
Patient teaching
• Urge patient not to smoke cigarettes because they may increase gastric acid secretion and worsen disease.
• Have patient report blood in stool or emesis.
• Warn patient to take drug as directed, even after pain subsides, to allow for adequate healing.
• Instruct users of OTC dose to report worsening symptoms to provider and not to exceed recommended dose without provider instruction.

N

☑ **Evaluation**
• Patient reports pain relief.
• Patient maintains normal cardiac output throughout drug therapy.
• Patient and family state understanding of drug therapy.

HIGH ALERT

norepinephrine bitartrate (levarterenol bitartrate, noradrenaline acid tartrate)
(nor-ep-ih-NEF-rin bigh-TAR-trayt)
Levophed

Pharmacologic class: adrenergic
Therapeutic class: vasopressor
Pregnancy risk category: C

Indications and dosages

▶ **To restore blood pressure in severe hypotension, shock, and during cardiac arrest.**
Adults: Initially, 8 to 12 mcg/minute by I.V. infusion, adjust to maintain low normal blood pressure (systolic blood pressure 80 to 100 mm Hg). Or 0.5 to 1 mcg/minute I.V. infusion, titrate to effect. Average maintenance dosage is 2 to 4 mcg/minute.
Children: 2 mcg/m²/minute or 2 mcg/minute by I.V. infusion; adjust dosage based on patient response. Or, initial I.V. infusion rate of 0.1 to 2 mcg/kg/minute, titrate to effect.

▶ **GI bleeding‡.** *Adults:* Give 8 mg in 250 ml normal saline solution intraperitoneally. Or give 8 mg in 100 ml of normal saline solution by NG tube every 1 hour for 6 to 8 hours and then every 2 hours for 4 to 6 hours. Frequency gradually reduced until discontinued.

▽ I.V. administration

• Prepare by adding 4 mg of drug to 1 L of 5% dextrose injection to equal a concentration of 4 mcg/ml.
• Never leave patient unattended during infusion.
• Use central venous catheter or large vein, such as in antecubital fossa, to minimize risk of extravasation. Dilute in dextrose 5% in normal saline solution for injection. Use continuous infusion pump to regulate flow rate and piggyback setup so I.V. line remains open if drug is stopped.

• Titrate infusion rate according to assessment findings and prescriber's guidelines. In previously hypertensive patients, don't raise blood pressure higher than 30 to 40 mm Hg below previous systolic pressure.
• Check site often for blanching and other signs of extravasation. If they occur, change infusion site immediately and call prescriber. Counteract effect by infiltrating area with 5 to 10 mg phentolamine and 10 to 15 ml of normal saline solution. Untreated extravasation can lead to tissue necrosis.
• If prolonged I.V. therapy is needed, change injection site often.
• Protect drug from light. Discard discolored solutions or solutions that contain precipitate. Drug solutions deteriorate after 24 hours.
⊗ **Incompatibilities**
Alkaline solutions, aminophylline, amobarbital, chlorothiazide, chlorpheniramine, iron salts, lidocaine, normal saline solution, oxidizing drugs, pentobarbital sodium, phenobarbital sodium, phenytoin sodium, ranitidine hydrochloride, sodium bicarbonate, streptomycin, thiopental, whole blood.

Contraindications and cautions

• Contraindicated in patients receiving cyclopropane or halothane anesthesia and in patients with mesenteric or peripheral vascular thrombosis, profound hypoxia, hypercapnia, or hypotension caused by blood volume deficits.
• Use cautiously in patients receiving MAO inhibitors, tricyclic antidepressants, or certain antihistamines and in patients with sulfite sensitivity.
⚠ **Lifespan:** In pregnant and breast-feeding women, drug is contraindicated. Use cautiously in elderly patients because of increased risk of vasoconstrictive adverse reactions.

Adverse reactions

CNS: anxiety, dizziness, fever, *headache,* insomnia, restlessness, tremor, weakness.
CV: *arrhythmias, bradycardia, decreased cardiac output,* marked increase in peripheral resistance, *severe hypertension.*
GU: decreased urine output.
Metabolic: hyperglycemia, increased glycogenolysis, *metabolic acidosis.*
Respiratory: *asthmatic episodes, respiratory difficulties.*

Reactions may be *common,* uncommon, *life-threatening,* or COMMON AND LIFE-THREATENING.

Other: *anaphylaxis,* swelling and enlargement of thyroid, tissue sloughing with extravasation.

Interactions

Drug-drug. *Alpha blockers:* May antagonize drug effects. Monitor patient.
Antihistamines, ergot alkaloids, guanethidine, methyldopa: May cause severe hypertension. Don't give together.
Bretylium: May cause arrhythmias. Monitor ECG closely.
Inhaled anesthetics: May increase risk of arrhythmias. Monitor ECG closely.
MAO inhibitors: May increase risk of hypertensive crisis. Monitor patient closely.
Tricyclic antidepressants: May increase the pressor response and cause arrhythmias. Use with caution.

Effects on lab test results

• May increase glucose level.

Pharmacokinetics

Absorption: Given I.V.
Distribution: Drug localizes in sympathetic nerve tissues.
Metabolism: Metabolized in liver and other tissues to inactive compounds.
Excretion: Excreted in urine. *Half-life:* About 1 minute.

Route	Onset	Peak	Duration
I.V.	Immediate	Immediate	1–2 min

Action

Chemical effect: Stimulates alpha- and beta$_1$-adrenergic receptors in sympathetic nervous system.
Therapeutic effect: Raises blood pressure.

Available forms

Injection: 1 mg/ml in 4-ml ampules

NURSING PROCESS

🔲 Assessment
• Assess patient's condition before starting therapy.
• During infusion, frequently monitor ECG, cardiac output, central venous pressure, pulmonary capillary wedge pressure, pulse rate, urine output, and color and temperature of limbs.

Also, check blood pressure every 2 minutes until stabilized; then check every 5 minutes.
• Be alert for adverse reactions and drug interactions.
• Monitor vital signs closely when therapy ends. Watch for sudden drop in blood pressure.
• Assess patient's and family's knowledge of drug therapy.

🔲 Nursing diagnoses
• Decreased cardiac output related to hypotension
• Risk for injury related to drug-induced adverse reactions
• Deficient knowledge related to drug therapy

🔲 Planning and implementation
• Drug isn't a substitute for blood or fluid volume deficit. If deficit exists, replace fluid before giving vasopressors.
• Keep emergency drugs on hand to reverse effects of norepinephrine: atropine for reflex bradycardia, phentolamine for injection to treat extravasation, and propranolol for arrhythmias.
• Immediately report to prescriber any decrease in urine output.
• When stopping drug, gradually slow infusion rate and report sudden drop in blood pressure.
Patient teaching
• Tell patient to immediately report discomfort at infusion site or difficulty breathing.

🔲 Evaluation
• Patient has normal cardiac output.
• Patient sustains no injuries from drug-induced adverse reactions.
• Patient and family state understanding of drug therapy.

N

norethindrone
(nor-ETH-in-drohn)
Camila, Errin, Jolivette, Micronor, Nora-BE, Nor-QD

norethindrone acetate
Aygestin

Pharmacologic class: progestin
Therapeutic class: contraceptive
Pregnancy risk category: X

Indications and dosages

▶ **Amenorrhea, abnormal uterine bleeding.**
Women: 2.5 to 10 mg norethindrone acetate P.O. daily for 5 to 10 days during second half of the theoretical menstrual cycle.
▶ **Endometriosis.** *Women:* 5 mg norethindrone acetate P.O. daily for 14 days; then increase by 2.5 mg daily every 2 weeks up to 15 mg daily.
▶ **To prevent pregnancy.** *Women:* Initially, 0.35 mg norethindrone P.O. on first day of menstruation; then 0.35 mg daily.

Contraindications and cautions

• Contraindicated in patients hypersensitive to the drug or any of its components; patients with thrombophlebitis, thromboembolic disorders, cerebrovascular insufficiency, or a history of these conditions; and patients with breast cancer, undiagnosed abnormal vaginal bleeding, severe hepatic disease, or missed abortion.
• Use cautiously in patients with diabetes mellitus, seizure disorder, migraine, cardiac or renal disease, asthma, or depression.
⚠ **Lifespan:** In pregnant women, drug is contraindicated. Breast-feeding woman may start taking progestin-only pills 6 weeks after delivery. A woman who is partially breast-feeding (supplementing with formula) can start taking drug by 3 weeks after delivery. In children, safety and effectiveness haven't been established.

Adverse reactions

CNS: depression, dizziness, lethargy, migraine, stroke.
CV: *edema*, hypertension, *pulmonary embolism, thromboembolism*, thrombophlebitis.
GI: abdominal cramps, nausea, vomiting.
GU: abnormal secretions, amenorrhea, breakthrough bleeding, cervical erosion, dysmenorrhea, uterine fibromas, vaginal candidiasis.
Hepatic: cholestatic jaundice.
Metabolic: hyperglycemia, weight changes.
Skin: acne, hirsutism, melasma, rash.
Other: breast tenderness, enlargement, or secretion; decreased libido.

Interactions

Drug-drug. *Barbiturates, carbamazepine, rifampin:* May decrease progestin effects. Monitor patient for lack of effect.
Bromocriptine: May cause amenorrhea, thus interfering with bromocriptine effects. Avoid use together.

Drug-food. *Caffeine:* May increase caffeine level. Monitor patient for caffeine effects.
Drug-lifestyle. *Smoking:* May increase risk of CV effects. If patient continues smoking, may need alternative therapy.

Effects on lab test results

• May increase glucose level.
• May increase liver function test values. May decrease T_3 uptake and glucose tolerance.

Pharmacokinetics

Absorption: Well absorbed from GI tract.
Distribution: Distributed widely. About 80% protein-bound.
Metabolism: Metabolized mainly in liver; undergoes extensive first-pass metabolism.
Excretion: Excreted primarily in feces. *Half-life:* 5 to 14 hours.

Route	Onset	Peak	Duration
P.O.	Unknown	1–2 hr	Unknown

Action

Chemical effect: Suppresses ovulation, possibly by inhibiting pituitary gonadotropin secretion, and forms thick cervical mucus.
Therapeutic effect: Prevents pregnancy and relieves symptoms of endometriosis, amenorrhea, and abnormal uterine bleeding.

Available forms

norethindrone
Tablets: 0.35 mg, 0.5 mg
norethindrone acetate
Tablets: 5 mg

NURSING PROCESS

⚗ Assessment
• Assess patient's condition before starting therapy and regularly thereafter to monitor drug effectiveness.
• Be alert for adverse reactions and drug interactions.
• Assess patient's and family's knowledge of drug therapy.
• Monitor blood pressure and edema.

⊕ Nursing diagnoses
• Ineffective health maintenance related to underlying condition

---

- Excess fluid volume related to drug-induced edema
- Deficient knowledge related to drug therapy

> **Planning and implementation**

⊛ **ALERT:** Norethindrone acetate is twice as potent as norethindrone. Don't use as contraception.
- Preliminary estrogen therapy is usually needed by patients with menstrual disorders.

⊛ **ALERT:** If visual disturbance, migraine, or headache occurs or if pulmonary emboli are suspected, withhold drug, notify prescriber, and provide supportive care.

⊛ **ALERT:** Don't confuse Micronor with Micro-K or Micronase.

Patient teaching
- If switching from combined hormonal contraceptives to progestin-only pill (POP), tell patient to take the first POP the day after the last active combined pill.
- If switching from POPs to combined pills, tell patient to take the first active combined pill on the first day of menstruation, even if the POPs pack isn't finished.
- Explain adverse effects of progestin and have patient read package insert before taking first dose.
- Tell patient to take drug at same time each day when used as a contraceptive. If she is more than 3 hours late or has missed a pill, tell her to take pill as soon as she remembers, to continue with her normal schedule, and to use backup contraception for the next 48 hours.
- Instruct patient to immediately report unusual symptoms such as prolonged episodes of bleeding, amenorrhea, or severe abdominal pain. Tell her to stop taking the drug and call prescriber if visual disturbance or migraine occurs.
- Teach patient how to perform routine monthly breast self-examination.
- Warn patient that edema and weight gain are likely. Advise her to restrict sodium intake.

☑ **Evaluation**
- Patient responds well to therapy.
- Patient's drug-induced edema is minimized with sodium restriction.
- Patient and family state understanding of drug therapy.

norfloxacin
(nor-FLOKS-uh-sin)
Noroxin

Pharmacologic class: fluoroquinolone
Therapeutic class: broad-spectrum antibiotic
Pregnancy risk category: C

Indications and dosages

▶ **UTI caused by susceptible strains of** *Escherichia coli, Enterococcus faecalis, Klebsiella, Enterobacter, Proteus, Pseudomonas aeruginosa, Citrobacter, Staphylococcus aureus, Staphylococcus epidermidis,* **and group D** *streptococci. Adults:* For uncomplicated infections, 400 mg P.O. b.i.d. for 7 to 10 days. For complicated infections, 400 mg b.i.d. for 10 to 21 days.

▶ **UTI caused by** *E. coli, K. pneumoniae,* **or** *Proteus mirabilis. Adults:* 400 mg P.O. b.i.d. for 3 days.

▶ **Acute, uncomplicated gonorrhea.** *Adults:* 800 mg P.O. as single dose, followed by doxycycline therapy to treat coexisting chlamydial infection.

▶ **Prostatitis from** *E. coli. Men:* 400 mg P.O. every 12 hours for 28 days.

▶ **Gastroenteritis‡.** *Adults:* 400 mg P.O. b.i.d. for 5 days.

▶ **Traveler's diarrhea‡.** *Adults:* 400 mg P.O. b.i.d. for 3 days.

◳ **Adjust-a-dose:** For patients with renal impairment, if creatinine clearance is less than 30 ml/minute, give 400 mg once daily.

Contraindications and cautions

- Contraindicated in patients hypersensitive to fluoroquinolones. Contraindicated in patients with a history of tendonitis or tendon rupture associated with fluoroquinolones.
- Use cautiously in patients with conditions that may predispose them to seizure disorders, such as cerebral arteriosclerosis and epilepsy.

※ **Lifespan:** In pregnant women, breast-feeding women, adolescents, and children, safety and effectiveness haven't been established.

Adverse reactions

CNS: asthenia, dizziness, fatigue, fever, headache, *seizures,* somnolence.

N

GI: constipation, dry mouth, flatulence, heartburn, nausea.
GU: crystalluria.
Hematologic: eosinophilia.
Musculoskeletal: arthralgia, arthritis, joint swelling, myalgia.
Skin: photosensitivity reaction, rash.
Other: *anaphylactoid reactions,* hypersensitivity reaction, rash.

Interactions

Drug-drug. *Aluminum hydroxide, aluminum-magnesium hydroxide, calcium carbonate, magnesium hydroxide, multivitamins, or other products containing iron or zinc:* May decrease effects of norfloxacin. Give antacid at least 6 hours before or 2 hours after norfloxacin.
Antacids, sucralfate: May interfere with absorption. Give at least 2 hours apart.
Cimetidine: May interfere with norfloxacin elimination. Use cautiously.
Cyclosporine: May increase cyclosporine level. Monitor level.
Didanosine: May decrease norfloxacin absorption. Avoid use together.
Iron salts: May decrease norfloxacin absorption, reducing anti-infective response. Give at least 2 hours apart.
Nitrofurantoin: May decrease norfloxacin effectiveness. Don't use together.
NSAIDs: May increase risk of CNS stimulation and seizures. Monitor patient closely.
Oral anticoagulants: May increase anticoagulant effect. Monitor patient closely for bleeding; monitor PT and INR.
Probenecid: May increase norfloxacin level by decreasing its excretion. Monitor patient for toxicity.
Sucralfate: May decrease norfloxacin absorption, reducing anti-infective response. If use together can't be avoided, give at least 6 hours apart.
Theophylline: May impair theophylline metabolism, resulting in increased theophylline level and risk of toxicity. Monitor theophylline level closely.
Warfarin: May increase anticoagulant effect. Monitor patient and INR closely.
Drug-food. *Any food:* May decrease drug absorption. Give drug 1 hour before or 2 hours after meals or ingestion of milk or other dairy products.
Caffeine: May increase caffeine effects. Discourage caffeine use.

Drug-lifestyle. *Sunlight:* May cause photosensitivity reaction. Urge patient to avoid unprotected or prolonged sun exposure.

Effects on lab test results

• May increase BUN, creatinine, ALT, AST, and alkaline phosphatase levels. May decrease hemoglobin level and hematocrit.
• May increase eosinophil count. May decrease neutrophil count.

Pharmacokinetics

Absorption: About 30% to 40%. As dose increases, percentage absorbed decreases. Food and dairy products may reduce absorption.
Distribution: Into renal tissue, liver, gallbladder, prostatic fluid, testicles, seminal fluid, bile, and sputum. About 10% to 15% protein-bound.
Metabolism: Unknown.
Excretion: Mostly excreted by kidneys with about 30% appearing in feces. *Half-life:* 3 to 4 hours.

Route	Onset	Peak	Duration
P.O.	Unknown	1–2 hr	Unknown

Action

Chemical effect: Inhibits bacterial DNA synthesis, mainly by blocking DNA gyrase.
Therapeutic effect: Kills certain bacteria.

Available forms

Tablets: 400 mg

NURSING PROCESS

Assessment
• Assess patient's infection before starting therapy and regularly thereafter to monitor drug effectiveness.
• Obtain a sample for culture and sensitivity tests before starting therapy, and repeat as needed throughout therapy. May begin therapy pending test results.
• Be alert for adverse reactions and drug interactions.
• Assess patient's and family's knowledge of drug therapy.

Nursing diagnoses
• Risk for infection related to bacteria
• Risk for injury related to drug-induced adverse CNS reactions

---

Reactions may be *common,* uncommon, **life-threatening**, or COMMON AND LIFE-THREATENING.

• Deficient knowledge related to drug therapy

▷ Planning and implementation
• Give drug on empty stomach.
• Make sure patient is well hydrated before and during therapy to avoid crystalluria.
⊕ **ALERT:** Don't confuse Noroxin with Neurontin or Floxin.
Patient teaching
• Urge patient to take drug 1 hour before or 2 hours after meals to promote absorption.
• Warn patient not to exceed recommended dosage.
• Encourage patient to drink several glasses of water throughout the day to maintain hydration and adequate urine output.
• Warn patient to avoid hazardous activities until the drug's CNS effects are known.

☑ Evaluation
• Patient is free from infection.
• Patient has no injuries from drug-induced adverse CNS reactions.
• Patient and family state understanding of drug therapy.

nortriptyline hydrochloride
(nor-TRIP-teh-leen high-droh-KLOR-ighd)
Aventyl*, Pamelor*✐

Pharmacologic class: tricyclic antidepressant
Therapeutic class: antidepressant
Pregnancy risk category: D

Indications and dosages
▶ **Depression.** *Adults:* 25 mg P.O. t.i.d. or q.i.d.; gradually increase up to maximum of 150 mg daily. Or entire dosage may be given at bedtime.
▶ **Premenstrual symptoms**‡. *Adults:* 50 to 125 mg daily.
▶ **Dermatologic disorders (chronic urticaria, angioedema, nocturnal pruritus in atopic eczema)**‡. *Adults:* 20 to 75 mg/day.
⊠ **Adjust-a-dose:** For elderly and adolescent patients, give 30 mg to 50 mg P.O. once daily or in divided doses.

Contraindications and cautions
• Contraindicated in patients hypersensitive to the drug or any of its components, patients in acute recovery phase after MI, and patients who have taken an MAO inhibitor within 14 days.
• Use cautiously in patients taking thyroid drugs and patients with glaucoma, suicidal tendency, history of urine retention or seizures, CV disease, or hyperthyroidism.
⚘ **Lifespan:** In pregnant women, breast-feeding women, and children, don't use unless benefits outweigh risks. In elderly patients, use cautiously and at a lower dose.

Adverse reactions
CNS: confusion, *dizziness, drowsiness,* EEG changes, excitation, extrapyramidal reactions, headache, nervousness, **seizures, stroke, suicidal ideation,** tremor, weakness.
CV: ECG changes, **heart block,** hypertension, MI, tachycardia.
EENT: *blurred vision,* mydriasis, tinnitus.
GI: anorexia, *constipation,* dry mouth, nausea, paralytic ileus, vomiting.
GU: urine retention.
Hematologic: *agranulocytosis, bone marrow depression,* eosinophilia, *thrombocytopenia.*
Skin: diaphoresis, photosensitivity, rash, urticaria.
Other: hypersensitivity reaction.

Interactions
Drug-drug. *Anticholinergics:* May increase anticholinergic effect. Paralytic ileus may occur. Monitor patient.
Barbiturates, CNS depressants: May increase CNS depression. Avoid use together.
Bupropion, cimetidine, methylphenidate, SSRIs, valproic acid: May increase nortriptyline level. Monitor patient for adverse reactions.
Carbamazepine: May increase nortriptyline and carbamazepine levels, leading to toxicity. Use with caution.
Clonidine: May cause loss of blood pressure control with potentially life-threatening increases in blood pressure. Don't use together.
Epinephrine, norepinephrine: May increase hypertensive effect. Use together cautiously; monitor blood pressure.
MAO inhibitors: May cause severe excitation, hyperpyrexia, or seizures. Don't use together.
Quinolones: May increase the risk of life-threatening arrhythmias, including torsades de pointes. Don't use together.
Rifamycin: May decrease nortriptyline level. Monitor it for decreased effect.

Drug-herb. *SAMe, St. John's wort, yohimbe:* Use with some tricyclic antidepressants may increase serotonin levels. Discourage use together.
Drug-lifestyle. *Alcohol use:* May increase CNS depression. Discourage use together.
Smoking: May decrease nortriptyline level. Monitor patient for lack of drug effect.
Sun exposure: May increase risk of photosensitivity reaction. Urge patient to avoid unprotected or prolonged exposure to sunlight.

Effects on lab test results

• May increase or decrease glucose level.
• May increase liver function test values and eosinophil count. May decrease RBC, WBC, granulocyte, and platelet counts.

Pharmacokinetics

Absorption: No information available.
Distribution: Distributed widely into body, including CNS. 95% protein-bound.
Metabolism: Metabolized by liver; significant first-pass effect may account for variability of levels in different patients taking same dosage.
Excretion: One third of a dose is excreted in urine as metabolites; some in feces. *Half-life:* 16 to more than 90 hours.

Route	Onset	Peak	Duration
P.O.	Unknown	7–8½ hr	16–90 hr

Action

Chemical effect: Unknown; increases amount of norepinephrine, serotonin, or both in CNS by blocking their reuptake by presynaptic neurons.
Therapeutic effect: Relieves depression.

Available forms

Capsules: 10 mg, 25 mg, 50 mg, 75 mg
Oral solution: 10 mg/5 ml*
Tablets: 10 mg ◇, 25 mg ◇

NURSING PROCESS

Assessment

• Assess patient's depression before starting therapy and regularly thereafter to monitor drug effectiveness.
• Be alert for adverse reactions and drug interactions.
• If dosage is greater than 100 mg/day, monitor drug level and maintain a range of 50 to 150 nanograms/ml.

• Assess patient's and family's knowledge of drug therapy.

Nursing diagnoses

• Disturbed thought processes related to depression
• Risk for injury related to drug-induced adverse CNS reactions
• Deficient knowledge related to drug therapy

Planning and implementation

• Lower the dosage in elderly or debilitated patient.
ALERT: Drug may increase the risk of suicidal thinking and behavior in young adults ages 18 to 24 during the first 2 months of treatment. Monitor patient closely.
ALERT: Stopping long-term therapy abruptly may cause nausea, headache, and malaise.
ALERT: Because hypertensive episodes may occur during surgery in patients receiving tricyclic antidepressants, gradually stop therapy starting several days before surgery.
• If signs of psychosis occur or increase, reduce dosage.
ALERT: Don't confuse nortriptyline with amitriptyline.
Patient teaching
• Advise patient to take full dose at bedtime to reduce risk of orthostatic hypotension.
• Warn patient to avoid hazardous activities until CNS effects of drug are known. Drowsiness and dizziness usually subside after a few weeks.
• Tell patient to avoid alcohol during drug therapy.
• Advise patient and family to watch for mood changes and suicidal tendencies and to report these to prescriber immediately.
• Warn patient not to stop drug suddenly.
• Advise patient to consult prescriber before taking other prescription or OTC drugs.
• Advise patient to use sun block, wear protective clothing, and avoid prolonged exposure to sunlight to avoid photosensitivity.

Evaluation

• Patient's depression improves.
• Patient sustains no injuries from drug-induced adverse CNS reactions.
• Patient and family state understanding of drug therapy.

---

nystatin
(ny-STAT-in)
Mycostatin, Nilstat, Nystop

Pharmacologic class: polyene macrolide
Therapeutic class: antifungal
Pregnancy risk category: C

Indications and dosages

▶ **GI tract infections.** *Adults:* 500,000 to
1 million units as oral tablets P.O. t.i.d.
▶ **Oral infections caused by *Candida albicans*
and other *Candida* species.** *Adults and children:* 400,000 to 600,000 units suspension
P.O. q.i.d. Or 200,000 or 400,000 units (1 or
2 lozenges) 4 or 5 times daily.
Infants: 200,000 units suspension P.O. q.i.d.
▶ **Vaginal infections.** *Adults:* 100,000 units, as
vaginal tablets, inserted high into vagina, daily
for 14 days.
▶ **Cutaneous or mucocutaneous yeast infections.** *Adults:* Apply topical products to affected
areas b.i.d. to t.i.d.
▶ **Candidal diaper dermatitis‡.** *Infants:*
100,000 units suspension P.O. q.i.d. as an adjunct to topical nystatin therapy.

Contraindications and cautions

● Contraindicated in patients hypersensitive to
the drug or any of its components.
⚠ **Lifespan:** In pregnant women, use only
when benefits outweigh risks to the fetus. In
breast-feeding women, safety and effectiveness
haven't been established.

Adverse reactions

GI: diarrhea, transient nausea, vomiting.
Skin: rash.

Interactions

None significant.

Effects on lab test results

None reported.

Pharmacokinetics

Absorption: Not absorbed from GI tract, intact
skin, or mucous membranes.
Distribution: None.
Metabolism: None.

Excretion: Oral form excreted almost entirely
unchanged in feces. *Half-life:* Unknown.

Route	Onset	Peak	Duration
P.O., topical, vaginal	Unknown	Unknown	Unknown

Action

Chemical effect: Unknown; probably acts by
binding to sterols in fungal cell membrane, altering cell permeability and allowing leakage of
intracellular components.
Therapeutic effect: Kills susceptible yeasts and
fungi.

Available forms

Cream/ointment/powder: 100,000 units/g
Lozenges: 200,000 units
Oral suspension: 100,000 units/ml*
Tablets: 500,000 units
Tablets (vaginal): 100,000 units

NURSING PROCESS

🔍 Assessment
● Assess patient's infection before starting therapy and regularly thereafter to monitor drug effectiveness.
● Be alert for adverse reactions.
● If patient has adverse GI reactions, monitor
his hydration.
● Assess patient's and family's knowledge of
drug therapy.

⊕ Nursing diagnoses
● Risk for infection related to organisms
● Risk for deficient fluid volume related to
drug-induced adverse GI reactions
● Deficient knowledge related to drug therapy

▶ Planning and implementation
● Drug isn't effective against systemic infections.
● Treatment should be continued at least
48 hours after symptoms have abated and cultures are normal.
● When treating oral candidiasis (thrush), clean
food debris from patient's mouth and have patient hold suspension in mouth for several minutes before swallowing.
● When treating an infant, swab drug on oral
mucosa.

N

- Immunosuppressed patients with oral candidiasis are sometimes instructed by prescriber to suck on vaginal tablets (100,000 units) because doing so provides prolonged contact with oral mucosa.
- Pregnant patients can use vaginal tablets up to 6 weeks before term to treat infection that may cause thrush in neonates.

Patient teaching
- Advise patient to take drug for at least 2 days after symptoms disappear to prevent reinfection. Consult prescriber for duration of therapy.
- Tell patient not to chew or swallow lozenge (troche) but to allow it to dissolve slowly in the mouth.
- Tell patient to premoisten oral mucosa and maintain adequate hydration when using lozenge (troche) formulation.
- Instruct patient to continue therapy during menstruation.
- Instruct patient in oral hygiene techniques. Poorly fitting dentures and overuse of mouthwash may alter oral flora and promote infection.
- Explain that predisposing factors for vaginal infection include use of antibiotics, hormonal contraceptives, and corticosteroids; diabetes; reinfection by sexual partner; and tight-fitting undergarments. Encourage patient to wear cotton (not synthetic) underpants.
- Teach patient about hygiene for affected areas, including wiping perineal area from front to back.
- Advise patient to report redness, swelling, or irritation.

☑ Evaluation
- Patient is free from infection.
- Patient maintains adequate hydration throughout drug therapy.
- Patient and family state understanding of drug therapy.

octreotide acetate
(ok-TREE-oh-tighd AS-ih-tayt)
Sandostatin, Sandostatin LAR Depot

Pharmacologic class: synthetic polypeptide
Therapeutic class: somatotropic hormone
Pregnancy risk category: B

Indications and dosages

▶ **Flushing and diarrhea caused by carcinoid tumors.** *Adults:* 100 to 600 mcg daily subcutaneously in two to four divided doses for first 2 weeks (usual daily dosage 300 mcg). Subsequent dosage based on patient's response. Patients currently on Sandostatin can switch to Sandostatin LAR Depot 20 mg I.M. to gluteal area every 4 weeks for 2 months. Immediate-release injection should be continued at the previous dosage during at least the first 2 weeks of therapy with the long-acting form.

▶ **Watery diarrhea caused by vasoactive intestinal polypeptide secreting tumors (VIPomas).** *Adults:* 200 to 300 mcg daily subcutaneously in two to four divided doses for first 2 weeks of therapy. Subsequent dosage based on individual response; typically doesn't exceed 450 mcg daily. Patients currently on Sandostatin can switch to Sandostatin LAR Depot 20 mg I.M. to gluteal area every 4 weeks for 2 months.

▶ **Acromegaly.** *Adults:* Initially, 50 mcg subcutaneously t.i.d.; then adjust by somatomedin C (IGF-1) or growth hormone (GH) level every 2 weeks. Or, multiple growth hormone levels at 0 to 8 hours after giving acetate form. Usual effective dosage, 100 mcg subcutaneously t.i.d. Some patients may need up to 500 mcg subcutaneously t.i.d., but dosages higher than 300 mg t.i.d. often add no benefits. Switch patients on Sandostatin to 20 mg Sandostatin LAR Depot I.M. to gluteal area every 4 weeks for 3 months.

▶ **GI fistula**‡. *Adults:* 0.05 to 0.2 mg subcutaneously every 8 hours.

▶ **Variceal bleeding**‡. *Adults:* 0.025 to 0.05 mg/hour continuous I.V. infusion. Duration is from 18 hours to 5 days.

▶ **AIDS-related diarrhea‡.** *Adults:* 0.1 to 0.5 mg subcutaneously t.i.d.
▶ **Short bowel (ileostomy) syndrome‡.** *Adults:* 0.025 mg/hour continuous I.V. infusion or 0.05 mg subcutaneously b.i.d.
▶ **Chemotherapy- and radiation-induced diarrhea‡.** *Adults:* 0.05 to 0.1 mg subcutaneously t.i.d. for 1 to 3 days.
▶ **Pancreatic fistula‡.** *Adults:* 0.05 to 0.2 mg subcutaneously every 8 hours.
▶ **Irritable bowel syndrome‡.** *Adults:* 0.1 mg single dose to 0.125 mg subcutaneously b.i.d.
▶ **Dumping syndrome‡.** *Adults:* 0.05 to 0.15 mg subcutaneously daily.

Contraindications and cautions

• Contraindicated in patients hypersensitive to the drug or any of its components.
✿ **Lifespan:** In pregnant women, use cautiously. In breast-feeding women and in children, safety and effectiveness haven't been established.

Adverse reactions

CNS: dizziness, fatigue, headache, lightheadedness, pain.
CV: *arrhythmias, bradycardia,* flushing.
GI: *abdominal pain or discomfort, diarrhea,* fat malabsorption, gallbladder abnormalities, loose stools, nausea, vomiting.
Metabolic: *hyperglycemia, hypoglycemia,* hypothyroidism.
Skin: edema, erythema, pain, and wheal at injection site.
Other: burning at subcutaneous injection site.

Interactions

Drug-drug. *Beta blockers, calcium channel blockers or drugs to control fluid and electrolyte balance, insulin, oral hypoglycemics:* May require dosage adjustments of these drugs. Monitor carefully.
Bromocriptine: May increase availability. Monitor patient.
Cyclosporine: May decrease cyclosporine level. Monitor patient.
Quinidine, terfenadine: May decrease metabolic clearance of CYP3A4. Use with caution.
Drug-food. *Dietary fats:* Drug may alter the absorption of dietary fats.
Vitamin B$_{12}$: May decrease vitamin B$_{12}$ level. Monitor level.

Effects on lab test results

• May decrease T4 and thyroid-stimulating hormone levels. May increase or decrease glucose level.

Pharmacokinetics

Absorption: Rapid and complete after subcutaneous use.
Distribution: To plasma, where it binds to lipoprotein and albumin.
Metabolism: Not clearly defined.
Excretion: About 32% unchanged in urine.
Half-life: About 1½ hours.

Route	Onset	Peak	Duration
I.M., SubQ	≤ 30 min	30–60 min	12 hr–6 wk

Action

Chemical effect: Mimics action of naturally occurring somatostatin.
Therapeutic effect: Relieves flushing and diarrhea caused by certain tumors and treats acromegaly.

Available forms

Depot: 10 mg/5 ml, 20 mg/5 ml, 30 mg/5 ml
Injection: 0.05-mg, 0.1-mg, 0.5-mg ampules; 0.2-mg/ml, 1-mg/ml multidose vials

NURSING PROCESS

✎ Assessment

• Assess patient's condition before starting therapy, and regularly thereafter to monitor the drug's effectiveness.
• Monitor IGF-1 or GH level every 2 weeks. Base dosage on this level.
• Monitor laboratory tests, such as thyroid function tests, urine 5-hydroxyindoleacetic acid, serotonin, substance P (for carcinoid tumors), and vasoactive intestinal peptide levels (for VIPomas), at baseline and then periodically.
• Monitor fluid and electrolyte levels.
• Be alert for adverse reactions and drug interactions.
• Assess patient's and family's knowledge of drug therapy.

⊞ Nursing diagnoses

• Diarrhea related to condition
• Fatigue related to drug-induced adverse CNS reaction
• Deficient knowledge related to drug therapy

▶ Planning and implementation
- Give drug in divided doses for first 2 weeks of therapy; subsequent daily dosage depends on patient's response.
- Read drug labels carefully, and check dosage and strength.
- ⊛ ALERT: For LAR Depot injection, give drug I.M. only. Avoid deltoid muscle because of discomfort at site.
- Drug therapy may alter fluid and electrolyte balance and may require adjustment of other drugs.
- Adjust LAR Depot dosage every 3 months based on GH level; range for depot dosage, 10 to 40 mg at intervals no sooner than 4 weeks.

Patient teaching
- Tell patient to report signs of gallbladder disease such as abdominal discomfort. Drug may be linked to cholelithiasis.
- Inform patient that laboratory tests are needed during therapy.
- Advise diabetic patient to monitor glucose level closely. Antidiabetics may need dosage adjustment.

☑ Evaluation
- Patient's bowel pattern is normal.
- Patient uses energy-saving measures to combat fatigue.
- Patient and family state understanding of drug therapy.

ofloxacin
(oh-FLOKS-eh-sin)
Floxin, Floxin Otic, Ocuflox

Pharmacologic class: fluoroquinolone
Therapeutic class: antibiotic
Pregnancy risk category: C

Indications and dosages

▶ **Lower respiratory tract infections caused by susceptible strains of** *Haemophilus influenzae* **or** *Streptococcus pneumoniae*. *Adults:* 400 mg P.O. every 12 hours for 10 days.

▶ **Cervicitis or urethritis caused by** *Chlamydia trachomatis* **or** *Neisseria gonorrhoeae*. *Adults:* 300 mg P.O. every 12 hours for 7 days.

▶ **Acute pelvic inflammatory disease.** *Adults:* 400 mg P.O. every 12 hours for 10 to 14 days.

▶ **Acute uncomplicated gonorrhea.** *Adults:* 400 mg P.O. as single dose.

▶ **Mild to moderate skin and skin-structure infections caused by susceptible strains of** *Staphylococcus aureus, Staphylococcus epidermidis, Streptococcus pyogenes,* **or** *Proteus mirabilis*. *Adults:* 400 mg P.O. every 12 hours for 10 days.

▶ **Cystitis caused by** *Escherichia coli* **or** *Klebsiella pneumoniae*. *Adults:* 200 mg P.O. every 12 hours for 3 days.

▶ **UTIs caused by susceptible strains of** *Citrobacter diversus, Enterobacter aerogenes, E. coli, P. mirabilis,* **or** *Pseudomonas aeruginosa*. *Adults:* 200 mg P.O. every 12 hours for 7 days. Complicated infections may need 10 days of therapy.

▶ **Prostatitis caused by** *E. coli*. *Adults:* 300 mg P.O. every 12 hours for 6 weeks.

▶ **Bacterial conjunctivitis.** *Adults and children age 1 year and older:* 1 or 2 drops every 2 to 4 hours in the affected eye on days 1 and 2, then 1 or 2 drops q.i.d. on days 3 through 7.

▶ **Otitis externa (swimmer's ear).** *Adults and children age 13 and older:* 10 drops (or 2 single-dispensing containers) into affected ear b.i.d. for 7 days.
Children 6 months to 12 years: 5 drops (or 1 single-dispensing container) into affected ear daily for 7 days.

▶ **Otitis media with tympanostomy tubes.** *Children ages 1 to 12:* Give 1 single-dispensing container into affected ear daily for 10 days.

▶ **Chronic suppurative otitis media with perforated tympanic membranes.** *Adults and children age 12 and older:* 2 dispensing-containers in affected ear b.i.d. for 14 days.

▶ **Adjunct for** *Brucella* **infections‡.** *Adults:* 400 mg P.O. daily for 6 weeks.

▶ **Typhoid fever‡.** *Adults:* 200 to 400 mg P.O. every 12 hours for 7 to 14 days.

▶ **Tuberculosis adjunct ‡.** *Adults:* 300 mg P.O. daily.

▶ **Postoperative sternotomy or soft tissue wounds caused by** *Mycobacterium fortuitum‡*. *Adults:* 300 or 600 mg P.O. daily for 3 to 6 months.

▶ **Acute Q fever pneumonia‡.** *Adults:* 600 mg P.O. daily for up to 16 days.

▶ **Mediterranean spotted fever‡.** *Adults:* 200 mg P.O. every 12 hours for 7 days.

▶ **Traveler's diarrhea‡.** *Adults:* 300 mg P.O. b.i.d. for 3 days.

▶ **Inhalational anthrax postexposure prophylaxis/treatment‡.** *Adults:* 400 mg P.O. b.i.d. for 60 days.

▶ **Legionnaire disease‡.** *Adults:* 400 mg P.O. every 12 hours for 2 to 3 weeks.

🔲 **Adjust-a-dose:** For patients with renal impairment, if creatinine clearance is 20 to 50 ml/minute, give usual recommended dose every 24 hours; if creatinine clearance is less than 20 ml/minute, give one-half of recommended dose every 24 hours.

For patients with hepatic impairment, maximum daily dosage is 400 mg.

Contraindications and cautions

• Contraindicated in patients hypersensitive to drug or other fluoroquinolones.
• Use cautiously in patients with renal impairment, history of seizures, or other CNS diseases such as cerebral arteriosclerosis.

⚖ **Lifespan:** In pregnant women, use cautiously. In breast-feeding women and in infants younger than age 1, safety and effectiveness haven't been established.

Adverse reactions

CNS: dizziness, drowsiness, fatigue, fever, *headache,* insomnia, lethargy, lightheadedness, malaise, nervousness, seizures, sleep disorders.
CV: chest pain.
EENT: visual disturbances.
GI: abdominal pain or discomfort, anorexia, diarrhea, dry mouth, dysgeusia, flatulence, nausea, vomiting.
GU: genital pruritus, vaginal discharge, vaginitis.
Hematologic: anemia, eosinophilia, leukocytosis, *leukopenia, lymphocytopenia, neutropenia.*
Metabolic: hyperglycemia, *hypoglycemia.*
Musculoskeletal: myalgia, transient arthralgia, trunk pain.
Skin: photosensitivity reaction, pruritus, rash.
Other: *anaphylaxis,* hypersensitivity reactions.

Interactions

Drug-drug. *Aluminum hydroxide, aluminum-magnesium hydroxide, calcium carbonate, magnesium hydroxide:* May decrease ofloxacin effects. Don't give these drugs within 2 hours of ofloxacin.
Cimetidine: May interfere with ofloxacin elimination. Monitor patient for toxicity.
Divalent or trivalent cations (such as zinc), or didanosine (chewable or buffered tablets or pe-

diatric powder for oral solution): May interfere with GI absorption of ofloxacin. Give these drugs at least 2 hours before or 2 hours after taking oral ofloxacin.
Iron salts: May decrease ofloxacin absorption, reducing anti-infective response. Give at least 2 hours apart.
NSAIDs: May increase risk of CNS stimulation and convulsive seizures. Avoid using together. Monitor patient for tremors and seizures if used together.
Oral anticoagulants: May increase anticoagulant effect. Monitor patient for bleeding and altered PT and INR.
Procainamide: May increase procainamide level. Monitor procainamide level; adjust dosage accordingly.
Sucralfate: May decrease absorption of oral ofloxacin, reducing anti-infective response. If use together can't be avoided, give at least 2 hours apart.
Theophylline: Some fluoroquinolones may decrease theophylline clearance. Monitor theophylline level.
Drug-food. *Any food:* May decrease oral drug absorption. Give drug on an empty stomach.
Drug-lifestyle. *Sun exposure:* May cause photosensitivity reactions. Urge patient to avoid unprotected or prolonged sun exposure.

Effects on lab test results

• May increase ALT, AST, and alkaline phosphatase levels. May decrease hemoglobin level and hematocrit. May increase or decrease glucose level.
• May increase eosinophil count. May decrease neutrophil and lymphocyte counts. May increase or decrease WBC count.
• May produce false-positive opiate assay results.

Pharmacokinetics

Absorption: Good.
Distribution: Wide.
Metabolism: Pyridobenzoxazine ring decreases extent.
Excretion: 68% to 90% unchanged in urine; less than 5% in feces. *Half-life:* 4 to 7½ hours.

Route	Onset	Peak	Duration
P.O.	Unknown	1–2 hr	Unknown
Topical	Unknown	Unknown	Unknown

Action

Chemical effect: May inhibit bacterial DNA gyrase and prevent DNA replication in susceptible bacteria.
Therapeutic effect: Kills susceptible aerobic gram-positive and gram-negative organisms.

Available forms

Ophthalmic solution: 0.3% in 5 ml, 10 ml
Otic solution: 0.3% in 0.25-ml single-dispensing containers, 5 ml, 10 ml
Tablets: 200 mg, 300 mg, 400 mg

NURSING PROCESS

Assessment

• Assess patient's infection before starting therapy and regularly thereafter to monitor the drug's effectiveness.
• Monitor regular blood studies and hepatic and renal function tests during long-term therapy.
• Give serologic test for syphilis to patient treated for gonorrhea. Drug isn't effective against syphilis, and treating gonorrhea may mask or delay symptoms of syphilis.
• Be alert for adverse reactions and drug interactions.
• If patient has an adverse GI reaction, monitor his hydration.
• Assess patient's and family's knowledge of drug therapy.

Nursing diagnoses

• Risk for infection related to presence of bacteria
• Risk for deficient fluid volume related to drug-induced adverse GI reactions
• Deficient knowledge related to drug therapy

Planning and implementation

• Give oral drug on empty stomach.
• **ALERT:** If patient develops restlessness, tremor, confusion, or hallucinations, stop giving the drug and notify prescriber. Take seizure precautions.
• **ALERT:** Ophthalmic and otic forms both come in 3% strengths. Don't confuse them; they're not interchangeable.

Patient teaching

• Advise patient to take oral drug with plenty of fluids but not with meals. Also, tell patient to avoid antacids, sucralfate, and products containing iron or zinc for at least 2 hours before and after each dose.
• Advise patient to complete full course of antibiotics, as directed.
• Warn patient to avoid hazardous tasks until the drug's CNS effects are known.
• Advise patient to use sun block and protective clothing to avoid photosensitivity reactions.
• Tell patient to stop taking the drug and notify prescriber if rash or other signs of hypersensitivity reactions develop.
• Tell patient to warm ear drops before instilling by holding the bottle in his hands for 1 or 2 minutes; this will avoid dizziness that may occur following instillation of cold solution.
• Give the patient these instructions for using eardrops: lie down with the affected ear upward and drop in the prescribed amount of drops. Remain lying down for 5 minutes to allow the drug to reach the ear canal. If treating middle ear infections, press the cartilage by the opening of the ear four times to help drug get to the middle ear.
• Advise patient using ear drops or eye drops to avoid contaminating the tip of the multidose container with his fingers, infectious material or other sources.

Evaluation

• Patient is free from infection.
• Patient maintains adequate hydration throughout drug therapy.
• Patient and family state understanding of drug therapy.

olanzapine

(oh-LAN-za-peen)
Zyprexa, Zyprexa Intramuscular, Zyprexa Zydis

Pharmacologic class: thienobenzodiazepine derivative
Therapeutic class: atypical antipsychotic
Pregnancy risk category: C

Indications and dosages

▶ **Short-term therapy for acute manic episodes related to bipolar I disorder.** *Adults:* Initially, 10 or 15 mg P.O. daily. Adjust dosage as needed by increments of 5 mg daily at inter-

vals of 24 hours or more. Maximum, 20 mg P.O. daily. Therapy lasts 3 or 4 weeks.

▶ **Short-term therapy for acute manic episodes of bipolar I disorder, given with lithium or valproate.** *Adults:* 10 mg P.O. once daily. Dosage range, 5 to 20 mg daily. Therapy lasts for 6 weeks.

▶ **Long-term therapy for bipolar I disorder.** *Adults:* 5 to 20 mg P.O. daily.

▶ **Agitation from schizophrenia and bipolar I mania.** *Adults:* 2.5 to 10 mg I.M. Maximum daily dosage, 30 mg I.M., in no more than 3 divided doses.

▶ **Long-term therapy for schizophrenia.** *Adults:* Initially, 5 to 10 mg P.O. daily. Goal, 10 mg P.O. daily within several days of starting therapy. Increase dosage weekly in increments of 5 mg daily to a maximum of 20 mg daily.

⬛ **Adjust-a-dose:** For patients who are debilitated, are predisposed to hypotensive reactions, have risk factors for slower drug metabolism (nonsmoking women older than age 65), or may be more pharmacodynamically sensitive to drug, the recommended starting dosage is 5 mg P.O. or 2.5 to 5 mg I.M. daily. In these patients, increase dosage with caution.

Contraindications and cautions

• Contraindicated in patients hypersensitive to the drug or any of its components.
• Use cautiously in patients with heart disease, cerebrovascular disease, diabetes, conditions that predispose patient to hypotension, history of seizures or conditions that might lower the seizure threshold, or hepatic impairment. Also use cautiously in patients with a history of paralytic ileus and in those at risk for aspiration pneumonia, prostatic hyperplasia, or angle-closure glaucoma.

⚠ **Lifespan:** In pregnant women, use drug only if benefits outweigh risks to the fetus. Breast-feeding women should stop breast-feeding or use another drug. In children younger than age 18, safety and effectiveness haven't been established. In elderly people with dementia, don't use; such patients may have an increased risk of stroke while using this drug.

Adverse reactions

CNS: abnormal gait, akathisia, *asthenia, dizziness,* extrapyramidal events, fever, *insomnia, neuroleptic malignant syndrome, parkinsonism,* personality disorder, *somnolence,* speech impairment, *suicide attempt* (P.O.), tardive dyskinesia.
CV: chest pain, hypertension, orthostatic hypotension, peripheral edema, tachycardia.
EENT: amblyopia, conjunctivitis, pharyngitis, rhinitis.
GI: *constipation, dry mouth, dyspepsia,* increased appetite, increased salivation and thirst, vomiting.
GU: amenorrhea, hematuria, metrorrhagia, urinary incontinence, UTI, vaginitis.
Hematologic: *leukopenia.*
Metabolic: *hyperglycemia,* weight gain.
Musculoskeletal: back pain, extremity pain, hypertonia, joint pain, joint stiffness and twitching.
Respiratory: dyspnea, increased cough.
Skin: ecchymosis, injection site pain, sweating.
Other: dental pain, flulike syndrome, injury.

Interactions

Drug-drug. *Antihypertensives:* May increase hypotensive effects. Monitor blood pressure closely.
Carbamazepine, omeprazole, rifampin: May increase olanzapine clearance. Monitor patient.
Diazepam: May increase CNS effects. Monitor patient closely.
Dopamine agonists, levodopa: May antagonize these drugs. Monitor patient.
Fluvoxamine: May decrease olanzapine clearance. Consider lower olanzapine dosage.
Drug-herb. *Nutmeg:* May reduce effectiveness of or interfere with drug therapy. Discourage using together.
Drug-lifestyle. *Alcohol use:* May increase CNS effects. Discourage using together.

Effects on lab test results

• May increase AST, ALT, GGT, CK, triglyceride, total cholesterol, and prolactin levels.

Pharmacokinetics

Absorption: Food doesn't affect rate or extent. About 40% of dose is limited by first-pass metabolism.
Distribution: Extensive, with a volume of distribution of about 1,000 L. About 93% protein-bound, mainly to albumin and alpha$_1$-acid glycoprotein.
Metabolism: By direct glucuronidation and cytochrome P-450–mediated oxidation.

Excretion: About 57% in urine and 30% in feces as metabolites. Only 7% of dose is recovered in urine unchanged. *Half-life:* 21 to 54 hours.

Route	Onset	Peak	Duration
P.O.	Unknown	6 hr	Unknown
I.M.	Rapid	15–45 min	Unknown

Action

Chemical effect: Binds to dopamine and serotonin receptors; may antagonize adrenergic, muscarinic, and histaminergic receptors.
Therapeutic effect: Relieves signs and symptoms of psychosis.

Available forms

Powder for injection: 10 mg
Tablets: 2.5 mg, 5 mg, 7.5 mg, 10 mg, 15 mg, 20 mg
Tablets (orally-disintegrating): 5 mg, 10 mg, 15 mg, 20 mg

NURSING PROCESS

Assessment
• Obtain history of patient's underlying condition before starting therapy, and reassess regularly thereafter to monitor drug's effectiveness.
• Obtain baseline and periodic liver function tests and lipid profiles.
• Monitor patient for signs of neuroleptic malignant syndrome (hyperpyrexia, muscle rigidity, altered mental condition, autonomic instability), which is rare but fatal. If patient has symptoms, stop drug immediately, notify prescriber, and treat symptoms.
• Monitor patient for tardive dyskinesia, which may occur after prolonged use. It may not appear until months or years later, and it may disappear spontaneously or persist for life despite stopping therapy.
• Monitor patient for abnormal body temperature regulation, especially if patient is exercising strenuously, exposed to extreme heat, receiving anticholinergics, or at risk for dehydration.
⚠ ALERT: Hyperglycemia is more likely to occur with olanzapine than with other antipsychotics. If patient has diabetes, check blood glucose level regularly. If patient has risk factors for diabetes, check fasting blood glucose level at baseline and periodically thereafter. In some cases,

hyperglycemia is reversible when antipsychotic therapy is stopped.
• Monitor patient for symptoms of hyperglycemia, including polydipsia, polyuria, polyphagia, and weakness; if symptoms develop, test fasting glucose level.
• Monitor patient for weight gain during treatment.
• Regularly reevaluate the drug's long-term effectiveness, especially in patients taking more than 20 mg daily.
• Assess patient's and family's knowledge of drug therapy.

⊕ Nursing diagnoses
• Disturbed thought processes related to underlying condition
• Risk for injury related to drug-induced adverse CNS reactions
• Deficient knowledge related to drug therapy

▷ Planning and implementation
• Start with a 5-mg dose in a patient who is debilitated, predisposed to hypotension, sensitive to drug, or affected by altered metabolism caused by smoking, gender, or age.
• Orally-disintegrating tablets contain phenylalanine.
• Inspect I.M. solution for particulate matter and discoloration before administration.
• Store vials at 68° to 77° F (20° to 25° C). Protect from light and don't freeze. To reconstitute I.M. injection, dissolve contents of 1 vial with 2.1 ml of sterile water for injection to yield a 5 mg/ml solution that is clear and yellow in appearance. Store at room temperature and administer within 1 hour of reconstitution. Discard any unused solution.
• Postural hypotension and bradycardia may be lessened after I.M. injection by keeping patient recumbent.
⚠ ALERT: Don't confuse olanzapine with olsalazine or ondansetron. Don't confuse Zyprexa with Zyrtec or Celexa.
⚠ ALERT: May increase the risk for suicidal thinking and behavior in young adults ages 18 to 24 during first 2 months of treatment.
Patient teaching
• Drug can be taken with or without food.
• Tell patient to avoid hazardous tasks until the drug's CNS effects are known.

• Warn patient against exposure to extreme heat; drug may impair body's ability to reduce core temperature.
• Tell patient not to drink alcohol during therapy.
• Tell patient to rise slowly to avoid effects of orthostatic hypotension.
• Instruct patient to relieve dry mouth with ice chips or sugarless candy or gum.
• Tell patient to monitor weight closely because olanzapine may cause weight gain.
• Advise patient that routine blood tests will be needed during therapy.
• Advise woman to notify prescriber if she becomes pregnant or intends to become pregnant during drug therapy. Advise her not to breast-feed during therapy.

☑ Evaluation
• Patient's behavior and communication show improved thought processes.
• Patient sustains no injury from adverse CNS reactions.
• Patient and family state understanding of drug therapy.

olmesartan medoxomil
(ol-meh-SAHR-tan me-DOKS-oh-mil)
Benicar

Pharmacologic class: angiotensin II receptor antagonist
Therapeutic class: antihypertensive
Pregnancy risk category: C (first trimester) and D (second and third trimesters)

Indications and dosages

▶ **Hypertension.** *Adults:* 20 mg P.O. daily in patients who aren't volume-contracted. If blood pressure isn't reduced after 2 weeks of therapy, increase dosage to 40 mg P.O. once daily.
⬧ Adjust-a-dose: In patients whose intravascular volume may be depleted, consider lower starting dose.

Contraindications and cautions

• Contraindicated in patients hypersensitive to drug or any of its components.
• Use cautiously in patients who are volume- or salt-depleted, in those whose renal function depends on the renin-angiotensin-aldosterone sys-

tem (such as patients with severe heart failure), and in those with renal artery stenosis.
☆ Lifespan: In pregnant women, drug isn't recommended; if woman becomes pregnant, stop drug immediately. Breast-feeding women should either stop breast-feeding or use another drug. In children, safety and effectiveness haven't been established. In elderly patients, use cautiously because they may have greater sensitivity to drug.

Adverse reactions

CNS: headache, dizziness.
EENT: pharyngitis, rhinitis, sinusitis.
GI: diarrhea.
GU: hematuria.
Metabolic: hyperglycemia, hypertriglyceridemia.
Musculoskeletal: back pain.
Respiratory: bronchitis, cough, upper respiratory tract infection.
Other: accidental injury, flulike symptoms.

Interactions

None reported.

Effects on lab test results

• May increase glucose, triglyceride, uric acid, liver enzyme, bilirubin, cholesterol, potassium, and CK levels. May decrease hemoglobin level and hematocrit.

Pharmacokinetics

Absorption: Rapid and complete. Steady-state level occurs within 3 to 5 days.
Distribution: 99% protein-bound.
Metabolism: None.
Excretion: In the urine and feces. *Half-life:* 13 hours.

Route	Onset	Peak	Duration
P.O.	Rapid	1–2 hr	24 hr

Action

Chemical effect: Blocks the vasoconstrictor and aldosterone-secreting effects of angiotensin II by selectively blocking the binding of angiotensin II to the angiotensin receptor in the vascular smooth muscle.
Therapeutic effect: Lowers blood pressure.

Available forms

Tablets: 5 mg, 20 mg, 40 mg

NURSING PROCESS

⚚ Assessment
• Monitor patients with heart failure closely for oliguria, azotemia, and acute renal impairment.
• Monitor BUN and creatinine levels in patients with renal artery stenosis.
• Be alert for adverse reactions.
• Assess patient's and family's knowledge of drug therapy.

⊕ Nursing diagnoses
• Risk for injury related to presence of hypertension
• Sleep deprivation related to drug-induced cough
• Deficient knowledge related to drug therapy

▶ Planning and implementation
• Symptomatic hypotension may occur in patients who are volume- or salt-depleted, especially those being treated with high doses of a diuretic. If hypotension occurs, place patient supine and treat supportively. When blood pressure is stabilized, therapy can continue.
• If blood pressure isn't adequately controlled, a diuretic or other antihypertensive may be added.
Patient teaching
• Tell patient to take drug exactly as prescribed and not to stop even if he feels better.
• Tell patient that drug may be taken with or without food.
• Tell patient to immediately report adverse reactions, especially light-headedness and syncope, to prescriber.
• Advise a woman of childbearing age to immediately report pregnancy to prescriber.
• Inform diabetic patient that glucose readings may become higher, and the dosage of their antidiabetics may need adjustment.
• Warn patient that reduced fluid volume from inadequate fluid intake, excessive perspiration, diarrhea, or vomiting may cause a drop in blood pressure, leading to lightheadedness and fainting.
• Inform patient that other antihypertensives can have additive or synergistic effects. Patient should inform prescriber of all drugs (including OTC) that he's taking.

☑ Evaluation
• Patient's blood pressure is normal.

• Patient's sleep patterns are undisturbed throughout therapy.
• Patient and family state understanding of drug therapy.

olsalazine sodium
(olh-SAL-uh-zeen SOH-dee-um)
Dipentum

Pharmacologic class: salicylate, non-aspirin
Therapeutic class: Gastrointestinal anti-inflammatory
Pregnancy risk category: C

Indications and dosages
▶ **Maintenance of remission of ulcerative colitis in patients intolerant of sulfasalazine.**
Adults: 500 mg P.O. b.i.d. with meals.

Contraindications and cautions
• Contraindicated in patients hypersensitive to salicylates.
• Use cautiously in patients with renal disease. Renal tubular damage may result from absorbed drug or its metabolites.
🕮 **Lifespan:** In pregnant women, use cautiously. In breast-feeding women, use cautiously; it's unknown if the drug appears in breast milk. In children, safety and effectiveness haven't been established.

Adverse reactions
CNS: depression, dizziness, headache, vertigo, fatigue, drowsiness, lethargy, insomnia.
GI: abdominal pain, *diarrhea,* heartburn, nausea, cramps, dyspepsia, bloating, anorexia, vomiting, stomatitis, rectal bleeding.
Musculoskeletal: arthralgia.
Respiratory: upper respiratory infection.
Skin: itching, rash.

Interactions
Drug-drug. *Anticoagulants, coumarin derivatives:* May increase anticoagulant effects. Monitor patient closely for bleeding.

Effects on lab test results
• May increase AST and ALT levels.

Pharmacokinetics
Absorption: About 2%.

Reactions may be *common,* uncommon, *life-threatening,* or COMMON AND LIFE-THREATENING.

Distribution: Liberated mesalamine is absorbed slowly from colon, resulting in very high local level.
Metabolism: 0.1% in liver; remainder reaches colon, where it's rapidly converted to mesalamine by colonic bacteria.
Excretion: About 80% in feces; less than 1% in urine. *Half-life:* About 1 hour.

Route	Onset	Peak	Duration
P.O.	Unknown	1 hr	Unknown

Action

Chemical effect: May convert to 5-aminosalicylic acid (5-ASA or mesalamine) in colon, where it has local anti-inflammatory effect.
Therapeutic effect: Prevents flare-up of ulcerative colitis.

Available forms

Capsules: 250 mg

NURSING PROCESS

Assessment
• Assess patient's condition before starting therapy and regularly thereafter to monitor drug's effectiveness.
• Monitor BUN and creatinine levels and urinalysis in patient with renal disease.
• Be alert for adverse reactions.
• Assess patient's and family's knowledge of drug therapy.

Nursing diagnoses
• Impaired tissue integrity related to ulcerative colitis
• Diarrhea related to drug's adverse effect on GI tract
• Deficient knowledge related to drug therapy

Planning and implementation
• To decrease GI irritation, give drug in evenly divided doses with food.
• Report diarrhea to prescriber. Although diarrhea appears dose-related, it's difficult to distinguish from worsening of disease symptoms. Worsening of disease has been noted with similar drugs.
⚠ ALERT: Don't confuse olsalazine with olanzapine.

Patient teaching
• Tell patient to take drug in evenly divided doses, with food, to minimize GI irritation.
• Urge patient to notify prescriber about adverse reactions, especially diarrhea or increased pain.

☑ Evaluation
• Patient has no evidence of ulcerative colitis.
• Patient is free from diarrhea.
• Patient and family state understanding of drug therapy.

omalizumab
(oh-mah-LIZZ-uh-mahb)
Xolair

Pharmacologic class: monoclonal antibody
Therapeutic class: antasthmatic
Pregnancy risk category: B

Indications and dosages

▶ **Moderate to severe persistent asthma in patients with positive skin test or in vitro reactivity to a seasonal allergen and whose symptoms are inadequately controlled with inhaled corticosteroids.** *Adults and children age 12 and older:* Dosage is determined by total immunoglobulin E (IgE) level (international unit/ml) measured before the start of therapy and by body weight (kg). See tables on this page. Divide doses greater than 150 mg and use more than one injection site. Inject subcutaneously every 2 or 4 weeks.

Contraindications and cautions

• Contraindicated in patients hypersensitive to the drug or any of its components.
⚖ Lifespan: In pregnant women, use only when potential benefits outweigh risks to the fetus. In breast-feeding women, use cautiously; it's unclear if drug appears in breast milk. In children younger than age 12, safety and effectiveness of drug haven't been established.

Adverse reactions

CNS: dizziness, fatigue, headache, pain.
EENT: earache, *pharyngitis,* sinusitis.
Musculoskeletal: arm pain, arthralgia, fracture, leg pain.
Respiratory: *upper respiratory tract infection.*
Skin: dermatitis, pruritus.

Other: *anaphylaxis* (immediate or delayed), hypersensitivity reaction, *injection site reaction, malignancy, viral infections.*

Interactions

None reported.

Effects on lab test results

• May increase IgE level for up to 1 year after therapy.

Pharmacokinetics

Absorption: Slow, with a bioavailability of about 62%.
Distribution: None specified.
Metabolism: Unknown.
Excretion: In liver and bile. *Half-life:* About 26 days.

Route	Onset	Peak	Duration
SubQ	Unknown	7–8 days	Unknown

Action

Chemical effect: Inhibits binding of IgE to a high-affinity receptor on the surface of mast cells and basophils. Reducing IgE limits the release of mediators of the allergic response and reduces the number of receptors on basophils.
Therapeutic effect: Treats asthma symptoms.

Available forms

Powder for injection: 150 mg/1.2 ml

NURSING PROCESS

Assessment

• Assess patient's respiratory condition before starting therapy and regularly thereafter to monitor drug's effectiveness.
• Be alert for adverse reactions.
ALERT: Observe patient after injection, and have drugs available to treat severe hypersensitivity reactions. If a severe hypersensitivity reaction occurs, stop therapy.
• Assess patient's and family's knowledge of drug therapy.

Nursing diagnoses

• Impaired gas exchange related to bronchospasm
• Acute pain related to drug-induced headache
• Deficient knowledge related to drug therapy

Planning and implementation

ALERT: Don't use for acute bronchospasm or status asthmaticus.
ALERT: Life-threatening anaphylactic reactions have occurred, usually within 2 hours of subcutaneous injection, but reaction can be delayed 2 to 24 hours or longer. Administration should only occur in health care setting under direct medical supervision for anaphylaxis for at least 2 hours after each Xolair injection and a patient medication guide must be given with each dose.
• Don't abruptly stop giving systemic or inhaled corticosteroids when starting this drug. Gradually decrease corticosteroids with prescriber nearby.
• Because the solution is slightly viscous, it may take 5 to 10 seconds to inject.
• Patient may have injection site reactions, including bruising, redness, warmth, burning, stinging, itching, hives, pain, induration, and inflammation. Most reactions occur within 1 hour of injection, last less than 8 days, and decrease in frequency with subsequent injections.
• Total IgE level may elevate during therapy and remain elevated for up to 1 year after therapy stops; testing IgE level during therapy can't be used as a guide to determine dosage. If therapy has been stopped for less than 1 year, use IgE level from the original dosage determination. If therapy has been stopped for 1 year or more, retest total IgE level.

Patient teaching
• Tell patient not to decrease the dosage or stop taking his other antasthmatics unless directed by prescriber.
• Tell patient not to expect immediate improvement in his asthma after starting therapy.
• Give patient medication guide with each dose.

Evaluation

• Patient exhibits normal breathing pattern.
• Patient states that drug-induced headache is relieved by analgesic.
• Patient and family state understanding of drug therapy.

omega-3-acid ethyl esters
(oh-MAY-gah THREE ASS-id ETH-ill ESS-turs)
Lovaza

Pharmacologic class: ethyl ester
Therapeutic class: lipid regulator
Pregnancy risk category: C

Indications and dosages

▶ **Adjunct to diet to reduce triglyceride level of 500 mg/dl or more.** *Adults:* 4 g P.O. once daily or divided equally b.i.d.

Contraindications and cautions

• Contraindicated in patients hypersensitive to drug or any of its components.
• Use cautiously in patients sensitive to fish.
⚘ **Lifespan:** In pregnant women, use only if benefits outweigh risks to the fetus. In breast-feeding women, use cautiously. Safety and effectiveness in children haven't been established.

Adverse reactions

CNS: pain.
CV: angina pectoris.
GI: altered taste, belching, dyspepsia.
Musculoskeletal: back pain.
Skin: rash.
Other: flulike syndrome, infection.

Interactions

Drug-drug. *Anticoagulants:* May prolong bleeding time. Monitor patient.

Effects on lab test results

• May increase ALT and LDL levels.

Pharmacokinetics

Absorption: Good.
Distribution: Unknown.
Metabolism: Unknown.
Excretion: Unknown.

Route	Onset	Peak	Duration
P.O.	Unknown	Unknown	Unknown

Action

Chemical effect: May be a poor substrate for the enzymes needed for triglyceride synthesis. Blocks formation of other fatty acids.
Therapeutic effect: Decreases triglyceride level.

Available forms

Capsules: 1 g

NURSING PROCESS

🔍 Assessment
• Before therapy, assess patient for conditions that increase triglyceride level, such as diabetes and hypothyroidism.
• Assess patient's current history for drugs known to sharply increase triglyceride level, including estrogen therapy, thiazide diuretics, and beta blockers. Drug made not be needed after stopping these drugs.
• Monitor patient for adverse drug effects.
• Assess patient's and family's knowledge of drug therapy.

🔷 Nursing diagnoses
• Ineffective health maintenance related to elevated triglyceride level
• Risk for injury related to very high triglyceride level
• Deficient knowledge related to drug therapy

▶ Planning and implementation
• Start therapy only after diet and lifestyle modifications have proven unsuccessful.
• Obtain baseline triglyceride level to confirm that they're consistently abnormal before therapy; then recheck periodically during therapy. If patient has an inadequate response after 2 months, stop drug.
• Monitor LDL level to make sure it doesn't increase excessively during therapy.
Ⓢ **ALERT:** Don't confuse Lovaza with lorazepam.
Patient teaching
• Explain that drug doesn't reduce the importance of following the recommended diet and exercise plan.
• Remind patient of the need for follow-up blood work to evaluate progress.
• Advise patient to notify prescriber about bothersome side effects.
• Advise patient to take with food.
• Tell patient to report planned or suspected pregnancy.

☑ Evaluation
• Patient reduces triglyceride level with diet, exercise, lifestyle modifications, and drug therapy.
• Patient has reduced triglyceride level.

O

• Patient and family state understanding of drug therapy.

omeprazole
(oh-MEH-pruh-zohl)
Prilosec◆, Prilosec OTC†, Zegerid

Pharmacologic class: substituted benzimidazole
Therapeutic class: proton pump inhibitor
Pregnancy risk category: C

Indications and dosages

▶ **Erosive esophagitis; symptomatic, poorly responsive gastroesophageal reflux disease (GERD).** *Adults with GERD who are unresponsive to H₂-receptor antagonist:* 20 mg P.O. daily for 4 to 8 weeks. May increase dosage to 40 mg daily if needed and extend therapy up to 12 weeks.
Children 2 to 16 years weighing less than 20 kg: 10 mg P.O. daily.
Children 2 to 16 years weighing 20 kg or more: 20 mg P.O. daily.
▶ **GERD without erosive esophagitis.** *Adults:* 20 mg P.O. daily for 4 weeks.
▶ **Pathologic hypersecretory conditions (such as Zollinger-Ellison syndrome).** *Adults:* Initially, 60 mg P.O. daily; adjust to patient's response. If daily amount exceeds 80 mg, give in divided doses. Dosages up to 120 mg t.i.d. may be given.
▶ **Duodenal ulcer (short-term therapy).** *Adults:* 20 mg P.O. daily for 4 to 8 weeks.
▶ **Gastric ulcer.** *Adults:* 40 mg P.O. daily for 4 to 8 weeks.
▶ *Helicobacter pylori* **eradication to reduce risk of duodenal ulcer recurrence as part of triple therapy with clarithromycin and amoxicillin.** *Adults:* 20 mg P.O. with 500 mg clarithromycin P.O. and 1,000 mg amoxicillin P.O., each given b.i.d. for 10 days. For patients with ulcers when therapy starts, another 18 days of 20 mg omeprazole P.O. once daily is recommended.
▶ *H. pylori* **eradication to reduce risk of duodenal ulcer recurrence as part of dual therapy with clarithromycin.** *Adults:* 40 mg P.O. once daily with clarithromycin 500 mg, P.O., t.i.d. for 14 days. For patients with ulcers pres-

ent at the start of therapy, give 20 mg omeprazole P.O. once daily for 14 more days.
▶ **Heartburn on 2 or more days per week.** *Adults:* 20 mg P.O. (Prilosec OTC) daily before breakfast for 14 days. May repeat the 14-day course every 4 months.
▶ **Posterior laryngitis‡.** *Adults:* 40 mg at bedtime for 6 to 24 weeks.

Contraindications and cautions

• Contraindicated in patients hypersensitive to the drug or any of its components.
⚖ **Lifespan:** In pregnant women, use cautiously. In breast-feeding women, use cautiously; it's unknown if the drug appears in breast milk. In children ages 2 to 16 years, drug may be used to treat GERD, erosive esophagitis, and for maintenance of healing in erosive esophagitis (tablets and capsules only).

Adverse reactions

CNS: dizziness, headache.
GI: abdominal pain, constipation, diarrhea, flatulence, nausea, vomiting.
Musculoskeletal: back pain.
Respiratory: cough.
Skin: rash.

Interactions

Drug-drug. *Ampicillin esters, iron derivatives, ketoconazole:* May decrease absorption. Give separately.
Clarithromycin: May increase level of either drug. Monitor patient for drug toxicity.
Diazepam, phenytoin, warfarin: May decrease hepatic clearance of these drugs, possibly leading to increased levels. Monitor patient closely.
Sucralfate: May delay absorption and reduce omeprazole bioavailability. Separate administration times by 30 minutes or more.
Drug-herb. *Male fern:* May inactivate herb. Discourage using together.
Pennyroyal: May change the rate at which toxic metabolites of herb form. Discourage using together.

Effects on lab test results

None reported.

Pharmacokinetics

Absorption: Rapid, but bioavailability is about 40% because of instability in gastric acid as

well as substantial first-pass effect. Bioavailability increases slightly with repeated doses.
Distribution: 95% protein-bound.
Metabolism: Mainly in liver.
Excretion: Mainly in urine. *Half-life:* 30 to 60 minutes.

Route	Onset	Peak	Duration
P.O.	≤ 1 hr	30 min–2 hr	< 3 days

Action

Chemical effect: Inhibits acid (proton) pump and binds to hydrogen-potassium adenosine triphosphatase on secretory surface of gastric parietal cells to block formation of gastric acid.
Therapeutic effect: Relieves symptoms caused by excessive gastric acid.

Available forms

Capsules (delayed-release): 10 mg, 20 mg, 40 mg
Capsule (Zegerid): 20 mg, 40 mg
Powder for oral suspension (Zegerid): 20 mg, 40 mg
Tablets (delayed-release): 20 mg

NURSING PROCESS

Assessment
• Assess patient's condition before starting therapy and regularly thereafter to monitor drug's effectiveness.
• Be alert for adverse reactions and drug interactions.
• If adverse GI reaction occurs, monitor patient's hydration.
• Assess patient's and family's knowledge of drug therapy.

Nursing diagnoses
• Impaired tissue integrity related to upper gastric disorder
• Risk for deficient fluid volume related to drug-induced adverse GI reactions
• Deficient knowledge related to drug therapy

Planning and implementation
• Give tablets or capsules 30 minutes before meals; powder for oral suspension 1 hour before meals.
• Zegerid powder for oral suspension may be used for short-term treatment of duodenal ulcers, GERD, and maintenance of healing of ero-

sive esophagitis; don't use in children younger than age 18.
• Use 2 tbs of water to mix 1 packet of powder for oral suspension; don't use any other liquids or food.
• Powder for oral suspension contains 460 mg of sodium per dose and 20 mEq of sodium bicarbonate.
• Lower doses aren't needed for patients with renal or hepatic impairment.
🛇 **ALERT:** Don't confuse Prilosec with Prozac, prilocaine, or Prinivil.
Patient teaching
• Explain importance of taking drug exactly as prescribed.
• Warn patient not to crush or chew tablets or capsules.
• Explain to patient how to reconstitute powder for oral suspension: Empty packet contents into a small cup containing 2 tbs of water; stir well and drink immediately. Refill cup with water and drink.
• Advise patient that OTC drug isn't intended for immediate relief of heartburn or to treat occasional heartburn (one episode of heartburn a week or less).
• Inform patient that OTC drug may require 1 to 4 days for full effect, although some patients may get complete relief of symptoms within 24 hours.

Evaluation
• Patient responds well to therapy.
• Patient maintains adequate hydration throughout drug therapy.
• Patient and family state understanding of drug therapy.

ondansetron hydrochloride
(on-DAN-seh-tron high-droh-KLOR-ighd)
Zofran, Zofran ODT

Pharmacologic class: serotonin receptor antagonist
Therapeutic class: antiemetic
Pregnancy risk category: B

Indications and dosages

▶ **To prevent nausea and vomiting caused by moderately emetogenic chemotherapy.**
Adults and children age 12 and older: 8 mg P.O.

30 minutes before start of chemotherapy. Follow with 8 mg P.O. 8 hours after first dose. Then follow with 8 mg every 12 hours for 1 to 2 days. Or, three doses of 0.15 mg/kg I.V. Give first dose 30 minutes before chemotherapy; give subsequent doses 4 and 8 hours after first dose. Infuse drug over 15 minutes. Or, adults may receive a single dose of 32 mg I.V. infused over 15 minutes, 30 minutes before chemotherapy. Don't repeat this dose.

Children ages 4 to 11: Give 4 mg P.O. 30 minutes before start of chemotherapy. Follow with 4 mg P.O. 4 and 8 hours after first dose. Then follow with 4 mg every 8 hours for 1 to 2 days. *Children ages 6 months to 18 years:* Three doses of 0.15 mg/kg I.V. Give first dose 30 minutes before chemotherapy; give subsequent doses 4 and 8 hours after first dose. Infuse drug over 15 minutes.

▶ **To prevent nausea and vomiting caused by highly emetogenic chemotherapy.** *Adults:* 24 mg P.O. 30 minutes before start of chemotherapy.

▶ **To prevent postoperative nausea and vomiting.** *Adults:* 4 mg I.V. (undiluted) over 2 to 5 minutes immediately before induction of anesthesia or postoperatively. Or, 4 mg I.M. as a single injection immediately before induction of anesthesia or postoperatively. Or, 16 mg P.O. 1 hour before induction of anesthesia.

Children ages 1 month to 12 years who weigh 40 kg (88 lb) or less: 0.1 mg/kg I.V. Give dose over 2 to 5 minutes as a single dose.

Children ages 1 month to 12 years who weigh more than 40 kg: Give 4 mg I.V. over 2 to 5 minutes as a single dose.

▶ **To prevent nausea and vomiting from radiation therapy—total body irradiation, a single high-dose fraction, or daily fractions to the abdomen.** *Adults:* 8 mg P.O. t.i.d.

⧈ **Adjust-a-dose:** For patients with severe liver impairment, don't exceed total daily dosage of 8 mg P.O. or a single maximum dose of 8 mg I.V. over 15 minutes.

▼ I.V. administration

- Dilute drug in 50 ml of D_5W injection or normal saline solution for injection before giving.
- Infuse drug over 15 minutes.
- Drug is stable for up to 48 hours after dilution in 5% dextrose and normal saline injection, 5% dextrose in half-normal saline injection, and 3% saline injection.

⊗ **Incompatibilities**
Acyclovir sodium, allopurinol, aminophylline, amphotericin B, ampicillin sodium, ampicillin sodium and sulbactam sodium, cefepime, cefoperazone, dexamethasone sodium phosphate, droperidol, fluorouracil, furosemide, ganciclovir, lorazepam, meropenem, methylprednisolone sodium succinate, piperacillin sodium, sargramostim, sodium bicarbonate.

Contraindications and cautions

- Contraindicated in patients hypersensitive to the drug or any of its components.
- Use cautiously and at a lower dose in patients with liver failure.

⚖ **Lifespan:** In pregnant women, use cautiously. In breast-feeding women, use cautiously; it's unknown if the drug appears in breast milk. In children, safety and effectiveness of the 24-mg tablet or the use of oral forms of drug for postoperative nausea and vomiting or radiation-induced nausea and vomiting haven't been established. In infants younger than age 1 month who are undergoing surgery, information on safety and effectiveness of drug is limited.

Adverse reactions

CNS: extrapyramidal syndrome, *headache, fatigue, malaise.*
CV: *arrhythmias, bradycardia,* chest pain, hypotension.
GI: *constipation,* diarrhea.
Skin: pruritus, rash.

Interactions

Drug-drug. *Drugs that alter hepatic drug-metabolizing enzymes (such as cimetidine, phenobarbital):* May alter pharmacokinetics of ondansetron. No dosage adjustment is needed.
Rifampin: May reduce ondansetron level, decreasing antiemetic effect. Monitor patient for adequate antiemetic effect; adjust dosage.

Effects on lab test results

- May increase ALT and AST levels.

Pharmacokinetics

Absorption: Variable; bioavailability is 50% to 60%.
Distribution: 70% to 76% protein-bound.
Metabolism: Extensive.
Excretion: Mainly in urine. *Half-life:* 4 hours.

Route	Onset	Peak	Duration
P.O., I.V.	Unknown	Unknown	Unknown

Action

Chemical effect: Blocking action may take place in CNS at chemoreceptor trigger zone and in peripheral nervous system on terminals of vagus nerve.
Therapeutic effect: Prevents nausea and vomiting from emetogenic chemotherapy or surgery.

Available forms

Injection: 2 mg/ml
Oral solution: 4 mg/5 ml
Tablets: 4 mg, 8 mg, 24 mg
Tablets (orally-disintegrating): 4 mg, 8 mg

NURSING PROCESS

📖 Assessment
• Assess patient's condition before starting therapy and regularly thereafter to monitor drug's effectiveness.
• Be alert for adverse reactions and drug interactions.
• Assess patient's and family's knowledge of drug therapy.

🔷 Nursing diagnoses
• Risk for deficient fluid volume related to nausea and vomiting
• Acute pain related to drug-induced headache
• Deficient knowledge related to drug therapy

▶ Planning and implementation
🚫 **ALERT:** Don't confuse Zofran with Zantac or Zosyn.
🚫 **ALERT:** Don't confuse Zofran with Precedex. These vials appear very similar.
🚫 **ALERT:** Don't confuse ondansetron with olanzapine.
Patient teaching
• Instruct patient when to take drug.
• Tell patient to report adverse reactions.
• Advise patient to report discomfort at I.V. site.

✓ Evaluation
• Patient maintains adequate hydration.
• Patient has no drug-induced headaches.
• Patient and family state understanding of drug therapy.

orlistat
(OR-lih-stat)
Alli†, Xenical

Pharmacologic class: lipase inhibitor
Therapeutic class: antiobesity drug
Pregnancy risk category: B

Indications and dosages

▶ **Management of obesity, including weight loss and weight maintenance, given with a reduced-calorie diet; reduction of risk of weight regain after weight loss.** *Adults:* 120 mg Xenical P.O. t.i.d. with each main meal containing fat (during or up to 1 hour after the meal). Or, 60 mg Alli with each meal containing fat, not to exceed 3 capsules per day.

Contraindications and cautions

• Contraindicated in patients hypersensitive to the drug or any of its components and in patients with chronic malabsorption syndrome or cholestasis.
• Use cautiously in patients with a history of hyperoxaluria or calcium oxalate nephrolithiasis, patients who are at risk for anorexia nervosa or bulimia, and patients who are receiving cyclosporine therapy because of changes in cyclosporine absorption related to variations in diet.
⚖ **Lifespan:** In pregnant and breast-feeding women, drug isn't recommended. In children, safety and effectiveness haven't been established.

Adverse reactions

CNS: anxiety, depression, dizziness, fatigue, *headache,* sleep disorder.
CV: pedal edema.
EENT: otitis.
GI: *abdominal pain, fatty or oily stool,* fecal incontinence, *fecal urgency, flatus with discharge, increased defecation,* infectious diarrhea, nausea, *oily evacuation, oily spotting,* **pancreatitis,** rectal pain, *vomiting.*
GU: menstrual irregularity, UTI, vaginitis.
Musculoskeletal: arthritis, *back pain,* joint disorder, leg pain, myalgia, tendinitis.
Respiratory: *influenza,* lower respiratory tract infection, *upper respiratory tract infection.*
Skin: dry skin, rash.
Other: gingival and tooth disorders.

0

Interactions

Drug-drug. *Cyclosporine:* May alter cyclosporine absorption. Monitor cyclosporine level.
Fat-soluble vitamins such as vitamin E, beta-carotene: May decrease vitamin absorption. Separate doses by 2 hours.
Pravastatin: May slightly increase pravastatin level and lipid-lowering effects. Monitor patient.
Warfarin: May change coagulation parameters. Monitor INR.

Effects on lab test results

• May decrease vitamin D, beta-carotene, LDL, and total cholesterol levels.

Pharmacokinetics

Absorption: Only a small amount.
Distribution: More than 99% protein-bound. Lipoproteins and albumin are major binding proteins.
Metabolism: Mainly in GI wall.
Excretion: Mostly unchanged in feces. *Half-life:* 1 to 2 hours.

Route	Onset	Peak	Duration
P.O.	Unknown	Unknown	Unknown

Action

Chemical effect: Binds with the active site of gastric and pancreatic lipases. These inactivated enzymes are thus unavailable to hydrolyze dietary fat, in the form of triglycerides, into absorbable free fatty acids and monoglycerides. Because the undigested triglycerides aren't absorbed, the resulting caloric deficit may help with weight control. The recommended dosage of 120 mg t.i.d. inhibits dietary fat absorption by about 30%.
Therapeutic effect: Weight loss and weight maintenance.

Available forms

Capsules: 60 mg†, 120 mg

NURSING PROCESS

Assessment

• Obtain history of patient's underlying condition before starting therapy; reassess regularly thereafter to monitor the drug's effectiveness.
• Screen patient for anorexia nervosa or bulimia; as with any weight-loss drug, drug can be misused.

• Organic causes of obesity, such as hypothyroidism, must be ruled out before patient starts orlistat therapy.
• In diabetic patient, monitor glucose level frequently during weight loss. Dose of oral antidiabetic or insulin may need to be reduced.
• Assess patient's and family's knowledge of drug therapy.

Nursing diagnoses

• Imbalanced nutrition: More than body requirements related to obesity
• Disturbed body image related to obesity
• Deficient knowledge related to drug therapy

Planning and implementation

ALERT: Pancreatitis has occurred with use of drug. Monitor patient closely.
• Use drug for a patient with an initial body mass index of 30 kg/m^2 or more (27 kg/m^2 or more if patient has other risk factors, such as hypertension, diabetes, or dyslipidemia).
• It's unknown whether drug is safe and effective to use longer than 2 years.
• Tell patient to follow dietary guidelines. GI effects may increase when patient takes drug with high-fat foods—specifically, when more than 30% of total daily calories come from fat.
• Drug reduces absorption of some fat-soluble vitamins and beta-carotene.
ALERT: Don't confuse Xenical with Xeloda.
Patient teaching
• Advise patient to follow a nutritionally balanced, reduced-calorie diet that derives only 30% of its calories from fat. Daily intake of fat, carbohydrate, and protein should be distributed over three main meals. If a meal is occasionally missed or contains no fat, tell patient that dose can be skipped.
• To ensure adequate nutrition, advise patient to take a daily multivitamin supplement that contains fat-soluble vitamins no sooner than within 2 hours of taking drug, such as at bedtime.
• Tell patient with diabetes that weight loss may improve glycemic control, so his oral antidiabetic or insulin dosage may need to be reduced.
• Tell woman to inform prescriber if she is pregnant, plans to become pregnant, or is breast-feeding.

Evaluation

• Patient's nutritional intake is adequate according to proper dietary guidelines.

- Patient reaches and maintains a stable weight.
- Patient and family state understanding of drug therapy.

oseltamivir phosphate
(ah-sul-TAM-ih-veer FOS-fayt)
Tamiflu

Pharmacologic class: neuraminidase inhibitor
Therapeutic class: antiviral
Pregnancy risk category: C

Indications and dosages

▶ **Uncomplicated, acute illness from influenza in patients who have been symptomatic for 2 days or less.** *Adults, children age 13 and older, and children age 1 and older who weigh more than 40 kg (88 lb):* 75 mg P.O. b.i.d. for 5 days.
Children age 1 and older who weigh 23 to 40 kg (51 to 88 lb): 60 mg oral suspension P.O. b.i.d. for 5 days.
Children age 1 and older who weigh 15 to 23 kg (33 to 51 lb): 45 mg oral suspension P.O. b.i.d. for 5 days.
Children age 1 and older who weigh 15 kg (33 lb) or less: 30 mg oral suspension P.O. b.i.d. for 5 days.
◼ **Adjust-a-dose:** For adults and adolescents with renal impairment, if creatinine clearance is 10 to 30 ml/minute, give 75 mg P.O. once daily for 5 days.

▶ **Prevention of influenza after close contact with infected person (beginning within 2 days of exposure).** *Adults and children age 13 and older, and children age 1 and older who weigh more than 40 kg (88 lb):* 75 mg P.O. once daily for at least 10 days.
Children age 1 and older who weigh 23 to 40 kg (51 to 88 lb): 60 mg oral suspension P.O. once daily for 10 days.
Children age 1 and older who weigh 15 to 23 kg (33 to 51 lb): 45 mg oral suspension P.O. once daily for 10 days.
Children age 1 and older who weigh 15 kg (33 lb) or less: 30 mg oral suspension P.O. once daily for 10 days.
◼ **Adjust-a-dose:** For adults and adolescents with renal impairment, if creatinine clearance is 10 to 30 ml/minute, give 75-mg capsule once every other day or 30 mg of oral suspension daily.

▶ **Prevention of influenza during a community outbreak.** *Adults and children age 13 and older:* 75 mg P.O. daily for up to 6 weeks.
◼ **Adjust-a-dose:** For patients with renal impairment, if creatinine clearance is 10 to 30 ml/minute, give 75 mg once every other day or 30 mg of oral suspension daily.

Contraindications and cautions

- Contraindicated in patients hypersensitive to the drug or any of its components.
⚘ **Lifespan:** In breast-feeding women, use only if benefits outweigh risks to the infant. In children younger than age 1, use for treatment or prevention of influenza hasn't been established.

Adverse reactions

CNS: dizziness, fatigue, headache, insomnia, vertigo.
GI: abdominal pain, diarrhea, nausea, vomiting.
Respiratory: bronchitis, cough.

Interactions

None significant.

Effects on lab test results

None reported.

Pharmacokinetics

Absorption: Good. More than 75% reaches systemic circulation as oseltamivir carboxylate.
Distribution: 3% to 42% protein-bound.
Metabolism: Extensive.
Excretion: Mostly in urine by glomerular filtration and tubular secretion. Less than 20% is eliminated in feces. *Half-life:* 1 to 10 hours.

Route	Onset	Peak	Duration
P.O.	Unknown	Unknown	Unknown

Action

Chemical effect: Inhibits the enzyme neuraminidase in influenza virus particles. This action may inhibit viral replication, possibly by interfering with viral particle aggregation and release from the host cell.
Therapeutic effect: Lessens the symptoms of influenza.

Available forms

Capsules: 30 mg, 45 mg, 75 mg
Oral suspension: 12 mg/ml after reconstitution

NURSING PROCESS

Assessment
- Obtain complete medical history before starting therapy.
- Assess renal function before giving drug, as directed.
- Assess patient's and family's knowledge of drug therapy.

Nursing diagnoses
- Risk for infection related to influenza virus
- Imbalanced nutrition: Less than body requirements related to drug's adverse GI effects
- Deficient knowledge related to drug therapy

Planning and implementation
- Drug is used mainly to treat symptoms and isn't a replacement for an annual influenza vaccination.
- No evidence supports use in treating other viral infections.
- Drug may be given with meals to decrease adverse GI effects.
- Safety and effectiveness of repeated courses of therapy haven't been established.

Patient teaching
- Tell patient to start drug within 2 days of start of symptoms.
- Inform patient that receiving this drug isn't a substitute for receiving the flu vaccination. Urge patient to continue receiving an annual vaccination.

Evaluation
- Patient recovers from influenza.
- Patient has no adverse GI effects and maintains adequate hydration.
- Patient and family state understanding of drug therapy.

oxaprozin potassium
(oks-uh-PROH-zin puh-TAH-see-um)
Daypro, Daypro ALTA

Pharmacologic class: NSAID
Therapeutic class: anti-inflammatory, analgesic
Pregnancy risk category: C

Indications and dosages

▶ **Osteoarthritis, rheumatoid arthritis.**
Adults: 1,200 mg P.O. once daily. Divide doses in patients unable to tolerate single doses. For osteoarthritis patients with low body weight and milder disease, give an initial dose of 600 mg once daily. Maximum daily dosage, 1,800 mg.
Adjust-a-dose: For patients with renal impairment and those undergoing hemodialysis, initial dose is 600 mg P.O. daily.

Contraindications and cautions
- Contraindicated in patients hypersensitive to the drug or any of its components and in those with syndrome of nasal polyps, angioedema, and bronchospastic reactions to aspirin or other NSAIDs.
- Use cautiously in patients with history of peptic ulcer disease, hepatic or renal dysfunction, hypertension, CV disease, or conditions that predispose to fluid retention.
Lifespan: In pregnant women, use cautiously. In breast-feeding women, use cautiously; it's unknown if the drug appears in breast milk. In children, safety and effectiveness haven't been established.

Adverse reactions
CNS: confusion, depression, sedation, sleep disturbances, somnolence.
EENT: tinnitus, visual disturbances.
GI: abdominal pain or distress, anorexia, *constipation, diarrhea, dyspepsia,* flatulence, **GI hemorrhage,** nausea, vomiting.
GU: dysuria, renal insufficiency, urinary frequency.
Skin: photosensitivity, rash.

Interactions
Drug-drug. *Antihypertensives, diuretics:* May decrease effect. Monitor patient closely, and adjust dosage.
Aspirin: May displace salicylates from protein-binding sites, increasing risk of salicylate toxicity. Avoid using together.
Aspirin, corticosteroids: May increase risk of adverse GI reactions. Avoid using together.
Cyclosporine: May increase risk of nephrotoxicity by both drugs. Monitor renal function tests.
Methotrexate: Increases risk of methotrexate toxicity. Avoid using together.

Oral anticoagulants: May increase risk of bleeding. Use together cautiously; monitor patient for bleeding.

Drug-herb. *Dong quai, feverfew, garlic, ginger, horse chestnut, red clover:* May increase risk of bleeding. Discourage using together.

St. John's wort: May increase risk of photosensitivity. Advise patient to avoid unprotected or prolonged exposure to sunlight.

Drug-lifestyle. *Alcohol use:* May increase risk of adverse GI reactions. Discourage using together.

Sun exposure: May cause photosensitivity reactions. Urge patient to avoid unprotected or prolonged exposure to sunlight.

Effects on lab test results

• May increase ALT, AST, BUN, and creatinine levels. May decrease hemoglobin level and hematocrit.
• May increase bleeding time.

Pharmacokinetics

Absorption: Bioavailability is 95%; food may reduce rate but not extent.
Distribution: About 99.9% protein-bound.
Metabolism: In liver.
Excretion: In urine (65%) and feces (35%).
Half-life: 42 to 50 hours.

Route	Onset	Peak	Duration
P.O.	Unknown	2 hr	Unknown

Action

Chemical effect: May inhibit prostaglandin synthesis.
Therapeutic effect: Relieves pain, fever, and inflammation.

Available forms

Caplets: 600 mg
Tablets: 600 mg

NURSING PROCESS

🗚 Assessment

• Assess patient's condition before starting therapy and regularly thereafter to monitor drug's effectiveness.
• Monitor liver function test results periodically during long-term therapy, and closely monitor patient with abnormal test results. Liver function values may be elevated. These abnormal

findings may persist, worsen, or resolve with continued therapy. Rarely, patient may progress to severe hepatic dysfunction.
• Be alert for adverse reactions and drug interactions.
• Assess patient's and family's knowledge of drug therapy.

🔟 Nursing diagnoses

• Chronic pain related to condition
• Impaired tissue integrity related to adverse GI effects of drug
• Deficient knowledge related to drug therapy

❯ Planning and implementation

• Give drug on empty stomach unless adverse GI reactions occur.
• Notify prescriber immediately about adverse reactions, especially GI symptoms.
🔅 **ALERT:** Don't confuse oxaprozin with oxazepam.

Patient teaching
• Tell patient experiencing adverse GI effects, to take drug with milk or meals.
• Explain that full therapeutic effects may be delayed for 2 to 4 weeks.
• Tell patient to report adverse visual or auditory reactions immediately.
• Teach patient to recognize and promptly report signs and symptoms of GI bleeding.
• Advise patient to use sunscreen, wear protective clothing, and avoid prolonged exposure to sunlight.
• Warn patient to avoid hazardous activities until CNS effects of drug are known.

✓ Evaluation

• Patient is free from pain.
• Patient maintains GI tissue integrity.
• Patient and family state understanding of drug therapy.

oxazepam
(oks-AZ-ih-pam)
Serax

Pharmacologic class: benzodiazepine
Therapeutic class: anxiolytic
Pregnancy risk category: D
Controlled substance schedule: IV

Indications and dosages

▶ **Alcohol withdrawal.** *Adults:* 15 to 30 mg P.O. t.i.d. or q.i.d.
▶ **Severe anxiety.** *Adults:* 15 to 30 mg P.O. t.i.d. or q.i.d.
▶ **Mild to moderate anxiety.** *Adults:* 10 to 15 mg P.O. t.i.d. or q.i.d.
▶ **Older patients with anxiety, tension, irritability, and agitation.** *Adults:* 10 mg P.O. t.i.d. May increase cautiously to 15 mg P.O. t.i.d. to q.i.d.

Contraindications and cautions

• Contraindicated in patients hypersensitive to the drug or any of its components.
• Use cautiously in patients with history of drug abuse and in those for whom a drop in blood pressure could lead to cardiac problems.
⚘ **Lifespan:** In pregnant and breast-feeding women, don't use. In children, safety and effectiveness haven't been established. In the elderly, use cautiously.

Adverse reactions

CNS: drowsiness, fainting, hangover, lethargy, *mental changes.*
CV: transient hypotension.
GI: abdominal discomfort, nausea, vomiting.
Hepatic: *hepatic dysfunction.*
Other: increased risk of falls.

Interactions

Drug-drug. *CNS depressants:* May increase CNS depression. Avoid using together.
Digoxin: May increase digoxin level, increasing toxicity. Monitor level closely.
Hormonal contraceptives: May increase oxazepam clearance. Monitor patient for decreased effect.
Lamotrigine: May decrease lamotrigine level. Adjust lamotrigine dosage as needed.
Phenytoin: May increase oxazepam clearance and phenytoin level. Monitor patient closely for phenytoin toxicity.
Drug-herb. *Catnip, kava, lady's slipper, lemon balm, passionflower, sassafras, skullcap, valerian:* May increase sedative effects. Discourage using together.
Drug-lifestyle. *Alcohol use:* May increase CNS depression. Discourage using together.
Smoking: May increase benzodiazepine clearance. Monitor patient for lack of drug effect.

Effects on lab test results

• May increase liver function test values.

Pharmacokinetics

Absorption: Good.
Distribution: Wide. 85% to 95% protein-bound.
Metabolism: In liver.
Excretion: In urine. *Half-life:* 5¾ to 10 hours.

Route	Onset	Peak	Duration
P.O.	Unknown	3 hr	Unknown

Action

Chemical effect: May stimulate GABA receptors in ascending reticular activating system.
Therapeutic effect: Relieves anxiety and promotes calmness.

Available forms

Capsules: 10 mg, 15 mg, 30 mg
Tablets: 10 mg, 15 mg, 30 mg

NURSING PROCESS

🜚 Assessment
• Assess patient's condition before starting therapy and regularly thereafter to monitor drug's effectiveness.
• Monitor liver, renal, and hematopoietic function studies periodically in patient receiving repeated or prolonged therapy.
• Be alert for adverse reactions and drug interactions.
• Assess patient's and family's knowledge of drug therapy.

🜚 Nursing diagnoses
• Disturbed thought processes related to condition
• Risk for injury related to drug-induced adverse CNS reactions
• Deficient knowledge related to drug therapy

▶ Planning and implementation
• Lower the dosage in an elderly or debilitated patient.
• Possibility of abuse and addiction exists. Don't abruptly stop giving the drug; withdrawal symptoms may occur.
🛈 ALERT: Don't confuse oxazepam with oxaprozin.

Patient teaching

• Warn patient to avoid hazardous activities until CNS effects of drug are known.
• Tell patient to avoid alcohol during therapy.
• Warn patient not to stop drug abruptly; withdrawal signs may occur.

☑ Evaluation

• Patient has less anxiety.
• Patient sustains no injury as result of drug therapy.
• Patient and family state understanding of drug therapy.

oxcarbazepine
(ox-car-BAY-zah-peen)
Trileptal

Pharmacologic class: carboxamide derivative
Therapeutic class: antiepileptic
Pregnancy risk category: C

Indications and dosages

▶ **Adjunctive therapy for partial seizures in patients with epilepsy.** *Adults:* Initially, 300 mg P.O. b.i.d. Increase by maximum of 600 mg daily (300 mg P.O. b.i.d.) at weekly intervals. Recommended daily dosage is 600 mg P.O. b.i.d.
Children ages 4 to 16: Initially, 4 to 5 mg/kg P.O. b.i.d., not to exceed 600 mg P.O. daily. Target maintenance dosage depends on patient weight. If patient weighs 20 to 29 kg (44 to 64 lb), target maintenance dosage is 900 mg daily. If 29.1 to 39 kg (64 to 86 lb), target maintenance dosage is 1,200 mg daily. If more than 39 kg (86 lb), target maintenance dosage is 1,800 mg daily. Achieve target dosage over 2 weeks.
▶ **Conversion to monotherapy for partial seizures in patients with epilepsy.** *Adults:* Initially, 300 mg P.O. b.i.d. with simultaneous reduction in dosage of other antiepileptics. Increase by a maximum of 600 mg daily at weekly intervals over 2 to 4 weeks. Recommended daily dosage is 2,400 mg P.O., divided b.i.d. Withdraw other antiepileptics completely over 3 to 6 weeks.
Children ages 4 to 16: Initially, 8 to 10 mg/kg P.O. daily divided b.i.d., with simultaneous reduction in dosage of other antiepileptics. Increase by a maximum of 10 mg/kg daily at

weekly intervals. Withdraw other antiepileptics completely over 3 to 6 weeks.
▶ **Initial monotherapy for partial seizures in patients with epilepsy.** *Adults:* Initially, 300 mg P.O. b.i.d. Increase by 300 mg daily every third day to a total daily dosage of 1,200 mg.
Children ages 4 to 16: Initially, 8 to 10 mg/kg P.O. daily divided b.i.d., increasing the dosage by 5 mg/kg daily every third day to the recommended daily dosage:
20 to 24 kg (44 to 54 lb): 600 to 900 mg
25 to 34 kg (55 to 76 lb): 900 to 1,200 mg
35 to 44 kg (77 to 98 lb): 900 to 1,500 mg
45 to 49 kg (99 to 109 lb): 1,200 to 1,500 mg
50 to 59 kg (110 to 131 lb): 1,200 to 1,800 mg
60 to 69 kg (132 to 153 lb): 1,200 to 2,100 mg
70 kg (154 lb): 1,500 to 2,100 mg.
⬧ **Adjust-a-dose:** For patients with renal impairment, if creatinine clearance is less than 30 ml/minute, therapy starts at 150 mg P.O. b.i.d. (one-half the usual starting dose) and increases slowly to achieve desired clinical response.

Contraindications and cautions

• Contraindicated in patients hypersensitive to the drug or any of its components.
• Use cautiously in patients who have had hypersensitivity reactions to carbamazepine.
⚖ **Lifespan:** Effects during pregnancy are unknown. Breast-feeding women should either stop breast-feeding or use another drug.

Adverse reactions

CNS: abnormal coordination, *abnormal gait, aggravated seizures,* agitation, amnesia, anxiety, asthenia, ataxia, confusion, *dizziness,* emotional lability, *fatigue,* feeling abnormal, fever, *headache,* hypoesthesia, impaired concentration, insomnia, nervousness, somnolence, speech disorder, tremor, vertigo.
CV: chest pain, edema, hypotension.
EENT: abnormal accommodation, *abnormal vision, diplopia,* epistaxis, *nystagmus,* pharyngitis, rhinitis, sinusitis.
GI: *abdominal pain,* anorexia, constipation, diarrhea, dry mouth, dyspepsia, gastritis, nausea, rectal hemorrhage, taste perversion, thirst, *vomiting.*
GU: urinary frequency, UTI, vaginitis.
Metabolic: hyponatremia, weight gain.
Musculoskeletal: back pain, muscle weakness.
Respiratory: bronchitis, chest infection, coughing, *upper respiratory tract infection.*

Skin: acne, bruising, increased sweating, purpura, rash, *Stevens–Johnson syndrome, toxic epidermal necrosis.*
Other: allergic reaction, hot flushes, toothache.

Interactions

Drug-drug. *Carbamazepine, valproic acid, verapamil:* May decrease level of the active metabolite of oxcarbazepine. Monitor patient and level closely.
Felodipine: May decrease felodipine level. Monitor patient closely.
Hormonal contraceptives: May decrease levels of ethinyl estradiol and levonorgestrel, which reduces contraceptive effect. Women of childbearing age should use other forms of contraception.
Lamotrigine: May decrease lamotrigine level. Adjust lamotrigine dosage as needed.
Phenobarbital: May decrease level of the active metabolite of oxcarbazepine and increase phenobarbital level. Monitor patient closely.
Phenytoin: May decrease level of the active metabolite of oxcarbazepine. Watch for reduced effect. May increase phenytoin level in adults receiving high doses of oxcarbazepine. Monitor phenytoin level closely when starting therapy in these patients.
Drug-lifestyle. *Alcohol use:* Increases CNS depression. Discourage using together.

Effects on lab test results

● May decrease sodium and T4 levels.

Pharmacokinetics

Absorption: Complete.
Distribution: About 40% of active metabolite is protein-bound, mostly to albumin.
Metabolism: Rapid; 4% of dose is oxidized to inactive metabolite.
Excretion: Mainly by the kidneys. *Half-life:* About 2 hours for drug, about 9 hours for active metabolite. Children younger than age 8 have about 30% to 40% increased clearance of drug.

Route	Onset	Peak	Duration
P.O.	Unknown	Variable	Unknown

Action

Chemical effect: May result from blockade of voltage-sensitive sodium channels, which causes stabilized hyperexcited neural membranes, inhibited repetitive neuronal firing, and reduced synaptic impulses. May stem from increased potassium conductance and modulation of high-voltage activated calcium channels.
Therapeutic effect: Controls partial seizures.

Available forms

Oral suspension: 60 mg/ml*
Tablets (film-coated): 150 mg, 300 mg, 600 mg

NURSING PROCESS

☒ Assessment
⊛ **ALERT:** Ask patient about history of hypersensitivity reaction to carbamazepine because 25% to 30% of affected patients may develop hypersensitivity to this drug. If signs or symptoms of hypersensitivity occur, stop drug immediately.
● Obtain history of patient's underlying condition before starting therapy, and reassess regularly thereafter to monitor the drug's effectiveness.
⊛ **ALERT:** Drug is linked to several adverse neurologic events, including psychomotor slowing, difficulty with concentration, speech or language problems, somnolence, fatigue, and abnormal coordination (including ataxia and gait disturbances). Monitor patient closely.
● Monitor patient for evidence of hyponatremia, including nausea, malaise, headache, lethargy, confusion, and decreased sensation.
● Assess patient's and family's knowledge of drug therapy.

⊕ Nursing diagnoses
● Risk for trauma related to seizures
● Risk for injury related to drug-induced adverse reactions
● Deficient knowledge related to drug therapy

▸ Planning and implementation
⊛ **ALERT:** Gradually stop giving the drug to minimize risk of increased seizure frequency.
● Correct hyponatremia as needed.
● Shake oral suspension well before giving. Suspension can be mixed with water or may be swallowed directly from the syringe. Oral suspension and tablets may be interchanged at equal doses. Suspension can be taken without regard to food.
● Serious skin reactions including Stevens-Johnson syndrome and toxic epidermal necrosis can occur.

Reactions may be *common*, uncommon, *life-threatening*, or COMMON AND LIFE-THREATENING.

Patient teaching
• Advise patient to tell prescriber if he has ever had a hypersensitivity reaction to carbamazepine.
• Tell patient that drug may be taken with or without food.
• Warn patient to avoid hazardous activities until the drug's CNS effects are known.
• Tell patient not to drink alcohol while taking drug.
• Advise patient not to interrupt therapy without consulting prescriber.
• Advise patient to immediately report skin rashes to his prescriber.
• Advise patient to report fever and swollen lymph nodes to his prescriber; multi-organ hypersensitivity reactions may occur, with diverse signs and symptoms.
• Advise patient to report signs and symptoms of hyponatremia, such as nausea, malaise, headache, lethargy, or confusion.
• Advise women using hormonal contraceptives to use a barrier method of birth control while taking drug.

☑ **Evaluation**
• Patient experiences no or fewer seizures during drug therapy.
• Patient sustains no injury from drug-induced adverse reactions.
• Patient and family state understanding of drug therapy.

oxybutynin chloride
(oks-ee-BYOO-tih-nin KLOR-ighd)
Ditropan, Ditropan XL, Oxytrol

Pharmacologic class: synthetic tertiary amine
Therapeutic class: urinary antispasmodic
Pregnancy risk category: B

Indications and dosages

▶ **Uninhibited or reflex neurogenic bladder.**
Adults: 5 mg P.O. b.i.d. to t.i.d., up to 5 mg q.i.d.
Children older than age 5: Give 5 mg P.O. b.i.d., up to 5 mg t.i.d.
▶ **Overactive bladder.** *Adults:* Initially, 5 mg Ditropan XL P.O. once daily. Adjust dosage weekly in 5-mg increments, as needed, to a maximum of 30 mg P.O. daily. Or, 1 transder-

mal patch (Oxytrol) twice weekly applied to dry, intact skin on abdomen, hip, or buttocks.

Contraindications and cautions

• Contraindicated in patients hypersensitive to the drug or any of its components, in debilitated patients with intestinal atony, in hemorrhaging patients with unstable CV condition, and in patients with myasthenia gravis, GI obstruction, glaucoma, adynamic ileus, megacolon, severe colitis, ulcerative colitis with megacolon, or obstructive uropathy.
• Use cautiously in patients with autonomic neuropathy, reflux esophagitis, or hepatic or renal disease. Use transdermal patch cautiously in patients with bladder outflow obstruction, gastroesophageal reflux, intestinal atony, and in those taking bisphosphonates.
⚖ **Lifespan:** In pregnant women, use cautiously. In breast-feeding women, use cautiously; it's unknown if the drug appears in breast milk. In the elderly, use cautiously. In the elderly who have intestinal atony, drug is contraindicated.

Adverse reactions

Oral form
CNS: dizziness, drowsiness, fever, impaired alertness, insomnia, restlessness.
CV: flushing, palpitations, tachycardia.
EENT: cycloplegia, mydriasis, transient blurred vision.
GI: bloated feeling, *constipation, dry mouth,* nausea, vomiting.
GU: impotence, urinary hesitancy, urine retention.
Skin: decreased diaphoresis, rash, urticaria.
Other: allergic reactions, suppressed lactation.
Transdermal form
CNS: fatigue, headache, somnolence.
CV: flushing.
EENT: abnormal vision.
GI: abdominal pain, diarrhea, *dry mouth,* flatulence, nausea.
GU: dysuria.
Musculoskeletal: back pain.
Skin: burns, erythema, macules, *pruritus,* rash, vesicles.

Interactions

Drug-drug. *Amantadine, anticholinergics:* May increase anticholinergic effects. Use together cautiously.

Atenolol, digoxin: May increase levels of these drugs. Monitor patient closely. Use of digoxin elixir or capsules may avoid the interaction.
CNS depressants: May increase CNS effects. Use cautiously.
Drug-lifestyle. *Alcohol use:* May increase CNS effects. Discourage using together.
Exercise, hot weather: May precipitate heatstroke. Urge patient to stay hydrated and to avoid exercise or increased activity during hot and humid weather.

Effects on lab test results

None reported.

Pharmacokinetics

Absorption: Rapid.
Distribution: Unknown. Transdermal system is widely distributed.
Metabolism: By liver. Transdermal system is metabolized by liver and gut wall by CYP3A4; bypasses first-pass metabolism.
Excretion: Mainly in urine. *Transdermal half-life:* 2 hours.

Route	Onset	Peak	Duration
P.O.	30–60 min	3–4 hr	6–10 hr
Transdermal	24–48 hr	Varies	96 hr

Action

Chemical effect: Produces direct spasmolytic effect and antimuscarinic (atropine-like) effect on smooth muscles of urinary tract, increasing bladder capacity and providing some local anesthesia and mild analgesia.
Therapeutic effect: Relieves bladder spasms.

Available forms

Syrup: 5 mg/5 ml
Tablets: 5 mg
Tablets (extended-release): 5 mg, 10 mg, 15 mg
Transdermal patch: 36-mg patch (delivers 3.9 mg/day)

NURSING PROCESS

Assessment

• Assess patient's bladder condition before starting therapy.
• Before giving drug, confirm neurogenic bladder by cystometry and rule out partial intestinal obstruction in patients with diarrhea, especially those with colostomy or ileostomy.
• Prepare patient for periodic cystometry to evaluate response to therapy.
• Watch geriatric patients for confusion and mental changes.
• Be alert for adverse reactions.
• Drug may aggravate symptoms of hyperthyroidism, coronary artery disease, heart failure, arrhythmias, tachycardia, hypertension, or prostatic hyperplasia.
• Assess patient's and family's knowledge of drug therapy.

Nursing diagnoses

• Acute pain related to bladder spasms
• Risk for injury related to drug-induced adverse CNS reactions
• Deficient knowledge related to drug therapy

Planning and implementation

• If patient has a UTI, give prescribed antibiotics.
• To minimize tendency toward tolerance, periodically stop therapy to determine whether patient can be weaned off drug.
ALERT: Don't confuse Ditropan with diazepam or Dithranol.
Patient teaching
• Warn patient to avoid hazardous activities until the drug's CNS effects are known.
• Tell patient not to drink alcohol during therapy.
• Advise patient that taking drug in hot weather raises the risk of fever or heatstroke, and urge patient to take precautions to avoid excessive heat and maintain adequate hydration.
• Instruct patient to change transdermal patch two times weekly and to avoid using the same site within 7 days. Also warn patient to wear only one patch at a time and to properly dispose of old patches to prevent accidental application or ingestion.
• Advise patient to store drug in tightly closed container at room temperature.

Evaluation

• Patient is free from bladder pain.
• Patient sustains no injuries from drug-induced adverse CNS reactions.
• Patient and family state understanding of drug therapy.

---

oxycodone hydrochloride
(oks-ee-KOH-dohn high-droh-KLOR-ighd)
**M-Oxy, OxyContin◆, OxyFAST, OxyIR,
Roxicodone*, Roxicodone Intensol**

Pharmacologic class: opioid
Therapeutic class: analgesic
Pregnancy risk category: B
Controlled substance schedule: II

Indications and dosages

▶ **Moderate to severe pain.** *Adults:* 5 mg P.O. every 6 hours, p.r.n.
▶ **Moderate to severe pain in patients not taking opioids who need a continuous around-the-clock analgesic for an extended period.** *Adults:* 10 mg extended-release tablets P.O. every 12 hours. May increase dosage every 1 to 2 days, as needed. The 80-mg and 160-mg forms are for opioid-tolerant patients only.
▧ **Adjust-a-dose:** For patients with impaired hepatic function, start extended-release tablets at one-third to one-half of usual dosage and adjust carefully. In patients with impaired renal function, if creatinine clearance is less than 60 ml/minute, reduce initial extended-release dose and adjust carefully.

Contraindications and cautions

• Contraindicated in patients hypersensitive to the drug or any of its components.
• Extended-release tablets are contraindicated in patients with known or suspected paralytic ileus.
• Use cautiously in debilitated patients and in those with head injury, increased intracranial pressure, seizures, asthma, COPD, prostatic hyperplasia, severe hepatic or renal disease, acute abdominal conditions, urethral stricture, hypothyroidism, Addison disease, or arrhythmias.
✽ **Lifespan:** In pregnant women, use cautiously. In breast-feeding women, use cautiously; it's unknown if the drug appears in breast milk. In children, drug isn't recommended. In the elderly, use cautiously due to increased risk of delayed renal excretion and of CNS effects.

Adverse reactions

CNS: *clouded sensorium, dizziness, euphoria,* sedation, somnolence.
CV: *bradycardia,* hypotension.
GI: *constipation,* ileus, nausea, *vomiting.*
GU: urine retention.
Respiratory: *respiratory depression.*
Other: physical dependence.

Interactions

Drug-drug. *Anticoagulants:* May increase anticoagulant effect if combination product with aspirin is used. Monitor PT and INR. Use together cautiously; monitor patient for bleeding.
CNS depressants, general anesthetics, hypnotics, MAO inhibitors, other opioid analgesics, protease inhibitors, sedatives, tranquilizers, tricyclic antidepressants: May have additive effects. Use together cautiously. Reduce oxycodone dosage as directed, and monitor patient response.
Drug-lifestyle. *Alcohol use:* May increase CNS depression. Discourage using together.

Effects on lab test results

• May increase amylase and lipase levels.

Pharmacokinetics

Absorption: Unknown.
Distribution: Unknown.
Metabolism: In liver.
Excretion: Mainly in urine. *Half-life:* 2 to 3 hours.

Route	Onset	Peak	Duration
P.O.	10–15 min	≤ 1 hr	3–6 hr
P.R.	Unknown	Unknown	Unknown

Action

Chemical effect: Binds with opiate receptors in CNS, altering response to pain by an unknown mechanism.
Therapeutic effect: Relieves pain.

Available forms

Capsules: 5 mg
Oral solution: 5 mg/5 ml, 20 mg/ml
Tablets: 5 mg, 10 mg, 15 mg, 20 mg, 30 mg
Tablets (extended-release): 10 mg, 20 mg, 40 mg, 80 mg

NURSING PROCESS

☞ Assessment
• Assess patient's pain before and after giving drug.
• Monitor circulation and respirations.
• Be alert for adverse reactions and drug interactions.

- Monitor patient for development of constipation.
- Assess patient's and family's knowledge of drug therapy.

✦ Nursing diagnoses
- Acute pain related to condition
- Ineffective breathing pattern related to drug-induced respiratory depression
- Deficient knowledge related to drug therapy

⟩ Planning and implementation
- Give drug with food or milk to avoid GI upset.
- ⚡ ALERT: Drug isn't intended for p.r.n. use or for immediate postoperative pain. Drug is only indicated for postoperative use if patient was receiving it before surgery or if pain is expected to persist for an extended length of time.
- For best results, give drug before patient has intense pain.
- Single-agent oxycodone solution or tablet is especially useful for patient who can't take aspirin or acetaminophen.
- ⚡ ALERT: If respirations are shallow or rate falls below 12 breaths/minute, withhold dose and notify prescriber.
- ⚡ ALERT: Don't confuse oxycodone immediate-release tablets with OxyContin extended-release tablets.
- ⚡ ALERT: Drug is addictive and abused as much as morphine. Chewing, crushing, snorting, or injecting it can lead to overdose and death.
- ⚡ ALERT: Don't confuse Roxicodone Intensol with other Intensol products manufactured by Roxane.

Patient teaching
- Instruct patient to take drug with food or milk to minimize GI upset.
- Tell patient to ask for drug before pain becomes intense.
- Tell patient not to chew or crush OxyIR or extended-release forms.
- Warn ambulatory patient about getting out of bed or walking. Warn outpatient to avoid hazardous activities until CNS effects of drug are known.

✓ Evaluation
- Patient is free from pain.
- Patient's respiratory rate and pattern remain within normal limits.
- Patient and family state understanding of drug therapy.

HIGH ALERT

oxymorphone hydrochloride
(oks-ee-MOR-fohn high-droh-KLOR-ighd)
Opana, Opana ER

Pharmacologic class: opioid
Therapeutic class: analgesic
Pregnancy risk category: C; D if used for prolonged periods or high doses at term
Controlled substance schedule: II

Indications and dosages

▶ **Moderate to severe pain.** *Adults:* 1 to 1.5 mg I.M. or subcutaneously every 4 to 6 hours, p.r.n. Or, 0.5 mg I.V. every 4 to 6 hours, p.r.n. Or, in opioid-naïve patients, give 10 to 20 mg P.O. every 4 to 6 hours. If needed, start with 5 mg P.O. and adjust based on patient response.
▶ **Moderate to severe pain in patients who need continuous, around-the-clock opioid treatment for an extended time.** *Opioid-naïve adults:* 5 mg extended-release form P.O. every 12 hours. Increase by 5 to 10 mg every 12 hours every 3 to 7 days as needed and tolerated. Patients taking Opana immediate-release tablets can be switched to extended-release Opana ER tablets by giving one-half the patient's total daily dosage of Opana as Opana ER every 12 hours.
◳ **Adjust-a-dose:** For patients with mild hepatic impairment or creatinine clearance less than 50 ml/minute, start with the lowest possible dose and increase slowly as tolerated.

▼ I.V. administration
- Give drug by direct I.V. injection. If needed, dilute in normal saline solution.
- To minimize hypotension, keep patient supine while giving drug.
⊗ **Incompatibilities**
None reported.

Contraindications and cautions
- Contraindicated in patients hypersensitive to drug and in those with acute asthma attacks, severe respiratory depression, upper airway obstruction, paralytic ileus, moderate to severe hepatic impairment, or pulmonary edema caused by a respiratory irritant.
- Use cautiously in debilitated patients and those with head injury, increased intracranial

---

pressure, seizures, asthma, COPD, acute abdominal conditions, biliary tract disease (including pancreatitis), acute alcoholism, delirium tremens, prostatic hyperplasia, renal or mild hepatic impairment, urethral stricture, respiratory depression, hypothyroidism, Addison disease, or arrhythmias.

※ **Lifespan:** In pregnant women, use cautiously. In breast-feeding women, use cautiously; it's unknown if the drug appears in breast milk. In the elderly, use cautiously due to increased risk of delayed renal excretion and of CNS effects. In children, drug is contraindicated.

Adverse reactions

CNS: *clouded sensorium, dizziness,* dysphoria, euphoria, hallucinations, headache, physical dependence, lightheadedness, restlessness, *sedation, seizures* (with large doses), *somnolence.*
CV: *bradycardia,* hypotension.
EENT: blurred vision, diplopia, miosis.
GI: *constipation,* ileus, *nausea, vomiting.*
GU: urine retention.
Respiratory: *respiratory depression.*
Skin: *increased sweating,* pruritus.

Interactions

Drug-drug. *Agonist/antagonist analgesics:* May reduce analgesic effect or cause withdrawal symptoms. Don't use together.
Anticholinergics: May increase risk of urine retention, severe constipation, and paralytic ileus. Monitor patient for abdominal pain or distention.
CNS depressants, general anesthetics, MAO inhibitors, tricyclic antidepressants: May have additive effects. Use together cautiously, and reduce opioid dosage.
Drug-lifestyle. *Alcohol use:* May have additive effects. Discourage using together.

Effects on lab test results

• May increase amylase and lipase levels.

Pharmacokinetics

Absorption: Good.
Distribution: Wide.
Metabolism: Mainly in liver.
Excretion: Mainly in urine. *Half-life:* For parenteral use, unknown. For ER tablets, 7 to 12 hours. For immediate-release tablets, 3 to 12 hours.

Route	Onset	Peak	Duration
I.V.	5–10 min	15–30 min	3–4 hr
I.M.	10–15 min	30–90 min	3–6 hr
P.O.	Variable	Variable	Variable
SubQ	10–15 min	60–90 min	3–6 hr

Action

Chemical effect: Binds with opiate receptors in CNS, altering response to pain by an unknown mechanism.
Therapeutic effect: Relieves pain.

Available forms

Injection: 1 mg/ml
Tablets: 5 mg, 10 mg
Tablets (extended-release): 5 mg, 10 mg, 20 mg, 40 mg

NURSING PROCESS

✍ Assessment
• Assess patient's pain before and after giving drug.
• Be alert for adverse reactions and drug interactions.
• Assess patient's and family's knowledge of drug therapy.

✡ Nursing diagnoses
• Acute pain related to condition
• Ineffective breathing pattern related to drug-induced respiratory depression
• Deficient knowledge related to drug therapy

▶ Planning and implementation
• Keep opioid antagonist (naloxone) and resuscitation equipment available.
• Use of this drug may worsen gallbladder pain.
• Drug isn't for mild pain. For better effect, give drug before patient has intense pain.
• Extended-release tablets aren't for p.r.n. use.
• Monitor CV and respiratory status. If respirations decrease or rate is below 12 breaths/minute, withhold dose and notify prescriber.
• Monitor bladder and bowel function. Patient may need a laxative.
⚠ **ALERT:** Don't confuse oxymorphone with oxymetholone or oxycodone.
Patient teaching
• Instruct patient to ask for drug before pain is intense. Make sure patient knows that extended-release tablets must be taken around-the-clock.

• When drug is used I.M. or I.V. after surgery, encourage patient to turn, cough, and deep-breathe and to use incentive spirometer to avoid lung problems.

• Caution ambulatory patient about getting out of bed or walking. Warn outpatient to avoid driving and other hazardous activities that require mental alertness until drug's CNS effects are known.

⊛ **ALERT:** Caution patient not to consume alcohol or take any prescription or OTC product containing alcohol with oral form of drug because doing so can lead to oxymorphone overdose.

⊛ **ALERT:** Warn patient not to crush, break, chew, or dissolve extended-release tablets; may lead to a fatal dose of oxymorphone.

• Instruct patient to take tablets 1 hour before or 2 hours after a meal.

• Instruct patient to keep oral form in a child-resistant container in a safe place. Accidental ingestion by a child can result in death.

• Advise patient or family to report a decreased respiratory rate.

• Teach patient about increasing fluid and fiber intake to prevent constipation.

☑ Evaluation

• Patient is free from pain.

• Patient's respiration is normal.

• Patient and family state understanding of drug therapy.

HIGH ALERT

oxytocin, synthetic injection
(oks-ih-TOH-sin)
Pitocin

Pharmacologic class: exogenous hormone
Therapeutic class: lactation stimulant, oxytocic
Pregnancy risk category: NR

Indications and dosages

▶ **To induce or stimulate labor.** *Adults:* Initially, 1-ml ampule (10 units) I.V. in 1,000 ml of D_5W, lactated Ringer's, or normal saline solution infused at 0.5 to 2 milliunits/minute. Increase rate in increments of no more than 1 to 2 milliunits/minute at 30- to 60-minute intervals until normal contraction pattern is established. Decrease rate when labor is firmly established. Rates exceeding 9 to 10 milliunits/minute rarely

are required; maximum dose 20 milliunits/minute.

▶ **To reduce postpartum bleeding after expulsion of placenta.** *Adults:* 10 to 40 units I.V. in 1,000 ml of D_5W or normal saline solution infused at rate that controls bleeding, usually 20 to 40 milliunits/minute. Give 10 units I.M. after delivery of placenta.

▶ **Incomplete or inevitable abortion.** *Adults:* 10 units I.V. in 500 ml of normal saline solution or dextrose 5% in normal saline solution or D_5W. Infuse at 10 to 20 milliunits/minute (20 to 40 gtt/minute).

▶ **Oxytocin challenge test to assess fetal distress in high-risk pregnancies greater than 31 weeks' gestation‡.** *Adults:* 5 to 10 units I.V. in 1 L of D_5W injection, yielding a solution of 5 to 10 milliunits per ml. Infuse 0.5 milliunits/minute, gradually increasing at 15-minute intervals to a maximum infusion of 20 milliunits/minute. Stop infusion when three moderate uterine contractions occur within a 10-minute period. Response of fetal heart rate may be used to evaluate prognosis.

▼ I.V. administration

• Give only by infusion.

• Give by piggyback infusion so drug can be stopped without interrupting I.V. line.

• Use an infusion pump.

⊗ **Incompatibilities**
Plasmin, norepinephrine bitartrate, Normosol-M with dextrose 5%, prochlorperazine, warfarin sodium.

Contraindications and cautions

• Contraindicated in patients hypersensitive to the drug or any of its components. Also contraindicated in cephalopelvic disproportion or delivery that requires conversion, as in transverse lie; in fetal distress when delivery isn't imminent; in prematurity; in other obstetric emergencies; and in severe toxemia, hypertonic uterine patterns, total placenta previa, or vasa previa.

• During first and second stages of labor, use cautiously because cervical laceration, uterine rupture, and maternal and fetal death may occur. In patients with grand multiparity, uterine sepsis, traumatic delivery, or overdistended uterus, use cautiously.

• Use cautiously in patients with invasive cervical carcinoma and in patients with history of cervical or uterine surgery.

⚖ **Lifespan:** Drug is only indicated for pregnant and postpartum women.

Adverse reactions

Maternal
CNS: *coma from water intoxication, seizures, subarachnoid hemorrhage from hypertension.*
CV: *arrhythmias; hypertension;* increased heart rate, systemic venous return, and cardiac output.
GI: nausea, vomiting.
GU: abruptio placentae, increased uterine motility, impaired uterine blood flow, pelvic hematoma, *postpartum hemorrhage,* tetanic uterine contractions, *uterine rupture.*
Hematologic: *fatal afibrinogenemia* (may be related to postpartum bleeding).
Other: *anaphylaxis,* hypersensitivity reactions.
Fetal
CNS: *Permanent CNS or brain damage, neonatal seizures.*
CV: *bradycardia,* PVCs, tachycardia.
Hematologic: hyperbilirubinemia.
Respiratory: *anoxia, asphyxia.*
Other: *fetal death.*

Interactions

Drug-drug. *Cyclopropane anesthetics:* May cause less pronounced tachycardia but more severe hypotension. May cause maternal sinus bradycardia with abnormal atrioventricular arrhythmias. Use together cautiously.
Thiopental anesthetics: May delay induction. Use together cautiously.
Vasoconstrictors: May cause severe hypertension in patients receiving caudal block anesthetic. Avoid using together.

Effects on lab test results

None reported.

Pharmacokinetics

Absorption: Unknown.
Distribution: Through extracellular fluid.
Metabolism: Rapid, in kidneys and liver. In early pregnancy, a circulating enzyme, oxytocinase, can inactivate drug.
Excretion: Small amounts in urine. *Half-life:* 3 to 5 minutes.

Route	Onset	Peak	Duration
I.V.	Immediate	Unknown	1 hr
I.M.	3–5 min	Unknown	2–3 hr

Action

Chemical effect: Causes potent and selective stimulation of uterine and mammary gland smooth muscle.
Therapeutic effect: Induces labor and milk ejection and reduces postpartum bleeding.

Available forms

Injection: 10 units/ml in ampule, vial, or syringe

NURSING PROCESS

🔧 Assessment
• Assess patient's condition before starting therapy and regularly thereafter.
• Monitor and record uterine contractions, heart rate, blood pressure, intrauterine pressure, fetal heart rate, and blood loss every 15 minutes.
• Be alert for adverse reactions and drug interactions.
• Monitor fluid intake and output. Antidiuretic effect may lead to fluid overload, seizures, and coma.
• Assess patient's and family's knowledge of drug therapy.

⊞ Nursing diagnoses
• Risk for deficient fluid volume related to postpartum bleeding
• Excessive fluid volume related to drug-induced antidiuretic effect
• Deficient knowledge related to drug therapy

▶ Planning and implementation
• Drug is used to induce or reinforce labor only when pelvis is known to be adequate, vaginal delivery is indicated, fetal maturity is ensured, and fetal position is favorable. Use only in hospital where critical care facilities and experienced clinician are immediately available.
• Drug isn't recommended for routine I.M. use, but 10 units may be given I.M. after delivery of placenta to control postpartum uterine bleeding.
• Never give oxytocin simultaneously by more than one route.
• Have 20% solution of magnesium sulfate available for relaxation of myometrium.
⚠ **ALERT:** If contractions are less than 2 minutes apart, if they're above 50 mm Hg, or if they last 90 seconds or longer, stop infusion, turn patient on her side, and notify prescriber.
⚠ **ALERT:** Don't confuse Pitocin with Pitressin.

O

---

⑤ **ALERT:** Don't confuse oxytocin with OxyContin.

Patient teaching
● Instruct patient to report unusual feelings or adverse effects at once.
● Instruct patient to remain lying down during administration.

☑ **Evaluation**
● Patient maintains adequate fluid balance with drug therapy.
● Patient doesn't develop edema.
● Patient and family state understanding of drug therapy.

HIGH ALERT

paclitaxel
(pak-lih-TAK-sil)
Onxol, Taxol

Pharmacologic class: antimitotic
Therapeutic class: antineoplastic
Pregnancy risk category: D

Indications and dosages

▶ **First-line and subsequent therapy for advanced ovarian cancer.** *Previously untreated adults:* 175 mg/m² over 3 hours every 3 weeks followed by cisplatin 75 mg/m² or 135 mg/m² over 24 hours followed by cisplatin 75 mg/m² every 3 weeks.
Previously treated adults: 135 or 175 mg/m² I.V. over 3 hours every 3 weeks.
▶ **Breast cancer that doesn't respond to combination chemotherapy for metastatic disease or relapse within 6 months of chemotherapy that included an anthracycline; node-positive breast cancer (after combination chemotherapy that includes doxorubicin).** *Adults:* 175 mg/m² I.V. over 3 hours every 3 weeks.
▶ **Initial therapy for advanced non–small-cell lung cancer in patients who aren't candidates for curative surgery or radiation.** *Adults:* 135 mg/m² I.V. infusion over 24 hours; follow with cisplatin 75 mg/m². Repeat cycle every 3 weeks.

⑤ **Adjust-a-dose:** For all indications, give subsequent courses when neutrophil count is at least 1,500/mm³ and platelet count is at least 100,000/mm³. For patients who experience severe neutropenia (neutrophil count less than 500/mm³ for at least 7 days) or severe peripheral neuropathy, reduce dose by 20% for subsequent courses.
▶ **AIDS-related Kaposi sarcoma.** *Adults:* 135 mg/m² I.V. over 3 hours every 3 weeks, or 100 mg/m² I.V. over 3 hours every 2 weeks. Don't give if baseline or subsequent neutrophil counts are less than 1,000/mm³.
⑤ **Adjust-a-dose:** In patients who experience severe neutropenia (neutrophil count less than 500/mm³ for a week or longer) or severe peripheral neuropathy, reduce dose by 20% for subsequent courses. In patients with elevated liver enzymes, toxicity increases. Adjust dosage.

▼ I.V. administration

● Preparing and giving drug are linked to carcinogenic, mutagenic, and teratogenic risks. Follow facility policy for safe handling.
● Dilute concentrate to 0.3 to 1.2 mg/ml before infusion. Compatible solutions include normal saline solution for injection, D_5W, dextrose 5% in normal saline for injection, and dextrose 5% in lactated Ringer's injection.
● Don't allow undiluted concentrate to come in contact with polyvinyl chloride I.V. bags or tubing. Prepare and store infusion solutions in glass containers. Store diluted solution in glass or polypropylene bottles, or use polypropylene or polyolefin bags. Administer through polyethylene-lined administration sets, and use in-line 0.22-micron filter.
● If extravasation occurs, stop infusion and notify prescriber.
● Diluted solutions are stable for 27 hours at room temperature. Prepared solution may appear hazy.
⊗ **Incompatibilities**
Amphotericin B, chlorpromazine, cisplatin, doxorubicin liposomal, hydroxyzine hydrochloride, methylprednisolone sodium succinate, mitoxantrone.

Contraindications and cautions

● Contraindicated in patients hypersensitive to the drug or to polyoxyethylated castor oil, a vehicle used in drug solution, and in patients with solid tumors with baseline neutrophil counts

---

below 1,500/mm³. When used to treat AIDS-related Kaposi sarcoma, contraindicated in patients with baseline neutrophil counts below 1,000/mm³.

• Use cautiously in patients who have received radiation therapy; they may have more frequent or severe myelosuppression.

⚕ Lifespan: In pregnant and breast-feeding women, drug isn't recommended. In children, safety and effectiveness haven't been established.

Adverse reactions

CNS: fever, peripheral neuropathy.
CV: abnormal ECG, *bradycardia,* hypotension.
GI: diarrhea, mucositis, nausea, vomiting.
Hematologic: anemia, *bleeding, leukopenia, neutropenia, thrombocytopenia.*
Musculoskeletal: arthralgia, myalgia.
Skin: *alopecia,* cellulitis at injection site, phlebitis.
Other: *anaphylaxis,* hypersensitivity reactions.

Interactions

Drug-drug. *Carbamazepine, phenobarbital:* May increase the metabolism of paclitaxel. Monitor patient for effectiveness.
Cisplatin: May have additive myelosuppressive effects. Use together cautiously.
Cyclosporine, dexamethasone, diazepam, estradiol, etoposide, ketoconazole, quinidine, retinoic acid, teniposide, testosterone, verapamil, vincristine: May inhibit paclitaxel metabolism. Use together cautiously.
Doxorubicin: May increase levels of doxorubicin and its metabolites. Dosage adjustments may be needed.

Effects on lab test results

• May increase alkaline phosphatase, AST, and triglyceride levels. May decrease hemoglobin level and hematocrit.
• May decrease neutrophil, WBC, and platelet counts.

Pharmacokinetics

Absorption: Given I.V.
Distribution: About 89% to 98% protein-bound.
Metabolism: May be metabolized in liver by CYP2C8 and CYP3A4.
Excretion: Unknown. *Half-life:* 2¼ to 5¾ hours.

Route	Onset	Peak	Duration
I.V.	Unknown	Unknown	Unknown

Action

Chemical effect: Inhibits normal reorganization of microtubule network needed for mitosis and other vital cellular functions.
Therapeutic effect: Stops ovarian and breast cancer cell activity.

Available forms

Injection: 6 mg/ml

NURSING PROCESS

Assessment
• Assess patient's condition before starting therapy and regularly thereafter to monitor drug's effectiveness.
• Continuously monitor patient for first 30 minutes of infusion. Monitor patient closely throughout infusion.
• Monitor blood counts and liver function test results frequently during therapy.
• Be alert for adverse reactions and drug interactions.
• Assess patient's and family's knowledge of drug therapy.

Nursing diagnoses
• Ineffective health maintenance related to cancer
• Ineffective protection related to drug-induced adverse hematologic reactions
• Deficient knowledge related to drug therapy

Planning and implementation
⚠ ALERT: Severe hypersensitivity reactions occur in about 4% of patients, usually within 2 or 3 minutes and almost always within 10 minutes.
• To reduce the risk of severe hypersensitivity, pretreat patient with corticosteroids, such as dexamethasone, and antihistamines. H₁-receptor antagonists, such as diphenhydramine, and H₂-receptor antagonists, such as cimetidine or ranitidine, may be used.
⚠ ALERT: Don't confuse paclitaxel with paroxetine. Don't confuse Taxol with Paxil or Taxotere.
Patient teaching
• Warn patient to watch for signs of bleeding and infection.
• Teach patient symptoms of peripheral neuropathy, such as tingling, burning, or numbness in

limbs, and urge him to report them immediately to prescriber. Dosage reduction may be needed.
• Warn patient that alopecia occurs in up to 82% of patients.
• Advise woman of childbearing age not to become pregnant during therapy. Recommend consulting prescriber before becoming pregnant.

☑ Evaluation
• Patient responds well to therapy.
• Patient develops no serious complications from drug-induced adverse hematologic reactions.
• Patient and family state understanding of drug therapy.

<hr>

HIGH ALERT

paclitaxel protein-bound particles
(pack-lih-TAK-sil)
Abraxane

Pharmacologic class: antimicrotubule drug
Therapeutic class: antineoplastic
Pregnancy risk category: D

Indications and dosages

▶ **Metastatic breast cancer after failure of combination chemotherapy or relapse within 6 months of adjuvant chemotherapy. Previous therapy should have included an anthracycline unless clinically contraindicated.**
Adults: 260 mg/m^2 I.V. over 30 minutes every 3 weeks.
▧ **Adjust-a-dose:** For patients with severe sensory neuropathy or a neutrophil count less than 500 cells/mm^3 for a week or longer, reduce dose to 220 mg/m^2. For recurrence of severe sensory neuropathy or severe neutropenia, reduce dose to 180 mg/m^2. For grade 3 sensory neuropathy, hold drug until condition improves to a grade 1 or 2; then resume drug at a reduced dosage for the duration of treatment.

▽ I.V. administration

• Because of the drug's cytotoxicity, handle it cautiously and wear gloves. If the drug contacts your skin, wash thoroughly with soap and water. If it contacts mucous membranes, flush them thoroughly with water.
• Reconstitute the vial with 20 ml of normal saline solution. Direct the stream slowly, over at least 1 minute, onto the inside wall of the vial to avoid foaming.
• Let the vial sit for 5 minutes to ensure proper wetting of the powder.
• Gently swirl or invert the vial for at least 2 minutes until completely dissolved. If foaming occurs, let the solution stand for 15 minutes for the foam to subside.
• If particles are visible, gently invert the vial again to ensure complete resuspension. The solution should be milky and uniform in appearance.
• Each reconstituted vial contains 5 mg/ml paclitaxel. Inject the dose into an empty polyvinyl chloride I.V. bag.
• Give the drug I.V. over 30 minutes.
• Store unopened vials at room temperature in the original package. Use the contents of reconstituted vials immediately, or, if needed, refrigerate at 36° to 46° F (2° to 8° C) for a maximum of 8 hours. If not used immediately, the vial should be protected from light.
• The suspension for infusion prepared as recommended in an infusion bag is stable at room temperature and ambient lighting for up to 8 hours.

⊗ **Incompatibilities**
None known.

Contraindications and cautions

• Contraindicated in patients with baseline neutrophil counts of less than 1,500/mm^3.
• Use hasn't been studied in patients with serum creatinine level more than 2 mg/dl or bilirubin level more than 1.5 mg/dl.
🍃 **Lifespan:** Women of childbearing age should avoid becoming pregnant during treatment. Women shouldn't breast-feed during treatment. In children, safety and effectiveness haven't been established.

Adverse reactions

CNS: *asthenia, sensory neuropathy.*
CV: *abnormal ECG,* **cardiac arrest, chest pain,** edema, hypertension, hypotension, *PE,* **supraventricular tachycardia, thromboembolism, thrombosis.**
EENT: *visual disturbances.*
GI: *diarrhea,* **intestinal obstruction, ischemic colitis,** mucositis, *nausea, oral candidiasis,* **pancreatitis, perforation,** *vomiting.*
Hematologic: *anemia,* bleeding, **NEUTROPENIA, thrombocytopenia.**

<hr>

Reactions may be *common,* uncommon, *life-threatening*, or COMMON AND LIFE-THREATENING.

Hepatic: *hepatic encephalopathy, hepatic necrosis.*
Musculoskeletal: *arthralgia, myalgia.*
Respiratory: cough, *dyspnea, pneumonia, respiratory tract infection.*
Skin: *alopecia,* injection site reactions.
Other: *anaphylaxis, angioedema,* hypersensitivity reactions, infections.

Interactions

Drug-drug. *Cytochrome P-450 inhibitors:* May decrease Abraxane metabolism. Use together cautiously.

Effects on lab test results

• May increase alkaline phosphatase, AST, bilirubin, creatinine, and GGT levels. May decrease hemoglobin level.
• May decrease neutrophil and platelet counts.

Pharmacokinetics

Absorption: Given I.V.
Distribution: 89% to 98% bound by serum proteins.
Metabolism: Heavily metabolized by several isoenzymes in the cytochrome P-450 pathway.
Excretion: 4% of drug recovered in urine unchanged. Less than 1% recovered in urine as metabolites. Fecal excretion 20% of the dose.
Half life: 27 hours.

Route	Onset	Peak	Duration
I.V.	Unknown	Unknown	Unknown

Action

Chemical effect: Prevents depolymerization of cellular microtubules, inhibiting reorganization of the microtubule network and disrupting mitosis and other vital cell functions.
Therapeutic effect: Inhibits breast cancer cell growth.

Available forms

Lyophilized powder for injection: 100 mg in single-use vial

NURSING PROCESS

Assessment
• Assess patient's condition before starting therapy and regularly thereafter to monitor drug's effectiveness.

• Assess the patient for symptoms of sensory neuropathy and severe neutropenia.
• Monitor liver and kidney function tests.
• Monitor infusion site closely.
• Assess patient's and family's knowledge of drug therapy.

Nursing diagnoses
• Risk for injury related to drug-induced hematologic reactions
• Ineffective health maintenance related to presence of neoplastic disease
• Deficient knowledge related to drug therapy

Planning and implementation
• Give only under the supervision of a practitioner experienced in using chemotherapy in a facility that can manage its complications.
ALERT: Don't substitute this drug for other forms of paclitaxel.
• Because Abraxane contains human albumin, there's a remote risk of transmitting viral disease and Creutzfeldt-Jakob disease.
• Complications of overdose may include bone marrow suppression, sensory neurotoxicity, and mucositis; there's no known antidote for overdose.

Patient teaching
• Advise male patients to avoid fathering children while taking this drug.
• Warn the patient that alopecia is common, but is reversible when treatment ends.
• Teach the patient to recognize signs of neuropathy, such as tingling, burning, and numbness in limbs.
• Tell the patient to report fever or other signs of infection, severe abdominal pain, or severe diarrhea.
• Advise the patient to contact her health care provider if nausea and vomiting persist or interfere with her ability to maintain nutrition. Reassure her that a drug can be prescribed that may help.
• Explain that many patients experience weakness and fatigue, so it's important to rest. Tiredness, paleness, and shortness of breath may result from low blood counts, and the patient may need a transfusion.
• To reduce or prevent mouth sores, remind the patient to perform proper oral hygiene.

☑ Evaluation
- Patient does not develop serious adverse hematologic reactions.
- Patient responds to pharmacologic therapy.
- Patient and family state understanding of drug therapy.

✳ **New Drug**

paliperidone
(pahl-ee-PEHR-ih-dohn)
Invega

Pharmacologic class: benzisoxazole derivative
Therapeutic class: antipsychotic
Pregnancy risk category: C

Indications and dosages

▶ **Schizophrenia.** *Adults:* 6 mg P.O. once daily in the morning. May increase or decrease dose in 3-mg increments to a range of 3 mg to 12 mg daily; don't exceed 12 mg/day.
🔲 **Adjust-a-dose:** In patients with creatinine clearance of 50 to 80 ml/minute, maximum dosage is 6 mg once daily; for patients with creatinine clearance of 10 to 49 ml/minute, maximum dosage is 3 mg once daily.

Contraindications and cautions

- Contraindicated in patients with known hypersensitivity to this drug or risperidone.
- Contraindicated for dementia-related psychosis because of increased risk for death.
- Contraindicated in patients with congenital long-QT syndrome or a history of cardiac arrhythmias.
- Contraindicated in patients with preexisting severe GI narrowing (esophageal motility disorders, small bowel inflammatory disease, short-gut syndrome).
- Use cautiously in patients with a history of seizures or diabetes; those at risk for aspiration pneumonia; those with bradycardia, hypokalemia, hypomagnesemia, known CV disease, cerebrovascular disease, dehydration, or hypovolemia; those taking antihypertensives, drugs that lower the seizure threshold.
- Use cautiously in patient with history of suicide attempts.
⚖ **Lifespan:** In pregnant women, use only if benefit justifies risk to fetus. Drug is found in breast milk; breast-feeding women shouldn't

use drug. In children younger than age 18, safety and effectiveness haven't been determined.

Adverse reactions

CNS: *akathisia,* anxiety, asthenia, dizziness, dystonia, extrapyramidal disorder, fatigue, *headache,* hypertonia, *Parkinsonism,* pyrexia, *somnolence,* tremor, dyskinesia, hyperkinesia.
CV: abnormal T waves, *AV block,* bundle branch block, hypertension, orthostatic hypotension, palpitations, *prolonged QTc interval,* sinus arrhythmia, tachycardia.
EENT: blurred vision.
GI: abdominal pain, dry mouth, dyspepsia, nausea, salivary hypersecretion.
Metabolic: blood insulin increases, hyperprolactemia.
Musculoskeletal: back pain, extremity pain.
Respiratory: cough.

Interactions

Drug-drug. *Anticholinergics:* May worsen side effects. Use together cautiously.
Antihypertensives: May exacerbate orthostatic hypotension. Use together cautiously.
Centrally-acting drugs: May worsen CNS side effects. Use together cautiously.
Levodopa, dopamine agonists: May antagonize effects of these drugs. Use together cautiously.
Drugs that prolong QTc interval such as antiarrhythmics (quinidine, procainamide, amiodarone, sotalol), antipsychotics (chlorpromazine, thioridazine), quinolone antibiotics (moxifloxacin): May further prolong QTc interval. Avoid use together.
Drug-lifestyle. *Alcohol use:* May worsen CNS effects. Avoid use together.

Effects on lab test results

- May increase insulin and prolactin levels.

Pharmacokinetics

Absorption: 28% absolute oral bioavailability; food may increase absorption.
Distribution: Unknown.
Metabolism: Cytochrome P-450 thought to have limited role.
Excretion: 59% excreted through urine as unchanged drug; 32% recovered as metabolites. *Half life:* 23 hours.

Route	Onset	Peak	Duration
P.O.	Unknown	24 hr	Unknown

Reactions may be *common,* uncommon, *life-threatening,* or **COMMON AND LIFE-THREATENING.**

Action

Chemical effect: May antagonize both central dopamine (D_2) and serotonin type 2 ($5\text{-}HT_{2A}$) receptors; also antagonizes $alpha_1$, $alpha_2$, and histamine$_1$ receptors. Drug is a major active metabolite of risperidone.
Therapeutic effect: Antipsychotic.

Available forms

Tablets (extended-release): 3 mg, 6 mg, 9 mg

NURSING PROCESS

Assessment
• Assess patient's psychosis before starting therapy and regularly thereafter to monitor drug's effectiveness.
• Assess blood pressure before staring therapy, and monitor regularly. Watch for orthostatic hypotension, especially during dosage adjustment.
• Monitor glucose level and renal fuction.
• Monitor for CV and neurologic changes.
• Be alert for adverse reactions and drug interactions.
• Assess patient's and family's knowledge of drug therapy.

Nursing diagnoses
• Disturbed thought process related to presence of psychosis
• Risk for injury related to drug-induced adverse reactions
• Deficient knowledge related to drug therapy

Planning and implementation
• Drug should be prescribed in small quantities due to inherent risk of suicide in psychotic patients.
• No antidote exists; use supportive care; commence CV and hemodynamic monitoring immediately.
• Don't crush or divide tablets; don't use if patient is unable to swallow tablets whole.
Patient teaching
• Inform the patient that the tablet shell will normally appear in feces.
• Tell patient to swallow the tablets whole, with liquids, and not to chew, crush, or divide tablets.
• Instruct the patient not to perform activities that require mental alertness until effects of this drug are known.
• Tell the patient to use caution in performing excessively strenuous activities as performing

this activity while on this drug may disrupt body temperature.
• Advise the patient that the drug may lower his blood pressure and to change positions slowly.
• Instruct the patient to contact the prescriber before taking any other drugs due to risk of interaction.
• Advise the patient to avoid alcohol while taking this drug.
• Advise woman to contact the prescriber if she becomes pregnant or plans to breast-feed.

Evaluation
• Patient behavior and communication indicate improved thought processes.
• Patient sustains no injury from drug-induced adverse reactions.
• Patient and family state understanding of drug therapy.

palivizumab
(pal-ih-VYE-zoo-mab)
Synagis

Pharmacologic class: monoclonal antibody
Therapeutic class: antiviral
Pregnancy risk category: C

Indications and dosages

▶ **To prevent serious lower respiratory tract disease caused by RSV in children at high risk.** *Infants and children:* 15 mg/kg I.M. monthly throughout RSV season, with first dose before RSV season.

Contraindications and cautions

• Contraindicated in children hypersensitive to the drug or any of its components.
• Use cautiously in children with thrombocytopenia or other coagulation disorders.
• **Lifespan:** Drug is only indicated in children.

Adverse reactions

CNS: nervousness, pain.
EENT: conjunctivitis, *otitis media,* pharyngitis, rhinitis, sinusitis.
GI: diarrhea, gastroenteritis, oral candidiasis, vomiting.
Hematologic: anemia.

Respiratory: *apnea, asthma,* bronchiolitis, bronchitis, cough, croup, dyspnea, pneumonia, *upper respiratory tract infection,* wheeze.
Skin: rash, fungal dermatitis, eczema, seborrhea.
Other: *anaphylaxis, failure to thrive,* flulike syndrome, hernia, hypersensitivity, injection site reaction, viral infection.

Interactions

None significant.

Effects on lab test results

• May increase ALT and AST levels. May decrease hemoglobin level and hematocrit.

Pharmacokinetics

Absorption: Absorbed well.
Distribution: Unknown.
Metabolism: Unknown.
Excretion: Unknown. *Half-life:* About 18 days.

Route	Onset	Peak	Duration
I.M.	Unknown	Unknown	Unknown

Action

Chemical effect: Inhibits RSV replication.
Therapeutic effect: Prevents RSV infection in high-risk children.

Available forms

Injection (single-use vial): 50 mg, 100 mg

NURSING PROCESS

⚡ Assessment

• Obtain accurate medical history before giving drug; ask if child has any coagulation disorders or liver dysfunction.
• Be alert for adverse reactions.
• Assess patient's and family's knowledge of drug therapy.

⊕ Nursing diagnoses

• Risk for infection related to RSV infection
• Risk for injury related to drug-induced adverse reactions
• Deficient knowledge related to drug therapy

▷ Planning and implementation

• Very rarely, nonfatal cases of anaphylaxis may occur following re-exposure to drug. Rare severe acute hypersensitivity reactions may occur

on initial exposure or re-exposure to drug. If a severe hypersensitivity reaction occurs, permanently stop drug. If milder hypersensitivity reactions occur, restart drug cautiously. If anaphylaxis or severe allergic reactions occur, give drug such as epinephrine and provide supportive care as needed.
• To reconstitute, slowly add 0.6 ml of sterile water for injection to the 50-mg vial or 1 ml of sterile water for injection into a 100-mg vial. Gently swirl vial for 30 seconds to avoid foaming; don't shake. Let reconstituted solution stand at room temperature for 20 minutes. Give within 6 hours of reconstitution. Only give drug I.M.
• Give drug in front thigh muscle, off to one side. Don't use gluteal muscle routinely as an injection site because of risk of damage to sciatic nerve. Divide injections larger than 1 ml.
• Give monthly doses throughout RSV season, even if RSV infection develops. In the northern hemisphere, RSV season typically lasts from November to April.
• For patients undergoing cardiopulmonary bypass, give dose immediately after the bypass, even if it's been less than a month since the last dose.

Patient teaching

• Explain to parent or caregiver that drug is used to prevent RSV and not to treat it.
• Advise parent that monthly injections are recommended throughout RSV season.
• Tell parent to immediately report adverse reactions or unusual bruising, bleeding, or weakness.

☑ Evaluation

• Patient doesn't develop RSV infection.
• Patient sustains no injury from drug-induced adverse reactions.
• Patient and family state understanding of drug therapy.

palonosetron hydrochloride
(pa-LOW-no-suh-tron high-droh-KLOHR-ighd)
Aloxi

Pharmacologic class: selective serotonin receptor antagonist
Therapeutic class: antiemetic
Pregnancy risk category: B

Reactions may be *common,* uncommon, *life-threatening*, or COMMON AND LIFE-THREATENING.

Indications and dosages

▶ **To prevent acute nausea and vomiting caused by moderately or highly emetogenic chemotherapy or delayed nausea and vomiting caused by moderately emetogenic chemotherapy.** *Adults:* 0.25 mg I.V. over 30 seconds; give 30 minutes before the start of chemotherapy. Give once per cycle, not more than every 7 days.

▽ I.V. administration

• Don't mix with other drugs.
• Give by either peripheral or central I.V. access.
• Give by rapid I.V. injection over 30 seconds. Flush I.V. line before and after with normal saline solution.
⊗ **Incompatibilities**
Don't mix (Y-site or otherwise) with other I.V. drugs.

Contraindications and cautions

• Contraindicated in patients hypersensitive to the drug or any of its components.
• Use cautiously in patients hypersensitive to other selective serotonin receptor antagonists; cross-sensitivity may occur. Also use cautiously in patients with cardiac conduction abnormalities, hypokalemia, or hypomagnesemia and in patients taking drugs that affect cardiac conduction.
☀ **Lifespan:** In pregnant women, use only if benefits outweigh risks to fetus. Breast-feeding women should stop breast-feeding or use a different antiemetic; it's unknown if drug appears in breast milk. In children, safety and effectiveness haven't been established.

Adverse reactions

CNS: anxiety, dizziness, headache, weakness.
CV: *bradycardia,* hypotension, *nonsustained ventricular tachycardia.*
GI: constipation, diarrhea.
Metabolic: *hyperkalemia.*

Interactions

Drug-drug. *Antiarrhythmics or other drugs that may prolong the QT interval, diuretics with potential for inducing electrolyte abnormalities, high doses of anthracycline:* May increase risk of prolonged QT interval. Use together cautiously.

Effects on lab test results

• May increase potassium level.

Pharmacokinetics

Absorption: Given I.V.
Distribution: Distributes well into tissues. 60% protein-bound.
Metabolism: 50% metabolized to inactive metabolites by CYP2D6 and, to a lesser extent, CYP3A4 and CYP1A2.
Excretion: 80% of drug and inactive metabolites is eliminated in the urine. *Half-life:* 40 hours.

Route	Onset	Peak	Duration
I.V.	30 min	Unknown	5 days

Action

Chemical effect: Binds to the 5-HT$_3$ receptor, which inhibits emesis caused by cytotoxic chemotherapy.
Therapeutic effect: Prevents vomiting from chemotherapy.

Available forms

Injection: 0.25 mg/5 ml (single-use vial)

NURSING PROCESS

⚗ Assessment

• Assess patient's condition before starting therapy and regularly thereafter to monitor drug's effectiveness.
• Obtain baseline potassium level.
• In patients with known cardiac conduction abnormalities, obtain baseline ECG.
• Be alert for adverse reactions and drug interactions.
• Assess patient's and family's knowledge of drug therapy.

⊕ Nursing diagnoses

• Risk for deficient fluid volume related to nausea and vomiting
• Acute pain related to drug-induced headache
• Deficient knowledge related to drug therapy

▶ Planning and implementation

• Give 30 minutes before chemotherapy on day 1 of each cycle.
• Consider giving with corticosteroids as part of the antiemetic therapy, particularly for patients receiving highly emetogenic chemotherapy.

• Give additional antiemetics for breakthrough nausea and vomiting.

Patient teaching

• Advise patients to take a different antiemetic for breakthrough nausea and vomiting, and tell patient to take it at the first sign of nausea and not to wait until symptoms are severe.

• Tell patients with a history of cardiac conduction abnormalities to report any changes in their drug regimen, such as the adding or stopping of antiarrhythmics.

☑ Evaluation

• Patient maintains adequate hydration.

• Patient doesn't experience drug-induced headaches.

• Patient and family state understanding of drug therapy.

pamidronate disodium
(pam-ih-DROH-nayt digh-SOH-dee-um)
Aredia

Pharmacologic class: bisphosphonate, pyrophosphate analogue
Therapeutic class: bone resorption inhibitor
Pregnancy risk category: D

Indications and dosages

▶ **Moderate to severe hypercalcemia related to malignancy (with or without metastases).** *Adults:* Dosage depends on severity of hypercalcemia. Calcium level is corrected for serum albumin as follows:

$$
\begin{aligned}
\text{Corrected serum} &= \text{serum} + 0.8\,(4 - \text{serum} \\
\text{calcium (cCa)} &\quad\ \text{calcium} \quad\ \text{albumin)} \\
\text{(in mg/dl)} &\quad\ \text{(in mg/dl)} \quad\ \text{(in g/dl)}
\end{aligned}
$$

Patients with moderate hypercalcemia (cCa level of 12 to 13.5 mg/dl) may receive 60 to 90 mg I.V. infusion as a single dose over 2 to 24 hours. Patients with severe hypercalcemia (cCa level higher than 13.5 mg/dl) may receive 90 mg over 2 to 24 hours. Wait at least 7 days to give repeat dose to allow for full response to initial dose.

▶ **Osteolytic bone lesions of multiple myeloma.** *Adults:* 90 mg I.V. over 4 hours once monthly.

▶ **Osteolytic bone lesions of breast cancer.** *Adults:* 90 mg I.V. over 2 hours every 3 to 4 weeks.

▶ **Moderate to severe Paget disease.** *Adults:* 30 mg I.V. as 4-hour infusion on 3 consecutive days for total dose of 90 mg. Cycle repeated, as needed.

▼ I.V. administration

• Reconstitute vial with 10 ml sterile water for injection. Once drug is completely dissolved, add to 250-ml (2-hour infusion), 500-ml (4-hour infusion), or 1,000-ml (up to 24-hour infusion) bag of half-normal or normal saline solution injection or D_5W. Inspect for precipitate before administering.

• Give drug only by I.V. infusion. Nephropathy may occur with rapid bolus injections.

• Infusions of longer than 2 hours may reduce the risk of renal toxicity, particularly in patients with renal insufficiency.

• Solution is stable for 24 hours at room temperature.

⊗ **Incompatibilities**
Calcium-containing infusion solutions, such as Ringer's injection or lactated Ringer's solution.

Contraindications and cautions

• Contraindicated in patients hypersensitive to the drug or to other bisphosphonates, such as etidronate.

• Use cautiously in patients with renal impairment.

⚹ **Lifespan:** In pregnant women, drug is contraindicated. In breast-feeding women, use cautiously; it's unknown if the drug appears in breast milk. In children, safety and effectiveness haven't been established.

Adverse reactions

CNS: *anxiety, fatigue, fever, headache, insomnia, pain, seizures.*
CV: *atrial fibrillation,* hypertension.
GI: *abdominal pain, anorexia, constipation, diarrhea, dyspepsia, GI hemorrhage, nausea, vomiting,*
GU: *renal failure, UTI.*
Hematologic: *anemia,* GRANULOCYTOPENIA, *leukopenia,* THROMBOCYTOPENIA.
Metabolism: hypocalcemia, *hypokalemia, hypomagnesemia,* hypophosphatemia.
Musculoskeletal: *arthralgia, bone pain, myalgia.*
Other: METASTASES.

Interactions

None significant.

Effects on lab test results

• May increase creatinine level. May decrease phosphate, potassium, magnesium, calcium, and hemoglobin levels and hematocrit.
• May decrease WBC and platelet counts.

Pharmacokinetics

Absorption: Given I.V.
Distribution: About 50% to 60% of dose is rapidly taken up by bone; drug is also taken up by kidneys, liver, spleen, teeth, and tracheal cartilage.
Metabolism: Unknown.
Excretion: By kidneys. *Half-life:* Alpha, 1½ hours; beta, 27¼ hours.

Route	Onset	Peak	Duration
I.V.	Unknown	Unknown	Unknown

Action

Chemical effect: Inhibits bone resorption. Adsorbs to hydroxyapatite crystals in bone and may directly block calcium phosphate dissolution.
Therapeutic effect: Lowers calcium level.

Available forms

Powder for injection: 30 mg/vial, 90 mg/vial
Solution for injection: 3 mg/ml, 6 mg/ml, 9 mg/ml in 10-ml vials

NURSING PROCESS

✍ Assessment

• Assess patient's condition before starting therapy and regularly thereafter to monitor drug's effectiveness.
• Assess hydration before therapy.
• Closely monitor electrolyte level, CBC and differential. Check creatinine level before each dose.
• Carefully monitor patient with anemia, leukopenia, or thrombocytopenia during first 2 weeks of therapy.
• Monitor patient's temperature. Fever is most likely 24 to 48 hours after therapy.
• Be alert for adverse reactions and drug interactions. Patients with renal impairment are at a greater risk for adverse reactions.

• Assess patient's and family's knowledge of drug therapy.

🔲 Nursing diagnoses

• Ineffective health maintenance related to hypercalcemia
• Risk for injury related to drug-induced hypocalcemia
• Deficient knowledge related to drug therapy

▶ Planning and implementation

• Use drug only after patient has been vigorously hydrated with saline solution. In patients with mild to moderate hypercalcemia, hydration alone may be sufficient.
• If patient has severe hypocalcemia, short-term administration of calcium may be needed.
• For a patient with multiple myeloma, limited information is available on those with creatinine level greater than 3 mg/dl. Before infusion, adequately hydrate patient with marked Bence Jones proteinuria and dehydration. Optimal duration of therapy is unknown, but may be 21 months.
⑤ **ALERT:** Because of the risk of renal dysfunction leading to renal failure, don't give single doses of more than 90 mg.
• In patient treated for bone metastases who has renal dysfunction, don't give the dose until renal function returns to baseline. Use in patient with severe renal impairment isn't recommended.
• In patient with breast cancer, optimal duration of therapy isn't known; may be 24 months for overall benefit.
⑤ **ALERT:** Don't confuse Aredia with Meridia.
Patient teaching
• Instruct patient to report unusual signs or symptoms at once.
• Inform patient of need for frequent tests to monitor effectiveness of drug and detect adverse reactions.

✅ Evaluation

• Patient's calcium level returns to normal.
• Patient doesn't develop hypocalcemia during drug therapy.
• Patient and family state understanding of drug therapy.

HIGH ALERT

pancuronium bromide
(pan-kyoo-ROH-nee-um BROH-mighd)

Pharmacologic class: nondepolarizing neuro-muscular blocker
Therapeutic class: skeletal muscle relaxant
Pregnancy risk category: C

Indications and dosages

▶ **Adjunct to anesthesia to induce skeletal muscle relaxation; to facilitate intubation; to lessen muscle contractions in pharmacologically or electrically induced seizures; to assist with mechanical ventilation. Dosage depends on anesthetic used, individual needs, and response. Dosages shown are representative; individualize dosage.**
Adults and children age 1 month and older: Initially, 0.04 to 0.1 mg/kg I.V.; then 0.01 mg/kg every 25 to 60 minutes.
Neonates younger than age 1 month: Individualize dosages. Give a test dose of 0.02 mg/kg to assess response.

▼ I.V. administration

• Mix drug only with fresh solutions.
• Store drug in refrigerator. Don't store in plastic containers or syringes, although plastic syringes may be used for administration.
⊗ **Incompatibilities**
Barbiturates, diazepam, other alkaline solutions.

Contraindications and cautions

• Contraindicated in patients hypersensitive to bromides, in those with tachycardia, and in those for whom even a minor increase in heart rate is undesirable.
• Use cautiously in debilitated patients and in those with respiratory depression, myasthenia gravis, myasthenic syndrome of lung cancer, bronchogenic carcinoma, dehydration, thyroid disorders, collagen diseases, porphyria, electrolyte disturbances, hyperthermia, toxemic states, or renal, hepatic, or pulmonary impairment.
⚖ **Lifespan:** In pregnant women undergoing cesarean section and in breast-feeding women, use large doses cautiously. In the elderly, use cautiously.

Adverse reactions

CV: increased blood pressure, tachycardia.

EENT: excessive salivation.
Musculoskeletal: residual muscle weakness.
Respiratory: *prolonged, dose-related respiratory insufficiency or apnea;* wheezing.
Skin: excessive diaphoresis, transient rashes.
Other: allergic or idiosyncratic hypersensitivity reactions, burning sensation.

Interactions

Drug-drug. *Amikacin, gentamicin, neomycin, streptomycin, tobramycin:* May increase the effects of nondepolarizing muscle relaxant, including prolonged respiratory depression. Use together only when needed. Dose of nondepolarizing muscle relaxant may need to be reduced.
Carbamazepine, phenytoin: May decrease the effects of pancuronium causing it to be less effective. May need to increase the dose of pancuronium.
Clindamycin; general anesthetics; kanamycin; ketamine; polymyxin antibiotics, such as polymyxin B sulfate and colistin; quinidine: May increase neuromuscular blockade, leading to an increase in skeletal muscle relaxation and prolonged effect. Use cautiously during surgical and postoperative periods.
Lithium, opioid analgesics, verapamil: May increase neuromuscular blockade, leading to an increase in skeletal muscle relaxation and respiratory paralysis. Use cautiously, and reduce pancuronium dose, as directed.
Succinylcholine: May increase intensity and duration of blockade. Allow succinylcholine effects to subside before giving pancuronium.
Theophylline: May reverse the neuromuscular blocking effects of pancuronium.

Effects on lab test results

None reported.

Pharmacokinetics

Absorption: Given I.V.
Distribution: About 87% bound to plasma proteins.
Metabolism: Unknown.
Excretion: Mainly in urine; some biliary. *Half-life:* About 2 hours.

Route	Onset	Peak	Duration
I.V.	30–45 sec	3–4½ min	35–45 min

Reactions may be *common,* uncommon, *life-threatening,* or COMMON AND LIFE-THREATENING.

Action

Chemical effect: Prevents acetylcholine from binding to receptors on muscle end plate, thus blocking depolarization.
Therapeutic effect: Relaxes skeletal muscles.

Available forms

Injection: 1 mg/ml, 2 mg/ml

NURSING PROCESS

Assessment

• Assess patient's condition before starting therapy and regularly thereafter to monitor drug's effectiveness.
• Monitor baseline electrolyte determinations (electrolyte imbalance can increase neuromuscular effects) and vital signs.
• Measure fluid intake and output; renal dysfunction may prolong duration of action because 25% of drug is unchanged before excretion.
• Monitor nerve stimulator and train-of-four to avoid overdosage and to confirm antagonism of neuromuscular blockade and recovery of muscle strength. Don't attempt reversal with neostigmine until you see signs of spontaneous recovery.
• Monitor respirations closely until patient fully recovers from neuromuscular blockade, as evidenced by tests of muscle strength (hand grip, head lift, and ability to cough).
• Be alert for adverse reactions and drug interactions.
• Assess patient's and family's knowledge of drug therapy.

Nursing diagnoses

• Ineffective health maintenance related to condition
• Ineffective breathing pattern related to drug's effect on respiratory muscles
• Deficient knowledge related to drug therapy

Planning and implementation

• Administer sedatives or general anesthetics before neuromuscular blockers. Neuromuscular blockers don't reduce consciousness or alter pain threshold. Give analgesics for pain.
• Give drug only if skilled in airway management.
• Have emergency respiratory support equipment (endotracheal equipment, ventilator, oxy-

gen, atropine, edrophonium, epinephrine, and neostigmine) immediately available.
• If giving with succinylcholine, allow succinylcholine effects to subside before giving this drug.
• Once spontaneous recovery starts, drug-induced neuromuscular blockade may be reversed with an anticholinesterase (such as neostigmine or edrophonium). Usually given with an anticholinergic such as atropine.
⑤ ALERT: Don't confuse pancuronium with pipecuronium.

Patient teaching
• Explain all events to patient because he can still hear.
• Reassure patient that he'll be monitored at all times and that pain drug will be provided, if appropriate.
• Tell patient that he may feel burning sensation at injection site.

Evaluation

• Patient's condition improves.
• Patient maintains adequate ventilation with mechanical assistance.
• Patient and family state understanding of drug therapy.

pantoprazole sodium

(pan-TOE-pra-zole SOH-dee-um)
Protonix, Protonix IV

Pharmacologic class: proton pump inhibitor
Therapeutic class: gastric acid suppressant
Pregnancy risk category: B

Indications and dosages

▶ **Short-term therapy for erosive esophagitis related to gastroesophageal reflux disease (GERD).** *Adults:* 40 mg P.O. once daily for up to 8 weeks. For those patients who haven't healed after 8 weeks of therapy, an additional 8-week course may be considered.
▶ **Patients with GERD who are unable to continue pantoprazole sodium delayed-release tablets.** *Adults:* 40 mg I.V. daily for 7 to 10 days. Switch to oral form as soon as patient is able to take oral drugs.
▶ **Long-term maintenance of healing erosive esophagitis and reduction in relapse rates of daytime and nighttime heartburn symptoms**

in patients with GERD. *Adults:* 40 mg P.O. once daily.

▶ **Pathological hypersecretion conditions related to Zollinger-Ellison syndrome or other neoplastic conditions.** *Adults:* Individualize dosage. Usual starting dose is 40 mg P.O. b.i.d. Adjust dosage to a maximum of 240 mg daily. Or, 80 mg I.V. every 12 hours for no more than 6 days. For those needing a higher dosage, 80 mg every 8 hours is expected to maintain acid output below 10 mEq/h. Maximum daily dose, 240 mg.

▼ I.V. administration

• Stop I.V. use as soon as P.O. use is possible.
• Reconstitute each vial with 10 ml of normal saline solution.
• Compatible diluents for infusion include 5% dextrose, normal saline solution, or lactated Ringer's injection.
• For GERD, further dilute with 100 ml of diluent to a final concentration of 0.4 mg/ml.
• For hypersecretion conditions, combine two reconstituted vials and further dilute with 80 ml of diluent to a total volume of 100 ml, with a final concentration of 0.8 mg/ml.
• Infuse diluted solutions I.V. over 15 minutes at no more than 3 mg/min (7 ml/min) for GERD and 6 mg/min (7 ml/min) for pathological hypersecretory conditions.
• Don't give another infusion simultaneously through the same line.
• Reconstituted solution may be stored for up to 6 hours at room temperature. Diluted solution may be stored for up to 24 hours at room temperature.
• Drug doesn't need protection from light.
⊗ **Incompatibilities**
Midazolam (Y-site), products or solutions containing zinc.

Contraindications and cautions

• Contraindicated in patients hypersensitive to the drug or any of its components.
⚖ **Lifespan:** Use in pregnancy only when clearly needed. In breast-feeding women, use cautiously. In children, safety and effectiveness haven't been established.

Adverse reactions

CNS: anxiety, asthenia, dizziness, headache, insomnia, migraine, pain.
CV: chest pain, peripheral edema.

EENT: pharyngitis, rhinitis, sinusitis.
GI: abdominal pain, constipation, diarrhea, dyspepsia, eructation, flatulence, gastroenteritis, GI disorder, nausea, vomiting.
GU: rectal disorder, urinary frequency, UTI.
Metabolic: hyperglycemia, hyperlipidemia.
Musculoskeletal: arthralgia, back pain, hypertonia, neck pain.
Respiratory: bronchitis, dyspnea, increased cough, upper respiratory tract infection.
Skin: rash.
Other: flulike symptoms, infection.

Interactions

Drug-drug. *Ampicillin esters, iron salts, ketoconazole:* May decrease absorption of these drugs. Monitor patient closely, and try to separate doses.
Drug-herb. *St. John's wort:* May increase risk of sunburn. Discourage use together.
Drug-food. *Food:* May delay absorption of pantoprazole for up to 2 hours, but the extent of absorption isn't affected. Give with or without meals.

Effects on lab test results

• May increase glucose, uric acid, and lipid levels.
• May increase or decrease liver function test values.
• May cause false-positive urine screen for tetrahydrocannabinol.

Pharmacokinetics

Absorption: Good, with an absolute bioavailability of 77%. Peak level occurs at 2½ hours. Food may delay absorption up to 2 hours, but the extent of absorption isn't affected.
Distribution: Mainly in the extracellular fluid; 98% protein-bound, mainly to albumin.
Metabolism: Extensive.
Excretion: About 71% in urine and 18% in feces through bile. *Half-life:* 1 hour.

Route	Onset	Peak	Duration
P.O.	Unknown	2½ hr	24 hr
I.V.	15–30 min	Unknown	24 hr

Action

Chemical effect: Inhibits the activity of the proton pump by binding to hydrogen-potassium adenosine triphosphatase, located at secretory surface of the gastric parietal cells.

Reactions may be *common,* uncommon, *life-threatening*, or COMMON AND LIFE-THREATENING.

Therapeutic effect: Suppresses gastric acid secretion.

Available forms

Granules for suspension: 40 mg unit dose packet
Injection: 40-mg vial
Tablets (delayed-release): 20 mg, 40 mg

NURSING PROCESS

⚡ Assessment
• Assess underlying condition before starting therapy and regularly thereafter to monitor drug's effectiveness.
• Assess patient for complaints of epigastric or abdominal pain and for bleeding (such as blood in stool or emesis).
• Be alert for adverse reactions and interactions.
• Assess patient's and family's knowledge of drug therapy.

⊕ Nursing diagnoses
• Risk for imbalanced fluid volume related to drug-induced adverse reactions
• Risk for aspiration related to underlying GI disorder
• Deficient knowledge related to pantoprazole therapy

▶ Planning and implementation
• Symptomatic response to therapy doesn't rule out gastric malignancy.
• **ALERT:** Don't confuse Protonix with Lotronex, Prilosec, Prozac, or Prevacid.
Patient teaching
• Instruct patient to take exactly as prescribed and at approximately the same time every day.
• Tell patient that drug can be taken with or without food.
• Inform patient that tablet is to be swallowed whole and not crushed, split, or chewed.
• Tell patient that antacids don't affect the absorption of pantoprazole.
• Instruct patient to report abdominal pain or signs of bleeding, such as tarry stool.
• Advise patient not to drink alcohol, eat food, or take other drugs (such as aspirin, NSAIDs) that could cause gastric irritation.

☑ Evaluation
• Patient maintains adequate hydration throughout therapy.

• Patient responds well to therapy and doesn't aspirate.
• Patient and family state understanding of pantoprazole therapy.

paroxetine hydrochloride
(par-OKS-eh-teen high-droh-KLOR-ighd)
Paxil, Paxil CR

Pharmacologic class: SSRI
Therapeutic class: antidepressant
Pregnancy risk category: D

Indications and dosages

▶ **Major depressive disorder.** *Adults:* Initially, 20 mg P.O. daily, preferably in morning, as directed. Increase by 10 mg daily at weekly intervals, to maximum of 50 mg daily, if needed. Or, initially, 25 mg Paxil CR P.O. as a single daily dose, usually in the morning, with or without food. May increase dosage at intervals of at least 1 week by 12.5 mg daily increments, up to a maximum of 62.5 mg daily.
▶ **Obsessive-compulsive disorder.** *Adults:* Initially, 20 mg P.O. daily, preferably in morning, as directed. Increase by 10 mg daily at weekly intervals to target dose of 40 mg daily. Maximum daily dose, 60 mg.
▶ **Panic disorder.** *Adults:* Initially, 10 mg P.O. daily. Increase by 10-mg increments at no less than weekly intervals to target dose of 40 mg daily. Maximum daily dose is 60 mg. Or, initially, 12.5 mg Paxil CR P.O. as a single daily dose, usually in the morning, with or without food. May increase dosage at intervals of at least 1 week by 12.5 mg daily increments, up to a maximum of 75 mg daily.
▶ **Generalized anxiety disorder.** *Adults:* Initially, 20 mg P.O. daily. Increase dosage by 10 mg daily at increments of at least 1 week. Maximum daily dose, 50 mg.
▶ **Posttraumatic stress disorder.** *Adults:* Initially, 20 mg P.O. daily. Increase dosage by 10 mg daily at intervals of at least 1 week. Maximum daily dosage, 50 mg.
▶ **Premenstrual dysphoric disorder (PMDD).** *Adults:* Initially, 12.5 mg P.O. (Paxil CR) once daily as a single daily dose, usually in the morning, with or without food. May increase to 25 mg daily after at least 1 week. May

be given either daily or limited to the luteal phase of the menstrual cycle.

► **Social anxiety disorder.** *Adults:* 20 mg P.O. (Paxil) once daily in the morning. Or, initially, 12.5 mg P.O (Paxil CR) once daily in the morning. Increase dosage at weekly intervals in increments of 12.5 mg/day, up to a maximum of 37.5 mg. daily.

▣ **Adjust-a-dose:** For geriatric or debilitated patients and patients with severe hepatic or renal disease, initially, give 10 mg P.O. (immediate-release) daily, preferably in morning. If patient doesn't respond, increase by 10-mg increments at weekly intervals to maximum daily dose of 40 mg. The recommended initial dose of Paxil CR is 12.5 mg daily. Don't exceed 50 mg daily.

► **Diabetic neuropathy‡.** *Adults:* 40 mg P.O. daily.

► **Headache‡.** *Adults:* 10 to 50 mg P.O daily for 3 to 9 months.

► **Premature ejaculation‡.** *Adults:* 20 mg P.O. 3 or 4 hours before planned intercourse, or 10 to 40 mg daily to increase ejaculatory latency time.

Contraindications and cautions

• Contraindicated in patients taking MAO inhibitors or thioridazine. Don't give drug within 14 days of an MAO inhibitor. Also, contraindicated in patients hypersensitive to the drug or any ingredient in the formulation.

• Use cautiously in patients with a history of seizures or mania; patients with severe, concomitant systemic illness; and patients at risk for volume depletion.

• Adults and children with major depressive disorders may experience suicidal ideation and behavior even while taking an antidepressant. Monitor patients for worsening depression or suicidal ideation, especially when therapy starts or dosage changes.

⚛ **Lifespan:** In pregnant women, use cautiously in first trimester because of risk of congenital malformations in the fetus. Neonates of women taking drug in the latter part of the third trimester may require prolonged hospitalization due to respiratory problems and feeding difficulties. In breast-feeding women, use cautiously; drug is distributed in breast milk. Not approved for use in children.

Adverse reactions

CNS: anxiety, *asthenia,* blurred vision, confusion, *dizziness, headache, insomnia,* nervousness, paresthesia, *somnolence, tremor.*
CV: orthostatic hypotension, palpitations, vasodilation.
EENT: dysgeusia, lump or tightness in throat.
GI: *bleeding, constipation, diarrhea, dry mouth,* dyspepsia, flatulence, increased or decreased appetite, *nausea,* taste perversion, vomiting.
GU: abnormal ejaculation, *female genital disorder (including anorgasmy, difficulty with orgasm), male genital disorders (including anorgasmy, erectile difficulties, delayed ejaculation or orgasm, impotence, and sexual dysfunction),* other urinary disorder, urinary frequency.
Metabolic: hyponatremia.
Musculoskeletal: myalgia, myopathy, myasthenia.
Skin: excessive sweating, rash.
Other: decreased libido, yawning.

Interactions

Drug-drug. *Buspirone, dextromethorphan, dihydroergotamine, isoniazid, lithium, meperidine, sumatriptan, tramadol, trazodone, tricyclic antidepressants:* May cause serotonin syndrome. Avoid use together.
Cimetidine: May decrease hepatic metabolism of paroxetine, leading to risk of toxicity. Dosage adjustments may be needed.
Digoxin: May decrease digoxin level. Monitor level closely.
NSAIDs, warfarin: May increase risk of bleeding. Use with caution; monitor patient closely for bleeding.
Phenelzine, selegiline, tranylcypromine: May cause serotonin syndrome, including CNS irritability, shivering, and altered consciousness. Don't give together. Wait at least 2 weeks after stopping an MAO inhibitor before giving any SSRI.
Phenobarbital, phenytoin: May alter pharmacokinetics of both drugs. Dosage adjustments may be needed.
Procyclidine: May increase procyclidine level. Monitor patient for excessive anticholinergic effects.
Sumatriptan: May cause weakness, hyperreflexia, and incoordination. Monitor patient.

Theophylline: Theophylline clearance may decrease threefold. Dosage reduction may be needed.

Thioridazine: May prolong QT interval and increase risk of serious ventricular arrhythmias, such as torsades de pointes and sudden death. Avoid use together.

Tricyclic antidepressants: May inhibit tricyclic antidepressant metabolism. Dose of tricyclic antidepressant may need to be reduced. Monitor patient closely.

Tryptophan: May increase risk of adverse reactions, such as nausea and dizziness. Avoid using together.

Drug-herb. *St. John's wort:* May result in sedative-hypnotic intoxication. Discourage using together.

Drug-lifestyle. *Alcohol use:* May alter psychomotor function. Discourage using together.

Effects on lab test results
• May decrease sodium level.
• May alter platelet count.

Pharmacokinetics
Absorption: Complete.
Distribution: Throughout body, including CNS; only 1% remains in plasma. About 93% to 95% protein-bound.
Metabolism: About 36%.
Excretion: About 64% in urine. *Half-life:* Immediate release, about 21 hours; controlled release, 15 to 20 hours.

Route	Onset	Peak	Duration
P.O.			
immediate-release	1–4 wk	2–8 hr	Unknown
controlled-release	Unknown	6–10 hr	Unknown

Action
Chemical effect: May inhibit CNS neuronal uptake of serotonin.
Therapeutic effect: Relieves depression.

Available forms
Suspension: 10 mg/5 ml
Tablets: 10 mg, 20 mg, 30 mg, 40 mg
Tablets (controlled-release): 12.5 mg, 25 mg, 37.5 mg

NURSING PROCESS

Assessment
• Assess patient's depression before starting therapy and regularly thereafter to monitor drug's effectiveness.
• Be alert for adverse reactions and drug interactions.
• Assess patient's and family's knowledge of drug therapy.
• For PMDD, the effectiveness of Paxil CR for longer than 3 menstrual cycles hasn't been established.
• Periodically reassess the need for continuing therapy.

Nursing diagnoses
• Disturbed thought processes related to depression
• Risk for injury related to drug-induced adverse CNS reactions
• Deficient knowledge related to drug therapy

Planning and implementation
• Don't give drug within 14 days of MAO inhibitor therapy.
• Don't crush CR tablet. If patient can't swallow a CR tablet whole, give a regular-release form.
• If signs of psychosis occur or increase, reduce dosage.
• Gradually reduce dosage to prevent withdrawal symptoms.
ALERT: May increase the risk for suicidal thinking and behavior in young adults ages 18 to 24 during the first 2 months of treatment. Monitor patient carefully.
ALERT: Don't confuse paroxetine with paclitaxel.
ALERT: Don't confuse Paxil with Doxil, Taxol, or Plavix.

Patient teaching
• Warn patient to avoid hazardous activities until the drug's CNS effects are known.
• Warn patient not to chew or crush Paxil CR tablet but to swallow it whole.
• Tell patient that he may notice improvement in 1 to 4 weeks but that he must continue with prescribed regimen to continue feeling benefits.
• Tell patient to abstain from alcohol during drug therapy.
ALERT: If patient wishes to switch from an SSRI to St. John's wort, tell him to wait a few weeks for the SSRI to fully leave his system be-

fore starting the herb. The exact time required will depend on which SSRI he takes.

☑ Evaluation
• Patient's depression improves.
• Patient sustains no injuries because of drug-induced adverse CNS reactions.
• Patient and family state understanding of drug therapy.

HIGH ALERT

pegfilgrastim
(peg-FILL-grass-tihm)
Neulasta

Pharmacologic class: colony-stimulating factor
Therapeutic class: neutrophil-growth stimulator
Pregnancy risk category: C

Indications and dosages

▶ **To reduce frequency of infection in patients with nonmyeloid malignancies taking myelosuppressive anticancer drugs that may cause febrile neutropenia.** *Adults:* 6 mg subcutaneously once per chemotherapy cycle. Don't give in the period between 14 days before and 24 hours after administration of cytotoxic chemotherapy.

Contraindications and cautions

• Contraindicated in patients hypersensitive to *Escherichia coli*–derived proteins, filgrastim, or any component of the drug.
• Don't use for peripheral blood progenitor cell mobilization.
• Use cautiously in patients with sickle cell disease, those receiving chemotherapy causing delayed myelosuppression, and those receiving radiation therapy.
⚠ **Lifespan:** In pregnant women, use drug only if benefits outweigh risks to the fetus. In breast-feeding women, use cautiously; it's unknown if the drug appears in breast milk. In infants, children, and adolescents who weigh less than 45 kg (99 lb), don't use the 6-mg single-use syringe dose. In children, safety and effectiveness haven't been established.

Adverse reactions

CNS: *dizziness, fatigue, fever, headache, insomnia.*

CV: *peripheral edema.*
GI: *abdominal pain, anorexia, constipation, diarrhea, dyspepsia, mucositis, nausea, stomatitis, taste perversion, vomiting.*
Hematologic: GRANULOCYTOPENIA, NEUTROPENIC FEVER, *splenic rupture.*
Musculoskeletal: *arthralgia, bone pain, generalized weakness, myalgia, skeletal pain.*
Respiratory: *acute respiratory distress syndrome (ARDS).*
Skin: *alopecia.*

Interactions

Drug-drug. *Lithium:* May increase the release of neutrophils. Monitor neutrophil counts closely.

Effects on lab test results

• May increase LDH, alkaline phosphatase, and uric acid levels.
• May increase WBC, granulocyte, and neutrophil counts.

Pharmacokinetics

Absorption: Unknown.
Distribution: Unknown.
Metabolism: Unknown.
Excretion: Unknown. *Half-life:* 15 to 80 hours.

Route	Onset	Peak	Duration
SubQ	Unknown	Unknown	Unknown

Action

Chemical effect: Binds cell receptors to stimulate proliferation, differentiation, commitment, and end-cell function of neutrophils. Pegfilgrastim and filgrastim have the same mechanism of action. Pegfilgrastim has a reduced renal clearance and therefore a longer half-life than filgrastim.
Therapeutic effect: Increases WBC count.

Available forms

Injection: 6 mg/0.6 ml single-use, preservative-free, prefilled syringes

---

NURSING PROCESS

⚕ Assessment
• Assess patient's underlying condition before starting therapy and regularly thereafter to monitor drug's effectiveness.

Reactions may be *common*, uncommon, *life-threatening*, or COMMON AND LIFE-THREATENING.

• Obtain CBC and platelet count before starting therapy.
• Monitor patient's hemoglobin level, hematocrit, and CBC and platelet count; as well as LDH, alkaline phosphatase, and uric acid levels during therapy.
• Assess patient's and family's knowledge of drug therapy.

Nursing diagnoses
• Acute pain related to adverse musculoskeletal effects of drug
• Risk for infection related to underlying condition and treatment
• Deficient knowledge related to pegfilgrastim therapy

Planning and implementation
• Store in the carton to protect from light.
• The maximum amount of filgrastim that can be given is unknown. Treat patient having symptomatic leukocytosis with leukapheresis.
ALERT: Splenic rupture may occur rarely with filgrastim use. Evaluate patient who experiences signs or symptoms of left upper abdominal or shoulder pain for an enlarged spleen or splenic rupture.
• Monitor patient for allergic reactions, including anaphylaxis, skin rash, and urticaria.
• Evaluate patient who develops fever, lung infiltrates, or respiratory distress for ARDS. If ARDS occurs, stop drug.
• Keep patient with sickle cell disease well hydrated, and monitor patient for symptoms of sickle cell crisis.
• Drug may act as a growth factor for tumors.
Patient teaching
• Inform patient of the drug's potential side effects.
• Advise patient to immediately report upper left abdominal or shoulder tip pain.
• Tell patient to report signs and symptoms of allergic reactions, fever, or breathing problems.
• Tell patient with sickle cell disease to maintain hydration and report signs or symptoms of sickle cell crisis.
• Instruct patient or caregiver how to give drug if it is to be given at home.
• Instruct patient or caregiver not to freeze drug. If accidentally frozen, thaw in refrigerator before administration. Tell them to discard if frozen twice.

Evaluation
• Patient states that pain management is adequate.
• Patient's WBC count is normal.
• Patient and family state understanding of drug therapy.

HIGH ALERT

peginterferon alfa-2a
(peg-inter-FEAR-on AL-fah TOO AY)
Pegasys

Pharmacologic class: biological response modifier
Therapeutic class: antiviral
Pregnancy risk category: C (X if used with ribavirin)

Indications and dosages

▶ **Chronic hepatitis C in patients with compensated liver disease and not previously treated with interferon alfa.** *Adults:* 180 mcg subcutaneously in abdomen or thigh, once weekly for 48 weeks, on the same day each week.
▶ **Chronic hepatitis C (regardless of genotype) in HIV-infected patients not previously treated with interferon.** *Adults:* 180 mcg subcutaneously weekly along with ribavirin (Copegus) 800 mg P.O. daily given in 2 divided doses for 48 weeks.
Adjust-a-dose: If patient has moderate to severe adverse reactions, decrease dosage to 135 mcg subcutaneously once a week; in some cases, decrease to 90 mcg subcutaneously once a week.

If patient has hematologic reactions and absolute neutrophil count (ANC) is less than 750/mm³, reduce dosage to 135 mcg subcutaneously once a week; if ANC is less than 500/mm³, stop drug until ANC exceeds 1,000/mm³ and restart at 90 mcg subcutaneously once a week. If platelet count is less than 50,000/mm³, reduce dosage to 90 mcg subcutaneously once a week; stop drug if platelet count drops below 25,000/mm³.

In patients on hemodialysis, decrease dosage to 135 mcg subcutaneously once a week.

In patients with ALT level increases above baseline, decrease dosage to 135 mcg subcutaneously once a week; if hepatic impairment

worsens or bilirubin level increases, stop therapy.

If patient develops mild depression, continue drug, but evaluate weekly. For moderate depression, reduce dosage to 135 mcg for 4 to 8 weeks and evaluate patient every week; in some cases, reduce to 90 mcg. If symptoms improve and remain stable for 4 weeks, continue at present dose or resume previous dose. If severe depression occurs, discontinue drug permanently.

Contraindications and cautions

- Contraindicated in patients hypersensitive to interferon alfa-2a or its components and in patients with autoimmune hepatitis or decompensated liver disease before or during therapy.
- Contraindicated in patients with Child Pugh score greater than 6 (class B and C).
- Use cautiously in patients with a history of depression, drug addiction, suicidal ideation, or suicide attempts. Also use cautiously in patients with baseline ANC less than 1,500/mm³, baseline platelet counts less than 90,000/mm³, or baseline hemoglobin level less than 10 g/dl. Use cautiously in patients with cardiac disease or hypertension, thyroid disease, autoimmune disorders, pulmonary disorders, colitis, pancreatitis, or ophthalmologic disorders. Also use cautiously in patients with creatinine clearance less than 50 ml/minute.
- Safety and effectiveness of drug haven't been established for hepatitis C in organ-transplant recipients, for patients with hepatitis C infected with hepatitis B, or in patients who haven't responded to other alpha interferon therapy.
- ⚱ Lifespan: In pregnant women, use only if benefits outweigh risks to the fetus; women of childbearing age must use effective contraception. In breast-feeding women, use cautiously; it's unknown whether drug appears in breast milk. In neonates and premature infants, don't use the drug because it contains benzyl alcohol. In children, safety and effectiveness of drug haven't been established. In the elderly, use cautiously because risk for adverse reactions increases.

Adverse reactions

CNS: aggressive behavior, anxiety, bipolar disorder, *cerebral hemorrhage, coma,* concentration and memory impairment, *depression, dizziness, drug overdose* and relapse of drug addiction, *insomnia, irritability, pain, suicide.*

CV: arrhythmias, hypotension, *myocardial infarction, pulmonary embolism.*
GI: *abdominal pain,* anorexia, *diarrhea,* dry mouth, *hemorrhagic* or ischemic colitis, nausea, *pancreatitis,* ulcerative colitis, vomiting.
Hematologic: *anemia, lymphopenia,* NEUTROPENIA, *thrombocytopenia.*
Metabolic: *diabetes mellitus,* hyper- or hypothyroidism, *hypoglycemia.*
Musculoskeletal: *arthralgia,* back pain, *myalgia.*
Respiratory: *interstitial pneumonitis,* pneumonia.
Skin: *alopecia,* dermatitis, increased sweating, *pruritus,* rash.
Other: *flulike symptoms, infection,* injection-site reaction.

Interactions

Drug-drug. *Ribavirin:* May increase risk of hematologic toxicity (neutropenia, anemia). The two drugs are commonly given together for additive therapeutic benefit, but laboratory values and symptoms must be monitored closely.
Theophylline: May increase theophylline level. Monitor theophylline level and adjust dosage as needed.

Effects on lab test results

- May increase ALT and triglyceride levels. May decrease hemoglobin level and hematocrit. May increase or decrease glucose level.
- May decrease ANC, WBC, and platelet counts. May increase or decrease thyroid function test values.

Pharmacokinetics

Absorption: Unknown.
Distribution: Unknown.
Metabolism: Possibly in liver and kidney.
Excretion: Unknown, about 30% is excreted by the kidneys. *Half-life:* 80 hours.

Route	Onset	Peak	Duration
SubQ	Unknown	3–4 days	≤ 1 wk

Action

Chemical effect: Binds to specific receptors on the cell surface, which causes rapid gene transcription that starts complex intracellular events and immunomodulation.

Reactions may be *common,* uncommon, *life-threatening,* or COMMON AND LIFE-THREATENING.

Therapeutic effect: Inhibits viral replication in infected cells and decreases cell proliferation.

Available forms

Injection: 180-mcg/ml single-dose vials, 180 mcg/0.5 ml prefilled syringes

NURSING PROCESS

Assessment

• Monitor patient weekly for psychiatric reactions, such as depression and thoughts of suicide, during the first 8 weeks of therapy. These symptoms may occur in a patient without earlier psychiatric illness. If moderate depression occurs and doesn't go away after decreasing dose, refer patient for psychiatric consultation. If severe depression occurs, immediately stop the drug and start psychiatric therapy.
• Obtain CBC and differential before starting therapy, and monitor it routinely thereafter. Stop giving the drug in the case of a large decrease in neutrophil or platelet counts.
• Obtain baseline eye examination and repeat periodically thereafter during therapy. If patient has a new or worsening eye disorder, stop the drug.
• Monitor lab values for kidney or liver impairment and for thyroid or glucose level changes that require therapy.

Nursing diagnoses

• Ineffective health maintenance related to underlying condition
• Risk for suicide related to adverse CNS effects of drug
• Deficient knowledge related to peginterferon alfa-2a therapy

Planning and implementation

• If uncontrollable thyroid disease, hyperglycemia, hypoglycemia, or diabetes mellitus occurs, stop giving the drug. Thyroid dysfunction may persist after drug is stopped.
• If persistent or unexplained pulmonary infiltrates or pulmonary dysfunction occur, stop giving the drug.
• If signs and symptoms of colitis (abdominal pain, bloody diarrhea, and fever) occur, stop giving the drug. Symptoms will resolve within 3 weeks.
• If signs and symptoms of pancreatitis or autoimmune hepatitis occur, stop giving the drug.

Patient teaching

• Teach patient proper technique for giving himself the drug and for properly disposing of needles and syringes.
• Tell patient to immediately report depression, mood or sleep changes, or thoughts of suicide.
• Tell patient to report signs and symptoms of pancreatitis, GI upset, eye disorders, flulike symptoms, or respiratory disorders.
• Instruct women of childbearing age who are taking drug or who are sexual partners of men taking drug to use two forms of effective contraception during therapy and for 6 months following the end of therapy.
• Inform patient, or partner of patient, who becomes pregnant during or for 6 months posttreatment, to notify prescriber immediately or call the Pregnancy Registry at 1-800-593-2214.
• Advise patient to avoid driving or operating machinery if dizziness, fatigue, confusion, or somnolence occur.

Evaluation

• Patient has improved health.
• Patient denies suicidal ideation.
• Patient and family state understanding of drug therapy.

HIGH ALERT

peginterferon alfa-2b
(pehg-in-ter-FEAR-ahn AL-fah TOO BEE)
PEG-Intron

Pharmacologic class: biological response modifier
Therapeutic class: antiviral
Pregnancy risk category: C (X if used with ribavirin)

Indications and dosages

▶ **Chronic hepatitis C in patients with compensated liver disease not previously treated with interferon alfa therapy.** *Adults:* Recommended regimen is about 1 mcg/kg subcutaneously once weekly for 48 weeks on the same day each week. Recommended doses are as follows:
37 to 45 kg (81 to 99 lb): 40 mcg (0.4 ml) of 100-mcg/ml strength
46 to 56 kg (100 to 123 lb): 50 mcg (0.5 ml) of 100-mcg/ml strength

57 to 72 kg (124 to 158 lb): 64 mcg (0.4 ml) of 160-mcg/ml strength
73 to 88 kg (159 to 194 lb): 80 mcg (0.5 ml) of 160-mcg/ml strength
89 to 106 kg (195 to 233 lb): 96 mcg (0.4 ml) of 240-mcg/ml strength
107 to 136 kg (234 to 299 lb): 120 mcg (0.5 ml) of 240-mcg/ml strength
137 to 160 kg (300 to 352 lb): 150 mcg (0.5 ml) of 300-mcg/ml strength

▶ **Chronic hepatitis C in patients not previously treated with interferon alpha, given with ribavirin.** *Adults:* Recommended regimen is about 1.5 mcg/kg subcutaneously once weekly for 48 weeks on same day each week. Specific doses are as follows:
Less than 40 kg (88 lb): 50 mcg (0.5 ml) of 100-mcg/ml strength
40 to 50 kg (88 to 110 lb): 64 mcg (0.4 ml) of 160-mcg/ml strength
51 to 60 kg (111 to 132 lb): 80 mcg (0.5 ml) of 160-mcg/ml strength
61 to 75 kg (133 to 165 lb): 96 mcg (0.4 ml) of 240-mcg/ml strength
76 to 85 kg (166 to 187 lb): 120 mcg (0.5 ml) of 240-mcg/ml strength
More than 85 kg (187 lb): 150 mcg (0.5 ml) of 300-mcg/ml strength

⧉ **Adjust-a-dose:** In patients with WBC counts less than 1,500/mm³, neutrophil counts less than 750/mm³, or platelet counts less than 80,000/mm³, decrease dosage by one-half. Oral ribavirin dose can be continued. If hemoglobin level is less than 10 g/dl, reduce oral ribavirin dosage by 200 mg daily. If hemoglobin level is less than 8.5 g/dl, WBC counts less than 1,000/mm³, neutrophil counts less than 500/mm³, or platelet counts less than 50,000/mm³, stop both drugs.

If patient develops mild depression, continue drug, but evaluate weekly. For moderate depression, reduce dosage by one-half for 4 to 8 weeks and evaluate patient every week. If symptoms improve and remain stable for 4 weeks, continue at present dose or resume previous dose. If severe depression occurs, stop drug.

For patients with stable CV disease whose hemoglobin level decreases more than 2 g/dl in any 4-week period, decrease peginterferon alfa-2b dosage by one-half and ribavirin dosage by 200 mg daily. If hemoglobin level is less than 12 g/dl after 4 weeks of reduced doses, stop both drugs.

Contraindications and cautions

● Contraindicated in patients hypersensitive to the drug or any of its components, and in patients with renal impairment (creatinine clearance below 50 ml/minute), pulmonary infiltrates, autoimmune hepatitis, or decompensated liver disease (Child-Pugh class B and C).
● Don't use drug in organ transplant recipients, patients who haven't responded to other alpha interferon therapy, or those with HIV or hepatitis B virus.
● Use cautiously in patients with psychiatric disorders; diabetes mellitus; CV disease; pulmonary function impairment; or autoimmune, ischemic, and infectious disorders.
⚠ **Lifespan:** In pregnant women and men whose sexual partners are pregnant, drug is contraindicated. Breast-feeding women should either stop breast-feeding or drug. In neonates and infants, drug is contraindicated because it contains benzyl alcohol. In children, safety and effectiveness haven't been established.

Adverse reactions

CNS: anxiety, *depression, dizziness,* emotional lability, *fatigue, fever, headache,* hypertonia, *insomnia,* irritability, malaise, **suicidal behavior.**
CV: flushing.
EENT: pharyngitis, sinusitis.
GI: *abdominal pain, anorexia,* colitis, *diarrhea,* dyspepsia, *nausea,* right upper quadrant pain, vomiting.
Hematologic: *neutropenia, thrombocytopenia.*
Hepatic: hepatomegaly.
Metabolic: hyperthyroidism, hypothyroidism, weight decrease.
Musculoskeletal: musculoskeletal pain.
Respiratory: cough.
Skin: *alopecia,* dry skin, increased sweating, pruritus, rash.
Other: *flulike symptoms,* injection site pain, injection site reaction (inflammation), rigors, viral infection.

Interactions

None reported.

Effects on lab test results

● May increase ALT, bilirubin, and uric acid levels. May increase or decrease TSH level.
● May decrease neutrophil and platelet counts.

Reactions may be *common,* uncommon, *life-threatening,* or COMMON AND LIFE-THREATENING.

Pharmacokinetics

Absorption: Slowed to mean of 4½ hours by pegylation of interferon alfa-2b.
Distribution: Unknown.
Metabolism: Unknown.
Excretion: Unknown, about 30% is excreted by the kidneys. *Half-life:* 40 hours.

Route	Onset	Peak	Duration
SubQ	Unknown	15–44 hr	48–72 hr

Action

Chemical effect: Binds to specific receptors on the cell surface, which causes rapid gene transcription that initiates complex intracellular events and various immunomodulating activities.
Therapeutic effect: Inhibits viral replication in infected cells, and decreases cell proliferation.

Available forms

Vials: 50 mcg/0.5 ml when reconstituted, 80 mcq/ml when reconstituted, 120 mcg/ml when reconstituted, 150 mcg/ml when reconstituted

NURSING PROCESS

Assessment
• Assess underlying condition before starting therapy and regularly thereafter to monitor drug's effectiveness.
• Assess patient for preexisting uncontrolled diabetes or thyroid disorder. Drug may aggravate hypothyroidism, hyperthyroidism, or diabetes.
• If patient has cardiac history, obtain ECG before starting therapy.
• Evaluate patient's volume and make sure patient is hydrated before starting therapy.
• Obtain eye examination in patients with diabetes or hypertension before starting therapy. Retinal hemorrhages, cotton wool spots, and retinal artery or vein obstruction may occur.
• Monitor CBC, platelet count, and AST, ALT, bilirubin, and TSH levels before starting therapy and periodically during therapy.
• Assess patient's and family's knowledge of drug therapy.

Nursing diagnoses
• Ineffective health maintenance related to underlying condition
• Risk for suicide related to adverse CNS effects of drug

• Deficient knowledge related to peginterferon alfa-2b therapy

Planning and implementation
• Drug may be used alone or with ribavirin for chronic hepatitis B.
• If patient has history of MI or arrhythmias, watch closely for hypotension, arrhythmias, tachycardia, cardiomyopathy, and MI.
ALERT: Alpha interferons may cause or aggravate life-threatening neuropsychiatric, autoimmune, ischemic, and infectious disorders. Monitor patient closely and periodically assess for them. Stop therapy in patient with persistently severe or worsening signs or symptoms of these disorders. In many cases, they resolve after stopping therapy.
• Monitor patient for depression and other psychiatric illness. If symptoms are severe, stop giving the drug and refer patient for psychiatric care.
• Monitor patient for signs and symptoms of colitis, such as abdominal pain, bloody diarrhea, and fever. If colitis occurs, stop giving the drug. Symptoms will resolve 1 to 3 weeks after stopping drug.
• Monitor patient for signs and symptoms of pancreatitis or hypersensitivity reactions. If these occur, stop giving the drug.
• Monitor patient with pulmonary disease for dyspnea, pulmonary infiltrates, pneumonitis, and pneumonia.
• If patient has renal disease, watch for signs and symptoms of toxicity.
• If patient has severe neutropenia or thrombocytopenia, stop giving the drug.
Patient teaching
• Explain appropriate use of the drug and its benefits and risks. Tell patient that adverse reactions may continue for several months after therapy is stopped.
• Advise patient that laboratory tests are required before therapy starts and periodically thereafter.
• Tell patient to take drug at bedtime and to use antipyretics to decrease the effect of flulike symptoms.
• Emphasize the importance of properly disposing of needles and syringes, and warn against reusing old needles and syringes.
• Tell patient that drug isn't known to prevent transmission of hepatitis C. It also isn't known whether drug cures hepatitis C or prevents cir-

rhosis, liver failure, or liver cancer that may result from hepatitis C.
• Advise patient to immediately report symptoms of depression or thoughts of suicide.

☑ **Evaluation**
• Patient has improved health.
• Patient reports no suicidal ideation.
• Patient and family state understanding of drug therapy.

penicillin G benzathine (benzylpenicillin benzathine)
(pen-ih-SIL-in gee BENZ-uh-theen)
Bicillin L-A, Permapen

Pharmacologic class: natural penicillin
Therapeutic class: long-acting antibiotic
Pregnancy risk category: B

Indications and dosages

▶ **Congenital syphilis.** *Children younger than age 2:* Give 50,000 units/kg I.M. as single dose.
▶ **Group A streptococcal upper respiratory tract infections.** *Adults:* 1.2 million units I.M. as single injection.
Children who weigh 27 kg (60 lb) or more: 900,000 units I.M. as single injection.
Children who weigh less than 27 kg (60 lb): 300,000 to 600,000 units I.M. as single injection.
▶ **To prevent poststreptococcal rheumatic fever and glomerulonephritis.** *Adults and children:* 1.2 million units I.M. once monthly or 600,000 units twice monthly.
▶ **Syphilis of less than 1 year's duration.**
Adults: 2.4 million units I.M. as single dose.
Children: 50,000 units/kg I.M. up to adult dosage as a single dose.
▶ **Syphilis of more than 1 year's duration.**
Adults: 2.4 million units I.M. weekly for 3 successive weeks.
Children: 50,000 units/kg I.M. up to adult dosage weekly for 3 successive weeks.
▶ **Yaws, bejel, and pinta.** *Adults:* 1.2 million units I.M. as a single dose.
▶ **To prevent diphtheria‡.** *Adults and children older than age 6 or weighing 30 kg (66 lb) or*
more: 1.2 million units I.M. as a single injection.
Children younger than age 6 or weighing less than 30 kg (66 lb): 600,000 units I.M. as a single dose.
▧ **Adjust-a-dose:** Decrease dose in patients with severe renal or hepatic disease.

Contraindications and cautions

• Contraindicated in patients hypersensitive to drug or other penicillins.
• Use cautiously in patients with other drug allergies, especially to cephalosporins.
⚘ **Lifespan:** In pregnant women, use cautiously. In breast-feeding women, don't use; drug appears in breast milk and may sensitize infant to drug, causing an adverse reaction.

Adverse reactions

CNS: neuropathy, pain, *seizures.*
Hematologic: eosinophilia, hemolytic anemia, *leukopenia, thrombocytopenia.*
Other: hypersensitivity reactions (*anaphylaxis,* chills, edema, fever, maculopapular and exfoliative dermatitis), sterile abscess at injection site.

Interactions

Drug-drug. *Aspirin, ethacrynic acid, furosemide, indomethacin, phenylbutazone, sulfonamides, thiazide diuretics:* May compete with penicillin G for renal tubular secretion and prolong penicillin half-life.
Heparin, oral anticoagulants: May increase risk of bleeding. Monitor PT, PTT, and INR. Monitor patient for bleeding.
Hormonal contraceptives: May decrease effectiveness of hormonal contraceptives and increase breakthrough bleeding. Advise patient to use another method during therapy.
Probenecid: May increase level of penicillin. Probenecid may be used for this purpose.

Effects on lab test results

• May decrease hemoglobin level and hematocrit.
• May increase eosinophil count. May decrease platelet, WBC, and granulocyte counts.
• May cause false-positive urine glucose test results.

Pharmacokinetics

Absorption: Slow.

Distribution: Wide. CSF penetration is poor but enhanced in patients with inflamed meninges. 45% to 68% protein-bound.
Metabolism: At injection site. 16% to 30% to inactive compounds.
Excretion: Mainly in urine. *Half-life:* 30 to 60 minutes.

Route	Onset	Peak	Duration
I.M.	Unknown	13–24 hr	1–4 wk

Action

Chemical effect: Inhibits cell wall synthesis during microorganism multiplication.
Therapeutic effect: Kills susceptible bacteria.

Available forms

Injection: 300,000 units/ml, 600,000 units/ml

NURSING PROCESS

Assessment
• Assess patient's infection before starting therapy and regularly thereafter to monitor drug's effectiveness.
• Before giving drug, ask the patient about allergic reactions to penicillin, cephalosporins, and cephamycins. Absence of past reactions is no guarantee against future allergic reactions.
• Obtain specimen for culture and sensitivity tests before giving first dose. If a sexually transmitted infection (STI) is suspected, obtain baseline venereal disease research laboratory (VDRL), and rapid plasma reagin (RPR), tests. Start therapy pending test results.
• Be alert for adverse reactions and drug interactions.
• Observe patient closely. Large doses and prolonged therapy raise the risk of bacterial or fungal superinfection, especially in an elderly, debilitated, or immunosuppressed patient.
• Assess patient's and family's knowledge of drug therapy.

Nursing diagnoses
• Risk for infection related to presence of bacteria
• Ineffective protection related to risk of hypersensitivity reactions to drug
• Deficient knowledge related to drug therapy

Planning and implementation
• Shake drug well before injection.

• Inject at a slow, steady rate to prevent needle from becoming blocked by suspended material in product.
⚡ **ALERT:** Never give drug I.V.; doing so has caused cardiac arrest and death.
• Inject deep into upper outer quadrant of buttocks in adult; in midlateral thigh in infant and young child. Avoid injection into or near major nerves or blood vessels to prevent severe neurovascular damage.
• If a high dose of penicillin is required for several days, change to an I.V. formulation (penicillin G potassium or penicillin G sodium) to avoid muscle fibrosis and atrophy from repeated I.M. injections (particularly in neonates and infants).
• Drug's extremely slow absorption makes allergic reactions difficult to treat. If patient develops signs of anaphylactic shock, such as rapidly developing dyspnea and hypotension, immediately stop giving the drug. Notify prescriber and immediately administer epinephrine, corticosteroids, antihistamines, or other resuscitative measures.
⚡ **ALERT:** Be aware of the various preparations of penicillin. They aren't interchangeable.
• Periodically monitor renal and hematopoietic function in patient receiving long-term therapy.
⚡ **ALERT:** Don't confuse penicillin with penicillamine. Don't confuse penicillin G potassium with penicillin G sodium, penicillin G procaine, or penicillin G benzathine.
⚡ **ALERT:** Bicillin L-A is the only penicillin G benzathine product indicated for the treatment of sexually transmitted infections, including syphilis. Don't substitute Bicillin C-R in its place as this may cause ineffective treatment.
Patient teaching
• Tell patient to call prescriber if rash, fever, or chills develop.
• Tell patient taking drug for active STI to take safe sex precautions, to reduce risks to fetus and neonate of syphilis during pregnancy, and to complete full drug course and follow-up testing.
• Instruct patient treated for active STI to bring partners in for therapy as well.
• Warn patient that injection may be painful but that ice applied to site may ease discomfort.

Evaluation
• Patient is free from infection.
• Patient shows no signs of allergy.

- Patient and family state understanding of drug therapy.

penicillin G potassium (benzylpenicillin potassium)
(pen-ih-SIL-in gee poh-TAH-see-um)
Pfizerpen

Pharmacologic class: natural penicillin
Therapeutic class: rapid-acting antibiotic
Pregnancy risk category: B

Indications and dosages

▶ **Moderate to severe systemic infection.**
Adults and children age 12 and older: Individualize dosage. 1 to 24 million units I.M. or I.V. daily in divided doses every 4 to 6 hours.
Children younger than age 12: Highly individualized; 25,000 to 400,000 units/kg I.M. or I.V. daily in divided doses every 4 to 6 hours.
▶ **Anthrax.** *Adults:* 5 to 20 million units I.V. daily in divided doses every 4 to 6 hours for at least 14 days after symptoms subside. Or, 80,000 units/kg in the first hour followed by a maintenance dose of 320,000 units/kg/day. Average adult dosage, 4 million units every 4 hours or 2 million units every 2 hours.
Children: 100,000 to 150,000 units/kg/day I.V. in divided doses every 4 to 6 hours for at least 14 days after symptoms subside.
▶ **Necrotizing ulcerative gingivitis.** *Adults:* 5 to 10 million units I.M. or I.V. daily.
▶ **Elimination of the diphtheria carrier-state.** *Adults:* 2 to 3 million units per day I.M. in divided doses every 4 to 6 hours for 10 to 12 days.
☒ **Adjust-a-dose:** For patients with renal impairment, if creatinine clearance is less than 10 ml/min, give full loading dose and then one-half of usual dose every 8 to 10 hours or usual dose every 12 to 18 hours; if creatinine clearance is more than 10 ml/minute, give full loading dose and then give one-half dose every 4 to 6 hours for additional doses.

▼ I.V. administration

- Use continuous I.V. infusion when large doses are required (10 million units or more). Otherwise, give by intermittent I.V. infusion over 1 to 2 hours.

⊗ **Incompatibilities**
Alcohol 5%, amikacin, aminoglycosides, aminophylline, amphotericin B sodium, chlorpromazine, dextran, dopamine, heparin sodium, hydroxyzine hydrochloride, lincomycin, metoclopramide, pentobarbital sodium, phenytoin sodium, prochlorperazine mesylate, promethazine hydrochloride, sodium bicarbonate, thiopental, vancomycin, vitamin B complex with C.

Contraindications and cautions

- Contraindicated in patients hypersensitive to the drug or other penicillins.
- Use cautiously in patients with other drug allergies, especially to cephalosporins and cephamycins.
🜂 **Lifespan:** In pregnant women, use cautiously. In breast-feeding women, don't use; drug appears in breast milk and may sensitize infant to penicillin and cause an adverse reaction.

Adverse reactions

CNS: *coma,* neuropathy, *seizures.*
CV: thrombophlebitis.
Hematologic: hemolytic anemia, *leukopenia, thrombocytopenia.*
Metabolic: *severe potassium poisoning.*
Other: hypersensitivity reactions (*anaphylaxis,* chills, edema, exfoliative dermatitis, fever, maculopapular eruptions, rash, urticaria), overgrowth of nonsusceptible organisms, pain at injection site.

Interactions

Drug-drug. *Aminoglycoside antibiotics:* May be synergistic with some penicillins but can deactivate some beta-lactam penicillins if mixed in same syringe or I.V. solution and administration set. May reduce oral aminoglycoside level when given with parenteral penicillins to renally impaired patients.
Aspirin, ethacrynic acid, furosemide, indomethacin, phenylbutazone, sulfonamides, thiazide diuretics: May compete with penicillin G for renal tubular secretion and prolong penicillin half-life.
Heparin, oral anticoagulants: May increase risk of bleeding. Monitor PT, PTT, and INR. Monitor patient for bleeding.
Hormonal contraceptives: May decrease effectiveness of hormonal contraceptives and in-

crease breakthrough bleeding. Advise patient to use another contraceptive during therapy.
Potassium-sparing diuretics: May increase risk of hyperkalemia. Don't use together.
Probenecid: May increase level of penicillin. Probenecid may be used for this purpose.

Effects on lab test results

• May increase potassium level. May decrease hemoglobin level and hematocrit.
• May increase eosinophil count. May decrease platelet, WBC, and granulocyte counts.

Pharmacokinetics

Absorption: Rapid from I.M. injection site.
Distribution: Wide. CSF penetration is poor but is enhanced in patients with inflamed meninges. 45% to 68% protein-bound.
Metabolism: At injection site.
Excretion: Mainly in urine. *Half-life:* 20 to 50 minutes.

Route	Onset	Peak	Duration
I.V.	Immediate	Immediate	4 hr
I.M.	Unknown	15–30 min	4 hr

Action

Chemical effect: Inhibits cell wall synthesis during microorganism multiplication.
Therapeutic effect: Kills susceptible bacteria.

Available forms

Injection (powder): 5 million units, 20 million units
Injection (premixed in dextrose): 1 million units, 2 million units, 3 million units

NURSING PROCESS

Assessment

• Assess patient's infection before starting therapy and regularly thereafter to monitor drug's effectiveness.
• Before giving, ask the patient about any allergic reactions to penicillin, cephalosporins, and cephamycins. Negative history of penicillin allergy is no guarantee against future allergic reactions.
• Obtain specimen for culture and sensitivity tests before first dose. Start therapy pending test results.
• Assess renal, cardiac, and vascular conditions with physical exams and laboratory testing be-

fore start of therapy. Drug contains 1.7 mEq potassium and 0.3 mEq sodium per 1 million units. If risk of fluid overload or electrolyte imbalance, decrease dosage and monitor electrolytes and renal tests frequently during therapy.
• Be alert for adverse reactions and drug interactions.
• Observe patient closely. Large doses and prolonged therapy raise the risk of neutropenia and bacterial or fungal superinfection especially in an elderly, debilitated, or immunosuppressed patient.
• Assess patient's and family's knowledge of drug therapy.

Nursing diagnoses

• Risk for infection related to presence of bacteria
• Ineffective protection related to risk of hypersensitivity reactions to drug
• Deficient knowledge related to drug therapy

Planning and implementation

• Reconstitute vials with sterile water for injection, D₅W, or normal saline solution for injection. Volume of diluent varies by manufacturer.
• Inject deep into upper outer quadrant of buttocks in adult and in midlateral thigh in infant and young child. Avoid injection into or near major nerves or blood vessels to prevent severe neurovascular damage.
ALERT: The various preparations of penicillin aren't interchangeable.
• Monitor level in patients taking large doses. A high level may lead to seizures. Take precautions and periodically monitor renal and hematopoietic function in patient receiving long-term therapy.
• Give drug I.M. deep into large muscle; warn patient that injection may be painful.
ALERT: Don't confuse penicillamine with penicillin. Don't confuse penicillin G potassium with penicillin G sodium, penicillin G procaine, or penicillin G benzathine.
Patient teaching
• Tell patient to call prescriber if rash, fever, or chills develop.
• Warn patient that I.M. injection may be painful but that ice applied to site may ease discomfort.

✓ **Evaluation**
• Patient is free from infection.
• Patient shows no signs of allergy.
• Patient and family state understanding of drug therapy.

penicillin G procaine
(benzylpenicillin procaine)
(pen-ih-SIL-in gee PROH-kayn)

Pharmacologic class: natural penicillin
Therapeutic class: long-acting antibiotic
Pregnancy risk category: B

Indications and dosages

▶ **Moderately severe infections of upper respiratory tract including pneumococcal pneumonia; tonsils; pharynx; and skin and soft tissues.** *Adults and children who weigh 27 kg (60 lb) or more:* 600,000 to 1 million units I.M. daily in 1 or 2 doses for at least 10 days.
Children who weigh less than 27 kg (60 lb): 300,000 units I.M. daily in single dose for at least 10 days.
▶ **Anthrax caused by** *Bacillus anthracis,* **including prophylaxis after exposure to inhalation anthrax.** *Adults:* 1.2 million units I.M. every 12 hours for up to 60 days.
Children: 25,000 units/kg I.M. (maximum, 1.2 million units) every 12 hours for up to 60 days.
▶ **Cutaneous anthrax.** *Adults:* 600,000 to 1 million units I.M. daily for 5 to 60 days depending on source of exposure.
▶ **Syphilis with negative CSF test.** *Adults and children older than age 12:* Give 600,000 units I.M. daily for 8 days.
▶ **Syphilis with no CSF test or positive CSF test.** *Adults and children older than age 12:* Give 600,000 units I.M. daily for 10 to 15 days.
▶ **Neurosyphilis.** *Adults and children older than age 12:* Give 2.4 million units I.M. daily with probenecid 500 mg P.O. q.i.d. for 10 to 14 days.
▶ **Congenital syphilis.** *Children less than 32 kg (70 lb):* Give 50,000 units/kg/day I.M. for 10 to 14 days.

Contraindications and cautions

• Contraindicated in patients hypersensitive to drug, other penicillins, or procaine.
• Use cautiously in patients with other drug allergies, especially to cephalosporins, and cephamycins.
⚠ **Lifespan:** In pregnant women, use cautiously. In breast-feeding women, don't use; drug appears in breast milk and drug use may sensitize infant to penicillin and cause adverse effects. Avoid use in newborns due to concern of sterile abscesses and procaine toxicity.

Adverse reactions

CNS: *seizures.*
Hematologic: hemolytic anemia, *leukopenia, thrombocytopenia.*
Musculoskeletal: arthralgia.
Other: hypersensitivity reactions (*anaphylaxis,* chills, edema, fever, prostration, rash, urticaria), overgrowth of nonsusceptible organisms.

Interactions

Drug-drug. *Aspirin, ethacrynic acid, furosemide, indomethacin, phenylbutazone, sulfonamides, thiazide diuretics:* May compete with penicillin G for renal tubular secretion and prolong penicillin half-life.
Heparin, oral anticoagulants: May increase risk of bleeding. Monitor PT, PTT, and INR. Monitor patient for bleeding.
Hormonal contraceptives: May decrease effectiveness of hormonal contraceptives and increase breakthrough bleeding. Advise patient to use alternative method during therapy.
Probenecid: May increase level of penicillin. Probenecid may be used for this purpose.

Effects on lab test results

• May decrease hemoglobin level and hematocrit.
• May increase eosinophil count. May decrease platelet, WBC, and granulocyte counts.

Pharmacokinetics

Absorption: Slow.
Distribution: Distributed widely. CSF penetration poor. 45% to 68% protein-bound.
Metabolism: Occurs at injection site. From 16% to 30% metabolized to inactive compounds.
Excretion: Mainly in urine. *Half-life:* About 12 hours.

Route	Onset	Peak	Duration
I.M.	Unknown	1–4 hr	1–2 days

Action

Chemical effect: Inhibits cell wall synthesis during microorganism multiplication.
Therapeutic effect: Kills susceptible bacteria.

Available forms

Injection: 600,000 units/ml

NURSING PROCESS

◪ Assessment

• Assess patient's infection before starting therapy and regularly thereafter to monitor drug's effectiveness.
• Before giving, ask patient about allergic reactions to penicillin, cephalosporins, and cephamycins. Negative history of penicillin allergy is no guarantee against future allergic reaction.
• Assess for allergy to drug. Give test dose of 0.1 ml of 1% or 2% intradermally and observe for erythema, wheal, flare, or eruption. If positive for sensitivity, drug is contraindicated.
• Obtain specimen for culture and sensitivity tests before giving first dose. Start therapy pending test results.
• Be alert for adverse reactions and drug interactions. Observe patient closely. Large doses and prolonged therapy raise the risk of neutropenia and bacterial or fungal superinfection, especially in a geriatric, debilitated, or immunosuppressed patient.
• Assess patient's and family's knowledge of drug therapy.

⊞ Nursing diagnoses

• Risk for infection related to presence of bacteria
• Ineffective protection related to risk of hypersensitivity reactions to drug
• Deficient knowledge related to drug therapy

▷ Planning and implementation

• Shake drug well before injection.
• Inject at a slow, steady rate to prevent needle from becoming blocked by suspended material in product.
• Inject deep into upper outer quadrant of buttocks in adults; in midlateral thigh in infants and small children. Avoid injection into or near ma-

jor nerves or blood vessels to prevent severe neurovascular damage.
⚉ **ALERT:** Never give I.V.; doing so has caused cardiac arrest and death.
• If high dose is required for several days, consider change to I.V. penicillin G potassium or penicillin G sodium to avoid muscle fibrosis and atrophy from repeated I.M. injections.
• In patients with renal insufficiency or those taking high doses of I.M. drug, give penicillin G procaine at least 1 hour before bacteriostatic oral antibiotics such as aminoglycosides because it may inactivate such oral drugs.
⚉ **ALERT:** Don't confuse penicillin G procaine, with penicillin G sodium, penicillin G potassium, or penicillin G benzathine.
• The drug's extremely slow absorption makes allergic reactions difficult to treat. If patient develops signs of anaphylactic shock, such as rapidly developing dyspnea and hypotension, immediately stop giving the drug. Notify prescriber and immediately administer epinephrine, corticosteroids, antihistamines, or other resuscitative measures.
• For a patient receiving long-term therapy, periodically monitor renal and hematopoietic function.
⚉ **ALERT:** Be aware of the various preparations of penicillin. They aren't interchangeable.
Patient teaching
• Tell patient to call prescriber if rash, fever, or chills develop.
• Warn patient that injection may be painful but that ice applied to site may ease discomfort.
• Teach patient taking drug for active sexually transmitted infection (STI) about safe sex practices, and address the risks of syphilis to fetus and neonate during pregnancy and the need to complete full drug course and follow-up testing.
• Instruct patient treated for active STI to bring partners in for treatment as well.

☑ Evaluation

• Patient is free from infection.
• Patient shows no signs of allergy.
• Patient and family state understanding of drug therapy.

P

---

penicillin G sodium
(benzylpenicillin sodium)
(pen-ih-SIL-in gee SOH-dee-um)
Crystapen ◆

Pharmacologic class: natural penicillin
Therapeutic class: rapid-acting antibiotic
Pregnancy risk category: B

Indications and dosages

▶ **Moderate to severe systemic infections.**
Adults and children age 12 and older: Highly
individualized; 1 to 24 million units daily I.M.
or I.V. in divided doses every 4 to 6 hours.
Children younger than age 12: Highly individualized; 25,000 to 400,000 units/kg daily I.M. or
I.V. in divided doses every 4 to 6 hours.
▶ **Bacterial endocarditis.** *Adults and children
age 12 and older:* 5 to 30 million units daily I.V.
in divided doses every 4 to 6 hours for 2 to 6
weeks depending on bacterial strain and severity
of infection.
Children younger than age 12: Give 50,000 to
250,000 units/kg daily I.M. or I.V. in divided
doses every 4 weeks.
▶ **Anthrax.** *Adults:* 5 to 20 million units I.V.
daily in divided doses every 4 to 6 hours, for at
least 14 days after symptoms subside. Or, 8 million units daily I.V. in divided doses every 6
hours. Higher doses may be required based on
organism's susceptibility.
Children: 100,000 to 150,000 units/kg/day I.V.
in divided doses every 4 to 6 hours for at least
14 days after symptoms lessen.
▶ **Neurosyphilis.** *Adults:* 18 to 24 million units
I.V. daily in divided doses every 4 hours for 10
to 14 days.
🔲 **Adjust-a-dose:** For patients with renal impairment, if creatinine clearance is less than 10 ml/
minute, give full loading dose and then half of
usual dose every 8 to 10 hours or usual dose
every 12 to 18 hours; if creatinine clearance is
more than 10 ml/minute, give full loading dose
and then give half dose every 4 to 6 hours.

▼ I.V. administration

● Reconstitute vials with sterile water for injection, normal saline solution for injection, or
D_5W. Volume of diluent varies with manufacturer and concentration needed.

● For patient receiving 10 million units of drug
or more daily, dilute in 1 to 2 L of compatible
solution and administer over 24 hours. Otherwise, give by intermittent I.V. infusion. Dilute
drug in 50 to 100 ml and give over 1 to 2 hours
every 4 to 6 hours.
● In a neonate or child, give divided doses, usually over 15 to 30 minutes.
⊗ **Incompatibilities**
Aminoglycosides, amphotericin B, bleomycin,
chlorpromazine, cytarabine, fat emulsions 10%,
heparin sodium, hydroxyzine hydrochloride,
invert sugar 10%, lincomycin, methylprednisolone sodium succinate, potassium chloride,
prochlorperazine mesylate, promethazine hydrochloride.

Contraindications and cautions

● Contraindicated in patients hypersensitive to
the drug or other penicillins.
● Use cautiously in patients with other drug allergies, especially to cephalosporins, and
cephamycins.
🔲 **Lifespan:** In pregnant women, use cautiously. In breast-feeding women, don't use; drug appears in breast milk and may sensitize infant to
penicillin and cause adverse effects.

Adverse reactions

CNS: neuropathy, *seizures.*
CV: thrombophlebitis.
Hematologic: hemolytic anemia, *leukopenia,
thrombocytopenia.*
Musculoskeletal: arthralgia.
Other: hypersensitivity reactions (*anaphylaxis,*
exfoliative dermatitis, urticaria), overgrowth of
nonsusceptible organisms, pain at injection site,
vein irritation,

Interactions

Drug-drug. *Aminoglycoside antibiotics:* May
deactivate some beta-lactam penicillins if mixed
in same syringe or I.V. solution and administration set. Oral aminoglycoside level may be reduced when given with parenteral penicillins to
a renally compromised patient.
*Aspirin, ethacrynic acid, furosemide, indo-
methacin, phenylbutazone, sulfonamides, thiazide diuretics:* May compete with penicillin G
for renal tubular secretion and prolong penicillin
half-life. Monitor patient.

Reactions may be *common,* uncommon, *life-threatening*, or COMMON AND LIFE-THREATENING.

Heparin, oral anticoagulants: May increase risk of bleeding. Monitor PT, PTT, and INR. Monitor patient for bleeding.

Hormonal contraceptives: May decrease effectiveness of hormonal contraceptives and increase breakthrough bleeding. Advise patient to use alternative contraception during therapy.

Probenecid: May increase level of penicillin. Probenecid may be used for this purpose.

Effects on lab test results

• May decrease hemoglobin level and hematocrit.
• May increase eosinophil count. May decrease platelet, WBC, and granulocyte counts.

Pharmacokinetics

Absorption: Rapid.
Distribution: Wide. CSF penetration is poor but is enhanced in patients with inflamed meninges. 45% to 68% protein-bound.
Metabolism: At injection site. 16% to 30% to inactive compounds.
Excretion: Mainly in urine. *Half-life:* 30 to 60 minutes.

Route	Onset	Peak	Duration
I.V.	Immediate	Immediate	4 hr
I.M.	Unknown	15–30 min	4 hr

Action

Chemical effect: Inhibits cell wall synthesis during microorganism multiplication.
Therapeutic effect: Kills susceptible bacteria.

Available forms

Injection: 5-million-unit vial

NURSING PROCESS

🗹 Assessment

• Assess patient's infection before starting therapy and regularly thereafter to monitor drug's effectiveness.
• Before giving, ask patient about allergic reactions to penicillin, cephalosporins, and cephamycins. Negative history of penicillin allergy is no guarantee against future allergic reaction.
• Obtain specimen for culture and sensitivity tests before first dose. Start therapy pending test results.
• Assess renal, cardiac, and vascular conditions with physical exams and laboratory testing be-

fore the start of therapy. Drug contains 2 mEq sodium per 1 million units. Assess risk of fluid overload or electrolyte imbalance; decrease dose and monitor electrolytes and renal tests frequently during therapy.
• Be alert for adverse reactions and drug interactions.
• Observe patient closely. Large doses and prolonged therapy raise the risk of neutropenia and bacterial or fungal superinfection, especially in geriatric, debilitated, or immunosuppressed patients.
• Assess patient's and family's knowledge of drug therapy.

🔹 Nursing diagnoses

• Risk for infection related to presence of bacteria
• Ineffective protection related to risk of hypersensitivity reactions to drug
• Deficient knowledge related to drug therapy

▷ Planning and implementation

• Give drug I.M. deep in upper outer quadrant of buttocks in adult; in midlateral thigh in young child. Don't massage injection site. Avoid injection near major nerves or blood vessels to prevent severe neurovascular damage.
• Give penicillin G sodium at least 1 hour before bacteriostatic antibiotics, and if given I.M., at different sites.
• Periodically monitor renal and hematopoietic function in patient receiving long-term therapy.
⏺ **ALERT:** Be aware of the various preparations of penicillin. They aren't interchangeable.
• Monitor level in patient taking large doses. A high level may lead to seizures. Take precautions.
⏺ **ALERT:** Don't confuse penicillamine with penicillin. Don't confuse penicillin G sodium with penicillin G potassium, penicillin G procaine, or penicillin G benzathine.
Patient teaching
• Tell patient to report discomfort at I.V. site.
• Warn patient that I.M. injection may be painful but that ice applied to site may ease discomfort.

🗹 Evaluation

• Patient is free from infection.
• Patient shows no signs of allergy.
• Patient and family state understanding of drug therapy.

penicillin V potassium (phenoxymethyl penicillin potassium)
Apo-Pen-VK♦, Novo-Pen-VK♦, Nu-Pen-VK♦, Penicillin VK, Veetids

Pharmacologic class: natural penicillin
Therapeutic class: antibiotic
Pregnancy risk category: B

Indications and dosages

▶ **Mild to moderately severe infections of upper respiratory tract (including pneumococcal pneumonia), oropharynx, sinuses, and skin and soft tissues; necrotizing ulcerative gingivitis.** *Adults and children older than age 12:* Give 125 mg to 500 mg (200,000 to 800,000 units) P.O. every 6 to 8 hours.
Children age 1 month to 12 years: Give 15 to 62.5 mg/kg (25,000 to 100,000 units/kg) P.O. daily, in divided doses every 4 to 8 hours.
▶ **Prophylaxis for rheumatic fever.** *Adults and children older than age 12:* Give 125 mg to 250 mg P.O. b.i.d.
▶ **Prophylaxis for pneumococcal infections in children with sickle cell anemia or splenectomy‡.** *Children age 5 and older:* 250 mg P.O. b.i.d.
Children 3 months to younger than age 5: Give 125 mg P.O. b.i.d.
▶ **Lyme disease‡.** *Adults:* 500 mg P.O. q.i.d. for 10 to 20 days.
▶ **Actinomycosis‡.** *Adults:* 10 to 20 mg/day penicillin G I.V. for 4 to 6 weeks, then 2 to 4 g/day penicillin V for 6 to 12 months.
▶ **Confirmed or suspected exposure to *Bacillus anthracis‡*.** *Adults:* 7.5 mg/kg P.O. q.i.d. Continue prophylaxis until exposure to *B. anthracis* has been ruled out. If exposure is confirmed and vaccine is available, continue prophylaxis for 4 weeks and until three doses of vaccine have been given or for 30 to 60 days if vaccine isn't available.
Children younger than age 9: Give 50 mg/kg P.O. daily in four divided doses. Continue prophylaxis until exposure to *B. anthracis* has been ruled out. If exposure is confirmed and vaccine is available, continue prophylaxis for 4 weeks and until three doses of vaccine have been given or for 30 to 60 days if vaccine isn't available.

Contraindications and cautions

• Contraindicated in patients hypersensitive to the drug or other penicillins.
• Use cautiously in patients with other drug allergies, especially to cephalosporins and cephamycins and in patients with hyperacidity of the GI tract since decreased pH can inactivate drug.
☀ **Lifespan:** In pregnant women, use cautiously. In breast-feeding women, don't use; drug appears in breast milk and use of drug may sensitize infant to penicillin and cause adverse effects.

Adverse reactions

CNS: neuropathy, *seizures.*
GI: diarrhea, *epigastric distress, nausea, vomiting.*
Hematologic: eosinophilia, hemolytic anemia, *leukopenia, thrombocytopenia.*
Other: hypersensitivity reactions (*anaphylaxis,* chills, edema, fever, rash, urticaria), overgrowth of nonsusceptible organisms.

Interactions

Drug-drug. *Beta blockers:* May increase risk of anaphylactic reactions to oral penicillins.
Contraceptives containing estrogen: May decrease effectiveness of hormonal contraceptive. Monitor patient for breakthrough bleeding. Advise patient to use alternative forms of birth control.
Methotrexate: May increase methotrexate level, increasing risk of toxicity. Monitor patient.
Oral neomycin: May reduce oral penicillin level. Monitor patient.
Probenecid: May increase level of penicillin. Probenecid may be used for this purpose.

Effects on lab test results

• May decrease hemoglobin level and hematocrit.
• May increase eosinophil count. May decrease platelet, WBC, and granulocyte counts.

Pharmacokinetics

Absorption: About 60% to 75%.
Distribution: Wide. CSF penetration is poor. 75% to 89% protein-bound.
Metabolism: Mainly in small intestine.
Excretion: Mainly in urine. *Half-life:* 30 minutes.

Route	Onset	Peak	Duration
P.O.	Unknown	30–60 min	6–8 hr

Action

Chemical effect: Inhibits cell wall synthesis during microorganism multiplication.
Therapeutic effect: Kills susceptible bacteria.

Available forms

Oral suspension: 125 mg/5 ml, 250 mg/5 ml (after reconstitution)
Tablets: 250 mg, 500 mg
Tablets (film-coated): 250 mg, 500 mg

NURSING PROCESS

☑ Assessment

• Assess patient's infection before starting therapy and regularly thereafter to monitor drug's effectiveness.
• Before giving drug, ask patient about any allergic reactions to penicillin, cephalosporins, and cephamycins. Negative history of penicillin allergy is no guarantee against future allergic reaction.
• Obtain specimen for culture and sensitivity tests before giving first dose. Start therapy pending test results.
• Periodically assess renal and hematopoietic function in patient receiving long-term therapy.
• Be alert for adverse reactions and drug interactions.
• If patient develops diarrhea during therapy, consider possibility of pseudomembranous colitis.
• Observe patient closely. Large doses and prolonged therapy raise the risk of bacterial or fungal superinfection, especially in geriatric, debilitated, or immunosuppressed patients.
• Assess patient's and family's knowledge of drug therapy.

✪ Nursing diagnoses

• Risk of infection related to presence of bacteria
• Ineffective protection related to risk of hypersensitivity reactions to drug
• Deficient knowledge related to drug therapy

▷ Planning and implementation

• Give drug at least 1 hour before bacteriostatic antibiotics.
• **ALERT:** Don't confuse penicillamine with penicillin.

Patient teaching

• Tell patient to take drug exactly as prescribed, even after he feels better.
• Tell patient that drug may be taken without regard to meals. If GI disturbances occur, drug may be taken with meals.
• Warn patient never to use leftover penicillin V for new illness or to share penicillin with family and friends.
• Inform patients using oral solution that any remaining solution must be discarded after 14 days.
• Drug of choice for endocarditis prophylaxis is amoxicillin.
• Tell patient to call prescriber if rash, fever, or chills develop.

☑ Evaluation

• Patient is free from infection.
• Patient shows no signs of allergy.
• Patient and family state understanding of drug therapy.

pentamidine isethionate

(pen-TAM-eh-deen ighs-eh-THIGH-oh-nayt)
NebuPent, Pentam 300

Pharmacologic class: diamidine derivative
Therapeutic class: antiprotozoal
Pregnancy risk category: C

Indications and dosages

▶ **Pneumocystis jiroveci (carinii) pneumonia.**
Adults and children older than age 4 months:
4 mg/kg I.V. or I.M. once daily for 14 to 21 days.
▶ **Prevention of P. jiroveci (carinii) pneumonia in high-risk patients.** *Adults:* 300 mg by inhalation (using Respirgard II jet nebulizer) once every 4 weeks.

▼ I.V. administration

• Reconstitute drug with 3 to 5 ml of sterile water for injection; then dilute in 50 to 250 ml of D_5W. Infuse over 1 to 2 hours.
• To minimize hypotension, infuse drug slowly with patient lying down.
⊗ **Incompatibilities**
Aldesleukin, cephalosporins, fluconazole, foscarnet.

P

Contraindications and cautions

• Contraindicated in patients with history of anaphylactic reaction to drug.
• Use cautiously in patients with diabetes, hypertension, hypotension, hyperglycemia, hypoglycemia, hypocalcemia, leukopenia, thrombocytopenia, anemia, pancreatitis, hepatic or renal dysfunction or history of ventricular tachycardia or Stevens-Johnson syndrome.

※ **Lifespan:** In pregnant women, use cautiously. In breast-feeding women, drug isn't recommended.

Adverse reactions

Parenteral form
CNS: confusion, dizziness, fever, hallucinations, neuralgia.
CV: cardiac arrhythmias, facial flushing, hypotension, *ventricular tachycardia.*
GI: abdominal discomfort, anorexia, diarrhea, metallic taste, nausea, *pancreatitis,* vomiting.
GU: *acute renal failure, renal toxicity.*
Hematologic: anemia, *leukopenia, thrombocytopenia.*
Metabolic: hyperglycemia, hyperkalemia, hypocalcemia, *hypoglycemia.*
Respiratory: *bronchospasm,* cough.
Skin: pruritus, rash, *Stevens-Johnson syndrome.*
Other: *anaphylactoid reactions, pain and induration at injection site* with I.M. route, phlebitis, tissue necrosis or sloughing from extravasation with I.V. route, *sterile abscess.*

Aerosol form
CNS: confusion, decreased taste or smell, *dizziness, fatigue,* fever, headache, tremors.
CV: *chest pain,* hypertension, hypotension.
GI: abdominal discomfort, anorexia, diarrhea, *metallic taste,* nausea, *pancreatitis, pharyngitis,* vomiting.
Hematologic: anemia, *leukopenia, thrombocytopenia.*
Metabolic: hyperglycemia, hypocalcemia, *hypoglycemia.*
Respiratory: BRONCHOSPASM, *chest congestion, cough, shortness of breath.*
Skin: *rash.*
Other: *chills, night sweats.*

Interactions

Drug-drug. *Aminoglycosides, amphotericin B, capreomycin, cisplatin, colistin, foscarnet, methoxyflurane, polymyxin B, vancomycin:* In-creases risk of nephrotoxicity. Monitor patient closely.

Effects on lab test results

• May increase BUN, creatinine, potassium, and liver enzyme levels. May decrease calcium and hemoglobin levels and hematocrit. May increase or severely decrease glucose level.
• May decrease WBC and platelet counts.

Pharmacokinetics

Absorption: Limited after aerosol use. Well absorbed after I.M. use.
Distribution: Drug appears to be extensively tissue-bound. CNS penetration is poor. Extent of protein-binding is unknown.
Metabolism: Unknown.
Excretion: Excreted unchanged in urine. *Half-life:* Varies according to route of administration; 9 to 13¼ hours for I.M., about 6¼ hours for I.V., unknown for aerosol.

Route	Onset	Peak	Duration
I.V.	Unknown	Immediate	Unknown
I.M.	Unknown	30 min–1 hr	Unknown
Aerosol	Unknown	Unknown	Unknown

Action

Chemical effect: Interferes with infectious organism's biosynthesis of DNA, RNA, phospholipids, and proteins.
Therapeutic effect: Hinders growth of susceptible organisms.

Available forms

Aerosol: 300-mg vial
Injection: 300-mg vial

NURSING PROCESS

Ⓡ **Assessment**
• Assess patient's infection before starting therapy and regularly thereafter to monitor drug's effectiveness.
Ⓢ **ALERT:** Monitor glucose level before therapy, daily during parenteral administration, and regularly afterwards. Glucose level may decrease initially, and hypoglycemia may be severe. Hyperglycemia and insulin-dependent diabetes mellitus may follow months after therapy ends and may be permanent.
• Monitor CBC, platelet count, calcium, liver function tests, potassium, and renal function

tests before, during, and after therapy. Monitor BUN, creatinine, calcium, and potassium levels daily during parenteral therapy due to risks of acute renal failure, hypocalcemia, and hyperkalemia.
• Closely monitor blood pressure during I.V. administration.
⊛ **ALERT:** Screen and treat patient for tuberculosis (TB) before using inhaled form. The risk of spreading TB to health care personnel and family members increases with high-pressure nebulizer use due to cough and droplet spread. If you're pregnant or plan to become pregnant, have another staff member care for this patient. Standard personal protection equipment is ineffective. Use care in choosing a room for patient using inhaled form.
• Be alert for adverse reactions and drug interactions.
• Assess patient's and family's knowledge of drug therapy.

🔁 **Nursing diagnoses**
• Risk for infection related to presence of organisms
• Risk for injury related to drug-induced adverse CNS reactions
• Deficient knowledge related to drug therapy

▷ **Planning and implementation**
• For I.M. use, reconstitute drug with 3 ml of sterile water to make solution containing 100 mg/ml; administer deeply using Z-track technique. Expect pain and induration at site.
• In patient with AIDS, this drug may produce less severe adverse reactions than co-trimoxazole and may be drug of choice.
• Give aerosol form only by Respirgard II jet nebulizer manufactured by Marquest (flow rate of 5 to 7 liters/minute from 40 to 50 pounds per square inch [psi] compressor). Dosage is based on particle size and delivery rate of this device; don't change to low-pressure (below 20 psi) compressors.
• To use aerosol, mix contents of one vial in 6 ml of sterile water for injection. Don't use normal saline solution; it will cause precipitation.
• Don't mix with other drugs.
• Inhaling drug may induce bronchospasm or cough, especially in patients with a history of smoking or asthma.

Patient teaching
• Instruct patient to use aerosol device until chamber is empty, which may take up to 45 minutes.
• Advise patient with significant cough and bronchospasm to report effects to prescriber. Aerosol bronchodilator may be prescribed for use just before therapy.
• Warn patient that I.M. injection is painful. Application of warm soaks is helpful.
• Tell patient to report lightheadedness or signs and symptoms of hypoglycemia immediately.

☑ **Evaluation**
• Patient is free from infection.
• Patient sustains no injuries because of drug-induced adverse CNS reactions.
• Patient and family state understanding of drug therapy.

HIGH ALERT

pentazocine hydrochloride and acetaminophen
Talacen

pentazocine and naloxone hydrochlorides
Talwin NX

pentazocine lactate
Talwin

Pharmacologic class: opioid partial agonist, opioid agonist-antagonist
Therapeutic class: analgesic, adjunct to anesthesia
Pregnancy risk category: C
Controlled substance schedule: IV

Indications and dosages

▶ **Moderate to severe pain.** *Adults:* 50 to 100 mg Talwin NX P.O. every 3 to 4 hours, p.r.n. Maximum oral dose, 600 mg daily. Or, 1 tablet Talacen P.O. every 4 hours, up to 6 tablets daily. Or, 30 mg I.M., I.V., or subcutaneously every 3 to 4 hours, p.r.n. Maximum total parenteral dose is 360 mg in 24 hours. Single doses above 30 mg I.V. or 60 mg I.M. or subcutaneously aren't recommended.

▶ **Labor.** *Women:* 30 mg I.M. as a single dose or 20 mg I.V. every 2 to 3 hours when contractions become regular.

▼ I.V. administration

• Give drug by direct I.V. injection.
• Administer slowly.
⊗ **Incompatibilities**
Aminophylline, amobarbital, glycopyrrolate, heparin sodium, nafcillin sodium, pentobarbital sodium, phenobarbital sodium, sodium bicarbonate.

Contraindications and cautions

• Contraindicated in patients hypersensitive to the drug or any of its components.
• Use cautiously in patients with hepatic or renal disease, acute MI, head injury, increased intracranial pressure, or respiratory depression.
☆ **Lifespan:** In pregnant women, use cautiously. In breast-feeding women, use cautiously; it's unknown if the drug appears in breast milk. In children younger than age 12, drug isn't recommended. In the elderly, use cautiously because they may be more sensitive to the drug's CNS effects.

Adverse reactions

CNS: confusion, *dizziness,* drowsiness, *euphoria,* hallucinations, headache, *lightheadedness,* psychotomimetic effects, *sedation,* visual disturbances.
CV: flushing, hypertension, hypotension, *shock,* tachycardia.
EENT: dry mouth, dysgeusia.
GI: constipation, nausea, vomiting.
GU: urine retention.
Respiratory: *respiratory depression.*
Skin: diaphoresis, induration, nodules, pruritus, rash, sloughing, and sclerosis of injection site.
Other: hypersensitivity reactions *(anaphylaxis),* physical and psychological dependence.

Interactions

Drug-drug. *CNS depressants:* May have additive effects. Use together cautiously.
Fluoxetine: May cause diaphoresis, ataxia, flushing, and tremor suggestive of serotonin syndrome. Use together cautiously.
Opioid analgesics: May decrease analgesic effect. Avoid using together.
Drug-lifestyle. *Alcohol use:* May have additive effects. Discourage using together.

Smoking: May increase requirements for pentazocine. Monitor drug's effectiveness; urge patient to stop smoking.

Effects on lab test results

• May interfere with laboratory tests for urinary 17-hydroxycorticosteroids.

Pharmacokinetics

Absorption: Well absorbed after P.O. or parenteral use, although P.O. form undergoes first-pass metabolism in liver and less than 20% of dose reaches systemic circulation unchanged. Bioavailability is increased in patients with hepatic dysfunction; patients with cirrhosis absorb 60% to 70% of drug.
Distribution: Appears to be wide.
Metabolism: In liver; may be prolonged in patients with impaired hepatic function.
Excretion: Mainly in urine, with very small amounts in feces. *Half-life:* 2 to 3 hours.

Route	Onset	Peak	Duration
P.O.	15–30 min	60–90 min	2–3 hr
I.V.	2–3 min	15–30 min	2–3 hr
I.M., SubQ	15–20 min	15–60 min	4–6 hr

Action

Chemical effect: Binds with opiate receptors at many sites in CNS, altering pain response by unknown mechanism.
Therapeutic effect: Relieves pain.

Available forms

pentazocine hydrochloride and acetaminophen
Tablets: 25 mg pentazocine hydrochloride and 650 mg acetaminophen
pentazocine and naloxone hydrochlorides
Tablets: 50 mg pentazocine hydrochloride and 0.5 mg naloxone hydrochloride
pentazocine lactate
Injection: 30 mg/ml

NURSING PROCESS

📝 Assessment

• Assess patient's pain before and after giving the drug.
• Monitor vital signs closely, especially respirations.
• Be alert for adverse reactions and drug interactions.

- Assess patient's and family's knowledge of drug therapy.

✛ Nursing diagnoses
- Acute pain related to condition
- Ineffective breathing pattern related to drug-induced respiratory depression
- Deficient knowledge related to drug therapy

❯ Planning and implementation
- Talwin NX, the oral pentazocine available in the U.S., contains the opioid antagonist naloxone, which prevents illicit use.
- ⚕ **ALERT:** Talwin NX is for P.O. use only. Severe, potentially fatal reaction may occur if given by injection.
- When giving I.M. or subcutaneously, rotate injection sites to minimize tissue irritation. If possible, avoid giving subcutaneously.
- Drug has opioid antagonist properties. May precipitate withdrawal syndrome in an opioid-dependent patient.
- Dependence may occur with prolonged use.
- ⚕ **ALERT:** If respiratory rate drops significantly, hold drug and notify prescriber. Have naloxone readily available to reverse respiratory depression.

Patient teaching
- Warn ambulatory patient about getting out of bed or walking. Warn outpatient to avoid hazardous activities until the drug's CNS effects are known.
- Inform patient about the risk of dependence.

✅ Evaluation
- Patient is free from pain.
- Patient maintains respiratory rate and pattern within normal limits.
- Patient and family state understanding of drug therapy.

pentetate calcium trisodium (Ca-DTPA)
(PEN-tuh-tayt KAL-see-um try-SOE-dee-um)

pentetate zinc trisodium (Zn-DTPA)

Pharmacologic class: chelate
Therapeutic class: radiation emergency drug

Pregnancy risk category: C (Ca-DTPA); B (Zn-DTPA)

Indications and dosages

▶ **To increase the rate of plutonium, americium, or curium elimination in patients with internal contamination.** *Adults and children age 12 and older:* Initially, 1 g Ca-DTPA by slow I.V. push over 3 to 4 minutes (or dilute in 100 to 250 ml D_5W, Ringer's lactate, or normal saline solution and infuse over 30 minutes) within the first 24 hours of exposure. Then, 1 g once daily of Zn-DTPA by slow I.V. push over 3 to 4 minutes (or dilute in 100 to 250 ml D_5W, Ringer's lactate, or normal saline solution and infuse over 30 minutes) until radioactive substances are removed. If patient was exposed by inhalation, give solution by nebulizer at a ratio of 1:1 with sterile water or saline.
Children younger than age 12: Initially, 14 mg/kg Ca-DTPA (maximum dose, 1 g) by slow I.V. push over 3 to 4 minutes within the first 24 hours of exposure. Then, 14 mg/kg once daily of Zn-DTPA by slow I.V. push over 3 to 4 minutes (maximum dose, 1 g) until radioactive substances are removed.

▽ I.V. administration
- Use a sterile filter if particles appear after ampule is opened.
- Administer by slow I.V. push over 3 to 4 minutes or dilute in 100 to 250 ml of D_5W, lactated Ringer's solution, or normal saline solution and infuse over 30 minutes.
- Store at room temperature.
- ⊗ **Incompatibilities**
None reported.

Contraindications and cautions
- Use cautiously in patients with severe hemochromatosis. Use inhalation route cautiously in patients with asthma.
- ⚘ **Lifespan:** In pregnant women, start and continue with Zn-DTPA unless patient has a high level of internal radioactive contamination. If the level of contamination is high, start with a single dose of Ca-DTPA and vitamin or mineral supplements containing zinc. Breast-feeding women should stop breast-feeding or use a different drug; it's unknown if drug appears in breast milk, but radiocontaminants do. Patient shouldn't breast-feed during therapy and should take precautions when discarding breast milk. In

P

children, safety and effectiveness of inhaled form haven't been established.

Adverse reactions

CNS: headache, lightheadedness.
CV: chest pain.
GI: diarrhea, metallic taste, nausea.
Skin: dermatitis, injection site reactions.
Other: allergic reaction.

Interactions

None known.

Effects on lab test results

• May decrease manganese, magnesium, and zinc levels with prolonged therapy.

Pharmacokinetics

Absorption: Unknown, not in GI system, organs, erythrocytes; 20% in lungs with inhalational route.
Distribution: Rapid, throughout extracellular space after I.V. use.
Metabolism: Minimal.
Excretion: Almost exclusively in urine by glomerular filtration. *Half-life:* About 7 hours.

Route	Onset	Peak	Duration
I.V., inhalation	1½ min	Unknown	< 24 hr

Action

Chemical effect: Forms stable complexes with metal ions by exchanging calcium or zinc ions for radioactive plutonium, americium, or curium ions. The complexes are excreted into urine faster than the unbound radioactive contaminants, thus speeding removal from the body.
Therapeutic effect: Reduces the effects of exposure to radioactive plutonium, americium, or curium.

Available forms

Injection: 200 mg/ml in 5-ml single-use vials

NURSING PROCESS

Assessment

• Obtain history of patient's radiation exposure before therapy.
• Obtain baseline CBC, zinc, BUN, and electrolyte levels, urinalysis, and blood and urine radioassays before starting therapy.

• During therapy, measure the radioactivity of blood, urine, and feces weekly.
• Regularly monitor urinalysis, CBC, BUN, and electrolyte levels during therapy.
• Assess patient's and family's knowledge of drug therapy.

Nursing diagnoses

• Risk for injury related to internal radioactive contamination
• Ineffective protection related to drug-induced depletion of endogenous trace metals
• Deficient knowledge related to drug therapy

Planning and implementation

• The binding capacity of Ca-DTPA is greatest in the first 24 hours after exposure.
ALERT: If patient needs further therapy after Ca-DTPA, switch to Zn-DTPA to avoid mineral depletion. If Zn-DTPA isn't available, continue Ca-DTPA as long as the patient receives supplemental zinc, magnesium, and manganese.
• When the route of contamination is unknown or if contamination occurs by multiple routes, use I.V. drug.
• If contamination occurs only by inhalation and within 24 hours, use nebulizer. Dilute drug 1:1 with sterile water or saline solution.
• The elimination rate is based on the quantity of radioactivity taken in.

Patient teaching
• Instruct patient to drink plenty of fluids so he urinates often.
• Remind patient that drug eliminates radioactivity through urine, which may make urine highly radioactive and dangerous to others.
• Instruct patient to flush the toilet several times after each use and to wash hands thoroughly after urinating.
• If the patient is coughing, tell him to dispose of phlegm carefully and not to swallow it, if possible.
• Tell parents of a young child to dispose of dirty diapers properly and to avoid handling urine, feces, or phlegm.

Evaluation

• The effects of radiation contamination are reduced.
• Patient experiences minimal loss of trace metals or receives mineral supplements as appropriate.

Reactions may be *common*, uncommon, *life-threatening*, or COMMON AND LIFE-THREATENING.

- Patient and family state understanding of drug therapy.

pentobarbital (pentobarbitone)
(pen-toh-BAR-beh-tol)

pentobarbital sodium
Nembutal Sodium

Pharmacologic class: barbiturate
Therapeutic class: anticonvulsant, sedative-hypnotic
Pregnancy risk category: D
Controlled substance schedule: II (oral and parenteral); III (rectal)

Indications and dosages

▶ **Sedation.** *Adults:* 20 to 40 mg P.O. b.i.d., t.i.d., or q.i.d.
Children: 2 to 6 mg/kg daily P.O. or P.R. t.i.d. Maximum dose, 100 mg daily.
▶ **Short-term therapy for insomnia.** *Adults:* 100 to 200 mg P.O. at bedtime or 150 to 200 mg I.M. Or, 120 to 200 mg P.R. Or, initially, 100 mg I.V. with additional small doses, to a total of 500 mg.
Children: 2 to 6 mg/kg I.M. Maximum dose is 100 mg. Or, for children ages 2 months to 1 year, give 30 mg P.R.; for children ages 1 to 4 years, give 30 or 60 mg P.R.; for children ages 5 to 12 years, give 60 mg P.R.; for children ages 12 to 14 years, give 60 or 120 mg P.R.
▶ **Preoperative sedation.** *Adults:* 150 to 200 mg I.M.
Children: 5 mg/kg P.O. or I.M. In children younger than age 10, the dose is usually given rectally.

▽ I.V. administration

- I.V. use of barbiturates may cause severe respiratory depression, laryngospasm, or hypotension. Have emergency resuscitation equipment available.
- To minimize deterioration, use I.V. injection solution within 30 minutes after opening container. Don't use cloudy solution.
- Reserve I.V. injection for emergencies and give under close supervision. Give slowly (50 mg/minute or less).
- Parenteral solution is alkaline. Local tissue reactions and injection site pain may result. Moni-

tor site for irritation and infiltration; extravasation can lead to tissue damage and necrosis. Assess patency of I.V. site before and during administration.
⊗ **Incompatibilities**
Other I.V. drugs or solutions.

Contraindications and cautions

- Contraindicated in patients with porphyria or hypersensitivity to barbiturates.
- Use cautiously in debilitated patients and in those with acute or chronic pain, depression, suicidal tendencies, history of drug abuse, or renal or hepatic impairment.
- ⚖ **Lifespan:** In pregnant and breast-feeding women, drug isn't recommended. In the elderly, use cautiously because of possible delayed renal excretion.

Adverse reactions

CNS: *drowsiness, hangover, lethargy,* paradoxical excitement in elderly patients.
GI: nausea, vomiting.
Hematologic: worsening of porphyria.
Respiratory: *respiratory depression.*
Skin: rash, *Stevens-Johnson syndrome,* urticaria.
Other: *angioedema.*

Interactions

Drug-drug. *CNS depressants, including opioid analgesics:* May cause excessive CNS and respiratory depression. Use together cautiously.
Corticosteroids, doxycycline, estrogens and hormonal contraceptives, oral anticoagulants, quinidine, theophylline, verapamil: May enhance metabolism of these drugs. Monitor patient for decreased effect.
MAO inhibitors: May inhibit barbiturate metabolism and prolong CNS depression. Reduce barbiturate dosage.
Metoprolol, propranolol: May reduce the effects of these drugs. Increase beta blocker dosage.
Rifampin: May decrease barbiturate level. Monitor patient for decreased effect.
Drug-lifestyle. *Alcohol use:* May impair coordination, increase CNS effects, and cause death. Strongly discourage use together.

Effects on lab test results

None reported.

Pharmacokinetics

Absorption: Rapid after P.O. use. Unknown after I.M. use.
Distribution: Wide. About 35% to 45% protein-bound.
Metabolism: In liver.
Excretion: 99% in urine. *Half-life:* 35 to 50 hours.

Route	Onset	Peak	Duration
P.O.	≤ 15 min	30–60 min	1–4 hr
I.V.	Immediate	Immediate	15 min
I.M.	10–25 min	Unknown	Unknown

Action

Chemical effect: May interfere with transmission of impulses from thalamus to cortex of brain.
Therapeutic effect: Promotes sleep and calmness.

Available forms

Capsules: 50 mg, 100 mg
Elixir: 18.2 mg/5 ml
Injection: 50 mg/ml
Suppositories: 30 mg, 60 mg, 120 mg, 200 mg

NURSING PROCESS

⚕ Assessment
• Assess patient's condition before starting therapy and regularly thereafter to monitor drug's effectiveness.
• An elderly patient may be more sensitive to the drug's CNS effects.
• Inspect patient's skin. Skin eruptions may precede life-threatening reactions to barbiturate therapy.
• Be alert for adverse reactions and drug interactions.
• Assess patient's and family's knowledge of drug therapy.

⊕ Nursing diagnoses
• Sleep deprivation related to condition
• Risk for injury related to drug-induced adverse CNS reactions
• Deficient knowledge related to drug therapy

▷ Planning and implementation
• Give I.M. injection deep into muscle. Superficial injection may cause pain, sterile abscess, and sloughing.

⑤ **ALERT:** If skin reactions occur, stop drug and notify prescriber. In some patients, high fever, stomatitis, headache, or rhinitis may precede skin reactions.
• Drug has no analgesic effect and may cause restlessness or delirium in a patient with pain.
⑤ **ALERT:** Long-term use isn't recommended; drug loses its effectiveness in promoting sleep after 14 days of continued use. Long-term high doses may cause dependence and may lead to withdrawal symptoms if drug is suddenly stopped. Gradually stop giving barbiturates.
⑤ **ALERT:** Don't confuse pentobarbital with phenobarbital.

Patient teaching
• Warn patient about performing activities that require alertness or physical coordination. For an acute care inpatient, particularly an elderly patient, supervise walking and raise bed rails.
• Inform patient that morning hangover is common after hypnotic dose, which suppresses REM sleep. Patient's dreams may increase after therapy stops.
• Tell woman who uses hormonal contraceptives to use barrier-method birth control because drug may decrease contraceptive effect.

✓ Evaluation
• Patient reports satisfactory sleep.
• Patient sustains no injuries from drug-induced adverse CNS reactions.
• Patient and family state understanding of drug therapy.

pentoxifylline
(pen-tok-SIH-fi-lin)
Pentoxil, Trental

Pharmacologic class: xanthine derivative
Therapeutic class: hemorheologic
Pregnancy risk category: C

Indications and dosages

▶ **Intermittent claudication caused by chronic occlusive vascular disease.** *Adults:* 400 mg P.O. t.i.d. with meals for at least 8 weeks.

Contraindications and cautions

• Contraindicated in patients who are intolerant of methylxanthines, such as caffeine and the-

ophylline, and in those with recent cerebral or retinal hemorrhage.

☀ **Lifespan:** In pregnant women, use cautiously. In breast-feeding women, drug isn't recommended. In children, safety and effectiveness haven't been established.

Adverse reactions

CNS: dizziness, headache.
GI: dyspepsia, nausea, vomiting.

Interactions

Drug-drug. *Anticoagulants:* May increase anticoagulant effect. Monitor PT and INR, and adjust anticoagulant dosage as needed.
Antihypertensives: May increase hypotensive effect. Adjust dosage; monitor patient's blood pressure closely.
Theophylline: May increase theophylline level. Monitor level; adjust theophylline dosage.
Drug-lifestyle. *Smoking:* May cause vasoconstriction. Advise patient to avoid smoking because it may worsen his condition.

Effects on lab test results

None reported.

Pharmacokinetics

Absorption: Rapid and almost completely absorbed by the GI tract.
Distribution: Bound by erythrocyte membrane.
Metabolism: Extensively by erythrocytes and liver.
Excretion: Mainly in urine. *Half-life:* About 30 to 45 minutes.

Route	Onset	Peak	Duration
P.O.	Unknown	1 hr	Unknown

Action

Chemical effect: May increase RBC flexibility and lower blood viscosity.
Therapeutic effect: Improves capillary blood flow.

Available forms

Tablets (controlled-release): 400 mg
Tablets (extended-release): 400 mg

NURSING PROCESS

✍ Assessment
• Assess patient's condition before starting therapy and regularly thereafter to monitor drug's effectiveness.
• Be alert for adverse reactions and drug interactions.
• In patients with other risk factors complicated by hemorrhage (recent surgery, peptic ulceration), assess for bleeding, and obtain hemoglobin level and hematocrit.
• In an elderly patient, watch for increased CNS effects.
• If adverse GI reaction occurs, monitor patient's hydration.
• Assess patient's and family's knowledge of drug therapy.

Nursing diagnoses
• Ineffective peripheral tissue perfusion related to condition
• Risk for deficient fluid volume related to drug-induced adverse GI reactions
• Deficient knowledge related to drug therapy

Planning and implementation
• Drug is useful in patient who isn't a good surgical candidate.
• Report adverse reactions to prescriber; dosage may need to be lowered.
• Monitor blood pressure for hypotension, particularly in patients also on antihypertensive therapy.
⚠ **ALERT:** Don't confuse Trental with Trendar or Trandate.
Patient teaching
• Advise patient to take drug with meals to minimize GI upset.
• Instruct patient to swallow drug whole, without breaking, crushing, or chewing.
• Tell patient to report adverse GI or CNS reactions.
• Advise patient not to smoke because nicotine causes vasoconstriction that can worsen his condition.
• Advise patient that effects of drug may not be seen for 2 to 4 weeks.
• Tell patient not to stop taking the drug during first 8 weeks of therapy unless directed by prescriber.

☑ Evaluation
• Patient has adequate peripheral tissue perfusion.
• Patient maintains adequate hydration throughout therapy.
• Patient and family state understanding of drug therapy.

perphenazine
(per-FEN-uh-zeen)

Pharmacologic class: phenothiazine (piperazine derivative)
Therapeutic class: antiemetic, antipsychotic
Pregnancy risk category: C

Indications and dosages

▶ **Psychosis in nonhospitalized patients.**
Adults: Initially, 4 to 8 mg P.O. t.i.d. Reduce to minimum effective dosage as soon as possible.
Children older than age 12: Lowest adult dosage.

▶ **Psychosis in hospitalized patients.** *Adults:*
Initially, 8 to 16 mg P.O. b.i.d., t.i.d., or q.i.d., increase to 64 mg daily, as needed.
Children older than age 12: Lowest adult dosage.

▶ **Severe nausea and vomiting.** *Adults:* 8 to 16 mg P.O. daily in divided doses. Occasionally, 24 mg may be necessary.

Contraindications and cautions

• Contraindicated in patients hypersensitive to the drug or any of its components; in comatose patients; in patients with CNS depression, blood dyscrasia, bone marrow depression, liver damage, or subcortical damage; and in those taking large doses of CNS depressants and itraconazole.
• Use cautiously with other CNS depressants or anticholinergics. Also use cautiously in debilitated patients and patients with alcohol withdrawal, depression, suicidal tendency, severe adverse reactions to other phenothiazines, impaired renal function, or respiratory disorders.
• ☀ Lifespan: In pregnant women, use cautiously; a neonate whose mother uses drug during pregnancy may have prolonged jaundice, extrapyramidal signs, hyperreflexia or hyporeflexia. In breast-feeding women, drug appears in breast milk; avoid using unless the benefit outweighs the risk to the infant. In children age 12 and younger, safety and effectiveness haven't been established. In the elderly, use cautiously because of risk of increased effects.

Adverse reactions

CNS: dizziness, EEG changes, *extrapyramidal reaction*, **neuroleptic malignant syndrome,** pseudoparkinsonism, sedation, **seizures,** *tardive dyskinesia.*
CV: *cardiac arrest,* ECG changes, orthostatic hypotension, tachycardia.
EENT: blurred vision, ocular changes.
GI: constipation, dry mouth.
GU: dark urine, inhibited ejaculation, menstrual irregularities, *urine retention.*
Hematologic: *agranulocytosis, hemolytic anemia,* hyperprolactinemia, *thrombocytopenia, transient leukopenia.*
Hepatic: cholestatic jaundice.
Metabolic: increased appetite, weight gain.
Skin: *mild photosensitivity reaction,* sterile abscess.
Other: allergic reactions, gynecomastia.

Interactions

Drug-drug. *Antacids:* May inhibit oral phenothiazine absorption. Administer drugs separately.
Anticonvulsants: May lower the seizure threshold. Monitor patient.
Barbiturates: May decrease phenothiazine effect. Observe patient closely.
Bromocriptine: May decrease bromocriptine effectiveness. Monitor patient for effect.
CNS depressants: May increase CNS depression. Avoid using together.
Lithium: May cause severe neurological toxicity with encephalitis-like syndrome; decreased therapeutic response to perphenazine. Don't use together.
Drug-herb. *Dong quai, St. John's wort:* May increase photosensitivity. Discourage using together.
Evening primrose oil: May increase risk of seizures. Discourage using together.
Kava: May increase risk of dystonic reactions. Discourage using together.
Milk thistle: May decrease liver toxicity caused by phenothiazines. Monitor liver enzyme level.
Yohimbe: May increase risk of yohimbe toxicity. Discourage using together.

Reactions may be *common,* uncommon, *life-threatening*, or COMMON AND LIFE-THREATENING.

Drug-lifestyle. *Alcohol use:* May increase CNS depression, particularly psychomotor skills. Strongly discourage use together.
Sun exposure: May increase photosensitivity reaction. Urge patient to avoid unprotected or prolonged exposure to sunlight.

Effects on lab test results

• May increase prolactin level. May decrease hemoglobin level and hematocrit.
• May increase liver function test values and eosinophil count. May decrease WBC, granulocyte, and platelet counts.
• May produce false-positive phenylketonuria or pregnancy test results.

Pharmacokinetics

Absorption: Rate and extent vary. Erratic and variable for P.O. tablet; much more predictable for P.O. concentrate.
Distribution: Wide. 91% to 99% protein-bound.
Metabolism: Extensive in liver.
Excretion: Mainly in urine; some in feces.
Half-life: 9 to 12 hours.

Route	Onset	Peak	Duration
P.O.	Varies	1–3 hr	Unknown

Action

Chemical effect: Probably blocks postsynaptic dopamine receptors in brain and inhibits medullary chemoreceptor trigger zone.
Therapeutic effect: Relieves signs and symptoms of psychosis; also relieves nausea and vomiting.

Available forms

Oral concentrate: 16 mg/5 ml
Tablets: 2 mg, 4 mg, 8 mg, 16 mg

NURSING PROCESS

Assessment
• Assess patient's condition before starting therapy and regularly thereafter to monitor drug's effectiveness.
• Obtain baseline blood pressure before starting therapy, and monitor it regularly. Watch for orthostatic hypotension.
• Test bilirubin level weekly during first month, and obtain periodic blood tests (CBC and liver function) and ophthalmic tests (long-term use).

• Be alert for adverse reactions and drug interactions.
• Monitor patient for tardive dyskinesia, which may occur after prolonged use. It may not appear until months or years later and may disappear spontaneously or persist for life despite no longer using the drug.
• If drug is used for nausea and vomiting, monitor patient's hydration.
• Assess patient's and family's knowledge of drug therapy.

Nursing diagnoses
• Disturbed thought processes related to psychosis
• Risk for deficient fluid volume related to nausea or vomiting
• Deficient knowledge related to drug therapy

Planning and implementation
• Dilute with fruit juice, milk, carbonated beverage, or semisolid food just before giving.
• Concentrate causes turbidity or precipitation in colas, black coffee, grape or apple juice, or tea. Don't mix with them.
• Prevent contact dermatitis by keeping drug away from skin and clothes. Wear gloves when preparing liquid forms.
• Protect drug from light. Slight yellowing concentrate doesn't affect potency. Discard markedly discolored solutions.
ALERT: When given with amitriptyline for depression, there's increased risk for suicidal thinking and behavior in young adults ages 18 to 24 during the first 2 months of treatment. Monitor patient carefully.
• Don't abruptly stop giving the drug unless severe adverse reaction occurs. After abruptly stopping long-term therapy, patient may experience gastritis, nausea, vomiting, dizziness, tremors, feeling of warmth or cold, diaphoresis, tachycardia, headache, or insomnia.
• If patient develops jaundice, symptoms of blood dyscrasia (fever, sore throat, infection, cellulitis, weakness), or extrapyramidal reactions that last longer than a few hours, withhold dose and notify prescriber.
• Acute dystonic reactions may be treated with diphenhydramine.
ALERT: Don't confuse perphenazine with prochlorperazine.

P

Patient teaching
- Advise patient to change positions slowly to minimize orthostatic hypotension.
- Teach patient which fluids are appropriate for diluting concentrate.
- Warn patient to avoid hazardous activities until the drug's CNS effects are known. Drowsiness and dizziness usually subside after a few weeks.
- Tell patient to avoid alcohol during drug therapy.
- Advise patient to report urine retention or constipation.
- Tell patient to use sunblock and to wear protective clothing to avoid photosensitivity reactions.
- Tell patient to relieve dry mouth with sugarless gum or hard candy.

☑ **Evaluation**
- Patient's thought processes are normal.
- Patient maintains adequate hydration throughout drug therapy.
- Patient and family state understanding of drug therapy.

phenazopyridine hydrochloride (phenylazo diamino pyridine hydrochloride)
(fen-eh-soh-PEER-eh-deen high-droh-KLOR-ighd)
Azo-Dine, Azo-Gesic, Azo-Standard†, Baridium†, Geridium, Phenazo† ♦, Prodium†, Pyridiate, Pyridium, Pyridium Plus, Re-Azo†, Urogesic, UTI Relief

Pharmacologic class: azo dye
Therapeutic class: urinary analgesic
Pregnancy risk category: B

Indications and dosages
▶ **Relief of symptoms of urinary tract irritation or infection.** *Adults:* 200 mg P.O. t.i.d. *Children ages 6 to 12 years:* 12 mg/kg P.O. daily divided into three equal doses.

Contraindications and cautions
- Contraindicated in patients with glomerulonephritis, severe hepatitis, uremia, or renal insufficiency.
⚕ **Lifespan:** In pyelonephritis during pregnancy, drug is contraindicated. In breast-feeding

women, safety and effectiveness haven't been established. In children younger than age 12, don't use.

Adverse reactions
CNS: headache, vertigo.
EENT: staining of contact lenses.
GI: mild GI disturbance, nausea.
Skin: pruritus, rash.

Interactions
None significant.

Effects on lab test results
- May alter urine glucose results when Clinistix or Tes-Tape is used. May interfere with urinalysis based on spectrometry or color reactions.

Pharmacokinetics
Absorption: Unknown.
Distribution: Unknown.
Metabolism: In liver.
Excretion: 65% in urine unchanged. *Half-life:* Unknown.

Route	Onset	Peak	Duration
P.O.	Unknown	Unknown	Unknown

Action
Chemical effect: Unknown; has local anesthetic effect on urinary mucosa.
Therapeutic effect: Relieves urinary tract pain.

Available forms
Tablets: 95 mg†, 97.2 mg, 100 mg†, 200 mg

NURSING PROCESS

⚗ **Assessment**
- Assess patient's pain before and after giving drug.
- Be alert for adverse reactions.
- If nausea occurs, monitor patient's hydration.
- Assess patient's and family's knowledge of drug therapy.

✢ **Nursing diagnoses**
- Acute pain related to underlying urinary tract condition
- Risk for deficient fluid volume related to drug-induced nausea
- Deficient knowledge related to drug therapy

⬚ Planning and implementation
• Administer drug with food to minimize nausea.
⑤ **ALERT:** Don't confuse Pyridium with pyridoxine, pyrimethamine, or pyridine.
Patient teaching
• Advise patient that taking drug with meals may minimize nausea.
• Tell patient to stop taking drug and notify prescriber if skin or sclera becomes yellow-tinged.
• Warn patient that drug colors urine red or orange. Drug may stain fabrics and contact lenses.
• Tell patient to notify prescriber if urinary tract pain persists after 2 days and the patient isn't also taking an antibiotic. If using drug with an antibiotic, stop drug after 2 days because it has no additional effectiveness. Drug isn't for long-term use.

✅ Evaluation
• Patient is free from pain.
• Patient maintains adequate hydration.
• Patient and family state understanding of drug therapy.

HIGH ALERT

phenobarbital (phenobarbitone)
(feen-oh-BAR-bih-tol)
Solfoton

phenobarbital sodium (phenobarbitone sodium)
Luminal Sodium

Pharmacologic class: barbiturate
Therapeutic class: anticonvulsant, sedative-hypnotic
Pregnancy risk category: D
Controlled substance schedule: IV

Indications and dosages

▶ **All forms of epilepsy except absence seizures; febrile seizures in children.** *Adults:* 60 to 200 mg P.O. daily in divided doses. Or 100 mg to 320 mg slow I.V. injection to a maximum dose of 600 mg daily.
Children: Loading dose of 15 to 20 mg/kg P.O. followed by 3 to 6 mg/kg/day P.O. in divided doses or once daily, usually at bedtime.

▶ **Status epilepticus.** *Adults:* 200 to 600 mg by slow I.V. injection; may repeat in 6 hours, if needed.
Children: 15 to 20 mg/kg by slow I.V. injection.
▶ **Sedation.** *Adults:* 30 to 120 mg P.O. daily in two or three divided doses.
Children: 8 to 32 mg P.O. daily in divided doses t.i.d.
▶ **Insomnia.** *Adults:* 100 to 200 mg P.O. or I.M. at bedtime.
▶ **Preoperative sedation.** *Adults:* 100 to 200 mg I.M. 60 to 90 minutes before surgery.
Children: 1 to 3 mg/kg I.V. or I.M. 60 to 90 minutes before surgery.
▶ **Prevention and treatment of hyperbilirubinemia‡.** *Neonates:* 7 mg/kg P.O. daily from the 1st to 5th days after birth. Or, 5 mg/kg I.M. on day 1 and then 5 mg/kg P.O. on the 2nd through 7th days after birth.
▶ **To lower serum bilirubin or serum lipid levels in the treatment of chronic cholestasis‡.** *Adults:* 90 to 180 mg P.O. daily in two or three divided doses.
Children younger than age 12: Give 3 to 12 mg/kg P.O. daily in two to three divided doses.

▼ I.V. administration
• Injection is reserved for emergencies because patients respond differently.
• Have resuscitation equipment available.
• If injectable solution contains precipitate, don't use.
• Observe patient with status epilepticus for decrease of seizures; stop drug when convulsions cease.
• Don't give more than 60 mg/minute because respiratory depression may occur. Monitor respirations closely.
⊗ **Incompatibilities**
Acidic solutions, amphotericin B, chlorpromazine, cimetadine, clindamycin, dimenhydrinate, diphenhydramine, droperidol, ephedrine, hydralazine, hydrocortisone sodium succinate, hydromorphone, hydroxyzine, insulin, kanamycin, levorphanol, meperidine, morphine, norepinephrine, pancuronium, penicillin G, pentazocine lactate, phenytoin, procaine, prochlorperazine mesylate, promethazine hydrochloride, ranitidine hydrochloride, streptomycin, vancomycin.

P

Contraindications and cautions

• Contraindicated in patients hypersensitive to barbiturates and in those with hepatic dysfunction, respiratory disease with dyspnea or obstruction, nephritis, or a history of manifest or latent porphyria.
• Use cautiously in debilitated patients and in patients with acute or chronic pain, depression, suicidal tendencies, history of drug abuse, altered blood pressure, CV disease, shock, or uremia.

⚠ Lifespan: In pregnant and breast-feeding women, drug isn't recommended. In the elderly, use cautiously; drug may cause paradoxical excitement in these patients.

Adverse reactions

CNS: drowsiness, hangover, lethargy.
CV: *bradycardia,* hypotension, thrombophlebitis.
GI: nausea, vomiting.
Hematologic: exacerbation of porphyria.
Respiratory: *apnea, respiratory depression.*
Skin: *erythema multiforme,* rash, *Stevens-Johnson syndrome,* urticaria.
Other: *angioedema;* necrosis, nerve injury at injection site, pain, swelling.

Interactions

Drug-drug. *Carbamazepine, corticosteroids, digitoxin, doxorubicin, doxycycline, estrogens and hormonal contraceptives, oral anticoagulants, quinidine, theophylline, tricyclic antidepressants, verapamil:* May enhance metabolism of these drugs. Monitor for decreased effect.
Chloramphenicol, MAO inhibitors, valproic acid: May increase barbiturate effect. Monitor patient for increased CNS and respiratory depression.
CNS depressants, including opioid analgesics: May increase CNS depression. Use together cautiously.
Diazepam: May increase effects of both drugs. Use together cautiously.
Griseofulvin: May decrease griseofulvin absorption. Administer drug separately.
Mephobarbital, primidone: May increase phenobarbital level. Monitor patient closely.
Metoprolol, propranolol: May reduce the effects of these drugs. Increase beta blocker dosage.
Rifampin: May decrease barbiturate level. Monitor patient for decreased effect.

Drug-lifestyle. *Alcohol use:* May impair coordination, increase CNS effects, and cause death. Strongly discourage use together.

Effects on lab test results

• May decrease bilirubin level.

Pharmacokinetics

Absorption: Good after P.O. use. 100% from I.M. injection.
Distribution: Wide. About 20% to 60% protein-bound.
Metabolism: In liver.
Excretion: In urine. *Half-life:* 1½ to 5 days.

Route	Onset	Peak	Duration
P.O.	20–60 min	8–12 hr	10–12 hr
I.V.	5 min	15 min	10–20 hr
I.M.	> 60 min	Unknown	10–12 hr

Action

Chemical effect: Unknown; may depress CNS synaptic transmission and increase seizure activity threshold in motor cortex. As sedative, may interfere with transmission of impulses from thalamus to brain cortex.
Therapeutic effect: Prevents and stops seizure activity; promotes calmness and sleep.

Available forms

Capsules: 16 mg
Elixir*: 15 mg/5 ml, 20 mg/5 ml
Injection: 30 mg/ml, 60 mg/ml, 65 mg/ml, 130 mg/ml
Tablets: 15 mg, 16 mg, 30 mg, 60 mg, 90 mg, 100 mg

NURSING PROCESS

Assessment
• Assess patient's condition before starting therapy and regularly thereafter to monitor drug's effectiveness.
• Monitor drug level closely. Therapeutic level is 15 to 40 mcg/ml.
• Be alert for adverse reactions and drug interactions.
• Assess patient's and family's knowledge of drug therapy.

Nursing diagnoses
• Risk for trauma related to seizures

Reactions may be *common,* uncommon, *life-threatening*, or COMMON AND LIFE-THREATENING.

• Risk for injury related to drug-induced adverse CNS reactions
• Deficient knowledge related to drug therapy

> ### Planning and implementation
• Don't abruptly stop giving the drug; seizures may worsen. If adverse reaction occurs, immediately notify prescriber.
• Give drug by deep I.M. injection. Superficial injection may cause pain, sterile abscess, and tissue sloughing.
⑤ ALERT: Don't confuse phenobarbital with pentobarbital.

Patient teaching
• Tell patient that phenobarbital is available in different strengths and sizes. Advise him to check prescription and refills closely.
• Inform patient that full effects don't occur for 2 to 3 weeks except when loading dose is used.
• Advise patient to avoid hazardous activities until the drug's CNS effects are known.
• Warn patient and parents not to abruptly stop taking the drug.
• Tell patient using hormonal contraceptives to use barrier-method birth control.

✓ Evaluation
• Patient is free from seizure activity.
• Patient has no injury from drug-induced adverse CNS reactions.
• Patient and family state understanding of drug therapy.

phentermine hydrochloride
(FEN-ter-meen high-droh-KLOR-ighd)
Adipex-P, Ionamin, Pro-Fast HS, Pro-Fast SA, Pro-Fast SR

Pharmacologic class: indirect-acting sympathomimetic amine
Therapeutic class: anorexigenic
Pregnancy risk category: C
Controlled substance schedule: IV

Indications and dosages

▶ **Short-term monotherapy in exogenous obesity as an adjunct to exercise, behavioral modification, and caloric restriction.** *Adults:* 8 mg P.O. t.i.d. 30 minutes before meals. Or, 15 to 37.5 mg daily before breakfast or 10 to 14 hours before bedtime. Give Pro-Fast HS or Pro-Fast SR capsules 2 hours after breakfast. Give Adipex-P before breakfast or 1 to 2 hours after breakfast.

Contraindications and cautions

• Contraindicated in agitated patients, patients hypersensitive to sympathomimetic amines, patients who have idiosyncratic reactions to them, patients who have taken an MAO inhibitor within 14 days, and patients with hyperthyroidism, moderate to severe hypertension, advanced arteriosclerosis, symptomatic CV disease, or glaucoma.
• Use cautiously in patients with mild hypertension.
⚖ Lifespan: In pregnant and breast-feeding women, drug isn't recommended. Use in children younger than 16 years of age isn't recommended.

Adverse reactions

CNS: dizziness, dysphoria, euphoria, headache, insomnia, overstimulation.
CV: increased blood pressure, palpitations, *pulmonary hypertension,* tachycardia.
EENT: blurred vision, eye irritation, mydriasis.
GI: constipation, diarrhea, dry mouth, dysgeusia, other GI disturbances.
GU: impotence.
Skin: urticaria.
Other: altered libido.

Interactions

Drug-drug. *Acetazolamide, antacids, sodium bicarbonate:* May increase renal reabsorption. Monitor patient.
Ammonium chloride, ascorbic acid: May decrease level and increase renal excretion of phentermine. Monitor patient for decreased effects.
Furazolidone, MAO inhibitors: May cause severe hypertension and hypertensive crisis. Don't use within 14 days of an MAO inhibitor.
Guanethidine: May decrease hypotensive effect. Monitor blood pressure closely.
Haloperidol, phenothiazines, tricyclic antidepressants: May increase CNS effects. Avoid using together.
Insulin, oral antidiabetics: May alter antidiabetic requirements. Monitor glucose level.
SSRIs: May increase sensitivity to phentermine with risk of serotonin syndrome.

Drug-food. *Caffeine:* May increase CNS stimulation. Discourage using together.

Effects on lab test results

None reported.

Pharmacokinetics

Absorption: Absorbed readily from GI tract.
Distribution: Throughout body.
Metabolism: Unknown.
Excretion: In urine. *Half-life:* 19 to 24 hours.

Route	Onset	Peak	Duration
P.O.	Unknown	Unknown	12–14 hr

Action

Chemical effect: Unknown; probably works by releasing stored norepinephrine from nerve terminals in the brain (primarily in the cerebral cortex and reticular activating system), thus promoting nerve impulse transmission.
Therapeutic effect: Depresses appetite.

Available forms

Capsules: 15 mg, 18.75 mg, 30 mg, 37.5 mg
Capsules (extended-release): 15 mg, 30 mg
Tablets: 8 mg, 15 mg, 18.75 mg, 30 mg, 37.5 mg

NURSING PROCESS

Assessment
• Weigh patient before starting therapy and regularly thereafter to monitor drug's effectiveness.
• Be alert for adverse reactions and drug interactions.
• Monitor patient for habituation and tolerance.
• Assess patient's and family's knowledge of drug therapy.

Nursing diagnoses
• Imbalanced nutrition: more than body requirements related to food intake
• Sleep deprivation related to drug-induced insomnia
• Deficient knowledge related to drug therapy

Planning and implementation
• Give drug at least 6 hours before bedtime to avoid insomnia.
• Make sure patient is following a weight-reduction program.

⑤ ALERT: Don't confuse phentermine with phentolamine.

Patient teaching
• Instruct patient to take drug at least 6 hours before bedtime to avoid sleep interference.
• Warn patient to avoid hazardous activities until the drug's CNS effects are known.
• Instruct patient that drug is meant to suppress appetite while patient maintains a reducing diet and that he shouldn't use the drug for longer than 3 to 4 weeks.
• Tell patient to avoid caffeine because it increases the effects of amphetamines and related amines.
• Tell patient to report signs of excessive stimulation.
• Inform patient that fatigue may result as drug effects wear off.

Evaluation
• Patient loses weight.
• Patient doesn't have insomnia.
• Patient and family state understanding of drug therapy.

HIGH ALERT

phenylephrine hydrochloride
(fen-il-EF-rin high-droh-KLOR-ighd)
Neo-Synephrine

Pharmacologic class: adrenergic
Therapeutic class: vasoconstrictor
Pregnancy risk category: C

Indications and dosages

▶ **Hypotensive emergencies during spinal anesthesia.** *Adults:* Initially, 0.1 to 0.2 mg I.V., followed by 0.1 to 0.2 mg, p.r.n.
▶ **Maintenance of blood pressure during spinal or inhalation anesthesia.** *Adults:* 2 to 3 mg subcutaneously or I.M. 3 or 4 minutes before anesthesia.
Children: 0.044 to 0.088 mg/kg subcutaneously or I.M.
▶ **Prolongation of spinal anesthesia.** *Adults:* 2 to 5 mg added to anesthetic solution.
▶ **Vasoconstrictor for regional anesthesia.** *Adults:* 1 mg phenylephrine added to 20 ml local anesthetic.
▶ **Mild to moderate hypotension.** *Adults:* 2 to 5 mg subcutaneously or I.M.; repeated in 1 to 2 hours as needed and tolerated. Maximum first

dose, 5 mg. Or, 0.1 to 0.5 mg slow I.V., no more than every 10 to 15 minutes.
Children: 0.1 mg/kg I.M. or subcutaneously; repeated in 1 to 2 hours as needed and tolerated.
▶ **Severe hypotension and shock (including drug-induced).** *Adults:* 0.1 to 0.18 mg/minute I.V. infusion. After blood pressure stabilizes, maintain at 0.04 to 0.06 mg/minute and adjust to patient response.
▶ **Paroxysmal supraventricular tachycardia.** *Adults:* Initially, 0.5 mg rapid I.V. Increase later doses by 0.1 to 0.2 mg. Maximum dose, 1 mg.

▽ I.V. administration

• For direct injection, dilute 10 mg (1 ml) with 9 ml sterile water for injection to provide solution containing 1 mg/ml.
• Prepare I.V. infusions by adding 10 mg of drug to 500 ml of D_5W or normal saline solution for injection.
• Initial infusion rate is usually 100 to 180 mcg/minute; maintenance rate is usually 40 to 60 mcg/minute.
• Use central venous catheter or large vein, as in antecubital fossa, to minimize risk of extravasation.
• Use continuous infusion pump to regulate flow rate.
• During infusion, frequently monitor ECG, blood pressure, cardiac output, central venous pressure, pulmonary capillary wedge pressure, pulse rate, urine output, and color and temperature of limbs. Titrate infusion rate according to findings and prescriber's guidelines.
• To treat extravasation, infiltrate site promptly with 10 to 15 ml of normal saline solution for injection that contains 5 to 10 mg phentolamine. Use a fine needle.
• After prolonged I.V. infusion, avoid abrupt withdrawal.
• Store at room temperature and protect from light.
⊗ **Incompatibilities**
Alkaline solutions, butacaine sulfate, iron salts, other metals, phenytoin sodium, thiopental sodium.

Contraindications and cautions

• Contraindicated in patients hypersensitive to the drug or any of its components, and in patients with severe hypertension or ventricular tachycardia.

• Use cautiously in patients with heart disease, hyperthyroidism, severe atherosclerosis, bradycardia, partial heart block, myocardial disease, or sulfite sensitivity.
• Correct blood volume depletion before using phenylephrine.
✹ **Lifespan:** In pregnant women, use cautiously. In breast-feeding women, use cautiously; it's unknown if the drug appears in breast milk. In the elderly, use cautiously.

Adverse reactions

CNS: *headache, lightheadedness, restlessness, weakness.*
CV: angina, ***arrhythmias, bradycardia,*** decreased cardiac output, hypertension, palpitations.
EENT: blurred vision.
GI: vomiting.
Respiratory: *asthma attacks.*
Skin: feeling of coolness, pilomotor response.
Other: ***anaphylaxis,*** *decreased organ perfusion with prolonged use,* tachyphylaxis, tissue sloughing with extravasation.

Interactions

Drug-drug. *Alpha blockers, phenothiazines:* May decrease vasopressor response. Monitor patient closely.
Bretylium: May increase risk of arrhythmias. Monitor ECG.
Guanethidine, oxytocics: May increase pressor response and cause severe, persistent hypertension. Monitor patient and blood pressure closely.
Halogenated hydrocarbon anesthetics: May lead to serious arrhythmias. Use with caution.
MAO inhibitors: May potentiate cardiac and pressor effects. Avoid use together.
Phenelzine, tranylcypromine: May cause severe headache, hypertension, fever, and hypertensive crisis. Avoid using together.
Tricyclic antidepressants: May increase the pressor response and cause arrhythmias. Use cautiously.

Effects on lab test results

None reported.

Pharmacokinetics

Absorption: Unknown.
Distribution: Rapid into peripheral tissue.
Metabolism: In liver and intestine.

Excretion: Mainly in urine. *Half-life:* 2 to 3 hours.

Route	Onset	Peak	Duration
I.V.	Immediate	Unknown	15–20 min
I.M.	10–15 min	Unknown	½–2 hr
SubQ	10–15 min	Unknown	50–60 min

Action

Chemical effect: Mainly stimulates alpha-adrenergic receptors in sympathetic nervous system.
Therapeutic effect: Raises blood pressure and stops paroxysmal supraventricular tachycardia.

Available forms

Injection: 10 mg/ml (1%)

NURSING PROCESS

⚡ Assessment
• Assess patient's condition before starting therapy and regularly thereafter to monitor drug's effectiveness.
• Monitor blood pressure often; avoid severe increase.
• Monitor ECG throughout therapy.
• Be alert for adverse reactions and drug interactions.
• Assess patient's and family's knowledge of drug therapy.

⊕ Nursing diagnoses
• Ineffective tissue perfusion (cerebral, cardiopulmonary, peripheral, GI, renal) related to underlying condition
• Decreased cardiac output related to drug-induced adverse reaction
• Deficient knowledge related to drug therapy

▷ Planning and implementation
• Maintain blood pressure slightly below patient's normal level. In previously normotensive patient, maintain systolic pressure at 80 to 100 mm Hg; in previously hypertensive patient, maintain systolic pressure at 30 to 40 mm Hg below usual level.
Patient teaching
• Tell patient to immediately report discomfort at infusion site.

☑ Evaluation
• Patient maintains tissue perfusion and cellular oxygenation.
• Patient maintains adequate cardiac output.
• Patient and family state understanding of drug therapy.

phenytoin (diphenylhydantoin)
(FEN-uh-toyn)
Dilantin-125, Dilantin Infatabs

phenytoin sodium (extended)
Dilantin Kapseals✦, Phenytek

phenytoin sodium (prompt)
Dilantin

Pharmacologic class: hydantoin derivative
Therapeutic class: anticonvulsant
Pregnancy risk category: D

Indications and dosages

▶ **Control of tonic-clonic (grand mal) and complex partial (temporal lobe) seizures.**
Adults: Highly individualized. Initially, 100 mg P.O. t.i.d. Increase in increments of 100 mg P.O. every 2 to 4 weeks until desired response is obtained. Usual range is 300 to 600 mg daily. If patient is stabilized with extended-release capsules, may give once-daily dose with 300-mg extended-release capsules.
Children: 5 mg/kg or 250 mg/m² P.O. extended-release capsules divided b.i.d. or t.i.d. Maximum daily dose is 300 mg.
▶ **For patient requiring a loading dose.**
Adults: Initially, 1 g P.O. daily divided into three doses and administered at 2-hour intervals. Or, 10 to 15 mg/kg I.V. at a rate not exceeding 50 mg/minute. Normal maintenance dose is started 24 hours later with frequent level determinations.
Children: Initially, 5 mg/kg P.O. daily in two or three equally divided doses with subsequent dose individualized to maximum of 300 mg daily. Usual dose is 4 to 8 mg/kg P.O. daily. Children older than age 6 may require the minimum adult dosage (300 mg daily).
▶ **To prevent and treat seizures during neurosurgery.** *Adults:* 100 to 200 mg I.M or I.V. every 4 hours during surgery and continued in the immediate postoperative period.

Reactions may be *common*, uncommon, *life-threatening*, or COMMON AND LIFE-THREATENING.

▶ **Status epilepticus.** *Adults:* Loading dose of 10 to 15 mg/kg I.V. (1 to 1.5 g may be needed) at a rate not exceeding 50 mg/minute; then maintenance dosage of 100 mg P.O. or I.V. every 6 to 8 hours.
Children: Loading dose of 15 to 20 mg/kg I.V., at a rate not exceeding 1 to 3 mg/kg/minute; then highly individualized maintenance dosages.

▶ **Alternative to magnesium sulfate for severe preeclampsia‡.** *Women:* 15 mg/kg I.V. given as 10 mg/kg initially and 5 mg/kg 2 hours later.

▶ **Cardiac glycoside–induced arrhythmias‡.** *Adults:* 100 mg I.V. every 5 minutes to a total of 1 g. Or, oral dose of 200 to 400 mg/day P.O.

◩ **Adjust-a-dose:** Elderly patients may need lower doses.

▽ I.V. administration

• Check patency of I.V. catheter before giving drug. Extravasation may cause severe local tissue damage.
• Never use cloudy solution.
• Avoid giving phenytoin by I.V. push into veins on back of hand to avoid discoloration known as purple glove syndrome. Inject into larger veins or central venous catheter.
• Give drug slowly (50 mg/minute) as an I.V. bolus.
• If giving as infusion, don't mix drug with D_5W because it will precipitate. Clear I.V. tubing first with normal saline solution. May mix with normal saline solution if needed and infuse over 30 to 60 minutes when possible.
• Infusion must begin within 1 hour after preparation and run through in-line filter.
• Discard 4 hours after preparation.

⊗ **Incompatibilities**
Amikacin, aminophylline, amphotericin B, bretylium, cephapirin, ciprofloxacin, D_5W, diltiazem, dobutamine, enalaprilat, fat emulsions, hydromorphone, insulin (regular), levorphanol, lidocaine, lincomycin, meperidine, morphine sulfate, nitroglycerin, norepinephrine, other I.V. drugs or infusion solutions, pentobarbital sodium, potassium chloride, procaine, propofol, streptomycin, sufentanil citrate, theophylline, vitamin B complex with C.

Contraindications and cautions

• Contraindicated in patients hypersensitive to hydantoin. I.V. use is contraindicated in patients with sinus bradycardia, SA block, second- or third-degree AV block, or Adams-Stokes syndrome.
• Use cautiously in debilitated patients, patients taking other hydantoin derivatives, and patients with hepatic dysfunction, hypotension, myocardial insufficiency, diabetes, or respiratory depression.
• Don't stop drug in pregnant women using the drug to prevent major seizures. An increase in seizure activity may occur in pregnant woman due to changes in drug absorption or metabolism, so monitor level carefully.

⚘ **Lifespan:** In pregnant women, drug isn't recommended; infants born to mothers taking phenytoin may have bleeding defects. Give vitamin K to the mother 1 month before and during delivery and to the neonate immediately after birth. In breast-feeding women, drug isn't recommended. In the elderly, use cautiously; they tend to metabolize drug slowly and may need lower doses.

Adverse reactions

CNS: *ataxia, confusion,* dizziness, headache, insomnia, nervousness, *slurred speech,* twitching.
CV: hypotension.
EENT: blurred vision, diplopia, gingival hyperplasia, nystagmus.
GI: nausea, vomiting.
Hematologic: *agranulocytosis,* anemia, *leukopenia,* macrocythemia, megaloblastic lymphadenopathy, *pancytopenia, thrombocytopenia.*
Hepatic: *toxic hepatitis.*
Metabolic: hyperglycemia.
Musculoskeletal: osteomalacia.
Skin: bullous, exfoliative, or purpuric dermatitis; *hirsutism;* hypertrichosis; photosensitivity reaction; scarlatiniform or morbilliform rash; *Stevens-Johnson syndrome; toxic epidermal necrolysis.*
Other: lupus erythematosus; pain, necrosis, or inflammation at injection site; periarteritis nodosa.

Interactions

Drug-drug. *Amiodarone, allopurinol, antihistamines, chloramphenicol, cimetidine, clonazepam, cycloserine, diazepam, disulfiram, fluconazole, ibuprofen, influenza vaccine, isoniazid, metronidazole, omeprazole, phenylbutazone, phenothiazines, salicylates, sulfamethizole, tri-*

P

cyclic antidepressants, valproate: May increase therapeutic effects of phenytoin. Monitor patient for toxicity.

Antacids, carbamazepine, dexamethasone, diazoxide, folic acid, phenobarbital, rifampin, theophylline: May decrease phenytoin activity. Monitor patient closely.

Atracurium, cisatracurium, doxacurium, mivacurium, pancuronium, rocuronium, vecuronium: May decrease the effects of nondepolarizing muscle relaxant causing it to be less effective. May need to increase the dosage of the nondepolarizing muscle relaxant.

Lithium: May increase toxicity. Monitor lithium level.

Meperidine: May increase toxic effects of meperidine while decreasing analgesic effect. Monitor patient for decreased effect and toxicity.

Warfarin: May displace warfarin. Monitor patient for bleeding complications.

Drug-herb. *Milk thistle:* May decrease risk of liver toxicity. Monitor patient.

Drug-food. *Enteral nutrition therapy:* May reduce orally administered phenytoin concentrations. Consider giving phenytoin 2 hours before starting enteral feeding, or wait 2 hours after stopping enteral feeding to administer phenytoin.

Drug-lifestyle. *Alcohol use:* May decrease phenytoin activity. Discourage using together.

Effects on lab test results

• May increase alkaline phosphatase, GGT, and glucose levels. May decrease protein-bound iodine, free thyroxine, urinary 17-hydroxysteroid, 17-ketosteroid, and hemoglobin levels and hematocrit.
• May increase urine 6-hydroxycortisol excretion. May decrease platelet, WBC, RBC, and granulocyte counts.
• May decrease dexamethasone suppression and metyrapone test values.

Pharmacokinetics

Absorption: Slow after P.O. use. Formulation-dependent; bioavailability may differ among products. Erratic from I.M. site.
Distribution: Wide throughout body. About 90% protein-bound.
Metabolism: In liver.
Excretion: In urine, with dose-dependent (zero-order) elimination kinetics. Above certain

dosage level, small increases in dose disproportionately increase level. *Half-life:* Varies with dose and concentration changes.

Route	Onset	Peak	Duration
P.O.	Unknown	½–2 hr	Unknown
P.O. extended-release	Unknown	4–12 hr	Unknown
I.V.	Immediate	1–2 hr	Unknown
I.M.	Unknown	Unknown	Unknown

Action

Chemical effect: Unknown; probably limits seizure activity by either increasing efflux or decreasing influx of sodium ions across cell membranes in motor cortex during generation of nerve impulses.
Therapeutic effect: Prevents and stops seizure activity.

Available forms

phenytoin
Oral suspension: 125 mg/5 ml
Tablets (chewable): 50 mg
phenytoin sodium (extended)
Capsules: 30 mg (27.6-mg base), 100 mg (92-mg base), 200 mg (184-mg base), 300 mg (276-mg base)
phenytoin sodium (prompt)
Capsules: 100 mg (92-mg base)
Injection: 50 mg/ml (46-mg base)

NURSING PROCESS

Assessment
• Assess patient's condition before starting therapy and regularly thereafter to monitor drug's effectiveness.
• Monitor phenytoin level; therapeutic level is 10 to 20 mcg/ml.
• Monitor CBC and calcium level every 6 months, and periodically monitor hepatic function.
• Check vital signs, blood pressure, and ECG during I.V. administration.
• Be alert for adverse reactions and drug interactions.
• Mononucleosis may decrease phenytoin level. Monitor patient for increased seizure activity.
• Assess patient's and family's knowledge of drug therapy.

✛ Nursing diagnoses

• Risk for trauma related to seizures
• Impaired oral mucous membrane related to gingival hyperplasia
• Deficient knowledge related to drug therapy

▷ Planning and implementation

• Use only clear or slightly yellow solution for injection. Don't refrigerate.
• Divided doses given with or after meals may decrease adverse GI reactions.
• Dilantin capsule is only P.O. form that can be given once daily. If any other brand or form is given once daily, toxic level may result.
• Don't give drug I.M. unless dosage adjustments are made. Drug may precipitate at site, cause pain, and be erratically absorbed.
• If rash appears, stop giving the drug. If rash is scarlatiniform or morbilliform, drug may be resumed after rash clears. If rash reappears, stop giving the drug. If rash is exfoliative, purpuric, or bullous, don't resume.
• Don't abruptly stop giving the drug; seizures may worsen. If adverse reaction occurs, immediately notify prescriber.
• If patient has megaloblastic anemia, prescriber may order folic acid and vitamin B_{12}.
⑬ **ALERT:** Don't confuse phenytoin with Mephyton or fosphenytoin.
⑬ **ALERT:** Don't confuse Dilantin with Dilaudid.

Patient teaching
• Advise patient to avoid hazardous activities until the drug's CNS effects are known.
• Advise patient not to change brand, dose, or form.
• Warn patient and parents not to abruptly stop taking the drug.
• Promote oral hygiene and regular dental examinations. Gingivectomy may be needed periodically if dental hygiene is poor.
• Inform patient that drug may color urine pink, red, or red-brown.
• Tell patient that heavy alcohol use may diminish drug's benefits.

✓ Evaluation

• Patient is free from seizure activity.
• Patient expresses importance of good oral hygiene and regular dental examinations.
• Patient and family state understanding of drug therapy.

physostigmine salicylate (eserine salicylate)
(fiz-oh-STIG-meen sa-LIS-il-ayt)
Antilirium

Pharmacologic class: cholinesterase inhibitor
Therapeutic class: antimuscarinic antidote
Pregnancy risk category: C

Indications and dosages

▶ **To reverse CNS toxicity caused by anticholinergics.** *Adults:* 0.5 to 2 mg I.M. or slow I.V. injection (1 mg/minute or slower). If coma, seizures, or arrhythmias recur, dose may be repeated.
Children: 0.02 mg/kg I.M. or slow I.V. injection (0.5 mg/minute or slower). Repeat every 5 to 10 minutes until patient responds. Maximum dose, 2 mg. Drug is only for life-threatening situations.

▽ I.V. administration

• Use only clear solution. Darkening of solution may indicate loss of potency.
• Give drug I.V. at controlled rate; use direct injection at no more than 1 mg/minute. Rapid administration may cause bradycardia and hypersalivation, leading to respiratory difficulties and seizures.
⊗ **Incompatibilities**
None reported.

Contraindications and cautions

• Contraindicated in patients taking choline esters or depolarizing neuromuscular blockers and in patients with mechanical obstruction of intestine or urogenital tract, asthma, gangrene, diabetes, CV disease, or vagotonia.
• Use cautiously in patients with sensitivity or allergy to sulfites.
☀ **Lifespan:** In pregnant women, use cautiously. In breast-feeding women, safety and effectiveness haven't been established. In children, use only in life-threatening situations.

Adverse reactions

CNS: ataxia, *excitability,* hallucinations, muscle twitching, muscle weakness, *restlessness, seizures, sweating.*
CV: *bradycardia,* hypotension, irregular pulse, palpitations.

P

EENT: miosis.
GI: *diarrhea,* epigastric pain, *excessive salivation,* nausea, vomiting.
GU: urinary urgency.
Respiratory: bronchial constriction, ***bronchospasm,*** dyspnea.

Interactions

Drug-drug. *Anticholinergics, atropine, procainamide, quinidine:* May reverse cholinergic effects. Observe patient for lack of drug effect.
Drug-herb. *Jaborandi tree, pill-bearing spurge:* May have additive effects and increase risk of toxicity. Discourage using together.

Effects on lab test results

None reported.

Pharmacokinetics

Absorption: Absorbed well from injection site.
Distribution: Wide, including across blood-brain barrier.
Metabolism: Cholinesterase hydrolyzes physostigmine relatively quickly.
Excretion: Primary mode unknown; small amount excreted in urine. *Half-life:* 1 to 2 hours.

Route	Onset	Peak	Duration
I.V.	3–5 min	≤ 5 min	30–60 min
I.M.	3–5 min	20–30 min	30–60 min

Action

Chemical effect: Inhibits destruction of acetylcholine released from parasympathetic and somatic efferent nerves. Acetylcholine accumulates, promoting increased stimulation of receptor.
Therapeutic effect: Reverses anticholinergic signs and symptoms.

Available forms

Injection: 1 mg/ml

NURSING PROCESS

Assessment
• Assess patient's condition before starting therapy and regularly thereafter. Effect is often immediate and dramatic, but may be transient and require repeated doses.
• Monitor vital signs often, especially respirations.
• Be alert for adverse reactions and drug interactions.

• Assess patient's and family's knowledge of drug therapy.

Nursing diagnoses
• Ineffective health maintenance related to underlying condition
• Risk for injury related to drug-induced adverse CNS reactions
• Deficient knowledge related to drug therapy

Planning and implementation
• Position patient to ease breathing. If hypersensitivity or cholinergic crisis occurs, have atropine injection readily available and give 0.5 mg subcutaneously or slow I.V. push. Provide respiratory support p.r.n. Best administered in presence of prescriber.
• If patient becomes restless or hallucinates, raise side rails of bed. Adverse reaction may indicate drug toxicity. Notify prescriber.
• If patient has excessive salivation or emesis, frequent urination, or diarrhea, stop the drug.
• If patient has excessive sweating or nausea, lower dose.
Patient teaching
• Tell patient to report adverse reactions, especially pain at the I.V. site.

Evaluation
• Patient responds well to therapy.
• Patient doesn't experience injury from adverse CNS reactions.
• Patient and family state understanding of drug therapy.

phytonadione (vitamin K₁)

(figh-toh-neh-DIGH-ohn)
Mephyton

Pharmacologic class: synthetic analogue of vitamin K
Therapeutic class: blood coagulation modifier
Pregnancy risk category: C

Indications and dosages

▶ **RDA.** *Infants age 6 months and younger:* 5 mcg.
Infants ages 6 months to 1 year: 10 mcg.
Children ages 1 to 3: Give 15 mcg.
Children ages 4 to 6: Give 20 mcg.
Children ages 7 to 10: Give 30 mcg.

Children ages 11 to 14: Give 45 mcg.
Adolescent males ages 15 to 18: Give 65 mcg.
Men ages 19 to 24: Give 70 mcg.
Men age 25 and older: Give 80 mcg.
Adolescent females ages 15 to 18: Give 55 mcg.
Women ages 19 to 24: Give 60 mcg.
Women age 25 and older, and pregnant or breast-feeding women: Give 65 mcg.

▶ **Hypoprothrombinemia secondary to vitamin K malabsorption, drug therapy, or excessive vitamin A.** *Adults:* Depending on severity, 2.5 to 25 mg P.O., subcutaneously, or I.M.; repeat and increase up to 50 mg, if needed.

▶ **Hypoprothrombinemia secondary to effect of oral anticoagulants.** *Adults:* 2.5 to 10 mg P.O., subcutaneously, or I.M. based on PT; repeat if needed within 12 to 48 hours after P.O. dose or within 6 to 8 hours after parenteral dose.

▶ **To prevent hemorrhagic disease of newborns.** *Neonates:* 0.5 to 1 mg I.M. or subcutaneously within 1 hour after birth.

▶ **Hemorrhagic disease of newborns.** *Neonates:* 1 mg subcutaneously or I.M. based on laboratory tests. Higher doses may be needed if mother has been taking oral anticoagulants.

▼ I.V. administration

⑤ **ALERT:** Severe reactions, including fatalities, may occur with I.V. injection. Use I.V. route only if other routes aren't available and when benefits outweigh serious risks.

• Dilute drug with normal saline solution for injection, D₅W, or 5% dextrose in normal saline solution for injection.
• Protect parenteral products from light. Wrap infusion container with aluminum foil.
⊗ **Incompatibilities**
Dobutamine, phenytoin sodium, ranitidine.

Contraindications and cautions

• Contraindicated in patients hypersensitive to the drug or any of its components.
☙ **Lifespan:** In pregnant women, use cautiously. In breast-feeding women, use cautiously; it's unknown if the drug appears in breast milk. In neonates, use cautiously and don't exceed recommended dosage.

Adverse reactions

CNS: dizziness, seizurelike movements.
CV: cardiac irregularities, flushing, rapid and weak pulse, transient hypotension after I.V. administration.

Skin: diaphoresis, erythema.
Other: *anaphylaxis and anaphylactoid reactions* (usually after rapid I.V. administration); cramplike pain; pain, swelling, and hematoma at injection site.

Interactions

Drug-drug. *Anticoagulants:* May cause temporary resistance to prothrombin-depressing anticoagulants, especially when larger doses of phytonadione are used. Monitor patient closely.
Cholestyramine resin, mineral oil: May inhibit GI absorption of oral vitamin K. Administer separately.

Effects on lab test results

• May decrease PT and INR.

Pharmacokinetics

Absorption: Requires bile salts for GI absorption after P.O. use. Unknown after I.M. or subcutaneous use.
Distribution: Concentrates briefly in liver.
Metabolism: Rapid, in liver.
Excretion: Unclear. *Half-life:* Unknown.

Route	Onset	Peak	Duration
P.O.	6–12 hr	Unknown	12–14 hr
I.V., I.M., SubQ	1–2 hr	Unknown	12–14 hr

Action

Chemical effect: An antihemorrhagic factor that promotes hepatic formation of active prothrombin.
Therapeutic effect: Controls abnormal bleeding.

Available forms

Injection (aqueous colloidal solution): 2 mg/ml, 10 mg/ml
Tablets: 5 mg

NURSING PROCESS

⟅ Assessment

• Assess patient's condition before starting therapy and regularly thereafter to monitor drug's effectiveness.
• Monitor PT to determine dosage effectiveness.
• Failure to respond to vitamin K may indicate coagulation defects.

- Be alert for adverse reactions and drug interactions.
- If adverse GI reactions occur, monitor patient's hydration.
- Assess patient's and family's knowledge of drug therapy.

🌐 Nursing diagnoses
- Ineffective protection related to underlying vitamin K deficiency
- Risk for deficient fluid volume related to adverse GI reactions
- Deficient knowledge related to drug therapy

▷ Planning and implementation
- Check brand name labels for administration route restrictions.
- Subcutaneous is the preferred route of administration.
- Give drug I.M. in upper outer quadrant of buttocks in an adult; inject in infant's outer thigh.
- If severe bleeding occurs, don't delay other therapy, such as fresh frozen plasma or whole blood.
- Does not counteract the anticoagulant effects of heparin or low–molecular-weight heparin.

Patient teaching
- Explain drug's purpose.
- Instruct patient to report adverse reactions.

☑ Evaluation
- Patient achieves normal PT level with drug therapy.
- Patient maintains adequate hydration throughout drug therapy.
- Patient and family state understanding of drug therapy.

pimecrolimus
(py-meck-roh-LY-muhs)
Elidel

Pharmacologic class: topical immunomodulator
Therapeutic class: topical skin product
Pregnancy risk category: C

Indications and dosages
▶ **Short-term and intermittent long-term therapy for mild to moderate atopic dermatitis in nonimmunocompromised patients for** whom the use of alternative, conventional therapies is deemed inadvisable or for patients who aren't adequately responding to or are intolerant of conventional therapies.
Adults and children age 2 and older: Apply a thin layer to the affected skin b.i.d. and rub in gently and completely.

Contraindications and cautions
- Contraindicated in patients hypersensitive to the drug or any of the cream's components.
- Don't use on areas of active cutaneous viral infections or infected atopic dermatitis.
- Not recommended for use in patients with Netherton syndrome or in immunocompromised patients.
- Use cautiously in patients with varicella zoster virus infection, herpes simplex virus infection, or eczema herpeticum.
- ⚖ **Lifespan:** In pregnant women, safety and effectiveness haven't been established. Breast-feeding women should stop breast-feeding or use another drug. In children younger than age 2, drug isn't recommended. In patients age 65 and older, safety and effectiveness haven't been established.

Adverse reactions
CNS: *headache.*
EENT: conjunctivitis, earache, epistaxis, eye infection, nasal congestion, *nasopharyngitis,* otitis media, pharyngitis, rhinitis, rhinorrhea, sinus congestion, sinusitis.
GI: abdominal pain, constipation, diarrhea, gastroenteritis, loose stools, nausea, sore throat, tonsillitis, toothache, vomiting.
GU: dysmenorrhea.
Musculoskeletal: arthralgias, back pain.
Respiratory: asthma, *bronchitis,* cough, dyspnea, *pneumonia, upper respiratory tract infections,* wheezing.
Skin: acne, folliculitis, impetigo, molluscum contagiosum, skin infections, skin papilloma, urticaria, varicella.
Other: *application site reaction* (burning, irritation, erythema, pruritus), bacterial infection, flu-like illness, herpes simplex, hypersensitivity reaction, *influenza, pyrexia,* staphylococcal infection, viral infection.

Interactions
Drug-drug. *CYP3A family of inhibitors (erythromycin, itraconazole, ketoconazole, flucona-*

zole, calcium channel blockers): May have an effect on metabolism of pimecrolimus. Use together cautiously.

Drug-lifestyle. *Natural or artificial sunlight:* Drug may shorten the time to skin tumor formation. Avoid or minimize exposure to sunlight.

Effects on lab test results

None reported.

Pharmacokinetics

Absorption: Low systemic absorption.
Distribution: 74% to 87% protein-bound.
Metabolism: No evidence of skin-mediated drug metabolism exists.
Excretion: After a single oral radiolabeled dose, about 81% of radioactivity can be recovered, mainly in feces (78.4%), as metabolites. Less than 1% of radioactivity in feces is from unchanged drug. *Half-life:* Unknown.

Route	Onset	Peak	Duration
Topical	Unknown	Unknown	Unknown

Action

Chemical effect: Unknown. May inhibit T cell activation by blocking the transcription of early cytokines. May also prevent the release of inflammatory cytokines and mediators from mast cells in vitro after stimulation by antigen/immunoglobulin E.
Therapeutic effect: Improves skin integrity.

Available forms

Cream: 1% in tubes of 30 g, 60 g and 100 g (Base contains the following alcohols: benzyl alcohol, cetyl alcohol, oleyl alcohol, and stearyl alcohol.)

NURSING PROCESS

☑ Assessment

• Assess underlying skin condition before starting therapy and regularly thereafter to monitor drug's effectiveness. Clear up infections at disease sites before use.
• Assess patient's and family's knowledge of drug therapy.

⊕ Nursing diagnoses

• Risk for situational low self-esteem related to skin disorder

• Impaired skin integrity related to underlying skin condition
• Deficient knowledge related to pimecrolimus therapy

▶ Planning and implementation

• May be used on all skin surfaces, including the head, neck, and intertriginous areas.
• Use only after other treatments have failed because of risk of cancer with its use.
• If disease resolves, stop giving the drug.
• If symptoms persist beyond 6 weeks, reevaluate patient.
⏱ **ALERT:** Don't use with occlusive dressing; this may promote systemic exposure.
• May cause local symptoms such as skin burning. Most local reactions start within 1 to 5 days, are mild to moderately severe, and last no longer than 5 days.
• Monitor patient for lymphadenopathy. If the cause isn't clear or the patient has acute infectious mononucleosis, consider stopping drug.
• Papillomas or warts may occur. If skin papillomas worsen or don't respond to conventional therapy, consider stopping drug.

Patient teaching
• Instruct patient to use as directed; this drug is for external use on the skin only. Tell patient to report any signs or symptoms of adverse reactions.
• Tell patient not to use drug with an occlusive dressing.
• Instruct patient to wash hands after application if hands aren't being treated.
• Tell patient to stop using the drug after signs and symptoms of atopic dermatitis have resolved. Tell patient to contact prescriber if symptoms persist beyond 6 weeks.
• Advise patient to resume therapy at the first signs or symptoms of recurrence.
• Instruct patient to minimize or avoid exposure to natural or artificial sunlight (including tanning beds and ultraviolet A and B therapy) while using this drug.
• Tell patient that application site reactions are expected, but to notify prescriber if reaction is severe or persists for longer than 1 week.

☑ Evaluation

• Patient has improved self-esteem as skin condition clears.

• Patient has improved skin condition.
• Patient and family state understanding of drug therapy.

HIGH ALERT

pioglitazone hydrochloride
(pigh-oh-GLIH-tah-zohn high-droh-KLOR-ighd)
Actos

Pharmacologic class: thiazolidinedione
Therapeutic class: antidiabetic
Pregnancy risk category: C

Indications and dosages

▶ **Monotherapy adjunct to diet and exercise to improve glycemic control in patients with type 2 diabetes mellitus, or combination therapy with a sulfonylurea, metformin, or insulin when diet, exercise, and the single drug don't yield adequate glycemic control.** *Adults:* Initially, 15 or 30 mg P.O. once daily. For patients who respond inadequately to initial dose, increase in increments; maximum daily dose is 45 mg. If used in combination therapy, don't exceed 30 mg daily.

Contraindications and cautions

• Contraindicated in patients hypersensitive to the drug or any of its components. Not recommended for New York Heart Association Class III and IV cardiac patients.
• Also contraindicated in patients with type 1 diabetes mellitus or diabetic ketoacidosis, patients with evidence of active liver disease, patients with ALT level more than 2½ times the upper limit of normal, and patients who experienced jaundice while taking troglitazone.
• There is an increased risk for fractures in females receiving long-term treatment.
⚖ **Lifespan:** In pregnant women, use only if benefits outweigh risks to the fetus; insulin is the preferred antidiabetic for use during pregnancy. Potentially excreted in breast milk. Avoid use if breast-feeding. Safety has not been established in children younger than 18.

Adverse reactions

CNS: headache.
CV: edema, *heart failure.*
EENT: pharyngitis, sinusitis.
Hematologic: anemia.

Metabolic: *aggravated diabetes mellitus, hypoglycemia with combination therapy,* weight gain.
Musculoskeletal: myalgia.
Respiratory: upper respiratory tract infection.
Other: tooth disorder.

Interactions

Drug-drug. *Atorvastatin, midazolam, nifedipine:* May reduce levels of these drugs. Monitor patient.
Hormonal contraceptives: May reduce level of hormonal contraceptives, resulting in less effective contraception. Advise patients taking pioglitazone and hormonal contraceptives to consider additional birth control measures.
Ketoconazole and other CYP3A4 inhibitors: May inhibit pioglitazone metabolism. Monitor patient's glucose level more frequently.
Drug-herb. *Aloe, bilberry leaf, bitter melon, burdock, dandelion, fenugreek, garlic, ginseng:* May improve blood glucose control and allow reduction of antidiabetic dosage. Advise patient to discuss herbal remedies with prescriber before using them.

Effects on lab test results

• May increase liver enzyme and HDL levels. May decrease glucose, triglyceride, and hemoglobin levels and hematocrit.

Pharmacokinetics

Absorption: On an empty stomach, rapidly absorbed and measurable in serum within 30 minutes; level peaks within 2 hours. Food slightly delays time to peak level (3 to 4 hours), but doesn't affect overall extent of absorption.
Distribution: Drug and its metabolites are more than 98% protein-bound, mainly to albumin.
Metabolism: Extensive, by the liver. Three metabolites, M-II, M-III, and M-IV, are pharmacologically active.
Excretion: About 15% to 30% of dose is recovered in urine, mainly as metabolites and their conjugates. Most of P.O. dose is excreted in bile and eliminated in feces. *Half-life:* 3 to 7 hours.

Route	Onset	Peak	Duration
P.O.	Unknown	< 2 hr	Unknown

Action

Chemical effect: Decreases insulin resistance in the periphery and in the liver, resulting in decreased glucose output by the liver.
Therapeutic effect: Lowers glucose level.

Available forms

Tablets: 15 mg, 30 mg, 45 mg

NURSING PROCESS

Assessment
• Obtain history of patient's underlying condition before starting therapy and regularly thereafter to monitor drug's effectiveness.
• Assess patient for excessive fluid volume. Monitor patient with heart failure for increased edema.
• Measure liver enzymes at start of therapy, every 2 months for the first year of therapy, and periodically thereafter. Obtain liver function test results in patients who develop evidence of liver dysfunction, such as nausea, vomiting, abdominal pain, fatigue, anorexia, or dark urine.
• Monitor hemoglobin level and hematocrit, especially during the first 4 to 12 weeks of therapy.
• Monitor glucose level regularly, especially during situations of increased stress, such as infection, fever, surgery, and trauma.
• Check glycosylated hemoglobin level periodically to evaluate therapeutic response to drug.
• Assess patient's and family's knowledge of drug therapy.

Nursing diagnoses
• Ineffective health maintenance related to hyperglycemia
• Risk for injury related to drug-induced hyperglycemia
• Deficient knowledge related to drug therapy

Planning and implementation
ALERT: Monitor patient for signs and symptoms of heart failure. If signs and symptoms occur, reconsider thiazolidinedione therapy. Drug shouldn't be used in patients with severe heart failure or those who have limited mobility or are confined to bed.
• If patient develops jaundice or if results of liver function tests show ALT elevations greater than three times the upper limit of normal, notify prescriber and stop giving the drug.

• Watch for hypoglycemia in patients taking pioglitazone with insulin or a sulfonylurea. Dosage adjustments of these drugs may be needed.
• Premenopausal, anovulatory women with insulin resistance may need contraception because ovulation may resume.

Patient teaching
• Tell patient to control his diet in order to manage type 2 diabetes because calorie restrictions, weight loss, and exercise improve insulin sensitivity and make drug therapy more effective.
• Instruct patient to adhere to dietary instructions and to have glucose and glycosylated hemoglobin level tested regularly.
• Inform patient taking drug with insulin or an oral antidiabetic about the signs and symptoms of hypoglycemia.
• Tell patient to notify prescriber about periods of stress, such as fever, trauma, infection, or surgery, because drug requirements may change.
• Inform patient that blood tests for liver function will be performed before the start of therapy, every 2 months for the first year, and periodically thereafter.
• Tell patient to report unexplained nausea, vomiting, abdominal pain, fatigue, anorexia, or dark urine immediately because these signs and symptoms may indicate liver problems.
• Advise patient to contact prescriber if he has signs or symptoms of heart failure (unusually rapid increase in weight or edema, shortness of breath).
• Inform patient that pioglitazone can be taken with or without meals.
• If patient misses a dose, warn against doubling the dose the following day.
• Advise premenopausal, anovulatory woman with insulin resistance that drug may restore ovulation; recommend that she consider contraception as needed.

Evaluation
• Patient's glucose level is normal with drug therapy.
• Patient doesn't experience hypoglycemia.
• Patient and family state understanding of drug therapy.

piperacillin sodium and tazobactam sodium

(pigh-PER-uh-sil-in SOH-dee-um and taz-oh-BAK-tem SOH-dee-um)
Zosyn

Pharmacologic class: beta-lactamase inhibitor, extended-spectrum penicillin
Therapeutic class: antibiotic
Pregnancy risk category: B

Indications and dosages

▶ **Moderate to severe infections caused by piperacillin-resistant, piperacillin and tazobactam–susceptible, beta-lactamase–producing strains of microorganisms in the following conditions: appendicitis (complicated by rupture or abscess) and peritonitis caused by** *Escherichia coli, Bacteroides fragilis, Bacteroides ovatus, Bacteroides thetaiotaomicron, Bacteroides vulgatus;* **skin and skin-structure infections caused by** *Staphylococcus aureus;* **postpartum endometritis or pelvic inflammatory disease caused by** *E. coli;* **moderately severe community-acquired pneumonia caused by** *Haemophilus influenzae. Adults:* 3.375 g (3 g piperacillin and 0.375 g tazobactam) every 6 hours as a 30-minute I.V. infusion for 7 to 10 days.
🔲 **Adjust-a-dose:** For patients with renal impairment, if creatinine clearance is 20 to 40 ml/minute, give 2.25 g (2 g piperacillin and 0.25 g tazobactam) every 6 hours; if clearance is less than 20 ml/minute, give same dose every 8 hours.

In patients undergoing continuous ambulatory peritoneal dialysis (CAPD), give same dose every 12 hours. In hemodialysis patients, give same dose every 12 hours with a supplemental dose of 0.75 g (0.67 g piperacillin and 0.08 g tazobactam) after each dialysis period.
▶ **Moderate to severe nosocomial pneumonia caused by piperacillin-resistant, beta-lactamase–producing strains of** *S. aureus* **and by piperacillin and tazobactam–susceptible** *Acinetobacter baumannii, H. influenzae, Klebsiella pneumoniae,* **and** *Pseudomonas aeruginosa. Adults:* 4.5 g (4 g piperacillin and 0.5 g tazobactam) every 6 hours given with an aminoglycoside for 7 to 14 days. For patients with *P. aeruginosa,* continue aminoglycoside therapy; if

P. aeruginosa isn't isolated, may stop aminoglycoside therapy.
🔲 **Adjust-a-dose:** For patients with renal impairment, if creatinine clearance is 20 to 40 ml/minute, give 3.375 g (3 g piperacillin and 0.375 g tazobactam) every 6 hours; if clearance is less than 20 ml/minute, give 2.25 g (2 g piperacillin and 0.25 g tazobactam) every 6 hours. In CAPD patients, give 2.25 g (2 g piperacillin and 0.25 g tazobactam) every 8 hours.

▼ I.V. administration

● Reconstitute each gram of drug with 5 ml of diluent, such as sterile or bacteriostatic water for injection, normal saline solution for injection, bacteriostatic normal saline solution for injection, D₅W, 5% dextrose in normal saline solution for injection, or dextran 6% in normal saline solution for injection. Shake until dissolved. Further dilute to final volume of 50 ml before infusion.
● Infuse drug over at least 30 minutes. Stop other primary infusions during administration if possible. Aminoglycoside antibiotics (such as gentamicin and tobramycin) are chemically incompatible with drug. Don't mix in same I.V. container.
● Use drug immediately after reconstitution. Discard unused drug in single-dose vials after 24 hours if held at room temperature; after 48 hours if refrigerated. Diluted drug is stable in I.V. bags for 24 hours at room temperature or 1 week if refrigerated.
● Change I.V. site every 48 hours.
⊗ **Incompatibilities**
Acyclovir sodium, aminoglycosides, amphotericin B, chlorpromazine, cisatracurium, cisplatin, dacarbazine, daunorubicin, dobutamine, doxorubicin, doxycycline hyclate, droperidol, famotidine, ganciclovir, gemcitabine, haloperidol lactate, hydroxyzine hydrochloride, idarubicin, lactated Ringer's solution, minocycline, mitomycin, mitoxantrone, nalbuphine, prochlorperazine edisylate, promethazine hydrochloride, streptozocin, vancomycin.

Contraindications and cautions

● Contraindicated in patients hypersensitive to the drug or other penicillins.
● Use cautiously in patients with other drug allergies, especially to cephalosporins (risk of

cross-sensitivity), and in those with bleeding tendencies, uremia, or hypokalemia.

☙ **Lifespan:** In pregnant women, use cautiously. In breast-feeding women, use cautiously; it's unknown if the drug appears in breast milk. In children younger than age 12, safety and effectiveness haven't been established.

Adverse reactions

CNS: agitation, anxiety, dizziness, fever, *headache, insomnia,* pain.
CV: chest pain, edema, hypertension, tachycardia.
EENT: rhinitis.
GI: abdominal pain, *constipation, diarrhea,* dyspepsia, *nausea,* stool changes, vomiting.
Hematologic: *thrombocytopenia.*
Respiratory: dyspnea.
Skin: pruritus, rash (including bullous, eczematoid, maculopapular, and urticarial).
Other: *anaphylaxis,* candidiasis, inflammation and phlebitis at I.V. site.

Interactions

Drug-drug. *Anticoagulants:* May increase risk of bleeding. Monitor PT, PTT, and INR, and monitor patient for bleeding.
Hormonal contraceptives: May decrease effectiveness of hormonal contraceptives. Advise alternative barrier method during therapy.
Probenecid: May increase level of piperacillin. Probenecid may be used for this purpose.
Vecuronium: May prolong neuromuscular blockage. Monitor patient closely.

Effects on lab test results

• May increase AST, ALT, alkaline phosphatase, bilirubin, BUN, and creatinine levels. May decrease hemoglobin level and hematocrit. May increase or decrease sodium, potassium and calcium levels.
• May increase PT, PTT, and eosinophil count. May decrease WBC and platelet counts.

Pharmacokinetics

Absorption: Given I.V.
Distribution: Both drugs are about 30% protein-bound.
Metabolism: Piperacillin is metabolized to a minor, microbiologically active desethyl metabolite. Tazobactam is metabolized to a single metabolite that lacks pharmacologic and antibacterial activities.

Excretion: In urine and bile. *Half-life:* Piperacillin, 40 minutes; tazobactam, 70 minutes.

Route	Onset	Peak	Duration
I.V.	Immediate	Immediate	Unknown

Action

Chemical effect: Piperacillin inhibits cell wall synthesis during microorganism multiplication; tazobactam increases piperacillin effectiveness by inactivating beta-lactamases, which destroy penicillins.
Therapeutic effect: Kills susceptible bacteria.

Available forms

Powder for injection: 2 g piperacillin and 0.25 g tazobactam per vial, 3 g piperacillin and 0.375 g tazobactam per vial, 4 g piperacillin and 0.5 g tazobactam per vial

NURSING PROCESS

🕮 Assessment
• Before giving drug, ask patient about previous allergic reactions to this drug or other penicillins. Negative history of penicillin allergy doesn't guarantee future safety.
• Assess patient's infection before starting therapy and regularly thereafter to monitor drug's effectiveness.
• Obtain specimen for culture and sensitivity tests before first dose. Start therapy pending test results.
• Be alert for adverse reactions and drug interactions. If adverse GI reaction occurs, monitor patient's hydration.
• Assess patient's and family's knowledge of drug therapy.

🕮 Nursing diagnoses
• Risk for infection related to presence of bacteria
• Risk of deficient fluid volume related to adverse GI reactions
• Deficient knowledge related to drug therapy

▶ Planning and implementation
• Because hemodialysis removes 6% of piperacillin dose and 21% of tazobactam dose, supplemental doses may be needed after hemodialysis.
Patient teaching
• Tell patient to report pain or discomfort at I.V. site.

P

• Advise patient to limit salt intake while taking drug because piperacillin contains 1.98 mEq of sodium per gram.
• Tell patient to report adverse reactions.

☑ **Evaluation**
• Patient is free from infection.
• Patient maintains adequate hydration.
• Patient and family state understanding of drug therapy.

polyethylene glycol and electrolyte solution
(pol-ee-ETH-ih-leen GLIGH-kohl and ee-LEK-troh-light soh-LOO-shun)
CoLyte, GoLYTELY, MoviPrep, NuLYTELY, OCL, TriLyte

Pharmacologic class: polyethylene glycol (PEG) 3350 nonabsorbable solution
Therapeutic class: laxative and bowel evacuant
Pregnancy risk category: C

Indications and dosages

▶ **Bowel preparation before GI examination.**
Adults: 240 ml P.O. every 10 minutes until 4 L are consumed. Typically, give 4 hours before examination, allowing 3 hours for drinking and 1 hour for bowel evacuation.
▶ **Management of acute iron overdose‡.**
Children older than age 3: Give 2,953 ml/kg over 5 days.

Contraindications and cautions

• Contraindicated in patients with GI obstruction or perforation, gastric retention, toxic colitis, or megacolon.
🜲 **Lifespan:** In pregnant women, use cautiously. In breast-feeding women, use cautiously; it's unknown if the drug appears in breast milk.

Adverse reactions

GI: bloating, cramps, nausea, vomiting.

Interactions

Drug-drug. *Oral drugs:* May decrease absorption if given within 1 hour of starting therapy. Don't give with other oral drugs.

Effects on lab test results
None reported.

Pharmacokinetics
Absorption: None.
Distribution: Not applicable; drug isn't absorbed.
Metabolism: Not applicable; drug isn't absorbed.
Excretion: In GI tract. *Half-life:* None.

Route	Onset	Peak	Duration
P.O.	≤ 1 hr	Varies	Varies

Action

Chemical effect: Acts as an osmotic agent. Sodium sulfate greatly reduces sodium absorption. The electrolyte concentration causes virtually no net absorption or secretion of ions.
Therapeutic effect: Cleanses bowel.

Available forms

Oral solution: PEG 3350 (6 g), sodium sulfate decahydrate (1.29 g), sodium chloride (146 mg), potassium chloride (75 mg), sodium bicarbonate (168 mg), polysorbate 80 (30 mg) per 100 ml (OCL)
Powder for oral solution: PEG 3350 (240 g), sodium sulfate (22.72 g), sodium chloride (5.84 g), potassium chloride (2.98 g), sodium bicarbonate (6.72 g) per 4 L (CoLyte); PEG 3350 (236 g), sodium sulfate (22.74 g), sodium bicarbonate (6.74 g), sodium chloride (5.86 g), potassium chloride (2.97 g) per 4 L (GoLYTELY); PEG 3350 (420 g), sodium bicarbonate (5.72 g), sodium chloride (11.2 g), potassium chloride (1.48 g) per 4 L (NuLYTELY); PEG 3350 (100 g), sodium sulfate (7.5 g), sodium chloride (2.691 g), potassium chloride (1.015 g) per 1 L (MoviPrep)

NURSING PROCESS

Assessment
• Assess patient's condition before starting therapy and regularly thereafter to monitor drug's effectiveness.
• Be alert for adverse reactions and drug interactions.
• Assess patient's and family's knowledge of drug therapy.

🖼 Nursing diagnoses

• Health-seeking behavior (testing) related to need to determine cause of underlying GI problem
• Risk for deficient fluid volume related to adverse GI reactions
• Deficient knowledge related to drug therapy

▷ Planning and implementation

• Use tap water to reconstitute powder. Shake vigorously to make sure all powder is dissolved. Refrigerate solution but use within 48 hours.
• **ALERT:** Don't add flavoring or additional ingredients to solution or administer chilled solution. Hypothermia has developed after ingestion of large amounts of chilled solution.
• If patient is scheduled for midmorning examination, give solution early in morning. Oral solution induces diarrhea in 30 to 60 minutes that rapidly cleans bowel, usually within 4 hours.
• When used as preparation for barium enema, give solution the evening before examination, to avoid interfering with barium coating of colonic mucosa.
• If giving to adult via NG tube infuse at 20 to 30 ml/minute.
• If given to semiconscious patient or to patient with impaired gag reflex, take care to prevent aspiration.
• No major shifts in fluid or electrolyte balance have been reported.
Patient teaching
• Tell patient to fast for 4 hours before taking solution and to ingest only clear fluids until examination is complete.
• Warn patient about adverse GI reactions to drug.
• Advise patient that rapid drinking of each portion is preferred to drinking small amounts continuously.

☑ Evaluation

• Patient is able to have examination.
• Patient maintains adequate fluid volume.
• Patient and family state understanding of drug therapy.

posaconazole
(poss-uh-KAHN-uh-zohl)
Noxafil

Pharmacologic class: triazole antifungal
Therapeutic class: anti-infective
Pregnancy risk category: C

Indications and dosages

▶ **Prevention of invasive *Aspergillus* and *Candida* infections in high-risk immuno-compromised patients.** *Adults and children age 13 and older:* 200 mg (5 ml) P.O. t.i.d. with a full meal or liquid nutritional supplement.

Contraindications and cautions

• Contraindicated in patients hypersensitive to drug or its components and in patients taking astemizole, cisapride, ergot derivatives, pimozide, quinidine, or terfenadine.
• Use cautiously in patients hypersensitive to other azole antifungals, patients with potentially proarrhythmic conditions, and patients with hepatic or renal insufficiency.
⚕ **Lifespan:** Use drug in pregnant or breast-feeding women only if the benefits outweigh the risks. Use not indicated in children younger than age 13.

Adverse reactions

CNS: *anxiety, dizziness, fatigue, fever, headache, insomnia, weakness.*
CV: *edema, hypertension, hypotension, tachycardia.*
EENT: altered taste, blurred vision, epistaxis, *pharyngitis.*
GI: *abdominal pain, constipation, diarrhea, dyspepsia, mucositis, nausea, vomiting.*
GU: *vaginal hemorrhage.*
Hematologic: *anemia,* FEBRILE NEUTROPENIA, NEUTROPENIA, *petechiae,* THROMBOCYTOPENIA.
Hepatic: *bilirubinemia.*
Metabolic: *hyperglycemia,* hypocalcemia, *hypokalemia,* **hypomagnesemia.**
Musculoskeletal: *arthralgia, back pain, pain.*
Respiratory: *cough, dyspnea,* upper respiratory tract infection.
Other: *anorexia, bacteremia, cytomegalovirus infection, herpes simplex, rigors.*

Interactions

Drug-drug. *Calcium channel blockers, cyclosporine, HMG-CoA reductase inhibitors, midazolam, phenytoin, sirolimus, tacrolimus, vinca alkaloids:* May increase levels of these drugs. Reduce doses, increase monitoring of levels, and observe patient for adverse effects.
Cimetidine, phenytoin: May decrease level and effectiveness of posaconazole. Avoid use together.
Rifabutin: May decrease level and efficacy of posaconazole while increasing rifabutin level and risk of toxicity. Avoid use together. If unavoidable, monitor patient for uveitis, leukopenia, and other adverse effects.
Drug-food. *Food, liquid nutritional supplements:* May greatly enhance absorption of drug. Always give drug with liquid supplement or food.

Effects on lab test results

• May increase AST, ALT, bilirubin, creatinine, alkaline phosphatase, and glucose levels. May decrease potassium, magnesium, and calcium levels.
• May decrease WBC, RBC, and platelet counts.

Pharmacokinetics

Absorption: Greatly improved when drug is taken with food or a nutritional supplement.
Distribution: Extensive into extravascular space and body tissues. More than 98% protein-bound, mainly to albumin.
Metabolism: Via the liver by glucuronidation.
Excretion: Mainly in feces, and much less in urine. *Half-life:* 35 hours.

Route	Onset	Peak	Duration
P.O.	Unknown	3–5 hr	Unknown

Action

Chemical effect: Drug blocks the synthesis of ergosterol, a vital component of the fungal cell membrane.
Therapeutic effect: Protects high-risk patients from *Aspergillus* and *Candida* infections.

Available forms

Oral suspension: 40 mg/ml

NURSING PROCESS

⚗ Assessment

• Assess patient for fungal infection before starting therapy, and reassess regularly.
• Correct electrolyte imbalances, especially potassium, magnesium, and calcium imbalances, before therapy starts.
• Be alert for adverse reactions and drug interactions.
• If adverse GI reactions occur, monitor patient's hydration.
• Assess patient's and family's knowledge of drug therapy.

⊕ Nursing diagnoses

• Risk for infection related to immunosuppression
• Risk for deficient fluid volume related to adverse GI reactions
• Deficient knowledge related to drug therapy

❯ Planning and implementation

• Obtain baseline liver function tests, including bilirubin level, before therapy starts and periodically during treatment. Notify prescriber if patient develops signs or symptoms of hepatic dysfunction.
• Monitor patient for signs and symptoms of electrolyte imbalance including a slow, weak or irregular pulse; ECG change; nausea; neuromuscular irritability; and tetany.
• Give drug with a full meal or a liquid nutritional supplement.
• Monitor patient who has severe vomiting or diarrhea for breakthrough fungal infection.
Patient teaching
• If patient can't eat or take a liquid supplement, instruct him to notify prescriber. A different anti-infective may be needed, or monitoring may need to be increased.
• Tell patient to notify prescriber about an irregular heartbeat, fainting, or severe diarrhea or vomiting.
• Explain the signs and symptoms of liver dysfunction, including abdominal pain, yellowing skin or eyes, pale stools, and dark urine.
• Urge patient to contact the prescriber or pharmacist before taking other prescription or OTC drugs, and herbal or dietary supplements.
• Tell patient to shake the suspension well before taking it.

Reactions may be *common*, uncommon, *life-threatening*, or COMMON AND LIFE-THREATENING.

• Instruct patient to measure doses using the spoon provided with the drug. Household spoons vary in size and may yield an incorrect dose.
• Point out that the calibrated spoon has two markings, one for 2.5 ml and one for 5 ml. Make sure patient understands which mark to use for his prescribed dose.
• To ensure a full dose, tell patient to fill the spoon with water and drink it after taking a dose. Urge him to clean the spoon with water before putting it away.
• Tell patient to store oral solution at room temperature.

☑ Evaluation
• Patient remains free from infection.
• Patient maintains adequate hydration.
• Patient and family state understanding of drug therapy.

potassium acetate
(poh-TAS-ee-um AS-ih-tayt)

Pharmacologic class: potassium supplement
Therapeutic class: electrolyte
Pregnancy risk category: C

Indications and dosages

▶ **Hypokalemia.** *Adults:* For potassium level above 2.5 mEq/L, no more than 10 mEq I.V. hourly at a concentration of 40 mEq/L or less. Maximum daily dose is 200 mEq. For potassium level less than 2 mEq/L, no more than 40 mEq I.V. hourly at a concentration of 80 mEq/L or less. Maximum daily dose is 400 mEq. Monitor ECG and perform frequent potassium tests with potassium replacement. Use I.V. route only for life-threatening hypokalemia or when oral replacement isn't feasible.
▶ **To prevent hypokalemia.** *Adults:* Dose is individualized to patient's needs, not to exceed 150 mEq daily. Give as an additive to I.V. infusions. Usual dose is 20 mEq/L infused at no more than 20 mEq/hour.
Children: Individualized dose not to exceed 3 mEq/kg daily. Give as an additive to I.V. infusions.

▼ I.V. administration
• Give drug only by I.V. infusion, never by I.V. push or I.M. route.
• Dilute drug before administration and give slowly; life-threatening hyperkalemia may result from a rapid infusion.
• Watch for pain and redness at infusion site. Large-bore needle reduces local irritation.
⊗ **Incompatibilities**
Calcium, phosphate, and sulfate solutions.

Contraindications and cautions
• Contraindicated in patients with severe renal impairment with oliguria, anuria, or azotemia; those with untreated Addison disease or adrenocortical insufficiency; and those with acute dehydration, heat cramps, hyperkalemia, hyperkalemic form of familial periodic paralysis, and conditions related to extensive tissue breakdown.
• Use cautiously in patients with cardiac disease or renal impairment.
❀ **Lifespan:** In pregnant women, use cautiously. In breast-feeding women, use cautiously; it's unknown if the drug appears in breast milk.

Adverse reactions
CNS: flaccid paralysis, listlessness, mental confusion, paresthesia of limbs, weakness or heaviness of legs.
CV: *arrhythmias, cardiac arrest,* ECG changes, *heart block.*
GI: abdominal pain, diarrhea, nausea, vomiting.
GU: oliguria.
Respiratory: *respiratory paralysis.*
Skin: cold skin, gray pallor.
Other: pain, redness at infusion site.

Interactions
Drug-drug. *ACE inhibitors, potassium-sparing diuretics:* May increase risk of hyperkalemia. Use cautiously.
Drug-herb. *Cascara, licorice:* May antagonize effects of potassium supplements. Discourage using together.
Drug-food. *Salt substitutes:* May increase risk of hyperkalemia. Don't use together.

Effects on lab test results
• May increase potassium level.

Pharmacokinetics
Absorption: Given I.V.

Distribution: Throughout body.
Metabolism: None significant.
Excretion: Mainly by kidneys. *Half-life:* Unknown.

Route	Onset	Peak	Duration
I.V.	Immediate	Immediate	Unknown

Action

Chemical effect: Aids in transmitting nerve impulses, contracting cardiac and skeletal muscle, and maintaining intracellular tonicity, cellular metabolism, acid-base balance, and normal renal function.
Therapeutic effect: Replaces and maintains potassium level.

Available forms

Injection: 2 mEq/ml in 20-ml, 50-ml, 100-ml vials; 4 mEq/ml in 50-ml vial

NURSING PROCESS

⚙ Assessment

• Assess patient's condition before starting therapy and regularly thereafter to monitor drug's effectiveness.
• During therapy, monitor ECG, renal function, fluid intake and output, and potassium, creatinine, and BUN levels.
• Be alert for adverse reactions and drug interactions.
• Assess patient's and family's knowledge of drug therapy.

⊕ Nursing diagnoses

• Ineffective health maintenance related to presence of hypokalemia
• Risk for injury related to drug-induced hyperkalemia
• Deficient knowledge related to drug therapy

▶ Planning and implementation

• Don't give potassium postoperatively until urine flow is established.
• ⚠ ALERT: Potassium preparations aren't interchangeable. Verify preparation before giving.
Patient teaching
• Inform patient of need for potassium supplementation.
• Tell patient that drug will be given through an I.V. line.
• Instruct patient to report adverse reactions.

✓ Evaluation

• Patient's potassium level returns to normal with drug therapy.
• Patient doesn't develop hyperkalemia as result of drug therapy.
• Patient and family state understanding of drug therapy.

potassium bicarbonate
(poh-TAS-ee-um bigh-KAR-buh-nayt)
K+ Care ET, K-Lyte, Klor Con/EF

Pharmacologic class: potassium supplement
Therapeutic class: mineral
Pregnancy risk category: C

Indications and dosages

▶ **Hypokalemia.** *Adults:* 25 to 50 mEq dissolved in 4 to 8 oz (120 to 240 ml) of water and given P.O. once daily to b.i.d. Maximum 150 mEq daily.

Contraindications and cautions

• Contraindicated in patients with untreated Addison disease, acute dehydration, heat cramps, hyperkalemia, hyperkalemic form of familial periodic paralysis, other conditions linked to extensive tissue breakdown, or severe renal impairment with oliguria, anuria, or azotemia.
• Use cautiously in patients with cardiac disease or renal impairment.
⚖ **Lifespan:** In pregnant women, use cautiously. In breast-feeding women, use cautiously; it's unknown if the drug appears in breast milk. In children, safety and effectiveness haven't been established.

Adverse reactions

CNS: flaccid paralysis, listlessness, mental confusion, paresthesia of limbs, weakness or heaviness of legs.
CV: *arrhythmias, cardiac arrest,* ECG changes (prolonged PR interval, widened QRS complex, ST-segment depression, and tall, tented T waves), *heart block.*
GI: abdominal pain, diarrhea, *hemorrhage,* nausea, *obstruction, perforation,* ulcerations, vomiting.

Reactions may be *common,* uncommon, *life-threatening,* or **COMMON AND LIFE-THREATENING**.

Interactions

Drug-drug. *ACE inhibitors, potassium-sparing diuretics:* May increase risk of hyperkalemia. Use cautiously.
Drug-food. *Salt substitutes:* May increase risk of hyperkalemia. Don't use together.

Effects on lab test results

• May increase potassium level.

Pharmacokinetics

Absorption: Well absorbed from GI tract.
Distribution: Throughout body.
Metabolism: None significant.
Excretion: Mainly by kidneys. *Half-life:* Unknown.

Route	Onset	Peak	Duration
P.O.	Unknown	≤ 4 hr	Unknown

Action

Chemical effect: Aids in transmitting nerve impulses, contracting cardiac and skeletal muscle, and maintaining intracellular tonicity, cellular metabolism, acid-base balance, and normal renal function.
Therapeutic effect: Replaces and maintains potassium level.

Available forms

Tablets (effervescent): 6.5 mEq, 25 mEq

NURSING PROCESS

Assessment

• Assess patient's condition before starting therapy, and regularly thereafter to monitor the drug's effectiveness.
• During therapy, monitor ECG, renal function, fluid intake and output, and potassium, creatinine, and BUN levels.
• Be alert for adverse reactions and drug interactions.
• Assess patient's and family's knowledge of drug therapy.

Nursing diagnoses

• Ineffective health maintenance related to presence of hypokalemia
• Risk for injury related to potassium-induced hyperkalemia
• Deficient knowledge related to drug therapy

Planning and implementation

• Dissolve potassium bicarbonate tablets completely in 6 to 8 oz of cold water to minimize GI irritation.
• Ask patient's flavor preference. Available in lime, fruit punch, and orange flavors.
• Have patient take with meals and sip slowly over 5 to 10 minutes.
• Don't give potassium supplements postoperatively until urine flow has been established.
ALERT: Potassium preparations aren't interchangeable. Verify preparation before giving.
Patient teaching
• Inform patient about need for potassium supplementation.
• Teach patient how to prepare and take drug.
• Instruct patient to report adverse reactions.

Evaluation

• Patient's potassium level returns to normal.
• Patient doesn't develop hyperkalemia as result of drug therapy.
• Patient and family state understanding of drug therapy.

HIGH ALERT

potassium chloride

(poh-TAS-ee-um KLOR-ighd)
Cena-K, Gen-K, K+ 8, K+ 10, Kaochlor, Kaon-Cl, Kaon-Cl-10, Kaon-Cl 20%*, Kay Ciel*, K+ Care, K-Dur 10, K-Dur 20⬧, K-Lor, Klor-Con, Klor-Con EF, Klor-Con 8, Klor-Con M10, Klor-Con M15, Klor-Con M25, Klorvess, Klotrix, K-Lyte/Cl, K-Tab, K-Vescent, Micro-K Extencaps, Micro-K 10 Extencaps, Micro-K LS, Potasalan, Slow-K

Pharmacologic class: potassium supplement
Therapeutic class: mineral
Pregnancy risk category: C

Indications and dosages

▶ **Prevention of hypokalemia.** *Adults and children:* Initially, 20 mEq P.O. daily in divided doses. Adjust dosage, as needed, based on potassium level.
▶ **Hypokalemia.** *Adults and children:* 40 to 100 mEq P.O. daily divided into two to four doses. Use I.V. potassium chloride when oral replacement isn't feasible. Maximum dosage of diluted I.V. potassium chloride is 20 mEq/hour of 40 mEq/L solution. Further doses based on

potassium level. Don't exceed 150 mEq P.O. daily in adults and 3 mEq/kg P.O. daily in children. Further doses are based on potassium level and blood pH. Monitor ECG and obtain potassium level frequently when giving I.V. potassium replacement.

▶ **Severe hypokalemia.** *Adults and children:* Dilute potassium chloride in a suitable I.V. solution to 80 mEq/L or less and give at no more than 40 mEq/hour. Base next dose on potassium level. Don't exceed 150 mEq I.V. daily in adults and 3 mEq/kg I.V. daily or 40 mEq/m² daily for children.

▶ **Acute MI‡.** *Adults:* High dose—80 mEq/L at 1.5 ml/kg/hour for 24 hours with an I.V. infusion of 25% dextrose and 50 units/L regular insulin. Low dose—40 mEq/L at 1 ml/kg/hour for 24 hours, with an I.V. infusion of 10% dextrose and 20 units/L regular insulin.

▼ I.V. administration

• Give parenteral drug only by infusion, never by I.V. push or I.M. route.
• Give slowly as dilute solution; life-threatening hyperkalemia may result from a rapid infusion.
⊗ **Incompatibilities**
Amikacin, amphotericin B, diazepam, dobutamine, ergotamine, fat emulsion 10%, methylprednisolone sodium succinate, penicillin G sodium, phenytoin sodium, promethazine hydrochloride.

Contraindications and cautions

• Contraindicated in patients with untreated Addison disease, adrenocortical insufficiency, acute dehydration, heat cramps, hyperkalemia, hyperkalemic form of familial periodic paralysis, other conditions linked to extensive tissue breakdown, or severe renal impairment with oliguria, anuria, or azotemia.
• Use cautiously in patients with cardiac disease or renal impairment.
❀ **Lifespan:** In pregnant women, use cautiously. In breast-feeding women, use cautiously; it's unknown if the drug appears in breast milk.

Adverse reactions

CNS: flaccid paralysis, listlessness, mental confusion, paresthesia of limbs, weakness or heaviness of limbs.
CV: *arrhythmias, cardiac arrest,* ECG changes (prolonged PR interval, widened QRS complex,

ST-segment depression, and tall, tented T waves), *heart block.*
GI: abdominal pain, diarrhea, GI ulcerations (stenosis, *hemorrhage, obstruction, perforation*), nausea, vomiting.
GU: oliguria.
Respiratory: *respiratory paralysis.*
Skin: cold skin, gray pallor, phlebitis.

Interactions

Drug-drug. *ACE inhibitors, potassium-sparing diuretics:* May increase risk of hyperkalemia. Use cautiously.
Drug-herb. *Cascara, licorice:* May antagonize effects of potassium supplements. Discourage using together.
Drug-food. *Salt substitutes:* May increase risk of hyperkalemia. Don't use together.

Effects on lab test results

• May increase potassium level.

Pharmacokinetics

Absorption: Well absorbed.
Distribution: Throughout body.
Metabolism: None significant.
Excretion: Mainly by kidneys; small amounts may be excreted by skin and intestinal tract, but intestinal potassium is usually reabsorbed. *Half-life:* Unknown.

Route	Onset	Peak	Duration
P.O.	Unknown	≤ 4 hr	Unknown
I.V.	Immediate	Immediate	Unknown

Action

Chemical effect: Aids in transmitting nerve impulses, contracting cardiac and skeletal muscle, and maintaining intracellular tonicity, cellular metabolism, acid-base balance, and normal renal function.
Therapeutic effect: Replaces and maintains potassium level.

Available forms

Capsules (controlled-release): 8 mEq, 10 mEq
Injection concentrate: 2 mEq/ml vials or premixed bags
Injection for I.V. infusion: 0.1 mEq/ml, 0.2 mEq/ml, 0.3 mEq/ml, 0.4 mEq/ml
Oral liquid: 20 mEq/15 ml*, 40 mEq/15 ml*

Powder for oral administration: 15 mEq/packet, 20 mEq/packet, 25 mEq/packet
Tablets (controlled-release): 8 mEq, 10 mEq, 20 mEq
Tablets (effervescent): 10 mEq, 20 mEq, 25 mEq, 50 mEq
Tablets (extended-release): 8 mEq, 10 mEq, 15 mEq, 20 mEq

NURSING PROCESS

☞ Assessment
• Assess patient's condition before starting therapy and regularly thereafter to monitor drug's effectiveness.
• During therapy, monitor ECG, renal function, fluid intake and output, and potassium, creatinine, and BUN levels.
• Be alert for adverse reactions and drug interactions.
• Assess patient's and family's knowledge of drug therapy.

⊕ Nursing diagnoses
• Ineffective health maintenance related to presence of hypokalemia
• Risk for injury related to drug-induced hyperkalemia
• Deficient knowledge related to drug therapy

▷ Planning and implementation
• When giving I.V. potassium replacement, monitor ECG and take potassium level frequently.
• Give cautiously because different potassium supplements deliver varying amounts of potassium. Never switch products without prescriber's order.
• Make sure powders are completely dissolved before giving.
• Don't crush sustained-release potassium products.
• Give potassium with or after meals with full glass of water or fruit juice to lessen GI distress.
• If tablet or capsule passage is likely to be delayed, as in GI obstruction, use sugar-free liquid (Kaochlor S-F 10%). Have patient sip slowly to minimize GI irritation.
• Enteric-coated tablets increase risk of GI bleeding and small-bowel ulcerations; use cautiously.
• Tablets in wax matrix sometimes lodge in esophagus and cause ulceration in cardiac pa-

tients who have esophageal compression from enlarged left atrium. Use liquid form in such patients and in those with esophageal stasis or obstruction.
• Drug is commonly given with potassium-wasting diuretics to maintain potassium level.
Ⓢ **ALERT:** Potassium preparations aren't interchangeable. Verify preparation before giving.
Ⓢ **ALERT:** Don't give potassium postoperatively until urine flow is established.
Patient teaching
• Tell patient that controlled-release tablets may appear in stool but that the drug has already been absorbed.
• Instruct patient to report adverse reactions and pain at the I.V. site.

☑ Evaluation
• Patient's potassium level returns to normal.
• Patient doesn't develop hyperkalemia.
• Patient and family state understanding of drug therapy.

potassium gluconate
(poh-TAS-ee-um GLOO-kuh-nayt)
Kaon, Kaylixir*, K-G Elixir*

Pharmacologic class: potassium supplement
Therapeutic class: mineral
Pregnancy risk category: C

Indications and dosages
▶ **Hypokalemia.** *Adults:* 40 to 100 mEq P.O. daily in three or four divided doses; 20 mEq P.O. daily for prevention. Further doses based on potassium level determinations.

Contraindications and cautions
• Contraindicated in patients with untreated Addison disease, acute dehydration, heat cramps, hyperkalemia, hyperkalemic form of familial periodic paralysis, other conditions related to extensive tissue breakdown, or severe renal impairment with oliguria, anuria, or azotemia.
• Use cautiously in patients with cardiac disease or renal impairment.
≋ **Lifespan:** In pregnant women, use cautiously. In breast-feeding women, use cautiously; it's unknown if the drug appears in breast milk. In

children, safety and effectiveness haven't been established.

Adverse reactions

CNS: flaccid paralysis, listlessness, mental confusion, paresthesia of limbs, weakness or heaviness of legs.
CV: *arrhythmias,* ECG changes (prolonged PR interval, widened QRS complex, ST-segment depression, and tall, tented T waves).
GI: *abdominal pain;* diarrhea; *GI ulcerations* that may be accompanied by stenosis, *hemorrhage, obstruction or perforation* (with oral products, especially enteric-coated tablets); nausea and vomiting.

Interactions

Drug-drug. *ACE inhibitors, potassium-sparing diuretics:* May increase risk of hyperkalemia. Use cautiously.
Drug-food. *Salt substitutes:* May increase risk of hyperkalemia. Don't use together.

Effects on lab test results

• May increase potassium level.

Pharmacokinetics

Absorption: Well absorbed from GI tract.
Distribution: Throughout body.
Metabolism: None significant.
Excretion: Mainly by kidneys; small amounts may be excreted by skin and intestinal tract, but intestinal potassium is usually reabsorbed. *Half-life:* Unknown.

Route	Onset	Peak	Duration
P.O.	Unknown	≤ 4 hr	Unknown

Action

Chemical effect: Aids in transmitting nerve impulses, contracting cardiac and skeletal muscle, and maintaining intracellular tonicity, cellular metabolism, acid-base balance, and normal renal function.
Therapeutic effect: Replaces and maintains potassium level.

Available forms

Liquid: 20 mEq/15 ml*
Tablets: 500 mg†, 595 mg† (83.45 mg and 99 mg potassium, respectively)

NURSING PROCESS

✍ Assessment
• Assess patient's condition before starting therapy and regularly thereafter to monitor drug's effectiveness.
• During therapy, monitor ECG, renal function, fluid intake and output, and potassium, creatinine, and BUN levels.
• Be alert for adverse reactions and drug interactions.
• Assess patient's and family's knowledge of drug therapy.

⊕ Nursing diagnoses
• Ineffective health maintenance related to presence of hypokalemia
• Risk for injury related to potassium-induced hyperkalemia
• Deficient knowledge related to drug therapy

▶ Planning and implementation
• Give cautiously because different potassium supplements deliver varying amounts of potassium. Never switch products without prescriber's order.
• Give drug with or after meals with glass of water or fruit juice.
• Have patient sip liquid potassium slowly to minimize GI irritation.
• Enteric-coated tablets aren't recommended because of increased risk of GI bleeding and small-bowel ulcerations.
⚠ **ALERT:** Potassium preparations aren't interchangeable. Verify preparation before giving.
⚠ **ALERT:** Don't give potassium supplements postoperatively until urine flow is established.
Patient teaching
• Inform patient of need for potassium supplementation.
• Teach patient how to take drug.
• Instruct patient to report adverse reactions.

☑ Evaluation
• Patient's potassium level returns to normal.
• Patient doesn't develop hyperkalemia as result of drug therapy.
• Patient and family state understanding of drug therapy.

---

potassium iodide
(poh-TAS-ee-um IGH-uh-dighd)
Iosat†, Pima, Thyrosafe†, ThyroShield†

potassium iodide, saturated solution (SSKI)

strong iodine solution (Lugol's solution)

Pharmacologic class: antithyroid
Therapeutic class: radiation protectant
Pregnancy risk category: D

Indications and dosages

▶ **Preparation for thyroidectomy.** *Adults and children:* 0.1 to 0.3 ml (2 to 6 drops) strong iodine solution P.O. t.i.d. for 10 days before surgery.
▶ **Thyrotoxic crisis.** *Adults and children:* 500 mg P.O. every 4 hours (about 10 drops of 1 g/ml solution).
▶ **Radiation protectant for thyroid gland.** *Adults:* 130 mg P.O. daily for 10 days after radiation exposure. Start no later than 3 to 4 hours after acute exposure.
Children ages 3 to 18: Give 65 mg P.O. daily for 10 days after exposure. Start no later than 3 to 4 hours after acute exposure.
Children ages 1 month to 3 years: 32.5 mg P.O. daily for 10 days after exposure. Start no later than 3 to 4 hours after acute exposure.
Infants from birth to age 1 month: 16.25 mg P.O. daily for 10 days after exposure. Start no later than 3 to 4 hours after acute exposure.
▶ **Hyperthyroidism.** *Adults and children:* 50 to 250 mg (1 to 5 drops of 1 g/ml solution) potassium iodide t.i.d. for 10 to 14 days before surgery. Or, 0.1 to 0.3 strong iodine solution (3 to 5 drops) t.i.d.
▶ **As an expectorant in chronic pulmonary diseases.** *Adults:* 325 to 650 mg P.O. t.i.d. *Children:* 162.5 to 325 mg P.O. t.i.d.

Contraindications and cautions

• Contraindicated in patients with tuberculosis, acute bronchitis, iodide hypersensitivity, impaired renal function, or hyperkalemia. Some forms contain sulfites, which may cause allergic reactions in hypersensitive people.

• Use cautiously in patients with hypocomplementemic vasculitis, goiter, or autoimmune thyroid disease.
☀ **Lifespan:** In pregnant and breast-feeding women, drug isn't recommended.

Adverse reactions

CNS: fever, frontal headache.
EENT: acute rhinitis, conjunctivitis, hyperemia, inflammation of salivary glands, periorbital edema.
GI: burning, diarrhea (sometimes bloody), irritation, *metallic taste, nausea*, vomiting.
Metabolic: *potassium toxicity* (confusion, irregular heart beat, numbness, tingling, pain or weakness in hands and feet, tiredness).
Skin: acneiform rash, mucous membrane ulceration.
Other: hypersensitivity reactions, tooth discoloration.

Interactions

Drug-drug. *ACE inhibitors, potassium-sparing diuretics:* May increase risk of hyperkalemia. Avoid using together.
Antithyroid drugs: May increase hypothyroid or goitrogenic effects. Monitor effects closely.
Lithium carbonate: May cause hypothyroidism. Use together cautiously.
Drug-food. *Salt substitutes:* May increase risk of hyperkalemia. Don't use together.

Effects on lab test results

• May increase potassium level.
• May increase or decrease thyroid function test results.

Pharmacokinetics

Absorption: Unknown.
Distribution: Unknown.
Metabolism: Unknown.
Excretion: Unknown. *Half-life:* Unknown.

Route	Onset	Peak	Duration
P.O.	≤ 24 hr	10–15 days	Unknown

Action

Chemical effect: Inhibits thyroid hormone formation by blocking iodotyrosine and iodothyronine synthesis, limits iodide transport into thyroid gland, and blocks thyroid hormone release.
Therapeutic effect: Lowers thyroid hormone level.

Available forms

potassium iodide
Oral solution: 65 mg/ml
Scored tablets: 65 mg, 130 mg
Syrup: 325 mg/5 ml
potassium iodide, saturated solution
Oral solution: 1 g/ml
strong iodine solution
Oral solution: iodine 50 mg/ml and potassium iodide 100 mg/ml

NURSING PROCESS

Assessment

• Assess patient's condition before starting therapy and regularly thereafter to monitor drug's effectiveness.
• Be alert for adverse reactions and drug interactions.
• Earliest signs of delayed hypersensitivity reactions caused by iodides are irritation and swelling of eyelids.
• Assess patient's and family's knowledge of drug therapy.

Nursing diagnoses

• Ineffective health maintenance related to underlying thyroid condition
• Ineffective protection related to hypersensitivity reactions
• Deficient knowledge related to drug therapy

Planning and implementation

• Potassium iodide is usually given with other antithyroid drugs.
• Dilute oral doses in water, milk, or fruit juice to hydrate patient and mask salty taste; give drug after meals to prevent gastric irritation.
• Give iodide through straw to prevent tooth discoloration.
• Store drug in light-resistant container.
Patient teaching
• Warn patient that suddenly stopping the drug may cause thyroid crisis.
• Tell patient to ask prescriber whether he can use iodized salt or eat shellfish.
• Tell patient to report adverse reactions.

Evaluation

• Patient's thyroid hormone level is lower with potassium iodide therapy.
• Patient doesn't experience hypersensitivity reactions.

• Patient and family state understanding of drug therapy.

pralidoxime chloride (2-pyridinealdoxime methochloride; 2-PAM chloride)
(pral-ih-DOKS-eem KLOR-ighd)
Protopam Chloride

Pharmacologic class: quaternary ammonium oxime
Therapeutic class: antidote
Pregnancy risk category: C

Indications and dosages

▶ **Antidote for organophosphate poisoning.**
Adults: 1 to 2 g in 100 ml of saline solution by I.V. infusion over 15 to 30 minutes. If infusion not practical or patient has pulmonary edema, give as 5% solution in water for injection by slow I.V. push over at least 5 minutes. Repeat in 1 hour if muscle weakness persists; may give further doses cautiously. Use I.M. or subcutaneous injection if I.V. route isn't feasible.
▶ **Anticholinesterase overdose.** *Adults:* 1 to 2 g I.V., followed by 250 mg I.V. every 5 minutes.

I.V. administration

• Give I.V. preparation slowly as diluted solution. Dilute with unpreserved sterile water.
• To lessen muscarinic effects and block accumulation of acetylcholine from organophosphate poisoning, give atropine 2 to 6 mg I.V. along with pralidoxime unless patient has cyanosis. (If he is cyanotic, give atropine I.M.) Give atropine every 5 to 60 minutes in adults until muscarinic signs and symptoms disappear; if they reappear, repeat the dose. Maintain atropinization for at least 48 hours.
• Infuse slowly since tachycardia, laryngospasm, muscle rigidity, and worsening of cholinergic symptoms may occur with rapid administration. Maximum injection rate is 200 mg/minute.
⊗ **Incompatibilities**
None reported.

Contraindications and cautions

• Use cautiously in patients with myasthenia gravis; overdose may cause myasthenic crisis.

pralidoxime chloride **1023**

Also use cautiously and with reduced dosage in patients with renal impairment.

⚖ **Lifespan:** In pregnant women, use cautiously. In breast-feeding women and in children, safety and effectiveness haven't been established.

Adverse reactions

CNS: dizziness, drowsiness, excitement, headache, manic behavior after recovery of consciousness.
CV: increased blood pressure, tachycardia.
EENT: blurred vision, diplopia, impaired accommodation.
GI: nausea.
Musculoskeletal: muscle rigidity, muscle weakness.
Respiratory: hyperventilation.
Skin: rash.
Other: pain at injection site.

Interactions

Drug-drug. *Atropine:* May cause flushing, tachycardia, dry mouth. Monitor patient.
Barbiturates: May increase the effects of barbiturates. Use together cautiously.

Effects on lab test results

• May increase AST, ALT, and CK levels.

Pharmacokinetics

Absorption: Unknown after I.M. or subcutaneous use.
Distribution: Throughout extracellular fluid. Drug isn't appreciably protein-bound, and it doesn't readily pass into CNS.
Metabolism: Unknown, but hepatic metabolism is likely.
Excretion: Rapid, in urine. *Half-life:* 1½ hours.

Route	Onset	Peak	Duration
I.V.	Unknown	5–15 min	Unknown
I.M.	Unknown	10–20 min	Unknown
SubQ	Unknown	Unknown	Unknown

Action

Chemical effect: Reactivates cholinesterase that has been inactivated by organophosphorus pesticides and related compounds, permitting degradation of accumulated acetylcholine and facilitating normal functioning of neuromuscular junctions.

Therapeutic effect: Alleviates signs and symptoms of organophosphate poisoning and cholinergic crisis in myasthenia gravis.

Available forms

Injection: 1 g/20 ml in 20-ml vial without diluent or syringe; 1 g/20 ml in 20-ml vial with diluent, syringe, needle, and alcohol swab (emergency kit); 600 mg/2 ml autoinjector (may contain benzyl alcohol), parenteral

NURSING PROCESS

Assessment
• Assess patient's condition before starting therapy and regularly thereafter. Drug relieves paralysis of respiratory muscles but is less effective in relieving depression of respiratory center.
• Drug isn't effective against poisoning caused by phosphorus, inorganic phosphates, or organophosphates that have no anticholinesterase activity.
• If poison was ingested, observe patient for 48 to 72 hours. Absorption from lower bowel may be delayed. It's difficult to distinguish between toxic effects produced by atropine or organophosphate compounds and those resulting from this drug.
• Watch for signs of rapid weakening in patient with myasthenia gravis who was treated for overdose of cholinergics. Patient can pass quickly from cholinergic crisis to myasthenic crisis and may need more cholinergic drugs to treat myasthenia. Keep edrophonium (Tensilon) available in such situations for establishing differential diagnosis.
• Be alert for adverse reactions.
• Assess patient's and family's knowledge of drug therapy.

Nursing diagnoses
• Ineffective health maintenance related to underlying condition
• Risk for injury related to adverse CNS reactions
• Deficient knowledge related to drug therapy

Planning and implementation
• Use drug only in hospitalized patients; have respiratory and other supportive measures available. If possible, obtain accurate medical history and chronology of poisoning. Give drug as soon

Rapid onset *Liquid form contains alcohol. ◆Canada †OTC ✐Photoguide ‡Off-label use

as possible; it's most effective when started within 24 hours.

● Remove secretions, maintain patent airway, and start artificial ventilation if needed. After dermal exposure to organophosphate, remove patient's clothing and wash his skin and hair with sodium bicarbonate, soap, water, and alcohol immediately. A second washing may be needed. When washing patient, wear protective gloves and clothes to avoid exposure.

● Draw blood for cholinesterase level before giving drug.

⚡ ALERT: Don't confuse pralidoxime with pramoxine or pyridoxine.

Patient teaching

● Tell patient to report adverse reactions immediately.

● Advise patient treated for organophosphate poisoning to avoid contact with insecticides for several weeks.

☑ Evaluation

● Patient responds well to therapy.

● Patient sustains no injury from adverse CNS reactions.

● Patient and family state understanding of drug therapy.

---

pramipexole dihydrochloride
(pram-ih-PEKS-ohl digh-high-droh-KLOR-ighd)
Mirapex

Pharmacologic class: dopamine agonist
Therapeutic class: antiparkinsonian
Pregnancy risk category: C

Indications and dosages

▶ **Signs and symptoms of idiopathic Parkinson disease.** *Adults:* Initially, 0.375 mg P.O. daily in three divided doses; don't increase more often than every 5 to 7 days. Maintenance daily dosage range is 1.5 to 4.5 mg in three divided doses.

⬛ Adjust-a-dose: For patients with renal impairment, if creatinine clearance is greater than 60 ml/minute, initial dose is 0.125 mg P.O. t.i.d., up to 1.5 mg t.i.d. If creatinine clearance is 35 to 59 ml/minute, initial dose is 0.125 mg P.O. b.i.d. up to 1.5 mg b.i.d. If creatinine clearance is 15 to 34 ml/minute, initial dose is 0.125 mg P.O. daily, up to 1.5 mg daily.

Contraindications and cautions

● Contraindicated in patients hypersensitive to the drug or any of its components.

● Use cautiously in patients with renal impairment; adjust dosage if needed.

☆ Lifespan: Use during pregnancy only if benefits outweigh risks to the fetus. In breastfeeding women, use cautiously. In children, safety and effectiveness haven't been established. In the elderly, use cautiously.

Adverse reactions

CNS: akathisia, amnesia, *asthenia, confusion,* delusions, *dizziness, dream abnormalities, dyskinesia,* dystonia, *extrapyramidal syndrome,* fever, gait abnormalities, *hallucinations,* hypertonia, hypoesthesia, *insomnia,* malaise, myoclonus, paranoid reaction, sleep disorders, *somnolence,* thought abnormalities.

CV: chest pain, general edema, *orthostatic hypotension,* peripheral edema.

EENT: accommodation abnormalities, diplopia, rhinitis, vision abnormalities.

GI: anorexia, *constipation,* dry mouth, dysphagia, *nausea.*

GU: impotence, urinary frequency, urinary incontinence, UTI.

Metabolic: weight loss.

Musculoskeletal: arthritis, bursitis, myasthenia, twitching.

Respiratory: dyspnea, pneumonia.

Skin: skin disorders.

Other: *accidental injury,* decreased libido.

Interactions

Drug-drug. *Butyrophenones, metoclopramide, phenothiazines, thiothixenes:* May diminish pramipexole effectiveness. Monitor patient closely.

Cimetidine, diltiazem, quinidine, quinine, ranitidine, triamterene, verapamil: May decrease pramipexole clearance. Adjust dosage.

Levodopa: May increase adverse effects of levodopa. Decrease levodopa dose, as directed.

Drug-herb. *Black horehound:* May have additive dopaminergic effects. Discourage using together.

Kava: May decrease dopaminergic effects. Discourage use together.

Effects on lab test results

None reported.

Pharmacokinetics

Absorption: Rapid. Absolute bioavailability exceeds 90%.
Distribution: Extensive throughout body.
Metabolism: 90% unchanged in urine.
Excretion: Mainly urinary. *Half-life:* 8 to 12 hours.

Route	Onset	Peak	Duration
P.O.	Rapid	2 hr	8–12 hr

Action

Chemical effect: Precise mechanism is unknown, but drug probably stimulates dopamine receptors in striatum.
Therapeutic effect: Relieves symptoms of idiopathic Parkinson disease.

Available forms

Tablets: 0.125 mg, 0.25 mg, 0.5 mg, 1 mg, 1.5 mg

NURSING PROCESS

🔲 Assessment
• Monitor vital signs carefully because drug may cause orthostatic hypotension, especially during dosage escalation.
• Assess patient's risk for physical injury from adverse CNS effects of drug (dyskinesia, dizziness, hallucinations, and somnolence).
• Assess patient's response to drug therapy, and adjust dosage.
• Assess patient's and family's knowledge of drug therapy.

🔲 Nursing diagnoses
• Impaired physical mobility related to underlying Parkinson disease
• Disturbed thought processes related to drug-induced CNS adverse reactions
• Deficient knowledge related to drug therapy

🔲 Planning and implementation
• Institute safety precautions.
🔲 **ALERT:** Don't abruptly stop giving the drug. Adjust dosage gradually according to patient's response and tolerance.
• Provide ice chips, drinks, or hard, sugarless candy to relieve dry mouth. Increase fluid and fiber intake to prevent constipation.

Patient teaching
• Instruct patient not to rise rapidly after sitting or lying down because of risk of orthostatic hypotension.
• Warn patient to avoid hazardous activities until the drug's CNS effects are known.
• Tell patient to contact prescriber before taking this drug with other drugs.
• Tell patient—especially geriatric patient—that hallucinations may occur.
• If nausea develops, advise patient to take drug with food.
• If woman is breast-feeding or intends to do so, tell her to notify prescriber.

🔲 Evaluation
• Patient has improved mobility and reduced muscle rigidity and tremor.
• Patient remains mentally alert.
• Patient and family state understanding of drug therapy.

HIGH ALERT

pramlintide acetate
(PRAM-lihn-tighd AS-ih-tayt)
Symlin

Pharmacologic class: human amylin analogue
Therapeutic class: antidiabetic
Pregnancy risk category: C

Indications and dosages

▶ **Adjunct to insulin in patients with type 1 diabetes who haven't achieved the desired glucose control.** *Adults:* Initially, 15 mcg subcutaneously immediately before major meals (more than 250 calories or 30 g of carbohydrates). Reduce preprandial rapid-acting or short-acting insulin dose, including fixed-mix insulin such as 70/30, by 50%. Increase pramlintide dose by 15-mcg increments every 3 days as long as no nausea has occurred, to a maintenance dose of 30 to 60 mcg. Adjust insulin dosage as needed.
▶ **Adjunct to insulin in patients with type 2 diabetes who haven't achieved the desired glucose control, with or without a sulfonylurea or metformin.** *Adults:* Initially, 60 mcg subcutaneously immediately before major meals. Reduce preprandial rapid-acting or short-acting insulin dose, including fixed-mix insulin,

by 50%. Increase pramlintide dose to 120 mcg when no significant nausea has occurred for 3 to 7 days. Adjust insulin dosage as needed.

Contraindications and cautions

• Contraindicated in patients hypersensitive to drug or its components, including metacresol, and in patients with gastroparesis or hypoglycemia unawareness. Don't use drug in patients noncompliant with current insulin and glucose monitoring regimen, patients with a glycosylated hemoglobin (HbA1c) level greater than 9%, patients with severe hypoglycemia during the previous 6 months, and patients who take drugs that stimulate GI motility.

☀ **Lifespan:** Use during pregnancy only if benefits outweigh risks to the fetus. Use cautiously in breast-feeding women; it isn't known whether drug appears in breast milk. Safety and effectiveness haven't been established in children. Use cautiously in elderly patients; drug seems to have similar effects on elderly and younger adults, but some older adults may have greater sensitivity to it.

Adverse reactions

CNS: dizziness, fatigue, *headache.*
EENT: pharyngitis.
GI: abdominal pain, *anorexia, nausea, vomiting.*
Metabolic: *hypoglycemia.*
Musculoskeletal: arthralgia.
Respiratory: cough.
Skin: injection site reaction.
Other: allergic reaction, *inflicted injury.*

Interactions

Drug-drug. *ACE inhibitors, disopyramide, fibrates, fluoxetine, MAO inhibitors, oral antidiabetics, pentoxifylline, propoxyphene, salicylates, sulfonamide antibiotics:* May increase the risk of hypoglycemia. Monitor blood glucose level closely.
Alpha glucosidase inhibitors (such as acarbose) and anticholinergics (such as atropine, benztropine, tricyclic antidepressants): May alter GI motility. Avoid using together.
Beta blockers, clonidine, guanethidine, reserpine: May mask signs of hypoglycemia. Monitor blood glucose level closely.
Oral drugs dependent on rapid onset of action (such as analgesics): May delay absorption because of slowed gastric emptying. If rapid effect

is needed, give oral drug 1 hour before or 2 hours after pramlintide.

Effects on lab test results

None reported.

Pharmacokinetics

Absorption: 30% to 40% bioavailable.
Distribution: Not extensively bound to blood cells or albumin.
Metabolism: Mainly renal.
Excretion: *Half-life of parent drug and active metabolite:* About 48 minutes each.

Route	Onset	Peak	Duration
SubQ	Unknown	19–21 min	Unknown

Action

Chemical effect: Slows the rate at which food leaves the stomach, reducing the initial postprandial increase in plasma glucose level. Drug also reduces postprandial glucagon concentrations, which decreases hyperglycemia, and reduces total caloric intake by modulating appetite.
Therapeutic effect: Lowers glucose level.

Available forms

Injection: 0.6 mg/ml in 5-ml vials

NURSING PROCESS

Assessment
• Before starting drug, review patient's HbA1c level, recent blood glucose monitoring data, history of insulin-induced hypoglycemia, current insulin regimen, and body weight.
• Monitor patient's glucose level.
• Assess patient for signs of hypoglycemia including dizziness, restlessness, diaphoresis, tremor, nausea, irritability, and poor concentration.
• Monitor patient for severe nausea and vomiting. Dosage reduction may be needed.
• Assess patient's and family's knowledge of drug therapy.

Nursing diagnoses
• Risk for injury related to drug-induced hypoglycemia
• Ineffective health maintenance related to hyperglycemia
• Deficient knowledge related to drug therapy

▶ Planning and implementation

• To give drug, use a U-100 insulin syringe, preferably a 0.3-ml size.

• Don't mix drug with any type of insulin, and give it as a separate injection.

• Give each dose subcutaneously into the abdomen or thigh. Rotate injection sites, and use a site separate from the insulin site used at the same time.

⚠ **ALERT:** Pramlintide may increase the risk of insulin-induced severe hypoglycemia, particularly in patients with type 1 diabetes.

• The risk of severe, drug-related hypoglycemia is highest within the first 3 hours after an injection.

• Symptoms of hypoglycemia may be masked in patients with a long history of diabetes, diabetic nerve disease, or intensified diabetes control.

• Stop drug if patient has persistent nausea or recurrent, unexplained hypoglycemia that requires medical assistance. Also stop drug if patient doesn't comply with blood glucose monitoring or drug dosage adjustments.

Patient teaching

• Teach patient how to take drug exactly as prescribed, immediately before mealtimes. Explain that it doesn't replace daily insulin but may lower the amount of insulin needed, especially before meals.

• Explain that a major meal contains more than 250 calories or 30 g of carbohydrates.

• Caution patient not to mix drug with insulin; instruct him to give the injections at separate sites.

• Instruct patient not to change doses of pramlintide or insulin without consulting the prescriber.

• Tell patient to refrain from driving, operating heavy machinery, or performing other risky activities where he could hurt himself or others, until drug's effects on his blood glucose are known.

• Caution patient about the possibility of severe hypoglycemia, particularly within 3 hours of injection.

• Teach patient and family members the signs and symptoms of hypoglycemia, including hunger, headache, sweating, tremor, irritability, and trouble concentrating.

• Instruct patient and family members what to do if hypoglycemia occurs.

• Tell patient to report severe nausea and vomiting.

• Advise woman of child-bearing potential to tell the prescriber if she is, could be, or is planning to become pregnant.

• Teach patient how to handle unusual situations, such as illness or stress, an inadequate or omitted insulin dose, inadvertent use of too much insulin or pramlintide, inadequate food intake, or missed meals.

• Tell patient to refrigerate vials. Contents of opened vials should be used within 28 days and contents of unopened vials before expiration date.

☑ Evaluation

• Patient does not experience hypoglycemia and sustains no injury.

• Patient's glucose level is normal with drug therapy.

• Patient and family state understanding of drug therapy.

pravastatin sodium (eptastatin)
(PRAH-vuh-stat-in SOH-dee-um)
Pravachol✦

Pharmacologic class: HMG-CoA reductase inhibitor
Therapeutic class: antilipemic
Pregnancy risk category: X

Indications and dosages

▶ **Primary hypercholesterolemia and mixed dyslipidemia; primary and secondary prevention of coronary events; hyperlipidemia; homozygous familial hypercholesterolemia.**
Adults: Initially, 40 mg P.O. once daily at the same time each day, with or without food. Adjust dosage every 4 weeks based on patient tolerance and response; maximum daily dose, 80 mg.

▶ **Heterozygous familial hypercholesterolemia.** *Children ages 14 to 18:* Give 40 mg P.O. once daily.
Children ages 8 to 13: Give 20 mg P.O. once daily.

☒ **Adjust-a-dose:** For patients with renal or hepatic impairment, start with 10 mg P.O. daily.

For patients also taking immunosuppressants, start with 10 mg P.O. at bedtime and adjust to

P

higher doses cautiously. Most patients given combination will receive maximum daily dose of 20 mg.

Contraindications and cautions

• Contraindicated in patients hypersensitive to the drug or any of its components, and in patients with active liver disease or unexplained persistent elevations of transaminase level.
• Use cautiously in patients who consume large quantities of alcohol or have a history of liver disease.
⚠ **Lifespan:** In pregnant women, breast-feeding women, and women of childbearing age (unless they have no risk of pregnancy), drug is contraindicated. In children younger than age 8, safety and effectiveness haven't been established.

Adverse reactions

CNS: dizziness, fatigue, headache.
CV: chest pain.
EENT: rhinitis.
GI: diarrhea, heartburn, nausea, vomiting.
GU: *renal failure* secondary to myoglobinuria.
Musculoskeletal: localized muscle pain, myalgia, myopathy, myositis, *rhabdomyolysis.*
Respiratory: cough.
Skin: rash.
Other: flulike symptoms.

Interactions

Drug-drug. *Cholestyramine, colestipol:* May decrease pravastatin level. Give pravastatin 1 hour before or 4 hours after these drugs.
Drugs that decrease level or activity of endogenous steroids (such as cimetidine, spironolactone): May increase risk of endocrine dysfunction. No intervention needed. Take complete drug history in patients who develop endocrine dysfunction.
Erythromycin, fibric acid derivatives (such as clofibrate, gemfibrozil), high doses of niacin, immunosuppressants: May increase risk of rhabdomyolysis. Don't use together.
Fluconazole, itraconazole, ketoconazole: May increase level and adverse effects of pravastatin. Consider reduced dose of pravastatin.
Gemfibrozil: May decrease protein-binding and urinary clearance of pravastatin. Avoid using together.
Hepatotoxic drugs: May increase risk of hepatotoxicity. Avoid using together.

Drug-herb. *Kava:* May increase risk of hepatotoxicity. Discourage using together.
Red yeast rice: May increase the risk of adverse events or toxicity because herb contains components similar to those of statin drugs. Discourage using together.
Drug-lifestyle. *Alcohol use:* May increase risk of hepatotoxicity. Discourage using together.

Effects on lab test results

• May increase ALT, AST, CK, alkaline phosphatase, and bilirubin levels.
• May alter thyroid function test values.

Pharmacokinetics

Absorption: Rapid. Although food reduces bioavailability, drug effects are the same if drug is taken with or 1 hour before meals.
Distribution: About 50% protein-bound. Drug undergoes extensive first-pass extraction, possibly because of active transport system into hepatocytes.
Metabolism: In liver, into at least six metabolites. Some are active.
Excretion: By liver and kidneys. *Half-life:* $1\frac{1}{4}$ to $2\frac{1}{4}$ hours.

Route	Onset	Peak	Duration
P.O.	Unknown	1 hr	Unknown

Action

Chemical effect: Inhibits HMG-CoA reductase, which is an early and rate-limiting step in the synthesis of cholesterol.
Therapeutic effect: Lowers LDL and total cholesterol levels in some patients.

Available forms

Tablets: 10 mg, 20 mg, 40 mg, 80 mg

NURSING PROCESS

⚕ **Assessment**

• Assess patient's condition before starting therapy and regularly thereafter to monitor drug's effectiveness.
• Obtain liver function tests at start of therapy and periodically thereafter. If elevations persist, arrange for patient to have a liver biopsy.
• Be alert for adverse reactions and drug interactions.
• Monitor patient for signs of rhabdomyolysis, such as muscle aches and weakness.

- If adverse GI reaction occurs, monitor patient's hydration.
- Assess patient's and family's knowledge of drug therapy.

⊕ Nursing diagnoses
- Risk for injury related to elevated cholesterol level
- Risk for deficient fluid volume related to adverse GI reactions
- Deficient knowledge related to drug therapy

⟩ Planning and implementation
- Begin only after diet and other nondrug therapies have proved ineffective.

Patient teaching
- Instruct patient to take recommended dosage in evening, preferably at bedtime.
- Teach patient about proper cholesterol-lowering diet (restricting total fat and cholesterol), and how to control other cardiac disease risk factors. Recommend weight control, exercise, and smoking cessation programs.
- Inform woman that drug is contraindicated during pregnancy. Advise her to notify prescriber immediately if she becomes pregnant.

☑ Evaluation
- Patient's LDL and total cholesterol levels are within normal range.
- Patient maintains adequate hydration.
- Patient and family state understanding of drug therapy.

prazosin hydrochloride
(PRAH-zoh-sin high-droh-KLOR-ighd)
Minipress

Pharmacologic class: alpha blocker
Therapeutic class: antihypertensive
Pregnancy risk category: C

Indications and dosages
▶ **Mild to moderate hypertension, alone or with diuretic or other antihypertensive.**
Adults: Initial dosage is 1 mg P.O. b.i.d. to t.i.d. Increase slowly; maximum daily dose is 20 mg. Maintenance dosage is 6 to 15 mg daily in three divided doses. Some patients need larger doses (up to 40 mg daily). If other antihypertensives

or diuretics are added, decrease to 1 to 2 mg t.i.d. and readjust.
▶ **BPH‡.** *Adults:* Initially, 2 mg P.O. b.i.d. Daily dose may range from 1 to 9 mg.

Contraindications and cautions
- Use cautiously in patients taking other antihypertensives.
- ⚖ **Lifespan:** In pregnant women, use cautiously. In breast-feeding women, drug isn't recommended. In children, safety and effectiveness haven't been established.

Adverse reactions
CNS: depression, *dizziness,* drowsiness, *first-dose syncope,* headache, weakness.
CV: edema, orthostatic hypotension, palpitations.
EENT: blurred vision, epistaxis, nasal congestion, reddened sclera.
GI: abdominal cramps, constipation, diarrhea, dry mouth, *nausea,* vomiting.
GU: impotence, priapism, urinary frequency.
Respiratory: dyspnea.
Skin: rash.

Interactions
Drug-drug. *Acebutolol, atenolol, betaxolol, carteolol, esmolol, metoprolol, nadolol, pindolol, propranolol, sotalol, timolol:* May increase risk of orthostatic hypotension in the early phases of use together. Assist patient to stand slowly until effects of drug are known.
Clonidine: May decrease antihypertensive effect of clonidine. Monitor blood pressure.
Diuretics: May increase risk of syncope with loss of consciousness.
Indomethacin: May decrease antihypertensive action of prazosin. Monitor blood pressure.
Verapamil: May increase prazosin level and increase risk of postural hypotension. Advise patient to sit or lie down if dizziness occurs.
Drug-herb. *Saw palmetto:* May have additive effect when used together for BPH.
Yohimbe: May antagonize antihypertensive effects. Discourage using together.

Effects on lab test results
- May increase BUN and uric acid levels.
- May increase liver function test values.

Pharmacokinetics

Absorption: Variable.
Distribution: Throughout body. About 97% protein-bound.
Metabolism: Extensive in liver.
Excretion: More than 90% in feces by bile; remainder in urine. *Half-life:* 2 to 4 hours.

Route	Onset	Peak	Duration
P.O.	30–90 min	2–4 hr	7–10 hr

Action

Chemical effect: Unknown; effects probably stem from alpha blocking activity.
Therapeutic effect: Lowers blood pressure.

Available forms

Capsules: 1 mg, 2 mg, 5 mg

NURSING PROCESS

⚡ Assessment

• Assess patient's condition before starting therapy and regularly thereafter to monitor drug's effectiveness.
• Frequently monitor patient's blood pressure and pulse rate.
• An elderly patient may be more sensitive to hypotensive effects of drug.
• Be alert for adverse reactions and drug interactions.
• Assess patient's and family's knowledge of drug therapy.

🔅 Nursing diagnoses

• Risk for injury related to presence of hypertension
• Sexual dysfunction related to drug-induced impotence
• Deficient knowledge related to drug therapy

▷ Planning and implementation

• If first dose is larger than 1 mg, severe syncope with loss of consciousness may occur (first-dose syncope).
• 🔅 ALERT: Don't stop therapy abruptly.
• If you suspect compliance problems, discuss twice-daily dose with prescriber.
Patient teaching
• Tell patient not to abruptly stop taking drug, but to call prescriber if unpleasant adverse reactions occur.

• Advise patient to minimize effects of orthostatic hypotension by rising slowly and avoiding sudden position changes.
• Dry mouth can be relieved with sugarless chewing gum, sour hard candy, or ice chips.
• Inform male patient of the possibility of impotence, and advise him to seek counseling to learn how to cope with this adverse effect.

✅ Evaluation

• Patient's blood pressure is normal.
• Patient seeks counseling for alternative methods of sexual gratification because of drug-induced impotence.
• Patient and family state understanding of drug therapy.

prednisolone (systemic)
(pred-NIS-uh-lohn)
Prelone

prednisolone sodium phosphate
Orapred, Orapred ODT, Pediapred

Pharmacologic class: glucocorticoid, mineralocorticoid
Therapeutic class: anti-inflammatory, immunosuppressant
Pregnancy risk category: C

Indications and dosages

▶ **Severe inflammation, modification of body's immune response to disease.** *Adults:* 2.5 to 15 mg prednisolone P.O. b.i.d., t.i.d., or q.i.d. Or, 5 to 60 mg prednisolone sodium phosphate P.O. daily.
Children: Initially, 0.14 to 2 mg/kg prednisolone P.O. or 4 to 60 mg/m^2 prednisolone P.O. daily in four divided doses. Or, initially, 0.14 to 2 mg/kg prednisolone sodium phosphate or 4 to 60 mg/m^2 prednisolone sodium phosphate P.O. daily in three or four divided doses.
▶ **Acute exacerbations of multiple sclerosis.** *Adults:* 200 mg prednisolone sodium phosphate P.O. daily for 1 week, followed by 80 mg every other day.
▶ **Nephrotic syndrome.** *Children:* 60 mg/m^2 prednisolone sodium phosphate P.O. daily in three divided doses for 4 weeks, followed by 4 weeks of single-dose, alternate-day therapy at 40 mg/m^2.

Reactions may be *common*, uncommon, *life-threatening*, or COMMON AND LIFE-THREATENING.

▶ **Uncontrolled asthma in patients taking inhaled corticosteroids and long-acting bronchodilators.** *Children:* 1 to 2 mg/kg prednisolone sodium phosphate P.O. daily in single or divided doses. Short course or "burst" therapy should continue until a child achieves a peak expiratory flow rate of 80% of his personal best or symptoms resolve. This usually requires 3 to 10 days of therapy, although it can take longer. No evidence shows that tapering the dosage after improvement will prevent a relapse.

Contraindications and cautions

• Contraindicated in patients hypersensitive to the drug or any of its components, and in those with fungal infections.
• Use cautiously in patients with recent MI, GI ulcer, renal disease, hypertension, osteoporosis, diabetes mellitus, hypothyroidism, cirrhosis, diverticulitis, nonspecific ulcerative colitis, recent intestinal anastomoses, thromboembolic disorders, seizures, myasthenia gravis, heart failure, tuberculosis, ocular herpes simplex, emotional instability, or psychotic tendencies.
⚖ Lifespan: In pregnant women, use cautiously. In breast-feeding women, high doses aren't recommended.

Adverse reactions

Most reactions to corticosteroids are dose- or duration-dependent.
CNS: euphoria, insomnia, pseudotumor cerebri, psychotic behavior, *seizures.*
CV: edema, *heart failure,* hypertension, *thromboembolism.*
EENT: cataracts, glaucoma.
GI: GI irritation, increased appetite, *pancreatitis, peptic ulceration.*
Metabolic: carbohydrate intolerance, growth suppression in children, hyperglycemia, hypokalemia.
Musculoskeletal: muscle weakness, osteoporosis.
Skin: acne, delayed wound healing, hirsutism, various skin eruptions.
Other: *acute adrenal insufficiency with increased stress (infection, surgery, or trauma) or abrupt withdrawal after long-term therapy;* susceptibility to infections.

Interactions

Drug-drug. *Antihypertensives:* May counteract effect of antihypertensives. Adjust dosage of antihypertensive as needed.
Aspirin, indomethacin, other NSAIDs: Increases risk of GI distress and bleeding. Avoid using together.
Azole antifungals (ketoconazole): May increase corticosteroid effects. Decrease corticosteroid dosage.
Barbiturates, phenytoin, rifampin: May decrease corticosteroid effect. Increase corticosteroid dosage.
Nondepolarizing muscle relaxants: May potentiate or counteract neuromuscular blocking action. Monitor patient closely.
Oral anticoagulants: May alter dosage requirements. Monitor PT and INR closely.
Potassium-depleting drugs (such as thiazide diuretics): May enhance potassium-wasting effects of prednisolone. Monitor potassium level.
Skin-test antigens: May decrease skin-test response. Defer skin testing until therapy is completed.
Toxoids, vaccines: May decrease antibody response and increase risk of neurologic complications. Check with prescriber about when to reschedule vaccine, if possible.

Effects on lab test results

• May increase glucose and cholesterol levels. May decrease potassium and calcium levels.

Pharmacokinetics

Absorption: Absorbed readily after P.O. use; variable with other routes.
Distribution: To muscle, liver, skin, intestine, and kidneys. Extensively protein-bound. Only unbound portion is active.
Metabolism: In liver.
Excretion: Inactive metabolites and small amounts of unmetabolized drug in urine; insignificant amount in feces. *Half-life:* 2 to 4 hours.

Route	Onset	Peak	Duration
P.O.	Rapid	1–2 hr	30–36 hr

Action

Chemical effect: Not clearly defined; decreases inflammation, mainly by stabilizing leukocyte lysosomal membranes; suppresses immune re-

sponse; stimulates bone marrow; and influences protein, fat, and carbohydrate metabolism.
Therapeutic effect: Relieves inflammation and induces immunosuppression.

Available forms

prednisolone
Oral liquid: 5 mg/5 ml, 15 mg/5 ml
Syrup: 15 mg/5 ml
Tablets: 5 mg
prednisolone sodium phosphate
Oral liquid: 5 mg/5 ml, 15 mg/5 ml
Syrup: 5 mg/5 ml, 15 mg/5 ml
Tablets (orally-disintegrating): 10 mg, 15 mg, 30 mg

NURSING PROCESS

Assessment
• Assess patient's condition before starting therapy and regularly thereafter to monitor drug's effectiveness.
• Monitor patient's weight, blood pressure, and electrolyte level.
• Watch for depression or psychotic episodes, especially with high dose.
• Monitor glucose level in a diabetic patient; he may need increase in insulin.
• Monitor patient's stress level; a dosage adjustment may be needed.
• Assess for adequate calcium supplementation.
• Be alert for adverse reactions and drug interactions.
• Assess patient's and family's knowledge of drug therapy.

Nursing diagnoses
• Ineffective health maintenance related to underlying condition
• Ineffective protection related to drug-induced adverse reactions
• Deficient knowledge related to drug therapy

Planning and implementation
• Always adjust to lowest effective dose, which may need to be increased during times of physiologic stress (such as surgery, trauma, or infection).
• Drug may be used for alternate-day therapy.
• Give dose with food when possible to reduce GI irritation.
• Refrigerate Orapred at 36° to 46° F (2° to 8° C).

• Unless contraindicated, give low-sodium diet high in potassium and protein. Give potassium supplements, as needed.
• Notify prescriber immediately if serious adverse reactions occur, and give supportive care.
• After long-term therapy, reduce dose gradually. Abrupt withdrawal may cause rebound inflammation, fatigue, weakness, arthralgia, fever, dizziness, lethargy, depression, fainting, orthostatic hypotension, dyspnea, anorexia, or hypoglycemia. Sudden withdrawal after prolonged use may be fatal.
⑤ **ALERT:** Don't confuse prednisolone with prednisone.

Patient teaching
• Tell patient not to stop drug without the prescriber's knowledge.
• Tell patient that if he misses a dose, he should take it as soon as possible unless it is near the time for his next dose. Tell him not to attempt to make up missed doses that are long overdue.
• Advise patient to take oral form with meals to minimize GI reactions.
⑤ **ALERT:** Tell patient not to cut, crush, or chew the orally-disintegrating tablets.
• Instruct patient to wait to remove the orally disintegrating tablet from the blister pack until he's ready to take it. The tablet can be swallowed whole or allowed to dissolve on the tongue with or without water.
• Warn patient receiving long-term therapy about cushingoid symptoms.
• Teach signs of early adrenal insufficiency: fatigue, muscle weakness, joint pain, fever, anorexia, nausea, dyspnea, dizziness, and fainting.
• Instruct patient to wear or carry medical identification that indicates his need for systemic glucocorticoids during stress.
• Tell patient to report slow healing, sudden weight gain, or swelling.
• Advise patient receiving long-term therapy to exercise or have physical therapy and to ask prescriber about vitamin D or calcium supplements.

Evaluation
• Patient responds well to therapy.
• Patient has no serious adverse reactions.
• Patient and family state understanding of drug therapy.

---

prednisone

(PRED-nih-sohn)

Deltasone, Meticorten, Orasone, Panasol-S, Prednisone Intensol*, Sterapred, Winpred ◆

Pharmacologic class: adrenocorticoid
Therapeutic class: anti-inflammatory, immunosuppressant
Pregnancy risk category: C

Indications and dosages

▶ **Severe inflammation or immunosuppression.** *Adults:* 5 to 60 mg P.O. daily in single or divided doses. Maximum, 250 mg daily. Maintenance dose given once daily or every other day. Dosage must be individualized.
Children: 0.14 to 2 mg/kg P.O. daily in four divided doses.
▶ **Acute exacerbations of multiple sclerosis.** *Adults:* 200 mg P.O. daily for 1 week; then 80 mg P.O. every other day for 1 month.

Contraindications and cautions

• Contraindicated in patients hypersensitive to the drug or any of its components, and in those with systemic fungal infections.
• Use cautiously in patients with GI ulcer, renal disease, hypertension, osteoporosis, diabetes mellitus, hypothyroidism, cirrhosis, diverticulitis, nonspecific ulcerative colitis, recent intestinal anastomoses, thromboembolic disorders, seizures, myasthenia gravis, heart failure, tuberculosis, ocular herpes simplex, emotional instability, or psychotic tendencies.
⚕ **Lifespan:** In pregnant women, use cautiously. In breast-feeding women, high doses aren't recommended.

Adverse reactions

Most reactions are dose- or duration-dependent.
CNS: *euphoria, insomnia,* pseudotumor cerebri, psychotic behavior, *seizures.*
CV: edema, *heart failure,* hypertension, *thromboembolism.*
EENT: cataracts, glaucoma.
GI: GI irritation, increased appetite, *peptic ulceration, pancreatitis.*
Metabolic: carbohydrate intolerance, growth suppression in children, hyperglycemia, hypokalemia.

Musculoskeletal: muscle weakness, osteoporosis.
Skin: acne, delayed wound healing, hirsutism, various skin eruptions.
Other: susceptibility to infections.

Interactions

Drug-drug. *Antihypertensives:* May counteract effect of antihypertensives. Adjust dosage of antihypertensive as needed.
Aspirin, indomethacin, other NSAIDs: May increase risk of GI distress and bleeding. Give together cautiously.
Barbiturates, phenytoin, rifampin: May decrease corticosteroid effect. Increase corticosteroid dosage.
Ketoconazole: May increase steroid effects. Decrease glucocorticoid dosage.
Oral anticoagulants: May alter dosage requirements. Monitor PT and INR closely.
Potassium-depleting drugs (such as thiazide diuretics): May enhance potassium-wasting effects of prednisone. Monitor potassium level.
Skin-test antigens: May decrease skin test response. Defer skin testing until therapy is completed.
Toxoids, vaccines: May decrease antibody response and increases risk of neurologic complications. Don't give together.

Effects on lab test results

• May increase ALT, AST, alkaline phosphatase, glucose, and cholesterol levels. May decrease potassium and calcium levels.

Pharmacokinetics

Absorption: Absorbed readily after P.O. use.
Distribution: To muscle, liver, skin, intestine, and kidneys. Extensively protein-bound. Only unbound portion is active.
Metabolism: In liver.
Excretion: Inactive metabolites and small amounts of unmetabolized drug in urine; insignificant amounts in feces. *Half-life:* 1 hour.

Route	Onset	Peak	Duration
P.O.	Varies	Varies	Varies

Action

Chemical effect: Not clearly defined; decreases inflammation; suppresses immune response; stimulates bone marrow; and influences protein, fat, and carbohydrate metabolism.

Therapeutic effect: Relieves inflammation and induces immunosuppression.

Available forms

Oral solution: 5 mg/5 ml*, 5 mg/ml (concentrate)*
Syrup: 5 mg/5 ml*
Tablets: 1 mg, 2.5 mg, 5 mg, 10 mg, 20 mg, 50 mg

NURSING PROCESS

⚡ Assessment
• Assess patient's condition before starting therapy and regularly thereafter to monitor drug's effectiveness.
• Monitor patient's weight, blood pressure, and electrolyte level.
• Watch for depression or psychotic episodes, especially when given in high doses.
• Monitor glucose level in a diabetic patient; he may need an increase in insulin.
• Monitor patient's stress level; dosage adjustment may be needed.
• Be alert for adverse reactions and drug interactions.
• Assess patient's and family's knowledge of drug therapy.

⊕ Nursing diagnoses
• Ineffective health maintenance related to underlying condition
• Ineffective protection related to drug-induced adverse reactions
• Deficient knowledge related to drug therapy

▷ Planning and implementation
• Always adjust to lowest effective dosage, which may need to be increased during times of physiologic stress (such as surgery, trauma, or infection).
• Drug may be used for alternate-day therapy.
• For better results and less toxicity, give once-daily dose in morning.
• Give oral dose with food to reduce GI irritation.
• After long-term therapy, reduce dosage gradually. Abruptly stopping the drug may cause rebound inflammation, fatigue, weakness, arthralgia, fever, dizziness, lethargy, depression, fainting, orthostatic hypotension, dyspnea, anorexia, or hypoglycemia. After long-term therapy, increased stress or abrupt withdrawal may cause acute adrenal insufficiency. Sudden withdrawal after prolonged use may be fatal.
• Unless contraindicated, give low-sodium diet high in potassium and protein. Give potassium supplements, as needed.
• If serious adverse reactions occur, notify prescriber immediately and give supportive care.
⚠ **ALERT:** Don't confuse prednisone with prednisolone.

Patient teaching
• Tell patient not to stop taking the drug without prescriber's knowledge.
• Advise patient to take oral form with meals to minimize GI reactions.
• Tell patient to report sudden weight gain, swelling, or slow healing.
• Advise patient receiving long-term therapy to exercise or have physical therapy, to ask prescriber about vitamin D or calcium supplements, and to have periodic eye examinations.
• Instruct patient to wear or carry medical identification that indicates his need for systemic glucocorticoids during stress.
• Warn patient receiving long-term therapy about cushingoid symptoms.
• Teach signs of early adrenal insufficiency: fatigue, muscular weakness, joint pain, fever, anorexia, nausea, dyspnea, dizziness, and fainting.

✓ Evaluation
• Patient responds well to therapy.
• Patient doesn't experience serious adverse reactions.
• Patient and family state understanding of drug therapy.

pregabalin
(preh-GAH-bah-linn)
Lyrica

Pharmacologic class: CNS drug
Therapeutic class: analgesic, anticonvulsant
Pregnancy risk category: C
Controlled substance schedule: V

Indications and dosages

▶ **Diabetic peripheral neuropathy.** *Adults:* Initially, 50 mg P.O. t.i.d. May increase to 100 mg P.O. t.i.d. within 1 week.
▶ **Fibromyalgia.** *Adults:* 75 mg P.O. b.i.d. May increase to 150 mg P.O. b.i.d. within 1 week

based upon patient response. Maximum dosage, 450 mg/day.

▶ **Postherpetic neuralgia.** *Adults:* Initially, 75 mg P.O. b.i.d. or 50 mg P.O. t.i.d. May increase to 300 mg/day in two or three equally divided doses within 1 week. If pain relief is insufficient after 2 to 4 weeks, may increase to 300 mg b.i.d. or 200 mg t.i.d.

▶ **Adjunctive treatment of partial onset seizures.** *Adults:* Initially, 75 mg P.O. b.i.d. or 50 mg P.O. t.i.d. Range, 150 to 600 mg/day.

▧ **Adjust-a-dose:** In patients with renal impairment, if creatinine clearance is 30 to 60 ml/minute, give 75 to 300 mg/day in two to three divided doses. If clearance is 15 to 30 ml/minute, give 25 to 150 mg/day in one dose or divided into two doses. If clearance is less than 15 ml/minute, give 25 to 75 mg/day in one dose.

If patient undergoes hemodialysis, give one supplemental dose according to these guidelines. If patient takes 25 mg daily, give 25 or 50 mg. If patient takes 25 to 50 mg daily, give 50 or 75 mg. If patient takes 75 mg daily, give 100 or 150 mg.

Contraindications and cautions

• Contraindicated in patients hypersensitive to pregabalin or any of its components.
• Use cautiously in patients with New York Heart Association Class III or Class IV heart failure.

♨ **Lifespan:** Use drug in pregnancy only if benefits outweigh risks to the fetus. It isn't known whether drug appears in breast milk. Patient should either stop breast-feeding or stop drug. Safety and effectiveness haven't been established in pediatric patients. Older adults may be more sensitive to side effects.

Adverse reactions

CNS: abnormal gait, abnormal thinking, amnesia, anxiety, asthenia, *ataxia,* confusion, depersonalization, *dizziness,* euphoria, headache, hypesthesia, hypertonia, incoordination, myoclonus, nervousness, nystagmus, paresthesia, somnolence, stupor, tremor, twitching, vertigo.
CV: edema, PR interval prolongation.
EENT: blurred or abnormal vision, conjunctivitis, diplopia, eye disorder, otitis media, tinnitus.
GI: abdominal pain, constipation, dry mouth, flatulence, gastroenteritis, vomiting.
GU: anorgasmia, impotence, urinary frequency, urinary incontinence.

Metabolic: HYPOGLYCEMIA, increased or decreased appetite, *weight gain.*
Musculoskeletal: arthralgia, back and chest pain, leg cramps, myalgia, myasthenia, neuropathy.
Respiratory: bronchitis, dyspnea.
Skin: ecchymosis, pruritus.
Other: accidental injury, *allergic reaction,* decreased libido, flu syndrome, infection, pain.

Interactions

Drug-drug. *CNS depressants:* May have additive effects on cognitive and gross motor function. Monitor patient for increased dizziness and somnolence.
Pioglitazone, rosiglitazone: May cause additive fluid retention and weight gain. Monitor patient closely.
Drug-lifestyle. *Alcohol use:* May have additive depressant effects on cognitive and gross motor function. Discourage alcohol use.

Effects on lab test results

• May increase CK level.
• May decrease platelet count.

Pharmacokinetics

Absorption: Well absorbed. Bioavailability exceeds 90%. Rate but not extent of absorption is decreased when drug is taken with food.
Distribution: Steady state is achieved in 24 to 48 hours. Not plasma protein–bound.
Metabolism: Negligible.
Excretion: Nearly proportional to creatinine clearance. About 90% eliminated via the kidneys as unchanged drug. *Half-life:* 6½ hours.

Route	Onset	Peak	Duration
P.O.	Unknown	1½–3 hr	Unknown

Action

Chemical effect: Drug may contribute to analgesic and anticonvulsant effects by binding to sites in CNS.
Therapeutic effect: Prevents seizure activity; relieves nerve pain caused by diabetic peripheral neuropathy or postherpetic neuralgia.

Available forms

Capsules: 25 mg, 50 mg, 75 mg, 100 mg, 150 mg, 200 mg, 225 mg, 300 mg

NURSING PROCESS

Assessment
• Assess patient's seizure disorder or diabetic peripheral neuropathy or postherpetic neuralgia prior to therapy and regularly thereafter.
• Monitor patient's weight and fluid status, especially if he has heart failure.
• Check for changes in vision.
• Watch for signs of rhabdomyolysis, such as dark, red, or cola-colored urine; muscle tenderness; generalized weakness; or muscle stiffness or aching.
• Evaluate patient's and family's knowledge of drug therapy.

Nursing diagnoses
• Risk for injury related to seizure disorder
• Acute pain related to diabetic peripheral neuropathy or postherpetic neuralgia
• Deficient knowledge related to drug therapy

Planning and implementation
• Taper drug gradually over at least 1 week. Stopping abruptly may result in increased seizure frequency, insomnia, headache, nausea, and diarrhea.
• In the case of overdose, treatment is supportive. Four hours of hemodialysis removes about 50% of drug. Contact poison control center.
Patient teaching
• Explain that drug may be taken with or without food.
• Warn patient not to stop drug abruptly.
• Caution patient to avoid hazardous activities until drug's effects are known.
• Instruct patient to watch for weight changes and water retention.
• Advise patient to report vision changes and malaise or fever accompanied by muscle pain, tenderness, or weakness.
• Inform a woman of childbearing age to immediately report planned or suspected pregnancy to prescriber.
• Tell a man who plans to father a child to consult prescriber about risks to fetus.
• If patient has diabetes, urge him to inspect his skin closely for ulcer formation.

Evaluation
• Patient does not experience seizures while taking drug.
• Patient reports pain relief.

• Patient and family state understanding of drug therapy.

primidone
(PRIH-mih-dohn)
Mysoline

Pharmacologic class: barbiturate analogue
Therapeutic class: anticonvulsant
Pregnancy risk category: D

Indications and dosages

▶ **Generalized tonic-clonic, focal, and complex-partial (psychomotor) seizures.**
Adults and children age 8 and older: Initially, 100 to 125 mg P.O. at bedtime on days 1 to 3; then 100 to 125 mg P.O. b.i.d. on days 4 to 6; then 100 to 125 mg P.O. t.i.d. on days 7 to 9; followed by maintenance dose of 250 mg P.O. t.i.d. to q.i.d.; maximum dose, 2 g daily.
Children younger than age 8: Initially, 50 mg P.O. at bedtime for 3 days; then 50 mg P.O. b.i.d. for 4 to 6 days; then 100 mg P.O. b.i.d. for 7 to 9 days; followed by maintenance dosage of 125 to 250 mg P.O. t.i.d., or 10 to 25 mg/kg daily in divided doses.
▶ **Benign familial tremor (essential tremor).**
Adults: 750 mg P.O. daily.
Adjust a dose: In patients receiving other anticonvulsants, primidone should be started at 100 mg to 125 mg at bedtime and gradually increased. This should be continued until satisfactory drug levels are achieved for combination or the other medication is discontinued. When primidone alone is the objective, the transition should be completed in less than 2 weeks.

Contraindications and cautions

• Contraindicated in patients with phenobarbital hypersensitivity or porphyria.
Lifespan: In pregnant and breast-feeding women, drug is contraindicated.

Adverse reactions

CNS: *ataxia, drowsiness,* emotional disturbances, fatigue, hyperirritability, vertigo.
CV: edema.
EENT: *diplopia,* edema of eyelids, nystagmus.
GI: anorexia, nausea, thirst, vomiting.
GU: impotence, polyuria.

Reactions may be *common,* uncommon, *life-threatening,* or **COMMON AND LIFE-THREATENING.**

Hematologic: eosinophilia, *leukopenia, thrombocytopenia.*
Skin: alopecia, morbilliform rash.

Interactions

Drug-drug. *Acetazolamide:* May decrease primidone level. Monitor patient for effect.
Anticoagulants: May decrease anticoagulant effects. Adjust anticoagulant dosage as needed.
Carbamazepine: May decrease primidone level and increase carbamazepine level. Observe patient for lack of effect or carbamazepine toxicity.
Corticosteroids: May decrease corticosteroid effects. Avoid use together, if possible.
Doxycycline: May decrease doxycycline effects. Consider alternative tetracycline.
Estrogen, oral contraceptives: May decrease contraceptive effectiveness. Recommend alternative contraceptive method.
Felodipine, methadone, metronidazole, nifedipine, quinidine, theophylline: May decrease effectiveness of these drugs. Consider increased dosage.
Isoniazid, nicotinamide: May increase primidone level. Monitor patient for toxicity.
Metoprolol, propranolol: May reduce the effects of these drugs. Consider an increased beta blocker dosage.
Phenytoin: May increase conversion of primidone to phenobarbital. Observe patient for increased phenobarbital effect.
Valproic acid: May increase primidone level. Consider decreased primidone dosage.
Drug-herb. *Glutamate:* May antagonize anticonvulsant effects of drug. Discourage using together.
Drug-lifestyle. *Alcohol use:* May impair coordination, increase CNS effects, and cause death. Strongly discourage use together.

Effects on lab test results

• May decrease hemoglobin level and hematocrit.
• May increase eosinophil count. May decrease WBC and platelet counts.

Pharmacokinetics

Absorption: Absorbed readily.
Distribution: Wide.
Metabolism: Slow, by liver, to phenylethylmalonamide (PEMA) and phenobarbital; PEMA is the major metabolite.
Excretion: In urine. *Half-life:* 5 to 15 hours.

Route	Onset	Peak	Duration
P.O.	Unknown	3–4 hr	Unknown

Action

Chemical effect: Unknown; some activity may be caused by PEMA and phenobarbital.
Therapeutic effect: Prevents seizures.

Available forms

Oral suspension: 250 mg/5 ml
Tablets: 50 mg, 250 mg

NURSING PROCESS

Assessment
• Assess patient's condition before starting therapy and regularly thereafter to monitor drug's effectiveness.
• Monitor blood drug level. Therapeutic primidone level is 5 to 12 mcg/ml. Therapeutic phenobarbital level is 15 to 40 mcg/ml.
• Monitor CBC and routine blood chemistry every 6 months.
• Monitor patient's hydration throughout drug therapy.
• Assess patient's and family's knowledge of drug therapy.

Nursing diagnoses
• Risk for trauma related to seizures
• Risk for deficient fluid volume related to adverse reactions
• Deficient knowledge related to drug therapy

Planning and implementation
• Shake liquid suspension well.
• Don't abruptly stop giving the drug, because seizures may worsen.
• Call prescriber immediately if adverse reactions develop.
ALERT: Don't confuse primidone with prednisone.
Patient teaching
• Advise patient to avoid hazardous activities until the drug's CNS effects are known.
• Warn patient and parents not to stop drug suddenly.
• Tell patient that full therapeutic response may take 2 weeks or longer.

Evaluation
• Patient is free from seizure activity.

• Patient maintains adequate hydration throughout drug therapy.
• Patient and family state understanding of drug therapy.

probenecid
(proh-BEN-uh-sid)

Pharmacologic class: sulfonamide derivative
Therapeutic class: uricosuric
Pregnancy risk category: B

Indications and dosages

▶ **Adjunct to penicillin therapy.** *Adults and children older than age 14 or who weigh more than 50 kg (110 lb):* 500 mg P.O. q.i.d.
Children ages 2 to 14 or who weigh 50 kg or less: Initially, 25 mg/kg P.O.; then 40 mg/kg in divided doses q.i.d.
▶ **Gonorrhea.** *Adults:* 3.5 g ampicillin P.O. with 1 g probenecid P.O. given together. Or, 1 g probenecid P.O. 30 minutes before 4.8 million units of aqueous penicillin G procaine I.M., injected at two different sites.
▶ **Hyperuricemia of gout, gouty arthritis.**
Adults: 250 mg P.O. b.i.d. for first week; then 500 mg b.i.d., to maximum of 3 g daily. Reevaluate maintenance dosage every 6 months and reduce in increments of 500 mg.
▶ **To diagnose parkinsonian syndrome or mental depression‡.** *Adults:* 500 mg P.O. every 12 hours for 5 doses.
▧ **Adjust-a-dose:** For patients with renal impairment with a GFR of 30 ml/minute or greater, dosage may need to be increased. Increases can be made in 0.5 g increments every 4 weeks. Usual daily dose is 2 g or less.

Contraindications and cautions

• Contraindicated in patients hypersensitive to the drug or any of its components, and in patients with uric acid kidney stones, blood dyscrasias, or acute gout attack.
• Use cautiously in patients with history of allergy to sulfa drugs; peptic ulcer or renal impairment.
⚘ **Lifespan:** In pregnant women, use cautiously. In breast-feeding women, use cautiously; it's unknown if the drug appears in breast milk. In children younger than age 2, drug is contraindicated.

Adverse reactions

CNS: dizziness, fever, headache.
CV: flushing, hypotension.
GI: anorexia, *gastric distress,* nausea, sore gums, vomiting.
GU: renal colic, urinary frequency.
Hematologic: *aplastic anemia,* hemolytic anemia, *leukopenia.*
Hepatic: *hepatic necrosis.*
Skin: alopecia, dermatitis, pruritus.
Other: *anaphylaxis,* hypersensitivity reaction.

Interactions

Drug-drug. *Methotrexate:* May impair excretion of methotrexate, causing increased level, effects, and toxicity. Monitor level closely and adjust dosage accordingly.
NSAIDs: May increase NSAID level and increase risk of toxicity. Adjust dosage, as needed.
Oral antidiabetics: May enhance hypoglycemic effect. Monitor glucose level closely. Dosage adjustment may be needed.
Rifampin: May decrease rifampin level. Monitor patient for lack of effect.
Salicylates: May inhibit uricosuric effect of probenecid, causing urate retention. Don't use together.
Sulfonamides: May decrease sulfonamide excretion. Monitor patient for signs of toxicity.
Sulfonylureas: May increase half-life of these drugs. Monitor blood glucose.
Zidovudine: May increase absorption of zidovudine. Monitor patient for cutaneous drug eruption, malaise, myalgia, and fever.
Drug-lifestyle. *Alcohol use:* May increase urate level. Discourage using together.

Effects on lab test results

• May decrease hemoglobin level and hematocrit.
• May falsely elevate theophylline level. May cause false-positive glucose test results with Benedict's solution or Clinitest.

Pharmacokinetics

Absorption: Complete.
Distribution: Throughout body. About 75% protein-bound.
Metabolism: In liver to active metabolites, with some uricosuric effect.
Excretion: Drug and metabolites in urine; probenecid is actively reabsorbed but metabo-

lites aren't. *Half-life:* 3 to 8 hours after 500-mg dose, 6 to 12 hours after larger doses.

Route	Onset	Peak	Duration
P.O.	Unknown	2–4 hr	8 hr

Action

Chemical effect: Blocks renal tubular reabsorption of uric acid, increasing excretion, and inhibits active renal tubular secretion of many weak organic acids, such as penicillins and cephalosporins.
Therapeutic effect: Lowers uric acid and prolongs penicillin action.

Available forms

Tablets: 500 mg

NURSING PROCESS

Assessment
• Assess patient's condition before starting therapy and regularly thereafter to monitor drug's effectiveness.
• Periodically monitor BUN and renal function tests in patient on long-term therapy.
• Be alert for adverse reactions and drug interactions.
• If adverse GI reactions occur, monitor patient's hydration.
• Assess patient's and family's knowledge of drug therapy.

Nursing diagnoses
• Ineffective health maintenance related to underlying condition
• Risk for deficient fluid volume related to adverse GI reactions
• Deficient knowledge related to drug therapy

Planning and implementation
• Drug is ineffective in patients with chronic renal insufficiency and a GFR less than 30 ml/minute.
• Give drug with milk, food, or antacids to minimize GI distress. Continued disturbances may indicate need to lower dosage.
• Encourage patient to drink to maintain minimum daily output of 2 L of water a day. Alkalinize urine with sodium bicarbonate or potassium citrate. These measures will prevent hematuria, renal colic, urate stone development, and costovertebral pain.

• Therapy doesn't start until acute attack subsides. Drug contains no analgesic or anti-inflammatory drug and isn't useful during acute gout attacks.
• Drug may increase frequency, severity, and duration of acute gout attacks during first 6 to 12 months of therapy. Prophylactic colchicine or another anti-inflammatory is given during first 3 to 6 months.
ALERT: Don't confuse probenecid with Procanbid.
Patient teaching
• Instruct patient to take drug with food or milk to minimize GI distress.
• Advise patient with gout to avoid all drugs that contain aspirin, which may precipitate gout. Acetaminophen may be used for pain.
• Tell patient with gout to avoid alcohol during drug therapy; it increases urate level.
• Tell patient with gout to limit intake of foods high in purine, such as anchovies, liver, sardines, kidneys, sweetbreads, peas, and lentils.
• Instruct patient and family that drug must be taken regularly or gout attacks may result. Tell patient to visit prescriber regularly so uric acid can be monitored and dosage adjusted, if needed. Lifelong therapy may be required in patients with hyperuricemia.

Evaluation
• Patient responds positively to therapy.
• Patient maintains adequate hydration.
• Patient and family state understanding of drug therapy.

HIGH ALERT

procainamide hydrochloride
(proh-KAYN-uh-mighd high-droh-KLOR-ighd)
Pronestyl

Pharmacologic class: procaine derivative
Therapeutic class: antiarrhythmic
Pregnancy risk category: C

Indications and dosages

▶ **Symptomatic PVCs; life-threatening ventricular tachycardia.** *Adults:* 100 mg every 5 minutes by slow I.V. push, no faster than 25 to 50 mg/minute, until arrhythmias disappear, adverse effects develop, or 500 mg have been given. Or, give a loading dose of 500 to 600 mg I.V. infusion over 25 to 30 minutes. Maximum

total dose is 1 g. When arrhythmias disappear, give continuous infusion of 2 to 6 mg/minute. If arrhythmias recur, repeat bolus and increase infusion rate. For I.M. administration, give 50 mg/kg/day divided every 3 to 6 hours; for arrhythmias during surgery, 100 to 500 mg I.M. For oral therapy, start with 50 mg/kg P.O. of conventional tablets or capsules in divided doses every 3 hours until therapeutic level is reached. For the maintenance dosage, substitute sustained-release form every 6 hours or extended-release form (Procanbid) at dose of 50 mg/kg P.O. in two divided doses every 12 hours.

Children‡: Dosage not established. Recommendations include 10 to 15 mg/kg I.V. over 15 minutes or 1 mg/kg every 3 to 5 minutes up to a total of 15 mg/kg over 1 hour. Recommended maintenance dosage is 50 mg to 100 mg/kg over 24 hours in divided doses every 4 hours or continuous infusion at 20 to 80 mEq/kg/min, not exceeding 100 mg/kg dose or 2 g in 24 hours.

Adjust-a-dose: For patients with renal or hepatic dysfunction, decrease dose or give at longer intervals.

▶ **To maintain normal sinus rhythm after conversion of atrial flutter‡.** *Adults:* 0.5 to 1 g P.O. of conventional tablets or capsules every 4 to 6 hours.

▶ **Loading dose to prevent atrial fibrillation or paroxysmal atrial tachycardia‡.** *Adults:* 1.25 g P.O. of conventional tablets or capsules. If arrhythmias persist after 1 hour, give additional 750 mg. If no change occurs, give 500 mg to 1 g P.O. every 2 hours until arrhythmias disappear or adverse effects occur. Maintenance dose is 1 g extended release every 6 hours.

▶ **Malignant hyperthermia‡.** *Adults:* 200 to 900 mg I.V., followed by an infusion.

▼ I.V. administration

• Vials for I.V. injection contain 1 g of drug: 100 mg/ml (10 ml) or 500 mg/ml (2 ml).
• Use infusion control device to give infusion precisely.
• Keep patient in supine position during I.V. use. If drug is given too rapidly, hypotension can occur. Watch closely for adverse reactions during infusion, and notify prescriber if they occur.
• Patient receiving infusions must be monitored at all times.
• If solution becomes discolored, check with pharmacy and expect to discard.

⊗ Incompatibilities

Bretylium, esmolol, ethacrynate, milrinone, phenytoin sodium.

Contraindications and cautions

• Contraindicated in patients hypersensitive to procaine and related drugs; in those with complete, second-, or third-degree heart block in absence of artificial pacemaker; and in those with myasthenia gravis or systemic lupus erythematosus. Also contraindicated in patients with atypical ventricular tachycardia (torsades de pointes) because procainamide may aggravate this condition.
• Use cautiously to treat ventricular tachycardia during coronary occlusion. Also use cautiously in patients with hepatic or renal insufficiency, blood dyscrasias, bone marrow suppression, heart failure, or other conduction disturbances, such as bundle-branch heart block, sinus bradycardia, or digoxin intoxication.

Lifespan: In pregnant women, use cautiously. In breast-feeding women, drug isn't recommended. In children, safety and effectiveness haven't been established.

Adverse reactions

CNS: confusion, depression, dizziness, fever, hallucinations.
CV: AV block, bradycardia, *heart failure*, hypotension, *ventricular asystole, ventricular fibrillation* after parenteral use.
GI: anorexia, bitter taste with large doses, diarrhea, nausea, vomiting.
Hematologic: *agranulocytosis*, hemolytic anemia, *neutropenia* (especially with sustained-release forms), *thrombocytopenia*.
Musculoskeletal: *myalgia*.
Skin: maculopapular rash, urticaria, pruritus.
Other: *lupuslike syndrome* (especially after prolonged use).

Interactions

Drug-drug. *Amiodarone:* May increase procainamide level and toxicity with additive effects on QT interval and QRS complex. Avoid using together.
Anticholinergics: May have additive anticholinergic effects. Monitor patient closely.
Anticholinesterases: May decrease anticholinesterase effect. Anticholinesterase dose may need to be increased.

Cimetidine: May increase procainamide level. Avoid this combination if possible. Monitor procainamide level closely and adjust the dosage as needed.

Lidocaine: May have additive cardiodepressant effects. Monitor ECG.

Neuromuscular skeletal muscle relaxants: May increase skeletal muscle relaxant effects. Monitor patient.

Propranolol, ranitidine: May increase procainamide level. Monitor patient for toxicity.

Quinidine, trimethoprim: May elevate procainamide and N-acetylprocainamide (NAPA) levels. Monitor patient for toxicity.

Quinolones: May increase procainamide level and risk of life threatening arrhythmias. Adjust dosage as needed.

Drug-herb. *Jimson weed:* May adversely affect CV function. Discourage using together.

Licorice: May prolong QT interval and be additive. Discourage using together.

Drug-lifestye. *Alcohol:* May alter action of procanamide. Discourage use together.

Effects on lab test results

• May increase ALT, AST, alkaline phosphatase, LDH, and bilirubin levels. May decrease hemoglobin level and hematocrit.

• May increase antinuclear antibody titer. May decrease neutrophil, granulocyte, and platelet counts.

Pharmacokinetics

Absorption: Usually 75% to 95% of P.O. dose. Rapid after I.M. dose.

Distribution: Wide in most body tissues, including CSF, liver, spleen, kidneys, lungs, muscles, brain, and heart. About 15% to 20% protein-bound.

Metabolism: In liver.

Excretion: In urine. *Half-life:* About 2½ to 4¾ hours.

Route	Onset	Peak	Duration
P.O.	Unknown	1–2 hr	Unknown
I.V.	Immediate	Immediate	Unknown
I.M.	10–30 min	15–60 min	Unknown

Action

Chemical effect: Class IA antiarrhythmic that decreases excitability, conduction velocity, automaticity, and membrane responsiveness with prolonged refractory period. Larger doses may induce AV block.

Therapeutic effect: Restores normal sinus rhythm.

Available forms

Capsules: 250 mg, 375 mg, 500 mg
Injection: 500 mg/ml
Tablets: 375 mg, 500 mg
Tablets (extended-release): 250 mg, 500 mg, 750 mg, 1,000 mg

NURSING PROCESS

℞ Assessment

• Assess patient's condition before starting therapy and regularly thereafter to monitor drug's effectiveness.

• Monitor level of procainamide and its active metabolite, NAPA. To suppress ventricular arrhythmias, therapeutic level of procainamide is 4 to 8 mcg/ml; therapeutic level of NAPA is 10 to 30 mcg/ml.

• Monitor QT interval closely in patient with renal impairment.

• Hypokalemia predisposes patient to arrhythmias; monitor electrolytes, especially potassium level.

• Monitor blood pressure and ECG continuously during I.V. use. Watch for prolonged QT intervals and QRS complexes, heart block, or increased arrhythmias.

• Monitor CBC frequently during first 3 months, particularly in patient taking sustained-release form.

• Be alert for adverse reactions and drug interactions.

• Assess patient's and family's knowledge of drug therapy.

⊕ Nursing diagnoses

• Decreased cardiac output related to presence of arrhythmia

• Ineffective protection related to adverse hematologic reactions

• Deficient knowledge related to drug therapy

▷ Planning and implementation

⚡ **ALERT:** Some drug products contain tartrazine and sulfites. Ask if patient is allergic to these agents.

⑤ **ALERT:** If blood pressure changes significantly or ECG changes occur, withhold drug, obtain rhythm strip, and notify prescriber immediately.
⑤ **ALERT:** Don't confuse procainamide with probenecid.

• Positive antinuclear antibody titer occurs in about 60% of patients without lupuslike symptoms. This response seems to be related to prolonged use, not to dosage. May progress to systemic lupus erythematosus if drug isn't stopped.

Patient teaching

• Instruct patient to report fever, rash, muscle pain, diarrhea, bleeding, bruises, or pleuritic chest pain.

• Stress importance of taking drug exactly as prescribed. This may require use of alarm clock for nighttime doses.

• Inform patient taking extended-release form that wax-matrix "ghost" from tablet may be passed in stool. Assure patient that drug is completely absorbed before this occurs.

• Tell patient not to crush or break sustained-release or extended-release tablets.

☑ Evaluation

• Patient regains normal cardiac output after drug stops abnormal heart rhythm.

• Patient maintains normal CBC.

• Patient and family state understanding of drug therapy.

HIGH ALERT

procarbazine hydrochloride
(proh-KAR-buh-zeen high-droh-KLOR-ighd)
Matulane

Pharmacologic class: alkylating agent
Therapeutic class: antineoplastic
Pregnancy risk category: D

Indications and dosages

▶ **Hodgkin lymphoma, non-Hodgkin lymphoma‡, brain tumors‡, small-cell lung cancer‡, melanoma‡, mycosis fungoides‡, and multiple myeloma‡.** *Adults:* 2 to 4 mg/kg P.O. daily in single dose or divided doses for first week. Then, 4 to 6 mg/kg daily until WBC count decreases to less than 4,000/mm³ or platelet count decreases to less than 100,000/mm³. If hematologic toxicity occurs, resume at 1 to 2 mg/kg daily.

Children: 50 mg/m² P.O. daily for first week; then 100 mg/m² until response or toxicity occurs. Maintenance dosage is 50 mg/m² P.O. daily after bone marrow recovery.

Contraindications and cautions

• Contraindicated in patients hypersensitive to the drug or any of its components and in those with inadequate bone marrow reserve as shown by bone marrow aspiration.

• Use cautiously in patients with impaired hepatic or renal function.

🜲 **Lifespan:** In pregnant and breast-feeding women, drug isn't recommended.

Adverse reactions

CNS: *coma,* confusion, depression, *hallucinations,* insomnia, nervousness, neuropathy, nightmares, paresthesia, *seizures.*
CV: *hypotension, tachycardia, syncope.*
EENT: nystagmus, photophobia, retinal hemorrhage.
GI: anorexia, constipation, diarrhea, dry mouth, dysphagia, nausea, stomatitis, *vomiting.*
GU: *urinary frequency, nocturia.*
Hematologic: anemia, *bleeding tendency, leukopenia, thrombocytopenia.*
Hepatic: *hepatotoxicity.*
Respiratory: *pleural effusion,* pneumonitis.
Skin: dermatitis, reversible alopecia.

Interactions

Drug-drug. *CNS depressants:* May have additive depressant effects. Avoid using together.
Digoxin: May decrease digoxin level. Monitor level closely.
Levodopa: May cause flushing and a significant rise in blood pressure within 1 hour of levodopa use. Separate administration times; monitor patient's blood pressure closely.
Local anesthetics, sympathomimetics, tricyclic antidepressants: May cause tremors, palpitations, and increased blood pressure. Monitor patient closely.
Opioids: May cause severe hypotension and death. Don't give together.
Drug-food. *Caffeine:* May result in arrhythmias, severe hypertension. Discourage caffeine intake.
Foods high in tyramine (cheese, red wine): May cause tremors, palpitations, and increased blood pressure. Monitor patient closely.

Drug-lifestyle. *Alcohol use:* May cause mild disulfiram-like reaction. Warn patient to avoid alcohol.

Effects on lab test results

• May increase liver enzyme level. May decrease hemoglobin level and hematocrit.
• May increase eosinophil count. May decrease platelet, WBC, and RBC counts.

Pharmacokinetics

Absorption: Rapid and complete.
Distribution: Wide; throughout body tissues, with highest levels in liver, kidneys, intestinal wall, and skin. Drug crosses blood-brain barrier.
Metabolism: Extensive in liver; some metabolites have cytotoxic activity.
Excretion: Drug and metabolites excreted mainly in urine. *Half-life:* Unknown.

Route	Onset	Peak	Duration
P.O.	Unknown	1 hr	Unknown

Action

Chemical effect: Unknown; thought to inhibit DNA, RNA, and protein synthesis.
Therapeutic effect: Kills selected cancer cells.

Available forms

Capsules: 50 mg

NURSING PROCESS

Assessment
• Assess patient's condition before starting therapy and regularly thereafter to monitor drug's effectiveness.
• Monitor CBC and platelet counts.
• Be alert for adverse reactions and drug interactions.
• Assess patient's and family's knowledge of drug therapy.

Nursing diagnoses
• Ineffective health maintenance related to presence of neoplastic disease
• Ineffective protection related to adverse hematologic reactions
• Deficient knowledge related to drug therapy

Planning and implementation
• Give drug at bedtime to lessen nausea.

⑤ ALERT: If patient becomes confused or if paresthesia or other neuropathies develop, stop giving the drug and notify prescriber.

Patient teaching
• Advise patient to take drug at bedtime and in divided doses.
• Warn patient to watch for signs of infection (fever, sore throat, fatigue) and bleeding (easy bruising, nosebleeds, bleeding gums, melena). Tell him to take his temperature daily.
• Warn patient not to drink alcohol during therapy.
• Tell patient to stop taking the drug and immediately notify the prescriber if disulfiram-like reaction occurs (chest pains, rapid or irregular heartbeat, severe headache, stiff neck).
• Tell patient to avoid foods high in tyramine, such as cheese, yogurt, and bananas.
• Warn patient to avoid hazardous activities until the drug's CNS effects are known.
• Advise woman of childbearing age not to become pregnant during therapy, and to consult with prescriber before becoming pregnant.

☑ Evaluation
• Patient responds well to therapy.
• Patient develops no serious adverse hematologic reactions.
• Patient and family state understanding of drug therapy.

prochlorperazine
(proh-klor-PER-ah-zeen)
Compazine, Compro

prochlorperazine edisylate
Compazine, Compazine Syrup

prochlorperazine maleate
Compazine, Compazine Spansule

Pharmacologic class: phenothiazine (piperazine derivative)
Therapeutic class: antiemetic, antipsychotic, anxiolytic
Pregnancy risk category: C

Indications and dosages

▶ **Preoperative nausea control.** *Adults:* 5 to 10 mg I.M. 1 to 2 hours before induction of anesthesia; repeat once in 30 minutes, if needed.

Or, 5 to 10 mg I.V. 15 to 30 minutes before induction of anesthesia; repeat once if needed. Or, 20 mg/L D$_5$W or normal saline solution by I.V. infusion. Begin infusion 15 to 30 minutes before induction of anesthesia.

► **Severe nausea and vomiting.** *Adults:* 5 to 10 mg P.O., t.i.d. or q.i.d. Or, 15 mg P.O. (sustained-release) on arising. Or, 10-mg sustained-release form P.O. every 12 hours. Or, 25 mg P.R., b.i.d. Or, 5 to 10 mg I.M. repeated every 3 to 4 hours, p.r.n. Or, 2.5 to 10 mg may be given I.V. Maximum parenteral dose is 40 mg daily.

Children who weigh 18 to 39 kg (40 to 85 lb): 2.5 mg P.O. or P.R., t.i.d. Or, 5 mg P.O. or P.R., b.i.d. Maximum dose is 15 mg daily. Or, give 0.132 mg/kg by deep I.M. injection. Control usually is obtained with one dose.

Children who weigh 14 to 18 kg (30 to 39 lb): 2.5 mg P.O. or P.R., b.i.d. or t.i.d. Maximum dose, 10 mg daily. Or give 0.132 mg/kg by deep I.M. injection. Control usually is obtained with one dose.

Children who weigh 9 to 13 kg (20 to 29 lb): 2.5 mg P.O. or P.R. once daily or b.i.d. Maximum dose, 7.5 mg daily. Or give 0.132 mg/kg by deep I.M. injection. Control usually is obtained with one dose.

► **To manage symptoms of psychotic disorders.** *Adults and children age 12 and older:* 5 to 10 mg P.O., t.i.d. or q.i.d.

Children ages 2 to 12: Give 2.5 mg P.O. or P.R., b.i.d. or t.i.d. Don't exceed 10 mg on day 1. Increase dosage gradually to recommended maximum, if needed. In children ages 2 to 5, maximum daily dose is 20 mg. In children ages 6 to 12, maximum daily dose is 25 mg.

► **To manage symptoms of severe psychoses.** *Adults and children age 12 and older:* 10 to 20 mg I.M. repeated in 1 to 4 hours, if needed. Rarely, patients may require 10 to 20 mg every 4 to 6 hours. Institute P.O. therapy after symptoms are controlled.

Children ages 2 to 12: Give 0.13 mg/kg I.M. then switch to oral dose.

► **Nonpsychotic anxiety.** *Adults:* 5 mg P.O., t.i.d. or q.i.d. Or, give 15-mg extended-release capsule once daily or 10-mg extended-release capsule every 12 hours.

▼ I.V. administration

• Drug may be given undiluted or diluted in an isotonic solution.

• Don't give faster than 5 mg/minute. Don't give by bolus injection.

⊗ **Incompatibilities**
Aldesleukin, allopurinol, amifostine, aminophylline, amphotericin B, ampicillin sodium, aztreonam, calcium gluconate, chloramphenicol sodium succinate, chlorothiazide, dexamethasone sodium phosphate, dimenhydrinate, etoposide, filgrastim, fludarabine, foscarnet, furosemide, gemcitabine, heparin sodium, hydrocortisone sodium succinate, hydromorphone, ketorolac, solutions containing methylparabens, midazolam hydrochloride, morphine, penicillin G potassium, penicillin G sodium, pentobarbital, phenobarbital sodium, phenytoin sodium, piperacillin sodium and tazobactam sodium, solutions containing propylparabens, thiopental, vitamin B complex with C.

Contraindications and cautions

• Contraindicated in patients hypersensitive to phenothiazines, patients with CNS depression (including coma), patients undergoing pediatric surgery, patients taking adrenergic blockers, and patients under the influence of alcohol.

• Use cautiously in patients who have been exposed to extreme heat and patients with impaired CV function, glaucoma, or seizure disorders.

▲ **Lifespan:** In pregnant women, drug is contraindicated except in cases of continuous nausea and vomiting when benefits outweigh risk to the fetus. In breast-feeding women, use cautiously; it's unknown if the drug appears in breast milk. In acutely ill children, use cautiously. In children younger than age 2 who weigh less than 9 kg (20 lb), drug is contraindicated. In the elderly, use cautiously, and gradually increase the dosage.

Adverse reactions

CNS: dizziness, EEG changes, *extrapyramidal reactions,* **neuroleptic malignant syndrome,** pseudoparkinsonism, sedation, tardive dyskinesia.
CV: ECG changes, *orthostatic hypotension,* tachycardia.
EENT: blurred vision, ocular changes.
GI: constipation, dry mouth.
GU: dark urine, inhibited ejaculation, menstrual irregularities, *urine retention.*
Hematologic: *agranulocytosis,* hyperprolactinemia, *transient leukopenia.*
Hepatic: cholestatic jaundice.

Reactions may be *common*, uncommon, *life-threatening*, or COMMON AND LIFE-THREATENING.

Metabolic: increased appetite, weight gain.
Skin: exfoliative dermatitis, *mild photosensitivity.*
Other: allergic reactions, gynecomastia.

Interactions

Drug-drug. *Antacids:* May inhibit absorption of oral phenothiazines. Separate antacid doses by at least 2 hours.
Anticholinergics, including antidepressants and antiparkinsonian drugs: May increase anticholinergic activity and aggravated parkinsonian symptoms. Use together cautiously.
Anticonvulsants: Phenothiazines may lower the seizure threshold. Adjust anticonvulsant dosage as needed.
Barbiturates: May decrease phenothiazine effect. Monitor patient for decreased effect.
CNS depressants: May cause additive CNS effects. Use together cautiously.
Lithium: May cause disorientation, unconsciousness, and extrapyramidal symptoms. Monitor patient closely.
Drug-herb. *Dong quai, St. John's wort:* May increase photosensitivity reactions. Discourage using together.
Ginkgo: May decrease effects of phenothiazines. Monitor patient.
Kava: May increase risk of dystonic reactions. Discourage using together.
Milk thistle: May decrease liver toxicity caused by phenothiazines. Monitor liver enzyme level if used together.
Yohimbe: May increase risk for yohimbe toxicity when used together. Discourage using together.
Drug-lifestyle. *Alcohol use:* May increase CNS depression, particularly decreasing psychomotor skills. Strongly discourage alcohol use.
Sun exposure: May cause photosensitivity reaction. Urge patient to avoid unprotected or prolonged sun exposure.

Effects on lab test results

• May decrease WBC and granulocyte counts. May alter liver function test values.
• May cause false-positive results for PKU, urobilinogen, amylase, uroporphyrins, porphobilinogens, and 5-hydroxyindolacetic acid levels. May cause false-positive pregnancy test.

Pharmacokinetics

Absorption: Erratic and variable with P.O. tablets; more predictable with P.O. concentrate. Unknown for P.R. use. Rapid for I.M. use.
Distribution: Widely into body. 91% to 99% protein-bound.
Metabolism: Extensively by liver, but no active metabolites are formed.
Excretion: Mainly in urine; some in feces.
Half-life: Unknown.

Route	Onset	Peak	Duration
P.O.	30–40 min	Unknown	3–12 hr
I.V.	Immediate	Immediate	Unknown
I.M.	10–20 min	Unknown	3–4 hr
P.R.	60 min	Unknown	3–4 hr

Action

Chemical effect: Acts on chemoreceptor trigger zone to inhibit nausea and vomiting; in larger doses, partially depresses vomiting center.
Therapeutic effect: Relieves nausea and vomiting, signs and symptoms of psychosis, and anxiety.

Available forms

prochlorperazine
Injection: 5 mg/ml
Suppositories: 2.5 mg, 5 mg, 25 mg
Tablets: 5 mg, 10 mg
prochlorperazine edisylate
Injection: 5 mg/ml
Syrup: 5 mg/5 ml
prochlorperazine maleate
Capsules (sustained-release): 10 mg, 15 mg
Tablets: 5 mg, 10 mg

NURSING PROCESS

Assessment

• Assess patient's condition before starting therapy and regularly thereafter to monitor drug's effectiveness.
• Watch for orthostatic hypotension, especially when giving drug by I.V. route.
• Monitor CBC and liver function test results during long-term therapy.
• Be alert for adverse reactions and drug interactions.
• Assess patient's and family's knowledge of drug therapy.

⊕ Nursing diagnoses
- Risk for deficient fluid volume related to nausea and vomiting
- Disturbed thought processes related to presence of psychosis
- Deficient knowledge related to drug therapy

▶ Planning and implementation
- Dilute solution with tomato or fruit juice, milk, coffee, carbonated beverage, tea, water, or soup; or mix with pudding.
- Inject I.M. deep into upper outer quadrant of gluteal region.
- Don't give subcutaneously or mix in syringe with another drug.
- Avoid getting concentrate or injection solution on hands or clothing.
- Drug is used only if vomiting can't be otherwise controlled or if only a few doses are needed. If more than four doses are needed in 24 hours, notify prescriber.
- Store drug in light-resistant container. Slight yellowing doesn't affect potency; discard extremely discolored solutions.

Patient teaching
- Tell patient to mix oral solution with flavored liquid to mask taste.
- Advise patient to wear protective clothing when exposed to sunlight.
- Tell patient to notify prescriber about adverse reactions.

☑ Evaluation
- Patient's nausea and vomiting are relieved.
- Patient's behavior and communication show better thought processes.
- Patient and family state understanding of drug therapy.

promethazine hydrochloride
(proh-METH-uh-zeen high-droh-KLOR-ighd)
Phenadoz, Phenergan*

Pharmacologic class: phenothiazine derivative
Therapeutic class: antiemetic, antihistamine, sedative
Pregnancy risk category: C

Indications and dosages

▶ **Motion sickness.** *Adults:* Give 25 mg P.O. or P.R. b.i.d. Take initial dose 30 to 60 minutes before anticipated travel, and repeat in 8 to 12 hours, p.r.n.
Children older than age 2: Give 12.5 to 25 mg P.O. or P.R. or 0.5 mg/kg.

▶ **Nausea and vomiting.** *Adults:* Give 12.5 to 25 mg P.O., I.M., or P.R. every 4 hours, p.r.n.
Children older than age 2: Give 0.5 mg/kg.

▶ **Rhinitis, allergy symptoms.** *Adults:* Give 12.5 mg P.O. or P.R. q.i.d. (before meals and at bedtime). Or, 25 mg P.O. or P.R. at bedtime.
Children older than age 2: Give 6.25 to 12.5 mg P.O. or P.R. t.i.d. Or, 25 mg P.O. or P.R. at bedtime.

▶ **Sedation.** *Adults:* Give 25 to 50 mg P.O., P.R., or I.M. at bedtime or p.r.n.
Children older than age 2: Give 12.5 to 25 mg P.O., I.M., or P.R. at bedtime.

▶ **Routine preoperative or postoperative sedation or adjunct to analgesics.** *Adults:* Give 25 to 50 mg I.M., I.V., P.R., or P.O.
Children older than age 2: Give 0.5 to 1.1 mg/ kg I.M., P.R., or P.O. or 12.5 mg to 25 mg.

▶ **Prevention of blood transfusion reactions.** *Adults:* Give 25 mg before or during blood transfusion.

▼ I.V. administration

- Don't give in concentration greater than 25 mg/ml or at rate exceeding 25 mg/minute.
- Shield I.V. solution from direct light.

⊗ **Incompatibilities**
Aldesleukin, allopurinol, aminophylline, amphotericin B, cephalosporins, chloramphenicol sodium succinate, chloroquine phosphate, chlorothiazide, diatrizoate meglumine (34.3%) and diatrizoate sodium (35%), diatrizoate meglumine (52%) and diatrizoate sodium (8%), diatrizoate sodium (75%), dimenhydrinate, doxorubicin liposomal, foscarnet, furosemide, heparin sodium, hydrocortisone sodium succinate, iodipamide meglumine (52%), iothalamate meglumine (60%), iothalamate sodium (80%), ketorolac, methohexital, morphine, nalbuphine, penicillin G potassium and sodium, pentobarbital sodium, phenobarbital sodium, phenytoin sodium, thiopental, vitamin B complex.

Contraindications and cautions

- Contraindicated in patients hypersensitive to the drug or any of its components, and in those with intestinal obstruction, prostatic hyperplasia, bladder-neck obstruction, seizure disorders,

coma, CNS depression, or stenosing peptic ulcerations.
• Use cautiously in patients with pulmonary, hepatic, or CV disease or asthma.
• Avoid combining drug with other respiratory depressants.
🏃 **Lifespan:** In pregnant women, safety and effectiveness haven't been established. In breast-feeding women, neonates, premature neonates, and acutely ill or dehydrated children, drug is contraindicated. Don't use in children for nausea and vomiting when the cause of the vomiting is unknown. In children younger than age 2, drug is contraindicated. Use with caution in children ages 2 and older, using the lowest effective dose and watch for respiratory depressant effects. In the elderly, use cautiously.

Adverse reactions

CNS: confusion, *drowsiness* (especially geriatric patients), extrapyramidal reactions, restlessness, sedation, tremors.
CV: ECG changes, hypotension.
EENT: nasal congestion, transient myopia.
GI: anorexia, constipation, *dry mouth,* nausea, vomiting.
GU: urine retention.
Hematologic: *agranulocytosis, leukopenia, thrombocytopenia.*
Respiratory: *respiratory depression* (in children).
Skin: photosensitivity, venous thrombosis at injection site.

Interactions

Drug-drug. *CNS depressants:* May increase sedation. Use together cautiously.
Epinephrine: May block or reverse effects of epinephrine. Use another vasopressor.
Levodopa: May decrease antiparkinsonian action of levodopa. Avoid using together.
Lithium: May reduce GI absorption or enhance renal elimination of lithium. Avoid using together.
MAO inhibitors: May increase extrapyramidal effects. Don't use together.
Drug-herb. *Dong quai, St. John's wort:* May increase photosensitivity reactions. Discourage using together.
Kava: May increase risk of dystonic reactions. Discourage using together.
Yohimbe: May increase risk of yohimbe toxicity when used together. Discourage using together.

Drug-lifestyle. *Alcohol use:* May increase sedation. Discourage using together.
Sun exposure: May cause photosensitivity reaction. Urge patient to avoid unprotected or prolonged sun exposure.

Effects on lab test results

• May increase glucose and hemoglobin levels and hematocrit.
• May decrease WBC, platelet, and granulocyte counts.
• May cause false-positive immunologic urine pregnancy test using Gravindex and false-negative results using Prepurex or Dap tests. May interfere with blood typing of ABO group.

Pharmacokinetics

Absorption: Well absorbed after P.O. use; fairly rapid after P.R. or I.M. use.
Distribution: Widely throughout body.
Metabolism: In liver.
Excretion: In urine and feces. *Half-life:* Unknown.

Route	Onset	Peak	Duration
P.O.	15–60 min	Unknown	≤ 12 hr
I.V.	3–5 min	Unknown	≤ 12 hr
I.M., P.R.	20 min	Unknown	≤ 12 hr

Action

Chemical effect: Competes with histamine for H4-receptor sites on effector cells. Prevents, but doesn't reverse, histamine-mediated responses.
Therapeutic effect: Prevents motion sickness and relieves nausea, nasal congestion, and allergy symptoms. Also promotes calmness.

Available forms

promethazine hydrochloride
Injection: 25 mg/ml, 50 mg/ml (I.M. use only)
Suppositories: 12.5 mg, 25 mg, 50 mg
Syrup: 6.25 mg/5 ml*
Tablets: 12.5 mg, 25 mg, 50 mg
promethazine theoclate
Tablets: 25 mg†

NURSING PROCESS

🔍 Assessment

• Assess patient's condition before starting therapy and regularly thereafter to monitor drug's effectiveness.

- Be alert for adverse reactions and drug interactions.
- Assess patient's and family's knowledge of drug therapy.

Nursing diagnoses
- Ineffective health maintenance related to underlying condition
- Risk for injury related to drug's sedating effects
- Deficient knowledge related to drug therapy

❯ Planning and implementation
- Pronounced sedative effect limits use in many ambulatory patients.
- Drug is used as adjunct to analgesics (usually to increase sedation); it has no analgesic activity.
- Give drug with food or milk to reduce GI distress.
- **ALERT:** Phenergan brand ampules contain sulfite. Check patient for sulfite allergy before administering Phenergan I.M.
- Inject I.M. deep into large muscle mass. Rotate injection sites.
- Don't give subcutaneously.
- Drug may be safely mixed with meperidine (Demerol) in same syringe.
- In patient scheduled for myelogram, stop drug 48 hours before procedure and don't resume giving the drug until 24 hours after the procedure, because of risk of seizures.
- **ALERT:** Caution should be used in children age 2 and older. This includes using the lowest effective dose, monitoring for respiratory depressant effects and avoiding combining promethazine hydrochloride with other drugs that are known to depress the respiratory system.

Patient teaching
- When treating for motion sickness, tell patient to take first dose 30 to 60 minutes before travel. Tell him to take dose after rising and with evening meal on next days of travel.
- Warn patient not to drink alcohol or engage in hazardous activities until the drug's CNS effects are known.
- Tell patient that coffee or tea may reduce drowsiness. Sugarless gum, sugarless sour hard candy, or ice chips may relieve dry mouth.
- Warn patient about photosensitivity and precautions to avoid it.
- Advise patient to stop drug 4 days before allergy skin tests.

☑ Evaluation
- Patient responds well to therapy.
- Patient doesn't experience injury from adverse reactions.
- Patient and family state understanding of drug therapy.

propafenone hydrochloride
(proh-puh-FEE-nohn high-droh-KLOR-ighd)
Rythmol, Rythmol SR

Pharmacologic class: sodium channel antagonist
Therapeutic class: antiarrhythmic (class IC)
Pregnancy risk category: C

Indications and dosages

❯ **Suppression of life-threatening ventricular arrhythmias, such as sustained ventricular tachycardia; prevention of supraventricular tachycardia associated with disabling symptoms and for disabling paroxysmal atrial fibrillation/flutter.** *Adults:* Initially, 150 mg P.O. every 8 hours. May increase dose at 3- to 4-day intervals to 225 mg every 8 hours. If needed, increase dosage to 300 mg every 8 hours. Maximum daily dosage is 900 mg.
Adjust-a-dose: For patients with hepatic failure, manufacturer recommends dosage reduction of 20% to 30%.

Contraindications and cautions

- Contraindicated in patients hypersensitive to the drug or any of its components, and in those with severe or uncontrolled heart failure, cardiogenic shock, bradycardia, marked hypotension, bronchospastic disorders, electrolyte imbalance, or SA, AV, or intraventricular disorders of impulse conduction in absence of pacemaker.
- Use cautiously in patients with heart failure because propafenone can have negative inotropic effect. Also use cautiously in patients taking other cardiac depressant drugs and in those with hepatic or renal impairment.
- **Lifespan:** In pregnant women, safety and effectiveness haven't been established. In breast-feeding women, drug isn't recommended. In children, safety and effectiveness haven't been established.

Adverse reactions

CNS: anxiety, ataxia, dizziness, drowsiness, fatigue, headache, insomnia, syncope, tremor, weakness.

CV: atrial fibrillation, *bradycardia*, bundle branch block, *heart failure*, chest pain, edema, first-degree AV block, hypotension, increased QRS duration, intraventricular conduction delay, palpitations, *proarrhythmic events (ventricular tachycardia, PVCs)*.

EENT: blurred vision.

GI: abdominal pain or cramps, anorexia, constipation, diarrhea, dry mouth, dyspepsia, flatulence, nausea, unusual taste, vomiting.

Musculoskeletal: joint pain.

Respiratory: dyspnea.

Skin: diaphoresis, rash.

Interactions

Drug-drug. *Antiarrhythmics:* May increase risk of heart failure. Monitor patient closely.

Cimetidine: May decrease metabolism of propafenone. Monitor patient for toxicity.

Cyclosporine, theophylline: May increase concentrations of these drugs. Monitor for toxicity.

Digoxin, oral anticoagulants: May increase levels of these drugs by about 35% to 85%, resulting in toxicity. Monitor patient's PT, INR, and digoxin level closely.

Local anesthetics: May increase risk of CNS toxicity. Monitor patient closely.

Metoprolol, propranolol: May slow metabolism of these drugs. Monitor patient for toxicity.

Quinidine: May slow propafenone metabolism. Avoid using together.

Rifampin: May increase propafenone clearance. Monitor patient for lack of effect.

Ritonavir, SSRIs: May increase propafenone level. Avoid using together.

Effects on lab test results

• May cause positive ANA titers.

Pharmacokinetics

Absorption: Good. Because of significant first-pass effect, bioavailability is limited, but it increases with dosage.

Distribution: 97% protein-bound.

Metabolism: In liver.

Excretion: Mainly in feces; some in urine.

Half-life: 2 to 32 hours.

Route	Onset	Peak	Duration
P.O.	Unknown	≤ 3½ hr	Unknown

Action

Chemical effect: Reduces inward sodium current in Purkinje and myocardial cells. Decreases excitability, conduction velocity, and automaticity in AV nodal, His-Purkinje, and intraventricular tissue; causes slight but significant prolongation of refractory period in AV nodal tissue.

Therapeutic effect: Restores normal sinus rhythm.

Available forms

Capsules (extended-release): 225 mg, 325 mg, 425 mg

Tablets: 150 mg, 225 mg, 300 mg

NURSING PROCESS

Assessment

• Assess patient's condition before starting therapy and regularly thereafter to monitor drug's effectiveness.

• Continuous cardiac monitoring is recommended at start of therapy and during dosage adjustments.

• Be alert for adverse reactions and drug interactions.

• Assess patient's and family's knowledge of drug therapy.

Nursing diagnoses

• Decreased cardiac output related to presence of arrhythmia

• Ineffective protection related to drug-induced proarrhythmias

• Deficient knowledge related to drug therapy

Planning and implementation

• Give drug with food to minimize adverse GI reactions.

⚠ **ALERT:** If PR interval or QRS complex increases by more than 25%, notify prescriber because reduction in dose may be needed.

• During use with digoxin, monitor ECG and digoxin level frequently.

Patient teaching

• Tell patient to take drug with food.

• Stress importance of taking drug exactly as ordered.

• Warn patient to avoid hazardous activities if adverse CNS disturbances occur.

P

☑ **Evaluation**
• Patient regains adequate cardiac output when arrhythmia is corrected.
• Patient doesn't develop any proarrhythmic events.
• Patient and family state understanding of drug therapy.

propoxyphene hydrochloride (dextropropoxyphene hydrochloride)

(proh-POK-sih-feen high-droh-KLOR-ighd)
642 ◆ , Darvon

propoxyphene napsylate (dextropropoxyphene napsylate)

Darvon-N

Pharmacologic class: opioid
Therapeutic class: analgesic
Pregnancy risk category: C
Controlled substance schedule: IV

Indications and dosages

▶ **Mild to moderate pain.** *Adults:* 65 mg propoxyphene hydrochloride P.O. every 4 hours, p.r.n. Maximum, 390 mg P.O. daily. Or, 100 mg propoxyphene napsylate P.O. every 4 hours, p.r.n. Maximum, 600 mg P.O. daily.

Contraindications and cautions

• Contraindicated in patients hypersensitive to the drug or any of its components, and in patients who are suicidal or addiction-prone.
• Use cautiously in patients with hepatic or renal disease, emotional instability, or history of drug or alcohol abuse.
☆ **Lifespan:** In pregnant women, use cautiously. In breast-feeding women, use cautiously; drug is found in breast milk, although no adverse reactions have occurred in infants receiving breast milk. In children, safety and effectiveness haven't been established.

Adverse reactions

CNS: *dizziness,* euphoria, headache, insomnia, paradoxical excitement, sedation.
GI: constipation, nausea, vomiting.
Respiratory: *respiratory depression.*
Other: physical and psychological dependence.

Interactions

Drug-drug. *Barbiturate anesthetics:* May increase respiratory and CNS depression. Use together cautiously.
Carbamazepine: May increase carbamazepine level. Monitor level closely.
CNS depressants: May have additive effects. Use together cautiously.
Protease inhibitors: May increase CNS and respiratory depression. Monitor patient.
Warfarin: May increase anticoagulant effect. Monitor PT and INR and patient for bleeding.
Drug-lifestyle. *Alcohol use:* May have additive effects. Discourage using together.

Effects on lab test results

• May increase or decrease liver function test values.
• May cause false decreases in urinary steroid excretion tests.

Pharmacokinetics

Absorption: Mainly in upper small intestine.
Distribution: Drug enters CSF.
Metabolism: In liver; about one-quarter of dose is metabolized to norpropoxyphene, an active metabolite.
Excretion: In urine. *Half-life:* 6 to 12 hours.

Route	Onset	Peak	Duration
P.O.	15 min–1 hr	2–2½ hr	4–6 hr

Action

Chemical effect: Binds with opioid receptors in CNS, altering both perception of and emotional response to pain through unknown mechanism.
Therapeutic effect: Relieves pain.

Available forms

propoxyphene hydrochloride
Capsules: 65 mg
propoxyphene napsylate
Tablets: 100 mg

NURSING PROCESS

🔍 **Assessment**
• Assess patient's pain before and after giving drug.
• Be alert for adverse reactions and drug interactions.
• If adverse GI reaction occurs, monitor patient's hydration.

Reactions may be *common,* uncommon, *life-threatening,* or COMMON AND LIFE-THREATENING.

• Assess patient's and family's knowledge of drug therapy.

⚕ Nursing diagnoses
• Acute pain related to underlying condition
• Risk for deficient fluid volume related to GI upset
• Deficient knowledge related to drug therapy

⟫ Planning and implementation
• Give with food to minimize adverse GI reactions.
• Consider giving laxative to prevent constipation.
• Drug can be considered a mild opioid analgesic, but pain relief is equivalent to that provided by aspirin. Tolerance and physical dependence have been observed. Typically used with aspirin or acetaminophen to maximize analgesia.
⚠ **ALERT:** A dose of 65 mg of propoxyphene hydrochloride equals 100 mg of propoxyphene napsylate.
Patient teaching
• Advise patient to take drug with food or milk to minimize GI upset.
⚠ **ALERT:** Warn patient not to exceed recommended dosage. Respiratory depression, hypotension, profound sedation, and coma may result if used in excess or with other CNS depressants. Products that contain propoxyphene alone or with other drugs are major cause of drug-related overdose and death.
• Advise patient not to drink alcohol during therapy.
• Warn ambulatory patient about getting out of bed or walking. Warn outpatient to avoid driving and other hazardous activities until drug's CNS effects are known.

☑ Evaluation
• Patient is free from pain.
• Patient maintains adequate hydration.
• Patient and family state understanding of drug therapy.

---

propranolol hydrochloride
(proh-PRAH-nuh-lohl high-droh-KLOR-ighd)
Inderal, Inderal LA, InnoPran XL, Novopranol ♦

Pharmacologic class: beta blocker
Therapeutic class: antianginal, antiarrhythmic, antihypertensive
Pregnancy risk category: C

Indications and dosages

▶ **Angina pectoris.** *Adults:* Total daily dosages of 80 to 320 mg P.O. when given b.i.d., t.i.d., or q.i.d. Or, one 80-mg extended-release capsule daily.
▶ **Mortality reduction after MI.** *Adults:* 180 to 240 mg P.O. daily in divided doses beginning 5 to 21 days after MI. Usually given t.i.d. or q.i.d.
▶ **Supraventricular, ventricular, and atrial arrhythmias; tachyarrhythmias caused by excessive catecholamine action during anesthesia.** *Adults:* 1 to 3 mg by slow I.V. push, not to exceed 1 mg/minute. After 3 mg have been given, another dose may be given in 2 minutes; subsequent doses, no sooner than every 4 hours. May be diluted and infused slowly. Usual maintenance dosage is 10 to 30 mg P.O. t.i.d. to q.i.d.
▶ **Hypertension.** *Adults:* Initially, 80 mg P.O. daily in two to four divided doses or extended-release form once daily. Increase at 3- to 7-day intervals to maximum daily dose of 640 mg. Usual maintenance dosage is 120 to 240 mg daily in two or three divided doses or 120 to 160 mg sustained-release once daily. Or, 80 mg InnoPran XL P.O. once daily at bedtime. Take consistently with or without food. Adjust to maximum of 120 mg daily if needed.
Children‡: Begin with 1 mg/kg. Usual dosage is 2 mg to 4 mg/kg in 2 equally divided doses.
▶ **Prevention of frequent, severe, uncontrollable, or disabling migraine or vascular headache.** *Adults:* Initially, 80 mg P.O. daily in divided doses or one extended-release capsule daily. Usual maintenance dosage is 160 to 240 mg daily.
▶ **Essential tremor.** *Adults:* 40 mg (tablets, solution) P.O. b.i.d. Usual maintenance dosage is 120 to 320 mg daily in three divided doses.
▶ **Hypertrophic subaortic stenosis.** *Adults:* 20 mg to 40 mg P.O. t.i.d. or q.i.d. before meals

P

---

and at bedtime or 80 to 160 mg extended-release capsule daily.

▶ **Adjunct therapy in pheochromocytoma.**
Adults: 60 mg P.O. daily in divided doses with alpha blocker 3 days before surgery.

▼ I.V. administration

• Drug is compatible with D_5W, half-normal and normal saline solutions, and lactated Ringer's solution.
• Give drug by direct injection into large vessel or I.V. line containing free-flowing, compatible solution; continuous I.V. infusion generally isn't recommended.
• Or dilute drug with normal saline solution and give by intermittent infusion over 10 to 15 minutes in 0.1- to 0.2-mg increments.
⊗ **Incompatibilities**
Amphotericin B, diazoxide.

Contraindications and cautions

• Contraindicated in patients with bronchial asthma, sinus bradycardia, heart block greater than first-degree, cardiogenic shock, or overt cardiac failure (unless failure is secondary to tachyarrhythmia that can be treated with propranolol).
• Use cautiously in patients taking other antihypertensives and in those with renal impairment, nonallergic bronchospastic diseases, Wolff-Parkinson-White syndrome, hepatic disease, diabetes mellitus (drug blocks some symptoms of hypoglycemia), or thyrotoxicosis (drug may mask some signs of that disorder).
※ **Lifespan:** In pregnant women, use cautiously. Small placenta and congenital anomalies in babies have occurred when mothers received propranolol. In breast-feeding women, drug isn't recommended.

Adverse reactions

CNS: dizziness (InnoPran XL), *fatigue,* fever, hallucinations, lethargy, mental depression, vivid dreams.
CV: *bradycardia, heart failure,* hypotension, intermittent claudication.
GI: constipation (InnoPran XL), diarrhea, nausea, vomiting.
Hematologic: *agranulocytosis.*
Musculoskeletal: arthralgia.
Respiratory: increased airway resistance.
Skin: rash.

Interactions

Drug-drug. *Aminophylline, theophylline:* May act antagonistically reducing the effects of one or both drugs. May reduce theophylline elimination. Monitor theophylline level and patient closely.
Amiodarone, fluconazole, fluoxetine, isoniazid, paroxetine, ritonavir, rizatriptan, zolmitriptan: May increase propranolol level. Use together cautiously.
Amobarbital, aprobarbital, butabarbital, butalbital, mephobarbital, pentobarbital, phenobarbital, primidone, secobarbital: May reduce propranolol effects. Increase beta blocker dose.
Cimetidine: May increase pharmacologic effects of beta blocker. Consider a different H_2-agonist or decrease the beta blocker dose.
Digoxin, diltiazem, verapamil: May cause hypotension, bradycardia, and increased depressant effect on myocardium. Use together cautiously.
Epinephrine: May cause an initial hypertensive episode followed by bradycardia. Stop the beta blocker 3 days before anticipated epinephrine use. Monitor patient closely.
Glucagon, isoproterenol: May antagonize propranolol effect. May be used therapeutically and in emergencies.
Hydralazine: May increase levels and pharmacologic effects of both drugs. Monitor patient closely. Dosage adjustment of either drug may be needed.
Insulin: May mask symptoms of hypoglycemia (such as tachycardia) as a result of beta blockade. Use cautiously in patients with diabetes.
Lidocaine I.V.: May reduce hepatic metabolism of lidocaine, increasing the risk of toxicity. Give bolus doses of lidocaine at a slower rate and monitor lidocaine level closely.
Oral antidiabetics: May alter requirements for these drugs in previously stabilized diabetic patients. Monitor patient for hypoglycemia.
Prazosin: May increase the risk of orthostatic hypotension in the early phases of use together. Assist patient to stand slowly until effects are known.
Verapamil: May increase the effects of both drugs. Monitor cardiac function closely and decrease dosages as needed.
Drug-herb. *Ginkgo:* May alter drug level. Discourage use of herb.
Melatonin: May reverse the negative effects of drug on nocturnal sleep. Advise patient to discuss use with prescriber.

Reactions may be *common,* uncommon, *life-threatening,* or COMMON AND LIFE-THREATENING.

Drug-lifestyle. *Alcohol:* May increase drug level. Use together cautiously.
Cocaine use: May increase angina-inducing potential of cocaine. Inform patient of this potentially dangerous combination.

Effects on lab test results

• May increase BUN, transaminase, alkaline phosphatase, and LDH levels.
• May decrease granulocyte count.
• May interfere with glaucoma screening test.

Pharmacokinetics

Absorption: Almost complete, and enhanced when given with food. Food increases the lag time and the time to maximum concentration of InnoPran XL.
Distribution: Widely throughout body. More than 90% protein-bound.
Metabolism: Almost totally in liver. P.O. form undergoes extensive first-pass metabolism.
Excretion: About 96% to 99% in urine as metabolites; remainder in feces as unchanged drug and metabolites. *Half-life:* About 4 hours; 8 hours for InnoPran XL.

Route	Onset	Peak	Duration
P.O.	30 min	60–90 min	12 hr
P.O. extended-release	Unknown	12–14 hr	24 hr
I.V.	≤1 min	≤1 min	< 5 min

Action

Chemical effect: Reduces cardiac oxygen demand by blocking catecholamine-induced increases in heart rate, blood pressure, and force of myocardial contraction. Depresses renin secretion and prevents vasodilation of cerebral arteries.
Therapeutic effect: Relieves anginal and migraine pain, lowers blood pressure, restores normal sinus rhythm, and helps limit MI damage.

Available forms

Capsules (extended-release): 60 mg, 80 mg, 120 mg, 160 mg
Injection: 1 mg/ml
Oral solution: 4 mg/ml, 8 mg/ml, 80 mg/ml (concentrate)
Tablets: 10 mg, 20 mg, 40 mg, 60 mg, 80 mg, 90 mg

NURSING PROCESS

Assessment
• Assess patient's condition before starting therapy and regularly thereafter to monitor drug's effectiveness.
• Frequently monitor blood pressure, ECG, and heart rate and rhythm, especially when giving by I.V. route.
• Be alert for adverse reactions and drug interactions.
• Assess patient's and family's knowledge of drug therapy.

Nursing diagnoses
• Ineffective health maintenance related to underlying condition
• Impaired gas exchange related to airway resistance
• Deficient knowledge related to drug therapy

Planning and implementation
• Check patient's apical pulse before therapy. If extremes in pulse rate occur, don't give the drug and immediately call the prescriber.
⑨ **ALERT:** Don't confuse Inderal with Inderide or Isordil.
• Double-check dose and route. I.V. doses are much smaller than oral doses.
• Give oral drug with meals. Food may increase absorption.
• Don't stop giving the drug before surgery for pheochromocytoma. Before any surgical procedure, notify anesthesiologist that patient is taking propranolol.
• If patient develops severe hypotension, notify prescriber; vasopressor may be prescribed.
• In an elderly patient, adverse reactions may increase and he may need an adjusted dose.
• Don't abruptly stop giving the drug.
• For overdose, give I.V. isoproterenol, I.V. atropine, or glucagon; refractory cases may require pacemaker.
Patient teaching
• Teach patient how to check pulse rate, and tell him to do so before each dose. Tell him to notify prescriber if rate changes significantly.
• Tell patient that taking drug twice a day or as extended-release capsule may improve compliance. Advise him to check with prescriber.
• Advise patient to continue taking drug as prescribed, even when he's feeling well. Tell him

P

not to stop drug suddenly because doing so can worsen angina and MI.

☑ Evaluation
- Patient responds well to therapy.
- Patient maintains adequate gas exchange.
- Patient and family state understanding of drug therapy.

propylthiouracil (PTU)
(proh-pil-thigh-oh-YOOR-uh-sil)
Propyl-Thyracil ◆

Pharmacologic class: thyroid hormone antagonist
Therapeutic class: antithyroid agent
Pregnancy risk category: D

Indications and dosages

▶ **Hyperthyroidism.** *Adults:* 300 to 400 mg P.O. daily in divided doses. Patients with severe hyperthyroidism or very large goiters may need initial doses of 600 to 900 mg daily. Continue until patient is euthyroid; then start maintenance dose of 100 mg to 150 mg P.O. daily.
Children age 10 and older: Initially, 150 to 300 mg P.O. daily in divided doses. Continue until patient is euthyroid. Individualize maintenance dosage.
Children ages 6 to 10: Initially, 50 to 150 mg P.O. daily in divided doses every 8 hours. Continue until patient is euthyroid. Individualize maintenance dosage.
Neonates and children: 5 to 7 mg/kg P.O. daily in divided doses every 8 hours, or give according to age as above.
▶ **Thyrotoxic crisis.** *Adults:* 200 mg P.O. every 4 to 6 hours on first day; after symptoms are under control, gradually reduce dosage to usual maintenance level.
▶ **To reduce mortality caused by alcoholic liver disease‡.** *Adults:* 300 mg/day.

Contraindications and cautions

- Contraindicated in patients hypersensitive to the drug or any of its components.
- ☀ **Lifespan:** In pregnant women, use cautiously. Pregnant women may need a lower dose as pregnancy progresses; monitor thyroid function studies closely. In breast-feeding women, drug is contraindicated.

Adverse reactions

CNS: drowsiness, headache, vertigo.
CV: vasculitis.
EENT: visual disturbances.
GI: diarrhea, loss of taste, *nausea,* salivary gland enlargement, *vomiting* (may be dose-related).
Hematologic: *agranulocytosis, aplastic anemia, leukopenia,* lymphadenopathy, *thrombocytopenia.*
Hepatic: jaundice, *hepatotoxicity.*
Metabolic: dose-related hypothyroidism (mental depression; cold intolerance; hard, nonpitting edema).
Musculoskeletal: arthralgia, myalgia.
Skin: pruritus, rash, skin discoloration, urticaria.
Other: drug-induced fever.

Interactions

Drug-drug. *Aminophylline, oxtriphylline, theophylline:* May decrease drug clearance. Dosage may need adjustment.
Anticoagulants: May increase anticoagulant effects. Monitor PT, PTT, and INR and monitor patient for bleeding.
Beta blockers: May decrease T_3 level and alter the action of beta blockers. Monitor patient closely.
Digoxin: May increase glycoside level. May need to decrease dosage.
Potassium iodide: May decrease response to drug. May need to increase dosage of antithyroid drug.

Effects on lab test results

- May increase liver enzyme level. May decrease hemoglobin level and hematocrit.
- May decrease granulocyte, WBC, and platelet counts.

Pharmacokinetics

Absorption: About 80% of drug is absorbed rapidly and readily from GI tract.
Distribution: Appears to be concentrated in thyroid gland. About 75% to 80% protein-bound.
Metabolism: Rapidly in liver.
Excretion: About 35% in urine. *Half-life:* 1 to 2 hours.

Route	Onset	Peak	Duration
P.O.	Unknown	1–1½ hr	Unknown

Reactions may be *common*, uncommon, *life-threatening*, or COMMON AND LIFE-THREATENING.

Action

Chemical effect: Inhibits oxidation of iodine in thyroid gland, blocking iodine's ability to combine with tyrosine to form T_4, and may prevent coupling of monoiodotyrosine and diiodotyrosine to form T_4 and T_3.

Therapeutic effect: Lowers thyroid hormone level.

Available forms

Tablets: 50 mg, 100 mg ♦

NURSING PROCESS

⚸ Assessment
• Assess patient's condition before starting therapy and regularly thereafter to monitor drug's effectiveness.
• Watch for signs of hypothyroidism (depression; cold intolerance; hard, nonpitting edema); adjust dosage as directed.
• Monitor CBC to detect impending leukopenia, thrombocytopenia, and agranulocytosis.
• Be alert for adverse reactions.
• If adverse GI reaction occurs, monitor patient's hydration.
• Assess patient's and family's knowledge of drug therapy.

⊕ Nursing diagnoses
• Ineffective health maintenance related to thyroid condition
• Risk for deficient fluid volume related to adverse GI reaction
• Deficient knowledge related to drug therapy

▷ Planning and implementation
• Give drug with meals to reduce adverse GI reaction.
• If patient develops severe rash or enlarged cervical lymph nodes, stop giving the drug and notify prescriber.
• Maintenance daily dosage is about ⅓ to ⅔ of initial daily dose.
• Store drug in light-resistant container.
• **ALERT:** Don't confuse propylthiouracil with Purinethol.
Patient teaching
• Tell patient to report skin eruptions (sign of hypersensitivity), fever, sore throat, or mouth sores (early signs of agranulocytosis).
• Instruct patient to ask prescriber whether he can use iodized salt and eat shellfish.

• Warn patient against OTC cough medicines because many contain iodine.

☑ Evaluation
• Patient's thyroid hormone level is normal.
• Patient maintains adequate hydration.
• Patient and family state understanding of drug therapy.

protamine sulfate
(PROH-tuh-meen SUL-fayt)

Pharmacologic class: antidote
Therapeutic class: heparin antagonist
Pregnancy risk category: C

Indications and dosages

▶ **Heparin overdose.** *Adults:* Dosage based on venous blood coagulation studies, usually 1 mg for each 90 to 115 units of heparin. Give by slow I.V. injection over 10 minutes, not to exceed 50 mg.

▽ I.V. administration
• May be given without further dilution or diluted in D_5W or normal saline solution.
• Give by slow injection over 10 minutes.
• Refrigerate at 15° to 30° C.
• Don't store diluted solutions; they contain no preservatives.
⊗ Incompatibilities
Cephalosporins, diatrizoate meglumine 52% and diatrizoate sodium 8%, diatrizoate sodium 60%, ioxaglate meglumine 39.3% and ioxaglate sodium 19.6%, penicillins.

Contraindications and cautions
• Contraindicated in patients hypersensitive to the drug or any of its components.
• Use cautiously after cardiac surgery.
🔥 Lifespan: In pregnant women, use cautiously. In breast-feeding women, use cautiously; it's unknown if the drug appears in breast milk. In children, safety and effectiveness haven't been established.

Adverse reactions

CV: *bradycardia, circulatory collapse,* drop in blood pressure, transitory flushing.
Respiratory: *acute pulmonary hypertension,* dyspnea, *pulmonary edema.*

Other: *anaphylactoid reactions, anaphylaxis,* feeling of warmth.

Interactions
None significant.

Effects on lab test results
None reported.

Pharmacokinetics
Absorption: Given I.V.
Distribution: Unknown.
Metabolism: Unknown, although it appears to be partially degraded, with release of some heparin.
Excretion: Unknown. *Half-life:* Shorter than heparin.

Route	Onset	Peak	Duration
I.V.	30–60 sec	Unknown	2 hr

Action
Chemical effect: Forms inert complex with heparin sodium.
Therapeutic effect: Blocks heparin's effects.

Available forms
Injection: 10 mg/ml

NURSING PROCESS

Assessment
• Assess patient's heparin overdose before therapy.
• Continually monitor patient; frequently check vital signs.
• Assess patient for fish allergy, vasectomized or infertile males and patients who have received protamine-containing insulin or previous protamine sulfate therapy; hypersensitivity reactions to protamine may develop.
• Watch for spontaneous bleeding (heparin rebound), especially in patients undergoing dialysis and in those who have undergone cardiac surgery. Protamine sulfate may act as anticoagulant in very high doses.
• Assess patient's and family's knowledge of drug therapy.

Nursing diagnoses
• Ineffective protection related to heparin overdose
• Risk for injury related to anaphylaxis

• Deficient knowledge related to drug therapy

Planning and implementation
• Calculate dosage carefully. One milligram of drug neutralizes no less than 100 units of heparin depending on salt (heparin calcium or heparin sodium) and source of heparin (beef or pork).
• Give drug slowly by direct injection. Treat shock.
⚠ ALERT: Don't confuse protamine with Protopam.
Patient teaching
• Instruct patient to report adverse reactions immediately.

Evaluation
• Patient doesn't experience injury.
• Patient and family state understanding of drug therapy.

pseudoephedrine hydrochloride
(soo-doh-eh-FED-rin high-droh-KLOR-ighd)
Cenafed, Children's Sudafed Liquid†, Decofed†, DeFed-60†, Dimetapp†, Dorcol Children's Decongestant†, Drixoral Non-Drowsy Formula†, Eltor 120◆†, Genaphed†, Halofed†, Halofed Adult Strength†, Maxenal◆† Myfedrine†, Novafed†, PediaCare Infants' Oral Decongestant Drops†, Pseudo 60†, Pseudofrin◆, Pseudogest†, Robidrine†, Sudafed†, Sudafed 12 Hour†, Sudafed 60†, Sufedrin†, Triaminic†

pseudoephedrine sulfate
Afrin†, Drixoral†, Drixoral 12 Hour Non-Drowsy Formula†

Pharmacologic class: sympathomimetic
Therapeutic class: decongestant
Pregnancy risk category: C

Indications and dosages
▶ **Nasal and eustachian tube decongestion.**
Adults and children age 12 and older: 60 mg P.O. every 4 to 6 hours; or 120 mg P.O. extended-release tablet every 12 hours; or 240 mg P.O. controlled-release tablet daily. Maximum dose is 240 mg daily.

Children ages 6 to 11: Give 30 mg P.O. every 4 to 6 hours. Maximum dose, 120 mg daily.
Children ages 2 to 5: Give 15 mg P.O. every 4 to 6 hours. Maximum dose, 60 mg daily, or 4 mg/kg or 125 mg/m² P.O. divided q.i.d.
Children younger than age 2: Consult a prescriber for specific dosage.

▶ **Prevention of otitic barotraumas during air travel or underwater diving‡.** *Adults:* 120-mg extended-release tablet P.O. 30 minutes before air travel or 60 mg P.O. 30 minutes before underwater diving.

Contraindications and cautions

• Contraindicated in patients taking MAO inhibitors and in patients with severe hypertension or severe coronary artery disease.
• Use cautiously in patients with hypertension, cardiac disease, diabetes, glaucoma, hyperthyroidism, or prostatic hyperplasia.
⚖ **Lifespan:** Use cautiously during pregnancy and breast-feeding. In children younger than age 12, extended-release forms are contraindicated.

Adverse reactions

CNS: *anxiety,* dizziness, headache, *insomnia, nervousness,* transient stimulation, tremor.
CV: *arrhythmias,* hypertension, *palpitations,* tachycardia.
GI: anorexia, dry mouth, nausea, vomiting.
GU: difficulty urinating.
Respiratory: burning, drying, stinging of nasal mucosa; excessive nasal discharge with topical drug forms; *respiratory difficulty;* sneezing.
Skin: pallor.

Interactions

Drug-drug. *Antihypertensives:* May attenuate hypotensive effect. Monitor blood pressure.
Phenelzine, tranylcypromine: May cause severe headache, hypertension, fever, and hypertensive crisis. Avoid using together.
Sympathomimetic agents: May cause additive effects and increased toxicity. Use with extreme caution or avoid using together.
Drug-herb. *Bitter orange:* May increase risk of hypertension and adverse CV effects. Discourage using together.

Effects on lab test results

None reported.

Pharmacokinetics

Absorption: Unknown.
Distribution: Wide, throughout body.
Metabolism: Incomplete in liver to inactive compounds.
Excretion: In urine; rate is accelerated with acidic urine. *Half-life:* 3 to 16 hours, depending on urine pH.

Route	Onset	Peak	Duration
P.O.	15–30 min	30–60 min	3–12 hr

Action

Chemical effect: Stimulates alpha-adrenergic receptors in upper respiratory tract, resulting in vasoconstriction.
Therapeutic effect: Relieves congestion of nasal passages and eustachian tube.

Available forms

pseudoephedrine hydrochloride
Capsules†: 60 mg
Capsules (liquid gel)†: 30 mg
Liquid†: 7.5 mg/0.8 ml, 15 mg/5 ml, 30 mg/5 ml
Tablets†: 30 mg, 60 mg
Tablets (chewable)†: 15 mg
Tablets (controlled-release)†: 240 mg (60-mg immediate, 180-mg delayed release)
Tablets (extended-release)†: 120 mg
pseudoephedrine sulfate
Tablets (extended-release)†: 120 mg (60-mg immediate, 60-mg delayed release)

NURSING PROCESS

🔖 **Assessment**
• Assess patient's condition before starting therapy and regularly thereafter to monitor drug's effectiveness.
• Be alert for adverse reactions and drug interactions.
• Elderly patients are more sensitive to drug's effects.
• Some OTC topical preparations contain sulfites. Determine patient allergy to sulfites before therapy.
• Assess patient's and family's knowledge of drug therapy.

🔖 **Nursing diagnoses**
• Ineffective health maintenance related to congestion

• Sleep deprivation related to drug-induced insomnia
• Deficient knowledge related to drug therapy

▷ Planning and implementation
• Don't crush or break extended-release forms.
• Give last dose at least 2 hours before bedtime to minimize insomnia.

Patient teaching
• Teach patient to read OTC drug labels so he can avoid using products containing other sympathomimetics or sulfites (if allergic).
• Tell patient not to take immediate-release drug within 2 hours of bedtime because it can cause insomnia.
• Tell patient to relieve dry mouth with sugarless gum or hard candy.
• Instruct patient to stop drug if he becomes unusually restless and to notify prescriber promptly.
• Inform patient about risk of overuse of nasal sprays and consequent rebound congestion. Warn against exceeding recommended dosage and using longer than 3 days unless instructed to do so by a physician.
• Instruct patient to stop drug and call prescriber if no improvement with oral dose within 7 days.
• Inform patient of risks of overdosing if he exceeds recommended daily dosage.
• Teach patient proper administration of sprays, drops, and inhalers, as needed.

☑ Evaluation
• Patient's congestion is relieved.
• Patient has no insomnia.
• Patient and family state understanding of drug therapy.

pyridostigmine bromide
(peer-ih-doh-STIG-meen BROH-mighd)
Mestinon*, Mestinon SR ♦

Pharmacologic class: cholinesterase inhibitor
Therapeutic class: muscle stimulant
Pregnancy risk category: C

Indications and dosages

▶ **Antidote for nondepolarizing neuromuscular blockers.** *Adults:* 10 to 20 mg I.V. preceded by atropine sulfate 0.6 to 1.2 mg I.V.

▶ **Myasthenia gravis.** *Adults:* 60 to 120 mg P.O. t.i.d. Usual dose is 600 mg daily, but a higher dose may be needed (up to 1,500 mg daily). For I.M. or I.V. use, give ⅓₀ of oral dose. Adjust dosage for each patient, depending on response and tolerance. Or, 180 to 540 mg sustained-release tablets (1 to 3 tablets) P.O. daily to b.i.d., with at least 6 hours between doses.
▶ **Prophylaxis against the lethal effects of the nerve agent Soman.** *Adults in the military:* 30 mg P.O. every 8 hours starting about 8 hours before Soman exposure. Discontinue at first sign of nerve gas poisoning and treat with atropine and pralidoxime immediately.

▽▼ I.V. administration
• Give I.V. injection no faster than 1 mg/minute. If administration is too rapid, bradycardia and seizures may result.
⊗ **Incompatibilities**
Alkaline solutions.

Contraindications and cautions
• Contraindicated in patients hypersensitive to anticholinesterases, in those with mechanical obstruction of the intestine or urinary tract, and in those with history of a reaction to bromides.
• Use cautiously in patients with bronchial asthma, bradycardia, or arrhythmias.
• Use cautiously in patients with renal impairment; lower doses may be required.
⚖ **Lifespan:** In pregnant and breast-feeding women, safety and effectiveness haven't been established. In neonates, Regonol is contraindicated because it contains benzyl alcohol.

Adverse reactions
CNS: headache with large doses, *seizures,* sweating, weakness.
CV: *bradycardia,* hypotension, *thrombophlebitis.*
EENT: miosis.
GI: abdominal cramps, diarrhea, excessive salivation, nausea, vomiting.
Musculoskeletal: muscle cramps, muscle fasciculations.
Respiratory: *bronchoconstriction, bronchospasm,* increased bronchial secretions.
Skin: rash.

Interactions
Drug-drug. *Aminoglycosides:* May increase response to drug. Use together cautiously.

Anesthetics, anticholinergics, atropine, cortico-steroids, magnesium, procainamide, quinidine: May antagonize cholinergic effects. Observe patient for lack of drug effect.
Ganglionic blockers: May increase risk of hypotension. Monitor patient closely.

Effects on lab test results

None reported.

Pharmacokinetics

Absorption: Poor.
Distribution: Unknown.
Metabolism: Unknown.
Excretion: In urine. *Half-life:* 1 to 3 hours, depending on route.

Route	Onset	Peak	Duration
P.O.	20–60 min	1–2 hr	3–12 hr
I.V.	2–5 min	Unknown	2–3 hr
I.M.	15 min	Unknown	2–3 hr

Action

Chemical effect: Inhibits destruction of acetylcholine released from parasympathetic and somatic efferent nerves. This allows acetylcholine to accumulate.
Therapeutic effect: Reverses effect of nondepolarizing neuromuscular blockers and myasthenia gravis.

Available forms

Injection: 5 mg/ml in 2-ml ampules or 5-ml vials
Syrup: 60 mg/5 ml
Tablets: 60 mg
Tablets (military use only): 30 mg
Tablets (sustained-release): 180 mg

NURSING PROCESS

Assessment
• Assess patient's condition before starting therapy and regularly thereafter to monitor drug's effectiveness.
• Monitor and document patient's response after each dose; optimum dose is difficult to judge.
• Monitor patient's vital signs, especially respirations.
• Be alert for adverse reactions and drug interactions.
• Assess patient's and family's knowledge of drug therapy.

Nursing diagnoses
• Impaired physical mobility related to underlying condition
• Ineffective breathing pattern related to adverse respiratory reactions
• Deficient knowledge related to drug therapy

Planning and implementation
• Stop all other cholinergics before giving drug.
• Don't crush extended-release tablets.
• When using sweet syrup for patient who has difficulty swallowing, pour over ice chips if he can't tolerate flavor.
• Position patient to ease breathing. Have atropine injection readily available, and provide respiratory support as needed.
• If patient's muscle weakness is severe, prescriber will determine if it's caused by drug-induced toxicity or worsening of myasthenia gravis. Test dose of edrophonium I.V. will aggravate drug-induced weakness but will temporarily relieve weakness caused by disease.
• The U.S. formulation of Regonol contains benzyl alcohol preservative, which may cause toxicity in neonates if given in large doses. The Canadian formulation of this drug doesn't contain benzyl ethanol.
• If appropriate, obtain prescriber's order for hospitalized patient to have bedside supply of tablets. Patients with long-standing disease often insist on self-administration.
⚠ **ALERT:** If drug is taken immediately before or during Soman exposure, drug may be ineffective against Soman, and may worsen the effects of Soman.
⚠ **ALERT:** Don't confuse Mestinon with Mesantoin or Metatensin.
Patient teaching
• When giving drug for myasthenia gravis, stress the importance of taking it exactly as ordered, on time, in evenly spaced doses. If prescriber has ordered extended-release tablets, tell patient to take tablets at same time each day, at least 6 hours apart. Tell him that he may have to take drug for life.
• Advise patient to wear or carry medical identification at all times.

Evaluation
• Patient has improved physical mobility.
• Patient maintains adequate respiratory pattern.
• Patient and family state understanding of drug therapy.

pyridoxine hydrochloride (vitamin B₆)

(peer-ih-DOKS-een high-droh-KLOR-ighd)
Aminoxin†, Nestrex†, Pyri 500, Rodex, Vitabee-6

Pharmacologic class: water-soluble vitamin
Therapeutic class: nutritional supplement
Pregnancy risk category: A

Indications and dosages

▶ **RDA**
Males and females 14 to 50 years of age: Give 1.2 to 1.3 mg/day.
Males and females > 50 years of age: Give 1.5 to 1.7 mg/day.
Pregnant females: Give 1.9 mg daily.
Lactating females: Give 2 mg daily.
Children ages 9 to 13: Give 1 mg.
Children ages 4 to 8: Give 0.6 mg.
Children ages 1 to 3: Give 0.5 mg.
Infants ages 6 months to 1 year: Give 0.6 mg.
Neonates and infants up to age 6 months: Give 0.3 mg.
▶ **Dietary vitamin B₆ deficiency.** *Adults:* 2.5 to 10 mg P.O. daily for 3 weeks; then 2 to 5 mg daily as supplement to proper diet.
▶ **Seizures related to vitamin B₆ deficiency or dependency.** *Adults and children:* 10 to 100 mg I.M. or I.V. in single dose.
▶ **Vitamin B₆–responsive anemias or dependency syndrome (inborn errors of metabolism).** *Adults:* Up to 600 mg I.M., P.O., or I.V. daily until symptoms subside; then 30 mg daily for life.
▶ **Prevention of vitamin B₆ deficiency during drug therapy.** *Adults:* 6 to 100 mg P.O. daily for isoniazid therapy.
▶ **Drug-induced vitamin B₆ deficiency.** *Adults:* 100 to 200 mg P.O. daily for 3 weeks, followed by 25 to 100 mg P.O. daily to prevent relapse.
▶ **Antidote for isoniazid poisoning.** *Adults:* 1 to 4 g I.V., followed by 1 g I.M. every 30 minutes until amount of pyridoxine given equals amount of isoniazid ingested.
▶ **Premenstrual syndrome‡.** *Adults:* 40 to 500 mg P.O., I.M., or I.V. daily.
▶ **Carpal tunnel syndrome‡.** *Adults:* 100 to 200 mg P.O. daily for 12 weeks or longer.

▶ **Hyperoxaluria type I‡.** *Adults:* 25 to 300 mg P.O. daily.
▶ **Adjunctive treatment in toxicity of *Gyromitra* mushroom poisoning.** *Adults:* 25 mg/kg I.V. over 15 to 30 minutes, repeated as needed up to 15 to 20 g daily.

▼ I.V. administration

• Protect drug from light. Don't use solution if it contains precipitate, although slight darkening is acceptable.
• Inject undiluted drug into I.V. line containing free-flowing compatible solution. Or, infuse diluted drug over prescribed duration for intermittent infusions. Don't use for continuous infusion.
⊗ **Incompatibilities**
Alkaline solutions, erythromycin estolate, iron salts, kanamycin, oxidizers, riboflavin phosphate sodium, streptomycin.

Contraindications and cautions

• Contraindicated in patients hypersensitive to the drug or any of its components, and in patients with heart disease.
⚕ **Lifespan:** No considerations reported.

Adverse reactions

CNS: drowsiness, paresthesia, somnolence, unstable gait.

Interactions

Drug-drug. *Levodopa:* May decrease levodopa effectiveness. Avoid using pyridoxine with levodopa. Pyridoxine has little or no effect on the combination drug levodopa and carbidopa.
Phenobarbital, phenytoin: May decrease anticonvulsant level, increasing risk of seizures. Monitor level closely; institute seizure precautions.
Drug-lifestyle. *Alcohol use:* May increase risk of delirium and lactic acidosis. Discourage using together.

Effects on lab test results

• May increase AST level. May decrease folic acid level.

Pharmacokinetics

Absorption: Drug and its substituents are absorbed readily from GI tract. May be diminished in patients with malabsorption syndromes or following gastric resection.

Distribution: Drug is stored mainly in liver.
Metabolism: In liver.
Excretion: In erythrocytes, pyridoxine is converted to pyridoxal phosphate and pyridoxamine is converted to pyridoxamine phosphate. The phosphorylated form of pyridoxine is transaminated to pyridoxal and pyridoxamine, which is phosphorylated rapidly. Conversion of pyridoxine phosphate to pyridoxal phosphate requires riboflavin. *Half-life:* 15 to 20 days.

Route	Onset	Peak	Duration
P.O., I.V., I.M.	Unknown	Unknown	Unknown

Action

Chemical effect: Vitamin B_6 stimulates various metabolic functions, including amino acid metabolism.
Therapeutic effect: Raises pyridoxine level, prevents and relieves seizure activity related to pyridoxine deficiency or dependency, and blocks effects of isoniazid poisoning.

Available forms

Capsules: 150 mg, 500 mg
Injection: 100 mg/ml
Tablets: 10 mg†, 25 mg†, 50 mg†, 100 mg†, 200 mg†, 250 mg†, 500 mg†
Tablets (enteric-coated): 20 mg†
Tablets (extended-release): 200 mg

NURSING PROCESS

⚎ Assessment
• Assess patient before starting therapy and regularly thereafter to monitor drug's effectiveness.
• Be alert for adverse CNS reactions and drug interactions. Patient taking high dose (2 to 6 g daily) may have difficulty walking because of reduced proprioceptive and sensory function.
• Monitor patient's diet. Excessive protein intake increases daily drug requirements.
• Assess patient's and family's knowledge of drug therapy.

⚎ Nursing diagnoses
• Ineffective health maintenance related to underlying condition
• Risk for injury related to drug-induced adverse CNS reactions
• Deficient knowledge related to drug therapy

▶ Planning and implementation
• When using drug to treat isoniazid toxicity, give anticonvulsants.
• If sodium bicarbonate is required to control acidosis in isoniazid toxicity, don't mix in same syringe with pyridoxine.
⚕ ALERT: Don't confuse pyridoxine with pralidoxime, pyrimethamine, or Pyridium.
Patient teaching
• Advise patient taking levodopa alone to avoid multivitamins containing pyridoxine because of decreased levodopa effect.
• If prescribed for maintenance therapy to prevent recurrence of deficiency, stress importance of compliance and good nutrition. Explain that pyridoxine with isoniazid has specific therapeutic purpose and isn't just a vitamin.

✓ Evaluation
• Patient responds well to therapy.
• Patient doesn't experience injury from adverse CNS reactions.
• Patient and family state understanding of drug therapy.

pyrimethamine
(peer-ih-METH-uh-meen)
Daraprim

pyrimethamine with sulfadoxine
Fansidar

Pharmacologic class: folic acid antagonist
Therapeutic class: antimalarial
Pregnancy risk category: C

Indications and dosages

▶ **Malaria prophylaxis and transmission control.** *Adults and children older than age 10:* Give 25 mg pyrimethamine P.O. weekly.
Children ages 4 to 10: Give 12.5 mg pyrimethamine P.O. weekly.
Children younger than age 4: Give 6.25 mg pyrimethamine P.O. weekly.
    Continued in all age groups at least 10 weeks after leaving endemic area.
▶ **Acute attacks of malaria.** *Adults and children older than age 10:* Give 25 mg pyrimethamine P.O. daily for 2 days when used with faster-acting antimalarials; when used alone, 50 mg P.O. daily for 2 days.

Children ages 4 to 10: Give 25 mg pyrimethamine P.O. daily for 2 days.

▶ **Acute attacks of malaria.** *Adults:* Give 2 to 3 tablets pyrimethamine with sulfadoxine as single dose, either alone or in sequence with quinine.

Children ages 9 to 14: Give 2 tablets pyrimethamine with sulfadoxine.

Children ages 4 to 8: Give 1 tablet pyrimethamine with sulfadoxine.

Children younger than age 4: Give ½ tablet pyrimethamine with sulfadoxine.

▶ **Malaria prophylaxis.** *Adults:* Give 1 tablet pyrimethamine with sulfadoxine weekly, or 2 tablets every 2 weeks.

Children ages 9 to 14: Give ¾ tablet pyrimethamine with sulfadoxine weekly, or 1½ tablets every 2 weeks.

Children ages 4 to 8: Give ½ tablet pyrimethamine with sulfadoxine weekly, or 1 tablet every 2 weeks.

Children younger than age 4: Give ½ tablet pyrimethamine with sulfadoxine weekly, or ½ tablet every 2 weeks.

▶ **Toxoplasmosis.** *Adults:* Initially, 50 to 75 mg pyrimethamine P.O. daily with 1 to 4 g of sulfadoxine for 1 to 3 weeks, then reduce both doses by 50% and continue therapy for an additional 4 to 5 weeks.

Children: Initially, 1 mg/kg pyrimethamine P.O. daily (not to exceed 100 mg) in two equally divided doses for 2 to 4 days; then 0.5 mg/kg daily for 4 weeks along with 100 mg sulfadiazine/kg P.O. daily, divided every 6 hours.

▶ **Isosporiasis‡.** *Adults:* 50 to 75 mg pyrimethamine P.O. daily.

Contraindications and cautions

● Contraindicated in patients hypersensitive to the drug or any of its components, and in those with megaloblastic anemia caused by folic acid deficiency. Pyrimethamine with sulfadoxine is contraindicated in patients with porphyria because it contains sulfadoxine, a sulfonamide.

● Repeated use of pyrimethamine with sulfadoxine is contraindicated in patients hypersensitive to pyrimethamine or sulfonamides, and in patients with severe renal insufficiency, marked liver parenchymal damage or blood dyscrasias, or megaloblastic anemia caused by folate deficiency.

● Use cautiously in patients with impaired hepatic or renal function, severe allergy or bron-

chial asthma, or G6PD deficiency; in those with seizure disorders (smaller doses may be needed); and in those treated with chloroquine.

⚖ **Lifespan:** In pregnant women at term, infants younger than age 2 months, and breastfeeding women, repeated use of pyrimethamine with sulfadoxine is contraindicated.

Adverse reactions

CNS: *seizures,* stimulation.
GI: anorexia, atrophic glossitis, diarrhea, vomiting.
Hematologic: *agranulocytosis, aplastic anemia, bone marrow suppression, leukopenia,* megaloblastic anemia, *pancytopenia, thrombocytopenia.*
Skin: *erythema multiforme,* rash, *Stevens-Johnson syndrome, toxic epidermal necrolysis.*

Interactions

Drug-drug. *Co-trimoxazole, methotrexate, sulfonamides, zidovudine:* May increase risk of bone marrow suppression. Don't use together. *Folic acid, PABA:* May decrease antitoxoplasmic effects. May require dosage adjustment. *Lorazepam:* May cause mild hepatotoxicity. Monitor liver enzymes.

Effects on lab test results

● May decrease hemoglobin level and hematocrit.
● May decrease granulocyte, WBC, platelet, and RBC counts.

Pharmacokinetics

Absorption: Well absorbed from intestinal tract.
Distribution: To kidneys, liver, spleen, and lungs. About 80% protein-bound.
Metabolism: To several unidentified compounds.
Excretion: In urine. *Half-life:* 4 days.

Route	Onset	Peak	Duration
P.O.	Unknown	1½–8 hr	Unknown

Action

Chemical effect: Inhibits enzyme dihydrofolate reductase, impeding reduction of this enzyme to tetrahydrofolic acid. Sulfadoxine competitively inhibits use of PABA.

Therapeutic effect: Prevents malaria and treats malaria and toxoplasmosis infections. Spectrum of activity includes asexual erythrocytic forms of susceptible *plasmodia* and *Toxoplasma gondii.*

Available forms

pyrimethamine
Tablets: 25 mg
pyrimethamine with sulfadoxine
Tablets: pyrimethamine 25 mg, sulfadoxine 500 mg

NURSING PROCESS

Assessment
• Assess patient's condition before starting therapy and regularly thereafter to monitor drug's effectiveness.
• Obtain twice-weekly blood counts, including platelets, for patients with toxoplasmosis because doses used approach toxic levels.
• Be alert for adverse reactions and drug interactions.
• Assess patient's and family's knowledge of drug therapy.

Nursing diagnoses
• Risk for infection related to presence of susceptible organism
• Ineffective protection related to adverse hematologic reactions
• Deficient knowledge related to drug therapy

Planning and implementation
• Give drug with meals to minimize GI distress.
• If signs of folic acid or folinic acid deficiency develop, reduce dosage or stop drug while patient receives parenteral folinic acid (leucovorin) until blood counts become normal.
• For toxoplasmosis, patients with AIDS may need lifelong drug therapy and suppressive therapy.
• Leucovorin should be administered concomitantly when drug is used for the treatment of toxoplasmosis.
• **ALERT:** Because of possibly severe skin reactions, use pyrimethamine with sulfadoxine only in regions where chloroquine-resistant malaria is prevalent and only when traveler plans to stay in region longer than 3 weeks.
Patient teaching
• Advise patient to take drug with food.

• Teach patient to watch for and immediately report signs of folic or folinic acid deficiency and acute toxicity.
• Warn patient taking pyrimethamine with sulfadoxine to stop drug and notify prescriber at first sign of rash.
• Instruct patient to take first prophylactic dose of pyrimethamine with sulfadoxine 1 to 2 days before traveling to endemic area.

Evaluation
• Patient is free from infection.
• Patient maintains normal hematologic parameters.
• Patient and family state understanding of drug therapy.

quetiapine fumarate
(KWET-ee-uh-peen FY00-muh-rayt)
Seroquel, Seroquel XR

Pharmacologic class: dibenzothiazepine derivative
Therapeutic class: antipsychotic
Pregnancy risk category: C

Indications and dosages

▶ **Schizophrenia.** *Adults:* For Seroquel, initially, 25 mg P.O. b.i.d.; increase in increments of 25 to 50 mg b.i.d. or t.i.d. on days 2 and 3, as tolerated. Target dosage range is 300 to 400 mg daily, divided into two or three daily doses by day 4. Make further dosage adjustments at intervals of not less than 2 days. Dosages can be increased or decreased by 25 to 50 mg b.i.d. based on response. Safety of doses above 800 mg daily hasn't been evaluated. Or, 300 mg Seroquel XR in the evening. Effective dosage range is 400 to 800 mg. Increase at intervals as short as 1 day and in increments up to 300 mg/day as tolerated.
▶ **Monotherapy and adjunct therapy with lithium or divalproex for the short-term treatment of acute manic episodes associated with bipolar I disorder.** *Adults:* Initially, 50 mg P.O. b.i.d. Increase dosage in increments of 100 mg/day in 2 divided doses, to 200 mg P.O.

b.i.d. on day 4. May increase dosage in increments not greater than 200 mg/day, up to 800 mg/day by day 6. Usual dosage, 400 to 800 mg daily.

▶ **Depression in bipolar disorder.** *Adults:* On day 1, give 50 mg P.O. On day 2, give 100 mg. On day 3, give 200 mg. On day 4 and thereafter, give 300 mg daily. Give drug at bedtime.

▧ **Adjust-a-dose:** For patients with hepatic impairment, initially give 25 mg P.O. daily. Increase in increments of 25 to 50 mg daily to an effective dose, depending on the patient's response and tolerance.

Elderly patients should be adjusted on immediate-release formula. The patient may be switched to Seroquel XR when stabilized on 200 mg/day. Patients with hepatic impairment should be slowly adjusted on immediate-release formula and be switched to Seroquel XR when stabilized on 200 mg/day.

Contraindications and cautions

• Contraindicated in patients hypersensitive to the drug or any of its components.
• Use cautiously in patients with CV or cerebrovascular disease or conditions that predispose them to hypotension; in those with history of seizures or conditions that lower seizure threshold; in those at risk for aspiration pneumonia; and in those who could experience conditions in which core body temperature may be elevated. Also use cautiously in patients who are debilitated.

⚗ **Lifespan:** In pregnant women, use only if benefits outweigh risks to the fetus. In breast-feeding women, stop breast-feeding or use a different drug. In children, safety and effectiveness haven't been established. In elderly patients, use cautiously and at a lower dose.

Adverse reactions

CNS: asthenia, *dizziness,* dysarthria, dyskinesia, fever, *headache,* hypertonia, **neuroleptic malignant syndrome, seizures,** somnolence, tardive extrapyramidal symptoms.
CV: orthostatic hypotension, palpitations, peripheral edema, tachycardia.
EENT: cataracts, ear pain, nasal congestion, pharyngitis, rhinitis, sinusitis.
GI: abdominal pain, anorexia, constipation, dry mouth, dyspepsia.
GU: urine retention.
Hematologic: *leukopenia.*

Metabolic: hyperglycemia, hypothyroidism, *weight gain.*
Musculoskeletal: back pain.
Respiratory: dyspnea, increased cough.
Skin: rash, sweating.
Other: flulike syndrome.

Interactions

Drug-drug. *Antihypertensives:* May increase drug effects. Monitor blood pressure.
Carbamazepine, glucocorticoids, phenobarbital, phenytoin, rifampin, thioridazine: May increase quetiapine clearance. Increase quetiapine dosage, if needed.
Cimetidine, erythromycin, fluconazole, itraconazole, ketoconazole: May decrease quetiapine clearance. Use together cautiously.
CNS depressants: May increase CNS effects. Use together cautiously.
Dopamine agonists, levodopa: May antagonize effects of these drugs. Monitor patient for effects.
Lorazepam: May reduce lorazepam clearance. Monitor patient.
Drug-lifestyle. *Alcohol use:* May increase CNS effects. Discourage use together.

Effects on lab test results

• May increase glucose, liver enzyme, cholesterol, and triglyceride levels. May decrease T_4 and thyroid-stimulating hormone levels.
• May decrease WBC count.

Pharmacokinetics

Absorption: Rapid. 100% bioavailability.
Distribution: Wide. 83% protein-bound.
Metabolism: Extensive.
Excretion: About 73% in urine, 20% in feces.
Half-life: 6 hours.

Route	Onset	Peak	Duration
P.O.	Unknown	1½ hr	Unknown

Action

Chemical effect: May block dopamine D_2 receptors and serotonin 5-HT_2 receptors in the brain. It also may act at histamine H_1 receptors and alpha$_1$-adrenergic receptors.
Therapeutic effect: Reduces symptoms of psychotic disorders.

Available forms

Tablets: 25 mg, 50 mg, 100 mg, 200 mg, 300 mg, 400 mg

Reactions may be *common,* uncommon, *life-threatening*, or COMMON AND LIFE-THREATENING.

Tablets (extended-release): 200 mg, 300 mg, 400 mg

⚡ Assessment

• Monitor patient for tardive dyskinesia. Condition may not appear until months or years after starting drug and may disappear spontaneously or persist for life, despite stopping the drug.
• Monitor patient's vital signs carefully, especially during the 3- to 5-day period of initial use and when restarting or increasing the dose.
• Assess patient's risk of physical injury from adverse CNS effects.
• Be alert for adverse reactions and drug interactions.
• Assess patient's and family's knowledge of drug therapy.

🔷 Nursing diagnoses

• Risk for imbalanced body temperature related to drug-induced hyperpyrexia
• Impaired physical mobility related to drug-induced adverse CNS effects
• Deficient knowledge related to drug therapy

▷ Planning and implementation

• An elderly or debilitated patient or a patient with hepatic impairment or tendency for hypotensive reactions usually needs a lower initial dose and more gradual dosage adjustment.
⚠️ **ALERT:** Elderly patients with dementia-related psychosis are at increased risk of death when treated with atypical antipsychotics.
⚠️ **ALERT:** May increase risk for suicidal thinking and behavior in young adults ages 18 to 24 during the first 2 months of treatment. Monitor patient carefully.
• Effectiveness for longer than 3 weeks hasn't been thoroughly studied. Periodically reevaluate the long-term usefulness of drug.
⚠️ **ALERT:** If symptoms of neuroleptic malignant syndrome (hyperpyrexia, muscle rigidity, altered mental status, or autonomic instability) occur, stop the drug and notify prescriber.
• Provide ice chips, drinks, or sugarless hard candy to help relieve dry mouth.
• Don't split XR tablet; have patient swallow whole.
⚠️ **ALERT:** Drug may cause hyperglycemia. Monitor patient with diabetes regularly. For patients with risk factors for diabetes, test fasting glucose

level at baseline and periodically during therapy. Monitor all patients for symptoms of hyperglycemia, including excessive hunger or thirst, frequent urinating, and weakness; if symptoms develop, test fasting glucose level. Hyperglycemia may reverse once drug is stopped.

Patient teaching

• Warn patient about risk of orthostatic hypotension, especially during initial use or after a dose increase.
• Tell patient to avoid becoming overheated or dehydrated during therapy.
• Tell patient not to cut, crush, or chew tablets.
• Advise patient to avoid activities that require mental alertness until the drug's CNS effects are known.
• Remind patient to have eye examination before starting drug therapy and every 6 months during therapy to check for cataract formation.
• Tell patient to notify prescriber of other prescription or OTC drugs he is taking or plans to take.
• Tell woman to notify prescriber if she becomes pregnant or intends to become pregnant during therapy. Advise her not to breast-feed during therapy.
• Advise patient not to drink alcohol during therapy.
• Tell patient that drug may be taken with or without food.

☑ Evaluation

• Patient maintains normal body temperature.
• Patient maintains physical mobility and doesn't experience extrapyramidal effects of drug.
• Patient and family state understanding of drug therapy.

quinapril hydrochloride
(KWIN-eh-pril high-droh-KLOR-ighd)
Accupril✐

Pharmacologic class: ACE inhibitor
Therapeutic class: antihypertensive
Pregnancy risk category: C (D in second and third trimesters)

Indications and dosages

▶ **Hypertension.** *Adults younger than age 65:* Initially, 10 to 20 mg P.O. daily. Adjust dosage

based on patient response at intervals of about 2 weeks. Most patients are controlled at 20, 40, or 80 mg daily as a single dose or in two divided doses.

Adults age 65 and older: Initially 10 mg P.O. once daily. Adjust dosage based on patient's response and tolerance.

▌**Adjust-a-dose:** For patients with renal impairment, if creatinine clearance exceeds 60 ml/minute, maximum initial dose is 10 mg P.O.; if clearance is 30 to 60 ml/minute, 5 mg; and if clearance is 10 to 30 ml/minute, 2.5 mg. No dosage recommendations are available for creatinine clearance less than 10 ml/minute.

▶ **Heart failure.** *Adults:* Initially, 10 mg P.O. daily. Increase dosage at weekly intervals. Usual effective dosage is 20 to 40 mg daily in equally divided doses.

▌**Adjust-a-dose:** For patients with renal impairment, if creatinine clearance exceeds 30 ml/minute, the recommended initial dose is 5 mg P.O.; if clearance is 10 to 30 ml/minute, 2.5 mg. No dosage recommendations are available for creatinine clearance less than 10 ml/minute.

Contraindications and cautions

• Contraindicated in patients hypersensitive to ACE inhibitors, in those with a history of angioedema during previous ACE inhibitor therapy, and in those with renal artery stenosis.
• Use cautiously in patients with impaired kidney function and increased potassium level.

⚜ **Lifespan:** In pregnant women in the second or third trimester, drug isn't recommended. In breast-feeding women, use cautiously; it's unknown if the drug appears in breast milk. In children, safety and effectiveness haven't been established.

Adverse reactions

CNS: depression, lightheadedness, malaise, nervousness, somnolence, syncope, vertigo.
CV: angina, *arrhythmias, hypertensive crisis,* orthostatic hypotension, palpitations, tachycardia, vasodilation.
EENT: dry throat.
GI: abdominal pain, constipation, dry mouth, *GI hemorrhage.*
Metabolic: hyperkalemia.
Musculoskeletal: back pain.
Respiratory: dry, persistent, tickling, nonproductive cough.

Skin: exfoliative dermatitis, diaphoresis, *photosensitivity reaction,* pruritus.
Other: *angioedema.*

Interactions

Drug-drug. *Digoxin:* May increase digoxin level. Monitor level.
Diuretics, other antihypertensives: May increase the risk of excessive hypotension. Expect to stop diuretic or lower dosage.
Lithium: May increase lithium level and lithium toxicity. Avoid using together.
Potassium-sparing diuretics: May increase risk of hyperkalemia. Monitor patient, ECG, and potassium level closely.
Quinolones, tetracyclines, and other drugs that interact with magnesium: May decrease absorption of these drugs. Monitor patient.
Drug-herb. *Licorice:* May cause sodium retention and increase blood pressure, interfering with the therapeutic effects of ACE inhibitors. Discourage using together.
Drug-food. *High-fat foods:* May impair absorption. Discourage using together.
Sodium substitutes containing potassium: May increase risk of hyperkalemia. Discourage using together; monitor patient closely.

Effects on lab test results

• May increase BUN, creatinine and potassium level.
• May increase liver function test values.

Pharmacokinetics

Absorption: At least 60%; rate and extent drop by 25% to 30% when given with high-fat meal.
Distribution: About 97% of drug and active metabolite are protein-bound.
Metabolism: 38% of dose de-esterified in liver to active metabolite.
Excretion: Mainly in urine. *Elimination half-life:* 2 hours; *terminal half-life:* 25 hours.

Route	Onset	Peak	Duration
P.O.	≤ 1 hr	2–4 hr	24 hr

Action

Chemical effect: Inhibits conversion of angiotensin I to angiotensin II, which lowers peripheral arterial resistance and decreases aldosterone secretion.
Therapeutic effect: Lowers blood pressure.

Reactions may be *common,* uncommon, *life-threatening,* or COMMON AND LIFE-THREATENING.

Available forms
Tablets: 5 mg, 10 mg, 20 mg, 40 mg

NURSING PROCESS

⏱ Assessment
• Assess patient's blood pressure before therapy and regularly thereafter. Take blood pressure just before giving a dose and then again 2 to 6 hours after dose to make sure blood pressure is controlled.
• Assess kidney and liver function before starting therapy and regularly thereafter.
• Monitor potassium level.
• Other ACE inhibitors have been linked to agranulocytosis and neutropenia. Monitor CBC with differential before therapy, every 2 weeks for first 3 months of therapy, and periodically thereafter.
• Be alert for adverse reactions and drug interactions.
• Assess patient's and family's knowledge of drug therapy.

⊕ Nursing diagnoses
• Risk for injury related to presence of hypertension
• Sleep deprivation related to drug-induced cough
• Deficient knowledge related to drug therapy

▷ Planning and implementation
• If patient has renal impairment, give a lower dose.
• Give drug on empty stomach. High-fat meals can impair absorption.
Patient teaching
• Advise patient to report evidence of infection, such as fever and sore throat.
• Tell patient to immediately report evidence of angioedema (breathing difficulty and swelling of face, eyes, lips, or tongue), especially after first dose.
• Warn patient that lightheadedness can occur, especially at start of therapy. Tell him to rise slowly, stop taking the drug, and notify prescriber if he experiences blackouts.
• Inadequate fluid intake, vomiting, diarrhea, and excessive perspiration can lead to lightheadedness and syncope. Tell patient to maintain adequate hydration/fluid intake and to use caution in hot weather and during exercise.

• Warn patient not to take potassium supplements or use sodium substitutes that contain potassium during therapy.
• Tell women to notify prescriber about suspected or confirmed pregnancy. Drug will need to be stopped.

☑ Evaluation
• Patient's blood pressure is normal.
• Patient's sleep patterns are undisturbed throughout therapy.
• Patient and family state understanding of drug therapy.

HIGH ALERT

quinidine gluconate (62% quinidine base)
(KWIN-ih-deen)

quinidine sulfate (83% quinidine base)

Pharmacologic class: cinchona alkaloid
Therapeutic class: antiarrhythmic, antimalarial
Pregnancy risk category: C

Indications and dosages

▶ **Atrial flutter or fibrillation.** *Adults:* 200 mg quinidine sulfate or equivalent base P.O. every 2 to 3 hours for five to eight doses, with subsequent daily increases until sinus rhythm is restored or toxic effects develop. Drug is given only after digitalization to avoid increasing AV conduction. Maximum dosage, 3 to 4 g daily. Or 300 mg Quinidex Extentabs P.O. (extended-release) every 8 to 12 hours.
▶ **Paroxysmal supraventricular tachycardia.** *Adults:* 400 to 600 mg quinidine sulfate P.O. every 2 to 3 hours until toxic adverse reactions develop or arrhythmia subsides.
▶ **Premature atrial and ventricular contractions; paroxysmal AV junctional rhythm; paroxysmal atrial tachycardia; paroxysmal ventricular tachycardia; maintenance after cardioversion of atrial fibrillation or flutter.** *Adults:* Test dose—200 mg quinidine sulfate or equivalent base P.O., then 200 to 300 mg P.O. every 4 to 6 hours. Or give a test dose of 200 mg quinidine gluconate I.M., then initial dose of 600 mg I.M., followed by 400 mg I.M. every 2 hours, p.r.n. Adjust each dose by the ef-

---

fect of the previous. Or, 300 to 600 mg quinidine sulfate or gluconate sustained-release tablets P.O. every 8 or 12 hours. Or, 800 mg quinidine gluconate I.V. diluted in 40 ml of D_5W and infused at 1 ml/minute.
Children: Test dose—2 mg/kg; then 30 mg/kg P.O. daily or 900 mg/m² P.O. daily in five divided doses.

▶ **Severe *Plasmodium falciparum* malaria.**
Adults: 6.25 mg/kg diluted in 5 ml/kg of normal saline I.V. infusion over 1 to 2 hours followed by a continuous maintenance infusion of 12.5 mcq/kg/minute for at least 24 hours and until parasitemia is reduced to less than 1%. Alternatively, 15 mg/kg diluted in 250 ml of normal saline infused over 4 hours, followed by maintenance infusion of 7.5 mg/kg I.V. infusion over 4 hours at 8 hour intervals until 3 maintenance doses have been administered and parasitemia is less than 1%.

▽ I.V. administration

• Use drug I.V. only for malaria or acute arrhythmias.
• Mix 10 ml (800 mg) of quinidine gluconate with 40 ml of D_5W and infuse at a slow rate of 1 ml/minute for maximum safety.
• Never use discolored (brownish) solution.
⊗ **Incompatibilities**
Alkalies, amiodarone, atracurium besylate, furosemide, heparin sodium, iodides.

Contraindications and cautions

• Contraindicated in patients hypersensitive to quinidine or related cinchona derivatives; in patients with idiosyncratic reactions to them; and in patients with intraventricular conduction defects, complete heart block, left bundle branch block, history of drug-induced torsades de pointes or prolonged QT interval, digitalis toxicity with grossly impaired AV conduction, or abnormal rhythms caused by escape mechanisms.
• Use cautiously in patients with asthma, muscle weakness, or infection with fever (hypersensitivity reactions to drug may be masked). Also use cautiously in patients with hepatic, renal, or cardiac impairment.
⚖ Lifespan: In pregnant women, use cautiously. In breast-feeding women, drug isn't recommended. In children, safety and effectiveness haven't been established.

Adverse reactions

CNS: cold sweats, confusion, dementia, fainting, fever, *headache, lightheadedness,* pallor, restlessness, *vertigo.*
CV: *aggravated heart failure, cardiotoxicity,* ECG changes (widening of QRS complex, notched P waves, *widened QT interval,* ST-segment depression), hypotension, *PVCs, SA and AV block, severe hypotension, torsades de pointes,* tachycardia, *ventricular fibrillation, ventricular tachycardia.*
EENT: blurred vision, *tinnitus.*
GI: abdominal pain, anorexia, *diarrhea,* excessive salivation, *nausea,* petechial hemorrhage of buccal mucosa, *vomiting.*
Hematologic: *agranulocytosis,* hemolytic anemia, *thrombocytopenia.*
Hepatic: *hepatotoxicity.*
Respiratory: *acute asthma attack, respiratory arrest.*
Skin: pruritus, rash.
Other: *angioedema,* cinchonism, hypersensitivity reaction, lupus erythematosus.

Interactions

Drug-drug. *Acetazolamide, antacids, sodium bicarbonate, thiazide diuretics:* May increase quinidine level because of alkaline urine. Monitor patient for increased effect.
Amiodarone: May increase quinidine level, producing potentially fatal cardiac arrhythmias. If use together can't be avoided, monitor quinidine level closely. Adjust quinidine as needed.
Antiarrhythmics (such as lidocaine, procainamide, propranolol): May increase risk of toxicity. Use together cautiously.
Anticoagulants: May increase anticoagulant effect. Monitor patient closely for bleeding.
Barbiturates, nifedipine, phenytoin, rifampin: May decrease level of quinidine. Monitor patient for decreased quinidine effect.
Cimetidine: May increase quinidine level. Monitor patient for increased effect.
Digoxin: May increase digoxin level after quinidine therapy starts. Monitor patient closely for digitalis toxicity.
Nondepolarizing neuromuscular blockers, succinylcholine: May increase neuromuscular blockade. Avoid using together.
Propafenone: May increase propafenone level and its effects. Use together cautiously.
Sucralfate: May decrease quinidine level. Adjust dosage.

Reactions may be *common,* uncommon, *life-threatening,* or COMMON AND LIFE-THREATENING.

Verapamil: May cause hypotension, bradycardia, or AV block. Monitor blood pressure and heart rate.

Drug-herb. *Jimson weed:* May adversely affect CV function. Discourage using together.
Licorice: May prolong the QT interval. Discourage using together.

Drug-food. *Grapefruit:* May delay absorption and onset of action of drug. Advise patient to avoid eating grapefruit or drinking its juice.

Effects on lab test results

• May increase liver enzyme level. May decrease hemoglobin level and hematocrit.
• May decrease platelet and granulocyte counts.

Pharmacokinetics

Absorption: Although all salts are well absorbed, levels vary greatly among individuals.
Distribution: Well distributed in all tissues except brain. About 80% protein-bound.
Metabolism: About 60% to 80% metabolized in liver to two metabolites.
Excretion: 10% to 30% in urine. Urine acidification increases excretion; alkalinization decreases it. *Half-life:* 5 to 12 hours.

Route	Onset	Peak	Duration
P.O.	1–3 hr	1–2 hr	6–8 hr
I.V.	Immediate	Immediate	Unknown
I.M.	Unknown	Unknown	Unknown

Action

Chemical effect: Has direct and indirect (anticholinergic) effects on cardiac tissue. Automaticity, conduction velocity, and membrane responsiveness are decreased. The effective refractory period is prolonged. Anticholinergic action reduces vagal tone.
Therapeutic effect: Restores normal sinus rhythm and relieves signs and symptoms of malaria infection.

Available forms

quinidine gluconate
Injection: 80 mg/ml
Tablets (sustained-release): 324 mg
quinidine sulfate
Tablets: 200 mg, 300 mg
Tablets (sustained-release): 300 mg

NURSING PROCESS

📝 Assessment

• Assess patient's arrhythmia before starting therapy and regularly thereafter to monitor drug's effectiveness.
• Monitor drug level. Therapeutic level for arrhythmias is 2 to 5 mcg/ml.
• Check apical pulse rate and blood pressure before starting therapy. Hypotension may occur, usually with parenteral use.
• Monitor liver function test results during first 4 to 8 weeks of therapy.
• Be alert for adverse reactions and drug interactions.
• Assess patient's and family's knowledge of drug therapy.

🔲 Nursing diagnoses

• Decreased cardiac output related to presence of arrhythmia
• Risk for deficient fluid volume related to drug-induced adverse GI reactions
• Deficient knowledge related to drug therapy

▷ Planning and implementation

• Give anticoagulant before starting therapy in a patient with long-standing atrial fibrillation because restoration of normal sinus rhythm may dislodge thrombi from atrial wall, causing thromboembolism.
• If patient develops unexplained fever or elevated hepatic enzyme level, monitor him for hepatotoxicity.
• If patient develops symptoms of cardiotoxicity, such as increased PR and QT intervals, 50% widening of the QRS complex, ventricular tachyarrhythmias, frequent ventricular ectopic beats, or tachycardia, stop drug immediately.
• Don't crush sustained-release tablets.
🔔 **ALERT:** Sustained-release preparations aren't interchangeable.
🔔 **ALERT:** Don't confuse quinidine with clonidine.

Patient teaching
• Tell patient to take drug with meals.
• Tell patient to report evidence of toxicity, including ringing in ears, visual disturbances, dizziness, headache, nausea, rash, or shortness of breath.
• Stress importance of follow-up care.

Q

☑ **Evaluation**
• Patient regains normal cardiac output with resolution of arrhythmia.
• Patient maintains adequate hydration throughout therapy.
• Patient and family state understanding of drug therapy.

quinupristin and dalfopristin

(KWIN-uh-pris-tin and DALF-oh-pris-tin)
Synercid

Pharmacologic class: streptogramin
Therapeutic class: antibiotic
Pregnancy risk category: B

Indications and dosages

▶ **Serious or life-threatening infections linked to vancomycin-resistant** *Enterococcus faecium* **bacteremia.** *Adults and children age 16 and older:* 7.5 mg/kg I.V. infusion over 1 hour every 8 hours. Length of therapy determined by site and severity of infection.

▶ **Complicated skin and skin-structure infections caused by** *Staphylococcus* **aureus (methicillin susceptible) or** *Streptococcus pyogenes.* *Adults and children age 16 and older:* 7.5 mg/kg by I.V. infusion over 1 hour every 12 hours for at least 7 days.

▽ I.V. administration

• Flush line with D_5W before and after each dose.
• Reconstitute powder for injection by adding 5 ml of sterile water for injection or D_5W. Gently swirl vial to dissolve powder completely; to limit foaming, don't shake the vial. Reconstituted solutions must be further diluted within 30 minutes.
• Add dose of reconstituted solution to 250 ml of D_5W; maximum concentration, 2 mg/ml. Diluted solution is stable for 5 hours at room temperature or 54 hours when refrigerated.
• Fluid-restricted patient with a central venous catheter may receive dose in 100 ml of D_5W. This concentration isn't recommended for peripheral venous administration.
• Give all doses by I.V. infusion over 1 hour. Use an infusion pump or device to control rate of infusion.

• If moderate to severe peripheral venous irritation occurs, consider increasing infusion volume to 500 or 750 ml, changing injection site, or infusing by central venous catheter.
⊗ **Incompatibilities**
Saline and heparin solutions.

Contraindications and cautions

• Contraindicated in patients hypersensitive to the drug or other streptogramin antibiotics.
⚖ **Lifespan:** In pregnant women, use only if benefits outweigh risks to the fetus. In breast-feeding women, use cautiously; it's unknown if the drug appears in breast milk. In children younger than age 16, safety and effectiveness haven't been established.

Adverse reactions

CNS: headache, pain.
CV: thrombophlebitis.
GI: diarrhea, nausea, vomiting.
Musculoskeletal: arthralgia, myalgia.
Skin: *edema, inflammation, and pain at infusion site;* pruritus; rash.

Interactions

Drug-drug. *Cyclosporine:* May decrease metabolism of cyclosporine and increase level. Monitor cyclosporine level.
Drugs metabolized by CYP3A4 (carbamazepine, delavirdine, diazepam, diltiazem, disopyramide, docetaxel, indinavir, lidocaine, lovastatin, methylprednisolone, midazolam, nevirapine, nifedipine, paclitaxel, ritonavir, tacrolimus, verapamil, vinblastine, and others): May increase levels, therapeutic effects, and adverse reactions of these drugs. Use together cautiously.
Drugs metabolized by CYP3A4 that may prolong the QT interval (such as quinidine): May decrease metabolism of these drugs and prolong QT interval. Avoid using together.

Effects on lab test results

• May increase AST, ALT, and bilirubin levels.

Pharmacokinetics

Absorption: Given I.V.
Distribution: Protein-binding is moderate.
Metabolism: Quinupristin and dalfopristin are converted to several active major metabolites by nonenzymatic reactions.

Excretion: About 75% of both drugs and their metabolites excreted in feces. About 15% of quinupristin and 19% of dalfopristin excreted in urine. *Half-life:* About 1 hour for quinupristin; about 15 minutes for dalfopristin.

Route	Onset	Peak	Duration
I.V.	Unknown	Unknown	Unknown

Action

Chemical effect: Inhibit or destroy susceptible bacteria through combined inhibition of protein synthesis in bacterial cells. Dalfopristin inhibits the early phase of protein synthesis in the bacterial ribosome, and quinupristin inhibits the late phase of protein synthesis.

Therapeutic effect: Inactivation or death of bacterial cells.

Available forms

Injection: 500 mg/10 ml (150 mg quinupristin and 350 mg dalfopristin)

NURSING PROCESS

Assessment
• Obtain history of patient's underlying condition before starting therapy, and reassess regularly thereafter to monitor drug's effectiveness.
• Overgrowth of nonsusceptible organisms may occur. Monitor patient closely for signs and symptoms of superinfection.
• Monitor liver function during therapy.
• Assess patient's and family's knowledge of drug therapy.

Nursing diagnoses
• Risk for infection related to presence of bacteria
• Diarrhea related to drug-induced adverse effect
• Deficient knowledge related to drug therapy

Planning and implementation
ALERT: Drug isn't active against *Enterococcus faecalis*. Make sure cultures are drawn to avoid misidentifying *E. faecalis* as *E. faecium*.
• To reduce adverse reactions, such as arthralgia and myalgia, decrease dose interval to every 12 hours.
• If patient develops diarrhea during or after therapy, notify prescriber because mild to life-threatening pseudomembranous colitis may occur.

Patient teaching
• Advise patient to immediately report irritation at I.V. site, pain in joints or muscles, and diarrhea.
• Tell patient to report persistent or worsening signs and symptoms of infection, such as pain and erythema.

Evaluation
• Patient is free from infection.
• Patient has no diarrhea.
• Patient and family state understanding of drug therapy.

rabeprazole sodium
(rah-BEH-pruh-zohl SOH-dee-um)
AcipHex

Pharmacologic class: proton pump inhibitor
Therapeutic class: antiulcerative
Pregnancy risk category: B

Indications and dosages

▶ **Erosive or ulcerative gastroesophageal reflux disease (GERD).** *Adults:* 20 mg P.O. daily for 4 to 8 weeks. Additional 8-week course may be considered, if needed.
▶ **To maintain healing of erosive or ulcerative GERD.** *Adults:* 20 mg P.O. daily.
▶ **Duodenal ulcers.** *Adults:* 20 mg P.O. daily after morning meal for up to 4 weeks.
▶ **Pathological hypersecretory conditions, including Zollinger-Ellison syndrome.** *Adults:* 60 mg P.O. daily; increase as needed to 100 mg P.O. daily or 60 mg P.O. b.i.d.
▶ **Symptomatic GERD, including daytime and nighttime heartburn.** *Adults:* 20 mg P.O. daily for 4 weeks. Additional 4-week course may be considered, if needed.
▶ *Helicobacter pylori* **eradication to reduce the risk of duodenal ulcer recurrence.** *Adults:* Three drug regimen: rabeprazole 20 mg P.O. b.i.d. given with amoxicillin 1,000 mg P.O.

b.i.d. and clarithromycin 500 mg P.O. b.i.d. for a total of 7 days.

Contraindications and cautions

• Contraindicated in patients hypersensitive to drug, other benzimidazoles (such as lansoprazole or omeprazole), or components in these formulations. For *H. pylori* eradication, clarithromycin is contraindicated in patients hypersensitive to any macrolide antibiotic and in those taking pimozide. Amoxicillin is contraindicated in patients hypersensitive to any penicillin.
• Use cautiously in patients with severe hepatic impairment.
⚱ Lifespan: In pregnant women, clarithromycin is contraindicated for *H. pylori* eradication. In children, safety and effectiveness haven't been established.

Adverse reactions

CNS: headache.

Interactions

Drug-drug. *Clarithromycin:* May increase level of rabeprazole. Monitor patient closely.
Cyclosporine: May inhibit cyclosporine metabolism. Use together cautiously.
Digoxin, ketoconazole, other gastric pH–dependent drugs: May decrease or increase drug absorption at increased pH values. Monitor patient closely.
Sucralfate: May delay rabeprazole absorption. Give rabeprazole at least 30 minutes before sucralfate.
Warfarin: May inhibit warfarin metabolism and increase PT and INR. Monitor patient closely.
Drug-herb. *St. John's wort:* May increase risk of sunburn. Discourage using together; urge patient to avoid unprotected or prolonged sun exposure.

Effects on lab test results

None reported.

Pharmacokinetics

Absorption: Acid labile; enteric coating allows drug to pass through the stomach relatively intact. Level peaks over a period of 2 to 5 hours.
Distribution: 96.3% protein-bound.
Metabolism: Extensive, in the liver, to inactive compounds.

Excretion: 90% in urine as metabolites. Remaining 10% of metabolites in feces. *Half-life:* 1 to 2 hours.

Route	Onset	Peak	Duration
P.O.	< 1 hr	2–5 hr	> 24 hr

Action

Chemical effect: Blocks activity of the acid (proton) pump by inhibiting gastric hydrogen-potassium adenosine triphosphatase at the secretory surface of gastric parietal cells, thereby blocking gastric acid secretion.
Therapeutic effect: Promotes healing of gastric erosion or ulceration by stopping gastric acid secretion.

Available forms

Tablets (delayed-release): 20 mg

NURSING PROCESS

✍ Assessment

• Obtain history of patient's underlying condition before starting therapy, and reassess regularly thereafter to monitor drug's effectiveness.
• Be alert for adverse reactions and drug interactions.
• Assess patient's and family's knowledge of drug therapy.

⊕ Nursing diagnoses

• Acute pain related to underlying condition
• Risk for injury related to drug-induced adverse reactions
• Deficient knowledge related to drug therapy

▶ Planning and implementation

• Don't crush, split, or allow patient to chew tablets.
• If duodenal ulcer or GERD isn't healed after first course of therapy, additional courses of therapy may be needed.
⚠ ALERT: Symptomatic response to therapy doesn't rule out presence of gastric malignancy.
• In patient who doesn't respond to therapy for *H. pylori*, test for susceptibility. If resistance to clarithromycin occurs or susceptibility testing isn't possible, give a different antimicrobial.
⚠ ALERT: For *H. pylori* eradication, pseudomembranous colitis may occur with nearly all antibacterials, including clarithromycin and amoxicillin. Monitor patient closely.

Reactions may be *common*, uncommon, *life-threatening*, or COMMON AND LIFE-THREATENING.

Patient teaching
- Explain importance of taking drug exactly as prescribed.
- Tell patient to swallow delayed-release tablets whole and not crush, chew, or split them.
- Tell patient that drug may be taken without regard to meals, unless patient is being treated for *H. pylori*; then all three drugs should be taken twice daily with the morning and evening meals.

☑ Evaluation
- Patient reports decreased pain with drug therapy.
- Patient sustains no injury as a result of drug-induced adverse reactions.
- Patient and family state understanding of drug therapy.

rabies immune globulin
(RAY-bees ih-MYOON GLOH-byoo-lin, HYOO-mun)
HyperRAB S/D, Imogam Rabies-HT

Pharmacologic class: immune serum
Therapeutic class: rabies prevention drug
Pregnancy risk category: C

Indications and dosages
▶ **Rabies exposure.** *Adults and children:* 20 international units/kg at time of first dose of rabies vaccine. If feasible, infiltrate the full dose in the area around and in the wounds. Give remainder, if any, I.M. separate from rabies vaccine injection site.

Contraindications and cautions
- Give only one dose to prevent interference with effectiveness of vaccine.
- Use cautiously in patients hypersensitive to thimerosal, in patients with a history of systemic allergic reactions after using human immunoglobulin, and in patients with immunoglobulin A deficiency.
- ⚘ **Lifespan:** In pregnant women, use cautiously. In breast-feeding women, safety and effectiveness haven't been established.

Adverse reactions
CV: malaise, slight fever, slight headache.
GU: nephrotic syndrome.

Skin: induration at injection site, pain, *rash,* redness.
Other: *anaphylaxis, angioedema.*

Interactions
Drug-drug. *Corticosteroids, immunosuppressive drugs:* May interfere with the active antibody response, predisposing patient to rabies. Avoid these drugs during postexposure immunization period.
Live-virus vaccines: May interfere with response to vaccine. Delay immunization.
Rabies vaccine: May partially suppress the antibody response to rabies immune globulin. Give full dose of immune globulin into wound, if feasible.

Effects on lab test results
None reported.

Pharmacokinetics
Absorption: Slow.
Distribution: Unknown.
Metabolism: Unknown.
Excretion: Unknown. *Half-life:* About 24 days.

Route	Onset	Peak	Duration
I.M.	Unknown	2–13 days	Unknown

Action
Chemical effect: Provides passive immunity to rabies.
Therapeutic effect: Prevents rabies.

Available forms
Injection: 150 units/ml in 2-ml, 10-ml vials

NURSING PROCESS

☲ Assessment
- Obtain history of animal bites, allergies, and immunization reactions.
- Ask patient when he last received a tetanus immunization. Prescriber may order booster.
- Be alert for adverse reactions and drug interactions.
- Assess patient's and family's knowledge of drug therapy.

⊕ Nursing diagnoses
- Risk for injury related to rabies exposure
- Ineffective protection related to drug-induced hypersensitivity reaction

• Deficient knowledge related to drug therapy

❯ Planning and implementation
• Use only with rabies vaccine and immediate local treatment of wound. Don't give in same syringe or at same site as rabies vaccine. Give drug regardless of interval between exposure and start of therapy.
• Don't give live-virus vaccines within 3 months of this drug.
🏶 **ALERT:** Drug provides passive immunity. Don't confuse with rabies vaccine, which is suspension of attenuated or killed microorganisms used to give active immunity. The two drugs usually are given together for prophylaxis after exposure to known or suspected rabid animals.
🏶 **ALERT:** Have epinephrine 1:1,000 immediately available to treat any acute anaphylactic reactions.
🏶 **ALERT:** Don't give more than 5 ml at one I.M. injection site; instead, divide I.M. doses larger than 5 ml and give at different sites. Use a large muscle, such as the gluteus.
Patient teaching
• Tell patient he may develop a slight fever and pain and redness at injection site.
• Explain that tetanus booster may be needed.
• Instruct patient to report signs of hypersensitivity immediately.

✅ Evaluation
• Patient has passive immunity to rabies.
• Patient shows no signs of hypersensitivity after receiving drug.
• Patient and family state understanding of drug therapy.

raloxifene hydrochloride
(rah-LOKS-ih-feen high-droh-KLOR-ighd)
Evista

Pharmacologic class: selective estrogen receptor modulator (SERM)
Therapeutic class: antiosteoporotic
Pregnancy risk category: X

Indications and dosages
▶ **To prevent and treat osteoporosis and to reduce the risk for invasive breast cancer in postmenopausal women with osteoporosis or who are at high risk for invasive breast cancer.** *Postmenopausal women:* 60 mg P.O. daily.

Contraindications and cautions
• Contraindicated in women hypersensitive to the drug or any of its components, and in those with current or past venous thromboembolic events, including deep vein thrombosis (DVT), pulmonary embolism, or retinal vein thrombosis.
• Use with hormone replacement therapy or systemic estrogen isn't recommended.
• Use cautiously in women with severe hepatic impairment.
🔥 **Lifespan:** In women who are pregnant or planning to become pregnant, in breast-feeding women, and in children, drug is contraindicated. In men, safety and effectiveness haven't been evaluated.

Adverse reactions
CNS: depression, fever, insomnia, migraine.
CV: chest pain, peripheral edema.
EENT: laryngitis, pharyngitis, *sinusitis.*
GI: abdominal pain, dyspepsia, flatulence, gastroenteritis, GI disorder, nausea, vomiting.
GU: cystitis, endometrial disorder, leukorrhea, UTI, vaginal bleeding, vaginitis.
Metabolic: weight gain.
Musculoskeletal: *arthralgia,* arthritis, leg cramps, myalgia,
Respiratory: increased cough, pneumonia.
Skin: rash, sweating.
Other: breast pain, flulike syndrome, hot flushes, infection.

Interactions
Drug-drug. *Cholestyramine:* May significantly reduce raloxifene absorption. Don't give these drugs together.
Highly protein-bound drugs, such as clofibrate, diazepam, diazoxide, ibuprofen, indomethacin, lidocaine, naproxen: May interfere with binding sites. Use together cautiously.
Warfarin: May decrease PT. Monitor PT and INR closely.

Effects on lab test results
• May increase calcium, inorganic phosphate, total protein, albumin, hormone-binding globulin, and apolipoprotein A levels. May decrease total cholesterol, low-density lipoprotein cholesterol, and apolipoprotein B levels.

Reactions may be *common,* uncommon, *life-threatening,* or COMMON AND LIFE-THREATENING.

Pharmacokinetics

Absorption: Rapid, with about 60% of dose absorbed after P.O. use.
Distribution: Wide. Extensively protein-bound.
Metabolism: Extensive first-pass metabolism to glucuronide conjugates.
Excretion: Mainly in feces, with less than 0.2% unchanged in urine. *Half-life:* 27½ hours.

Route	Onset	Peak	Duration
P.O.	Unknown	Unknown	24 hr

Action

Chemical effect: Reduces resorption of bone and decreases overall bone turnover by selectively activating and blocking estrogen receptors, resulting in increased bone mineral density.
Therapeutic effect: Prevents bone breakdown in postmenopausal women.

Available forms

Tablets: 60 mg

NURSING PROCESS

📠 Assessment

• Obtain history of patient's condition before starting therapy, and reassess regularly thereafter to monitor drug's effectiveness.
• Monitor patient for signs of blood clots. The greatest risk of thromboembolic events is during the first 4 months of therapy.
• Monitor patient for breast abnormalities.
• Monitor lipid level, blood pressure, body weight, and liver function.
• Assess patient's and family's knowledge of drug therapy.

⊕ Nursing diagnoses

• Ineffective peripheral tissue perfusion related to potential DVT formation
• Imbalanced nutrition: less than body requirements related to drug-induced adverse GI reactions
• Deficient knowledge related to drug therapy

▷ Planning and implementation

⊛ **ALERT:** Stop drug at least 72 hours before prolonged immobilization, and resume only after patient is fully mobile.
• If you suspect thromboembolic event, stop giving the drug and notify prescriber.

• Report unexplained uterine bleeding immediately to prescriber.
• Effect on bone mineral density with more than 2 years of drug therapy isn't known.
Patient teaching
• Advise patient to avoid long periods of restricted movement (such as during traveling) because it increases the risk of venous thromboembolic events.
• Inform patient that hot flashes or flushing may occur and that drug doesn't aid in reducing them.
• Instruct patient to take other bone-loss prevention measures, including taking supplemental calcium and vitamin D if dietary intake is inadequate, performing weight-bearing exercises, and stopping alcohol consumption and smoking.
• Tell patient that drug may be taken with or without food.
• Advise patient to report any unexplained uterine bleeding or breast abnormalities.
• Explain drug's adverse effects; instruct patient to read package insert before starting therapy and each time prescription is renewed.

☑ Evaluation

• Patient has no pain, redness, or swelling in legs.
• Patient maintains normal dietary intake.
• Patient and family state understanding of drug therapy.

✳ New Drug

raltegravir
(rahl-TEH-gruh-veer)
Isentress

R

Pharmacologic class: HIV integrase strand transfer inhibitor
Therapeutic class: antiretroviral
Pregnancy risk category: C

Indications and dosages

▶ **HIV-1 infection with other antiretrovirals in treatment-experienced patients who have continued HIV-1 replication despite antiretroviral therapy.** *Adults:* 400 mg P.O. b.i.d.

Contraindications and cautions

• Contraindicated in patients who are hypersensitive to drug or its components.

• Use cautiously in patients taking drugs known to cause myopathy or rhabdomyolysis, such as statins.

⚱ **Lifespan:** For pregnant women, give drug only if the potential benefit justifies the risk to the fetus. Register pregnant women for monitoring of maternal-fetal outcomes by calling the Antiretroviral Pregnancy Registry at 1-800-258-4263. Advise breast-feeding women that drug isn't recommended during therapy. For children younger than age 16, safety and efficacy haven't been established. Use cautiously in elderly patients, especially those with hepatic, renal, and cardiac insufficiency.

Adverse reactions

CNS: *headache,* fever, fatigue, dizziness.
GI: *diarrhea, nausea,* abdominal pain, vomiting.
Hematologic: *neutropenia,* anemia, ***thrombocytopenia.***
Metabolic: hyperglycemia.
Musculoskeletal: asthenia, myopathy, ***rhabdomyolysis.***
Skin: lipodystrophy.

Interactions

Drug-drug. *Atazanavir:* May increase raltegravir levels.
UGT1A1 inhibitors, such as rifampin: May decrease raltegravir levels. Use together cautiously.

Effects on lab test results

• May increase bilirubin, AST, ALT, alkaline phosphatase, amylase, lipase, glucose, creatine kinase levels. May decrease hemoglobin level.
• May decrease neutrophil and platelet counts.

Pharmacokinetics

Absorption: Reaches steady state within 2 days of administration.
Distribution: About 83% bound to human plasma protein.
Metabolism: Via UGT1A1-mediated glucuronidation pathway.
Excretion: 51% excreted in feces; 32% in urine. *Half-life:* About 9 hours.

Route	Onset	Peak	Duration
P.O.	Rapid	3 hrs	Unknown

Action

Chemical effect: Inhibits HIV-1 integrase, an enzyme required for HIV-1 viral replication.
Therapeutic effect: Reduces symptoms of HIV.

Available forms

Tablets: 400 mg

NURSING PROCESS

🔬 Assessment

• Monitor adverse reactions and drug interactions.
• Perform laboratory tests, including CBC, platelet count, and liver function studies, before therapy and regularly throughout.
• Assess patient's and family's knowledge of drug therapy.

⊕ Nursing diagnoses

• Risk for infection related to presence of virus
• Risk for injury related to adverse reactions
• Deficient knowledge related to drug therapy

▶ Planning and implementation

• Use drug with at least one other antiretroviral.
• Drug should be reserved for patients who demonstrate resistance to other regimens.
• Monitor patient for signs of myopathy.
Patient teaching
• Inform patient that drug doesn't cure HIV infection. He may continue to develop opportunistic infections and other complications of HIV infection and that transmission of HIV to others through sexual contact or blood contamination is still possible.
• Advise patient to use barrier protection during sexual intercourse.
• Advise patient to immediately report worsening symptoms or unexplained muscle pain, tenderness, or weakness while taking the drug.
• To decrease the risk of developing HIV resistance, instruct patient to avoid missing doses.
• Tell patient that if a dose is missed, he should take the next dose as soon as possible. If a dose is skipped he shouldn't double the next dose.
• Advise patient to report use of other drugs, including OTC drugs; this drug interacts with other drugs.
• Tell patient that drug may be taken without regard to meals.

Reactions may be *common,* uncommon, ***life-threatening***, or COMMON AND LIFE-THREATENING.

✓ Evaluation

• Patient's health improves, and signs and symptoms of underlying condition diminish with use of drug.
• Patient is free from injury from adverse reactions.
• Patient and family state understanding of drug therapy.

ramelteon
(rah-MEHL-tee-on)
Rozerem

Pharmacologic class: melatonin receptor agonist
Therapeutic class: hypnotic
Pregnancy risk category: C

Indications and dosages

▶ **Insomnia characterized by trouble falling asleep.** *Adults:* 8 mg P.O. within 30 minutes of bedtime. Don't give with or immediately after a high-fat meal.

Contraindications and cautions

• Contraindicated with hypersensitivity to the drug or its components. Don't use in patients taking fluvoxamine or in those with severe hepatic impairment, sleep apnea, or COPD.
• Use cautiously in patients with depression or moderate hepatic impairment.
🕮 **Lifespan:** Use drug in pregnancy only if benefits outweigh risks to the fetus. In breastfeeding women, avoid use. In children, safety and effectiveness haven't been established.

Adverse reactions

CNS: complex sleep disorders, depression, dizziness, fatigue, headache, somnolence, worsened insomnia.
GI: diarrhea, impaired taste, nausea.
Musculoskeletal: arthralgia, myalgia.
Respiratory: upper respiratory tract infection.
Other: *anaphylaxis, angioedema,* flulike syndrome.

Interactions

Drug-drug. *CNS depressants:* May cause excessive CNS depression. Use together cautiously.

Fluconazole (strong CYP2C9 inhibitor), keto-conazole (strong CYP3A4 inhibitor), weak CYP1A2 inhibitors: May increase ramelteon level. Use together cautiously.
Fluvoxamine (strong CYP1A2 inhibitor): May increase ramelteon level. Avoid use together.
Rifampin (strong cytochrome P-450 enzyme inducer): May decrease ramelteon level. Monitor patient for lack of effect.
Drug-food. *Food (especially high-fat meals):* May delay time to peak drug effect. Tell patient to take drug on an empty stomach.
Drug-lifestyle. *Alcohol use:* May cause excessive CNS depression. Discourage alcohol use.

Effects on lab test results

• May increase prolactin level. May alter blood cortisol and testosterone levels.

Pharmacokinetics

Absorption: Rapid. Oral bioavailability is 1.8%. Food consumption decreases and delays peak level by 45 minutes.
Distribution: 82% protein-bound; 70% to serum albumin. Tissue distribution is substantial.
Metabolism: Rapid, first pass metabolism mainly by CYP1A2 (also by CYP2C and CYP3A4), with four active metabolites formed.
Excretion: 84% in urine, 4% in feces. Less than 0.1% as the parent compound. Elimination complete 96 hours after dose. *Half-life:* Parent compound, 1 to 2½ hours; metabolite M-II, 2 to 5 hours.

Route	Onset	Peak	Duration
P.O.	Rapid	½–½ hr	Unknown

Action

Chemical effect: Acts on receptors believed to maintain the circadian rhythm underlying the normal sleep-wake cycle.
Therapeutic effect: Promotes sleep.

Available forms

Tablets: 8 mg

✐ Assessment

• Thoroughly evaluate the cause of insomnia before starting drug.
• Assess patient for behavioral or cognitive disorders.

• Evaluate patient's and family's knowledge of drug therapy.

🖝 Nursing diagnoses
• Sleep deprivation related to presence of insomnia
• Risk for injury related to drug-induced adverse CNS effects
• Deficient knowledge related to drug therapy

▷ Planning and implementation
• Give drug on an empty stomach to prevent delays in peak effect.
• Drug doesn't cause physical dependence.
• In cases of overdose, consider the possibility of multiple drug ingestion, and contact a poison control center. Treat symptomatically.

Patient teaching
• Instruct patient to take dose within 30 minutes of bedtime.
• Tell patient not to take drug with or after a heavy meal.
• Warn patient about possible complex sleep-related behaviors.
• Caution against performing activities that require mental alertness or physical coordination after taking drug.
• Caution patient to avoid alcohol while taking ramelteon.
• Tell patient to consult prescriber if insomnia worsens or behavior changes.
• Urge woman to consult prescriber if menses stops, libido decreases, or breast discharge or fertility problems develop.

✓ Evaluation
• Patient reports that drug effectively promotes sleep.
• Patient sustains no injury from adverse CNS effects.
• Patient and family state understanding of drug therapy.

ramipril
(reh-MIH-pril)
Altace

Pharmacologic class: ACE inhibitor
Therapeutic class: antihypertensive
Pregnancy risk category: C (D in second and third trimesters)

Indications and dosages
▶ **Hypertension.** *Adults not receiving a diuretic:* Initially, 2.5 mg P.O. daily.
Adults receiving a diuretic: Initially, 1.25 mg P.O. once daily. Adjust dosage based on blood pressure response. Usual maintenance dosage is 2.5 to 20 mg daily as a single dose or in two equal doses.
⧅ **Adjust-a-dose:** For patients with renal impairment, if creatinine clearance is less than 40 ml/minute (creatinine higher than 2.5 mg/dl), recommended initial dose is 1.25 mg daily, adjusted upward to maximum dose of 5 mg based on blood pressure response.
In patients receiving diuretic therapy, symptomatic hypotension may occur. To minimize this, stop diuretic, if possible, 2 to 3 days before starting ramipril. When this isn't possible, give initial dose of 1.25 mg.
▶ **Heart failure post-MI.** *Adults:* Initially, 2.5 mg P.O. b.i.d. Adjust to target dosage of 5 mg P.O. b.i.d.
⧅ **Adjust-a-dose:** For patients with renal impairment, start therapy with 1.25 mg P.O. once daily, and increase to 1.25 mg b.i.d. Maximum dosage is 2.5 mg b.i.d.
▶ **Reduction in risk of MI, stroke, and death from CV causes.** *Adults age 55 and older:* 2.5 mg P.O. once daily for 1 week, then 5 mg P.O. once daily for 3 weeks. Increase as tolerated to maintenance dosage of 10 mg P.O. once daily.
⧅ **Adjust-a-dose:** For patients with renal impairment, if creatinine clearance is less than 40 ml/minute, give one-quarter of recommended dose.

Contraindications and cautions
• Contraindicated in patients hypersensitive to ACE inhibitors, in those with history of angioedema during previous therapy with ACE inhibitor, and in those with renal artery stenosis.
• Use cautiously in patients with renal impairment.
☀ **Lifespan:** In pregnant and breast-feeding women, drug isn't recommended. In children, safety and effectiveness haven't been established.

Adverse reactions
CNS: amnesia, anxiety, asthenia, depression, dizziness, fatigue, headache, insomnia, syncope, lightheadedness, malaise, nervousness, neural-

gia, neuropathy, paresthesia, *seizures,* somnolence, tremors, vertigo.
CV: angina, *arrhythmias,* chest pain, edema, *MI,* orthostatic hypotension, palpitations.
EENT: epistaxis, tinnitus.
GI: abdominal pain, anorexia, constipation, diarrhea, dry mouth, dyspepsia, gastroenteritis, nausea, vomiting.
GU: impotence.
Metabolic: *hyperkalemia,* weight gain.
Musculoskeletal: arthralgia, arthritis, myalgia.
Respiratory: dry, persistent, tickling, nonproductive cough; dyspnea.
Skin: dermatitis, increased diaphoresis, photosensitivity reaction, pruritus, rash.
Other: *angioedema,* hypersensitivity reactions.

Interactions

Drug-drug. *Diuretics:* May cause excessive hypotension, especially at start of therapy. Stop diuretic at least 3 days before starting ramipril, increase sodium intake, or reduce starting dose of ramipril.
Insulin, oral antidiabetics: May increase risk of hypoglycemia, especially at start of ramipril therapy. Monitor patient closely.
Lithium: May increase lithium level. Use together cautiously, and monitor lithium level for toxicity.
Potassium-sparing diuretics, potassium supplements: May increase risk of hyperkalemia because ramipril attenuates potassium loss. Monitor potassium level closely.
Drug-herb. *Capsaicin:* May increase risk of cough. Discourage using together.
Licorice: May cause sodium retention and increase blood pressure, interfering with therapeutic effects of ACE inhibitors. Discourage using together.
Drug-food. *Salt substitutes containing potassium:* May increase risk of hyperkalemia because ramipril attenuates potassium loss. Monitor potassium level closely.

Effects on lab test results

• May increase BUN, creatinine, bilirubin, liver enzyme, glucose, and potassium levels. May decrease hemoglobin level and hematocrit.

Pharmacokinetics

Absorption: 50% to 60%.
Distribution: 73% protein-bound; ramiprilat (metabolite), 58%.

Metabolism: Almost completely converted to ramiprilat, which is six times more potent than parent drug.
Excretion: 60% in urine; 40% in feces. *Half-life:* 9 to 18 hours.

Route	Onset	Peak	Duration
P.O.	1–2 hr	3–6 hr	24 hr

Action

Chemical effect: May inhibit conversion from angiotensin I to angiotensin II, a potent vasoconstrictor. This decreases peripheral arterial resistance, thus decreasing aldosterone secretion.
Therapeutic effect: Lowers blood pressure.

Available forms

Capsules: 1.25 mg, 2.5 mg, 5 mg, 10 mg

NURSING PROCESS

Assessment
• Assess patient's blood pressure before starting therapy and regularly thereafter to monitor drug's effectiveness.
• Assess kidney function closely during first few weeks of therapy. Regularly assess creatinine and BUN levels. Patient with severe heart failure whose kidney function depends on angiotensin-aldosterone system may experience acute renal impairment during therapy. Hypertensive patient with renal artery stenosis also may show signs of worsening kidney function at start of therapy.
• Monitor CBC before therapy, every 2 weeks for first 3 months of therapy, and periodically thereafter.
• Monitor potassium level. Risk factors for hyperkalemia include renal insufficiency, diabetes, and use of drugs that raise potassium level.
• Be alert for adverse reactions and drug interactions.
• Assess patient's and family's knowledge of drug therapy.

Nursing diagnoses
• Risk for injury related to presence of hypertension
• Sleep deprivation related to drug-induced cough
• Deficient knowledge related to drug therapy

Planning and implementation

- Stop diuretic 2 to 3 days before starting therapy, if possible.
- If patient has trouble swallowing pills whole, capsule may be opened and the contents sprinkled onto 4 ounces of applesauce or mixed in 4 ounces (118 ml) of water or apple juice. These mixtures may be stored at room temperature for up to 24 hours, or refrigerated for up to 48 hours.

Patient teaching

- Instruct patient not to use salt substitutes or potassium supplements during therapy.
- If patient has trouble swallowing, tell him to open capsules and sprinkle contents on food.
- Tell patient to rise slowly to avoid initial lightheadedness. If syncope occurs, tell him to stop taking the drug and notify the prescriber.
- Tell patient not to abruptly stop therapy.
- Advise patient to report signs of angioedema and laryngeal edema, which may occur after first dose.
- Tell patient to report signs of infection.
- Tell woman to report pregnancy. Drug will need to be stopped.

Evaluation

- Patient's blood pressure is normal.
- Patient's sleep patterns are undisturbed throughout therapy.
- Patient and family state understanding of drug therapy.

---

ranitidine hydrochloride
(ruh-NIH-tuh-deen high-droh-KLOR-ighd)
Nu-Ranit ◆ , Zantac*, Zantac EFFERdose, Zantac 75†, Zantac 150 Maximum Strength†

Pharmacologic class: H$_2$-receptor antagonist
Therapeutic class: antiulcerative
Pregnancy risk category: B

Indications and dosages

▶ **Intractable duodenal ulcer; pathologic hypersecretory conditions, such as Zollinger-Ellison syndrome; short-term therapy for patients unable to tolerate oral forms (I.V. only).** *Adults:* 150 mg P.O. b.i.d. or 300 mg at bedtime. Or, 50 mg I.V. or I.M. every 6 to 8 hours. Parenteral dose should not exceed 400 mg daily. Patients with Zollinger-Ellison

syndrome may need up to 6 g P.O. daily. Or, for Zollinger-Ellison syndrome, 1 mg/kg/hour for 4 hours; then increase in increments of 0.5 mg/kg/hour if needed, to a maximum of 2.5 mg/kg/hour.

▶ **Duodenal and gastric ulcer.** *Children ages 1 month to 16 years:* 2 to 4 mg/kg P.O. b.i.d. to a maximum of 300 mg/day. Maintenance dosage is 2 to 4 mg/kg P.O. once daily to a maximum of 150 mg daily or 2 to 4 mg/kg I.V. daily in divided doses every 6 to 8 hours.
Neonates less than 1 month of age receiving extracorporeal membrane oxygenation (called ECMO): 2 mg/kg I.V. every 12 to 24 hours or as a continuous infusion.

▶ **Maintenance therapy for duodenal ulcer.** *Adults:* 150 mg P.O. at bedtime.

▶ **Gastroesophageal reflux disease.** *Adults:* 150 mg P.O. b.i.d.
Children age 1 month and older: 5 to 10 mg/kg P.O. daily in two divided doses.

▶ **Erosive esophagitis.** *Adults:* 150 mg P.O. q.i.d.; maintenance dosage, 150 mg P.O. b.i.d.
Children age 1 month and older: 5 to 10 mg/kg P.O. daily in 2 divided doses.

▶ **Self-medication for occasional heartburn, acid indigestion, and sour stomach.** *Adults and children age 12 and older:* 75 mg to 150 mg once or twice daily; maximum daily dosage, 150 mg.

Adjust-a-dose: For patients with renal impairment, if creatinine clearance is less than 50 ml/min, give 150 mg P.O. every 24 hours or 50 mg I.M. or I.V. every 18 to 24 hours.

I.V. administration

- To prepare I.V. injection, dilute 2 ml (50 mg) with compatible I.V. solution to a total volume of 20 ml, and inject over at least 5 minutes. Compatible solutions include sterile water for injection, normal saline solution for injection, D$_5$W, and lactated Ringer's injection.
- To give drug by intermittent I.V. infusion, dilute 50 mg (2 ml) in 100 ml compatible solution and infuse at a rate of 5 to 7 ml/minute. The premixed solution is 50 ml and doesn't need further dilution. Infuse over 15 to 20 minutes. After dilution, solution is stable for 48 hours at room temperature.
- For premixed I.V. infusion, give by slow I.V. drip (over 15 to 20 minutes). Don't add other drugs to solution. If used with primary I.V. fluid system, stop primary solution during infusion.

- Store I.V. vial at 39° to 86° F (4° to 30° C). Store premixed containers at 36° F to 77° F (2° C to 25° C).
⊗ **Incompatibilities**
Amphotericin B, atracurium, cefazolin, cefoxitin, ceftazidime, cefuroxime, chlorpromazine, clindamycin phosphate, diazepam, ethacrynate sodium, hetastarch, hydroxyzine, insulin, methotrimeprazine, midazolam, norepinephrine, pentobarbital sodium, phenobarbital, phytonadione.

Contraindications and cautions

- Contraindicated in patients hypersensitive to the drug or any of its components.
- Use cautiously in patients with hepatic dysfunction. Adjust dosage in patients with impaired kidney function.
☀ **Lifespan:** In pregnant women, use cautiously. In breast-feeding women, use cautiously; it's unknown if the drug appears in breast milk. In children, safety and effectiveness haven't been established for pathological hypersecretory conditions or the maintenance of healing duodenal ulcer. In neonates younger than 1 month, safety and effectiveness haven't been established. In elderly patients, use cautiously.

Adverse reactions

CNS: malaise, vertigo.
EENT: blurred vision.
GI: abdominal discomfort, constipation, diarrhea, nausea, vomiting.
Hematologic: *pancytopenia, reversible leukopenia, thrombocytopenia.*
Hepatic: jaundice.
Skin: rash.
Other: *anaphylaxis, angioedema,* burning and itching at injection site.

Interactions

Drug-drug. *Antacids:* May interfere with ranitidine absorption. Stagger doses.
Diazepam: May decrease diazepam absorption. Monitor patient for decreased effectiveness; adjust dosage.
Glipizide: May increase hypoglycemic effect. Adjust glipizide dosage.
Procainamide: May decrease renal clearance of procainamide. Monitor patient for procainamide toxicity.
Warfarin: May interfere with warfarin clearance. Monitor patient closely for bleeding.

Drug-lifestyle. *Smoking:* May increase gastric acid secretion and worsen disease. Discourage using together.

Effects on lab test results

- May increase creatinine and ALT levels.
- May decrease RBC, WBC, and platelet counts.
- May cause false-positive test for urine protein using Multistix.

Pharmacokinetics

Absorption: About 50% to 60% of P.O. dose; rapid from parenteral sites after I.M. dose.
Distribution: To many body tissues and CSF; about 10% to 19% protein-bound.
Metabolism: In liver.
Excretion: In urine and feces. *Half-life:* 2 to 3 hours.

Route	Onset	Peak	Duration
P.O.	≤ 1 hr	1–3 hr	≤ 13 hr
I.V., I.M.	Unknown	Unknown	≤ 13 hr

Action

Chemical effect: Competitively inhibits action of H_2 at receptor sites of parietal cells, decreasing gastric acid secretion.
Therapeutic effect: Relieves GI discomfort.

Available forms

Capsules: 150 mg, 300 mg
Granules (effervescent): 150 mg
Infusion: 1 mg/ml in 50-ml containers
Injection: 25 mg/ml
Syrup: 15 mg/ml*
Tablets: 75 mg†, 150 mg†, 300 mg
Tablets (effervescent): 25 mg, 150 mg

NURSING PROCESS

Assessment
- Assess patient's GI condition before starting therapy and regularly thereafter to monitor drug's effectiveness.
- Zantac EFFERdose contains phenylalanine.
- Be alert for adverse reactions and drug interactions.
- Assess patient's and family's knowledge of drug therapy.

R

✣ Nursing diagnoses
• Impaired tissue integrity related to underlying GI condition
• Risk for injury related to drug-induced adverse CNS reactions
• Deficient knowledge related to drug therapy

❯ Planning and implementation
• Don't use aluminum-based needles or equipment when mixing or giving drug parenterally because drug is incompatible with aluminum.
• No dilution is needed when giving drug I.M.
• The effervescent tablet may be dissolved in 5 ml of water and given with an oral syringe or in a medicine cup.
Ⓢ **ALERT:** Don't confuse ranitidine with rimantadine.
Ⓢ **ALERT:** Don't confuse Zantac with Xanax or Zyrtec.
Patient teaching
• Remind patient taking drug once daily to take it at bedtime.
• Instruct patient to take drug with or without food.
• Urge patient not to smoke cigarettes; smoking may increase gastric acid secretion and worsen disease.

✓ Evaluation
• Patient states that GI discomfort is relieved.
• Patient sustains no injury as result of drug-induced adverse CNS reactions.
• Patient and family state understanding of drug therapy.

ranolazine
(rah-NOH-lah-zeen)
Ranexa✦

Pharmacologic class: fatty acid oxidation inhibitor
Therapeutic class: antianginal
Pregnancy risk category: C

Indications and dosages
❯ **Chronic angina, given with amlodipine, beta blockers, or nitrates, in patients who haven't achieved an adequate response with other antianginals.** *Adults:* Initially, 500 mg P.O. b.i.d. Increase as needed to maximum of 1,000 mg b.i.d.

Contraindications and cautions
• Contraindicated in patients taking QT interval–prolonging drugs or CYP3A inhibitors (including diltiazem) and in patients with ventricular tachycardia, hepatic impairment, or a prolonged QT interval.
• Use cautiously in patients with renal impairment.
⚖ **Lifespan:** In pregnant women, use only if benefit to mother outweighs risk to fetus. It isn't known whether drug appears in breast milk. In children, safety and efficacy haven't been established. In elderly patients, start at the low end of the dosage range and adjust slowly.

Adverse reactions
CNS: dizziness, headache.
CV: palpitations, peripheral edema, syncope.
EENT: tinnitus, vertigo.
GI: abdominal pain, constipation, dry mouth, nausea, vomiting.
Respiratory: dyspnea.

Interactions
Drug-drug. *Antipsychotics or tricyclic antidepressants metabolized by CYP2D6:* May increase levels of these drugs. Dosage reduction may be needed.
Cyclosporine, paroxetine, ritonavir: May increase ranolazine level. Use cautiously together, and monitor patient for increased adverse effects.
Digoxin: May increase digoxin level. Monitor digoxin level periodically; digoxin dosage may need to be reduced.
Diltiazem, macrolide antibiotics (azithromycin, erythromycin), protease inhibitors, verapamil: May increase ranolazine level and prolong QT interval. Avoid use together.
Drugs that prolong the QT interval; antiarrhythmics, such as dofetilide, quinidine, and sotalol; antipsychotics; such as chlorpromazine and ziprasidone: May increase the risk of prolonged QT interval. Avoid use together.
Potent CYP3A inhibitors, such as ketoconazole: May increase ranolazine level. Use together is contraindicated.
Simvastatin: May increase simvastatin level. Monitor patient for adverse effects, and decrease simvastatin dosage as needed.
Drug-food. *Grapefruit:* May increase ranolazine level and prolong QT interval. Avoid use together.

Reactions may be *common*, uncommon, *life-threatening*, or COMMON AND LIFE-THREATENING.

Effects on lab test results
• May increase serum creatinine and BUN levels. May decrease hematocrit level.
• May decrease eosinophil count.

Pharmacokinetics
Absorption: Highly variable. Steady state occurs within 3 days.
Distribution: 62% bound by plasma proteins.
Metabolism: Rapid and extensive in liver and intestine, mainly by CYP3A and CYP2D6, to four metabolites.
Excretion: 75% in urine; 25% in feces. *Half-life:* 7 hours.

Route	Onset	Peak	Duration
P.O.	Rapid	2–5 hr	Unknown

Action
Chemical effect: Unknown. May result from increased efficiency of myocardial oxygen use when myocardial metabolism is shifted away from fatty acid oxidation toward glucose oxidation. Antianginal and anti-ischemic properties don't decrease heart rate or blood pressure and don't increase myocardial work.
Therapeutic effect: Relieves chronic angina.

Available forms
Tablets (extended-release): 500 mg

NURSING PROCESS

Assessment
• Obtain history of patient's underlying condition before therapy, and reassess regularly thereafter.
• Monitor ECG for prolonged QT interval and measure the QTc interval regularly.
• If patient has renal insufficiency, monitor blood pressure closely.

Nursing diagnoses
• Ineffective health maintenance related to underlying condition
• Decreased cardiac output related to drug-induced adverse reactions
• Deficient knowledge related to drug therapy

Planning and implementation
⚠ ALERT: Ranolazine prolongs the QT interval in a dose-related manner. If ranolazine is given with other drugs that prolong the QTc interval,

torsades de pointes or sudden death may occur. Don't exceed maximum dosage.
• Drug may be taken without regard to meals.
• Don't crush or cut tablets.
Patient teaching
• Educate patient about drug's potential to cause an irregular heartbeat. Advise patient to immediately report palpitations or fainting and to tell prescriber about all other prescription or OTC drugs or herbal supplements he takes.
• Tell patient that he should keep taking other drugs prescribed for angina.
• Explain that drug won't stop a sudden anginal attack; advise him to keep other treatments, such as S.L. nitroglycerin, readily available.
• Tell patient that drug may be taken with or without food.
• Advise patient to avoid grapefruit juice while taking this drug.
• Warn patient that drug must be swallowed whole and not crushed, broken, or chewed.
• Tell patient to avoid activities that require mental alertness until effects of the drug are known.

✓ Evaluation
• Patient shows improvement in underlying condition.
• Patient maintains adequate cardiac output throughout therapy.
• Patient and family state understanding of drug therapy.

rasagiline mesylate
(reh-SAH-jih-leen MEH-sih-layt)
Azilect⌀

Pharmacologic class: irreversible, selective MAO inhibitor type B
Therapeutic class: antiparkinsonian
Pregnancy risk category: C

Indications and dosages
▶ **Idiopathic Parkinson disease, as monotherapy or with levodopa.** *Adults:* As monotherapy, 1 mg P.O. once daily. With levodopa, 0.5 mg P.O. once daily, increased to 1 mg once daily if needed. If patient taking both drugs has hallucinations or dyskinesia, levodopa dosage may be reduced.

⬕ **Adjust-a-dose:** If patient has mild hepatic impairment or takes a CYP1A2 inhibitor, such as ciprofloxacin, give 0.5 mg once daily.

Contraindications and cautions

• Contraindicated in patients with pheochromocytoma, and patients taking amphetamines, cold products, dextromethorphan, ephedrine, MAO inhibitors, meperidine, methadone, phenylephrine, propoxyphene, pseudoephedrine, sympathomimetic amines, or tramadol.
• Use cautiously in patients with mild hepatic impairment.
⚖ **Lifespan:** Use cautiously in pregnant or breast-feeding women. In geriatric patients, safety of drug is similar to that in younger adults.

Adverse reactions

Monotherapy
CNS: depression, *dizziness, falls,* fever, hallucinations, *headache,* malaise, paresthesia, syncope, vertigo.
CV: angina pectoris, *chest pain,* postural hypotension.
EENT: gingivitis.
GI: anorexia, diarrhea, dyspepsia, gastroenteritis, vomiting.
GU: albuminuria, impotence.
Hematologic: *leukopenia.*
Musculoskeletal: arthralgia, arthritis, neck pain.
Respiratory: asthma, rhinitis.
Skin: alopecia, *carcinoma,* ecchymosis, vesiculobullous rash.
Other: allergic reaction, decreased libido, flu-like syndrome.
Combined with levodopa
CNS: abnormal dreams, amnesia, ataxia, confusion, *dyskinesia,* dystonia, *falls,* hallucinations, *headache,* paresthesia, somnolence, *stroke,* sweating.
CV: bundle branch block, postural hypotension.
EENT: epistaxis, gingivitis.
GI: abdominal pain, anorexia, constipation, diarrhea, dry mouth, dyspepsia, dysphagia, *nausea,* vomiting, weight loss.
GU: albuminuria.
Hematologic: anemia, *hemorrhage.*
Musculoskeletal: arthralgia, arthritis, bursitis, hernia, leg cramps, myasthenia, neck pain, tenosynovitis.
Respiratory: dyspnea.

Skin: *carcinoma,* ecchymosis, pruritus, rash, ulcer.
Other: infection.

Interactions

Drug-drug. *Ciprofloxacin and other CYP1A2 inhibitors:* May double rasagiline level. Decrease rasagiline dosage to 0.5 mg daily.
Levodopa: May increase rasagiline level. Watch for dyskinesia, dystonia, hallucinations, and hypotension, and reduce levodopa dosage if needed.
Serotonin-norepinephrine reuptake inhibitors, SSRIs, tricyclic antidepressants: May cause severe or fatal CNS toxicity. Stop rasagiline for at least 14 days before starting an antidepressant. Stop fluoxetine for 5 weeks before starting rasagiline.
Drug-food. *Tyramine-rich foods and supplements:* May cause hypertensive crisis. Urge patient to avoid tyramine-rich foods, such as aged meat, salami, pickled herring, aged cheese, unpasteurized beer, red wine, fava beans, sauerkraut, soybean products, and concentrated yeast extract.
Drug-herb. *St. John's wort:* May cause severe reaction. Discourage use together.

Effects on lab test results

• May increase liver enzyme levels.
• May decrease WBC count.

Pharmacokinetics

Absorption: Rapidly absorbed after P.O. use.
Distribution: Wide. 88% to 94% bound to plasma proteins.
Metabolism: Almost completely metabolized in the liver by CYP1A2.
Excretion: Mainly in urine as glucuronide conjugates, with small amounts in feces. *Half-life:* 3 hours.

Route	Onset	Peak	Duration
P.O.	Variable	1 hr	1 wk

Action

Chemical effect: Unknown. Inhibition of MAO type B may increase extracellular dopamine level in the CNS, improving neurotransmission.
Therapeutic effect: Relieves the signs and symptoms of Parkinson disease.

Available forms

Tablets: 0.5 mg, 1 mg

NURSING PROCESS

🗓 Assessment

• Assess patient's condition before starting therapy and regularly thereafter to monitor drug's effectiveness.
• Be alert for drug interactions.
• If patient takes levodopa with rasagiline, watch for adverse effects; a reduced dosage of levodopa may be needed.
• Assess patient's and family's knowledge of drug therapy.

⊕ Nursing diagnoses

• Impaired physical mobility related to underlying condition
• Risk for injury related to drug-induced adverse CNS reactions
• Deficient knowledge related to drug therapy

⊠ Planning and implementation

• Protect patient from falls; postural hypotension may occur during first 2 months of therapy.
• Examine the patient's skin periodically for possible melanoma.
• Drug should be stopped at least 14 days before elective surgery.
• Evidence of overdose may not appear for 12 hours and may include cool and clammy skin, diaphoresis, drowsiness, hallucinations, hyperpyrexia, hypertension or hypotension, severe headache, and respiratory depression or failure.
• In case of overdose, hospitalize immediately and give supportive care. Provide respiratory support, monitor body temperature, manage hyperoxia, and maintain fluid and electrolyte balance for at least 2 days.

Patient teaching
• Explain the risk of hypertensive crisis if patient ingests tyramine while taking rasagiline. Give patient a list of tyramine-containing foods and products.
• Tell patient to contact prescriber if hallucinations occur.
• Urge patient to watch for skin changes that could suggest melanoma and to have periodic skin examinations by a health professional.
• Instruct patient to maintain his usual dosage schedule if he misses a dose and not to double the next dose to make up for a missed one.

☑ Evaluation

• Patient has improved physical mobility.
• Patient sustains no injury from adverse CNS reactions.
• Patient and family state understanding of drug therapy.

HIGH ALERT

repaglinide

(reh-PAG-lih-nighd)
Prandin

Pharmacologic class: meglitinide
Therapeutic class: antidiabetic
Pregnancy risk category: C

Indications and dosages

▶ **Adjunct to diet and exercise to lower glucose level in patients with type 2 diabetes mellitus (non–insulin-dependent diabetes mellitus) whose hyperglycemia can't be controlled satisfactorily by diet and exercise alone; adjunct to diet, exercise, and metformin, rosiglitazone, or pioglitazone.** *Adults:* For patients not previously treated or whose glycosylated hemoglobin (HbA1c) is below 8%, start dose at 0.5 mg P.O. given 15 minutes before meal; however, time may vary from immediately before to as long as 30 minutes before meal. For patients previously treated with glucose-lowering drugs and whose HbA1c is 8% or more, initial dose is 1 to 2 mg P.O. with each meal. Recommended dosage range is 0.5 to 4 mg with meals b.i.d., t.i.d., or q.i.d. Maximum, 16 mg daily. Base dosage on glucose-level response. May double dosage up to 4 mg with each meal until satisfactory glucose-level response is achieved. Allow at least 1 week between dosage adjustments to assess response to each dose.

🔲 **Adjust-a-dose:** For patients with severe renal impairment, starting dose is 0.5 mg P.O. with meals.

Contraindications and cautions

• Contraindicated in patients hypersensitive to the drug or any of its components and in those with insulin-dependent diabetes mellitus or diabetic ketoacidosis with or without coma.
• Use cautiously in patients with hepatic insufficiency. Reduced metabolism may increase drug level and cause hypoglycemia. Also use cau-

tiously in debilitated and malnourished patients and in those with adrenal or pituitary insufficiency because they're more susceptible to the hypoglycemic effect of glucose-lowering drugs.

🔆 **Lifespan:** In pregnant women and breast-feeding women, don't use. In children, safety and effectiveness haven't been established. In the elderly, use cautiously.

Adverse reactions

CNS: *headache,* paresthesia.
CV: angina, chest pain.
EENT: rhinitis, sinusitis.
GI: constipation, diarrhea, dyspepsia, nausea, vomiting.
GU: UTI.
Metabolic: hyperglycemia, HYPOGLYCEMIA.
Musculoskeletal: arthralgia, back pain.
Respiratory: bronchitis, upper respiratory infection.
Other: tooth disorder.

Interactions

Drug-drug. *Barbiturates, carbamazepine, rifampin:* May increase repaglinide metabolism. Monitor glucose level.
Beta blockers, chloramphenicol, coumarins, MAO inhibitors, NSAIDs, other drugs that are highly protein-bound, probenecid, salicylates, sulfonamides: May increase hypoglycemic action of repaglinide. Monitor glucose level.
Calcium channel blockers, corticosteroids, estrogens, hormonal contraceptives, isoniazid, nicotinic acid, phenothiazines, phenytoin, sympathomimetics, thiazides and other diuretics, thyroid products: May produce hyperglycemia and loss of glycemic control. Monitor glucose level.
Erythromycin, gemfibrozil, inhibitors of CYP3A4, ketoconazole, miconazole: May inhibit repaglinide metabolism. Monitor glucose level and avoid using gemfibrozil and repaglinide together.
Levonorgestrel and ethinyl estradiol, simvastatin: May increase repaglinide level. Monitor glucose level.
Drug-herb. *Aloe, bilberry leaf, bitter melon, burdock, dandelion, fenugreek, garlic, ginseng:* May improve glucose control so that antidiabetic dosage needs to be reduced. Advise patient to discuss the use of herbal remedies before taking drug.

Effects on lab test results

• May increase or decrease glucose level.

Pharmacokinetics

Absorption: Rapid and complete. Absolute bioavailability is 56%.
Distribution: More than 98% protein-bound.
Metabolism: Completely metabolized by oxidative biotransformation and direct conjugation with glucuronic acid.
Excretion: About 90% is recovered in feces and 8% in urine. *Half-life:* 1 hour.

Route	Onset	Peak	Duration
P.O.	Rapid	1 hr	Unknown

Action

Chemical effect: Stimulates the release of insulin from beta cells in the pancreas.
Therapeutic effect: Lowers glucose level.

Available forms

Tablets: 0.5 mg, 1 mg, 2 mg

NURSING PROCESS

🔲 Assessment
• Monitor glucose level before starting therapy, and regularly thereafter to monitor drug's effectiveness.
• Be alert for adverse reactions and drug interactions.
• Monitor elderly patients and patients taking beta blockers carefully because hypoglycemia may be difficult to recognize in these patients.
• Assess patient's and family's knowledge of drug therapy.

� Nursing diagnoses
• Imbalanced nutrition: more than body requirements related to patient's underlying condition
• Risk for injury related to drug-induced hypoglycemic episode
• Deficient knowledge related to drug therapy

🔷 Planning and implementation
• Increase dosage carefully in a patient with renal impairment who needs dialysis.
• If repaglinide alone is inadequate, metformin may be added.
• Loss of glycemic control can occur during stress, such as fever, trauma, infection, or surgery. Stop giving the drug and give insulin.

Reactions may be *common,* uncommon, *life-threatening,* or COMMON AND LIFE-THREATENING.

• Oral antidiabetics have been linked to increased CV mortality compared to changing diet alone.
• Give drug immediately or up to 30 minutes before meals.
⑤ **ALERT:** Don't confuse Prandin with Avandia.
Patient teaching
• Teach patient about importance of diet and exercise along with drug therapy.
• Discuss symptoms of hypoglycemia with patient and family.
• Advise patient to monitor glucose level periodically to determine minimum effective dose.
• Encourage patient to keep regular medical appointments and have glucose level checked to monitor long-term glucose control.
• Tell patient to take drug before meals, usually 15 minutes before start of meal; however, time can vary from immediately to up to 30 minutes before meal.
• Tell patient to skip dose if he skips a meal and to add dose if he adds a meal.
• Teach patient how to monitor glucose level carefully and what to do when he is ill, undergoing surgery, or under added stress.

☑ **Evaluation**
• Patient's glucose level is controlled and an adequate nutritional balance is maintained.
• Patient has no severe decreases in glucose level.
• Patient and family state understanding of drug therapy.

✳ New Drug

retapamulin
(reh-teh-PAM-ue-lin)
Altabax

Pharmacologic class: pleuromutilin
Therapeutic class: antibiotic
Pregnancy risk category: B

Indications and dosages

▶ **Impetigo caused by susceptible strains of** *Streptococcus pyogenes* **or methicillin-susceptible** *Staphylococcus aureus.* *Adults and children age 9 months and older:* Apply a thin layer to affected area (up to 100 cm² total body surface area in adults or 2% total body surface area in children) b.i.d. for 5 days.

Contraindications and cautions

• Contraindicated in patients hypersensitive to drug or its components.
⚖ **Lifespan:** In pregnant women, safety and effectiveness are unknown; use only if benefits outweigh risks. In breast-feeding women, safety and effectiveness are unknown; use cautiously. In children younger than age 9 months, safety and effectiveness haven't been established.

Adverse reactions

CNS: headache, pyrexia.
GI: diarrhea, nausea.
Respiratory: nasopharyngitis.
Skin: application site irritation, pruritus, eczema.

Interactions

None known.

Effects on lab test results

• May increase CPK levels.

Pharmacokinetics

Absorption: Low potential for systemic absorption.
Distribution: 94% bound to plasma proteins.
Metabolism: Mostly in the liver through mono- and dioxygenation into multiple metabolites. CYP3A4 is the major enzyme involved.
Excretion: Unknown. *Half-life:* Unknown.

Route	Onset	Peak	Duration
Transdermal	Within 24 hr	Unknown	Unknown

Action

Chemical effect: Inhibits bacterial protein synthesis.
Therapeutic effect: Bacteriostatic or bactericidal (depending on concentration) against methicillin-susceptible *S. aureus* or *S. pyogenes.*

Available forms

1% ointment: 5-, 10-, or 15-g tubes

NURSING PROCESS

📋 **Assessment**
• Assess patient for signs of infection and monitor periodically during therapy.
• Monitor CPK level.
• Assess patient's and family's knowledge of drug therapy.

R

⊕ Nursing diagnoses
- Risk for infection related to underlying disease process
- Deficient knowledge related to drug therapy

▶ Planning and implementation
- Notify prescriber if patient's condition does not improve in 3 or 4 days or if a local reaction develops.
- Wash hands before and after application or use a glove.
- To reduce development of resistance or superinfection, only treat infections proven to be susceptible to this drug.
- The affected area may be covered with a sterile bandage or gauze, if needed.
- Monitor the site for local irritation; if the reaction is severe, wipe the drug off the skin and don't reapply.
- Don't apply the drug to mucous membranes.

Patient teaching
- Tell patient to wash his hands before and after application or use a glove.
- Tell patient to notify his prescriber if his condition doesn't improve in 3 or 4 days or if a local reaction develops.
- Advise patient to continue using the drug throughout the entire course of therapy.
- Warn patient that the drug is for external use only.

✓ Evaluation
- Patient is free from infection.
- Patient has no adverse reactions to therapy.
- Patient and family state understanding of drug therapy.

HIGH ALERT

reteplase
(REE-teh-plays)
Retavase

Pharmacologic class: recombinant plasminogen activator
Therapeutic class: thrombolytic
Pregnancy risk category: C

Indications and dosages

▶ **Acute MI; massive pulmonary embolism.**
Adults: Double-bolus injection of 10 + 10 units. Give each bolus I.V. over 2 minutes. If compli-

cations don't occur after first bolus, give second bolus 30 minutes after start of first.

▽ I.V. administration
- Reconstitute drug according to manufacturer's instructions.

⊗ **Incompatibilities**
Other I.V. drugs.

Contraindications and cautions

- Contraindicated in patients with active internal bleeding, bleeding diathesis, history of stroke, recent intracranial or intraspinal surgery or trauma, severe uncontrolled hypertension, intracranial neoplasm, arteriovenous malformation, or aneurysm.
- Use cautiously in patients who've had major surgery, obstetric delivery, organ biopsy, or trauma within 10 days and in those with previous puncture of noncompressible vessel, cerebrovascular disease, recent GI or GU bleeding, or heart disease.

⚠ **Lifespan:** Use in pregnancy only if benefits outweigh risks to the fetus. In breast-feeding women, use cautiously; it's unknown if the drug appears in breast milk. In children, safety and effectiveness haven't been established.

Adverse reactions

CNS: *intracranial hemorrhage.*
CV: *arrhythmias, cholesterol embolization, hemorrhage.*
GI: *hemorrhage.*
GU: hematuria.
Hematologic: anemia, *bleeding tendency.*
Other: bleeding at puncture sites.

Interactions

Drug-drug. *Heparin, oral anticoagulants, platelet inhibitors (abciximab, aspirin, dipyridamole):* May increase risk of bleeding. Use together cautiously.

Effects on lab test results

- May decrease plasminogen, fibrinogen, and hemoglobin level and hematocrit.
- May cause unreliable results of coagulation tests or measurements of fibrinolytic activity.

Pharmacokinetics

Absorption: Given I.V.
Distribution: Rapid distribution.
Metabolism: Unknown.

Reactions may be *common*, uncommon, *life-threatening*, or COMMON AND LIFE-THREATENING.

Excretion: In urine and feces. *Half-life:* 13 to 16 minutes.

Route	Onset	Peak	Duration
I.V.	Unknown	Unknown	Unknown

Action

Chemical effect: Enhances cleavage of plasminogen to generate plasmin.
Therapeutic effect: Dissolves and breaks up clots.

Available forms

Injection: 10.4 units (18.1 mg)/vial. Supplied in kit with components for reconstitution for 2 single-use vials. Also available in half kits with 1 single-use vial.

NURSING PROCESS

Assessment
• Monitor ECG.
• Monitor patient for bleeding. Avoid I.M. injections, invasive procedures, and unneeded handling of patient.
• Assess patient's and family's knowledge of drug therapy.

Nursing diagnoses
• Ineffective cardiopulmonary tissue perfusion related to underlying condition
• Risk for injury related to adverse effects of drug
• Deficient knowledge related to drug therapy

Planning and implementation
• Reteplase is given I.V. as double-bolus injection. If bleeding or allergic reaction occurs after first bolus, notify prescriber.
• Avoid noncompressible pressure sites during therapy. If an arterial puncture is needed, use a vessel in the arm that can be compressed manually. Apply pressure for at least 30 minutes; then apply a pressure dressing. Check site often for bleeding.
Patient teaching
• Teach patient and family about drug.
• Tell patient to report adverse reactions immediately.

Evaluation
• Patient's cardiopulmonary assessment findings show improved perfusion.

• Patient has no serious adverse reactions to therapy.
• Patient and family state understanding of drug therapy.

Rh$_O$ (D) immune globulin, human
(ARR AITCH OH DEE ih-MYOON GLOH-byoo-lin, HYOO-mun)

Rh$_O$(D) immune globulin, human (Rh$_O$[D] IGIM)
BayRho-D Full Dose, RhoGAM

Rh$_O$(D) immune globulin, human (Rh$_O$[D] IGIV)
Rhophylac, WinRho SDF

Rh$_O$(D) immune globulin, human, microdose (Rh$_O$[D] IG microdose)
HyperRHO S/D Mini-Dose, MICRhoGAM

Pharmacologic class: immune serum
Therapeutic class: anti-Rh$_O$(D)-positive prevention drug
Pregnancy risk category: C

Indications and dosages

▶ **Rh exposure (postabortion, postmiscarriage, ectopic pregnancy, postpartum, or threatened abortion 13 weeks or later).**
Women: Transfusion unit or blood bank determines fetal packed RBC volume entering patient's blood. Give one vial I.M. if fetal packed RBC volume is below 15 ml. More than one vial I.M. may be required if large fetomaternal hemorrhage occurs. Must be given within 72 hours after delivery or miscarriage.
▶ **Transfusion accident.** *Adults and children:* Usually, 600 mcg I.V. every 8 hours or 1,200 mcg I.M. every 12 hours until total dose given. Total dose depends on volume of packed RBCs or whole blood infused. Consult blood bank or transfusion unit at once. Must be given within 72 hours.
▶ **Postabortion or postmiscarriage to prevent Rh antibody formation up to and including 12 weeks' gestation.** *Women:* Consult transfusion unit or blood bank. One microdose

R

vial suppresses immune reaction to 2.5 ml Rh$_O$(D)-positive RBCs. Should be given within 3 hours but may be given up to 72 hours after abortion or miscarriage.

▶ **Amniocentesis or abdominal trauma during pregnancy.** *Women:* Base dose on extent of fetomaternal hemorrhage.

▶ **Idiopathic thrombocytopenia purpura.** *Adults and children:* 250 units/kg (50 mcg/kg) I.V. as single dose or in two divided doses given on separate days. If patient responded to initial dose, maintenance dose is 125 to 300 units/kg (25 to 60 mcg/kg) based on platelet count and hemoglobin level. If patient had inadequate response to initial dose and hemoglobin level is more than 10 g/dl, maintenance dose is 250 to 300 units/kg (50 to 60 mcg/kg); for those with hemoglobin level of 8 to 10 g/dl, maintenance dose is 125 to 200 units/kg (25 to 40 mcg/kg).

▽ I.V. administration

• Reconstitute only with normal saline solution. For WinRho SDF, use 0.8% saline supplied by manufacturer: 2.5 ml for the 120-mcg and 300-mcg vials and 8.5 ml for the 1,000-mcg vial. Slowly inject diluent into vial and gently swirl vial until dissolved. Don't shake vial.
• Give injection over 3 to 5 minutes.
• Refrigerate drug at 36° to 46° F (2° to 8° C).
⊗ **Incompatibilities**
Other I.V. drugs.

Contraindications and cautions

• Contraindicated in Rh$_O$(D)-positive or Du-positive patients, those previously immunized to Rh$_O$(D) blood factor, those with anaphylactic or severe systemic reaction to human globulin, and those with immunoglobulin A deficiency.
• Use cautiously in patients with thrombocytopenia or bleeding disorders.
⚠ **Lifespan:** In pregnant women, use cautiously. Drug doesn't appear in breast milk. Microdose must not be used for any indication with continuation of pregnancy.

Adverse reactions

CNS: slight fever.
Hematologic: *intravascular hemolysis.*
Other: *anaphylaxis,* discomfort at injection site.

Interactions

Drug-drug. *Live-virus vaccines:* May interfere with response to Rh$_O$(D) immune globulin. Delay immunization for 3 months.

Effects on lab test results

None reported.

Pharmacokinetics

Absorption: Unknown.
Distribution: Unknown.
Metabolism: Unknown.
Excretion: Unknown. *Half-life:* 24 to 30 days.

Route	Onset	Peak	Duration
I.V., I.M.	Unknown	Unknown	Unknown

Action

Chemical effect: Suppresses active antibody response and formation of anti-Rh$_O$(D) in Rh$_O$(D)-negative, Du-negative people exposed to Rh-positive blood.
Therapeutic effect: Blocks adverse effects of Rh-positive exposure.

Available forms

I.M. injection: Single-dose syringes with 5% gamma globulin or 15% to 18% protein
I.V. infusion: 120 mcg, 300 mcg, 500 mcg, 1,000 mcg; 3,000 mcg

NURSING PROCESS

🗹 Assessment

• Obtain history of Rh-negative patient's Rh-positive exposure, allergies, and reactions to immunizations.
• Assess patient's and family's knowledge of drug therapy.

🔁 Nursing diagnoses

• Risk for injury related to Rh-positive exposure
• Ineffective protection related to drug-induced anaphylaxis
• Deficient knowledge related to drug therapy

▷ Planning and implementation

• Inject I.M. into the anterolateral aspect of the upper thigh or deltoid muscle.
• If administering 1,000 mcg, don't give entire dose in one muscle; divide dose between several different sites.

- Make sure epinephrine 1:1,000 is available in case of anaphylaxis.
- After delivery, have neonate's cord blood typed and crossmatched; confirm if mother is Rh$_O$(D)-negative and Du-negative. Give to mother only if infant is Rh$_O$(D)-positive or Du-positive.
- Drug gives passive immunity to woman exposed to Rh$_O$(D)-positive fetal blood during pregnancy and prevents formation of maternal antibodies, which would endanger future Rh$_O$(D)-positive pregnancies.
- Defer vaccination with live-virus vaccines for 3 months after giving drug.
- MICRhoGAM is recommended for every woman having an abortion or miscarriage up to 12 weeks' gestation unless she is Rh$_O$(D)-positive or Du-positive, she has Rh antibodies, or father or fetus is Rh-negative.

Patient teaching
- Explain how drug protects future Rh$_O$(D)-positive fetuses.

✔ Evaluation
- Patient shows evidence of passive immunity to exposure to Rh$_O$(D)-positive blood.
- Patient doesn't develop anaphylaxis after drug administration.
- Patient and family state understanding of drug therapy.

ribavirin
(ry-beh-VY-rihn)
Copegus, Rebetol, Riba Pak, Ribasphere, Ribatab, Virazole

Pharmacologic class: synthetic nucleoside
Therapeutic class: antiviral
Pregnancy risk category: X

Indications and dosages
▸ **Hospitalized patients infected by RSV.** *Infants and young children:* 20-mg/ml solution delivered by small particle aerosol generator (SPAG-2) and mechanical ventilator or oxygen hood, face mask, or oxygen tent at about 12.5 L of mist per minute. Therapy lasts 12 to 18 hours daily for 3 to 7 days.
▸ **Chronic hepatitis C.** *Adults weighing 75 kg (165 lb) or less:* 1,000 mg Rebetol P.O. daily in divided doses (400 mg in morning, 600 mg in evening) with interferon alfa-2b 3 million units

subcutaneously three times weekly. Or, 1,000 mg Copegus with 180 mcg of Pegasys (peginterferon alfa-2a).
Adults weighing more than 75 kg: 1,200 mg Rebetol P.O. divided b.i.d. (600 mg in morning, 600 mg in evening) with interferon alfa-2b, 3 million units subcutaneously three times weekly. Or, 1,200 mg Copegus with 180 mcg of Pegasys.
▸ **Chronic hepatitis C (regardless of genotype) in HIV-infected patients who have not previously been treated with interferon.** *Adults:* 800 mg (Copegus) P.O. daily given in two divided doses with peginterferon alfa-2a (Pegasys) 180 mcg subcutaneously weekly for 48 weeks.

Contraindications and cautions
- Contraindicated in patients hypersensitive to the drug or any of its components, and in those with creatinine clearance less than 50 ml/minute, history of significant or unstable cardiac disease, Child-Pugh class B or C, or hemoglobinopathies, such as sickle cell anemia and thalassemia.
- Contraindicated with concomitant use of peginterferon alfa or interferon alfa in patients with autoimmune hepatitis.
- Contraindicated in patients with a history of significant or unstable heart disease.
- Avoid use in patients with evidence of pancreatitis.
- Use cautiously in patients with renal impairment.
⚠ **Lifespan:** In women who are or may become pregnant and in men whose sexual partners are pregnant, drug is contraindicated. Breast-feeding women should stop breast-feeding or use another drug, taking into consideration the importance of the drug. In children, capsules and tablets are contraindicated. In elderly patients, use cautiously.

Adverse reactions
CNS: anxiety, asthenia, *depression,* dizziness, fatigue, headache, insomnia, *seizures, suicide.*
CV: *cardiac arrest,* chest pains, hypotension.
EENT: conjunctivitis, lacrimation, pharyngitis, rash or erythema of eyelids, rhinitis.
GI: nausea.
Hematologic: hemolytic anemia, *neutropenia,* reticulocytosis, *severe anemia, thrombocytopenia.*

Musculoskeletal: arthralgia, myalgia.
Respiratory: apnea, bacterial pneumonia, *bronchospasms, pneumothorax, worsening of respiratory state.*
Skin: rash.
Other: *flulike syndrome,* weight decrease.

Interactions

Drug-drug. *Antacids containing aluminum, magnesium, or simethicone:* May affect drug level. Monitor patient.
Didanosine: May increase toxicity. Avoid using together.
Stavudine, zidovudine: May decrease antiretroviral activity. Use together cautiously.

Effects on lab test results

● May increase bilirubin, AST, and ALT levels. May decrease hemoglobin level and hematocrit.
● May increase reticulocyte count. May decrease platelet and WBC counts.

Pharmacokinetics

Absorption: Some ribavirin is absorbed systemically after inhalation. Rapid and extensive absorption with P.O. use.
Distribution: Concentrates in bronchial secretions.
Metabolism: Metabolized to 1,2,4-triazole-3-carboxamide (deribosylated ribavirin).
Excretion: Most of drug in urine. *Half-life:* First phase, 9¼ hours; second phase, 40 hours; after a single P.O. dose, 120 to 170 hours.

Route	Onset	Peak	Duration
P.O.	Unknown	2 hr	Unknown
Inhalation	Immediate	Immediate	Unknown

Action

Chemical effect: Inhibits viral activity by unknown mechanism, possibly by inhibiting RNA and DNA synthesis by depleting intracellular nucleotide pools.
Therapeutic effect: Inhibits RSV activity.

Available forms

Capsules: 200 mg
Oral solution: 40 mg/ml
Powder to be reconstituted for inhalation: 6 g in 100-ml glass vial
Tablets: 200 mg, 400 mg, 600 mg

NURSING PROCESS

▧ Assessment

● Assess patient's respiratory infection before starting therapy, and regularly thereafter to monitor drug's effectiveness.
● Monitor ventilator function. Drug may precipitate in ventilator apparatus, causing equipment malfunction with serious consequences.
● Watch for anemia in patient taking drug longer than 1 to 2 weeks.
● Be alert for adverse reactions.
● Assess patient's and family's knowledge of drug therapy.

⊕ Nursing diagnoses

● Risk for infection related to presence of RSV
● Risk for injury related to drug-induced adverse CV reactions
● Deficient knowledge related to drug therapy

▶ Planning and implementation

⊛ ALERT: Assess patient for underlying cardiac disease before initiating ribavirin. Fatal and nonfatal myocardial infarctions have been reported.
● Aerosol form is indicated only for severe lower respiratory tract infection caused by RSV. Start therapy pending test results, but existence of RSV infection must be documented.
● Most infants and children with RSV infection don't need treatment. Infants with underlying conditions, such as prematurity or cardiopulmonary disease, benefit most from using aerosol form of drug.
● Give drug by SPAG-2 only. Don't use any other aerosol generator.
● For reconstitution, use sterile USP water for injection, not bacteriostatic water. Water used to reconstitute this drug must not contain an antimicrobial.
● Discard solutions placed in SPAG-2 unit at least every 24 hours before adding newly reconstituted solution.
● Avoid unneeded occupational exposure to drug. Adverse effects reported in health care personnel exposed to aerosolized drug include eye irritation and headache.
● Capsules and tablets aren't effective as monotherapy for chronic hepatitis C.
● Store reconstituted solutions at room temperature for 24 hours.
● Stop drug at first sign of pancreatitis.

Reactions may be *common,* uncommon, *life-threatening,* or COMMON AND LIFE-THREATENING.

⊛ ALERT: Don't confuse ribavirin with ribo-flavin.

Patient teaching

• Inform parents of children with RSV infection of need for drug therapy, and answer their questions.

• Advise patient to use correct device.

• Explain to women of childbearing age and men with sexual partners of childbearing age the effects of drug on a fetus and the need to inform the prescriber immediately if pregnancy occurs.

• Reinforce the importance of avoiding pregnancy during and for 6 months after therapy. Recommend two reliable forms of contraception.

☑ Evaluation

• Patient is free from infection.

• Patient develops no adverse CV reactions after drug administration.

• Parents state understanding of drug therapy.

rifabutin

(rif-uh-BYOO-tin)
Mycobutin

Pharmacologic class: semisynthetic ansamycin
Therapeutic class: antituberculotic
Pregnancy risk category: B

Indications and dosages

▶ **To prevent disseminated** *Mycobacterium avium* **complex (MAC) in patients with advanced HIV infection.** *Adults:* 300 mg P.O. daily as single dose or divided b.i.d.

Contraindications and cautions

• Contraindicated in patients hypersensitive to drug or other rifamycin derivatives (such as rifampin).

• Use cautiously in patients with neutropenia and thrombocytopenia.

⚘ Lifespan: Use during pregnancy only when clearly needed. In breast-feeding women, drug isn't recommended. In children, safety and effectiveness haven't been established.

Adverse reactions

CNS: fever, headache.
CV: ECG changes.

EENT: uveitis.
GI: abdominal pain, diarrhea, dyspepsia, eructation, flatulence, nausea, vomiting.
GU: discolored urine.
Hematologic: anemia, eosinophilia, LEUKOPENIA, NEUTROPENIA, *thrombocytopenia.*
Musculoskeletal: myalgia.
Skin: *rash.*

Interactions

Drug-drug. *Corticosteroids:* May decrease corticosteroid effects. Double dose of corticosteroids, if needed.
Cyclosporine: May reduce immunosuppressive effects. Don't use together.
Delavirdine, indinavir: May decrease level of these drugs and increase concentration of rifabutin. Avoid use together.
Drugs metabolized by the liver, benzodiazepines, beta blockers, buspirone, doxycycline, hydantoins, indinavir, losartan, macrolides, methadone, morphine, nelfinavir, quinidine, theophylline, tricyclic antidepressants, zidovudine: May decrease level of these drugs. Because rifabutin, like rifampin, induces liver enzymes, it may lower levels of many other drugs as well. Monitor patient for effect.
Hormonal contraceptives: May decrease effectiveness. Instruct patient to use an additional form of birth control.
Warfarin: May decrease anticoagulant effect. Monitor INR, and increase anticoagulant dosage as needed.
Drug-food. *High-fat foods:* May slow absorption of drug. Discourage taking drug with high-fat meals.

Effects on lab test results

• May increase alkaline phosphatase, AST, and ALT levels. May decrease hemoglobin level and hematocrit.

• May increase eosinophil count. May decrease neutrophil, WBC, and platelet counts.

Pharmacokinetics

Absorption: Readily absorbed from GI tract.
Distribution: Because of its high lipophilicity, drug has high propensity for distribution and intracellular tissue uptake. About 85% protein-bound.
Metabolism: In liver.

R

Excretion: Mainly in urine; about 30% in feces. *Half-life:* 45 hours.

Route	Onset	Peak	Duration
P.O.	Unknown	1¼–4 hr	Unknown

Action

Chemical effect: Blocks bacterial protein synthesis by inhibiting DNA-dependent RNA polymerase in susceptible bacteria.
Therapeutic effect: Prevents disseminated MAC in patients with advanced HIV infection.

Available forms

Capsules: 150 mg

NURSING PROCESS

⚡ Assessment
• Assess patient's condition before starting therapy, and regularly thereafter to monitor drug's effectiveness.
• Perform baseline hematologic studies and repeat periodically.
• Be alert for adverse reactions and drug interactions.
• Assess patient's and family's knowledge of drug therapy.

✪ Nursing diagnoses
• Risk for infection related to immune system dysfunction
• Ineffective protection related to drug-induced adverse hematologic reactions
• Deficient knowledge related to drug therapy

▷ Planning and implementation
• High-fat meals slow rate but not extent of absorption.
• Give drug with food. Mix with soft foods for patient who has difficulty swallowing.
• No evidence exists that drug will provide effective prophylaxis against *Mycobacterium tuberculosis*. Patients requiring prophylaxis against both *M. tuberculosis* and MAC may require rifampin and rifabutin.
• Don't use as monotherapy in patients with active tuberculosis. Doing so may foster tuberculosis that's resistant to both rifabutin and rifampin.
ⓢ **ALERT:** Don't confuse rifabutin, rifampin, and rifapentine.

Patient teaching
• Tell patient that drug may turn urine, feces, sputum, saliva, tears, and skin brownish-orange. Tell him not to wear soft contacts because they may be permanently stained.
• Instruct patient to report photophobia, excessive lacrimation, or eye pain. Drug may rarely cause uveitis.

✓ Evaluation
• Patient doesn't develop disseminated MAC.
• Patient maintains normal hematologic values throughout therapy.
• Patient and family state understanding of drug therapy.

rifampin (rifampicin)
(rih-FAM-pin)
Rifadin, Rimactane, Rofact ◆

Pharmacologic class: rifamycin derivative antibiotic
Therapeutic class: antituberculotic
Pregnancy risk category: C

Indications and dosages

▶ **Tuberculosis.** *Adults:* 10 mg/kg P.O. or I.V. daily in single dose. Maximum, 600 mg daily. *Children older than age 5:* Give 10 to 20 mg/kg P.O. or I.V. daily in single dose. Maximum, 600 mg daily. Use with other antituberculotics is recommended.
▶ **Meningococcal carriers.** *Adults:* 600 mg P.O. or I.V. b.i.d. for 2 days or once daily for 4 days.
Children ages 1 month or older: 10 mg/kg P.O. or I.V. b.i.d. for 2 days or once daily for 4 days. Maximum, 600 mg daily.
Neonates: 5 mg/kg P.O. or I.V. b.i.d. for 2 days.
▶ **Prophylaxis of *Haemophilus influenzae* type B.** *Adults and children:* 20 mg/kg P.O. daily for 4 days. Maximum, 600 mg daily.
▶ **Leprosy‡.** *Adults:* 600 mg P.O. once monthly, usually with other drugs.
Children 10 to 14 years: 450 mg P.O. once monthly, usually with other drugs.

▼ I.V. administration

• Reconstitute vial with 10 ml of sterile water for injection to make solution containing 60 mg/ml.

• Add to 100 ml of D_5W and infuse over 30 minutes, or add to 500 ml of D_5W and infuse over 3 hours.
• When dextrose is contraindicated, drug may be diluted with normal saline solution for injection.

⊗ **Incompatibilities**
Diltiazem, minocycline, I.V. solutions other than dextrose or normal saline.

Contraindications and cautions

• Contraindicated in patients hypersensitive to the drug or any of its components.
• Use cautiously and under strict medical supervision in patients with liver disease.
⚖ **Lifespan:** In pregnant women, use only when benefits outweigh risks to the fetus. During the last 2 weeks of pregnancy, use of the drug may lead to postnatal hemorrhage in the mother or infant. Monitor clotting factors closely. In breast-feeding women, decide whether to discontinue drug or breast-feeding based on importance of drug to mother; drug appears in breast milk.

Adverse reactions

CNS: ataxia, behavioral changes, confusion, dizziness, drowsiness, fatigue, generalized numbness, headache.
CV: *shock.*
EENT: exudative conjunctivitis, visual disturbances.
GI: abdominal pain, anorexia, diarrhea, epigastric distress, flatulence, nausea, *pancreatitis, pseudomembranous colitis,* sore mouth and tongue, vomiting.
GU: *acute renal failure,* hematuria, hemoglobinuria, menstrual disturbances.
Hematologic: eosinophilia, hemolytic anemia, *thrombocytopenia, transient leukopenia.*
Hepatic: *hepatotoxicity,* worsening of porphyria.
Metabolic: hyperuricemia.
Musculoskeletal: osteomalacia.
Respiratory: shortness of breath, wheezing.
Skin: pruritus, rash, urticaria.
Other: discoloration of body fluids, flulike syndrome.

Interactions

Drug-drug. *ACE inhibitors, analgesics, antiarrhythmics, anticoagulants, anticonvulsants, antifungals, barbiturates, benzodiazepines, beta blockers, buspirone, chloramphenicol, corticosteroids, cyclosporine, digoxin, doxycycline, estrogens, fluoroquinolones, haloperidol, hormonal contraceptives, hydantoids, macrolides, narcotic, progestins, protease inhibitors, quinine derivatives, sulfonylureas, tacrolimus, thyroid hormones, theophylline, tricyclic antidepressants, verapamil, zidovudine, zolpidem:* May reduce effectiveness of these drugs. Monitor patient carefully.
Halothane: May increase risk of hepatotoxicity in both drugs. Monitor liver function closely.
Ketoconazole, para-aminosalicylate sodium: May interfere with absorption of rifampin. Give these drugs 8 to 12 hours apart.
Drug-herb. *Kava:* May increase the risk of hepatotoxicity. Discourage use.
Drug-lifestyle. *Alcohol use:* May increase risk of hepatotoxicity. Discourage using together.

Effects on lab test results

• May increase ALT, AST, alkaline phosphatase, bilirubin, BUN, creatinine, and uric acid levels. May decrease hemoglobin level and hematocrit.
• May increase eosinophil count. May decrease platelet and WBC counts.

Pharmacokinetics

Absorption: Complete. Food delays absorption.
Distribution: Wide. 84% to 91% protein-bound.
Metabolism: Extensive.
Excretion: Mainly in bile; drug, but not metabolite, is reabsorbed. Some in urine. *Half-life:* 1¼ to 5 hours.

Route	Onset	Peak	Duration
P.O.	Unknown	2–4 hr	Unknown
I.V.	Unknown	Unknown	Unknown

Action

Chemical effect: Kills bacteria by inhibiting DNA-dependent RNA polymerase, thus impairing RNA synthesis.
Therapeutic effect: Kills susceptible bacteria.

Available forms

Capsules: 150 mg, 300 mg
Injection: 600 mg

NURSING PROCESS

⏣ Assessment
• Assess patient's infection before starting therapy, and regularly thereafter to monitor drug's effectiveness.
• Monitor liver function, hematopoiesis, and uric acid level.
• Be alert for adverse reactions and drug interactions.
• Watch closely for signs of hepatic impairment.
• If adverse GI reaction occurs, monitor hydration.
• Assess patient's and family's knowledge of drug therapy.

⊕ Nursing diagnoses
• Risk for infection related to presence of susceptible bacteria
• Risk for deficient fluid volume related to drug-induced adverse reactions
• Deficient knowledge related to drug therapy

▷ Planning and implementation
• Give drug 1 hour before or 2 hours after meals for optimal absorption; if GI irritation occurs, patient may take with meals.
• Drug may inhibit standard assays for folate and vitamin B_{12}. Consider alternative assay method.
• Giving at least one additional antituberculotic is recommended.
⊛ **ALERT:** Don't confuse rifampin, rifabutin, and rifapentine. Don't confuse Rifadin with Ritalin.
Patient teaching
• Warn patient about drowsiness and red-orange discoloration of urine, feces, saliva, sweat, sputum, and tears. Soft contact lenses may be permanently stained.
• Advise patient not to drink alcohol while taking the drug.
• Recommend taking drug with a full glass of water to maintain adequate hydration.

☑ Evaluation
• Patient is free from infection.
• Patient maintains adequate hydration throughout therapy.
• Patient and family state understanding of drug therapy.

rifapentine
(rif-ah-PEN-teen)
Priftin

Pharmacologic class: rifamycin derivative antibiotic
Therapeutic class: antituberculotic
Pregnancy risk category: C

Indications and dosages

▶ **Pulmonary tuberculosis, with at least one other antituberculotic to which the isolate is susceptible.** *Adults:* During intensive phase of short-course therapy, 600 mg P.O. twice weekly for 2 months in conjunction with other appropriate antituberculotics (isoniazid, pyrazinamide, ethambutol, streptomycin), with an interval between doses of not less than 3 days (72 hours). During the continuation phase of short-course therapy, 600 mg P.O. once weekly for 4 months with isoniazid.

Contraindications and cautions

• Contraindicated in patients hypersensitive to rifamycin (rifapentine, rifampin, or rifabutin).
• Use drug cautiously and with frequent monitoring in patients with liver disease.
⚖ **Lifespan:** During last 2 weeks of pregnancy, drug may lead to postnatal hemorrhage in mother or infant; monitor clotting parameters closely. Use with caution in breast-feeding women. It isn't known if drug appears in breast milk.

Adverse reactions

CNS: dizziness, headache, pain.
CV: hypertension.
GI: anorexia, diarrhea, dyspepsia, nausea, *pseudomembranous colitis,* vomiting.
GU: hematuria, proteinuria, pyuria, urinary casts.
Hematologic: anemia, *leukopenia, lymphopenia, neutropenia, thrombocytosis.*
Metabolic: *hyperuricemia.*
Musculoskeletal: arthralgia.
Respiratory: hemoptysis.
Skin: rash, acne, maculopapular rash, pruritus.

Interactions

Drug-drug. *Antiarrhythmics, antibiotics, anticonvulsants, antifungals, barbiturates, benzodiazepines, beta blockers, calcium channel block-*

Reactions may be *common*, uncommon, *life-threatening*, or COMMON AND LIFE-THREATENING.

ers, corticosteroids, digoxin, haloperidol, HIV protease inhibitors, hormonal contraceptives, immunosuppressants, levothyroxine, opioid analgesics (methadone), oral anticoagulants, oral hypoglycemics, progestins, quinine, reverse transcriptase inhibitors, sildenafil, theophylline, tricyclic antidepressants: May increase metabolism and decrease the activity of these drugs. Dosage adjustments may be needed.

Effects on lab test results

- May increase uric acid, ALT, and AST levels. May decrease hemoglobin level and hematocrit.
- May increase platelet count. May decrease neutrophil and WBC counts.

Pharmacokinetics

Absorption: Relative bioavailability is 70%.
Distribution: About 98% protein-bound.
Metabolism: Hydrolyzed by an esterase enzyme to the microbiologically active 25-desacetyl rifapentine. Rifapentine contributes 62% to drug's activity and 25-desacetyl contributes 38%.
Excretion: About 17% in urine and 70% in feces. *Half-life:* 13 hours.

Route	Onset	Peak	Duration
P.O.	Unknown	5–6 hr	Unknown

Action

Chemical effect: Kills susceptible strains of *Mycobacterium tuberculosis,* both inside and outside cells, by inhibiting DNA-dependent RNA polymerase. Rifapentine and rifampin share similar antimicrobial action.
Therapeutic effect: Kills susceptible bacteria.

Available forms

Tablets (film-coated): 150 mg

NURSING PROCESS

▨ Assessment
- Assess patient's condition before starting therapy and regularly thereafter to monitor drug's effectiveness.
- Assess patient's understanding of disease and stress importance of strict compliance with drug and daily companion medications, as well as needed follow-up visits and laboratory tests.
- Monitor liver function, CBC, and uric acid level.

- Monitor patient for persistent or severe diarrhea and notify prescriber if it occurs.
- Assess patient's and family's knowledge of drug therapy.

⊞ Nursing diagnoses
- Risk for infection related to patient's underlying condition
- Noncompliance related to long-term therapeutic regimen
- Deficient knowledge related to drug therapy

▷ Planning and implementation
- Give pyridoxine (vitamin B_6) during rifapentine therapy to a malnourished patient, a patient predisposed to neuropathy (alcoholic, diabetic), or an adolescent.
- Drug must be given with appropriate daily companion drugs. Compliance with all drugs, especially with daily companion drugs on the days when rifapentine isn't given, is crucial for early sputum conversion and protection from tuberculosis relapse.
- ⊛ **ALERT:** Don't confuse rifampin, rifabutin, and rifapentine.

Patient teaching
- Stress importance of strict compliance with regimen of drug and daily companion drugs, as well as needed follow-up visits and laboratory tests.
- Advise patient to use barrier-method of birth control.
- Tell patient to take drug with food if nausea, vomiting, or GI upset occurs.
- Instruct patient to notify prescriber if any of the following occur: fever, loss of appetite, malaise, nausea, vomiting, darkened urine, yellowish discoloration of skin and eyes, pain or swelling of joints, and excessive loose stools or diarrhea.
- Instruct patient to protect pills from excessive heat.
- Tell patient that drug can turn body fluids red-orange. Contact lenses can become permanently stained.

✓ Evaluation
- Patient experiences sputum conversion and recovers from tuberculosis.
- Patient complies with therapeutic regimen.
- Patient and family state understanding of drug therapy.

R

riluzole
(RIGH-loo-zohl)
Rilutek

Pharmacologic class: benzothiazole, glutamate antagonist
Therapeutic class: neuroprotector
Pregnancy risk category: C

Indications and dosages

▶ **Amyotrophic lateral sclerosis (ALS).**
Adults: 50 mg P.O. every 12 hours on empty stomach.

Contraindications and cautions

• Contraindicated in patients hypersensitive to the drug or any of its components.
• Use cautiously in patients with hepatic or renal dysfunction. Also use cautiously in women and Japanese patients (who may have a lower metabolic capacity to eliminate riluzole compared with men and white patients, respectively).
⚠ **Lifespan:** In pregnant patients, use only if benefits outweigh risks; risks specific to fetus aren't known. In breast-feeding women, drug isn't recommended. In children, safety and effectiveness haven't been established. In elderly patients, use cautiously.

Adverse reactions

CNS: aggravation reaction, *asthenia,* circumoral paresthesia, depression, dizziness, headache, hypertonia, insomnia, malaise, somnolence, vertigo.
CV: hypertension, orthostatic hypotension, palpitations, peripheral edema, tachycardia.
EENT: rhinitis, sinusitis.
GI: abdominal pain, anorexia, dry mouth, dyspepsia, diarrhea, flatulence, *nausea,* oral candidiasis, stomatitis, vomiting.
GU: dysuria, UTI.
Hematologic: *neutropenia.*
Metabolic: weight loss.
Musculoskeletal: arthralgia, back pain.
Respiratory: *decreased lung function,* increased cough.
Skin: alopecia, eczema, exfoliative dermatitis, pruritus.
Other: phlebitis, tooth disorder.

Interactions

Drug-drug. *Inducers of CYP1A2 (omeprazole, rifampicin):* May increase riluzole elimination. Monitor patient for loss of therapeutic effect. *Potential inhibitors of CYP1A2 (amitriptyline, phenacetin, quinolones, theophylline):* May decrease riluzole elimination. Monitor patient closely for toxicity.
Drug-food. *Any food:* May decrease drug bioavailability. Give 1 hour before or 2 hours after meals.
Caffeine: May decrease drug elimination. Monitor patient for adverse reactions.
Charbroiled foods: May increase drug elimination. Discourage patient from eating these foods while on drug therapy.
Drug-lifestyle. *Alcohol use:* May increase risk of hepatotoxicity. Discourage using together.
Smoking: May increase drug elimination. Urge patient to stop smoking.

Effects on lab test results

• May increase AST, ALT, bilirubin, and GGT levels.
• May decrease neutrophil count.

Pharmacokinetics

Absorption: Well absorbed from GI tract, with average absolute oral bioavailability of about 60%. High-fat meal decreases absorption.
Distribution: 96% protein-bound.
Metabolism: Extensive in liver.
Excretion: Mainly in urine, with small amount in feces. *Half-life:* 12 hours with repeated doses.

Route	Onset	Peak	Duration
P.O.	Unknown	Unknown	Unknown

Action

Chemical effect: Unknown.
Therapeutic effect: Improves signs and symptoms of ALS.

Available forms

Tablets: 50 mg

NURSING PROCESS

⚕ Assessment
• Obtain history of patient's ALS.
• Obtain liver and renal function studies and CBC before and during therapy.

Reactions may be *common*, uncommon, *life-threatening*, or COMMON AND LIFE-THREATENING.

• Monitor patient carefully because rare but severe cases of neutropenia have occurred.
• Assess patient's and family's knowledge of drug therapy.

🔷 Nursing diagnoses
• Impaired physical mobility related to ALS
• Risk for deficient fluid volume related to adverse GI reactions
• Deficient knowledge related to drug therapy

▷ Planning and implementation
• If baseline liver function test results (especially bilirubin level) rise, don't use drug. Drug may increase aminotransferase level. If level exceeds 10 times upper limit of normal, or if jaundice develops, notify prescriber.
• Give drug at least 1 hour before or 2 hours after a meal.
Patient teaching
• Tell patient to take drug at same time each day. If he misses a dose, instruct him not to double the dose but to take the next dose as scheduled.
• Instruct patient to report febrile illness; check his WBC count.
• Warn patient to avoid hazardous activities until drug's CNS effects are known.
• Advise patient to limit alcohol intake during therapy.
• Tell patient to store drug at room temperature, protected from bright light and out of children's reach.

☑ Evaluation
• Patient responds well to therapy.
• Patient maintains adequate hydration.
• Patient and family state understanding of drug therapy.

risedronate sodium
(ri-SEH-droe-nate SOE-dee-um)
Actonel◆

Pharmacologic class: bisphosphonate
Therapeutic class: antiresorptive
Pregnancy risk category: C

Indications and dosages
▶ **To prevent and treat postmenopausal osteoporosis.** *Adults:* 5-mg tablet P.O. once dai-

ly, or 35-mg tablet once weekly or 75 mg P.O. on 2 consecutive days for a total of two tablets each month when fewer dosing days are desirable. Give at least 30 minutes before first food or drink (except water) of the day.
▶ **Glucocorticoid-induced osteoporosis in patients who are either starting or continuing glucocorticoid therapy at 7.5 mg or more of prednisone or equivalent daily.** *Adults:* 5 mg P.O. daily.
▶ **Paget disease.** *Adults:* 30 mg P.O. daily for 2 months. If relapse occurs or alkaline phosphatase level doesn't normalize, give same dose for 2 months or longer after first course.
▶ **To increase bone mass in men with osteoporosis.** *Adults:* 35-mg tablet P.O. once weekly. Give at least 30 minutes before first food or drink (except water) of the day.

Contraindications and cautions
• Contraindicated in patients hypersensitive to the drug or any of its components, and in patients who are hypocalcemic or unable to stand or sit upright for 30 minutes after administration.
• Drug isn't recommended for patients with severe renal impairment (creatinine clearance below 30 ml/minute).
• Use cautiously in patients with upper GI disorders such as dysphagia, esophagitis, and esophageal or gastric ulcers.
⚠ Lifespan: In pregnant women, use only when benefits outweigh risks to the fetus. In breast-feeding women, use cautiously. It isn't known if drug appears in breast milk. In children, safety and effectiveness of drug haven't been established.

Adverse reactions
CNS: anxiety, asthenia, depression, dizziness, *headache,* hypertonia, insomnia, neuralgia, *pain,* paresthesia, vertigo.
CV: chest pain, CV disorder, *hypertension,* peripheral edema.
EENT: amblyopia, cataract, conjunctivitis, pharyngitis, otitis media, rhinitis, sinusitis, tinnitus.
GI: abdominal pain, constipation, diarrhea, esophageal irritation and ulceration, flatulence, gastritis, nausea, rectal disorder.
GU: cystitis, *UTI.*
Hematologic: anemia.

Musculoskeletal: *arthralgia, back pain,* bone pain, bursitis, leg cramps, myalgia, neck pain, tendon disorder.
Respiratory: bronchitis, dyspnea, pneumonia.
Skin: *carcinoma,* ecchymosis, pruritus, *rash.*
Other: *infection,* tooth disorder.

Interactions

Drug-drug. *Calcium supplements, antacids that contain calcium, magnesium, or aluminum:* May interfere with risedronate absorption. Advise patient to separate administration times.
Drug-food. *Any food:* May interfere with drug absorption. Advise patient to take drug at least 30 minutes before first food or drink of the day (other than water).

Effects on lab test results

● May decrease calcium, phosphorus, and hemoglobin levels and hematocrit.

Pharmacokinetics

Absorption: Absorbed via the GI tract. Steady state occurs in 57 days. Mean absolute oral bioavailability of 30-mg tablet is 0.63%. Because food alters absorption, give drug at least 30 minutes before breakfast.
Distribution: About 60% distributed to bone. About 24% protein-bound.
Metabolism: No evidence of systemic metabolism.
Excretion: About 50% in urine within 24 hours. Unabsorbed drug is eliminated unchanged in feces. *Half-life:* 20 days.

Route	Onset	Peak	Duration
P.O.	Unknown	1 hr	Unknown

Action

Chemical effect: Reverses the loss of bone mineral density by reducing bone turnover and bone resorption by inhibiting osteoclasts. In patients with Paget disease, drug causes bone turnover to return to normal.
Therapeutic effect: Reverses the loss of bone mineral density.

Available forms

Tablets: 5 mg, 30 mg, 35 mg

NURSING PROCESS

☑ Assessment

● Assess underlying condition before starting therapy and regularly thereafter to monitor drug's effectiveness.
● Evaluate renal function before beginning therapy. Drug isn't recommended for patients with creatinine clearance below 30 ml/minute.
● Assess patient for the following risk factors for the development of osteoporosis: family history, previous fracture, smoking, a decrease in bone mineral density below the premenopausal mean, a thin body frame, white or Asian race, and early menopause.
● Assess patient's and family's knowledge of drug therapy.

⊕ Nursing diagnoses

● Risk for injury related to decreased bone mass
● Ineffective health maintenance related to underlying disease
● Deficient knowledge related to risedronate sodium therapy

▶ Planning and implementation

⑤ **ALERT:** Follow dosage instructions carefully because benefits of the drug may be compromised by failure to take it according to instructions. Give drug at least 30 minutes before patient's first food or drink (other than water) of the day.
● Give drug with 6 to 8 oz plain water to facilitate delivery to the stomach. Don't allow patient to lie down for 30 minutes after taking drug.
⑤ **ALERT:** Bisphosphonates have been linked to such GI disorders as dysphagia, esophagitis, and esophageal or gastric ulcers. Monitor patient for symptoms of esophageal disease (such as dysphagia, retrosternal pain, or severe persistent or worsening heartburn).
● If patient's dietary intake of calcium and vitamin D is inadequate, give supplements. However, because calcium supplements and drugs containing calcium, aluminum, or magnesium may interfere with absorption, separate doses.
● Store drug at 68° to 77° F (20° to 25° C).
● Bisphosphonates can interfere with bone-imaging agents.
Patient teaching
● Explain that drug is used to replace bone lost as a result of certain disease processes.

- Instruct patient to adhere to dosage instructions.
- Tell patient to take drug at least 30 minutes before the first food or drink (other than water) of the day. Tell patient to take drug with 6 to 8 oz of water while sitting or standing. Warn against lying down for 30 minutes after taking drug.
- Advise patient not to chew or suck the tablet because doing so could cause mouth irritation.
- Advise patient to notify the prescriber immediately if symptoms of esophageal disease (difficulty or pain when swallowing, retrosternal pain, or severe heartburn) develop.
- Advise patient to take calcium and vitamin D if dietary intake is inadequate, but to take them at a different time than risedronate.
- Advise patient to stop smoking and drinking alcohol, as appropriate. Also, instruct patient to perform weight-bearing exercise.
- Tell patient to store drug in a cool (room temperature), dry place and away from children.
- Urge patient to read the patient information guide before starting therapy.
- Tell patient if he misses a dose of the 35-mg tablet, he should take 1 tablet on the morning after he remembers and return to taking 1 tablet once a week, as originally scheduled on his chosen day. Patients shouldn't take 2 tablets on the same day.
- Tell woman to inform prescriber if she is pregnant or breast-feeding or plans to become pregnant.

☑ Evaluation

- Patient sustains no injury related to decreased bone mass.
- Patient shows improvement in underlying condition.
- Patient and family state understanding of drug therapy.

risperidone
(ris-PER-ih-dohn)
Risperdal✐, **Risperdal Consta, Risperdal M-Tab**✐

Pharmacologic class: benzisoxazole derivative
Therapeutic class: antipsychotic
Pregnancy risk category: C

Indications and dosages

▶ **Short-term therapy for schizophrenia.**
Adults: Initially, 1 mg P.O. b.i.d. Increase in increments of 1 mg b.i.d. on days 2 and 3 to a target dosage of 3 mg b.i.d. Or, 1 mg P.O. on day 1, increase to 2 mg once daily on day 2, and 4 mg once daily on day 3. Wait at least 1 week before adjusting dosage further. Adjust doses by 1 to 2 mg. Maximum, 8 mg daily. Once tolerance to P.O. formulation has been established, patient may be switched to I.M. formulation, if appropriate. Give 25 mg by deep I.M. gluteal injection every 2 weeks; alternating injections between the two buttocks. Adjust dosage no sooner than every 4 weeks. Maximum, 50 mg I.M. every 2 weeks. Continue oral antipsychotic for 3 weeks after first I.M. injection. Then stop oral therapy.

📉 Adjust-a-dose: For patients with hepatic or renal impairment, slowly adjust to 2 mg P.O.; if tolerated, give 25 mg I.M. every 2 weeks or alternatively give initial dose of 12.5 mg I.M. Continue oral antipsychotic for 3 weeks after first injection to maintain therapeutic drug levels.

▪▪ **NEW INDICATION: Schizophrenia in adolescents.** *Adolescents ages 13 to 17:* Initially, 0.5 mg P.O. daily. Adjust by 0.5 mg to 1 mg daily to target dosage of 3 mg daily. Maximum, 6 mg daily.

▪▪ **NEW INDICATION: Short-term treatment of bipolar mania associated with bipolar I disorder in children and adolescents.** *Children and adolescents ages 10 to 17:* Initially, 0.5 mg P.O. daily. Adjust by 0.5 mg to 1 mg daily to target dosage of 2.5 mg daily. Maximum, 6 mg daily.

▶ **Delaying relapse in long-term therapy for schizophrenia.** *Adults:* Initially, 1 mg P.O. on day 1, increase to 2 mg once daily on day 2, and 4 mg once daily on day 3. Dosage range, 2 to 8 mg daily.

▶ **Monotherapy or combination therapy with lithium or valproate for short-term (3-week) treatment of acute manic or mixed episodes in bipolar I disorder.** *Adults:* 2 to 3 mg P.O. once daily. Adjust dose by 1 mg daily. Dosage range, 1 to 6 mg daily.

📉 Adjust-a-dose: For elderly or debilitated patients, hypotensive patients, or patients with severe renal or hepatic impairment, initially give 0.5 mg P.O. b.i.d. Increase dosage in increments

R

of 0.5 mg b.i.d. Increase dosages beyond 1.5 mg b.i.d. at intervals of at least 1 week. Subsequent switches to once-daily doses may be made after patient has received a twice-daily regimen for 2 or 3 days at the target dose.

▶ **Irritability, including aggression, self-injury, mood swings, and temper tantrums, in autistic disorders.** *Adolescents and children age 5 and older who weigh 20 kg (44 lb) or more:* Initially, 0.5 mg P.O. once daily or divided b.i.d. After 4 days, increase to 1 mg. If needed, may increase in 0.5-mg increments at intervals of at least 2 weeks.

Children age 5 and older who weigh less than 20 kg: Initially, 0.25 mg P.O. once daily or divided b.i.d. After 4 days, increase to 0.5 mg. If needed, may increase in 0.25-mg increments at intervals of at least 2 weeks. Increase cautiously in children who weigh less than 15 kg (33 lb).

Contraindications and cautions

• Contraindicated in patients hypersensitive to the drug or any of its components.
• Use cautiously in patients with prolonged QT interval, CV disease, cerebrovascular disease, dehydration, hypovolemia, history of seizures, exposure to extreme heat, or conditions that could affect metabolism or hemodynamic responses. Also use cautiously in patients at risk for aspiration pneumonia.
• Use I.M. injection cautiously in those with hepatic or renal impairment. Stabilize patient on oral drug before switching to I.M. injection.
⚖ **Lifespan:** In pregnant women, use cautiously. In breast-feeding women, drug is contraindicated. In elderly patients with dementia, drug is contraindicated.

Adverse reactions

CNS: abnormal thinking and dreaming, aggressiveness, agitation, akathisia, anxiety, depression, dizziness, extrapyramidal reactions, fatigue, fever, hallucination, headache, hypoesthesia, insomnia, nervousness (I.M.), *neuroleptic malignant syndrome,* pain, parkinsonism, somnolence, *suicide attempt,* tardive dyskinesia, *transient ischemic attack or stroke in elderly patients with dementia,* tremor.
CV: chest pain, hypertension (I.M.), orthostatic hypotension, peripheral edema, *prolonged QT interval,* syncope, tachycardia.

EENT: abnormal vision; ear disorder (I.M.), pharyngitis, *rhinitis,* sinusitis.
GI: *abdominal pain, anorexia, constipation,* diarrhea (I.M.), dry mouth, *dyspepsia,* increased saliva, *nausea,* tooth ache, tooth disorder, *vomiting.*
Hematologic: anemia.
Metabolic: *hyperglycemia;* weight decrease (I.M.), *weight gain.*
Musculoskeletal: arthralgia, back pain; leg pain, myalgia (I.M.).
Respiratory: coughing, upper respiratory infection.
Skin: acne, dry skin, injection site pain (I.M.), photosensitivity, rash.

Interactions

Drug-drug. *Antihypertensives:* May enhance hypotensive effects. Monitor blood pressure.
Carbamazepine: May increase risperidone clearance, leading to decreased effectiveness. Monitor patient closely.
Clozapine: May decrease risperidone clearance, increasing toxicity. Monitor patient closely.
CNS depressants: May cause additive CNS depression. Monitor patient closely.
Dopamine agonists, levodopa: May antagonize the effects of these drugs. Monitor patient closely.
Fluoxetine, paroxetine: May increase risperidone level, increasing the risk of adverse reactions, including serotonin syndrome. Monitor patient closely and adjust risperidone dosage as needed.
Drug-lifestyle. *Alcohol use:* May cause additive CNS depression. Discourage using together.
Sun exposure: May increase photosensitivity reactions. Discourage prolonged or unprotected sun exposure.

Effects on lab test results

• May increase glucose and prolactin levels. May decrease hemoglobin level and hematocrit.

Pharmacokinetics

Absorption: Well absorbed; absolute oral bioavailability is 70%. Slowly absorbed via I.M. injection.
Distribution: Risperidone about 90% protein-bound; major active metabolite about 77% protein-bound.
Metabolism: Extensive in liver.

Excretion: Metabolite in urine. *Half-life:* 3 to 20 hours.

Route	Onset	Peak	Duration
P.O.	Unknown	1 hr	Unknown
I.M.	3 wk	4–6 wk	7 wk

Action

Chemical effect: Blocks dopamine and serotonin receptors as well as alpha$_1$, alpha$_2$, and H$_1$ receptors in the CNS.
Therapeutic effect: Relieves signs and symptoms of psychosis.

Available forms

Oral solution: 1 mg/ml
Powder for I.M. injection: 12.5 mg, 25 mg, 37.5 mg, 50 mg
Tablets: 0.25 mg, 0.5 mg, 1 mg, 2 mg, 3 mg, 4 mg
Tablets (orally-disintegrating): 0.5 mg, 1 mg, 2 mg, 3 mg, 4 mg

NURSING PROCESS

Assessment
• Assess patient's psychosis before starting therapy and regularly thereafter to monitor drug's effectiveness.
• Assess blood pressure before starting therapy, and monitor regularly. Watch for orthostatic hypotension, especially during dosage adjustment.
• Monitor CBC, liver functions tests, ECG, serum prolactin, and routine chemistry during prolonged administration.
• Be alert for adverse reactions and drug interactions.
ALERT: Watch for tardive dyskinesia. It may occur after prolonged use; it may not appear until months or years later and may disappear spontaneously or persist for life despite stopping the drug.
• Assess patient's and family's knowledge of drug therapy.

Nursing diagnoses
• Disturbed thought processes related to presence of psychosis
• Risk for injury related to drug-induced adverse CNS reactions
• Deficient knowledge related to drug therapy

Planning and implementation
ALERT: Fatal hyperglycemia may occur in a patient taking atypical antipsychotics. Monitor patient with diabetes regularly. For patients with risk factors for diabetes, perform fasting glucose testing at baseline and periodically. Monitor all patients for symptoms of hyperglycemia, including excessive thirst, hunger, frequent urinating, and weakness; if symptoms develop, perform fasting glucose testing. Hyperglycemia may resolve once therapy is stopped.
• When restarting therapy for patient who has been off drug, follow 3-day dose initiation schedule.
• When switching patient to drug from another antipsychotic, stop other drug immediately when risperidone therapy starts.
• When switching from a depot antipsychotic to oral risperidone, start risperidone at the time of the next scheduled injection.
• Orally-disintegrating tablets contain phenylalanine; 3-mg tablet contains 0.63 mg phenylalanine and 4-mg tablet contains 0.84 mg phenylalanine.
• Give oral antipsychotic for the first 3 weeks of I.M. injection therapy because of injection's prolonged onset of action. Then stop oral therapy.
• To reconstitute I.M. injection, remove dose pack from the refrigerator and allow it to reach room temperature. Inject premeasured diluent into vial and shake vigorously for at least 10 seconds. Suspension will appear uniform, thick, and milky; particles will be visible, but no dry particles remain. Manufacturer recommends that drug be used immediately; suspension must be used within 6 hours of reconstitution. If more than 2 minutes pass before injection, shake vigorously again. See manufacturer's package insert for more detailed instructions.
• Before reconstitution, store I.M. injection kit in refrigerator and protect from light. Drug can be stored at temperatures less than 77° F (25° C) for no more than 7 days before administration.
• Oral solution may be mixed with water, coffee, orange juice, or low-fat milk. It isn't compatible with cola or tea.
ALERT: Fatal cerebrovascular adverse events, such as stroke or transient ischemic attacks, may occur in elderly patients with dementia.
Patient teaching
• Warn patient to rise slowly, avoid hot showers, and use extra caution during first few days of therapy to avoid fainting.

R

• Warn patient to avoid activities that require alertness until the drug's CNS effects are known. Drowsiness and dizziness usually subside after a few days.

• Tell patient not to drink alcohol and to avoid prolonged exposure to sunlight during therapy.

• Tell patient to use sun block and to wear protective clothing in sunlight.

• Advise patient to use caution in hot weather to prevent heatstroke; drug may affect the body's ability to regulate temperature.

• Tell woman to notify prescriber if she is or plans to become pregnant during therapy and for at least 12 weeks after last I.M. injection.

• Warn patient not to breast-feed during treatment and for at least 12 weeks after last I.M. injection.

• Inform patient that drug may be taken with or without food.

• Tell patient not to remove the orally-disintegrating tablets from blister pack until just before use. Explain that he should peel the foil apart to expose the tablet rather than pushing the tablet through the foil. Then, tell him to dissolve the tablet on his tongue.

• Tell patient not to split or chew the orally-disintegrating tablets.

☑ **Evaluation**

• Patient behavior and communication indicate improved thought processes.

• Patient sustains no injury from drug-induced adverse CNS reactions.

• Patient and family state understanding of drug therapy.

ritonavir
(rih-TOH-nuh-veer)
Norvir

Pharmacologic class: protease inhibitor
Therapeutic class: antiretroviral
Pregnancy risk category: B

Indications and dosages

▶ **HIV infection.** *Adults:* 600 mg P.O. b.i.d. with meals. If adverse events occur, may give 300 mg b.i.d.; then increase at 2- to 3-day intervals by 100 mg b.i.d. If given with saquinavir, reduce saquinavir to 400 mg P.O. b.i.d. and ritonavir to 400 or 600 mg P.O. b.i.d.

Children age 1 month and older as part of combination therapy: Initially, 250 mg/m² P.O. b.i.d. Increase by 50 mg/m² b.i.d. at 2- to 3-day intervals to target dose of 400 mg/m² b.i.d. Do not exceed 600 mg b.i.d.

Contraindications and cautions

• Contraindicated in patients hypersensitive to the drug or any of its components, and in those who are taking dihydroergotamine or ergotamine drugs. Also contraindicated with alfuzosin, amiodarone, cisapride, ergot derivatives, flecainide, lovastatin, midazolam, propafenone, quinidine, simvastatin, triazolam, and voriconazole.

⚘ **Lifespan:** Use in pregnancy only if benefits outweigh risks to fetus. If used during pregnancy, contact the antiretroviral pregnancy registry at 800-258-4263 or www.APRegistry.com. In breast-feeding women, use cautiously. It isn't known if drug appears in breast milk.

Adverse reactions

CNS: anxiety, *asthenia,* circumoral paresthesia, confusion, depression, dizziness, *generalized tonic-clonic seizure,* fever, headache, insomnia, malaise, pain, paresthesia, peripheral paresthesia, somnolence, thinking abnormality.

CV: syncope, vasodilation.

EENT: pharyngitis.

GI: abdominal pain, anorexia, constipation, diarrhea, dyspepsia, flatulence, *nausea, pancreatitis, pseudomembranous colitis,* taste perversion, vomiting.

Hematologic: *leukopenia, thrombocytopenia.*

Hepatic: *hepatitis.*

Metabolic: *diabetes mellitus,* weight loss.

Musculoskeletal: arthralgia, myalgia.

Skin: rash, sweating.

Other: fat redistribution/accumulation, *hypersensitivity reactions.*

Interactions

Drug-drug. *Alfuzosin, amiodarone, cisapride, ergot derivatives, flecainide, midazolam, propafenone, quinidine, triazolam, voriconazole:* May cause serious and life-threatening adverse reactions. Use together is contraindicated.
Atovaquone, divalproex, lamotrigine, phenytoin, warfarin: May decrease levels of these drugs. Use together cautiously and monitor drug levels closely, if appropriate.
Beta blockers, disopyramide, fluoxetine, mexiletine, nefazodone: May increase levels of these

---

Reactions may be *common,* uncommon, *life-threatening,* or COMMON AND LIFE-THREATENING.

drugs, causing cardiac and neurologic events. Use together with caution.

Bupropion, buspirone, calcium channel blockers, carbamazepine, clonazepam, clorazepate, cyclosporine, dexamethasone, diazepam, dronabinol, estazolam, ethosuximide, flurazepam, lidocaine, methamphetamine, metoprolol, perphenazine, prednisone, propoxyphene, quinine, risperidone, SSRIs, tacrolimus, tricyclic antidepressants, thioridazine, timolol, tramadol, zolpidem: May increase levels of these drugs. Use cautiously together and consider decreasing the dosage of these drugs by almost 50%.

Clarithromycin: May increase clarithromycin level. Patients with impaired renal function require 50% reduction in clarithromycin if creatinine clearance is 30 to 60 ml/minute, and a 75% reduction if it's below 30 ml/minute.

Delavirdine: Increases ritonavir level. Use together cautiously. Dosage recommendations not established for combined use.

Didanosine: May decrease didanosine absorption. Separate doses by 2½ hours.

Disulfiram, metronidazole: May increase risk of disulfiram-like reactions since ritonavir formulations contain alcohol. Monitor patient.

Ethinyl estradiol: May decrease ethinyl estradiol level. Use a different or another method of birth control.

Fluticasone: May increase fluticasone exposure leading to significantly decreased serum cortisol concentrations, which may lead to systemic corticosteroid effects (including Cushing syndrome). Don't use together, if possible.

HMG-CoA reductase inhibitors: May cause a large increase in statin level, causing myopathy. Avoid use with lovastatin and simvastatin. Use cautiously with atorvastatin. Consider using fluvastatin or pravastatin.

Indinavir: May increase indinavir level. Use together cautiously.

Itraconazole, ketoconazole: May increase levels of these drugs. Don't exceed 200 mg per day of these drugs.

Meperidine: May decrease level of meperidine and its metabolite. Dosage increase and long-term use of meperidine with ritonavir not recommended because of CNS effects. Use cautiously together.

Methadone: May decrease methadone level. Consider increasing methadone dosage.

Phosphodiesterase type 5 (PDE 5) inhibitors (sildenafil, tadalafil, vardenafil): May increase level of PDE 5 inhibitor causing potentially fatal hypotension, syncope, visual changes, or prolonged erection. Use together cautiously and with increased monitoring for adverse reactions. Tell patient not to exceed 25 mg of sildenafil in a 48-hour period, 10 mg of tadalafil in a 72-hour period, or 2.5 mg of vardenafil in a 72-hour period.

Rifabutin: May increase rifabutin level. Monitor patient and reduce rifabutin daily dosage by at least 75% of usual dose.

Rifampin: May decrease ritonavir level. Consider using rifabutin in place of rifampin.

Saquinavir: May increase saquinavir level. Adjust dosage by giving 400 mg saquinavir b.i.d. and 400 mg ritonavir b.i.d.

Theophylline: May decrease theophylline level. Increase dosage based on level.

Trazodone: May increase trazodone level causing nausea, dizziness, hypotension, and syncope. Avoid use together. If unavoidable, use cautiously with a lower dose of trazodone.

Drug-herb. *St. John's wort:* May substantially reduce drug level. Discourage use together.

Drug-food. *Any food:* May increase drug absorption. Give drug with food.

Drug-lifestyle. *Smoking:* May decrease level of ritonavir. Discourage smoking.

Effects on lab test results

• May increase ALT, AST, GGT, glucose, triglyceride, lipid, CPK, and uric acid levels. May decrease hemoglobin level and hematocrit.
• May decrease WBC, RBC, platelet, and neutrophil counts.

Pharmacokinetics

Absorption: Enhanced by food.
Distribution: Absolute bioavailability unknown. 98% to 100% albumin-bound.
Metabolism: In liver and kidneys.
Excretion: In urine and feces. *Half-life:* Unknown.

Route	Onset	Peak	Duration
P.O.	Unknown	2–4 hr	Unknown

Action

Chemical effect: HIV protease inhibitor with activity against HIV-1 and HIV-2 proteases; binds to protease-active site and inhibits enzyme activity.

Therapeutic effect: Prevents cleavage of viral polyproteins, resulting in formation of immature noninfectious viral particles.

Available forms

Capsules: 100 mg
Oral solution: 80 mg/ml

NURSING PROCESS

⚕ Assessment
• Use cautiously in patients with hepatic insufficiency.
• Assess patient's and family's knowledge of drug therapy.

⊕ Nursing diagnoses
• Risk for infection related to presence of virus
• Deficient knowledge related to drug therapy

▷ Planning and implementation
⚠ ALERT: Don't confuse Norvir with Norvasc. Don't confuse ritonavir with Retrovir.
Patient teaching
• Inform patient that drug doesn't reduce the risk of HIV transmission or cure HIV infection or the illnesses it may cause.
• Tell patient that the taste of oral solution may be improved by mixing with flavored milk within 1 hour of dose.
• Tell patient to take drug with meal.
• If patient misses a dose, instruct him to take next dose at once. He shouldn't take double doses.
• Advise patient to report use of other drugs, including OTC drugs.
• Advise patient taking PDE 5 inhibitors about an increased risk of adverse events, including hypotension, visual changes, and prolonged erection. He should promptly report any symptoms to his prescriber. Tell patient not to exceed 25 mg of sildenafil in a 48-hour period, 10 mg of tadalafil in a 72-hour period, or 2.5 mg of vardenafil in a 72-hour period.
• To prevent transmission of disease, HIV-positive women shouldn't breast-feed.

☑ Evaluation
• Patient's infection is controlled.
• Patient and family state understanding of drug therapy.

rivastigmine tartrate
(riv-uh-STIG-meen TAR-trayt)
Exelon

Pharmacologic class: cholinesterase inhibitor
Therapeutic class: Alzheimer disease drug
Pregnancy risk category: B

Indications and dosages

▶ **Mild to moderate dementia of the Alzheimer type.** *Adults:* Initially, 1.5 mg P.O. b.i.d. with food. If tolerated, may be increased to 3 mg b.i.d. after 2 weeks. Further increases to 4.5 mg b.i.d. and 6 mg b.i.d. may be given as tolerated after 2 weeks on the previous dose. Effective dosage range is 6 to 12 mg daily, with maximum recommended dosage of 12 mg daily. Or initially apply one 4.6 mg/24 hours patch daily to back, chest, or upper arm. If tolerated for a minimum of 4 weeks, increase to maintenance dosage of 9.5 mg/24 hours. Restart at the lower dosage if interrupted for longer than a few days.
▶ **Mild to moderate dementia in Parkinson disease.** *Adults:* Initially, 1.5 mg P.O. b.i.d. May increase, as tolerated, to 3 mg b.i.d., then to 4.5 mg b.i.d., and finally to 6 mg b.i.d. after at least 4 weeks at each dose. Or, initially apply one 4.6 mg/24 hours patch daily to back, chest, or upper arm. If tolerated for a minimum of 4 weeks, increase to maintenance dosage of 9.5 mg/24 hours. Restart at the lower dosage if interrupted for longer than a few days.

Contraindications and cautions

• Contraindicated in patients hypersensitive to the drug, any of its components, or other carbamate derivatives.
• Use cautiously in patients who take NSAIDs and who have a history of ulcers or GI bleeding and in patients with sick sinus syndrome or other supraventricular cardiac conditions, asthma or obstructive pulmonary disease, or seizures.
☀ Lifespan: Use in pregnancy if benefits outweigh risks to the fetus. In breast-feeding women, use cautiously because it isn't known if drug appears in breast milk.

Adverse reactions

CNS: aggressive reaction, agitation, anxiety, asthenia, confusion, delusion, depression, *dizziness,* fatigue, hallucination, *headache,* insom-

nia, malaise, nervousness, pain, paranoid reaction, somnolence, syncope, tremor, vertigo.
CV: chest pain, hypertension, peripheral edema.
EENT: pharyngitis, rhinitis.
GI: *abdominal pain, anorexia,* constipation, *diarrhea,* dyspepsia, eructation, flatulence, GI bleeding, *nausea, vomiting.*
GU: urinary incontinence, urinary obstruction, UTI.
Metabolic: weight loss.
Musculoskeletal: arthralgia, back pain, bone fracture.
Respiratory: bronchitis, cough, upper respiratory tract infection.
Skin: increased sweating, rash.
Other: *accidental trauma,* flulike symptoms.

Interactions

Drug-drug. *Anticholinergics:* May interfere with anticholinergic activity. Monitor patient closely.
Bethanechol, succinylcholine, and other neuromuscular blockers or cholinergic antagonists: May have synergistic effect. Monitor patient closely.
Drug-lifestyle. *Smoking:* May increase rivastigmine clearance. Monitor patient closely.

Effects on lab test results

None reported.

Pharmacokinetics

Absorption: Rapid, with level peaking in about 1 hour. Although drug is given with food, it delays peak level by about 1½ hours. Absolute bioavailability is 36%.
Distribution: Wide, throughout body; drug crosses the blood-brain barrier. About 40% protein-bound.
Metabolism: Rapid and extensive.
Excretion: Mainly through the kidneys. *Half-life:* About 1½ hours in patients with normal renal function.

Route	Onset	Peak	Duration
P.O.	Unknown	1 hr	12 hr

Action

Chemical effect: Thought to increase acetylcholine level by reversibly inhibiting its hydrolysis by cholinesterase. Acetylcholine is probably the primary neurotransmitter that is depleted in Alzheimer disease.

Therapeutic effect: Improves cognitive function.

Available forms

Capsules: 1.5 mg, 3 mg, 4.5 mg, 6 mg
Solution: 2 mg/ml
Transdermal patch: 4.6 mg/24 hours, 9.5 mg/24 hours

NURSING PROCESS

⚖ Assessment
• Assess underlying condition before starting therapy and regularly thereafter to monitor drug's effectiveness.
• Perform complete health history, and carefully monitor for adverse effects any patient with a history of GI bleeding, NSAID use, arrhythmias, seizures, or pulmonary conditions.
• Assess patient's and family's knowledge of drug therapy.

⊕ Nursing diagnoses
• Acute or chronic confusion related to underlying disease
• Risk for imbalanced fluid volume related to drug-induced GI effects
• Deficient knowledge related to rivastigmine tartrate therapy

▶ Planning and implementation
• Expect significant GI adverse effects, such as nausea, vomiting, and anorexia; they're less common during maintenance.
• Monitor patient for dehydration and weight loss due to GI adverse effects.
• ⊛ **ALERT:** Severe vomiting may occur in patient who resumes therapy after an interruption. If therapy is interrupted for longer than several days, resume therapy at 1.5 mg b.i.d. to maintenance level.
• Dramatic memory improvement is unlikely. As disease progresses, the benefits of drug may decline.
• Monitor patient for symptoms of active or occult GI bleeding.
• Monitor patients weighing less than 50 kg carefully with use of transdermal patch. They are more likely to experience side effects.
Patient teaching
• Advise patient to report any episodes of nausea, vomiting, or diarrhea.

R

• Inform patient and caregiver that memory improvement may be subtle and that a more likely result of therapy is a slower decline in memory loss.

• Tell patient to take with food in the morning and evening.

• Instruct patient to consult prescriber before taking OTC drugs.

• Tell patient to place patch on back, chest, or upper arm and to rotate sites.

☑ Evaluation

• Patient's cognition improves and he experiences less confusion.

• Patient and family state that adverse GI effects haven't occurred or have been managed effectively.

• Patient and family state understanding of drug therapy.

rizatriptan benzoate
(rih-zah-TRIP-tin BEN-zoh-ayt)
Maxalt, Maxalt-MLT

Pharmacologic class: selective 5-hydroxytryptamine (5-HT$_1$) receptor agonist
Therapeutic class: antimigraine drug
Pregnancy risk category: C

Indications and dosages

▶ **Acute migraine headaches with or without aura.** *Adults:* Initially, 5 to 10 mg P.O. If first dose is ineffective, another dose can be given at least 2 hours after first dose. Maximum, 30 mg daily. For patients taking propranolol, 5 mg P.O., up to maximum of three doses (15 mg total) in 24 hours.

Contraindications and cautions

• Contraindicated in patients hypersensitive to the drug or any of its components and in the management of hemiplegic or basilar migraines. Also contraindicated in patients with ischemic heart disease (angina pectoris, history of MI, or documented silent ischemia) or those with evidence of ischemic heart disease, coronary artery vasospasm (Prinzmetal variant angina), or other significant underlying CV disease. Also contraindicated in patients with uncontrolled hypertension and within 24 hours of another 5-HT$_1$ agonist or ergotamine-containing or ergot-type

drug, such as dihydroergotamine or methysergide.

• Don't use within 14 days of an MAO inhibitor.

• Use cautiously in patients with hepatic or renal impairment. Also use cautiously in patients with risk factors for coronary artery disease (hypertension, hypercholesterolemia, smoking, obesity, diabetes, strong family history of coronary artery disease, women with surgical or physiologic menopause, or men older than age 40), unless a cardiac evaluation provides evidence that patient is free from cardiac disease.

⚠ **Lifespan:** Use in pregnancy only if benefits clearly outweigh risks to the fetus. In breastfeeding women, don't use drug because the effects on infants are unknown. In children, safety and effectiveness haven't been established.

Adverse reactions

CNS: asthenia, decreased mental acuity, dizziness, euphoria, fatigue, headache, hypesthesia, pain, paresthesia, somnolence, tremor.
CV: chest pain, *coronary artery vasospasm,* flushing, pressure or heaviness, palpitations, *MI, transient myocardial ischemia, ventricular fibrillation, ventricular tachycardia.*
EENT: neck, throat, and jaw heaviness, pain, or pressure.
GI: diarrhea, dry mouth, nausea, vomiting.
Respiratory: dyspnea.
Other: hot flushes, warm or cold sensations.

Interactions

Drug-drug. *Ergot-containing or ergot-type drugs (dihydroergotamine, methysergide), other 5-HT$_1$ agonists:* May prolong vasospastic reactions. Don't use within 24 hours of rizatriptan.
MAO inhibitors: May increase rizatriptan level. Don't use together. Allow at least 14 days between stopping an MAO inhibitor and giving rizatriptan.
Propranolol: May increase rizatriptan level. Reduce rizatriptan dose to 5 mg.
SNRIs, SSRIs: May cause serotonin syndrome (diarrhea, fever, hallucinations, labile blood pressure, nausea, weakness, hyperreflexia, incoordination, tachycardia, vomiting). Monitor patient.

Effects on lab test results

None reported.

Pharmacokinetics

Absorption: Complete, with an absolute bio-availability of 45%.
Distribution: Wide. 14% protein-bound.
Metabolism: Mainly by oxidative deamination by MAO-A.
Excretion: 82% in urine. *Half-life:* 2 to 3 hours.

Route	Onset	Peak	Duration
P.O.	Unknown	1–1½ hr	Unknown

Action

Chemical effect: Believed to exert its effect by acting as an agonist at serotonin receptors on extracerebral intracranial blood vessels, which results in vasoconstriction of the affected vessels, inhibition of neuropeptide release, and reduction of pain transmission in the trigeminal pathways.
Therapeutic effect: Relieves migraine pain.

Available forms

Tablets: 5 mg, 10 mg
Tablets (disintegrating): 5 mg, 10 mg

NURSING PROCESS

🗹 Assessment
• Use drug only after a definite diagnosis of migraine is established.
• Assess patient for history of coronary artery disease, hypertension, arrhythmias, or presence of risk factors for coronary artery disease.
• Perform baseline and periodic CV evaluation in patients who develop risk factors for coronary artery disease.
• Monitor renal and liver function tests before starting therapy, and report abnormalities.
• Assess patient's and family's knowledge of drug therapy.

🔁 Nursing diagnoses
• Acute pain related to presence of migraine headache
• Risk for activity intolerance related to adverse drug reactions
• Deficient knowledge related to drug therapy

▶ Planning and implementation
• Don't give to patient with hemiplegic migraine, basilar migraine, or cluster headaches.
⚠ ALERT: Don't give drug within 24 hours of a drug containing ergot or 5-HT₁ agonist or within 14 days of an MAO inhibitor.

• For patient with cardiac risk factors who has had a satisfactory cardiac evaluation, give first dose while monitoring ECG and have emergency equipment readily available.
• If patient develops palpitations or neck, throat, or jaw pain, pressure, or heaviness, stop giving the drug and notify prescriber.
• Safety of treating more than four headaches in a 30-day period, on average, hasn't been established.
• Drug contains phenylalanine.
Patient teaching
• Inform patient that drug doesn't prevent headache.
• For Maxalt-MLT, tell patient to remove blister pack from sachet and to remove drug from blister pack immediately before use. Tell him not to pop tablet out of blister pack but to carefully peel pack away with dry hands, place tablet on tongue, and let it dissolve. Tablet is then swallowed with saliva. No water is needed or recommended. Tell patient that dissolving tablet doesn't provide more rapid headache relief.
• Advise patient that if headache returns after first dose, a second dose may be taken with medical approval at least 2 hours after the first dose. Don't take more than 30 mg in a 24-hour period.
• Tell patient that food may delay onset of drug action.
• Advise patient to notify prescriber if pregnancy occurs or is suspected.

🗹 Evaluation
• Patient has relief from migraine headache.
• Patient maintains baseline activity level.
• Patient and family state understanding of drug therapy.

ropinirole hydrochloride
(roh-PIN-er-ohl high-droh-KLOR-ighd)
Requip

Pharmacologic class: nonergoline dopamine agonist
Therapeutic class: antiparkinsonian
Pregnancy risk category: C

Indications and dosages

▶ **Idiopathic Parkinson disease.** *Adults:* Initially, 0.25 mg P.O. t.i.d. Dosages can be adjust-

R

ed weekly. After week 4, dosage may be increased by 1.5 mg daily on a weekly basis up to dosage of 9 mg daily, and then increased weekly by up to 3 mg daily to maximum daily dose of 24 mg.

▶ **Moderate to severe restless leg syndrome.** *Adults:* Initially, 0.25 mg P.O. 1 to 3 hours before bedtime. May increase dosage, as needed and tolerated after 2 days to 0.5 mg, then to 1 mg by the end of the first week. May further increase dosage as needed and tolerated as follows: week 2, give 1 mg once daily. Week 3, give 1.5 mg once daily. Week 4, give 2 mg once daily. Week 5, give 2.5 mg once daily. Week 6, give 3 mg once daily. And week 7, give 4 mg once daily. All doses should be taken 1 to 2 hours before bedtime.

Contraindications and cautions

- Contraindicated in patients hypersensitive to the drug or any of its components.
- Use cautiously in patients with severe hepatic or renal impairment.

⚓ **Lifespan:** Use during pregnancy only if benefits outweigh risks to fetus. In nursing mothers, decision should be made whether to stop nursing or to stop drug. In patients older than age 65, clearance is reduced; dosage is individually adjusted to response.

Adverse reactions

Early Parkinson disease (without levodopa)
CNS: aggravated Parkinson disease, amnesia, asthenia, confusion, *dizziness,* fatigue, hallucinations, headache, hyperkinesia, hypesthesia, impaired concentration, malaise, pain, somnolence, syncope, vertigo.
CV: atrial fibrillation, chest pain, edema, extrasystoles, flushing hypertension, hypotension, orthostatic symptoms, palpitations, peripheral ischemia, tachycardia.
EENT: abnormal vision, eye abnormality, pharyngitis, rhinitis, sinusitis, xerophthalmia.
GI: abdominal pain, anorexia, constipation, dry mouth, *dyspepsia,* flatulence, *nausea, vomiting.*
GU: UTI, impotence (male).
Respiratory: bronchitis, dyspnea.
Skin: increased sweating.
Other: viral infection, yawning.
Advanced Parkinson disease (with levodopa)
CNS: abnormal dreaming, aggravated parkinsonism, amnesia, anxiety, confusion, *dizziness, hallucinations, headache,* insomnia, nervous-

ness, pain, paresthesia, *somnolence,* syncope, tremor.
CV: hypotension.
EENT: diplopia, increased saliva.
GI: abdominal pain, constipation, diarrhea, dry mouth, dysphagia, flatulence, *nausea,* vomiting.
GU: UTI, pyuria, urinary incontinence.
Hematologic: anemia.
Metabolic: weight loss.
Musculoskeletal: arthralgia, arthritis, *dyskinesia,* hypokinesia, paresis.
Respiratory: dyspnea, upper respiratory infection.
Skin: increased sweating.
Other: *falls,* injury, viral infection.
Restless leg syndrome
CNS: dizziness, fatigue, paresthesia, somnolence, vertigo.
CV: peripheral edema.
EENT: nasal congestion, *nasopharyngitis.*
GI: diarrhea, dry mouth, dyspepsia, *nausea, vomiting.*
Musculoskeletal: arthralgia, extremity pain, muscle cramps,
Respiratory: cough.
Skin: increased sweating.
Other: influenza.

Interactions

Drug-drug. *CNS depressants:* May increase CNS effects. Use together cautiously.
Dopamine antagonists (butyrophenones, metoclopramide, phenothiazines, thioxanthenes): May decrease ropinirole effectiveness. Monitor patient closely.
Estrogens: May decrease ropinirole clearance. If estrogens are started or stopped during therapy, adjust ropinirole dosage.
Inhibitors or substrates of CYP1A2 (cimetidine, ciprofloxacin, diltiazem, erythromycin, fluvoxamine, tacrine): May decrease ropinirole clearance. If these drugs are started or stopped during therapy, adjust ropinirole dosage.
Drug-lifestyle. *Alcohol use:* May increase sedative effects. Discourage using together.
Smoking: May increase drug clearance. Urge patient to stop smoking, especially during drug therapy.

Effects on lab test results

- May increase BUN and alkaline phosphatase levels. May decrease hemoglobin level and hematocrit.

Reactions may be *common,* uncommon, *life-threatening*, or COMMON AND LIFE-THREATENING.

Pharmacokinetics

Absorption: Rapid, with an absolute bioavailability of 55%.
Distribution: Wide. About 40% protein-bound.
Metabolism: Extensive by the liver to inactive metabolites.
Excretion: Less than 10%, unchanged in urine.
Half-life: 6 hours.

Route	Onset	Peak	Duration
P.O.	Unknown	1–2 hr	Unknown

Action

Chemical effect: Unknown. A dopamine agonist thought to stimulate postsynaptic dopamine D2 receptors in the brain.
Therapeutic effect: Improves physical mobility in patients with parkinsonism.

Available forms

Tablets: 0.25 mg, 0.5 mg, 1 mg, 2 mg, 3 mg, 4 mg, 5 mg

NURSING PROCESS

⚷ Assessment
• Assess patient before starting therapy and frequently thereafter to monitor the drug's effectiveness.
• Monitor patient carefully for orthostatic hypotension, especially during dose escalation.
• Assess patient for adequate nutritional intake.
• Assess patient's and family's knowledge of drug therapy.

⊕ Nursing diagnoses
• Impaired physical mobility related to underlying Parkinson disease
• Disturbed thought processes related to drug-induced CNS adverse reactions
• Deficient knowledge related to drug therapy

⊠ Planning and implementation
• Give drug with food to decrease nausea.
• Drug may increase the risk of dopaminergic adverse effects of levodopa and may cause or worsen dyskinesia. Decrease levodopa dosage if needed.
• Don't abruptly stop drug. Withdraw gradually over 7 days to avoid hyperpyrexia and confusion.
• When used for restless leg syndrome, no dose taper is needed when stopping therapy.

Patient teaching
• Tell patient to take drug with food if nausea occurs.
• Explain that hallucinations may occur, particularly in an elderly patient.
• To minimize effects of orthostatic hypotension, instruct patient not to rise rapidly after sitting or lying down, especially when therapy starts or dosage changes.
• Advise patient to avoid hazardous activities until the drug's CNS effects are known.
• Tell patient not to drink alcohol during therapy.
• Tell woman to notify prescriber if pregnancy is suspected or planned, or if she is breast-feeding.

☑ Evaluation
• Patient has improved mobility and reduced muscle rigidity and tremor.
• Patient remains mentally alert.
• Patient and family state understanding of drug therapy.

HIGH ALERT

rosiglitazone maleate
(roh-sih-GLIH-tah-zohn MAL-ee-ayt)
Avandia◆

Pharmacologic class: thiazolidinedione
Therapeutic class: antidiabetic
Pregnancy risk category: C

Indications and dosages

▶ **Adjunct to diet and exercise (as monotherapy) to improve glycemic control in patients with type 2 diabetes mellitus, or (as combination therapy) with sulfonylurea, metformin, or insulin when diet, exercise, and a single drug don't result in adequate glycemic control.** *Adults:* Initially, 4 mg P.O. daily in the morning or in divided doses b.i.d. in the morning and evening. If fasting glucose level doesn't improve after 12 weeks, increase to 8 mg P.O. daily or in divided doses b.i.d. Maximum dose is 8 mg daily, except in patients taking insulin. For patients stabilized on insulin, continue insulin dose when therapy starts. Doses greater than 4 mg daily with insulin aren't indicated.
⧈ Adjust-a-dose: If patient reports hypoglycemia or if fasting glucose level decreases to less

R

---

than 100 mg/dl, decrease insulin dosage by 10% to 25%. Base further adjustments on response.

Contraindications and cautions

• Contraindicated in patients hypersensitive to the drug or any of its components, and in patients with New York Heart Association Class III or IV cardiac status unless expected benefits outweigh risks. Also contraindicated in patients who developed jaundice while taking troglitazone and in patients with active liver disease, increased baseline liver enzyme level (ALT level is greater than three times the upper limit of normal), type 1 diabetes, or diabetic ketoacidosis.
• Combination therapy with metformin and rosiglitazone is contraindicated in patients with renal impairment. Rosiglitazone can be used as monotherapy in patients with renal impairment.
• Use cautiously in patients with edema or heart failure.
⚠ Lifespan: Drug isn't recommended for pregnant or breast-feeding women.

Adverse reactions

CNS: headache, fatigue.
CV: edema, *heart failure,* peripheral edema.
EENT: sinusitis.
GI: *diarrhea,* weight gain.
Hematologic: anemia.
Metabolic: hyperglycemia, *hypoglycemia.*
Musculoskeletal: back pain.
Respiratory: *upper respiratory tract infection.*
Other: injury.

Interactions

Drug-drug. *Gemfibrozil:* May increase rosiglitazone level. May need to decrease rosiglitazone dosage if gemfibrozil is added.
Rifamycins (rifabutin, rifampin, rifapentine): May increase rosiglitazone clearance and decrease glucose control. Monitor blood glucose level carefully when starting or stopping rosiglitazone therapy.
Drug-herb. *Bitter melon, fenugreek, ginseng:* May improve glucose control. Patient may need reduced antidiabetic dosage. Discourage using together.

Effects on lab test results

• May increase ALT, HDL, LDL, total cholesterol, and glucose levels. May decrease free fatty acid, glucose, and hemoglobin levels and hematocrit.

Pharmacokinetics

Absorption: Level peaks about 1 hour after a dose. Absolute bioavailability is 99%.
Distribution: About 99.8% protein-bound, mainly to albumin.
Metabolism: Extensive, with no unchanged drug in urine. Mainly through N-demethylation and hydroxylation.
Excretion: About 64% in urine and 23% in feces. *Half-life:* 3 to 4 hours.

Route	Onset	Peak	Duration
P.O.	Unknown	1 hr	Unknown

Action

Chemical effect: Lowers glucose level by improving insulin sensitivity. Highly selective and potent agonist for receptors in key target areas for insulin action, such as adipose tissue, skeletal muscle, and liver.
Therapeutic effect: Lowers glucose level.

Available forms

Tablets: 2 mg, 4 mg, 8 mg

NURSING PROCESS

Assessment

• Obtain history of patient's underlying condition before starting therapy, and reassess regularly thereafter to monitor drug's effectiveness.
• Check liver enzyme level before therapy starts. Don't use drug in patients with increased baseline liver enzyme level. In patients with normal baseline liver enzyme level, monitor level every 2 months for the first 12 months and periodically afterward. If ALT level is elevated, recheck level as soon as possible. If level remains elevated, notify prescriber and stop drug.
• Monitor glucose level regularly and glycosylated hemoglobin level periodically to determine therapeutic response to drug.
• If patient has heart failure, watch for increased edema during rosiglitazone therapy.
• Assess patient's and family's knowledge of drug therapy.

Nursing diagnoses

• Ineffective health maintenance related to hyperglycemia

- Risk for injury related to drug-induced hypoglycemia
- Deficient knowledge related to drug therapy

▶ Planning and implementation
- Before starting drug, treat patient for other causes of poor glycemic control, such as infection.
- Because calorie restriction, weight loss, and exercise help improve insulin sensitivity and make drug therapy effective, these measures are essential.
- ⓢ **ALERT:** May increase incidence of bone fractures in women, most commonly in the arms, hands, and feet.
- For patients inadequately controlled with a maximum dose of a sulfonylurea or metformin, add this drug to current regimen; don't switch therapies.
- ⓢ **ALERT:** This drug alone or with insulin can cause fluid retention that may lead to or worsen heart failure. Observe patient for signs or symptoms of heart failure, such as rapid weight gain, shortness of breath, and edema. If cardiac health deteriorates, stop drug. Risk for MI is increased in patients at high risk for MI.
- Macular edema may occur or worsen during therapy. If patient reports vision problems, obtain ophthalmic examination.
- Because ovulation may resume in premenopausal, anovulatory woman with insulin resistance, contraceptive measures may need to be considered.
- ⓢ **ALERT:** Don't confuse Avandia with Prandin.

Patient teaching
- Advise patient that drug can be taken with or without food.
- Inform patient that blood will be tested to check liver function before therapy starts, every 2 months for the first 12 months, and periodically thereafter.
- Tell patient to immediately report unexplained signs or symptoms—such as nausea, vomiting, abdominal pain, fatigue, anorexia, or dark urine—because they may indicate liver problems.
- Instruct patient to contact prescriber if he has signs or symptoms of heart failure, such as unusually rapid increase in weight, edema, or shortness of breath.
- Urge patient to report vision changes or problems.

- Inform premenopausal, anovulatory woman with insulin resistance that ovulation may resume and that she may want to consider contraceptive measures.
- Advise patient that diabetes management must include diet control because calorie restriction, weight loss, and exercise improve insulin sensitivity and make drug therapy effective.

✓ Evaluation
- Patient's glucose level is normal with drug therapy.
- Patient doesn't have hypoglycemia.
- Patient and family state understanding of drug therapy.

rosuvastatin calcium
(ro-SOO-va-stat-in KAL-see-uhm)
Crestor✔

Pharmacologic class: HMG-CoA reductase inhibitor
Therapeutic class: antihyperlipidemic
Pregnancy risk category: X

Indications and dosages

▶ **Adjunct to diet to reduce total cholesterol, LDL, apolipoprotein B (ApoB), non-HDL, and triglyceride levels, as well as to increase HDL level in primary hypercholesterolemia (heterozygous familial and nonfamilial), mixed dyslipidemia (Fredrickson Type IIA and IIB); adjunct to diet to treat elevated triglyceride level (Fredrickson Type IV); with diet, to slow atherosclerosis progression in patients with high total and LDL cholesterol.**
Adults: Initially, 10 mg P.O. daily. Increase dosage, if needed, to a maximum of 40 mg daily. Increase every 2 to 4 weeks based on lipid level. If aggressive lipid lowering is needed, drug may be started at 20 mg once daily.
▶ **Adjunct to other lipid-lowering therapies to reduce LDL, ApoB, and total cholesterol levels in homozygous familial hypercholesterolemia.** *Adults:* Initially, 20 mg once daily. Maximum, 40 mg daily.
▨ **Adjust-a-dose:** For patients with renal impairment, if creatinine clearance is less than 30 ml/minute, start with 5 mg once daily; don't exceed 10 mg once daily. In patients taking 40 mg who develop unexplained persistent pro-

R

teinuria, reduce dosage. For patients taking gemfibrozil with rosuvastatin, don't exceed 10 mg once daily. For patients requiring less aggressive treatment, those at risk for myopathy, Asian patients, or patients also taking cyclosporine, initial dose is 5 mg.

Contraindications and cautions

● Contraindicated in patients hypersensitive to the drug or any of its components, and in patients with active liver disease or unexplained persistent elevations in transaminases.
● Use cautiously in patients who drink substantial amounts of alcohol and in patients with a history of liver disease. Also use cautiously in patients at increased risk for developing myopathies, such as patients 65 or older or those with renal impairment or hypothyroidism.
● Use with gemfibrozil only when the benefit clearly outweighs the risk. Don't exceed recommended dosage.
⚠ **Lifespan:** In pregnant women, drug is contraindicated. In breast-feeding women, use cautiously; it's unknown if the drug appears in breast milk. In children, safety and effectiveness haven't been established.

Adverse reactions

CNS: anxiety, asthenia, depression, dizziness, headache, hypertonia, insomnia, neuralgia, pain, paresthesia, vertigo.
CV: chest pain, hypertension, palpitation, vasodilation.
EENT: pharyngitis, rhinitis, sinusitis.
GI: abdominal pain, constipation, diarrhea, dyspepsia, nausea, flatulence, gastritis, gastroenteritis, periodontal abscess, vomiting.
GU: proteinuria, UTI.
Hematologic: anemia.
Metabolic: *diabetes mellitus.*
Musculoskeletal: arthritis, back pain, myalgia, *myopathy,* neck pain, pathological fracture, pelvic pain, *rhabdomyolysis.*
Respiratory: *asthma,* bronchitis, dyspnea, increased cough, pneumonia.
Skin: ecchymosis, pruritus, rash.
Other: accidental injury, flulike syndrome.

Interactions

Drug-drug. *Antacids:* May decrease level of rosuvastatin. Give antacids 2 hours after rosuvastatin.

Cyclosporine: May increase rosuvastatin level and increase risk of myopathy or rhabdomyolysis. Don't exceed 5 mg daily. Monitor patient for signs and symptoms of toxicity.
Gemfibrozil: May increase rosuvastatin level and increase risk of myopathy or rhabdomyolysis. Don't exceed 10 mg daily. Monitor patient for signs and symptoms of toxicity.
Oral contraceptives: May increase plasma concentrations of ethinyl estradiol and norgestrel. Use together cautiously.
Warfarin: Doesn't change warfarin plasma concentration but may increase PT and INR. Monitor INR and look for signs of increased bleeding.
Drug-lifestyle. *Alcohol use:* May increase risk of hepatotoxicity. Avoid using together.

Effects on lab test results

● May increase CK, transaminase, glucose, glutamyl transpeptidase, alkaline phosphatase, and bilirubin levels.
● May increase thyroid function test values.
● May cause dipstick-positive proteinuria and microscopic hematuria tests.

Pharmacokinetics

Absorption: About 20%; peak level occurs within 3 to 5 hours. Rate of absorption is decreased by food, but the extent of absorption is unaffected. The drug may be given at any time of day without any change in level.
Distribution: About 88% protein-bound, mainly to albumin.
Metabolism: About 10%.
Excretion: 90% in feces. *Half-life:* About 19 hours.

Route	Onset	Peak	Duration
P.O.	Unknown	3–5 hr	Unknown

Action

Chemical effect: Inhibits HMG-CoA reductase, which is an early and rate-limiting step in the synthetic pathway of cholesterol.
Therapeutic effect: Lowers total cholesterol, LDL, ApoB, non-HDL, and triglyceride levels.

Available forms

Tablets: 5 mg, 10 mg, 20 mg, 40 mg

NURSING PROCESS

⚕ Assessment
• Assess patient's condition before starting therapy and regularly thereafter to monitor drug's effectiveness.
• Perform liver function tests before therapy and again at 12 weeks. Repeat liver function tests 12 weeks following a dosage increase and then twice a year thereafter. If CK level increases to greater than 10 times the upper limit of normal, stop drug.
• Be alert for adverse reactions and drug interactions.
• If adverse GI reactions occur, monitor hydration.
• Assess patient's and family's knowledge of drug therapy.

⊕ Nursing diagnoses
• Risk for injury related to elevated cholesterol level
• Risk for deficient fluid volume related to adverse GI reactions
• Deficient knowledge related to drug therapy

▷ Planning and implementation
• Begin drug only after diet and other nondrug therapies have proven ineffective. Give standard low-cholesterol diet during therapy.
• Withhold drug temporarily with any condition, such as sepsis, hypotension, major surgery, trauma, uncontrolled seizures, and severe metabolic, endocrine, and electrolyte disorders that may predispose patient to the development of myopathy or rhabdomyolysis.
⊕ ALERT: Asian patients are at a greater risk of elevated drug level.
Patient teaching
• Instruct patient to take drug exactly as prescribed.
• Teach patient about restricting total fat and cholesterol intake, and recommend weight control, exercise, and smoking cessation programs.
• Tell patient to immediately report any signs of unexplained muscle pain, tenderness, or weakness, especially if accompanied by malaise or fever.
• Instruct patient that antacids containing aluminum or magnesium should be taken at least 2 hours after this drug.

• Inform woman that drug is contraindicated during pregnancy. Advise her to notify prescriber immediately if she becomes pregnant.

✓ Evaluation
• Patient's LDL and total cholesterol levels are within normal range.
• Patient maintains adequate hydration.
• Patient and family state understanding of drug therapy.

✻ New Drug

HIGH ALERT
rotigotine transdermal system
(roh-TIG-oh-teen)
Neupro

Pharmacologic class: dopamine agonist
Therapeutic class: antiparkinsonian
Pregnancy risk category: C

Indications and dosages
▶ **Parkinson disease.** *Adults:* Initially, 2 mg/24 hours applied transdermally; titrate weekly by 2 mg/24 hours, based on patient response and tolerance, to a maximum of 6 mg/24 hours.

Contraindications and cautions
• Contraindicated in patients hypersensitive to rotigotine or components of the transdermal system.
• Use cautiously in patients hypersensitive to sulfite; this product contains sodium metabisulfite, a sulfite that may cause allergic-type reactions (including anaphylaxis and asthmatic episodes) in susceptible individuals.
• Use cautiously in patients with a history of somnolence, in those with sleep disorders, and in those taking sedatives; patients may fall asleep during activities of daily living, including operating motor vehicles, resulting in accidents.
• Use with caution in patients with severe CV disease.
⚘ Lifespan: In pregnant women, drug hasn't been studied. In breast-feeding women, breast-feeding may be inhibited because drug decreases prolactin secretion. It isn't known if drug is found in breast milk. In children, safety and effectiveness haven't been established. In elderly patients older than age 80, there may be in-

creased drug levels because of skin changes associated with aging.

Adverse reactions

CNS: asthenia, *dizziness,* fatigue, fever, *headache,* vertigo, *somnolence,* insomnia, hallucinations, depression, tremor, anxiety, syncope, paresthesia, confusion, ataxia, abnormal gait, neuralgia, hypoesthesia, hypertonia.
CV: edema, hypertension, chest pain, orthostatic hypotension, tachycardia.
EENT: abnormal vision.
GI: dry mouth, *nausea, vomiting,* constipation, diarrhea, anorexia, dyspepsia, abdominal pain.
GU: UTI.
Hematologic: purpura.
Metabolic: weight gain.
Musculoskeletal: back pain, arthralgia, leg pain.
Respiratory: upper respiratory infections, coughing.
Skin: *application site reactions,* sweating, pruritus.
Other: fatigue, sinusitis, rhinitis, flulike symptoms.

Interactions

Drug-drug. *Dopamine antagonists:* May reduce the effectiveness of rotigotine. Monitor patient response.
Sedatives and other CNS depressants: May increase drowsiness. Use together cautiously.
Drug-lifestyle. *Alcohol:* May increase the risk of drowsiness. Discourage use together.

Effects on lab test results

• May increase BUN and GGT levels. May decrease albumin, glucose, and hemoglobin levels.

Pharmacokinetics

Absorption: Through the skin; about 45% of drug released from the patch within 24 hours.
Distribution: About 90% protein-bound.
Metabolism: Mostly by hepatic conjugation and N-dealkylation.
Excretion: Primarily in urine (71%) as inactive metabolites, with some excretion in feces (11%); nondialyzable. *Half-life:* 5 to 7 hours.

Route	Onset	Peak	Duration
Transdermal	3 hr	Unknown	24 hr

Action

Chemical effect: Unknown; may be related to its ability to stimulate dopamine receptors in the brain.
Therapeutic effect: Decreases symptoms of Parkinson disease.

Available forms

Transdermal system: 2 mg/24 hours, 4 mg/24 hours, and 6 mg/24 hours

NURSING PROCESS

Assessment
• Obtain history of patient's condition before starting therapy and reassess regularly thereafter to monitor the drug's effectiveness.
• Be alert for signs of excessive somnolence including daytime sleepiness.
• Monitor BUN, GGT, and hemoglobin levels.
• Assess patient's and family's knowledge of drug therapy.

Nursing diagnoses
• Impaired physical mobility related to underlying parkinsonism
• Risk for injury related to drug-induced adverse reactions
• Deficient knowledge related to drug therapy

Planning and implementation
• Ask patients about sulfite sensitivity, particularly patients with asthma because they have a higher incidence of sulfite sensitivity.
• Apply patch to a clean, dry area, free from topical products.
• Provide patient with contact information for parkinsonism support groups.
• Don't cut the patch into smaller pieces.
⑨ **ALERT:** Monitor the patient for drowsiness; patient may fall asleep during activities of daily living, including operating a vehicle.
• Watch for signs and symptoms of postural hypotension, especially while increasing the dosage.
• Monitor blood pressure and heart rate.
• Monitor patient for peripheral edema and weight gain.
• Monitor the application site for redness, edema, or pruritus. Daily rotation of application sites will reduce the incidence of application site reactions.
• Regularly monitor patient for melanomas.

Reactions may be *common,* uncommon, *life-threatening,* or COMMON AND LIFE-THREATENING.

• Monitor the patient for new or worsening dyskinesia.

• Because the back layer of the patch contains aluminum, to avoid burns the patch should be removed before MRI or cardioversion.

• Neuroleptic malignant syndrome has been reported with rapid dose reduction, withdrawal of, or changes in antiparkinsonism treatment. At the end of treatment, the dosage should be tapered slowly, reducing the daily dosage by 2 mg/24 hours every other day until withdrawal is complete.

Patient Teaching

• Warn patient to remove the back layer of the patch before MRI or cardioversion. The back layer contains aluminum, which may cause burns.

• Advise the patient to store patches in the sealed storage pouch.

• Teach the patient not to cut or touch the medicated side of the patch prior to application and to wash his hands after applying the patch.

• Tell the patient to apply the patch to clean, dry, and intact skin on his abdomen, thigh, hip, flank, shoulder, or upper arm. Teach him to avoid skin folds and areas that could be rubbed with tight clothing or waistbands.

• Teach the patient to avoid applying creams, lotions, and other topical products to the area where the patch will be placed. Tell him to avoid applying heat to the patch. Instruct the patient to rotate application sites daily to reduce the risk of skin reactions.

• Tell the patient to wear the patch continuously for 24 hours; removal of one patch should be followed immediately by reapplication of a new one.

• Advise patient about possible drowsiness, including somnolence and the potential for falling asleep while engaged in activities of daily living. Warn patient not to drive a car or engage in other dangerous activities until effects of the drug are known.

• Discuss common side effects with patient (nausea and vomiting are more common during initial therapy).

• Advise the patient to avoid alcohol and to discuss with his provider the use of sedatives during therapy.

☑ **Evaluation**

• Patient reports drug's effectiveness by decreasing symptoms.

• Patient does not sustain injury from adverse side effects.

• Patient and family state understanding of drug therapy.

salmeterol xinafoate
(sal-MEE-ter-ohl zee-neh-FOH-ayt)
Serevent Diskus

Pharmacologic class: selective beta$_2$ agonist
Therapeutic class: bronchodilator
Pregnancy risk category: C

Indications and dosages

▶ **Long-term maintenance therapy for asthma; to prevent bronchospasm in patients with nocturnal asthma or reversible obstructive airway disease who need regular short-acting beta agonists.** *Adults and children older than age 4:* Give 1 inhalation (50 mcg) every 12 hours, morning and evening.

▶ **To prevent exercise-induced bronchospasm.** *Adults and children age 4 and older:* 1 inhalation (50 mcg) at least 30 minutes before exercise.

▶ **Maintenance therapy for bronchospasm with COPD (including emphysema and chronic bronchitis).** *Adults:* 1 inhalation (50 mcg) every 12 hours, morning and evening.

Contraindications and cautions

• Contraindicated in patients hypersensitive to drug or any of its components.

• Use cautiously in patients who are unusually responsive to sympathomimetics and patients with coronary insufficiency, arrhythmias, hypertension or other CV disorders, thyrotoxicosis, or seizure disorders.

⚠ **Lifespan:** In pregnant women, use cautiously. Don't use in breast-feeding women. In children younger than age 4, safety and effectiveness haven't been established.

Adverse reactions

CNS: dizziness, *headache,* nervousness, sinus headache, tremor.

CV: palpitations, tachycardia, *ventricular arrhythmias.*
EENT: nasal cavity or sinus disorder, *nasopharyngitis,* sore throat.
GI: diarrhea, heartburn, nausea, vomiting.
Musculoskeletal: joint and back pain, myalgia.
Respiratory: *bronchospasm,* cough, lower respiratory tract infection, upper respiratory tract infection, *worsening of asthma.*
Other: *anaphylaxis,* hypersensitivity reactions.

Interactions

Drug-drug. *Beta agonists, methylxanthines, theophylline:* May cause adverse cardiac effects with excessive use. Monitor patient closely.
Beta blockers: May negate the beta agonist effects of salmeterol, resulting in severe bronchospasm. Use alternative to beta blocker, if possible. If beta blocker use can't be avoided, use a cardioselective beta blocker and monitor patient closely.
MAO inhibitors, tricyclic antidepressants: May cause severe adverse CV effects. Don't use within 14 days of MAO or tricyclic therapy.

Effects on lab test results

None reported.

Pharmacokinetics

Absorption: Low or undetectable because of low therapeutic dose.
Distribution: Local to lungs. 94% to 99% protein-bound.
Metabolism: Extensive.
Excretion: Primarily in feces. *Half-life:* 5½ hours.

Route	Onset	Peak	Duration
Inhalation	10–20 min	3 hr	12 hr

Action

Chemical effect: Unclear; selectively activates beta$_2$-adrenergic receptors, which results in bronchodilation and blocks release of allergic mediators from mast cells in respiratory tract.
Therapeutic effect: Improves breathing.

Available forms

Inhalation powder: 50 mcg/blister

NURSING PROCESS

Assessment
• Assess patient's respiratory condition before starting therapy and regularly thereafter to monitor drug's effectiveness.
• Assess peak flow readings before starting therapy and periodically thereafter.
• Be alert for adverse reactions and drug interactions.
• Assess patient's and family's knowledge of drug therapy.

Nursing diagnoses
• Ineffective breathing pattern related to respiratory condition
• Acute pain related to drug-induced headache
• Deficient knowledge related to drug therapy

Planning and implementation
• Don't give drug for acute bronchospasm.
• Report insufficient relief or worsening condition.
• If headache occurs, give mild analgesic.
⚠ ALERT: A serious asthma episode or asthma-related death may occur, with black patients at greatest risk. Use only in patients not adequately controlled on inhaled corticosteroids.
⚠ ALERT: Don't confuse Serevent with Serentil.
Patient teaching
• Tell patient to take drug at about 12-hour intervals, even if he is feeling better.
• Tell patient to prevent exercise-induced bronchospasm by taking drug 30 to 60 minutes before exercise.
⚠ ALERT: Instruct patient not to use for acute bronchospasm; have them use a short-acting beta agonist (such as albuterol) instead.
• Tell patient to contact prescriber if short-acting beta agonist no longer provides sufficient relief or if taking more than 4 inhalations daily. Tell patient not to increase the dosage.
• If patient is using an inhaled corticosteroid, he should continue. Warn him not to take other drugs without prescriber's consent.
• Instruct patient not to exhale into Diskus, and to only use Diskus in a level, horizontal position.

Evaluation
• Patient exhibits normal breathing pattern.
• Patient states that drug-induced headache is relieved after analgesic administration.

• Patient and family state understanding of drug therapy.

saquinavir mesylate
(suh-KWIN-uh-veer MEH-sih-layt)
Invirase

Pharmacologic class: protease inhibitor
Therapeutic class: antiretroviral
Pregnancy risk category: B

Indications and dosages

▶ **Adjunct therapy for advanced HIV infection in selected patients.** *Adults and children older than age 16:* Give 1,000 mg P.O. b.i.d. with 100 mg ritonavir. Or 1,000 mg P.O. b.i.d. with 100 mg ritonavir and 400 mg lopinavir.

Contraindications and cautions

• Contraindicated in patients hypersensitive to the drug and its components, and in patients taking terfenadine, rifampin, astemizole, pimozide, triazolam, midazolam, ergot derivatives, or cisapride.
• Use cautiously in patients with liver impairment.
⚖ **Lifespan:** In pregnant women, breastfeeding women, and children younger than age 16, safety and effectiveness haven't been established.

Adverse reactions

CNS: asthenia, dizziness, headache, paresthesia.
CV: chest pain.
GI: abdominal pain, constipation, diarrhea, mouth ulcers, *nausea, pancreatitis.*
Hematologic: *pancytopenia, thrombocytopenia.*
Hepatic: *cirrhosis,* elevated liver enzymes, *portal hypertension.*
Metabolic: hyperglycemia, lipodystrophy, *new-onset diabetes mellitus.*
Musculoskeletal: musculoskeletal pain.
Respiratory: bronchitis, cough, influenza, pneumonia, sinusitis.
Skin: dry lips/skin, eczema, pruritus, rash.
Other: adipogenic effects.

Interactions

Drug-drug. *Amitriptyline, imipramine:* May increase levels of these drugs. Monitor drug levels and adjust dosage as needed.
Amlodipine, diltiazem, felodipine, isradipine, nicardipine, nifedipine, nimodipine, nisoldipine, verapamil: May increase levels of these drugs. Use together cautiously.
Antiarrhythmics (amiodarone, bepridil, flecainide, propafenone, quinidine): May cause serious or life-threatening reactions. Avoid using together.
Carbamazepine, phenobarbital, phenytoin: May decrease saquinavir level. Use together cautiously.
Cyclosporine, rapamycin, tacrolimus: May increase levels of these drugs. Monitor drug levels.
Delavirdine: May increase saquinavir level. Use cautiously, and monitor hepatic enzymes. Decrease dosage when used together.
Dexamethasone: May decrease saquinavir level. Use together cautiously.
Efavirenz: May decrease level of both drugs. Don't use together.
Ergot derivatives (dihydroergotamine, ergonovine, ergotamine, methylergonovine): May cause serious or life-threatening reactions such as ergot toxicity characterized by peripheral vasospasm and ischemia of the arms and legs and other tissues. Avoid using together.
Ethinyl estradiol: May decrease level of contraceptive. Recommend additional contraceptive during therapy.
HMG-CoA reductase inhibitors (atorvastatin, lovastatin, simvastatin): May increase levels of these drugs, which increases risk of myopathy, including rhabdomyolysis. Avoid using together.
Indinavir, lopinavir and ritonavir, nelfinavir, ritonavir: May increase level of saquinavir. Use together cautiously.
Lidocaine: May increase antiarrhythmic level. Use together cautiously and monitor level.
Loperamide: May increase loperamide level while decreasing saquinavir level. Avoid use together.
Macrolide antibiotics such as clarithromycin: May increase level of both drugs. Use together cautiously. Reduce antibiotic dose in patients with renal impairment.
Methadone: May decrease methadone level. Increase methadone dosage as needed.

S

Midazolam, triazolam: May cause serious or life-threatening reactions such as prolonged or increased sedation or respiratory depression. Avoid using together.

Nevirapine: May decrease saquinavir level. Monitor patient.

Phosphodiesterase type 5 inhibitors (sildenafil, tadalafil, vardenafil): May increase peak level and exposure of these drugs. Use together cautiously. Reduce dose of sildenafil to 25 mg, dose of vardenafil to 2.5 mg and dose of tadalafil to 10 mg when given with saquinavir.

Rifabutin, rifampin: May reduce the steady-state level of saquinavir. Use rifabutin and saquinavir together cautiously. Don't use with rifampin.

Warfarin: May affect warfarin level. Monitor INR.

Drug-herb. *Garlic supplements:* May decrease drug level by half. Discourage using together.

St. John's wort: May substantially reduce level of drug, causing loss of therapeutic effect. Discourage using together.

Drug-food. *Any food:* May increase drug absorption. Advise patient to take drug within 2 hours after eating a meal.

Grapefruit juice: May increase drug level. Give with another liquid.

Effects on lab test results

- May increase liver enzyme level.
- May decrease WBC, RBC, and platelet counts.

Pharmacokinetics

Absorption: Poor.
Distribution: More than 98% protein-bound.
Metabolism: Rapid.
Excretion: Mainly in feces. *Half-life:* 1 to 2 hours.

Route	Onset	Peak	Duration
P.O.	Unknown	Unknown	7 hr

Action

Chemical effect: Inhibits HIV protease and prevents cleavage of HIV polyproteins, which are essential for HIV maturation.
Therapeutic effect: Hinders HIV activity.

Available forms

Capsules (hard gelatin): 200 mg
Tablets (film-coated): 500 mg

NURSING PROCESS

⚕ Assessment
- Obtain history of patient's HIV infection.
- Monitor CBC and platelet counts and electrolyte, uric acid, liver enzyme, and bilirubin levels before and during therapy.
- Be alert for adverse reactions and drug interactions, including those caused by adjunct therapy (zidovudine or zalcitabine).
- If patient has an adverse GI reaction, monitor his hydration.
- Watch for adipogenic side effects with prolonged therapy (redistribution or accumulation of body fat, dorsocervical fat enlargement, peripheral wasting, breast enlargement, and cushingoid appearance).
- Assess patient's and family's knowledge of drug therapy.

⊕ Nursing diagnoses
- Risk for infection related to presence of HIV
- Risk for deficient fluid volume related to adverse GI reactions
- Deficient knowledge related to drug therapy

▶ Planning and implementation
⚠ **ALERT:** If severe toxicity occurs, stop drug until cause is identified or toxicity resolves. Therapy may resume with no dosage change.
- Notify prescriber of adverse reactions, and obtain an order for a mild analgesic, antiemetic, or antidiarrheal, if needed.
⚠ **ALERT:** Don't confuse saquinavir with Sinequan.
Patient teaching
- Tell patient to take drug with meals or within 2 hours after a full meal.
- Urge patient to report adverse reactions.
- Reinforce need for adequate protection of sexual partners. Drug doesn't prevent transmission of HIV.
- Inform patient that drug is usually given with other AIDS-related antiviral drugs.
⚠ **ALERT:** Advise patient taking sildenafil, tadalafil, or vardenafil about an increased risk of adverse effects, including hypotension, visual changes, and priapism, and the need to report them promptly. Tell patient not to exceed 25 mg of sildenafil in 48 hours; 10 mg of tadalafil in 72 hours; or 2.5 mg of vardenafil in 72 hours.

☑ Evaluation
- Patient responds well to therapy.
- Patient maintains adequate hydration.
- Patient and family state understanding of drug therapy.

HIGH ALERT

sargramostim (granulocyte macrophage colony-stimulating factor, GM-CSF)
(sahr-GRAH-moh-stihm)
Leukine

Pharmacologic class: biological response modifier
Therapeutic class: hematopoietic growth factor
Pregnancy risk category: C

Indications and dosages

▶ **To accelerate hematopoiesis after autologous bone marrow transplantation (BMT) in patients with malignant lymphoma, acute lymphoblastic leukemia, or chemotherapeutically treated Hodgkin lymphoma.** *Adults:* 250 mcg/m² daily as 2-hour I.V. infusion beginning 2 to 4 hours after BMT and no less than 24 hours after last dose of chemotherapy or radiation. Patient's post-BMT absolute neutrophil count (ANC) must be less than 500/mm³. Continue until ANC exceeds 1,500/mm³ for 3 consecutive days.

▶ **BMT failure or engraftment delay.** *Adults:* 250 mcg/m² as 2-hour I.V. infusion daily for 14 days. May repeat after taking 7 days off from therapy. If engraftment still hasn't occurred, a third course of 500 mcg/m² I.V. daily for 14 days may be tried after another 7 days off therapy.

▶ **Neutrophil recovery following chemotherapy in acute myelogenous leukemia.** *Adults:* 250 mcg/m² I.V. infusion over 4 hours daily. Start therapy about day 11 or 4 days after end of induction therapy.

▶ **To mobilize hematopoietic progenitor cells into peripheral blood for collection by leukapheresis; to accelerate myeloid engraftment after autologous peripheral blood progenitor cell (PBPC) transplantation.** *Adults:* 250 mcg/m² by continuous I.V. infusion over 24 hours or subcutaneously once daily. After PBPC, continue until the ANC exceeds 1,500/mm³ for 3 consecutive days.

▼ I.V. administration

- Reconstitute drug with 1 ml of sterile water for injection. Direct stream of sterile water against side of vial and gently swirl contents to minimize foaming. Avoid excessive or vigorous agitation or shaking.
- Dilute in normal saline solution. If final level is less than 10 mcg/ml, add human albumin at final level of 0.1% to saline solution before adding drug to prevent adsorption to components of delivery system. For final level of 0.1% human albumin, add 1 mg human albumin per 1 ml saline solution.
- Give as soon as possible and no later than 6 hours after reconstituting.
- Don't use an in-line membrane filter since adsorption of the drug could occur.
- Vials are for single-dose use and contain no preservatives. Discard unused portion.
- Refrigerate sterile powder, reconstituted solution, and diluted solution for injection. Don't freeze or shake.
⊗ **Incompatibilities**
Other I.V. drugs, unless specific compatibility data are available.

Contraindications and cautions

- Contraindicated in patients hypersensitive to the drug or any of its components or to yeast-derived products. Also contraindicated in patients with excessive leukemic myeloid blasts in bone marrow or peripheral blood, and within 24 hours preceding or following chemotherapy or radiotherapy.
- Use cautiously in patients with cardiac disease, hypoxia, fluid retention, pulmonary infiltrates, heart failure, or impaired kidney or liver function.
☀ **Lifespan:** In pregnant women, use cautiously. In breast-feeding women, use cautiously; it's unknown if the drug appears in breast milk. In children, safety and effectiveness haven't been established.

Adverse reactions

CNS: asthenia, CNS disorders, fever, malaise.
CV: edema, pericardial effusion, *supraventricular arrhythmia.*
EENT: mucous membrane disorder.

GI: anorexia, diarrhea, GI disorder, *hemorrhage,* nausea, stomatitis, vomiting.
GU: abnormal kidney function, *urinary tract disorder.*
Hematologic: *blood dyscrasias, hemorrhage.*
Hepatic: *liver damage.*
Respiratory: *dyspnea, lung disorders,* pleural effusion.
Skin: alopecia, rash.
Other: SEPSIS.

Interactions

Drug-drug. *Corticosteroids, lithium:* May increase myeloproliferative effects of sargramostim. Use together cautiously.

Effects on lab test results

• May increase BUN, creatinine, AST, ALT, and bilirubin levels.

Pharmacokinetics

Absorption: Given I.V.
Distribution: Bound to specific receptors on target cells.
Metabolism: Unknown.
Excretion: Unknown. *Half-life:* About 2 hours.

Route	Onset	Peak	Duration
I.V.	≤ 30 min	2 hr	6 hr
SubQ	Rapid	1–4 hr	Unknown

Action

Chemical effect: Differs from natural human GM-CSF. Induces cellular responses by binding to specific receptors on surfaces of target cells.
Therapeutic effect: Stimulates formation of granulocytes (neutrophils, eosinophils) and macrophages.

Available forms

Liquid: 500 mcg*
Powder for injection: 250 mcg

NURSING PROCESS

Assessment
• Assess patient's condition before starting therapy and regularly thereafter to monitor drug's effectiveness.
• Monitor CBC with differential biweekly, including examination for presence of blast cells.

• Be alert for adverse reactions and drug interactions.
• Monitor patient's hydration throughout drug therapy.
• Assess patient's and family's knowledge of drug therapy.

Nursing diagnoses
• Ineffective health maintenance related to underlying condition
• Risk for deficient fluid volume related to drug-induced adverse effects
• Deficient knowledge related to drug therapy

Planning and implementation
• Drug's effect may be lessened in patient who has received extensive radiotherapy to hematopoietic sites in abdomen or chest or who has been exposed to multiple drugs (alkylating, anthracycline antibiotics, antimetabolites) before autologous BMT.
• Drug is effective in accelerating myeloid recovery in patients receiving bone marrow purged from monoclonal antibodies.
• Drug can act as growth factor for tumors, particularly myeloid cancers.
• Blood counts return to normal or baseline level within 3 to 7 days after stopping therapy.
• If severe adverse reaction occurs, notify prescriber. Dosage may need to be reduced by half or stopped temporarily. Resume therapy when reaction decreases. Transient rashes and local reactions at injection site may occur; serious allergic or anaphylactic reaction isn't common.
• Stimulation of marrow precursors may result in rapid rise of WBC count. If blast cells appear or increase to 10% or more of WBC count or if underlying disease progresses, stop drug. If ANC is more than 20,000/mm^3 or if platelet count is more than 50,000/mm^3, temporarily stop drug or reduce dosage by half.
ALERT: Don't confuse Leukine with Leukeran.
Patient teaching
• Inform patient and family about need for therapy and frequent blood tests.
• Advise patient to report adverse reactions immediately.

Evaluation
• Patient exhibits positive response to drug therapy.
• Patient maintains adequate hydration throughout therapy.

Reactions may be *common,* uncommon, *life-threatening,* or COMMON AND LIFE-THREATENING.

• Patient and family state understanding of drug therapy.

scopolamine (hyoscine)
(skoh-POL-uh-meen)
Transderm-Scōp, Transderm-V ◆

scopolamine hydrobromide (hyoscine hydrobromide)
Scopace

scopolamine N-butylbromide (hyoscine N-butylbromide)
Buscopan ◆

Pharmacologic class: anticholinergic
Therapeutic class: antiemetic, antivertigo drug, adjunct to anesthesia
Pregnancy risk category: C

Indications and dosages

▶ **Spastic states.** *Adults:* 0.4 to 0.8 mg Scopace P.O. daily. Or, 0.32 to 0.65 mg scopolamine hydrobromide subcutaneously, I.M. or I.V. t.i.d. or q.i.d.

▶ **To reduce secretions preoperatively.**
Adults: 0.2 to 0.6 mg scopolamine hydrobromide I.M. 30 to 60 minutes before induction of anesthesia.
Children ages 8 to 12: Give 0.3 mg scopolamine hydrobromide I.M. 45 minutes before induction of anesthesia.
Children ages 3 to 8: Give 0.2 mg scopolamine hydrobromide I.M. 45 minutes before induction of anesthesia.
Children ages 7 months to 3 years: 0.15 mg scopolamine hydrobromide I.M. 45 minutes before induction of anesthesia.
Infants ages 4 to 7 months: 0.1 mcg scopolamine hydrobromide I.M. 45 minutes before induction of anesthesia.

▶ **To prevent nausea and vomiting from motion sickness.** *Adults:* 1 Transderm-Scōp patch (a circular flat unit), which delivers 1 mg over 3 days (72 hours). Apply to skin behind ear at least 4 hours before antiemetic is needed. Or 0.3 to 0.6 mg scopolamine hydrobromide subcutaneously, I.M., or I.V. Or 0.25 to 0.8 mg P.O 1 hour before exposure to motion; subsequent

doses of 0.25 to 0.8 mg may be given t.i.d. if needed.
Children: 0.006 mg/kg or 0.2 mg/m^2 scopolamine hydrobromide subcutaneously, I.M., or I.V.

▼ I.V. administration

• Intermittent and continuous infusions aren't recommended.
• For direct injection, dilute with sterile water and inject through patent I.V. line.
• Protect I.V. solutions from freezing and light; store at room temperature.
⊗ **Incompatibilities**
Alkalies, anticholinergics, methohexital.

Contraindications and cautions

• Contraindicated in patients with angle-closure glaucoma, obstructive uropathy, obstructive disease of GI tract, asthma, chronic pulmonary disease, myasthenia gravis, paralytic ileus, intestinal atony, unstable CV status in acute hemorrhage, or toxic megacolon.
• Transderm-Scōp is contraindicated in patients allergic to scopolamine and other belladonna alkaloids.
• Use cautiously in patients with autonomic neuropathy, hyperthyroidism, coronary artery disease, arrhythmias, heart failure, hypertension, hiatal hernia with reflux esophagitis, hepatic or renal disease, or ulcerative colitis. Also use cautiously in patients in hot or humid environments because of drug-induced heatstroke.
• Use Transderm-Scōp cautiously in patients with liver or renal impairment, pyloric obstruction, or urinary bladder and neck obstruction.
☀ **Lifespan:** In pregnant women and children younger than age 6, use cautiously. In breast-feeding women, don't use. In children, Transderm-Scōp is contraindicated. In the elderly, use Transderm-Scōp cautiously.

Adverse reactions

CNS: confusion, delirium, disorientation, drowsiness, dizziness, fever, hallucinations, headache, irritability, restlessness.
CV: flushing, palpitations, *paradoxical bradycardia,* tachycardia.
EENT: blurred vision, difficulty swallowing, dilated pupils, increased intraocular pressure, photophobia.
GI: constipation, dry mouth, epigastric distress, nausea, vomiting.

S

GU: urinary hesitancy, urine retention.
Respiratory: bronchial plugging, *depressed respirations.*
Skin: contact dermatitis, dryness, rash with transdermal patch.

Interactions

Drug-drug. *Centrally acting anticholinergics (antihistamines, phenothiazines, tricyclic antidepressants):* May increase risk of adverse CNS reactions. Monitor patient closely.
CNS depressants: May increase risk of CNS depression. Monitor patient closely.
Drug-herb. *Jaborandi tree:* May decrease effects of drug. Discourage using together.
Pill-bearing spurge: May decrease effects of drug. Discourage using together.
Squaw vine: May decrease metabolic breakdown of drug. Discourage using together.
Drug-lifestyle. *Alcohol use:* May increase risk of CNS depression. Discourage using together.

Effects on lab test results

None reported.

Pharmacokinetics

Absorption: Good with P.O. and transdermal use. Rapid with I.M. or subcutaneous use.
Distribution: Wide. Probably crosses blood-brain barrier.
Metabolism: Extensively metabolized by the liver.
Excretion: May be in urine as metabolites.
Half-life: 8 hours.

Route	Onset	Peak	Duration
P.O.	30–60 min	1 hr	4–6 hr
I.V., I.M., SubQ	30 min	Unknown	4 hr
Transdermal	3–6 hr	24 hr	72 hr

Action

Chemical effect: Inhibits muscarinic actions of acetylcholine. It also may affect neural pathways originating in the labyrinth (inner ear) to inhibit nausea and vomiting.
Therapeutic effect: Relieves spasticity, nausea, and vomiting; reduces secretions; and blocks cardiac vagal reflexes.

Available forms

scopolamine
Transdermal patch: 1.5 mg

scopolamine hydrobromide
Injection: 0.3, 0.4, 0.5, 0.86, and 1 mg/ml in 1-ml vials and ampules; 0.4 mg/ml and 0.86 mg/ml in 0.5-ml ampules
Tablets (soluble): 0.4 mg
scopolamine N-butylbromide ◆
Injection: 20 mg/ml
Tablets: 10 mg

NURSING PROCESS

Assessment
- Assess patient's condition before starting therapy and regularly thereafter to monitor drug's effectiveness.
- Be alert for adverse reactions and drug interactions.
- Assess patient's and family's knowledge of drug therapy.

Nursing diagnoses
- Risk for deficient fluid volume related to nausea and vomiting
- Risk for injury related to drug-induced adverse CNS reactions
- Deficient knowledge related to drug therapy

Planning and implementation
- In therapeutic doses, drug may produce amnesia, drowsiness, and euphoria; patient may need to be reoriented.
- Raise side rails of bed as a precaution because some patients become temporarily excited or disoriented. Symptoms disappear when sedative effect is complete.
- Tolerance may develop when given for a long time.
- Apply patch the night before patient's expected travel.
- **ALERT:** Overdose may cause curarelike effects such as respiratory paralysis.
Patient teaching
- Advise patient to apply patch the night before planned trip. Transdermal form releases controlled amount of drug. Transderm-Scōp is effective when applied 2 or 3 hours before travel but is more effective when applied 12 hours before.
- Advise patient to wash and dry hands thoroughly before applying transdermal patch. After removing patch, he should discard it and wash hands and application site thoroughly, especial-

---

Reactions may be *common*, uncommon, *life-threatening*, or COMMON AND LIFE-THREATENING.

ly before touching eyes. Otherwise, pupils may dilate.
- Inform patient that discarded patch should be folded in half with sticky sides together and disposed out of reach of children and pets.
- Tell patient that if patch becomes displaced, he should remove it and replace it with another patch on fresh site.
- Advise patient not to cut the patch, because this will lead to increased absorption and possible toxicity.
- Alert patient to risk of withdrawal symptoms (nausea, vomiting, headache, dizziness) if transdermal patch is used longer than 72 hours.
- Tell patient to ask pharmacist for the brochure that comes with transdermal patch.
- Advise patient to refrain from activities that require alertness until drug's CNS effects are known.
- Instruct patient to report signs of urinary hesitancy or urine retention.
- Recommend use of sugarless gum or hard candy to help minimize dry mouth.

✓ Evaluation
- Patient responds well to therapy.
- Patient doesn't experience injury from adverse CNS reactions.
- Patient and family state understanding of drug therapy.

HIGH ALERT

secobarbital sodium
(sek-oh-BAR-bih-tohl SOH-dee-um)
Seconal Sodium

Pharmacologic class: barbiturate
Therapeutic class: anticonvulsant, sedative-hypnotic
Pregnancy risk category: D
Controlled substance schedule: II

Indications and dosages
▶ **Preoperative sedation.** *Adults:* 200 to 300 mg P.O. 1 to 2 hours before surgery. *Children:* 2 to 6 mg/kg P.O. 1 to 2 hours before surgery. Maximum single dose, 100 mg.
▶ **Insomnia.** *Adults:* 100 mg P.O. at bedtime.

Contraindications and cautions
- Contraindicated in patients hypersensitive to barbiturates and in patients with marked liver

impairment, porphyria, or respiratory disease in which dyspnea or obstruction is evident.
- Use cautiously in patients with acute or chronic pain, depression, suicidal tendencies, history of drug abuse, or hepatic impairment.
☀ **Lifespan:** In pregnant or breast-feeding women, drug isn't recommended.

Adverse reactions
CNS: complex sleep disorders, *drowsiness, hangover, lethargy,* paradoxical excitement in geriatric patients, somnolence.
GI: constipation, nausea, vomiting.
Hematologic: exacerbation of porphyria.
Respiratory: *respiratory depression.*
Skin: rash, *Stevens-Johnson syndrome,* urticaria.
Other: *anaphylaxis, angioedema,* physical or psychological dependence.

Interactions
Drug-drug. *Chloramphenicol, MAO inhibitors, valproic acid:* May inhibit barbiturate metabolism; may cause prolonged CNS depression. Reduce barbiturate dosage.
CNS depressants, including opioid analgesics: May cause excessive CNS and respiratory depression. Use together cautiously.
Corticosteroids, doxycycline, estrogens, hormonal contraceptives, oral anticoagulants, theophylline, tricyclic antidepressants, verapamil: May enhance metabolism of these drugs. Monitor patient for decreased effect.
Griseofulvin: May decrease absorption of griseofulvin. Monitor patient for decreased griseofulvin effectiveness.
Metoprolol, propranolol: May reduce the effects of these drugs. Consider an increased beta blocker dose.
Rifampin: May decrease barbiturate level. Monitor patient for decreased effect.
Warfarin: May decrease the anticoagulant effects of warfarin. Monitor INR and adjust warfarin dosage as needed.
Drug-lifestyle. *Alcohol use:* May impair coordination, increase CNS effects, and cause death. Strongly discourage alcohol use with this drug.

Effects on lab test results
- May increase AST and ALT levels.

Pharmacokinetics
Absorption: Rapid and almost complete.

S

Distribution: Rapid. About 30% to 45% protein-bound.
Metabolism: Oxidized in liver to inactive metabolites.
Excretion: In urine. *Half-life:* About 30 hours.

Route	Onset	Peak	Duration
P.O.	15 min	5–30 min	1–4 hr

Action

Chemical effect: Probably interferes with transmission of impulses from thalamus to cortex of brain.
Therapeutic effect: Promotes pain relief and calmness and relieves acute seizures.

Available forms

Capsules: 100 mg

NURSING PROCESS

Assessment
• Assess patient's condition before starting therapy and regularly thereafter to monitor drug's effectiveness.
• Assess mental status before therapy. An elderly patient is more sensitive to the drug's CNS effects.
• Be alert for adverse reactions and drug interactions.
• Assess patient's and family's knowledge of drug therapy.

Nursing diagnoses
• Sleep deprivation related to underlying condition
• Risk for injury related to drug-induced adverse CNS reactions
• Deficient knowledge related to drug therapy

Planning and implementation
• Make sure a patient who is depressed, suicidal, or drug-dependent or who has a history of drug abuse isn't hoarding drug or planning an intentional overdose.
• Skin eruptions may precede a fatal reaction. If skin reactions occur, stop giving the drug and notify the prescriber. In some patients, high fever, stomatitis, headache, or rhinitis may precede skin reactions.
• Long-term use isn't recommended because drug loses effectiveness after 14 days of use.
• **ALERT:** Don't confuse Seconal with Sectral.

Patient teaching
• Warn patient about possible complex sleep-related behaviors.
• Warn patient to avoid activities that require mental alertness or physical coordination. For inpatient, supervise walking and raise bed rails, particularly for an elderly patient.
• Inform patient that morning hangover is common after hypnotic dose, which suppresses REM sleep. Patient may experience increased dreaming after drug is stopped.
• Advise woman who uses a hormonal contraceptive to use a barrier method because drug may enhance the metabolism of a hormonal contraceptive and decrease its effect.

Evaluation
• Patient states that drug effectively induces sleep.
• Patient doesn't experience injury from adverse CNS reactions.
• Patient and family state understanding of drug therapy.

selegiline
(seh-LEJ-eh-leen)
Emsam

selegiline hydrochloride
(L-deprenyl hydrochloride)
Eldepryl, Emsam, Zelapar

Pharmacologic class: MAO inhibitor
Therapeutic class: antidepressant, antiparkinsonian
Pregnancy risk category: C

Indications and dosages

▶ **Adjunctive treatment with levodopa and carbidopa in managing signs and symptoms of Parkinson disease.** *Adults:* 10 mg P.O. daily divided as 5 mg at breakfast and 5 mg at lunch. After 2 or 3 days, levodopa and carbidopa dosage may need gradual decrease. If using Zelapar, begin with 1.25 mg P.O. once daily before breakfast, without liquid. After 6 weeks, increase to 2.5 mg once daily if needed and tolerated. Don't allow patient to eat or drink for 5 minutes after taking the drug.

Reactions may be *common*, uncommon, *life-threatening*, or COMMON AND LIFE-THREATENING.

▶ **Major depressive disorder.** *Adults:* Apply one patch daily to dry, intact skin on the upper torso, upper thigh, or upper arm. Initially, give 6 mg/24 hours. Increase as needed in increments of 3 mg/24 hours at intervals of 2 or more weeks. Maximum dosage, 12 mg/24 hours. *Elderly patients:* 6 mg/24 hours.

Contraindications and cautions

• Contraindicated in patients hypersensitive to drug, in patients with pheochromocytoma, and in those taking bupropion, carbamazepine, cyclobenzaprine, dextromethorphan, duloxetine, methadone, meperidine, mirtazapine, MAO inhibitors, oxcarbazepine, propoxyphene, SSRIs, sympathomimetics, tramadol, tricyclic antidepressants, venlafaxine. Don't use oral drug with the transdermal system.

⚕ **Lifespan:** In pregnant women, use cautiously. In breast-feeding women, safety and effectiveness haven't been established. In children, drug isn't approved for use.

Adverse reactions

Transdermal form
CNS: headache, insomnia.
CV: chest pain, low blood pressure, orthostatic blood pressure.
GI: diarrhea, dry mouth, dyspepsia.
Metabolic: weight gain, weight loss.
Skin: application site reaction, rash.
Oral form
CNS: behavioral changes, chorea, confusion, *dizziness,* dyskinesia, facial grimacing, fatigue, hallucinations, headache, increased apraxia, increased bradykinesia, increased tremors, involuntary movements, loss of balance, malaise, restlessness, stiff neck, syncope, twitching, vivid dreams.
CV: angina, *arrhythmias,* hypertension, hypotension, orthostatic hypotension, palpitations, peripheral edema, tachycardia.
EENT: blepharospasm.
GI: abdominal pain, anorexia or poor appetite, constipation, diarrhea, dry mouth, dysphagia, heartburn, *nausea,* vomiting.
GU: prostatic hyperplasia, sexual dysfunction, slow urination, transient nocturia, urinary frequency, urinary hesitancy, urine retention.
Metabolic: weight loss.
Skin: *application site reactions,* diaphoresis, hair loss, rash.

Interactions

Drug-drug. *Adrenergics:* May increase pressor response, particularly in patients who have taken overdose of selegiline. Use together cautiously.
Bupropion; cold products and weight loss preparations containing vasoconstrictors; cyclobenzaprine; dextromethorphan; MAO inhibitors; meperidine; methadone; mirtazapine; propoxyphene; sympathomimetic amines including amphetamines; tramadol; tricyclic antidepressants: May cause hypertensive crisis. Separate use by at least 2 weeks.
Carbamazepine, oxcarbazepine: May increase selegiline level. Use together is contraindicated.
Citalopram, duloxetine, fluoxetine, fluvoxamine, nefazodone, paroxetine, sertraline, venlafaxine: May cause serotonin syndrome involving CNS irritability, shivering, and altered consciousness. Don't give together. Wait at least 2 weeks after stopping an MAO inhibitor before giving any SSRI.
Meperidine: May cause stupor, muscle rigidity, severe agitation, and elevated temperature. Avoid using together.
Drug-herb. *Cacao tree:* May have vasopressor effects. Discourage using together.
Ginseng: May increase risk of adverse reactions, including headache, tremor, and mania. Discourage using together.
St. John's wort: May cause increased serotonergic effects. Warn patient against use together.
Drug-food. *Foods high in tyramine:* May cause hypertensive crisis. Monitor patient's blood pressure; instruct patient to avoid these foods.

Effects on lab test results

• May cause false-positive result for amphetamine on urine drug screen.

Pharmacokinetics

Absorption: Rapid.
Distribution: Unknown.
Metabolism: Three metabolites include N-desmethyldeprenyl, L-amphetamine, and L-methamphetamine.
Excretion: 45% in urine as metabolite. *Half-life:* selegiline, 2 to 10 hours; N-desmethyldeprenyl, 2 hours; L-amphetamine, 17¾ hours; L-methamphetamine, 20½ hours.

Route	Onset	Peak	Duration
P.O.	Unknown	30 min–2 hr	Unknown
Transdermal	Unknown	Unknown	24 hr

S

Action

Chemical effect: May act by selectively inhibiting MAO type B (found mostly in brain). Also may directly increase dopaminergic activity by decreasing reuptake of dopamine into nerve cells. Amphetamine and methamphetamine (active metabolites) may contribute to this effect.
Therapeutic effect: Improves physical mobility and elevates mood.

Available forms

Capsules: 5 mg
Tablets: 5 mg
Tablets (orally-disintegrating): 1.25 mg
Transdermal system: 6 mg/24 hours, 9 mg/24 hours, 12 mg/24 hours

NURSING PROCESS

⚗ Assessment

• Assess patient's condition before starting therapy and regularly thereafter to monitor drug's effectiveness.
• Monitor patients with major depressive disorder for worsening of symptoms and for suicidal behavior, especially during the first few weeks of treatment and whenever dosage changes.
• Be alert for adverse reactions and drug interactions.
• Assess patient's and family's knowledge of drug therapy.

🔄 Nursing diagnoses

• Impaired physical mobility related to underlying condition
• Risk for injury related to depression or drug-induced adverse CNS reactions
• Deficient knowledge related to drug therapy

➤ Planning and implementation

• Some patients experience increased adverse reactions to levodopa and need a 10% to 30% reduction of levodopa and carbidopa dosage.
⑤ ALERT: Drug may increase the risk of suicidal thinking in children and adolescents. May increase the risk for suicidal thinking and behavior in young adults ages 18 to 24 during the first 2 months of treatment; monitor patient carefully. Drug isn't approved for use in children.
⑤ ALERT: Don't confuse selegiline with Stelazine or Eldepryl with enalapril or Elavil.

Patient teaching

• Advise patient not to take more than 10 mg daily because greater amount of drug won't improve effectiveness and may increase adverse reactions.
• Tell the patient to take Zelapar capsules and tablets with food.
• Tell the patient Zelapar disintegrating tablets should be taken in the morning before breakfast and without liquid. Tell patient the tablet will disintegrate on top of the tongue within seconds and to avoid eating or drinking for 5 minutes after taking the tablet.
• Warn patient to move cautiously or change positions slowly at start of therapy because he may become dizzy or lightheaded.
• Caution patient to avoid driving and other hazardous activities that require mental alertness until the drug's effects are known.
• Advise patient not to overindulge in tyramine-rich foods or beverages. If using a 9-mg/24-hour or higher transdermal system, urge him to avoid these products altogether.
⑤ ALERT: Warn patient about the many drugs including OTC drugs that may interact with this drug and about the need to consult a pharmacist or his prescriber before using them.
• Teach patient and family the signs and symptoms of hypertensive crisis including severe headache, sore or stiff neck, nausea, vomiting, sweating, rapid heart beat, dilated pupils, and photophobia.
⑤ ALERT: Advise family members to watch patient for anxiety, agitation, insomnia, irritability, hostility, and aggressiveness and to report these immediately to prescriber.
• Tell patient not to cut the transdermal system into smaller pieces.
• When disposing of used patch, tell patient to fold sticky sides together and dispose out of reach of children and pets.
• Advise patient to wash hands thoroughly after touching patch.
• Tell patient to avoid exposing transdermal system to direct external heat sources such as heating pads, electric blankets, hot tubs, heated waterbeds, and prolonged sunlight.
• Tell patient to stop using the transdermal system 10 days before having surgery requiring general anesthesia.
• Advise woman planning pregnancy or breast-feeding to first contact her prescriber.

☑ Evaluation

• Patient exhibits improved physical mobility.
• Patient doesn't experience depression or injury from adverse CNS reactions.
• Patient and family state understanding of drug therapy.

---

sertraline hydrochloride
(SER-truh-leen high-droh-KLOR-ighd)
Zoloft✍

Pharmacologic class: SSRI
Therapeutic class: antidepressant
Pregnancy risk category: C

Indications and dosages

▶ **Depression.** *Adults:* 50 mg P.O. daily. Adjust dosage as tolerated and needed, at intervals of no less than 1 week. Maximum dosage, 200 mg daily.
▶ **Post-traumatic stress disorder, social anxiety disorder, obsessive compulsive disorder, panic disorder.** *Adults:* Initially, 25 mg P.O. once daily. Increase dosage to 50 mg P.O. once daily after 1 week of therapy. Dosage may be increased at weekly intervals to a maximum of 200 mg daily. Maintain patient on lowest effective dosage.
Children ages 13 to 17: Give 50 mg once daily.
Children ages 6 to 12: Give 25 mg once daily.
▶ **Premenstrual dysphoric disorder.** *Women:* Initially, 50 mg daily P.O. continuously, or limited to the luteal phase of the menstrual cycle. Patients not responding may benefit from dose increases at 50-mg increments per menstrual cycle up to 150 mg daily when taken daily throughout the menstrual cycle, or 100 mg daily when taken during the luteal phase of the menstrual cycle. If a 100-mg daily dose has been established with luteal-phase regimen, a 50-mg daily adjustment step for 3 days should be used at the beginning of each luteal phase.
▶ **Premature ejaculation‡.** *Adults:* 25 to 50 mg P.O. daily or p.r.n.
⧄ **Adjust-a-dose:** Give lower or less frequent doses with hepatic impairment.

Contraindications and cautions

• Contraindicated in patients hypersensitive to the drug or any of its components, and in patients receiving pimozide.
• Contraindicated with use of MAO inhibitors.
• Use cautiously in patients at risk for suicide and in those with seizure disorder, major affective disorder, or diseases or conditions that affect metabolism or hemodynamic responses.
• Drug should not be discontinued abruptly.
⚘ **Lifespan:** In pregnant women, use cautiously. In breast-feeding women, use cautiously; it's unknown if the drug appears in breast milk. In children younger than age 18, drug isn't approved for use in treatment of major depressive disorder due to possible increased risk of suicidal behavior.

Adverse reactions

CNS: anxiety, confusion, *dizziness, fatigue, headache,* hyperesthesia, hypertonia, hypesthesia, *insomnia,* nervousness, paresthesia, *somnolence, tremor,* twitching.
CV: chest pain, flushing, hot flushes, palpitations.
GI: abdominal pain, anorexia, constipation, *diarrhea, dry mouth, dyspepsia,* flatulence, increased appetite, *loose stools, nausea,* thirst, vomiting.
GU: decreased libido, male sexual dysfunction.
Musculoskeletal: myalgia.
Skin: *diaphoresis,* pruritus, rash.

Interactions

Drug-drug. *Benzodiazepines (except lorazepam and oxazepam), phenytoin, tolbutamide:* May decrease clearance of these drugs. Monitor patient for increased drug effects.
Cimetidine: May decrease sertraline clearance. Monitor patient for toxicity.
Clozapine: May increase clozapine level. Monitor and adjust clozapine dosage as needed.
Disulfiram: May cause a disulfiram reaction because oral concentrate contains alcohol. Avoid using together.
MAO inhibitors: May cause serotonin syndrome, including rapid fluctuation in vital signs, CNS irritability, shivering, and altered consciousness. Don't give together. Wait at least 2 weeks after stopping an MAO inhibitor before giving any SSRI.
Pimozide: May increase pimozide level and cause bradycardia. Avoid using together.

S

SNRIs, triptans: May cause serotonin syndrome (weakness, hyperreflexia, incoordination). Monitor patient closely.

Tricyclic antidepressants (TCAs): May inhibit TCA metabolism. Reduce TCA dosage. Monitor patient closely.

Warfarin, other highly protein-bound drugs: May increase level of warfarin or other highly bound drug. Monitor patient, PT, and INR closely.

Drug-herb. *St. John's wort:* May cause additive effects and serotonin syndrome, including CNS irritability, shivering, and altered consciousness. Discourage use together.

Drug-lifestyle. *Alcohol use:* May enhance CNS effects. Advise patient to avoid alcohol use.

Effects on lab test results

• May increase ALT, AST, cholesterol, and triglyceride levels. May decrease uric acid level.

Pharmacokinetics

Absorption: Well absorbed from GI tract. Rate and extent enhanced when taken with food.
Distribution: More than 98% protein-bound.
Metabolism: Probably hepatic.
Excretion: Mainly as metabolites in urine and feces. *Half-life:* 26 hours.

Route	Onset	Peak	Duration
P.O.	2–4 wk	4½–8½ hr	Unknown

Action

Chemical effect: Unknown; may be linked to inhibited neuronal uptake of serotonin in CNS.
Therapeutic effect: Relieves depression.

Available forms

Oral concentrate: 20 mg/ml
Tablets: 25 mg, 50 mg, 100 mg

NURSING PROCESS

Assessment

• Assess patient's condition before starting therapy and regularly thereafter to monitor drug's effectiveness.
• Assess patient for risk factors for suicide.
• Be alert for adverse reactions and drug interactions.
• Assess patient's and family's knowledge of drug therapy.

Nursing diagnoses

• Disturbed thought processes related to presence of depression
• Risk for injury related to drug-induced adverse CNS reactions
• Deficient knowledge related to drug therapy

Planning and implementation

• Give drug once daily, either morning or evening. Drug may be given with or without food.
• Don't give within 14 days of MAO inhibitor therapy.

ALERT: Drug may increase the risk of suicidal thinking in children and adolescents. May increase the risk for suicidal thinking and behavior in young adults ages 18 to 24 during the first 2 months of treatment; monitor patient carefully.

• In a patient with a latex allergy, don't use the rubber oral concentrate dropper.
• Don't discontinue drug abruptly. Taper gradually over several weeks, and monitor the patient carefully for SSRI discontinuation syndrome.

ALERT: Don't confuse sertraline with selegiline or Serentil. Don't confuse Zoloft with Zocor.

Patient teaching
• Advise patient to use caution when performing hazardous tasks that require alertness and not to drink alcohol or take other drugs that affect CNS while taking this drug.
• Instruct patient to check with prescriber or pharmacist before taking OTC drugs.
• Advise patient to mix the oral concentrate with 4 oz of water, ginger ale, or lemon-lime soda only, and to take the dose right away.
• Instruct patient that sudden discontinuation will cause unpleasant side effects.

Evaluation

• Patient behavior and communication indicate improved thought processes.
• Patient doesn't experience injury from adverse CNS reactions.
• Patient and family state understanding of drug therapy.

sevelamer carbonate

(seh-VEL-ah-mer KAR-buh-nayt)
Renvela

sevelamer hydrochloride

Renagel

Pharmacologic class: polymeric phosphate binder
Therapeutic class: antihyperphosphatemic
Pregnancy risk category: C

Indications and dosages

▶ **To reduce phosphorus level in patients with end-stage renal disease who are undergoing hemodialysis.** *Adults:* Depends on severity of hyperphosphatemia. Gradually adjust dosage based on phosphorus level, with goal of lowering phosphorus to 6 mg/dl or less. If phosphorus level is 9 mg/dl or more, start with 1.6 g P.O. t.i.d. with meals; if phosphorus level is between 7.5 and 9 mg/dl, 1.2 g Renagel P.O. t.i.d. or 1.6 g Renvela P.O. t.i.d. with meals; if phosphorus level is between 5.5 and 7.5 mg/dl, 800 mg P.O. t.i.d. with meals.

Dosage may be increased or decreased by one tablet per meal at 2-week intervals according to the patient's serum phosphorus level. If serum phosphorous level is greater than 6 mg/dl, increase by 1 tablet per meal. If serum phosphorous level is less than 3.5 mg/dl, decrease by 1 tablet per meal.

Contraindications and cautions

• Contraindicated in patients hypersensitive to the drug or any of its components, and in those with hypophosphatemia or bowel obstruction.
• Use cautiously in patients with dysphagia, swallowing disorders, severe GI motility disorders, or major GI tract surgery.
• Safety and efficacy haven't been studied in patients on dialysis.
⚠ **Lifespan:** Use in pregnancy only if benefits clearly outweigh potential risks to the fetus. In breast-feeding women, use cautiously; it's unknown if the drug appears in breast milk. In children, safety and effectiveness haven't been established.

Adverse reactions

CNS: headache, pain.
CV: hypertension, hypotension, *thrombosis.*
GI: constipation, *diarrhea, dyspepsia,* flatulence, *nausea, vomiting.*
Respiratory: cough.
Skin: *pruritus.*
Other: infection.

Interactions

Drug-drug. *Antiarrhythmics, anticonvulsants:* May interact. Give drug at least 1 hour before or 3 hours after giving these drugs and monitor levels of these drugs.
Ciprofloxacin: May reduce the bioavailability of ciprofloxacin. Give 1 hour before or 3 hours after sevelamer.

Effects on lab test results

• May increase alkaline phosphatase level.

Pharmacokinetics

Absorption: Unknown.
Distribution: Binds bile acids in the intestines forming a nonabsorbable complex with phosphorus.
Metabolism: None.
Excretion: In feces. *Half-life:* Unknown.

Route	Onset	Peak	Duration
P.O.	Unknown	Unknown	Unknown

Action

Chemical effect: Inhibits intestinal phosphate absorption.
Therapeutic effect: Decreases phosphorus level.

Available forms

Sevelamer carbonate
Tablets: 800 mg
Sevelamer hydrochloride
Tablets: 400 mg, 800 mg

NURSING PROCESS

Assessment

• Obtain history of patient's underlying condition before starting therapy, and reassess regularly thereafter to monitor the drug's effectiveness.

S

- Monitor calcium, bicarbonate, and chloride levels.
- Watch for symptoms of thrombosis (numbness or tingling of limbs, chest pain, shortness of breath), and notify prescriber if they occur.
- Assess patient's and family's knowledge of drug therapy.

⊕ Nursing diagnoses
- Ineffective tissue perfusion (cardiopulmonary or peripheral) related to potential drug-induced thrombosis
- Imbalanced nutrition: less than body requirements related to drug-induced adverse GI effects
- Deficient knowledge related to drug therapy

⊳ Planning and implementation
- Don't crush or break capsules or tablets, and give only with meals.
- Drug may bind to other drugs given at the same time and decrease their bioavailability. Give other drugs 1 hour before or 3 hours after sevelamer.
- **⚠ ALERT:** Drug may reduce vitamins D, E, and K and folic acid. Give a multivitamin supplement.
Patient teaching
- Instruct patient to take with meals and adhere to prescribed diet.
- Inform patient that drug must be taken whole because contents expand in water; tell him not to open or chew capsules.
- Tell patient to take other drugs as directed, but they must be taken either 1 hour before or 3 hours after sevelamer.
- Inform patient about common adverse reactions and instruct him to report them immediately. Teach patient signs and symptoms of thrombosis (numbness, tingling limbs, chest pain, changes in level of consciousness).

☑ Evaluation
- Patient doesn't develop a thrombus.
- Patient maintains adequate nutrition.
- Patient and family state understanding of drug therapy.

sibutramine hydrochloride monohydrate
(sigh-BYOO-truh-meen high-droh-KLOR-ighd mah-noh-HIGH-drayt)
Meridia

Pharmacologic class: dopamine, norepinephrine, and serotonin reuptake inhibitor
Therapeutic class: anorexic
Pregnancy risk category: C
Controlled substance schedule: IV

Indications and dosages
▶ **To manage obesity.** *Adults:* 10 mg P.O. once daily with or without food. If weight loss isn't adequate after 4 weeks, increase dosage to 15 mg P.O. daily. Patients who don't tolerate the 10-mg dose may receive 5 mg P.O. daily. Doses above 15 mg daily aren't recommended.

Contraindications and cautions
- Contraindicated in patients hypersensitive to the drug or any of its components, those taking MAO inhibitors or other centrally acting appetite suppressants, and those with anorexia nervosa. Don't use drug in patients with severe renal or hepatic dysfunction, history of hypertension, seizures, coronary artery disease, heart failure, arrhythmias, or stroke.
- Use cautiously in patients with angle-closure glaucoma, and in patients predisposed to bleeding events or taking drugs that affect hemostasis or platelet function.
- Use not recommended for longer than 2 years.
- **⚘ Lifespan:** In pregnant and breast-feeding women, use isn't recommended. Women of childbearing age should use adequate contraception and notify prescriber promptly if they become pregnant. In children younger than age 16, safety and effectiveness haven't been established.

Adverse reactions
CNS: anxiety, asthenia, CNS stimulation, decrease or loss of hearing, depression, dizziness, emotional lability, *headache, insomnia,* migraine, nervousness, paresthesia, somnolence, tinnitus.
CV: chest pain, generalized edema, hypertension, palpitations, tachycardia, vasodilation.

EENT: ear disorder, ear pain, laryngitis, *pharyngitis,* sinusitis, thirst, *rhinitis.*
GI: abdominal pain, *anorexia, constipation, dry mouth,* dyspepsia, gastritis, increased appetite, nausea, rectal disorder, taste perversion, vomiting.
GU: dysmenorrhea, metrorrhagia, UTI, vaginal candidiasis.
Musculoskeletal: arthralgia, joint disorder, myalgia, neck or back pain, tenosynovitis.
Respiratory: cough.
Skin: acne, rash, sweating.
Other: accident, allergic reaction, flulike syndrome, herpes simplex, injury.

Interactions

Drug-drug. *Cimetidine, erythromycin, ketoconazole:* May result in small increases in sibutramine metabolites. Use cautiously together.
CNS depressants: May enhance CNS depression. Use cautiously.
Dextromethorphan, dihydroergotamine, fentanyl, fluoxetine, fluvoxamine, lithium, MAO inhibitors, meperidine, paroxetine, pentazocine, sertraline, sumatriptan, tryptophan, venlafaxine: May cause hyperthermia, tachycardia, and loss of consciousness. Don't use together.
Ephedrine, pseudoephedrine: May increase blood pressure or heart rate. Use cautiously.
Drug-lifestyle. *Alcohol use:* May enhance CNS depression. Discourage using together.

Effects on lab test results

• May increase ALT, AST, GGT, LDH, alkaline phosphatase, and bilirubin levels.

Pharmacokinetics

Absorption: Rapid. About 77% of dose is absorbed.
Distribution: Rapid and extensive. Active metabolites are extensively protein-bound.
Metabolism: Extensive in the first pass by the liver to two active metabolites, M1 and M2.
Excretion: About 77% in urine. *Half-life:* M1 is 14 hours and M2 is 16 hours.

Route	Onset	Peak	Duration
P.O.	Unknown	3–4 hr	Unknown

Action

Chemical effect: Inhibits reuptake of norepinephrine, serotonin, and dopamine.
Therapeutic effect: Facilitates weight loss.

Available forms

Capsules: 5 mg, 10 mg, 15 mg

NURSING PROCESS

Assessment
• Monitor patient for adverse reactions and drug interactions.
• Assess patient for organic causes of obesity before starting therapy.
• Assess patient's dietary intake.
• Measure blood pressure and pulse before starting therapy, with dosage changes, and at regular intervals during therapy.
• Assess patient's and family's knowledge of drug therapy.

Nursing diagnoses
• Imbalanced nutrition: more than body requirements related to increased caloric intake
• Sleep deprivation related to drug-induced insomnia
• Deficient knowledge related to drug therapy

Planning and implementation
• Don't give drug within 14 days of MAO inhibitor therapy.
• Give patient ice chips or sugarless hard candy to relieve dry mouth.
• Make sure patient follows appropriate diet regimen.
Patient teaching
• Advise patient to immediately report rash, hives, or other allergic reactions.
• Instruct patient to inform prescriber if he is taking or plans to take other prescription or OTC drugs.
• Advise patient to have blood pressure and pulse monitored at regular intervals. Stress importance of regular follow-up visits with prescriber.
• Advise patient to use drug with reduced calorie diet.
• Tell patient that weight loss can cause gallstones. Teach patient about signs and symptoms and the need to report them to prescriber promptly.

Evaluation
• Patient achieves nutritional balance with the use of drugs and a reduced-calorie diet.
• Patient experiences normal sleep patterns.

S

• Patient and family state understanding of drug therapy.

sildenafil citrate

(sil-DEN-ah-fil SIGH-trayt)
Revatio

Pharmacologic class: cyclic guanosine monophosphate (cGMP)–specific phosphodiesterase type 5 (PDE5) inhibitor
Therapeutic class: vasodilator
Pregnancy risk category: B

Indications and dosages

▶ **To improve exercise ability in patients with World Health Organization group I pulmonary arterial hypertension.** *Adults:* 20 mg P.O. t.i.d., 4 to 6 hours apart.

Contraindications and cautions

• Contraindicated in patients hypersensitive to drug or its components and in those taking organic nitrates.
• Don't use in patients with pulmonary venoocclusive disease.
• Use cautiously in patients with resting hypotension, severe left ventricular outflow obstruction, autonomic dysfunction, and volume depletion.
• Use cautiously in patients with hepatic or severe renal impairment, retinitis pigmentosa, bleeding disorders, or active peptic ulcer disease; those who have had an MI, a stroke, or a life-threatening arrhythmia in last 6 months; those with history of coronary artery disease causing unstable angina or uncontrolled high or low blood pressure; those with deformation of the penis and conditions that may cause priapism (such as sickle cell anemia, multiple myeloma, or leukemia); and those taking bosentan.
⚠ Lifespan: In pregnant women, use cautiously. Use cautiously in breast-feeding women; it isn't known whether drug appears in breast milk. Safety and effectiveness haven't been established in children. Use cautiously in elderly patients because they have an increased risk of impaired renal, hepatic, and cardiac function and of concurrent disease.

Adverse reactions

CNS: dizziness, fever, *headache.*
CV: flushing, hypotension, *MI, sudden cardiac death, stroke, transient ischemic attack, ventricular arrhythmias.*
EENT: blurred vision, burning, epistaxis, impaired color discrimination, photophobia, rhinitis, sinusitis.
GI: diarrhea, dyspepsia, gastritis.
Musculoskeletal: myalgia.
Skin: erythema.

Interactions

Drug-drug. *Alpha blockers:* May cause symptomatic hypotension. Use together cautiously.
Amlodipine: May further reduce blood pressure. Monitor blood pressure closely.
Bosentan: May decrease sildenafil level. Monitor patient.
Cytochrome P-450 inducers, rifampin: May reduce sildenafil level. Monitor effect.
Hepatic isoenzyme inhibitors (such as cimetidine, erythromycin, itraconazole, ketoconazole): May increase sildenafil level. Avoid using together.
Isosorbide, nitroglycerin: May cause severe hypotension. Use of nitrates in any form is contraindicated during therapy.
Protease inhibitors: May significantly increase sildenafil level. Don't use together.
Vitamin K antagonists: May increase risk of bleeding (primarily epistaxis). Monitor patient.
Drug-food. *Grapefruit:* May increase drug level and delay absorption. Advise patient to avoid using together.

Effects on lab test results

None reported.

Pharmacokinetics

Absorption: Rapid. Absolute bioavailability is 40%.
Distribution: Extensively into body tissues. About 96% protein-bound.
Metabolism: Mainly in the liver to an active metabolite with properties similar to those of parent drug.
Excretion: About 80% in feces and 13% in urine. *Half-life:* 4 hours.

Route	Onset	Peak	Duration
P.O.	15–30 min	30 min–2 hr	4 hr

Action

Chemical effect: Increases cyclic guanosine monophosphate level by preventing its breakdown by phosphodiesterase, prolonging smooth muscle relaxation of the pulmonary vasculature, which leads to vasodilation.

Therapeutic effect: Improved exercise tolerance in patients with World Health Organization group I pulmonary arterial hypertension.

Available forms

Tablets: 20 mg

NURSING PROCESS

⚕ Assessment
• Assess patient for underlying conditions that could be adversely affected by vasodilatory effects of the drug including resting hypotension (blood pressure below 90/50 mm Hg), fluid depletion, severe ventricular outflow obstruction, or autonomic dysfunction.
• Monitor patient's vital signs carefully at start of treatment.
• Monitor patient for evidence of pulmonary edema; if it occurs, consider pulmonary venoocclusive disease.
• Monitor patient for development of visual disturbances such as photophobia, impaired color discrimination, blurred vision, and burning.
• Assess patient's and family's knowledge of drug therapy.

✪ Nursing diagnoses
• Ineffective tissue perfusion (cardiopulmonary) related to underlying condition
• Activity intolerance related to underlying medical condition
• Deficient knowledge related to drug therapy

▶ Planning and implementation
⚟ **ALERT:** Don't substitute Viagra for Revatio because there isn't an equivalent dose.
⚟ **ALERT:** Sudden loss or decrease of hearing, along with tinnitus and dizziness, may occur.
• Patients with pulmonary arterial hypertension caused by connective tissue disease are more prone to epistaxis during therapy than those with primary pulmonary hypertension.
• The serious CV events linked to this drug's use in erectile dysfunction mainly involve patients with underlying CV disease who are at in-creased risk for cardiac effects related to sexual activity.

Patient teaching
• Warn patient that drug should never be used with nitrates.
• Advise patient to rise slowly from lying down.
• Inform patient that drug can be taken with or without food.
• Warn patient that discrimination between colors such as blue and green may become impaired during therapy; warn him to avoid hazardous activities that rely on recognizing colors.
• Instruct patient to notify prescriber of decrease or loss of hearing, tinnitus, visual changes, dizziness, or fainting.
• Caution patient to take drug only as prescribed.

☑ Evaluation
• Patient's pulmonary artery pressure decreases, and patient reaches pulmonary hemodynamic stability.
• Patient experiences improved exercise tolerance with drug therapy.
• Patient and family state understanding of drug therapy.

sildenafil citrate
(sil-DEN-ah-fil SIGH-trayt)
Viagra⌀

Pharmacologic class: phosphodiesterase type 5 (PDE 5) inhibitor
Therapeutic class: erectile dysfunction drug
Pregnancy risk category: B

Indications and dosages

▶ **Erectile dysfunction.** *Men younger than age 65:* Initially, 50 mg P.O., p.r.n., about 1 hour before sexual activity. Dosage range is 25 to 100 mg, based on effectiveness and tolerance. Maximum, 1 dose daily.
▧ **Adjust-a-dose:** Men age 65 and older or those with hepatic or severe renal impairment or those taking potent CYP3A4 inhibitors (erythromycin, itraconazole, ketoconazole, saquinavir) should take 25 mg P.O. about 1 hour before sexual activity. Base dose on patient response. Maximum, 1 dose daily.

Contraindications and cautions

- Contraindicated in patients hypersensitive to the drug or any of its components, those with underlying CV disease, and those using organic nitrates at any frequency and in any form.
- Use cautiously in patients with hepatic or severe renal impairment; those with anatomic deformation of the penis; those with conditions that may predispose them to priapism (such as sickle cell anemia, multiple myeloma, leukemia), retinitis pigmentosa, bleeding disorders, or active peptic ulcer disease; those who have had an MI, stroke, or life-threatening arrhythmia during previous 6 months; and those with history of cardiac failure, coronary artery disease, or uncontrolled high or low blood pressure.

⚜ **Lifespan:** In men age 65 and older, use cautiously. Not indicated for use in women or children.

Adverse reactions

CNS: anxiety, dizziness, *headache, seizures,* somnolence, tinnitus, vertigo.
CV: *cerebrovascular hemorrhage, flushing,* hypotension, *MI, sudden cardiac death, transient ischemic attack, ventricular arrhythmia.*
EENT: abnormal vision (photophobia, color-tinged vision, blurred vision), decrease or loss of hearing, decreased vision, diplopia, increased intraocular pressure, ocular burning, ocular redness or bloodshot appearance, ocular swelling or pressure, perimacular edema, retinal bleeding, retinal vascular disease, temporary vision loss, vitreous detachment or traction.
GI: diarrhea, dyspepsia.
GU: hematuria, priapism, UTI.
Musculoskeletal: arthralgia, back pain.
Respiratory: respiratory tract infection.
Skin: rash.
Other: flulike syndrome.

Interactions

Drug-drug. *Alpha blockers:* May cause hypotension or syncope. Caution patient not to take 50- to 100-mg doses of sildenafil within 4 hours of an alpha blocker. A dose of 25 mg may be taken at any time.
Azole antifungals (itraconazole, ketoconazole): May increase sildenafil level. Reduce starting dose of sildenafil to 25 mg.
CYP3A4 inducers, rifampin: May decrease sildenafil level. Monitor drug effect.

Delavirdine, protease inhibitors: May increase sildenafil level and sildenafil-related adverse events, including hypotension, visual changes, and priapism. Tell patient not to exceed 25 mg of sildenafil in a 48-hour period.
Hepatic isoenzyme inhibitors (such as cimetidine, erythromycin, itraconazole, ketoconazole): May reduce sildenafil clearance. Avoid using together, or reduce dosage to 25 mg.
Isosorbide, nitroglycerin, other nitrates: May cause severe hypotension. Use of nitrates in any form with sildenafil is contraindicated.
Drug-food. *Grapefruit:* May increase level and delay absorption. Advise patient to avoid consuming grapefruit products.
High-fat meals: Reduces rate of absorption and decreases peak level. Tell patient to separate dose from meals.

Effects on lab test results

None reported.

Pharmacokinetics

Absorption: Rapid. Absolute bioavailability is 40%.
Distribution: Extensively into body tissues. About 96% protein-bound.
Metabolism: Mainly in the liver to an active metabolite with properties similar to those of parent drug.
Excretion: About 80% in feces and 13% in urine. *Half-life:* 4 hours.

Route	Onset	Peak	Duration
P.O.	30 min	30 min–2 hr	4 hr

Action

Chemical effect: Enhances the effect of nitric oxide (NO) by inhibiting PDE 5. When sexual stimulation causes local release of NO, inhibition of PDE 5 causes increased level of cyclic guanosine monophosphate in the corpus cavernosum, resulting in smooth muscle relaxation and inflow of blood.
Therapeutic effect: Causes erection.

Available forms

Tablets: 25 mg, 50 mg, 100 mg

NURSING PROCESS

℞ Assessment

• Discuss patient's history of erectile dysfunction to establish need for drug versus other therapies.
• Assess patient for CV risk factors because serious events have been reported with drug, and report risk factors to prescriber.
• Assess patient's and family's knowledge of drug therapy.

🔅 Nursing diagnoses

• Sexual dysfunction related to patient's underlying condition
• Ineffective tissue perfusion (cardiopulmonary) related to drug-induced effects on blood pressure and cardiac output
• Deficient knowledge related to drug therapy

▷ Planning and implementation

🔅 **ALERT:** Serious CV events, including MI, sudden cardiac death, ventricular arrhythmia, cerebrovascular hemorrhage, transient ischemic attack, and hypertension, may occur in patients during or shortly after sexual activity.
🔅 **ALERT:** Drug's systemic vasodilation causes transient decreases in supine blood pressure and cardiac output about 2 hours after use. Together with the cardiac risk of sexual activity, the risk for patients with underlying CV disease is increased.
🔅 **ALERT:** Sudden loss or decrease of hearing, along with tinnitus and dizziness, may occur.
🔅 **ALERT:** Don't confuse Viagra with Allegra.
Patient teaching
• Explain that drug is contraindicated with regular or intermittent use of nitrates.
• Warn patient about cardiac risk with sexual activity, especially if he has CV risk factors. If patient has symptoms such as angina pectoris, dizziness, or nausea at the start of sexual activity, instruct him to notify prescriber and refrain from further sexual activity.
• Warn patient that erections lasting longer than 4 hours and priapism (painful erections longer than 6 hours) may occur and should be reported immediately. If priapism isn't treated immediately, penile tissue damage and permanent loss of potency may result.
• Inform patient that drug doesn't protect against sexually transmitted diseases and that

protective measures, such as condoms, should be used.
• Instruct patient to take drug 30 minutes to 4 hours before sexual activity; maximum benefit can be expected less than 2 hours after ingesting drug.
• Advise patient that drug is most rapidly absorbed if taken on an empty stomach.
• Inform patient to avoid potentially hazardous activities that rely on color discrimination because blue and green discrimination may be impaired.
• Instruct patient to notify prescriber if visual or hearing changes occur.
• Advise patient that drug is effective only with sexual stimulation.
• Tell patient to take drug only as prescribed.
• Advise patient taking HIV drugs or alpha blockers about an increased risk of sildenafil-related adverse events, including hypotension, visual changes, and priapism, and he should promptly report any symptoms to his prescriber. Tell him not to exceed 25 mg of sildenafil in a 48-hour period.

☑ Evaluation

• Sexual activity improves with drug therapy.
• Patient doesn't experience adverse CV events.
• Patient and family state understanding of drug therapy.

simvastatin

(sim-vuh-STAT-in)
Zocor∕

Pharmacologic class: HMG-CoA reductase inhibitor
Therapeutic class: antihyperlipidemic
Pregnancy risk category: X

Indications and dosages

▶ **To reduce risk of CAD mortality and CV events in patients at high risk, hyperlipidemia.** *Adults:* Initially, 20 to 40 mg P.O. daily in evening. Dosage adjusted every 4 weeks based on patient tolerance and response. Maximum, 80 mg daily.
▶ **To reduce total cholesterol and LDL levels in patients with homozygous familial hypercholesterolemia.** *Adults:* 40 mg daily in evening; or 80 mg daily in three divided doses

of 20 mg in morning, 20 mg in afternoon, and 40 mg in evening.

▶ **Heterozygous familial hypercholesterolemia.** *Children ages 10 to 17:* Give 10 mg P.O. once daily in the evening. Maximum, 40 mg daily.

🔋 **Adjust-a-dose:** For patients taking cyclosporine, initially give 5 mg P.O. daily; don't exceed 10 mg daily. For patients taking fibrates or niacin, maximum is 10 mg P.O. daily. For patients taking amiodarone or verapamil, maximum is 20 mg P.O. daily. For patients with severe renal insufficiency, initially give 5 mg P.O. daily.

Contraindications and cautions

● Contraindicated in patients hypersensitive to the drug or any of its components, and in those with active liver disease or conditions that have unexplained persistent elevations of transaminase level.
● Use cautiously in patients who consume substantial quantities of alcohol or have a history of liver disease.
🔆 **Lifespan:** In pregnant women, breast-feeding women, and women of childbearing age, drug is contraindicated.

Adverse reactions

CNS: asthenia, headache.
GI: abdominal pain, constipation, diarrhea, dyspepsia, flatulence, nausea.
Hepatic: *cirrhosis, hepatitis, hepatic necrosis.*
Musculoskeletal: myalgia.
Respiratory: upper respiratory tract infection.

Interactions

Drug-drug. *Amiodarone, verapamil:* May increase risk of myopathy and rhabdomyolysis. Don't exceed 20 mg simvastatin daily.
Clarithromycin, erythromycin, HIV protease inhibitors, nefazodone: May increase risk of myopathy and rhabdomyolysis. Avoid using together, or suspend therapy during treatment with clarithromycin or erythromycin.
Cyclosporine, danazol, fibrates, niacin: May increase risk of myopathy and rhabdomyolysis. Monitor patient closely if use together can't be avoided. Don't exceed 10 mg simvastatin daily.
Digoxin: May elevate digoxin level slightly. Closely monitor at the start of therapy.
Fluconazole, itraconazole, ketoconazole: May increase level and adverse effects of simvastatin.

Avoid this combination. If they must be given together, reduce dosage of simvastatin.
Hepatotoxic drugs: May increase risk of hepatotoxicity. Avoid using together.
Non-nucleoside reverse transcriptase inhibitors (delavirdine, efavirenz, nevirapine): May increase or decrease simvastatin level. Monitor patient for unexplained muscle pain.
Warfarin: May enhance anticoagulant effect. Monitor PT and INR at the start of therapy and during dosage adjustment.
Drug-herb. *Red yeast rice:* May increase the risk of adverse events or toxicity. Discourage using together.
St. John's wort: May increase clearance of simvastatin, resulting in reduced effectiveness. Avoid using together.
Drug-food. *Grapefruit juice:* May increase drug level and risk of adverse effects, including myopathy and rhabdomyolysis. Advise patient against drinking grapefruit juice.
Drug-lifestyle. *Alcohol use:* May increase the risk of hepatotoxicity. Discourage using together.

Effects on lab test results

● May increase liver enzyme and CPK levels.

Pharmacokinetics

Absorption: Good, but extensive hepatic extraction limits availability of active inhibitors to 5% of dose or less.
Distribution: More than 95% protein-bound.
Metabolism: Hydrolysis occurs in liver; at least three major metabolites have been identified.
Excretion: Mainly in bile. *Half-life:* 3 hours.

Route	Onset	Peak	Duration
P.O.	Unknown	1½–2½ hr	Unknown

Action

Chemical effect: Inhibits HMG-CoA reductase. This enzyme is an early (and rate-limiting) step in synthetic pathway of cholesterol.
Therapeutic effect: Lowers LDL and total cholesterol level.

Available forms

Tablets: 5 mg, 10 mg, 20 mg, 40 mg, 80 mg
Tablets (orally-disintegrating): 10 mg, 20 mg, 40 mg, 80 mg

Reactions may be *common*, uncommon, *life-threatening*, or COMMON AND LIFE-THREATENING.

NURSING PROCESS

🔆 Assessment
• Obtain history of patient's LDL and total cholesterol level before starting therapy, and reassess regularly thereafter to monitor the drug's effectiveness.
• Obtain liver function test results before starting therapy and periodically thereafter. If enzyme level elevations persist, a liver biopsy may be performed.
• Monitor patient for myalgia or muscle weakness and for elevated CK level, during treatment. Rhabdomyolysis with and without acute renal insufficiency has been reported.
• Be alert for adverse reactions and drug interactions.
• Assess patient's dietary fat intake.
• Assess patient's and family's knowledge of drug therapy.

🔆 Nursing diagnoses
• Risk for injury related to presence of elevated cholesterol level
• Constipation related to drug-induced adverse GI reactions
• Deficient knowledge related to drug therapy

🔆 Planning and implementation
• Drug therapy starts only after diet and other nondrug therapies have proven ineffective.
• Make sure patient follows a standard low-cholesterol diet during therapy.
• Give drug with evening meal for enhanced effectiveness.
• If cholesterol level falls below target range, dosage may be reduced.
🔆 ALERT: Don't confuse Zocor with Cozaar.
Patient teaching
• Tell patient to take drug with evening meal to enhance absorption and cholesterol biosynthesis.
• Teach patient dietary management of lipids (restricting total fat and cholesterol intake) and measures to control other cardiac disease risk factors. If appropriate, suggest weight control, exercise, and smoking cessation programs.
• Tell patient to inform prescriber about adverse reactions, particularly muscle aches and pains.
🔆 ALERT: Inform woman that drug is contraindicated during pregnancy. Advise her to notify prescriber immediately if pregnancy occurs.

☑ Evaluation
• Patient's LDL and total cholesterol level are within normal limits.
• Patient regains and maintains normal bowel pattern throughout therapy.
• Patient and family state understanding of drug therapy.

sirolimus
(sir-AH-lih-mus)
Rapamune

Pharmacologic class: macrocyclic lactone
Therapeutic class: immunosuppressant
Pregnancy risk category: C

Indications and dosages

▶ **Prophylaxis of organ rejection in patients receiving renal transplants.** *Adults and children age 13 and older who weigh 40 kg (88 lb) or more:* Initially, 6 mg P.O. as a one-time loading dose as soon as possible after transplantation; then maintenance dose of 2 mg P.O. once daily. Give 4 hours after cyclosporine and corticosteroids. Maximum daily dose is 40 mg. If a daily dose exceeds 40 mg because of loading dose, give the loading dose over 2 days. Monitor trough level at least 3 to 4 days after loading dose.
Children age 13 and older who weigh less than 40 kg: Initially, 3 mg/m^2 P.O. as a one-time loading dose after transplantation; then maintenance dose of 1 mg/m^2 P.O. once daily.

🔆 **Adjust-a-dose:** For patients with hepatic impairment, reduce maintenance dosage by one-third. Adjusting loading dosage isn't needed.

Contraindications and cautions

• Contraindicated in patients hypersensitive to the drug or any of its derivatives or components.
• Use cautiously in patients with hyperlipidemia or impaired liver or renal function.
• Risk for angioedema, particularly when combined with ACE inhibitors.
• Safety and effectiveness haven't been established in liver and lung transplant patients; therefore, such use isn't recommended.
🔆 **Lifespan:** In pregnant women, use only if benefits outweigh risks to the fetus. In breastfeeding women, drug is contraindicated. Women of childbearing age should use contraception

S

before therapy, during, and for 12 weeks after therapy. In children younger than age 13, safety and effectiveness haven't been established.

Adverse reactions

CNS: *anxiety, asthenia,* confusion, *depression,* dizziness, emotional lability, *fever, headache,* hypertonia, hypesthesia, hypotonia, *insomnia,* malaise, neuropathy, paresthesia, *pain,* somnolence, syncope, *tremor.*
CV: atrial fibrillation, *chest pain, edema,* facial edema, *heart failure, hemorrhage,* hypertension, hypotension, palpitations, *peripheral edema,* peripheral vascular disorder, tachycardia, thrombophlebitis, *thrombosis,* vasodilation.
EENT: abnormal vision, cataracts, conjunctivitis, deafness, ear pain, epistaxis, otitis media, *pharyngitis,* rhinitis, sinusitis, tinnitus.
GI: *abdominal pain,* anorexia, ascites, *constipation, diarrhea, dyspepsia,* dysphagia, enlarged abdomen, eructation, esophagitis, flatulence, gastritis, gastroenteritis, gingivitis, gum hyperplasia, hernia, ileus, mouth ulcerations, *nausea,* oral candidiasis, *peritonitis,* stomatitis, *vomiting.*
GU: albuminuria, bladder pain, dysuria, glycosuria, hematuria, hydronephrosis, impotence, kidney pain, nocturia, oliguria, pelvic pain, pyuria, scrotal edema, testis disorder, *toxic nephropathy, tubular necrosis,* urinary frequency, urinary incontinence, urine retention, *UTI.*
Hematologic: *anemia,* leukocytosis, *leukopenia,* lymphadenopathy, polycythemia, THROMBOCYTOPENIA, *thrombotic thrombocytopenic purpura.*
Hepatic: *hepatic artery thrombosis.*
Metabolic: *acidosis,* Cushing syndrome, dehydration, *diabetes mellitus,* hypercalcemia, *hypercholesteremia,* hyperglycemia, HYPERKALEMIA, *hyperlipidemia,* hyperphosphatemia, hypervolemia, hypocalcemia, *hypoglycemia, hypokalemia, hypomagnesemia,* hyponatremia, *hypophosphatemia, weight gain,* weight loss.
Musculoskeletal: *arthralgia,* arthrosis, *back pain,* bone necrosis, leg cramps, myalgia, osteoporosis, tetany.
Respiratory: *asthma,* atelectasis, bronchitis, cough, dyspnea, *hypoxia, lung edema,* pleural effusion, pneumonia, upper respiratory tract infection.
Skin: *acne,* ecchymoses, fungal dermatitis, hirsutism, pruritus, *rash,* skin hypertrophy, skin ulcer, sweating.

Other: abscess, abnormal healing, *angioedema,* cellulitis, chills, flulike syndrome, infection, *sepsis.*

Interactions

Drug-drug. *Aminoglycosides, amphotericin, other nephrotoxic drugs:* May increase risk of nephrotoxicity. Use cautiously.
Bromocriptine, cimetidine, clarithromycin, clotrimazole, danazol, erythromycin, fluconazole, indinavir, itraconazole, metoclopramide, nicardipine, ritonavir, verapamil, other drugs that inhibit CYP3A4: May decrease sirolimus metabolism and increase sirolimus level. Monitor patient for toxicity and elevated liver enzymes.
Carbamazepine, phenobarbital, phenytoin, rifabutin, rifapentine, other drugs that induce CYP3A4: May increase sirolimus metabolism and decrease sirolimus level. Monitor patient closely.
Cyclosporine: May inhibit sirolimus metabolism, increasing levels and toxicity risk. Give sirolimus 4 hours after cyclosporine to prevent variations in sirolimus concentration.
Diltiazem: May increase sirolimus level. Monitor and reduce dosage of sirolimus as needed.
Erythromycin, ketoconazole: May increase rate and extent of sirolimus absorption. Avoid using together.
Rifampin: May decrease sirolimus level. Consider alternatives to rifampin.
Tacrolimus: May increase risk of hepatic artery thrombosis. Don't use together.
Vaccines: May reduce effectiveness of vaccination. Avoid live vaccines.
Drug-herb. *St. John's wort:* May reduce sirolimus concentrations. Avoid using together.
Drug-food. *All food:* May affect bioavailability. Drug should be taken consistently either with or without food to minimize variability.
Grapefruit juice: May decrease drug metabolism. Discourage dilution of drug with juice.
Drug-lifestyle. *Sun exposure:* May increase risk of skin cancer. Tell patient to take precautions.

Effects on lab test results

• May increase BUN, creatinine, liver enzyme, cholesterol, and lipid levels. May decrease sodium, magnesium, and hemoglobin levels and hematocrit. May increase or decrease phosphate, potassium, glucose, and calcium levels.

Reactions may be *common,* uncommon, *life-threatening,* or COMMON AND LIFE-THREATENING.

• May increase RBC count. May decrease platelet count. May increase or decrease WBC count.

Pharmacokinetics

Absorption: Rapid, with mean peak level occurring in about 1 to 3 hours. Oral bioavailability is about 14% for the oral solution. Food decreases peak level and increases time to peak level.
Distribution: Extensive. About 92% protein-bound.
Metabolism: Extensive, by the mixed function oxidase system, mainly CYP3A4. Seven major metabolites have been identified in whole blood.
Excretion: 91% in feces and 2.2% in urine.
Half-life: About 62 hours.

Route	Onset	Peak	Duration
P.O.	Unknown	1–3 hr	Unknown

Action

Chemical effect: An immunosuppressant that inhibits T-lymphocyte activation and proliferation that occur in response to antigenic and cytokine stimulation. Also inhibits antibody formation.
Therapeutic effect: Immunosuppression in patients receiving renal transplants.

Available forms

Oral solution: 1 mg/ml
Tablets: 1 mg, 2 mg

NURSING PROCESS

🔯 Assessment
• Obtain history of patient's organ transplantation before starting therapy.
• Monitor patient's liver and renal function, and triglyceride level, before starting therapy.
• Monitor drug level in children who weigh less than 40 kg (88 lb), patients with hepatic impairment, patients taking drugs that induce or inhibit CYP3A4, and patients whose cyclosporine dosage has been drastically reduced or stopped.
• Monitor patient for infection and development of lymphoma, which may result from immunosuppression.
• Watch for development of rhabdomyolysis if patient is taking sirolimus and cyclosporine is started as an HMG-CoA reductase inhibitor.

• Assess patient's and family's knowledge of drug therapy.

🔯 Nursing diagnoses
• Risk for injury related to potential for organ rejection
• Ineffective protection related to drug-induced immunosuppression
• Deficient knowledge related to drug therapy

▶ Planning and implementation
• Give drug consistently with or without food.
• 🟢 **ALERT:** In patient with mild to moderate hepatic impairment, reduce maintenance dosage by about one-third. Loading dose doesn't need to be reduced.
• Dilute oral solution before giving. After dilution, use it immediately.
• When diluting drug, empty correct amount into glass or plastic container filled with at least 2 oz (60 ml) of water or orange juice. Don't use grapefruit juice or any other liquid. Stir vigorously and have patient drink immediately. Refill container with at least 4 oz (120 ml) of water or orange juice, stir again, and have patient drink all contents.
• After opening bottle, use contents within 1 month. If needed, bottles and pouches may be stored at room temperature (up to 77° F [25° C]) for several days. Drug can be kept in oral syringe for 24 hours at room temperature or refrigerated at 36° to 46° F (2° to 8° C).
• A slight haze may develop during refrigeration, but this won't affect quality of drug. If haze develops, bring drug to room temperature and shake gently until haze disappears.
• Use drug in a regimen with cyclosporine and corticosteroids. This drug should be taken 4 hours after cyclosporine dose.
• Two to four months following transplantation, patient with low to moderate risk of graft rejection should be tapered off cyclosporine over 4 to 8 weeks. During the taper, adjust sirolimus dosage every 1 to 2 weeks to obtain level between 12 to 24 nanograms/ml. Dosage adjustments should also be based on condition, tissue biopsies, and laboratory findings.
• After transplantation, give antimicrobials for 1 year as directed to prevent *Pneumocystis jiroveci (carinii)* pneumonia and for 3 months as directed to prevent CMV infection.
• If patient has hyperlipidemia, start additional interventions, such as diet, exercise, and lipid-

S

lowering drugs. Use with lipid-lowering drugs is common.
• Don't withdraw cyclosporine in patients with high risk of graft rejection, including patients with Banff grade III acute rejection or vascular rejection before cyclosporine withdrawal, a creatinine level greater than 4.5 mg/dl, or a high panel of reactive antibodies; those who have had retransplants or multi-organ transplants; and those who are dialysis-dependent or who are black.

Patient teaching
• Show patient how to store, dilute, and take drug properly.
• Tell patient to take drug consistently with or without food to minimize absorption variability.
• Advise patient to take drug 4 hours after taking cyclosporine.
• Tell patient to wash area with soap and water if solution touches skin or mucous membranes; tell him to rinse eyes with plain water if solution gets in eyes.
• Inform woman of childbearing age of risks during pregnancy. Tell her to use effective contraception before and during therapy and for 12 weeks after stopping the drug.
• Advise patient to take precautions against sun exposure.

☑ Evaluation
• Patient doesn't experience organ rejection.
• Patient is free from infection and serious bleeding episodes throughout drug therapy.
• Patient and family state understanding of drug therapy.

HIGH ALERT

sitagliptin phosphate
(SIGH-tuh-glip-ten FOSS-fayt)
Januvia⬦

Pharmacologic class: dipeptidyl peptidase-4 (DPP-4) enzyme inhibitor
Therapeutic class: antidiabetic
Pregnancy risk category: B

Indications and dosages

▶ **To improve glycemic control in type 2 diabetes, alone or with metformin or a thiazolidinedione when the single drug alone with diet and exercise doesn't provide adequate control.** *Adults:* 100 mg P.O. once daily, with or without food.
🔄 **Adjust-a-dose:** For patients with renal impairment, if creatinine clearance is 30 to 50 ml/minute, give 50 mg once daily. If clearance is less than 30 ml/minute or patient has end-stage renal disease with hemodialysis or peritoneal dialysis, give 25 mg once daily. Drug may be taken without regard to timing of dialysis session.

Contraindications and cautions

• Contraindicated in patients with type 1 diabetes or diabetic ketoacidosis and in patients hypersensitive to sitagliptin.
• Use cautiously in patients with moderate to severe renal insufficiency and in those taking other antidiabetics.
🔆 **Lifespan:** In breast-feeding women, use cautiously. It's unknown if drug appears in breast-milk. In children, safety and effectiveness aren't known. In elderly patients, assess renal function before therapy and periodically throughout. Adjust dosage carefully because these patients are more likely to have decreased renal function.

Adverse reactions

CNS: headache.
EENT: nasopharyngitis.
GI: abdominal pain, diarrhea, nausea.
Metabolic: *hypoglycemia.*
Respiratory: upper respiratory tract infection.
Skin: exfoliative skin conditions including *Stephens-Johnson syndrome.*
Other: *anaphylaxis, angioedema.*

Interactions

None significant.

Effects on lab test results

• May increase creatinine level.
• May increase WBC count.

Pharmacokinetics

Absorption: Rapidly absorbed with 87% bioavailability.
Distribution: Mean volume is about 198 L. 38% bound by plasma proteins.
Metabolism: Minimal.
Excretion: Mainly renal, with a small amount via feces. *Half-life:* 12½ hours.

Route	Onset	Peak	Duration
P.O.	Rapid	1–4 hr	Unknown

Action

Chemical effect: Inhibits DPP-4, an enzyme that rapidly inactivates incretin hormones, which play a part in the body's regulation of glucose. By increasing and prolonging active incretin level, drug helps to increase insulin release and decrease circulating glucose.
Therapeutic effect: Stabilizes blood glucose level.

Available forms

Tablets: 25 mg, 50 mg, 100 mg

NURSING PROCESS

Assessment
• Obtain history of patient's underlying condition before starting therapy, and reassess regularly.
• In patients at risk for renal insufficiency, periodically assess renal function.
• Monitor glycosylated hemoglobin level periodically to assess long-term glycemic control.
• Assess patient's and family's knowledge of drug therapy.

Nursing diagnoses
• Ineffective health maintenance related to hyperglycemia
• Risk for injury related to drug-induced hypoglycemia
• Deficient knowledge related to drug therapy

Planning and implementation
• Management of type 2 diabetes should include exercise and diet control. Because caloric restrictions, weight loss, and exercise help improve insulin sensitivity and help make drug therapy effective, these measures are essential for proper diabetes management.
• Watch for hypoglycemia, especially in patients receiving combination therapy.
Patient teaching
• Tell patient that drug isn't a substitute for diet and exercise and that it's important to follow a prescribed diet and physical activity routine. Urge patient to monitor his glucose level.
• Inform patient and family members of the signs and symptoms of hyperglycemia and hypoglycemia and the steps to take if these symptoms occur.
• Provide patient with information on complications associated with diabetes and ways to assess for them.
• Tell patient to notify prescriber during periods of stress, such as fever, infection, or surgery; dosage may need adjustment.
• Tell patient drug may be taken without regard to food or meals.

Evaluation
• Patient's blood glucose level is within normal limits.
• Patient doesn't experience hypoglycemic reactions.
• Patient and family state understanding of drug therapy.

sodium bicarbonate
(SOH-dee-um bigh-KAR-buh-nayt)
**Arm and Hammer Pure Baking Soda†,
Bell/ans†**

Pharmacologic class: alkalinizer
Therapeutic class: ion buffer, oral antacid
Pregnancy risk category: C

Indications and dosages

▶ **Adjunct to advanced CV life support during cardiopulmonary resuscitation (no longer routinely recommended).** *Adults:* Inject either 300 to 500 ml of a 5% solution or 200 to 300 mEq of a 7.5% or 8.4% solution as rapidly as possible. Base further doses on subsequent blood gas values. Or, 1-mEq/kg dose, then repeat 0.5 mEq/kg every 10 minutes.
Children age 2 and younger: 1 mEq/kg I.V. or intraosseous injection of a 4.2% to 8.4% solution. Give slowly. Don't exceed daily dose of 8 mEq/kg.
▶ **Severe metabolic acidosis.** *Adults:* Dosage depends on blood carbon dioxide content, pH, and patient's condition. Generally, give 90 to 180 mEq/L I.V. during first hour, then adjust as needed.
▶ **Less urgent metabolic acidosis.** *Adults and children age 12 and older:* 2 to 5 mEq/kg as a 4- to 8-hour I.V. infusion.

S

▶ **Urine alkalization.** *Adults:* 48 mEq (4 g) P.O. initially; then 12 to 24 mEq (1 to 2 g) every 4 hours. May need doses of 30 to 48 mEq (2.5 to 4 g) every 4 hours, up to 192 mEq (16 g) daily.
Children: 1 to 10 mEq (84 to 840 mg)/kg P.O. daily.
▶ **Antacid.** *Adults:* 300 mg to 2 g P.O. one to four times daily.

▼ I.V. administration

● Sodium bicarbonate inactivates such catecholamines as norepinephrine and dopamine and forms precipitate with calcium. Don't mix sodium bicarbonate with solutions of these drugs; flush line adequately.
● Usually given by infusion. For immediate treatment, drug may be given by direct, rapid injection; however, in neonates and children younger than age 2, slow administration is preferred to avoid hypernatremia, decreased CSF pressure, and intracranial hemorrhage.
⊗ **Incompatibilities**
Alcohol 5% in dextrose 5%; allopurinol; amiodarone; amphotericin B; amino acids; ascorbic acid injection; bupivacaine; calcium salts; carboplatin; carmustine; cefotaxime; ciprofloxacin; cisatracurium; cisplatin; corticotropin; dextrose 5% in lactated Ringer's injection; diltiazem; dobutamine; dopamine; doxorubicin liposomal; epinephrine hydrochloride; fat emulsion 10%; glycopyrrolate; hydromorphone; idarubicin; imipenem-cilastatin sodium; Ionosol B, D, or G with invert sugar 10%; isoproterenol; labetalol; lactated Ringer's injection; levorphanol; leucovorin calcium; lidocaine; magnesium sulfate; meperidine; meropenem; methylprednisolone sodium succinate; metoclopramide; midazolam; morphine sulfate; nalbuphine; norepinephrine bitartrate; ondansetron; oxacillin; penicillin G potassium; pentazocine lactate; pentobarbital sodium; procaine; Ringer's injection; sargramostim; 1/6 M sodium lactate; streptomycin; succinylcholine; thiopental; ticarcillin disodium and clavulanate potassium; vancomycin; verapamil; vinca alkaloids; vitamin B complex with vitamin C.

Contraindications and cautions

● Contraindicated in patients with metabolic or respiratory alkalosis; patients who are losing chlorides from vomiting or continuous GI suc-

tion; patients taking diuretics known to produce hypochloremic alkalosis; and patients with hypocalcemia in which alkalosis may produce tetany, hypertension, seizures, or heart failure. Oral sodium bicarbonate is contraindicated in patients with acute ingestion of strong mineral acids.
● Use cautiously in patients with hypertension, heart failure or other edematous or sodium-retaining conditions or renal insufficiency.
❈ **Lifespan:** In pregnant women, use cautiously. In breast-feeding women, use cautiously; it's unknown if the drug appears in breast milk.

Adverse reactions

GI: belching, flatulence, gastric distention.
Metabolic: hypernatremia, hyperosmolarity (with overdose), hypokalemia, *metabolic alkalosis.*
Other: irritation and pain at injection site.

Interactions

Drug-drug. *Anorexigenics, flecainide, mecamylamine, quinidine, sympathomimetics:* May increase urine alkalization, decrease renal clearance, and increase pharmacologic or toxic effects. Monitor patient for toxicity.
Chlorpropamide, lithium, methotrexate, salicylates, tetracycline: May increase renal clearance of these drugs, possibly resulting in decreased pharmacologic effects. Monitor patient for lack of effect.

Effects on lab test results

● May increase sodium and lactate levels. May decrease potassium level.

Pharmacokinetics

Absorption: Good.
Distribution: Confined to systemic circulation.
Metabolism: None.
Excretion: Filtered and reabsorbed by kidneys; less than 1% of filtered drug is excreted. *Half-life:* Unknown.

Route	Onset	Peak	Duration
P.O.	Unknown	Unknown	Unknown
I.V.	Immediate	Immediate	Unknown

Action

Chemical effect: Restores body's buffering capacity and neutralizes excess acid.

Reactions may be *common*, uncommon, *life-threatening*, or COMMON AND LIFE-THREATENING.

Therapeutic effect: Restores normal acid-base balance and relieves acid indigestion.

Available forms

Injection: 4% (2.4 mEq/5 ml), 4.2% (5 mEq/10 ml), 5% (297.5 mEq/500 ml), 7.5% (8.92 mEq/10 ml, 44.6 mEq/50 ml, and 179 mEq/200 ml), 8.4% (10 mEq/10 ml, and 50 mEq/50 ml)
Tablets†: 325 mg, 650 mg

NURSING PROCESS

⚕ Assessment
• Assess patient's condition before starting therapy and regularly thereafter to monitor drug's effectiveness.
• To avoid risk of alkalosis, obtain blood pH, Pao_2, $Paco_2$, and electrolyte level.
• If sodium bicarbonate is being used to produce alkaline urine, monitor urine pH (should be greater than 7) every 4 to 6 hours.
• Be alert for adverse reactions and drug interactions.
• Assess patient's and family's knowledge of drug therapy.

☺ Nursing diagnoses
• Ineffective health maintenance related to underlying condition
• Risk for injury related to drug-induced adverse reactions
• Deficient knowledge related to drug therapy

▷ Planning and implementation
• Drug isn't routinely recommended for use in cardiac arrest because it may produce paradoxical acidosis from CO_2 production. It shouldn't be routinely given during early stages of resuscitation unless acidosis is clearly present.
• Drug may be used after such interventions as defibrillation, cardiac compression, and administration of first-line drugs.
• Give drug with water, not milk; drug may cause hypercalcemia, alkalosis, or possibly renal calculi.
• Inform prescriber of laboratory results.
Patient teaching
• Tell patient not to take with milk.
• Discourage use as antacid. Offer nonabsorbable antacid if it's to be used repeatedly.

☑ Evaluation
• Patient regains normal acid-base balance.
• Patient doesn't experience injury from drug-induced adverse reactions.
• Patient and family state understanding of drug therapy.

HIGH ALERT

sodium chloride
(SOH-dee-um KLOR-ighd)

Pharmacologic class: electrolyte
Therapeutic class: chloride and sodium replacement
Pregnancy risk category: C

Indications and dosages

▶ **Fluid and electrolyte replacement in hyponatremia caused by severe electrolyte loss, severe salt depletion or dehydration.** *Adults:* Dosage is highly individualized. The 3% and 5% solutions are used only with frequent electrolyte determination and given only by slow I.V. With half-normal saline solution: 3% to 8% of body weight, according to deficiencies, over 18 to 24 hours. With normal saline solution: 2% to 6% of body weight, according to deficiencies, over 18 to 24 hours.

▽ I.V. administration
• Infuse 3% and 5% solutions very slowly and cautiously to avoid pulmonary edema. Use only for critical situations, and observe patient continually.
• When infusing peripherally, avoid infiltration and use a large vein.
⊗ **Incompatibilities**
Amphotericin B, chlordiazepoxide, diazepam, fat emulsion, mannitol, methylprednisolone sodium succinate, phenytoin sodium.

Contraindications and cautions
• Contraindicated in patients with conditions in which giving sodium and chloride is detrimental. The 3% and 5% saline solution injections are contraindicated in patients with increased, normal, or only slightly decreased electrolyte level.
• Use cautiously in postoperative patients and patients with heart failure, circulatory insufficiency, renal dysfunction, or hypoproteinemia.

S

⚖ **Lifespan:** In pregnant women, use cautiously. In breast-feeding women, use cautiously; it's unknown if the drug appears in breast milk. In the elderly, use cautiously.

Adverse reactions

CV: *aggravation of heart failure,* edema if given too rapidly or in excess, thrombophlebitis.
Metabolic: *aggravation of existing metabolic acidosis* with excessive infusion, electrolyte disturbances, hypernatremia, hypokalemia.
Respiratory: *pulmonary edema* if given too rapidly or in excess.
Skin: abscess, local tenderness, tissue necrosis at injection site.

Interactions

None significant.

Effects on lab test results

• May increase sodium and chloride levels. May decrease potassium and bicarbonate levels.

Pharmacokinetics

Absorption: Without hesitation.
Distribution: Wide.
Metabolism: None significant.
Excretion: Mainly in urine; some in sweat, tears, and saliva. *Half-life:* Unknown.

Route	Onset	Peak	Duration
P.O.	Unknown	Unknown	Unknown
I.V.	Immediate	Immediate	Unknown

Action

Chemical effect: Replaces and maintains sodium and chloride levels.
Therapeutic effect: Restores normal sodium and chloride levels.

Available forms

Injection: *Half-normal saline solution:* 25 ml, 50 ml, 150 ml, 250 ml, 500 ml, 1,000 ml
Normal saline solution: 2 ml, 3 ml, 5 ml, 10 ml, 20 ml, 25 ml, 30 ml, 50 ml, 100 ml, 150 ml, 250 ml, 500 ml, 1,000 ml
3% saline solution: 500 ml
5% saline solution: 500 ml
14.6% saline solution: 20 ml, 40 ml, 200 ml
23.4% saline solution: 30 ml, 50 ml, 100 ml, 200 ml

Tablets (enteric-coated): 650 mg, 1 g, 2.25 g
Tablets (slow-release): 600 mg

NURSING PROCESS

🩺 Assessment

• Obtain history of patient's sodium and chloride levels before starting therapy, and reassess regularly thereafter to monitor drug's effectiveness.
• Monitor other electrolyte levels.
• Assess patient's fluid status.
• Be alert for adverse reactions.
• Assess patient's and family's knowledge of drug therapy.

🔃 Nursing diagnoses

• Imbalanced nutrition: less than body requirements related to subnormal levels of sodium and chloride
• Excess fluid volume related to the saline solution's water-drawing power
• Deficient knowledge related to drug therapy

▶ Planning and implementation

• Give tablet with glass of water.
• 🔔 **ALERT:** Don't confuse concentrates (14.6% and 23.4%) available to add to parenteral nutrient solutions with normal saline solution injection, and never give without diluting. Read label carefully.
Patient teaching
• Tell patient to report adverse reactions promptly.

☑ Evaluation

• Patient's sodium and chloride levels are normal.
• Patient doesn't exhibit signs and symptoms of fluid retention.
• Patient and family state understanding of drug therapy.

sodium ferric gluconate complex
(SOH-dee-um FEH-rik GLOO-kuh-nayt KOM-pleks)
Ferrlecit

Pharmacologic class: macromolecular iron complex
Therapeutic class: hematinic
Pregnancy risk category: B

Reactions may be *common,* uncommon, *life-threatening,* or COMMON AND LIFE-THREATENING.

Indications and dosages

▶ **Iron deficiency anemia in patients undergoing long-term hemodialysis and receiving supplemental erythropoietin therapy.** *Adults and children older than age 15:* Give 10 ml (125 mg elemental iron) diluted in 100 ml normal saline solution I.V. over 1 hour. May also be given undiluted as a slow I.V. infusion at 12.5 mg/minute. Most patients need a minimum cumulative dose of 1 g elemental iron given at more than eight sequential dialysis treatments to achieve a favorable hemoglobin level or hematocrit response. May be given during dialysis session.
Children ages 6 to 15: Give 0.12 ml/kg (1.5 mg/kg elemental iron) diluted in 25 ml 0.9% sodium chloride I.V. infusion over 1 hour at eight sequential dialysis sessions. Maximum dose, 125 mg.

▼ I.V. administration

• Don't add sodium ferric gluconate complex to parenteral nutrition solutions for I.V. infusion.
• Use immediately after dilution in normal saline solution.
• Dilute in 100 ml normal saline solution and give over 1 hour. Don't exceed 2.1 mg/minute.
• Patient may develop profound hypotension with flushing, lightheadedness, malaise, fatigue, weakness, or severe chest, back, flank, or groin pain after rapid I.V. administration of iron. These reactions don't indicate hypersensitivity and may result from rapid administration of drug. Monitor patient closely during infusion.
⊗ Incompatibilities
Other I.V. drugs.

Contraindications and cautions

• Contraindicated in patients hypersensitive to the drug or any of its components (such as benzyl alcohol), and in patients with anemia not linked to iron deficiency. Don't give to patients with iron overload.
☀ Lifespan: In breast-feeding women, use cautiously; it's unknown if the drug appears in breast milk. In children younger than age 6, safety and effectiveness haven't been established. In the elderly, begin treatment at lowest dose and observe closely.

Adverse reactions

CNS: asthenia, headache, fatigue, malaise, dizziness, paresthesia, agitation, insomnia, somnolence, syncope, pain, fever.
CV: hypotension, hypertension, tachycardia, *bradycardia,* angina, chest pain, *MI,* edema, flushing.
EENT: conjunctivitis, abnormal vision, rhinitis.
GI: nausea, vomiting, diarrhea, rectal disorder, dyspepsia, eructation, flatulence, melena, abdominal pain.
GU: UTI.
Hematologic: abnormal erythrocytes, anemia, lymphadenopathy.
Metabolic: *hyperkalemia,* hypervolemia, *hypoglycemia,* hypokalemia.
Musculoskeletal: arm pain, arthralgia, back pain, cramps, myalgia.
Respiratory: coughing, dyspnea, pneumonia, *pulmonary edema,* upper respiratory tract infections.
Skin: increased sweating, pruritus, rash.
Other: *carcinoma,* chills, flulike syndrome, *hypersensitivity reactions,* infection, injection site reaction, rigors, *sepsis.*

Interactions

Drug-drug. *ACE inhibitors (enalapril):* May increase adverse effects of I.V. iron. Use together cautiously.
Oral iron supplements: May decrease absorption of oral iron preparations. Monitor patient.

Effects on lab test results

• May increase or decrease potassium level. May decrease glucose and hemoglobin levels and hematocrit.

Pharmacokinetics

Absorption: Given I.V.
Distribution: Unknown.
Metabolism: Unknown.
Excretion: Unknown. *Half-life:* 1 hour in otherwise healthy adults.

Route	Onset	Peak	Duration
I.V.	Unknown	Unknown	Unknown

Action

Chemical effect: Drug restores total body iron content, which is critical for normal hemoglobin synthesis and oxygen transport.

Therapeutic effect: Restores total body iron content.

Available forms

Injection: 62.5 mg elemental iron (12.5 mg/ml) in 5-ml ampules

NURSING PROCESS

Assessment
• Obtain history of patient's underlying condition before starting therapy, and reassess regularly to monitor drug's effectiveness.
• Find out about other sources of iron patient may be taking, such as nonprescription iron preparations and iron-containing multivitamin and mineral supplements.
• Monitor hematocrit and hemoglobin, MCV, ferritin, and iron saturation levels during therapy.
• Assess patient's and family's knowledge of drug therapy.

Nursing diagnoses
• Risk for injury related to drug-induced adverse reactions
• Activity intolerance related to underlying condition
• Deficient knowledge related to drug therapy

Planning and implementation
• Dose is expressed in milligrams of elemental iron.
• Don't give drug to patient with iron overload, which commonly occurs in hemoglobinopathy and other refractory anemia.
• **ALERT:** Life-threatening hypersensitivity reactions (characterized by CV collapse, cardiac arrest, bronchospasm, oral or pharyngeal edema, dyspnea, angioedema, urticaria, or pruritus sometimes linked with pain and muscle spasm of chest or back) may occur during infusion. Have adequate supportive measures readily available. Monitor patient closely.
• Some adverse reactions in hemodialysis patients may be related to dialysis itself or to chronic renal impairment.
• **ALERT:** Drug contains benzyl alcohol and may cause "gasping syndrome" in neonates.
• **ALERT:** Don't confuse Ferrlecit with Ferralet.
Patient teaching
• Advise to immediately report signs or symptoms of iron poisoning, which include abdominal pain, diarrhea, vomiting, drowsiness, or hyperventilation.

Evaluation
• Patient doesn't experience injury as a result of drug-induced adverse reactions.
• Patient experiences improved activity tolerance.
• Patient and family state understanding of drug therapy.

sodium phosphate
(SOH-dee-um FOS-fayt)
Fleet Enema, Fleet Pediatric Enema, Fleet Phospho-soda†

Pharmacologic class: acid salt
Therapeutic class: mineral, saline laxative
Pregnancy risk category: C (I.V.), NR (P.R.)

Indications and dosages

▶ **Constipation, cleansing following or preparation before a bowel procedure.** *Adults and children age 12 and older:* 20 to 45 ml of solution mixed with 120 ml of cold water P.O. Or, 120 ml P.R. (as enema).
Children ages 10 to 11: Give 10 to 20 ml of solution mixed with 120 ml of cold water P.O.
Children ages 5 to 9: Give 5 to 10 ml of solution mixed with 120 ml of cold water P.O.
Children older than age 2: Give 60 ml P.R.
▶ **Total parenteral nutrition (TPN).** *Adults and children:* Doses are highly individualized. Usually 10 to 15 millimoles (mM) per liter of TPN solution I.V.; titrate per phosphate level. Normal range 3 to 4.5 mg/dl for adults, 4 to 7 mg/dl for children.
Infants receiving TPN: Usually 1.5 to 2 mM/kg I.V. daily; titrate per phosphate level.

I.V. administration

• To avoid errors, drug should be prescribed in terms of millimoles (mM) of phosphorous.
• Dilute and mix with larger volume of fluid.
• To avoid toxicity, infuse slowly.
• Infusions with high concentrations of phosphate may cause hypocalcemia. Monitor calcium level.
⊗ **Incompatibilities**
None reported.

Reactions may be *common*, uncommon, **life-threatening**, or COMMON AND LIFE-THREATENING.

Contraindications and cautions

• Contraindicated in patients on sodium-restricted diets and in patients with intestinal obstruction or perforation, edema, heart failure, megacolon, impaired renal function, or symptoms of appendicitis or acute surgical abdomen, such as abdominal pain, nausea, and vomiting.
• I.V. sodium phosphate contraindicated in patients with hypernatremia, high phosphate level, or low calcium level.
• Use cautiously in patients with large hemorrhoids or anal abrasions.
• Use I.V. sodium phosphate cautiously in patients with cardiac disease, renal impairment, adrenal insufficiency, and cirrhosis.
☀ **Lifespan:** In pregnant women, use cautiously. In breast-feeding women, use cautiously because it's unknown if the drug appears in breast milk. In children younger than age 4, use only as directed by prescriber.

Adverse reactions

GI: abdominal cramps.
Metabolic: fluid and electrolyte disturbances (such as hypernatremia, hyperphosphatemia, hypocalcemia) with daily use.
Other: hypocalcemic tetany, laxative dependence with long-term or excessive use.

Interactions

None significant.

Effects on lab test results

• May increase sodium and phosphate levels. May decrease electrolyte level with prolonged use.

Pharmacokinetics

Absorption: About 1% to 20% of P.O. dose absorbed; unknown after P.R. administration. About 80% of I.V. dose reabsorbed through the renal tubules for homeostasis.
Distribution: Unknown.
Metabolism: Unknown.
Excretion: Renal for I.V. route. *Half-life:* Unknown.

Route	Onset	Peak	Duration
P.O.	30 min–3 hr	Varies	Varies
P.R.	5–10 min	Varies	Ends with evacuation
I.V.	Unknown	Unknown	Unknown

Action

Chemical effect: Oral and rectal use produces osmotic effect in small intestine by drawing water into intestinal lumen. I.V. use maintains body's normal phosphate level.
Therapeutic effect: Relieves constipation. Prevents hypophosphatemia.

Available forms

Enema: 160 mg/ml sodium phosphate and 60 mg/ml sodium biphosphate
I.V. infusion: 3 mM phosphate and 4 mEq sodium/L in 10-, 15-, 30-, 50-ml vials
Liquid: 2.4 g/5 ml sodium phosphate and 900 mg/5 ml sodium biphosphate

NURSING PROCESS

✥ Assessment

• Assess patient's condition before starting therapy and regularly thereafter to monitor drug's effectiveness.
• Before giving drug for constipation, determine whether patient has adequate fluid intake, exercise, and diet.
• Be alert for adverse reactions.
• Assess for signs of overdose during I.V. therapy, including paresthesias of extremities, confusion, paralysis, cardiac arrhythmias.
Ⓢ **ALERT:** Up to 10% of sodium content of drug may be absorbed.
• Assess patient's and family's knowledge of drug therapy.

✥ Nursing diagnoses

• Constipation related to underlying condition
• Acute pain related to drug-induced abdominal cramping
• Deficient knowledge related to drug therapy

▶ Planning and implementation

• Dilute drug with water before giving. Follow administration with full glass of water.
• Make sure that patient has easy access to bathroom facilities, commode, or bedpan.
Ⓢ **ALERT:** Severe electrolyte imbalances may occur if recommended dosage is exceeded.
Patient teaching
• Teach patient about dietary sources of bulk, which include bran and other cereals, fresh fruit, and vegetables.

• Tell patient to maintain adequate fluid intake of at least 6 to 8 glasses of water or juices daily unless contraindicated.

✓ Evaluation
• Patient's constipation is relieved.
• Patient's abdominal cramping ceases.
• Patient and family state understanding of drug therapy.

sodium phosphate monohydrate
(SOE-dee-um FOS-fate maw-no-HIGH-drate)

sodium phosphate dibasic anhydrous
(SOE-dee-um FOS-fate die-BAY-sick an-HIGH-drus)
Osmo-Prep, Visicol

Pharmacologic class: osmotic laxative
Therapeutic class: bowel evacuant
Pregnancy risk category: C

Indications and dosages
▶ **To cleanse the bowel before colonoscopy.**
Adults: 40 tablets taken in the following manner: The evening before the procedure, 3 tablets P.O. with at least 8 oz of clear liquid every 15 minutes for a total of 20 tablets. The last dose will be only 2 tablets. The day of the procedure, 3 tablets P.O. with at least 8 oz of clear liquid every 15 minutes for a total of 20 tablets, starting 3 to 5 hours before the procedure. The last dose will be only 2 tablets.

Contraindications and cautions
• Contraindicated in patients hypersensitive to the drug or any of its components. Avoid giving drug to patients with heart failure, ascites, unstable angina, gastric retention, ileus, acute intestinal obstruction, pseudo-obstruction, severe chronic constipation, bowel perforation, acute colitis, toxic megacolon, or hypomotility syndrome (hypothyroidism, scleroderma).
• Use cautiously in patients with a history of electrolyte abnormalities, current electrolyte abnormalities, or impaired renal function. Also, use cautiously in patients who take drugs that can induce electrolyte abnormalities or prolong the QT interval.

≋ **Lifespan:** In children, safety and effectiveness haven't been established. In elderly patients, use cautiously because of greater sensitivity to drug.

Adverse reactions
CNS: dizziness, headache.
GI: abdominal bloating, abdominal pain, nausea, vomiting.

Interactions
Drug-drug. *Oral drugs:* May reduce absorption of these drugs because of rapid peristalsis and diarrhea induced by sodium phosphate monohydrate and sodium phosphate dibasic anhydrous. Separate administration times.

Effects on lab test results
• May increase phosphorus level. May decrease potassium and calcium levels.

Pharmacokinetics
Absorption: Rapid. Duration of action is 1 to 3 hours after administration.
Distribution: Unknown.
Metabolism: Not expected to be metabolized by the liver.
Excretion: Almost entirely via the kidneys.
Half-life: Unknown.

Route	Onset	Peak	Duration
P.O.	Unknown	3 hr	1–3 hr

Action
Chemical effect: The primary mechanism probably is thought the osmotic action of sodium, which causes large amounts of water to be drawn into the colon.
Therapeutic effect: Cleanses the colon.

Available forms
Tablets: 1.5 g sodium phosphate (1.102 g sodium phosphate monohydrate and 0.398 g sodium phosphate dibasic anhydrous)

NURSING PROCESS

✍ Assessment
• Assess underlying condition before starting therapy, and reassess regularly thereafter to monitor drug's effectiveness.

• Obtain laboratory studies before starting therapy and correct electrolyte imbalances before giving drug.
• Assess patient's and family's knowledge of drug therapy.

🔹 **Nursing diagnoses**
• Acute pain related to abdominal discomfort
• Risk for deficient fluid volume related to adverse GI effects
• Deficient knowledge related to drug therapy

▷ **Planning and implementation**
• Undigested or partially digested tablets and other drugs may be seen in the stool or during colonoscopy.
• As with other sodium phosphate cathartic preparations, this drug may induce colonic mucosal ulceration.
• Monitor patient for signs of dehydration.
• Don't repeat administration within 7 days.
• No enema or laxative is needed with drug.
🔹 **ALERT:** Giving with other products containing sodium phosphate may result in death from significant fluid shifts, electrolyte abnormalities, and cardiac arrhythmias. A patient with an electrolyte disturbance has an increased risk of prolonged QT interval. Use drug cautiously in those taking other drugs known to prolong the QT interval.
Patient teaching
• Instruct patient to drink at least 8 oz of clear liquid with each dose. Inadequate fluid intake may lead to excessive fluid loss and hypovolemia.
• Tell patient to drink only clear liquids for at least 12 hours before starting the purgative regimen.
• Warn patient against taking an additional enema or laxative, particularly one that contains sodium phosphate.
• Tell patient that undigested or partially digested tablets and other drugs may appear in the stool.

✅ **Evaluation**
• Patient states that pain management methods are effective.
• Patient maintains adequate hydration.
• Patient and family state understanding of therapy.

sodium polystyrene sulfonate
(SOH-dee-um pol-ee-STIGH-reen SUL-fuh-nayt)
Kayexalate, Kionex, SPS

Pharmacologic class: cation-exchange resin
Therapeutic class: potassium-removing resin
Pregnancy risk category: C

Indications and dosages

▶ **Hyperkalemia.** *Adults:* 15 g P.O. daily to q.i.d. in water or sorbitol (3 to 4 ml/g of resin). Or mix powder with appropriate medium—aqueous suspension or diet appropriate for renal impairment—and instill into NG tube. Or, 30 to 50 g every 6 hours as warm emulsion deep into sigmoid colon (20 cm), retained for 30 minutes. In persistent vomiting or paralytic ileus, high-retention enema of sodium polystyrene sulfonate (30 g) suspended in 200 ml of 10% methylcellulose, 10% dextrose, or 25% sorbitol solution may be given.
Children: 1 g of resin P.O. or P.R. for each mEq of potassium to be removed. Or, 1 g/kg every 6 hours. P.O. route preferred because drug should stay in intestine for at least 6 hours.

Contraindications and cautions

• Contraindicated in patients hypersensitive to the drug or any of its components, and in those with hypokalemia.
• Use cautiously in patients with severe heart failure, severe hypertension, or marked edema.
🔹 **Lifespan:** In pregnant women, use cautiously. In breast-feeding women, use cautiously; it's unknown if the drug appears in breast milk.

Adverse reactions

GI: anorexia, *constipation, diarrhea* with sorbitol emulsions, fecal impaction in elderly patients, gastric irritation, nausea, vomiting.
Metabolic: hypocalcemia, hypokalemia, *hypomagnesemia,* sodium retention.

Interactions

Drug-drug. *Nonabsorbable, cation-donating antacids and laxatives including magnesium hydroxide:* May cause systemic alkalosis and reduced potassium exchange capability. Don't use together.

S

Effects on lab test results

• May increase sodium level. May decrease potassium, calcium, and magnesium levels.

Pharmacokinetics

Absorption: None.
Distribution: None.
Metabolism: None.
Excretion: Unchanged in feces. *Half-life:* Unknown.

Route	Onset	Peak	Duration
P.O., P.R.	2–12 hr	Unknown	Unknown

Action

Chemical effect: Exchanges sodium ions for potassium ions in intestine. Much of exchange capacity is used for cations other than potassium (calcium and magnesium) and, possibly, fats and proteins.
Therapeutic effect: Lowers potassium level.

Available forms

Powder: 1-lb jar (3.5 g/5 ml)
Suspension (1.25 g/5 ml): 60 ml*, 120 ml*, 480 ml*

NURSING PROCESS

⚷ Assessment

• Obtain history of patient's potassium level before starting therapy.
• Monitor potassium level regularly. Treatment may result in potassium deficiency. Treatment usually stops when potassium level declines to 4 or 5 mEq/L.
• **ALERT:** Watch for other signs of hypokalemia, such as irritability, confusion, arrhythmias, ECG changes, severe muscle weakness and paralysis, and cardiotoxicity in patient taking digitalis.
• Monitor patient for symptoms of other electrolyte deficiencies (magnesium, calcium) because drug is nonselective. In patient receiving therapy for longer than 3 days, monitor calcium level. Supplementary calcium may be needed.
• Watch for sodium overload. Drug contains about 100 mg of sodium/g. About one-third of sodium in resin is retained.
• Be alert for adverse reactions and drug interactions.
• Watch for constipation with P.O. use.
• Assess patient's and family's knowledge of drug therapy.

⊕ Nursing diagnoses

• Ineffective health maintenance related to presence of hyperkalemia
• Constipation related to drug-induced adverse GI reactions
• Deficient knowledge related to drug therapy

▷ Planning and implementation

• Don't heat resin because it will impair drug's effectiveness.
• Mix resin only with water or sorbitol for P.O. use. Never mix with orange juice (high potassium content) to disguise taste.
• Chill oral suspension for greater palatability.
• If sorbitol is given, mix with resin suspension.
• Consider solid form. Resin cookie and candy recipes are available. Ask pharmacist or dietitian to supply.
• To prevent constipation, use sorbitol (10 to 20 ml of 70% syrup every 2 hours, p.r.n.) to produce one or two watery stools daily.
• Premixed forms are available (SPS and others) for P.R. use.
• If preparing manually, mix polystyrene resin only with water and sorbitol for P.R. use. Don't use mineral oil for P.R. administration to prevent impaction. Ion exchange requires aqueous medium. Sorbitol content prevents impaction.
• Prepare P.R. dose at room temperature. Stir emulsion gently during administration.
• Use #28F rubber tube. Insert tube 20 cm into sigmoid colon and tape in place. Or, consider indwelling urinary catheter with 30-ml balloon inflated distal to anal sphincter to aid in retention. This is especially helpful for patients with poor sphincter control (for example, after stroke). Use gravity flow. Drain returns constantly through Y-tube connection. Place patient in knee-chest position or with hips on pillow for a while if back leakage occurs.
• After P.R. administration, flush tubing with 50 to 100 ml of nonsodium fluid to ensure delivery of all drug. Flush rectum to remove resin.
• Prevent fecal impaction in geriatric patient by giving resin P.R. Give cleansing enema before P.R. administration. The patient will need to retain enema, ideally for 6 to 10 hours, but 30 to 60 minutes is acceptable.
• If hyperkalemia is severe, prescriber won't depend solely on polystyrene resin to lower potassium level. Dextrose 50% with regular insulin may be given by I.V. push.

Patient teaching
- Explain importance of following prescribed low-potassium diet.
- Explain need to retain enema, ideally for 6 to 10 hours, but 30 to 60 minutes is acceptable.
- Tell patient to report adverse reactions.

☑ Evaluation
- Patient's potassium level is normal.
- Patient doesn't develop constipation.
- Patient and family state understanding of drug therapy.

solifenacin succinate
(sohl-ih-FEN-ah-sin SUC-sin-eight)
VESIcare

Pharmacologic class: muscarinic receptor antagonist
Therapeutic class: urinary tract antispasmodic
Pregnancy risk category: C

Indications and dosages
▶ **Overactive bladder with urinary urgency, frequency, and urge incontinence.** *Adults:* 5 mg P.O. once daily. May increase to 10 mg once daily if 5-mg dose is well tolerated.
🔲 Adjust-a-dose: If creatinine clearance is less than 30 ml/minute or the patient has moderate liver impairment (Child-Pugh score B), maintain the dose at 5 mg.

Contraindications and cautions
- Contraindicated in patients hypersensitive to drug or any of its components and in patients with urine or gastric retention or uncontrolled narrow-angle glaucoma. Don't use in patients with severe hepatic impairment.
- Use cautiously in patients with a history of prolonged QT interval, those being treated for angle-closure glaucoma, and those with bladder outflow obstruction, decreased GI motility, renal insufficiency, or moderate liver impairment.
⚖ **Lifespan:** In pregnant women, use only if benefits outweigh potential risks to the fetus. Women shouldn't breast-feed while taking drug. Safety and effectiveness in children hasn't been established. In elderly patients, level and half-life may increase though safety and effectiveness are similar to those for younger adults.

Adverse reactions
CNS: depression, dizziness, fatigue.
CV: hypertension, leg swelling.
EENT: blurred vision, dry eyes, pharyngitis.
GI: *constipation, dry mouth,* dyspepsia, nausea, upper abdominal pain, vomiting.
GU: urine retention, UTI.
Respiratory: cough.
Other: influenza.

Interactions
Drug-drug. *Drugs that prolong the QT interval:* May increase the risk of serious cardiac arrhythmias. Monitor patient and ECG closely. *Potent CYP3A4 inhibitors (such as ketoconazole):* May increase solifenacin level. Don't exceed solifenacin dose of 5 mg daily when used together.

Effects on lab test results
None reported.

Pharmacokinetics
Absorption: Absolute bioavailability is about 90%.
Distribution: Wide, except in CNS. About 98% bound by plasma proteins.
Metabolism: Extensive, mainly by CYP3A4.
Excretion: Mainly in urine and, to a lesser extent, feces. *Half-life:* 2 or 3 days.

Route	Onset	Peak	Duration
P.O.	Unknown	3–8 hr	Unknown

Action
Chemical effect: Relaxes smooth muscle of the bladder by competitively antagonizing the muscarinic receptors.
Therapeutic effect: Relieves symptoms of overactive bladder.

Available forms
Tablets (film-coated): 5 mg, 10 mg

NURSING PROCESS

🔲 Assessment
- Assess bladder function, and monitor drug effects.
- Monitor patient for decreased gastric motility and constipation.

- Evaluate patient's and family's knowledge of drug therapy.

⊞ Nursing diagnoses
- Impaired urinary elimination related to underlying medical condition
- Constipation related to drug-induced adverse effects
- Deficient knowledge related to drug therapy

▣ Planning and implementation
- If patient has bladder outlet obstruction, watch for urine retention.
- If the patient has urinary retention, notify prescriber and prepare for urinary catheterization.
- Dry mouth and constipation are the most frequently reported adverse effects of drug therapy.
- Chronic overdose may result in fixed, dilated pupils, blurred vision, dry skin, tremors, and inability to perform the heel-to-toe exam. These effects should subside when drug is stopped.

Patient teaching
- Explain that drug may blur vision. Tell patient to use caution when performing hazardous activities or tasks that require clear vision until effects of the drug are known.
- Discourage use of other drugs that may cause dry mouth, constipation, urine retention, or blurred vision.
- Urge patient to notify prescriber about abdominal pain or constipation that lasts 3 days or longer.
- Tell patient that drug decreases the ability to sweat normally, and advise cautious use in hot environments or during strenuous activity.
- Tell patient to swallow tablet whole with liquid.
- Inform patient that drug may be taken with or without food.

☑ Evaluation
- Patient experiences improved bladder function with drug therapy.
- Patient maintains normal bowel regimen.
- Patient and family state understanding of drug therapy.

somatropin
(soh-muh-TROH-pin)
Genotropin, Genotropin MiniQuick, Humatrope, Norditropin, Nutropin, Nutropin AQ, Saizen, Serostim, Tev-Tropin, Zorbtive

Pharmacologic class: anterior pituitary hormone
Therapeutic class: human growth hormone (GH)
Pregnancy risk category: C

Indications and dosages

▶ **Long-term therapy for growth failure in patients with inadequate secretion of endogenous GH.** *Children:* 0.18 to 0.3 mg/kg Humatrope subcutaneously or I.M. weekly, divided equally and given either 3 alternate days, six times weekly, or daily. Or, up to 0.3 mg/kg Nutropin or Nutropin AQ subcutaneously weekly in daily divided doses. Or, 0.06 mg/kg Saizen I.M. or subcutaneously three times weekly. Or, 0.024 to 0.034 mg/kg Norditropin subcutaneously, six to seven times weekly. Or 0.16 to 0.24 mg/kg Genotropin subcutaneously weekly, divided into five to seven doses. Or 1.5 mg/kg somatropin depot subcutaneously once monthly or 0.75 mg/kg subcutaneously twice monthly on the same days of each month.

▶ **Growth failure from chronic renal insufficiency up to time of kidney transplant.** *Children:* Weekly dosage of up to 0.35 mg/kg Nutropin or Nutropin AQ subcutaneously divided into daily doses.

▶ **Long-term therapy for short stature related to Turner syndrome.** *Children:* Up to 0.375 mg/kg Humatrope, Nutropin, or Nutropin AQ subcutaneously weekly, divided into equal doses given three to seven times weekly. Up to 0.067 mg/kg Norditropin subcutaneously daily.

▶ **Short stature related to Noonan syndrome.** *Children:* Up to 0.066 mg/kg Norditropin subcutaneously daily.

▶ **Long-term therapy for growth failure in children with Prader-Willi syndrome (PWS) diagnosed by genetic testing.** *Children:* 0.24 mg/kg Genotropin subcutaneously weekly, divided into six to seven doses.

▶ **To replace endogenous GH in patients with GH deficiency.** *Adults:* Initially, not more than 0.006 mg/kg Humatrope, Nutropin, or Nu-

tropin AQ subcutaneously daily. Humatrope may be increased to maximum of 0.0125 mg/kg daily. Nutropin and Nutropin AQ may be increased to maximum of 0.025 mg/kg daily in patients younger than age 35 or 0.0125 mg/kg daily in patients older than age 35. With Genotropin, starting dose isn't more than 0.04 mg/kg subcutaneously weekly, divided into six to seven doses. Dose may be increased at 4- to 8-week intervals to a maximum dose of 0.08 mg/kg subcutaneously weekly, divided into six to seven doses. With Saizen, starting dose isn't more than 0.005 mg/kg/day. May increase after 4 weeks to maximum of 0.01 mg/kg/day based on patient tolerance and clinical response.

▶ **AIDS wasting or cachexia.** *Adults and children weighing more than 55 kg (121 lb):* 6 mg Serostim subcutaneously at bedtime.
Adults and children weighing 45 to 55 kg (99 to 121 lb): 5 mg Serostim subcutaneously at bedtime.
Adults and children weighing 35 to 45 kg (77 to 99 lb): 4 mg Serostim subcutaneously at bedtime.
Adults and children weighing less than 35 kg: 0.1 mg/kg Serostim subcutaneously daily at bedtime.

▶ **Long-term treatment of growth failure in children born small for gestational age who don't achieve catch-up growth by age 2.** *Children:* 0.48 mg/kg Genotropin subcutaneously weekly, divided into five to seven doses.
▶ **Idiopathic short stature.** *Children:* Up to 0.37 mg/kg Humatrope subcutaneously weekly, divided into equal doses given 6 to 7 times per week.

Contraindications and cautions

• Contraindicated in patients with closed epiphyses or active underlying intracranial lesion.
• Don't reconstitute Humatrope with supplied diluent for patients with known sensitivity to either m-cresol or glycerin.
• Genotropin is contraindicated in patients with PWS who are severely obese or have severe respiratory impairment.
☀ **Lifespan:** In pregnant and breast-feeding women, drug isn't indicated. In children with hypothyroidism and in those with GH deficiency caused by an intracranial lesion, use cautiously; these children should be examined frequently for progression or recurrence of underlying disease.

Adverse reactions

CNS: headache, weakness.
CV: mild, transient edema.
Hematologic: *leukemia.*
Metabolic: hypothyroidism, mild hyperglycemia.
Musculoskeletal: localized muscle pain.
Other: *antibodies to GH,* injection site pain.

Interactions

Drug-drug. *Corticosteroids, corticotropin:* May inhibit growth response to GH with long-term use. Monitor patient.

Effects on lab test results

• May increase glucose, inorganic phosphorus, alkaline phosphatase, and parathyroid hormone levels.

Pharmacokinetics

Vary by formulation.
Absorption: About 80% bioavailable after subcutaneous injection.
Distribution: Unknown.
Metabolism: About 90% in liver.
Excretion: About 0.1% unchanged in urine.
Half-life: ½ to 3 hours.

Route	Onset	Peak	Duration
I.M, SubQ	Unknown	7½ hr	12–48 hr

Action

Chemical effect: Purified GH of recombinant DNA origin that stimulates linear, skeletal muscle, and organ growth.
Therapeutic effect: Stimulates growth.

Available forms

Genotropin injection: 5.8 mg (about 17.4 international units/vial), 13.8 mg (about 41.4 international units/vial)
Genotropin MiniQuick injection: 0.2 mg/vial, 0.4 mg/vial, 0.6 mg/vial, 0.8 mg/vial, 1 mg/vial, 1.2 mg/vial, 1.4 mg/vial, 1.6 mg/vial, 1.8 mg/vial, 2 mg/vial
Humatrope injection: 5 mg (about 15 international units/vial), 6 mg (18 international units/cartridge), 12 mg (36 international units/cartridge), 24 mg (72 international units/cartridge)
Norditropin injection: 4 mg (about 12 international units/ml), 8 mg (about 24 international units/ml), 5 mg/1.5 ml cartridges, 10 mg/1.5 ml cartridges, 15 mg/1.5 ml cartridges

Nutropin AQ injection: 10 mg (about 30 international units/vial)
Nutropin injection: 5 mg (about 15 international units/vial), 10 mg (about 30 international units/vial)
Saizen injection: 5 mg (about 15 international units/vial)
Serostim injection: 4 mg (about 12 international units/vial), 5 mg (about 15 international units/vial), 6 mg (about 18 international units/vial)
Somatropin depot injection: 13.5 mg/vial, 18 mg/vial, 22.5 mg/vial
Tev-Tropin injection: 5 mg (about 15 international units/vial)
Zorbtive injection: 4 mg (about 12 international units/vial), 5 mg (about 15 international units/vial), 6 mg (about 18 international units/vial), 8.8 mg (about 26.4 international units/vial)

NURSING PROCESS

🔍 Assessment
• Assess child's growth before therapy and regularly thereafter to monitor drug's effectiveness.
• Ensure adults taking Saizen for GH replacement have GH deficiency alone or with multiple hormone deficiencies (result of pituitary or hypothalamic disease, surgery, radiation, or trauma) or had GH deficiency during childhood and confirmed deficiency as an adult.
• Be alert for adverse reactions.
• Toxicity in neonates may occur from exposure to benzyl alcohol used in drug as preservative.
• Conduct regular checkup with monitoring of height, blood, and radiologic studies.
• Observe patient for signs of glucose intolerance and hyperglycemia.
• Monitor patient's periodic thyroid function tests for hypothyroidism, which may require treatment with thyroid hormone.
• Assess patient's and family's knowledge of drug therapy.

Nursing diagnoses
• Delayed growth and development related to lack of adequate endogenous GH
• Ineffective health maintenance related to adverse metabolic reactions
• Deficient knowledge related to drug therapy

⮞ Planning and implementation
• To prepare solution, inject supplied diluent into vial containing drug by aiming stream of liquid against glass wall of vial. Then swirl vial with gentle rotary motion until contents are completely dissolved; don't shake vial.
• After reconstitution, solution should be clear. Don't inject solution if it's cloudy or contains particles.
• The subcutaneous route is preferred. Rotate injection sites to reduce the risk of lipoatrophy.
• Store reconstituted drug in refrigerator; use within 14 days.
• If sensitivity to diluent develops, drugs may be reconstituted with sterile water for injection. When drug is reconstituted in this manner, use only one reconstituted dose per vial, refrigerate solution if it isn't used immediately after reconstitution, use reconstituted dose within 24 hours, and discard unused portion.
• If final height is achieved, or epiphyseal fusion occurs, do not continue therapy.
• Excessive glucocorticoid therapy inhibits growth-promoting effect of somatropin. In patient with corticotropin deficiency, adjust glucocorticoid-replacement dosage carefully to avoid growth inhibition.
⏺ **ALERT:** Don't confuse somatropin with somatrem or sumatriptan.
Patient teaching
• Inform parents that child with endocrine disorders (including GH deficiency) may develop slipped capital epiphyses. Tell them to notify prescriber if child begins limping.

☑ Evaluation
• Patient exhibits growth.
• Patient's thyroid function studies and glucose level are normal.
• Patient and family state understanding of drug therapy.

HIGH ALERT

sorafenib
(soar-uh-PHEN-ihb)
Nexavar✑

Pharmacologic class: multi-kinase inhibitor
Therapeutic class: antineoplastic
Pregnancy risk category: D

Indications and dosages

NEW INDICATION: Unresectable hepatocellular carcinoma. *Adults:* 400 mg P.O. b.i.d. without food. Dosage may be reduced to 400 mg per day or every other day if adverse reactions such as toxic skin effects occur.

▶ **Advanced renal cell carcinoma.** *Adults:* 400 mg P.O. b.i.d. at least 1 hour before or 2 hours after eating. Continue until disease progresses or unacceptable toxicity occurs.

Adjust-a-dose: If patient develops grade 2 skin toxicity (pain and swelling with normal activities), continue treatment and use topical therapy to relieve symptoms. If symptoms don't improve in 1 week or if they occur a second or third time, stop treatment until toxicity resolves to grade 0 or 1 (able to perform daily activities). Resume treatment at 400 mg daily or every other day. At fourth occurrence of grade 2 toxicity, stop treatment.

If patient develops grade 3 skin toxicity (ulceration, blistering, severe pain of hands and feet, leaving patient unable to perform daily activities) or a second occurrence, stop treatment until toxicity resolves to grade 0 or 1. Resume treatment at 400 mg daily or every other day. At third occurrence of grade 3 toxicity, stop treatment.

Contraindications and cautions

• Contraindicated in patients severely hypersensitive to drug or its components.
• Use cautiously in patients with bleeding disorders, healing wounds, current or previous hand-foot skin reactions, or liver, renal, or cardiac disease, such as hypertension, cardiac ischemia, or a history of MI.

Lifespan: Drug may cause serious birth defects or fetal death. Warn women of childbearing potential to avoid pregnancy during and for 2 weeks following treatment. Mothers shouldn't breast-feed during treatment. In children, safety and effectiveness haven't been established. Elderly patients may be more sensitive to adverse effects.

Adverse reactions

CNS: *asthenia,* depression, *fatigue, headache, neuropathy.*
CV: hypertension.
EENT: hoarseness.

GI: abdominal pain, anorexia, constipation, diarrhea, dyspepsia, dysphagia, mucositis, nausea, stomatitis, vomiting.
GU: erectile dysfunction.
Hematologic: anemia, *bleeding, **hemorrhage, leukopenia, lymphopenia, neutropenia, thrombocytopenia.***
Metabolic: *hypophosphatemia,* hypothyroidism, *weight loss.*
Musculoskeletal: *arthralgia, joint pain, myalgia.*
Respiratory: *cough, dyspnea.*
Skin: acne, *alopecia, dry skin,* erythema, exfoliative dermatitis, flushing, *hand-foot reaction, pruritus, rash.*
Other: flulike illness, pyrexia.

Interactions

Drug-drug. *CYP2B6 or CYP2C8 substrates:* May increase levels of these drugs. Use cautiously together.
CYP3A4 inducers (such as carbamazepine, dexamethasone, phenobarbital, phenytoin, rifampin): May increase sorafenib metabolism and decrease its effects. Monitor patient.
Doxorubicin, drugs metabolized by the UGT1A1 pathway (such as irinotecan): May increase levels of these drugs. Use cautiously together.
Warfarin: May increase the risk of bleeding. Monitor PT, INR, and patient for bleeding.
Drug-herb. *St. John's wort:* May decrease drug effects. Discourage use together.

Effects on lab test results

• May increase TSH, lipase, amylase, transaminase, and bilirubin levels. May decrease phosphate level.
• May decrease RBC, WBC, and platelet counts.

Pharmacokinetics

Absorption: Well absorbed; food reduces bioavailability.
Distribution: 99.5% bound by plasma proteins.
Metabolism: In the liver by CYP3A4 and by glucuronidation mediated by UGT1A9.
Excretion: 77% in feces, 19% in urine. *Half-life:* 25 to 48 hours.

Route	Onset	Peak	Duration
P.O.	Unknown	3 hr	Unknown

Action

Chemical effect: Decreases tumor cell proliferation by interacting with multiple intracellular and cell-surface kinases that may influence growth of new blood vessels into a tumor.
Therapeutic effect: Slows carcinoma growth.

Available forms

Tablets: 200 mg

NURSING PROCESS

Assessment
• Assess neoplastic disease before starting therapy, and reassess regularly.
• To avoid serious drug interactions, take a careful drug history.
• Monitor patient closely for hand-foot skin reaction, especially during the first 6 weeks of treatment.
• Monitor patient for cardiac ischemia.
• Assess patient for unusual bruising or bleeding.
• Assess patient's and family's knowledge of drug therapy.

Nursing diagnoses
• Ineffective health maintenance related to neoplastic disease
• Risk for falls related to drug-induced adverse reactions
• Deficient knowledge related to drug therapy

Planning and implementation
• Measure blood pressure weekly during the first 6 weeks of treatment to check for hypertension.
• Stop therapy in patients undergoing major surgery. Before restarting therapy, monitor incision for adequate healing.
• Provide patient with contact information for cancer support groups and instructions for managing adverse effects.
Patient teaching
• Tell patient to swallow tablet whole, 1 hour before or 2 hours after a meal, with water.
• Remind patient to have his blood pressure checked weekly for the first 6 weeks of treatment and as needed throughout therapy.
• Explain that hair loss, nausea, vomiting, diarrhea, and fatigue are common.
• Inform patient that mild to moderate skin reactions are common. Tell him to notify pre-

scriber if they occur. If they're severe, treatment may have to be stopped or dosage reduced. Urge patient to report pain, redness, blisters, or skin ulceration to prescriber immediately.
• Tell patient to report bleeding episodes right away.
• Tell patient to notify prescriber if he develops chest pain or other serious heart problem.
⚠ **ALERT:** Advise women to avoid pregnancy during treatment and for at least 2 weeks afterward. Men and women should both use effective contraception during this time.
• Tell patient to keep an up-to-date list of all medications he takes and to tell all health care providers, including dentists, that he takes this drug.

Evaluation
• Patient shows positive response to drug therapy on follow-up studies.
• Patient doesn't experience falls.
• Patient and family state understanding of drug therapy.

sotalol hydrochloride
(SOH-tuh-lol high-droh-KLOR-ighd)
Betapace, Betapace AF, Rylosol ◆

Pharmacologic class: beta blocker
Therapeutic class: antianginal, antiarrhythmic, antihypertensive
Pregnancy risk category: B

Indications and dosages

▶ **Documented, life-threatening ventricular arrhythmias.** *Adults:* Initially, 80 mg Betapace P.O. b.i.d. Dosage is increased every 2 to 3 days as needed and tolerated; most patients respond to 160 to 320 mg daily. A few patients with refractory arrhythmias have received as much as 640 mg daily.
Adjust-a-dose: For patients with renal impairment, if creatinine clearance is 30 to 60 ml/minute, interval is increased to every 24 hours; if clearance is 10 to 30 ml/minute, give every 36 to 48 hours; if clearance is less than 10 ml/minute, individualize dosage.
▶ **To maintain normal sinus rhythm (delayed recurrence of atrial fibrillation or flutter) in patients with symptomatic atrial fibrillation or flutter who are currently in sinus rhythm.**

Reactions may be *common*, uncommon, *life-threatening*, or COMMON AND LIFE-THREATENING.

Adults: Initially, 80 mg Betapace AF P.O. b.i.d. If initial dose doesn't reduce the frequency of relapses of atrial fibrillation or flutter and patient has a QTc interval of less than 520 msec, may increase to 120 mg P.O. b.i.d. after 3 days. Maximum, 160 mg P.O. b.i.d.

⧄ **Adjust-a-dose:** For patients with renal impairment, if creatinine clearance is 40 to 60 ml/ minute, give once daily.

Contraindications and cautions

• Contraindicated in patients hypersensitive to the drug or any of its components, and patients with severe sinus node dysfunction, sinus bradycardia, second- or third-degree AV block in absence of an artificial pacemaker, congenital or acquired long-QT interval syndrome, cardiogenic shock, uncontrolled heart failure, or bronchial asthma. Don't give to patients with a creatinine clearance less than 40 ml/minute.
• Use cautiously in patients with renal impairment, sick sinus syndrome, or diabetes mellitus.
⚖ **Lifespan:** In pregnant women, use cautiously. In breast-feeding women and in children, safety and effectiveness haven't been established.

Adverse reactions

CNS: asthenia, dizziness, fatigue, headache, lightheadedness, sleep problems, weakness.
CV: *arrhythmias, AV block, bradycardia,* chest pain, ECG abnormalities, edema, *heart failure,* hypotension, palpitations, *proarrhythmic events (ventricular tachycardia, PVCs, ventricular fibrillation).*
GI: diarrhea, dyspepsia, *nausea,* vomiting.
Respiratory: *bronchospasm,* dyspnea.

Interactions

Drug-drug. *Antacids containing aluminum oxide or magnesium hydroxide:* May decrease effect of sotalol. Stagger dosing by 2 hours.
Antiarrhythmics: May have additive effects. Avoid using together.
Antihypertensives, catecholamine-depleting drugs (such as guanethidine, haloperidol, and reserpine): May enhance hypotensive effects. Monitor patient closely.
Calcium channel blockers: May enhance myocardial depression. Monitor patient carefully.
Clonidine: May enhance rebound effect seen after withdrawal of clonidine. May cause life-threatening or fatal increases in blood pressure.

Stop sotalol several days before withdrawing clonidine.
General anesthetics: May cause additional myocardial depression. Monitor patient closely.
Insulin, oral antidiabetics: May cause hyperglycemia and mask its symptoms. Adjust dosage.
Macrolide antibiotics, quinolones: May increase risk of arrhythmias. Use together cautiously.
Prazosin: May increase the risk of orthostatic hypotension in the early phases of use together. Assist patient to stand slowly until effects are known.

Effects on lab test results

• May increase glucose level.

Pharmacokinetics

Absorption: Well absorbed, with bioavailability of 90% to 100%. Food may interfere.
Distribution: Unknown. Doesn't bind to proteins and crosses blood-brain barrier poorly.
Metabolism: Not metabolized.
Excretion: Mainly in urine in unchanged form.
Half-life: 12 hours.

Route	Onset	Peak	Duration
P.O.	Unknown	2½–4 hr	Unknown

Action

Chemical effect: Depresses sinus heart rate, slows AV conduction, decreases cardiac output, and lowers systolic and diastolic blood pressure.
Therapeutic effect: Restores normal sinus rhythm, lowers blood pressure, and relieves angina.

Available forms

Tablets: 80 mg, 120 mg, 160 mg, 240 mg

NURSING PROCESS

⊥ Assessment

• Assess patient's condition before starting therapy and regularly thereafter to monitor drug's effectiveness.
• Monitor patient's electrolyte level and ECG regularly, especially if patient is taking diuretics. Electrolyte imbalances, such as hypokalemia and hypomagnesemia, may enhance QT interval prolongation and increase risk of serious arrhythmias such as torsades de pointes.
• Be alert for adverse reactions and drug interactions.

- Assess patient's and family's knowledge of drug therapy.

◈ Nursing diagnoses
- Ineffective health maintenance related to underlying condition
- Fatigue related to adverse reactions
- Deficient knowledge related to drug therapy

▷ Planning and implementation
- Because proarrhythmic events may occur at start of therapy and during dosage adjustments, patient should be hospitalized for a minimum of 3 days on the maintenance dose. Facilities and personnel should be available to monitor cardiac rhythm and interpret ECG.
- Although patient receiving I.V. lidocaine can start therapy with sotalol without ill effect, other antiarrhythmics should be stopped before starting therapy. Therapy typically is delayed until 2 or 3 half-lives have elapsed. After withdrawal of amiodarone, sotalol shouldn't be given until QT interval normalizes.
- Adjust dosage slowly, allowing 2 to 3 days between dose increases for adequate monitoring of QT intervals and for drug level to reach steady-state level.
- ⊛ **ALERT:** The baseline QTc interval must be 450 msec or less in order to start a patient on Betapace AF. During initiation and adjustment, monitor QT interval 2 to 4 hours after each dose. If the QTc interval is 500 msec or longer, reduce dosage or stop drug.
- ⊛ **ALERT:** Don't confuse sotalol with Stadol. Don't substitute Betapace AF for Betapace.

Patient teaching
- Explain importance of taking drug as prescribed, even when feeling well. Instruct patient not to stop drug suddenly.
- Tell patient that drug may be taken without regard to meals, but should be taken the same way consistently.
- Tell patient to take antacids two hours after sotalol to avoid interfering with absorption.
- Teach patient how to check his pulse rate.

☑ Evaluation
- Patient responds well to therapy.
- Patient states energy-conserving measures to combat fatigue.
- Patient and family state understanding of drug therapy.

spironolactone
(spih-ron-uh-LAK-tohn)
Aldactone, Novo-spiroton

Pharmacologic class: mineralocorticoid receptor antagonist
Therapeutic class: potassium-sparing diuretic
Pregnancy risk category: C

Indications and dosages
▶ **Edema.** *Adults:* 25 to 200 mg P.O. daily or in divided doses.
Children: 3.3 mg/kg P.O. daily or in divided doses.
▶ **Essential hypertension.** *Adults:* 50 to 100 mg P.O. daily or in divided doses.
Children: 1 to 2 mg/kg P.O. b.i.d.
▶ **Diuretic-induced hypokalemia.** *Adults:* 25 to 100 mg P.O. daily when P.O. potassium supplements are contraindicated.
▶ **Diagnosis of primary hyperaldosteronism.** *Adults:* 400 mg P.O. daily for 4 days (short test) or 3 to 4 weeks (long test). If hypokalemia and hypertension are corrected, presumptive diagnosis of primary hyperaldosteronism is made.
▶ **To manage primary hyperaldosteronism.** *Adults:* 100 to 400 mg P.O. daily. In patients unwilling or unable to undergo surgery, start with 400 mg daily and then maintain at lowest possible dose.
▶ **Hirsutism‡.** *Adults:* 50 to 200 mg P.O. daily.
▶ **Premenstrual syndrome‡.** *Adults:* 25 mg P.O. q.i.d. beginning on day 14 of menstrual cycle.
▶ **Heart failure in patients taking an ACE inhibitor and a loop diuretic with or without digoxin‡.** *Adults:* Initially, 12.5 to 25 mg P.O. daily.
▶ **To decrease risk of metrorrhagia‡.** *Adults:* 50 mg P.O. b.i.d. on days 4 through 21 of menstrual cycle.
▶ **Acne vulgaris‡.** *Adults:* 100 mg P.O. daily.

Contraindications and cautions
- Contraindicated in patients with anuria, acute or progressive renal insufficiency, rapidly deteriorating renal function, or hyperkalemia.
- Contraindicated in patients taking amiloride or triamterene concomitantly.

- Use cautiously in patients with fluid or electrolyte imbalances, impaired kidney function, or hepatic disease.

☀ **Lifespan:** In pregnant women, use cautiously. In breast-feeding women, safety and effectiveness haven't been established.

Adverse reactions

CNS: ataxia, confusion, drowsiness, headache, lethargy.
GI: cramping, diarrhea, gastric bleeding, gastritis, ulceration, vomiting.
GU: impotence, menstrual disturbances.
Hematologic: *agranulocytosis.*
Metabolic: dehydration, *hyperkalemia,* hyponatremia, mild acidosis.
Skin: erythematous rash, hirsutism, maculopapular eruptions, urticaria.
Other: *anaphylaxis, angioedema,* breast soreness, drug fever, gynecomastia.

Interactions

Drug-drug. *ACE inhibitors, indomethacin, other potassium-sparing diuretics, potassium supplements:* May increase risk of hyperkalemia. Don't use together, especially in patients with renal impairment.
Aspirin, other salicylates: May block diuretic effect of spironolactone. Antihypertensive effect of drug not affected. Monitor edema, ascites, fluid overload.
Barbiturates and narcotics: May increase risk of orthostatic hypotension. Use cautiously together.
Corticosteroids, ACTH: May intensify electrolyte depletion, causing hypokalemia. Monitor potassium levels.
Digoxin: May alter digoxin clearance, increasing risk of digoxin toxicity. Monitor digoxin level.
Lithium: May increase risk of lithium toxicity. Don't use together.
Warfarin, other anticoagulants: May decrease effectiveness of anticoagulants. Monitor PT and INR; increase dosage as needed.
Drug-food. *Potassium-containing salt substitutes, potassium-rich foods (such as citrus fruits, tomatoes):* May increase risk of hyperkalemia. Tell patient to use low-potassium salt substitutes and to eat high-potassium foods cautiously.

Drug-lifestyle. *Alcohol:* May increase risk of orthostatic hypotension. Discourage use together.

Effects on lab test results

- May increase BUN, creatinine, and potassium levels. May decrease sodium level.
- May decrease granulocyte count.
- May falsely increase digoxin level.

Pharmacokinetics

Absorption: About 90%.
Distribution: More than 90% protein-bound.
Metabolism: Rapid and extensive.
Excretion: Canrenone and other metabolites mainly in urine, minimally in feces. *Half-life:* 1¼ to 2 hours.

Route	Onset	Peak	Duration
P.O.	Unknown	1–2 hr	Unknown

Action

Chemical effect: Antagonizes aldosterone in distal tubule.
Therapeutic effect: Promotes water and sodium excretion and hinders potassium excretion, lowers blood pressure, and helps to diagnose primary hyperaldosteronism.

Available forms

Tablets: 25 mg, 50 mg, 100 mg

NURSING PROCESS

Assessment
- Assess patient's condition before starting therapy and regularly thereafter to monitor drug's effectiveness. Maximum antihypertensive response may be delayed up to 2 weeks.
- Monitor electrolyte level, fluid intake and output, weight, and blood pressure.
- Be alert for adverse reactions and drug interactions.
- Assess patient's and family's knowledge of drug therapy.

Nursing diagnoses
- Excess fluid volume related to presence of edema
- Impaired urinary elimination related to diuretic therapy
- Deficient knowledge related to drug therapy

▷ Planning and implementation
● Give drug with meals to enhance absorption.
● Protect drug from light.
● Inform laboratory that patient is taking spironolactone because it may interfere with some laboratory tests that measure digoxin level.
⑤ **ALERT:** Don't confuse Aldactone with Aldactazide.

Patient teaching
⑤ **ALERT:** To prevent serious hyperkalemia, warn patient not to eat large amounts of potassium-rich foods and not to use potassium-containing salt substitutes or potassium supplements.
● Tell patient to take drug with meals and, if possible, early in day to avoid interruption of sleep by nocturia.

☑ Evaluation
● Patient shows no signs of edema.
● Patient demonstrates adjustment of lifestyle to deal with altered patterns of urinary elimination.
● Patient and family state understanding of drug therapy.

stavudine (2,3-didehydro-3-deoxythymidine, d4T)
(stay-VYOO-deen)
Zerit, Zerit XR

Pharmacologic class: nucleoside reverse transcriptase inhibitor
Therapeutic class: antiretroviral
Pregnancy risk category: C

Indications and dosages

▶ **Patients with advanced HIV infection who are intolerant of or unresponsive to other antivirals.** *Adults and children who weigh 60 kg (132 lb) or more:* 40 mg P.O. every 12 hours, or 100 mg P.O. extended-release daily.
Adults and children who weigh more than 30 kg (66 lb) but less than 60 kg: 30 mg P.O. every 12 hours, or 75 mg P.O. extended-release daily.
Children who weigh less than 30 kg: 1 mg/kg every 12 hours if at least age 14 days. If age 13 days or less, give 0.5 mg/kg every 12 hours.
⑤ **Adjust-a-dose:** For patients with renal impairment adjust dosage as follows. If creatinine clearance is 26 to 50 ml/minute, give 20 mg

every 12 hours if patient weighs 60 kg or more or 15 mg every 12 hours if patient weighs less than 60 kg. If creatinine clearance is 10 to 25 ml/minute, give 20 mg every 24 hours if patient weighs 60 kg or more or 15 mg every 24 hours if patient weighs less than 60 kg. For adults undergoing hemodialysis, give 20 mg every 24 hours if patient weighs 60 kg or more or 15 mg every 24 hours if patient weighs less than 60 kg. Give dose after hemodialysis.

Contraindications and cautions
● Contraindicated in patients hypersensitive to the drug or any of its components.
● Don't use Zerit XR in patients with creatinine clearance of 50 ml/minute or less.
● Lactic acidosis and severe hepatomegaly with steatosis, including fatal cases, have been reported with the use of nucleoside analogues alone or in combination, including stavudine.
● Use cautiously in patients with renal impairment or a history of peripheral neuropathy.
≋ **Lifespan:** In pregnant women, use cautiously. In breast-feeding women, safety and effectiveness haven't been established.

Adverse reactions
CNS: anxiety, asthenia, depression, dizziness, fever, headache, insomnia, malaise, nervousness, peripheral neuropathy.
CV: chest pain.
EENT: conjunctivitis.
GI: abdominal pain, anorexia, constipation, diarrhea, dyspepsia, nausea, *pancreatitis,* vomiting, weight loss.
Hematologic: anemia, *leukopenia, neutropenia, thrombocytopenia.*
Hepatic: *hepatotoxicity,* severe hepatomegaly with steatosis.
Metabolic: *lactic acidosis.*
Musculoskeletal: *arthralgia, back pain,* myalgia.
Respiratory: *dyspnea.*
Skin: diaphoresis, maculopapular rash, pruritus, rash.
Other: breast enlargement, *chills,* redistribution or accumulation of body fat.

Interactions
Drug-drug. *Didanosine, hydroxyurea:* May increase risk of lactic acidosis, hepatotoxicity, pancreatitis, peripheral neuropathy. Monitor patient closely.

Reactions may be *common,* uncommon, *life-threatening*, or COMMON AND LIFE-THREATENING.

Doxorubicin, ribavirin: May increase risk of toxicities. Use together cautiously.
Ketoconazole, ritonavir: May increase stavudine level. Monitor patient closely.
Methadone: May decrease stavudine absorption. Avoid using together.
Myelosuppressants: May cause additive myelosuppression. Avoid using together.
Zidovudine: May inhibit stavudine phosphorylation. Don't use together.

Effects on lab test results

• May increase liver enzyme level. May decrease hemoglobin level and hematocrit.
• May decrease neutrophil and platelet counts.

Pharmacokinetics

Absorption: Rapid with mean absolute bioavailability of 86.4% for immediate release; slower and less bioavailability with extended-release form.
Distribution: Equal, between RBCs and plasma. Binds poorly to proteins.
Metabolism: Not extensive.
Excretion: About 40% renal. *Half-life:* 1 to 2 hours.

Route	Onset	Peak	Duration
P.O.	Unknown	1 hr	8 hr
P.O. extended-release	Unknown	3 hr	24 hr

Action

Chemical effect: Prevents replication of HIV by interfering with enzyme reverse transcriptase.
Therapeutic effect: Inhibits HIV infection.

Available forms

Capsules: 15 mg, 20 mg, 30 mg, 40 mg
Capsules (extended-release): 37.5 mg, 50 mg, 75 mg, 100 mg
Powder for oral solution: 1 mg/ml

NURSING PROCESS

☰ Assessment

• Assess patient's condition before starting therapy and regularly thereafter to monitor drug's effectiveness.
• Periodically monitor CBC and levels of creatinine, AST, ALT, and alkaline phosphatase.

• Be alert for adverse reactions and drug interactions.
• Assess patient's and family's knowledge of drug therapy.

⊞ Nursing diagnoses

• Risk for infection related to presence of HIV
• Disturbed sensory perception (peripheral) related to drug-induced peripheral neuropathy
• Deficient knowledge related to drug therapy

▶ Planning and implementation

③ **ALERT:** Peripheral neuropathy appears to be major dose-limiting adverse effect. If it occurs, temporarily stop giving the drug; then resume at 50% of recommended dose.
• Dose is calculated based on patient's weight.
③ **ALERT:** Don't confuse drug with other antivirals that may use initials for identification.
• Motor weakness that mimics Guillain-Barré syndrome (including respiratory failure) may occur in HIV-positive patient taking this drug with other antiretrovirals, usually in those with lactic acidosis. Monitor patient for evidence of lactic acidosis, including generalized fatigue, GI problems, tachypnea, or dyspnea. Symptoms may continue or worsen when stopping drug. In patients with these symptoms, promptly stop antiretroviral therapy and perform a full medical workup immediately. Permanently stopping drug should be considered.
• Monitor patient for pancreatitis, especially when this drug is used with didanosine or hydroxyurea. Use caution when restarting drug after confirmed diagnosis of pancreatitis.
• If patient has trouble swallowing capsule, mix contents of the capsule in applesauce or yogurt. Instruct patient not to chew or crush the beads while swallowing.
Patient teaching
• Tell patient that drug may be taken with or without food.
• Tell patient to shake oral solution vigorously before taking it, to store it in the refrigerator, and to discard unused solution after 30 days.
• Advise patient that he can't take drug if he developed peripheral neuropathy while taking other nucleoside analogues or if his treatment plan includes cytotoxic antineoplastics.
• Warn patient not to take any other drugs for HIV or AIDS (especially street drugs) unless prescriber has approved them.

- Explain that drug doesn't prevent transmission of virus; tell patient to use a barrier method of contraception.
- Teach patient signs and symptoms of peripheral neuropathy—pain, burning, aching, weakness, or pins and needles in limbs—and tell him to report these immediately.
- Tell patient to report symptoms of lactic acidosis, including fatigue, GI problems, dyspnea, and tachypnea.
- Tell patient to report symptoms of pancreatitis, including abdominal pain, nausea, vomiting, weight loss or fatty stools.

☑ **Evaluation**
- Patient's infection is controlled.
- Patient maintains normal peripheral neurologic function.
- Patient and family state understanding of drug therapy.

HIGH ALERT

streptokinase
(strep-toh-KIGH-nayz)
Streptase

Pharmacologic class: plasminogen activator
Therapeutic class: thrombolytic enzyme
Pregnancy risk category: C

Indications and dosages

▶ **Arteriovenous cannula occlusion.** *Adults:* 250,000 international units in 2 ml I.V. solution by I.V. pump infusion into each occluded limb of cannula over 25 to 35 minutes. Clamp cannula for 2 hours. Then aspirate contents of cannula, flush with saline solution, and reconnect.
▶ **Venous thrombosis, pulmonary embolism, arterial thrombosis and embolism.** *Adults:* Loading dose is 250,000 international units by I.V. infusion over 30 minutes. Sustaining dose is 100,000 international units/hour by I.V. infusion for 72 hours for deep vein thrombosis and 100,000 international units/hour over 24 hours by I.V. infusion pump for pulmonary embolism.
▶ **Lysis of coronary artery thrombi after acute MI.** *Adults:* I.V. infusion preferred using 1,500,000 international units infused over 60 minutes. Or, if using intracoronary infusion, the total dose for intracoronary infusion is 140,000 international units. Loading dose is 15,000 to 20,000 international units by coronary

catheter over 15 seconds to 2 minutes, followed by infusion of maintenance dose of 2,000 international units/minute for 60 minutes.

▼ I.V. administration

- Reconstitute each drug vial with 5 ml of normal saline solution for injection. Further dilute to 45 ml.
- Don't shake; roll gently to mix. Some precipitate may be present; discard if large amounts appear. Filter solution with 0.8-micron or larger filter. Use within 8 hours.
- Administer with a controlled infusion device.
- Store powder at room temperature and refrigerate after reconstitution.
⊗ **Incompatibilities**
Dextrans, other I.V. drugs.

Contraindications and cautions

- Contraindicated in patients with ulcerative wounds, active internal bleeding, uncontrolled hypercoagulation, chronic pulmonary disease with cavitation, subacute bacterial endocarditis or rheumatic valvular disease, visceral or intracranial malignant neoplasms, ulcerative colitis, diverticulitis, severe hypertension, acute or chronic hepatic or renal insufficiency, recent stroke, recent trauma with possible internal injuries, or recent cerebral embolism, thrombosis, or hemorrhage.
- Also contraindicated within 10 days after intra-arterial diagnostic procedure or any surgery, including liver or kidney biopsy, lumbar puncture, thoracentesis, paracentesis, or extensive or multiple venous cut downs.
- I.M. injections and other invasive procedures are contraindicated during streptokinase therapy.
- Use cautiously when treating arterial embolism that originates from left side of heart because of danger of cerebral infarction.
⚖ **Lifespan:** In pregnant women, use cautiously. In breast-feeding women and in children, safety and effectiveness haven't been established.

Adverse reactions

CNS: fever, headache, polyradiculoneuropathy.
CV: flushing, hypotension, *reperfusion arrhythmias,* vasculitis.
EENT: periorbital edema.
GI: nausea.
Hematologic: *bleeding.*
Musculoskeletal: musculoskeletal pain.

Reactions may be *common*, uncommon, *life-threatening*, or COMMON AND LIFE-THREATENING.

Respiratory: *bronchospasm,* minor breathing difficulty, *pulmonary edema.*
Skin: pruritus, urticaria.
Other: *angioedema, delayed hypersensitivity reactions* (interstitial nephritis, vasculitis, serum-sickness–like reactions), *hypersensitivity reactions (anaphylaxis),* phlebitis or bleeding at injection site.

Interactions

Drug-drug. *Anticoagulants:* May increase risk of bleeding. Monitor patient closely.
Antifibrinolytics, such as aminocaproic acid: May inhibit and reverse streptokinase activity. Use only when indicated during streptokinase therapy.
Aspirin, dipyridamole, drugs that affect platelet activity, indomethacin, phenylbutazone: May increase risk of bleeding. Monitor patient closely. Combined therapy with low-dose aspirin (162.5 mg) or dipyridamole has improved acute and long-term results.

Effects on lab test results

• May decrease hemoglobin level and hematocrit.
• May increase PT, PTT, and INR.

Pharmacokinetics

Absorption: Given I.V.
Distribution: Unknown
Metabolism: Insignificant.
Excretion: Removed from circulation by antibodies and reticuloendothelial system. *Half-life:* First phase, 18 minutes; second phase, 83 minutes.

Route	Onset	Peak	Duration
I.V.	Immediate	20 min–2 hr	4 hr

Action

Chemical effect: Activates plasminogen in two steps. Plasminogen and streptokinase form a complex that exposes plasminogen-activating site. Plasminogen is then converted to plasmin by cleavage of peptide bond.
Therapeutic effect: Dissolves blood clots.

Available forms

Injection: 250,000 international units, 750,000 international units, and 1.5 million international units in vials for reconstitution

NURSING PROCESS

Assessment

• Assess patient's condition before starting therapy and regularly thereafter to monitor drug's effectiveness.
• Assess patient for increased risk of bleeding (such as from recent surgery, stroke, trauma, or hypertension) before starting therapy.
• Before starting therapy, draw blood to determine PTT and PT. Rate of I.V. infusion depends on thrombin time and streptokinase resistance. Then repeat studies often and keep laboratory flow sheet on patient's chart to monitor PTT, PT, hemoglobin level, and hematocrit.
• Monitor patient for excessive bleeding every 15 minutes for first hour, every 30 minutes for second through eighth hours, then once every shift.
• Assess pulses, color, and sensation of limbs every hour.
• Be alert for adverse reactions and drug interactions.
• Assess patient's and family's knowledge of drug therapy.

Nursing diagnoses

• Ineffective cardiopulmonary tissue perfusion related to condition
• Risk for deficient fluid volume related to potential for bleeding
• Deficient knowledge related to drug therapy

Planning and implementation

• Only prescriber with experience in thrombotic disease management and in a setting where close monitoring can be performed should use drug.
• Before using streptokinase to clear an occluded arteriovenous cannula, try flushing with heparinized saline solution.
ALERT: Streptokinase may cause life-threatening side effects when used to clear occluded I.V. catheters. Use only if clearly needed.
ALERT: To check for hypersensitivity reactions, give 100 international units I.D.; wheal and flare response within 20 minutes means patient is probably allergic. Monitor vital signs frequently.
• If patient has had either recent streptococcal infection or recent treatment with streptokinase, higher loading dose may be needed.
• If bleeding occurs, stop therapy and notify prescriber. Pretreatment with heparin or drugs

S

affecting platelets causes high risk of bleeding but may improve long-term results.
• Have aminocaproic acid available to treat bleeding and corticosteroids to treat allergic reactions.
• Have typed and crossmatched packed RBCs ready to treat hemorrhage.
• Keep involved limb in straight alignment to prevent bleeding from infusion site.
• Avoid unnecessary handling of patient, and pad side rails. Bruising is more likely during therapy.
• Keep venipuncture sites to minimum; use pressure dressing on puncture sites for at least 15 minutes.
⊛ **ALERT:** Immediately notify prescriber if hypersensitivity occurs. Antihistamines or corticosteroids may be used to treat mild reactions. If severe reaction occurs, stop infusion and notify prescriber.
• Heparin by continuous infusion is usually started within 1 hour after stopping streptokinase. Use infusion pump to give heparin.
• In patient with acute MI, thrombolytic therapy may decrease infarct size, improve ventricular function, and decrease risk of heart failure. Drug must be given within 6 hours of onset of symptoms for optimal effect, but benefits have been reported up to 24 hours.
Patient teaching
• Tell patient to report oozing, bleeding, or signs of hypersensitivity immediately.

☑ **Evaluation**
• Patient responds well to therapy.
• Patient maintains adequate fluid balance.
• Patient and family state understanding of drug therapy.

streptomycin sulfate
(strep-toh-MIGH-sin SUL-fayt)

Pharmacologic class: aminoglycoside
Therapeutic class: antibiotic
Pregnancy risk category: D

Indications and dosages

▶ **Streptococcal endocarditis.** *Adults:* 1 g I.M. every 12 hours for 1 week, and then 500 mg every 12 hours for 1 week, given with penicillin.

Adults older than age 60: Give 500 mg I.M. every 12 hours for 14 days.
▶ **Primary and adjunct treatment in tuberculosis.** *Adults:* 1 g or 15 mg/kg I.M. (up to 1 g) daily or 25 to 30 mg/kg (up to 1.5 g) two or three times weekly.
Children: 20 to 40 mg/kg (up to 1 g) I.M. daily in divided doses injected deep into large muscle mass or 25 to 30 mg/kg (up to 1 g) two or three times weekly. Given with other antituberculotics but not with capreomycin. Continue until sputum specimen becomes negative.
▶ **Enterococcal endocarditis.** *Adults:* 1 g I.M. every 12 hours for 2 weeks, and then 500 mg every 12 hours for 4 weeks, given with penicillin.
▶ **Tularemia.** *Adults:* 1 to 2 g I.M. daily in divided doses injected deep into upper outer quadrant of buttocks. Continue for 7 to 14 days until patient is afebrile for 5 to 7 days.
▤ **Adjust-a-dose:** For patients with renal impairment, initial dose is the same as for normal renal function. Later doses and frequency determined by renal function study results and blood level. If creatinine clearance is 50 to 80 ml/minute, give 7.5 mg/kg every 24 hours. If it's 10 to 50 ml/minute, give 7.5 mg/kg every 24 to 72 hours. If it's less than 10 ml/minute, give 7.5 mg/kg every 72 to 96 hours.

Contraindications and cautions

• Contraindicated in patients hypersensitive to the drug or other aminoglycosides and patients with labyrinthine disease.
• Use cautiously in patients with impaired kidney function or neuromuscular disorders.
☗ **Lifespan:** In pregnant women, drug is contraindicated. In breast-feeding women and in the elderly, use cautiously.

Adverse reactions

CNS: *neuromuscular blockade.*
EENT: ototoxicity.
GI: nausea, vomiting.
GU: *nephrotoxicity.*
Hematologic: eosinophilia, *leukopenia, thrombocytopenia.*
Respiratory: *apnea.*
Skin: exfoliative dermatitis.
Other: *anaphylaxis, angioedema,* hypersensitivity reactions.

Interactions

Drug-drug. *Acyclovir, aminoglycosides, amphotericin B, cisplatin, methoxyflurane, vancomycin:* May increase risk of nephrotoxicity. Monitor patient.

Atracurium, doxacurium, mivacurium, pancuronium, rocuronium, tubocurarine, vecuronium: May increase the effects of nondepolarizing muscle relaxant, including prolonged respiratory depression. Use together only when necessary. Dose of nondepolarizing muscle relaxant may need to be reduced.

Cephalosporins: May increase risk of nephrotoxicity. Use together cautiously.

Dimenhydrinate: May mask symptoms of streptomycin-induced ototoxicity. Use together cautiously.

I.V. loop diuretics (such as furosemide): May increase ototoxicity. Use together cautiously.

Effects on lab test results

• May increase BUN, creatinine, and nonprotein nitrogen levels. May decrease hemoglobin level and hematocrit.
• May increase eosinophil count. May decrease WBC and platelet counts.

Pharmacokinetics

Absorption: Unknown after I.M. use.
Distribution: Wide, although CSF penetration is low. 36% protein-bound.
Metabolism: None.
Excretion: Mainly in urine; less in bile. *Half-life:* 2 to 3 hours; up to 100 hours with renal impairment.

Route	Onset	Peak	Duration
I.M.	Unknown	1–2 hr	Unknown

Action

Chemical effect: Inhibits bacterial protein synthesis by binding directly to 30S ribosomal subunit.
Therapeutic effect: Kills bacteria.

Available forms

Injection: 400 mg/ml in 2.5-ml ampules
Powder for injection: 200 mg/ml in 1-g vials

NURSING PROCESS

Assessment
• Assess patient's infection before starting therapy and regularly thereafter to monitor drug's effectiveness.
• Obtain specimen for culture and sensitivity tests before first dose except when treating tuberculosis. Start therapy pending test results.
ALERT: Obtain blood for peak streptomycin level 1 to 2 hours after I.M. injection; for trough level, draw blood just before next dose. Don't use heparinized tube because heparin is incompatible with aminoglycosides.
• Evaluate patient's hearing before therapy, during therapy, and 6 months after therapy ends.
• Be alert for adverse reactions and drug interactions.
• Assess patient's and family's knowledge of drug therapy.

Nursing diagnoses
• Risk for infection related to presence of susceptible bacteria
• Disturbed sensory perception (auditory) related to drug-induced adverse reactions
• Deficient knowledge related to drug therapy

Planning and implementation
• Protect hands when preparing drug because drug is irritating.
• Inject drug deep into upper outer quadrant of buttocks. Rotate injection sites.
ALERT: Never give streptomycin I.V.
• Encourage adequate fluid intake. Patient should be well hydrated while taking drug to minimize chemical irritation of renal tubules.
• In primary treatment of tuberculosis, stop drug when sputum becomes negative.
Patient teaching
• Warn patient that injection may be painful.
• Emphasize the need to drink at least 2,000 ml daily (if not contraindicated) during therapy.
• Instruct patient to report hearing loss, roaring noises, or fullness in ears or dizziness immediately.

Evaluation
• Patient is free from infection.
• Patient's auditory function remains normal.
• Patient and family state understanding of drug therapy.

S

succimer
(SUK-sih-mer)
Chemet

Pharmacologic class: heavy metal antagonist
Therapeutic class: chelate
Pregnancy risk category: C

Indications and dosages

▶ **Lead poisoning in children with blood lead levels above 45 mcg/dl.** *Children:* 10 mg/kg or 350 mg/m² every 8 hours for 5 days. Round dose to nearest 100 mg (see table). For next 2 weeks, decrease interval to every 12 hours.

Weight (kg)	Dose (mg)
8–15	100
16–23	200
24–34	300
35–44	400
≥ 45	500

Contraindications and cautions

• Contraindicated in patients hypersensitive to the drug or any of its components.
• Use cautiously in patients with compromised kidney function.
• Monitor patient for neutropenia. If absolute neutrophil count falls below 1,200/mm³, stop drug.
⚠ **Lifespan:** None reported.

Adverse reactions

CNS: dizziness, drowsiness, headache, paresthesia, sensory motor neuropathy, sleepiness.
CV: *arrhythmias.*
EENT: cloudy film in eyes, nasal congestion, otitis media, plugged ears, rhinorrhea, sore throat, watery eyes.
GI: abdominal cramps, diarrhea, hemorrhoidal symptoms, loose stools, loss of appetite, metallic taste, nausea, stomach pain, vomiting.
GU: decreased urination, difficult urination, *flank pain,* proteinuria.
Hematologic: intermittent eosinophilia, *neutropenia.*
Musculoskeletal: back, leg, kneecap, or rib pain.
Respiratory: cough, head cold.

Skin: herpetic rash, mucocutaneous eruptions, papular rash, pruritus.
Other: candidiasis, *flulike syndrome.*

Interactions

None reported.

Effects on lab test results

• May increase AST, ALT, alkaline phosphatase, and cholesterol levels.
• May increase eosinophil and platelet counts.
• May cause false-positive results for ketones in urine using nitroprusside reagents (Ketostix) and falsely decreased uric acid and CK levels.

Pharmacokinetics

Absorption: Rapid but variable.
Distribution: Unknown.
Metabolism: Rapid and extensive.
Excretion: 39% in feces unchanged; remainder mainly in urine. *Half-life:* 48 hours.

Route	Onset	Peak	Duration
P.O.	Unknown	1–2 hr	Unknown

Action

Chemical effect: Forms water-soluble complexes with lead and increases its excretion in urine.
Therapeutic effect: Relieves signs and symptoms of lead poisoning.

Available forms

Capsules: 100 mg

NURSING PROCESS

Assessment
• Assess child's condition before starting therapy and regularly thereafter to monitor drug's effectiveness.
• Measure severity by initial blood lead level and by rate and degree of rebound of blood lead level. Use severity as guide for more frequent blood lead monitoring.
• Monitor transaminase level and neutrophil count before starting therapy, and at least weekly during therapy. Transient, mild elevations of transaminase level may occur. Monitor patient with history of hepatic disease more closely.
• Monitor patient at least once weekly for rebound lead level. Elevated lead level and associ-

ated symptoms may return rapidly after drug is stopped because of redistribution of lead from bone to soft tissues and blood.
• Be alert for adverse reactions.
• If adverse GI reactions occur, monitor patient's hydration.
• Evaluate parents' knowledge of drug therapy.

Nursing diagnoses
• Ineffective health maintenance related to presence of lead poisoning
• Risk for deficient fluid volume related to drug-induced adverse GI reactions
• Deficient knowledge related to drug therapy

Planning and implementation
• Course of treatment lasts 19 days. Repeated courses may be needed if indicated by weekly monitoring of blood lead level.
• A minimum of 2 weeks between courses is recommended unless high blood lead level indicates need for immediate therapy.
ALERT: Administration of succimer with other chelates isn't recommended. Patient who has received edetate calcium disodium with or without dimercaprol may use succimer as subsequent therapy after 4-week interval.
• Maintain adequate fluid intake.
Patient teaching
• Tell parents of child who can't swallow capsule to open it and sprinkle contents on small amount of soft food. Or, medicated beads from capsule may be poured on spoon and followed with flavored beverage such as a fruit drink.
• Help parents identify and remove sources of lead in child's environment. Chelation therapy isn't a substitute for preventing further exposure.
• Tell parents to consult prescriber if rash occurs. Consider possibility of allergic or other mucocutaneous reactions each time drug is used.

Evaluation
• Patient responds well to therapy.
• Patient maintains adequate hydration.
• Parents state understanding of drug therapy.

HIGH ALERT

succinylcholine chloride (suxamethonium chloride)
(SUK-seh-nil-KOH-leen KLOR-ighd)
Anectine, Anectine Flo-Pack, Quelicin

Pharmacologic class: depolarizing neuromuscular blocker
Therapeutic class: skeletal muscle relaxant
Pregnancy risk category: C

Indications and dosages

▶ **Adjunct to anesthesia to induce skeletal muscle relaxation; to facilitate intubation and assist with mechanical ventilation or orthopedic manipulations (drug of choice); to lessen muscle contractions in pharmacologically or electrically induced seizures.** *Adults:* Dosage depends on anesthetic used, individual needs, and response. Give 0.6 mg/kg I.V. over 10 to 30 seconds; then give 2.5 mg/minute, p.r.n. Or, 2.5 to 4 mg/kg I.M. up to maximum of 150 mg I.M. in deltoid muscle. For short procedures, the optimum dose range is 0.3 to 1.1 mg/kg. The average dose is 0.6 mg/kg. Maximum paralysis occurs in 2 minutes. Recovery time is in 4 to 6 minutes. For long procedures, the average rate for adults is 2.5 to 4.3 mg/minute. For prolonged muscular relaxation, give intermittent I.V. injections of 0.3 to 1.1 mg/kg, then 0.04 to 0.07 mg/kg.
Children: 1 to 2 mg/kg I.V. or 2.5 to 4 mg/kg I.M. Maximum I.M. dose is 150 mg.

I.V. administration
• Use immediately after reconstitution.
• Store injectable form in refrigerator. Store powder form at room temperature in tightly closed container.
• Solutions of 0.1% to 0.2% are common for I.V. infusions (1 to 2 mg/ml).
⊗ **Incompatibilities**
Barbiturates, nafcillin, sodium bicarbonate, thiopental sodium, or any solutions with pH above 8.5.

Contraindications and cautions
• Contraindicated in patients hypersensitive to the drug or any of its components and in patients with abnormally low pseudocholines-

S

---

terase level, angle-closure glaucoma, personal or family history of malignant hyperthermia, or penetrating eye injury.

• Use cautiously in debilitated patients, those taking quinidine or digoxin therapy, and those with severe burns or trauma, electrolyte imbalances, hyperkalemia, paraplegia, spinal neuraxis injury, stroke, degenerative or dystrophic neuromuscular disease, myasthenia gravis, myasthenic syndrome of lung cancer, bronchogenic carcinoma, dehydration, thyroid disorders, collagen diseases, porphyria, fractures, muscle spasms, eye surgery, pheochromocytoma, respiratory depression, or hepatic, renal, or pulmonary impairment.

⚖ Lifespan: In women undergoing cesarean section and in breast-feeding women, use large doses cautiously. In the elderly, use cautiously.

Adverse reactions

CV: *arrhythmias, bradycardia, cardiac arrest,* flushing, hypertension, hypotension, tachycardia.
EENT: increased intraocular pressure.
Musculoskeletal: muscle fasciculation, myoglobinemia, *postoperative muscle pain.*
Respiratory: *apnea, bronchoconstriction, prolonged respiratory depression.*
Other: allergic or idiosyncratic hypersensitivity reactions *(anaphylaxis),* excessive salivation, *malignant hyperthermia.*

Interactions

Drug-drug. *Aminoglycoside antibiotics, including amikacin, gentamicin, kanamycin, neomycin, and streptomycin; anticholinesterases, such as echothiophate, edrophonium, neostigmine, physostigmine, and pyridostigmine; general anesthetics, such as enflurane, halothane, and isoflurane; polymyxin antibiotics, such as colistin and polymyxin B sulfate:* May increase neuromuscular blockade, leading to increased skeletal muscle relaxation and potentiation of effect. Use cautiously during surgical and postoperative periods.
Cyclophosphamide, lithium, MAO inhibitors: May cause prolonged apnea. Avoid using together; monitor patient closely.
Digoxin: May cause arrhythmias. Use together cautiously.
Methotrimeprazine, opioid analgesics: May increase neuromuscular blockade, leading to in-

creased skeletal muscle relaxation and, possibly, respiratory paralysis. Use cautiously.
Parenteral magnesium sulfate: May potentiate neuromuscular blockade, leading to increased skeletal muscle relaxation and, possibly, respiratory paralysis. Use cautiously, preferably with reduced doses.
Drug-herb. *Melatonin:* May potentiate blocking properties of succinylcholine. Discourage using together.

Effects on lab test results

• May increase myoglobin and potassium levels.

Pharmacokinetics

Absorption: Unknown.
Distribution: In extracellular fluid and rapid to site of action.
Metabolism: Rapid, by plasma pseudocholinesterase.
Excretion: About 10% unchanged in urine.
Half-life: Unknown.

Route	Onset	Peak	Duration
I.V.	≤ 1 min	1–2 min	4–10 min
I.M.	2–3 min	Unknown	10–30 min

Action

Chemical effect: Prolongs depolarization of muscle end plate.
Therapeutic effect: Relaxes skeletal muscles.

Available forms

Injection: 20 mg/ml, 50 mg/ml
Powder for infusion: 500-mg and 1-g vials

NURSING PROCESS

📋 **Assessment**
• Assess patient's condition before starting therapy and regularly thereafter to monitor the drug's effectiveness.
• Monitor baseline and ongoing electrolyte level and vital signs (check respiratory rate every 5 to 10 minutes during infusion).
• Monitor respiratory rate and pulse oximetry closely until patient is fully recovered from neuromuscular blockade, as evidenced by tests of muscle strength (hand grip, head lift, and ability to cough).

- Be alert for adverse reactions and drug interactions.
- Assess patient's and family's knowledge of drug therapy.

⊞ Nursing diagnoses
- Ineffective health maintenance related to underlying condition
- Ineffective breathing pattern related to drug's effect on respiratory muscles
- Deficient knowledge related to drug therapy

⟩ Planning and implementation
⚡ ALERT: Drug should only be given by a practitioner skilled in airway management.
- The drug of choice for procedures less than 3 minutes and for orthopedic manipulations—use caution in fractures or dislocations.
- Give sedatives or general anesthetics before neuromuscular blockers. Neuromuscular blockers don't induce unconsciousness or alter pain threshold.
- Keep airway clear. Have emergency respiratory support equipment immediately available.
⚡ ALERT: Careful drug calculation is essential. Always verify with another professional.
- To evaluate patient's ability to metabolize drug, give 10-mg I.M. or I.V. test dose after patient is anesthetized. No respiratory depression or transient depression for up to 5 minutes indicates drug may be given. Don't give subsequent doses if patient develops respiratory paralysis sufficient to permit endotracheal intubation. (Recovery within 30 to 60 minutes.)
- Give deep I.M., preferably high into deltoid muscle.
- Give analgesics.
⚡ ALERT: Don't use reversing drugs. Unlike with nondepolarizing drugs, giving neostigmine or edrophonium with this depolarizing drug may worsen neuromuscular blockade.
- Repeated or continuous infusions of succinylcholine aren't advised, because they may reduce response or prolong muscle relaxation and apnea.
⚡ ALERT: Rarely, cardiac arrest may occur within minutes of succinylcholine administration in children. Carefully monitor ECG for peaked T-waves, which may be an early sign of arrhythmias.
Patient teaching
- Explain all events and happenings to patient because he can still hear.

- Reassure patient that he is being monitored at all times.
- Inform patient that postoperative stiffness is normal and will soon subside.

✓ Evaluation
- Patient responds well to therapy.
- Patient maintains adequate respiratory patterns with mechanical assistance.
- Patient and family state understanding of drug therapy.

sucralfate
(SOO-krahl-fayt)
Carafate, Sulcrate ◆

Pharmacologic class: pepsin inhibitor
Therapeutic class: antiulcerative
Pregnancy risk category: B

Indications and dosages
▶ **Maintenance therapy for duodenal ulcer.**
Adults: 1 g P.O. b.i.d., before meals.
▶ **Therapy for up to 8 weeks for duodenal ulcer; gastric ulcer‡.** *Adults:* 1 g P.O. q.i.d. 1 hour before meals and at bedtime.

Contraindications and cautions
- Use cautiously in patients with chronic renal impairment.
⚘ Lifespan: In pregnant women, use cautiously. In breast-feeding women, use cautiously; it's unknown if the drug appears in breast milk. In children, safety and effectiveness haven't been established.

Adverse reactions
CNS: dizziness, headache, sleepiness, vertigo.
GI: bezoar formation, constipation, diarrhea, dry mouth, flatulence, gastric discomfort, indigestion, nausea, vomiting.
Musculoskeletal: back pain.
Skin: pruritus, rash.

Interactions
Drug-drug. *Antacids:* May decrease binding of drug to gastroduodenal mucosa, impairing effectiveness. Don't give within 30 minutes of each other.

S

Cimetidine, digoxin, phenytoin, ranitidine, tetracycline, theophylline: May decrease absorption. Separate doses by at least 2 hours. *Ciprofloxacin, lomefloxacin, moxifloxacin, norfloxacin, ofloxacin:* May decrease absorption of the quinolone, reducing anti-infective response. If use together can't be avoided, give at least 2 hours apart.

Effects on lab test results

None reported.

Pharmacokinetics

Absorption: About 3% to 5%. Acts locally.
Distribution: To GI tract and small amount to tissues.
Metabolism: None.
Excretion: About 90% in feces; absorbed drug excreted unchanged in urine. *Half-life:* 6 to 20 hours.

Route	Onset	Peak	Duration
P.O.	Unknown	≤ 6 hr	6 hr

Action

Chemical effect: May adhere to and protect ulcer's surface by forming barrier.
Therapeutic effect: Aids in duodenal ulcer healing.

Available forms

Suspension: 1 g/10 ml
Tablets: 1 g

NURSING PROCESS

Assessment
• Assess patient's GI symptoms before starting therapy and regularly thereafter to monitor drug's effectiveness.
• Be alert for adverse reactions and drug interactions.
• Monitor patient for severe, persistent constipation.
• Assess patient's and family's knowledge of drug therapy.

Nursing diagnoses
• Impaired tissue integrity related to presence of duodenal ulcer

• Constipation related to drug-induced adverse GI reactions
• Deficient knowledge related to drug therapy

Planning and implementation
• Give drug on an empty stomach for best results.
• Don't give I.V.
• Antacids may be used to relieve symptoms but should be separated from sucralfate doses by at least 30 minutes.
ALERT: Don't confuse sucralfate with salsalate or Carafate with Cafergot.
Patient teaching
• Instruct patient to take drug 1 hour before each meal and bedtime.
• Tell patient to continue on prescribed regimen to ensure complete healing. Pain and ulcerative symptoms may subside within first few weeks of therapy.
• Urge patient to avoid cigarette smoking because it may increase gastric acid secretion and worsen disease. Also tell patient to avoid alcohol, chocolate, and spicy foods.
• Tell patient to sleep with head of bed elevated.
• Tell patient to avoid large meals within 2 hours of bedtime.

Evaluation
• Patient's ulcer pain is gone.
• Patient maintains normal bowel elimination patterns.
• Patient and family state understanding of drug therapy.

sulfasalazine (salazosulfapyridine, sulphasalazine)

(sul-fuh-SAL-uh-zeen)
Azulfidine, Azulfidine EN-Tabs, Salazopyrin ♦, Salazopyrin EN-Tabs ♦

Pharmacologic class: sulfonamide
Therapeutic class: anti-inflammatory
Pregnancy risk category: B

Indications and dosages

▶ **Mild to moderate ulcerative colitis, adjunct therapy in severe ulcerative colitis.**

Adults: Initially, 3 to 4 g P.O. daily in evenly divided doses. May begin with a lower dose of 1 to 2 g/day to avoid GI intolerance; usual maintenance dosage is 1 to 2 g P.O. daily in divided doses every 6 hours. Dosage may be started with 1 to 2 g, with gradual increase to minimize adverse effects.

Children older than age 2: Initially, 40 to 60 mg/kg P.O. daily, divided into three to six doses; then 30 mg/kg daily in four doses. If GI intolerance occurs, reduce dosage.

▶ **Rheumatoid arthritis in patients who have responded inadequately to salicylates or other NSAIDs.** *Adults:* 2 g P.O. daily b.i.d. in evenly divided doses. Dosage may be started at 0.5 to 1 g daily and be gradually increased over 3 weeks to reduce GI intolerance.

▶ **Patients with polyarticular-course juvenile rheumatoid arthritis who have responded inadequately to salicylates or other NSAIDs.** *Children age 6 and older:* 30 to 50 mg/kg P.O. daily in two divided doses (as delayed-release tablet). Maximum dose is 2 g daily. To reduce GI intolerance, start with one-fourth to one-third of planned maintenance dosage and increase weekly until maintenance dosage is reached at 1 month.

▶ **Crohn disease‡.** *Adults:* 3 to 6 g P.O. daily in divided doses for active disease. 1.5 to 3 g P.O. daily in divided doses for maintenance therapy.

Contraindications and cautions

• Contraindicated in patients hypersensitive to the drug or its metabolites, and patients with porphyria or intestinal or urinary obstruction.
• Use cautiously and in reduced dosages in patients with impaired liver or kidney function, severe allergy, bronchial asthma, or G6PD deficiency.

⚕ **Lifespan:** In pregnant women, use cautiously. In breast-feeding women, use cautiously; it's unknown if the drug appears in breast milk. In infants younger than age 2, drug is contraindicated.

Adverse reactions

CNS: depression, hallucinations, headache, *seizures.*
GI: abdominal pain, anorexia, *diarrhea, nausea,* stomatitis, *vomiting.*

GU: crystalluria, hematuria, infertility, oligospermia, *toxic nephrosis with oliguria and anuria.*
Hematologic: *agranulocytosis, aplastic anemia,* hemolytic anemia, *leukopenia,* megaloblastic anemia, *thrombocytopenia.*
Hepatic: *hepatotoxicity,* jaundice.
Skin: *epidermal necrolysis, erythema multiforme,* exfoliative dermatitis, generalized skin eruption, photosensitivity reactions, pruritus, *Stevens-Johnson syndrome,* urticaria.
Other: hypersensitivity reactions (*anaphylaxis,* drug fever, serum sickness).

Interactions

Drug-drug. *Antibiotics:* May alter action of sulfasalazine by altering internal flora. Monitor patient closely.
Digoxin: May reduce digoxin absorption. Monitor patient closely.
Folic acid: May decrease absorption. No intervention needed.
Hormonal contraceptives: May decrease contraceptive effectiveness and increases risk of breakthrough bleeding. Suggest nonhormonal contraceptive.
Iron: May lower sulfasalazine level by iron chelation. Monitor patient closely.
Methotrexate: May increase risk of methotrexate-induced bone marrow suppression. Monitor for hematologic toxicity.
Oral anticoagulants: May increase anticoagulant effect. Monitor patient for bleeding.
Oral antidiabetics: May increase hypoglycemic effect. Monitor glucose level.
Drug-herb. *Dong quai, St. John's wort:* May increase risk of photosensitivity. Discourage using together.

Effects on lab test results

• May increase AST and ALT levels. May decrease hemoglobin level and hematocrit.
• May decrease granulocyte, platelet, RBC, and WBC counts.

Pharmacokinetics

Absorption: Poor. 70% to 90% transported to colon, where intestinal flora metabolize drug to its active ingredients, which exert their effects locally. One metabolite, sulfapyridine, is absorbed from colon, but only small portion of metabolite 5-aminosalicylic acid is absorbed.

Distribution: Distributed locally in colon. Distribution of absorbed metabolites is unknown.
Metabolism: Divided by intestinal flora in colon.
Excretion: Mainly in urine. *Half-life:* 6 to 8 hours.

Route	Onset	Peak	Duration
P.O.			
parent drug	Unknown	1½–6 hr	Unknown
metabolites	Unknown	12–24 hr	Unknown

Action

Chemical effect: Unknown.
Therapeutic effect: Relieves inflammation in GI tract.

Available forms

Oral suspension: 250 mg/5 ml
Tablets (with or without enteric coating): 500 mg

NURSING PROCESS

Assessment
• Assess patient's condition before starting therapy and regularly thereafter to monitor drug's effectiveness.
• Monitor CBC and liver function tests at baseline, every other week for first 3 months, monthly for next 3 months, then as needed.
• Be alert for adverse reactions and drug interactions.
• Monitor patient's hydration throughout drug therapy.
• Assess patient's and family's knowledge of drug therapy.

Nursing diagnoses
• Acute pain related to inflammation of GI tract
• Risk for deficient fluid volume related to drug-induced adverse GI reactions
• Deficient knowledge related to drug therapy

Planning and implementation
• Minimize adverse GI reaction by spacing doses evenly and giving after food intake.
• Drug colors alkaline urine orange-yellow.
• **ALERT:** If patient shows evidence of hypersensitivity, stop immediately and notify prescriber.
• **ALERT:** Don't confuse sulfasalazine with sulfisoxazole, salsalate, or sulfadiazine.

Patient teaching
• Instruct patient to take drug after meals and to space doses evenly.
• Warn patient that drug may cause skin and urine to turn orange-yellow and may permanently stain soft contact lenses yellow.
• Warn patient to avoid direct sunlight and ultraviolet light, to prevent photosensitivity reaction.
• Instruct patient to notify physician immediately with complaints of pallor, sore throat, purpura, or jaundice.

Evaluation
• Patient is free from pain.
• Patient maintains adequate hydration.
• Patient and family state understanding of drug therapy.

sulfinpyrazone
(sul-fin-PEER-uh-zohn)
Anturane

Pharmacologic class: uricosuric
Therapeutic class: platelet aggregation inhibitor, uricolytic
Pregnancy risk category: NR

Indications and dosages

▶ **Intermittent or chronic gouty arthritis.**
Adults: Initially, 100 mg to 200 mg P.O. b.i.d. during the first week; then 200 mg to 400 mg P.O. b.i.d. Maximum dosage, 800 mg daily. After urate level is controlled, dosage can sometimes be reduced to 200 mg daily in divided doses.
▶ **Prophylaxis of thromboembolic disorders, including angina, MI, transient (cerebral) ischemic attacks, and presence of prosthetic heart valves**. *Adults:* 600 to 800 mg P.O. daily in divided doses to decrease platelet aggregation.

Contraindications and cautions

• Contraindicated in patients hypersensitive to pyrazole derivatives (including oxyphenbutazone and phenylbutazone) and patients with active peptic ulcer, symptoms of GI inflammation or ulceration, or blood dyscrasias.
• Use cautiously in patients with healed peptic ulcer.

Reactions may be *common,* uncommon, *life-threatening*, or COMMON AND LIFE-THREATENING.

⚓ **Lifespan:** In pregnant women, use cautiously. In breast-feeding women and in children, safety and effectiveness haven't been established.

Adverse reactions

GI: *dyspepsia,* epigastric pain, *nausea,* reactivation of peptic ulcerations.
Hematologic: *agranulocytosis, aplastic anemia,* anemia, *blood dyscrasias, leukopenia, thrombocytopenia.*
Respiratory: *bronchoconstriction* in patients with aspirin-induced asthma.
Skin: rash.

Interactions

Drug-drug. *Aspirin, niacin, salicylates:* May inhibit uricosuric effect of sulfinpyrazone. Don't use together.
Cholestyramine: May bind and delay absorption of sulfinpyrazone. Give sulfinpyrazone at least 1 hour before or 4 to 6 hours after cholestyramine.
Oral anticoagulants: May increase anticoagulant effect and risk of bleeding. Use together cautiously.
Oral antidiabetics: May increase effects. Monitor glucose level closely.
Probenecid: May inhibit renal excretion of sulfinpyrazone. Use together cautiously.
Protein-bound drugs: May cause interaction. Monitor patient for toxicity.
Theophylline: May increase theophylline clearance. Monitor level.
Verapamil: May decrease verapamil effect. Monitor patient.
Drug-lifestyle. *Alcohol use:* May decrease drug effectiveness. Discourage using together.

Effects on lab test results

• May increase BUN and creatinine levels. May decrease hemoglobin level and hematocrit.
• May decrease RBC, WBC, granulocyte, and platelet counts.

Pharmacokinetics

Absorption: Complete.
Distribution: 98% to 99% protein-bound.
Metabolism: Rapid.
Excretion: In urine, about 50% unchanged.
Half-life: 3 hours.

Route	Onset	Peak	Duration
P.O.	Unknown	1–2 hr	4–6 hr

Action

Chemical effect: Blocks renal tubular reabsorption of uric acid, increasing excretion, and inhibits platelet aggregation.
Therapeutic effect: Relieves signs and symptoms of gouty arthritis.

Available forms

Capsules: 200 mg
Tablets: 100 mg

NURSING PROCESS

📖 **Assessment**
• Assess patient's condition before starting therapy and regularly thereafter to monitor drug's effectiveness.
• Monitor BUN level, CBC, and kidney function studies periodically during long-term use.
• Monitor fluid intake and output. Therapy may lead to renal colic and formation of uric acid stones until acid level are normal (about 6 mg/dl).
• Be alert for adverse reactions and drug interactions.
• Assess patient's and family's knowledge of drug therapy.

💬 **Nursing diagnoses**
• Ineffective health maintenance related to presence of gouty arthritis
• Risk for injury related to drug-induced adverse CNS reactions
• Deficient knowledge related to drug therapy

▶ **Planning and implementation**
• Give drug with milk, food, or antacids to minimize GI disturbances.
• Encourage patient to drink fluids to maintain minimum daily output of 2 to 3 L. Alkalinize urine with sodium bicarbonate or other agent. Keep in mind that alkalinizers are used therapeutically to increase drug activity, preventing urolithiasis.
• Drug is recommended for patient unresponsive to probenecid. Suitable for long-term use; neither cumulative effects nor tolerance develops.
• Drug contains no anti-inflammatory or analgesic and is of no value during acute gout attacks.
• Drug may increase frequency, severity, and length of acute gout attacks during first 6 to

S

12 months of therapy. Give prophylactic colchicine or another anti-inflammatory during first 3 to 6 months.
• Lifelong therapy may be needed in patient with hyperuricemia.
• Drug decreases urinary excretion of aminohippuric acid, interfering with laboratory test results.
⚠ **ALERT:** Don't confuse Anturane with Artane or Antabuse.

Patient teaching
• Warn patient with gout not to take aspirin-containing drugs because they may precipitate gout. Acetaminophen may be used for pain.
• Tell patient to take drug with food, milk, or antacid. Also instruct him to drink plenty of water.
• Instruct patient with gout to avoid foods high in purine, such as anchovies, liver, sardines, kidneys, sweetbreads, peas, and lentils.
• Inform patient and family that drug must be taken regularly or gout attacks may result. Tell patient to see prescriber regularly so blood level can be monitored and dosage adjusted if needed.

☑ **Evaluation**
• Patient regains and maintains normal uric acid level.
• Patient doesn't experience injury from adverse CNS reactions.
• Patient and family state understanding of drug therapy.

sulindac
(SUL-in-dak)
Apo-Sulin ♦ , Clinoril, Novo-Sundac ♦

Pharmacologic class: NSAID
Therapeutic class: analgesic, anti-inflammatory
Pregnancy risk category: B (D in third trimester)

Indications and dosages

▶ **Osteoarthritis, rheumatoid arthritis, ankylosing spondylitis.** *Adults:* Initially, 150 mg P.O. b.i.d.; increase to 200 mg b.i.d., as needed.
▶ **Acute subacromial bursitis or supraspinatus tendinitis, acute gouty arthritis.** *Adults:*
200 mg P.O. b.i.d. for 7 to 14 days. Reduce dosage as symptoms subside.

Contraindications and cautions

• Contraindicated in patients hypersensitive to the drug or any of its components, and in patients for whom aspirin or NSAIDs precipitate asthma, rhinitis, urticaria, nasal polyps, angioedema, bronchospasm, or other allergic or anaphylactoid symptoms. Contraindicated for treatment of perioperative pain associated with coronary artery bypass graft surgery.
• Use cautiously in patients with history of ulcers and GI bleeding, renal dysfunction, hepatic dysfunction, compromised cardiac function or hypertension, or conditions predisposing to fluid retention.
⚖ **Lifespan:** In pregnant women, drug isn't recommended. In breast-feeding women and in children, safety and effectiveness haven't been established.

Adverse reactions

CNS: dizziness, headache, nervousness, psychosis.
CV: edema, *heart failure,* hypertension, palpitations.
EENT: tinnitus, transient visual disturbances.
GI: anorexia, constipation, dyspepsia, *epigastric distress,* flatulence, **GI bleeding,** nausea, occult blood loss, ***pancreatitis,*** peptic ulceration.
GU: interstitial nephritis, nephrotic syndrome, ***renal failure.***
Hematologic: *agranulocytosis, aplastic anemia,* hemolytic anemia, *neutropenia, thrombocytopenia.*
Skin: pruritus, *rash.*
Other: *anaphylaxis, angioedema,* drug fever, hypersensitivity syndrome.

Interactions

Drug-drug. *ACE inhibitors:* May decrease antihypertensive effects of these drugs. Monitor blood pressure.
Anticoagulants: May increase risk of bleeding. Monitor PT closely.
Cyclosporine: May increase nephrotoxicity of cyclosporine. Monitor renal function.
Diflunisal, dimethyl sulfoxide (DMSO): May decrease metabolism of sulindac to its active metabolite, reducing its effectiveness. Topical DMSO used with sulindac has caused severe peripheral neuropathy. Don't use together.

Reactions may be *common,* uncommon, *life-threatening,* or COMMON AND LIFE-THREATENING.

Diuretics: May increase effects of regular diuretics on blood pressure, but decrease effects of potassium-sparing diuretics. Monitor blood pressure and electrolytes.

Lithium: May decrease lithium level. Monitor patient and blood level carefully.

Methotrexate: May increase methotrexate toxicity. Avoid using together.

NSAIDs: May decrease sulindac level and increase risk of adverse GI reactions. Avoid using together.

Probenecid: May increase level of sulindac and its active metabolite. Monitor patient for toxicity.

Sulfonamides, sulfonylureas, other highly protein-bound drugs: May displace these drugs from protein-binding sites, leading to increased toxicity. Monitor patient closely for toxicity.

Effects on lab test results

- May increase BUN, creatinine, liver enzyme, and potassium levels. May decrease hemoglobin level and hematocrit.
- May increase bleeding time. May decrease platelet, neutrophil, and granulocyte counts.

Pharmacokinetics

Absorption: 90%.
Distribution: Extensively protein-bound.
Metabolism: In liver to an active sulfide metabolite.
Excretion: In urine. *Half-life:* Parent drug, 8 hours; active metabolite, about 16 hours.

Route	Onset	Peak	Duration
P.O.	Unknown	2–4 hr	Unknown

Action

Chemical effect: Unknown; produces antiinflammatory, analgesic, and antipyretic effects, possibly by inhibiting prostaglandin synthesis.
Therapeutic effect: Relieves pain and inflammation.

Available forms

Tablets: 150 mg, 200 mg

NURSING PROCESS

🔲 Assessment

- Assess patient's condition before starting therapy and regularly thereafter to monitor the drug's effectiveness.

- Periodically monitor liver and kidney function and CBC in patient taking long-term therapy.
- Be alert for adverse reactions and drug interactions.
- Assess patient's and family's knowledge of drug therapy.

🔲 Nursing diagnoses

- Acute pain related to presence of arthritis
- Impaired tissue integrity related to drug's adverse effect on GI mucosa
- Deficient knowledge related to drug therapy

▶ Planning and implementation

- Notify prescriber of adverse reactions.

⚡ **ALERT:** Don't confuse Clinoril with Clozaril.

Patient teaching

- Tell patient to take drug with food, milk, or antacids to reduce adverse GI reactions.
- Advise patient to refrain from driving or performing other hazardous activities that require mental alertness until the drug's CNS effects are known.
- Teach patient signs and symptoms of GI bleeding, and tell him to contact prescriber immediately if they occur. Serious GI toxicity, including peptic ulceration and bleeding, can occur in patient taking NSAIDs despite absence of GI symptoms.

⚡ **ALERT:** Tell patient to notify prescriber immediately if easy bruising or prolonged bleeding occurs.

- Instruct patient to report any edema and to have his blood pressure checked monthly. Drug causes sodium retention but may not affect kidneys as much as other NSAIDs.
- Instruct patient not to take aspirin, aspirin-containing products, or other NSAIDs with sulindac.
- Tell patient to notify prescriber and undergo complete eye examination if visual disturbances occur.

☑ Evaluation

- Patient is free from pain.
- Patient doesn't experience adverse GI reactions.
- Patient and family state understanding of drug therapy.

S

sumatriptan succinate
(soo-muh-TRIP-ten SEK-seh-nayt)
Imitrex

Pharmacologic class: selective 5-hydroxytryptamine (5-HT$_1$) receptor agonist
Therapeutic class: antimigraine drug
Pregnancy risk category: C

Indications and dosages

▶ **Acute migraine attacks (with or without aura).** *Adults:* 6 mg subcutaneously. Maximum recommended dosage is two 6-mg injections in 24 hours, separated by at least 1 hour. Or, 25 to 100 mg P.O. initially. If response isn't achieved in 2 hours, may give second dose of 25 to 100 mg. Additional doses may be used in at least 2-hour intervals. Maximum daily oral dose, 200 mg. Or, 5 mg, 10 mg, or 20 mg administered once in one nostril. May repeat once after 2 hours for maximum daily inhalation dose of 40 mg. For 10-mg dose, give a single 5-mg dose in each nostril.

▶ **Acute treatment of cluster headache episodes.** *Adults:* 6 mg subcutaneously. Maximum recommended dosage is two 6-mg injections in 24 hours, separated by at least 1 hour.
▣ **Adjust-a-dose:** For patients with hepatic impairment, don't exceed maximum single oral dose of 50 mg.

Contraindications and cautions

• Contraindicated in patients hypersensitive to the drug or any of its components, and in patients with history, symptoms, or signs of ischemic cardiac, cerebrovascular (stroke, transient ischemic attack), or peripheral vascular (ischemic bowel disease) syndromes, or MI.
• Contraindicated in patients with uncontrolled hypertension, severe hepatic impairment (oral form), and hemiplegic or basilar migraines.
• Contraindicated within 24 hours of another 5-HT agonist or ergotamine-containing drug and within 14 days of MAO inhibitor therapy (oral form only; decrease dosage of sumatriptan if given by injection while patient is on an MAO inhibitor).
• Don't give drug I.V.; it can cause coronary vasospasms.

• Use cautiously in patients who may have unrecognized coronary artery disease (CAD), such as postmenopausal women, men older than age 40, and patients with risk factors for CAD.
✹ **Lifespan:** In pregnant women and women who intend to become pregnant, use cautiously. In breast-feeding women and in children, safety and effectiveness haven't been established.

Adverse reactions

CNS: anxiety, *dizziness,* drowsiness, fatigue, headache, malaise, *vertigo.*
CV: *atrial fibrillation, coronary artery vasospasm,* hypertension, *MI,* pressure or tightness in chest, *transient myocardial ischemia, ventricular fibrillation, ventricular tachycardia.*
EENT: altered vision; discomfort of jaw, mouth, nasal cavity, sinus, throat, or tongue.
GI: abdominal discomfort, diarrhea, dysphagia, nausea, unusual or bad taste (nasal spray), vomiting.
Musculoskeletal: muscle cramps, myalgia, neck pain.
Respiratory: dyspnea and upper respiratory inflammation (P.O.).
Skin: diaphoresis.
Other: cold sensation; flushing, *tingling,* or *injection site reaction* (subcutaneous); heaviness, pressure, or tightness; numbness; tight feeling in head; *warm, hot, or burning sensation.*

Interactions

Drug-drug. *Ergot and ergot derivatives, other serotonin$_{1B/1D}$ agonists:* May prolong vasospastic effects. Don't use within 24 hours of sumatriptan therapy.
MAO inhibitors: May reduce sumatriptan clearance. Avoid using sumatriptan tablets or nasal spray within 2 weeks of stopping MAO inhibitor. Use injection cautiously in patients and decrease sumatriptan dosage.
SNRIs, SSRIs: May cause weakness, hyperreflexia, and incoordination. Monitor patient closely if use together is warranted.
Drug-herb. *Horehound:* May enhance serotonergic effects. Discourage using together.

Effects on lab test results

• May increase liver enzyme levels.

Pharmacokinetics

Absorption: Rapid after P.O. and intranasal use but with low absolute bioavailability (about 15% and 17% respectively); absorbed well from injection site after subcutaneous use.

Distribution: Wide, into body tissues. About 14% to 21% protein-bound.

Metabolism: About 80%, in liver.

Excretion: Mainly in urine. *Half-life:* About 2 hours.

Route	Onset	Peak	Duration
P.O.	30 min	2–4 hr	Unknown
SubQ	10–20 min	1–2 hr	Unknown
Intranasal	Rapid	1–2 hr	Unknown

Action

Chemical effect: Unknown; thought to selectively activate vascular serotonin (5-HT) receptors. Stimulation of specific receptor subtype 5-HT$_1$, present on cranial arteries and the dura mater, causes vasoconstriction of cerebral vessels but has minimal effects on systemic vessels, tissue perfusion, and blood pressure.

Therapeutic effect: Relieves acute migraine pain.

Available forms

Injection: 6 mg/0.5 ml (12 mg/ml) in 0.5-ml prefilled syringes and vials
Nasal spray: 5 mg/spray, 20 mg/spray
Tablets: 25 mg, 50 mg, 100 mg (base) ◆

NURSING PROCESS

Assessment

• Assess patient's condition before starting therapy and regularly thereafter to monitor the drug's effectiveness.
• Be alert for adverse reactions and drug interactions.
• Assess patient's and family's knowledge of drug therapy.

Nursing diagnoses

• Acute pain related to presence of acute migraine attack
• Risk for injury related to drug-induced adverse reactions
• Deficient knowledge related to drug therapy

▶ Planning and implementation

• If patient has risk of unrecognized CAD, give first dose with prescriber present.
• Give single tablet whole with fluids as soon as patient complains of migraine symptoms. Give second tablet if symptoms come back, but no sooner than 2 hours after first tablet.
• Maximum recommended subcutaneous dosage in 24-hour period is two 6-mg injections separated by at least 1 hour. If patient doesn't experience relief, notify prescriber.
• Patient will most likely experience relief within 1 to 2 hours.
• Redness or pain at injection site should subside within 1 hour after injection.

ALERT: Serious adverse cardiac effects can follow administration of this drug, but such events are rare.

• If patient doesn't experience relief, notify prescriber.

ALERT: Don't confuse sumatriptan with somatropin.

Patient teaching

• Make sure patient understands that drug is intended only to treat migraine attack, not to prevent or reduce number of attacks.
• Tell patient that drug may be given at any time during migraine attack but should be given as soon as symptoms appear.
• Drug is available in spring-loaded injector system that makes it easy for the patient to give injection to himself. Review detailed information with patient. Make sure patient understands how to load injector, give injection, and dispose of used syringes.
• Instruct patient taking P.O. form when and how often to take drug. Warn patient not to take more than 200 mg within 24 hours.
• Instruct patient to use intranasal spray in one nostril. (If giving 10 mg, 1 spray into each nostril.) A second spray may be used if headache returns, but not before 2 hours has elapsed from the first use.
• Tell patient who experiences persistent or severe chest pain to call prescriber immediately. Patient who experiences pain or tightness in throat, wheezing, heart throbbing, rash, lumps, hives, or swollen eyelids, face, or lips should stop using drug and call prescriber.
• Tell woman who is pregnant or intends to become pregnant not to take this drug.

S

☑ **Evaluation**

• Patient is free from pain.
• Patient doesn't experience injury from adverse CV reactions.
• Patient and family state understanding of drug therapy.

HIGH ALERT

sunitinib malate
(soo-NIH-tih-nib MAH-layt)
Sutent✲

Pharmacologic class: multi-kinase inhibitor
Therapeutic class: antineoplastic
Pregnancy risk category: D

Indications and dosages

▶ **GI stromal tumor that's progressing despite imatinib therapy or because patient is intolerant of imatinib and advanced renal cell carcinoma.** *Adults:* 50 mg P.O. once daily for 4 weeks, followed by a 2-week rest period off the drug. Repeat cycle.
⧄ **Adjust-a-dose:** Increase or decrease dosage in 12.5-mg increments based on individual safety and tolerability.

Contraindications and cautions

• Contraindicated in patients who are hypersensitive to the drug or any of its components. Don't use in patients with non–small-cell lung cancer.
• Use cautiously in patients with a history of hypertension, MI, angina, coronary artery bypass graft, symptomatic heart failure, stroke, TIA, or pulmonary embolism.
※ **Lifespan:** Drug inhibits angiogenesis, a critical component of embryonic and fetal development; tell women of childbearing age to avoid becoming pregnant during treatment. Mothers should either stop breast-feeding or stop the drug. In children, safety and efficacy haven't been established.

Adverse reactions

CNS: *asthenia, dizziness, fatigue, fever, headache, peripheral neuropathy.*
CV: *decreased left ventricular ejection fraction,* hypertension, peripheral edema, *thromboembolic events.*
EENT: increased lacrimation, periorbital edema.

GI: abdominal pain, altered taste, anorexia, appetite disturbance, burning sensation in mouth, constipation, diarrhea, dyspepsia, flatulence, *GI perforation,* mucositis, nausea, oral pain, *pancreatitis,* stomatitis, vomiting.
Hematologic: *anemia, bleeding, leukopenia, lymphopenia,* NEUTROPENIA, THROMBOCYTOPENIA.
Metabolic: *dehydration,* hyperkalemia, *hypernatremia, hyperuricemia, hypokalemia,* hyponatremia, hypophosphatemia, hypothyroidism.
Musculoskeletal: *arthralgia, back pain, limb pain, myalgia.*
Respiratory: *cough, dyspnea.*
Skin: *alopecia, dry skin, hair color changes, hand-foot syndrome, rash,* skin blistering, *skin discoloration.*
Other: *adrenal insufficiency.*

Interactions

Drug-drug. *CYP3A4 inducers (such as carbamazepine, dexamethasone, phenobarbital, phenytoin, rifabutin, rifampin, rifapentine):* May decrease sunitinib level and effects. If use together can't be avoided, increase sunitinib dosage to 87.5 mg daily.
Strong CYP3A4 inhibitors (such as atazanavir, clarithromycin, indinavir, itraconazole, ketoconazole, nefazodone, nelfinavir, ritonavir, saquinavir, telithromycin, voriconazole): May increase sunitinib level and toxicity. If use together can't be avoided, decrease sunitinib dosage to 37.5 mg daily.
Drug-food. *Grapefruit:* May increase drug level. Tell patient to avoid grapefruit.
Drug-herb. *St. John's wort:* May cause an unpredictable decrease in drug level. Discourage use together.

Effects on lab test results

• May increase AST, ALT, alkaline phosphatase, total and indirect bilirubin, amylase, lipase, creatinine, uric acid, and TSH levels. May decrease phosphorus and hemoglobin levels and hematocrit. May increase or decrease potassium and sodium levels.
• May decrease RBC, neutrophil, lymphocyte, leukocyte, and platelet counts.

Pharmacokinetics

Absorption: Unaffected by food. Reaches steady-state level in 10 to 14 days.

Distribution: 95% plasma protein–bound. Metabolite is 90% plasma protein–bound.
Metabolism: Mainly in the liver through the CYP3A4 pathway.
Excretion: Via feces (61%) and urine (16%).
Half-life: 40 to 60 hours; *primary metabolite:* 80 to 110 hours.

Route	Onset	Peak	Duration
P.O.	Rapid	6–12 hr	Unknown

Action

Chemical effect: A multi-kinase inhibitor targeting several receptor tyrosine kinases, which are involved in tumor growth, pathologic angiogenesis, and metastatic progression of cancer.
Therapeutic effect: Slows carcinoma growth.

Available forms

Capsules: 12.5 mg, 25 mg, 50 mg

NURSING PROCESS

Assessment
• Assess neoplastic disease before starting therapy, and reassess regularly.
• Monitor patient's blood pressure, and treat hypertension as needed. If severe hypertension occurs, stop treatment until blood pressure is adequately controlled.
• Monitor patient for signs and symptoms of heart failure, especially if he has a history of heart disease.
• Notify prescriber if patient develops signs or symptoms of heart failure.
• If patient has seizures, consider reversible posterior leukoencephalopathy syndrome. Signs and symptoms include hypertension, headache, decreased alertness, altered mental functioning, and vision loss. Notify prescriber immediately.
• If patient will be undergoing surgery or suffers trauma or severe infection, assess him for adrenal insufficiency (muscle weakness, weight loss, depression, salt craving, low blood pressure).
• Assess patient's and family's knowledge of drug therapy.

Nursing diagnoses
• Ineffective health maintenance related to neoplastic disease

• Risk for falls related to drug-induced adverse reactions
• Deficient knowledge related to drug therapy

Planning and implementation
• Obtain baseline weight before starting therapy, and then weigh patient daily. Evaluate and treat unexpected and rapid weight gain.
• Obtain CBC with platelet count and serum chemistries, including phosphate level, before each treatment cycle.
• Obtain baseline evaluation of ejection fraction in all patients before treatment. If patient had a cardiac event in the year preceding treatment, check ejection fraction periodically.
• Patients with an ejection fraction less than 50% and more than 20% below baseline will need a decreased dosage or interruption of treatment.
• Provide antiemetics or antidiarrheals as needed for adverse GI effects.
Patient teaching
• Advise patient to keep appointments for blood tests before each treatment cycle and, if needed, periodic heart function evaluations.
• Tell patient about common adverse effects, such as diarrhea, nausea, vomiting, fatigue, mouth pain, and taste disturbance.
• Inform patient about changes that may occur in skin and hair, including color changes and dry, red, blistering skin of the hands and feet.
• Urge patient to tell health care providers about all prescribed and OTC drugs or herbal supplements he takes.
• Warn patient not to consume grapefruit products during therapy.
• Tell patient to notify his prescriber about unusual bleeding, trouble breathing, wheezing, severe or prolonged diarrhea or vomiting, or swelling of the hands or lower legs.

Evaluation
• Patient shows positive response to drug therapy on follow-up studies.
• Patient doesn't experience falls.
• Patient and family state understanding of drug therapy.

S

T

tacrine hydrochloride
(TAK-reen high-droh-KLOR-ighd)
Cognex

Pharmacologic class: centrally acting reversible anticholinesterase
Therapeutic class: psychotherapeutic for Alzheimer disease
Pregnancy risk category: C

Indications and dosages

▶ **Mild to moderate dementia of Alzheimer type.** *Adults:* Initially, 10 mg P.O. q.i.d. After 4 weeks, if patient tolerates drug and transaminase level isn't elevated, increase dosage to 20 mg q.i.d. After another 4 weeks, increase dosage to 30 mg q.i.d. If still tolerated, increase to 40 mg q.i.d. after another 4 weeks.

▧ **Adjust-a-dose:** For patients with ALT level three to five times the upper limit of normal (ULN) range, reduce dosage by 40 mg daily and monitor ALT level weekly until normal. If ALT is more than five times ULN, stop therapy and monitor patient for signs and symptoms of hepatitis. May rechallenge when ALT returns to normal. With rechallenge doses, monitor ALT weekly for 16 weeks, then monthly for 2 months, then every 3 months thereafter.

Contraindications and cautions

• Contraindicated in patients hypersensitive to the drug or acridine derivatives, and in those who have previously developed drug-related jaundice and been confirmed with elevated total bilirubin level of more than 3 mg/dl.
• Use cautiously in patients with sick sinus syndrome or bradycardia; those at risk for peptic ulceration (including patients taking NSAIDs or those with history of peptic ulcer); those with history of hepatic disease; and those with renal disease, asthma, prostatic hyperplasia, or other urinary outflow impairment.
⚘ **Lifespan:** In pregnant and breast-feeding women, drug isn't recommended. In children, drug isn't indicated.

Adverse reactions

CNS: abnormal thinking, agitation, anxiety, ataxia, confusion, depression, *dizziness,* fatigue, *headache,* insomnia, somnolence.
CV: chest pain, facial flushing.
EENT: rhinitis.
GI: anorexia, changes in stool color, constipation, *diarrhea,* dyspepsia, loose stools, *nausea, vomiting.*
Hepatic: jaundice.
Metabolic: weight loss.
Musculoskeletal: myalgia.
Respiratory: cough, upper respiratory tract infection.
Skin: rash.

Interactions

Drug-drug. *Anticholinergics:* May decrease effectiveness of anticholinergics. Monitor patient closely.
Anticholinesterases, cholinergics (such as bethanechol): May have additive effects. Monitor patient for toxicity.
Cimetidine: May increase tacrine level. Monitor patient for toxicity.
Fluvoxamine: May increase tacrine level. Monitor patient.
Succinylcholine: May enhance neuromuscular blockade and prolong duration of action. Monitor patient.
Theophylline: May increase theophylline level and prolong theophylline half-life. Carefully monitor theophylline level, and adjust dosage.
Drug-food. *Any food:* May decrease drug absorption. Tell patient to take drug on empty stomach.
Drug-lifestyle. *Smoking:* May decrease level of drug. Monitor response.

Effects on lab test results

• May increase ALT and AST levels.

Pharmacokinetics

Absorption: Rapid, with absolute bioavailability of about 17%. Food reduces bioavailability by 30% to 40%.
Distribution: About 55% bound to plasma proteins.
Metabolism: Undergoes first-pass metabolism, which is dose-dependent. Extensively metabolized.
Excretion: In urine. *Half-life:* 2 to 4 hours.

Route	Onset	Peak	Duration
P.O.	Unknown	30 min–3 hr	Unknown

Action

Chemical effect: Reversibly inhibits enzyme cholinesterase in CNS, allowing buildup of acetylcholine.
Therapeutic effect: Improves thinking in patients with Alzheimer disease.

Available forms

Capsules: 10 mg, 20 mg, 30 mg, 40 mg

NURSING PROCESS

Assessment
• Assess patient's cognitive ability before starting therapy and regularly thereafter to monitor drug's effectiveness.
• Check ALT level every other week from at least week 4 to week 16 of therapy. If ALT is twice the ULN range, check weekly. If no problems occur, decrease frequency of testing to every 3 months. Whenever dosage is increased, resume monitoring every other week.
• Assess patient's and family's knowledge of drug therapy.

Nursing diagnoses
• Disturbed thought processes related to Alzheimer disease
• Diarrhea related to drug-induced adverse GI reactions
• Deficient knowledge related to drug therapy

Planning and implementation
• Stop drug if patient has evidence of jaundice, increase in total serum bilirubin, or hypersensitivity. Don't resume therapy.
• If patient doesn't improve in 3 to 6 months, consider stopping the drug.
• Give drug between meals. If GI upset becomes a problem, give drug with meals, although level may drop by 30% to 40%.
• If drug is stopped for 4 weeks or longer, restart at the basic dosage and adjust according to the schedule, as if the patient were being started on drug for the first time.
• Obtain order for antidiarrheal, if indicated.
Patient teaching
• Inform patient and family that drug doesn't alter underlying degenerative disease. Instead, it may alleviate symptoms of Alzheimer disease.

• Explain to patient and family that the effect of therapy depends on taking the drug at regular intervals.
🔔 **ALERT:** Instruct caregivers when to give drug. Explain that dosage adjustment is integral to safe use. Abruptly stopping or reducing daily dose by 80 mg or more may trigger behavioral disturbances and cognitive decline.
• Advise patient and caregivers to report immediately any significant adverse effects or changes in status.

☑ Evaluation
• Patient exhibits improved cognitive ability.
• Patient or caregiver states that drug-induced diarrhea hasn't occurred.
• Patient and family state understanding of drug therapy.

tacrolimus
(tek-roh-LYE-mus)
Prograf

Pharmacologic class: macrolide
Therapeutic class: immunosuppressant
Pregnancy risk category: C

Indications and dosages

▶ **To prevent organ rejection in allogenic liver, kidney, or heart transplant.** *Adults:* Give with adrenal corticosteroid therapy. For patients unable to take drug orally, give 0.03 to 0.05 mg/kg/day (liver or kidney) or 0.01 mg/kg/day (heart) I.V. as continuous infusion no sooner than 6 hours after transplant. Switch to oral therapy as soon as possible, with first dose given 8 to 12 hours after stopping I.V. infusion. For renal transplant, give oral dose within 24 hours of transplantation after renal function has recovered. Recommended initial P.O. dosages are as follows: For liver transplant, give 0.1 to 0.15 mg/kg daily in two divided doses every 12 hours. For kidney transplant, give 0.2 mg/kg daily in two divided doses every 12 hours. For heart transplant, give 0.075 mg/kg daily in two divided doses every 12 hours. Adjust dosages based on patient's response.
Children (liver transplant only): Initially, 0.03 to 0.05 mg/kg daily I.V.; then 0.15 to

T

0.2 mg/kg daily P.O. on schedule similar to that of adults, adjusted as needed.

▧ **Adjust-a-dose:** Give lowest recommended P.O. and I.V. dosages to patients with renal or hepatic impairment.

▶ **Crohn disease‡.** *Adults and children age 12 and older:* 200 mcg/kg P.O. daily in 2 divided doses for 10 weeks.

▽ I.V. administration

• Dilute drug with normal saline solution injection or D_5W injection to 0.004 to 0.02 mg/ml before use.
• Each required daily dose of diluted drug is infused continuously over 24 hours.
• Monitor patient continuously during first 30 minutes of infusion; then check often for anaphylaxis.
• Keep epinephrine 1:1,000 available to treat anaphylaxis.
• Store diluted solution for no more than 24 hours in glass or polyethylene containers. Don't store drug in polyvinyl chloride container.

⊗ **Incompatibilities**
Solutions or I.V. drugs with a pH above 9, such as acyclovir and ganciclovir.

Contraindications and cautions

• Contraindicated in patients hypersensitive to the drug or any of its components. I.V. form contraindicated in patients hypersensitive to castor oil derivatives.
• Use cautiously in patients with renal or hepatic impairment.

✹ **Lifespan:** In pregnant or breast-feeding women, drug isn't recommended.

Adverse reactions

CNS: asthenia, *coma,* delirium, fever, *headache,* insomnia, *neurotoxicity,* pain, *paresthesia, tremor.*
CV: *chest pain, hypertension,* peripheral edema.
GI: *abdominal pain, anorexia,* ascites, *constipation, diarrhea,* nausea, *vomiting.*
GU: *abnormal kidney function,* **nephrotoxicity,** *oliguria,* UTI.
Hematologic: *anemia,* leukocytosis, THROMBOCYTOPENIA.
Metabolic: *hyperglycemia,* **hyperkalemia,** *hypokalemia,* HYPOMAGNESEMIA.
Musculoskeletal: *back pain.*
Respiratory: atelectasis, *dyspnea, pleural effusion.*

Skin: photosensitivity reactions.
Other: *anaphylaxis.*

Interactions

Drug-drug. *Bromocriptine, cimetidine, clarithromycin, clotrimazole, cyclosporine, danazol, diltiazem, erythromycin, ethinyl estradiol, fluconazole, itraconazole, ketoconazole, methylprednisolone, metoclopramide, nefazodone, nicardipine, nifedipine, omeprazole, protease inhibitors, verapamil:* May increase tacrolimus level. Monitor patient for adverse effects.
Carbamazepine, phenobarbital, phenytoin, rifabutin, rifampin: May decrease tacrolimus level. Monitor tacrolimus effectiveness.
Cyclosporine: May increase risk of excess nephrotoxicity. Don't give together.
Immunosuppressants (except adrenocorticosteroids): May oversuppress immune system. Monitor patient closely, especially during times of stress.
Inducers of cytochrome P-450 enzyme system: May increase tacrolimus metabolism and decrease drug level. Dosage adjustment may be needed.
Inhibitors of cytochrome P-450 enzyme system: May decrease tacrolimus metabolism and increase drug level. Dosage adjustment may be needed.
Nephrotoxic drugs (such as aminoglycosides, amphotericin B, cisplatin, cyclosporine): May cause additive or synergistic effects. Monitor patient closely.
Viral vaccines: May interfere with immune response to live-virus vaccines.
Drug-herb. *St. John's wort:* May decrease tacrolimus level. Monitor effectiveness of tacrolimus.
Drug-food. *Any food:* May inhibit drug absorption. Tell patient to take drug on an empty stomach.
Grapefruit juice: May increase drug level in liver transplant patients. Discourage use together.

Effects on lab test results

• May increase glucose, creatinine, and BUN levels. May decrease magnesium and hemoglobin levels and hematocrit. May increase or decrease potassium level.
• May increase liver function test values and WBC and platelet counts.

Pharmacokinetics

Absorption: Variable. Food reduces absorption and bioavailability of drug.
Distribution: Distribution between whole blood and plasma depends on several factors, such as hematocrit, temperature of separation of plasma, drug level, and protein level. Drug is 75% to 99% protein-bound.
Metabolism: Extensive.
Excretion: Mainly in bile. *Half-life:* 33 to 56 hours.

Route	Onset	Peak	Duration
P.O., I.V.	Unknown	1½–3½ hr	Unknown

Action

Chemical effect: Unknown; may inhibit T-lymphocyte activation, which results in immunosuppression.
Therapeutic effect: Prevents organ rejection.

Available forms

Capsules: 0.5 mg, 1 mg, 5 mg
Injection: 5 mg/ml

NURSING PROCESS

Assessment
• Obtain history of patient's organ transplant before starting therapy, and reassess regularly to monitor the drug's effectiveness.
• Monitor patient for signs of neurotoxicity and nephrotoxicity, especially in those receiving high dosage or those with renal dysfunction.
• Obtain potassium and glucose levels regularly. Monitor patient for hyperglycemia.
• Drug increases risk of infections, lymphomas, and other cancers.
• Be alert for adverse reactions and drug interactions.
• Assess patient's and family's knowledge of drug therapy.

Nursing diagnoses
• Risk for injury related to organ transplant rejection
• Ineffective protection related to drug-induced immunosuppression
• Deficient knowledge related to drug therapy

Planning and implementation
• Child with normal kidney and liver function may need a higher dose than an adult.

• Patient with hepatic or renal dysfunction needs lowest possible dosage.
• Black renal transplant patients may require higher doses.
• Use with adrenal corticosteroids for all indications. For heart transplant patients, also use with azathioprine or mycophenolate mofetil.
• Give oral drug on empty stomach.
🜄 **ALERT:** The use of sirolimus with tacrolimus may increase the risk of wound healing complications, renal impairment, and posttransplant type 1 diabetes mellitus in heart transplant patients. Don't use together.
• Because of risk of anaphylaxis, use injection only in patient who can't take oral form.
• Don't use other immunosuppressants (except adrenocorticosteroids) during therapy.
• Avoid potassium-sparing diuretics during therapy.
• Hepatic transplant trough levels are best maintained at 5 to 20 nanograms/ml 1 to 2 months posttransplant. Renal transplant trough levels are best maintained at 7 to 20 nanograms/ml between posttransplant months 1 to 3, and then 1 to 5 nanograms/ml for posttransplant months 4 to 12.

Patient teaching
• Instruct patient to take drug on empty stomach and not to take it with grapefruit juice.
• Explain need for repeated tests during therapy to monitor adverse reactions and drug effectiveness.
• Advise woman of childbearing age to notify prescriber if she becomes pregnant or plans to do so.
• Instruct patient to check with prescriber before taking other drugs.

Evaluation
• Patient has no signs and symptoms of organ rejection.
• Patient develops no serious complications from drug-induced adverse reactions.
• Patient and family state understanding of drug therapy.

T

tacrolimus (topical)
(tack-row-LYE-mus)
Protopic

Pharmacologic class: macrolide
Therapeutic class: immunosuppressant
Pregnancy risk category: C

Indications and dosages

▶ **Moderate to severe atopic dermatitis in patients unresponsive to other therapies or unable to use other therapies because of risks.** *Adults:* Apply thin layer of 0.03% or 0.1% strength to affected areas b.i.d. and rub in completely. Continue for 1 week after affected area clears.
Children ages 2 to 15: Apply thin layer of 0.03% strength to affected areas b.i.d. and rub in completely. Continue for 1 week after affected area clears.

Contraindications and cautions

• Contraindicated in patients hypersensitive to the drug or any of its components.
• Don't use in patients with Netherton syndrome or generalized erythroderma, or in immunocompromised patients.
⚠ **Lifespan:** In pregnant women, use only if benefits to the patient outweigh risks to the fetus. In breast-feeding women, the drug appears in breast milk; weigh benefits to the mother against risks to the infant. In children ages 2 to 15, use only 0.03% ointment.

Adverse reactions

CNS: asthenia, *fever, headache,* hyperesthesia, insomnia, pain.
CV: facial edema, peripheral edema.
EENT: conjunctivitis, *otitis media, pharyngitis,* rhinitis, sinusitis.
GI: abdominal pain, diarrhea, dyspepsia, gastroenteritis, nausea, vomiting.
GU: dysmenorrhea.
Hematologic: lymphadenopathy, *lymphoma.*
Musculoskeletal: back pain, myalgia.
Respiratory: *asthma,* bronchitis, *increased cough,* pneumonia.
Skin: acne, benign skin neoplasm, contact dermatitis, dry skin, eczema, eczema herpeticum, exfoliative dermatitis, *folliculitis,* fungal dermatitis, herpes zoster, maculopapular rash, pus-

tular rash, *pruritus,* rash, *skin burning, skin cancer,* skin disorder, *skin erythema, skin infection,* sunburn, tingling, urticaria, vesiculobullous rash.
Other: accidental injury, alcohol intolerance, allergic reaction, cyst, flulike symptoms, herpes simplex, infection, lack of drug effect, periodontal abscess.

Interactions

Drug-drug. *CYP3A4 inhibitors (erythromycin, fluconazole, itraconazole, ketoconazole):* May interfere with effects of tacrolimus. Use together cautiously.
Drug-lifestyle. *Sun exposure:* May cause risk of phototoxicity. Tell patient to avoid or minimize exposure to artificial or natural sunlight.

Effects on lab test results

None reported.

Pharmacokinetics

Absorption: Immediate, with no systemic accumulation.
Distribution: Unknown.
Metabolism: Unknown.
Excretion: Unknown. *Half-life:* Unknown.

Route	Onset	Peak	Duration
Topical	Unknown	Unknown	Unknown

Action

Chemical effect: May inhibit T-lymphocyte activation in the skin, which causes immunosuppression. Also inhibits the release of mediators from mast cells and basophils in skin.
Therapeutic effect: Improves skin condition.

Available forms

Ointment: 0.03%, 0.1%

NURSING PROCESS

📝 **Assessment**

• Assess patient's underlying condition before starting therapy, and reassess regularly to monitor the drug's effectiveness.
• Assess patient with infected atopic dermatitis; clear infections at treatment site before using drug.
• Assess patient's and family's knowledge of drug therapy.

⊞ Nursing diagnoses

- Impaired skin integrity related to underlying skin condition
- Acute pain related to drug-induced adverse effects
- Deficient knowledge related to tacrolimus therapy

▷ Planning and implementation

- Drug is used only for short-term or intermittent therapy. Avoid long-term use.
- Limit application to areas of involvement with atopic dermatitis.
- Only 0.03% ointment is indicated for use in children ages 2 to 15.
- Use only after other treatments have failed because of a possible risk of cancer with Protopic.
- ⚠ ALERT: Don't use occlusive dressings over drug. This may promote systemic absorption.
- Drug may increase the risk of varicella zoster, herpes simplex virus, and eczema herpeticum.
- Assess all cases of lymphadenopathy to determine etiology. If a clear etiology is unknown or acute mononucleosis is diagnosed, consider stopping drug.
- Monitor all cases of lymphadenopathy until resolution.
- Local adverse effects are most common during the first few days of therapy.

Patient teaching

- Tell patient to wash hands before and after applying drug and to avoid applying drug to wet skin. Skin should be completely dry before applying drug.
- Instruct patient not to use bandages or other occlusive dressings.
- Tell patient not to bathe, shower, or swim immediately after application because doing so could wash the ointment off.
- Advise patient to avoid or minimize exposure to natural or artificial sunlight.
- Tell patient that, if he needs to be outdoors after applying drug, he should wear loose-fitting clothing that covers the treated area. Check with prescriber regarding sunscreen use.
- Tell patient not to use drug for any disorder other than that for which it was prescribed.
- Instruct patient to report adverse reactions.
- Tell patient to store the ointment at room temperature.

☑ Evaluation

- Patient has improved skin condition.

- Patient states that pain management techniques are effective.
- Patient and family state understanding of drug therapy.

tadalafil
(tah-DAH-lah-phil)
Cialis

Pharmacologic class: phosphodiesterase type 5 inhibitor
Therapeutic class: erectile dysfunction drug, vasodilator
Pregnancy risk category: B

Indications and dosages

▶ **Erectile dysfunction.** *Men:* 10 mg P.O. as a single dose, p.r.n., before sexual activity. Range is 5 to 20 mg based on effectiveness and tolerance. Maximum, one dose daily. Or, 2.5 mg P.O. daily without regard to sexual activity. May increase to 5 mg daily based on patient response.

⧄ **Adjust-a-dose:** For patients with renal impairment, if creatinine clearance is 31 to 50 ml/minute, starting dosage is 5 mg once daily and maximum dosage is 10 mg taken once every 48 hours; if 30 ml/minute or less, maximum dosage is 5 mg once every 72 hours. For patients with mild to moderate hepatic impairment (Child-Pugh class A or B), dosage shouldn't exceed 10 mg daily. For patients taking potent CYP3A4 inhibitors (such as erythromycin, itraconazole, ketoconazole, ritonavir), don't exceed one 10-mg dose every 72 hours.

Contraindications and cautions

- Contraindicated in patients hypersensitive to the drug or any of its components, and in those taking nitrates or alpha blockers (other than tamsulosin 0.4 mg once daily). Drug isn't recommended for patients with severe hepatic impairment (Child-Pugh class C), MI within 90 days, New York Heart Association Class II or greater heart failure within 6 months, stroke within 6 months, uncontrolled arrhythmias, blood pressure lower than 90/50 mm Hg or higher than 170/100 mm Hg, unstable angina, or angina that occurs during sexual intercourse. Drug also isn't recommended for patients whose cardiac status makes sexual activity inadvisable and for those with hereditary degenerative retinal disorders.

T

• Use cautiously in patients taking potent CYP3A4 inhibitors and in patients with bleeding disorders, significant peptic ulceration, or renal or hepatic impairment. Use cautiously in patients with conditions that predispose them to priapism (such as sickle cell anemia, multiple myeloma, or leukemia), anatomical penis abnormalities, or left ventricular outflow obstruction.
❈ **Lifespan:** Drug is for men only. In elderly men, consider a lower dose because they may be more sensitive to drug effects.

Adverse reactions

CNS: dizziness, headache.
CV: flushing.
EENT: decrease or loss of hearing, nasal congestion, tinnitus, vision loss.
GI: dyspepsia.
Musculoskeletal: back pain, limb pain, myalgia.

Interactions

Drug-drug. *Alpha blockers (except tamsulosin 0.4 mg daily), nitrates:* May enhance hypotensive effects. Avoid using together.
Potent CYP3A4 inhibitors (such as erythromycin, itraconazole, ketoconazole, ritonavir): May increase tadalafil level. Patient shouldn't exceed 10 mg every 72 hours.
Rifampin and other CYP3A4 inducers: May decrease tadalafil level. Monitor patient closely.
Drug-food. *Grapefruit:* May increase drug level. Discourage use together. Monitor patient closely.
Drug-lifestyle. *Alcohol use:* May increase risk of headache, dizziness, orthostatic hypotension, and increased heart rate. Discourage use together.

Effects on lab test results

None reported.

Pharmacokinetics

Absorption: Median effect occurs in 2 hours.
Distribution: Distributed into tissues. 94% protein-bound.
Metabolism: Mainly through CYP3A4 isoenzymes.
Excretion: In feces and urine. *Half-life:* 17½ hours.

Route	Onset	Peak	Duration
P.O.	30 min	30 min–6 hr	Up to 1 day

Action

Chemical effect: Prevents breakdown of cyclic guanosine monophosphate (cGMP) by phosphodiesterase, thus increasing cGMP level.
Therapeutic effect: Prolongs smooth muscle relaxation and promotes blood flow into the corpus cavernosum.

Available forms

Tablets (film-coated): 2.5 mg, 5 mg, 10 mg, 20 mg

NURSING PROCESS

🔖 Assessment

🕲 **ALERT:** Sexual activity may increase cardiac risk. Assess patient's cardiac risk before he starts drug.
• Before patient starts drug, assess for underlying causes of erectile dysfunction.
• Assess patient's and family's knowledge of drug therapy.

🌐 Nursing diagnoses

• Sexual dysfunction related to patient's underlying condition
• Risk for injury related to potential for prolonged erections or priapism
• Deficient knowledge related to drug therapy

▶ Planning and implementation

• Drug may cause transient decreases in supine blood pressure.
• Drug increases risk of prolonged erections and priapism.
Patient teaching
• Warn patient that taking drug with nitrates or alpha blockers could cause a serious drop in blood pressure, raising the risk of heart attack or stroke.
• Tell patient to seek immediate medical attention if he develops chest pain, hearing, or vision problems after taking the drug.
• Urge patient to seek emergency medical care if his erection lasts longer than 4 hours.
• Tell patient to take drug about 60 minutes before anticipated sexual activity. Explain that drug has no effect without sexual stimulation.
• Warn patient not to change dose unless directed by prescriber.
• Caution patient against drinking large amounts of alcohol while taking drug.

Reactions may be *common*, uncommon, *life-threatening*, or COMMON AND LIFE-THREATENING.

☑ **Evaluation**

• Sexual activity improves with drug therapy.
• Patient sustains no injury from prolonged erection or priapism.
• Patient and family state understanding of drug therapy.

HIGH ALERT

tamoxifen citrate

(teh-MOKS-uh-fen SIGH-trayt)

Apo-Tamox♦ , Nolvadex-D♦ , Soltamox, Tamofen♦

Pharmacologic class: nonsteroidal antiestrogen
Therapeutic class: antineoplastic
Pregnancy risk category: D

Indications and dosages

▶ **Advanced postmenopausal breast cancer.**
Women: 20 to 40 mg P.O. daily. Give doses greater than 20 mg/day in divided doses (morning and evening).
▶ **Adjunct treatment for breast cancer.**
Adults: 20 to 40 mg P.O. daily for no more than 5 years. Give doses greater than 20 mg/day in divided doses (morning and evening).
▶ **Reduction of breast cancer risk.** *Women at high risk:* 20 mg P.O. daily for 5 years.
▶ **Ductal carcinoma in situ (DCIS).** *Adults:* 20 mg P.O. daily for 5 years.
▶ **Stimulation of ovulation‡.** *Women:* 5 to 40 mg P.O. b.i.d. for 4 days.

Contraindications and cautions

• Contraindicated in patients hypersensitive to the drug or any of its components, in women receiving coumarin-type anticoagulants, and in those with history of deep vein thrombosis or pulmonary emboli.
• Use cautiously in patients with leukopenia or thrombocytopenia.
♨ **Lifespan:** In pregnant or breast-feeding women, drug isn't recommended. Patient should avoid pregnancy for at least 2 months after stopping drug. In children, safety and effectiveness haven't been established.

Adverse reactions

CNS: confusion, headache, sleepiness, *stroke,* weakness.
CV: hot flushes.
EENT: cataracts, corneal changes, retinopathy.

GI: diarrhea, nausea, vomiting.
GU: amenorrhea, *endometrial cancer,* irregular menses, vaginal discharge and bleeding, *uterine sarcoma.*
Hematologic: *leukopenia, thrombocytopenia.*
Hepatic: cholestasis, fatty liver, *hepatic necrosis.*
Metabolic: fluid retention, hypercalcemia, weight changes.
Musculoskeletal: brief exacerbation of pain from osseous metastases.
Respiratory: *pulmonary embolism.*
Skin: rash, skin changes.
Other: temporary bone or tumor pain.

Interactions

Drug-drug. *Antacids:* May affect absorption of enteric-coated tablet. Don't use within 2 hours of tamoxifen dose.
Bromocriptine: May elevate tamoxifen level. Monitor patient for toxicity.
Coumadin-type anticoagulants: May cause significant increase in anticoagulant effect. Monitor patient, PT, and INR closely.
Cytotoxic drugs (fluorouracil, methotrexate): May increase risk of thromboembolic events. Monitor patient, PT, and INR closely.

Effects on lab test results

• May increase BUN, creatinine, calcium, and liver enzyme levels.
• May decrease WBC and platelet counts.

Pharmacokinetics

Absorption: Appears to be well absorbed.
Distribution: Widely in total body water.
Metabolism: Extensive by the liver.
Excretion: Drug and metabolites mainly in feces, mostly as metabolites. *Half-life:* More than 7 days.

Route	Onset	Peak	Duration
P.O.	Unknown	5 hr	Unknown

Action

Chemical effect: Exact antineoplastic action is unknown; acts as estrogen antagonist.
Therapeutic effect: Hinders function of breast cancer cells.

Available forms

Oral solution: 10 mg/5 ml

T

Tablets: 10 mg, 20 mg
Tablets (enteric-coated): 10 mg, 20 mg

NURSING PROCESS

⚕ Assessment
• Assess patient's breast cancer before starting therapy and regularly thereafter to monitor drug's effectiveness.
• Monitor CBC closely in patient with leukopenia or thrombocytopenia.
• Monitor lipid level during long-term therapy in patient with hyperlipidemia.
• Monitor calcium level in early stages of therapy; drug may compound hypercalcemia related to bone metastases.
• Be alert for adverse reactions.
• Monitor patient's hydration status if adverse GI reaction occurs.
• Assess patient's and family's knowledge of drug therapy.

⚕ Nursing diagnoses
• Ineffective health maintenance related to presence of breast cancer
• Risk for deficient fluid volume related to drug-induced adverse GI reactions
• Deficient knowledge related to drug therapy

▷ Planning and implementation
• Make sure patient swallows enteric-coated tablets whole.
⚖ **ALERT:** Serious events (including uterine cancer, stroke, DVT, and pulmonary embolism) are linked to use in women at high risk for cancer and women with DCIS. Prescribers should discuss potential benefits and risks with women considering drug to reduce risk of developing breast cancer. The benefits outweigh risks in women already diagnosed with breast cancer.
Patient teaching
• Tell patient to use oral solution within 3 months of opening and not to freeze or refrigerate.
• Instruct patient to report symptoms of pulmonary embolism (chest pain, difficulty breathing, rapid breathing, sweating or fainting).
• Tell patient to report symptoms of stroke (headache, vision changes, confusion, difficulty speaking or walking, and weakness of face, arm or leg, especially on one side of the body).
• Reassure patient that acute bone pain during drug therapy usually means that drug will produce good response. Tell her to take an analgesic for pain.
• Encourage patient who is taking or has taken drug to have regular gynecologic examinations because of increased risk of uterine cancer.
• If patient is taking drug to reduce risk of breast cancer, teach proper technique for breast self-examination.
• Tell patient that annual mammograms are important.
• Advise patient to use barrier form of contraception because short-term therapy induces ovulation in premenopausal women.
• Advise woman of childbearing age to avoid becoming pregnant during therapy and for at least 2 months following discontinuation of therapy. Tell her to consult with prescriber before becoming pregnant.

⚕ Evaluation
• Patient responds well to drug.
• Patient maintains adequate hydration.
• Patient and family state understanding of drug therapy.

tamsulosin hydrochloride
(tam-SOO-loh-sin high-droh-KLOR-ighd)
Flomax

Pharmacologic class: alpha$_{1A}$ antagonist
Therapeutic class: BPH drug
Pregnancy risk category: B

Indications and dosages
▶ **BPH.** *Men:* 0.4 mg P.O. once daily, given 30 minutes after same meal each day. If no response after 2 to 4 weeks, increase dosage to 0.8 mg P.O. once daily.

Contraindications and cautions
• Contraindicated in patients hypersensitive to the drug or any of its components.
• Use cautiously in patients who have experienced hepatic or renal insufficiency, priapism, sulfa allergy, or orthostasis.
⚖ **Lifespan:** Drug is indicated for men only.

Adverse reactions
CNS: asthenia, *dizziness, headache,* insomnia, somnolence, syncope, vertigo.
CV: chest pain, orthostatic hypotension.

EENT: amblyopia, pharyngitis, *rhinitis,* sinusitis.
GI: diarrhea, nausea.
GU: abnormal ejaculation.
Musculoskeletal: back pain.
Respiratory: cough.
Other: decreased libido, *infection,* tooth disorder.

Interactions

Drug-drug. *Alpha blockers:* May interact with tamsulosin. Avoid using together.
Cimetidine: May decrease tamsulosin clearance. Use cautiously.
Warfarin: Study results are inconclusive. Use together cautiously.

Effects on lab test results

None reported.

Pharmacokinetics

Absorption: More than 90%. Food increases bioavailability by 30%.
Distribution: Into extracellular fluids. 94% to 99% protein-bound.
Metabolism: Mainly by cytochrome P-450 enzymes in the liver.
Excretion: 76% in urine; 21% in feces. *Half-life:* 9 to 13 hours.

Route	Onset	Peak	Duration
P.O.	Unknown	4–5 hr	9–15 hr

Action

Chemical effect: Selectively blocks alpha receptors in the prostate, leading to relaxation of smooth muscles in the bladder neck and prostate, which improves urine flow and reduces symptoms of BPH.
Therapeutic effect: Improves urine flow.

Available forms

Capsules: 0.4 mg

NURSING PROCESS

Assessment
• Assess patient for signs of prostatic hyperplasia, including frequency of urination, nocturnal urination, and urinary hesitancy.
• Monitor patient for decreases in blood pressure and notify prescriber.
• Assess patient's and family's knowledge of drug therapy.

Nursing diagnoses
• Risk for injury related to decreased blood pressure and resulting syncope
• Impaired urinary elimination related to underlying prostatic hyperplasia
• Deficient knowledge related to drug therapy

Planning and implementation
• Symptoms of BPH and cancer of the prostate are similar; cancer should be ruled out before therapy starts.
• If therapy is interrupted for several days or more, restart therapy at one capsule daily.
• Drug may cause a sudden drop in blood pressure, especially after the first dose or when changing doses.
⚠ **ALERT:** Advise patient considering cataract surgery to inform the ophthalmologist that he is taking the drug. Floppy iris syndrome may occur during surgery.
⚠ **ALERT:** Don't confuse Flomax with Fosamax.
Patient teaching
• Instruct patient not to crush, chew, or open capsules.
• Tell patient to get up slowly from chair or bed when therapy starts and to avoid situations where injury could occur because of syncope. Advise him that drug may cause a sudden drop in blood pressure, especially after the first dose or when changing doses.
• Instruct patient not to drive or perform hazardous tasks for 12 hours after the initial dose or a change in dose, until response can be monitored.
• Tell patient to take drug about 30 minutes after same meal each day.
• If patient needs cataract surgery, urge him to tell surgeon that he takes tamsulosin.

Evaluation
• Patient has no sudden decreases in blood pressure.
• Patient has normal urinary elimination patterns.
• Patient and family state understanding of drug therapy.

telbivudine

(tehl-BIV-yoo-deen)

Sebivo ◆ , Tyzeka

Pharmacologic class: synthetic thymidine nucleoside analogue
Therapeutic class: antiviral
Pregnancy risk category: B

Indications and dosages

▶ **Chronic hepatitis B.** *Adults and children age 16 or older:* 600 mg P.O. daily.
⊠ **Adjust-a-dose:** For patients with renal insufficiency: If creatinine clearance is 30 to 49 ml/minute, give 600 mg every 48 hours; if clearance is less than 30 ml/minute and patient doesn't need dialysis, give 600 mg every 72 hours. For patients with end-stage renal disease, give 600 mg every 96 hours, after hemodialysis.

Contraindications and cautions

• Contraindicated in patients who are hypersensitive to the drug or its components.
• Use cautiously in patients with renal impairment, in elderly patients because they're more likely to have renal insufficiency and increased sensitivity to adverse drug reactions, and in those with lamivudine-resistant hepatitis B infection.
❧ **Lifespan:** For pregnant women, the drug should be used only if maternal benefit outweighs risk to an unborn baby. Register patients in the Antiretroviral Pregnancy Registry by calling 1-800-258-4263 to monitor fetal outcomes. Breast-feeding women should choose a different means for feeding the baby; the drug may appear in breast milk. For children younger than age 16, safety and effectiveness haven't been established.

Adverse reactions

CNS: fatigue, headache, malaise, pyrexia.
Hematologic: *neutropenia.*
Musculoskeletal: muscle-related symptoms, myopathy.
Respiratory: nasopharyngitis, *upper respiratory tract infection.*
Other: flu and flulike symptoms.

Interactions

Drug-drug. *Other drugs that alter renal function (aminoglycosides, cyclosporine, NSAIDs, tacrolimus, vancomycin):* May increase risk of nephrotoxicity and cause decreased telbivudine elimination. Monitor renal function closely and adjust dosage if necessary.

Effects on lab test results

• May increase CK, ALT, AST, lipase, creatinine, and lactate levels.
• May increase neutrophil count.

Pharmacokinetics

Absorption: Steady state achieved in 5 to 7 days.
Distribution: Wide. Only 3.3% bound to plasma proteins.
Metabolism: Extensively by CYP3A4 and CYP3A5.
Excretion: Mostly in urine. *Half-life:* 40 to 49 hours.

Route	Onset	Peak	Duration
P.O.	Immediate	1–4 hr	Unknown

Action

Chemical effect: Inhibits HBV replication by interrupting HBV DNA polymerase activity.
Therapeutic effect: Works as antiviral.

Available forms

Tablets: 600 mg

NURSING PROCESS

▩ **Assessment**
• Assess patient's condition before therapy and regularly thereafter.
• Assess patient's and family's knowledge of drug therapy.

⊕ **Nursing diagnoses**
• Risk for injury secondary to adverse drug effects
• Ineffective therapeutic regimen management secondary to long-term drug therapy
• Deficient knowledge related to drug therapy

▷ **Planning and implementation**
• Monitor hepatic and renal function test results.
⊛ **ALERT:** The patient may develop lactic acidosis and severe hepatomegaly with steatosis during treatment. Risk factors include female gender, obesity, and concurrent antiretroviral therapy.

Reactions may be *common*, uncommon, *life-threatening*, or COMMON AND LIFE-THREATENING.

• Monitor patient for symptoms of myopathy.
• Register pregnant women in the Antiretroviral Pregnancy Registry.
• Stopping telbivudine may cause severe worsening of hepatitis B. Monitor hepatic function closely during therapy and for several months after stopping the drug. If appropriate, therapy may need to be resumed.

Patient teaching
• Teach patient the signs and symptoms of lactic acidosis, such as weakness, muscle pain, difficulty breathing, nausea and vomiting, coldness in the arms and legs, dizziness, lightheadedness, and fast or irregular heartbeat. Tell patient to immediately report any of these to his health care provider.
• Advise patient not to change the dose or stop the drug because his symptoms may worsen.
• Teach patient the signs and symptoms of worsening liver disease, such as jaundice, dark urine, light-colored stool, decreased appetite, nausea, and stomach pain.
• Remind patient that telbivudine doesn't cure hepatitis B and doesn't prevent spreading it to others.
• Tell patient that the drug may be taken without regard to food.

✓ Evaluation
• Patient remains free from injury during therapy.
• Patient maintains therapeutic regimen as shown by improvement of hepatitis B viral infection.
• Patient and family state understanding of drug therapy.

telithromycin
(teh-lith-roh-MY-sin)
Ketek

Pharmacologic class: ketolide
Therapeutic class: antibiotic
Pregnancy risk category: C

Indications and dosages

➤ **Mild to moderate community-acquired pneumonia caused by** *Streptococcus pneumoniae* **(including multi–drug-resistant isolates),** *Haemophilus influenzae, Moraxella catarrhalis, Chlamydophila pneumoniae,* **or** *Mycoplasma pneumoniae. Adults:* 800 mg P.O. once daily for 7 to 10 days.

⧈ Adjust-a-dose: For patient with renal impairment and a creatinine clearance less than 30 ml/minute, including patients on dialysis, give 600 mg P.O. once daily. On dialysis days, give after session complete. For patient who also has hepatic impairment, give 400 mg once daily.

Contraindications and cautions

• Contraindicated in patients hypersensitive to telithromycin or any macrolide antibiotic, and in patients with myasthenia gravis or a history of hepatitis or jaundice caused by drug. Don't give to patients with congenitally prolonged QTc interval, patients with ongoing proarrhythmic conditions (such as uncorrected hypokalemia or hypomagnesemia or significant bradycardia), or patients who are taking Class IA antiarrhythmics (such as quinidine, procainamide), Class III antiarrhythmics (such as dofetilide), cisapride, or pimozide.

⚘ Lifespan: In pregnant or breast-feeding women, use cautiously. In children, safety and effectiveness haven't been established.

Adverse reactions

CNS: dizziness, headache, transient loss of consciousness.
CV: *prolonged QTc interval, torsades de pointes, ventricular arrhythmias,* vagal syndrome.
EENT: blurred vision, difficulty focusing, diplopia.
GI: *diarrhea,* loose stools, nausea, *pseudomembranous colitis,* taste disturbance, vomiting.
Hepatic: hepatic dysfunction, *hepatitis, hepatotoxicity.*

Interactions

Drug-drug. *Atorvastatin, lovastatin, simvastatin:* May increase levels of these drugs, increasing the risk of myopathy. Avoid use together.
Benzodiazepines (midazolam): May increase benzodiazepine level. Monitor patient closely, and consider adjusting benzodiazepine dosage.
Cisapride: May increase QTc level. Avoid use together.

T

CYP3A4 inducers (carbamazepine, phenobarbital, phenytoin): May decrease telithromycin level. Avoid use together.
CYP3A4 inhibitors (itraconazole, ketoconazole): May increase telithromycin level. Monitor patient closely.
Digoxin: May increase digoxin level. Monitor digoxin level.
Drugs metabolized by the cytochrome P-450 system (such as carbamazepine, cyclosporine, hexobarbital, phenytoin, sirolimus, tacrolimus): May increase serum levels of these drugs, increasing or prolonging their effects. Use together cautiously, and monitor patient closely.
Ergot alkaloid derivatives (such as ergotamine): May increase the risk of ergot toxicity, characterized by severe peripheral vasospasm and dysesthesia. Avoid use together.
Metoprolol: May increase metoprolol level. Use together cautiously.
Oral anticoagulants: May increase the effects of the anticoagulant. Monitor PT and INR during co-administration.
Pimozide: May increase pimozide level. Use together is contraindicated.
Rifampin: May decrease telithromycin level significantly. Avoid use together.
Sotalol: May decrease sotalol level. Monitor patient for lack of effect.
Theophylline: May increase theophylline level and cause nausea and vomiting. Separate telithromycin and theophylline doses by 1 hour.

Effects on lab test results
• May increase AST and ALT levels.
• May increase platelet count.

Pharmacokinetics
Absorption: Bioavailability is about 57%.
Distribution: 60% to 70% protein-bound.
Metabolism: About 50% by CYP3A4.
Excretion: 13% unchanged in urine, and 7% unchanged in feces. *Half-life:* 10 hours.

Route	Onset	Peak	Duration
P.O.	Unknown	1 hr	Unknown

Action
Chemical effect: Inhibits bacterial protein synthesis.
Therapeutic effect: Hinders or kills susceptible bacteria.

Available forms
Tablets: 300 mg, 400 mg

NURSING PROCESS

Assessment
• Assess patient's history of allergies, especially to macrolides, before starting therapy.
• Obtain patient's medical history before starting therapy, including a list of drugs he's taking.
• Obtain sample for culture and sensitivity tests before giving the first dose. Start therapy pending test results.
• Be alert for adverse reactions and drug interactions.
• Assess patient for diarrhea during therapy; patients with diarrhea may have pseudomembranous colitis.
• Assess patient's and family's knowledge of drug therapy.

Nursing diagnoses
• Risk for injury related to adverse effects of drug
• Risk for deficient fluid volume related to potential for drug-induced adverse GI reactions
• Deficient knowledge related to drug therapy

Planning and implementation
• Monitor electrolyte level before starting therapy and periodically thereafter. Electrolyte imbalances must be corrected before or during therapy to avoid proarrhythmic conditions.
• Obtain hematologic, renal, and hepatic studies before starting therapy and during therapy.
 ALERT: Monitor patient for evidence of acute liver failure, including fatigue, nausea, jaundice, pale stools, darkened urine, abdominal pain, and enlarged liver. Fatal liver failure has occurred in patients taking drug. Notify prescriber immediately if signs and symptoms occur.
• Drug may cause visual disturbances including blurred vision, difficulty focusing, and diplopia, particularly in women and patients younger than age 40. Adverse visual effects occur most often after the first or second dose, last several hours, and sometimes return with later doses. For some patients, the symptoms will resolve during treatment; for others, they'll continue until treatment is complete.
 ALERT: Drug may prolong the QTc interval. Rarely, an irregular heartbeat may cause the patient to faint.

⑤ **ALERT:** Drug may cause transient loss of consciousness, including instances of associated vagal syndrome.

Patient teaching
• Urge patient to take drug exactly as prescribed until all of the tablets are gone, even if he feels better before the prescription is finished.
• Tell patient that drug can be taken with or without food.
• Warn patient that this drug may cause vision disturbances, liver problems, or fainting. Caution patient to avoid hazardous activities during therapy.
• Tell patient to report diarrhea or any episodes of fainting that occur while taking this drug.
• Tell patient to store tablets at room temperature.
• Tell patient to report new onset of weakness, abdominal pain, or other symptoms of liver problems.

☑ **Evaluation**
• Patient is free from injury.
• Patient maintains adequate hydration with therapy.
• Patient and family state understanding of drug therapy.

telmisartan
(tel-mih-SAR-tan)
Micardis

Pharmacologic class: angiotensin II receptor antagonist
Therapeutic class: antihypertensive
Pregnancy risk category: C (D in second and third trimesters)

Indications and dosages

▶ **Hypertension (used alone or with other antihypertensives).** *Adults:* 40 mg P.O. daily. Blood pressure response is dose-related between 20 and 80 mg daily.

Contraindications and cautions

• Contraindicated in patients hypersensitive to the drug or any of its components.
• Use cautiously in patients with renal and hepatic insufficiency and in those with an activated renin-angiotensin system, such as volume- or salt-depleted patients (those being treated with high doses of diuretics, for example).
☀ **Lifespan:** In pregnant women, don't use. If pregnancy is suspected, notify prescriber because drug should be stopped. Breast-feeding women should stop breast-feeding or use another drug, taking into account importance of drug therapy. In children, safety and effectiveness haven't been established.

Adverse reactions

CNS: dizziness, fatigue, headache, pain.
CV: chest pain, hypertension, peripheral edema.
EENT: pharyngitis, sinusitis.
GI: abdominal pain, diarrhea, dyspepsia, nausea.
GU: UTI.
Musculoskeletal: back pain, myalgia.
Respiratory: cough, upper respiratory tract infection.
Other: flulike symptoms.

Interactions

Drug-drug. *Digoxin:* May increase digoxin level. Monitor digoxin level closely.
Warfarin: May slightly decrease warfarin level. Monitor INR.

Effects on lab test results

• May increase liver enzyme and creatinine levels. May decrease hemoglobin level and hematocrit.

Pharmacokinetics

Absorption: Readily absorbed. Absolute bioavailability is dose-dependent.
Distribution: Extensively protein-bound; volume of distribution is about 500 L.
Metabolism: Metabolized by conjugation to an inactive metabolite.
Excretion: Mainly unchanged in feces. *Half-life:* 24 hours.

Route	Onset	Peak	Duration
P.O.	Unknown	30 min–1 hr	24 hr

Action

Chemical effect: Blocks the vasoconstrictive and aldosterone-secreting effects of angiotensin II by selectively blocking the binding of angiotensin II to the AT_1 receptor in many tissues, such as vascular smooth muscle and adrenal glands.
Therapeutic effect: Lowers blood pressure.

Available forms

Tablets: 20 mg, 40 mg, 80 mg

NURSING PROCESS

⚡ Assessment
• In patient whose renal function may depend on activity of the renin-angiotensin-aldosterone system, such as those with severe heart failure, use of ACE inhibitors and angiotensin-receptor antagonists may be related to oliguria or progressive azotemia and (rarely) to acute renal failure or death.
• In patient with biliary obstruction, drug level may elevate because of inability to excrete drug.
• Drug isn't removed by hemodialysis; orthostatic hypotension may develop in patient undergoing dialysis. Closely monitor blood pressure.
• Assess patient's and family's knowledge of drug therapy.

⊕ Nursing diagnoses
• Risk for injury related to presence of hypertension
• Ineffective cerebral and cardiopulmonary tissue perfusion related to drug-induced hypotension
• Deficient knowledge related to drug therapy

▷ Planning and implementation
• Most of the antihypertensive effect is present within 2 weeks. Maximal blood pressure reduction is generally attained after 4 weeks. If blood pressure isn't controlled by drug alone, a diuretic may be added.
• If hypotension occurs, place patient in supine position and give normal saline solution I.V. if needed.
Patient teaching
• Inform patient that drug may be taken without regard to meals.
• Inform woman of childbearing age of consequences of second- and third-trimester exposure to drug. Instruct patient to immediately report suspected pregnancy to prescriber.
• Tell patient that transient hypotension may occur. Instruct him to lie down if feeling dizzy and to climb stairs slowly and rise slowly to standing position.
• Instruct patient with heart failure to notify prescriber about decreased urine output.

• Teach patient other means to reduce blood pressure, such as diet control, exercise, smoking cessation, and stress reduction.
• Inform patient that drug shouldn't be removed from blister-sealed packet until immediately before use.

☑ Evaluation
• Patient sustains no injury from underlying disease.
• Patient has no hypotension and maintains adequate tissue perfusion.
• Patient and family state understanding of drug therapy.

HIGH ALERT

temazepam
(teh-MAZ-ih-pam)
Restoril

Pharmacologic class: benzodiazepine
Therapeutic class: sedative-hypnotic
Pregnancy risk category: X
Controlled substance schedule: IV

Indications and dosages

▶ **Short-term therapy for insomnia.** *Adults:* 15 to 30 mg P.O. 30 minutes before bedtime. In some patients, 7.5 mg to 15 mg may be sufficient.
Elderly or debilitated patients: Start with 7.5 mg P.O. at bedtime until response is determined.

Contraindications and cautions

• Contraindicated in patients hypersensitive to benzodiazepines.
• Use cautiously in patients with chronic pulmonary insufficiency, impaired liver or kidney function, severe or latent depression, suicidal tendencies, or history of drug abuse.
⚖ **Lifespan:** In pregnant women, drug is contraindicated. In breast-feeding women, drug isn't recommended. In children, safety and effectiveness haven't been established.

Adverse reactions

CNS: anxiety, confusion, depression, *dizziness, drowsiness,* disturbed coordination, daytime sedation, euphoria, fatigue, headache, *lethargy,* nervousness, nightmares, complex sleep disorders, vertigo, weakness.
CV: hypotension, palpitations.

Reactions may be *common*, uncommon, *life-threatening*, or COMMON AND LIFE-THREATENING.

EENT: blurred vision.
GI: diarrhea, dry mouth, nausea.
Respiratory: dyspnea.
Other: *anaphylaxis, angioedema,* physical or psychological dependence.

Interactions

Drug-drug. *CNS depressants, including opioid analgesics:* May increase CNS depression. Use together cautiously.
Drug-herb. *Calendula, catnip, hops, lady's slipper, lemon balm, passion flower, sassafras, skullcap, valerian, yerba mate:* May increase sedative effects. Monitor patient closely; discourage use together.
Kava: May cause excessive sedation. Discourage use together.
Drug-lifestyle. *Alcohol use:* May cause additive CNS effects. Strongly discourage use together.

Effects on lab test results

• May increase liver enzyme level.

Pharmacokinetics

Absorption: Good.
Distribution: Wide, throughout body. 98% protein-bound.
Metabolism: In liver, mainly to inactive metabolites.
Excretion: As metabolites in urine. *Half-life:* 10 to 17 hours.

Route	Onset	Peak	Duration
P.O.	Unknown	1–2 hr	Unknown

Action

Chemical effect: May act on limbic system, thalamus, and hypothalamus of CNS to produce hypnotic effects.
Therapeutic effect: Promotes sleep.

Available forms

Capsules: 7.5 mg, 15 mg, 22.5 mg, 30 mg

NURSING PROCESS

Assessment
• Assess patient's sleeping disorder before starting therapy and regularly thereafter to monitor drug's effectiveness.
• Assess mental status before starting therapy. An elderly patient is more sensitive to drug's adverse CNS effects.

• Be alert for adverse reactions and drug interactions.
• Assess patient's and family's knowledge of drug therapy.

Nursing diagnoses
• Insomnia related to underlying disorder
• Risk for injury related to drug-induced adverse CNS reactions
• Deficient knowledge related to drug therapy

Planning and implementation
• Before leaving the bedside, make sure patient who is depressed, suicidal, or drug-dependent, or who has history of drug abuse has swallowed the capsule to prevent hoarding.
• Use drug on an as-needed basis.
• Supervise walking and bed safety, particularly for elderly patients.
⊗ **ALERT:** Don't confuse Restoril with Vistaril.
Patient teaching
• Warn patient to avoid activities that require mental alertness or physical coordination.
• Warn patient about possible complex sleep disorders.

Evaluation
• Patient states that drug induces sleep.
• Patient doesn't experience injury from adverse CNS reactions.
• Patient and family state understanding of drug therapy.

HIGH ALERT

tenecteplase
(te-NEK-te-plase)
TNKase

Pharmacologic class: recombinant tissue plasminogen activator
Therapeutic class: thrombolytic
Pregnancy risk category: C

Indications and dosages

▶ **Reduction of mortality from acute MI.**
Adults weighing less than 60 kg (132 lb): Give 30 mg (6 ml) by I.V. bolus over 5 seconds.
Adults weighing 60 to 69 kg (132 to 152 lb): Give 35 mg (7 ml) by I.V. bolus over 5 seconds.
Adults weighing 70 to 79 kg (153 to 174 lb): Give 40 mg (8 ml) by I.V. bolus over 5 seconds.

T

Adults weighing 80 to 89 kg (175 to 196 lb):
Give 45 mg (9 ml) by I.V. bolus over 5 seconds.
Adults weighing 90 kg (197 lb) or more: Give
50 mg (10 ml) by I.V. bolus over 5 seconds.
Maximum dose is 50 mg.

▼ I.V. administration

• Use syringe prefilled with sterile water for injection, and inject entire contents into drug vial.
Don't use bacteriostatic water for injection.
• Gently swirl solution once mixed. Don't
shake. Make sure contents are completely dissolved.
• Draw up the appropriate dose needed from the
reconstituted vial with the syringe and discard
any unused portion.
• Give drug immediately once reconstituted, or
refrigerate and use within 8 hours.
• Give drug in a designated line.
• Give heparin with tenecteplase, but not in the
same I.V. line.
⊗ **Incompatibilities**
Solutions containing dextrose.

Contraindications and cautions

• Contraindicated in patients with active internal bleeding; history of stroke; intracranial or
intraspinal surgery or trauma during previous
2 months; intracranial neoplasm, aneurysm, or
arteriovenous malformation; severe uncontrolled hypertension; or known bleeding diathesis.
• Use cautiously in patients who have had recent major surgery (such as coronary artery bypass grafting), organ biopsy, or obstetrical delivery, or previous puncture of noncompressible
vessels. Also use cautiously in patients with recent trauma, recent GI or GU bleeding, high
risk of left ventricular thrombus, acute pericarditis, hypertension (systolic 180 mm Hg or
above, diastolic 110 mm Hg or above), severe
hepatic dysfunction, hemostatic defects, subacute bacterial endocarditis, septic thrombophlebitis, diabetic hemorrhagic retinopathy, or
cerebrovascular disease.
☀ **Lifespan:** In pregnant women, use cautiously. In breast-feeding women, use cautiously; it's
unknown if the drug appears in breast milk. In
children, safety and effectiveness haven't been
established. In patients age 75 and older, give
cautiously; weigh drug benefits against the risk
of increased adverse effects.

Adverse reactions

CNS: fever, *intracranial hemorrhage, stroke.*
CV: *cholesterol embolism, coronary reperfusion arrhythmias, major hematoma,* minor
hematoma.
EENT: epistaxis, pharyngeal bleeding.
GI: *GI bleeding,* nausea, vomiting.
GU: *hematuria.*
Hematologic: *bleeding at puncture sites.*

Interactions

Drug-drug. Anticoagulants *(heparin, vitamin K
antagonists), drugs that alter platelet function
(acetylsalicylic acid, dipyridamole, glycoprotein
IIb/IIIa inhibitors):* May increase risk of bleeding when used before, during, or after therapy
with tenecteplase. Use cautiously.

Effects on lab test results

• May increase PT, PTT, and INR.

Pharmacokinetics

Absorption: Given I.V.
Distribution: Related to weight and is an approximation of plasma volume.
Metabolism: Mainly hepatic.
Excretion: Unknown. *Half-life:* 20 minutes to
2 hours.

Route	Onset	Peak	Duration
I.V.	Immediate	Immediate	20–24 min

Action

Chemical effect: Binds to fibrin and converts
plasminogen to plasmin. Specificity to fibrin decreases systemic activation of plasminogen and
the resulting breakdown of circulating fibrinogen.
Therapeutic effect: Dissolves blood clots.

Available forms

Injection: 50 mg

NURSING PROCESS

⚕ Assessment
• Assess underlying condition before starting
therapy, and reassess regularly to monitor drug's
effectiveness.
• Monitor ECG for reperfusion arrhythmias.
• Assess pain before therapy, and reassess regularly.

Reactions may be *common*, uncommon, *life-threatening*, or COMMON AND LIFE-THREATENING.

- Assess patient's and family's knowledge of drug therapy.

✥ **Nursing diagnoses**
- Ineffective tissue perfusion, coronary, related to presence of blood clots
- Acute pain related to MI
- Deficient knowledge related to tenecteplase therapy

▷ **Planning and implementation**
- Minimize arterial and venous punctures during therapy.
- Avoid noncompressible arterial punctures and internal jugular and subclavian venous punctures.
- Monitor patient for bleeding. If serious bleeding occurs, immediately stop giving heparin and antiplatelet drugs.
- Cholesterol embolism is rarely related to thrombolytic use, but may be lethal. Signs and symptoms may include livedo reticularis, "purple toe" syndrome, acute renal failure, gangrenous digits, hypertension, pancreatitis, MI, cerebral infarction, spinal cord infarction, retinal artery occlusion, bowel infarction, and rhabdomyolysis.
Patient teaching
- Inform patient about proper dental care to avoid excessive gum bleeding.
- Advise patient to immediately report any adverse effects or excessive bleeding.
- Explain use of drug to patient and family.

☑ **Evaluation**
- Patient regains tissue perfusion with dissolution of blood clots.
- Patient is relieved of pain.
- Patient and family state understanding of drug therapy.

HIGH ALERT

teniposide (VM-26)
(teh-NIP-uh-sighd)
Vumon

Pharmacologic class: podophyllotoxin
Therapeutic class: antineoplastic
Pregnancy risk category: D

Indications and dosages

▶ **Refractory childhood acute lymphoblastic leukemia.** *Children:* Optimum dosage hasn't been established. One protocol is 165 mg/m^2 I.V. twice weekly for eight or nine doses, usually with other drugs.
⬣ **Adjust-a-dose:** Consider dosage adjustments in patients with renal and hepatic insufficiency. Patients with Down syndrome may have increased sensitivity to the drug; begin therapy with a reduced dose, and monitor patient.

▼ **I.V. administration**
- Preparation and administration have carcinogenic, mutagenic, and teratogenic risks. Follow institutional policy to reduce risks.
- Dilute drug in D$_5$W or normal saline solution injection to concentration of 0.1, 0.2, 0.4, or 1 mg/ml. Don't agitate vigorously; precipitation may form. Discard cloudy solutions.
- Don't give drug through membrane-type in-line filter because diluent may dissolve filter.
- Infuse over 30 to 60 minutes to prevent hypotension. If hypotension occurs, stop infusion.
- Ensure proper placement of catheter. Extravasation can cause local tissue necrosis or sloughing.
- Prepare and store in glass containers. Solutions containing 0.5 to 1 mg/ml of drug are stable for 4 hours; those containing 0.1 to 0.2 mg/ml are stable for 6 hours at room temperature.
⊗ **Incompatibilities**
Heparin, idarubicin. Don't mix with other drugs or solutions.

Contraindications and cautions

- Contraindicated in patients hypersensitive to the drug or to polyoxyethylated castor oil (an injection vehicle).
- Use cautiously in patients with myelosuppression.
- Severe hypersensitivity reactions may occur with initial dose or after repeated exposure.
⚘ **Lifespan:** In pregnant and breast-feeding women, drug isn't recommended.

Adverse reactions

CV: hypotension from rapid infusion.
GI: diarrhea, nausea, mucositis, vomiting.
Hematologic: *anemia, leukopenia,* myelosuppression, *neutropenia, thrombocytopenia.*
Skin: alopecia, tissue necrosis, sloughing, or phlebitis at injection site.
Other: *hypersensitivity reactions (bronchospasm,* chills, dyspnea, fever, hypotension, flushing, tachycardia, urticaria).

Interactions

Drug-drug. *Methotrexate:* May increase clearance and intracellular level of methotrexate. Monitor patient closely.
Sodium salicylate, sulfamethizole, tolbutamide: May displace teniposide from protein-binding sites and increase toxicity. Monitor patient closely.

Effects on lab test results

• May increase uric acid level. May decrease hemoglobin level and hematocrit.
• May decrease RBC, WBC, platelet, and neutrophil counts.

Pharmacokinetics

Absorption: Given I.V.
Distribution: Mainly in liver, kidneys, small intestine, and adrenals. Drug crosses blood-brain barrier to limited extent. Extensively bound to plasma proteins.
Metabolism: Extensive, in liver.
Excretion: About 40% through kidneys as unchanged drug or metabolites. *Half-life:* 5 hours.

Route	Onset	Peak	Duration
I.V.	Unknown	Unknown	Unknown

Action

Chemical effect: Acts in late S or early G2 phase of cell cycle, thus preventing cells from entering mitosis.
Therapeutic effect: Prevents reproduction of leukemic cells.

Available forms

Injection: 50 mg/5 ml

NURSING PROCESS

Assessment

• Assess patient's condition before starting therapy and regularly thereafter to monitor drug's effectiveness.
• Obtain baseline blood counts and kidney and liver function tests; then monitor periodically.
• Monitor blood pressure before therapy and at 30-minute intervals during infusion.
• Be alert for adverse reactions and drug interactions.
• Assess patient's and family's knowledge of drug therapy.

Nursing diagnoses

• Ineffective health maintenance related to presence of leukemia
• Ineffective protection related to drug-induced immunosuppression
• Deficient knowledge related to drug therapy

Planning and implementation

• Some prescribers may decide to use drug despite patient's history of hypersensitivity because therapeutic benefits may outweigh risks. Give antihistamines and corticosteroids to these patients before infusion begins, and monitor them closely during drug administration.
ALERT: Have diphenhydramine, hydrocortisone, epinephrine, and appropriate emergency equipment available to establish airway in case of anaphylaxis.
ALERT: Report systolic blood pressure below 90 mm Hg, and stop infusion.
Patient teaching
• Tell patient to immediately report discomfort at the I.V. site.
• Encourage adequate fluid intake to increase urine output and facilitate excretion of uric acid.
• Review infection-control and bleeding precautions to take during therapy.
• Reassure patient that hair should grow back after therapy stops.
• Instruct patient and parents to notify prescriber if adverse reactions occur.

Evaluation

• Patient responds well to drug.
• Patient doesn't develop serious complications from immunosuppression.
• Patient and family state understanding of drug therapy.

tenofovir disoproxil fumarate
(teh-NAH-fuh-veer dy-soh-PRAHK-sul FOO-mah-rayt)
Viread

Pharmacologic class: nucleotide reverse transcriptase inhibitor
Therapeutic class: antiviral
Pregnancy risk category: B

Indications and dosages

▶ **HIV-1 infection, with other antiretrovirals.**
Adults: 300 mg P.O. once daily without regard

Reactions may be *common,* uncommon, *life-threatening,* or **COMMON AND LIFE-THREATENING.**

to food. When given with didanosine, give 2 hours before or 1 hour after didanosine.

⧈ **Adjust-a-dose:** For patients with renal impairment, if creatinine clearance is 30 to 49 ml/minute, give 300 mg every 48 hours. If creatinine clearance is 10 to 29 ml/minute, give 300 mg twice weekly.

For hemodialysis patients, give 300 mg every 7 days or after a total of 12 hours of hemodialysis.

Contraindications and cautions

• Contraindicated in patients hypersensitive to the drug or any of its components.
• Use cautiously in patients with hepatic impairment or risk factors for liver disease, and in patients with renal impairment.
⚖ **Lifespan:** In pregnant women, use only if benefits to the woman outweigh risks to the fetus. Breast-feeding women should stop breast-feeding or use another drug. In children, safety and effectiveness haven't been established. In the elderly, use cautiously because they are more likely to have renal impairment and to be receiving other drug therapy.

Adverse reactions

CNS: asthenia, depression, fever, headache, insomnia, peripheral neuropathy.
CV: chest pain.
GI: abdominal pain, anorexia, *diarrhea,* dyspepsia, flatulence, *nausea,* vomiting.
GU: glycosuria, *renal toxicity.*
Hematologic: *neutropenia.*
Hepatic: *hepatomegaly with steatosis, hepatotoxicity.*
Metabolic: hyperglycemia, *lactic acidosis,* weight loss.
Musculoskeletal: back pain, decreased bone density, myalgias.
Skin: fat accumulation and redistribution, rash, sweating.

Interactions

Drug-drug. *Acyclovir, cidofovir, ganciclovir, valacyclovir, valganciclovir (drugs that reduce renal function or compete for renal tubular secretion):* May increase level of tenofovir or other renally eliminated drugs. Monitor patient for adverse effects.
Atazanavir: May decrease atazanavir level, causing resistance. Give both drugs with ritonavir.

Didanosine (buffered formulation): May increase didanosine bioavailability. Monitor patient for didanosine-related adverse effects, such as bone marrow suppression, GI distress, and peripheral neuropathy. Give tenofovir 2 hours before or 1 hour after didanosine.

Effects on lab test results

• May increase amylase, AST, ALT, creatinine kinase, serum and urine glucose, and triglyceride levels. May decrease HIV-1 RNA level.
• May decrease neutrophil and CD4 cell counts.

Pharmacokinetics

Absorption: In fasting patients, poor (bioavailability 25%) with peak level in about 1 hour. A high-fat meal delays peak by 1 hour but increases bioavailability to 40%.
Distribution: Minimally bound to plasma proteins.
Metabolism: Not by liver enzymes, including cytochrome P-450 enzymes.
Excretion: Renal, through glomerular filtration and active tubular secretion. *Half-life:* About 17 hours after single dose.

Route	Onset	Peak	Duration
P.O.	Unknown	1–2 hr	Unknown

Action

Chemical effect: Tenofovir disoproxil fumarate is hydrolyzed to produce tenofovir. Tenofovir undergoes sequential phosphorylations to yield tenofovir diphosphate. Tenofovir diphosphate is a competitive antagonist of HIV reverse transcriptase.
Therapeutic effect: Inhibits HIV replication.

Available forms

Tablets: 300 mg as the fumarate salt (equivalent to 245 mg of tenofovir disoproxil)

NURSING PROCESS

🕮 **Assessment**

• Assess patient's viral infection before starting therapy and regularly thereafter to monitor drug's effectiveness.
• Assess patient for risk of severe adverse reactions. Antiretrovirals, alone or combined, have been linked to lactic acidosis and severe (including fatal) hepatomegaly with steatosis. These effects may occur without elevated transaminase

level. Risk is increased for women, obese patients, and those exposed to antiretrovirals long-term. Monitor all patients for hepatotoxicity, including lactic acidosis and hepatomegaly with steatosis.
● Assess patient's and family's knowledge of drug therapy.

Nursing diagnoses
● Noncompliance related to long-term therapy
● Risk for infection related to presence of HIV
● Deficient knowledge related to drug therapy

Planning and implementation
● Antiretrovirals have been linked to the accumulation and redistribution of body fat, resulting in central obesity, peripheral wasting, and development of a buffalo hump. The long-term effects of these changes are unknown. Monitor patients for changes in body fat.
● Tenofovir may be linked to bone abnormalities (osteomalacia and decreased bone mineral density) and renal toxicity (increased creatinine and phosphaturia levels). Monitor patient carefully during long-term therapy.
● Drug may lead to decreased HIV-1 RNA level and CD4 cell counts.
● The effects on the progression of HIV infection are unknown.
● Because of a high rate of early virologic resistance, triple antiretroviral therapy with abacavir, lamivudine, and tenofovir shouldn't be used as a new therapy regimen for untreated or pretreated patients. Monitor patients currently controlled with this drug combination and those who use this combination in addition to other antiretroviral drugs, and consider modifying therapy.
● Because of a high rate of early virologic failure and emergence of resistance, therapy with tenofovir with didanosine and lamivudine isn't recommended as a new treatment regimen for therapy-naïve or therapy-experienced patients with HIV infection. Patients currently on this regimen should be considered for treatment modification.
Patient teaching
● Instruct patient to take tenofovir with a meal to enhance bioavailability.
● Tell patient to report adverse effects, including nausea, vomiting, diarrhea, flatulence, and headache.

Evaluation
● Patient complies with therapy regimen.
● Patient has reduced signs and symptoms of infection.
● Patient and family state understanding of drug therapy.

terazosin hydrochloride
(ter-uh-ZOH-sin high-droh-KLOR-ighd)
Hytrin

Pharmacologic class: selective alpha$_1$ blocker
Therapeutic class: antihypertensive
Pregnancy risk category: C

Indications and dosages
▶ **Hypertension.** *Adults:* Initially, 1 mg P.O. at bedtime, increased gradually based on response. Usual dosage range is 1 to 5 mg daily. Maximum, 20 mg daily.
▶ **Symptomatic BPH.** *Adults:* Initially, 1 mg P.O. at bedtime. Dosage increased in stepwise manner to 2 mg, 5 mg, and 10 mg once daily to achieve optimal response. Most patients require 10 mg daily for optimal response.

Contraindications and cautions
● Contraindicated in patients hypersensitive to the drug or any of its components.
⚜ **Lifespan:** In pregnant women, use cautiously. In breast-feeding women, use cautiously; it's unknown if the drug appears in breast milk. In children, safety and effectiveness haven't been established.

Adverse reactions
CNS: *asthenia, dizziness, headache,* nervousness, paresthesia, somnolence.
CV: atrial fibrillation, palpitations, orthostatic hypotension, *peripheral edema,* tachycardia.
EENT: blurred vision, nasal congestion, sinusitis.
GI: nausea.
GU: impotence, priapism.
Hematologic: *thrombocytopenia.*
Musculoskeletal: back pain, muscle pain.
Respiratory: dyspnea.
Other: decreased libido.

Interactions

Drug-drug. *Antihypertensives:* May cause excessive hypotension. Use together cautiously. *Clonidine:* May decrease antihypertensive effect of clonidine. Monitor patient.
Drug-herb. *Butcher's broom:* May cause diminished effect. Discourage using together.

Effects on lab test results

• May decrease total protein, albumin, and hemoglobin levels and hematocrit.
• May decrease platelet and WBC counts.

Pharmacokinetics

Absorption: Rapid, with about 90% of dose bioavailable.
Distribution: About 90% to 94% bound to plasma proteins.
Metabolism: In liver.
Excretion: About 40% in urine, 60% in feces, mostly as metabolites. Up to 30% may be unchanged. *Half-life:* About 12 hours.

Route	Onset	Peak	Duration
P.O.	≤ 15 min	2–3 hr	24 hr

Action

Chemical effect: Decreases blood pressure by vasodilation produced in response to blockade of alpha$_1$-adrenergic receptors. Improves urine flow by blocking alpha$_1$ receptors in smooth muscle of bladder neck and prostate, thus relieving urethral pressure and reestablishing urine flow.
Therapeutic effect: Lowers blood pressure and relieves symptoms of BPH.

Available forms

Capsules: 1 mg, 2 mg, 5 mg, 10 mg

NURSING PROCESS

Assessment

• Assess patient's condition before starting therapy and regularly thereafter to monitor drug's effectiveness.
• Assess and monitor patient for prostate cancer because it may resemble BPH.
• Monitor blood pressure often.
• Be alert for adverse reactions and drug interactions.
• Assess patient's and family's knowledge of drug therapy.

Nursing diagnoses

• Risk for injury related to presence of hypertension
• Sexual dysfunction related to drug-induced impotence
• Deficient knowledge related to drug therapy

Planning and implementation

• Use cautiously with initial dose, and monitor patient—especially elderly patient—for postural hypotension.
⚠ **ALERT:** If drug is stopped for several days, begin again at the initial dose and adjust regimen.
Patient teaching
• Tell patient not to stop drug but to call prescriber if adverse reaction occurs.
• Tell patient to take the first dose at bedtime. If he must get up, he should do so slowly to prevent dizziness or blackouts.
• Warn patient to avoid activities that require mental alertness for 12 hours after first dose.
• Teach patient other means to reduce blood pressure, such as diet control, exercise, smoking cessation, and stress reduction.

Evaluation

• Patient's blood pressure is normal.
• Patient develops and maintains positive attitude toward his sexuality despite impotence.
• Patient and family state understanding of drug therapy.

terbutaline sulfate
(ter-BYOO-tuh-leen SUL-fayt)
Brethine, Bricanyl

Pharmacologic class: beta$_2$ agonist
Therapeutic class: bronchodilator
Pregnancy risk category: B

Indications and dosages

▶ **Bronchospasm in patients with reversible obstructive airway disease.** *Adults and children older than age 15:* Initially, 2.5 mg P.O. t.i.d. or q.i.d. Increase to 5 mg P.O. t.i.d. at 6-hour intervals while awake. Maximum, 15 mg daily. Or, 0.25 mg subcutaneously. May repeat in 15 to 30 minutes. Maximum, 0.5 mg every 4 hours.
Children ages 12 to 15: Give 2.5 mg P.O. t.i.d. Maximum, 7.5 mg daily.

▶ **Premature labor‡.** *Women:* Initially, 2.5 to 10 mcg/minute I.V.; increase dosage gradually as tolerated in 10- to 20-minute intervals until desired effects are achieved. Maximum dosages range from 17.5 to 30 mcg/minute, although dosages of up to 80 mcg/minute have been used cautiously. Continue infusion for at least 12 hours after uterine contractions stop. Maintenance therapy, 2.5 to 10 mg P.O. every 4 to 6 hours.

▼ I.V. administration

• Protect injection from light. If discolored, don't use.
• Monitor uterine response, maternal blood pressure, and maternal and fetal heart rates. Also monitor patient for circulatory overload and pulmonary edema.
⊗ **Incompatibility**
Bleomycin.

Contraindications and cautions

• Contraindicated in patients hypersensitive to the drug or any of its components, or to sympathomimetic amines.
• Use cautiously in patient with CV disorders, hyperthyroidism, diabetes, or seizure disorders.
⚖ **Lifespan:** In pregnant women, use cautiously. In breast-feeding women, use cautiously; it's unknown if the drug appears in breast milk. In children age 11 and younger, safety and effectiveness haven't been established.

Adverse reactions

CNS: dizziness, drowsiness, headache, nervousness, tremor, weakness.
CV: *arrhythmias,* chest discomfort, flushing, hypertension, *palpitations,* tachycardia.
EENT: tinnitus.
GI: heartburn, nausea, *vomiting.*
Metabolic: hypokalemia.
Respiratory: dyspnea, *paradoxical bronchospasm.*
Skin: diaphoresis.

Interactions

Drug-drug. *CNS stimulants:* May increase CNS stimulation. Avoid use together.
Cyclopropane, digoxin, halogenated inhaled anesthetics, levodopa: May increase risk of arrhythmias. Monitor patient closely.
MAO inhibitors: May cause severe hypertension (hypertensive crisis). Don't use together.

Propranolol, other beta blockers: May block bronchodilating effects of terbutaline. Avoid use together.
Sympathomimetics: May cause additive CV effects. Avoid use together.
Theophylline derivatives: May increase risk of cardiotoxic effects. Avoid use together.

Effects on lab test results

• May increase liver enzyme level. May decrease potassium level.

Pharmacokinetics

Absorption: 33% to 50% of P.O. dose; unknown for subcutaneous route.
Distribution: Widely distributed throughout body.
Metabolism: Partially metabolized in liver to inactive compounds.
Excretion: Excreted primarily in urine. *Half-life:* Unknown.

Route	Onset	Peak	Duration
P.O.	30 min	2–3 hr	4–8 hr
SubQ	≤ 15 min	30–60 min	1½–4 hr

Action

Chemical effect: Relaxes bronchial smooth muscle by acting on beta$_2$-adrenergic receptors.
Therapeutic effect: Improves breathing ability.

Available forms

Injection: 1 mg/ml
Tablets: 2.5 mg, 5 mg

NURSING PROCESS

☑ Assessment

• Assess patient's condition before starting therapy and regularly thereafter to monitor drug's effectiveness.
• Monitor patient closely for toxicity.
• Assess patient's and family's knowledge of drug therapy.

⊕ Nursing diagnoses

• Ineffective breathing pattern related to underlying respiratory condition
• Acute pain related to drug-induced headache
• Deficient knowledge related to drug therapy

Reactions may be *common*, uncommon, *life-threatening*, or COMMON AND LIFE-THREATENING.

⧓ Planning and implementation
● For subcutaneous administration, inject in lateral deltoid area.
● If bronchospasm develops during therapy, notify prescriber immediately.
● Mild analgesic may be used to treat drug-induced headache.
⑤ **ALERT:** Don't confuse terbutaline with tolbutamide or terbinafine.

Patient teaching
● Explain to patient and family why drug is needed.
● Instruct patient to report paradoxical bronchospasm, and tell him to stop drug if it happens.
● Warn patient that tolerance may develop with prolonged use.

☑ Evaluation
● Patient's breathing is improved.
● Patient's headache is relieved with mild analgesic.
● Patient and family state understanding of drug therapy.

teriparatide (rDNA origin)
(tehr-ih-PAHR-uh-tighd)
Forteo

Pharmacologic class: recombinant human parathyroid hormone (PTH)
Therapeutic class: antiosteoporotic
Pregnancy risk category: C

Indications and dosages

▶ **Osteoporosis in postmenopausal women at high risk for fracture; to increase bone mass in men with primary or hypogonadal osteoporosis who are at high risk for fracture.**
Adults: 20 mcg subcutaneously in thigh or abdominal wall once daily.

Contraindications and cautions

● Contraindicated in patients hypersensitive to the drug or any of its components. Don't give to patients who have had radiation to the skeleton, those with Paget disease or unexplained alkaline phosphatase elevations, or those at increased risk for osteosarcoma such as children. Don't give drug to patients with bone metastases, a history of skeletal malignancies, or metabolic bone diseases other than osteoporosis. Avoid

use in patients with hypercalcemia or primary hyperparathyroidism. Don't continue therapy beyond 2 years.
● Use cautiously in patients with active or recent urolithiasis and in patients with hepatic, renal, or cardiac disease.
⚘ **Lifespan:** In pregnant and breast-feeding women, drug isn't recommended. In children, safety and effectiveness haven't been established.

Adverse reactions

CNS: asthenia, depression, dizziness, headache, insomnia, *pain,* syncope, vertigo.
CV: angina pectoris, hypertension, orthostatic hypotension.
EENT: pharyngitis, rhinitis.
GI: constipation, diarrhea, dyspepsia, nausea, tooth disorder, vomiting.
Metabolic: hypercalcemia.
Musculoskeletal: *arthralgia,* leg cramps, neck pain.
Respiratory: cough, dyspnea, pneumonia.
Skin: rash, sweating.

Interactions

Drug-drug. *Calcium supplements:* May increase urinary calcium excretion. Dosage may need adjustment.
Digoxin: Hypercalcemia may predispose patient to digitalis toxicity. Use together cautiously.

Effects on lab test results

● May increase calcium and uric acid levels. May decrease phosphorus level.
● May increase urinary calcium and phosphorus excretion.

Pharmacokinetics

Absorption: Rapid and extensive, with level peaking after about 30 minutes. Availability is about 95%.
Distribution: Unknown.
Metabolism: Unknown for drug, but PTH is metabolized in the liver.
Excretion: Unknown for drug, but PTH is excreted by the kidneys. Elimination is rapid.
Half-life: 1 hour.

Route	Onset	Peak	Duration
SubQ	Rapid	30 min	3 hr

Action

Chemical effect: Regulates calcium and phosphorus metabolism in bones and kidneys, increases calcium, and decreases phosphorus level.

Therapeutic effect: Decreases risk of fractures in patients with osteoporosis.

Available forms

Injection: 750 mcg/3 ml in a prefilled pen

NURSING PROCESS

⚡ Assessment

⚠ **ALERT:** Because of the risk of osteosarcoma, give drug only to patient for whom benefits outweigh risks.

• If patient could have urolithiasis or hypercalciuria, measure urinary calcium excretion before therapy.

• Assess patient's and family's knowledge of drug therapy.

⊕ Nursing diagnoses

• Risk for falls related to presence of osteoporosis

• Chronic pain related to adverse drug effects

• Deficient knowledge related to drug therapy

▶ Planning and implementation

• Monitor patient for orthostatic hypotension, which may occur within 4 hours after a dose.

• Track calcium level. If patient develops persistent hypercalcemia, stop drug and evaluate its possible cause.

• Safety and effectiveness haven't been established for use beyond 2 years.

Patient teaching

• Instruct patient on the proper use and disposal of the prefilled pen.

• Tell patient not to share pen with others.

• Advise patient to sit or lie down if drug causes a fast heartbeat, lightheadedness, or dizziness. Tell patient to report persistent or worsening symptoms.

• Instruct patient to report persistent symptoms of hypercalcemia (nausea, vomiting, constipation, lethargy, and muscle weakness).

☑ Evaluation

• Patient doesn't fall.

• Patient reports no pain or states that pain is controlled by therapy.

• Patient and family state understanding of drug therapy.

testolactone
(tes-tuh-LAK-tohn)
Teslac

Pharmacologic class: aromatase inhibitor
Therapeutic class: antineoplastic
Pregnancy risk category: C
Controlled substance schedule: III

Indications and dosages

▶ **Advanced postmenopausal breast cancer.**
Women: 250 mg P.O. q.i.d. Some patients may benefit from 2 g per day. Therapy should continue for at least 3 months unless disease actively progresses.

Contraindications and cautions

• Contraindicated in patients hypersensitive to the drug or any of its components, and in men with breast cancer.

🌂 **Lifespan:** In pregnant women, use cautiously. In breast-feeding women, drug isn't recommended. In children, drug isn't indicated.

Adverse reactions

CNS: paresthesia, peripheral neuropathy.
CV: edema, increased blood pressure.
GI: anorexia, diarrhea, glossitis, nausea, vomiting.
Skin: alopecia, erythema, nail changes.
Other: hot flashes.

Interactions

Drug-drug. *Oral anticoagulants:* May increase pharmacologic effects. Monitor patient carefully.

Effects on lab test results

• May increase calcium level. May decrease estradiol level.

• May increase 24-hour urinary excretion of creatine.

Pharmacokinetics

Absorption: Good.
Distribution: Wide.
Metabolism: Extensive.

Reactions may be *common*, uncommon, *life-threatening*, or COMMON AND LIFE-THREATENING.

Excretion: Mainly in urine. *Half-life:* Unknown.

Route	Onset	Peak	Duration
P.O.	6–12 wk	Unknown	Unknown

Action

Chemical effect: Unknown; may change tumor's hormonal environment and alter neoplastic process.
Therapeutic effect: Hinders breast cancer cell activity.

Available forms

Tablets: 50 mg

NURSING PROCESS

☑ Assessment
• Assess patient's breast cancer before starting therapy and regularly thereafter to monitor drug's effectiveness.
• Monitor fluid and electrolyte levels, especially calcium level.
• Assess patient's and family's knowledge of drug therapy.

✛ Nursing diagnoses
• Ineffective health maintenance related to presence of breast cancer
• Disturbed sensory perception (tactile) related to drug-induced paresthesia and peripheral neuropathy
• Deficient knowledge related to drug therapy

▶ Planning and implementation
• Encourage patient to drink fluids to aid calcium excretion, and encourage exercise to prevent hypercalcemia. Immobilized patient is prone to hypercalcemia.
• Higher-than-recommended doses don't promote remission.
• Continue therapy for at least 3 months unless disease actively progresses.
Patient teaching
• Inform patient that therapeutic response isn't immediate; it may take up to 3 months for benefit to be noted.
• Encourage patient to exercise and drink plenty of fluids to help prevent hypercalcemia.
• Tell patient to report adverse effects.

☑ Evaluation
• Patient responds well to drug.
• Patient lists ways to protect against risk of injury caused by diminished tactile sensation.
• Patient and family state understanding of drug therapy.

testosterone
(tess-TOSS-teh-rohn)
Striant, Testopel Pellets

testosterone cypionate
Depo-Testosterone

testosterone enanthate
Delatestryl

testosterone propionate

Pharmacologic class: androgen
Therapeutic class: antineoplastic, hormone replacement
Pregnancy risk category: X
Controlled substance schedule: III

Indications and dosages

▶ **Hypogonadism.** *Men:* 50 to 400 mg testosterone cypionate or testosterone enanthate I.M. every 2 to 4 weeks. Or, 10 to 25 mg testosterone propionate I.M. two to three times weekly. Another alternative is 75 to 150 mg of testosterone cypionate or enanthate I.M. every 7 to 10 days. Or, 150 to 450 mg (two to six pellets) implanted subcutaneously every 3 to 6 months. Or, apply one 30 mg buccal tablet to the gum area above the incisor tooth on either side of the mouth, b.i.d. in the morning and evening about 12 hours apart. Alternate sides of the mouth with each application.
▶ **Delayed puberty.** *Boys:* 25 to 50 mg testosterone propionate I.M. two or three times weekly for up to 6 months. Or, two 75-mg pellets implanted subcutaneously for each 25 mg of testosterone propionate needed each week. Pellets last 3 to 6 months.
▶ **Metastatic breast cancer 1 to 5 years after menopause.** *Women:* 50 to 100 mg testosterone propionate I.M. three times weekly. Or, 200 to 400 mg testosterone cypionate or testosterone enanthate I.M. every 2 to 4 weeks.

▶ **Postpartum breast pain and engorgement.**
Women: 25 to 50 mg testosterone propionate
I.M. daily for 3 to 4 days.

Contraindications and cautions

• Contraindicated in men with breast or prostate
cancer; women, patients with hypercalcemia;
and those with cardiac, hepatic, or renal decompensation.

⚜ **Lifespan:** In pregnant and breast-feeding
women, drug is contraindicated. In children, use
cautiously because of risk of accelerated bone
maturation leading to short stature. In the elderly, use cautiously.

Adverse reactions

CNS: anxiety, depression, headache, paresthesia, sleep apnea syndrome.
CV: edema.
GI: nausea.
GU: bladder irritability; excessive hormonal effects in boys and men (prepubertal: *acne,
growth of body and facial hair,* phallic enlargement, premature epiphyseal closure, priapism;
postpubertal: decreased ejaculatory volume,
epididymitis, gynecomastia, impotence, oligospermia, testicular atrophy); hypoestrogenic effects in women (*acne;* clitoral enlargement; decreased or increased libido; diaphoresis; *edema;*
flushing; *hirsutism; hoarseness;* menstrual irregularities; *oily skin; weight gain;* vaginitis, including burning, drying, and itching; vaginal
bleeding).
Hematologic: polycythemia, suppression of
clotting factors.
Hepatic: *cholestatic hepatitis,* reversible jaundice.
Metabolic: hypercalcemia.
Skin: hypersensitivity skin signs and symptoms,
local edema.
Other: pain and induration at injection site.

Interactions

Drug-drug. *Hepatotoxic drugs:* May increase
risk of hepatotoxicity. Monitor patient closely.
Insulin, oral antidiabetics: May alter dosage requirements. Monitor glucose level in diabetic
patients.
Oral anticoagulants: May alter dosage requirements. Monitor PT and INR.

Effects on lab test results

• May increase sodium, potassium, phosphate,
cholesterol, liver enzyme, calcium, and creatinine levels. May decrease thyroxine-binding
globulin and total T_4 levels.
• May increase RBC count and resin uptake of
T_3 and T_4.

Pharmacokinetics

Absorption: Unknown.
Distribution: 98% to 99% protein-bound,
mainly to testosterone–estradiol-binding globulin.
Metabolism: In liver.
Excretion: In urine. *Half-life:* 10 to 100 minutes.

Route	Onset	Peak	Duration
Buccal	Unknown	10–12 hr	2–4 hr
I.M.	Unknown	10–100 min	Unknown
SubQ	Unknown	Unknown	3–6 mo

Action

Chemical effect: Stimulates target tissues to develop normally in androgen-deficient men. Drug
may have some antiestrogen properties, making
it useful to treat certain estrogen-dependent
breast cancers. Its action in postpartum breast
engorgement isn't known because drug doesn't
suppress lactation.
Therapeutic effect: Increases testosterone level, inhibits some estrogen activity, and relieves
postpartum breast pain and engorgement.

Available forms

testosterone
Buccal tablet (extended-release): 30 mg
Pellets (subcutaneous implant): 75 mg
testosterone cypionate
Injection (in oil): 100 mg/ml, 200 mg/ml
testosterone enanthate
Injection (in oil): 200 mg/ml
testosterone propionate
Injection (in oil): 100 mg/ml

NURSING PROCESS

📝 **Assessment**

• Assess patient's condition before starting therapy and regularly thereafter to monitor drug's
effectiveness.
• Periodically monitor calcium level and liver
function test results.

• Monitor hemoglobin and hematocrit for poly-cythemia.
• Monitor prepubertal boys by X-ray for rate of bone maturation.
• Be alert for adverse reactions and drug inter-actions.
• Assess patient's and family's knowledge of drug therapy.

🔷 Nursing diagnoses
• Ineffective health maintenance related to un-derlying condition
• Disturbed body image related to drug-induced adverse androgenic reactions
• Deficient knowledge related to drug therapy

▶ Planning and implementation
• Give daily dose requirement in divided doses for best results.
• Store preparations at room temperature. If crystals appear, warm and shake bottle to dis-perse them.
• Inject deep into upper outer quadrant of gluteal muscle. Rotate sites to prevent muscle atrophy. Report soreness at site because of pos-sibility of postinfection furunculosis.
• Unless contraindicated, use with diet high in calories and protein taken in small, frequent meals.
• Report signs of virilization in woman.
• Edema generally can be controlled with sodi-um restriction or diuretics.
🔔 ALERT: Therapeutic response in breast cancer usually appears within 3 months. If signs of dis-ease progression appear, stop giving the drug. In metastatic breast cancer, hypercalcemia usually signals progression of bone metastases. Report signs of hypercalcemia.
• Androgens may alter results of laboratory studies during therapy and for 2 to 3 weeks after therapy ends.
🔔 ALERT: Testosterone and methyltestosterone aren't interchangeable. Don't confuse testos-terone with testolactone.
Patient teaching
• Tell patient to use effective barrier-method contraception during therapy.
• Instruct man to report priapism, reduced ejac-ulatory volume, and gynecomastia. Drug may need to be stopped.
• Inform woman that virilization may occur. Tell her to report androgenic effects immediate-ly. Stopping drug will prevent further andro-

genic changes but probably won't reverse those already present.
• Teach patient to recognize and report signs of hypoglycemia.
• Instruct patient to follow dietary measures to combat drug-induced adverse reactions.
• Teach patient to place the buccal tablet to his gum just above the incisor tooth on either side of his mouth and to alternate sides with each dose.

☑ Evaluation
• Patient responds well to drug.
• Patient states acceptance of altered body im-age.
• Patient and family state understanding of drug therapy.

testosterone transdermal system
(tess-TOSS-teh-rohn tranz-DER-mal SIHS-tum)
Androderm, AndroGel, Testim

Pharmacologic class: androgen
Therapeutic class: hormone replacement
Pregnancy risk category: X
Controlled substance schedule: III

Indications and dosages

▶ **Primary or hypogonadotropic hypogo-nadism.** *Men:* 5 mg Androderm daily either as two 2.5-mg systems or one 5-mg system applied at bedtime to clean, dry skin on back, abdomen, upper arms, or thighs. Or, 5 g, 7.5 g, or 10 g AndroGel applied to upper arms, shoulders, and abdomen daily. Or, 5 or 10 g Testim, applied to upper arms and shoulders daily, preferably in the morning.

Contraindications and cautions

• Contraindicated in patients hypersensitive to the drug or any of its components, in women, and in patients with known or suspected breast or prostate cancer.
• Use cautiously in patients with renal, hepatic, or cardiac disease.
🔷 **Lifespan:** In children, drug isn't indicated. In elderly men, use cautiously because they may be at greater risk for prostatic hyperplasia or prostate cancer.

T

Adverse reactions

CV: depression, headache, *stroke.*
GI: GI bleeding.
GU: prostate abnormalities, prostatitis, UTI.
Skin: acne, allergic contact dermatitis, burning, *blister under system,* induration (at application site), irritation, *pruritus.*
Other: breast tenderness, gynecomastia.

Interactions

Drug-drug. *Antidiabetics:* May alter antidiabetic dosage requirements. Monitor glucose level.
Oral anticoagulants: May alter anticoagulant dosage requirements. Monitor PT and INR.
Oxyphenbutazone: May elevate oxyphenbutazone level. Monitor patient for adverse reactions.

Effects on lab test results

• May increase sodium, potassium, phosphate, cholesterol, liver enzyme, calcium, and creatinine levels.
• May increase RBC count.

Pharmacokinetics

Absorption: Continual, over 24 hours.
Distribution: Chiefly bound to sex–hormone-binding globulin.
Metabolism: In liver.
Excretion: In urine. *Half-life:* 10 to 100 minutes.

Route	Onset	Peak	Duration
Transdermal	Unknown	2–4 hr	2 hr after removal

Action

Chemical effect: Stimulates target tissues to develop normally in androgen-deficient men.
Therapeutic effect: Increases testosterone in androgen-deficient men.

Available forms

1% gel: 2.5 g and 5 g packets, 75 g nonaerosol metered pump, 5 g tube
Transdermal system: 2.5 mg/day, 5 mg/day

NURSING PROCESS

Assessment

• Assess patient's condition before starting therapy and regularly thereafter to monitor drug's effectiveness.

• Because long-term use of systemic androgens is linked to polycythemia, monitor hematocrit and hemoglobin values periodically in patient on long-term therapy.
• Periodically assess liver function tests, lipid profiles, and prostatic acid phosphatase and prostate-specific antigen levels.
• Be alert for adverse reactions and drug interactions.
• Assess patient's and family's knowledge of drug therapy.

Nursing diagnoses

• Sexual dysfunction related to androgen deficiency
• Risk for impaired skin integrity related to drug-induced irritation at application site
• Deficient knowledge related to drug therapy

Planning and implementation

• Apply Androderm to clean, dry skin on back, abdomen, upper arms, or thighs.
• Apply gel by rubbing entire dose into skin, then don't allow patient to bathe for 2 to 6 hours.
• Wash hands immediately with soap and water after applying Androgel.
Patient teaching
• Teach patient how to apply transdermal system.
• Tell patient to fully prime the AndroGel pump by depressing the pumping mechanism three times before first use and discarding that portion. For 5 g dose, he should pump 5 times, for 7.5 g, 6 times, and for 10 g, 8 times. The gel can be pumped into the palm of the hand then applied to application sites.
• Tell patient that topical testosterone preparations can cause virilization in women sexual partners. Advise these women to report acne or changes in body hair. Tell patient to wear a shirt during close physical contact or to wash site if applied within 2 to 6 hours of contact.
• Advise patient to report to prescriber persistent erections, nausea, vomiting, changes in skin color, or ankle edema.

Evaluation

• Patient states that he can resume normal sexual activity.
• Patient maintains normal skin integrity.
• Patient and family state understanding of drug therapy.

tetanus immune globulin, human
(TET-nuss ih-MYOON GLOH-byoo-lin)
BayTet, HyperTET

Pharmacologic class: immune serum
Therapeutic class: tetanus prevention and treatment agent
Pregnancy risk category: C

Indications and dosages

▶ **Tetanus exposure.** *Adults and children age 7 and older:* 250 units I.M.
Children younger than age 7: Give 4 units/kg I.M.

▶ **Tetanus.** *Adults and children:* Single doses of 3,000 to 6,000 units I.M. according to infection severity. Optimal dosage hasn't been established.

Contraindications and cautions

● In patients with thrombocytopenia or coagulation disorders, I.M. injection is contraindicated unless potential benefits outweigh risks.
⚖ **Lifespan:** In pregnant women, use cautiously. In breast-feeding women, use cautiously; it's unknown if the drug appears in breast milk.

Adverse reactions

CNS: slight fever.
GU: nephrotic syndrome.
Other: *anaphylaxis, angioedema,* erythema, pain, stiffness at injection site; hypersensitivity reactions.

Interactions

Drug-drug. *Live-virus vaccines:* May interfere with response. Defer live-virus vaccines for approximately 3 months after tetanus immune globulin.
Measles, mumps, polio, rubella, and varicella vaccines: Tetanus antibodies may interfere with immune response. Separate vaccines by 3 months.

Effects on lab test results

None reported.

Pharmacokinetics

Absorption: Slow.
Distribution: Unknown.
Metabolism: Unknown.

Excretion: Unknown. *Half-life:* About 23 days.

Route	Onset	Peak	Duration
I.M.	Unknown	2–3 days	4 wk

Action

Chemical effect: Provides passive immunity to tetanus.
Therapeutic effect: Prevents tetanus, and treats active tetanus infection.

Available forms

Injection: 250 units per vial or syringe

NURSING PROCESS

⚡ Assessment

● Obtain history of injury, tetanus immunizations, last tetanus toxoid injection, allergies, and reaction to immunizations.
● Antibodies remain at effective level for about 4 weeks (several times the duration of antitoxin-induced antibodies), which protects patient for incubation period of most tetanus cases.
● Be alert for adverse reactions and drug interactions.
● Assess patient's and family's knowledge of drug therapy.

⊕ Nursing diagnoses

● Risk for injury related to potential for tetanus to occur
● Deficient knowledge related to drug therapy

▶ Planning and implementation

⑤ **ALERT:** Have epinephrine 1:1,000 available to treat hypersensitivity reactions.
● Use drug if wound is more than 24 hours old or if patient has had fewer than two tetanus toxoid injections.
● Keep drug refrigerated.
● Thoroughly clean wound and remove all foreign matter.
● Inject drug into deltoid muscle for adult or child age 3 and older and into anterolateral aspect of thigh in neonate or child younger than age 3.
⑤ **ALERT:** Don't confuse drug with tetanus toxoid. Tetanus immune globulin isn't a substitute for tetanus toxoid, which should be given at same time to produce active immunization. Don't give at same site as toxoid.

T

Patient teaching

• Warn patient that pain and tenderness at injection site may occur. Suggest mild analgesic for pain relief.
• Tell patient to document date of tetanus immunization, and encourage him to keep immunization current.

✓ Evaluation

• Patient doesn't develop tetanus.
• Patient and family state understanding of drug therapy.

---

tetracycline hydrochloride
(tet-ruh-SIGH-kleen high-droh-KLOR-ighd)
Achromycin†, Apo-Tetra◆, Nu-Tetra◆, Sumycin, Topicycline

Pharmacologic class: tetracycline
Therapeutic class: antibiotic
Pregnancy risk category: D

Indications and dosages

▶ **Infections caused by sensitive gram-negative and gram-positive organisms, including *Chlamydia, Mycoplasma, Rickettsia,* and organisms that cause trachoma.** *Adults:* 1 to 2 g P.O. daily divided into two to four doses for 10 to 14 days.
Children older than age 8: Give 25 to 50 mg/kg P.O. daily divided into four doses.

▶ **Uncomplicated urethral, endocervical, or rectal infection caused by *Chlamydia trachomatis*.** *Adults:* 500 mg P.O. q.i.d. for at least 7 days.

▶ **Brucellosis.** *Adults:* 500 mg P.O. every 6 hours for 3 weeks combined with 1 g of streptomycin I.M. every 12 hours first week and daily the second week.

▶ **Gonorrhea in patients sensitive to penicillin.** *Adults:* Initially, 1.5 g P.O.; then 500 mg every 6 hours for 4 days.

▶ **Syphilis.** *Nonpregnant women who are sensitive to penicillin:* 500 mg P.O. q.i.d. for 15 days.

▶ **Acne.** *Adults and adolescents:* Initially, 125 to 250 mg P.O. every 6 hours; then 125 to 500 mg daily or every other day. Or, apply 3% ointment or 2.2% solution to affected areas daily or b.i.d.

▶ **Lyme disease‡.** *Adults:* 250 to 500 mg P.O. q.i.d. for 10 to 30 days.

▶ **Adjunct therapy for acute transmitted epididymitis (children older than age 8); pelvic inflammatory disease; and infection with *Helicobacter pylori*‡.** *Adults:* 500 mg P.O. q.i.d. for 10 to 14 days.

▶ **Malaria‡.** *Adults:* 250 mg P.O. q.i.d. for 7 days with quinine sulfate.
Children older than age 8: Give 25 mg/kg daily in 4 divided doses for 7 days with quinine sulfate.

Contraindications and cautions

• Contraindicated in patients hypersensitive to tetracyclines.
• Use cautiously in patients with impaired kidney or liver function.
⚠ **Lifespan:** In women in the last half of pregnancy and in children younger than age 8, use cautiously, if at all, because drug may cause permanent discoloration of teeth, enamel defects, and bone-growth retardation. In breast-feeding women, drug isn't recommended.

Adverse reactions

CNS: dizziness, headache, intracranial hypertension (pseudotumor cerebri).
CV: pericarditis.
EENT: dysphagia, glossitis, sore throat.
GI: anorexia, *diarrhea,* enterocolitis, *epigastric distress,* esophagitis, inflammatory lesions in anogenital region, oral candidiasis, *nausea,* stomatitis, vomiting.
Hematologic: eosinophilia, *neutropenia, thrombocytopenia.*
Musculoskeletal: retardation of bone growth (children younger than age 9).
Skin: *candidal superinfection,* increased pigmentation, maculopapular and erythematous rashes, photosensitivity reactions, urticaria.
Other: enamel defects, *hypersensitivity reactions,* permanent discoloration of teeth.

Interactions

Drug-drug. *Antacids (including sodium bicarbonate); antidiarrheals containing bismuth subsalicylate, kaolin, or pectin; laxatives containing aluminum, calcium, or magnesium:* May decrease antibiotic absorption. Give tetracyclines 1 hour before or 2 hours after these drugs.
Ferrous sulfate, other iron products, zinc: May decrease antibiotic absorption. Give tetracyclines 2 hours before or 3 hours after iron.

Hormonal contraceptives: May decrease contraceptive effectiveness and increase risk of breakthrough bleeding. Recommend nonhormonal form of birth control.

Lithium carbonate: May alter lithium level. Monitor patient.

Methoxyflurane: May cause severe nephrotoxicity with tetracyclines. Monitor patient carefully.

Oral anticoagulants: May potentiate anticoagulant effects. Monitor PT and adjust anticoagulant dosage.

Penicillins: May interfere with bactericidal action of penicillins. Avoid using together.

Drug-food. *Milk, other dairy products, other foods:* May decrease drug absorption. Give drug 1 hour before or 2 hours after these products.

Drug-lifestyle. *Sun exposure:* May cause photosensitivity reactions. Urge patient to avoid prolonged or unprotected exposure to sunlight.

Effects on lab test results

- May increase BUN and liver enzyme levels.
- May increase eosinophil count. May decrease platelet and neutrophil counts.
- May cause false-negative reading with glucose enzymatic tests (Diastix).

Pharmacokinetics

Absorption: 75% to 80%. Food or milk products significantly reduces.

Distribution: Wide in body tissues and fluids. CSF penetration is poor. 20% to 67% protein-bound.

Metabolism: None.

Excretion: Mainly unchanged in urine. *Half-life:* 6 to 11 hours.

Route	Onset	Peak	Duration
P.O.	Unknown	2–4 hr	Unknown

Action

Chemical effect: Unknown; may act by binding to 30S ribosomal subunit of microorganisms, thus inhibiting protein synthesis.

Therapeutic effect: Hinders bacterial activity.

Available forms

Capsules: 250 mg, 500 mg
Ointment†: 3%
Oral suspension: 125 mg/5 ml
Topical solution: 2.2 mg/ml

NURSING PROCESS

⚗ Assessment

- Assess patient's infection before starting therapy and regularly thereafter to monitor drug's effectiveness.
- Obtain specimen for culture and sensitivity tests before giving the first dose. Start therapy pending test results.
- If adverse GI reaction occurs, monitor hydration.
- Be alert for adverse reactions and drug interactions.
- Assess patient's and family's knowledge of drug therapy.

Nursing diagnoses

- Risk for infection related to presence of susceptible bacteria
- Risk for deficient fluid volume related to drug-induced adverse GI reactions
- Deficient knowledge related to drug therapy

▶ Planning and implementation

⚠ ALERT: Check expiration date. Outdated or deteriorated tetracyclines have been linked to reversible nephrotoxicity (Fanconi syndrome).

- Give drug on empty stomach.
- Don't expose drug to light or heat.

Patient teaching

- Tell patient to take drug with full glass of water on empty stomach, at least 1 hour before or 2 hours after meals. Also, tell him to take drug at least 1 hour before bedtime to prevent esophagitis. Explain that effectiveness of drug is reduced when taken with milk or other dairy products, food, antacids, or iron products.
- Tell patient to take drug exactly as prescribed, even after he feels better, and to take entire amount prescribed.
- Warn patient to avoid direct sunlight and ultraviolet light. Recommend sunscreen to help prevent photosensitivity reactions. Tell patient that photosensitivity persists after drug is stopped.
- Advise patient that topical forms of the drug may stain skin and clothing.
- Tell patient using topical preparation to wash, rinse, and thoroughly dry the affected area before applying the drug. Also, advise patient to avoid getting it in his eyes, nose, mouth, or other mucous membranes.

☑ Evaluation

- Patient is free from infection.
- Patient maintains adequate hydration.
- Patient and family state understanding of drug therapy.

theophylline
(thee-OFF-ih-lin)

Immediate-release liquids
Elixophyllin*

Immediate-release tablets and capsules
Theolair

Timed-release capsules
Theo-24

Timed-release tablets
Theochron, Uniphyl

Pharmacologic class: xanthine derivative
Therapeutic class: bronchodilator
Pregnancy risk category: C

Indications and dosages

▶ **Oral theophylline for acute bronchospasm in patients not already receiving theophylline.** *Adults (nonsmokers):* Loading dose of 6 mg/kg P.O.; then 3 mg/kg every 6 hours for two doses. Maintenance dosage is 3 mg/kg every 8 hours.
Children ages 9 to 16 and young adult smokers: Loading dose of 6 mg/kg P.O.; then 3 mg/kg every 4 hours for three doses; then 3 mg/kg every 6 hours.
Children ages 6 months to 9 years: Loading dose of 6 mg/kg P.O.; then 4 mg/kg every 4 hours for three doses; then 4 mg/kg every 6 hours.
Older adults or those with cor pulmonale: Loading dose of 6 mg/kg P.O.; then 2 mg/kg every 6 hours for two doses; then 2 mg/kg every 8 hours.
⊠ Adjust-a-dose: For adults with heart failure or liver disease, give loading dose of 6 mg/kg P.O.; then 2 mg/kg every 8 hours for two doses; then 1 to 2 mg/kg every 12 hours.
▶ **Parenteral theophylline for patients not receiving theophylline.** *Adults (nonsmokers):* Loading dose of 4.7 mg/kg given slow I.V.; then

maintenance infusion of 0.55 mg/kg/hour I.V. for 12 hours; then 0.39 mg/kg/hour.
Adults (otherwise healthy smokers): Loading dose of 4.7 mg/kg given slow I.V.; then maintenance infusion of 0.79 mg/kg/hour I.V. for 12 hours; then 0.63 mg/kg/hour.
Older adults or those with cor pulmonale: Loading dose of 4.7 mg/kg given slow I.V.; then maintenance infusion of 0.47 mg/kg/hour I.V. for 12 hours; then 0.24 mg/kg/hour.
Adults with heart failure or liver disease: Loading dose of 4.7 mg/kg given slow I.V.; then maintenance infusion of 0.39 mg/kg/hour I.V. for 12 hours; then 0.08 to 0.16 mg/kg/hour.
Children ages 9 to 16: Loading dose of 4.7 mg/kg given slow I.V.; then maintenance infusion of 0.79 mg/kg/hour I.V. for 12 hours; then 0.63 mg/kg/hour.
Children ages 6 months to 9 years: Loading dose of 4.7 mg/kg given slow I.V.; then maintenance infusion of 0.95 mg/kg/hour I.V. for 12 hours; then 0.79 mg/kg/hour.
▶ **Oral and parenteral theophylline for acute bronchospasm in patients receiving theophylline.** *Adults and children:* Each 0.5 mg/kg I.V. or P.O. (loading dose) increases plasma level by 1 mcg/ml. Ideally, dose is based on current theophylline level. In emergencies, some prescribers use 2.5 mg/kg P.O. dose of rapidly absorbed form if no obvious signs of theophylline toxicity are present.
▶ **Chronic bronchospasm.** *Adults and children:* 16 mg/kg or 400 mg P.O. daily (whichever is less) given in three or four divided doses at 6-to 8-hour intervals. Or, 12 mg/kg or 400 mg P.O. daily (whichever is less) using extended-release preparation given in two or three divided doses at 8- or 12-hour intervals. Dosage increased as tolerated at 2- to 3-day intervals to maximum dosage as follows:
Adults and children age 16 and older: Give 13 mg/kg or 900 mg P.O. daily (whichever is less) in divided doses.
Children ages 12 to 16: Give 18 mg/kg P.O. daily in divided doses.
Children ages 9 to 12: Give 20 mg/kg P.O. daily in divided doses.
Children ages 1 to 9: Give 24 mg/kg P.O. daily in divided doses.
Children younger than age 1¼: Loading dose is 1 mg/kg P.O. or I.V. for each 2-mcg/ml increase in theophylline level desired. Maintenance dosage for premature neonates up to 40 weeks

postconception age is 1 mg/kg every 12 hours. Maintenance dosage for term neonates up to age 4 weeks is 1 to 2 mg/kg every 12 hours; 1 to 2 mg/kg every 8 hours in those age 4 to 8 weeks; and 1 to 3 mg/kg every 6 hours in those older than age 8 weeks.

▶ **Cystic fibrosis‡.** *Infants:* 10 to 20 mg/kg I.V. daily.

▶ **Promotion of diuresis; Cheyne-Stokes respirations; paroxysmal nocturnal dyspnea‡.** *Adults:* 200 to 400 mg I.V. bolus as a single dose.

▽ I.V. administration

• Use commercially available infusion solution, or mix drug in D₅W.
• Use infusion pump for continuous infusion.
⊗ **Incompatibilities**
Ascorbic acid, ceftriaxone, cimetidine, hetastarch, phenytoin.

Contraindications and cautions

• Contraindicated in patients with active peptic ulcer or seizure disorders and in those who are hypersensitive to xanthine compounds (caffeine, theobromine).
• Don't use extended-release forms for acute bronchospasm.
• Use cautiously in patients with COPD, cardiac failure, cor pulmonale, cardiac arrhythmias, renal or hepatic disease, peptic ulceration, hyperthyroidism, diabetes mellitus, glaucoma, severe hypoxemia, hypertension, compromised cardiac or circulatory function, angina, acute MI, or sulfite sensitivity.
⚘ **Lifespan:** In pregnant women, use cautiously. In breast-feeding women, use is discouraged; infants of breast-feeding women may exhibit irritability, insomnia, or fretting. In young children, infants, neonates, and the elderly, use cautiously.

Adverse reactions

CNS: *dizziness,* headache, *insomnia,* irritability, muscle twitching, *restlessness, seizures.*
CV: *arrhythmias,* extrasystoles, flushing, *marked hypotension,* palpitations, sinus tachycardia.
GI: diarrhea, epigastric pain, *nausea, vomiting.*
Respiratory: increased respiratory rate, *respiratory arrest.*

Interactions

Drug-drug. *Adenosine:* May decrease antiarrhythmic effectiveness. Higher doses of adenosine may be needed.
Allopurinol, certain macrolide antibiotics (such as erythromycin), cimetidine, contraceptives, fluoroquinolones (such as ciprofloxacin), influenza virus vaccine, mexiletine, propafenone: May decrease hepatic clearance of theophylline and elevate theophylline level. Monitor patient for toxicity.
Barbiturates, carbamazepine, phenytoin, rifampin: May enhance metabolism and decrease theophylline blood level. Monitor patient for decreased effect.
Carteolol, pindolol, propranolol, timolol: May act antagonistically, reducing the effects of one or both drugs. The elimination of theophylline may also be reduced. Monitor theophylline level and patient closely.
Nadolol: May antagonize drug; may cause bronchospasm in sensitive patients. Use together cautiously.
Drug-herb. *Cacao tree:* May inhibit drug metabolism. Discourage use together.
Cayenne: May increase drug absorption. Discourage use together.
St. John's wort: May decrease drug effectiveness. Discourage use together.
Drug-food. *Any food:* May accelerate absorption. Give drug on an empty stomach.
Caffeine: May decrease hepatic clearance of theophylline and elevate theophylline level. Monitor patient for toxicity.
Drug-lifestyle. *Smoking:* May increase drug elimination, increasing dosage requirements. Monitor drug response and level.

Effects on lab test results

• May increase free fatty acid level.

Pharmacokinetics

Absorption: Good. Food may further alter rate of absorption, especially of some extended-release preparations.
Distribution: Throughout extracellular fluids. About 50% protein-bound, equilibrium between fluid and tissues occurs within 1 hour of I.V. loading dose.
Metabolism: In liver to inactive compounds.
Excretion: About 10% excreted unchanged in urine. *Half-life:* Adults, 7 to 9 hours; smokers,

4 to 5 hours; children, 3 to 5 hours; premature infants, 20 to 30 hours.

Route	Onset	Peak	Duration
P.O.			
regular	15–60 min	1–2 hr	Unknown
enteric-coated	15–60 min	1–2 hr	5 hr
extended-release	15–60 min	1–2 hr	4–7 hr
I.V.	15 min	15–30 min	Unknown

Action

Chemical effect: Inhibits phosphodiesterase, the enzyme that degrades cAMP, and relaxes smooth muscle of bronchial airways and pulmonary blood vessels.
Therapeutic effect: Improves breathing ability.

Available forms

Capsules (extended-release): 100 mg, 125 mg, 200 mg, 300 mg, 400 mg
D₅W injection: 200 mg in 50 ml or 100 ml; 400 mg in 100 ml, 250 ml, 500 ml, or 1,000 ml; 800 mg in 500 ml or 1,000 ml
Elixir: 27 mg/5 ml, 80 mg/15 ml*
Tablets: 125 mg, 250 mg, 300 mg
Tablets (extended-release): 100 mg, 200 mg, 300 mg, 400 mg, 450 mg, 600 mg

NURSING PROCESS

⚎ Assessment
• Assess patient's condition before starting therapy and regularly thereafter to monitor drug's effectiveness.
• Monitor vital signs; measure fluid intake and output. Expect effects such as improvement in quality of pulse and respirations.
• Metabolism rate varies among individuals; dosage is determined by monitoring response, tolerance, pulmonary function, and drug level. Therapeutic level is 10 to 20 mcg/ml in adults and 5 to 15 mcg/ml in children.
• Be alert for adverse reactions and drug interactions.
⚡ **ALERT:** Monitor patient for signs and symptoms of toxicity, including tachycardia, anorexia, nausea, vomiting, diarrhea, restlessness, irritability, and headache. The presence of any of these signs or symptoms in a patient taking theophylline warrants checking theophylline level and adjusting dosage as indicated.

• If adverse GI reaction occurs, monitor hydration.
• Assess patient's and family's knowledge of drug therapy.

⊕ Nursing diagnoses
• Impaired gas exchange related to presence of bronchospasm
• Risk for deficient fluid volume related to drug-induced adverse GI reactions
• Deficient knowledge related to drug therapy

▶ Planning and implementation
• Give oral drug around the clock, using sustained-release product at bedtime.
⚡ **ALERT:** Don't confuse sustained-release form with standard-release form.
• Dose may need to be increased in a cigarette smoker or a habitual marijuana smoker; smoking causes drug to be metabolized faster.
• Daily dose may need to be decreased in a patient with heart failure or hepatic disease, or in an elderly patient, because metabolism and excretion may be decreased.
⚡ **ALERT:** Don't confuse Theolair with Thyrolar.
Patient teaching
• Instruct patient not to dissolve, crush, or chew sustained-release products. For child unable to swallow capsules, sprinkle contents of capsules over soft food and tell patient to swallow without chewing.
• Supply instructions for home care and dosage schedule.
• Tell patient to relieve GI symptoms by taking oral drug with full glass of water after meals, although food in stomach delays absorption.
• Instruct patient to take drug regularly, as directed.
• Inform elderly patient that dizziness may occur at start of therapy.
• Have patient change position slowly and avoid hazardous activities.
• Tell patient to check with prescriber before taking other drugs, including OTC drugs. OTC drugs may contain ephedrine with theophylline salts; excessive CNS stimulation may result.
• If patient's dose is stabilized while he is smoking and he then quits smoking, tell patient to notify his prescriber; the dosage may need to be reduced.

☑ Evaluation

• Patient demonstrates improved gas exchange, exhibited in arterial blood gas values and respiratory status.
• Patient maintains adequate hydration.
• Patient and family state understanding of drug therapy.

thiamine hydrochloride (vitamin B₁)

(THY-eh-min hy-droh-KLOR-ighd)
Thiamilate†

Pharmacologic class: water-soluble vitamin
Therapeutic class: nutritional supplement
Pregnancy risk category: A

Indications and dosages

▶ **RDA.** *Men age 19 and older:* Give 1.2 mg P.O. daily.
Boys ages 14 to 18: Give 1.2 mg P.O. daily.
Women age 19 and older: Give 1.1 mg P.O. daily.
Girls ages 14 to 18: Give 1 mg P.O. daily.
Pregnant women: Give 1.4 mg P.O. daily.
Breast-feeding women: Give 1.5 mg P.O. daily.
Children ages 9 to 13: Give 0.9 mg P.O. daily.
Children ages 4 to 8: Give 0.6 mg P.O. daily.
Children ages 1 to 3: Give 0.5 mg P.O. daily.
Infants age 6 months to 1 year: Give 0.3 mg P.O. daily.
Neonates and infants younger than age 6 months: Give 0.2 mg P.O. daily.
▶ **Beriberi.** *Adults:* Depending on severity, 10 to 20 mg I.M. t.i.d. for 2 weeks, followed by dietary correction and multivitamin supplement containing 5 to 10 mg of thiamine daily for 1 month.
Children: Depending on severity, 10 to 50 mg I.M. daily for several weeks with adequate diet.
▶ **Wet beriberi with myocardial failure.** *Adults and children:* 10 to 30 mg I.V. for emergency therapy.
▶ **Wernicke encephalopathy.** *Adults:* Initially, 100 mg I.V.; then 50 to 100 mg I.V. or I.M. daily until patient is consuming regular balanced diet.

▼ I.V. administration

• Keep epinephrine available to treat anaphylaxis; give large I.V. doses cautiously.
• If patient has history of hypersensitivity reactions, apply skin test before starting therapy.
• Dilute drug before administration.
⊗ **Incompatibilities**
Alkali carbonates, barbiturates, citrates, erythromycin estolate, kanamycin, streptomycin, sulfites. Don't use with materials that yield alkaline solutions. Unstable in alkaline solutions.

Contraindications and cautions

• Contraindicated in patients hypersensitive to thiamine products.
☀ **Lifespan:** In pregnant women, use cautiously if dose exceeds RDA.

Adverse reactions

CNS: restlessness, weakness.
CV: *CV collapse,* cyanosis.
EENT: tightness of throat.
GI: nausea, *hemorrhage.*
Respiratory: *pulmonary edema.*
Skin: diaphoresis, feeling of warmth, pruritus, urticaria.
Other: *anaphylactic shock,* hypersensitivity reactions, tenderness and induration after I.M. use.

Interactions

None significant.

Effects on lab test results

None reported.

Pharmacokinetics

Absorption: Absorbed readily after small P.O. doses; after large P.O. dose, total amount absorbed is limited. In alcoholics and patients with cirrhosis or malabsorption, GI absorption is decreased. When given with meals, rate of absorption decreases, but total absorption remains same. After I.M. dose, rapid and complete.
Distribution: Wide. When intake exceeds minimal requirements, tissue stores become saturated.
Metabolism: In liver.
Excretion: In urine. *Half-life:* Unknown.

Route	Onset	Peak	Duration
P.O., I.V., I.M.	Unknown	Unknown	Unknown

Action

Chemical effect: Combines with adenosine triphosphate to form coenzyme needed for carbohydrate metabolism.
Therapeutic effect: Restores normal thiamine level.

Available forms

Injection: 100 mg/ml, 200 mg/ml
Tablets: 5 mg†, 10 mg†, 25 mg†, 50 mg†, 100 mg†, 250 mg†, 500 mg†
Tablets (enteric-coated): 20 mg†

NURSING PROCESS

Assessment
• Assess patient's condition before starting therapy and regularly thereafter to monitor drug's effectiveness.
• Be alert for adverse reactions.
• Assess patient's and family's knowledge of drug therapy.

Nursing diagnoses
• Imbalanced nutrition: less than body requirements related to the presence of thiamine deficiency
• Diarrhea related to drug-induced adverse GI reactions
• Deficient knowledge related to drug therapy

Planning and implementation
• Use parenteral route only when P.O. route isn't feasible.
• For treating alcoholic patient, give thiamine before dextrose infusions to prevent encephalopathy.
• Drug malabsorption is most likely in a patient with alcoholism, cirrhosis, or GI disease.
• Significant deficiency can occur in about 3 weeks of thiamine-free diet. Thiamine deficiency usually requires simultaneous therapy for multiple deficiencies.
• If breast-fed infant develops beriberi, give drug to both mother and child.
⚠ ALERT: Don't confuse thiamine with Thorazine.
Patient teaching
• Stress proper nutritional habits to prevent recurrence of deficiency.

Evaluation
• Patient regains normal thiamine level.

• Patient maintains normal bowel pattern.
• Patient and family state understanding of drug therapy.

thioridazine hydrochloride
(thigh-oh-RIGH-duh-zeen high-droh-KLOR-ighd)

Pharmacologic class: phenothiazine (piperidine derivative)
Therapeutic class: antipsychotic
Pregnancy risk category: C

Indications and dosages

▶ **Schizophrenia in patients who don't respond to treatment with other antipsychotics.** *Adults:* Initially, 50 to 100 mg P.O. t.i.d., with gradual, incremental increases up to 800 mg daily in divided doses, if needed. Dosage varies. *Children:* Initially, 0.5 mg/kg P.O. daily in divided doses. Increase dose gradually to optimum therapeutic effect. Maximum dose is 3 mg/kg/day.

Contraindications and cautions

• Contraindicated in patients hypersensitive to the drug or any of its components, and in those with CNS depression, severe hypertensive or hypotensive cardiac disease, coma, reduced level of CYP2D6 isoenzyme, congenital long-QT syndrome, or a history of cardiac arrhythmias.
• Don't give to patients taking fluvoxamine, propranolol, pindolol, fluoxetine, or drugs that inhibit the CYP2D6 enzyme or that prolong the QT interval.
• Use cautiously in debilitated patients and in patients with hepatic disease, CV disease, respiratory disorder, hypocalcemia, seizure disorder, severe reactions to insulin or electroconvulsive therapy, and exposure to extreme heat or cold (including antipyretic therapy) or organophosphate insecticides.
Lifespan: In pregnant women, use cautiously. In breast-feeding women, use cautiously; it's unknown if the drug appears in breast milk. In elderly patients, use cautiously.

Adverse reactions

CNS: dizziness, EEG changes, extrapyramidal reactions, *neuroleptic malignant syndrome,* sedation, tardive dyskinesia.

CV: ECG changes, *orthostatic hypotension,* tachycardia.
EENT: blurred vision, ocular changes, retinitis pigmentosa.
GI: constipation, dry mouth.
GU: dark urine, inhibited ejaculation, menstrual irregularities, *urine retention.*
Hematologic: *agranulocytosis,* hyperprolactinemia, transient leukopenia.
Hepatic: cholestatic jaundice.
Metabolic: increased appetite, weight gain.
Skin: mild photosensitivity reactions.
Other: allergic reaction, gynecomastia.

Interactions

Drug-drug. *Antacids:* May inhibit absorption of oral phenothiazines. Separate doses by at least 2 hours.
Barbiturates, lithium: May decrease phenothiazine effect. Monitor patient.
Centrally-acting antihypertensives: May decrease antihypertensive effect. Monitor blood pressure.
CNS depressants: May increase CNS depression. Use together cautiously.
Drugs that inhibit the CYP2D6 enzyme system, drugs that prolong the QT interval, fluoxetine, fluvoxamine, pindolol, propranolol: May increase risk of serious or fatal cardiac arrhythmias. Don't use together.
Drug-herb. *Dong quai, St. John's wort:* May increase photosensitivity reactions. Discourage use together.
Kava: May increase risk of dystonic reactions. Discourage use together.
Milk thistle: May decrease liver toxicity caused by phenothiazines. If drug and herb are used together, monitor liver enzyme level.
Yohimbe: May increase risk for yohimbe toxicity. Discourage use together.
Drug-lifestyle. *Alcohol use:* May increase CNS depression, particularly psychomotor skills. Strongly discourage use.
Sun exposure: May increase photosensitivity reactions. Advise patient to avoid prolonged or unprotected exposure to sunlight.

Effects on lab test results

• May increase liver enzyme and prolactin levels.
• May decrease granulocyte and WBC counts.

Pharmacokinetics

Absorption: Erratic and variable, although P.O. concentrates and syrups are more predictable than tablets.
Distribution: Wide. 91% to 99% protein-bound.
Metabolism: Extensive, by liver by the CYP2D6 enzyme system.
Excretion: Mainly as metabolites in urine, some in feces. *Half-life:* 20 to 40 hours.

Route	Onset	Peak	Duration
P.O.	Varies	Unknown	Unknown

Action

Chemical effect: Unknown; probably blocks postsynaptic dopamine receptors in brain.
Therapeutic effect: Manages symptoms of schizophrenia.

Available forms

Oral concentrate: 30 mg/ml, 100 mg/ml* (3% to 4.2% alcohol)
Tablets: 10 mg, 15 mg, 25 mg, 50 mg, 100 mg, 150 mg, 200 mg

NURSING PROCESS

🔖 Assessment

• Assess patient's condition before starting therapy and regularly thereafter to monitor drug's effectiveness.
• Monitor patient for tardive dyskinesia. It may occur after prolonged use or months or years later. It may disappear spontaneously or persist for life, despite stopping the drug.
• Monitor therapy with weekly bilirubin tests during first month, periodic blood tests (CBC and liver function), and ophthalmologic tests (long-term therapy).
⊛ ALERT: Monitor patient for symptoms of neuroleptic malignant syndrome (extrapyramidal effects, hyperthermia, autonomic disturbance), which is rare but can be fatal. It may not relate to length of drug use or type of neuroleptic; however, more than 60% of patients are men.
• Before starting therapy, perform baseline ECG and measure potassium level. Don't give drug to a patient with a QTc interval longer than 450 msec. Stop drug in patients with a QTc longer than 500 msec.
• Assess patient's and family's knowledge of drug therapy.

⊞ Nursing diagnoses

• Disturbed thought processes related to underlying condition
• Risk for injury related to drug-induced adverse CNS reactions
• Deficient knowledge related to drug therapy

▶ Planning and implementation

⊛ **ALERT:** Different liquid formulations have different concentrations. Check dosage.
⊛ **ALERT:** Drug prolongs the QTc interval in a dose-related manner.
• Prevent contact dermatitis by keeping drug away from skin and clothes. Wear gloves when preparing liquid forms.
• Dilute liquid concentrate with water or fruit juice just before giving.
• Shake suspension well before using.
• Don't abruptly stop giving the drug unless the patient experiences a severe adverse reaction. Abruptly stopping long-term therapy may cause gastritis, nausea, vomiting, dizziness, tremors, feeling of warmth or cold, diaphoresis, tachycardia, headache, or insomnia.
• Report jaundice, symptoms of blood dyscrasia (fever, sore throat, infection, cellulitis, weakness), or persistent extrapyramidal reactions (longer than a few hours), especially in pregnant women and in children, and withhold drug.
• Acute dystonic reactions may be treated with diphenhydramine.
⊛ **ALERT:** Don't confuse thioridazine with Thorazine.

Patient teaching
• Warn patient to avoid activities that require alertness until the drug's CNS effects are known. Drowsiness and dizziness usually subside after a few weeks.
• Tell patient to watch for orthostatic hypotension, especially with parenteral administration. Advise patient to change position slowly.
• Tell patient not to drink alcohol while taking drug.
• Instruct patient to report urine retention or constipation.
• Inform patient that drug may discolor urine.
• Tell patient to watch for and notify prescriber of blurred vision.
• Advise patient to relieve dry mouth with sugarless gum or hard candy.
• Tell patient to use sunblock and to wear protective clothing to avoid photosensitivity reactions.

☑ Evaluation

• Patient's behavior and communication exhibit improved thought processes.
• Patient doesn't experience injury from adverse CNS reactions.
• Patient and family state understanding of drug therapy.

HIGH ALERT

thiotepa
(thy-oh-TEE-puh)
Thioplex

Pharmacologic class: alkylating drug
Therapeutic class: antineoplastic
Pregnancy risk category: D

Indications and dosages

▶ **Breast and ovarian cancers, lymphoma, Hodgkin lymphoma.** *Adults and children older than age 12:* Give 0.3 to 0.4 mg/kg I.V. every 1 to 4 weeks or 0.2 mg/kg for 4 to 5 days at intervals of 2 to 4 weeks.
▶ **Bladder tumor.** *Adults and children older than age 12:* Give 60 mg in 30 to 60 ml of normal saline solution instilled in bladder for 2 hours once weekly for 4 weeks.
▶ **Neoplastic effusions.** *Adults and children older than age 12:* Give 0.6 to 0.8 mg/kg intracavitarily or intratumor every 1 to 4 weeks.
▶ **Malignant meningeal neoplasm‡.** *Adults:* 1 to 10 mg/m^2 intrathecally, once to twice weekly.

▼ I.V. administration

• Follow facility policy to minimize risks. Preparation and administration of parenteral form are linked to mutagenic, teratogenic, and carcinogenic risks to personnel.
• Reconstitute drug with 1.5 ml of sterile water for injection. Don't reconstitute with other solutions.
• Further dilute solution with normal saline solution injection, D$_5$W, dextrose 5% in normal saline solution for injection, Ringer's injection, or lactated Ringer's injection.
• Drug may be given rapid I.V. in doses of 0.3 to 0.4 mg/kg at intervals of 1 to 4 weeks.
• If pain occurs at insertion site, dilute further or use local anesthetic. Make sure drug doesn't infiltrate.
• Refrigerate and protect dry powder from direct sunlight.

Reactions may be *common,* uncommon, *life-threatening,* or COMMON AND LIFE-THREATENING.

- Solutions are stable for up to 5 days if refrigerated. Solution should be clear to slightly opaque. Discard if solution appears very opaque or contains precipitate.

⊗ **Incompatibilities**
Cisplatin, filgrastim, minocycline, vinorelbine.

Contraindications and cautions

- Contraindicated in patients hypersensitive to the drug or any of its components and in those with severe bone marrow, hepatic, or renal dysfunction.
- Use cautiously in patients with mild bone marrow suppression or renal or hepatic dysfunction.

⚫ **Lifespan:** In pregnant and breast-feeding women, drug isn't recommended. In children age 12 and younger, safety and effectiveness haven't been established.

Adverse reactions

CNS: dizziness, fatigue, fever, headache, weakness.
EENT: blurred vision, conjunctivitis, *laryngeal edema.*
GI: abdominal pain, anorexia, stomatitis, *nausea, vomiting.*
GU: amenorrhea, decreased spermatogenesis, dysuria, hemorrhagic cystitis, urine retention.
Hematologic: anemia, *leukopenia, neutropenia, thrombocytopenia.*
Respiratory: *asthma.*
Skin: alopecia, dermatitis, rash, urticaria.
Other: *anaphylaxis,* hypersensitivity reactions, pain at injection site.

Interactions

Drug-drug. *Alkylating drugs, radiation therapy:* May intensify toxicity rather than enhance therapeutic response. Avoid using together.
Anticoagulants, aspirin: May increase bleeding risk. Avoid using together.
Neuromuscular blockers: May prolong muscular paralysis. Monitor patient closely.
Succinylcholine: May increase apnea. Monitor patient closely.

Effects on lab test results

- May increase uric acid level. May decrease pseudocholinesterase and hemoglobin levels and hematocrit.
- May decrease lymphocyte, platelet, WBC, RBC, and neutrophil counts.

Pharmacokinetics

Absorption: Absorption from bladder after instillation ranges from 10% to 100% of instilled dose; also variable after intracavitary use. Increased by certain pathologic conditions.
Distribution: Crosses blood-brain barrier.
Metabolism: Extensive, in liver.
Excretion: Drug and metabolites in urine. *Half-life:* 2¼ hours.

Route	Onset	Peak	Duration
I.V., bladder instillation, intracavitary	Unknown	Unknown	Unknown

Action

Chemical effect: Cross-links strands of cellular DNA and interferes with RNA transcription, causing growth imbalance that leads to cell death.
Therapeutic effect: Kills certain cancer cells.

Available forms

Injection: 15-mg vials

NURSING PROCESS

Assessment
- Assess patient's condition before starting therapy and regularly thereafter to monitor drug's effectiveness.
- Adverse GU reactions are reversible in 6 to 8 months.
- Monitor CBC weekly for at least 3 weeks after giving the last dose.
- Monitor uric acid level.
- Be alert for adverse reactions and drug interactions.
- Assess patient's and family's knowledge of drug therapy.

Nursing diagnoses
- Ineffective health maintenance related to presence of neoplastic disease
- Ineffective protection related to drug-induced immunosuppression
- Deficient knowledge related to drug therapy

Planning and implementation
- Drug can be given by all parenteral routes, including direct injection into tumor.
- Dehydrate patient 8 to 10 hours before bladder instillation. Instill drug into bladder by

catheter; ask patient to retain solution for
2 hours. If discomfort is too great with 60 ml,
reduce volume to 30 ml. Reposition patient
every 15 minutes for maximum area contact.
• When intracavitary use is needed, for neoplastic effusions, mix drug with 2% procaine hydrochloride or epinephrine hydrochloride 1:1,000.
• Report WBC count below 3,000/mm³ or
platelet count below 150,000/mm³ and stop
drug.
• To prevent hyperuricemia with resulting uric
acid nephropathy, allopurinol may be used with
adequate hydration.
Patient teaching
• Tell patient to watch for signs of infection
(fever, sore throat, fatigue) and bleeding (easy
bruising, nosebleeds, bleeding gums, melena).
Tell patient to take temperature daily and to report even mild infections.
• Instruct patient to avoid OTC products containing aspirin.
• Advise woman of childbearing age to avoid
becoming pregnant during therapy and to consult with prescriber if pregnancy is suspected.

☑ Evaluation
• Patient responds well to drug.
• Patient doesn't develop serious complications
from drug-induced immunosuppression.
• Patient and family state understanding of drug
therapy.

thiothixene
(thy-oh-THIKS-een)
Navane

thiothixene hydrochloride
Navane*

Pharmacologic class: thioxanthene
Therapeutic class: antipsychotic
Pregnancy risk category: C

Indications and dosages
▶ **Mild to moderate psychosis.** *Adults and
children age 12 and older:* Initially, 2 mg P.O.
t.i.d. Increase gradually to 15 mg daily.
▶ **Severe psychosis.** *Adults and children age
12 and older:* Initially, 5 mg P.O. b.i.d. Increase
gradually to 20 to 30 mg daily. Maximum recommended dosage is 60 mg daily.

Contraindications and cautions
• Contraindicated in patients hypersensitive to
the drug or any of its components and in those
with circulatory collapse, coma, CNS depression, or blood dyscrasia.
• Use cautiously in patients with history of
seizure disorder or during alcohol withdrawal.
Also use cautiously in debilitated patients and in
patients with CV disease (may cause sudden
drop in blood pressure), glaucoma, prostatic hyperplasia, or exposure to extreme heat.
⚖ Lifespan: In pregnant women, use cautiously. In breast-feeding women, use cautiously; it's
unknown if the drug appears in breast milk. In
children younger than age 12, drug isn't recommended. In the elderly, use cautiously.

Adverse reactions
CNS: agitation, dizziness, EEG changes, extrapyramidal reactions (pseudoparkinsonism,
dystonias, akathisia), insomnia, *neuroleptic ma-
lignant syndrome,* restlessness, sedation, tar-
dive dyskinesia.
CV: ECG changes, *orthostatic hypotension,*
tachycardia.
EENT: *blurred vision,* ocular changes, nasal
congestion.
GI: constipation, dry mouth.
GU: inhibited ejaculation, menstrual irregulari-
ties, *urine retention.*
Hematologic: *agranulocytosis,* leukocytosis,
transient leukopenia.
Hepatic: jaundice.
Metabolic: weight gain.
Skin: mild photosensitivity reactions.
Other: allergic reaction, gynecomastia.

Interactions
Drug-drug. *Anticholinergics:* May potentiate
anticholinergic effects. Use together cautiously.
Antihypertensives: May potentiate antihypertensive effects. Use together cautiously.
Other CNS depressants: May increase CNS depression. Avoid using together.
Drug-herb. *Nutmeg:* May cause a loss of symptom control or interfere with therapy for psychiatric illnesses. Discourage using together.
Drug-lifestyle. *Alcohol use:* May increase CNS
depression. Discourage using together.
Sun exposure: May increase photosensitivity reactions. Advise patient to avoid prolonged or
unprotected exposure to sunlight.

Effects on lab test results
- May increase liver enzyme level.
- May decrease granulocyte count. May increase or decrease WBC count.

Pharmacokinetics
Absorption: Rapid.
Distribution: Wide, throughout body. 91% to 99% protein-bound.
Metabolism: Minimal.
Excretion: Mainly as parent drug in feces.
Half-life: 20 to 40 hours.

Route	Onset	Peak	Duration
P.O.	Several wk	Unknown	Unknown

Action
Chemical effect: Unknown; probably blocks postsynaptic dopamine receptors in brain.
Therapeutic effect: Relieves signs and symptoms of psychosis.

Available forms
thiothixene
Capsules: 1 mg, 2 mg, 5 mg, 10 mg, 20 mg
thiothixene hydrochloride
Oral concentrate: 5 mg/ml*

NURSING PROCESS

Assessment
- Assess patient's psychosis before starting therapy and regularly thereafter to monitor drug's effectiveness.
- Watch for orthostatic hypotension; monitor blood pressure.
- Monitor patients, especially children, for tardive dyskinesia. It may occur after prolonged use or may not appear until months or years later. It may disappear spontaneously or persist for life, despite stopping the drug.
- Monitor therapy with weekly bilirubin tests during first month, periodic blood tests (CBC and liver function), and ophthalmologic tests for those in long-term therapy.
- **ALERT:** Monitor patient for symptoms of neuroleptic malignant syndrome (extrapyramidal effects, hyperthermia, autonomic disturbance), which is rare but can be fatal. It isn't necessarily related to length of drug use or type of neuroleptic; however, more than 60% of patients are men.

- Be alert for adverse reactions and drug interactions.
- Assess patient's and family's knowledge of drug therapy.

Nursing diagnoses
- Disturbed thought processes related to presence of psychosis
- Risk for injury related to drug-induced adverse CNS reactions
- Deficient knowledge related to drug therapy

Planning and implementation
- Prevent contact dermatitis by keeping drug away from skin and clothes. Wear gloves when preparing liquid form.
- Dilute liquid concentrate with water or fruit juice just before giving.
- Slight yellowing of concentrate is common and doesn't affect potency. Discard markedly discolored solutions.
- Don't abruptly stop giving the drug unless warranted by a severe adverse reaction. Abruptly stopping long-term therapy may cause gastritis, nausea, vomiting, dizziness, tremors, feeling of warmth or cold, diaphoresis, tachycardia, headache, or insomnia.
- Report jaundice, symptoms of blood dyscrasia (fever, sore throat, infection, cellulitis, weakness), or persistent extrapyramidal reactions (longer than a few hours), especially in pregnant woman or in child, and withhold dose.
- Acute dystonic reactions may be treated with diphenhydramine.
- **ALERT:** Don't confuse Navane with Nubain or Norvasc.
Patient teaching
- Warn patient to avoid activities that require alertness until the drug's CNS effects are known. Drowsiness and dizziness usually subside after a few weeks.
- Tell patient not to drink alcohol while taking drug.
- If urine retention or constipation occurs, instruct patient to notify prescriber.
- Tell patient to relieve dry mouth with sugarless gum or hard candy.
- To avoid photosensitivity reactions, tell patient to use sunblock and wear protective clothing.
- Tell patient to watch for orthostatic hypotension; advise patient to change position slowly.

T

☑ Evaluation
- Patient's behavior and communication exhibit improved thought processes.
- Patient doesn't experience injury from adverse CNS reactions.
- Patient and family state understanding of drug therapy.

tiagabine hydrochloride
(ty-AG-ah-been hy-droh-KLOR-ighd)
Gabitril

Pharmacologic class: GABA uptake inhibitor
Therapeutic class: anticonvulsant
Pregnancy risk category: C

Indications and dosages

▶ **Adjunctive therapy in partial seizures.**
Adults: Initially, 4 mg P.O. once daily. Total daily dosage may be increased by 4 to 8 mg at weekly intervals until response is noted or up to 56 mg daily. Divide dosage b.i.d. to q.i.d.
Children ages 12 to 18: Initially, 4 mg P.O. once daily. Total daily dosage may be increased by 4 mg at the beginning of week 2 and by 4 to 8 mg/week until response is noted or up to 32 mg daily. Divide dose b.i.d. to q.i.d.
▣ **Adjust-a-dose:** Dosage may be decreased in patients with hepatic insufficiency.

Contraindications and cautions
- Contraindicated in patients hypersensitive to the drug or any of its components.
⚕ **Lifespan:** In pregnant women, use only if clearly needed. In breast-feeding women, use cautiously; it's unknown if drug appears in breast milk. In children younger than age 12, safety and effectiveness haven't been established.

Adverse reactions
CNS: abnormal gait, agitation, *asthenia,* ataxia, confusion, depression, difficulty with memory, *dizziness,* difficulty with concentration and attention, emotional lability, generalized weakness, hostility, insomnia, language problems, *nervousness,* pain, paresthesia, *somnolence,* speech disorder, tremor.
CV: vasodilation.
EENT: nystagmus, pharyngitis.

GI: abdominal pain, diarrhea, increased appetite, mouth ulcerations, *nausea,* vomiting.
Musculoskeletal: myasthenia.
Respiratory: increased cough.
Skin: pruritus, rash.

Interactions
Drug-drug. *Carbamazepine, phenobarbital, primidone, phenytoin:* May increase tiagabine clearance. Monitor patient for loss of therapeutic effect. May need to increase tiagabine dose. *CNS depressants:* May increase CNS effects. Use cautiously.
Drug-lifestyle. *Alcohol use:* May increase CNS effects. Discourage using together.

Effects on lab test results
None reported.

Pharmacokinetics
Absorption: Rapid and more than 95%. Absolute bioavailability is 90%.
Distribution: About 96% bound to plasma proteins.
Metabolism: Likely to be metabolized by CYP3A isoenzymes.
Excretion: About 25% is in urine; 63% in feces. *Half-life:* 7 to 9 hours.

Route	Onset	Peak	Duration
P.O.	Rapid	45 min	7–9 hr

Action
Chemical effect: Unknown; may enhance the activity of GABA, the major inhibitory neurotransmitter in the CNS. It binds to recognition sites related to the GABA uptake carrier and may thus permit more GABA to be available for binding to receptors on postsynaptic cells.
Therapeutic effect: Prevents partial seizures.

Available forms
Tablets: 2 mg, 4 mg, 12 mg, 16 mg

NURSING PROCESS

✐ Assessment
- Assess patient's seizure disorder before starting therapy and regularly thereafter to monitor drug's effectiveness.
- Assess patient's compliance with therapy at each follow-up visit.

ALERT: Monitor patient carefully for status epilepticus, because sudden death may occur in patient taking an anticonvulsant.
• Assess patient for adverse reactions and drug interactions.
• Assess patient's and family's knowledge of drug therapy.

Nursing diagnoses
• Risk for injury related to seizure disorder
• Impaired physical mobility related to drug-induced generalized weakness
• Deficient knowledge related to drug therapy

Planning and implementation
• In patient with impaired liver function, lower initial and maintenance doses or longer dosage intervals may be needed.
ALERT: Never abruptly stop giving the drug, because seizure frequency may increase. Gradually stop giving the drug unless safety concerns require a more rapid withdrawal.
ALERT: Drug may cause seizures and status epilepticus in patients without a history of epilepsy. Nonepileptic patients who develop seizures should stop drug and be evaluated for underlying seizure disorder. Prescribers are discouraged from using the drug for off-label indications.
• Patient who isn't receiving at least one enzyme-inducing antiepileptic when starting therapy may require lower dose or slower dosage adjustments.
• Report breakthrough seizure activity to prescriber.
ALERT: Don't confuse tiagabine with tizanidine; both have 4-mg starting doses.
Patient teaching
• Advise patient to take drug only as prescribed.
• Advise patient to take drug with food.
• Warn patient that drug may cause dizziness, somnolence, and other symptoms and signs of CNS depression. Advise patient to avoid driving and other potentially hazardous activities that require mental alertness until the drug's CNS effects are known.
• Tell woman to notify prescriber if she becomes pregnant or plans to become pregnant during therapy.
• Tell woman to notify prescriber if planning to breast-feed because drug may appear in breast milk.

Evaluation
• Patient is free from seizure activity.
• Patient receives therapeutic dose and doesn't experience muscle weakness.
• Patient and family state understanding of drug therapy.

ticarcillin disodium
(tigh-kar-SIL-in digh-SOH-dee-um)

Pharmacologic class: alpha-carboxypenicillin, extended-spectrum penicillin
Therapeutic class: antibiotic
Pregnancy risk category: B

Indications and dosages
▶ **Severe systemic infections caused by susceptible strains of gram-positive and especially gram-negative organisms (including *Pseudomonas* and *Proteus*).** *Adults and children older than age 1 month:* 200 to 300 mg/kg I.V. daily in divided doses every 4 to 6 hours.
▶ **Uncomplicated UTI.** *Adults and children weighing 40 kg (88 lb) or more:* 1 g I.V. or I.M. every 6 hours.
Infants and children older than age 1 month and weighing less than 40 kg: 50 to 100 mg/kg I.V. or I.M. daily in divided doses every 6 to 8 hours.
▶ **Complicated UTI.** *Adults:* 150 to 200 mg/kg I.V. daily in divided doses every 4 or 6 hours.
Adjust-a-dose: For patients with renal impairment, give the initial loading dose of 3 g I.V.; then base I.V. doses on creatinine clearance. If creatinine clearance is 30 to 60 ml/minute, dosage is 2 g I.V. every 4 hours; if clearance is 10 to 29 ml/minute, 2 g I.V. every 8 hours; if below 10 ml/minute, 2 g every 12 hours or 1 g I.M. every 6 hours; and if below 10 ml/minute with hepatic dysfunction, 2 g every 24 hours or 1 g I.M. every 12 hours.

I.V. administration
• Reconstitute drug in vials using D₅W, normal saline solution injection, sterile water for injection, or other compatible solution.
• Reconstitute 3-g piggyback vials with a minimum of 30 ml compatible solution; if diluting with 50 ml diluent, dilute to 60 mg/ml. If diluting with 100 ml diluent, dilute to 30 mg/ml.
• Add 4 ml of diluent for each gram of drug to obtain 200 mg/ml. May dilute further, if desired.

• For direct injection, give slowly to avoid vein irritation. For intermittent infusion, give over 30 minutes to 2 hours. Infusing with a concentration of 50 mg/ml may reduce vein irritation.
• Continuous infusion may cause vein irritation. Change site every 48 hours.

⊗ **Incompatibilities**
Aminoglycosides, amphotericin B, ciprofloxacin, doxapram, fluconazole, gentamicin, methylprednisolone sodium succinate, vancomycin.

Contraindications and cautions

• Contraindicated in patients hypersensitive to penicillins.
• Use cautiously in patients with other drug allergies, especially to cephalosporins (possible cross-sensitivity), and those with impaired kidney function, hemorrhagic conditions, hypokalemia, or sodium restrictions (contains 5.2 to 6.5 mEq sodium/g).
※ **Lifespan:** In pregnant women and breastfeeding women, use cautiously.

Adverse reactions

CNS: asterixis, lethargy, neuromuscular excitability, *seizures,* stupor.
CV: phlebitis, vein irritation.
GI: diarrhea, nausea, vomiting.
Hematologic: eosinophilia, *granulocytopenia,* hemolytic anemia, *leukopenia, neutropenia, thrombocytopenia.*
Metabolic: hypokalemia.
Other: *hypersensitivity reactions, anaphylaxis,* overgrowth of nonsusceptible organisms, pain at injection site.

Interactions

Drug-drug. *Hormonal contraceptives:* May decrease effectiveness of hormonal contraceptives. Recommend an additional form of contraception during penicillin therapy.
Lithium: May alter renal elimination of lithium. Monitor lithium level closely.
Methotrexate: May decrease renal clearance of methotrexate. Monitor patient carefully.
Probenecid: May increase level of ticarcillin and other penicillins. Probenecid may be used for this purpose.

Effects on lab test results

• May increase ALT, AST, alkaline phosphatase, LDH, and sodium levels. May decrease potassium and hemoglobin levels and hematocrit.

• May increase eosinophil count. May decrease platelet, WBC, neutrophil, and granulocyte counts.
• May cause false-positive urine protein result.

Pharmacokinetics

Absorption: Unknown after I.M. use.
Distribution: Distributed widely. Penetrates minimally into CSF with non-inflamed meninges. 45% to 65% protein-bound.
Metabolism: About 13% metabolized by hydrolysis to inactive compounds.
Excretion: Mainly in urine; also in bile. *Half-life:* About 1 hour.

Route	Onset	Peak	Duration
I.V.	Immediate	Immediate	Unknown
I.M.	Unknown	30–75 min	Unknown

Action

Chemical effect: Inhibits cell-wall synthesis during microorganism multiplication; bacteria resist penicillins by producing penicillinase enzymes that convert penicillins to inactive penicilloic acid. Drug resists these enzymes.
Therapeutic effect: Kills bacteria.

Available forms

Injection: 3 g

NURSING PROCESS

🔖 **Assessment**

• Assess patient's infection before starting therapy and regularly thereafter to monitor drug's effectiveness.
• Before giving drug, find out if patient is allergic to penicillin. Negative history of penicillin allergy is no guarantee against future allergic reaction.
• Obtain specimen for culture and sensitivity tests before giving the first dose. Start therapy pending test results.
• Monitor potassium level.
• Monitor CBC and platelet count.
• Monitor INR in patient taking warfarin therapy because drug may prolong PT.
• Be alert for adverse reactions and drug interactions.
• If adverse GI reaction occurs, monitor patient's hydration.
• Assess patient's and family's knowledge of drug therapy.

Reactions may be *common,* uncommon, *life-threatening,* or COMMON AND LIFE-THREATENING.

⊕ Nursing diagnoses
• Risk for infection related to presence of susceptible bacteria
• Risk for deficient fluid volume related to drug-induced adverse GI reactions
• Deficient knowledge related to drug therapy

▷ Planning and implementation
• Lower the dose in a patient with renal impairment.
• Reconstitute drug for I.M. use in vials with sterile water for injection, normal saline solution injection, or lidocaine 1% (without epinephrine). Use 2 ml of diluent per gram of drug.
• Inject I.M. dose deep into large muscle. Don't exceed 2 g per injection.
• Give drug at least 1 hour before bacteriostatic antibiotics.
• Drug is typically used with another antibiotic, such as gentamicin.
⊛ ALERT: Institute seizure precautions. Patient with high drug level may develop seizures.
Patient teaching
• Instruct patient to report adverse reactions.

✓ Evaluation
• Patient is free from infection.
• Patient maintains adequate hydration.
• Patient and family state understanding of drug therapy.

---

ticarcillin disodium and clavulanate potassium
(ty-kar-SIL-in dy-SOH-dee-um and KLAV-yoo-lan-nayt poh-TAH-see-um)
Timentin

Pharmacologic class: beta-lactamase inhibitor, extended-spectrum penicillin
Therapeutic class: antibiotic
Pregnancy risk category: B

Indications and dosages
▶ **Systemic septicemia; lower respiratory tract, bone and joint, skin and skin structure, intra-abdominal, and urinary tract infections.** *Adults weighing 60 kg (132 lb) or more:* 3.1 g (3 g ticarcillin and 100 mg clavulanic acid) I.V. every 4 to 6 hours.

▶ **Moderate gynecologic infections.** *Adults weighing 60 kg or more:* 200 mg of ticarcillin/kg daily I.V. in divided doses every 6 hours.
▶ **Severe gynecologic infections.** *Adults weighing 60 kg or more:* 300 mg of ticarcillin/kg daily I.V. in divided doses every 4 hours.
▶ **Systemic, urinary tract, and gynecologic infections.** *Adults weighing less than 60 kg:* 200 to 300 mg/kg I.V. daily (based on ticarcillin content) in divided doses every 4 to 6 hours.
Children age 3 months and older and weighing less than 60 kg: For mild to moderate infections, 200 mg of ticarcillin/kg I.V. daily in divided doses every 6 hours. For severe infections, 300 mg/kg daily in divided doses every 4 hours.
Children age 3 months and older weighing 60 kg or more: For mild to moderate infections, 3.1 g (3 g ticarcillin and 100 mg clavulanic acid) I.V. every 6 hours; for severe infections, 3.1 g every 4 hours.
◨ **Adjust-a-dose:** For patients with renal impairment, if creatinine clearance is greater than 60 ml/minute, give 3.1 g every 4 hours; if 30 to 60 ml/minute, give 2 g every 4 hours; if 10 to 30 ml/minute, give 2 g every 8 hours; if less than 10 ml/minute, give 2 g every 12 hours; and if less than 10 ml/minute and the patient has hepatic dysfunction, give 2 g every 24 hours. If the patient is on peritoneal dialysis, give 3.1 g every 12 hours and if the patient is on hemodialysis, give 2 g every 12 hours and 3.1 g after hemodialysis.

▽ I.V. administration
• Reconstitute drug with 13 ml of sterile water for injection or normal saline solution injection.
• Further dilute to maximum of 10 to 100 mg/ml (based on ticarcillin component). In fluid-restricted patient, dilute to maximum of 48 mg/ml if using D_5W, 43 mg/ml if using normal saline solution injection, or 86 mg/ml if using sterile water for injection.
• Infuse over 30 minutes.
⊗ Incompatibilities
Aminoglycosides, amphotericin B, cisatracurium, other anti-infectives, sodium bicarbonate, vancomycin.

Contraindications and cautions
• Contraindicated in patients hypersensitive to penicillins.

• Use cautiously in patients with other drug allergies, especially to cephalosporins (possible cross-sensitivity), and those with impaired kidney function, hemorrhagic condition, hypokalemia, or sodium restrictions (contains 4.5 mEq sodium/g).

☀ **Lifespan:** In pregnant women, use cautiously. In breast-feeding women, use cautiously; it's unknown if the drug appears in breast milk.

Adverse reactions

CNS: asterixis, giddiness, headache, lethargy, neuromuscular excitability, *seizures,* stupor.
CV: phlebitis, vein irritation.
GI: diarrhea, epigastric pain, flatulence, nausea, *pseudomembranous colitis,* stomatitis, taste and smell disturbances, vomiting.
Hematologic: anemia, eosinophilia, *granulocytopenia,* hemolytic anemia, *leukopenia, neutropenia, thrombocytopenia.*
Metabolic: hypokalemia.
Other: *anaphylaxis, hypersensitivity reactions,* overgrowth of nonsusceptible organisms, pain at injection site.

Interactions

Drug-drug. *Hormonal contraceptives:* May decrease effectiveness of hormonal contraceptives. Recommend an additional form of contraception during ticarcillin therapy.
Lithium: May alter renal elimination of lithium. Monitor level closely.
Methotrexate: May decrease renal clearance of methotrexate. Monitor level.
Probenecid: May increase blood level of ticarcillin. Probenecid may be used for this purpose.

Effects on lab test results

• May increase ALT, AST, alkaline phosphatase, LDH, and sodium levels. May decrease potassium and hemoglobin levels and hematocrit.
• May increase eosinophil count. May decrease platelet, WBC, neutrophil, and granulocyte counts.
• May cause false-positive urine protein result.

Pharmacokinetics

Absorption: Given I.V.
Distribution: Ticarcillin disodium distributed widely. Penetrates minimally into CSF with noninflamed meninges. Clavulanic acid penetrates pleural fluid, lungs, and peritoneal fluid.

Metabolism: About 13% of ticarcillin dose metabolized by hydrolysis to inactive compounds; clavulanic acid is thought to undergo extensive metabolism but its fate is unknown.
Excretion: Ticarcillin mainly in urine; also in bile. Clavulanate metabolites in urine. *Half-life:* About 1 hour.

Route	Onset	Peak	Duration
I.V.	Immediate	Immediate	Unknown

Action

Chemical effect: Inhibits cell wall synthesis during microorganism replication; clavulanic acid increases ticarcillin's effectiveness by inactivating beta lactamases, which destroy ticarcillin.
Therapeutic effect: Kills susceptible bacteria.

Available forms

Injection: 3 g ticarcillin and 100 mg clavulanic acid

NURSING PROCESS

⚕ Assessment

• Assess patient's infection before starting therapy and regularly thereafter to monitor drug's effectiveness.
• Before giving drug, find out if patient is allergic to penicillin. Negative history of penicillin allergy is no guarantee against future allergic reaction.
• Obtain specimen for culture and sensitivity tests before giving the first dose. Start therapy pending test results.
• Monitor CBC and platelet count.
• Be alert for adverse reactions and drug interactions.
• If adverse GI reactions occur, monitor patient's hydration.
• Assess patient's and family's knowledge of drug therapy.

⚕ Nursing diagnoses

• Risk for infection related to presence of susceptible bacteria
• Risk for deficient fluid volume related to drug-induced adverse GI reactions
• Deficient knowledge related to drug therapy

⟩ Planning and implementation

• Lower the dose in patient with renal impairment.

• Give drug at least 1 hour before bacteriostatic antibiotics.
Patient teaching
• Instruct patient to report adverse reactions immediately.

☑ **Evaluation**
• Patient is free from infection.
• Patient maintains adequate hydration.
• Patient and family state understanding of drug therapy.

ticlopidine hydrochloride
(tu-KLOH-peh-deen hy-droh-KLOR-ighd)
Ticlid

Pharmacologic class: platelet aggregation inhibitor
Therapeutic class: antithrombotic
Pregnancy risk category: B

Indications and dosages

▶ **To reduce risk of thrombotic stroke in patients with history of stroke or stroke precursors in patients intolerant or allergic to aspirin, or who have failed aspirin therapy.**
Adults: 250 mg P.O. b.i.d. with meals.
▶ **Prevention of coronary artery stent thrombosis.** *Adults:* 250 mg P.O. b.i.d. taken with food together with antiplatelet doses of aspirin for up to 30 days.

Contraindications and cautions

• Contraindicated in patients hypersensitive to the drug or any of its components and in those with hematopoietic disorders (such as neutropenia, thrombocytopenia, or disorders of hemostasis), active pathologic bleeding (such as peptic ulceration or active intracranial bleeding), or severe hepatic impairment.
• Drug is reserved for patients intolerant to aspirin.
⚠ **Lifespan:** In pregnant women, use cautiously. In breast-feeding women, drug isn't recommended. In children, safety and effectiveness haven't been established.

Adverse reactions

CNS: dizziness, *intracerebral bleeding.*
CV: vasculitis.
EENT: conjunctival hemorrhage, epistaxis.

GI: *abdominal pain,* anorexia, *bleeding, diarrhea,* dyspepsia, flatulence, nausea, vomiting.
GU: dark-colored urine, hematuria, nephrotic syndrome.
Hematologic: *agranulocytosis, immune thrombocytopenia, neutropenia, pancytopenia.*
Hepatic: cholestatic jaundice, *hepatitis.*
Metabolic: hyponatremia.
Musculoskeletal: arthropathy, myositis.
Respiratory: allergic pneumonitis.
Skin: ecchymoses, pruritus, purpura, *thrombocytopenic purpura, rash,* urticaria.
Other: *hypersensitivity reactions, postoperative bleeding,* serum sickness, systemic lupus erythematosus.

Interactions

Drug-drug. *Antacids:* May decrease ticlopidine level. Separate administration times by at least 2 hours.
Aspirin and other NSAIDs: May potentiate effects of aspirin or other NSAIDs on platelets. Use together cautiously and for no longer than 30 days with aspirin.
Cimetidine: May decrease clearance of ticlopidine and increase risk of toxicity. Avoid using together.
Digoxin: May slightly decrease digoxin level. Monitor level.
Heparin, oral anticoagulants: Safety of combined use hasn't been established. Stop these drugs before starting ticlopidine.
Theophylline: May decrease theophylline clearance and risk of toxicity. Monitor patient closely, and adjust theophylline dosage.
Drug-herb. *Red clover:* May increase risk of bleeding. Caution against using together.

Effects on lab test results

• May increase ALT, AST, alkaline phosphatase and bilirubin levels. May decrease sodium level.
• May decrease neutrophil, WBC, RBC, platelet, and granulocyte counts.

Pharmacokinetics

Absorption: Rapid and extensive; enhanced by food.
Distribution: 98% protein- and lipoprotein-bound.
Metabolism: Extensive, in liver. More than 20 metabolites have been identified; unknown if parent drug or active metabolites are responsible for pharmacologic activity.

Excretion: 60% in urine; 23% in feces. *Half-life:* 1¼ hours after single dose; 4 to 5 days after multiple doses.

Route	Onset	Peak	Duration
P.O.	Unknown	2 hr	Unknown

Action

Chemical effect: Unknown; may block adenosine diphosphate-induced platelet-fibrinogen and platelet-platelet binding.
Therapeutic effect: Prevents blood clots from forming.

Available forms

Tablets: 250 mg

NURSING PROCESS

Assessment
• Assess patient's condition before starting therapy and regularly thereafter to monitor drug's effectiveness.
• Obtain baseline liver function tests before starting therapy. Monitor test results closely, especially during first 4 months of therapy, and repeat when liver dysfunction is suspected.
• Determine baseline CBC and WBC differentials, repeat at second week of therapy and every 2 weeks until end of third month. If patient shows signs of declining neutrophil count, or if count falls 30% below baseline, test more frequently. After first 3 months, obtain CBC and WBC differential counts only in patient showing signs of infection.
• Be alert for adverse reactions and drug interactions.
• Assess patient's and family's knowledge of drug therapy.

Nursing diagnoses
• Impaired cerebral tissue perfusion related to stroke potential or history
• Ineffective protection related to drug-induced adverse hematologic reactions
• Deficient knowledge related to drug therapy

Planning and implementation
• Thrombocytopenia may occur rarely. Report platelet count of 80,000/mm³ or less, and stop giving the drug. Give 20 mg of methylprednisolone I.V. to normalize bleeding time within 2 hours. Platelet transfusions also may be used.

• When used preoperatively, drug may decrease risk of graft occlusion in patient receiving coronary artery bypass grafts and reduce severity of drop in platelet count in patient receiving extracorporeal hemoperfusion during open heart surgery.

Patient teaching
• Tell patient to take drug with meals; this substantially increases bioavailability and improves GI tolerance.
• Tell patient being treated for stroke to avoid aspirin-containing products and to check with prescriber before taking OTC drugs.
• Explain that drug prolongs bleeding time, but that patient should report unusual or prolonged bleeding. Advise patient to tell dentist and other health care providers that he is taking this drug.
• Stress importance of regular blood tests.
• Because neutropenia can increase risk of infection, tell patient to promptly report such signs as fever, chills, and sore throat.
• If drug is substituted for a fibrinolytic or anticoagulant, tell patient to stop those drugs before starting ticlopidine.
• Advise patient to stop drug 10 to 14 days before elective surgery.
• Tell patient to report yellow skin or sclera, severe or persistent diarrhea, rashes, subcutaneous bleeding, light-colored stools, and dark urine.

Evaluation
• Patient maintains adequate cerebral perfusion.
• Patient doesn't develop serious complications.
• Patient and family state understanding of drug therapy.

tigecycline
(tigh-geh-SY-kleen)
Tygacil

Pharmacologic class: glycylcycline antibacterial
Therapeutic class: antibiotic
Pregnancy risk category: D

Indications and dosages

▶ **Complicated skin and skin structure infections; complicated intra-abdominal infections.** *Adults:* Initially 100 mg I.V.; then 50 mg every 12 hours for 5 to 14 days. Infuse drug over 30 to 60 minutes.

§ **Adjust-a-dose:** For patients with severe hepatic impairment, give initial dose of 100 mg I.V. and then 25 mg I.V. every 12 hours.

▽ I.V. administration

- Reconstitute powder with 5.3 ml of normal saline solution or D_5W to yield 10 mg/ml.
- Gently swirl the vial until the powder dissolves.
- Immediately withdraw the dose from the vial and add it to 100 ml of normal saline solution or D_5W. The maximum concentration is 1 mg/ml.
- Inspect the I.V. solution for particulates and discoloration (green or black) before giving it. Reconstituted solution should be yellow to orange.
- Immediately dilute reconstituted drug for I.V. infusion.
- Use a dedicated I.V. line or a Y-site, and flush the line with normal saline or D_5W before and after infusion.
- Infuse the drug over 30 to 60 minutes.
- Store unopened vials at room temperature in the original package. Store diluted solution at room temperature for up to 6 hours, or refrigerate for up to 24 hours.

⊗ **Incompatibilities**
Amphotericin B, chlorpromazine, methylprednisolone, voriconazole.

Contraindications and cautions

- Contraindicated in patients hypersensitive to tigecycline.
- Use cautiously in patients with severe hepatic impairment and in those hypersensitive to tetracycline antibiotics. Also use cautiously as monotherapy in patients with complicated intra-abdominal infections caused by intestinal perforation.
- ⚖ **Lifespan:** In pregnant women, use drug only if benefits to patient outweigh risks to fetus. In breast-feeding women, use cautiously; it isn't known if drug appears in breast milk. In children, safety and effectiveness haven't been established. Older adults may be more sensitive to drug's adverse effects.

Adverse reactions

CNS: asthenia, dizziness, fever, headache, insomnia, pain, *pseudotumor cerebri.*
CV: hypertension, hypotension, peripheral edema.

GI: abdominal pain, constipation, *diarrhea,* dyspepsia, *nausea, vomiting.*
Hematologic: anemia, leukocytosis, ***thrombocytopenia.***
Metabolic: hyperglycemia, hypokalemia, hypoproteinemia.
Musculoskeletal: back pain.
Respiratory: cough, dyspnea.
Skin: local reaction, phlebitis, pruritus, rash, sweating.
Other: abscess, abnormal healing, allergic reaction, infection, ***sepsis.***

Interactions

Drug-drug. *Hormonal contraceptives:* May decrease contraceptive effectiveness. Advise patient to use nonhormonal form of contraception during treatment.
Warfarin: May increase risk of bleeding. Monitor INR.

Effects on lab test results

- May increase alkaline phosphatase, amylase, bilirubin, BUN, creatinine, LDH, AST, and ALT levels. May decrease potassium, protein, calcium, sodium, and hemoglobin levels and hematocrit. May increase or decrease blood glucose level.
- May increase INR, PT, PTT, and WBC count. May decrease platelet count.

Pharmacokinetics

Absorption: Given I.V.
Distribution: Extensive in tissues. About 70% to 90% bound to serum proteins.
Metabolism: Not extensively metabolized in the liver.
Excretion: Mainly through bile and feces as unchanged drug and metabolites; lesser amount via kidneys. *Half life:* 27 to 42 hours.

Route	Onset	Peak	Duration
I.V.	Unknown	Unknown	Unknown

Action

Chemical effect: Inhibits protein translation in bacteria by binding to the 30S ribosomal unit.
Therapeutic effect: Kills susceptible bacteria.

Available forms

Lyophilized powder: 50-mg vials

NURSING PROCESS

⚡ Assessment
- Assess patient for tetracycline allergy before giving drug.
- Obtain specimen for culture and sensitivity tests before giving first dose. Therapy may begin pending test results.
- If patient develops diarrhea, monitor patient closely for pseudomembranous colitis.
- If patient has abdominal infection caused by intestinal perforation, monitor him for sepsis.
- Evaluate patient's and family's knowledge of drug therapy.

⊕ Nursing diagnoses
- Ineffective protection related to presence of susceptible bacteria
- Risk for deficient fluid volume related to drug-induced adverse GI reactions
- Deficient knowledge related to drug therapy

▷ Planning and implementation
- Be alert for potentially dangerous toxicities of tetracyclines, such as photosensitivity, pseudotumor cerebri, pancreatitis and anti-anabolic action (increased BUN level, azotemia, acidosis, and hypophosphatemia).
- Excessive doses may increase the risk of nausea and vomiting. Drug isn't removed by hemodialysis.

Patient teaching
- Tell patient that drug is used to treat only bacterial infections, not viral infections.
- Explain that it's common to feel better after a few days of therapy. Stress that patient will need to finish the full course of treatment even if he feels better before it's finished.
- Tell patient to report burning or pain at the I.V. site.
- Tell women of childbearing age to avoid becoming pregnant during treatment. Urge those who use hormonal contraception to also use barrier contraception during treatment.
- Advise patient to notify a health care provider if pregnancy is suspected or confirmed.

☑ Evaluation
- Patient is free from infection.
- Patient maintains adequate hydration.
- Patient and family state understanding of drug therapy.

tinidazole
(ty-NIH-duh-zohl)
Tindamax

Pharmacologic class: antiprotozoal
Therapeutic class: anti-infective
Pregnancy risk category: C (X in first trimester)

Indications and dosages
▶ **Bacterial vaginosis.** *Non-pregnant women:* 2 g once daily for 2 days with food, or 1 g once daily for 5 days with food.
▶ **Trichomoniasis caused by** *Trichomonas vaginalis. Adults:* 2 g P.O. as a single dose taken with food. Sexual partners should be treated at the same time with the same dose.
▶ **Giardiasis caused by** *Giardia lamblia (G. duodenalis). Adults:* 2 g P.O. as a single dose taken with food.
Children older than age 3: Give 50 mg/kg (up to 2 g) as a single dose taken with food.
▶ **Intestinal amebiasis caused by** *Entamoeba histolytica. Adults:* 2 g P.O. daily for 3 days, taken with food.
Children older than age 3: Give 50 mg/kg (up to 2 g) P.O. daily for 3 days, taken with food.
▶ **Amebic liver abscess (amebiasis).** *Adults:* 2 g P.O. daily for 3 to 5 days, taken with food.
Children older than age 3: Give 50 mg/kg (up to 2 g) P.O. daily for 3 to 5 days, taken with food.
▣ **Adjust-a-dose:** For patients on hemodialysis, give an additional dose equal to one-half the recommended dose after the hemodialysis session.

Contraindications and cautions
- Contraindicated in patients hypersensitive to the drug, its components, or other nitroimidazole derivatives.
- Use cautiously in patients with CNS disorders and in those with blood dyscrasias or hepatic dysfunction.
- ⚘ **Lifespan:** In pregnant women, drug is contraindicated during the first trimester; during the second and third trimesters, use if benefits to the patient outweigh risks to the fetus. Breastfeeding women should stop breast-feeding or use another drug; they should wait 3 days after the last dose before resuming breast-feeding. In children age 3 and younger, safety and effec-

tiveness haven't been established. In elderly patient, dose selection should reflect the possibility of decreased liver or kidney function and other medical conditions or drug therapies.

Adverse reactions

CNS: dizziness, fatigue, headache, malaise, peripheral neuropathy, *seizures,* weakness.
GI: anorexia, constipation, cramps, dyspepsia, metallic taste, nausea, vomiting.
Other: hypersensitivity reactions.

Interactions

Drug-drug. *Cholestyramine:* May decrease oral bioavailability of tinidazole. Separate doses to minimize this effect.
Cyclosporine, tacrolimus: May increase cyclosporine and tacrolimus levels. Monitor patient closely for toxicity, including headache, nausea, vomiting, nephrotoxicity, and electrolyte abnormalities.
Cytochrome P-450 inducers, such as fosphenytoin, phenobarbital, phenytoin, and rifampin: May increase tinidazole elimination. Monitor patient.
Cytochrome P-450 inhibitors, such as cimetidine and ketoconazole: May prolong tinidazole half-life and decrease clearance. Monitor patient.
Disulfiram: May increase abdominal cramping, nausea, vomiting, headaches, and flushing. If patient took disulfiram during previous 2 weeks, don't give tinidazole.
Fluorouracil: May decrease fluorouracil clearance, increasing adverse effects without added benefit. Monitor patient for rash, nausea, vomiting, stomatitis, and leukopenia.
Fosphenytoin, phenytoin: May prolong phenytoin half-life and decrease clearance of I.V. drug. Monitor patient for toxicity.
Lithium: May increase lithium level. Monitor patient and serum lithium and creatinine levels.
Oxytetracycline: May antagonize tinidazole. Assess patient for lack of effect.
Warfarin and other oral anticoagulants: May increase anticoagulant effect. Anticoagulant dosage may need adjustment and for up to 8 days after tinidazole therapy.
Drug-herb. *St. John's wort:* May increase or decrease tinidazole level. Discourage use together.
Drug-lifestyle. *Alcohol and alcohol-containing products:* May increase abdominal cramping,

nausea, vomiting, headaches, and flushing. Discourage use together and for 3 days after stopping tinidazole.

Effects on lab test results
• May increase AST, ALT, glucose, LDH, and triglyceride levels.
• May decrease WBC count.

Pharmacokinetics
Absorption: Rapid, complete, and unaffected by food.
Distribution: Into body tissues, fluids, and breast milk. Crosses the blood-brain and placental barriers. About 12% bound to plasma proteins.
Metabolism: Mainly by CYP3A4 enzymes and partially by oxidation, hydroxylation, and conjugation in the liver.
Excretion: By liver and kidneys, with 20% to 25% in urine and 12% in feces. *Half-life:* About 12 to 14 hours.

Route	Onset	Peak	Duration
P.O.	Unknown	1½ hr	Unknown

Action

Chemical effect: Against *Trichomonas,* action may result from reduction of the compound's nitro group into a free nitro radical. Mechanism of action against *Giardia* and *Entamoeba* is unknown.
Therapeutic effect: Hinders growth of susceptible organisms.

Available forms

Tablets: 250 mg, 500 mg

NURSING PROCESS

Assessment
• Assess patient's infection before starting therapy and regularly thereafter to monitor drug's effectiveness.
• Children should be monitored closely if therapy exceeds 3 days.
• Be alert for adverse reactions and drug interactions.
ALERT: Stop giving the drug immediately if abnormal neurologic signs or symptoms occur, such as seizures or numbness of the limbs.
• Assess patient's and family's knowledge of drug therapy.

⚙ Nursing diagnoses
- Risk for injury related to drug-induced adverse neurologic reactions
- Risk for deficient fluid volume related to drug-induced adverse GI reactions
- Deficient knowledge related to drug therapy

▷ Planning and implementation
- For patients unable to swallow tablets, a suspension may be made by grinding 2 g of tinidazole into a powder and mixing with 10 ml of cherry syrup. Transfer to a graduated amber container with several rinses of cherry syrup to a final volume of 30 ml.
- Drug is stable for 7 days at room temperature. Shake well.
- Give drug with food to minimize adverse GI effects.
- If candidiasis develops during therapy, give an antifungal.

Patient teaching
- Tell patient to take drug with food.
- Warn patient not to drink alcohol or use alcohol-containing products while taking tinidazole and for 3 days afterward.
- Advise patient to immediately report pregnancy.
- If patient is being treated for a sexually transmitted disease, explain that sexual partners should be treated at the same time.

☑ Evaluation
- Patient has no adverse neurological effects.
- Patient maintains adequate hydration during drug therapy.
- Patient and family state understanding of drug therapy.

HIGH ALERT

tinzaparin sodium
(TIN-zuh-pehr-in SOE-dee-um)
Innohep

Pharmacologic class: low–molecular-weight heparin (LMWH)
Therapeutic class: anticoagulant
Pregnancy risk category: B

Indications and dosages

▶ **Adjunct treatment (with warfarin sodium) of symptomatic deep vein thrombosis with or without pulmonary embolism.** *Adults:* 175 an-

tifactor Xa international units per kg of body weight subcutaneously once daily for at least 6 days and until the patient is adequately anticoagulated with warfarin (INR at least 2) for 2 consecutive days. Begin warfarin when appropriate, usually within 1 to 3 days after tinzaparin starts. The volume to be given may be calculated as follows:

$$\frac{\text{Patient weight}}{\text{in kg}} \times 0.00875 \text{ ml/kg} = \frac{\text{volume to be}}{\text{given (in ml)}}$$

▶ **Deep vein thrombosis prophylaxis‡.**
Adults: 3,500 antifactor Xa international units or 50 antifactor Xa international units/kg daily for patients at moderate to high risk, respectively. Start 1 to 2 hours before surgery, and continue for 5 to 10 days. For prophylaxis in orthopedic procedures: 75 antifactor Xa international units/kg daily starting 12 to 24 hours postoperatively. Alternative: 4,500 antifactor Xa international units 12 hours before orthopedic surgery followed by 4,500 antifactor Xa international units daily.

Contraindications and cautions
- Contraindicated in patients hypersensitive to the drug or to heparin, sulfites, benzyl alcohol, or pork products. Also contraindicated in patients with active major bleeding and patients with current or previous heparin-induced thrombocytopenia.
- Use cautiously in patients with increased risk of hemorrhage, such as those with thrombocytopenia, bacterial endocarditis, uncontrolled hypertension, diabetic retinopathy, or congenital or acquired bleeding disorders (such as hepatic failure, amyloidosis, GI ulceration, or hemorrhagic stroke). Also use cautiously in patients being treated with platelet inhibitors, in patients who have recently undergone brain, spinal, or ophthalmologic surgery, and in patients with renal insufficiency.
- Use cautiously in patients with neuraxial (spinal or epidural) anesthesia or spinal puncture because these patients have an increased risk of neurologic injury and epidural or spinal hematoma.
- Use cautiously in patients with severe renal impairment and creatinine clearance less than 30 ml/minute.
- ☀ **Lifespan:** In pregnant women, use cautiously and only when clearly needed. Vaginal bleeding has been reported in pregnant women re-

ceiving tinzaparin; use only if benefits outweigh risks. In breast-feeding women, use cautiously; it's unknown if the drug appears in breast milk. In children, safety and effectiveness haven't been established. In the elderly, use cautiously because they may have reduced elimination of drug.

Adverse reactions

CNS: *cerebral or intracranial bleeding,* confusion, dizziness, fever, headache, insomnia, pain.
CV: angina pectoris, *arrhythmias,* chest pain, dependent edema, hypertension, hypotension, *MI, thromboembolism,* tachycardia.
EENT: epistaxis, ocular hemorrhage.
GI: anorectal bleeding, constipation, dyspepsia, flatulence, hematemesis, hemarthrosis, *GI hemorrhage,* melena, nausea, *retroperitoneal or intra-abdominal bleeding,* vomiting.
GU: dysuria, hematuria, urine retention, UTI, *vaginal hemorrhage.*
Hematologic: *agranulocytosis,* anemia, *hemorrhage,* pancytopenia, *thrombocytopenia.*
Musculoskeletal: back pain.
Respiratory: dyspnea, pneumonia, *pulmonary embolism,* respiratory disorder.
Skin: bullous eruption, cellulitis, *injection site hematoma,* pruritus, purpura, rash, skin necrosis, wound hematoma.
Other: allergic reaction, congenital anomaly, *fetal death, fetal distress, hypersensitivity reactions,* impaired healing, infection, spinal or *epidural hematoma.*

Interactions

Drug-drug. *Oral anticoagulants, platelet inhibitors (such as dextran, dipyridamole, NSAIDs, salicylates, sulfinpyrazone), thrombolytics:* May increase the risk of bleeding. Use together cautiously, and monitor patient.

Effects on lab test results

• May increase AST and ALT levels. May decrease hemoglobin level and hematocrit.
• May increase granular leukocyte count. May decrease granulocyte, platelet, RBC, and WBC counts.

Pharmacokinetics

Absorption: Plasma level peaks in 4 to 5 hours.
Distribution: The volume of distribution is similar in magnitude to that of blood volume, which suggests that distribution is limited to the central compartment.
Metabolism: Partially metabolized by desulfation and depolymerization, similar to that of other LMWHs.
Excretion: Mainly renal. *Half-life:* 3 to 4 hours.

Route	Onset	Peak	Duration
SubQ	2–3 hr	4–5 hr	Unknown

Action

Chemical effect: Inhibits reactions that lead to blood clotting, including the formation of fibrin clots. The drug also acts as a potent coinhibitor of several activated coagulation factors, especially factors Xa and IIa (thrombin). It also induces release of tissue factor pathway inhibitor, which may contribute to the antithrombotic effect.
Therapeutic effect: Reduces the ability of blood to clot.

Available forms

Injection: 20,000 anti-Xa international units per ml in 2-ml vials

NURSING PROCESS

⚚ Assessment
• Assess patient's condition before starting therapy and regularly thereafter to monitor drug's effectiveness.
• Monitor platelet count during therapy. If platelet count falls below 100,000/mm^3, stop drug.
• Periodically monitor CBC and stool tests for occult blood during therapy.
• Drug may affect PT and INR levels. Patients who also receive warfarin should have blood drawn for PT and INR tests just before the next scheduled dose of this drug.
• Drug contains sodium metabisulfite, which may cause allergic reactions in susceptible people.
• Weigh patient before starting therapy to calculate accurate dosage.
• Assess patient's and family's knowledge of drug therapy.

⊞ Nursing diagnoses
• Ineffective protection related to increased risk of bleeding

T

• Ineffective tissue perfusion, peripheral, related to deep vein thrombosis
• Deficient knowledge related to tinzaparin sodium therapy

▷ Planning and implementation
• Dose is based on actual body weight.
• If patient develops serious bleeding or receives a large overdose, replace volume and hemostatic blood elements (such as RBCs, fresh frozen plasma, and platelets), as needed. If this treatment is ineffective, consider giving protamine sulfate.
⑤ **ALERT:** Don't give I.M. or I.V., and don't mix with other injections or infusions.
⑤ **ALERT:** Drug can't be interchanged (unit for unit) with heparin or other LMWHs.
• While giving the drug, have the patient lie or sit down. Give drug by deep subcutaneous injection into the abdominal wall. Insert the whole length of the needle into a skin fold held between your thumb and forefinger. Hold the skin fold throughout the injection. To minimize bruising, don't rub the injection site after administration.
• Rotate injection sites between the right and left anterolateral and posterolateral abdominal wall.
• Use an appropriate calibrated syringe to ensure withdrawal of the correct volume of drug from vial.
⑤ **ALERT:** When neuraxial anesthesia (epidural or spinal anesthesia) or spinal puncture is used, the patient is at risk for spinal hematoma, which can result in long-term or permanent paralysis. Watch for evidence of neurologic impairment. Consider the risks and benefits of neuraxial intervention in patients being anticoagulated with LMWHs or heparinoids.
• Store drug at room temperature.
Patient teaching
• Inform patient that coadministration of warfarin will begin within 1 to 3 days of tinzaparin administration. Explain the importance of warfarin therapy.
• Stress the importance of laboratory monitoring to ensure effectiveness and safety of therapy.
• Instruct patient to take safety measures to prevent cuts and bruises (such as using a soft toothbrush and an electric razor).
• Review the warning signs of bleeding, and instruct the patient to report evidence of bleeding immediately.

• Gasping syndrome may occur in premature infants who receive large amounts of benzyl alcohol. Warn women about the risks to the fetus if she becomes pregnant during therapy.

☑ Evaluation
• Patient states appropriate bleeding precautions to take.
• Patient's peripheral neurovascular status returns to baseline.
• Patient and family state understanding of tinzaparin sodium therapy.

tiotropium bromide
(tee-oh-TROPE-ee-um BROH-mighd)
Spiriva

Pharmacologic class: long-acting anticholinergic (antimuscarinic)
Therapeutic class: bronchodilator
Pregnancy risk category: C

Indications and dosages

▶ **Maintenance therapy for bronchospasm in COPD, including chronic bronchitis and emphysema.** *Adults:* One capsule (18 mcg) inhaled orally once daily using the HandiHaler inhalation device.

Contraindications and cautions

• Contraindicated in patients hypersensitive to atropine, its derivatives, ipratropium, or any component of the product.
• Use cautiously in patients with creatinine clearance of 50 ml/minute or less and patients with angle-closure glaucoma, prostatic hyperplasia, or bladder neck obstruction.
⚘ **Lifespan:** In pregnant women, use cautiously. In breast-feeding women, use cautiously; it's unknown if the drug appears in breast milk. In children, safety and effectiveness haven't been established.

Adverse reactions

CNS: depression, paresthesia.
CV: *angina pectoris,* chest pain, edema.
EENT: cataract, dysphonia, epistaxis, glaucoma, laryngitis, pharyngitis, rhinitis, *sinusitis.*
GI: abdominal pain, constipation, *dry mouth,* dyspepsia, gastroesophageal reflux, stomatitis, vomiting.

Reactions may be *common,* uncommon, *life-threatening,* or COMMON AND LIFE-THREATENING.

GU: UTI.
Metabolic: hypercholesterolemia, hyperglyce-mia.
Musculoskeletal: arthritis, leg pain, myalgia, skeletal pain.
Respiratory: cough, *paradoxical broncho-spasm, upper respiratory tract infection.*
Skin: rash.
Other: *accidental injury, angioedema,* allergic reaction, candidiasis, flulike syndrome, herpes zoster, infections.

Interactions

Drug-drug. *Anticholinergics:* May increase the risk of adverse reactions. Avoid using together.

Effects on lab test results

• May increase cholesterol and glucose levels.

Pharmacokinetics

Absorption: Poorly absorbed from GI tract; absolute bioavailability is 19.5% after inhaling dry powder. Plasma level peaks 3 hours after inhalation.
Distribution: Extensively bound to tissues and 72% bound to plasma proteins.
Metabolism: Small amounts by CYP2D6 and CYP3A4 pathways.
Excretion: About 14% in urine, the rest in feces. *Half-life:* 5 to 6 days.

Route	Onset	Peak	Duration
Inhalation	30 min	3 hr	> 24 hr

Action

Chemical effect: Competitive, reversible inhibition of muscarinic receptors leads to bronchodilation.
Therapeutic effect: Improves breathing.

Available forms

Capsules for inhalation: 18 mcg

NURSING PROCESS

☰ Assessment

• Obtain baseline assessment of patient's respiratory status before starting therapy, and assess frequently thereafter to monitor the drug's effectiveness.
• Be alert for adverse reactions; eye pain, blurred vision, visual halos, colored images, or

red eyes may be signs of acute narrow-angle glaucoma.
⚠ **ALERT:** Watch for evidence of hypersensitivity (especially angioedema) and paradoxical bronchospasm.
• Assess patient's and family's knowledge of drug therapy.

☰ Nursing diagnoses

• Impaired gas exchange related to underlying respiratory condition
• Risk for activity intolerance related to underlying pulmonary condition
• Deficient knowledge related to drug therapy

▷ Planning and implementation

• Drug is for maintenance treatment of COPD, not for acute bronchospasm.
• Capsules aren't for oral ingestion. Give them only by oral inhalation and only with the Handi-Haler device.
• Capsules may be stored at room temperature prior to use. Remove capsule for oral inhalation from blister card just before use. Capsules should not be stored in the HandiHaler device.
• To give, place the capsule in the center chamber of the HandiHaler device. Close the mouthpiece until it clicks, but leave the dust cap open. Press the piercing button one time. Instruct the patient to breathe out completely, raise Handi-Haler device to his mouth, and close his lips tightly around the mouthpiece. The patient should keep his head upright and inhale slowly and deeply at a rate sufficient to hear the capsule vibrate. After the patient has inhaled until his lungs are full, have him hold his breath for as long as is comfortable while simultaneously taking the HandiHaler device out of his mouth; he then should resume normal breathing. The patient shouldn't ever breathe into the mouthpiece. The patient should inhale again to ensure a full dose of the drug.
• After taking the daily dose, dispose of the capsule and close the HandiHaler mouthpiece and dust cap for storage.
• Signs of overdose include dry mouth, bilateral conjunctivitis, altered mental state, tremors, abdominal pain, and severe constipation. Alert prescriber if overdose is suspected, and provide supportive care.
⚠ **ALERT:** Don't confuse Spiriva with Inspra.

T

Patient teaching

- Inform patient that drug is for maintenance treatment of COPD and not for immediate relief of breathing problems.
- Explain that capsules are for inhalation and shouldn't be swallowed.
- Provide full instructions for the HandiHaler device.
- Tell patient not to get the powder in his eyes.
- Review the signs and symptoms of hypersensitivity (especially angioedema) and paradoxical bronchospasm. Tell patient to stop the drug and contact the prescriber if they arise.
- Advise patient to report eye pain, blurred vision, visual halos, colored images, or red eyes immediately.
- Tell patient to keep capsules in sealed blisters and to remove each capsule just before use. Caution against storing capsules in the Handi-Haler device.
- Instruct patient to store capsules at 77° F (25° C) and not to expose them to extreme temperatures or moisture.

☑ Evaluation

- Patient's respiratory signs and symptoms improve.
- Patient's activity intolerance improves.
- Patient and family state understanding of drug therapy.

tipranavir
(tih-PRAN-uh-veer)
Aptivus

Pharmacologic class: nonpeptidic protease inhibitor
Therapeutic class: antiretroviral
Pregnancy risk category: C

Indications and dosages

▶ **HIV-1 in patients with viral replication who are highly treatment-experienced or have HIV-1 strains resistant to multiple protease inhibitors.** *Adults:* 500 mg P.O. b.i.d. with 200 mg of ritonavir. Give with food.

Contraindications and cautions

- Contraindicated in patients hypersensitive to any ingredients of the product, patients with moderate (Child-Pugh class B) and severe

(Child-Pugh class C) hepatic insufficiency, and patients taking drugs that depend on CYP3A for clearance, such as amiodarone, astemizole, bepridil, cisapride, dihydroergotamine, ergonovine, ergotamine, flecainide, methylergonovine, midazolam, pimozide, propafenone, quinidine, terfenadine, and triazolam.
- Use cautiously in patients with sulfonamide allergy, diabetes, liver disease, hepatitis B or C, or hemophilia A or B.
☆ **Lifespan:** In pregnant women, use only if benefits to the patient outweigh risks to the fetus. If patient is pregnant or becomes pregnant and is exposed to drug, register her with the Antiretroviral Pregnancy Registry at 1-800-258-4263. Breast-feeding isn't recommended during treatment. In children, safety and effectiveness haven't been established. In elderly patients, use cautiously because these patients are more likely to have decreased organ function, multidrug therapy, and multiple illnesses.

Adverse reactions

CNS: asthenia, depression, dizziness, fatigue, headache, insomnia, pyrexia, malaise, peripheral neuropathy, sleep disorder, somnolence.
GI: abdominal distention, abdominal pain, *diarrhea,* dyspepsia, flatulence, GERD, nausea, *pancreatitis,* vomiting.
GU: renal insufficiency.
Hematologic: anemia, *neutropenia, thrombocytopenia.*
Hepatic: *hepatic failure, hepatitis.*
Metabolic: anorexia, decreased appetite, dehydration, *diabetes mellitus,* facial wasting, hyperglycemia, weight loss.
Musculoskeletal: muscle cramps, myalgia.
Respiratory: bronchitis, cough, dyspnea.
Skin: acquired lipodystrophy, exanthem, lipoatrophy, lipohypertrophy, pruritus, *rash.*
Other: flulike syndrome, hypersensitivity, reactivation of herpes simplex and varicella zoster.

Interactions

Drug-drug. *Amiodarone, bepridil, flecainide, propafenone, quinidine:* May increase levels of these drugs and risk of serious or life-threatening arrhythmias. Avoid use together.
Astemizole, cisapride, pimozide, terfenadine: May cause serious or life-threatening arrhythmias. Avoid use together.

Reactions may be *common,* uncommon, *life-threatening,* or **COMMON AND LIFE-THREATENING.**

Atorvastatin: May increase levels of both drugs. Start with lowest dose of atorvastatin, and monitor patient closely or consider other drugs.
Clarithromycin: May increase levels of both drugs. If patient's creatinine clearance is 30 to 60 ml/minute, decrease clarithromycin dosage by 50%. If creatinine clearance is less than 30 ml/minute, decrease clarithromycin dosage by 75%.
Cyclosporine, sirolimus, tacrolimus: May cause unpredictable interaction. Monitor drug level closely until they've stabilized.
Desipramine: May increase desipramine level. Decrease dosage and monitor desipramine level.
Dihydroergotamine, ergonovine, ergotamine, methylergonovine: May cause acute ergot toxicity, including peripheral vasospasm and ischemia of extremities. Avoid use together.
Diltiazem, felodipine, nicardipine, nisoldipine, verapamil: May cause unpredictable interaction. Use together cautiously, and monitor patient closely.
Disulfiram, metronidazole: May cause disulfiram reaction. Use together cautiously.
Estrogen-based hormone therapy: May decrease estrogen level, and rash may occur. Monitor patient carefully. Advise using nonhormonal contraception.
Fluoxetine, paroxetine, sertraline: May increase levels of these drugs. Adjust dosages as needed.
Glimepiride, glipizide, glyburide, pioglitazone, repaglinide, tolbutamide: May affect glucose level. Monitor glucose level carefully.
Lovastatin, simvastatin: May increase risk of myopathy and rhabdomyolysis. Avoid use together.
Meperidine: May increase normeperidine metabolite. Avoid use together.
Methadone: May decrease methadone level by 50%. Consider increased methadone dose.
Midazolam, triazolam: May cause prolonged or increased sedation or respiratory depression. Avoid use together.
Rifabutin: May increase rifabutin level. Decrease rifabutin dosage by 75%.
Rifampin: May lead to loss of virologic response and resistance to tipranavir and other protease inhibitors. Avoid use together.
Sildenafil, tadalafil, vardenafil: May increase levels of these drugs. Tell patient to use together cautiously. Tell him not to exceed 25 mg of sildenafil in 48 hours, 10 mg of tadalafil in 72 hours, or 2.5 mg of vardenafil in 72 hours.

Warfarin: May cause unpredictable reaction. Check INR often.
Drug-herb. *St. John's wort:* May lead to loss of virologic response and resistance to drug and class. Warn patient to avoid use together.

Effects on lab test results

• May increase total cholesterol, triglyceride, blood glucose, amylase, lipase, ALT, and AST levels.
• May decrease WBC count.

Pharmacokinetics

Absorption: Limited; bioavailability is increased when taken with a high-fat meal.
Distribution: 99.9% bound to plasma proteins.
Metabolism: Mediated by cytochrome P-450; few plasma metabolites found.
Excretion: Mostly unchanged in feces; some in urine. *Half life:* 4¾ to 6 hours.

Route	Onset	Peak	Duration
P.O.	Unknown	3 hr	Unknown

Action

Chemical effect: Inhibits virus-specific processing of polyproteins in HIV-1 infected cells, thus preventing formation of mature virions.
Therapeutic effect: Produces immature, noninfectious virus.

Available forms

Capsules: 250 mg

NURSING PROCESS

Assessment
• Carefully obtain patient's drug history. Many drugs may interact with tipranavir.
• Obtain liver function tests at start of treatment and often during treatment.
• Obtain cholesterol and triglyceride levels at start of and periodically during therapy.
• If patient has diabetes, monitor glucose level closely. Hyperglycemia may occur.
• Monitor patient for evidence of hepatitis, such as fatigue, malaise, anorexia, nausea, jaundice, bilirubinemia, acholic stools, liver tenderness, and hepatomegaly.
• Monitor patient for cushingoid symptoms, such as central obesity, buffalo hump, peripheral wasting, facial wasting, and breast enlargement.

T

• Evaluate patient's and family's knowledge of drug therapy.

⊕ Nursing diagnoses
• Risk for injury related to potential for many drugs to interact with tipranavir
• Ineffective protection related to drug-induced adverse hematologic reactions
• Deficient knowledge related to drug therapy

⟩ Planning and implementation
⊛ **ALERT:** Don't give this drug to treatment-naïve patients.
• To be effective, drug must be given with 200 mg of ritonavir and other antiretrovirals.
⊛ **ALERT:** Patients who have chronic hepatitis B or C have an increased risk of hepatotoxicity.
• If patient has indicators of hepatitis, stop drug.
Patient teaching
• Explain that drug doesn't cure HIV infection and doesn't reduce the risk of transmitting the virus to others.
⊛ **ALERT:** Warn patient that many drugs may interfere with tipranavir. Urge patient to tell prescriber about all prescription drugs, OTC drugs, and herbal products he takes.
• Tell patient that drug is effective only when taken with ritonavir and other antiretrovirals.
• Instruct patient to take drug with food.
• Urge patient to stop drug and contact prescriber if he has evidence of hepatitis, such as fatigue, malaise, anorexia, nausea, jaundice, bilirubinemia, acholic stools, or liver tenderness.
• If patient uses hormonal contraceptives, advise additional or alternative contraception during treatment.
• Tell patient that redistribution or accumulation of body fat may occur.

✓ Evaluation
• Patient has no drug interactions.
• Patient has no serious adverse hematologic effects.

tobramycin sulfate
(toh-bruh-MIGH-sin SUL-fayt)
Tobi

Pharmacologic class: aminoglycoside
Therapeutic class: antibiotic
Pregnancy risk category: D

Indications and dosages
▶ **Serious infections caused by sensitive strains of *Citrobacter, Enterobacter, Escherichia coli, Klebsiella, Proteus, Providencia, Pseudomonas, Serratia*, and *Staphylococcus aureus*.** *Adults and children with normal renal function:* 3 mg/kg I.M. or I.V. daily divided every 8 hours. Up to 5 mg/kg daily divided every 6 to 8 hours for life-threatening infections.
Neonates younger than age 1 week or premature infants: Up to 4 mg/kg I.V. or I.M. daily in two equal doses every 12 hours.
▶ **Bronchopulmonary *Pseudomonas aeruginosa* in cystic fibrosis patients.** *Adults and children 6 years and older:* 300 mg by oral inhalation every 12 hours. Intervals should never be less than 6 hours apart, and cycle should be for 28 days, followed by at least 28 days off.

▽ I.V. administration
• Dilute in 50 to 100 ml of normal saline solution or D_5W for adults and in less volume for children.
• Infuse over 20 to 60 minutes. After I.V. infusion, flush line with normal saline solution or D_5W.
⊗ **Incompatibilities**
Allopurinol; amphotericin B; beta lactam antibiotics; dextrose 5% in Isolyte E, M, or P; heparin sodium; hetastarch; indomethacin; I.V. solutions containing alcohol; other I.V. drugs; propofol; sargramostim.

Contraindications and cautions
• Contraindicated in patients hypersensitive to aminoglycosides.
• Use cautiously in patients with impaired kidney function or neuromuscular disorders.
⚖ **Lifespan:** In pregnant and breast-feeding women, drug isn't recommended. In the elderly, use cautiously.

Adverse reactions
CNS: confusion, disorientation, headache, lethargy.
EENT: ototoxicity.
GI: diarrhea, nausea, vomiting.
GU: *nephrotoxicity.*
Hematologic: *agranulocytosis,* anemia, eosinophilia, *leukopenia, thrombocytopenia.*
Other: *anaphylaxis,* hypersensitivity reactions.

Reactions may be *common*, uncommon, *life-threatening*, or COMMON AND LIFE-THREATENING.

Interactions

Drug-drug. *Acyclovir, amphotericin B, cephalothin, cisplatin, methoxyflurane, other aminoglycosides, vancomycin:* May increase nephrotoxicity. Use together cautiously.
Atracurium, pancuronium, rocuronium, vecuronium: May increase the effects of nondepolarizing muscle relaxant, including prolonged respiratory depression. Use together only when necessary. Dose of nondepolarizing muscle relaxant may need to be reduced.
Dimenhydrinate: May mask symptoms of ototoxicity. Use cautiously.
General anesthetics: May potentiate neuromuscular blockade. Monitor patient closely.
I.V. loop diuretics (such as furosemide): May increase ototoxicity. Use together cautiously.
Parenteral penicillins (such as ticarcillin): May inactivate tobramycin. Don't mix.

Effects on lab test results

• May increase BUN, creatinine, and nonprotein nitrogen and nitrogenous compound levels. May decrease calcium, magnesium, potassium, and hemoglobin levels and hematocrit.
• May increase eosinophil count. May decrease WBC, platelet, and granulocyte counts.

Pharmacokinetics

Absorption: Unknown.
Distribution: Wide, although CSF penetration is low, even in patients with inflamed meninges. Minimally protein-bound.
Metabolism: None.
Excretion: Mainly in urine; small amount may be excreted in bile. Oral inhalation form is excreted in sputum. *Half-life:* 2 to 3 hours.

Route	Onset	Peak	Duration
I.V.	Immediate	Immediate	8 hr
I.M.	Unknown	30–90 min	8 hr
Inhalation	Unknown	10 min	Unknown

Action

Chemical effect: Inhibits protein synthesis by binding directly to 30S ribosomal subunit.
Therapeutic effect: Kills susceptible bacteria.

Available forms

Injection: 40 mg/ml, 10 mg/ml (pediatric)
Powder for injection: 30 mg/ml after reconstitution

Premixed parenteral injection for I.V. infusion: 60 mg or 80 mg in normal saline solution
Solution for nebulization: 300 mg/5 ml

NURSING PROCESS

Assessment

• Assess patient's infection before starting therapy and regularly thereafter to monitor drug's effectiveness.
• Obtain specimen for culture and sensitivity tests before giving the first dose. Start therapy pending test results.
• Weigh patient and review baseline kidney function studies before starting therapy.
• Assess patient's hearing before starting therapy and during therapy. Report tinnitus, vertigo, or hearing loss.
• Monitor kidney function (output, specific gravity, urinalysis, BUN and creatinine levels, and creatinine clearance).
• Be alert for adverse reactions and drug interactions.
• Assess patient's and family's knowledge of drug therapy.

Nursing diagnoses

• Risk for infection related to susceptible bacteria
• Risk for injury related to potential for drug-induced nephrotoxicity
• Deficient knowledge related to drug therapy

Planning and implementation

• Don't use commercially packaged products in normal saline solution for I.M. injection. For I.M. injection, use multidose vial or prefilled syringes.
• Draw blood for peak level 1 hour after I.M. injection and 30 minutes to 1 hour after infusion ends; draw blood for trough level just before next dose. Don't collect blood in heparinized tube because heparin is incompatible with drug.
ALERT: Peak level higher than 12 mcg/ml and trough level higher than 2 mcg/ml may be linked to increased risk of toxicity.
• Nebulizer treatment for inhaled drug should last 15 minutes. Drug shouldn't be diluted or admixed with other drugs.
• Notify prescriber of signs of decreasing kidney function.
• Keep patient well hydrated during therapy to minimize chemical irritation of renal tubules.

T

• If no response occurs in 3 to 5 days, therapy may be stopped and new specimens obtained for culture and sensitivity testing.

⑤ **ALERT:** Don't confuse tobramycin with Trobicin.

Patient teaching

• Emphasize need to drink 2 L of fluid each day.

• Instruct patient to report adverse reactions.

☑ **Evaluation**

• Patient is free from infection.

• Patient maintains normal kidney function.

• Patient and family state understanding of drug therapy.

tolcapone
(TOHL-cah-pohn)
Tasmar

Pharmacologic class: COMT inhibitor
Therapeutic class: antiparkinsonian
Pregnancy risk category: C

Indications and dosages

▶ **Adjunct to levodopa and carbidopa for signs and symptoms of idiopathic Parkinson disease.** *Adults:* Initially, 100 mg P.O. t.i.d. (with levodopa and carbidopa), although 200 mg P.O. t.i.d. may be given if the anticipated benefit is justified. If starting therapy with 200 mg t.i.d. and dyskinesia occurs, reduce dosage of levodopa. Maximum, 600 mg daily.

Contraindications and cautions

• Contraindicated in patients hypersensitive to the drug or any of its components and in patients with liver disease, elevated ALT or AST values, or history of nontraumatic rhabdomyolysis, hyperpyrexia, or confusion possibly related to drug. Also contraindicated in patients withdrawn from drug because of evidence of drug-induced hepatocellular injury.

• Use cautiously in patients with severe renal impairment.

⚜ **Lifespan:** In pregnant women, use only if benefits to patient outweigh risks to fetus. In breast-feeding women, use cautiously.

Adverse reactions

CNS: agitation, balance loss, *confusion,* depression, *dizziness, dyskinesia, dystonia, excessive dreaming,* falling, fatigue, fever, *hallucinations, headache,* hyperactivity, hyperkinesia, hypertonia, hypokinesia, irritability, paresthesia, mental deficiency, *sleep disorder, somnolence,* speech disorder, syncope, tremor.

CV: chest discomfort, chest pain, hypotension, *orthostatic complaints,* palpitations.

EENT: pharyngitis, sinus congestion, tinnitus.

GI: abdominal pain, *anorexia,* constipation, *diarrhea,* dry mouth, dyspepsia, flatulence, *nausea, vomiting.*

GU: hematuria, impotence, micturition disorder, urinary incontinence, urine discoloration, UTI.

Hematologic: *bleeding.*

Hepatic: *hepatic failure.*

Musculoskeletal: arthritis, *muscle cramps,* neck pain, stiffness.

Respiratory: bronchitis, dyspnea, upper respiratory tract infection.

Skin: increased sweating, rash.

Other: burning, influenza.

Interactions

Drug-drug. *CNS depressants:* May enhance sedative effects. Use cautiously.

Nonselective MAO inhibitors (phenelzine, tranylcypromine): May increase risk of hypertensive crisis. Don't use together.

Effects on lab test results

• May increase liver function test values.

Pharmacokinetics

Absorption: Rapid. Absolute bioavailability is 65%.

Distribution: Not widely distributed into tissues. 99.9% bound to plasma proteins.

Metabolism: Almost complete, mainly by glucuronidation.

Excretion: 60% in urine; 40% in feces. *Half-life:* 2 to 3 hours.

Route	Onset	Peak	Duration
P.O.	Unknown	2 hr	Unknown

Action

Chemical effect: Unknown; may reversibly inhibit human erythrocyte COMT when given with levodopa and carbidopa, resulting in a decrease in levodopa clearance and a twofold increase in levodopa bioavailability. Decreased clearance of levodopa prolongs half-life of levodopa from 2 to 3½ hours.

Therapeutic effect: Improves physical mobility in patients with parkinsonism.

Available forms

Tablets: 100 mg, 200 mg

NURSING PROCESS

Assessment

• Assess patient's history of Parkinson disease before starting therapy, and reassess during therapy to monitor drug's effectiveness.

• Monitor liver function test results before starting therapy, every 2 to 4 weeks for the first 6 months, then as clinically indicated. If the dose is increased to 200 mg t.i.d., resume monitoring as described. Stop drug if AST or ALT exceed 2 times the upper limit of normal or if patient shows signs or symptoms of hepatic dysfunction.

• Assess patient's risk for physical injury because of drug's adverse CNS effects.

• Monitor patient for orthostatic hypotension and syncope.

• Assess patient's and family's knowledge of drug therapy.

Nursing diagnoses

• Impaired physical mobility related to underlying Parkinson disease

• Disturbed thought processes related to drug-induced CNS adverse reactions

• Deficient knowledge related to drug therapy

Planning and implementation

⚠ **ALERT:** Be sure patient has provided written informed consent before drug is used. Give drug only to patient taking levodopa and carbidopa who doesn't respond to, or who isn't an appropriate candidate for, other adjunctive therapies because of risk of liver toxicity.

• Give first dose of the day with first daily dose of levodopa and carbidopa.

• Patient with severe renal dysfunction may need a lower dose.

• Don't give the drug, and notify prescriber, if hepatic transaminases are elevated or if patient appears jaundiced or complains of nausea, upper right quadrant pain, fatigue, lethargy, anorexia, pruritus, or dark urine.

• Because of risk of liver toxicity, stop giving the drug if patient shows no benefit within 3 weeks.

• Because of highly protein-bound nature of drug, dialysis doesn't significantly remove drug.

• If severe diarrhea linked to therapy occurs, notify prescriber.

Patient teaching

• Advise patient to take drug exactly as prescribed.

• Teach patient signs of liver dysfunction (jaundice, fatigue, loss of appetite, persistent nausea, pruritus, dark urine, or right upper quadrant tenderness) and instruct him to report them immediately.

• Warn patient about risk of orthostatic hypotension; tell him to use caution when rising from a seated or lying position.

• Instruct patient to avoid hazardous activities until the drug's CNS effects are known.

• Tell patient nausea may occur at the start of therapy.

• Inform patient about risk of increased dyskinesia or dystonia.

• Tell patient to report planned, suspected, or known pregnancy during therapy.

• Instruct patient to report adverse effects to prescriber, including diarrhea and hallucinations.

• Inform patient that drug may be taken without regard to meals.

Evaluation

• Patient exhibits improved mobility with reduction of muscular rigidity and tremor.

• Patient remains mentally alert.

• Patient and family state understanding of drug therapy.

tolterodine tartrate
(tohl-TER-oh-deen TAR-trate)
Detrol, Detrol LA

Pharmacologic class: muscarinic receptor antagonist
Therapeutic class: anticholinergic
Pregnancy risk category: C

Indications and dosages

▶ **Overactive bladder in patients with symptoms of urinary frequency, urgency, or urge incontinence.** *Adults:* 2 mg P.O. b.i.d. Dosage may be lowered to 1 mg P.O. b.i.d. based on patient response and tolerance. Or, 4 mg of

extended-release capsule P.O. daily; may be decreased to 2 mg P.O. daily.

Adjust-a-dose: For patients with significantly reduced hepatic or renal function and patients taking drug that inhibits CYP3A4 isoenzyme system, give 1 mg P.O. b.i.d. or 2 mg P.O. daily of extended-release capsules.

Contraindications and cautions

• Contraindicated in patients hypersensitive to the drug or any of its components and in those with uncontrolled angle-closure glaucoma or urine or gastric retention.
• Use cautiously in patients with significant bladder outflow obstruction, GI obstructive disorders (such as pyloric stenosis), controlled angle-closure glaucoma, or hepatic or renal impairment.
Lifespan: In pregnant women, use only if benefits outweigh risks. Breast-feeding women should either stop breast-feeding or use another drug. In children, safety and effectiveness haven't been established.

Adverse reactions

CNS: dizziness, fatigue, *headache,* nervousness, paresthesia, somnolence, vertigo.
CV: chest pain, hypertension.
EENT: abnormal vision, pharyngitis, rhinitis, sinusitis, xerophthalmia.
GI: abdominal pain, constipation, diarrhea, *dry mouth,* dyspepsia, flatulence, nausea, vomiting.
GU: dysuria, micturition frequency, urine retention, UTI.
Metabolic: weight gain.
Musculoskeletal: arthralgia, back pain.
Respiratory: bronchitis, cough, upper respiratory tract infection.
Skin: dry skin, erythema, pruritus, rash.
Other: falls, flulike syndrome, fungal infection, infection.

Interactions

Drug-drug. *Antifungals (itraconazole, ketoconazole, miconazole), cyclosporine, CYP3A4 inhibitors (such as macrolide antibiotics clarithromycin and erythromycin), vinblastine, vincristine:* May increase tolterodine concentration. Don't give tolterodine doses above 1 mg b.i.d. (2 mg daily of extended-release capsules) with these drugs.

Effects on lab test results

None reported.

Pharmacokinetics

Absorption: Well absorbed with about 77% bioavailability. Peak level occurs within 1 to 2 hours after administration. Food increases bioavailability of immediate release form by 53%.
Distribution: Volume of distribution is about 113 L. 96% protein-bound.
Metabolism: Mainly by oxidation by the CYP2D6 pathway and forms an active 5-hydroxymethyl metabolite.
Excretion: Mainly in urine, the rest in feces. Less than 1% of dose is recovered as unchanged drug, and 5% to 14% is recovered as the active metabolite. *Half-life:* 1¾ to 3½ hours for immediate-release form, and about 8 hours for extended-release form.

Route	Onset	Peak	Duration
P.O.	Unknown	1–2 hr	Unknown

Action

Chemical effect: A competitive muscarinic receptor antagonist. Both urinary bladder contraction and salivation are mediated via cholinergic muscarinic receptors.
Therapeutic effect: Relieves symptoms of overactive bladder.

Available forms

Capsules (extended-release): 2 mg, 4 mg
Tablets: 1 mg, 2 mg

NURSING PROCESS

Assessment
• Assess baseline bladder function before starting therapy, and reassess frequently to monitor drug's effectiveness.
• Be alert for adverse reactions and drug interactions.
• Assess patient's and family's knowledge of drug therapy.

Nursing diagnoses
• Impaired urinary elimination related to underlying medical condition
• Urinary retention related to drug-induced adverse effects
• Deficient knowledge related to drug therapy

Planning and implementation
• Food increases the absorption of drug, but no dosage adjustment is needed.

- If patient has urine retention, notify prescriber and prepare for urinary catheterization.
- Dry mouth is the most common adverse reaction.

Patient teaching
- Tell patient that sugarless gum, hard candy, or saliva substitute may help relieve dry mouth.
- Advise patient to avoid driving or other potentially hazardous activities until visual effects of drug are known.
- Instruct patient to immediately report signs of infection, urine retention, or GI problems.

☑ Evaluation
- Patient experiences improved bladder function with drug therapy.
- Patient doesn't experience urine retention.
- Patient and family state understanding of drug therapy.

topiramate
(toh-PEER-uh-mayt)
Topamax

Pharmacologic class: sulfamate-substituted monosaccharide
Therapeutic class: antiepileptic
Pregnancy risk category: C

Indications and dosages

▶ **Adjunctive therapy for partial seizures, primary generalized tonic-clonic seizures, or Lennox-Gastaut syndrome.** *Adults:* For partial onset seizures, 200 to 400 mg P.O. daily in two divided doses. For primary generalized tonic-clonic seizures, 400 mg P.O. daily in two divided doses. Start at 25 to 50 mg daily, and adjust to an effective dosage in increments of 25 to 50 mg weekly.
Children ages 2 to 16: Give 5 to 9 mg/kg P.O. daily in two divided doses. Begin dosage adjustment at 1 to 3 mg/kg nightly for 1 week. Then increase at 1- to 2-week intervals by 1 to 3 mg/kg daily in two divided doses to achieve optimal response.

▶ **Prevention of migraine headaches.** *Adults:* Week one, 25 mg P.O. every p.m. for 7 days. Week two, 25 mg P.O. b.i.d. for 7 days. Week three, 25 mg P.O. every a.m. and 50 mg P.O. every p.m. for 7 days. Maintenance dosage

50 mg P.O. b.i.d. If needed, may use longer intervals between dosage adjustments.

▶ **Initial monotherapy in patients with partial onset or primary generalized tonic-clonic seizures.** *Adults and children age 10 or older:* The recommended daily dosage is 400 mg P.O. divided b.i.d. (morning and evening). To achieve this dosage, adjust as follows: The first week, give 25 mg P.O. b.i.d. The second week, give 50 mg P.O. b.i.d. The third week, give 75 mg P.O. b.i.d. The fourth week, give 100 mg P.O. b.i.d. The fifth week, give 150 mg P.O. b.i.d. The sixth week, give 200 mg P.O. b.i.d.
⎗ Adjust-a-dose: For patients with creatinine clearance less than 70 ml/minute, reduce dosage by 50%. For patients on hemodialysis, may need to give supplemental doses to avoid rapid drops in drug level during prolonged dialysis treatment.

Contraindications and cautions

- Contraindicated in patients hypersensitive to the drug or any of its components.
- Use cautiously in patients with hepatic or renal impairment. Also use cautiously with other drugs that predispose patients to heat-related disorders, including other carbonic anhydrase inhibitors and anticholinergics.
⚖ Lifespan: In pregnant and breast-feeding women, use cautiously.

Adverse reactions

CNS: abnormal coordination; agitation; aggression; apathy; asthenia; *ataxia; confusion;* depression; depersonalization; difficulty with attention, concentration, language, or *memory; dizziness;* emotional lability; euphoria; *fatigue;* fever; **generalized tonic-clonic seizures;** hallucinations; hyperkinesias; hypertonia; hypesthesia; hypokinesia; insomnia; malaise; mood problems; *nervousness; nystagmus; paresthesia;* personality disorder; *psychomotor slowing;* psychosis; *somnolence; speech disorders;* stupor; *suicide attempts; tremor;* vertigo.
CV: chest pain, edema, hot flushes, palpitations.
EENT: *abnormal vision,* conjunctivitis, *diplopia,* eye pain, hearing problems, pharyngitis, sinusitis, tinnitus.
GI: abdominal pain, *anorexia,* constipation, diarrhea, dry mouth, dyspepsia, flatulence, gastroenteritis, gingivitis, *nausea,* taste perversion, vomiting.
GU: amenorrhea, dysuria, dysmenorrhea, hematuria, impotence, intermenstrual bleeding, leuk-

orrhea, menorrhagia, menstrual disorder, micturition frequency, renal calculi, urinary incontinence, UTI, vaginitis.
Hematologic: anemia, epistaxis, *leukopenia.*
Metabolic: weight loss.
Musculoskeletal: arthralgia, back or leg pain, muscular weakness, myalgia, rigors.
Respiratory: bronchitis, cough, dyspnea, *upper respiratory tract infection.*
Skin: acne, alopecia, increased sweating, pruritus, rash.
Other: body odor, breast pain, decreased libido, flulike syndrome.

Interactions

Drug-drug. *Carbamazepine:* May decrease topiramate level. Monitor patient.
Carbonic anhydrase inhibitors (acetazolamide, dichlorphenamide): May increase risk of renal calculus formation. Avoid use together.
CNS depressants: May increase risk of topiramate-induced CNS depression and other adverse cognitive and neuropsychiatric events. Use cautiously.
Hormonal contraceptives: May decrease effectiveness. Report changes in bleeding patterns; urge patient to use nonhormonal contraceptive.
Phenytoin: May decrease topiramate level and increase phenytoin level. Monitor levels.
Valproic acid: May decrease valproic acid and topiramate levels. Monitor patient.
Drug-lifestyle. *Alcohol use:* May increase risk of topiramate-induced CNS depression and other adverse cognitive and neuropsychiatric events. Discourage use together.

Effects on lab test results

• May increase liver enzyme level. May decrease bicarbonate and hemoglobin levels and hematocrit.
• May decrease WBC count.

Pharmacokinetics

Absorption: Rapid.
Distribution: 15% to 41% bound to plasma proteins.
Metabolism: Not extensive.
Excretion: Mainly unchanged in urine. *Half-life:* 21 hours.

Route	Onset	Peak	Duration
P.O.	Unknown	2 hr	Unknown

Action

Chemical effect: May block action potential, suggestive of a sodium channel blocking action. May also potentiate activity of GABA and antagonize ability of kainate to activate the amino acid (glutamate) receptor.
Therapeutic effect: Prevents partial-onset seizures.

Available forms

Capsules, sprinkle: 15 mg, 25 mg
Tablets: 25 mg, 50 mg, 100 mg, 200 mg

NURSING PROCESS

⚖ Assessment
• Assess patient's seizure disorder before starting therapy and regularly thereafter to monitor drug's effectiveness.
• Carefully monitor patient taking topiramate with other antiepileptic drugs; dosage adjustment may be needed to achieve optimal response.
• Oligohidrosis and hyperthermia have been infrequently reported, mainly in children. Monitor patient closely, especially in hot weather.
• Because Topamax inhibits carbonic anhydrase, it may cause hyperchloremic, non-anion gap metabolic acidosis from renal bicarbonate. Usually, this occurs early in treatment, although it may happen at any time. Assess patient for factors that may predispose him to acidosis, such as renal disease, severe respiratory disorders, status epilepticus, diarrhea, surgery, ketogenic diet, or drugs.
• Monitor patient for serious symptoms of acute and chronic metabolic acidosis, which include abnormal heart rhythms and stupor. Less severe complications include fatigue, anorexia, and hyperventilation. Left untreated, the acidosis can cause kidney damage, osteoporosis, or osteomalacia—also called rickets, in children.
• Assess patient's compliance with therapy at each follow-up visit.
• Assess patient's and family's knowledge of drug therapy.

✛ Nursing diagnoses
• Risk for injury related to seizure disorder
• Acute pain related to increased risk of renal calculi formation
• Deficient knowledge related to drug therapy

Reactions may be *common*, uncommon, *life-threatening*, or COMMON AND LIFE-THREATENING.

▶ Planning and implementation

• Renal insufficiency requires a lower dosage. For hemodialysis patients, supplemental doses may be needed to avoid rapid drops in drug level during prolonged dialysis.

• Measure baseline and periodic bicarbonate levels during treatment. If metabolic acidosis develops and persists, consider reducing the dosage or stopping drug (using dose tapering). If patient continues on drug despite persistent acidosis, alkali treatment should be considered.

⚠ **ALERT:** If an ocular adverse event occurs, characterized by acute myopia and secondary angle-closure glaucoma, stop drug.

⚠ **ALERT:** Don't confuse Topamax with Toprol-XL, Tegretol, or Tegretol-XR.

Patient teaching

• Tell patient to maintain adequate fluid intake during therapy to minimize risk of forming renal calculi.

• Advise patient not to drive or operate hazardous machinery until the drug's CNS effects are known.

• Tell patient that drug may decrease effectiveness of hormonal contraceptives, and suggest barrier-method birth control.

• Tell patient to avoid crushing or breaking tablets because of bitter taste.

• Tell patient that drug can be taken without regard to food.

• Tell patient to notify prescriber immediately if he experiences changes in vision.

☑ Evaluation

• Patient is free from seizure activity.

• Patient maintains adequate hydration to prevent renal calculus formation.

• Patient and family state understanding of drug therapy.

HIGH ALERT

topotecan hydrochloride
(toh-poh-TEE-ken hy-droh-KLOR-ighd)
Hycamtin

Pharmacologic class: antitumor drug
Therapeutic class: antineoplastic
Pregnancy risk category: D

Indications and dosages

▶ **Metastatic carcinoma of ovary after failure of initial or subsequent chemotherapy;**
small-cell lung cancer after failure of first-line chemotherapy. *Adults:* 1.5 mg/m^2 by I.V. infusion over 30 minutes, daily for 5 consecutive days, starting on day 1 of a 21-day cycle, for minimum of four cycles in absence of tumor progression.

▶ **With cisplatin, to treat stage IV-B, recurrent or persistent cervical cancer unresponsive to surgery or radiation.** *Adults:* 0.75 mg/m^2 by I.V. infusion over 30 minutes on days 1, 2, and 3, followed by 50 mg/m^2 cisplatin by I.V. infusion on day 1. Repeat cycle every 21 days. Base subsequent doses of each drug on hematologic toxicities.

⬛ **Adjust-a-dose:** For patients with renal impairment, if creatinine clearance is 20 to 39 ml/minute, decrease dosage to 0.75 mg/m^2. If severe neutropenia occurs, reduce dosage by 0.25 mg/m^2 for subsequent courses. Or, in severe neutropenia, give granulocyte-colony stimulating factor (GSF) after subsequent course (before resorting to dosage reduction) starting from day 6 of the course (24 hours after topotecan administration).

⬛ **NEW INDICATION: Relapsed small-cell lunger cancer after complete or partial response and at least 45 days from end of first-line chemotherapy.** *Adults:* 2.3 mg/m^2 (rounded to nearest 0.25 mg) P.O. once daily for 5 consecutive days starting on day 1 of a 21-day cycle.

⬛ **Adjust-a-dose:** For patients with grade 3 or 4 diarrhea or severe or prolonged neutropenia, reduce dosage by 0.4 mg/m^2/day.

▼ I.V. administration

• Prepare drug under a vertical laminar flow hood while wearing gloves and protective clothing. If drug contacts skin, wash immediately and thoroughly with soap and water. If mucous membranes are affected, flush with water.

• Reconstitute drug in each 4-mg vial with 4 ml sterile water for injection.

• Dilute appropriate volume of reconstituted solution in normal saline solution or D$_5$W before use.

• Infuse over 30 minutes.

• Protect unopened vials of drug from light. Reconstituted vials stored at 68° to 77° F (20° to 25° C) and exposed to ambient lighting are stable for 24 hours.

⊗ **Incompatibilities**
Dexamethasone, mitomycin.

Contraindications and cautions

• Contraindicated in patients hypersensitive to the drug or any of its components and in patients with severe bone marrow depression.
※ **Lifespan:** In pregnant and breast-feeding women, drug is contraindicated.

Adverse reactions

CNS: asthenia, fatigue, fever, headache, paresthesia.
GI: abdominal pain, anorexia, constipation, diarrhea, stomatitis, nausea, vomiting.
Hematologic: *anemia, leukopenia, neutropenia, thrombocytopenia.*
Respiratory: dyspnea, *cough.*
Skin: *alopecia,* rash.
Other: *sepsis.*

Interactions

Drug-drug. *Cisplatin:* May increase severity of myelosuppression. Use together very cautiously.
Filgrastim (6-GCSF): May prolong duration of neutropenia. Don't give GCSF until day 6 of regimen, 24 hours after completion of topotecan therapy.

Effects on lab test results

• May increase ALT, AST, and bilirubin levels. May decrease hemoglobin level and hematocrit.
• May decrease WBC, platelet, and neutrophil counts.

Pharmacokinetics

Absorption: Given I.V.
Distribution: About 35% bound to plasma proteins.
Metabolism: In liver.
Excretion: 30% in urine. *Half-life:* For I.V., 2 to 3 hours; for P.O., 3 to 6 hours.

Route	Onset	Peak	Duration
I.V.	Unknown	Unknown	Unknown
P.O.	Unknown	1–2 hr	Unknown

Action

Chemical effect: Results from damage to DNA produced during DNA synthesis when replication enzymes interact with the complex formed.
Therapeutic effect: Kills certain cancer cells.

Available forms

Capsules: 0.25 mg, 1 mg
Injection: 4-mg single-dose vial

NURSING PROCESS

⚖ Assessment
• Assess patient's and family's knowledge of drug therapy.
• Assess patient's underlying condition before and often during therapy.
• Monitor patient's CBC often during therapy.
• Be alert for adverse reactions and drug interactions.

⊕ Nursing diagnoses
• Ineffective health maintenance related to neoplastic disease
• Deficient knowledge related to drug therapy

▷ Planning and implementation
⚑ ALERT: Patient must have a baseline neutrophil count of more than 1,500/mm^3 and platelet count of more than 100,000/mm^3 before therapy can start.
• Frequent monitoring of peripheral blood cell count is critical. Don't give repeated doses until neutrophil count is more than 1,000/mm^3, platelet count is more than 100,000/mm^3, and hemoglobin is more than 9 mg/dl.
Patient teaching
• Instruct patient to promptly report sore throat, fever, chills, or unusual bleeding or bruising.
• Advise woman of childbearing age not to become pregnant, and not to breast-feed, during therapy.
• Tell patient and family about need for close monitoring of blood cell counts.

☑ Evaluation
• Patient shows positive response to drug.
• Patient and family state understanding of drug therapy.

torsemide
(TOR-seh-mighd)
Demadex

Pharmacologic class: loop diuretic
Therapeutic class: antihypertensive, diuretic
Pregnancy risk category: B

Indications and dosages

▶ **Diuresis in patients with heart failure.**
Adults: Initially, 10 to 20 mg P.O. or I.V. once

daily. If response is inadequate, double dose until response is obtained. Maximum, 200 mg daily.

▶ **Diuresis in patients with chronic renal impairment.** *Adults:* Initially, 20 mg P.O. or I.V. once daily. If response is inadequate, double dose until response is obtained. Maximum, 200 mg daily.

▶ **Diuresis in patients with hepatic cirrhosis.** *Adults:* Initially, 5 to 10 mg P.O. or I.V. once daily with aldosterone antagonist or potassium-sparing diuretic. If response is inadequate, double dose until response is obtained. Maximum, 40 mg daily.

▶ **Hypertension.** *Adults:* Initially, 5 mg P.O. daily. Increase to 10 mg in 4 to 6 weeks if needed and tolerated. If response is still inadequate, add another antihypertensive.

▼ I.V. administration

• Drug may be given by direct injection over at least 2 minutes. Rapid injection may cause ototoxicity. Don't give more than 200 mg at a time.
• Switch to oral form as soon as possible.
⊗ **Incompatibilities**
None reported.

Contraindications and cautions

• Contraindicated in patients hypersensitive to the drug or other sulfonylurea derivatives and in those with anuria.
• Use cautiously in patients with hepatic disease, cirrhosis, or ascites; sudden changes in fluid and electrolyte balance may precipitate hepatic coma.
⚱ **Lifespan:** In pregnant women, use cautiously. In breast-feeding women, use cautiously; it's unknown if the drug appears in breast milk. In children, safety and effectiveness haven't been established. In elderly patients, use cautiously.

Adverse reactions

CNS: asthenia, dizziness, headache, nervousness, insomnia, syncope.
CV: chest pain, ECG abnormalities, edema, orthostatic hypotension, *ventricular tachycardia.*
EENT: rhinitis, sore throat.
GI: constipation, diarrhea, dyspepsia, *hemorrhage,* nausea.
GU: excessive urination, impotence.
Metabolic: *alkalosis, dehydration,* electrolyte imbalances, including hyperglycemia and hypocalcemia, *hypokalemia, hypomagnesemia,* hyperuricemia; *hypochloremia.*

Musculoskeletal: arthralgia, myalgia.
Respiratory: cough.
Other: excessive thirst, gout.

Interactions

Drug-drug. *Chlorothiazide, chlorthalidone, hydrochlorothiazide, indapamide, metolazone:* May cause excessive diuretic response resulting in serious electrolyte abnormalities or dehydration. Adjust doses carefully and monitor patient for this effect.
Cholestyramine: May decrease absorption of torsemide. Separate administration times by at least 3 hours.
Indomethacin: May decrease diuretic effectiveness in sodium-restricted patients. Avoid use together.
Lithium, ototoxic drugs (such as aminoglycosides, ethacrynic acid): May increase toxicity of these drugs. Avoid use together.
NSAIDs: May potentiate nephrotoxicity of NSAIDs. Use together cautiously.
Probenecid: May decrease diuretic effectiveness. Avoid use together.
Salicylates: May decrease excretion, possibly leading to salicylate toxicity. Avoid use together.
Spironolactone: May decrease renal clearance of spironolactone. Dosage adjustments aren't needed.
Drug-herb. *Licorice:* May cause rapid potassium loss. Discourage use together.

Effects on lab test results

• May increase glucose, BUN, creatinine, cholesterol, and uric acid levels. May decrease calcium, potassium, and magnesium levels.

Pharmacokinetics

Absorption: Little first-pass metabolism.
Distribution: 99% bound to plasma proteins.
Metabolism: 80% in liver.
Excretion: 22% to 34% unchanged in urine.
Half-life: 3½ hours.

Route	Onset	Peak	Duration
P.O.	1 hr	1–2 hr	6–8 hr
I.V.	≤ 10 min	≤ 1 hr	6–8 hr

Action

Chemical effect: Enhances excretion of sodium, chloride, and water by acting on ascending portion of loop of Henle.

Therapeutic effect: Promotes water and sodium excretion and lowers blood pressure.

Available forms

Injection: 10 mg/ml
Tablets: 5 mg, 10 mg, 20 mg, 100 mg

NURSING PROCESS

Assessment
● Assess patient's condition before starting therapy and regularly thereafter to monitor drug's effectiveness.
● Monitor an elderly patient, who is especially susceptible to excessive diuresis, with potential for circulatory collapse and thromboembolic complications.
● During rapid diuresis and routinely with long-term use, monitor fluid intake and output, electrolyte level, blood pressure, weight, and pulse rate. Drug may cause profound diuresis and water and electrolyte depletion.
● Watch for signs of hypokalemia, such as muscle weakness and cramps.
● Be alert for adverse reactions and drug interactions.
● Assess patient's and family's knowledge of drug therapy.

Nursing diagnoses
● Excess fluid volume related to presence of edema
● Risk for injury related to presence of hypertension
● Deficient knowledge related to drug therapy

Planning and implementation
● Give oral drug in morning to prevent nocturia.
● Make sure patient is on a high-potassium diet; refer patient to a dietitian for guidance. Foods rich in potassium include citrus fruits, tomatoes, bananas, dates, and apricots.
ALERT: Don't confuse torsemide with furosemide.
Patient teaching
● Tell patient to take drug in the morning to prevent sleep interruption.
● Advise patient to change position slowly to prevent dizziness.
● Advise patient to immediately report ringing in ears because it may indicate toxicity.
● Tell patient to check with prescriber or pharmacist before taking OTC drugs.

Evaluation
● Patient shows no signs of edema.
● Patient's blood pressure is normal.
● Patient and family state understanding of drug therapy.

tramadol hydrochloride
(TRAM-uh-dohl high-droh-KLOR-ighd)
Ultram, Ultram ER

Pharmacologic class: opioid agonist
Therapeutic class: analgesic
Pregnancy risk category: C

Indications and dosages
▶ **Moderate to moderately severe pain.**
Adults: 50 to 100 mg P.O. every 4 to 6 hours, p.r.n. Maximum dosage is 400 mg daily; or 100 mg P.O. of extended-release tablet once daily and titrated as necessary by 100 mg increments every 5 days to response or maximum dose of 300 mg daily.
Adjust-a-dose: Maximum dosage in patients older than age 75 is 300 mg daily. For patients with cirrhosis, give 50 mg P.O. every 12 hours. For patients with renal impairment, if creatinine clearance is less than 30 ml/minute, give dose every 12 hours. Maximum, 200 mg daily. Hemodialysis patients can receive their regular dose on same day of dialysis. Extended-release form should not be used if creatinine clearance is less than 30 ml/minute or with severe liver impairment (Child-Pugh class C).

Contraindications and cautions
● Contraindicated in patients hypersensitive to the drug or any of its components, and in those with acute intoxication from alcohol, hypnotics, centrally-acting analgesics, opioids, or psychotropic drugs.
● Use cautiously in patients at risk for seizures or respiratory depression; patients with increased intracranial pressure or head injury, acute abdominal conditions, or renal or hepatic impairment; and patients physically dependent on opioids.
Lifespan: In pregnant women and in children, safety and effectiveness haven't been established. In breast-feeding women, drug isn't recommended. Use with caution in the elderly.

Adverse reactions

CNS: anxiety, *asthenia, CNS stimulation,* confusion, coordination disturbance, *dizziness,* euphoria, *headache,* malaise, nervousness, *seizures,* sleep disorder, *somnolence, vertigo.*
CV: vasodilation.
EENT: visual disturbances.
GI: abdominal pain, anorexia, *constipation,* diarrhea, dry mouth, dyspepsia, flatulence, *nausea, vomiting.*
GU: menopausal symptoms, urinary frequency, urine retention.
Musculoskeletal: hypertonia.
Respiratory: *respiratory depression.*
Skin: *pruritus,* rash, sweating.

Interactions

Drug-drug. *Carbamazepine:* May increase tramadol metabolism. Patients receiving long-term carbamazepine therapy at dosage of up to 800 mg daily may require up to twice the recommended dose of tramadol. Concomitant use of tramadol extended release is not recommended.
CNS depressants: May have additive effects. Use together cautiously. Dosage of tramadol may need to be reduced.
MAO inhibitors, SSRIs: May increase risk of seizures. Monitor patient closely.
Quinidine: May increase tramadol exposure by up to 60%. Avoid use together.
Drug-herb. *5-hydroxytryptophan (5-HTP), SAMe, St. John's wort:* May increase serotonin level. Discourage use together.

Effects on lab test results

• May increase liver enzyme level. May decrease hemoglobin level and hematocrit.

Pharmacokinetics

Absorption: Rapid and almost complete.
Distribution: About 20% bound to plasma proteins.
Metabolism: Extensively metabolized.
Excretion: 30% in urine as unchanged drug and 60% as metabolites. *Half-life:* 6 to 7 hours.

Route	Onset	Peak	Duration
P.O.	Unknown	2 hr	Unknown

Action

Chemical effect: Unknown; centrally acting synthetic analgesic compound not chemically related to opioids that is thought to bind to opioid receptors and inhibit reuptake of norepinephrine and serotonin.
Therapeutic effect: Relieves pain.

Available forms

Tablets: 50 mg
Tablets (extended-release): 100 mg, 200 mg, 300 mg

NURSING PROCESS

Assessment
• Assess patient's pain before starting therapy and regularly thereafter to monitor drug's effectiveness.
• Monitor CV and respiratory status.
ALERT: Closely monitor patient at risk for seizures; drug may reduce seizure threshold.
• Monitor patient for drug dependence. Drug can produce dependence similar to that of codeine or dextropropoxyphene and thus has potential to be abused.
• Be alert for adverse reactions and drug interactions.
• Assess patient's and family's knowledge of drug therapy.

Nursing diagnoses
• Acute pain related to underlying condition
• Risk for constipation related to drug-induced adverse GI reactions
• Deficient knowledge related to drug therapy

Planning and implementation
• For better analgesic effect, give drug before onset of intense pain.
• If respiratory rate decreases or falls below 12 breaths/minute, withhold dose and notify prescriber.
• Because constipation is a common adverse effect, anticipate need for laxative therapy.
ALERT: Don't confuse tramadol with trazodone or trandolapril.
Patient teaching
• Instruct patient to take drug only as prescribed and not to increase dosage or dosage interval unless instructed by prescriber.
• Tell patient to swallow tablet whole, and do not crush, swallow or split.
• Tell ambulatory patient to be careful when getting out of bed and walking. Warn outpatient to refrain from driving and performing other po-

tentially hazardous activities that require mental alertness until drug's CNS effects are known.
• Instruct patient to check with prescriber before taking OTC drugs; drug interactions can occur.

☑ **Evaluation**
• Patient is free from pain.
• Patient regains normal bowel pattern.
• Patient and family state understanding of drug therapy.

trandolapril
(tran-DOH-luh-pril)
Mavik

Pharmacologic class: ACE inhibitor
Therapeutic class: antihypertensive
Pregnancy risk category: C (D in second and third trimesters)

Indications and dosages

▶ **Hypertension.** *Adults:* For patient not receiving a diuretic, initially 1 mg for a nonblack patient and 2 mg for a black patient P.O. once daily. If response isn't adequate, dose may be increased at intervals of at least 1 week. Maintenance dosage is 2 to 4 mg daily for most patients. Some patients receiving 4-mg once-daily doses may need b.i.d. doses. For patient also receiving diuretic, initial dose is 0.5 mg P.O. once daily. Subsequent doses adjusted based on blood pressure response.

▶ **Heart failure or left ventricular dysfunction after acute MI.** *Adults:* Start therapy 3 to 5 days after MI with 1 mg P.O. daily. Adjust as tolerated to target dosage of 4 mg daily.

Contraindications and cautions

• Contraindicated in patients hypersensitive to the drug or any of its components and in patients with a history of angioedema with previous therapy with ACE inhibitor.
• Use cautiously in patients with impaired renal function, heart failure, or renal artery stenosis.
⚠ **Lifespan:** In pregnant women, drug is contraindicated. Breast-feeding women should stop breast-feeding or stop the drug. In children, safety and effectiveness haven't been established.

Adverse reactions

CNS: anxiety, dizziness, drowsiness, fatigue, headache, insomnia, paresthesia, vertigo.
CV: *bradycardia,* chest pain, edema, first-degree AV block, flushing, hypotension, palpitations.
EENT: epistaxis, throat irritation.
GI: abdominal distention, abdominal pain or cramps, constipation, diarrhea, dyspepsia, *pancreatitis,* vomiting.
GU: *acute renal failure,* impotence, urinary frequency.
Hematologic: *leukopenia, neutropenia.*
Metabolic: *hyperkalemia,* hyponatremia.
Respiratory: dry, persistent, tickling, non-productive cough; dyspnea; upper respiratory tract infection.
Skin: pemphigus, pruritus, rash.
Other: *anaphylaxis, angioedema,* decreased libido.

Interactions

Drug-drug. *Diuretics:* May increase risk of excessive hypotension. Monitor blood pressure closely.
Lithium: May increase lithium level and lithium toxicity. Avoid use together; monitor lithium level.
NSAIDs: May reduce hypotensive effect of trandolapril. Monitor blood pressure.
Potassium-sparing diuretics, potassium supplements: May increase risk of hyperkalemia. Monitor potassium level closely.
Drug-herb. *Licorice:* May increase sodium retention and blood pressure. Discourage use together.
Drug-food. *Salt substitutes containing potassium:* May increase risk of hyperkalemia. Monitor potassium level closely.

Effects on lab test results

• May increase BUN, creatinine, potassium, uric acid, and liver enzyme levels. May decrease sodium level.
• May decrease neutrophil and WBC counts.

Pharmacokinetics

Absorption: Food slows absorption.
Distribution: 80% protein-bound.
Metabolism: In liver.
Excretion: In urine and feces. *Half-life:* 5 to 10 hours. Longer in patients with renal impairment.

Reactions may be *common,* uncommon, *life-threatening*, or COMMON AND LIFE-THREATENING.

Route	Onset	Peak	Duration
P.O.			
drug	Unknown	1 hr	Unknown
metabolite	4–10 hr	1 hr	Unknown

Action

Chemical effect: Inhibits circulating and tissue ACE activity, which reduces angiotensin II formation, decreases vasoconstriction and aldosterone secretion, and increases plasma renin.
Therapeutic effect: Lowers blood pressure.

Available forms

Tablets: 1 mg, 2 mg, 4 mg

NURSING PROCESS

Assessment
• Monitor patient's blood pressure, renal function, and potassium level before and during therapy.
• Monitor patient for hypotension. If possible, stop diuretic therapy 2 to 3 days before starting drug.
• Monitor patient for jaundice, and immediately alert prescriber if it occurs.
• Monitor patient's compliance with therapy.
• Assess patient's and family's knowledge of drug therapy.

Nursing diagnoses
• Risk for injury related to hypertension
• Deficient knowledge related to drug therapy

Planning and implementation
• Prevent or minimize orthostatic hypotension.
• Maintain patient's nondrug therapies, such as sodium restriction, stress management, smoking cessation, and exercise program.
ALERT: Angioedema that involves the tongue, glottis, or larynx may be fatal because of airway obstruction. Have resuscitation equipment readily available for maintaining a patent airway; give appropriate therapy, including epinephrine 1:1,000 (0.3 to 0.5 ml) subcutaneously.
Patient teaching
• Advise patient to report infection and other adverse reactions.
• Tell patient to avoid salt substitutes.
• Tell patient to use caution in hot weather and during exercise.

• Tell woman to immediately report suspected pregnancy.
• Advise patient about to undergo surgery or anesthesia to inform prescriber of use of drug.

Evaluation
• Patient's blood pressure is normal.
• Patient and family state understanding of drug therapy.

HIGH ALERT

trastuzumab
(trahs-TOO-zuh-mab)
Herceptin

Pharmacologic class: monoclonal antibody
Therapeutic class: antineoplastic
Pregnancy risk category: B

Indications and dosages

▶ **Monotherapy for patients with metastatic breast cancer whose tumors overexpress the human epidermal growth factor receptor 2 (HER2) protein and who have received one or more chemotherapy regimens for their metastatic disease; or with paclitaxel for metastatic breast cancer in patients whose tumors overexpress the HER2 protein and who haven't received chemotherapy for their metastatic disease.** *Adults:* Initial loading dose of 4 mg/kg I.V. over 90 minutes. If the initial loading dose is well tolerated, maintenance dosage is 2 mg/kg I.V. weekly as a 30-minute I.V. infusion.

I.V. administration

• Reconstitute drug in each vial with 20 ml of bacteriostatic water for injection, USP, 1.1% benzyl alcohol preserved, as supplied, to yield a multidose solution containing 21 mg/ml. Immediately after reconstitution, label vial for drug expiration 28 days from date of reconstitution.
• If patient is hypersensitive to benzyl alcohol, drug must be reconstituted with sterile water for injection. Drug reconstituted with sterile water for injection must be used immediately; unused portion must be discarded. Avoid other reconstitution diluents.
• Determine dose (milligrams) of drug needed, based on loading dose of 4 mg/kg or maintenance dose of 2 mg/kg. Calculate volume of 21-mg/ml solution and withdraw amount from

T

---

vial; add it to an infusion bag containing 250 ml of normal saline solution.
- Don't give as an I.V. push or bolus.
- Vials of drug are stable at 36° to 46° F (2° to 8° C) before reconstitution. Discard reconstituted solution after 28 days. Store drug solution diluted in normal saline solution for injection at 36° to 46° F before use; it's stable for up to 24 hours.
⊗ **Incompatibilities**
Other I.V. drugs or dextrose solutions.

Contraindications and cautions

- Use cautiously in patients with cardiac dysfunction. Watch closely for ventricular dysfunction and heart failure, and stop drug if signs of decreased left ventricular dysfunction develop.
- Use cautiously in patients hypersensitive to drug or its components. Severe hypersensitivity reactions, infusion reactions, and pulmonary events can develop. Hypersensitivity reaction typically occurs during or within 24 hours of administration.
⚖ **Lifespan:** In pregnant women, use only if clearly needed. Breast-feeding women should stop breast-feeding during therapy and for 6 months after the last dose, or they should use another drug. In children, safety and effectiveness haven't been established. In elderly patients, use cautiously.

Adverse reactions

CNS: *asthenia,* depression, *dizziness, fever, headache, insomnia,* neuropathy, *pain,* paresthesia, peripheral neuritis.
CV: edema*, **heart failure, left ventricular dysfunction,*** peripheral edema, tachycardia.
EENT: pharyngitis, rhinitis, sinusitis.
GI: abdominal pain, anorexia, diarrhea, nausea, vomiting.
GU: UTI.
Hematologic: anemia, ***leukopenia.***
Musculoskeletal: arthralgia, *back pain,* bone pain.
Respiratory: *cough, dyspnea.*
Skin: acne, *rash.*
Other: allergic reaction, ANAPHYLAXIS, chills, infection, flulike syndrome, herpes simplex, ***hypersensitivity reactions.***

Interactions

Drug-drug. *Anthracyclines, cyclophosphamide:* May increase risk of cardiotoxic effects. Monitor patient closely.

Paclitaxel: May decrease clearance of trastuzumab. Monitor patient closely.

Effects on lab test results

- May decrease hemoglobin level and hematocrit.
- May decrease WBC count.

Pharmacokinetics

Absorption: Given I.V.
Distribution: Volume is 44 ml/kg.
Metabolism: Unknown.
Excretion: Unknown. *Half-life:* 1 to 32 days.

Route	Onset	Peak	Duration
I.V.	Unknown	Unknown	Unknown

Action

Chemical effect: Recombinant DNA-derived monoclonal antibody that selectively binds to HER2. Inhibits proliferation of human tumor cells that overexpress HER2.
Therapeutic effect: Hinders function of specific breast cancer tumor cells that overexpress HER2.

Available forms

Injection: lyophilized sterile powder containing 440 mg per vial

NURSING PROCESS

🔖 **Assessment**

- Before therapy starts, make sure patient has had a thorough baseline cardiac assessment, including history, physical examination, and evaluation, to determine risk for developing cardiotoxicity.
- Use drug only in patients with metastatic breast cancer whose tumors have HER2 protein overexpression.
- Assess patient for chills and fever, especially during the first infusion.
- Monitor patient closely for signs and symptoms of cardiac dysfunction, especially if also receiving anthracyclines and cyclophosphamide.
- Monitor patient for dyspnea, increased cough, paroxysmal nocturnal dyspnea, peripheral edema, and S3 gallop. Monitor patients also receiving chemotherapy closely for cardiac dysfunction or failure, anemia, leukopenia, diarrhea, and infection.
- Assess patient's and family's knowledge of drug therapy.

Reactions may be *common*, uncommon, *life-threatening*, or COMMON AND LIFE-THREATENING.

✠ Nursing diagnoses
• Imbalanced nutrition: less than body requirements related to drug-induced GI adverse effects
• Decreased cardiac output related to drug-induced decreased left ventricular function
• Deficient knowledge related to drug therapy

▶ Planning and implementation
• Treat first-dose, infusion-related symptoms with acetaminophen, diphenhydramine, and meperidine (with or without reducing the rate of infusion).
• If patient has a significant decrease in cardiac function, notify prescriber.

Patient teaching
• Tell patient about possibility of first-dose, infusion-related adverse effects.
• Instruct patient to notify prescriber immediately if signs and symptoms of cardiac dysfunction develop, such as shortness of breath, increased cough, or peripheral edema.
• Instruct patient to report adverse effects to prescriber.

☑ Evaluation
• Patient has no adverse GI effects (nausea, vomiting, diarrhea).
• Patient has no dyspnea, increased cough, paroxysmal nocturnal dyspnea, peripheral edema, or S_3 gallop as result of drug-induced cardiac dysfunction.
• Patient and family state understanding of drug therapy.

travoprost
(TRA-voe-prost)
Travatan, Travatan Z

Pharmacologic class: prostaglandin analogue
Therapeutic class: antiglaucoma drug, ocular antihypertensive
Pregnancy risk category: C

Indications and dosages

▶ **Reduction of elevated intraocular pressure (IOP) in patients with open-angle glaucoma or ocular hypertension who are intolerant of other IOP-lowering drugs, or in patients who have had insufficient responses to other IOP-lowering drugs.** *Adults:* 1 drop in conjunctival sac of affected eye once daily in evening.

Contraindications and cautions
• Contraindicated in patients hypersensitive to the drug, benzalkonium chloride, or other components.
• Use cautiously in patients with renal or hepatic impairment, active intraocular inflammation (iritis, uveitis), or risk factors for macular edema. Also use cautiously in aphakic patients and pseudophakic patients with a torn posterior lens capsule.
• Don't use in patients with angle-closure glaucoma or inflammatory or neovascular glaucoma.
⚜ **Lifespan:** In pregnant women and in women attempting to become pregnant, drug isn't recommended. In breast-feeding women, use cautiously; it's unknown if the drug appears in breast milk. In children, safety and effectiveness haven't been established.

Adverse reactions
CNS: anxiety, depression, headache, pain.
CV: angina pectoris, *bradycardia,* chest pain, hypertension, hypotension.
EENT: abnormal vision, blepharitis, blurred vision, cataracts, conjunctival hyperemia, conjunctivitis, *decreased visual acuity,* dry eyes, *eye discomfort,* eye disorders, *eye pain, eye pruritus, foreign body sensation,* iris discoloration, keratitis, lid margin crusting, *ocular hyperemia,* photophobia, sinusitis, subconjunctival hemorrhage, tearing.
GI: dyspepsia, GI disorder.
GU: prostate disorder, urinary incontinence, UTI.
Metabolic: hypercholesterolemia.
Musculoskeletal: arthritis, back pain.
Respiratory: bronchitis, sinusitis.
Other: accidental injury, cold syndrome, infection.

Interactions
Drug-herb. *Areca, jaborandi:* May cause additive effects. Discourage use together.

Effects on lab test results
• May increase cholesterol level.

Pharmacokinetics
Absorption: Absorbed through the cornea.
Distribution: Level peaks within 30 minutes.
Metabolism: Hydrolyzed by esterases in the cornea to its active free acid. The liver primarily

metabolizes the active acid of drug reaching the systemic circulation.

Excretion: Within 1 hour. *Half-life:* 45 minutes.

Route	Onset	Peak	Duration
Ophthalmic	Unknown	30 min	Unknown

Action

Chemical effect: May increase uveoscleral outflow.

Therapeutic effect: Reduces IOP.

Available forms

Ophthalmic solution: 0.004%

NURSING PROCESS

⚂ Assessment

• Assess patient's condition before starting therapy and regularly thereafter to monitor drug's effectiveness.

• If a pregnant woman or a woman attempting to become pregnant accidentally comes in contact with drug, immediately cleanse the exposed area thoroughly with soap and water.

• Assess patient's and family's knowledge of drug therapy.

⊕ Nursing diagnoses

• Acute pain related to adverse EENT effects of drug

• Risk for activity intolerance related to decreased visual acuity

• Deficient knowledge related to travoprost therapy

▷ Planning and implementation

• Have patient remove contact lenses before you give the drug. Lenses may be reinserted 15 minutes afterward.

• If multiple ophthalmic drugs are being used, separate doses by at least 5 minutes.

• Temporary or permanent increased pigmentation of the iris and eyelid may occur as well as increased pigmentation and growth of the eyelashes.

Patient teaching

• Teach patient to instill drops, and advise him to wash hands before and after doing so. Warn him not to touch dropper or tip to eye or surrounding tissue.

• Advise patient to apply light pressure on lacrimal sac for 1 minute after instillation to minimize systemic absorption of drug.

• Tell patient to remove contact lenses before instilling solution and to leave them out for 15 minutes afterward.

• Advise patient that, if more than one ophthalmic drug is being used, the drugs should be given at least 5 minutes apart.

• Tell patient receiving treatment to only one eye about the potential for increased brown pigmentation of the iris, eyelid skin darkening, and increased length, thickness, pigmentation, or number of lashes in the treated eye.

• Tell patient that, if eye trauma or infection occurs or if eye surgery is needed, he should seek medical advice before continuing to use the multidose container.

• Advise patient to immediately report conjunctivitis or lid reactions.

• Stress importance of compliance with recommended therapy.

• Tell pregnant woman or woman attempting to become pregnant that, if she accidentally comes in contact with drug, she should immediately cleanse the exposed area with soap and water.

☑ Evaluation

• Patient denies pain.

• Patient's activity level improves.

• Patient and family state understanding of travoprost therapy.

trazodone hydrochloride
(TRAYZ-oh-dohn high-droh-KLOR-ighd)

Pharmacologic class: triazolopyridine derivative

Therapeutic class: antidepressant

Pregnancy risk category: C

Indications and dosages

▶ **Depression.** *Adults:* Initially, 150 mg P.O. daily in divided doses. Increase by 50 mg daily every 3 to 4 days, as needed. Average daily dose ranges from 150 to 400 mg. Maximum, 600 mg daily for inpatients; 400 mg daily for outpatients.

▶ **Aggressive behavior‡.** *Adults:* 50 mg P.O. b.i.d.

▶ **Panic disorder‡.** *Adults:* 300 mg P.O. daily.

▶ **Insomnia‡.** *Adults:* 25 to 75 mg P.O. with an SSRI.

Contraindications and cautions

• Contraindicated in patients in initial recovery phase of MI and in patients hypersensitive to drug.
• Use cautiously in patients with cardiac disease and in those at risk for suicide.
⚖ **Lifespan:** In pregnant women, breast-feeding women, and children, safety and effectiveness haven't been established.

Adverse reactions

CNS: anger, confusion, *dizziness, drowsiness,* fatigue, headache, hostility, insomnia, nervousness, nightmares, *suicidal thinking,* syncope, tremor, vivid dreams, weakness.
CV: hypertension, orthostatic hypotension, shortness of breath, tachycardia.
EENT: blurred vision, nasal congestion, tinnitus.
GI: anorexia, constipation, dry mouth, dysgeusia, nausea, vomiting.
GU: hematuria, priapism, urine retention.
Hematologic: anemia.
Skin: diaphoresis, rash, urticaria.
Other: decreased libido.

Interactions

Drug-drug. *Antihypertensives:* May increase hypotensive effect of trazodone. Monitor blood pressure; antihypertensive dosage may have to be decreased.
Clonidine, CNS depressants: May increase CNS depression. Avoid use together.
CYP3A4 inducers (carbamazepine): May reduce trazodone level. Monitor patient closely; trazodone dosage may need to be increased.
CYP3A4 inhibitors (indinavir, ketoconazole, and ritonavir): May slow the clearance of trazodone and increase trazodone level. May cause nausea, hypotension, and fainting. Consider decreasing trazodone dosage.
Digoxin, phenytoin: May increase levels of these drugs. Monitor patient for toxicity.
MAO inhibitors: May cause an unknown interaction. Use together cautiously.
Phenothiazines: May increase trazodone level. Monitor toxic effects.
SSRIs, venlafaxine: May cause serotonin syndrome. Use together cautiously.

Drug-herb. *St. John's wort:* May cause serotonin syndrome. Discourage use together.
Drug-lifestyle. *Alcohol use:* May increase CNS depression. Discourage use together.

Effects on lab test results

• May increase ALT and AST levels. May decrease hemoglobin level and hematocrit.

Pharmacokinetics

Absorption: Well absorbed from GI tract. Food delays absorption but increases amount of drug absorbed by 20%.
Distribution: Wide in body; not concentrated in any particular tissue.
Metabolism: In liver.
Excretion: About 75% in urine; remainder in feces. *Half-life:* First phase, 3 to 6 hours; second phase, 5 to 9 hours.

Route	Onset	Peak	Duration
P.O.	Unknown	1–2 hr	Unknown

Action

Chemical effect: Unknown, although it inhibits serotonin uptake in brain; not a tricyclic derivative.
Therapeutic effect: Relieves depression.

Available forms

Tablets: 50 mg, 100 mg, 150 mg, 300 mg

NURSING PROCESS

🜰 Assessment

• Assess patient's condition before starting therapy and regularly thereafter to monitor drug's effectiveness.
• Be alert for adverse reactions and drug interactions.
• Assess patient's and family's knowledge of drug therapy.

⊕ Nursing diagnoses

• Disturbed thought processes related to presence of depression
• Risk for injury related to drug-induced adverse CNS reactions
• Deficient knowledge related to drug therapy

T

▷ Planning and implementation

● Give after meal or light snack for optimal absorption and to decrease risk of dizziness.
● Don't abruptly stop giving the drug, but stop it at least 48 hours before surgery.
⑨ **ALERT:** Drug may increase risk for suicidal thinking and behavior in young adults ages 18 to 24 during the first 2 months of treatment. Monitor patient closely.
● If an adverse reaction occurs, notify prescriber.
⑨ **ALERT:** Don't confuse trazodone with tramadol.

Patient teaching
● Instruct patient to take drug after a meal or light snack.
⑨ **ALERT:** Advise patient to notify prescriber immediately if priapism (prolonged, painful erection unrelated to sexual stimulation) occurs; emergency interventions are needed within 6 hours to prevent permanent erectile dysfunction.
● Warn patient to avoid activities that require alertness and good psychomotor coordination until the drug's CNS effects are known; drowsiness and dizziness usually subside after first few weeks.
● Teach patient's family how to recognize signs of suicidal tendency or suicidal ideation and to report such behaviors immediately.

☑ Evaluation

● Patient's behavior and communication exhibit improved thought processes.
● Patient doesn't experience adverse CNS reactions.
● Patient and family state understanding of drug therapy.

treprostinil sodium
(treh-PROSS-ti-nil soh-DEE-uhm)
Remodulin

Pharmacologic class: vasodilator
Therapeutic class: antihypertensive
Pregnancy risk category: B

Indications and dosages

▷ **New York Heart Association Class II to IV pulmonary arterial hypertension (PAH) to reduce symptoms caused by exercise.** *Adults:* Initially, 1.25 nanograms/kg/minute by continuous subcutaneous or I.V. infusion. If initial

dose isn't tolerated, reduce infusion rate to 0.625 nanograms/kg/minute. Increase by increments of no more than 1.25 nanograms/kg/minute every week for the first 4 weeks, and then by no more than 2.5 nanograms/kg/minute every week for duration of infusion. Maximum infusion rate is 40 nanograms/kg/minute. To determine subcutaneous infusion rate in ml/hour, use this formula:

$$\text{Infusion rate (ml/hr)} = \frac{[\text{dosage (nanograms/kg/minute)} \times \text{body weight (kg)} \times 0.00006]}{\text{drug strength (mg/ml)}}$$

When using an appropriate infusion pump and reservoir, select a predetermined intravenous infusion rate to allow for a desired infusion period length of up to 48 hours between system changeovers. Typical intravenous infusion system reservoirs have volumes of 50 or 100 ml. With this selected intravenous infusion rate (ml/hr), the diluted intravenous Remodulin concentration (mg/ml) can be calculated using this formula:

$$\text{Diluted I.V. concentration (mg/ml)} = \frac{[\text{dosage (nanograms/kg/minute)} \times \text{weight (kg)} \times 0.00006]}{\text{I.V. infusion rate (ml/minute)}}$$

The amount of Remodulin injection needed to make the required diluted intravenous Remodulin concentration for the given reservoir size can then be calculated using this formula:

$$\text{Amount of Remodulin injection (ml)} = [\text{diluted I.V. concentration (mg/ml)} \div \text{vial strength (mg/ml)}] \times \text{total volume of diluted Remodulin solution in reservoir (ml)}$$

Add the calculated amount of Remodulin injection to the reservoir along with the sufficient volume of diluent to achieve the desired total volume in the reservoir.

▧ **Adjust-a-dose:** In patients with mild or moderate hepatic insufficiency, initial dose is 0.625 nanograms/kg of ideal body weight per minute; increase cautiously.

▷ **To diminish the rate of clinical deterioration in patients with pulmonary arterial hypertension (PAH) who are transitioning therapy from Flolan (epoprostenol).** *Adults:* Begin treprostinil infusion at a rate that's 10% of starting epoprostenol dose. Decrease epoprostenol in 20% increments while increasing treprostinil in

20% increments, always maintaining a total dose of 110% of epoprostenol starting dose. Once epoprostenol is at 20% of starting dose, and treprostinil is at 90%, decrease epoprostenol to 5% and increase treprostinil to 110%. Finally, stop epoprostenol and maintain treprostinil dose at 110% of epoprostenol starting dose plus an additional 5% to10% as needed. Change rate based on individual patient response. Treat worsening of PAH symptoms with increases in treprostinil doses. Treat adverse effects associated with prostacyclin and prostacyclin analogues with decreases in epoprostenol doses.

▼ I.V. administration

• Remodulin must be diluted with either sterile water for injection or normal saline solution injection.
• Drug must be administered through a surgically placed, indwelling central venous catheter.
• Diluted Remodulin is stable at ambient temperature for up to 48 hours at concentrations as low as 0.004 mg/ml (4,000 nanograms/ml).
• Patient must have access to a backup infusion pump and infusion sets.
⊗ Incompatibilities
Other I.V. drugs.

Contraindications and cautions

• Contraindicated in patients hypersensitive to the drug or to structurally related compounds.
• Use cautiously in patients with hepatic or renal impairment.
▲ Lifespan: In pregnant women, use only if clearly needed. In breast-feeding women, use cautiously; it's unknown if the drug appears in breast milk. In children, safety and effectiveness haven't been established; select dose cautiously. In the elderly, use cautiously.

Adverse reactions

CNS: dizziness, fatigue, *headache.*
CV: chest pain, edema, hypotension, ***right ventricular heart failure,*** vasodilation.
GI: diarrhea, nausea.
Respiratory: dyspnea.
Skin: pallor, pruritus, *rash.*
Other: *infusion site pain,* infusion site reaction, *jaw pain.*

Interactions

Drug-drug. *Anticoagulants:* May increase risk of bleeding. Monitor patient closely for bleeding.

Antihypertensives, diuretics, vasodilators: May enhance reduction in blood pressure. Monitor blood pressure.

Effects on lab test results

None reported.

Pharmacokinetics

Absorption: Rapid and complete. 100% bioavailable.
Distribution: 91% bound to plasma proteins.
Metabolism: By the liver. Five metabolites are known, but their activity isn't.
Excretion: In the urine, 4% as unchanged drug and 64% as metabolites. *Half-life:* 2 to 4 hours.

Route	Onset	Peak	Duration
I.V., SubQ	Unknown	Unknown	Unknown

Action

Chemical effect: Acts by direct vasodilation of pulmonary and systemic arterial vascular beds and inhibition of platelet aggregation.
Therapeutic effect: Reduces pulmonary artery pressure.

Available forms

Injection: 1 mg/ml, 2.5 mg/ml, 5 mg/ml, 10 mg/ml

NURSING PROCESS

Assessment
• Assess patient's condition before starting therapy and regularly thereafter to monitor drug's effectiveness.
• Make sure adequate monitoring and emergency care are available when starting therapy.
• Assess patient's ability to accept, place, and care for subcutaneous catheter and to use infusion pump.
• Assess patient's ability to accept and care for I.V. catheter and to use the infusion pump.
• Be alert for adverse reactions and drug interactions.
• Assess patient's and family's knowledge of drug therapy.

Nursing diagnoses
• Activity intolerance related to presence of pulmonary hypertension

- Acute pain related to adverse drug effect of headache
- Deficient knowledge related to drug therapy

▶ Planning and implementation

- Drug should be used only by prescribers experienced in the diagnosis and treatment of PAH.
- Give by continuous subcutaneous infusion via a self-inserted subcutaneous catheter, using an infusion pump designed for subcutaneous drug delivery. Or give by continuous I.V. infusion through an indwelling central venous catheter.
- The infusion pump should be small and light-weight; be adjustable to approximately 0.002 ml/hour; have occlusion or no-delivery, low-battery, programming-error, and motor-malfunction alarms; have delivery accuracy of ± 6% or better; and be positive-pressure driven.
- The reservoir should be made of polyvinyl chloride, polypropylene, or glass.
- A single syringe can be given up to 72 hours at 99° F (37° C).
- Use a single vial no longer than 14 days after the initial introduction into the vial.
- Inspect for particulate matter and discoloration before giving.
- Unopened vials are stable until the date indicated when stored at 59° to 77° F (15° to 25° C).
- If patient doesn't improve or if symptoms worsen, increase dosage. If patient has an excessive effect or unacceptable infusion site symptoms, decrease dosage.
- Don't abruptly stop giving the drug or reduce the dosage by a large amount; symptoms of PAH may worsen.

Patient teaching
- Tell patient drug is infused continuously through subcutaneous or I.V. catheter, via an infusion pump.
- Inform patient that therapy will be needed for prolonged period, possibly years.
- Inform patient that many side effects may be related to the underlying disease (dyspnea, fatigue, chest pain, right ventricular failure, pallor).
- Tell patient that the most common local reactions are pain, erythema, induration, and rash at the infusion site.

☑ Evaluation

- Patient states activity intolerance is improving.
- Patient doesn't have headache.
- Patient and family state understanding of drug therapy.

triamcinolone acetonide
(trigh-am-SIN-oh-lohn)
Kenalog-10, Kenalog-40

triamcinolone hexacetonide
Aristospan Intra-Articular, Aristospan Intralesional

Pharmacologic class: glucocorticoid
Therapeutic class: anti-inflammatory, immunosuppressant
Pregnancy risk category: C

Indications and dosages

▶ **Severe inflammation or immunosuppression.** *Adults:* Initially, 2.5 to 60 mg triamcinolone acetonide I.M. Additional doses of 20 to 100 mg may be given, if needed, at 6-week intervals. Or, 2.5 to 15 mg intra-articularly, or up to 1 mg intralesionally, as needed. Or, with triamcinolone hexacetonide, use up to 0.5 mg per square inch of affected skin intralesionally, or 2 to 20 mg intra-articularly every 3 to 4 weeks, as needed.
Children: Base dosage on the disease severity and the response instead of age and body weight or surface area. Taper to a stop as soon as possible.

Contraindications and cautions

- Contraindicated in patients hypersensitive to the drug or any of its components, and in those with systemic fungal infections.
- Use cautiously in patients with GI ulcer, renal disease, hypertension, osteoporosis, diabetes mellitus, hypothyroidism, cirrhosis, diverticulitis, nonspecific ulcerative colitis, recent intestinal anastomoses, thromboembolic disorders, seizures, myasthenia gravis, heart failure, tuberculosis, ocular herpes simplex, emotional instability, or psychotic tendencies.
- ⚖ Lifespan: In pregnant women, use cautiously. In breast-feeding women, use cautiously; it's unknown if the drug appears in breast milk.

Adverse reactions

CNS: *euphoria,* headache, *insomnia,* paresthesia, *pseudotumor cerebri,* psychotic behavior, *seizures,* vertigo.
CV: *arrhythmias,* edema, *heart failure,* hypertension, *thromboembolism,* thrombophlebitis.

Reactions may be *common,* uncommon, *life-threatening,* or COMMON AND LIFE-THREATENING.

EENT: cataracts, glaucoma.
GI: GI irritation, increased appetite, nausea, *pancreatitis, peptic ulceration,* vomiting.
GU: menstrual irregularities.
Metabolic: carbohydrate intolerance, hyperglycemia, hypokalemia.
Musculoskeletal: growth suppression in children, muscular weakness, osteoporosis.
Skin: acne, bruising, delayed wound healing, various skin eruptions, petechiae.
Other: *acute adrenal insufficiency* during times of increased stress; cushingoid state (moonface, buffalo hump, central obesity), hirsutism; susceptibility to infections.

Interactions

Drug-drug. *Aspirin, indomethacin, other NSAIDs:* May increase risk of GI distress and bleeding. Give together cautiously.
Barbiturates, phenytoin, rifampin: May decrease corticosteroid effect. Increase corticosteroid dosage.
Drugs that deplete potassium (such as thiazide diuretics): May increase potassium-wasting effects of triamcinolone. Monitor potassium level.
Oral anticoagulants: May alter dosage requirements. Monitor PT closely.
Skin-test antigens: May decrease response. Defer skin testing.
Toxoids, vaccines: May decrease antibody response and increase risk of neurologic complications. Avoid use together.

Effects on lab test results

• May increase glucose and cholesterol levels. May decrease potassium and calcium levels.

Pharmacokinetics

Absorption: Readily after P.O. use. Variable after other routes.
Distribution: To muscle, liver, skin, intestines, and kidneys. Extensively bound to plasma proteins; only unbound portion is active.
Metabolism: In liver.
Excretion: In urine; insignificant amount in feces. *Half-life:* 18 to 36 hours.

Route	Onset	Peak	Duration
I.M., intralesional, intra-articular, intrasynovial	Varies	Varies	Varies

Action

Chemical effect: Not clearly defined; decreases inflammation, mainly by stabilizing leukocyte lysosomal membranes; suppresses immune response; stimulates bone marrow; and influences protein, fat, and carbohydrate metabolism.
Therapeutic effect: Relieves inflammation and suppresses immune system function.

Available forms

triamcinolone acetonide
Injection (suspension): 3 mg/ml, 10 mg/ml, 40 mg/ml
triamcinolone hexacetonide
Injection (suspension): 5 mg/ml, 20 mg/ml

NURSING PROCESS

Assessment
• Assess patient before and after starting therapy; monitor weight, blood pressure, and electrolyte level.
• Watch for adverse reactions, drug interactions, depression, or psychotic episodes, especially with high doses.
• Assess patient's and family's knowledge of drug therapy.

Nursing diagnoses
• Ineffective health maintenance related to underlying condition
• Risk for injury related to drug-induced adverse reactions
• Deficient knowledge related to drug therapy

Planning and implementation
• Always adjust to lowest effective dosage.
• For adults, give I.M. injection deep into gluteal muscle; rotate injection sites to prevent muscle atrophy.
• Don't use 10-mg/ml strength for I.M. administration.
• Assist prescriber with intralesional, intra-articular, or intrasynovial administration.
• Don't use 40-mg/ml strength for I.D. or intralesional administration.
• **ALERT:** Parenteral form isn't for I.V. use; different salt formulations aren't interchangeable.
• Don't use diluents that contain preservatives; flocculation may occur.
• Unless contraindicated, give low-sodium diet high in potassium and protein. Give potassium supplements, as needed.

• Gradually reduce drug dosage after long-term therapy. After abruptly stopping the drug, the patient may experience rebound inflammation, fatigue, weakness, arthralgia, fever, dizziness, lethargy, depression, fainting, orthostatic hypotension, dyspnea, anorexia, or hypoglycemia. After prolonged use, sudden withdrawal may be fatal.

⊛ **ALERT:** Don't confuse triamcinolone with Triaminicin, Triaminic, or Triaminicol.

Patient teaching
• Teach patient signs of early adrenal insufficiency (fatigue, muscle weakness, joint pain, fever, anorexia, nausea, dyspnea, dizziness, and fainting).
• Instruct patient to wear or carry medical identification at all times.
• Warn patient receiving long-term therapy about cushingoid symptoms, and tell him to report sudden weight gain and swelling to prescriber.
• Tell patient to report slow healing.
• Advise patient receiving long-term therapy to consider exercise or physical therapy. Also tell patient to ask prescriber about vitamin D or calcium supplements.

☑ **Evaluation**
• Patient responds well to drug.
• Patient doesn't experience injury from adverse reactions.
• Patient and family state understanding of drug therapy.

triamcinolone acetonide
(trigh-am-SIN-oh-lohn as-EE-tuh-nighd)
Azmacort, Nasacort AQ

Pharmacologic class: glucocorticoid
Therapeutic class: anti-inflammatory, immunosuppressant
Pregnancy risk category: C

Indications and dosages

▶ **Corticosteroid-dependent asthma.** *Adults:* 2 inhalations t.i.d. or q.i.d. Maximum, 16 inhalations daily. In some patients, maintenance can be accomplished when total daily dose is given b.i.d.
Children ages 6 to 12: Give 1 or 2 inhalations t.i.d. or q.i.d. or 2 to 4 inhalations b.i.d. Maximum, 12 inhalations daily.

▶ **Treatment of nasal symptoms of seasonal and perennial allergic rhinitis.** *Adults and children age 12 years and older:* (Nasacort AQ) 2 sprays into each nostril once daily.
Children age 12 years and older: (Nasacort AQ) 1 spray into each nostril once daily.

Contraindications and cautions

• Contraindicated in patients hypersensitive to the drug or any of its components, and in those with status asthmaticus.
• Use cautiously, if at all, in patients with tuberculosis of respiratory tract; untreated fungal, bacterial, or systemic viral infections; or ocular herpes simplex. Also use cautiously in patients receiving systemic corticosteroids.
⚖ **Lifespan:** In pregnant women, use cautiously. In breast-feeding women, drug isn't recommended.

Adverse reactions

CNS: *headache* (Nasacort AQ).
CV: facial edema.
EENT: dry or irritated nose or throat, hoarseness; nasal irritation, rhinitis (Nasacort AQ), *sneezing.*
GI: dry or irritated tongue or mouth, *oral candidiasis.*
Respiratory: cough, wheezing.
Other: adrenal insufficiency, **hypothalamic-pituitary-adrenal function suppression.**

Interactions

None significant.

Effects on lab test results

None reported.

Pharmacokinetics

Absorption: Slow.
Distribution: Without spacer, about 10% to 25% of dose goes to airways; remainder goes to mouth and throat and is swallowed. Spacer may help a greater percentage reach lungs.
Metabolism: In liver. Some drug that reaches lungs may be metabolized locally.
Excretion: In urine and feces. *Half-life:* 18 to 36 hours; 5½ hours (HFA).

Route	Onset	Peak	Duration
Inhalation	1–4 wk	Unknown	Unknown
Intranasal	Unknown	4 hr	Unknown

Reactions may be *common*, uncommon, *life-threatening*, or COMMON AND LIFE-THREATENING.

Action

Chemical effect: May decrease inflammation by stabilizing leukocyte lysosomal membranes.
Therapeutic effect: Improves breathing ability.

Available forms

Inhalation aerosol: 75 mcg/metered dose
Nasal spray: 55 mcg/actuation

NURSING PROCESS

Assessment

• Assess patient's asthma or allergic rhinitis before starting therapy and regularly thereafter to monitor drug's effectiveness.
• Be alert for adverse reactions.
• Assess patient's and family's knowledge of drug therapy.

Nursing diagnoses

• Ineffective breathing pattern related to presence of asthma
• Impaired tissue integrity related to drug's adverse effect on oral mucosa
• Deficient knowledge related to drug therapy

Planning and implementation

• Patient who has recently been transferred to oral inhaled steroids from systemic administration of steroids may need to be placed back on systemic steroids during periods of stress or severe asthma attacks.
• Taper oral therapy slowly.
• If patient is also to receive bronchodilator by inhalation, give bronchodilator first, wait several minutes, and then give triamcinolone.
• If more than one inhalation is ordered for each dose, wait 1 minute between inhalations.
• Store drug between 36° and 86° F (2° and 30° C).
• **ALERT:** Don't confuse triamcinolone with Triaminicin, Triaminic, or Triaminicol.

Patient teaching
• Inform patient that inhaled steroids don't provide relief for emergency asthma attacks.
• Instruct patient to use drug as prescribed, even when feeling well.
• Advise patient to ensure delivery of proper dose by gently warming canister to room temperature before using and by using the spacer. Patient can carry canister in his pocket to keep it warm.

• Instruct patient requiring bronchodilator to use it several minutes before triamcinolone. Tell him to wait 1 minute before repeat inhalations and to hold his breath for a few seconds to enhance drug action.
• Teach patient to check mucous membranes frequently for signs of fungal infection.
• Tell patient to prevent oral fungal infections by gargling or rinsing mouth with water after each use of inhaler but not to swallow water.
• Tell patient to keep inhaler clean and unobstructed by washing it with warm water and drying it thoroughly after use.
• Instruct patient to contact prescriber if response to therapy decreases; prescriber may need to adjust dosage. Tell patient not to exceed recommended dosage on his own.
• Instruct patient to wear or carry medical identification at all times.

Evaluation

• Patient exhibits improved breathing ability.
• Patient maintains normal oral mucosa integrity.
• Patient and family state understanding of drug therapy.

triamterene
(trigh-AM-tuh-reen)
Dyrenium

Pharmacologic class: potassium-sparing diuretic
Therapeutic class: diuretic
Pregnancy risk category: C

Indications and dosages

▶ **Edema.** *Adults:* Initially, 100 mg P.O. b.i.d. after meals. Total daily dose shouldn't exceed 300 mg.

Contraindications and cautions

• Contraindicated in patients hypersensitive to the drug or any of its components, and in those with anuria, severe or progressive renal disease or dysfunction, severe hepatic disease, or hyperkalemia.
• Use cautiously in patients with impaired liver function or diabetes mellitus, and in debilitated patients.

⚖ **Lifespan:** In pregnant women, use cautiously. In breast-feeding women, safety and effectiveness haven't been established. In children, safety and effectiveness haven't been established. In elderly patients, use cautiously.

Adverse reactions

CNS: dizziness, fatigue, headache, weakness.
CV: hypotension.
GI: diarrhea, dry mouth, stomatitis, nausea, vomiting.
GU: azotemia, interstitial nephritis, nephrolithiasis.
Hematologic: *agranulocytosis,* megaloblastic anemia related to low folic acid level, *thrombocytopenia.*
Hepatic: jaundice.
Metabolic: *acidosis,* hyperglycemia, HYPERKALEMIA, hypokalemia, hyponatremia.
Musculoskeletal: muscle cramps.
Skin: photosensitivity reactions, rash.
Other: *anaphylaxis.*

Interactions

Drug-drug. *ACE inhibitors, potassium supplements:* May increase risk of hyperkalemia. Don't use together.
Amantadine: May increase risk of amantadine toxicity. Don't use together.
Lithium: May decrease lithium clearance, increasing risk of lithium toxicity. Monitor lithium level.
NSAIDs (indomethacin): May increase risk of nephrotoxicity. Avoid use together.
Quinidine: May interfere with some laboratory tests that measure quinidine level. Inform laboratory that patient is taking triamterene.
Drug-food. *Potassium-containing salt substitutes, potassium-rich foods:* May increase risk of hyperkalemia. Discourage use together.
Drug-lifestyle. *Sun exposure:* May increase risk of photosensitivity reactions. Urge patient to avoid prolonged or unprotected exposure to sunlight.

Effects on lab test results

• May increase BUN, creatinine, glucose, and uric acid levels. May decrease sodium and hemoglobin levels and hematocrit. May increase or decrease potassium level.
• May increase liver function test values. May decrease RBC, granulocyte, and platelet counts.

Pharmacokinetics

Absorption: Rapid; extent varies.
Distribution: About 67% protein-bound.
Metabolism: By hydroxylation and sulfation.
Excretion: In urine. *Half-life:* 100 to 150 minutes.

Route	Onset	Peak	Duration
P.O.	2–4 hr	6–8 hr	7–9 hr

Action

Chemical effect: Inhibits sodium reabsorption and potassium and hydrogen excretion by direct action on distal tubule.
Therapeutic effect: Promotes water and sodium excretion.

Available forms

Capsules: 50 mg, 100 mg

NURSING PROCESS

⚗ Assessment
• Assess patient's edema before starting therapy and regularly thereafter. Full effect of triamterene is delayed 2 to 3 days when used alone.
• Monitor blood pressure, and BUN and electrolyte levels.
• Watch for blood dyscrasia.
• Be alert for adverse reactions and drug interactions.
• Assess patient's and family's knowledge of drug therapy.

⊕ Nursing diagnoses
• Excess fluid volume related to underlying condition
• Ineffective health maintenance related to drug-induced hyperkalemia
• Deficient knowledge related to drug therapy

▷ Planning and implementation
• Give drug after meals, to minimize nausea.
⊕ ALERT: Withdraw drug gradually to minimize excessive rebound potassium excretion.
• Drug is less potent than thiazides and loop diuretics and is useful as adjunct to other diuretic therapy. Triamterene is usually used with potassium-wasting diuretics.
• When used with other diuretics, lower initial dose of each drug and adjust to individual requirements.

⊕ **ALERT:** Don't confuse triamterene with trimipramine.

Patient teaching
• Tell patient to take drug after meals.
⊕ **ALERT:** Warn patient to avoid excessive ingestion of potassium-rich foods, potassium-
containing salt substitutes, and potassium supplements to prevent serious hyperkalemia.
• Instruct patient to avoid direct sunlight, wear
protective clothing, and use sunblock to prevent
photosensitivity reactions.

☑ **Evaluation**
• Patient has no signs of edema.
• Patient's potassium level is normal.
• Patient and family state understanding of drug
therapy.

HIGH ALERT

triazolam
(trigh-AH-zoh-lam)
Apo-Triazo ♦ , Halcion

Pharmacologic class: benzodiazepine
Therapeutic class: sedative-hypnotic
Pregnancy risk category: X
Controlled substance schedule: IV

Indications and dosages

▶ **Insomnia.** *Adults:* 0.125 to 0.5 mg P.O. at
bedtime.
Adults older than age 65: Give 0.125 mg P.O. at
bedtime; increased, if needed, to 0.25 mg P.O. at
bedtime.

Contraindications and cautions

• Contraindicated in patients hypersensitive to
benzodiazepines.
• Use cautiously in patients with impaired liver
or kidney function, chronic pulmonary insufficiency, sleep apnea, depression, suicidal tendencies, or history of drug abuse.
☀ **Lifespan:** In pregnant women, drug is contraindicated. In breast-feeding women, drug
isn't recommended. In children, safety and effectiveness haven't been established.

Adverse reactions

CNS: amnesia, ataxia, complex sleep disorders,
confusion, depression, *dizziness, drowsiness,
headache,* lack of coordination, lightheadedness, nervousness, rebound insomnia.

GI: nausea, stomatitis, vomiting.
Other: *anaphylaxis, angioedema,* physical or
psychological abuse.

Interactions

Drug-drug. *Cimetidine, erythromycin, hormonal contraceptives, isoniazid, ranitidine:* May
prolong triazolam level. Monitor patient for increased sedation.
*CNS depressants, including anticonvulsants, an-
tihistamines, opioid analgesics, other psychotropic drugs:* May cause excessive CNS depression. Use together cautiously.
Diltiazem: May increase CNS depression and
prolong effects of triazolam. Use lower dose of
triazolam.
*Fluconazole, itraconazole, ketoconazole, mi-
conazole:* May increase and prolong drug level,
CNS depression, and psychomotor impairment.
Don't use together.
Potent CYP3A inhibitors, such as nefazodone:
May decrease clearance of triazolam. Don't use
together.
Drug-herb. *Calendula, catnip, hops, lady's
slipper, lemon balm, passion flower, sassafras,
skullcap, valerian, yerba maté:* May increase
risk of sedative effects. Monitor patient closely
if used together.
Kava: May cause excessive sedation. Discourage use together.
Drug-food. *Grapefruit juice:* May delay drug
onset and increase effects. Advise patient to
avoid use together.
Drug-lifestyle. *Alcohol use:* May cause additive
CNS effects. Strongly discourage use together.

Effects on lab test results

• May increase liver function test values.

Pharmacokinetics

Absorption: Good.
Distribution: Wide. 90% protein-bound.
Metabolism: In liver.
Excretion: In urine. *Half-life:* 1½ to 5½ hours.

Route	Onset	Peak	Duration
P.O.	Unknown	1–2 hr	Unknown

Action

Chemical effect: May act on limbic system,
thalamus, and hypothalamus of CNS to produce
hypnotic effects.
Therapeutic effect: Promotes sleep.

Available forms

Tablets: 0.125 mg, 0.25 mg

NURSING PROCESS

Assessment
• Assess patient before therapy and regularly thereafter to monitor drug's effectiveness.
• Assess mental status and neurologic function before starting therapy. An elderly patient is more sensitive to the drug's CNS effects.
• Be alert for adverse reactions and drug interactions.
• Assess patient's and family's knowledge of drug therapy.

Nursing diagnoses
• Insomnia related to underlying disorder
• Risk for injury related to drug-induced adverse CNS reactions
• Deficient knowledge related to drug therapy

Planning and implementation
• Make plans to prevent hoarding or intentional overdose by patient who's depressed, suicidal, drug-dependent, or has history of drug abuse.
• Store drug in cool, dry place away from light.
• Institute safety precautions once drug has been given.
ALERT: Don't confuse Halcion with Haldol or halcinonide.
Patient teaching
• Warn patient not to take more than prescribed amount because overdose can occur at total daily dosage of 2 mg (four times the highest recommended amount).
• Warn patient about performing activities that require mental alertness or physical coordination. For inpatient, supervise walking and raise bed rails, particularly for elderly patient.
• Warn patient about possible complex sleep disorders.
• Inform patient that drug is short-acting and has less tendency to cause morning drowsiness.
• Tell patient that rebound insomnia may develop for 1 or 2 nights after stopping therapy.

Evaluation
• Patient states that drug produces sleep.
• Patient sustains no injury from adverse CNS reactions.
• Patient and family state understanding of drug therapy.

trifluoperazine hydrochloride
(trigh-floo-oh-PER-eh-zeen high-droh-KLOR-ighd)

Pharmacologic class: phenothiazine (piperazine derivative)
Therapeutic class: antiemetic, antipsychotic
Pregnancy risk category: C

Indications and dosages
▶ **Anxiety.** *Adults:* 1 to 2 mg P.O. b.i.d. Maximum, 6 mg daily. Don't use for longer than 12 weeks.
▶ **Schizophrenia and other psychotic disorders.** *Adult outpatients:* 1 to 2 mg P.O. b.i.d., increased if needed.
Adult inpatients: 2 to 5 mg P.O. b.i.d.; may increase gradually to 40 mg daily.
Children ages 6 to 12 (hospitalized or under close supervision): 1 mg P.O. daily or b.i.d.; may increase gradually to 15 mg daily, if needed.

Contraindications and cautions
• Contraindicated in patients hypersensitive to phenothiazines and in patients experiencing coma, CNS depression, bone marrow suppression, or liver damage.
• Use cautiously in debilitated patients and in patients with CV disease (may cause drop in blood pressure), seizure disorder, glaucoma, or prostatic hyperplasia. Also use cautiously in patients exposed to extreme heat.
Lifespan: In pregnant or breast-feeding women and in children younger than age 6, safety and effectiveness haven't been established. In elderly patients, use cautiously.

Adverse reactions
CNS: dizziness, drowsiness, *extrapyramidal reactions*, fatigue, headache, insomnia, **neuroleptic malignant syndrome,** pseudoparkinsonism, *tardive dyskinesia.*
CV: ECG changes, *orthostatic hypotension,* tachycardia.
EENT: *blurred vision,* ocular changes.
GI: constipation, dry mouth, nausea.
GU: menstrual irregularities, *urine retention.*
Hematologic: *agranulocytosis, transient leukopenia.*
Hepatic: cholestatic jaundice.
Metabolic: weight gain.

Skin: *photosensitivity reactions,* rash.
Other: allergic reaction, gynecomastia, inhibited lactation.

Interactions

Drug-drug. *Antacids:* May inhibit absorption of oral phenothiazines. Separate doses by at least 2 hours.
Barbiturates, lithium: May decrease phenothiazine effect. Monitor patient.
Centrally-acting antihypertensives: May decrease antihypertensive effect. Monitor blood pressure.
CNS depressants: May increase CNS depression. Use together cautiously.
Propranolol: May increase levels of both propranolol and trifluoperazine. Monitor patient closely.
Warfarin: May decrease effect of oral anticoagulants. Monitor PT and INR.
Drug-herb. *Dong quai, St. John's wort:* May increase photosensitivity reactions. Discourage use together.
Ginkgo: May decrease adverse effects of thioridazine. Monitor patient.
Kava: May increase risk of dystonic reactions. Discourage use together.
Milk thistle: May decrease liver toxicity caused by phenothiazines. Discourage use together; monitor liver enzyme levels if used together.
Yohimbe: May increase risk of yohimbe toxicity. Discourage use together.
Drug-lifestyle. *Alcohol use:* May increase CNS depression, particularly psychomotor skills. Strongly discourage use together.
Sun exposure: May cause photosensitivity reactions. Urge patient to avoid prolonged or unprotected exposure to sunlight.

Effects on lab test results

• May increase liver enzyme levels.
• May decrease WBC and granulocyte counts.

Pharmacokinetics

Absorption: Variable with P.O. use.
Distribution: Wide. 91% to 99% protein-bound.
Metabolism: Extensively by liver.
Excretion: Mainly in urine; some in feces.
Half-life: 20 to 40 hours.

Route	Onset	Peak	Duration
P.O.	Up to several wk	Unknown	Unknown

Action

Chemical effect: Unknown; probably blocks postsynaptic dopamine receptors in brain.
Therapeutic effect: Relieves anxiety and signs and symptoms of psychotic disorders.

Available forms

Oral concentrate: 10 mg/ml
Tablets (regular and film-coated): 1 mg, 2 mg, 5 mg, 10 mg

NURSING PROCESS

🔬 Assessment
• Assess patient's condition before starting therapy and regularly thereafter to monitor drug's effectiveness.
• Watch for orthostatic hypotension, especially with parenteral use.
• Monitor patient for tardive dyskinesia, which may occur after prolonged use. It may not appear until months or years later and may disappear spontaneously or persist for life, despite stopping the drug.
• Monitor therapy with weekly bilirubin tests during first month, periodic blood tests (CBC and liver function), and ophthalmologic tests (long-term use).
🛇 **ALERT:** Monitor patient for symptoms of neuroleptic malignant syndrome (extrapyramidal effects, hyperthermia, autonomic disturbance), which is rare but can be fatal. It isn't necessarily related to length of drug use or type of neuroleptic; however, more than 60% of patients are men.
• Assess patient's and family's knowledge of drug therapy.

⊕ Nursing diagnoses
• Anxiety related to underlying condition
• Disturbed thought processes related to underlying psychotic disorder
• Deficient knowledge related to drug therapy

➤ Planning and implementation
• Although there's little likelihood of contact dermatitis, those sensitive to phenothiazine drugs should avoid direct contact. Wear gloves when preparing liquid forms.
• Dilute liquid concentrate with 60 ml of tomato or fruit juice, carbonated beverage, coffee, tea, milk, water, or semisolid food.

T

• Protect concentrate from light. Slight yellowing of drug is common; it doesn't affect potency. Discard markedly discolored solutions.

• Keep patient supine for 1 hour after drug administration, and advise him to change position slowly.

• Don't abruptly stop giving the drug unless a severe adverse reaction occurs. Abruptly stopping long-term therapy may cause gastritis, nausea, vomiting, dizziness, tremor, feeling of warmth or cold, diaphoresis, tachycardia, headache, insomnia, anorexia, muscle rigidity, altered mental status, or evidence of autonomic instability.

• Don't give the dose, and notify prescriber, if patient develops jaundice, symptoms of blood dyscrasia (fever, sore throat, infection, cellulitis, weakness), or extrapyramidal reactions longer than a few hours, especially in pregnant women and in children.

• Acute dystonic reactions may be treated with diphenhydramine.

🔺 ALERT: Don't confuse trifluoperazine with triflupromazine.

Patient teaching

• Teach patient or caregiver how to prepare oral form of drug.

• Warn patient to avoid activities that require alertness or good psychomotor coordination until drug's CNS effects are known; drowsiness and dizziness usually subside after a few weeks.

• Tell patient not to drink alcohol during therapy.

• Instruct patient to report urine retention or constipation.

• Tell patient to use sun block and wear protective clothing to avoid photosensitivity reactions.

• Tell patient to relieve dry mouth with sugarless gum or hard candy.

✓ **Evaluation**

• Patient's anxiety is reduced.

• Patient's behavior and communication exhibit improved thought processes.

• Patient and family state understanding of drug therapy.

trihexyphenidyl hydrochloride
(try-heks-eh-FEEN-ih-dil hy-droh-KLOR-ighd)
Apo-Trihex ♦ , Trihexy-2, Trihexy-5

Pharmacologic class: anticholinergic
Therapeutic class: antiparkinsonian
Pregnancy risk category: C

Indications and dosages

▶ **All forms of parkinsonism; adjunct with levodopa in managing parkinsonism.** *Adults:* 1 mg P.O. first day, increased by 2 mg every 3 to 5 days until total of 6 to 10 mg is given daily. Usually given t.i.d. with meals. Sometimes given q.i.d. (last dose at bedtime). Postencephalitic parkinsonism may require total daily dosage of 12 to 15 mg.

▶ **Drug-induced extrapyramidal reactions.** *Adults:* 5 to 15 mg P.O. daily. Initial dose of 1 mg may control some reactions.

Contraindications and cautions

• Contraindicated in patients hypersensitive to the drug or any of its components.

• Use cautiously in patients with glaucoma; cardiac, hepatic, or renal disorders; obstructive disease of the GI or GU tract; or prostatic hyperplasia.

⚠ **Lifespan:** In pregnant women, safety and effectiveness haven't been established. In breastfeeding women, drug isn't recommended. In children, safety and effectiveness haven't been established. In elderly patients, watch for mental confusion or disorientation.

Adverse reactions

CNS: dizziness, drowsiness, hallucinations, headache, nervousness, weakness.
CV: tachycardia.
EENT: blurred vision, increased intraocular pressure, mydriasis.
GI: constipation, *dry mouth, nausea,* vomiting.
GU: urinary hesitancy, urine retention.

Interactions

Drug-drug. *Amantadine:* May have additive anticholinergic reactions, such as confusion and hallucinations. Reduce dosage of trihexyphenidyl before giving it.
Levodopa: May increase drug effect. May require lower doses of both drugs.

Drug-lifestyle. *Alcohol use:* May increase sedative effects. Discourage use together.

Effects on lab test results

None reported.

Pharmacokinetics

Absorption: Readily absorbed.
Distribution: Unknown. Crosses blood-brain barrier.
Metabolism: Unknown.
Excretion: In urine. *Half-life:* 5½ to 10¾ hours.

Route	Onset	Peak	Duration
P.O.	1 hr	2–3 hr	6–12 hr

Action

Chemical effect: Unknown; blocks central cholinergic receptors, helping to balance cholinergic activity in basal ganglia.
Therapeutic effect: Improves physical mobility in patients with parkinsonism.

Available forms

Elixir: 2 mg/5 ml
Tablets: 2 mg, 5 mg

NURSING PROCESS

🗓 Assessment

• Assess patient's condition before starting therapy and regularly thereafter to monitor drug's effectiveness.
• **⊛ ALERT:** Gonioscopic ocular evaluation and monitoring of intraocular pressure are needed, especially if patient is older than age 40.
• Be alert for adverse reactions and drug interactions. Adverse reactions are dose-related and usually transient.
• Assess patient's and family's knowledge of drug therapy.

🔀 Nursing diagnoses

• Impaired physical mobility related to presence of parkinsonism
• Risk for injury related to drug-induced adverse CNS reactions
• Deficient knowledge related to drug therapy

▶ Planning and implementation

• Dosage may need to be increased gradually in a patient who develops drug tolerance.
• Give drug with meals.

Patient teaching

• Warn patient that drug may cause nausea if taken before meals.
• Tell patient to avoid activities that require alertness until the drug's CNS effects are known.
• Advise patient to report urinary hesitancy or urine retention.
• Tell patient to relieve dry mouth with cool drinks, ice chips, sugarless gum, or hard candy.

☑ Evaluation

• Patient has improved physical mobility.
• Patient sustains no injury from adverse reactions.
• Patient and family state understanding of drug therapy.

trimethobenzamide hydrochloride

(try-meth-oh-BEN-zuh-myd hy-droh-KLOR-ighd)
Tigan, Trimazide

Pharmacologic class: ethanolamine-related antihistamine
Therapeutic class: antiemetic
Pregnancy risk category: C

Indications and dosages

▶ **Nausea, vomiting.** *Adults:* 250 mg P.O. t.i.d. or q.i.d.; or 200 mg I.M. t.i.d. or q.i.d.
▶ **Prevention of postoperative nausea and vomiting.** *Adults:* 200 mg I.M. as single dose before or during surgery; if needed, repeat 3 hours after termination of anesthesia. Limit use to prolonged vomiting from known cause. *Children weighing 13 to 40 kg (28 to 88 lb):* 100 to 200 mg P.O. t.i.d. or q.i.d.

Contraindications and cautions

• Contraindicated in patients hypersensitive to the drug or any of its components.
🕯 **Lifespan:** In pregnant women, use cautiously. In breast-feeding women, safety and effectiveness haven't been established. In children, use cautiously. In children with viral illness, drug isn't recommended because it may contribute to development of Reye syndrome.

Adverse reactions

CNS: *coma,* depression, disorientation, dizziness, *drowsiness,* headache, parkinson-like symptoms, *seizures.*

CV: hypotension.
EENT: blurred vision.
GI: diarrhea.
Hepatic: jaundice.
Musculoskeletal: muscle cramps.
Skin: hypersensitivity reaction (burning, pain, redness, stinging, swelling at I.M. injection site).

Interactions

Drug-drug. *CNS depressants:* May cause additive CNS depression. Avoid use together.
Drug-lifestyle. *Alcohol use:* May cause additive CNS depression. Discourage use together.

Effects on lab test results

None reported.

Pharmacokinetics

Absorption: About 60% after P.O. use; unknown after I.M. use.
Distribution: Unknown.
Metabolism: About 50% to 70%, probably in liver.
Excretion: In urine and feces. *Half-life:* 7 to 9 hours.

Route	Onset	Peak	Duration
P.O.	10–20 min	Unknown	3–4 hr
I.M.	15–30 min	Unknown	2–3 hr

Action

Chemical effect: Unknown; may act on chemoreceptor trigger zone to inhibit nausea and vomiting.
Therapeutic effect: Prevents or relieves nausea and vomiting.

Available forms

Capsules: 100 mg, 250 mg
Injection: 100 mg/ml

NURSING PROCESS

Assessment
• Assess patient's condition before starting therapy and regularly thereafter to monitor drug's effectiveness.
• Be alert for adverse reactions and drug interactions.
• Assess patient's and family's knowledge of drug therapy.

Nursing diagnoses
• Risk for deficient fluid volume related to potential for or presence of nausea and vomiting
• Diarrhea related to drug-induced adverse GI reactions
• Deficient knowledge related to drug therapy

Planning and implementation
• Inject I.M. dose deep into upper outer quadrant of gluteal region to reduce pain and local irritation.
• If skin hypersensitivity reaction occurs, don't give the drug.
ALERT: Don't confuse Tigan with Ticar.
Patient teaching
• Advise patient of possibility of drowsiness and dizziness, and caution against driving or performing other activities requiring alertness until the drug's CNS effects are known.
• Warn patient that giving the drug I.M. may be painful.

Evaluation
• Patient maintains adequate hydration, and nausea and vomiting cease.
• Patient maintains normal bowel pattern.
• Patient and family state understanding of drug therapy.

trimethoprim
(try-METH-uh-prim)
Primsol, Proloprim, Trimpex

Pharmacologic class: synthetic folate antagonist
Therapeutic class: antibiotic
Pregnancy risk category: C

Indications and dosages

▶ **Acute otitis media caused by susceptible strains of *Streptococcus pneumoniae* and *Haemophilus influenzae*.** *Children age 6 months and older:* 10 mg/kg Primsol daily in divided doses every 12 hours for 10 days.
▶ **Uncomplicated UTI caused by *Escherichia coli, Proteus mirabilis, Klebsiella pneumoniae, Enterobacter* species, coagulase-negative *Staphylococcus* species (including *Staphylococcus saprophyticus*).** *Adults:* 100 mg (10 ml) every 12 hours, or 200 mg (20 ml) daily for 10 days.

Reactions may be *common*, uncommon, *life-threatening*, or COMMON AND LIFE-THREATENING.

▶ **Prophylaxis of chronic and recurrent UTI‡.** *Adults:* 100 mg P.O. at bedtime for 6 weeks to 6 months.

▶ **Traveler's diarrhea‡.** *Adults:* 200 mg P.O. b.i.d. for 3 to 5 days.

▶ *Pneumocystis jiroveci (carinii)* **pneumonia‡.** *Adults:* 5 mg/kg P.O. t.i.d. with dapsone 100 mg daily for 21 days.

▧ **Adjust-a-dose:** For patients with renal impairment, if creatinine clearance is 15 to 30 ml/minute, give half the recommended dose every 12 hours; if less than 15 ml/minute, don't use drug.

Contraindications and cautions

• Contraindicated in patients hypersensitive to the drug or any of its components, and in those with documented megaloblastic anemia caused by folate deficiency.
• Use cautiously in patients with hepatic impairment.
☀ **Lifespan:** In pregnant women, use cautiously. In breast-feeding women, drug isn't recommended. In children younger than age 12, safety and effectiveness (other than of Primsol) haven't been established.

Adverse reactions

CNS: fever.
GI: diarrhea, epigastric distress, glossitis, nausea, vomiting.
Hematologic: *leukopenia,* megaloblastic anemia, *methemoglobinemia, thrombocytopenia.*
Skin: exfoliative dermatitis, *pruritus, rash.*

Interactions

Drug-drug. *Phenytoin:* May decrease phenytoin metabolism and increase blood level. Monitor patient for toxicity.

Effects on lab test results

• May increase BUN, creatinine, bilirubin, and aminotransferase levels. May decrease hemoglobin level and hematocrit.
• May decrease platelet and WBC counts.

Pharmacokinetics

Absorption: Quick and complete.
Distribution: Wide. About 42% to 46% protein-bound.
Metabolism: Less than 20% in liver.
Excretion: Mainly in urine. *Half-life:* 8 to 11 hours.

Route	Onset	Peak	Duration
P.O.	Unknown	1–4 hr	Unknown

Action

Chemical effect: Interferes with action of dihydrofolate reductase, inhibiting bacterial synthesis of folic acid.
Therapeutic effect: Inhibits certain bacteria.

Available forms

Oral solution: 50 mg/5 ml
Tablets: 100 mg, 200 mg

NURSING PROCESS

▧ **Assessment**
• Assess patient's infection before starting therapy and regularly thereafter to monitor drug's effectiveness.
• Obtain urine specimen for culture and sensitivity tests before giving the first dose. Start therapy pending test results.
⊛ **ALERT:** Monitor CBC routinely. Signs and symptoms such as sore throat, fever, pallor, and purpura may be early indications of serious blood disorders. Prolonged use of trimethoprim at high doses may cause bone marrow suppression.
• Be alert for adverse reactions and drug interactions.
• If adverse GI reactions occur, monitor hydration.
• Assess patient's and family's knowledge of drug therapy.

▧ **Nursing diagnoses**
• Ineffective protection related to presence of susceptible bacteria
• Risk for deficient fluid volume related to drug-induced adverse GI reactions
• Deficient knowledge related to drug therapy

▧ **Planning and implementation**
• Because resistance to trimethoprim develops rapidly when drug is given alone, it's usually given with other drugs.
⊛ **ALERT:** Trimethoprim is also used with sulfamethoxazole; don't confuse the two.
Patient teaching
• Instruct patient to take drug as prescribed, even if he feels better.

T

✓ Evaluation

- Patient is free from infection.
- Patient maintains adequate hydration.
- Patient and family state understanding of drug therapy.

HIGH ALERT

triptorelin pamoate
(trip-TOE-reh-lin PAM-o-eight)
Trelstar Depot, Trelstar LA

Pharmacologic class: synthetic luteinizing hormone-releasing hormone (LHRH) analogue
Therapeutic class: antineoplastic
Pregnancy risk category: X

Indications and dosages

▶ **Palliative treatment of advanced prostate cancer.** *Men:* 3.75 mg Trelstar Depot I.M. given monthly as a single injection, or 11.25 mg Trelstar LA I.M. into either buttock every 12 weeks.

Contraindications and cautions

- Contraindicated in patients hypersensitive to the drug or any of its components, other LHRH agonists, or LHRH.
- Use cautiously in patients with metastatic vertebral lesions or upper or lower urinary tract obstruction during the first few weeks of therapy.
- Use cautiously in patients with hepatic and renal impairment; they have a level of exposure to drug two to four times higher than normal.
- ☀ **Lifespan:** Drug is used for men only. In boys, safety and effectiveness haven't been studied.

Adverse reactions

CNS: dizziness, emotional lability, fatigue, headache, insomnia, pain, *spinal cord compression.*
CV: hypertension.
GI: diarrhea, vomiting.
GU: impotence, urine retention, UTI.
Hematologic: anemia.
Musculoskeletal: leg pain, *skeletal pain.*
Skin: pruritus.
Other: *hot flushes,* pain at injection site.

Interactions

Drug-drug. *Hyperprolactinemic drugs:* May decrease pituitary gonadotropin-releasing hormone (GnRH) receptors. Don't use together.

Effects on lab test results

- May increase glucose, BUN, AST, ALT, and alkaline phosphatase levels. May transiently increase testosterone level. May decrease hemoglobin level and hematocrit.

Pharmacokinetics

Absorption: Maintains level over a period of a month.
Distribution: No evidence of protein-binding.
Metabolism: Unknown, but is unlikely to involve hepatic microsomal enzymes; no metabolites have been identified.
Excretion: By liver and kidneys. *Half-life:* 2 to 3 hours.

Route	Onset	Peak	Duration
I.M.	Unknown	Unknown	1 mo

Action

Chemical effect: Is a potent inhibitor of gonadotropin secretion. In men, testosterone declines to a level typically seen in surgically castrated men. As a result, tissues and functions that depend on these hormones become inactive.
Therapeutic effect: Decreases effects of sex hormones on tumor growth in the prostate gland.

Available forms

Injection: 3.75 mg, 11.25 mg

NURSING PROCESS

ᙎ Assessment

- Assess patient's condition before starting therapy and regularly thereafter to monitor drug's effectiveness.
- Monitor testosterone and prostate-specific antigen levels.
- Assess patient's and family's knowledge of drug therapy.

⊕ Nursing diagnoses

- Ineffective health maintenance related to underlying condition
- Acute pain related to adverse drug effects
- Deficient knowledge related to drug therapy

▶ Planning and implementation

- Give drug only under the supervision of an experienced prescriber.

🌡️ **ALERT:** Only sterile water may be used as a diluent.

- Reconstitute powder with 2 ml of sterile water for injection. Shake well until suspension appears milky. Use 20 G needle.
- Change the injection site periodically.
- Monitor patients with metastatic vertebral lesions or upper or lower urinary tract obstruction during the first few weeks of therapy.
- Initially, drug causes a transient increase in testosterone level. As a result, signs and symptoms of prostate cancer may worsen during the first few weeks of therapy.
- Patients may have worsening of symptoms or onset of new symptoms, including bone pain, neuropathy, hematuria, or urethral or bladder outlet obstruction.

🌡️ **ALERT:** Spinal cord compression, which can lead to paralysis and possibly death, may occur. If spinal cord compression or renal impairment develops, give standard treatment. In extreme cases, immediate orchiectomy is considered.
- If patient has an allergic reaction, immediately stop giving the drug, treat symptoms, and give supportive care.
- Diagnostic tests of pituitary-gonadal function conducted during and after therapy may be misleading.

Patient teaching
- Inform the patient about adverse reactions.
- Tell patient that symptoms (including bone pain, neuropathy, hematuria, or urethral or bladder outlet obstruction) may worsen during the first few weeks of therapy.
- Inform patient that a blood test will be used to monitor response to therapy.

☑️ **Evaluation**
- Patient responds well to drug.
- Patient denies pain.
- Patient and family state understanding of drug therapy.

trospium chloride
(TROSE-pee-uhm KLOHR-ighd)
Sanctura, Sanctura XL

Pharmacologic class: anticholinergic
Therapeutic class: antimuscarinic, antispasmodic
Pregnancy risk category: C

Indications and dosages

▶ **Overactive bladder with symptoms of urinary urge incontinence, urgency, and frequency.** *Adults younger than age 75:* Give 20 mg P.O. b.i.d. or 60 mg extended-release P.O. daily in the morning, taken on an empty stomach or at least 1 hour before a meal.
Adults age 75 and older: Based on patient tolerance, reduce dosage to 20 mg once daily.
📋 **Adjust-a-dose:** If patient's creatinine clearance is less than 30 ml/minute, give 20 mg P.O. once daily at bedtime. Extended-release form isn't recommended.

Contraindications and cautions

- Contraindicated in patients hypersensitive to the drug or any of its components and in patients with or at risk for urine retention, gastric retention, or uncontrolled narrow-angle glaucoma.
- Use cautiously in patients with significant bladder outflow obstruction, obstructive GI disorders, ulcerative colitis, intestinal atony, myasthenia gravis, severe renal insufficiency, moderate or severe hepatic impairment, or controlled narrow-angle glaucoma.
⚕️ **Lifespan:** In pregnant women, use only if benefits to the patient outweigh risks to the fetus. In breast-feeding women, use cautiously; it's unknown if the drug appears in breast milk. In children, safety and effectiveness haven't been established. In elderly patients, use a lower dose because they may have an increased risk of anticholinergic effects.

Adverse reactions

CNS: fatigue, headache.
EENT: dry eyes.
GI: abdominal pain, *constipation, dry mouth,* dyspepsia, flatulence.
GU: urine retention.

Interactions

Drug-drug. *Anticholinergics:* May increase dry mouth, constipation, or other adverse effects. Monitor patient.
Digoxin, metformin, morphine, pancuronium, procainamide, tenofovir, vancomycin: May alter elimination of these drugs or trospium, increasing level. Monitor patient closely.
Drug-food. *High-fat food:* May decrease absorption by up to 80%. Give trospium at least 1 hour before meals or on an empty stomach.

Drug-lifestyle. *Alcohol use:* May increase drowsiness. Discourage use together.

Effects on lab test results

None reported.

Pharmacokinetics

Absorption: Less than 10%. Taking drug after a high-fat meal significantly decreases absorption. It should be taken at least 1 hour before meals or on an empty stomach.
Distribution: Mostly in plasma. 50% to 85% protein-bound.
Metabolism: Not defined. Major pathway is most likely the liver.
Excretion: About 85% appears in feces and about 6% in urine. *Half-life:* About 20 hours.

Route	Onset	Peak	Duration
P.O.	Unknown	5–6 hr	Unknown

Action

Chemical effect: Opposes the effect of acetylcholine on muscarinic receptors, reducing smooth muscle tone in the bladder and increasing maximum bladder capacity and volume at first contraction.
Therapeutic effect: Relieves symptoms of overactive bladder.

Available forms

Capsules (extended-release): 60 mg
Tablets: 20 mg

NURSING PROCESS

Assessment
• Assess patient before starting therapy to determine baseline bladder function, and reassess during therapy to monitor drug's effectiveness.
• Monitor patient for decreased gastric motility and constipation.
• Assess patient's and family's knowledge of drug therapy.

Nursing diagnoses
• Impaired urinary elimination related to underlying medical condition
• Impaired oral mucous membrane related to drug-induced adverse effects
• Deficient knowledge related to drug therapy

Planning and implementation
• If the patient has bladder-outflow obstruction, watch for evidence of urine retention.
• If the patient has urine retention, notify prescriber and prepare for urinary catheterization.
• Dry mouth and constipation are the most frequently reported adverse effects.

Patient teaching
• Tell patient to take drug on an empty stomach, at least 1 hour before meals.
• Discourage use of other drugs that may cause dry mouth, constipation, blurred vision, or urine retention.
• Tell patient that alcohol may increase drowsiness and fatigue. Urge him not to drink alcohol to excess while taking drug.
• Explain that drug may decrease sweating and increase the risk of heatstroke when used in hot environments or during strenuous activities.
• Urge patient to avoid activities that are hazardous or require mental alertness until the drug's CNS effects are known.

Evaluation
• Patient's bladder function improves with drug therapy.
• Patient has no dry mouth or controls adverse effects with sugarless gum, hard candy, or saliva substitute.
• Patient and family state understanding of drug therapy.

HIGH ALERT

urokinase
(yoo-roh-KIGH-nays)
Abbokinase

Pharmacologic class: enzyme
Therapeutic class: thrombolytic
Pregnancy risk category: B

Indications and dosages

▶ **Lysis of acute massive pulmonary emboli and pulmonary emboli accompanied by unstable hemodynamics.** *Adults:* For I.V. infusion only by constant infusion pump. Priming dose: 4,400 international units/kg over 10 minutes,

followed with 4,400 international units/kg/hour
for 12 hours. Flush any drug remaining in the
I.V. tubing with a volume of compatible I.V.
solution about equal to that of the tubing at
15 ml/hour.

▶ **Venous catheter occlusion‡.** *Adults:* Instill
5,000 international units into occluded catheter.

▽ I.V. administration

• Add 5 ml of sterile water for injection to vial.
Don't use bacteriostatic water for injection to
reconstitute; it contains preservatives. Use im-
mediately after reconstitution.
• Dilute further with normal saline solution or
D₅W solution before infusion.
• Solution may be filtered through a 0.45 mi-
cron or smaller filter before administration.
• Give by infusion pump. Total volume of fluid
given shouldn't exceed 200 ml.
• Store powder at 36° to 46° F (2° to 8° C).
⊗ **Incompatibilities**
Other I.V. drugs.

Contraindications and cautions

• Contraindicated in patients with active internal bleeding; aneurysm; arteriovenous malformation; bleeding diathesis; visceral or intracranial cancer; ulcerative colitis; diverticulitis;
severe hypertension; hemostatic defects, including those secondary to severe hepatic or renal
insufficiency; uncontrolled hypocoagulation;
subacute bacterial endocarditis or rheumatic
valvular disease; history of stroke; recent trauma with possible internal injuries; or recent
cerebral embolism, thrombosis, or hemorrhage.
• Also contraindicated within 10 days after
intra-arterial diagnostic procedure or surgery
(liver or kidney biopsy, lumbar puncture, thoracentesis, paracentesis, or extensive or multiple
cutdowns); and within 2 months after intracranial or intraspinal surgery.
• I.M. injections and other invasive procedures
are contraindicated during urokinase therapy.
⚕ **Lifespan:** In pregnant women, drug should
be used only when clearly needed. Drug is contraindicated during the first 10 days postpartum.
In children, safety and effectiveness haven't
been established.

Adverse reactions

CNS: fever, hemiplegia, *stroke.*
CV: *reperfusion arrhythmias,* tachycardia,
transient hypotension or hypertension.

GI: nausea, vomiting.
Hematologic: *bleeding.*
Respiratory: *bronchospasm,* minor breathing
difficulties.
Skin: phlebitis, rash.
Other: *anaphylaxis,* chills.

Interactions

Drug-drug. *Anticoagulants:* May increase risk
of bleeding. Monitor patient closely.
*Aspirin, dipyridamole, indomethacin, phenylbu-
tazone, other drugs affecting platelet activity:*
May increase risk of bleeding. Monitor patient
closely.

Effects on lab test results

• May decrease hemoglobin level and hematocrit.
• May increase PT, PTT, and INR.

Pharmacokinetics

Absorption: Given I.V.
Distribution: Rapidly cleared from circulation.
Most of drug accumulates in kidneys and liver.
Metabolism: Rapid, in liver.
Excretion: Small amount in urine and bile.
Half-life: 10 to 20 minutes.

Route	Onset	Peak	Duration
I.V.	Immediate	20 min–2 hr	4 hr

Action

Chemical effect: Activates plasminogen by directly cleaving peptide bonds at two sites.
Therapeutic effect: Dissolves blood clots in
lungs, coronary arteries, and venous catheters.

Available forms

Injection: 250,000 international units/vial

NURSING PROCESS

℞ Assessment

• Assess patient's condition before starting therapy and regularly thereafter to monitor drug's
effectiveness.
• Assess patient for contraindications to therapy.
• Monitor patient for excessive bleeding every
15 minutes for first hour, every 30 minutes for
second through eighth hours, then once every
shift. Pretreatment with drugs affecting platelets
places patient at high risk for bleeding.

• Monitor pulse rates and color and sensation of limbs every hour.
• Keep laboratory flow sheet on patient's chart to monitor PTT, PT, INR, hemoglobin level, and hematocrit.
• Be alert for adverse reactions and drug interactions.
• Assess patient's and family's knowledge of drug therapy.

✪ Nursing diagnoses
• Ineffective tissue perfusion (cardiopulmonary, peripheral) related to presence of blood clot(s)
• Ineffective protection related to drug-induced bleeding
• Deficient knowledge related to drug therapy

❯ Planning and implementation
• Have typed and crossmatched RBCs and aminocaproic acid available to treat bleeding, and keep corticosteroids available to treat allergic reactions.
• Keep venipuncture sites to a minimum; use pressure dressing on puncture sites for at least 15 minutes.
• Keep limb being treated in alignment to prevent bleeding from infusion site.
• Don't handle the patient unnecessarily; pad side rails. Bruising is more likely during therapy.
• To prevent recurrent thrombosis, start heparin by continuous infusion when patient's thrombin time has decreased to less than twice the normal control value after urokinase has been stopped.
⑤ **ALERT:** Rarely, orolingual edema, urticaria, cholesterol embolization, and infusion reactions causing hypoxia, cyanosis, acidosis, and back pain may occur.
Patient teaching
• Instruct patient to report symptoms of bleeding and other adverse reactions.

☑ Evaluation
• Patient regains normal tissue perfusion with dissolution of blood clots.
• Patient doesn't experience serious complications from drug-induced bleeding.
• Patient and family state understanding of drug therapy.

---

ursodiol
(ur-sih-DIGH-al)
Actigall, URSO 250, URSO Forte

Pharmacologic class: bile acid
Therapeutic class: gallstone-dissolving drug
Pregnancy risk category: B

Indications and dosages
▶ **Dissolution of gallstones smaller than 20 mm in diameter in patients who are poor candidates for surgery or who refuse surgery.**
Adults: 8 to 10 mg/kg P.O. daily in two or three divided doses.
▶ **Prevention of gallstone formation in obese patients experiencing rapid weight loss.**
Adults: 300 mg P.O. b.i.d.

Contraindications and cautions
• Contraindicated in patients hypersensitive to the drug or other bile acids and in patients with chronic hepatic disease, unremitting acute cholecystitis, cholangitis, biliary obstruction, gallstone-induced pancreatitis, or biliary fistula. Capsules are contraindicated in patients with calcified cholesterol stones, radiopaque stones, or radiolucent bile pigment stones.
☀ **Lifespan:** In pregnant women, use cautiously. In breast-feeding women, use cautiously; it's unknown if the drug appears in breast milk. In children, safety and effectiveness haven't been established.

Adverse reactions
CNS: anxiety, depression, *dizziness,* fatigue, *headache,* sleep disorders.
EENT: rhinitis.
GI: *abdominal pain,* biliary pain, cholecystitis, *constipation, diarrhea, dyspepsia,* flatulence, metallic taste, *nausea,* stomatitis, *vomiting.*
GU: UTI.
Musculoskeletal: arthralgia, back pain, myalgia.
Respiratory: cough.
Skin: diaphoresis, dry skin, hair thinning, pruritus, rash, urticaria.

Interactions
Drug-drug. *Antacids that contain aluminum, cholestyramine, colestipol:* May bind ursodiol and prevent its absorption. Avoid use together.

Reactions may be *common,* uncommon, *life-threatening,* or COMMON AND LIFE-THREATENING.

Clofibrate, estrogens, hormonal contraceptives:
May increase hepatic cholesterol secretion; may
counteract effects of ursodiol. Avoid use together.

Effects on lab test results

• May decrease liver enzyme level in patients
with liver disease.

Pharmacokinetics

Absorption: About 90%.
Distribution: Conjugated and then secreted into
hepatic bile ducts. Drug in bile is concentrated
in gallbladder and expelled into duodenum in
gallbladder bile. A small amount appears in systemic circulation.
Metabolism: In liver. A small amount undergoes bacterial degradation with each cycle of
enterohepatic circulation.
Excretion: Mainly in feces; very small amount
in urine. *Half-life:* Unknown.

Route	Onset	Peak	Duration
P.O.	Unknown	1–3 hr	Unknown

Action

Chemical effect: Unknown; probably suppresses hepatic synthesis and secretion of cholesterol
as well as intestinal cholesterol absorption. After long-term administration, drug can solubilize
cholesterol from gallstones.
Therapeutic effect: Dissolves cholesterol gallstones.

Available forms

Capsules: 300 mg
Tablets: 250 mg, 300 mg

NURSING PROCESS

Assessment
• Assess patient's condition before starting therapy and regularly thereafter to monitor drug's
effectiveness.
• Usually, therapy is long-term and requires ultrasound images of gallbladder every 6 months.
If partial stone dissolution doesn't occur within
12 months, it's unlikely that complete dissolution will. Safety of use for longer than
24 months hasn't been established.
⊛ ALERT: Monitor liver function test results, including AST and ALT levels, at beginning of
therapy, after 1 month, after 3 months, and then
every 6 months during therapy. Abnormal test

results may indicate worsening of disease. A hepatotoxic metabolite of drug may form in some
patients.
• Be alert for adverse reactions and drug interactions.
• If adverse GI reaction occurs, monitor patient's hydration.
• Assess patient's and family's knowledge of
drug therapy.

Nursing diagnoses
• Risk for injury related to presence of gall-
stones
• Risk for deficient fluid volume related to
drug-induced adverse GI reactions
• Deficient knowledge related to drug therapy

Planning and implementation
• Gallstone dissolution requires months of therapy.
• Recurrence of stones within 5 years has been
observed in up to 50% of patients.
• Complete dissolution doesn't occur in all patients.
Patient teaching
• Tell patient about alternative therapies, including watchful waiting (with no intervention)
and cholecystectomy because relapse rate after
bile acid therapy may be as high as 50% after
5 years.
• Take with meals or snacks.

Evaluation
• Patient is free from gallstones.
• Patient maintains adequate hydration.
• Patient and family state understanding of drug
therapy.

valacyclovir hydrochloride
(val-ay-SIGH-kloh-veer high-droh-KLOR-ighd)
Valtrex

Pharmacologic class: synthetic purine nucleo-
side
Therapeutic class: antiviral
Pregnancy risk category: B

Indications and dosages

▶ **Herpes zoster (shingles) in immunocompetent patient.** *Adults:* 1 g P.O. t.i.d. for 7 days.

▨ **Adjust-a-dose:** For patient with renal impairment, if creatinine clearance is 30 to 49 ml/minute, give 1 g every 12 hours; if 10 to 29 ml/minute, give 1 g every 24 hours; if less than 10 ml/minute, give 500 mg every 24 hours.

▶ **Initial episodes of genital herpes in immunocompetent patient.** *Adults:* 1 g P.O. b.i.d. for 10 days.

▨ **Adjust-a-dose:** For patients with renal impairment, if creatinine clearance is 10 to 29 ml/minute, give 1 g every 24 hours; if less than 10 ml/minute, give 500 mg every 24 hours.

▶ **Recurrent genital herpes in immunocompetent patient.** *Adults:* 500 mg P.O. b.i.d. for 3 days.

▨ **Adjust-a-dose:** For patients with renal impairment, if creatinine clearance is 29 ml/minute or less, give 500 mg every 24 hours.

▶ **Chronic suppression of recurrent genital herpes.** *Adults:* 1 g P.O. once daily.

▨ **Adjust-a-dose:** For patients with renal impairment, if creatinine clearance is 29 ml/minute or less, give 500 mg every 24 hours.

▶ **Chronic suppression of genital herpes in patient with a history of 9 or fewer recurrences per year.** *Adults:* 500 mg P.O. daily.

▨ **Adjust-a-dose:** For patients with renal impairment, if creatinine clearance is 29 ml/minute or less, give 500 mg every 48 hours.

▶ **Chronic suppression of recurrent genital herpes in HIV-infected patient with CD4 count of 100/mm^3 or more.** *Adults:* 500 mg P.O. b.i.d. Safety and effectiveness of therapy beyond 6 months hasn't been established.

▨ **Adjust-a-dose:** For patients with renal impairment, if creatinine clearance is 29 ml/minute or less, give 500 mg every 24 hours.

▶ **Cold sores (herpes labialis).** *Adults:* 2 g P.O. for two doses, taken about 12 hours apart.

▨ **Adjust-a-dose:** For patient with renal impairment, if creatinine clearance is 30 to 49 ml/minute, give 1 g every 12 hours for two doses; if 10 to 29 ml/minute, give 500 mg every 12 hours for two doses; if less than 10 ml/minute, give 500 mg as a single dose.

Contraindications and cautions

• Contraindicated in patients hypersensitive to or intolerant of valacyclovir, acyclovir, and their components.

• Drug isn't recommended for immunocompromised patients. Thrombotic thrombocytopenic purpura and hemolytic uremic syndrome have been fatal in some patients with advanced HIV disease and in bone marrow transplant and renal transplant recipients.

• Use cautiously in patients with renal impairment and in those receiving other nephrotoxic drugs.

⚠ **Lifespan:** In pregnant women, use only if benefits to the patient outweigh risks to the fetus. In breast-feeding women, use cautiously; it's unknown if the drug appears in breast milk. In children, safety and effectiveness haven't been established. In elderly patients, a lower dose may be needed, depending on underlying renal status.

Adverse reactions

CNS: depression, dizziness, *headache.*
GI: abdominal pain, diarrhea, *nausea,* vomiting.
GU: dysmenorrhea.
Musculoskeletal: arthralgia.

Interactions

Drug-drug. *Cimetidine, probenecid:* May reduce rate (but not extent) of conversion from valacyclovir to acyclovir and reduce renal clearance of acyclovir, thereby increasing acyclovir level. Monitor patient for possible toxicity.

Effects on lab test results

• May increase AST, ALT, alkaline phosphatase, and creatinine levels. May decrease hemoglobin level and hematocrit.
• May decrease WBC and platelet counts.

Pharmacokinetics

Absorption: Rapid. Absolute bioavailability of about 54.5%.
Distribution: 13.5% to 17.9% protein-bound.
Metabolism: Rapid; nearly completely converted to acyclovir and L-valine by first-pass intestinal or hepatic metabolism.
Excretion: In urine and feces. *Half-life:* Averages 2½ to 3¼ hours.

Route	Onset	Peak	Duration
P.O.	30 min	Unknown	Unknown

Action

Chemical effect: Rapidly converted to acyclovir, which becomes incorporated into viral DNA and inhibits viral DNA polymerase, thereby inhibiting viral replication.
Therapeutic effect: Inhibits susceptible viral growth of herpes zoster.

Available forms

Caplets: 500 mg, 1,000 mg

NURSING PROCESS

⚒ Assessment

• Assess patient's infection before starting therapy.
• Assess patient's and family's knowledge of drug therapy.

🔅 Nursing diagnoses

• Risk for infection related to herpes zoster
• Deficient fluid volume related to adverse GI reactions
• Deficient knowledge related to drug therapy

⟩ Planning and implementation

• Although overdose hasn't been reported, precipitation of acyclovir in renal tubules may occur when solubility (2.5 mg/ml) is exceeded in the intratubular fluid. In the event of acute renal failure and anuria, the patient may benefit from hemodialysis until kidney function is restored.
🔔 **ALERT:** Don't confuse valacyclovir (Valtrex) with valganciclovir (Valcyte).
Patient teaching
• Inform patient that drug may be taken with or without food.
• Review signs and symptoms of herpes infection (rash, tingling, itching, and pain), and advise patient to notify prescriber immediately if they occur. Treatment should begin as soon as possible after symptoms appear, preferably within 48 hours.

☑ Evaluation

• Patient is free from infection.
• Patient maintains adequate hydration.
• Patient and family state understanding of drug therapy.

valganciclovir

(val-gan-SYE-kloh-veer)
Valcyte

Pharmacologic class: synthetic nucleoside
Therapeutic class: antiviral
Pregnancy risk category: C

Indications and dosages

▶ **Active CMV retinitis in patients with AIDS.** *Adults:* Induction dose is 900 mg (two 450-mg tablets) P.O. b.i.d. with food for 21 days; maintenance dose is 900 mg P.O. once daily with food.
▶ **Inactive CMV retinitis.** *Adults:* 900 mg P.O. once daily with food.
▶ **Prevention of CMV in kidney, heart, and pancreas-kidney transplants.** *Adults:* 900 mg P.O. daily with food 10 days before through 100 days after transplant.
◪ **Adjust-a-dose:** Patients with renal impairment need adjusted dosage. For creatinine clearance of 40 to 59 ml/minute, 450 mg b.i.d. for induction followed by 450 mg daily for maintenance. For creatinine clearance of 25 to 39 ml/minute, 450 mg daily for induction followed by 450 mg every two days for maintenance. For creatinine clearance of 10 to 24 ml/minute, 450 mg every other day for induction followed by 450 mg twice weekly for maintenance.

Contraindications and cautions

• Contraindicated in patients hypersensitive to valganciclovir or ganciclovir or in liver transplant patients. Safety and effectiveness in the prevention of CMV disease in other solid-organ transplant patients, such as lung transplant patients, haven't been established.
• Don't use in patients receiving hemodialysis.
• Use cautiously in patients with cytopenias and in those who have received immunosuppressants or radiation.
⚘ **Lifespan:** In pregnant women, use only if benefits to the woman outweigh risks to the fetus. In breast-feeding women, use cautiously; it's unknown if drug appears in breast milk. In children, safety and effectiveness haven't been established.

Adverse reactions

CNS: agitation, confusion, hallucinations, *headache, insomnia,* paresthesia, peripheral neuropathy, psychosis, *pyrexia, seizures.*

V

EENT: retinal detachment.
GI: *abdominal pain, diarrhea, nausea, vomiting.*
Hematologic: anemia, *aplastic anemia, bone marrow depression,* NEUTROPENIA, *pancytopenia, thrombocytopenia.*
Other: catheter-related infection, hypersensitivity reactions, local or systemic infections, *sepsis.*

Interactions

Drug-drug. *Didanosine:* May increase absorption of didanosine. Monitor patient closely for didanosine toxicity.
Immunosuppressants, zidovudine: May increase risk of neutropenia, anemia, thrombocytopenia, and bone marrow depression. Monitor CBC.
Mycophenolate mofetil: May increase level of both drugs in renally impaired patients. Use together carefully.
Probenecid: May decrease renal clearance of ganciclovir. Monitor patient for ganciclovir toxicity.
Drug-food. *Any food:* May increase absorption of drug. Give drug with food.

Effects on lab test results

• May increase creatinine level. May decrease hemoglobin level and hematocrit.
• May decrease RBC, WBC, neutrophil, and platelet counts.

Pharmacokinetics

Absorption: Well absorbed from GI tract. Higher when taken with food.
Distribution: Minimally protein-bound.
Metabolism: In intestinal wall and liver to ganciclovir.
Excretion: Renal. *Half-life:* 4 hours.

Route	Onset	Peak	Duration
P.O.	Unknown	1–3 hr	Unknown

Action

Chemical effect: Converted to ganciclovir, which inhibits replication of viral DNA synthesis of CMV.
Therapeutic effect: Inhibits CMV.

Available forms

Tablets: 450 mg

NURSING PROCESS

⚕ Assessment
• Assess patient's condition before starting therapy and regularly thereafter to monitor drug's effectiveness.
• Obtain baseline laboratory studies before starting therapy and reassess regularly.
• Assess patient's and family's knowledge of drug therapy.

Nursing diagnoses
• Risk for imbalanced fluid volume related to adverse GI effects
• Ineffective protection related to adverse hematologic reactions
• Deficient knowledge related to valganciclovir therapy

Planning and implementation
• Adhere to dosage guidelines for valganciclovir because ganciclovir and valganciclovir aren't interchangeable, and overdose may occur.
• Cytopenia may occur at any time during treatment and may increase with continued use. Cell counts usually recover 3 to 7 days after stopping the drug. Monitor patient's CBC closely and frequently throughout therapy.
• No drug interaction studies have been conducted; however, because drug is converted to ganciclovir, drug interactions probably are similar.
• Drug may cause temporary or permanent inhibition of spermatogenesis.
⚠ **ALERT:** Severe leukopenia, neutropenia, anemia, pancytopenia, bone marrow depression, aplastic anemia and thrombocytopenia may occur. If patient's absolute neutrophil count is less than 500/mm^3, platelet count is less than 25,000/mm^3, or hemoglobin level is less than 8 g/dl, don't use the drug.
• Overdose may cause severe or even fatal bone marrow depression and renal toxicity; if overdose occurs, maintain adequate hydration and consider hematopoietic growth factors. Dialysis may be used to reduce level.
⚠ **ALERT:** Don't confuse valganciclovir with valacyclovir or Valcyte with Valtrex.
Patient teaching
• Instruct women of childbearing age to use contraception during treatment. Instruct men to use barrier contraception during and for 90 days after treatment.

Reactions may be *common,* uncommon, *life-threatening*, or COMMON AND LIFE-THREATENING.

• Inform patient about infection control and bleeding precautions.
• Tell patient to take drug with food.

☑ Evaluation

• Patient remains well hydrated throughout therapy.
• Patient has no serious adverse hematologic reactions.
• Patient and family state understanding of drug therapy.

valproate sodium
(val-PROH-ayt SOH-dee-um)
Depacon, Depakene

valproic acid
Depakene

divalproex sodium
Depakote✐, Depakote ER, Depakote Sprinkle, Epival ♦

Pharmacologic class: carboxylic acid derivative
Therapeutic class: anticonvulsant
Pregnancy risk category: D

Indications and dosages

▶ **Simple and complex absence seizures, mixed seizure types (including absence seizures).** *Adults and children 10 years of age and older:* Initially, 10 to 15 mg/kg P.O. or I.V. daily; then increase by 5 to 10 mg/kg daily at weekly intervals up to maximum of 60 mg/kg daily. If total dose exceeds 250 mg, divide into two or more doses. Don't use Depakote ER in children younger than age 10.

▶ **Mania.** *Adults:* Initially, 750 mg divalproex sodium (delayed-release) P.O. daily in divided doses. Adjust dosage based on patient's response; maximum dosage is 60 mg/kg daily.

▶ **Prevention of migraine headache.** *Adults:* Initially, 250 mg divalproex sodium (delayed-release) P.O. b.i.d. Some patients may need up to 1,000 mg daily. Or, 500 mg Depakote ER P.O. daily for 1 week; then 1,000 mg P.O. daily.

▶ **Complex partial seizures.** *Adults and children age 10 and older:* 10 to 15 mg/kg P.O. or I.V. daily; then increase by 5 to 10 mg/kg daily at weekly intervals, up to 60 mg/kg daily.

⧉ **Adjust-a-dose:** For elderly patients, use lower initial dose and adjust more slowly.

▼ I.V. administration

• Dilute with at least 50 ml of a compatible diluent (D_5W, saline solution, lactated Ringer's injection).
• Give I.V. over 1 hour. Don't exceed 20 mg/minute.
• Use of I.V. therapy for longer than 14 days hasn't been studied.
⊗ **Incompatibilities**
None reported.

Contraindications and cautions

• Contraindicated in patients hypersensitive to the drug or any of its components and in patients with hepatic dysfunction or urea cycle disorder.
🌣 **Lifespan:** In pregnant and breast-feeding women, drug isn't recommended. In children younger than age 10, safety and effectiveness of Depakote ER haven't been established. In elderly patients, start at lower dose and adjust dosage more slowly.

Adverse reactions

CNS: aggressiveness, ataxia, behavioral deterioration, dizziness, emotional upset, depression, headache, hyperactivity, incoordination, muscle weakness, psychosis, *sedation,* tremor.
EENT: diplopia, nystagmus.
GI: abdominal cramps, anorexia, constipation, diarrhea, increased appetite and weight gain, *indigestion, nausea, pancreatitis, vomiting.*
Hematologic: *bone marrow suppression,* bruising, eosinophilia, *hemorrhage, leukopenia,* petechiae, *thrombocytopenia.*
Hepatic: *hepatotoxicity.*
Skin: alopecia, *erythema multiforme,* photosensitivity reactions, pruritus, rash, *Stevens-Johnson syndrome.*
Other: *flulike syndrome,* infection.

Interactions

Drug-drug. *Aspirin, chlorpromazine, cimetidine, felbamate:* May cause valproic acid toxicity. Use together cautiously and monitor levels.
Benzodiazepines, other CNS depressants: May cause excessive CNS depression. Avoid use together.

V

Carbamazepine: May result in carbamazepine CNS toxicity (acute psychotic reaction). Monitor level carefully.

Cholestyramine: May decrease valproate level. Monitor patient for decreased effect.

Erythromycin: May increase valproate level. Monitor patient for toxicity.

Lamotrigine: May inhibit lamotrigine metabolism. Decrease lamotrigine dosage when valproic acid therapy starts.

Phenobarbital: May increase phenobarbital level. Monitor patient closely.

Phenytoin: May increase or decrease phenytoin level and increase metabolism of valproic acid. Monitor patient closely.

Rifampin: May decrease valproate level. Monitor level.

Warfarin: May displace warfarin from binding sites. Monitor PT and INR.

Drug-herb. *Glutamine:* May increase risk of seizures. Discourage use together.

White willow: May increase risk of adverse effects because herb contains substances similar to aspirin. Discourage use together.

Drug-lifestyle. *Alcohol use:* May cause excessive CNS depression. Discourage use together.

Effects on lab test results

• May increase ALT, AST, and bilirubin levels.
• May increase eosinophil count and bleeding time. May decrease platelet and WBC counts.
• May produce false-positive test results for ketones in urine.

Pharmacokinetics

Absorption: Valproate sodium and divalproex sodium quickly convert to valproic acid, which is then quickly and almost completely absorbed.

Distribution: Throughout body. 80% to 95% protein-bound.

Metabolism: In liver.

Excretion: Mainly in urine; some excreted in feces and exhaled in air. *Half-life:* 6 to 16 hours.

Route	Onset	Peak	Duration
P.O.	Unknown	1–4 hr	Unknown
I.V.	Unknown	Unknown	Unknown

Action

Chemical effect: Unknown; may increase brain level of GABA, which transmits inhibitory nerve impulses in CNS.

Therapeutic effect: Prevents and treats certain types of seizure activity.

Available forms

valproate sodium
Injection: 100 mg/ml
Syrup: 250 mg/5 ml
valproic acid
Capsules: 250 mg
Syrup: 200 mg/5 ml ♦
Tablets (crushable): 100 mg ♦
Tablets (enteric-coated): 200 mg ♦ , 500 mg ♦
divalproex sodium
Capsules (containing coated particles): 125 mg
Tablets (delayed-release): 125 mg, 250 mg, 500 mg
Tablets (extended-release): 500 mg

NURSING PROCESS

⚡ Assessment

• Assess patient's condition before starting therapy and regularly thereafter to monitor drug's effectiveness.
• Monitor drug level; therapeutic level is 50 to 100 mcg/ml.
• Before starting drug and periodically thereafter, monitor liver function studies, platelet counts, and PT.
• Be alert for adverse reactions and drug interactions.
• Assess patient's and family's knowledge of drug therapy.

⊕ Nursing diagnoses

• Risk for trauma related to seizure activity
• Disturbed thought processes related to drug-induced adverse CNS reactions
• Deficient knowledge related to drug therapy

▷ Planning and implementation

• To switch adults and children ages 10 and older taking Depakote for seizures to Depakote ER, give dose of new drug that's 8% to 20% larger than previous drug dose.
• Don't give syrup to patient who needs sodium restriction. Check with prescriber.
• Give drug with food or milk to minimize adverse GI reaction.
• Suddenly stopping the drug may worsen seizures. If adverse reaction develops, call prescriber immediately.

Reactions may be *common*, uncommon, *life-threatening*, or COMMON AND LIFE-THREATENING.

⊛ **ALERT:** Serious or fatal hepatotoxicity may follow nonspecific symptoms, such as malaise, fever, and lethargy. If patient has suspected or apparently substantial hepatic dysfunction, notify prescriber immediately and stop giving the drug.

• Patients at high risk for developing hepatotoxicity include those with congenital metabolic disorders, mental retardation, or organic brain disease; those taking other anticonvulsants; and children younger than age 2.

• Divalproex sodium carries a lower risk of adverse GI effects than other drug forms.

• If tremors occur, notify prescriber. Dosage may need to be reduced.

⊛ **ALERT:** Fatal hyperammonemic encephalopathy may occur in patients with a urea cycle disorder, particularly ornithine transcarbamylase deficiency. Evaluate patients with risk factors for urea cycle disorders before starting therapy. If symptoms of unexplained hyperammonemic encephalopathy occur during therapy, stop drug; give prompt, appropriate treatment; and evaluate for underlying urea cycle disorder.

Patient teaching

• Tell patient that drug may be taken with food or milk to reduce adverse GI effects.

• Instruct patient not to chew capsules and not to crush or chew extended-release tablets.

• Tell patient and parents that syrup shouldn't be mixed with carbonated beverages.

• Tell patient and parents to keep drug out of children's reach.

• Warn patient and parents not to stop drug therapy abruptly.

• Advise patient to refrain from driving or performing other potentially hazardous activities that require mental alertness until drug's CNS effects are known.

☑ **Evaluation**

• Patient is free from seizure activity.

• Patient maintains normal thought processes.

• Patient and family state understanding of drug therapy.

valsartan
(val-SAR-tihn)
Diovan

Pharmacologic class: angiotensin II receptor blocker
Therapeutic class: antihypertensive
Pregnancy risk category: C (D in second and third trimesters)

Indications and dosages

▶ **Hypertension, used alone or with other antihypertensives.** *Adults:* Initially, 80 mg P.O. once daily. Expect a reduction in blood pressure in 2 to 4 weeks. If additional antihypertensive effect is needed, increase dosage to 160 or 320 mg daily, or add a diuretic. (Addition of a diuretic has a greater effect than dose increases above 80 mg.) Usual dosage range is 80 to 320 mg daily.
Children ages 6 to 16: Initially, 1.3 mg/kg P.O. daily, up to 40 mg. Adjust dosage according to patient response up to 2.7 mg/kg or 160 mg.

▶ **Heart failure (New York Heart Association classes II to IV).** *Adults:* Initially, 40 mg P.O. b.i.d. Increase as tolerated to 80 mg b.i.d. Maximum dosage is 160 mg b.i.d. Avoid using with ACE inhibitors or beta blockers.

▶ **To reduce CV death in stable post-MI patients with left ventricular failure or dysfunction.** *Adults:* 20 mg P.O. b.i.d. Initial dose may be given as soon as 12 hours following MI. Increase dosage to 40 mg b.i.d. within 7 days. Increase subsequent doses as tolerated to target dosage of 160 mg b.i.d.

Contraindications and cautions

• Contraindicated in patients hypersensitive to the drug or any of its components.

• Use cautiously in patients with severe renal or hepatic disease.

⚕ **Lifespan:** In pregnant women, drugs that act directly on the renin-angiotensin system can cause injury and even death to the developing fetus. When pregnancy is verified, drug should be stopped immediately. In children, drug isn't recommended for children younger than age 6 years, or for children with a glomerular filtration rate of less than 30 ml/minute/1.73 m².

V

Adverse reactions

CNS: *dizziness,* fatigue, headache, insomnia, vertigo.
CV: edema, hypotension, postural hypotension, syncope.
EENT: blurred vision, pharyngitis, rhinitis, sinusitis.
GI: abdominal pain, diarrhea, dyspepsia, nausea.
GU: renal impairment.
Hematologic: *neutropenia.*
Metabolic: *hyperkalemia.*
Musculoskeletal: arthralgia, back pain.
Respiratory: cough, upper respiratory tract infection.
Other: *angioedema,* viral infection.

Interactions

Drug-drug. *Other angiotensin II blockers, potassium-sparing diuretics, potassium supplements:* May increase potassium level. Avoid use together.
Drug-food. *Salt substitutes containing potassium:* May increase potassium level. In heart failure patients, may also increase creatinine level. Discourage use together.

Effects on lab test results

• May increase potassium level.
• May decrease neutrophil count.

Pharmacokinetics

Absorption: Bioavailability about 25%; food decreases absorption.
Distribution: Not extensive. 95% protein-bound.
Metabolism: In liver and kidneys.
Excretion: In urine and feces. *Half-life:* 6 hours.

Route	Onset	Peak	Duration
P.O.	< 2 hr	2–4 hr	24 hr

Action

Chemical effect: Blocks binding of angiotensin II to receptor sites in vascular smooth muscle and adrenal gland.
Therapeutic effect: Inhibits pressor effects of renin-angiotensin system.

Available forms

Tablets: 40 mg, 80 mg, 160 mg, 320 mg

NURSING PROCESS

Assessment
• Monitor patient for hypotension. Correct volume and sodium depletions before starting drug.
• Assess patient's and family's knowledge of drug therapy.

Nursing diagnoses
• Risk for injury related to presence of hypertension
• Deficient knowledge related to drug therapy

Planning and implementation
• Drug can be given with or without food.
• Request that the pharmacist prepare a suspension for children unable to swallow pills. Shake suspension at least 10 seconds before pouring.
• Suspension has greater availability than tablets and may require dosage adjustment if switched to tablets.
Patient teaching
• Tell woman to notify prescriber if she becomes pregnant.
• Teach patient other means of reducing blood pressure, including proper diet, exercise, smoking cessation, and stress reduction.

Evaluation
• Patient's blood pressure becomes normal.
• Patient and family state understanding of drug therapy.

vancomycin hydrochloride
(van-koh-MY-sin hy-droh-KLOR-ighd)
Vancocin, Vancoled

Pharmacologic class: glycopeptide
Therapeutic class: antibiotic
Pregnancy risk category: C (B for pulvules)

Indications and dosages

▶ **Severe staphylococcal infections when other antibiotics are ineffective or contraindicated.** *Adults:* 500 mg I.V. over 1 hour, every 6 hours, or 1 g every 12 hours.
Children: 40 mg/kg I.V. over 1 hour, daily in divided doses every 6 hours.
Neonates: Initially, 15 mg/kg; then 10 mg/kg I.V. daily, divided every 12 hours for first week

Reactions may be *common*, uncommon, *life-threatening*, or COMMON AND LIFE-THREATENING.

after birth; then every 8 hours up to age
1 month.

▶ **Endocarditis prophylaxis for dental proce-dures.** *Adults:* 1 g I.V. slowly over 1 hour, start-ing 1 hour before procedure.
Children: 20 mg/kg I.V. over 1 hour, starting
1 hour before procedure.
⬚ **Adjust-a-dose:** For patients with renal impair-ment, adjust I.V. dosage.

▶ **Antibiotic-related pseudomembranous and staphylococcal enterocolitis.** *Adults:* 125 to
500 mg P.O. every 6 hours for 7 to 10 days.
Children: 40 mg/kg P.O. daily in divided doses
every 6 to 8 hours for 7 to 10 days. Maximum,
2 g daily.

▼▼ I.V. administration

• Dilute in 200 ml of saline solution injection or
D_5W.
• Infuse over 60 minutes.
• Check site daily for phlebitis and irritation.
Watch for irritation and infiltration; extravasa-tion can cause tissue damage and necrosis.
• If red-man syndrome occurs because drug is
infused too rapidly, stop infusion and report to
prescriber.
• Refrigerate I.V. solution after reconstitution,
and use within 96 hours.
⊗ **Incompatibilities**
Albumin, alkaline solutions, aminophylline,
amobarbital, amphotericin B, aztreonam, cepha-losporins, chloramphenicol, chlorothiazide, cor-ticosteroids, dexamethasone sodium phosphate,
foscarnet, heavy metals, heparin, hydrocorti-sone, idarubicin, methotrexate, nafcillin, peni-cillin G potassium, pentobarbital, phenobarbital,
phenytoin, piperacillin, piperacillin sodium-tazobactam sodium, sargramostim, sodium bi-carbonate, ticarcillin disodium, ticarcillin di-sodium and clavulanate potassium, vitamin B
complex with C, warfarin.

Contraindications and cautions

• Contraindicated in patients hypersensitive to
the drug or any of its components.
• Use cautiously in patients receiving other neu-rotoxic, nephrotoxic, or ototoxic drugs; patients
older than age 60; and those with impaired liver
or kidney function, hearing loss, or allergies to
other antibiotics.
⚘ **Lifespan:** In pregnant women, use cautious-ly. In breast-feeding women, safety and effec-tiveness haven't been established.

Adverse reactions

CNS: fever, pain.
CV: hypotension.
EENT: ototoxicity, tinnitus.
GI: nausea, *pseudomembranous colitis.*
GU: *nephrotoxicity.*
Hematologic: eosinophilia, *leukopenia.*
Respiratory: dyspnea, wheezing.
Skin: red-man syndrome (maculopapular rash
on face, neck, trunk, and limbs with rapid I.V.
infusion; pruritus and hypotension with hista-mine release).
Other: *anaphylaxis,* chills, superinfection,
thrombophlebitis at injection site.

Interactions

Drug-drug. *Aminoglycosides, amphotericin B,
cisplatin, pentamidine:* May increase risk of
nephrotoxicity and ototoxicity. Monitor patient
closely.

Effects on lab test results

• May increase BUN and creatinine levels.
• May increase eosinophil count. May decrease
neutrophil and WBC counts.

Pharmacokinetics

Absorption: Minimal systemic absorption with
P.O. use. (Drug may accumulate in patients with
colitis or renal failure.)
Distribution: In body fluids. Achieves thera-peutic level in CSF if meninges inflamed.
Metabolism: Unknown.
Excretion: In urine with parenteral use; in feces
with P.O. use. *Half-life:* 6 hours.

Route	Onset	Peak	Duration
P.O.	Unknown	Unknown	Unknown
I.V.	Immediate	Immediate	Unknown

Action

Chemical effect: Hinders bacterial cell wall
synthesis, damaging bacterial plasma membrane
and making cell more vulnerable to osmotic
pressure.
Therapeutic effect: Kills susceptible bacteria.

Available forms

Powder for injection: 500-mg, 1-g vials
Powder for oral solution: 1-g, 10-g bottles
Pulvules: 125 mg, 250 mg

V

NURSING PROCESS

⚖ Assessment
● Assess patient's infection before starting therapy and regularly thereafter to monitor drug's effectiveness.
● Obtain urine specimen for culture and sensitivity tests before giving first dose. Start therapy pending test results.
● Obtain hearing evaluation and kidney function studies before starting therapy, and repeat during therapy.
● Check level regularly, especially in elderly patients, premature infants, and those with decreased renal function.
● Be alert for adverse reactions and drug interactions.
● Assess patient's and family's knowledge of drug therapy.

⊕ Nursing diagnoses
● Risk for infection related to presence of susceptible bacteria
● Risk for injury related to drug-induced adverse reactions
● Deficient knowledge related to drug therapy

▷ Planning and implementation
● In patient with renal dysfunction, use a lower dose.
● **ALERT:** Oral administration is ineffective for systemic infections, and I.V. administration is ineffective for pseudomembranous (*Clostridium difficile*) diarrhea.
● Oral form is stable for 2 weeks when refrigerated.
● Don't give drug I.M.
● When using drug to treat staphylococcal endocarditis, give for at least 4 weeks.
Patient teaching
● Tell patient to take entire amount of drug exactly as directed, even after he feels better.
● Tell patient to stop taking the drug and immediately report any adverse reactions, especially ringing in ears or fullness.

✓ Evaluation
● Patient is free from infection.
● Patient doesn't experience injury from adverse reactions.
● Patient and family state understanding of drug therapy.

vardenafil hydrochloride
(var-DEN-ah-phill high-droh-KLOR-ighd)
Levitra⊘

Pharmacologic class: selective inhibitor of cyclic guanosine monophosphate (cGMP)–specific phosphodiesterase type 5 (PDE5)
Therapeutic class: erectile dysfunction drug
Pregnancy risk category: B

Indications and dosages

▶ **Erectile dysfunction.** *Men:* 10 mg P.O. p.r.n., 1 hour before sexual activity. Dose range is 5 to 20 mg based on effectiveness and tolerance. Maximum, 1 dose daily.
Men age 65 and older: Initial dose is 5 mg P.O. p.r.n., 1 hour before sexual activity. Maximum, 1 dose daily.
⊠ **Adjust-a-dose:** For patients with moderate hepatic impairment (Child-Pugh class B), initial dose is 5 mg daily, p.r.n., not to exceed 10 mg daily. Patients taking ritonavir shouldn't exceed 2.5 mg in a 72-hour period. Patients taking itraconazole 400 mg daily or ketoconazole 400 mg daily shouldn't exceed 2.5 mg daily. Patients taking erythromycin, itraconazole 200 mg daily, or ketoconazole 200 mg daily shouldn't exceed 5 mg daily.

Contraindications and cautions

● Contraindicated in patients hypersensitive to the drug or any of its components and in those taking nitrates or alpha blockers.
● Use cautiously in patients with unstable angina; hypotension (systolic pressure lower than 90 mm Hg); uncontrolled hypertension (blood pressure higher than 170/110 mm Hg); stroke, life-threatening arrhythmia, or MI within past 6 months; severe cardiac failure; severe hepatic impairment (Child-Pugh class C); end-stage renal disease requiring dialysis; hereditary degenerative retinal disorders; hepatic or renal dysfunction; anatomical deformation of the penis; or prolonged QT interval. Also use cautiously in patients taking Class IA or Class III antiarrhythmics and in those with conditions that predispose them to priapism (sickle cell anemia, multiple myeloma, or leukemia).
⚖ Lifespan: Only indicated for men. Men age 65 and older have reduced drug clearance.

Adverse reactions

CNS: dizziness, *headache.*
CV: *flushing.*
EENT: decrease or loss of hearing, rhinitis, sinusitis, tinnitus, visual changes.
GI: dyspepsia, nausea.
Musculoskeletal: back pain.
Other: flulike syndrome.

Interactions

Drug-drug. *Alpha blockers:* May increase hypotensive effects. Don't use together.
Erythromycin, itraconazole 200 mg daily, ketoconazole 200 mg daily: May increase vardenafil level. Don't exceed 5 mg daily.
Itraconazole 400 mg daily, ketoconazole 400 mg daily: May increase vardenafil level. Don't exceed 2.5 mg daily.
Nitrates: May increase hypotensive effects. Don't use together.
Ritonavir: May increase vardenafil level. Don't exceed 2.5 mg in a 72-hour period.
Drug-food. *High-fat meals:* May decrease peak level of drug. Advise patient to take on an empty stomach.

Effects on lab test results

• May increase CK level.

Pharmacokinetics

Absorption: Rapid. Absolute bioavailability is 15%.
Distribution: Both drug and its major active metabolite are 95% protein-bound. Protein-binding is reversible and independent of drug level.
Metabolism: Mainly through CYP3A4, along with CYP3A5 and CYP2C isoenzymes. N-demethylation converts drug into the major metabolite, which accounts for 7% of drug.
Excretion: Mainly in feces. *Half-life:* 4 to 5 hours.

Route	Onset	Peak	Duration
P.O.	Immediate	30 min–2 hr	Unknown

Action

Chemical effect: Selectively inhibits cGMP-specific PDE5 and prevents the breakdown of cGMP by phosphodiesterase, leading to increased cGMP level and prolonged smooth muscle relaxation promoting the flow of blood into the corpus cavernosum.

Therapeutic effect: Stimulates penile erection.

Available forms

Tablets: 2.5 mg, 5 mg, 10 mg, 20 mg

NURSING PROCESS

Assessment
• Assess patient's erectile dysfunction before starting therapy and regularly thereafter to monitor drug's effectiveness.
• Be alert for adverse reactions and drug interactions.
• Assess patient's and family's knowledge of drug therapy.

Nursing diagnoses
• Sexual dysfunction related to process of erectile dysfunction
• Chronic low self-esteem related to erectile dysfunction
• Deficient knowledge related to drug therapy

Planning and implementation
ALERT: Because of cardiac risk during sexual activity, drug increases risk for patients with underlying CV disease.
Patient teaching
• Tell patient that drug doesn't protect against sexually transmitted diseases and that he should use protective measures to prevent infection.
• Advise patient that drug is most rapidly absorbed if taken on an empty stomach.
• Tell patient to notify prescriber of visual or auditory changes.
• Instruct patient to seek medical attention if erection persists for longer than 4 hours because of risk of permanent erectile dysfunction.
• Tell patient to take drug 60 minutes before anticipated sexual activity. The drug will have no effect in the absence of sexual stimulation.
• Tell patient not to take drug more than once per day.

Evaluation
• Patient reports improvement in sexual functioning.
• Patient demonstrates increased self-esteem.
• Patient and family state understanding of drug therapy.

varenicline tartrate
(vah-RENN-ih-kleen TAR-trayt)
Chantix✒

Pharmacologic class: nicotinic acetylcholine receptor partial agonist
Therapeutic class: smoking cessation aid
Pregnancy risk category: C

Indications and dosages

▶ **Smoking cessation.** *Adults:* Starting 1 week before patient plans to stop smoking, give 0.5 mg P.O. once daily on days 1 through 3. Days 4 through 7, give 0.5 mg P.O. b.i.d. Day 8 through the end of week 12, give 1 mg P.O. b.i.d. If patient successfully stops smoking, give an additional 12-week course of treatment to increase the likelihood of long-term success.
⊠ **Adjust-a-dose:** If patient has severe renal impairment, 0.5 mg P.O. once daily. Adjust as needed to maximum of 0.5 mg b.i.d. If patient has end-stage renal disease and is undergoing dialysis, 0.5 mg once daily.

Contraindications and cautions

• Use cautiously in patients with severe renal impairment.
⚖ **Lifespan:** In pregnant or breast-feeding women, use cautiously. In children, safety and effectiveness haven't been established. In elderly patients, use cautiously.

Adverse reactions

CNS: *abnormal dreams,* altered attention or emotions, anxiety, asthenia, depression, dizziness, fatigue, *headache, insomnia,* irritability, lethargy, malaise, nightmares, restlessness, sensory disturbance, sleep disorder, somnolence.
CV: chest pain, edema, hot flush, hypertension.
EENT: altered taste, epistaxis.
GI: abdominal pain, constipation, diarrhea, dry mouth, dyspepsia, flatulence, gingivitis, *nausea,* vomiting.
GU: menstrual disorder, polyuria.
Metabolic: decreased appetite, increased appetite, thirst.
Musculoskeletal: arthralgia, back pain, muscle cramps, myalgia.
Respiratory: dyspnea, upper respiratory tract disorder.

Skin: rash.
Other: flulike syndrome.

Interactions

Drug-drug. *Nicotine replacement therapy:* May increase nausea, vomiting, dizziness, dyspepsia, and fatigue. Monitor patient closely.

Effects on lab test results

• May increase liver function test values.

Pharmacokinetics

Absorption: Virtually complete after oral use with high systemic availability.
Distribution: Less than 20% bound to plasma proteins.
Metabolism: Minimal.
Excretion: Via the kidneys, mainly through glomerular filtration and active tubular secretion. *Half-life:* 24 hours.

Route	Onset	Peak	Duration
P.O.	4 days	3–4 hr	24 hr

Action

Chemical effect: Blocks the effects of nicotine by binding with high affinity and selectivity at $alpha_4beta_2$ neuronal nicotinic acetylcholine receptors. Drug also provides some of nicotine's effects to ease withdrawal symptoms.
Therapeutic effect: Helps patient quit smoking.

Available forms

Tablets: 0.5 mg, 1 mg

NURSING PROCESS

🔍 **Assessment**
• Assess patient's readiness and motivation to stop smoking.
• Be alert for adverse reactions.
⚠ **ALERT:** Monitor patient for behavior and mood changes including agitation, depression, suicidal ideation, and worsening of pre-existing psychological disorders.
• Assess patient's and family's knowledge of drug therapy.

⚙ **Nursing diagnoses**
• Risk for injury related to smoking habit
• Noncompliance related to drug-induced nausea
• Deficient knowledge related to drug therapy

Reactions may be *common,* uncommon, *life-threatening*, or COMMON AND LIFE-THREATENING.

⋙ Planning and implementation
• Patients who develop intolerable nausea may need dosage reduction.
• Because smoking affects the action of certain drugs—such as theophylline, warfarin, and insulin—these drug levels may need temporary monitoring after patient stops smoking. Dosage adjustment may be needed.

Patient teaching
• Provide patient with educational materials and needed counseling.
• Instruct patient to choose a date to stop smoking and to begin treatment 1 week before this date.
• Tell patient to use caution when driving or operating machinery until effects of drug are known.
• Instruct patient and his family to contact prescriber if behavior or mood changes occur.
• Advise patient to take each dose with a full glass of water after eating.
• Teach patient to gradually increase the dosage over the first week to a target of 1 mg in the morning and 1 mg in the evening.
• Explain that nausea and insomnia are common and usually temporary. Urge him to contact the prescriber if adverse effects are persistently troubling; a dosage reduction may help.
• Urge patient to continue trying to abstain from smoking if he has early lapses after successfully quitting.
• Tell patient that dosages of other drugs he takes may need adjustment when he stops smoking.
• If woman plans to become pregnant or to breast-feed, explain the risks of smoking and the risks and benefits of taking this drug to aid smoking cessation.

☑ Evaluation
• Patient remains free of injury.
• Patient remains compliant with drug therapy.
• Patient and family state understanding of drug therapy.

vasopressin (ADH)
(VAY-soh-preh-sin)
Pitressin

Pharmacologic class: posterior pituitary hormone
Therapeutic class: ADH, peristaltic stimulant
Pregnancy risk category: C

Indications and dosages

▶ **Neurogenic diabetes insipidus.** *Adults:* 5 to 10 units I.M. or subcutaneously b.i.d. to q.i.d., p.r.n. Range 5 to 60 units daily. Or, intranasally (aqueous solution used as spray or applied to cotton balls) in individualized doses, based on response.
Children: 2.5 to 10 units I.M. or subcutaneously b.i.d. to q.i.d., p.r.n. Or, intranasally (aqueous solution used as spray or applied to cotton balls) in individualized doses.
▶ **Postoperative abdominal distention.**
Adults: Initially, 5 units (aqueous) I.M.; then every 3 to 4 hours, increasing dose to 10 units, if needed. Reduce dosage proportionately for children.
▶ **To expel gas before abdominal X-ray.**
Adults: 10 units subcutaneously 2 hours before X-ray; then again 30 minutes later.
▶ **Provocative testing for growth hormone and corticotropin release‡.** *Adults:* 10 units I.M.
Children: 0.3 units/kg I.M.
▶ **GI hemorrhage‡.** *Adults:* 0.2 to 0.4 units/minute I.V. Increase up to 0.9 units/minute if needed. Or, 0.1 to 0.5 units/minute intra-arterially.
▶ **Pulseless arrest (ventricular fibrillation, rapid ventricular tachycardia, asystole, pulseless electrical activity)‡.** *Adults:* 40 units I.V. as a single one-time dose.

▽ I.V. administration
• Drug is used I.V. for GI hemorrhage and pulseless arrest only.
• For GI hemorrhage, dilute with normal saline solution or D_5W to 0.1 to 1 unit/ml.
• For pulseless arrest, give as bolus during advanced cardiac life support (ACLS).
⊗ **Incompatibilities**
None reported.

V

Contraindications and cautions

● Contraindicated in patients with chronic nephritis accompanied by nitrogen retention.

● Use cautiously in preoperative and postoperative polyuric patients and those with seizure disorders, migraine headache, asthma, CV disease, heart failure, renal disease, goiter with cardiac complications, arteriosclerosis, or fluid overload.

⚜ **Lifespan:** In pregnant women, use cautiously. In breast-feeding women, use cautiously; it's unknown if the drug appears in breast milk. In children and elderly patients, use cautiously.

Adverse reactions

CNS: headache, tremor, vertigo.
CV: angina in patients with vascular disease, *arrhythmias,* circumoral pallor, vasoconstriction, decreased cardiac output, *myocardial ischemia, cardiac arrest.*
GI: abdominal cramps, flatulence, nausea, vomiting.
Skin: cutaneous gangrene, diaphoresis.
Other: hypersensitivity reactions (*anaphylaxis, angioedema, bronchoconstriction,* urticaria), water intoxication (*coma,* confusion, drowsiness, headache, listlessness, *seizures,* weight gain).

Interactions

Drug-drug. *Carbamazepine, chlorpropamide, clofibrate, fludrocortisone, tricyclic antidepressants:* May increase antidiuretic response. Use together cautiously.
Demeclocycline, heparin, lithium, norepinephrine: May decrease antidiuretic activity. Use together cautiously.
Drug-lifestyle. *Alcohol use:* May decrease antidiuretic activity. Discourage use together.

Effects on lab test results

None reported.

Pharmacokinetics

Absorption: Unknown.
Distribution: Throughout extracellular fluid without evidence of protein-binding.
Metabolism: Most of drug is destroyed rapidly in liver and kidneys.
Excretion: In urine. *Half-life:* 10 to 20 minutes.

Route	Onset	Peak	Duration
I.V	Unknown	Unknown	Unknown
I.M., SubQ, intranasal	Unknown	Unknown	2–8 hr

Action

Chemical effect: Increases permeability of renal tubular epithelium to adenosine monophosphate and water; epithelium promotes reabsorption of water and produces concentrated urine (ADH effect).
Therapeutic effect: Promotes water reabsorption and stimulates GI motility.

Available forms

Injection: 0.5-, 1-, and 10-ml ampules (20 units/ml)

NURSING PROCESS

⚟ Assessment

● Assess patient's condition before starting therapy and regularly thereafter to monitor drug's effectiveness.

● Monitor specific gravity of urine, and fluid intake and output, to aid evaluation of drug effectiveness.

● To prevent possible seizures, coma, and death, observe patient closely for early signs of water intoxication.

● Monitor patient's blood pressure often; watch for hypertension or lack of response to drug, which may be indicated by hypotension. Also monitor daily weight.

● Be alert for adverse reactions and drug interactions.

● Assess patient's and family's knowledge of drug therapy.

⊕ Nursing diagnoses

● Risk for deficient fluid volume related to polyuria from diabetes insipidus
● Diarrhea related to drug-induced increased GI motility
● Deficient knowledge related to drug therapy

▷ Planning and implementation

● Drug may be used for transient polyuria resulting from ADH deficiency related to neurosurgery or head injury.

● To reduce adverse reactions, use minimum effective dosage.

Reactions may be *common,* uncommon, *life-threatening,* or COMMON AND LIFE-THREATENING.

• Give drug with one to two glasses of water to reduce adverse reactions and improve therapeutic response.
• A rectal tube facilitates gas expulsion after vasopressin injection.
⊛ **ALERT:** Never inject during first stage of labor; doing so may cause uterus to rupture.
• Aqueous solution can be used as a nasal spray or it can be applied to cotton balls. Follow the manufacturer's guidelines for intranasal use.
⊛ **ALERT:** Don't confuse vasopressin with desmopressin.
Patient teaching
• Instruct patient how to give drug. Tell patient taking drug subcutaneously to rotate injection sites to prevent tissue damage.
• Stress importance of monitoring fluid intake and output.
• Tell patient to immediately notify prescriber if an adverse reaction occurs.

☑ **Evaluation**
• Patient maintains adequate hydration.
• Patient has no diarrhea.
• Patient and family state understanding of drug therapy.

HIGH ALERT

vecuronium bromide
(veh-kyoo-ROH-nee-um BROH-mighd)

Pharmacologic class: nondepolarizing neuromuscular blocker
Therapeutic class: skeletal muscle relaxant
Pregnancy risk category: C

Indications and dosages

▶ **Adjunct to general anesthesia; to facilitate endotracheal intubation; to provide skeletal muscle relaxation during surgery or mechanical ventilation. Dosage depends on anesthetic used, individual needs, and response. Dosages are representative and must be adjusted.** *Adults and children age 10 and older:* Initially, 0.08 to 0.1 mg/kg I.V. bolus. During prolonged surgery, may give maintenance doses of 0.01 to 0.015 mg/kg within 25 to 40 minutes of initial dose. Maintenance doses may be given every 12 to 15 minutes in patients receiving balanced anesthesia. Or, drug may be given by continuous I.V. infusion of 1 mcg/kg/minute initially, then 0.8 to 1.2 mcg/kg/minute.

Children younger than age 10: May require slightly higher initial dose as well as supplementation slightly more often than adults.

▼ I.V. administration

• Give drug by rapid I.V. injection. Or, 10 to 20 mg may be added to 100 ml of compatible solution and given by I.V. infusion.
• Compatible solutions include D_5W, normal saline solution for injection, dextrose 5% in normal saline solution for injection, and lactated Ringer's injection.
• Store reconstituted solution in refrigerator. Discard after 24 hours.
⊗ **Incompatibilities**
Alkaline solutions, amphotericin B, diazepam, furosemide, thiopental.

Contraindications and cautions

• Contraindicated in patients hypersensitive to bromides.
• Use cautiously in patients with altered circulation caused by CV disease and edematous states and in patients with hepatic disease, severe obesity, bronchogenic carcinoma, electrolyte disturbances, or neuromuscular disease.
⚘ **Lifespan:** In pregnant woman, use cautiously. In breast-feeding women, use cautiously; it's unknown if the drug appears in breast milk. In the elderly, use cautiously.

Adverse reactions

Musculoskeletal: skeletal muscle weakness, prolonged paralysis.
Respiratory: *apnea, respiratory insufficiency.*

Interactions

Drug-drug. *Amikacin, gentamicin, neomycin, streptomycin, tobramycin:* May increase the effects of nondepolarizing muscle relaxant, including prolonged respiratory depression. Use together only if necessary. May need to reduce dosage of nondepolarizing muscle relaxant.
Bacitracin; clindamycin; general anesthetics, such as enflurane, halothane, isoflurane; kanamycin; other skeletal muscle relaxants; polymyxin antibiotics, such as colistin, polymyxin B sulfate; quinidine; tetracyclines: May potentiate neuromuscular blockade, leading to increased skeletal muscle relaxation and potentiation of effect. Use cautiously during surgical and postoperative periods.

V

Carbamazepine, phenytoin: May decrease the effects of vecuronium. May need to increase dosage of the vecuronium.

Effects on lab test results

None reported.

Pharmacokinetics

Absorption: Given I.V.
Distribution: In extracellular fluid; rapidly reaches its site of action (skeletal muscles). 60% to 90% protein-bound.
Metabolism: Hepatic; rapid and extensive.
Excretion: In feces and urine. *Half-life:* 20 minutes.

Route	Onset	Peak	Duration
I.V.	≤ 1 min	3–5 min	25–30 min

Action

Chemical effect: Prevents acetylcholine from binding to receptors on motor end plate, thus blocking depolarization.
Therapeutic effect: Relaxes skeletal muscle.

Available forms

Injection: 10-mg vial, 20-mg vial

NURSING PROCESS

📖 Assessment

• Assess patient's condition before starting therapy and regularly thereafter to monitor drug's effectiveness.
• Monitor respiratory rate closely until patient is fully recovered from neuromuscular blockade as evidenced by tests of muscle strength (hand grip, head lift, and ability to cough).
• Be alert for adverse reactions and drug interactions.
• Assess patient's and family's knowledge of drug therapy.

🔄 Nursing diagnoses

• Ineffective health maintenance related to underlying condition
• Ineffective breathing pattern related to drug's effect on respiratory muscles
• Deficient knowledge related to drug therapy

▶ Planning and implementation

• Keep airway clear. Have emergency respiratory support equipment available immediately.

• Drug should be used only by personnel skilled in airway management.
• Previous administration of succinylcholine may enhance neuromuscular blocking effect and duration of action.
• Give sedatives or general anesthetics before neuromuscular blockers. Neuromuscular blockers don't obtund consciousness or alter pain threshold.
• Give analgesics for pain.
• Nerve stimulator and train-of-four monitoring are recommended to confirm antagonism of neuromuscular blockade and recovery of muscle strength. Before attempting pharmacologic reversal with neostigmine, some evidence of spontaneous recovery should be seen.
⑤ **ALERT:** Careful dose calculation is essential. Always verify with another health care professional.
• Don't give by I.M. injection.
Patient teaching
• Explain all events and happenings to patient because he can still hear.
• Reassure patient that he is being monitored at all times.

☑ Evaluation

• Patient responds well to drug.
• Patient maintains effective breathing pattern with mechanical assistance.
• Patient and family state understanding of drug therapy.

venlafaxine hydrochloride
(ven-leh-FAKS-een high-droh-KLOR-ighd)
Effexor, Effexor XR*

Pharmacologic class: dopamine, neuronal serotonin, and norepinephrine reuptake inhibitor
Therapeutic class: antidepressant
Pregnancy risk category: C

Indications and dosages

▶ **Depression.** *Adults:* Initially, 75 mg P.O. daily in two or three divided doses, or 75 mg (extended-release) P.O. once daily with food. With both forms, increase dosage as tolerated and needed in increments of 75 mg daily at intervals of no less than 4 days. For moderately depressed outpatients, usual maximum dosage is

---

225 mg daily; in certain severely depressed patients, dosage may be as high as 350 mg daily.

▶ **Generalized or social anxiety disorder.** *Adults:* 75 mg extended-release capsules P.O. once daily. May increase as needed in increments of 75 mg daily at intervals of no less than 4 days to maximum of 225 mg daily.

▶ **Prevention of major depressive disorder relapse‡.** *Adults:* 100 to 200 mg P.O. daily, or 75 to 225 mg (extended-release) P.O. daily.

▶ **Panic disorder.** *Adults:* Initially, 37.5 mg (extended-release) P.O. daily for 1 week. Then, increase dose to 75 mg daily. If no response, increase by up to 75 mg daily in no less than weekly intervals, as needed, to a maximum dosage of 225 mg daily.

☐ **Adjust-a-dose:** For patients with hepatic impairment, reduce total daily dosage by one-half.

For patients with mild to moderate renal impairment (GFR of 10 to 70 ml/minute), reduce total daily dosage by one-quarter to one-half. In patients undergoing hemodialysis, don't give the dose until dialysis session is completed; reduce daily dosage by one-half.

Contraindications and cautions

• Contraindicated in patients hypersensitive to the drug or any of its components and in those who took an MAO inhibitor within 14 days.
• Use cautiously in patients with renal impairment or diseases, in those with conditions that could affect hemodynamic responses or metabolism, and in those with a history of mania or seizures.

⚜ **Lifespan:** In pregnant women, use cautiously. In breast-feeding women, use cautiously; it's unknown if the drug appears in breast milk. In children, safety and effectiveness haven't been established.

Adverse reactions

CNS: abnormal dreams, agitation, anxiety, *asthenia, dizziness, headache,* insomnia, *nervousness,* paresthesia, *somnolence,* tremor.
CV: hypertension.
EENT: blurred vision.
GI: *anorexia, constipation,* diarrhea, *dry mouth,* dyspepsia, flatulence, *nausea,* vomiting.
GU: *abnormal ejaculation,* impaired urination, impotence, urinary frequency.
Metabolic: weight loss.
Skin: rash, *diaphoresis.*
Other: chills, infection, yawning.

Interactions

Drug-drug. *Haloperidol:* May increase haloperidol level. Use together cautiously.
Phenelzine, selegiline, tranylcypromine: May cause serotonin syndrome, which includes CNS irritability, shivering, and altered consciousness. Don't give together. Wait at least 2 weeks after stopping an MAO inhibitor before giving any SSRI.
Trazodone: May cause serotonin syndrome. Avoid use together.
Drug-herb. *St. John's wort:* May increase sedative-hypnotic effects. Discourage use together.
Yohimbe: May cause additive stimulation. Discourage use together.

Effects on lab test results

• May increase serum cholesterol level.
• May decrease serum sodium level.

Pharmacokinetics

Absorption: About 92%.
Distribution: About 25% to 29% bound to plasma proteins.
Metabolism: Extensive in liver.
Excretion: In urine. *Half-life:* 5 hours.

Route	Onset	Peak	Duration
P.O.	Unknown	Unknown	Unknown

Action

Chemical effect: Blocks reuptake of norepinephrine and serotonin into neurons in CNS.
Therapeutic effect: Relieves depression.

Available forms

Capsules (extended-release): 37.5 mg, 75 mg, 150 mg
Tablets: 25 mg, 37.5 mg, 50 mg, 75 mg, 100 mg

NURSING PROCESS

℞ Assessment

• Assess patient's depression before starting therapy and regularly thereafter to monitor drug's effectiveness.
• Carefully monitor blood pressure. Drug is linked to sustained, dose-dependent increases in blood pressure. Greatest increases, averaging about 7 mm Hg above baseline, occur in patients taking 375 mg daily.

V

- Be alert for adverse reactions and drug interactions.
- Assess patient's and family's knowledge of drug therapy.

⊕ Nursing diagnoses
- Disturbed thought processes related to presence of depression
- Risk for injury related to drug-induced adverse CNS reactions
- Deficient knowledge related to drug therapy

▶ Planning and implementation
- Give drug with food.
- ⑤ **ALERT:** If given for 6 weeks or longer, don't abruptly stop giving the drug; taper dosage over a 2-week period.
- ⑤ **ALERT:** Drug may increase the risk for suicidal thinking and behavior in young adults ages 18 to 24 during the first 2 months of treatment.
- Closely monitor patients being treated for depression for signs and symptoms of worsening condition and suicidal ideation, especially when therapy starts or dosage is adjusted. Symptoms may include agitation, insomnia, anxiety, aggressiveness, and panic attacks.

Patient teaching
- Instruct patient to take drug with food.
- Warn patient to avoid hazardous activities until the drug's CNS effects are known.
- Caution woman not to become pregnant during treatment. Neonates exposed to drug late in the third trimester have developed complications requiring prolonged hospitalization, respiratory support, and tube feeding, possibly related to serotonin syndrome.
- Tell patient it may take several weeks before the full antidepressant effect is seen.
- Tell patient not to drink alcohol while taking drug and to notify prescriber before taking other medications, including OTC preparations, because of possible interactions.
- Instruct patient to notify prescriber if adverse reaction occurs.
- Urge family members to closely monitor the patient for signs of worsening condition and suicidal ideation.

☑ Evaluation
- Patient's behavior and communication show improved thought processes.
- Patient sustains no injury from adverse CNS reactions.

- Patient and family state understanding of drug therapy.

HIGH ALERT

verapamil hydrochloride
(veh-RAP-uh-mil high-droh-KLOR-ighd)
Apo-Verap ♦ , Calan⌀, Calan SR, Covera-HS, Isoptin SR, Novo-Veramil ♦ , Nu-Verap ♦ , Verelan, Verelan PM

Pharmacologic class: calcium channel blocker
Therapeutic class: antianginal, antiarrhythmic, antihypertensive
Pregnancy risk category: C

Indications and dosages

▶ **Vasospastic angina; classic chronic, stable angina pectoris; unstable angina; chronic atrial fibrillation.** *Adults:* Starting dose is 80 mg P.O. every 6 to 8 hours. Increase at weekly intervals, as needed. Some patients may need up to 480 mg daily. Or, 180 mg Covera-HS P.O. at bedtime; maximum, 480 mg P.O. daily at bedtime.

▶ **Supraventricular arrhythmias.** *Adults:* 0.075 to 0.15 mg/kg (5 to 10 mg) by I.V. push over 2 minutes with ECG and blood pressure monitoring. If no response occurs, give a second dose of 10 mg (0.15 mg/kg) 30 minutes after the initial dose.
Children ages 1 to 15: Give 0.1 to 0.3 mg/kg as I.V. bolus over 2 minutes. If no response, repeat in 30 minutes.
Children younger than age 1: Give 0.1 to 0.2 mg/kg as I.V. bolus over at least 2 minutes with continuous ECG monitoring. If no response, repeat in 30 minutes.

▶ **To prevent recurrent paroxysmal supraventricular tachycardia.** *Adults:* 240 to 480 mg P.O. daily in three or four divided doses.

▶ **To control ventricular rate in digitalized patients with chronic atrial flutter or atrial fibrillation.** *Adults:* 240 to 320 mg P.O. in three or four divided doses.

▶ **Hypertension.** *Adults:* Usual starting dose is 80 mg P.O. t.i.d. Daily dose may be increased to 360 to 480 mg. Initial dose of extended-release tablets or capsules is 120 to 240 mg daily in the morning. Initial dose of Covera-HS is 180 mg at bedtime and of Verelan PM is 200 mg at bedtime. Start therapy with sustained-release capsules at 180 mg (240 mg for Verelan) daily in

---

the morning. Adjust dosage based on effectiveness 24 hours after giving dose. Increase by 120 mg daily until a maximum dose of 480 mg daily is given. Sustained-release capsules should be given only once daily. Antihypertensive effects are usually seen within the first week of therapy. Most patients respond to 240 mg daily.

▼ I.V. administration

• Give drug by direct injection into vein or into tubing of free-flowing, compatible I.V. solution.
• Compatible solutions include D_5W, half-normal and normal saline solutions, and Ringer's and lactated Ringer's solutions.
• Give I.V. doses slowly over at least 2 minutes (3 minutes for elderly patients) to minimize risk of adverse reactions.
• Perform continuous ECG and blood pressure monitoring during administration.
⊗ **Incompatibilities**
Albumin, aminophylline, amphotericin B, ampicillin sodium, co-trimoxazole, dobutamine, hydralazine, nafcillin, oxacillin, propofol, sodium bicarbonate, solutions with a pH greater than 6.

Contraindications and cautions

• Contraindicated in patients hypersensitive to the drug or any of its components and in those with severe left ventricular dysfunction; cardiogenic shock; second- or third-degree AV block or sick sinus syndrome, except in presence of functioning pacemaker; atrial flutter or fibrillation and accessory bypass tract syndrome; severe heart failure (unless secondary to verapamil therapy); or severe hypotension.
• I.V. use is contraindicated in patients with ventricular tachycardia and in those receiving I.V. beta blockers.
• Use cautiously in patients with increased intracranial pressure or hepatic or renal disease.
� Lifespan: In pregnant women, use cautiously. In breast-feeding women, avoid drug; it appears in breast milk. In elderly patients, use cautiously.

Adverse reactions

CNS: asthenia, dizziness, headache.
CV: *AV block, bradycardia, heart failure,* peripheral edema, transient hypotension, *ventricular fibrillation, ventricular asystole.*
GI: constipation, nausea.
Respiratory: *pulmonary edema.*
Skin: rash.

Interactions

Drug-drug. *Acebutolol, atenolol, betaxolol, carteolol, esmolol, metoprolol, nadolol, penbutolol, pindolol, propranolol, timolol:* May increase the effects of both drugs. Monitor cardiac function closely, and decrease dosages as needed.
Antihypertensives, quinidine: May cause hypotension. Monitor blood pressure.
Carbamazepine, digoxin: May increase levels of these drugs. Monitor patient for toxicity.
Cyclosporine: May increase cyclosporine level. Monitor cyclosporine level.
Disopyramide, flecainide, propranolol, other beta blockers: May cause heart failure. Use together cautiously.
Lithium: May decrease lithium level. Monitor patient closely.
Rifampin: May decrease oral bioavailability of verapamil. Monitor patient for lack of effect.
Drug-herb. *Black catechu:* May cause additive effects. Tell patient to use together cautiously.
Yerba maté: May decrease clearance of yerba maté methylxanthines and cause toxicity. Discourage concomitant use.
Drug-food. *Any food:* May increase drug absorption. Tell patient to take drug with food.
Drug-lifestyle. *Alcohol use:* May enhance effects of alcohol. Discourage use together.

Effects on lab test results

• May increase ALT, AST, alkaline phosphatase, and bilirubin levels.

Pharmacokinetics

Absorption: Rapid and complete from GI tract after P.O. use; only about 20% to 35% reaches systemic circulation.
Distribution: About 90% of circulating drug is protein-bound.
Metabolism: In liver.
Excretion: In urine as unchanged drug and active metabolites. *Half-life:* 6 to 12 hours.

Route	Onset	Peak	Duration
P.O.	1–2 hr	1–9 hr	8–24 hr
I.V.	Rapid	Immediate	1–6 hr

Action

Chemical effect: Not clearly defined; inhibits calcium ion influx across cardiac and smooth-muscle cells, thus decreasing myocardial contractility and oxygen demand. Drug also dilates coronary arteries and arterioles.

Therapeutic effect: Relieves angina, lowers blood pressure, and restores normal sinus rhythm.

Available forms

Capsules (extended-release): 120 mg, 180 mg, 240 mg
Capsules (sustained-release): 80 mg, 120 mg, 200 mg, 240 mg, 360 mg
Injection: 2.5 mg/ml
Tablets: 40 mg, 80 mg, 120 mg
Tablets (extended-release): 100 mg, 120 mg, 180 mg, 200 mg, 240 mg, 300 mg
Tablets (sustained-release): 120 mg, 180 mg, 240 mg

NURSING PROCESS

Assessment
• Assess patient's condition before starting therapy and regularly thereafter to monitor drug's effectiveness.
• Monitor blood pressure at start of therapy and during dosage adjustments.
• Monitor liver function studies during long-term treatment.
• Be alert for adverse reactions and drug interactions.
• Assess patient's and family's knowledge of drug therapy.

Nursing diagnoses
• Acute pain related to presence of angina
• Decreased cardiac output related to presence of arrhythmia
• Deficient knowledge related to drug therapy

Planning and implementation
• Give lower doses to patient with severely compromised cardiac function or to a patient taking beta blockers.
• Give drug with food, but keep in mind that giving extended-release tablets with food may decrease rate and extent of absorption. It also produces smaller fluctuations of peak and trough levels.
• If drug is being used to terminate supraventricular tachycardia, prescriber may have patient perform vagal maneuvers after receiving drug.
• Assist patient with walking because dizziness may occur.

• If patient has signs of heart failure, such as swelling of hands and feet or shortness of breath, notify prescriber.
ALERT: Don't confuse Isoptin with Intropin; don't confuse Verelan with Vivarin, Voltaren, Ferralyn, or Virilon.

Patient teaching
• Instruct patient to take drug with food.
• If patient continues nitrate therapy during adjustment of oral verapamil dosage, urge continued compliance. S.L. nitroglycerin, especially, may be taken as needed when angina is acute.
• Advise patient to increase fluid and fiber intake to combat constipation. Give stool softener.
• Instruct patient to report adverse reactions, especially swelling of hands and feet and shortness of breath.

Evaluation
• Patient has reduced severity or frequency of angina.
• Patient regains normal cardiac output with restoration of normal sinus rhythm.
• Patient and family state understanding of drug therapy.

HIGH ALERT

vinblastine sulfate (VLB)
(vin-BLAH-steen SUL-fayt)
Velban

Pharmacologic class: vinca alkaloid
Therapeutic class: antineoplastic
Pregnancy risk category: D

Indications and dosages

▶ **Breast or testicular cancer, Hodgkin and non-Hodgkin lymphoma, choriocarcinoma, lymphosarcoma, mycosis fungoides, Kaposi sarcoma, histiocytosis.** *Adults:* 0.1 mg/kg or 3.7 mg/m^2 I.V. weekly or every 2 weeks. May be increased to maximum of 0.5 mg/kg or 18.5 mg/m^2 weekly according to response. If WBC count is less than 4,000/mm^3, don't repeat dose.
▶ **Letterer-Siwe disease (histiocytosis X).** *Children:* 6.5 mg/m^2. Adjust dosage by hematologic response.
▶ **Hodgkin lymphoma.** *Children:* 6 mg/m^2 with other drugs. Adjust dosage by hematologic response.

▶ **Testicular germ cell carcinoma.** *Children:* 3 mg/m² with other drugs. Adjust dosage by hematologic response.

◪ **Adjust-a-dose:** If bilirubin level is greater than 3 mg/dl, decrease dosage by half.

▽ I.V. administration

• Preparation and administration of parenteral form are linked to carcinogenic, mutagenic, and teratogenic risks. Follow facility policy to reduce risks.
• Reconstitute drug in 10-mg vial with 10 ml of saline solution injection or sterile water. This yields 1 mg/ml.
• Inject drug directly into vein or running I.V. line over 1 minute. Drug also may be given in 50 ml of D₅W or normal saline solution infused over 15 minutes.
• If extravasation occurs, stop infusion immediately and notify prescriber. Manufacturer recommends that moderate heat be applied to area of leakage. Local injection of hyaluronidase may help disperse drug. Some clinicians prefer to apply ice packs on and off every 2 hours for 24 hours, with local injection of hydrocortisone or normal saline solution.
• Refrigerate reconstituted solution. Discard after 30 days.
⊗ **Incompatibilities**
Cefepime, furosemide, heparin.

Contraindications and cautions

• Contraindicated in patients with severe leukopenia or bacterial infection.
• Use cautiously in patients with hepatic dysfunction.
⚘ **Lifespan:** In pregnant women, give only if clearly needed. In breast-feeding women, drug isn't recommended; it isn't known if drug appears in breast milk.

Adverse reactions

CNS: depression, headache, loss of deep tendon reflexes, numbness, paresthesia, peripheral neuropathy and neuritis, *seizures, stroke.*
CV: hypertension, *MI, phlebitis.*
EENT: pharyngitis.
GI: abdominal pain, anorexia, *bleeding,* constipation, diarrhea, ileus, nausea, stomatitis, ulcer, vomiting.
GU: aspermia, oligospermia, urine retention.

Hematologic: anemia, *leukopenia* (lowest results on days 4 to 10; lasts another 7 to 14 days), *thrombocytopenia.*
Metabolic: hyperuricemia, *weight loss.*
Musculoskeletal: *muscle pain and weakness,* uric acid nephropathy.
Respiratory: *acute bronchospasm,* shortness of breath.
Skin: cellulitis, necrosis with extravasation, reversible alopecia, vesiculation.

Interactions

Drug-drug. *Erythromycin, other drugs that inhibit cytochrome P-450 pathway:* May increase toxicity of vinblastine. Monitor patient closely.
Mitomycin: May increase risk of bronchospasm and shortness of breath. Monitor patient closely.
Phenytoin: May decrease phenytoin level. Monitor patient closely.

Effects on lab test results

• May increase uric acid level. May decrease hemoglobin level and hematocrit.
• May decrease WBC and platelet counts.

Pharmacokinetics

Absorption: Given I.V.
Distribution: Widely in body tissues. Crosses blood-brain barrier but doesn't achieve therapeutic level in CSF.
Metabolism: Partially in liver to active metabolite.
Excretion: Mainly in bile as unchanged drug; smaller portion excreted in urine. *Half-life:* Alpha phase, about 3¾ minutes; beta phase, 1½ hours; terminal phase, 25 hours.

Route	Onset	Peak	Duration
I.V.	Unknown	Unknown	Unknown

Action

Chemical effect: Arrests mitosis in metaphase, blocking cell division.
Therapeutic effect: Inhibits replication of certain cancer cells.

Available forms

Injection: 10-mg vials (lyophilized powder), 1 mg/ml in 10-ml vials

NURSING PROCESS

⚏ Assessment
• Assess patient's condition before starting therapy and regularly thereafter to monitor drug's effectiveness.
• Before therapy and each dose, monitor CBC. Leukopenic effects reach lowest point in 4 to 10 days, with recovery in 7 to 14 days.
⚕ **ALERT:** After giving drug, monitor patient for development of life-threatening acute bronchospasm. Reaction is most likely if patient also receives mitomycin.
• Be alert for adverse reactions and drug interactions.
• Assess patient for numbness and tingling in hands and feet. Assess gait for early evidence of foot drop. Drug is less neurotoxic than vincristine.
• Assess patient's and family's knowledge of drug therapy.

⚏ Nursing diagnoses
• Ineffective health maintenance related to presence of neoplastic disease
• Ineffective protection related to drug-induced adverse hematologic reactions
• Deficient knowledge related to drug therapy

⚏ Planning and implementation
• Give antiemetic before giving drug.
• Don't give drug into limb with compromised circulation.
⚕ **ALERT:** Drug is fatal if given intrathecally; it's for I.V. use only.
• If acute bronchospasm occurs after administration, notify prescriber immediately.
• Make sure patient maintains adequate fluid intake to facilitate excretion of uric acid.
• If stomatitis occurs, stop giving the drug and notify prescriber.
• Don't repeat dose more frequently than every 7 days to prevent severe leukopenia.
⚕ **ALERT:** Don't confuse vinblastine with vincristine or vindesine.
Patient teaching
• Teach patient about infection control and bleeding precautions.
• Warn patient that alopecia may occur, but that it's usually reversible.
• Tell patient to report adverse reactions promptly.

• Encourage adequate fluid intake to increase urine output and facilitate excretion of uric acid.

⚏ Evaluation
• Patient responds well to drug.
• Patient develops no serious complications from adverse hematologic reactions.
• Patient and family state understanding of drug therapy.

HIGH ALERT

vincristine sulfate (VCR, LCR)
(vin-KRIH-steen SUL-fayt)
Vincasar PFS

Pharmacologic class: vinca alkaloid
Therapeutic class: antineoplastic
Pregnancy risk category: D

Indications and dosages

▶ **Acute lymphoblastic and other leukemias, Hodgkin lymphoma, non-Hodgkin lymphoma, neuroblastoma, rhabdomyosarcoma, Wilms tumor; bladder, brain, breast and small cell lung cancers‡, idiopathic thrombocytopenia purpura‡, Kaposi sarcoma‡, multiple myeloma‡, chronic lymphocytic and myelocytic leukemias‡, autoimmune hemolytic anemia‡.** *Adults:* 1.4 mg/m² I.V. weekly. Maximum, 2 mg weekly.
Children weighing more than 10 kg (22 lb): 2 mg/m² I.V. weekly. Maximum single dose is 2 mg.
Children weighing 10 kg or less: 0.05 mg/kg I.V. once weekly.
⚏ **Adjust-a-dose:** If serum bilirubin level is greater than 3 mg/dl, decrease dose by half.

▼ I.V. administration

• Preparation and administration of parenteral form are linked to carcinogenic, mutagenic, and teratogenic risks. Follow facility policy to reduce risks.
• Inject drug directly into vein or running I.V. line slowly over 1 minute. Drug also may be given in 50 ml of D_5W or normal saline solution infused over 15 minutes.
• If drug extravasates, stop infusion immediately and notify prescriber. Apply heat on and off every 2 hours for 24 hours. Give 150 units of hyaluronidase to area of infiltrate.

Reactions may be *common*, uncommon, *life-threatening*, or COMMON AND LIFE-THREATENING.

• All vials (1-, 2-, and 5-ml) contain 1 mg/ml solution and should be refrigerated.

⊗ **Incompatibilities**

Cefepime, furosemide, idarubicin, sodium bicarbonate.

Contraindications and cautions

• Contraindicated in patients hypersensitive to the drug or any of its components and in those with demyelinating form of Charcot-Marie-Tooth syndrome. Don't give drug to patients who are receiving radiation therapy through sites that include the liver.

• Use cautiously in patients with hepatic dysfunction, neuromuscular disease, or infection.

⚞ **Lifespan:** In pregnant or breast-feeding women, drug isn't recommended.

Adverse reactions

CNS: acute uric acid neuropathy, ataxia, *coma,* cranial nerve palsies, fever, headache, hoarseness, jaw pain, loss of deep tendon reflexes, paresthesia, peripheral neuropathy, *permanent neurotoxicity, seizures,* sensory loss, wrist drop and foot drop, vocal cord paralysis.

CV: hypertension, hypotension, *phlebitis.*

EENT: diplopia, optic and extraocular neuropathy, ptosis, visual disturbances.

GI: anorexia, *constipation, cramps,* diarrhea, dysphagia, ileus that mimics surgical abdomen, *intestinal necrosis, nausea, stomatitis, vomiting.*

GU: dysuria, polyuria, urine retention,

Hematologic: anemia, *leukopenia, thrombocytopenia.*

Metabolic: hyperuricemia, hyponatremia, weight loss.

Musculoskeletal: muscle weakness and cramps.

Respiratory: *acute bronchospasm.*

Skin: cellulitis at injection site, rash, *reversible alopecia,* severe local reaction with extravasation.

Other: SIADH.

Interactions

Drug-drug. *Asparaginase:* May decrease hepatic clearance of vincristine. Monitor patient closely for toxicity.

Azole antifungals: May increase vincristine toxicity. If possible, avoid use together.

Calcium channel blockers: May increase vincristine accumulation. Monitor patient for toxicity.

Digoxin: May decrease digoxin effects. Monitor digoxin level.

Mitomycin: May increase frequency of bronchospasm and acute pulmonary reactions. Monitor patient closely.

Phenytoin: May decrease phenytoin level. Monitor patient closely.

Quinolone antibiotics: May decrease antimicrobial effect of quinolones. Monitor response.

Effects on lab test results

• May increase uric acid level. May decrease sodium and hemoglobin levels and hematocrit.

• May decrease WBC and platelet counts.

Pharmacokinetics

Absorption: Given I.V.

Distribution: Wide. Bound to erythrocytes and platelets. Crosses blood-brain barrier but doesn't achieve therapeutic level in CSF.

Metabolism: Extensive, in liver.

Excretion: Mainly in bile; smaller portion in urine. *Half-life:* First phase, 5 minutes; second phase, 2¼ hours; terminal phase, 85 hours.

Route	Onset	Peak	Duration
I.V.	Unknown	Unknown	Unknown

Action

Chemical effect: Arrests mitosis in metaphase, blocking cell division.

Therapeutic effect: Inhibits replication of certain cancer cells.

Available forms

Injection: 1 mg/ml in 1-, 2-, and 5-ml multiple-dose vials; 1 mg/ml in 1- and 2-ml preservative-free vials

NURSING PROCESS

V

⚕ Assessment

• Assess patient's condition before starting therapy and regularly thereafter to monitor drug's effectiveness.

⚚ **ALERT:** After giving drug, monitor patient for development of life-threatening acute bronchospasm. Reaction is most likely to occur if patient also receives mitomycin.

• Monitor patient for hyperuricemia, especially if he has leukemia or lymphoma.
• Be alert for adverse reactions and drug interactions.
• Check for depression of Achilles tendon reflex, numbness, tingling, footdrop or wristdrop, difficulty in walking, ataxia, and slapping gait. Also check ability to walk on heels.
• Monitor bowel function. Constipation may be early sign of neurotoxicity.
• Assess patient's and family's knowledge of drug therapy.

Nursing diagnoses
• Ineffective health maintenance related to presence of neoplastic disease
• Ineffective protection related to drug-induced adverse hematologic reactions
• Deficient knowledge related to drug therapy

Planning and implementation
• Give antiemetic before drug.
• Don't give drug to one patient as single dose. The 5-mg vials are for multiple-dose use.
• **ALERT:** Drug is fatal if given intrathecally; it's for I.V. use only.
• Because of risk of neurotoxicity, don't give drug more than once a week. Children are more resistant to neurotoxicity than adults. Neurotoxicity is dose-related and usually reversible.
• If acute bronchospasm occurs after giving the drug, immediately notify the prescriber.
• Maintain good hydration and give allopurinol to prevent uric acid nephropathy.
• If SIADH develops, fluid restriction may be needed.
• Give stool softener, laxative, or water before each dose to help prevent constipation.
• **ALERT:** Don't confuse vincristine with vinblastine or vindesine.
Patient teaching
• Instruct patient on infection control and bleeding precautions.
• Warn patient that alopecia may occur, but that it's usually reversible.
• Tell patient to report adverse reactions promptly.
• Encourage fluid intake to facilitate excretion of uric acid.
• Advise woman of childbearing age not to become pregnant during therapy. Also recommend that she consult with prescriber when planning a pregnancy.

Evaluation
• Patient responds well to drug.
• Patient doesn't develop serious complications from adverse hematologic reactions.
• Patient and family state understanding of drug therapy.

HIGH ALERT

vinorelbine tartrate
(vin-oh-REL-been TAR-trayt)
Navelbine

Pharmacologic class: semisynthetic vinca alkaloid
Therapeutic class: antineoplastic
Pregnancy risk category: D

Indications and dosages

▶ **Alone or as adjunct therapy with cisplatin for first-line treatment of ambulatory patients with nonresectable advanced non–small-cell lung cancer; alone or with cisplatin in stage IV of non–small-cell lung cancer; with cisplatin in stage III of non–small-cell lung cancer.** *Adults:* 30 mg/m^2 I.V. weekly. In combination treatment, same dosage used along with 120 mg/m^2 of cisplatin, given on days 1 and 29, and then every 6 weeks, or vinorelbine 25 mg/m^2 weekly with cisplatin 100 mg/m^2 given every 4 weeks.
▶ **Breast cancer‡.** *Adults:* 20 to 30 mg/m^2 I.V. infusion over 20 to 60 minutes weekly. Or, 30 mg/m^2 direct I.V. injection over 3 to 5 minutes weekly. If used in combination therapy, give 25 or 30 mg/m^2 I.V. in periodic doses. If used with mitoxantrone and ifosfamide, give 12 mg/m^2 I.V. in periodic doses.
Adjust-a-dose: Dosage adjustments are made according to hematologic toxicity or hepatic insufficiency, whichever results in lower dosage. If patient's granulocyte count falls between 1,000/mm^3 and 1,500/mm^3, reduce dosage by half. If three consecutive doses are skipped because of granulocytopenia, stop drug. If total bilirubin is 2.1 to 3 mg/dl, reduce dosage to 15 mg/m^2; if total bilirubin is greater than 3 mg/dl, reduce dosage to 7.5 mg/m^2.

▼ I.V. administration
• Drug must be diluted.

• Give drug I.V. over 6 to 10 minutes into side port of free-flowing I.V. line that is closest to I.V. bag.
• After the infusion, flush the line with 75 to 125 ml of D₅W or normal saline solution.

⊗ **Incompatibilities**

Acyclovir, allopurinol, aminophylline, amphotericin B, ampicillin sodium, cefazolin, cefoperazone, ceftriaxone, cefuroxime, fluorouracil, furosemide, ganciclovir, methylprednisolone, mitomycin, piperacillin, sodium bicarbonate, thiotepa, trimethoprim-sulfamethoxazole.

Contraindications and cautions

• Contraindicated in patients with pretreatment granulocyte counts below 1,000/mm³.
• Use cautiously in patients whose bone marrow may have been compromised by previous exposure to radiation therapy or chemotherapy or whose bone marrow is still recovering from previous chemotherapy. Also use cautiously in patients with hepatic impairment.

⚕ **Lifespan:** In pregnant and breast-feeding women, drug isn't recommended. In children, safety and effectiveness haven't been established.

Adverse reactions

CNS: asthenia, fatigue, peripheral neuropathy.
GI: anorexia, constipation, diarrhea, nausea, paralytic ileus, stomatitis, vomiting.
Hematologic: *anemia,* **bone marrow suppression, granulocytopenia,** LEUKOPENIA.
Hepatic: *bilirubinemia.*
Musculoskeletal: arthralgia, chest pain, jaw pain, loss of deep tendon reflexes, myalgia.
Respiratory: *ARDS,* dyspnea, pneumonia.
Skin: *alopecia,* rash.
Other: injection site pain or reaction, SIADH.

Interactions

Drug-drug. *Cisplatin:* May increase risk of bone marrow suppression when given with cisplatin. Monitor hematologic status closely.
Drugs that inhibit CYP3A isoenzymes: May inhibit metabolism of vinorelbine and cause an earlier onset or increased severity of adverse reactions. Exercise caution.
Mitomycin: May cause pulmonary reactions. Monitor patient's respiratory status closely.
Paclitaxel: May increase risk of neuropathy when given with vinorelbine. Monitor patient.

Effects on lab test results

• May increase bilirubin level. May decrease hemoglobin level and hematocrit.
• May decrease liver function test values and granulocyte, WBC, and platelet counts.

Pharmacokinetics

Absorption: Given I.V.
Distribution: Widely in body tissues. Bound to lymphocytes and platelets.
Metabolism: Extensive, in liver.
Excretion: Mainly in bile; smaller portion in urine. *Half-life:* 27¾ to 43½ hours.

Route	Onset	Peak	Duration
I.V.	Unknown	Unknown	Unknown

Action

Chemical effect: Arrests mitosis in metaphase, blocking cell division.
Therapeutic effect: Inhibits replication of selected cancer cells.

Available forms

Injection: 10 mg/ml, 50 mg/5 ml

NURSING PROCESS

⚖ **Assessment**

• Assess patient's condition before starting therapy and regularly thereafter to monitor drug's effectiveness.
• Monitor patient closely for hypersensitivity reactions.
• To determine dose before each treatment, monitor patient's peripheral blood count and bone marrow.
• Be alert for adverse reactions and drug interactions.
• Assess patient for numbness and tingling in hands and feet. Assess gait for early evidence of foot drop.
⚠ **ALERT:** Monitor patient's deep tendon reflexes; loss may indicate cumulative toxicity.
• Assess patient's and family's knowledge of drug therapy.

⊕ **Nursing diagnoses**

• Ineffective health maintenance related to presence of neoplastic disease
• Ineffective protection related to drug-induced adverse hematologic reactions
• Deficient knowledge related to drug therapy

V

▷ Planning and implementation

• Give antiemetic before giving drug.

• Check patient's granulocyte count before administration; it should be 1,000/mm³ or more. If it's less, don't give the dose, and notify the prescriber.

• Take care to avoid extravasation because drug can cause considerable irritation, localized tissue necrosis, and thrombophlebitis. If extravasation occurs, stop drug immediately and inject remaining portion of dose into a different vein.

⑤ **ALERT:** Drug is fatal if given intrathecally; it's for I.V. use only.

• Drug may be a contact irritant, and solution must be handled and given with care. Gloves are recommended. Avoid inhaling vapors and don't allow drug to contact skin or mucous membranes, especially those of eyes. In case of contact, wash with copious amounts of water for at least 15 minutes.

Patient teaching

• Instruct patient on infection control and bleeding precautions.

• Warn patient that alopecia may occur, but that it's usually reversible.

• Instruct patient not to take other drugs, including OTC preparations, unless approved by prescriber.

• Instruct patient to tell prescriber about signs and symptoms of infection (fever, chills, malaise) because drug has immunosuppressant activity.

✓ Evaluation

• Patient responds well to drug.

• Patient doesn't develop serious complications from adverse hematologic reactions.

• Patient and family state understanding of drug therapy.

vitamin A (retinol)
(VIGH-tuh-min ay)
Aquasol A, Palmitate-A 5000

Pharmacologic class: fat-soluble vitamin
Therapeutic class: vitamin
Pregnancy risk category: A (C at higher-than-recommended doses)

Indications and dosages

▶ **RDA.** RDAs are in retinol equivalents (RE).
1 RE has activity of 1 mcg of all-trans retinol,

6 mcg of beta carotene, or 12 mcg of carotenoid provitamins.

Men older than age 11: Give 1,000 mcg RE or 5,000 international units.

Pregnant women and women older than age 11: Give 800 mcg RE or 4,000 international units.

Breast-feeding women (first 6 months): Give 1,300 mcg RE or 6,500 international units.

Breast-feeding women (second 6 months): Give 1,200 mcg RE or 6,000 international units.

Children ages 7 to 10: Give 700 mcg RE or 3,500 international units.

Children ages 4 to 6: Give 500 mcg RE or 2,500 international units.

Children ages 1 to 3: Give 400 mcg RE or 2,000 international units.

Neonates and infants younger than age 1: Give 375 mcg RE or 1,875 international units.

▶ **Severe vitamin A deficiency.** *Adults and children older than age 8:* Give 100,000 international units I.M. or P.O. daily for 3 days, followed by 50,000 international units I.M. or P.O. daily for 2 weeks; then 10,000 to 20,000 international units P.O. daily for 2 months. Follow with adequate dietary nutrition and RE vitamin A supplements.

Children ages 1 to 8: Give 17,500 to 35,000 international units I.M. daily for 10 days.

Infants younger than age 1: Give 7,500 to 15,000 international units I.M. daily for 10 days.

▶ **Maintenance dosage to prevent recurrence of vitamin A deficiency.** *Children ages 1 to 8:* Give 5,000 to 10,000 international units P.O. daily for 2 months; then adequate dietary nutrition and RE vitamin A supplements.

Contraindications and cautions

• Contraindicated for oral administration in patients with malabsorption syndrome; if malabsorption is from inadequate bile secretion, oral route may be used with administration of bile salts (dehydrocholic acid). Also contraindicated in patients hypersensitive to other ingredients in product and in those with hypervitaminosis A.

• I.V. administration contraindicated except for special water-miscible forms intended for infusion with large parenteral volumes. I.V. push of vitamin A of any type is also contraindicated (anaphylaxis or anaphylactoid reactions and death have resulted).

⚘ **Lifespan:** In pregnant women, use cautiously. In breast-feeding women, use cautiously, avoiding doses exceeding RE.

Adverse reactions

CNS: fatigue, headache, *increased intracranial pressure,* irritability, lethargy, malaise.
EENT: exophthalmos, papilledema.
GI: anorexia, epigastric pain, polydipsia, vomiting.
GU: hypomenorrhea, polyuria.
Hepatic: *cirrhosis,* hepatomegaly, jaundice.
Metabolic: hypercalcemia.
Musculoskeletal: cortical thickening over radius and tibia, decalcification of bone, migratory arthralgia, periostitis, premature closure of epiphyses, slow growth.
Skin: alopecia; dry, cracked, scaly skin; erythema; increased pigmentation; inflamed tongue, lips, and gums; lip fissures; massive desquamation; night sweats, pruritus.
Other: *anaphylactic shock,* splenomegaly.

Interactions

Drug-drug. *Cholestyramine resin, mineral oil:* May decrease GI absorption of fat-soluble vitamins. If needed, give mineral oil at bedtime.
Hormonal contraceptives: May increase vitamin A level. Monitor patient.
Isotretinoin, multivitamins containing vitamin A: May increase risk of toxicity. Avoid use together.
Neomycin (oral): May decrease vitamin A absorption. Avoid use together.

Effects on lab test results

● May increase liver enzyme and calcium levels.

Pharmacokinetics

Absorption: Absorbed readily and completely if fat absorption is normal. Larger doses or regular dose in patients with fat malabsorption, low protein intake, or hepatic or pancreatic disease may be absorbed incompletely. Because vitamin A is fat soluble, absorption requires bile salts, pancreatic lipase, and dietary fat.
Distribution: Stored (mainly as palmitate) in liver. Normal adult liver stores are sufficient to provide vitamin A requirements for 2 years. Lesser amounts of retinyl palmitate are stored in kidneys, lungs, adrenal glands, retinas, and in-

traperitoneal fat. Vitamin A circulates bound to specific alpha$_1$, retinol-binding protein.
Metabolism: In liver.
Excretion: Retinol (fat-soluble) combines with glucuronic acid and is metabolized to retinal and retinoic acid. Retinoic acid undergoes biliary excretion in feces. Retinal, retinoic acid, and other water-soluble metabolites are excreted in urine and feces. *Half-life:* Unknown.

Route	Onset	Peak	Duration
P.O., I.M.	Unknown	3–5 hr	Unknown

Action

Chemical effect: Stimulates retinal function, bone growth, reproduction, and integrity of epithelial and mucosal tissues.
Therapeutic effect: Raises vitamin A level in body.

Available forms

Capsules: 10,000 international units, 15,000 international units, 25,000 international units, 50,000 international units
Injection: 2-ml vials (50,000 international units/ml with 0.5% chlorobutanol, polysorbate 80, butylated hydroxyanisole, and butylated hydroxytoluene)
Tablets: 5,000 international units

NURSING PROCESS

⚕ Assessment

● Assess patient's vitamin A intake from fortified foods, self-administered drugs, dietary supplements, and prescription drug sources before starting therapy, and reassess regularly thereafter to monitor drug's effectiveness.
● If dose is high, watch for adverse reactions. Acute toxicity may result from a single dose of 25,000 international units/kg; 350,000 international units in infants and over 2 million international units in adults may also be acutely toxic. Doses that don't exceed RE are usually nontoxic.
● Chronic toxicity in infants (age 3 to 6 months) may result from doses of 18,500 international units daily for 1 to 3 months. In adults, chronic toxicity has resulted from doses of 50,000 international units daily for more than 18 months; 500,000 international units daily for 2 months, and 1 million international units daily for 3 days.

V

- Be alert for drug interactions.
- Assess patient's and family's knowledge of drug therapy.

✤ Nursing diagnoses
- Imbalanced nutrition: less than body requirements related to inadequate intake
- Ineffective health maintenance related to vitamin A toxicity caused by excessive intake
- Deficient knowledge related to drug therapy

▶ Planning and implementation
- Adequate vitamin A absorption requires suitable protein, vitamin E, zinc intake, and bile secretion; give supplemental salts, if needed. Zinc supplements may be needed in patient receiving long-term total parenteral nutrition.
- Liquid preparations may be mixed with cereal or fruit juice to be given by NG tube.
- I.M. absorption is most rapid and complete with aqueous preparations, intermediate with emulsions, and slowest with oil suspensions.
- ⚠ **ALERT:** Give parenteral form by I.M. route or continuous I.V infusion in total parenteral nutrition. Never give as I.V. bolus.
- Protect drug from light.

Patient teaching
- Warn patient against taking megadoses of vitamins without specific indications. Also stress that he not share prescribed vitamins with others.
- Explain importance of avoiding prolonged use of mineral oil while taking this drug because it reduces vitamin A absorption.
- Review the signs and symptoms of vitamin A toxicity, and tell patient to report them immediately.
- Advise patient to consume adequate protein, vitamin E, and zinc, which, along with bile, are needed for vitamin A absorption.
- Instruct patient to store vitamin A in tight, light-resistant container.

✅ Evaluation
- Patient regains normal vitamin A level.
- Patient shows no signs or symptoms of vitamin A toxicity.
- Patient and family state understanding of drug therapy.

vitamin C (ascorbic acid)
(VIGH-tuh-min see)
Ascor L500, Cecon†, Cenolate†, Cevi-Bid†, Dull-C†, Fruit C†, N'ice Vitamin C Drops†, SunKist Vitamin C†, Vicks Vitamin C Drops†, Vita-C†

Pharmacologic class: water-soluble vitamin
Therapeutic class: vitamin
Pregnancy risk category: A (C at higher-than-recommended doses)

Indications and dosages

▶ **RDA.** *Men:* 90 mg.
Women: 75 mg.
Pregnant women ages 14 to 18: Give 80 mg.
Pregnant women ages 19 to 50: Give 85 mg.
Breast-feeding women ages 14 to 18: Give 115 mg.
Breast-feeding women ages 19 to 50: Give 120 mg.
Boys ages 9 to 13: Give 45 mg.
Boys ages 14 to 18: Give 75 mg.
Girls ages 9 to 13: Give 45 mg.
Girls ages 14 to 18: Give 65 mg.
Children ages 4 to 8: Give 25 mg.
Children ages 1 to 3: Give 15 mg.
Infants ages 6 months to 1 year: Give 50 mg.
Neonates and infants younger than age 6 months: Give 40 mg.
▶ **Frank and subclinical scurvy.** *Adults:* Depending on severity, 300 mg to 1 g P.O., subcutaneously, I.M., or I.V. daily; then at least 50 mg daily for maintenance.
Children: Depending on severity, 100 to 300 mg P.O., subcutaneously, I.M., or I.V. daily; then at least 30 mg daily for maintenance.
Premature infants: 75 to 100 mg P.O., I.M., I.V., or subcutaneously daily.
▶ **Extensive burns, delayed fracture or wound healing, postoperative wound healing, severe febrile or chronic disease states.**
Adults: 300 to 500 mg P.O., subcutaneously, I.M., or I.V. daily for 7 to 10 days. For extensive burns, 1 to 2 g daily.
Children: 100 to 200 mg P.O., subcutaneously, I.M., or I.V. daily.
▶ **Prevention of vitamin C deficiency in patients with poor nutritional habits or increased requirements.** *Adults:* 70 to 150 mg P.O., subcutaneously, I.M., or I.V. daily.

Reactions may be *common*, uncommon, *life-threatening*, or COMMON AND LIFE-THREATENING.

Pregnant or breast-feeding women: 70 to 150 mg P.O., subcutaneously, I.M., or I.V. daily.
Children: at least 40 mg P.O., subcutaneously, I.M., or I.V. daily.
Infants: at least 35 mg P.O., subcutaneously, I.M., or I.V. daily.
▶ **Potentiation of methenamine in urine acidification.** *Adults:* 4 to 12 g P.O. daily in divided doses.

▼ I.V. administration

• Avoid rapid I.V. administration. It may cause faintness or dizziness.
• Give I.V. infusion cautiously in patients with renal insufficiency.
• Protect solution from light and refrigerate ampules.
⊗ **Incompatibilities**
Many drugs.

Contraindications and cautions

⚖ **Lifespan:** In pregnant women, give only if clearly needed. In breast-feeding women, use cautiously.

Adverse reactions

CNS: dizziness with rapid I.V. delivery, faintness.
GI: diarrhea.
GU: acid urine, oxaluria, renal calculi.
Other: discomfort at injection site.

Interactions

Drug-drug. *Aspirin (high doses):* May increase risk of ascorbic acid deficiency. Monitor patient closely.
Estrogen, hormonal contraceptives: May increase level of estrogen. Monitor patient.
Oral iron supplements: May increase iron absorption. A beneficial drug interaction. Encourage use together.
Warfarin: May decrease anticoagulant effect. Monitor patient closely.
Drug-herb. *Bearberry:* May inactivate bearberry in urine. Discourage use together.

Effects on lab test results

• May cause false-negative urine glucose determinations with large doses (larger than 500 mg). May cause false-negative results if ingested 48 to 72 hours before amine-dependent stool occult blood tests.

Pharmacokinetics

Absorption: After P.O. use, absorbed readily; may be reduced with very large doses or in patients with diarrhea or GI diseases. Unknown for I.M and subcutaneous use.
Distribution: Wide, with high levels in liver, leukocytes, platelets, glandular tissues, and lens of eyes. Protein-binding is low.
Metabolism: In liver.
Excretion: In urine. Renal excretion is directly proportional to blood level. *Half-life:* Unknown.

Route	Onset	Peak	Duration
P.O., I.V., I.M., SubQ	Unknown	Unknown	Unknown

Action

Chemical effect: Stimulates collagen formation and tissue repair; involved in oxidation-reduction reactions throughout body.
Therapeutic effect: Raises vitamin C level in body.

Available forms

Capsules (timed-release): 250 mg†, 500 mg†, 1,000 mg†
Crystals: 1,000 mg/¼ tsp†
Injection: 222 mg/ml, 250 mg/ml, 500 mg/ml
Lozenges: 25 mg†, 60 mg†
Oral solution: 100 mg/ml†
Powder: 60 mg/¼ tsp†, 1,060 mg/¼ tsp†
Tablets: 100 mg†, 250 mg†, 500 mg†, 1,000 mg†
Tablets (chewable): 50 mg†, 60 mg†, 100 mg†, 200 mg†, 250 mg†, 500 mg†, 1,000 mg†
Tablets (timed-release): 500 mg†, 1,000 mg†, 1.5 g†

NURSING PROCESS

🔲 Assessment

• Assess patient's condition before starting therapy and regularly thereafter to monitor drug's effectiveness.
• When giving for urine acidification, check urine pH to ensure effectiveness.
• Be alert for adverse reactions and drug interactions.
• If adverse GI reactions occur, monitor patient's hydration.
• Assess patient's and family's knowledge of drug therapy.

V

⊕ Nursing diagnoses
- Imbalanced nutrition: less than body requirements related to inadequate intake
- Risk for deficient fluid volume related to drug-induced adverse GI reactions
- Deficient knowledge related to drug therapy

▶ Planning and implementation
- Give P.O. solution directly into mouth, or mix with food.
- Utilization of vitamin may be better with I.M. route, the preferred parenteral route.

Patient teaching
- Stress proper nutritional habits to prevent recurrence of deficiency.
- Advise patient with vitamin C deficiency to decrease or stop smoking.

☑ Evaluation
- Patient regains normal vitamin C level.
- Patient maintains adequate hydration.
- Patient and family state understanding of drug therapy.

vitamin D
(VIGH-tuh-min dee)

cholecalciferol (vitamin D₃)
(koh-lih-kal-SIF-eh-rol)
Delta-D, Vitamin D₃

ergocalciferol (vitamin D₂)
(er-goh-kal-SIF-er-ohl)
Calciferol, Drisdol

Pharmacologic class: fat-soluble vitamin
Therapeutic class: vitamin
Pregnancy risk category: A, C with doses over the RDA

Indications and dosages

▶ **RDA for cholecalciferol.** *Adolescents and adults:* 200 to 400 international units.
Children 4 to 10 years: 400 international units.
Infants and children (birth to 3 years): 300 to 400 international units.
Pregnant or breast-feeding women: 400 international units.

▶ **Rickets and other vitamin D deficiency diseases.** *Adults:* Initially, 12,000 international units P.O. daily; increase by response up to 500,000 international units daily. After correcting deficiency, patient should have adequate diet and take supplements.

▶ **Hypoparathyroidism.** *Adults and children:* 50,000 to 200,000 international units P.O. daily with calcium supplement.

▶ **Familial hypophosphatemia.** *Adults:* 10,000 to 80,000 international units P.O. daily with phosphorus supplement.

Contraindications and cautions

- Contraindicated in patients with hypercalcemia, hypervitaminosis D, or renal osteodystrophy with hyperphosphatemia.
- Use cautiously in cardiac patients, especially those receiving digoxin, and in patients with increased sensitivity to these drugs.
- Give ergocalciferol cautiously to patients with impaired kidney function, heart disease, renal calculi, or arteriosclerosis.

⚠ **Lifespan:** In pregnant women and breast-feeding women, use cautiously.

Adverse reactions

Adverse reactions listed are usually seen only in vitamin D toxicity.
CNS: headache, irritability, overt psychosis, somnolence, weakness.
CV: *arrhythmias,* calcifications of soft tissues including heart, hypertension.
EENT: conjunctivitis (calcific), photophobia, rhinorrhea.
GI: anorexia, constipation, dry mouth, metallic taste, nausea, polydipsia, vomiting.
GU: albuminuria, hypercalciuria, impaired kidney function, nocturia, polyuria, reversible azotemia.
Metabolic: hypercalcemia, hyperthermia, weight loss.
Musculoskeletal: bone demineralization, bone and muscle pain.
Skin: pruritus.
Other: decreased libido.

Interactions

Drug-drug. *Cholestyramine resin, mineral oil:* May inhibit GI absorption of oral vitamin D. Space doses. Use together cautiously.
Corticosteroids: May antagonize effect of vitamin D. Monitor vitamin D level closely.
Digoxin: May increase risk of arrhythmias. Monitor calcium level.

Phenobarbital, phenytoin: May increase vitamin D metabolism, which decreases half-life as well as drug's effectiveness. Monitor patient closely.
Thiazide diuretics: May cause hypercalcemia in patients with hypoparathyroidism. Monitor patient closely.
Verapamil: May increase risk of atrial fibrillation because of increased calcium. Monitor patient closely.

Effects on lab test results

• May increase BUN, creatinine, AST, ALT, urine urea, albumin, calcium, and cholesterol levels.

Pharmacokinetics

Absorption: From small intestine.
Distribution: Throughout body. Bound to proteins stored in liver.
Metabolism: In liver and kidneys.
Excretion: Mainly in bile; small amount in urine. *Half-life:* 24 hours.

Route	Onset	Peak	Duration
P.O.	2–24 hr	3–12 hr	Varies

Action

Chemical effect: Promotes absorption and utilization of calcium and phosphate, helping to regulate calcium homeostasis.
Therapeutic effect: Helps to maintain normal calcium and phosphate levels in body.

Available forms

Capsules: 1.25 mg (50,000 international units) D_2; 10,000 international units (D_3)†
Oral liquid: 8,000 international units/ml in 60-ml dropper bottle (D_2)†
Tablets: 400 international units (D_3)†, 1,000 international units (D_3)†

NURSING PROCESS

Assessment
• Assess patient's condition before starting therapy and regularly thereafter to monitor drug's effectiveness.
ALERT: Monitor patient's eating and bowel habits; dry mouth, nausea, vomiting, metallic taste, and constipation may be early evidence of toxicity.
• Monitor serum and urine calcium, potassium, and urea levels when high doses are used.

• Be alert for adverse reactions and drug interactions.
• Assess patient's and family's knowledge of drug therapy.

Nursing diagnoses
• Imbalanced nutrition: less than body requirements related to inadequate intake
• Ineffective health maintenance related to vitamin D toxicity
• Deficient knowledge related to drug therapy

Planning and implementation
• Doses of 60,000 international units a day can cause hypercalcemia.
• Malabsorption from inadequate bile or hepatic dysfunction may require addition of exogenous bile salts with oral form.
• Patient with hyperphosphatemia requires dietary phosphate restrictions and binding agents to avoid metastatic calcifications and renal calculus formation.
Patient teaching
• Warn patient of dangers of increasing dose without consulting prescriber. Vitamin D is fat soluble.
• Tell patient taking vitamin D to restrict his intake of magnesium-containing antacids.

Evaluation
• Patient regains normal vitamin D level.
• Patient doesn't develop vitamin D toxicity.
• Patient and family state understanding of drug therapy.

vitamin E (tocopherol)
(VIGH-tuh-min EE)
Aquasol E Drops†, Aquavit-E†, E-200 I.U. Softgels†, E-400 I.U. Softgels†, Mixed E 400 Softgels†, Mixed E 1000 Softgels†, Nutr-E-Sol†, Vitamin E with Mixed Tocopherols†, Vita-Plus E Softgels†

Pharmacologic class: fat-soluble vitamin
Therapeutic class: vitamin
Pregnancy risk category: A

Indications and dosages

▶ **RDA.** RDAs are in α-tocopherol equivalents (α-TE). One α-TE equals 1 mg of D-α tocopherol or 1.49 international units.

Adults, pregnant women: Give 15 α-TE.
Breast-feeding women: Give 19 α-TE.
Children ages 14 to 18: Give 15 α-TE.
Children ages 9 to 13: Give 11 α-TE.
Children ages 4 to 8: Give 7 α-TE.
Children ages 1 to 3: Give 6 α-TE.
Infants ages 7 to 12 months: Give 5 α-TE.
Infants age 6 months and younger: Give 4 α-TE.
▶ **Vitamin E deficiency in adults and in children with malabsorption syndrome.** *Adults:* Depending on severity, 60 to 75 international units P.O. daily.
Children: 1 international unit/kg P.O. daily.

Contraindications and cautions

None reported.
☀ **Lifespan:** In pregnant women, use cautiously. In breast-feeding women, use cautiously.

Adverse reactions

None reported at standard doses.

Interactions

Drug-drug. *Cholestyramine resin, mineral oil:* May inhibit GI absorption of oral vitamin E. Space doses. Use together cautiously.
Iron: May catalyze oxidation and increase daily requirements. Give separately.
Oral anticoagulants: May increase hypoprothrombinemic effects, possibly causing bleeding. Monitor patient closely.
Vitamin K: May antagonize effects of vitamin K with large doses of vitamin E. Avoid use together.

Effects on lab test results

None reported.

Pharmacokinetics

Absorption: GI absorption depends on presence of bile. Only 20% to 60% of vitamin obtained from dietary sources is absorbed. As dosage increases, fraction of vitamin E absorbed decreases.
Distribution: To all tissues and stored in adipose tissues.
Metabolism: In liver.
Excretion: Mainly in bile; small amount in urine. *Half-life:* Unknown.

Route	Onset	Peak	Duration
P.O.	Unknown	Unknown	Unknown

Action

Chemical effect: May act as an antioxidant and protect RBC membranes against hemolysis.
Therapeutic effect: Raises vitamin E level in body.

Available forms

Capsules: 100 international units†, 200 international units†, 400 international units†, 1,000 international units†
Drops: 15 international units/0.3 ml†
Liquid: 15 international units/30 ml, 798 international units/30 ml†
Oral solution: 50 international units/ml†
Tablets (chewable): 100 international units†, 200 international units†, 400 international units†, 500 international units†, 800 international units†, 1,000 international units†

NURSING PROCESS

⚖ Assessment
• Assess patient's condition before starting therapy and regularly thereafter to monitor drug's effectiveness.
• Monitor patient with liver or gallbladder disease for response to therapy. Adequate bile is essential for vitamin E absorption.
• Be alert for drug interactions.
• Assess patient's and family's knowledge of drug therapy.

⊕ Nursing diagnoses
• Imbalanced nutrition: less than body requirements related to inadequate intake
• Deficient knowledge related to drug therapy

▷ Planning and implementation
• Requirements increase with rise in dietary polyunsaturated acids.
• Make sure patient swallows tablets or capsules whole.
• Store drug in tightly closed, light-resistant container.
• If patient has malabsorption caused by lack of bile, give vitamin E with bile salts.
• Hypervitaminosis E symptoms include fatigue, weakness, nausea, headache, blurred vision, flatulence, diarrhea.
Patient teaching
• Tell patient not to crush tablets or open capsules. An oral solution and chewable tablets are commercially available.

• Discourage patient from taking megadoses, which can cause thrombophlebitis. Vitamin E is fat soluble.

☑ **Evaluation**
• Patient regains normal vitamin E level.
• Patient and family state understanding of drug therapy.

voriconazole
(vhor-i-KHAN-a-zawl)
Vfend

Pharmacologic class: synthetic triazole
Therapeutic class: antifungal
Pregnancy risk category: D

Indications and dosages

▶ **Invasive aspergillosis; serious infections caused by *Fusarium* species and *Scedosporium apiospermum* in patients intolerant of or refractory to other therapy.** *Adults:* Initially, 6 mg/kg I.V. every 12 hours for two doses; then 4 mg/kg I.V. every 12 hours for maintenance. Switch to P.O. form as tolerated, using the following maintenance dosages:
Adults weighing 40 kg (88 lb) or more: Maintenance dosage, 200 mg P.O. every 12 hours. May increase to 300 mg P.O. every 12 hours, if needed.
Adults weighing less than 40 kg: Maintenance dosage, 100 mg P.O. every 12 hours. May increase to 150 mg P.O. every 12 hours, if needed.
▶ **Candidemia in nonneutropenic patients; candida infections of the kidney, abdomen, bladder wall, wounds, and skin (disseminated).** *Adults:* Initially, 6 mg/kg I.V. every 12 hours for two doses; then 4 mg/kg I.V. every 12 hours for maintenance. If patient unable to tolerate maintenance dosage, decrease to 3 mg/kg. Switch to P.O. form as tolerated, using the maintenance dosages shown here.
Adults weighing 40 kg (88 lb) or more: 200 mg P.O. every 12 hours. May increase to 300 mg P.O. every 12 hours, if needed.
Adults weighing less than 40 kg: 100 mg P.O. every 12 hours. May increase to 150 mg P.O. every 12 hours, if needed.
▶ **Esophageal candidiasis.** *Adults weighing 40 kg or more:* 200 mg P.O. every 12 hours.

Treat for a minimum of 14 days and for at least 7 days following resolution of symptoms.
Adults weighing less than 40 kg: 100 mg P.O. every 12 hours. Treat for a minimum of 14 days and for at least 7 days following resolution of symptoms.
⬧ **Adjust-a-dose:** In patients with mild to moderate hepatic cirrhosis, decrease the maintenance dosage by one-half.

▼ I.V. administration
• Reconstitute powder with 19 ml of sterile water for injection to obtain a volume of 20 ml of clear concentrate containing 10 mg/ml of drug. If a vacuum doesn't pull the diluent into the vial, discard the vial. Shake vial until all the powder is dissolved.
• Further dilute the solution to a concentration of 5 mg/ml or less. Follow the manufacturer's instructions for diluting.
• Infuse over 1 to 2 hours, at a concentration of 5 mg/ml or less and a maximum of 3 mg/kg hourly.
• Infusion reactions, including flushing, fever, sweating, tachycardia, chest tightness, dyspnea, faintness, nausea, pruritus, and rash, may occur as soon as infusion starts. If reaction occurs, notify prescriber. Infusion may need to be stopped.
• Monitor creatinine level in patient with moderate to severe renal dysfunction (creatinine clearance less than 50 ml/minute). If creatinine level increases, consider changing to P.O. form.
• Store unreconstituted vials at controlled room temperature (59° to 86° F [15° to 30° C]). Use reconstituted solution immediately.
⊗ **Incompatibilities**
Blood products, electrolyte supplements, 4.2% sodium bicarbonate infusion.

Contraindications and cautions
• Contraindicated in patients hypersensitive to the drug or any of its components and in those with rare hereditary problems of galactose intolerance, Lapp lactase deficiency, or glucose-galactose malabsorption. Also contraindicated in patients taking rifampin, carbamazepine, long-acting barbiturates, sirolimus, rifabutin, ergot alkaloids, pimozide, quinidine, efavirenz, or ritonavir.
• Use cautiously in patients hypersensitive to other azoles. Use I.V. form cautiously in patients with creatinine clearance less than 50 ml/minute.

V

⚘ Lifespan: In pregnant women, don't use; drug can harm fetus. In breast-feeding women, use cautiously; it's unknown whether drug appears in breast milk. In children younger than age 12, safety and effectiveness haven't been established.

Adverse reactions

CNS: dizziness, hallucinations, headache, fever.
CV: hypertension, hypotension, peripheral edema, *prolonged QT interval,* tachycardia, vasodilation.
EENT: *abnormal vision,* chromatopsia, dry mouth, photophobia.
GI: abdominal pain, diarrhea, nausea, vomiting.
GU: *acute renal failure.*
Hepatic: cholestatic jaundice.
Metabolic: hypokalemia, *hypomagnesemia.*
Skin: pruritus, rash.
Other: chills.

Interactions

Drug-drug. *Benzodiazepines, calcium channel blockers, lovastatin, omeprazole, sulfonylureas, vinca alkaloids:* May increase levels of these drugs. Adjust dosages of these drugs, and monitor patient for adverse effects.
Carbamazepine, long-acting barbiturates, rifabutin, rifampin: May decrease voriconazole level. Avoid use together.
Coumarin anticoagulants, warfarin: May significantly increase PT. Monitor PT or other appropriate anticoagulant test results.
Cyclosporine, tacrolimus: May increase levels of these drugs. Reduce their dosages, and monitor levels. Adjust doses and monitor levels of these drugs when voriconazole is stopped.
Efavirenz: May significantly decrease voriconazole level and significantly increase efavirenz level. Avoid use together.
Ergot alkaloids (such as ergotamine), sirolimus: May increase levels of these drugs. Avoid use together.
HIV protease inhibitors (amprenavir, nelfinavir, saquinavir), nonnucleoside reverse transcriptase inhibitors (delavirdine): May increase levels of both drugs. Monitor patient for adverse effects.
Oral contraceptives containing ethinyl estradiol and norethindrone: May increase levels and adverse effects of these drugs. Monitor patient closely.

Phenytoin: May decrease voriconazole level and increase phenytoin level. Increase voriconazole maintenance dose, and monitor phenytoin level.
Pimozide, quinidine: May increase levels of these drugs, possibly leading to QT prolongation and torsades de pointes. Avoid use together.
Ritonavir: May significantly decrease voriconazole level. Avoid use together.
Drug-lifestyle. *Sun exposure:* May cause photosensitivity reaction. Tell patient to avoid excessive or unprotected sun exposure.

Effects on lab test results

• May increase AST, ALT, bilirubin, alkaline phosphatase, and creatinine levels. May decrease potassium, magnesium, and hemoglobin levels and hematocrit.
• May decrease platelet, WBC, and RBC counts.

Pharmacokinetics

Absorption: Oral bioavailability is about 96%.
Distribution: Extensive. 58% protein-bound.
Metabolism: By CYP2C19, CYP2C9, and CYP3A4.
Excretion: Via hepatic metabolism, with less than 2% unchanged in urine. *Half-life:* Depends on dose.

Route	Onset	Peak	Duration
P.O., I.V.	Immediate	1–2 hr	12 hr

Action

Chemical effect: Inhibits an essential step in fungal ergosterol biosynthesis.
Therapeutic effect: Kills susceptible fungi.

Available forms

Injection: 200 mg
Powder for oral suspension: 45 g (40 mg/ml after reconstitution)
Tablets: 50 mg, 200 mg

NURSING PROCESS

⚞ Assessment

• Assess patient's condition before starting therapy and regularly thereafter to monitor drug's effectiveness.
• Monitor liver function test results throughout therapy. Monitor patient who develops abnormal liver function test results for more severe hepatic dysfunction.

- Monitor renal function during treatment.
- If treatment lasts more than 28 days, monitor visual acuity, visual fields, and color perception.
- Assess patient's and family's knowledge of drug therapy.

⊕ Nursing diagnoses
- Risk for infection related to presence of fungus
- Risk for injury related to adverse CNS effects of drug
- Deficient knowledge related to drug therapy

▶ Planning and implementation
- Use oral form in patient with moderate to severe renal impairment unless benefits of I.V. use outweigh risks.
- Reconstitute powder for oral suspension with 46 ml of water. Shake the bottle vigorously for about 1 minute. Remove cap, push bottle adaptor into neck of the bottle, and replace cap. The reconstituted suspension should be shaken for about 10 seconds before each use. Administer using the supplied oral dispenser.
- The reconstituted oral suspension should not be mixed with any other medication or flavoring agent and should not be further diluted. Reconstituted suspension can be stored at a controlled room temperature (59° to 86° F [15 to 30° C]) for 14 days.
- If patient develops signs and symptoms of liver disease that may be caused by therapy, stop drug.

Patient teaching
- Tell patient to take oral drug at least 1 hour before or 1 hour after a meal.
- Advise patient to avoid driving or operating machinery while taking drug, especially at night, because vision changes, including blurring and photophobia, may occur.
- Tell patient to avoid strong, direct sunlight during therapy.
- Tell woman of childbearing potential to use effective contraception during treatment.

☑ Evaluation
- Infection is successfully treated.
- Patient sustains no injury.
- Patient and family state understanding of drug therapy.

HIGH ALERT

warfarin sodium
(WAR-feh-rin SOH-dee-um)
Coumadin✦, Jantoven

Pharmacologic class: coumarin derivative
Therapeutic class: anticoagulant
Pregnancy risk category: X

Indications and dosages

▶ **Pulmonary embolism related to deep vein thrombosis, MI, rheumatic heart disease with heart valve damage, prosthetic heart valves, chronic atrial fibrillation.** *Adults:* Initially, 2 to 5 mg P.O. or I.V daily for 2 to 4 days. Use PT and INR determinations to establish optimum dose. Usual maintenance dosage, 2 to 10 mg daily.

▼ I.V. administration

- Reconstitute by adding 2.7 ml of sterile water for injection to vial of 5 mg of warfarin. Resulting solution contains 2 mg/ml.
- Inject dose slowly over 1 to 2 minutes.
⊗ **Incompatibilities**
None reported.

Contraindications and cautions

- Contraindicated in patients with bleeding or hemorrhagic tendencies, GI ulcerations, severe hepatic or renal disease, severe uncontrolled hypertension, subacute bacterial endocarditis, polycythemia vera, or vitamin K deficiency. Also contraindicated in patients who have had recent eye, brain, or spinal cord surgery.
- Use cautiously in patients with diverticulitis, colitis, mild or moderate hypertension, mild or moderate hepatic or renal disease, drainage tubes in any orifice, or regional or lumbar block anesthesia. Also use cautiously if patient has any condition that increases the risk of hemorrhage.
- Patient's genetic make up may influence response to warfarin. Patients with genetic CYP2C9 or VKORC1 variations should start at a lower dose. Genetic testing may lower the risks of its use.
⚕ **Lifespan:** In pregnant women, drug is contraindicated. In breast-feeding women, use cautiously; it's unknown if the drug appears in breast

W

---

milk. Infants, especially neonates, may be more susceptible to anticoagulants because of vitamin K deficiency. In elderly patients, use a lower dose because they have an increased risk of bleeding.

Adverse reactions

CNS: asthenia, *fever,* headache, malaise.
GI: anorexia, cramps, *diarrhea,* melena, mouth ulcerations, nausea, sore mouth, vomiting.
GU: excessive menstrual bleeding, hematuria, priapism.
Hematologic: *hemorrhage.*
Hepatic: *hepatitis,* jaundice.
Skin: alopecia, dermatitis, gangrene, necrosis, *rash,* urticaria.

Interactions

Drug-drug. *Acetaminophen:* May increase bleeding with more than 2 weeks of acetaminophen therapy at dosages of more than 2 g/day. Monitor patient carefully.
Allopurinol, amiodarone, anabolic steroids, cephalosporins, chloramphenicol, cimetidine, clofibrate, danazol, diazoxide, diflunisal, disulfiram, erythromycin, ethacrynic acid, fluoroquinolones, glucagon, heparin, influenza virus vaccine, isoniazid, lovastatin, meclofenamate, methimazole, methylthiouracil, metronidazole, miconazole, nalidixic acid, neomycin (oral), pentoxifylline, propafenone, propoxyphene, quinidine, sulfonamides, tamoxifen, tetracyclines, thiazides, thrombolytics, thyroid drugs, tricyclic antidepressants, vitamin E: May increase PT. Monitor patient for bleeding. Reduce anticoagulant dosage.
Aminoglutethimide, atorvastatin, barbiturates, carbamazepine, corticosteroids, corticotropin, hormonal contraceptives containing estrogen, griseofulvin, mercaptopurine, methaqualone, nafcillin, pravastatin, rifampin, spironolactone, sucralfate, trazodone, vitamin K: May decrease PT/INR with reduced anticoagulant effect. Monitor patient carefully.
Anticonvulsants: May increase levels of phenytoin and phenobarbital. Monitor patient for toxicity.
Chloral hydrate, glutethimide, propylthiouracil, sulfinpyrazone: May increase or decrease PT. Avoid use, if possible. Monitor patient carefully.
Cholestyramine: May decrease response when given too close together. Give 6 hours after oral anticoagulants.

NSAIDs, salicylates: May increase PT and ulcerogenic effects. Don't use together.
Sulfonylureas (oral antidiabetics): May increase hypoglycemic response. Monitor glucose level.
Drug-herb. *Angelica:* May significantly prolong PT when used together. Discourage use together.
Arnica, ginkgo biloba, ginseng, motherwort, pau d'arco, red clover: May increase risk of bleeding. Discourage use together.
Drug-food. *Foods or enteral products containing vitamin K:* May impair anticoagulation. Tell patient to maintain consistent daily intake of leafy green vegetables.
Drug-lifestyle. *Alcohol use:* May increase anticoagulant effects. Discourage alcohol intake; however, one or two drinks daily are unlikely to affect warfarin response.

Effects on lab test results

- May increase ALT and AST levels.
- May increase INR, PT, and PTT.

Pharmacokinetics

Absorption: Rapid and complete.
Distribution: Extensively protein-bound; especially to albumin.
Metabolism: In liver.
Excretion: Metabolites reabsorbed from bile and excreted in urine. *Half-life:* 1 to 3 days.

Route	Onset	Peak	Duration
P.O.	½–3 days	Unknown	2–5 days
I.V.	Unknown	Unknown	2–5 days

Action

Chemical effect: Inhibits vitamin K–dependent activation of clotting factors II, VII, IX, and X, formed in liver.
Therapeutic effect: Reduces ability of blood to clot.

Available forms

Powder for injection: 5 mg
Tablets: 1 mg, 2 mg, 2.5 mg, 3 mg, 4 mg, 5 mg, 6 mg, 7.5 mg, 10 mg

NURSING PROCESS

Assessment
- Assess patient's condition before starting therapy and regularly thereafter to monitor drug's effectiveness.

Reactions may be *common,* uncommon, *life-threatening,* or COMMON AND LIFE-THREATENING.

• Draw blood to establish baseline coagulation parameters before starting therapy.

⚠ **ALERT:** INR determinations are essential for proper control. Clinicians typically try to maintain INR at two to three times normal; risk of bleeding is high when INR exceeds six times normal.

• Be alert for adverse reactions and drug interactions. An elderly patient or a patient with renal or hepatic failure is especially sensitive to warfarin effect.

• Regularly inspect patient for bleeding gums, bruises on arms or legs, petechiae, nosebleed, melena, tarry stools, hematuria, and hematemesis.

• Observe the breast-fed infant of a mother taking the drug for unexpected bleeding.

• Assess patient's and family's knowledge of drug therapy.

⊕ **Nursing diagnoses**
• Risk for injury related to potential for blood clot formation from underlying condition
• Ineffective protection related to increased risk of bleeding
• Deficient knowledge related to drug therapy

▶ **Planning and implementation**
• Give drug at same time each day.
• I.V. form may be obtained from manufacturer for rare patient who can't have oral therapy. Follow guidelines carefully to prepare and give the drug.
• Because onset of action is delayed, heparin sodium is commonly given during first few days of treatment. When heparin is given simultaneously, blood for PT shouldn't be drawn within 5 hours of intermittent I.V. heparin administration. Blood for PT may be drawn at any time during continuous heparin infusion.

⚠ **ALERT:** If patient has a fever and rash, notify the prescriber immediately and don't give the dose; these symptoms may signal severe adverse reactions.

• The drug's anticoagulant effect can be neutralized by vitamin K injections.
• Drug is best oral anticoagulant for patient taking antacids or phenytoin.

Patient teaching
• Stress importance of compliance with prescribed dosage and follow-up appointments. Patient should wear or carry medical identification that indicates his increased risk of bleeding.

• Instruct patient and family to watch for signs of bleeding and to immediately notify the prescriber if they occur.

• Warn patient to avoid OTC products containing aspirin, other salicylates, or drugs that may interact with warfarin.

• Tell patient to notify prescriber if menses are heavier than usual; dosage adjustment may be needed.

• Tell patient to use an electric razor when shaving, to avoid scratching skin, and to use soft toothbrush.

• Instruct patient to read food labels. Food and enteral feedings that contain vitamin K may impair anticoagulation.

• Tell patient to daily eat a consistent amount of leafy green vegetables that contain vitamin K. Eating varying amounts may alter anticoagulant effects.

✓ **Evaluation**
• Patient doesn't develop blood clots.
• Patient recounts appropriate bleeding precautions.
• Patient and family state understanding of drug therapy.

Z

zafirlukast
(zay-FEER-loo-kast)
Accolate

Pharmacologic class: synthetic, selective peptide leukotriene receptor antagonist
Therapeutic class: anti-inflammatory, bronchodilator
Pregnancy risk category: B

Indications and dosages

▶ **Prevention and long-term treatment of chronic asthma.** *Adults and children age 12 and older:* 20 mg P.O. b.i.d. taken 1 hour before or 2 hours after meals.
Children ages 5 to 11: Give 10 mg P.O. b.i.d. taken 1 hour before or 2 hours after meals.

▶ **Prevention of seasonal allergic rhinitis‡.**
Adults: 20 to 40 mg P.O. as a single dose before exposure to allergen.

Contraindications and cautions

• Contraindicated in patients hypersensitive to the drug or any of its components.
• Use cautiously in patients with hepatic impairment.
≋ **Lifespan:** In pregnant women, drug should be used only if clearly needed. In breast-feeding women, drug shouldn't be given because it appears in breast milk. In children younger than age 5, safety and effectiveness haven't been established. In elderly patients, use cautiously.

Adverse reactions

CNS: asthenia, dizziness, fever, *headache,* pain.
GI: abdominal pain, diarrhea, dyspepsia, nausea, vomiting.
Musculoskeletal: back pain, myalgia.
Other: accidental injury, infection.

Interactions

Drug-drug. *Aspirin:* May increase zafirlukast level. Monitor patient.
Erythromycin, theophylline: May decrease zafirlukast level. Monitor patient.
Warfarin: May increase PT. Monitor PT and INR levels, and adjust dosage of anticoagulant.
Drug-food. *Any food:* May reduce rate and extent of drug absorption. Give drug 1 hour before or 2 hours after meals.

Effects on lab test results

• May increase liver enzyme levels.

Pharmacokinetics

Absorption: Rapid.
Distribution: Unknown.
Metabolism: Extensive.
Excretion: Mainly in feces; 10% in urine. *Half-life:* 10 hours.

Route	Onset	Peak	Duration
P.O.	Unknown	3 hr	Unknown

Action

Chemical effect: Selectively competes for leukotriene receptor sites. Blocks inflammatory action and inhibits bronchoconstriction.
Therapeutic effect: Improves breathing.

Available forms

Tablets: 10 mg, 20 mg

NURSING PROCESS

✍ Assessment
• Assess patient's and family's understanding of drug therapy.

⊕ Nursing diagnoses
• Impaired gas exchange related to bronchospasm
• Deficient knowledge related to drug therapy

▷ Planning and implementation
⑤ **ALERT:** Don't use drug for reversing bronchospasm in acute asthma attack.
⑤ **ALERT:** Reducing dose may rarely cause eosinophilia, vasculitic rash, worsening pulmonary symptoms, cardiac complications, or neuropathy, such as Churg-Strauss syndrome.
Patient teaching
• Tell patient to keep taking drug even if symptoms disappear.
• Advise patient to continue taking other antiasthmatics.
• Instruct patient to take drug 1 hour before or 2 hours after meals.

☑ Evaluation
• Patient has improved gas exchange.
• Patient and family state understanding of drug therapy.

HIGH ALERT

zaleplon
(ZAL-eh-plon)
Sonata

Pharmacologic class: pyrazolopyrimidine
Therapeutic class: hypnotic
Pregnancy risk category: C
Controlled substance schedule: IV

Indications and dosages

▶ **Short-term treatment of insomnia.** *Adults:* 10 mg P.O. at bedtime; may increase dosage to 20 mg if needed. Low-weight adults may respond to 5-mg dose.
Elderly and debilitated patients: Initially, 5 mg P.O. at bedtime; doses over 10 mg aren't recommended.

⧈ **Adjust-a-dose:** For patients with mild to moderate hepatic impairment and those taking cimetidine, give 5 mg P.O. daily.

Contraindications and cautions

• Don't use in patients with severe hepatic impairment.
• Use cautiously in debilitated patients, in those with compromised respiratory function, and in those with signs and symptoms of depression.
☀ **Lifespan:** In pregnant and breast-feeding women, drug isn't recommended. In children, safety and effectiveness haven't been established. In elderly patients, use cautiously.

Adverse reactions

CNS: amnesia, anxiety, asthenia, complex sleep disorders, depersonalization, depression, difficulty concentrating, dizziness, fever, hallucinations, *headache,* hypertonia, hypesthesia, malaise, migraine, nervousness, paresthesia, somnolence, tremor, vertigo.
CV: chest pain, peripheral edema.
EENT: abnormal vision, conjunctivitis, ear pain, epistaxis, eye pain, hyperacusis, parosmia.
GI: abdominal pain, anorexia, colitis, constipation, dry mouth, dyspepsia, nausea.
GU: dysmenorrhea.
Musculoskeletal: arthritis, back pain, myalgia.
Respiratory: bronchitis.
Skin: photosensitivity reactions, pruritus, rash.
Other: *anaphylaxis, angioedema.*

Interactions

Drug-drug. *Cimetidine:* May cause pharmacokinetic interaction. For patient taking cimetidine, use an initial zaleplon dose of 5 mg.
CNS depressants (imipramine, thioridazine): May produce additive CNS effects. Use cautiously together.
CYP3A4 inducers (carbamazepine, phenobarbital, phenytoin, rifampin, others): May reduce zaleplon effectiveness. Consider a different hypnotic.
Drug-food. *Heavy meals, high-fat foods:* May prolong absorption, delaying peak zaleplon level by about 2 hours; sleep onset may be delayed. Separate drug from meals.
Drug-lifestyle. *Alcohol use:* May increase CNS effects. Discourage use together.

Effects on lab test results

None reported.

Pharmacokinetics

Absorption: Rapid and almost complete. Level peaks within 1 hour. Taking drug after a high-fat or heavy meal delays peak level by about 2 hours.
Distribution: Substantially into extravascular tissues. About 60% protein-bound.
Metabolism: Extensive, mainly by aldehyde oxidase and, to a lesser extent, CYP3A4 to inactive metabolites. Less than 1% of dose is excreted unchanged in urine.
Excretion: Rapid. *Half-life:* 1 hour.

Route	Onset	Peak	Duration
P.O.	1 hr	1 hr	3–4 hr

Action

Chemical effect: Has a chemical structure unrelated to benzodiazepines but interacts with the GABA and benzodiazepine receptor complex in the CNS. Modulation of this complex is hypothesized to be responsible for sedative, anxiolytic, muscle relaxant, and anticonvulsant effects of benzodiazepines.
Therapeutic effect: Promotes sleep.

Available forms

Capsules: 5 mg, 10 mg

NURSING PROCESS

⧈ **Assessment**
• Carefully assess patient because sleep disturbances may be a symptom of an underlying physical or psychiatric disorder.
• Closely monitor elderly or debilitated patient, or patient with compromised respiratory function because of illness.
• Monitor patient for drug abuse and dependence.
• Assess patient's and family's knowledge of drug therapy.

⧈ **Nursing diagnoses**
• Insomnia related to underlying disorder
• Risk for injury related to drug-induced adverse CNS reactions
• Deficient knowledge related to drug therapy

Z

Planning and implementation
● Don't give drug with or after a high-fat or heavy meal.
● Drug works rapidly; give right before bedtime or after patient has been unable to sleep.
● Adverse reactions are usually dose-related. Give lowest effective dose.
● Limit hypnotic use to 7 to 10 days. If hypnotics will be taken for more than 3 weeks, prescriber should reevaluate patient.
● To reduce the risk of drug abuse and dependence, drug shouldn't be given as more than a 1-month supply.

Patient teaching
● Advise patient that drug works rapidly and should be taken immediately before bedtime or after trying unsuccessfully to sleep.
● Advise patient to take drug only if he can sleep undisturbed for at least 4 hours.
● Warn patient that drowsiness, dizziness, light-headedness, and difficulty with coordination occur most often within 1 hour after taking drug.
● Warn patient about possibility of complex sleep disorders.
● Advise patient to avoid performing activities that require mental alertness until the drug's CNS effects are known.
● Advise patient not to drink alcohol while taking drug and to notify prescriber before taking any prescription or OTC drugs.
● Tell patient not to take drug after a high-fat or heavy meal.
● Advise patient to report any continued sleep problems despite use of drug.
● Tell patient that dependence can occur; drug is recommended for short-term use only.
● Warn patient not to abruptly stop drug because withdrawal symptoms, including discomfort, stomach and muscle cramps, vomiting, sweating, shakiness, and seizures, may occur.
● Tell patient that insomnia may recur for a few nights after stopping drug, but should resolve on its own.
● Advise patient that zaleplon may cause changes in behavior and thinking, including outgoing or aggressive behavior, loss of personal identity, confusion, strange behavior, performing complex activities while sleeping, agitation, hallucinations, worsening of depression, or suicidal thoughts. Tell patient to notify prescriber immediately if any of these problems occur.

Evaluation
● Patient states that drug effectively promotes sleep.
● Patient sustains no injury from drug-induced adverse CNS reactions.
● Patient and family state understanding of drug therapy.

zanamivir
(zah-NAM-ah-veer)
Relenza

Pharmacologic class: neuraminidase inhibitor
Therapeutic class: antiviral
Pregnancy risk category: C

Indications and dosages

▶ **Uncomplicated acute illness caused by influenza A and B virus in patients who have been symptomatic for no longer than 2 days.** *Adults and children age 7 and older:* Two oral inhalations (one 5-mg blister per inhalation for a total dose of 10 mg) b.i.d. using the Diskhaler inhalation device for 5 days. Give two doses on the first day of treatment with at least 2 hours between doses. Subsequent doses should be about 12 hours apart (in the morning and evening) at about the same time each day.
▶ **To prevent influenza in a household setting.** *Adults and children age 5 and older:* Two oral inhalations (one 5-mg blister per inhalation for total dose of 10 mg) once daily for 10 days.
▶ **To prevent influenza in a community setting.** *Adults and adolescents:* Two oral inhalations (one 5-mg blister per inhalation for total dose of 10 mg) once daily for 28 days.

Contraindications and cautions

● Contraindicated in patients hypersensitive to the drug or any of its components. Drug is not recommended for patients with underlying airway disease (such as asthma and COPD).
⚛ **Lifespan:** In pregnant women, use only if benefits outweigh risks. In breast-feeding women, use cautiously; it's unknown if the drug appears in breast milk. In children younger than age 5, safety and effectiveness haven't been established.

Adverse reactions

CNS: dizziness, headache.
EENT: ear, nose, and throat infections; nasal signs and symptoms; sinusitis.
GI: diarrhea, nausea, vomiting.
Hematologic: lymphopenia, *neutropenia*.
Respiratory: bronchitis, *bronchospasm*, cough.

Interactions

None reported.

Effects on lab test results

• May increase ALT, AST, and CK levels.
• May decrease lymphocyte and neutrophil counts.

Pharmacokinetics

Absorption: About 4% to 17%, with peak level occurring 1 to 2 hours following a 10-mg dose.
Distribution: Less than 10% protein-bound.
Metabolism: Not metabolized.
Excretion: In urine, unchanged, within 24 hours. Unabsorbed drug in feces. *Half-life:* 2½ to 5¼ hours.

Route	Onset	Peak	Duration
Inhalation	Unknown	1–2 hr	Unknown

Action

Chemical effect: Probably inhibits the enzyme neuraminidase on the surface of the influenza virus, possibly altering virus particle aggregation and release. When neuraminidase is inhibited, the virus can't escape from its host cell to attack others, thereby inhibiting the process of viral proliferation.
Therapeutic effect: Lessens the symptoms of influenza.

Available forms

Powder for inhalation: 5 mg per blister

NURSING PROCESS

⚡ Assessment
• Obtain accurate patient medical history before starting therapy.
• Lymphopenia, neutropenia, and a rise in liver enzyme and CK levels may occur during treatment. Monitor patient appropriately.

• Monitor patient for bronchospasm and decline in lung function. If they occur, stop giving the drug.
• Assess patient's and family's knowledge of drug therapy.

🔅 Nursing diagnoses
• Risk for infection related to influenza virus
• Imbalanced nutrition: less than body requirements related to drug's adverse GI effects
• Deficient knowledge related to drug therapy

▶ Planning and implementation
⑤ ALERT: Serious cases of bronchospasm, including death, have been reported during treatment. Stop drug in any patient who develops bronchospasm or a decline in respiratory function.
• Have patient exhale fully before inserting the mouthpiece. Then, keeping the Diskhaler level, have patient close his lips around the mouthpiece, and have him breathe in steadily and deeply. Instruct patient to hold his breath for a few seconds after inhaling to help keep the drug in his lungs.
• There is no information suggesting drug is effective when started more than 48 hours after symptoms appear.
Patient teaching
• Teach patient how to properly use the drug with the Diskhaler inhalation device, and tell him to carefully read the instructions.
• Advise patient to keep the Diskhaler level when loading and inhaling drug. Tell patient to check inside the mouthpiece of the Diskhaler before each use to make sure it's free of foreign objects.
• Instruct patient with respiratory disease who has an impending scheduled dose of inhaled bronchodilator to take it before taking zanamivir. Tell patient with asthma to have a fast-acting bronchodilator available in case of wheezing during therapy.
• Tell patient to finish the entire 5-day course even if he feels better and symptoms improve before the fifth day.
• Inform patient that zanamivir hasn't been shown to reduce the risk of transmitting influenza virus to others.

Z

☑ Evaluation

• Patient recovers from influenza.
• Patient has no adverse GI effects.
• Patient and family state understanding of drug therapy.

zidovudine (azidothymidine, AZT)
(zigh-DOH-vyoo-deen)
Novo-AZT ◆, Retrovir

Pharmacologic class: thymidine analogue
Therapeutic class: antiretroviral
Pregnancy risk category: C

Indications and dosages

▶ **HIV infection.** *Adults:* 600 mg P.O. daily in divided doses given with other antiretrovirals. Or, for patients who can't take the oral form, 1 mg/kg I.V. over 1 hour, every 4 hours around the clock until oral therapy can be used.
Children ages 6 weeks to 12 years: 160 mg/m^2 P.O. every 8 hours. Maximum, 200 mg every 8 hours. Give with other antiretrovirals.
▶ **Adjust-a-dose:** Patients with end-stage renal disease (creatinine clearance less than 15 ml/minute) maintained on dialysis should receive 1 mg/kg I.V. every 6 to 8 hours.
▶ **To prevent maternal-fetal HIV transmission.** *Pregnant women past 14 weeks' gestation:* 100 mg P.O. five times daily until the start of labor. Then, 2 mg/kg I.V. over 1 hour followed by a continuous I.V. infusion of 1 mg/kg/hour until the umbilical cord is clamped.
Neonates: 2 mg/kg P.O. every 6 hours starting within 12 hours after birth and continuing until age 6 weeks. Or, give 1.5 mg/kg via I.V. infusion over 30 minutes every 6 hours.
▶ **Adjust-a-dose:** For patients on hemodialysis or peritoneal dialysis, give 100 mg P.O. every 6 to 8 hours. For patients with mild to moderate hepatic dysfunction or liver cirrhosis, reduce daily dosage.
▶ **Prophylaxis after occupational or nonoccupational exposure to HIV‡.** *Adults:* 600 mg P.O. daily in two or three divided doses for 4 weeks given with other antiretrovirals. Prophylaxis should begin as soon as possible after exposure, preferably within hours.

▽ I.V. administration

• Dilute drug before use. Remove calculated dose from vial; add to D$_5$W to yield no more than 4 mg/ml.
• Adding solution to biological or colloidal fluids (such as blood products and protein solutions) isn't recommended.
• Infuse drug over 1 hour at constant rate; give every 4 hours around the clock. Avoid rapid infusion or bolus injection.
• Solution is physically and chemically stable for 24 hours at room temperature and for 48 hours if refrigerated at 36° to 46° F (2° to 8° C). Store undiluted vials at 59° to 77° F (15° to 25° C) and protect them from light.
⊗ **Incompatibilities**
Biological or colloidal solutions, such as blood products or protein-containing solutions; meropenem.

Contraindications and cautions

• Contraindicated in patients hypersensitive to the drug or any of its components.
• Use cautiously and with close monitoring in patients with advanced symptomatic HIV infection and in those with severe bone marrow depression. Also use cautiously in patients with hepatomegaly, hepatitis, or other known risk factors for hepatic disease.
※ **Lifespan:** In breast-feeding women, drug shouldn't be used. In elderly patients, use cautiously.

Adverse reactions

CNS: asthenia, dizziness, fever, headache, insomnia, malaise, paresthesia, *seizures,* somnolence.
GI: abdominal pain, anorexia, constipation, diarrhea, dyspepsia, nausea, taste perversion, vomiting.
Hematologic: *agranulocytosis,* anemia, *bone marrow suppression, thrombocytopenia.*
Metabolic: *lactic acidosis.*
Musculoskeletal: myalgia.
Skin: diaphoresis, *rash.*

Interactions

Drug-drug. *Atovaquone, fluconazole, methadone, probenecid, valproic acid:* May increase zidovudine level. Adjust dosage if needed.
Doxorubicin, ribavirin, stavudine: May antagonize zidovudine. Avoid use together.

Reactions may be *common,* uncommon, *life-threatening*, or COMMON AND LIFE-THREATENING.

Ganciclovir, interferon alfa, other bone marrow suppressants or cytotoxic drugs: May increase hematologic toxicity of zidovudine. Use cautiously as with other reverse transcriptase inhibitors.

Nelfinavir, rifampin, ritonavir: May decrease zidovudine bioavailability. Dosage adjustment isn't needed.

Phenytoin: May alter phenytoin level and decrease zidovudine clearance by 30%. Monitor patient closely.

Effects on lab test results

• May increase ALT, AST, alkaline phosphatase, and LDH levels. May decrease hemoglobin level and hematocrit.
• May decrease granulocyte and platelet counts.

Pharmacokinetics

Absorption: Rapid.
Distribution: Good CSF penetration. About 36% protein-bound.
Metabolism: Rapid, to inactive compound.
Excretion: In urine. *Half-life:* 1 hour.

Route	Onset	Peak	Duration
P.O.	Unknown	30–90 min	Unknown
I.V.	Immediate	30–90 min	Unknown

Action

Chemical effect: Prevents replication of HIV by inhibiting the enzyme reverse transcriptase.
Therapeutic effect: Reduces symptoms of HIV infection.

Available forms

Capsules: 100 mg
Injection: 10 mg/ml
Syrup: 50 mg/5 ml
Tablets: 300 mg

NURSING PROCESS

Assessment

• Assess patient's condition before starting therapy and regularly thereafter to monitor drug's effectiveness.
• Monitor CBC with differential and platelet counts every 2 weeks to detect anemia or agranulocytosis.
• Be alert for adverse reactions and drug interactions.
• Assess patient's and family's knowledge of drug therapy.

Nursing diagnoses

• Risk for infection related to presence of HIV
• Ineffective protection related to drug-induced adverse hematologic reactions
• Deficient knowledge related to drug therapy

Planning and implementation

• Drug temporarily decreases illness and risk of death in certain patients with AIDS or AIDS-related complex.
• Optimum duration of treatment and optimum dosage for effectiveness with minimum toxicity aren't yet known.
• **ALERT:** Notify prescriber of abnormal hematologic study results. Significant anemia (hemoglobin level of less than 7.5 g/dl or reduction of more than 25% of baseline) or significant neutropenia (granulocyte count of less than 750/mm³ or reduction of more than 50% from baseline) may warrant interrupting therapy until marrow begins to recover.

Patient teaching
• Advise patient that blood transfusions may be needed during treatment. Drug often causes low RBC count.
• Stress importance of compliance with every-4-hours dose. Suggest ways to avoid missing doses, perhaps by using an alarm clock.
• Warn patient not to take other drugs for AIDS (especially street drugs) unless approved by prescriber. Some supposed AIDS cures may interfere with drug's effectiveness.
• Advise pregnant HIV-infected women that drug therapy only reduces risk of HIV transmission to neonates. Long-term risks to infants are unknown.
• Advise patient considering drug as prophylaxis against HIV after exposure (such as after needle-stick injury) that its safety and effectiveness haven't been proven.

Evaluation

• Patient has reduced severity and frequency of symptoms linked to HIV infection.
• Patient doesn't develop complications from therapy.
• Patient and family state understanding of drug therapy.

Z

ziprasidone
(zi-PRAY-si-done)
Geodon

Pharmacologic class: atypical antipsychotic
Therapeutic class: psychotropic
Pregnancy risk category: C

Indications and dosages

▶ **Symptomatic schizophrenia.** *Adults:* Initially, 20 mg P.O. b.i.d. with food. Dosages are highly individualized. Dosage adjustments should occur no sooner than every 2 days, but to allow for lowest possible doses, the interval should be several weeks. Effective dosage range is usually 20 to 80 mg b.i.d. Maximum recommended dosage is 100 mg b.i.d.
▶ **Rapid control of acute agitation in schizophrenic patients.** *Adults:* 10 to 20 mg I.M. as a single dose. Doses of 10 mg may be given every 2 hours; doses of 20 mg may be given every 4 hours. Maximum cumulative dose is 40 mg daily.
▶ **Acute bipolar mania, including manic and mixed episodes, with or without psychotic features.** *Adults:* 40 mg P.O. b.i.d. on day 1. Increase to 60 or 80 mg P.O. b.i.d. on day 2 with subsequent adjustments based on patient response within the range of 40 to 80 mg b.i.d. Give with food.

Contraindications and cautions

• Contraindicated in patients hypersensitive to the drug or any of its components. Also contraindicated in patients taking drugs that prolong QT interval and in those who have a QTc interval longer than 500 msec. Contraindicated in patients with a history of QT-interval prolongation, congenital QT-interval syndrome, recent MI, and uncompensated heart failure.
• Use cautiously in patients with acute diarrhea and in patients with a history of bradycardia, hypokalemia, seizures, aspiration pneumonia, or hypomagnesemia.
• Give I.M. ziprasidone with caution to patients with impaired renal function.
⚠ **Lifespan:** In pregnant women, use only if benefits outweigh risks. Breast-feeding women should stop breast-feeding or shouldn't use the drug. In children, safety and effectiveness haven't been established. In elderly patients,

safety and effectiveness of I.M. use haven't been established.

Adverse reactions

P.O. use
CNS: dystonia.
CV: tachycardia.
EENT: abnormal vision.
Musculoskeletal: myalgia.
Respiratory: cough.
Skin: rash.
I.M. use
CNS: speech disorders.
CV: vasodilation.
GU: priapism.
Musculoskeletal: back pain.
Skin: sweating.
Other: flulike syndrome, tooth disorder.
Both routes
CNS: agitation, akathisia, anxiety, asthenia, cogwheel rigidity, dizziness, extrapyramidal symptoms, *headache*, hypertonia, insomnia, *neuroleptic malignant syndrome,* paresthesia, personality disorder, psychosis, *somnolence, suicide attempt.*
CV: *bradycardia,* hypertension, orthostatic hypotension.
EENT: rhinitis.
GI: abdominal pain, anorexia, constipation, diarrhea, dry mouth, dyspepsia, *nausea, rectal hemorrhage,* vomiting.
GU: dysmenorrhea.
Metabolic: hyperglycemia.
Skin: furunculosis, injection site pain.

Interactions

Drug-drug. *Antihypertensives:* May enhance hypotensive effects. Monitor blood pressure.
Carbamazepine: May decrease ziprasidone level. Higher ziprasidone doses may be needed to achieve desired effect.
Drugs that increase dopamine level, such as levodopa and dopamine agonists: May have antagonistic effect on ziprasidone. Use together cautiously.
Drugs that lower potassium and magnesium levels, such as diuretics: May increase risk of arrhythmias. If giving together, monitor potassium and magnesium levels.
Drugs that prolong QT interval, including arsenic trioxide, chlorpromazine, dofetilide, dolasetron mesylate, droperidol, halofantrine, levomethadyl acetate, mefloquine, mesoridazine,

---

Reactions may be *common,* uncommon, *life-threatening,* or COMMON AND LIFE-THREATENING.

moxifloxacin, pentamidine, pimozide, probucol, quinidine, sotalol, sparfloxacin, tacrolimus, thioridazine, or other class IA and III antiarrhythmics: May increase risk of arrhythmias when used together. Don't give together.
Itraconazole, ketoconazole: May increase ziprasidone level. Lower doses of ziprasidone may be needed to achieve desired effect.

Effects on lab test results
• May increase glucose level.

Pharmacokinetics
Absorption: Doubled when taken with food, which is recommended. Level peaks in about 6 to 8 hours.
Distribution: Extensively protein-bound.
Metabolism: Hepatic metabolism; no active metabolites. Less than one-third of drug is metabolized through cytochrome P-450 system, mainly via CYP3A4 and partly via CYP1A2.
Excretion: Unknown. *Half-life:* 2¼ to 7 hours.

Route	Onset	Peak	Duration
P.O.	1–3 days	6–8 hr	12 hr
I.M.	Unknown	1 hr	Unknown

Action
Chemical effect: May work by antagonizing dopamine and serotonin, the neurotransmitters usually targeted for treatment of positive and negative symptoms of schizophrenia. Blocking these neurotransmitters allows symptomatic improvement with minimal adverse effects in the extrapyramidal system.
Therapeutic effect: Relieves psychotic signs and symptoms of schizophrenia.

Available forms
Capsules: 20 mg, 40 mg, 60 mg, 80 mg
Injection: 20-mg/ml single-dose vials (after reconstitution)

NURSING PROCESS

Assessment
• Assess patient's condition before starting therapy and regularly thereafter to monitor drug's effectiveness.
• Assess and monitor patient who experiences dizziness, palpitations, or syncope.
• Drug may prolong QT interval. Other antipsychotics should be considered in patient with a

history of QT-interval prolongation, acute MI, congenital QT-interval syndrome, and other conditions that place the patient at risk for life-threatening arrhythmias. Don't give other drugs that prolong the QT interval with ziprasidone.
• Patient taking antipsychotics is at risk for developing neuroleptic malignant syndrome or tardive dyskinesia.
• Electrolyte disturbances, such as hypokalemia or hypomagnesemia, increase the risk of arrhythmias. Before starting therapy, monitor potassium and magnesium levels and correct imbalances.
• Assess patient's and family's knowledge of drug therapy.

Nursing diagnoses
• Disturbed thought processes related to underlying condition
• Risk for falls related to adverse CNS effects of drug
• Deficient knowledge related to ziprasidone therapy

Planning and implementation
• Don't adjust dosage sooner than every 2 days. Longer intervals may be needed because symptoms may take 4 to 6 weeks to respond.
• Monitor patient for prolonged QT interval during therapy. Further monitor patient with symptoms of arrhythmias. If QTc interval is greater than 500 msec, stop drug.
ALERT: Hyperglycemia may occur in patient taking drug. Regularly monitor patient with diabetes. Patient with risk factors for diabetes should undergo fasting blood glucose testing at baseline and periodically during therapy. Monitor every patient for symptoms of hyperglycemia including polydipsia, polyuria, polyphagia, and weakness; if symptoms develop, perform fasting blood glucose testing. Hyperglycemia may be reversible when antipsychotic is stopped.
• Immediately treat patient with symptoms of neuroleptic malignant syndrome, which can be life-threatening.
• Monitor patient for tardive dyskinesia.
• If long-term ziprasidone therapy is needed, switch to P.O. route as soon as possible. Effect of I.M. administration for more than 3 consecutive days isn't known.
• Don't give drug I.M. to schizophrenic patient already taking ziprasidone P.O.
• Give oral drug with food, which increases the effect.

• For I.M. use, add 1.2 ml of sterile water for injection to vial and shake vigorously until entire drug is dissolved.

• Don't mix I.M. injection with any other product besides sterile water for injection.

• Inspect for particulate matter and discoloration before administration, whenever solution and container permit.

• Store dry form at room temperature. Store reconstituted form for up to 24 hours at room temperature or up to 7 days refrigerated (36° to 46° F [2° to 8° C]). Protect from light.

Patient teaching

• Tell patient to take drug with food.

• Tell patient to immediately report to prescriber symptoms of dizziness, fainting, irregular heartbeat, or relevant cardiac problems.

• Advise patient to report to prescriber any recent episodes of diarrhea.

• Advise patient to report to prescriber abnormal movements.

• Tell patient to report to prescriber sudden fever, muscle rigidity, or change in mental status.

☑ Evaluation

• Patient has reduced psychotic symptoms with drug therapy.

• Patient doesn't fall.

• Patient and family state understanding of drug therapy.

zoledronic acid
(zoe-LEH-druh-nick ASS-id)
Reclast, Zometa

Pharmacologic class: bisphosphonate
Therapeutic class: antihypercalcemic
Pregnancy risk category: D

Indications and dosages

▶ **Hypercalcemia related to malignancy.**
Adults: 4 mg by I.V. infusion over at least 15 minutes. If albumin-corrected calcium level doesn't return to normal, consider retreatment with 4 mg. Allow at least 7 days to pass before retreatment to allow a full response to the initial dose.

▶ **Multiple myeloma and bone metastases of solid tumors (given with standard antineoplastic therapy).** *Adults:* 4 mg infused over at least 15 minutes every 3 to 4 weeks. Duration of treatment in studies was 15 months for prostate cancer, 12 months for breast cancer and multiple myeloma, and 9 months for other solid tumors. Prostate cancer should have progressed after treatment with at least one hormonal therapy.

▶ **Paget disease of bone.** *Adults:* 5 mg by I.V. infusion over at least 15 minutes. Administer through a vented infusion line. May repeat, if relapse occurs.

▶ **Postmenopausal osteoporosis.** *Adult women:* 5 mg by I.V. infusion over at least 15 minutes, once yearly.

⎙ Adjust-a-dose: For patients with creatinine clearance of 50 to 60 ml/minute, give 3.5 mg. If clearance is 40 to 49 ml/minute, give 3.3 mg. If clearance is 30 to 39 ml/minute, give 3 mg.

For patients with normal baseline creatinine level but an increase of 0.5 mg/dl during therapy, and in those with abnormal baseline creatinine level who have an increase of 1 mg/dl, withhold drug. Resume treatment only when creatinine level has returned to within 10% of baseline value.

▼ I.V. administration

• Reconstitute by adding 5 ml of sterile water to each vial. Powder must be completely dissolved.

• Withdraw 5 ml for 4 mg of drug and mix in 100 ml of normal saline solution or D_5W.

• To withdraw the appropriate dose for a patient with creatinine clearance 60 ml/minute or less: withdraw 4.4 ml for the 3.5 mg dose, 4.1 ml for the 3.3 mg dose, and 3.8 ml for the 3 mg dose.

• Inspect solution for particulate matter and discoloration before giving it.

• The drug must be given as an I.V. infusion over at least 15 minutes. Give drug as a single I.V. solution in a line separate from all other drugs.

• If not used immediately after reconstitution, solution must be refrigerated and given within 24 hours.

⊗ Incompatibilities
Other I.V. drugs; solutions that contain calcium, such as lactated Ringer's solution.

Contraindications and cautions

• Contraindicated in patients with clinically significant hypersensitivity to drug, other bisphosphonates, or ingredients in formulation.

Reactions may be *common*, uncommon, *life-threatening*, or COMMON AND LIFE-THREATENING.

• Not recommended in patients with hypercalcemia of malignancy with creatinine greater than 4.5 mg/dl. Not recommended in patients with bone metastases with creatinine greater than 3 mg/dl.

• Use cautiously in patients with aspirin-sensitive asthma because other bisphosphonates may cause bronchoconstriction in these patients.

⚖ **Lifespan:** In pregnant women, don't use. Women of childbearing age should avoid becoming pregnant. In breast-feeding women, use cautiously; it's unknown if the drug appears in breast milk. In children, safety and effectiveness haven't been established. In elderly patients, monitor renal function.

Adverse reactions

Hypercalcemia
CNS: agitation, anxiety, confusion, *depression, dizziness,* fever, *headache, insomnia,* somnolence.
CV: hypotension.
GI: abdominal pain, anorexia, constipation, diarrhea, dysphagia, nausea, vomiting.
GU: candidiasis, *renal failure,* UTI.
Hematologic: anemia, *granulocytopenia, pancytopenia, thrombocytopenia.*
Metabolic: dehydration.
Musculoskeletal: arthralgia, osteonecrosis of the jaw, *skeletal pain.*
Respiratory: *cough, dyspnea,* pleural effusion.
Other: infection, PROGRESSION OF CANCER.
Bone metastases
CNS: *anxiety, depression, dizziness,* fatigue, *fever, headache, hypoesthesia, insomnia, paresthesia,* weakness.
CV: hypotension, leg edema.
GI: *abdominal pain, anorexia, constipation, diarrhea, increased appetite, nausea, vomiting.*
GU: *renal failure, UTI.*
Hematologic: anemia, *neutropenia.*
Metabolic: dehydration, weight loss.
Musculoskeletal: *arthralgia, back pain, myalgia,* osteonecrosis of the jaw, *skeletal pain.*
Respiratory: *cough, dyspnea.*
Skin: alopecia, dermatitis.
Other: infection, PROGRESSION OF CANCER, rigors.

Interactions

Drug-drug. *Aminoglycosides, loop diuretics:* May have additive effects to lower calcium lev-

el. Give together cautiously, and monitor calcium level.
Thalidomide: May increase risk of renal dysfunction in multiple myeloma patients. Use together cautiously.

Effects on lab test results

• May increase creatinine level. May decrease calcium, phosphorus, magnesium, potassium, and hemoglobin levels and hematocrit.
• May decrease RBC, WBC, and platelet counts.

Pharmacokinetics

Absorption: Given I.V.
Distribution: About 22% protein-bound. Post-infusion decline of level is consistent with a triphasic process: Low level observed up to 28 days after a dose.
Metabolism: Doesn't inhibit cytochrome P-450 enzymes or undergo biotransformation in vivo.
Excretion: Mainly via kidneys. *Half-life:* Alpha is about 15 minutes; beta is 1¾ hours for early distribution. *Terminal half-life:* About 7 days.

Route	Onset	Peak	Duration
I.V.	Unknown	Unknown	7–28 days

Action

Chemical effect: Inhibits bone resorption, probably by inhibiting osteoclast activity and osteoclastic resorption of mineralized bone and cartilage, decreasing calcium release induced by the stimulatory factors produced by tumors.
Therapeutic effect: Lowers calcium level in malignant disease.

Available forms

Injection: 4 mg zoledronic acid, 220 mg mannitol, and 24 mg sodium citrate in 5 ml vials; 5 mg zoledronic acid, 4,950 mg mannitol, and 30 mg sodium citrate in 100 ml vials

NURSING PROCESS

▨ Assessment

• Assess patient's condition before starting therapy and regularly thereafter to monitor drug's effectiveness.
• Assess kidney function before and during therapy because drug is excreted mainly via the kidneys. The risk of adverse reactions may be greater in a patient with renal impairment. If pa-

Z

tient has renal impairment, give drug only if benefits outweigh risks, and at a lower dose.
• Measure creatinine level before each dose.
• Make sure patient is adequately hydrated before giving drug; urine output should be about 2 L daily.
• Assess patient's dental health before starting therapy. Make sure patient has had a dental exam with appropriate preventive dentistry before being treated with bisphosphonates, especially patients with cancer, those receiving chemotherapy or corticosteroids, and those with poor oral hygiene.
• Assess patient's and family's knowledge of drug therapy.

⊕ Nursing diagnoses
• Ineffective protection related to adverse hematologic effects
• Ineffective health maintenance related to underlying condition
• Deficient knowledge related to drug therapy

▷ Planning and implementation
⚡ **ALERT:** A significant decline in renal function could progress to renal failure; single doses shouldn't exceed 4 mg, and infusion should last at least 15 minutes.
⚡ **ALERT:** After giving drug, carefully monitor renal function and calcium, phosphate, magnesium, and creatinine levels.
• Other bisphosphonates have been linked to bronchoconstriction in patients with asthma and aspirin sensitivity.
• Give patient an oral calcium supplement of 500 mg and a multiple vitamin containing 400 international units of vitamin D daily.
Patient teaching
• Review use and administration of drug with patient and family.
• Instruct patient to report adverse effects promptly.
• Explain importance of periodic laboratory tests to monitor therapy and renal function.
• Advise patient to notify prescriber if she is pregnant.

☑ Evaluation
• Patient has no adverse hematologic reactions.
• Patient shows improvement in condition.
• Patient and family state understanding of drug therapy.

zolmitriptan
(zohl-muh-TRIP-tan)
Zomig, Zomig-ZMT

Pharmacologic class: selective 5-hydroxytryptamine (5-HT$_1$) receptor agonist
Therapeutic class: antimigraine drug
Pregnancy risk category: C

Indications and dosages

▶ **Acute migraine headache.** *Adults:* Initially, 2.5 mg or less P.O. increased to 5 mg per dose, if needed. If headache returns after initial dose, second dose may be given after 2 hours. Maximum dose is 10 mg in 24-hour period. Or, give 2.5 mg P.O. of orally-disintegrating tablets; don't break tablets in half. Or, 5 mg (one nasal spray) into one nostril. If headache returns after initial dose, a second dose may be given after 2 hours. Maximum dose is 10 mg in 24-hour period.
◨ **Adjust-a-dose:** For patients with liver disease, use doses lower than 2.5 mg. Also, don't use orally-disintegrating tablets; they shouldn't be split. Avoid use of nasal spray because doses lower than 5 mg can't be given.

Contraindications and cautions

• Contraindicated in patients hypersensitive to the drug or any of its components, in those with uncontrolled hypertension, and in those with symptoms or findings consistent with ischemic heart disease (angina pectoris, history of MI or documented silent ischemia), coronary artery vasospasm (including Prinzmetal variant angina), or other significant heart disease.
• Avoid use within 24 hours of other 5-HT$_1$ agonists or drugs containing ergot, or within 2 weeks of stopping MAO inhibitor therapy. Also avoid use in patients with hemiplegic or basilar migraine.
• Use cautiously in patients with liver disease and in patients who may be at risk for coronary artery disease, such as postmenopausal women, men older than age 40, or patients with hypertension, hypercholesterolemia, obesity, diabetes, smoking, or family history of coronary artery disease.
⚖ **Lifespan:** In pregnant women, use cautiously. In breast-feeding women, use cautiously; it's unknown if the drug appears in breast milk. In

---

Reactions may be *common*, uncommon, *life-threatening*, or COMMON AND LIFE-THREATENING.

children, safety and effectiveness haven't been established.

Adverse reactions

CNS: asthenia, *dizziness,* hypesthesia, pain, paresthesia, somnolence, vertigo.
CV: *coronary artery vasospasm; MI;* pain, tightness, pressure, or heaviness in chest; palpitations; *transient myocardial ischemia; ventricular fibrillation; ventricular tachycardia.*
EENT: pain, tightness, or pressure in the neck, throat, or jaw.
GI: dry mouth, dyspepsia, dysphagia, nausea.
Musculoskeletal: myalgia, myasthenia.
Skin: sweating.
Other: warm or cold sensations.

Interactions

Drug-drug. *Cimetidine:* May double zolmitriptan half-life. Monitor patient closely.
Ergot-containing drugs, serotonin$_{1B/1D}$ agonists: May cause vasospastic reactions. Avoid use within 24 hours of almotriptan.
Hormonal contraceptives: May increase zolmitriptan level. Monitor patient closely.
MAO inhibitors: May increase zolmitriptan level. Avoid using drug within 2 weeks of stopping MAO inhibitor therapy.
SSRIs: May cause additive serotonin effects, resulting in weakness, hyperreflexia, or incoordination. If given together, monitor patient closely.

Effects on lab test results

• May increase glucose level.

Pharmacokinetics

Absorption: Well absorbed following P.O. use; absolute bioavailability of 40%.
Distribution: 25% protein-bound.
Metabolism: Converted to active N-desmethyl metabolite.
Excretion: About 65% of dose is recovered in urine (8% unchanged) and 30% in feces. *Half-life:* 3 hours.

Route	Onset	Peak	Duration
P.O.	Unknown	2 hr	3 hr
P.O. orally-disintegrating	Unknown	2 hr	Unknown
Nasal spray	5 min	3 hr	Unknown

Action

Chemical effect: Selective serotonin receptor agonist causes constriction of cranial blood vessels and inhibits proinflammatory neuropeptide release.
Therapeutic effect: Relieves migraine headache pain.

Available forms

Nasal spray: 5 mg
Tablets: 2.5 mg, 5 mg
Tablets (orally-disintegrating): 2.5 mg, 5 mg

NURSING PROCESS

Assessment
• Assess patient's history of migraine headaches before starting therapy and regularly thereafter to monitor drug's effectiveness.
• Assess patient for history of coronary artery disease, hypertension, arrhythmias, or presence of risk factors for coronary artery disease.
• Monitor liver function test results before starting drug therapy, and report abnormalities.
• Use drug only when a clear diagnosis of migraine has been established.
• Assess patient's and family's knowledge of drug therapy.

Nursing diagnoses
• Acute pain related to presence of migraine headache
• Ineffective cardiopulmonary tissue perfusion related to drug-induced adverse cardiac events
• Deficient knowledge related to drug therapy

Planning and implementation
• Use a lower dose in a patient with moderate to severe hepatic impairment; don't give orally disintegrating tablets because they can't be split.
• Don't give drug to prevent migraine headaches or to treat hemiplegic migraines, basilar migraines, or cluster headaches.
⑤ **ALERT:** Don't give drug within 24 hours of ergot-containing drugs or within 2 weeks of MAO inhibitor.
Patient teaching
• Tell patient that drug is intended to relieve the symptoms of migraines, not to prevent them.
• Advise patient to take drug as prescribed. Caution against taking a second dose unless instructed by prescriber. Tell patient that if a sec-

Z

ond dose is indicated and permitted, he should take it at least 2 hours after initial dose.
• Advise patient to immediately report pain or tightness in chest or throat, heart throbbing, rash, skin lumps, or swelling of face, lips, or eyelids.
• Inform the patient that safety of treating an average of more than 3 headaches in 30 days with the tablets, or an average of more than 4 headaches in 30 days with the nasal spray hasn't been established.
• Tell woman not to take drug if she's planning or suspects a pregnancy.
• Instruct patient to remove the orally disintegrating tablet from the blister pack just before use and to let it dissolve on the tongue.
• Advise patient not to break the orally-disintegrating tablets in half.

☑ Evaluation
• Patient has relief from migraine headache.
• Patient has no pain or tightness in the chest or throat, arrhythmias, increases in blood pressure, or MI.
• Patient and family state understanding of drug therapy.

HIGH ALERT

zolpidem tartrate
(ZOHL-peh-dim TAR-trayt)
Ambien⊘, Ambien CR, Tovalt ODT

Pharmacologic class: imidazopyridine
Therapeutic class: hypnotic
Pregnancy risk category: C
Controlled substance schedule: IV

Indications and dosages
▶ **Short-term management of insomnia.**
Adults: 10 mg P.O. (immediate-release) or 12.5 mg P.O. (extended-release) immediately before bedtime.
⊠ **Adjust-a-dose:** *Elderly patients:* 5 mg P.O. (immediate-release) or 6.25 mg (extended-release) immediately before bedtime. Maximum daily dose is 10 mg (immediate-release) or 6.25 mg (extended-release).
Debilitated patients and those with hepatic insufficiency: 5 mg P.O. immediately before bedtime. Maximum daily dosage is 10 mg. If using the extended-release tablet, maximum daily dose is 6.25 mg.

Contraindications and cautions
• Use cautiously in patients with conditions that could affect metabolism or hemodynamic responses and in those with compromised respiratory status, because hypnotics may depress respiratory drive. Also use cautiously in patients with depression or history of alcohol or drug abuse.
⚜ **Lifespan:** In pregnant women, use only if benefits outweigh fetal risks. In breast-feeding women, drug isn't recommended. In children, safety and effectiveness haven't been established.

Adverse reactions
CNS: abnormal dreams, amnesia, daytime drowsiness, depression, dizziness, hangover effect, *headache,* lethargy, light-headedness, complex sleep disorders.
CV: chest discomfort, hypertension, palpitations.
EENT: pharyngitis, sinusitis.
GI: abdominal pain, constipation, diarrhea, dry mouth, dyspepsia, nausea, vomiting.
Musculoskeletal: arthralgia, back or chest pain, myalgia.
Skin: rash.
Other: *anaphylaxis, angioedema,* flulike syndrome, hypersensitivity reactions.

Interactions
Drug-drug. *Antifungals:* May decrease metabolism of zolpidem, increasing CNS depression; consider lower dose.
CNS depressants: May increase CNS depression. Use together cautiously.
Drug-food. *Any food:* May decrease rate and extent of absorption. Tell patient to take drug on an empty stomach.
Drug-lifestyle. *Alcohol use:* May cause excessive CNS depression. Discourage use together.

Effects on lab test results
None reported.

Pharmacokinetics
Absorption: Rapid. Food delays drug absorption.
Distribution: About 92.5% protein-bound.
Metabolism: In liver.
Excretion: Mainly in urine. *Half-life:* 2½ hours.

Route	Onset	Peak	Duration
P.O.	Rapid	30 min–2 hr	Unknown

Reactions may be *common*, uncommon, *life-threatening*, or COMMON AND LIFE-THREATENING.

Action

Chemical effect: Interacts with one of three identified GABA and benzodiazepine receptor complexes but isn't a benzodiazepine. Exhibits hypnotic activity but has no muscle relaxant or anticonvulsant properties.
Therapeutic effect: Promotes sleep.

Available forms

Tablets: 5 mg, 10 mg
Tablets (extended-release): 6.25 mg, 12.5 mg
Tablets (orally-disintegrating): 5 mg, 10 mg

NURSING PROCESS

◈ Assessment
• Assess patient's condition before starting therapy and regularly thereafter to monitor drug's effectiveness.
• Be alert for adverse reactions and drug interactions.
• Assess patient's and family's knowledge of drug therapy.

◈ Nursing diagnoses
• Insomnia related to underlying disorder
• Risk for injury related to drug-induced adverse CNS reactions
• Deficient knowledge related to drug therapy

◈ Planning and implementation
• Drug has a rapid onset of action; give when patient is ready to sleep.
• Use hypnotics only for short-term management of insomnia, usually 7 to 10 days. Persistent insomnia may indicate primary psychiatric or medical disorder.
• Because most adverse reactions are dose-related, use smallest effective dose in all patients, especially elderly or debilitated patients.
• Give drug at least 1 hour before meals or 2 hours after meals.
Ⓢ **ALERT:** Don't confuse Ambien with Amen.
Patient teaching
• Tell patient to take drug immediately before going to bed.
• For faster onset, instruct patient not to take drug with or immediately after a meal. Food decreases drug's absorption.
• Warn patient about possible complex sleep disorders.

Ⓢ **ALERT:** Tell patient not to crush, chew, or divide the extended-release or the orally-disintegrating tablets.
• Place the orally-disintegrating tablet in the mouth, allow the tablet to disintegrate, and then tell the patient to swallow. The tablet may be taken with or without water.
• Warn patient about performing activities that require mental alertness or physical coordination. For inpatient, supervise walking and raise bed rails, particularly for geriatric patient.

☑ Evaluation
• Patient states that drug effectively promotes sleep.
• Patient sustains no injury from adverse CNS reactions.
• Patient and family state understanding of drug therapy.

zoster vaccine, live
(ZOSS-tur vack-SEEN)
Zostavax

Pharmacologic class: vaccine, live attenuated
Therapeutic class: vaccine
Pregnancy risk category: C

Indications and dosages

▶ **Prevention of herpes zoster (shingles).**
Adults age 60 and older: One reconstituted vial subcutaneously as a single dose.

Contraindications and cautions

• Contraindicated in patients with a history of anaphylactic or anaphylactoid reactions to gelatin, neomycin, or any component of the vaccine; patients with primary or acquired immunodeficiency; patients taking immunosuppressive therapy or corticosteroids; patients with active, untreated tuberculosis; and pregnant women.
※ **Lifespan:** In pregnant patients, avoid use during and for 3 months after pregnancy. In breast-feeding patients, it isn't known if vaccine appears in breast milk; use cautiously. In children, Zostavax shouldn't be used; it can't be substituted for Varivax.

Adverse reactions

CNS: asthenia, fever, headache.
EENT: rhinitis.

Z

GI: diarrhea.
Musculoskeletal: polymyalgia rheumatica.
Respiratory: *asthma exacerbation,* respiratory disorder, respiratory infection.
Skin: hematoma, *injection site reactions (redness, pain, tenderness, swelling),* pruritus, skin disorder, warmth.
Other: flulike syndrome.

Interactions

Drug-drug. *Immunosuppressants, including corticosteroids.* May decrease immune response. Use together is contraindicated.

Effects on lab test results

None reported.

Pharmacokinetics

Absorption: Unknown.
Distribution: Unknown.
Metabolism: Unknown.
Excretion: Unknown.

Route	Onset	Peak	Duration
SubQ	6 wk	Unknown	4 yr

Action

Chemical effect: Stimulates active immunity to varicella-zoster virus.
Therapeutic effect: Protects against herpes zoster.

Available forms

Injection: Lyophilized vaccine in a single-dose vial with supplied diluent

NURSING PROCESS

Assessment
• Ask if patient has ever had a reaction to a vaccine. Keep epinephrine 1:1000 available for immediate use to treat anaphylaxis.
• Monitor patient for hypersensitivity reaction.
• Assess patient's and family's knowledge of drug therapy.

Nursing diagnoses
• Health-seeking behavior to protect against herpes zoster
• Deficient knowledge related to drug therapy

Planning and implementation
ALERT: Drug is given only by subcutaneous injection; don't give by I.V. route.
• Defer vaccination if patient has acute illness or a fever higher than 101.3° F (38.5° C).
• Inject diluent into the vial of lyophilized vaccine and gently agitate to mix thoroughly.
• Inject the total volume subcutaneously, immediately after reconstitution, into outer aspect of upper arm.
• If reconstituted vaccine isn't used within 30 minutes, discard it.
• Store frozen at 5° F (–15° C) or colder until ready to use.
Patient teaching
• Explain to patient the benefits and risks of the vaccine.
• Inform patient that injection site reactions are common and may include redness, pain, swelling, itching, and bruising.

Evaluation
• Patient gains immunity against herpes zoster.
• Patient and family state understanding of drug therapy.

Herbal medicines

aloe

Reported uses

• Externally as a topical gel for minor burns, sunburn, cuts, frostbite, skin irritation, and other wounds and abrasions
• Amenorrhea, asthma, colds, seizures, bleeding, and ulcers. Preparations also used to treat acne, AIDS, arthritis, blindness, bursitis, cancer, colitis, depression, diabetes, glaucoma, hemorrhoids, multiple sclerosis, peptic ulcers, and varicose veins

Cautions

• External preparations shouldn't be used by people hypersensitive to herb or those with a history of allergic reactions to plants in the Liliaceae family (such as garlic, onions, and tulips).
• Aloe shouldn't be taken orally by people with cardiac or kidney disease (because of risk of hypokalemia and disturbance of cardiac rhythm), by those with intestinal obstruction, and by those with Crohn disease or ulcerative colitis.
⚹ Lifespan: Pregnant women, breast-feeding women, and children shouldn't use.

Adverse reactions

CV: arrhythmias.
GI: damage to intestinal mucosa, harmless brown discoloration of intestinal mucous membranes, painful intestinal spasms, *severe hemorrhagic diarrhea.*
GU: kidney damage, red discoloration of urine, reflex stimulation of uterine musculature causing miscarriage or premature birth.
Metabolic: fluid and electrolyte loss, hypokalemia.
Musculoskeletal: accelerated bone deterioration, muscle weakness.
Skin: contact dermatitis, delayed healing of deep wounds.

Interactions

Herb-drug. *Antiarrhythmics, digoxin:* Oral form may lead to toxic reaction. Monitor patient closely.
Corticosteroids, diuretics: Increases potassium loss. Monitor patient for signs of hypokalemia.

Disulfiram: Tincture contains alcohol and could precipitate a disulfiram reaction. Discourage use together.
Herb-herb. *Licorice:* Increases risk of potassium deficiency. Discourage use together.

angelica

Reported uses

• Gynecologic disorders, postmenopausal symptoms, menstrual discomfort, anemia, and mild peptic discomfort, such as GI spasms, flatulence, bloating, colic, and loss of appetite; to strengthen the heart; to improve circulation in the limbs; and to relieve osteoporosis, hay fever, cough, asthma, bronchitis, acne, and eczema

Cautions

• People with diabetes should use caution because various species of this plant contain polysaccharides that may disrupt glucose control.
⚹ Lifespan: Pregnant or breast-feeding women shouldn't use angelica because it may have stimulant effects on the uterus.

Adverse reactions

CV: hypotension.
Skin: photodermatitis, phototoxicity.

Interactions

Herb-drug. *Antacids, H$_2$-receptor antagonists, proton pump inhibitors, sucralfate:* Herb may increase acid production in the stomach and may interfere with absorption of these drugs. Discourage use together.
Anticoagulants: Excessive amounts of herb may potentiate anticoagulant effects. Avoid use together.
Herb-lifestyle. *Sun exposure:* Photosensitivity reaction may occur. Advise a person taking angelica to avoid unprotected or prolonged exposure to sunlight.

---

*Liquid may contain alcohol.

bilberry

Reported uses

- Visual and circulatory problems, glaucoma, cataracts, diabetic retinopathy, macular degeneration, varicose veins, and hemorrhoids
- To improve night vision

Cautions

- Urge caution in those taking anticoagulants. Herb may be unsuitable for those with a bleeding disorder.
- **Lifespan:** Pregnant and breast-feeding women should avoid herb.

Adverse reactions

GI: nausea.
Metabolic: hypoglycemia.
Other: toxic reaction.

Interactions

Herb-drug. *Anticoagulants, antiplatelets:* Inhibits platelet aggregation, possibly increasing the risk of bleeding. Monitor patient.
Disulfiram: May cause disulfiram reaction if herbal preparation contains alcohol. Advise patient to avoid use together.

capsicum

Reported uses

- Bowel disorders, chronic laryngitis, and peripheral vascular disease
- Counterirritant and external analgesic
- Topical preparation FDA-approved for temporary relief of pain from rheumatoid arthritis, osteoarthritis, postherpetic neuralgia (shingles), and diabetic neuropathy.
- FDA-tested for psoriasis, intractable pruritus, vitiligo, phantom limb pain, mastectomy pain, Guillain-Barré syndrome, neurogenic bladder, vulvar vestibulitis, apocrine chromhidrosis, and reflex sympathetic dystrophy
- In personal defense sprays and for refractory pruritus and pruritus caused by renal failure

Cautions

- People hypersensitive to herb or chili pepper products should avoid capsicum. Those with irritable bowel syndrome should avoid it because capsicum has irritant and peristaltic effects.
- Those with asthma who use capsicum may experience more bronchospasms.
- **Lifespan:** Pregnant women should avoid capsicum because of possible uterine stimulant effects.

Adverse reactions

EENT: blepharospasm, extreme burning pain, lacrimation, conjunctival edema, hyperemia, burning pain in nose, sneezing, serous discharge.
GI: oral burning, diarrhea, gingival irritation, bleeding gums.
Respiratory: *bronchospasm,* cough, retrosternal discomfort.
Skin: transient skin irritation, itching, stinging, erythema without vesicular eruption, contact dermatitis.

Interactions

Herb-drug. *ACE inhibitors:* Increases risk of cough when applied topically. Monitor patient closely.
Anticoagulants: May alter anticoagulant effects. Monitor PT and INR closely; tell patient to avoid use together.
Antiplatelets, heparin and low–molecular-weight heparin, warfarin: Increases risk of bleeding. Advise patient to avoid use together. If used together, monitor patient for bleeding.
Aspirin, salicylic acid compounds: Reduces bioavailability of these drugs. Discourage use together.
MAO inhibitors: Herb increases catecholamine secretion and increases risk of hypertensive crisis. Discourage use together.
Theophylline: Herb increases theophylline absorption. Discourage use together.
Herb-herb. *Anticoagulant or antiplatelet herbs, such as feverfew, garlic, ginger, ginkgo, ginseng:* Increases anticoagulant effects of capsicum, and increases risk of bleeding. Discourage use together. Anyone who uses them together should be monitored closely for bleeding.

Bold italic type indicates that reaction may be life-threatening.

cat's claw

Reported uses

• GI problems, including inflammatory bowel disease (Crohn disease or ulcerative colitis) diverticulitis, gastritis, dysentery, ulcerations and hemorrhoids, and to enhance immunity
• Systemic inflammatory diseases such as arthritis and rheumatism
• By cancer patients for its antimutagenic effects
• With zidovudine to stimulate the immune system by patients with HIV infection
• As a contraceptive

Cautions

• Those who have had transplant surgery, and those who have an autoimmune disease, multiple sclerosis, or tuberculosis should avoid use.
• Anyone who has a coagulation disorder or takes an anticoagulant should also avoid use.
• People with a history of peptic ulcer disease or gallstones should use caution when taking this herb because it stimulates stomach acid secretion.
🌿 Lifespan: Women who are pregnant or breast-feeding shouldn't use this herb.

Adverse reactions

CV: hypotension.

Interactions

Herb-drug. Antihypertensives: May potentiate hypotensive effects. Discourage use together.
Immunosuppressants: May counteract therapeutic effects because herb has immunostimulant properties. Discourage use together.
Herb-food. Food: May enhance absorption of herb.

chamomile

Reported uses

• Sedation or relaxation (main use)
• Stomach disorders, such as GI spasms and other GI inflammatory conditions
• Insomnia

• Menstrual disorders, migraine, epidermolysis bullosa, eczema, eye irritation, throat discomfort, and hemorrhoids
• As a topical bacteriostat and mouthwash

Cautions

• May be an abortifacient, and some of its components may have teratogenic effects.
• Contraindicated in patients hypersensitive to ragweed pollens.
• Urge caution in those hypersensitive to components of volatile oils and in those at risk for contact dermatitis.
• Safety in people with liver or kidney disorders hasn't been established, and they should avoid use.
🌿 Lifespan: Discourage use by pregnant or breast-feeding women. Herb shouldn't be given to infants or children younger than age 2.

Adverse reactions

EENT: conjunctivitis, eyelid angioedema.
GI: nausea, vomiting.
Skin: contact dermatitis, eczema.
Other: anaphylaxis.

Interactions

Herb-drug. Anticoagulants: May potentiate effects. Discourage use together.
Other drugs: Potential for decreased absorption of drugs because of antispasmodic activity of herb in the GI tract. Discourage use together.

echinacea

Reported uses

• As a wound-healing agent for abscesses, burns, eczema, varicose ulcers of the leg, and other skin wounds
• As a nonspecific immunostimulant for the supportive treatment of upper respiratory tract infections, the common cold, and UTIs

Cautions

• Shouldn't be used by anyone with severe illness, such as HIV infection, collagen disease, leukosis, multiple sclerosis, tuberculosis, or autoimmune disease.
• People with chronic diseases such as diabetes, bronchial asthma, allergies, polyarthritis, organ

transplantation, inflammatory GI disease, impaired resorption, or respiratory disease should avoid use.
- Shouldn't be used with pneumonial, nonrespiratory infection; acute flu; or fungal infection.
☙ **Lifespan:** Discourage use by pregnant or breast-feeding women because effects of herb are unknown. Shouldn't be used in children because of increased risk of allergic reaction.

Adverse reactions

CNS: fever.
GI: nausea, minor GI symptoms, unpleasant taste, vomiting.
GU: diuresis.
Other: allergic reaction in patients allergic to plants belonging to the daisy family, tachyphylaxis.

Interactions

Herb-drug. *Disulfiram, metronidazole:* Herbal products that contain alcohol may cause a disulfiram reaction. Discourage use together.
Immunosuppressants such as cyclosporine: Decreases effectiveness of these drugs. Discourage use together.
Herb-lifestyle. *Alcohol use:* Echinacea preparations containing alcohol may enhance CNS depression. Discourage use together.

eucalyptus

Reported uses

- Internally and externally as an expectorant and for infections and fevers
- Topically to treat sore muscles and rheumatism

Cautions

- People who have had an allergic reaction to eucalyptus or its vapors should avoid use.
- Those who have liver disease or intestinal tract inflammation shouldn't use.
- Essential oil preparations shouldn't be applied to an infant's or child's face because of risk of severe bronchial spasm.
☙ **Lifespan:** Pregnant and breast-feeding women shouldn't use.

Adverse reactions

CNS: delirium, dizziness, *seizures.*
EENT: miosis.
GI: epigastric burning, nausea, vomiting.
Musculoskeletal: muscular weakness.
Respiratory: *asthma-like attacks.*

Interactions

Herb-drug. *Antidiabetics:* Enhances effects. Discourage use together.
Other drugs: Eucalyptus oil induces detoxication enzyme systems in the liver and may affect any drug metabolized in liver. Watch for intended drug effects and toxic reactions.
Herb-herb. *Other herbs that cause hypoglycemia (basil, glucomannan, Queen Anne's lace):* Decreases glucose level. Advise caution.

evening primrose

Reported uses

- Infusion for sedative and astringent properties
- Asthmatic coughs, GI disorders, whooping cough, psoriasis, multiple sclerosis, asthma, Raynaud disease, and Sjögren syndrome
- Poultices made from oil to speed wound healing
- Pruritic symptoms of atopic dermatitis, psoriasis, and eczema; breast pain and tenderness from premenstrual syndrome; benign breast disease; and diabetic neuropathy
- In rheumatoid arthritis, to improve symptoms and reduce the need for pain medication; also used to lower serum cholesterol, improve hypertension, and decrease platelet aggregation
- To calm hyperactive children

Cautions

- Urge caution or discourage use in people with schizophrenia and in those taking antiseizure drugs.
☙ **Lifespan:** In pregnant and breast-feeding women, discourage use; effects are unknown.

Adverse reactions

CNS: headache, *seizures.*
CV: thrombosis.
GI: nausea.
Skin: rash.
Other: *immunosuppression,* inflammation.

Bold italic type indicates that reaction may be life-threatening.

Interactions

Herb-drug. *Phenothiazines:* May increase risk of seizures. Discourage use together.

fennel

Reported uses

- To increase milk secretion, promote menses, facilitate birth, and increase libido
- As an expectorant to manage cough and bronchitis
- Mild spastic disorders of the GI tract, feelings of fullness, and flatulence
- Upper respiratory tract infections in children (syrup)

Cautions

- Should be used cautiously by people allergic to other members of the Umbelliferae family, such as celery, carrots, or mugwort.
- Discourage use in those with a history of seizures.
- ☀ **Lifespan:** In pregnant women, discourage use.

Adverse reactions

CNS: *seizures,* hallucinations.
GI: nausea, vomiting.
Respiratory: *pulmonary edema.*
Skin: contact dermatitis, photodermatitis.
Other: allergic reaction.

Interactions

Herb-drug. *Anticonvulsants, drugs that lower the seizure threshold:* Increases risk of seizure. Monitor patient very closely.
Herb-lifestyle. *Sun exposure:* Increases risk of photosensitivity reactions. Person taking fennel should wear protective clothing and sunscreen and should limit exposure to direct sunlight.

feverfew

Reported uses

- As an antipyretic
- Psoriasis, toothache, insect bites, rheumatism, asthma, stomachache, and menstrual problems

- Migraine prophylaxis

Cautions

- Shouldn't be taken internally by anyone allergic to members of the daisy, or Asteraceae, family—including yarrow, southernwood, wormwood, chamomile, marigold, goldenrod, ragweed, coltsfoot, and dandelion—or anyone who has had previous reaction to herb.
- Those taking anticoagulants such as warfarin and heparin should use herb cautiously.
- ☀ **Lifespan:** Pregnant women shouldn't use because of herb's potential abortifacient properties. Breast-feeding women shouldn't use. Children shouldn't use.

Adverse reactions

CNS: dizziness.
CV: tachycardia.
GI: GI upset, mouth ulcerations.
Skin: contact dermatitis.

Interactions

Herb-drug. *Anticoagulants, antiplatelet drugs including aspirin and thrombolytics:* Herb inhibits prostaglandin synthesis and platelet aggregation. Monitor patient for increased bleeding.
Iron supplements: May decrease iron absorption. Separate doses by 2 hours or more.

flax

Reported uses

- Constipation, functional disorders of the colon resulting from laxative abuse, irritable bowel syndrome, and diverticulitis
- As a supplement to decrease the risk of hypercholesterolemia and atherosclerosis
- As a poultice for areas of local inflammation

Cautions

- People with an ileus or esophageal stricture, and those experiencing an acute inflammatory illness of the GI tract, should avoid use.
- ☀ **Lifespan:** Pregnant and breast-feeding women, and women planning to become pregnant, shouldn't use.

Adverse reactions

GI: diarrhea, flatulence, nausea.

Interactions

Herb-drug. *Anticoagulants, antiplatelet drugs:* May cause additive effects and increased risk of bleeding. Discourage use together.
Antidiabetic drugs: May decrease serum glucose levels. Tell patient to monitor his glucose level.
Laxatives, stool softeners: Possible increase in laxative actions of herb. Discourage use together.
Oral drugs: Because of herb's fibrous content and binding potential, drug absorption may be altered or prevented. Advise patient to avoid taking herb within 2 hours of a drug.

garlic

Reported uses

• To decrease total cholesterol level, decrease triglyceride level, and increase HDL level
• To help prevent atherosclerosis because of its effect on blood pressure and platelet aggregation
• To decrease the risk of cancer, especially cancer of the GI tract; of stroke; and of MI
• Cough, colds, fevers, and sore throats
• Asthma, diabetes, heavy metal poisoning, constipation, and athlete's foot
• As an antimicrobial and to reduce symptoms in patients with AIDS

Cautions

• Shouldn't be used by anyone sensitive to garlic or other members of the Liliaceae family or by those with GI disorders, such as peptic ulcer or reflux disease.
⚕ **Lifespan:** Herb shouldn't be used by pregnant women because it has oxytocic effects.

Adverse reactions

CNS: dizziness, fatigue, headache.
CV: orthostatic hypertension, tachycardia.
GI: halitosis; irritation of mouth, esophagus, and stomach; nausea; vomiting.
Hematologic: decreased hemoglobin production and lysis of RBCs (with long-term use or excessive amounts).

Metabolic: hypothyroidism.
Respiratory: asthma, shortness of breath.
Skin: contact dermatitis, diaphoresis.
Other: allergic reaction, *anaphylaxis,* garlic odor.

Interactions

Herb-drug. *Anticoagulants, NSAIDs, prostacyclin:* May increase bleeding time. Discourage use together.
Antidiabetics: Glucose level may be decreased further. Advise caution if using together, and tell patient to monitor glucose level closely.
Drugs metabolized by the enzyme CYP2E1 (such as acetaminophen): Decreases metabolism of these drugs. Monitor patient for therapeutic effects and toxic reaction.
Herb-herb. *Herbs with anticoagulant effects:* Increases bleeding time. Discourage use together.
Herbs with antihyperglycemic effects: Glucose level may be further decreased. Advise caution and close monitoring of glucose level.

ginger

Reported uses

• As an antiemetic, GI protectant, anti-inflammatory for arthritis treatment, CV stimulant, antitumor agent, antioxidant, and as therapy for microbial and parasitic infestations
• Seasickness, morning or motion sickness, and postoperative nausea and vomiting, and to provide relief from pain and swelling caused by rheumatoid arthritis, osteoarthritis, or muscular discomfort

Cautions

• People with gallstones or with an allergy to herb should avoid use.
• Those with bleeding disorders should avoid using large amounts of herb.
• Anyone taking a CNS depressant or an antiarrhythmic should use ginger cautiously.
⚕ **Lifespan:** Pregnant women should avoid using large amounts of herb.

Adverse reactions

CNS: CNS depression.
CV: *arrhythmias.*

Bold italic type indicates that reaction may be life-threatening.

GI: heartburn.
Hematologic: increased bleeding time.

Interactions

Herb-drug. *Anticoagulants and other drugs that can increase bleeding time:* May further increase bleeding time. Discourage use together.
Herb-herb. *Herbs that may increase bleeding time:* May further increase bleeding time. Discourage use together.

ginkgo

Reported uses

- Primarily to manage cerebral insufficiency, dementia, and circulatory disorders such as intermittent claudication
- Headaches, asthma, colitis, impotence, depression, altitude sickness, tinnitus, cochlear deafness, vertigo, premenstrual syndrome, macular degeneration, diabetic retinopathy, and allergies
- In addition to physical therapy for Fontaine stage IIIB peripheral arterial disease to decrease pain during ambulation with a minimum of 6 weeks of treatment

Cautions

- People with a history of an allergic reaction to ginkgo or any of its components and those with increased risk of intracranial hemorrhage (hypertension, diabetes) should avoid use.
- Anyone taking an antiplatelet or an anticoagulant should avoid use because of the increased risk of bleeding.
- Herb should be avoided before surgery.
- **Lifespan:** Pregnant and breast-feeding women shouldn't use.

Adverse reactions

CNS: dizziness, headache, *seizures,* subarachnoid hemorrhage.
GI: diarrhea, flatulence, nausea, vomiting.
Skin: contact hypersensitivity reaction, dermatitis.

Interactions

Herb-drug. *Anticoagulants, antiplatelets, high-dose vitamin E:* May increase the risk of bleeding. Discourage use together.
MAO inhibitors: Theoretically, herb can potentiate the activity of these drugs. Advise patient to stop taking herb.
SSRIs: Herb extracts may reverse the sexual dysfunction caused by these drugs. Urge patient to consult prescriber before using together.
Warfarin: Possibly increases INR when taken together. Monitor INR.
Herb-herb. *Garlic and other herbs that increase bleeding time:* Potentiates anticoagulant effects. Advise caution.

ginseng

Reported uses

- To minimize or reduce the activity of the thymus gland
- As a sedative, demulcent (soothes irritated or inflamed internal tissues or organs), aphrodisiac, antidepressant, sleep aid, and diuretic
- To improve stamina, concentration, healing, stress resistance, vigilance, and work efficiency and to improve well-being in elderly people with debilitated or degenerative conditions
- To decrease fasting glucose and hemoglobin A1c levels and for hyperlipidemia, hepatic dysfunction, and impaired cognitive function

Cautions

- Should be used cautiously by anyone with CV disease, autoimmune diseases, allergic rhinitis, asthma, eczema, hypertension, hypotension, or diabetes, and by those receiving steroid therapy.
- **Lifespan:** In pregnant or breast-feeding women, discourage use; effects are unknown.

Adverse reactions

CNS: confusion, dizziness, drowsiness, headache, insomnia, nervousness.
CV: chest pain, hypotension, palpitations.
EENT: epistaxis.
GI: diarrhea, nausea, vomiting.
GU: diffuse mammary nodules, diuresis, impotence, vaginal bleeding.
Musculoskeletal: joint pain.

*Liquid may contain alcohol.

Skin: pruritus, skin eruptions (with ginseng abuse).
Other: breast pain.

Interactions

Herb-drug. *Antidiabetics, insulin:* Increases hypoglycemic effects. Monitor glucose level.
Drugs metabolized by CYP3A4: Herb may inhibit this enzyme system. Monitor patient for clinical effects and toxicity.
Phenelzine, other MAO inhibitors: May cause headache, irritability, visual hallucinations, and other interactions. Discourage use together.
Warfarin: Herb may decrease drug effect. Discourage using herb.

goldenseal

Reported uses

- GI disorders, gastritis, peptic ulceration, anorexia, postpartum hemorrhage, dysmenorrhea, eczema, pruritus, tuberculosis, cancer, mouth ulcerations, otorrhea, tinnitus, and conjunctivitis
- As a wound antiseptic, diuretic, laxative, and anti-inflammatory agent
- To shorten the duration of acute *Vibrio cholera* diarrhea and diarrhea caused by some species of *Giardia, Salmonella, Shigella,* and some *Enterobacteriaceae*
- To improve biliary secretion and function in hepatic cirrhosis

Cautions

- People with hypertension, heart failure, or arrhythmias, or severe renal or hepatic disease should avoid use.
- ⚹ Lifespan: Pregnant or breast-feeding women shouldn't use. Infants shouldn't use.

Adverse reactions

CNS: delirium, hallucinations, paralysis, paresthesia, reduced mental alertness, sedation.
CV: *asystole, heart block,* hypertension, hypotension.
GI: diarrhea, GI cramping, mouth ulcerations, nausea, vomiting,
Hematologic: *leukopenia,* megaloblastic anemia from decreased vitamin B absorption.

Respiratory: *respiratory depression.*
Skin: contact dermatitis.

Interactions

Herb-drug. *Anticoagulants:* May reduce anticoagulant effect. Discourage use together.
Antidiabetics, insulin: Increases hypoglycemic effects. Discourage use together; advise patient to monitor glucose level closely.
Antihypertensives: May reduce or enhance hypotensive effect. Discourage use together.
Beta blockers, calcium channel blockers, digoxin: May interfere with or enhance cardiac effects. Discourage use together.
Cephalosporins, disulfiram, metronidazole: May cause disulfiram-like reaction when taken with liquid herbal preparations. Discourage use together.
CNS depressants, such as benzodiazepines: May enhance sedative effects. Discourage use together.
Herb-lifestyle. *Alcohol use:* May enhance sedative effects. Discourage use together.

grapeseed

Reported uses

- As an antioxidant for circulatory disorders (hypoxia from atherosclerosis, inflammation, and cardiac or cerebral infarction)
- Pain, limb heaviness, and swelling from peripheral circulatory disorders and to treat inflammatory conditions, varicose veins, and cancer

Cautions

- People with liver dysfunction should use cautiously.
- ⚹ Lifespan: No considerations reported.

Adverse reactions

Hepatic: *hepatotoxicity.*

Interactions

None reported.

Bold italic type indicates that reaction may be life-threatening.

kava

Reported uses

- Nervous anxiety, insomnia, stress, and restlessness
- Orally as a sedative, to promote wound healing, and for headaches, seizure disorders, the common cold, respiratory tract infection, tuberculosis, and rheumatism
- Urogenital infections, including chronic cystitis, venereal disease, uterine inflammation, menstrual problems, and vaginal prolapse
- As an aphrodisiac
- As juice, for skin diseases, including leprosy
- As a poultice, for intestinal problems, otitis, and abscesses

Cautions

- People hypersensitive to herb or any of its components should avoid it. Depressed people should avoid herb because of possible sedative activity; those with endogenous depression should avoid it because of increased risk of suicide.
- People with renal disease, thrombocytopenia, or neutropenia should use cautiously.
- ☙ Lifespan: Pregnant women shouldn't use this herb because of possible loss of uterine tone. Breast-feeding women shouldn't use. Children shouldn't use.

Adverse reactions

CNS: mild euphoric changes characterized by feelings of happiness, fluent and lively speech, and increased sensitivity to sounds; morning fatigue, sedation, *suicidal thoughts.*
EENT: disorders of oculomotor equilibrium, pupil dilation, visual accommodation disorders.
GI: mild GI disturbances, mouth numbness.
Hepatic: *liver toxicity.*
Metabolic: increased HDL cholesterol; reduced levels of albumin, bilirubin, total protein, and urea.
Respiratory: pulmonary hypertension.
Skin: scaly rash.

Interactions

Herb-drug. *Antiplatelet drugs, type B MAO inhibitors:* Possible additive effects. Monitor patient closely.

Barbiturates, benzodiazepines: Kava lactones potentiate the effects of CNS depressants, leading to toxicity. Discourage use together.
Drugs metabolized by cytochrome P-450: May inhibit drug metabolism, causing increased drug levels and risk of toxicity. Discourage use together.
Hepatotoxic drugs: May cause additive effects. Discourage use together.
Levodopa: Possible reduced effectiveness of levodopa therapy in patients with Parkinson disease, apparently because of dopamine antagonism. Advise patient to use cautiously.
Herb-herb. *Calamus, calendula, California poppy, capsicum, catnip, celery, couch grass, elecampane, German chamomile, goldenseal, gotu kola, hops, Jamaican dogwood, lemon balm, sage, sassafras, shepherd's purse, Siberian ginseng, skullcap, stinging nettle, St. John's wort, valerian, wild lettuce, yerba maté:* Additive sedative effects may occur. Advise great caution.
Herb-lifestyle. *Alcohol use:* Increases risk of CNS depression and liver damage. Discourage use together.

milk thistle

Reported uses

- Dyspepsia, liver damage from chemicals, Amanita mushroom poisoning, support in inflammatory liver disease and cirrhosis, loss of appetite, and gallbladder and spleen disorders
- As a liver protectant

Cautions

- Herb shouldn't be used by people hypersensitive to it or to plants in the Asteraceae family. Use in decompensated cirrhosis isn't recommended.
- ☙ Lifespan: Pregnant and breast-feeding women shouldn't use.

Adverse reactions

CNS: headache.
GI: diarrhea, nausea, vomiting.
Skin: eczema, pruritus, rash, urticaria.

Interactions

Herb-drug. *Aspirin:* May improve aspirin metabolism in people with liver cirrhosis. Advise person to consult prescriber before use.
Cisplatin: May prevent kidney damage by cisplatin. Advise patient to consult prescriber before use.
Disulfiram: Herbal products that contain alcohol may cause a disulfiram-like reaction. Discourage use together.
Hepatotoxic drugs: May prevent liver damage from butyrophenones, phenothiazines, phenytoin, acetaminophen, and halothane. Advise patient to consult prescriber before use.
Tacrine: Silymarin, the active component of milk thistle, reduces adverse cholinergic effects when given together. Advise patient to consult prescriber before use.

nettle

Reported uses

- Allergic rhinitis, osteoarthritis, rheumatoid arthritis, kidney stones, asthma, and BPH
- As a diuretic, an expectorant, a general health tonic, a pain reliever and anti-inflammatory, and a lung tonic for ex-smokers
- Eczema, hives, bursitis, tendinitis, laryngitis, sciatica, and premenstrual syndrome
- Possibly hay fever and irrigation of the urinary tract
- Decrease postoperative blood loss, bacteremia, and inflammation

Cautions

⚱ Lifespan: Herb shouldn't be used by women who are pregnant or breast-feeding because of its diuretic and uterine stimulation properties. Children shouldn't use.

Adverse reactions

CV: edema.
GI: gastric irritation, gingivostomatitis.
GU: decreased urine formation, increased diuresis in patients with arthritic conditions and those with myocardial or chronic venous insufficiency, *oliguria.*
Skin: burning sensation, topical irritation.

Interactions

Herb-drug. *Disulfiram:* Possible disulfiram reaction if taken with liquid extract or tincture. Discourage use together.
Herb-lifestyle. *Alcohol use:* Possible additive effect from liquid extract and tincture. Discourage alcohol use.

passion flower

Reported uses

- As a sedative, a hypnotic, and an antispasmodic for treating muscle spasms
- As an analgesic for menstrual cramping, pain, or migraines
- For neuralgia, generalized seizures, nervous agitation, and insomnia
- Crushed leaves and flowers topically for cuts and bruises

Cautions

- Excessive amounts may cause sedation and may potentiate MAO inhibitor therapy.
- Those with liver disease or a history of alcoholism should avoid products that contain alcohol.
⚱ Lifespan: Women who are pregnant or breast-feeding shouldn't use.

Adverse reactions

CNS: agitation, confusion, drowsiness, flushing, headache, psychosis.
CV: hypotension, *shock,* tachycardia, *ventricular arrhythmias.*
GI: nausea, vomiting.
Respiratory: *asthma.*
Other: allergic reaction.

Interactions

Herb-drug. *Disulfiram, metronidazole:* Herbal products that contain alcohol may cause a disulfiram-like reaction. Discourage use together.
Hexobarbital: Increases sleeping time; other barbiturate effects may be potentiated. Monitor patient's level of consciousness carefully.
MAO inhibitors: Actions can be potentiated by herb. Discourage use together.

Bold italic type indicates that reaction may be life-threatening.

St. John's wort

Reported uses

- Depression, bronchial inflammation, burns, cancer, enuresis, gastritis, hemorrhoids, hypothyroidism, insect bites and stings, insomnia, kidney disorders, and scabies, and as a wound-healing agent
- HIV infection
- Topically for phototherapy of skin diseases, including psoriasis, cutaneous T-cell lymphoma, warts, and Kaposi sarcoma

Cautions

- Transplant patients maintained on cyclosporine or tacrolimus therapy should avoid this herb because of the risk of organ rejection.

⚠ Lifespan: Pregnant women and both men and women planning pregnancy shouldn't use this herb because of mutagenic risk to sperm cells and oocytes and adverse effects on reproductive cells. Breast-feeding women and children shouldn't use.

Adverse reactions

CNS: fatigue, headache, neuropathy, restlessness.
GI: abdominal pain, constipation, diarrhea, digestive complaints, dry mouth, fullness sensation, nausea.
Skin: photosensitivity reactions, pruritus.
Other: delayed hypersensitivity.

Interactions

Herb-drug. *Alprazolam, midazolam:* Decreases drug level. Monitor patient closely.
Amitriptyline, chemotherapeutics, cyclosporine, digoxin, drugs metabolized by the cytochrome P-450 enzyme system, hormonal contraceptives, protease inhibitors, theophylline, warfarin: Decreases effectiveness of these drugs. May require adjustment of drug dosage. Monitor patient closely; discourage use together.
Anesthetics: May have synergistic or unpredictable effects. Discourage use together.
Indinavir: Substantially reduces drug level, causing loss of therapeutic effects. Discourage use together.
MAO inhibitors, including phenelzine and tranylcypromine: May increase effects and

cause toxicity and hypertensive crisis. Discourage use together.
Opioids: Increases sedative effects. Discourage use together.
Reserpine: Antagonizes effects of reserpine. Discourage use together.
SSRIs, such as citalopram, fluoxetine, paroxetine, sertraline: Increases risk of serotonin syndrome. Discourage use together.
Herb-herb. *Herbs with sedative effects, such as calamus, calendula, California poppy, capsicum, catnip, celery, couch grass, elecampane, German chamomile, goldenseal, gotu kola, Jamaican dogwood, kava, lemon balm, sage, sassafras, shepherd's purse, Siberian ginseng, skullcap, stinging nettle, valerian, wild carrot, wild lettuce:* May enhance effects of herbs. Discourage use together.
Herb-food. *Tyramine-containing foods such as beer, cheese, dried meats, fava beans, liver, wine, and yeast:* May cause hypertensive crisis when used together. Advise person to separate food from herb.
Herb-lifestyle. *Alcohol use:* May increase sedative effects. Discourage use together.
Sun exposure: Increases risk of photosensitivity reaction. Advise person to avoid unprotected or prolonged exposure to sunlight.

saw palmetto

Reported uses

- As a mild diuretic
- GU problems such as BPH and to increase sperm production, breast size, and sexual vigor

Cautions

- Those with breast cancer or hormone-dependent illnesses other than BPH should avoid this herb.

⚠ Lifespan: Women of childbearing potential, women who are pregnant or breast-feeding, and children shouldn't use this herb.

Adverse reactions

CNS: headache.
CV: hypertension.
GI: abdominal pain, constipation, diarrhea, nausea.

GU: dysuria, impotence, urine retention, false negative PSA result.
Musculoskeletal: back pain.
Other: decreased libido.

Interactions

Herb-drug. *Adrenergics, hormones, hormone-like drugs:* May cause estrogen, androgen, and alpha-blocking effects. Drug dosages may need adjustment if patient takes this herb. Monitor patient closely.

valerian

Reported uses

• Menstrual cramps, restlessness and sleep disorders from nervous conditions, and other symptoms of psychological stress, such as anxiety, nervous headaches, and gastric spasms
• Topically as a bath additive for restlessness and sleep disorders

Cautions

• People with hepatic impairment shouldn't use this herb because of the risk of hepatotoxicity.
• People with acute or major skin injuries, fever, infectious diseases, cardiac insufficiency, or hypertonia shouldn't bathe with valerian products.
⚘ **Lifespan:** Women who are pregnant or breast-feeding and children shouldn't use this herb; its effects are unknown.

Adverse reactions

CNS: ataxia, dizziness, excitability, headache, insomnia.
CV: cardiac disturbance.
EENT: blurred vision.
GI: nausea.
Other: hypersensitivity reaction, hypothermia.

Interactions

Herb-drug. *Barbiturates, benzodiazepines:* May have additive effects. Monitor patient closely.
CNS depressants: May have additive effects. Discourage use together.
Disulfiram: Disulfiram reaction may occur if herbal extract or tincture contains alcohol. Discourage use together.

Herb-herb. *Herbs with sedative effects, such as catnip, hops, kava, passion flower, skullcap:* May increase sedative effects. Advise caution.
Herb-lifestyle. *Alcohol use:* May increase sedative effects. Discourage using together.

Bold italic type indicates that reaction may be life-threatening.

Appendices
and index

Glossary

Absorption: progress of a drug from the time it's administered, through the time it passes to the tissues, until it becomes available for use by the body.

Agranulocytosis: an abnormal blood condition characterized by a severe reduction in the number of granulocytes, basophils, eosinophils, and neutrophils that results in high fever, exhaustion, and bleeding ulcers of the throat, mucous membranes, and GI tract; an acute disease that may be an adverse reaction to drug or radiation therapy.

Allergic reaction: a local or general reaction after exposure to an allergen to which the patient has already been exposed and sensitized; may range from localized dermatitis to anaphylaxis.

Alopecia: absence or loss of hair.

Angioedema: a potentially life-threatening condition characterized by sudden swelling of tissue in the face, neck, lips, tongue, throat, hands, feet, genitals, or intestine.

Aplastic anemia: a deficiency of all of the formed elements of the blood related to bone marrow failure; caused by neoplastic bone marrow disease or by destruction of the bone marrow by exposure to toxic chemicals, radiation, or certain drugs; also known as *pancytopenia*.

Arthralgia: any pain that affects a joint.

Azotemia: a toxic condition caused by renal insufficiency and subsequent retention of urea in the blood; also called *uremia*.

Cushing syndrome: a metabolic disorder caused by increased production of adrenocorticotropic hormone from a tumor of the adrenal cortex or of the anterior lobe of the pituitary gland, or by excessive intake of glucocorticoids; characterized by central obesity, "moon face," glucose intolerance, growth suppression in children, and weakening of the muscles.

Disseminated intravascular coagulation (DIC): a life-threatening coagulopathy resulting from overstimulation of the body's clotting and anticlotting processes in response to disease, septicemia, neoplasms, obstetric emergencies, severe trauma, prolonged surgery, and hemorrhage.

Distribution: the process by which the drug is delivered to the tissues and fluids of the body.

Duration of action: length of time the drug produces its therapeutic effect.

Eosinophilia: an increase in the number of eosinophils in the blood accompanying many inflammatory conditions; substantial increases are considered a reflection of an allergic response.

Erythema: redness of the skin caused by dilation and congestion of the superficial capillaries, often a sign of inflammation or infection.

Excretion: the elimination of drugs from the body.

Gray baby syndrome: a life-threatening condition that can occur in newborns (especially premature one) who are given chloramphenicol for a bacterial infection such as meningitis; symptoms, usually appearing 2 to 9 days after therapy has begun, include vomiting, loose green stools, refusal to suck, hypotension, cyanosis, low body temperature, and CV collapse; the baby becomes limp and has a gray coloring.

Half-life: the time it takes for half of the drug to be eliminated by the body.

Hemolytic anemia: a disorder characterized by the premature destruction of RBCs; anemia may be minimal or absent, reflecting the ability of the bone marrow to increase production of RBCs.

Hepatitis: inflammation of the liver, usually from a viral infection but sometimes from toxic agents.

Hirsutism: excessive growth of dark, coarse body hair in a characteristically male pattern.

Hypercalcemia: greater-than-normal amounts of calcium in the blood; signs and symptoms include confusion, anorexia, abdominal pain, muscle pain, and weakness.

Hyperglycemia: greater-than-normal amounts of glucose in the blood; signs and symptoms include excessive hunger, thirst, frequent urination, fatigue, weight loss, blurred vision, and poor wound healing.

Hyperkalemia: greater-than-normal amounts of potassium in the blood; signs and symptoms include nausea, fatigue, weakness, and palpitations or irregular pulse.

Hypermagnesemia: greater-than-normal amounts of magnesium in the blood; toxic levels may cause cardiac arrhythmias and may depress deep tendon reflexes and respiration.

Hypernatremia: greater-than-normal amounts of sodium in the blood; signs and symptoms include confusion, seizures, coma, dysrhythmic muscle twitching, lethargy, tachycardia, and irritability.

Hyperplasia: an increase in the number of cells.

Hypersensitivity reaction: an abnormal and undesirable reaction in response to a foreign agent; classified by the mechanism involved and the time it takes to occur and assigned a rating of 1 through 4 (Types I, II, III, IV).

Hypocalcemia: less-than-normal amounts of calcium in the blood; signs and symptoms of severe hypocalcemia include cardiac arrhythmias and muscle cramping and twitching as well as numbness and tingling of the hands, feet, lips, and tongue.

Hypoglycemia: less-than-normal amounts of glucose in the blood; signs and symptoms include weakness, drowsiness, confusion, hunger, dizziness, pallor, irritability, tremor, sweating, headache, a cold and clammy feeling, rapid heart beat, and if left untreated, delirium, coma, and death.

Hypokalemia: less-than-normal amounts of potassium in the blood; signs and symptoms include palpitations, muscle weakness or cramping, paresthesias, frequent urination, delirium, depression, and GI complaints such as constipation, nausea, vomiting, and abdominal cramping.

Hypomagnesemia: less-than-normal amounts of magnesium in the blood; signs and symptoms include nausea, vomiting, muscle weakness, tremors, tetany, and lethargy.

Hyponatremia: less-than-normal amounts of sodium in the blood; signs and symptoms may range from mild anorexia, headache, or muscle cramps to obtundation, coma, or seizures.

Leukocytosis: an abnormal increase in the number of circulating WBCs; types are basophilia, eosinophilia, and neutrophilia.

Leukopenia: an abnormal decrease in the number of WBCs to fewer than $5,000/mm^3$.

Metabolism: the body's ability to change a drug from its dosage form to a more water-soluble form that can then be excreted.

Myalgia: diffuse muscle pain, usually occurring with malaise.

Nephrotic syndrome: an abnormal kidney condition characterized by marked proteinuria, hypoalbuminemia, and edema.

Neuroleptic malignant syndrome: the rarest and most serious of the neuroleptic-induced movement disorders, a neurologic emergency in most cases; signs and symptoms include fever, rigidity, tremor, drowsiness, and confusion progressing to stupor and coma, seizures, and cardiac arrhythmias.

Neutropenia: an abnormal decrease in the number of circulating neutrophils in the blood.

Onset of action: time interval that starts when the drug is administered and ends when the therapeutic effect begins.

Pancytopenia: a deficiency of all of the formed elements of the blood related to bone marrow failure caused by neoplastic bone marrow disease or by destruction of the bone marrow after exposure to toxic chemicals, radiation, or certain drugs; also known as *aplastic anemia*.

Peak concentration: reached when the absorption rate of a drug equals the elimination rate.

Pharmacodynamics: the study of drug action in the body at the tissue site; includes uptake, movement, binding, and interactions.

Pharmacokinetics: the study of the action of drugs within the body, including the routes and mechanisms of absorption and excretion, the rate at which a drug's action begins, the duration of effect, the biotransformation of the substance in the body, and the effects and routes of metabolite excretion.

Pruritus: itching.

Pseudomembranous colitis: a complication of antibiotic therapy that causes severe local tissue inflammation of the colon; signs and symptoms include watery diarrhea, abdominal pain or cramping, and low-grade fever.

Pseudotumor cerebri: benign intracranial hypertension, most common in women ages 20 to 50, caused by increased pressure within the brain; symptoms include headache, dizziness, nausea, vomiting, and ringing or rushing sound in the ears.

Psoriasis: a common skin disorder characterized by the eruption of red, silvery-scaled maculopapules, predominantly on the elbows, knees, scalp, and trunk.

Reye syndrome: an encephalopathy that affects children; linked to the use of aspirin and other salicylate-containing drug, as well as other causes; the syndrome may follow an upper respiratory infection or chicken pox; its onset is rapid, usually starting with irritable, combative behavior and vomiting, progressing to semiconsciousness, seizures, coma, and possibly death.

Serotonin syndrome: a typically mild, yet potentially serious drug-related condition most often reported in patients taking two or more drugs that increase CNS serotonin levels; the most common combinations involve MAO inhibitors, SSRIs, and tricyclic antidepressants; signs and symptoms include confusion, agitation, restlessness, rapid heart rate, muscle rigidity or twitching, tremors, and nausea.

Serum sickness: an immune complex disease appearing 1 or 2 weeks after infection of a foreign serum or serum protein, with local and systemic reactions, such as urticaria, fever, general lymphadenopathy, edema, arthritis, and occasionally albuminuria or severe nephritis.

Syncope: a brief loss of consciousness caused by oxygen deficiency to the brain, often preceded by a feeling of dizziness; have the patient lie down or place his head between his knees to prevent it.

Thrombocytopenia: an abnormal decrease in the number of platelets in the blood, predisposing the patient to bleeding disorders.

Thrombocytopenic purpura: a bleeding disorder characterized by a marked decrease in the number of platelets, causing multiple bruises, petechiae, and hemorrhage into the tissues.

Tinnitus: sound in one or both ears, such as buzzing, ringing, or whistling, occurring without external stimuli; it may be from many causes such as an ear infection, the use of certain drugs, a blocked auditory tube or canal, head trauma, or sensoryneuro changes.

Urticaria: an itchy skin condition characterized by pale wheals with well-defined red edges; this may be the result of an allergic response to insect bites, food, or drugs.

Preventing miscommunication

Although abbreviations can save time, they also raise the risk of misinterpretation, which can lead to potentially disastrous consequences, especially when dealing with drug administration. To help reduce the risk of being misunderstood, always take the time to write legibly and to spell out anything that could be misread. This caution extends to how you write numbers as well as drug names and other drug-related instructions.

Dosages

For instance, when writing a drug dosage, never add a zero after a decimal point and never fail to add a zero before a decimal point. If you write 1.0 mg instead of the correct 1 mg, the dosage easily could be misread as 10 mg. Likewise, if you write .5 mg instead of the correct 0.5 mg, the dosage could be misread as 5 mg.

Drug names

Be careful with drug names as well. For instance, If you write $MgSO_4$ as shorthand for magnesium sulfate, you could be misread as meaning morphine sulfate. The opposite is also true; if you write MS or MSO_4, meaning morphine sulfate, you could be misread as meaning magnesium sulfate. Instead, make sure to clearly write out all drug names, particularly those that could be easily confused or could be dangerous if confused.

Common dangerous abbreviations

Finally, try to avoid these common—and dangerous—abbreviations.

Abbreviation	Intended use	Potential misreading	Preferred use
BT	bedtime	May be read as "bid" or twice daily	Spell out "bedtime."
cc	cubic centimeters	May be read as "u" or units	Use milliliters, abbreviated as mL or ml.
D/C	discharge or discontinue	May lead to premature discontinuation of drug therapy or premature discharge	Spell out discharge or discontinue.
hs	bedtime	May be read as "half-strength"	Spell out bedtime.
HS	half-strength	May be read as "bedtime"	Spell out half-strength.
IJ	injection	May be read as "IV"	Spell out "injection."
IN	intranasal	May be read as "IM" or "IV"	Spell out "intranasal" or use "NAS."
IU	international unit	May be read as "IV" or "10"	Spell out "international unit."
μg	microgram	May be read as "mg"	Use "mcg."
o.d. or O.D.	once daily	May be read as "right eye"	Spell out "once daily."

Abbreviation	Intended use	Potential misreading	Preferred use
per os	by mouth	May be read as "left eye"	Use "PO" or spell out "orally."
q1d	once daily	May be read as "qid"	Spell out "once daily."
q.d. or QD	daily	May be read as "qid"	Spell out "daily."
qhs	every bedtime	May be read as "qhr" (every hour)	Spell out "nightly."
qn	every night	May be read as "qh" (every hour)	Spell out "nightly" or "at bedtime."
q.o.d. or QOD	every other day	May be read as "q.d." (daily) or "q.i.d." (four times daily)	Spell out "every other day."
SC, SQ	subcutaneous	May be read as "SL" (sublingual) or "5 every"	Spell out "subcutaneous" or use "subcut" or "SubQ."
U or u	unit	May be read as "0" (100 instead of 10U)	Spell out "unit."
x7d	for 7 days	May be read as "for seven doses"	Spell out "for 7 days."
°	hour	May be read as a zero	Spell out "hour" or use "hr."

Pregnancy risk categories

The FDA has assigned a pregnancy risk category to each drug based on available clinical and pre-clinical information. The five categories (A, B, C, D, X) reflect a drug's potential to cause birth defects. Although drugs should ideally be avoided during pregnancy, sometimes they're needed; this rating system permits rapid assessment of the risk-benefit ratio. Drugs in category A are generally considered safe to use in pregnancy; drugs in category X are generally contraindicated.

- A: Adequate studies in pregnant women haven't shown a risk to fetus.
- B: Animal studies haven't shown a risk to fetus, but controlled studies haven't been conducted in pregnant women; or animal studies have shown an adverse effect on fetus, but adequate studies in pregnant women haven't shown a risk to fetus.
- C: Animal studies have shown an adverse effect on fetus, but adequate studies haven't been conducted in pregnant women. The benefits from use in pregnant women may be acceptable despite risks.

- D: The drug may cause risk to fetus, but the potential benefits of use in pregnant women may be acceptable despite the risks (such as in a life-threatening situation or a serious disease for which safer drugs can't be used or are ineffective).
- X: Studies in animals or humans show fetal abnormalities, or adverse-reaction reports indicate evidence of fetal risk. The risks involved clearly outweigh potential benefits.
- NR: Not rated.

Controlled substance schedules

Drugs regulated under the jurisdiction of the Controlled Substances Act of 1970 are divided into the following groups or schedules:

- Schedule I (C-I): High abuse potential and no accepted medical use. Examples include heroin, cocaine, and LSD.
- Schedule II (C-II): High abuse potential with severe dependence liability. Examples include opioids, amphetamines, and some barbiturates.
- Schedule III (C-III): Less abuse potential than schedule II drugs and moderate dependence liability. Examples include nonbarbiturate sedatives, nonamphetamine stimulants, anabolic steroids, dronabinol, and limited amounts of certain opioids.
- Schedule IV (C-IV): Less abuse potential than schedule III drugs and limited dependence liability. Examples include some sedatives, anxiolytics, and non-opioid analgesics.

- Schedule V (C-V): Limited abuse potential. This category includes mainly small amounts of opioids, such as codeine, used as antitussives or antidiarrheals. Under federal law, limited quantities of certain C-V drugs may be purchased without a prescription directly from a pharmacist if allowed under specific state laws. The purchaser must be at least age 18 and must furnish suitable identification. All such transactions must be recorded by the dispensing pharmacist.

Combination drug products

Accuretic

Generic components
Tablets
10 mg quinapril and 12.5 mg hydrochlorothiazide
20 mg quinapril and 12.5 mg hydrochlorothiazide
20 mg quinapril and 25 mg hydrochlorothiazide

Indications and dosages
Hypertension
Adults: 1 tablet P.O. per day in the morning. Adjust drug using the individual products; then switch to appropriate dosage of the combination product.

Activella
femHRT

Generic components
Tablets
2.5 mcg ethinyl estradiol and 0.5 mg norethindrone acetate (femHRT)
5 mcg ethinyl estradiol and 1 mg norethindrone acetate (femHRT)
0.5 mg ethinyl estradiol and 0.1 mg norethindrone acetate (Activella)
1 mg ethinyl estradiol and 0.5 mg norethindrone acetate (Activella)

Indications and dosages
Signs and symptoms of menopause and prevention of osteoporosis
Women with intact uterus: 1 tablet P.O. daily.

ACTOPlus MET

Generic components
Tablets
15 mg pioglitazone hydrochloride and 500 mg metformin hydrochloride
15 mg pioglitazone hydrochloride and 850 mg metformin hydrochloride

Indications and dosages
Type 2 diabetes mellitus
Adults: For patients inadequately controlled on metformin alone or for patients who initially responded to pioglitazone alone but now require additional glycemic control, start with either the 15 mg/500 mg or 15 mg/850 mg combination P.O. once daily or b.i.d.; adjust dosage based on therapeutic response.

Adderall
Adderall XR
Controlled Substance Schedule (CSS) II

Generic components
Tablets
5 mg: 1.25 mg dextroamphetamine sulfate, 1.25 mg dextroamphetamine saccharate, and 1.25 mg amphetamine aspartate, 1.25 mg amphetamine sulfate
7.5 mg: 1.875 mg dextroamphetamine sulfate, 1.875 mg dextroamphetamine saccharate, 1.875 mg amphetamine aspartate, and 1.875 mg amphetamine sulfate
10 mg: 2.5 mg dextroamphetamine sulfate, 2.5 mg dextroamphetamine saccharate, 2.5 mg amphetamine aspartate, and 2.5 mg amphetamine sulfate
12.5 mg: 3.125 mg dextroamphetamine sulfate, 3.125 mg dextroamphetamine saccharate, 3.125 mg amphetamine aspartate, and 3.125 mg amphetamine sulfate
15 mg: 3.75 mg dextroamphetamine sulfate, 3.75 mg dextroamphetamine saccharate, 3.75 mg amphetamine aspartate, and 3.75 mg amphetamine sulfate
20 mg: 5 mg dextroamphetamine sulfate, 5 mg dextroamphetamine saccharate, 5 mg amphetamine aspartate, and 5 mg amphetamine sulfate
30 mg: 7.5 mg dextroamphetamine sulfate, 7.5 mg dextroamphetamine saccharate, 7.5 mg amphetamine aspartate, and 7.5 mg amphetamine sulfate
Capsules (extended-release)
5 mg: 1.25 mg dextroamphetamine sulfate, 1.25 mg dextroamphetamine saccharate, 1.25 mg amphetamine aspartate, and 1.25 mg amphetamine sulfate

10 mg: 2.5 mg dextroamphetamine sulfate, 2.5 mg dextroamphetamine saccharate, 2.5 mg amphetamine aspartate, and 2.5 mg amphetamine sulfate
15 mg: 3.75 mg dextroamphetamine sulfate, 3.75 mg dextroamphetamine saccharate, 3.75 mg amphetamine aspartate, and 3.75 mg amphetamine sulfate
20 mg: 5 mg dextroamphetamine sulfate, 5 mg dextroamphetamine saccharate, 5 mg amphetamine aspartate, and 5 mg amphetamine sulfate
25 mg: 6.25 mg dextroamphetamine sulfate, 6.25 mg dextroamphetamine saccharate, 6.25 mg amphetamine aspartate, and 6.25 mg amphetamine sulfate
30 mg: 7.5 mg dextroamphetamine sulfate, 7.5 mg dextroamphetamine saccharate, 7.5 mg amphetamine aspartate, and 7.5 mg amphetamine sulfate

Indications and dosages
Narcolepsy
Adults and children age 12 and older: Initially, 10 mg immediate-release tablet daily. Increase by 10 mg weekly to maximum dose of 60 mg in two or three divided doses every 4 to 6 hours.
Children ages 6 to 12: Initially, 5 mg immediate-release tablet P.O. daily. Increase by 5 mg at weekly intervals to maximum of 60 mg in divided doses.
Attention deficit hyperactivity disorder
Adults: 20 mg extended-release capsules P.O. daily.
Adolescents ages 13 to 17: Initially, 10 mg extended-release capsule P.O. daily. Increase after 1 week to 20 mg daily if needed.
Children age 6 and older: Initially, 5 mg immediate-release tablet P.O. daily or b.i.d. Increase by 5 mg at weekly intervals until expected response. Dosage should rarely exceed 40 mg.
Children ages 6 to 12: Initially, 10 mg extended-release capsule P.O. daily in a.m. Increase by 5 to 10 mg in weekly intervals to a maximum dose of 30 mg.
Children ages 3 to 5: Initially 2.5 mg immediate-release tablet P.O. daily. Increase by 2.5 mg at weekly intervals until optimal response. Divide total daily amount into two or three doses and give 4 to 6 hours apart.

Advicor

Generic components
Tablets
20 mg lovastatin and 500 mg niacin
20 mg lovastatin and 750 mg niacin
20 mg lovastatin and 1,000 mg niacin
40 mg lovastatin and 1,000 mg niacin

Indications and dosages
Hyperlipidemia
Adults: 1 tablet daily P.O. at night.

Aggrenox

Generic components
Capsules
25 mg aspirin and 200 mg dipyridamole

Indications and dosages
Stroke
Adults: To decrease risk of stroke, 1 capsule P.O. b.i.d. in the morning and evening. Swallow capsule whole; may be taken with or without food.

Aldactazide

Generic components
Tablets
25 mg spironolactone and 25 mg hydrochlorothiazide
50 mg spironolactone and 50 mg hydrochlorothiazide

Indications and dosages
Edema or hypertension
Adults: One to eight 25 mg spironolactone and 25 mg hydrochlorothiazide tablets daily. Or, one to four 50 mg spironolactone and 50 mg hydrochlorothiazide tablets daily.

Alor 5/500
Lortab ASA
Panasal 5/500
CSS III

Generic components
Tablets
500 mg aspirin and 5 mg hydrocodone bitartrate

Indications and dosages
Moderate to moderately severe pain
Adults: 1 or 2 tablets every 4 hours. Maximum dosage, 8 tablets in 24 hours.

Anexsia 5/325
Norco 5/325
CSS III

Generic components
Tablets
325 mg acetaminophen and 5 mg hydrocodone bitartrate

Indications and dosages
Moderate to moderately severe pain
Adults: 1 to 2 tablets every 4 to 6 hours. Maximum dosage, 12 tablets in 24 hours.

Anexsia 5/500
Co-Gesic
Lorcet HD
Lortab 5/500
Panacet 5/500
Vicodin
CSS III

Generic components
Tablets or capsules
500 mg acetaminophen and 5 mg hydrocodone bitartrate

Indications and dosages
Moderate to moderately severe pain
Adults: 1 to 2 tablets every 4 to 6 hours. Maximum dosage, 8 tablets in 24 hours.

Anexsia 7.5/325
Norco 7.5/325
CSS III

Generic components
Tablets
325 mg acetaminophen and 7.5 mg hydrocodone bitartrate

Indications and dosages
Moderate to moderately severe pain
Adults: 1 to 2 tablets every 4 to 6 hours. Maximum dosage, 12 tablets in 24 hours.

Anexsia 7.5/650
Lorcet Plus
CSS III

Generic components
Tablets
650 mg acetaminophen and 7.5 mg hydrocodone bitartrate

Indications and dosages
Arthralgia, bone pain, dental pain, headache, migraine, moderate pain
Adults: 1 to 2 tablets every 4 hours. Maximum dosage, 6 tablets in 24 hours.

Anexsia 10/660
Vicodin HP
CSS III

Generic components
Tablets
660 mg acetaminophen and 10 mg hydrocodone bitartrate

Indications and dosages
Arthralgia, bone pain, dental pain, headache, migraine, moderate pain
Adults: 1 tablet every 4 to 6 hours. Maximum dosage, 6 tablets in 24 hours.

Atacand HCT

Generic components
Tablets
16 mg candesartan and 12.5 mg hydrochlorothiazide
32 mg candesartan and 12.5 mg hydrochlorothiazide

Indications and dosages
Hypertension
Adults: 1 tablet P.O. daily in the morning.
Adjust dosage using the individual products;
then switch to appropriate dosage.

Atripla

Generic components
Tablets
600 mg efavirenz, 200 mg emtricitabine, and
300 mg tenofovir disoproxil fumarate

Indications and dosages
HIV infection
Adults: 1 tablet P.O. once daily on an empty
stomach. Taking at bedtime may lessen nervous
system symptoms.

Avalide

Generic components
Tablets
150 mg irbesartan and 12.5 mg hydrochlorothiazide
300 mg irbesartan and 12.5 mg hydrochlorothiazide
300 mg irbesartan and 25 mg hydrochlorothiazide

Indications and dosages
Hypertension
Adults: 1 tablet P.O. daily. Adjust dosage with
individual products; then switch to combination
product when patient's condition is stabilized.
Maximum daily dose, 300 mg irbesartan and
25 mg hydrochlorothiazide.

Avandamet

Generic components
Tablets
2 mg rosiglitazone hydrochloride and 500 mg
metformin hydrochloride
2 mg rosiglitazone hydrochloride and 1,000 mg
metformin hydrochloride
4 mg rosiglitazone hydrochloride and 500 mg
metformin hydrochloride
4 mg rosiglitazone hydrochloride and 1,000 mg
metformin hydrochloride

Indications and dosages
Type 2 diabetes mellitus
Adults: For drug-naive patients, as initial
therapy, give 2 mg/500 mg combination P.O.
once daily. For second-line treatment, give
4 mg/500 mg combination P.O. once daily or
2 mg/500 mg combination P.O. b.i.d. Adjust
dosages based on therapeutic response.

Benicar HCT

Generic components
Tablets
20 mg olmesartan and 12.5 mg hydrochlorothiazide
40 mg olmesartan and 12.5 mg hydrochlorothiazide
40 mg olmesartan and 25 mg hydrochlorothiazide

Indications and dosages
Hypertension
Adults: 1 tablet P.O. per day in the morning.
Adjust dosage using the individual products;
then switch to the combination product when
patient's adjustment schedule is stable.

BiDil

Generic components
Tablets
20 mg isosorbide dinitrate and 37.5 mg hydralazine

Indications and dosages
Heart failure
Adults: 1 to 2 tablets P.O. t.i.d.

Caduet

Generic components
Tablets
2.5 mg amlodipine and 10 mg atorvastatin
2.5 mg amlodipine and 20 mg atorvastatin
2.5 mg amlodipine and 40 mg atorvastatin
5 mg amlodipine and 10 mg atorvastatin
5 mg amlodipine and 20 mg atorvastatin
5 mg amlodipine and 40 mg atorvastatin
5 mg amlodipine and 80 mg atorvastatin
10 mg amlodipine and 10 mg atorvastatin
10 mg amlodipine and 20 mg atorvastatin
10 mg amlodipine and 40 mg atorvastatin
10 mg amlodipine and 80 mg atorvastatin

Indications and dosages
Hypertension and angina with hyperlipidemia
Adults: 5 to 10 mg with 10 to 80 mg atorvastatin P.O. once daily. Determine most effective dosage for each component, and then select most appropriate combination.

Capital with Codeine
Tylenol with Codeine Elixir
CSS V

Generic components
Elixir
120 mg acetaminophen and 12 mg codeine phosphate/5 ml

Indications and dosages
Mild to moderate pain
Adults: 15 ml every 4 hours.

Capozide

Generic components
Tablets
25 mg captopril and 15 mg hydrochlorothiazide
50 mg captopril and 15 mg hydrochlorothiazide
25 mg captopril and 25 mg hydrochlorothiazide
50 mg captopril and 25 mg hydrochlorothiazide

Indications and dosages
Hypertension
Adults: 1 to 2 tablets P.O. daily, in the morning. Adjust dosage using the individual products;

then switch to the combination product when patient's adjustment schedule is stable.

Clorpres

Generic components
Tablets
15 mg chlorthalidone and 0.1 mg clonidine hydrochloride
15 mg chlorthalidone and 0.2 mg clonidine hydrochloride
15 mg chlorthalidone and 0.3 mg clonidine hydrochloride

Indications and dosages
Hypertension
Adults: 1 to 2 tablets per day P.O. in the morning. Adjust dosage using the individual products; then switch to the combination product when patient's adjustment schedule is stable.

CombiPatch

Generic components
Transdermal patch
0.05 mg/day estradiol and 0.14 mg/day norethindrone
0.05 mg/day estradiol and 0.25 mg/day norethindrone

Indications and dosages
Signs and symptoms of menopause
Women: Change patch twice a week.

Combivent

Generic components
Metered-dose inhaler
18 mcg ipratropium bromide and 90 mcg albuterol

Indications and dosages
Bronchospasm with COPD in patients who require more than a single bronchodilator
Adults: Two inhalations q.i.d. Not for use during acute attack. Use caution with known sensitivity to atropine, soy, or peanuts.

Combivir

Generic components
Tablets
150 mg lamivudine and 300 mg zidovudine

Indications and dosages
HIV infection
Adults and children 12 and older who weigh more than 50 kg (110 lb): 1 tablet P.O. b.i.d.

Corzide

Generic components
Tablets
40 mg nadolol and 5 mg bendroflumethiazide
80 mg nadolol and 5 mg bendroflumethiazide

Indications and dosages
Hypertension
Adults: 1 tablet P.O. per day in the morning. Adjust dosage using the individual products; then switch to the combination product when patient's adjustment schedule is stable.

Darvocet-A500
CSS IV

Generic components
Tablets
500 mg acetaminophen and 100 mg propoxyphene napsylate

Indications and dosages
Mild to moderate pain
Adults: 1 tablet every 4 hours. Maximum dosage, 8 tablets in 24 hours.

Darvocet-N50
CSS IV

Generic components
Tablets
325 mg acetaminophen and 50 mg propoxyphene napsylate

Indications and dosages
Mild to moderate pain
Adults: 2 tablets every 4 hours. Maximum dosage, 12 tablets in 24 hours.

Darvocet-N100
CSS IV

Generic components
Tablets
650 mg acetaminophen and 100 mg propoxyphene napsylate

Indications and dosages
Mild to moderate pain
Adults: 1 tablet every 4 hours. Maximum dosage, 6 tablets in 24 hours.

Diovan HCT

Generic components
Tablets
80 mg valsartan and 12.5 mg hydrochlorothiazide
160 mg valsartan and 12.5 mg hydrochlorothiazide
160 mg valsartan and 25 mg hydrochlorothiazide
320 mg valsartan and 12.5 mg hydrochlorothiazide
320 mg valsartan and 25 mg hydrochlorothiazide

Indications and dosages
Hypertension
Adults: 1 tablet per day P.O. Not for initial therapy; start using each component first.

Duetact

Generic components
Tablets
30 mg pioglitazone and 2 mg glimepiride
30 mg pioglitazone and 4 mg glimepiride

Indications and dosages
Type 2 diabetes mellitus
Adults: For patients currently on glimepiride alone, start with either 30 mg/2 mg or 30 mg/4 mg combination P.O. once daily; adjust dosage based on therapeutic response.
Adults: For patients currently on pioglitazone alone, start with 30 mg/2 mg combination P.O. once daily; adjust dosage based on therapeutic response.

Dyazide

Generic components
Capsules
37.5 mg triamterene and 25 mg hydrochloro-thiazide

Indications and dosages
Edema or hypertension
Adults: 1 to 2 capsules daily.

Empirin with Codeine No. 3
CSS III

Generic components
Tablets
325 mg aspirin and 30 mg codeine phosphate

Indications and dosages
Fever and mild to moderate pain
Adults: 1 to 2 tablets every 4 hours. Maximum dosage, 12 tablets in 24 hours.

Empirin with Codeine No. 4
CSS III

Generic components
Tablets
325 mg aspirin and 60 mg codeine phosphate

Indications and dosages
Fever and mild to moderate pain
Adults: 1 tablet every 4 hours. Maximum dosage, 6 tablets in 24 hours.

Endocet 5/325
Percocet 5/325
Roxicet
CSS II

Generic components
Tablets
325 mg acetaminophen and 5 mg oxycodone hydrochloride

Endocet 7.5/325
Percocet 7.5/325
CSS II

Generic components
Tablets
325 mg acetaminophen and 7.5 mg oxycodone hydrochloride

Indications and dosages
Moderate to moderately severe pain
Adults: 1 tablet every 6 hours. Maximum dosage, 8 tablets in 24 hours.

Endocet 7.5/500
Percocet 7.5/500
CSS II

Generic components
Tablets
500 mg acetaminophen and 7.5 mg oxycodone hydrochloride

Indications and dosages
Moderate to moderately severe pain
Adults: 1 to 2 tablets every 4 to 6 hours. Maximum dosage, 8 tablets in 24 hours.

Endocet 10/325
Percocet 10/325
CSS II

Generic components
Tablets
325 mg acetaminophen and 10 mg oxycodone hydrochloride

Indications and dosages
Moderate to moderately severe pain
Adults: 1 tablet every 6 hours. Maximum dosage, 6 tablets in 24 hours.

Indications and dosages
Moderate to moderately severe pain
Adults: 1 tablet every 6 hours. Maximum dosage, 12 tablets in 24 hours.

Epzicom

Generic components
Tablets
600 mg abacavir with 300 mg lamivudine

Indications and dosages
HIV infection
Adults: 1 tablet daily, taken without regard to food and with other antiretrovirals.

Eryzole
Pediazole

Generic components
Granules for oral suspension
Erythromycin ethylsuccinate (equivalent of 200 mg erythromycin activity) and 600 mg sulfisoxazole per 5 ml when reconstituted according to manufacturer's directions

Indications and dosages
Acute otitis media
Children: 50 mg/kg/day erythromycin and 150 mg/kg/day sulfisoxazole in divided doses q.i.d. for 10 days. Give without regard to meals. Refrigerate after reconstitution; use within 14 days.

Fioricet with Codeine
CSS III

Generic components
Capsules
325 mg acetaminophen, 50 mg butalbital, 40 mg caffeine, and 30 mg codeine phosphate

Indications and dosages
Headache and mild to moderate pain
Adults and children age 12 and older: 1 to 2 capsules every 4 hours. Maximum dosage, 6 capsules in 24 hours.

Fiorinal with Codeine
CSS III

Generic components
Capsules
325 mg aspirin, 50 mg butalbital, 40 mg caffeine, and 30 mg codeine phosphate

Indications and dosages
Tension headache symptoms
Adults and children age 12 and older: 1 to 2 capsules every 4 hours. Maximum dosage, 6 capsules in 24 hours.

Hyzaar

Generic components
Tablets
50 mg losartan and 12.5 mg hydrochlorothiazide
100 mg losartan and 12.5 mg hydrochlorothiazide
100 mg losartan and 25 mg hydrochlorothiazide

Indications and dosages
Hypertension
Adults: 1 tablet per day P.O. in the morning. Not for initial therapy; start using each component and if desired effects are obtained, Hyzaar may be used.

Inderide

Generic components
Tablets
40 mg propranolol hydrochloride and 25 mg hydrochlorothiazide
80 mg propranolol hydrochloride and 25 mg hydrochlorothiazide

Indications and dosages
Hypertension
Adults: 1 tablet P.O. b.i.d. Adjust dosage using the individual products; then switch to the combination product when patient's adjustment schedule is stable. Maximum total daily dose shouldn't exceed 160 mg propranolol and 50 mg hydrochlorothiazide.

Lexxel

Generic components
Extended-release tablets
5 mg enalapril maleate and 2.5 mg felodipine
5 mg enalapril maleate and 5 mg felodipine

Indications and dosages
Hypertension
Adults: 1 tablet per day P.O. Adjust dosage using the individual products; then switch to the combination product when patient's adjustment schedule is stable. Make sure that patient swallows tablet whole. Don't cut, crush, or allow him to chew.

Limbitrol
Limbitrol DS

Generic components
Tablets
5 mg chlordiazepoxide and 12.5 mg amitriptyline
10 mg chlordiazepoxide and 25 mg amitriptyline

Indications and dosages
Severe depression
Adults: 10 mg chlordiazepoxide with 25 mg amitriptyline 3 to 4 times per day up to 6 times daily. For patients who don't tolerate the higher doses, 5 mg chlordiazepoxide with 12.5 mg amitriptyline 3 to 4 times per day. Reduce dosage after initial response.

Lopressor HCT

Generic components
Tablets
50 mg metoprolol and 25 mg hydrochlorothiazide
100 mg metoprolol and 25 mg hydrochlorothiazide
100 mg metoprolol and 50 mg hydrochlorothiazide

Indications and dosages
Hypertension
Adults: 1 tablet P.O. per day. Adjust dosage using the individual products; then switch to the

combination product when patient's adjustment schedule is stable.

Lorcet 10/650
CSS III

Generic components
Tablets
650 mg acetaminophen and 10 mg hydrocodone bitartrate

Indications and dosages
Moderate to moderately severe pain
Adults: 1 tablet every 4 to 6 hours. Maximum dosage, 6 tablets in 24 hours.

Lortab 2.5/500
CSS III

Generic components
Tablets
500 mg acetaminophen and 2.5 mg hydrocodone bitartrate

Indications and dosages
Moderate to moderately severe pain
Adults: 1 to 2 tablets every 4 to 6 hours. Maximum dosage, 8 tablets in 24 hours.

Lortab 7.5/500
CSS III

Generic components
Tablets
500 mg acetaminophen and 7.5 mg hydrocodone bitartrate

Indications and dosages
Moderate to moderately severe pain
Adults: 1 tablet every 4 to 6 hours. Maximum dosage, 8 tablets in 24 hours.

Lortab 10/500
CSS III

Generic components
Tablets
500 mg acetaminophen and 10 mg hydrocodone bitartrate

Indications and dosages
Moderate to moderately severe pain
Adults: 1 tablet every 4 to 6 hours. Maximum dosage, 6 tablets in 24 hours.

Lortab Elixir
CSS III

Generic components
Elixir
167 mg acetaminophen and 2.5 mg/5 ml hydrocodone bitartrate

Indications and dosages
Moderately severe pain
Adults: 15 ml every 4 to 6 hours. Maximum dosage, 90 ml/day.

Lotensin HCT

Generic components
Tablets
5 mg benazepril and 6.25 mg hydrochlorothiazide
10 mg benazepril and 12.5 mg hydrochlorothiazide
20 mg benazepril and 12.5 mg hydrochlorothiazide
20 mg benazepril and 25 mg hydrochlorothiazide

Indications and dosages
Hypertension
Adults: 1 tablet per day P.O. in the morning. Adjust dosage using the individual products; then switch to the combination product when patient's adjustment schedule is stable.

Lotrel

Generic components
Capsules
2.5 mg amlodipine and 10 mg benazepril
5 mg amlodipine and 10 mg benazepril
5 mg amlodipine and 20 mg benazepril
5 mg amlodipine and 40 mg benazepril
10 mg amlodipine and 20 mg benazepril
10 mg amlodipine and 40 mg benazepril

Indications and dosages
Hypertension
Adults: 1 capsule P.O. daily in the morning. Monitor patient for hypertension and adverse effects closely over first 2 weeks and regularly thereafter.

Maxzide

Generic components
Tablets
37.5 mg triamterene and 25 mg hydrochlorothiazide
75 mg triamterene and 50 mg hydrochlorothiazide

Indications and dosages
Edema or hypertension
Adults: 1 tablet daily.

Micardis HCT

Generic components
Tablets
40 mg telmisartan and 12.5 mg hydrochlorothiazide
80 mg telmisartan and 12.5 mg hydrochlorothiazide
80 mg telmisartan and 25 mg hydrochlorothiazide

Indications and dosages
Hypertension
Adults: 1 tablet P.O. per day; may be adjusted up to 160 mg telmisartan and 25 mg hydrochlorothiazide, based on patient's response.

Minizide

Generic components
Capsules
1 mg prazosin and 0.5 mg polythiazide
2 mg prazosin and 0.5 mg polythiazide
5 mg prazosin and 0.5 mg polythiazide

Indications and dosages
Hypertension
Adults: 1 capsule P.O. b.i.d. or t.i.d. Adjust drug using the individual products; then switch to appropriate dosage of the combination product.

Monopril-HCT

Generic components
Tablets
10 mg fosinopril and 12.5 mg hydrochlorothiazide
20 mg fosinopril and 12.5 mg hydrochlorothiazide

Indications and dosages
Hypertension
Adults: 1 tablet P.O. per day in the morning. Adjust dosage using the individual products, then switch to appropriate dosage of the combination product.

Norco 325/10
CSS III

Generic components
Tablets
325 mg acetaminophen and 10 mg hydrocodone bitartrate

Indications and dosages
Moderate to moderately severe pain
Adults: 1 tablet every 4 to 6 hours. Maximum dosage, 6 tablets in 24 hours.

Percocet 2.5/325
CSS II

Generic components
Tablets
325 mg acetaminophen and 2.5 mg oxycodone hydrochloride

Indications and dosages
Moderate to moderately severe pain
Adults: 1 to 2 tablets every 4 to 6 hours. Maximum dosage, 12 tablets in 24 hours.

Percocet 10/650
CSS II

Generic components
Tablets
650 mg acetaminophen and 10 mg oxycodone hydrochloride

Indications and dosages
Moderate to moderately severe pain
Adults: 1 tablet every 4 hours. Maximum dosage, 6 tablets in 24 hours.

Percodan
CSS II

Generic components
Tablets
325 mg aspirin, 4.5 mg oxycodone hydrochloride, and 0.38 mg oxycodone terephthalate

Indications and dosages
Moderate to moderately severe pain
Adults: 1 tablet every 6 hours. Maximum dosage, 12 tablets in 24 hours.

Perloxx
Roxicet 5/500
Roxilox
Tylox
CSS II

Generic components
Tablets
500 mg acetaminophen and 5 mg oxycodone hydrochloride

Indications and dosages
Moderate to moderately severe pain
Adults: 1 tablet every 6 hours.

Prefest

Generic components
Tablets
1 mg estradiol and 0.09 mg norgestimate

Indications and dosages
Moderate to severe symptoms of menopause and prevention of osteoporosis
Women with intact uterus: 1 tablet/day P.O. (3 days of pink tablets: estradiol alone; followed by 3 days of white tablets: estradiol and norgestimate combination; continue cycle uninterrupted).

Premphase

Generic components
Tablets
0.625 mg conjugated estrogens; 0.625 mg conjugated estrogens with 5 mg medroxyprogesterone

Indications and dosages
Moderate to severe symptoms of menopause and prevention of osteoporosis
Women with intact uterus: 1 tablet per day P.O. Use estrogen alone on days 1 to 14 and estrogen-medroxyprogesterone tablet on days 15 to 28.

Prempro

Generic components
Tablets
0.3 mg conjugated estrogen and 1.5 mg medroxyprogesterone
0.45 mg conjugated estrogen and 1.5 mg medroxyprogesterone
0.625 mg estrogen and 2.5 mg medroxyprogesterone
0.625 mg conjugated estrogen and 5 mg medroxyprogesterone

Indications and dosages
Signs and symptoms of menopause and prevention of osteoporosis
Women with intact uterus: 1 tablet per day P.O.

Prinzide
Zestoretic

Generic components
Tablets
10 mg lisinopril and 12.5 mg hydrochlorothiazide
20 mg lisinopril and 12.5 mg hydrochlorothiazide
20 mg lisinopril and 25 mg hydrochlorothiazide

Indications and dosages
Hypertension
Adults: 1 tablet per day P.O. taken in the morning. Adjust dosage using the individual products; then switch to the combination product when patient's adjustment schedule is stable.

Roxicet Oral Solution
CSS II

Generic components
Solution
325 mg acetaminophen and 5 mg/5 ml oxycodone hydrochloride

Indications and dosages
Moderate to moderately severe pain
Adults: 5 ml every 6 hours. Maximum dosage, 60 ml in 24 hours.

Symbicort

Generic components
Inhalation aerosol
80 mcg budesonide and 4.5 mcg formoterol fumarate dihydrate
160 mcg budesonide and 4.5 mcg formoterol fumarate dihydrate

Indications and dosages
Long-term maintenance of asthma
Adults and children age 12 and older: 2 inhalations b.i.d. (morning and evening) select dosage based on asthma severity and other drugs being taken. Maximum daily dosage, 640 mcg budesonide/18 mcg formoterol.

Symbyax

Generic components
Capsules
6 mg olanzapine and 25 mg fluoxetine
6 mg olanzapine and 50 mg fluoxetine
12 mg olanzapine and 25 mg fluoxetine
12 mg olanzapine and 50 mg fluoxetine

Indications and dosages
Bipolar disorder
Adults: 1 capsule daily in the evening. Begin with 6 mg/25 mg capsule and adjust according to efficacy and tolerability.

Talacen
CSS IV

Generic components
Tablets
650 mg acetaminophen and 25 mg pentazocine hydrochloride

Indications and dosages
Mild to moderate pain
Adults: 1 tablet every 4 hours. Maximum dosage, 6 tablets in 24 hours.

Talwin Compound
CSS IV

Generic components
Tablets
325 mg aspirin and 12.5 mg pentazocine hydrochloride

Indications and dosages
Moderate pain
Adults: 2 tablets every 6 to 8 hours. Maximum dosage, 8 tablets in 24 hours.

Talwin NX
CSS IV

Generic components
Tablets
0.5 mg naloxone and 50 mg pentazocine hydrochloride

Indications and dosages
Moderate to severe pain
Adults: 1 to 2 tablets every 3 to 4 hours. Maximum dosage, 12 tablets daily.

Tarka

Generic components
Tablets
1 mg trandolapril and 240 mg verapamil
2 mg trandolapril and 180 mg verapamil
2 mg trandolapril and 240 mg verapamil
4 mg trandolapril and 240 mg verapamil

Indications and dosages
Hypertension
Adults: 1 tablet P.O. per day, taken with food. Adjust dosage using the individual products; then switch to the combination product when patient's adjustment schedule is stable. Make sure that patient swallows tablet whole. Don't cut, crush, or allow him to chew.

Tenoretic

Generic components
Tablets
50 mg atenolol and 25 mg chlorthalidone
100 mg atenolol and 25 mg chlorthalidone

Indications and dosages
Hypertension
Adults: 1 tablet P.O. daily in the morning. Adjust dosage using the individual products; then switch to appropriate dosage.

Teveten HCT

Generic components
Tablets
600 mg eprosartan and 12.5 mg hydrochlorothiazide
600 mg eprosartan and 25 mg hydrochlorothiazide

Indications and dosages
Hypertension
Adults: 1 tablet P.O. each day. Establish dosage with each component alone before using the combination product; if blood pressure isn't controlled on 600 mg/25 mg tablet, 300 mg eprosartan may be added each evening.

Trizivir

Generic components
Tablets
300 mg abacavir sulfate, 300 mg zidovudine, and 150 mg lamivudine

Indications and dosages
HIV infection
Adults and adolescents who weigh more than 40 kg (88 lb): 1 tablet P.O. b.i.d. Carefully monitor patient for hypersensitivity reactions.

Truvada

Generic components
Tablets
200 mg emtricitabine with 300 mg tenofovir

Indications and dosages
HIV infection
Adults and adolescents weighing more than 40 kg (88 lb): 1 tablet daily, taken without regard to food and with other antiretrovirals.

Tylenol with Codeine No. 2
CSS III

Generic components
Tablets
300 mg acetaminophen and 15 mg codeine phosphate

Indications and dosages
Fever and mild to moderate pain
Adults: 1 to 2 tablets every 4 hours. Maximum dosage, 12 tablets in 24 hours.

Tylenol with Codeine No. 3
CSS III

Generic components
Tablets
300 mg acetaminophen and 30 mg codeine phosphate

Indications and dosages
Fever and mild to moderate pain
Adults: 1 to 2 tablets every 4 hours. Maximum dosage, 12 tablets in 24 hours.

Tylenol with Codeine No. 4
CSS III

Generic components
Tablets
300 mg acetaminophen and 60 mg codeine phosphate

Indications and dosages
Fever and mild to moderate pain
Adults: 1 tablet every 4 hours. Maximum dosage, 12 tablets in 24 hours.

Tylox 5/500
CSS II

Generic components
Tablets
500 mg acetaminophen and 5 mg oxycodone hydrochloride

Indications and dosages
Moderate to moderately severe pain
Adults: 1 capsule every 6 hours. Maximum dosage, 8 capsules in 24 hours.

Uniretic

Generic components
Tablets
7.5 mg moexipril and 12.5 mg hydrochlorothiazide
15 mg moexipril and 12.5 mg hydrochlorothiazide
15 mg moexipril and 25 mg hydrochlorothiazide

Indications and dosages
Hypertension
Adults: 0.5 to 2 tablets per day. Not for initial therapy. Adjust dose to maintain appropriate blood pressure.

Vaseretic

Generic components
Tablets
5 mg enalapril maleate and 12.5 mg hydrochlorothiazide
10 mg enalapril maleate and 25 mg hydrochlorothiazide

Indications and dosages
Hypertension
Adults: 1 to 2 tablets per day P.O. in the morning. Adjust dosage using the individual products; then switch to the combination product when patient's adjustment schedule is stable. Make sure that patient swallows tablet whole. Don't cut, crush, or allow him to chew.

Vicodin ES
CSS III

Generic components
Tablets
750 mg acetaminophen and 7.5 mg hydrocodone bitartrate

Indications and dosages
Moderate to moderately severe pain
Adults: 1 tablet every 4 to 6 hours. Maximum dosage, 5 tablets in 24 hours.

Vytorin

Generic components
Tablets
10 mg ezetimibe and 10 mg simvastatin
10 mg ezetimibe and 20 mg simvastatin
10 mg ezetimibe and 40 mg simvastatin
10 mg ezetimibe and 80 mg simvastatin

Indications and dosages
Hypercholesterolemia
Adults: 1 tablet daily, taken in the evening with a cholesterol-lowering diet and exercise. Dosage of simvastatin in the combination may be adjusted based on patient response. If given with a bile sequestrant, must be given at least 2 hours before or 4 hours after the bile sequestrant.

Ziac

Generic components
Tablets
2.5 mg bisoprolol and 6.25 mg hydrochlorothiazide
5 mg bisoprolol and 6.25 mg hydrochlorothiazide
10 mg bisoprolol and 6.25 mg hydrochlorothiazide

Indications and dosages
Hypertension
Adults: 1 tablet daily P.O. in morning. Initial dose is 2.5/6.25 mg tablet P.O. daily. Adjust dosage within 1 week; optimum antihypertensive effect may require 2 to 3 weeks.

Zydone 5/400
CSS III

Generic components
Tablets
400 mg acetaminophen and 5 mg hydrocodone bitartrate

Indications and dosages
Moderate to moderately severe pain
Adults: 1 to 2 tablets every 4 to 6 hours. Maximum dosage, 8 tablets in 24 hours.

Zydone 7.5/400
CSS III

Generic components
Tablets
400 mg acetaminophen and 7.5 mg hydrocodone bitartrate

Indications and dosages
Moderate to moderately severe pain
Adults: 1 tablet every 4 to 6 hours. Maximum dosage, 6 tablets in 24 hours.

Zydone 10/400
CSS III

Generic components
Tablets
400 mg acetaminophen and 10 mg hydrocodone bitartrate

Indications and dosages
Moderate to moderately severe pain
Adults: 1 tablet every 4 to 6 hours. Maximum dosage, 6 tablets in 24 hours.

Toxic drug–drug interactions

Interaction	Drugs	Interacting drugs
Decreased corticosteroid effects	*corticosteroids* (betamethasone, cortisone, dexamethasone, fludrocortisone, hydrocortisone, methylprednisolone, prednisolone, prednisone, triamcinolone)	*rifamycins* (rifabutin, rifampin, rifapentine)
Digoxin toxicity and arrhythmias	*digoxin*	*tetracyclines* (demeclocycline, doxycycline, minocycline, tetracycline) *thiazide diuretics* (chlorothiazide, hydrochlorothiazide, indapamide, methyclothiazide, metolazone, polythiazide, trichlormethiazide) verapamil
Hearing loss	*aminoglycosides* (amikacin, gentamicin, kanamycin, netilmicin, streptomycin, tobramycin)	*loop diuretics* (bumetanide, ethacrynic acid, furosemide, torsemide)
Increased bleeding	*warfarin* (Coumadin)	alteplase *androgens* [17-alkyl] (danazol, fluoxymesterone, methyltestosterone, oxandrolone) cimetidine cranberry juice *fibric acids* (clofibrate, fenofibrate, gemfibrozil) *salicylates* (aspirin, methylsalicylate) amiodarone *azole antifungals* (fluconazole, itraconazole, ketoconazole, miconazole, voriconazole) *macrolide antibiotics* (azithromycin, clarithromycin, erythromycin) metronidazole *quinine derivatives* (quinidine, quinine) *quinolones* (ciprofloxacin, levofloxacin, moxifloxacin, norfloxacin, ofloxacin) sulfinpyrazone *sulfonamides* (sulfasalazine, sulfisoxazole, trimethoprimsulfamethoxazole) *thyroid hormones* (levothyroxine, liothyronine, liotrix, thyroid) *vitamin E*
Increased potassium level	*potassium-sparing diuretics* (amiloride, spironolactone, triamterene)	*angiotensin-converting enzyme (ACE) inhibitors* (benazepril, captopril, enalapril, fosinopril, lisinopril, moexipril, perindopril, quinapril, ramipril, trandolapril) *angiotensin II receptor antagonists* (candesartan, eprosartan, irbesartan, losartan, olmesartan, telmisartan, valsartan) *potassium preparations* (potassium acetate, potassium bicarbonate, potassium chloride, potassium citrate, potassium gluconate, potassium iodine, potassium phosphate)

Nursing considerations

- Avoid use together, if possible.
- Effects may persist for 2 to 3 weeks after stopping therapy.

- Use together cautiously.
- Monitor serum digoxin levels. The therapeutic range for digoxin is 0.8 to 2 nanograms/ml.
- Effects of tetracyclines on digoxin may persist for several months after the antibiotic is stopped.
- Monitor serum potassium and magnesium levels if patient is taking both thiazide diuretics and digoxin.
- Monitor patient for evidence of digoxin toxicity, including arrhythmias (such as bradycardia, atrioventricular [AV] block, ventricular ectopy), lethargy, drowsiness, confusion, hallucinations, headache, syncope, vision disturbance, nausea, anorexia, vomiting, or diarrhea.

- Use together cautiously.
- Patients with renal insufficiency are at greater risk.
- Irreversible hearing loss is more likely with this combination than when either drug is used alone.

- Avoid use together, if possible.
- If drugs must be used together, monitor coagulation values carefully; the dosage requirements for warfarin will be decreased.
- Suggest taking a different histamine$_2$ antagonist.
- Aspirin doses of 500 mg or more daily cause a greater risk.

- Use together cautiously.
- Monitor prothrombin time and international normalized ratio closely when starting or stopping any of these drugs.
- Bleeding effects may persist after interacting drug is stopped.
- Typically, the warfarin dose needs to be reduced.
- Vitamin E doses of less than 400 mg daily may not have this effect.

- Use together cautiously.
- High-risk patients include those with renal impairment, type 2 diabetes, decreased renal perfusion, and those who are elderly.
- Don't use potassium preparations and potassium-sparing diuretics unless the patient has severe hypokalemia that isn't responding to either drug class alone.
- Monitor the patient's potassium level; also monitor patient for palpitations, chest pain, nausea and vomiting, paresthesias, and muscle weakness.

(continued)

Interaction	Drugs	Interacting drugs
Increased risk of pregnancy, breakthrough bleeding	*barbiturates* (amobarbital, butabarbital, pentobarbital, phenobarbital, primidone, secobarbital)	*hormonal contraceptives*
Life-threatening hypertension	*clonidine*	*beta blockers* (acebutolol, atenolol, betaxolol, carteolol, esmolol, metoprolol, nadolol, penbutolol, pindolol, propranolol, timolol)
		tricyclic antidepressants (amitriptyline, amoxapine, clomipramine, desipramine, doxepin, imipramine, nortriptyline, protriptyline, trimipramine)
	monoamine oxidase (MAO) inhibitors (isocarboxazid, phenelzine, tranylcypromine)	*anorexiants* (amphetamine, benzphetamine, dextroamphetamine, methamphetamine, phentermine)
		methylphenidate (dexmethylphenidate, Concerta)
Methotrexate toxicity	*methotrexate*	*nonsteroidal anti-inflammatory drugs (NSAIDs)* (diclofenac, etodolac, fenoprofen, flurbiprofen, ibuprofen, indomethacin, ketoprofen, ketorolac, meclofenamate, nabumetone, naproxen, oxaprozin, piroxicam, sulindac, tolmetin)
		penicillins (amoxicillin, ampicillin, carbenicillin, cloxacillin, dicloxacillin, oxacillin, penicillin G, penicillin V, piperacillin, ticarcillin)
Reduced penicillin effectiveness	*penicillins* (amoxicillin, ampicillin, carbenicillin, cloxacillin, dicloxacillin, nafcillin, penicillin G, penicillin V, piperacillin, ticarcillin)	*tetracyclines* (demeclocycline, doxycycline, minocycline, tetracycline)
Rhabdomyolysis and myopathy	*HMG-CoA reductase inhibitors* (atorvastatin, fluvastatin, lovastatin, pravastatin, rosuvastatin, simvastatin)	*cyclosporine* *gemfibrozil* *protease inhibitors* (amprenavir, atazanavir, indinavir, lopinavir with ritonavir, nelfinavir, ritonavir, saquinavir)
		macrolide antibiotics (azithromycin, clarithromycin, erythromycin)
Serious cardiac events	*quinidine*	*verapamil*
Serotonin syndrome	*selective serotonin reuptake inhibitors (SSRIs)* (fluoxetine, paroxetine, sertraline)	*risperidone*

Nursing considerations

- Use together cautiously.
- Suggest use of an alternative barrier form of contraception during therapy with both drugs.

- Use together cautiously.
- Monitor blood pressure closely when starting and stopping clonidine and beta blockers simultaneously; stop the beta blocker first.

- Use together is contraindicated.

- Avoid using these drugs together, if possible.
- Several deaths have occurred as a result of hypertensive crisis leading to cerebral hemorrhage.
- Monitor patient for hypertension, hyperpyrexia, and seizures.
- Hypertensive reaction may occur for several weeks after stopping an MAO inhibitor.

- Use together is contraindicated.

- Use together cautiously.
- Monitor patient for mouth sores, hematemesis, diarrhea with melena, nausea and weakness, and bone marrow suppression.
- Methotrexate toxicity is less likely to occur with weekly low-dose methotrexate regimens for rheumatoid arthritis and other inflammatory diseases.
- Longer leucovorin rescue should be considered when giving NSAIDs and methotrexate at antineoplastic doses.
- Obtain methotrexate levels twice weekly for the first 2 weeks of concurrent penicillin and methotrexate therapy.

- Avoid use together, if possible.

- Use of nelfinavir with simvastatin is contraindicated.
- Avoid use together, if possible.
- Monitor patient taking an HMG-CoA reductase inhibitor and gemfibrozil for signs of acute renal failure, including decreased urine output, elevated blood urea nitrogen and creatinine levels, edema, dyspnea, tachycardia, distended neck veins, nausea, vomiting, weakness, fatigue, confusion, and agitation.
- Monitor patient for fatigue, muscle aches and weakness, joint pain, unintentional weight gain, seizures, dramatically increased serum creatine kinase level, and dark, red, or cola-colored urine.

- Use together cautiously.
- Monitor patient for rhabdomyolysis, especially 5 to 21 days after starting the macrolide antibiotic.

- Use together only when there are no other alternatives.
- Monitor patient for hypotension, bradycardia, ventricular tachycardia, and AV block.
- Tell patient to report diaphoresis, dizziness, or blurred vision as well as palpitations, shortness of breath, dizziness or fainting, and chest pain.
- Complications of this interaction may be noticed after as little as 1 day or as long as 5 months of combined therapy.

- Monitor patient carefully if an SSRI is started or stopped or if dosage is changed during risperidone therapy. Risperidone levels may increase.
- Assess patient for central nervous system (CNS) irritability, increased muscle tone, muscle twitching or jerking, and changes in level of consciousness (LOC).
- Although average doses of fluoxetine and paroxetine may cause this interaction, higher doses of sertraline (greater than 100 mg daily) are needed.

(continued)

Interaction	Drugs	Interacting drugs
Serotonin syndrome *(continued)*	*SSRIs* (citalopram, fluoxetine, fluvoxamine, nefazodone, paroxetine, sertraline, venlafaxine)	*selective 5-HT₁ receptor agonists* (almotriptan, eletriptan, frovatriptan, naratriptan, rizatriptan, sumatriptan, zolmitriptan)
	serotonin reuptake inhibitors (citalopram, escitalopram, fluoxetine, fluvoxamine, nefazodone, paroxetine, sertraline, venlafaxine)	*MAO inhibitors* (isocarboxazid, phenelzine, selegiline, tranylcypromine)
		sibutramine *sympathomimetics* (amphetamine, dextroamphetamine, methamphetamine, phentermine)
Severe arrhythmias	*dofetilide*	*thiazide diuretics* (chlorothiazide, hydrochlorothiazide, indapamide, methyclothiazide, metolazone, polythiazide, trichlormethiazide) *verapamil*
	pimozide	*SSRIs* (citalopram, sertraline)
	quinolones (gatifloxacin, levofloxacin, moxifloxacin)	*antiarrhythmics* (amiodarone, bretylium, disopyramide, procainamide, quinidine, sotalol) *erythromycin* *phenothiazines* (chlorpromazine, fluphenazine, mesoridazine, perphenazine, prochlorperazine, promethazine, thioridazine) *tricyclic antidepressants* (amitriptyline, amoxapine, clomipramine, desipramine, doxepin, imipramine, nortriptyline, trimipramine)
		ziprasidone
	thioridazine	*fluoxetine*
Severe hypotension	*nitrates* (amyl nitrite, isosorbide dinitrate, isosorbide mononitrate, nitroglycerin)	*sildenafil* *tadalafil* *vardenafil*
	protease inhibitors (amprenavir, indinavir, nelfinavir, ritonavir, saquinavir)	*sildenafil* *tadalafil* *vardenafil*
Severe muscular depression	*cholinesterase inhibitors* (ambenonium, edrophonium, neostigmine, pyridostigmine)	*Corticosteroids* (betamethasone, corticotropin, cortisone, cosyntropin, dexamethasone, fludrocortisone, hydrocortisone, methylprednisolone, prednisolone, prednisone, triamcinolone)

Nursing considerations

- Avoid combining these drugs if possible.
- If concurrent use can't be avoided, start with the lowest dosages possible, and observe the patient closely.
- Stop the selective 5-HT$_1$ receptor agonist at the first sign of interaction. Begin an antiserotonergic drug such as cyproheptadine (Periactin).
- Some patients may note increased frequency of migraine and reduced effectiveness of antimigraine drugs if a serotonin reuptake inhibitor is begun.
- Monitor patient for evidence of serotonin syndrome, including CNS irritability, motor weakness, shivering, muscle twitching, and altered LOC.

- Don't use these drugs together.
- Allow 1 week after stopping nefazodone or venlafaxine before giving an MAO inhibitor.
- Allow 2 weeks after stopping citalopram, escitalopram, fluvoxamine, paroxetine, or sertraline before giving an MAO inhibitor.
- Allow 5 weeks after stopping fluoxetine before giving an MAO inhibitor.
- Allow 2 weeks after stopping an MAO inhibitor before giving any serotonin reuptake inhibitor.
- Serotonin syndrome effects include CNS irritability, motor weakness, shivering, myoclonus, and altered LOC.
- The selective MAO type-B inhibitor selegiline has been given with fluoxetine, paroxetine, or sertraline to patients with Parkinson disease without negative effects.

- Don't use these drugs together, if possible.
- If this combination must be used, carefully monitor the patent for adverse effects, which require immediate medical attention.
- Monitor the patient closely for increased CNS effects, such as anxiety, jitteriness, agitation and restlessness, plus dizziness, nausea, vomiting, motor weakness, shivering, myoclonus, and altered LOC.

- Use together is contraindicated.
- In the event of inadvertent use together, monitor electrocardiogram for excessive prolongation of the QTc interval or the development of ventricular arrhythmias.
- Use of a thiazide diuretic increases potassium excretion.
- Monitor renal function and QTc interval every 3 months during dofetilide and verapamil therapy.

- Use together is contraindicated.
- Life-threatening risk is from prolongation of the QTc interval.

- Use of class IA or III antiarrhythmics, erythromycin, phenothiazines, or tricyclic antidepressants with levofloxacin should be avoided.
- Moxifloxacin may be used with caution and increased monitoring with phenothiazines and tricyclic antidepressants but should be avoided with antiarrhythmics and erythromycin.

- Use together is contraindicated.

- Use together is contraindicated.
- Risk increases proportional to increased dose of thioridazine.

- Use together is contraindicated.
- Before giving a nitrate, find out if a patient with chest pain has taken a drug for erectile dysfunction during the previous 24 to 48 hours.

- Use together is contraindicated.
- Tell patient to take sildenafil exactly as prescribed. Dosage may be reduced to 25 mg and an interval of at least 48 hours between drugs may be needed.

- If given together in a patient with myasthenia gravis, watch for severe muscle deterioration unresponsive to cholinesterase inhibitor therapy.
- Be prepared to provide respiratory support and mechanical ventilation, as needed.
- Corticosteroid therapy may have long-term benefits in patients with myasthenia gravis.

Dialyzable drugs

The amount of a drug removed by dialysis differs among patients and depends on several factors, including the patient's condition, the drug's properties, length of dialysis and dialysate used, rate of blood flow or dwell time, and purpose of dialysis. This table indicates the effect of conventional hemodialysis on selected drugs.

Drug	Level reduced by hemodialysis?	Drug	Level reduced by hemodialysis?
acebutolol	Yes	bivalirudin	Yes
acetaminophen	Yes (may not influence toxicity)	bumetanide	No
		bupropion	No
acetazolamide	No	buspirone	No
acetylcysteine	Yes	busulfan	Yes
acyclovir	Yes	captopril	Yes
albuterol	No	carbamazepine	No
allopurinol	Yes	carbenicillin	Yes
alprazolam	No	carboplatin	Yes
amantadine	No	carisoprodol	Yes
amikacin	Yes	carmustine	No
amiodarone	No	carvedilol	No
amitriptyline	No	cefaclor	Yes
amlodipine	No	cefadroxil	Yes
amoxicillin	Yes	cefazolin	Yes
amoxicillin and clavulanate potassium	Yes	cefepime	Yes
		cefoperazone	Yes
amphotericin B	No	ceforanide	Yes
ampicillin	Yes	cefotaxime	Yes
ampicillin and sulbactam sodium	Yes	cefoxitin	Yes
aprepitant	No	cefpirome	Yes
arsenic trioxide	No	cefpodoxime	Yes
ascorbic acid	Yes	ceftazidime	Yes
aspirin	Yes	ceftibuten	Yes
atenolol	Yes	ceftizoxime	Yes
atorvastatin	No	ceftriaxone	No
atropine	No	cefuroxime	Yes
auranofin	No	cephalexin	Yes
azathioprine	Yes	cephradine	Yes
aztreonam	Yes	chloral hydrate	Yes

Drug	Level reduced by hemodialysis	Drug	Level reduced by hemodialysis
chlorambucil	No	dipyridamole	No
chloramphenicol	Yes (very small amount)	disopyramide	No
chlordiazepoxide	No	dopamine	No
chloroquine	No	doripenem	Yes
chlorpheniramine	Yes	doxazosin	No
chlorpromazine	No	doxepin	No
chlorthalidone	No	doxorubicin	No
cilastatin	Yes	doxycycline	No
cilazapril	Yes	drotrecogin alfa	Unknown
cimetidine	Yes	emtricitabine	Yes
ciprofloxacin	Yes (only by 10%)	enalapril	Yes
cisplatin	No	enoxaparin	No
clavulanic acid	Yes	epoetin alfa	No
clindamycin	No	erythromycin	Yes (only by 20%)
clofibrate	No	ethacrynic acid	No
clonazepam	No	ethambutol	Yes (only by 20%)
clonidine	No	ethosuximide	Yes
clorazepate	No	famciclovir	Yes
cloxacillin	No	famotidine	No
codeine	No	fenoprofen	No
colchicine	No	filgrastim	No
cortisone	No	flecainide	No
co-trimoxazole	Yes	fluconazole	Yes
cyclophosphamide	Yes	flucytosine	Yes
deferoxime	Yes	fluorouracil	No
desloratadine	No	fluoxetine	No
dexamethasone	No	flurazepam	No
diazepam	No	foscarnet	Yes
diazoxide	Yes	fosinopril	No
diclofenac	No	furosemide	No
dicloxacillin	No	gabapentin	Yes
didanosine	Yes	ganciclovir	Yes
digoxin	No	gemcitabine	Yes
digoxine immune Fab	No	gemfibrozil	No
diltiazem	No	gemifloxacin	Yes
diphenhydramine	No	gentamicin	Yes

Drug	Level reduced by hemodialysis	Drug	Level reduced by hemodialysis
glipizide	No	mannitol	Yes
gluthemide	No	maraviroc	Yes
glyburide	No	mechlorethamine	No
guanfacine	No	mefenamic acid	No
haloperidol	No	meperidine	No
heparin	No	meprobamate	Yes
hydralazine	No	mercaptopurine	Yes
hydrochlorothiazide	No	meropenem	Yes
hydroxyzine	No	mesalamine	Yes
ibuprofen	No	metformin	Yes
ifosfamide	Yes	methadone	No
imipramine	No	methicillin	No
indapamide	No	methotrexate	Yes
indomethacin	No	methyldopa	Yes
insulin	No	methylprednisolone	Yes
irbesartan	No	metoclopramide	No
iron dextran	No	metolazone	No
isoniazid	No	metoprolol	Yes
isosorbide	Yes	metronidazole	Yes
isradipine	No	mexiletine	Yes
kanamycin	Yes	miconazole	No
ketoconazole	No	midazolam	No
labetalol	No	minocycline	No
lamivudine	No	minoxidil	Yes
lansoprazole	No	misoprostol	No
lapatinib	No	morphine	No
levocetirizine	No	nabumetone	No
levofloxacin	No	nadolol	Yes
lidocaine	No	nafcillin	No
linezolid	Yes	nalmefene	No
lisinopril	Yes	naltrexone	No
lithium	Yes	naproxen	No
lomefloxacin	No	nelfinavir	No
lomustine	No	nicardipine	No
loratadine	No	nifedipine	No
lorazepam	No	nimodipine	No

Drug	Level reduced by hemodialysis	Drug	Level reduced by hemodialysis
nitazoxanide	No	pyridoxine	Yes
nitrofurantoin	Yes	quinapril	No
nitroglycerin	No	quinidine	No
nitroprusside	Yes	quinine	No
nizatidine	No	ramipril	No
norfloxacin	No	ranitidine	Yes
nortriptyline	No	rifampin	No
octreotide	Yes	ritodrine	Yes
ofloxacin	Yes	rituximab	No
olanzapine	No	rosiglitazone	No
omeprazole	No	salsalate	Yes
oxazepam	No	sertraline	No
paclitaxel	No	sotalol	Yes
paroxetine	No	stavudine	Yes
penicillin	Yes	streptomycin	Yes
pentamidine	No	sucralfate	No
pentazocine	Yes	sulbactam	Yes
pentobarbital	No	sulfamethoxazole	Yes
perindopril	Yes	sulfisoxazole	Yes
phenobarbital	Yes	sulindac	No
phenylbutazone	No	tazobactam	Yes
phenytoin	No	telbivudine	Yes (by 23%)
piperacillin	Yes	temazepam	No
piroxicam	No	theophylline	Yes
prazosin	No	ticarcillin	Yes
prednisone	No	ticarcillin and clavulanate	Yes
pregabalin	Yes	timolol	No
primidone	Yes	tirofiban	Yes
procainamide	Yes	tobramycin	Yes
promethazine	No	tocainide	Yes
propofol	Unknown	tolbutamide	No
propoxyphene	No	topiramate	Yes
propranolol	No	topotecan	Yes
protriptyline	No	torsemide	No
pseudoephedrine	No	tramadol	No
pyrazinamide	Yes	trandolapril	Yes

Drug	Level reduced by hemodialysis
trazodone	No
triazolam	No
trimethoprim	Yes
valacyclovir	Yes
valganciclovir	Yes
valproic acid	No
valsartan	No
vancomycin	Yes
venlafaxine	No
verapamil	No
vigabatrin	Yes
warfarin	No
zolpidem	No
zonisamide	Yes

Herb–drug interactions

Herb	Drug	Possible effects
aloe (dried juice from leaf [latex])	antiarrhythmics, digoxin	May lead to hypokalemia, which may potentiate digoxin and antiarrhythmics.
	oral drugs	May decrease drug absorption because of more rapid GI transit time.
	stimulant laxatives	May increase risk of potassium loss.
	thiazide diuretics, other potassium-wasting drugs, such as corticosteroids	May cause additive effect of potassium wasting.
bilberry	anticoagulants, antiplatelets	Decreases platelet aggregation.
	hypoglycemics, insulin	May increase insulin level, causing hypoglycemia; additive effect with antidiabetics.
capsicum	ACE inhibitors	May cause cough.
	anticoagulants, antiplatelets	Decreases platelet aggregation and increases fibrinolytic activity, prolonging bleeding time.
	antihypertensives	May interfere with antihypertensives by increasing catecholamine secretion.
	aspirin, NSAIDs	Stimulates GI secretions to help protect against NSAID-induced GI irritation.
	CNS depressants, such as barbiturates, benzodiazepines, opioids	Increases sedative effect.
	cocaine	May increase effects of drug and risk of adverse reactions, including death. Use together includes exposure to capsicum in pepper spray.
	H_2 blockers, proton-pump inhibitors	Decreases effects of the increased catecholamine secretion by herb.
	hepatically metabolized drugs	May increase hepatic metabolism of drugs by increasing G6PD and adipose lipase activity.
	MAO inhibitors	May decrease efficacy because of increased acid secretion by capsicum.
	theophylline	Increases absorption of theophylline, possibly leading to higher drug level or toxicity.
chamomile	anticoagulants	Warfarin constituents in herb may enhance drug therapy and prolong bleeding time.
	drugs requiring GI absorption	May delay drug absorption.

(continued)

1377

Herb	Drug	Possible effects
chamomile *(continued)*	drugs with sedative properties, such as benzodiazepines	May cause additive effects and adverse reactions.
	iron	Tannic acid content in herb may reduce iron absorption.
echinacea	hepatotoxic drugs	Hepatotoxicity may increase with drugs known to elevate liver enzyme levels.
	immunosuppressants	Herb may counteract drugs.
	warfarin	Increases bleeding time without increased INR.
evening primrose oil	anticoagulants, antiplatelets	Increases risk of bleeding and bruising.
	anticonvulsants	Lowers seizure threshold.
feverfew	anticoagulants, antiplatelets	May decrease platelet aggregation and increase fibrinolytic activity.
	methysergide	May potentiate drug.
garlic	anticoagulants, antiplatelets	Enhances platelet inhibition, leading to increased anticoagulation.
	antihyperlipidemics	May have additive lipid-lowering properties.
	antihypertensives	May cause additive hypotension.
	cyclosporine	May decrease efficacy of drug. May induce metabolism and decrease drug level to subtherapeutic; may cause rejection.
	hormonal contraceptives	May decrease efficacy of drugs.
	insulin, other drugs causing hypoglycemia	May increase insulin level, causing hypoglycemia, an additive effect with these drugs.
	nonnucleotide reverse transcriptase inhibitors (NNRTIs)	May affect metabolism of these drugs.
	saquinavir	Decreases drug level, causing therapeutic failure and increased viral resistance.
ginger	anticoagulants, antiplatelets	Inhibits platelet aggregation by antagonizing thromboxane synthetase and enhancing prostacyclin, leading to prolonged bleeding time.
	antidiabetics	May interfere with diabetes therapy because of hypoglycemic effects.
	antihypertensives	May antagonize drug effects.
	barbiturates	May enhance drug effects.

Herb	Drug	Possible effects
ginger *(continued)*	calcium channel blockers	May increase calcium uptake by myocardium, leading to altered drug effects.
	chemotherapy	May reduce nausea caused by chemotherapy.
	H$_2$ blockers, proton-pump inhibitors	May decrease efficacy because of increased acid secretion by herb.
ginkgo	anticoagulants, antiplatelets	May enhance platelet inhibition, leading to increased anti-coagulation.
	anticonvulsants	May decrease effectiveness of drugs.
	drugs known to lower seizure threshold	May further reduce seizure threshold.
	insulin	Ginkgo leaf extract can alter insulin secretion and metabolism, affecting glucose level.
	thiazide diuretics	Ginkgo leaf may increase blood pressure.
ginseng	alcohol	Increases alcohol clearance, possibly by increasing activity of alcohol dehydrogenase.
	anabolic steroids, hormones	May potentiate effects of drugs. Estrogenic effects of herb may cause vaginal bleeding and breast nodules.
	antibiotics	Herb may enhance effects of some antibiotics.
	anticoagulants, antiplatelets	Decreases platelet adhesiveness.
	antidiabetics	May enhance glucose-lowering effects.
	antipsychotics	Because of CNS stimulant activity, avoid use with these drugs.
	digoxin	May falsely elevate drug level.
	furosemide	May decrease diuretic effect with this drug.
	immunosuppressants	May interfere with drug therapy.
	MAO inhibitors	Potentiates action of MAO inhibitors. May cause insomnia, headache, tremors, and hypomania.
	stimulants	May potentiate drug effects.
	warfarin	Causes antagonism of warfarin, resulting in a decreased INR.

(continued)

Herb	Drug	Possible effects
goldenseal	antihypertensives	Large amounts of herb may interfere with blood pressure control.
	CNS depressants, such as barbiturates, benzodiazepines, opioids	Increases sedative effect.
	diuretics	Causes additive drug effect.
	general anesthetics	May potentiate hypotensive action of drugs.
	H₂ blockers, proton-pump inhibitors	May decrease efficacy because of increased acid secretion by herb.
	heparin	May counteract anticoagulant effect of drug.
grapeseed	warfarin	Increases effects and INR because of tocopherol content of herb.
green tea	acetaminophen, aspirin	May increase efficacy of these drugs by as much as 40%.
	adenosine	May inhibit hemodynamic effects of drug.
	albuterol, isoproterenol, metaproterenol, terbutaline	May increase the cardiac inotropic effect of these drugs.
	clozapine	May cause acute worsening of psychotic symptoms.
	disulfiram	Increases risk of adverse effects of caffeine; decreases clearance and increases half-life of caffeine.
	ephedrine	Increases risk of agitation, tremors, and insomnia.
	hormonal contraceptives	Decreases clearance by 40% to 65%. Increases effects and adverse effects.
	lithium	Abrupt caffeine withdrawal increases drug level; may cause lithium tremor.
	MAO inhibitors	Large amounts of herb may precipitate hypertensive crisis.
	mexiletine	Decreases caffeine elimination by 50%. Increases effects and adverse effects.
	verapamil	Increases caffeine level by 25%; increases effects and adverse effects.
	warfarin	Causes antagonism resulting from vitamin content of herb.
hawthorn berry	cardiovascular drugs	May potentiate or interfere with conventional therapies used for congestive heart failure, hypertension, angina, and arrhythmias.
	CNS depressants	Causes additive effects.

Herb	Drug	Possible effects
hawthorn berry (continued)	coronary vasodilators	Causes additive vasodilator effects when used with theophylline, caffeine, papaverine, sodium nitrate, adenosine, and epinephrine.
	digoxin	Causes additive positive inotropic effect, with potential for drug toxicity.
kava	alcohol	Potentiates depressant effect of alcohol and other CNS depressants.
	benzodiazepines	Use with these drugs may result in comalike states.
	CNS depressants or stimulants	May hinder therapy with CNS stimulants.
	hepatotoxic drugs	May increase risk of liver damage.
	levodopa	Decreases efficacy because of dopamine antagonism by herb.
licorice	antihypertensives	Decreases effect of drug therapy. Large amounts of herb cause sodium and water retention and hypertension.
	aspirin	May provide protection against aspirin-induced damage to GI mucosa.
	corticosteroids	Causes additive and enhanced effects of drugs.
	digoxin	Herb causes hypokalemia, which predisposes to drug toxicity.
	hormonal contraceptives	Increases fluid retention and potential for increased blood pressure resulting from fluid overload.
	hormones	Interferes with estrogen or antiestrogen therapy.
	insulin	Causes hypokalemia and sodium retention.
	spironolactone	Decreases effects of drug.
ma huang (ephedra)	amitriptyline	May decrease hypertensive effects of herb.
	antidiabetics	Decreases drug effect because of hyperglycemia caused by herb.
	caffeine	Increases risk of stimulatory adverse effects of ephedra and caffeine and risk of hypertension, myocardial infarction, stroke, and death.
	caffeine, CNS stimulants, theophylline	Causes additive CNS stimulation.
	dexamethasone	Increases clearance and decreases efficacy of drug.
	digoxin	Increases risk of arrhythmias.

(continued)

Herb	Drug	Possible effects
ma huang (ephedra) *(continued)*	MAO inhibitors	Potentiates drugs.
	oxytocin	May cause hypertension.
	theophylline	May increase risk of stimulatory adverse effects.
melatonin	CNS depressants, such as barbiturates, benzodiazepines, opioids	Increases sedative effect.
	fluoxetine	Improves sleep in some patients with major depressive disorder.
	fluvoxamine	May significantly increase melatonin level; may decrease melatonin metabolism.
	immunosuppressants	May stimulate immune function and interfere with drug therapy.
	isoniazid	May enhance effects of drug against some *Mycobacterium* species.
	nifedipine	May decrease efficacy of drug; increases heart rate.
	verapamil	Increases melatonin excretion.
milk thistle	drugs causing diarrhea	Increases bile secretion and often causes loose stools. May increase effect of other drugs commonly causing diarrhea.
	hepatotoxic drugs, such as acetaminophen, butyrophenones, ethanol, phenothiazines, phenytoin	May have liver membrane-stabilization and antioxidant effects, leading to protection from liver damage.
	indinavir	May decrease trough level of drug, reducing virologic response.
nettle	anticonvulsants	May increase sedative adverse effects; may increase risk of seizure.
	anxiolytics, hypnotics, opioids	May increase sedative adverse effects.
	iron	Tannic acid content of herb may reduce iron absorption.
	warfarin	Antagonism resulting from vitamin K content of aerial parts of herb.
passion flower	CNS depressants, such as barbiturates, benzodiazepines, opioids	Increases sedative effect.
St. John's wort	5-hydroxytriptamine$_1$ (5-HT$_1$) agonists (triptans)	Increases risk of serotonin syndrome.
	alcohol, opioids	Enhances the sedative effect of these drugs.
	anesthetics	May prolong effect of drugs.

Herb	Drug	Possible effects
St. John's wort (continued)	barbiturates	Decreases drug-induced sleep time.
	cyclosporine	Decreases drug level below therapeutic levels, threatening transplanted organ rejection.
	digoxin	May reduce drug level, which decreases therapeutic effects.
	human immunodeficiency virus (HIV) protease inhibitors, indinavir, NNRTIs	Induces cytochrome P-450 metabolic pathway, which may decrease therapeutic effects of drugs using this pathway for metabolism. Avoid use together because of the potential for subtherapeutic antiretroviral level and insufficient virologic response that could lead to resistance or class cross-resistance.
	hormonal contraceptives	Increases breakthrough bleeding; decreases level and efficacy of drugs.
	irinotecan	Decreases drug level by 50%.
	iron	Tannic acid content of herb may reduce iron absorption.
	MAO inhibitors, nefazodone, SSRIs, trazodone	Causes additive effects with MAO inhibitors, SSRIs, and other antidepressants, potentially leading to serotonin syndrome, especially when combined with SSRIs.
	photosensitizing drugs	Increases photosensitivity.
	reserpine	Antagonizes effects of drug.
	sympathomimetic amines, such as pseudoephedrine	Causes additive effects.
	theophylline	May decrease drug level, making the drug less effective.
	warfarin	May alter INR. Reduces efficacy of anticoagulant, requiring increased dosage of drug.
valerian	alcohol	May be risk of increased sedation.
	CNS depressants, sedative hypnotics	Enhances effects of these drugs.
	iron	Tannic acid content of herb may reduce iron absorption.

Dietary teaching for drug therapy

This table contains important dietary information that should be included when teaching patients about drug therapy.

Foods and dietary concerns	Representative foods
Calcium-rich foods (needed by children, patients with hypocalcemia, and post-menopausal women)	Bok choy Broccoli Calcium-fortified beverages, cereals, and breads Canned salmon Canned sardines Cheese Clams Collard greens Creamed soup Kale Milk Molasses Oysters Sardines Soy beans and other soy-based products Spinach Tofu Turnip greens Yogurt
High-sodium foods (should be avoided with CHF, fluid overload, and hypertension)	Beer Butter Buttermilk Canned seafood Canned soup Canned spaghetti Cookies Cured meat Fast food Pickles Prepackaged dinners Pretzels Salad dressings Sauces Sauerkraut Snack foods, such as cheese puffs, crackers, and potato chips Tomato ketchup
Iron-rich foods (helpful for maintaining RBCs)	Beets Cereals Dried beans and peas Dried fruit Enriched grains Leafy green vegetables Organ meats, such as heart, kidney, liver

Foods and dietary concerns	Representative foods
Low-sodium foods (patients with CHF, fluid overload, and hypertension should include in diet)	Egg yolks Fresh fruit Fresh vegetables Grits Honey Jam and jelly Lean meat Lima beans Macaroons Potatoes Poultry Pumpkin Red kidney beans Sherbet Unsalted nuts
Potassium-rich foods (should be eaten when taking potassium-wasting diuretics)	Avocados Bananas Broccoli Cantaloupe Dried fruit Grapefruit Lima beans Navy beans Nuts Oranges Peaches Potatoes Prunes Rhubarb Spinach Sunflower seeds Tomatoes
Purine-rich foods (should be avoided with gout)	Anchovies Kidneys Lentils Liver Sardines Sweetbreads
Tyramine-rich foods (should be avoided when taking MAO inhibitors and some antihypertensives)	Aged cheese Avocados Bananas Beer Bologna Caffeinated beverages Chocolate Liver Pepperoni Pickled fish Red wine (Chianti) Ripe fruit Salami

(continued)

Foods and dietary concerns	Representative foods
Tyramine-rich foods *(continued)*	Smoked fish Yeast Yogurt
Urine acidifiers (helpful for excretion of some drugs)	Cheese Cranberries Eggs Fish Grains Plums Poultry Prunes Red meat
Urine alkalinizers (helpful for excretion of some drugs)	Apples Berries Citrus fruit Milk Vegetables
Vitamin K-rich foods (should be avoided or strictly limited when taking anticoagulants)	Collard greens Kale Mustard greens Parsley (raw) Spinach Swiss chard Turnip greens

Table of equivalents and conversions

Metric system equivalents

Metric weight

1 kilogram (kg or Kg)	=	1,000 grams (g or gm)
1 gram	=	1,000 milligrams (mg)
1 milligram	=	1,000 micrograms (mcg)
0.6 g	=	600 mg
0.3 g	=	300 mg
0.1 g	=	100 mg
0.06 g	=	60 mg
0.03 g	=	30 mg
0.015 g	=	15 mg
0.001 g	=	1 mg

Metric volume

1 liter (l or L)	=	1,000 milliliters (ml)*
1 milliliter	=	1,000 microliters (mcl)

Household		Metric
1 teaspoon (tsp)	=	5 ml
1 tablespoon (T or tbs)	=	15 ml
2 tablespoons	=	30 ml
8 ounces	=	240 ml
1 pint (pt)	=	473 ml
1 quart (qt)	=	946 ml
1 gallon (gal)	=	3,785 ml

Weight conversions

1 oz = 30 g	1 lb = 453.6 g	2.2 lb = 1 kg

Temperature conversions

Centigrade degrees	Fahrenheit degrees	Centigrade degrees	Fahrenheit degrees	Centigrade degrees	Fahrenheit degrees
41.1	106.0	38.1	100.6	35.1	95.2
41.0	105.8	38.0	100.4	35.0	95.0
40.9	105.6	37.9	100.2	34.9	94.8
40.8	105.4	37.8	100.0	34.8	94.6
40.7	105.2	37.7	99.8	34.7	94.4
40.6	105.0	37.6	99.6	34.6	94.2
40.4	104.8	37.4	99.4	34.4	94.0
40.3	104.6	37.3	99.2	34.3	93.8
40.2	104.4	37.2	99.0	34.2	93.6
40.1	104.2	37.1	98.8	34.1	93.4
40.0	104.0	37.0	98.6	34.0	93.2
39.9	103.8	36.9	98.4	33.9	93.0
39.8	103.6	36.8	98.2	33.8	92.8
39.7	103.4	36.7	98.0	33.7	92.6
39.6	103.2	36.5	97.8	33.6	92.4
39.4	103.0	36.4	97.6	33.4	92.2
39.3	102.8	36.3	97.4	33.3	92.0
39.2	102.6	36.2	97.2	33.2	91.8
39.1	102.4	36.1	97.0	33.1	91.6
39.0	102.2	36.0	96.8	33.0	91.4
38.9	102.0	35.9	96.6	32.9	91.2
38.8	101.8	35.8	96.4	32.8	91.0
38.7	101.6	35.7	96.2	32.7	90.8
38.6	101.4	35.6	96.0	32.6	90.6
38.4	101.2	35.4	95.8	32.4	90.4
38.3	101.0	35.3	95.6	32.3	90.2
38.2	100.8	35.2	95.4	32.2	90.0

*1 ml = 1 cubic centimeter (cc); however, ml is the preferred measurement term.

Adverse reactions misinterpreted as age-related changes

In elderly patients, adverse drug reactions can easily be misinterpreted as the typical signs and symptoms of aging. The table below, which shows possible adverse reactions for common drug classifications, can help you avoid such misinterpretations.

Drug Classifications	Agitation	Anxiety	Arrhythmias	Ataxia	Changes in appetite	Confusion	Constipation	Depression
ACE inhibitors						●	●	●
Alpha₁ adrenergic blockers		●					●	●
Antianginals	●	●	●			●		
Antiarrhythmics			●					
Anticholinergics	●	●	●			●	●	●
Anticonvulsants	●		●	●	●	●	●	●
Antidepressants, tricyclic	●	●	●	●	●	●	●	
Antidiabetics, oral						●		
Antihistamines						●	●	●
Antilipemics							●	
Antiparkinsonians	●	●	●	●	●	●	●	●
Antipsychotics	●	●	●	●	●	●	●	●
Barbiturates	●	●	●			●		
Benzodiazepines	●			●	●	●	●	●
Beta blockers		●	●					●
Calcium channel blockers		●	●			●	●	
Corticosteroids	●					●	●	●
Diuretics			●			●		
NSAIDs		●				●	●	●
Opioids	●	●				●	●	●
Skeletal muscle relaxants	●	●		●		●		●
Thyroid hormones		●	●		●			

Drugs that shouldn't be crushed or chewed

Drug	Difficulty breathing	Disorientation	Dizziness	Drowsiness	Edema	Fatigue	Hypotension	Insomnia	Memory loss	Muscle weakness	Restlessness	Sexual dysfunction	Tremors	Urinary dysfunction	Visual changes
			●		●	●	●	●				●			●
			●	●	●	●	●	●				●	●	●	●
			●		●	●	●	●			●	●	●		●
	●		●		●	●									
		●	●	●					●	●	●		●		●
	●	●	●	●	●	●							●		●
	●	●	●	●	●	●					●				●
			●		●	●				●					
		●	●			●							●	●	●
			●			●		●			●	●		●	●
		●	●	●		●	●				●		●		●
			●	●		●	●				●	●	●		●
	●	●	●	●		●					●				
	●	●	●	●	●	●		●		●			●		●
	●		●			●		●				●	●		●
	●		●		●		●	●				●			●
				●	●		●	●				●			●
			●		●	●					●		●		
			●	●	●	●		●			●				●
	●	●	●	●		●	●		●		●		●	●	●
			●	●		●	●	●					●		
								●					●		

Drugs that shouldn't be crushed or chewed

Slow-release, enteric-coated, encapsulated-bead, wax-matrix, sublingual, and buccal drug forms are made to release their active ingredients over a certain period of time or at preset points after administration. Crushing these drug forms can dramatically affect their absorption rate and increase the risk of adverse reactions.

Other reasons not to crush some drug forms include taste, tissue irritation, and unusual formulation—for example, a capsule within a capsule, a liquid within a capsule, or a multiple-compressed tablet. Some drugs shouldn't be crushed because they're teratogenic. Avoid crushing the following brand-name drugs, for the reasons noted beside them.

Accutane (irritant)

Aciphex (delayed release)

Actifed 12-Hour (sustained release)

Adalat CC (sustained release)

Advicor (extended release)

Aggrenox (extended release)

Allegra D (extended release)

Allerest 12 Hour (sustained release)

Altocor (extended release)

Ambien CR (extended release)

Amnesteem (irritant)

Ansaid (taste)

Aricept ODT (orally disintegrating)

Arthrotec (delayed release)

Asacol (delayed release)

Aspirin (enteric coated)

Atrohist LA (long acting)

Augmentin XR (extended release)

Avinza (extended release)

Avodart (irritant)

Azulfidine EN-tabs (enteric coated)

Biaxin XL (extended release)

Biohist LA (long acting)

Bisacodyl (enteric coated)

Bontril Slow-Release (slow release)

Bromfed (slow release)

Bromfed-PD (slow release)

Bronkodyl SR (slow release)

Calan SR (sustained release)

Carbatrol (extended release)

Cardizem CD, LA (slow release)

Cartia XT (extended release)

Ceclor CD (slow release)

Ceftin (strong, persistent taste)

Cellcept (teratogenic)

Chloral Hydrate (liquid within a capsule, taste)

Chlor-Trimeton Allergy 8-hour and 12-hour (slow release)

Choledyl SA (slow release)

Cipro XR (extended release)

Citalopram HBr (orally disintegrating)

Claritin-D 12-hour (slow release)

Claritin-D 24-hour (slow release)

Cleocin (taste)

Colace (liquid within a capsule)

Colazal (granules within capsules must reach colon intact)

Colestid (protective coating)

Compazine Spansules (slow release)

Concerta (extended release)

Contac 12 Hour, Maximum Strength 12 Hour (slow release)

Cotazym-S (enteric coated)

Covera-HS (extended release)

Creon (enteric coated)

Cytovene (irritant)

Cytoxan (toxic)

Dallergy, Dallergy-Jr (slow release)

Deconamine SR (slow release)

Depakene (slow release, mucous membrane irritant)

Depakote (enteric coated)

Depakote ER (extended release)

Dexedrine Spansule (slow release)

Diamox Sequels (slow release)

Dilacor XR (extended release)

Dilatrate-SR (slow release)

Dilt XR (extended release)

Diltia XT (extended release)

Dimetane Extentabs (extended release)

Dimetapp Extentabs (slow release)

Ditropan XL (slow release)

Dolobid (irritant)

Donnatel Extentabs (extended release)

Doxidan Liquigels (liquid within capsule)

Drisdol (liquid filled)

Dristan (protective coating)

Drixoral (slow release)

Dulcolax (enteric coated)

Dynabac (slow release)

DynaCirc CR (slow release)

Easprin (enteric coated)

Ecotrin (enteric coated)

Ecotrin Maximum Strength (enteric coated)

E.E.S. 400 Filmtab (enteric coated)

Effexor XR (extended release)

Emend (hard gelatin capsule)

E-Mycin (enteric coated)

Entex LA (slow release)

Entex PSE (slow release)

Equanil (extended release)

Ergostat (sublingual)

Eryc (enteric coated)

Ery-Tab (enteric coated)

Erythrocin Stearate (enteric coated)

Erythromycin Base (enteric coated)

Eskalith CR (slow release)

Extendryl JR, SR (slow release)

Feldene (mucous membrane irritant)

Feosol (enteric coated)

Feratab (enteric coated)

Fergon (slow release)

Fero-Folic 500 (slow release)

Fero-Grad-500 (slow release)

Ferro-Sequel (slow release)

Feverall Children's Capsules, Sprinkle (taste)

Flomax (slow release)

Focalin XR (extended release)

Fumatinic (slow release)

Geocillin (taste)

Glucophage XR (extended release)

Glucotrol XL (slow release)

Glumetza (extended release)

Guaifed (slow release)

Guaifed-PD (slow release)

Guaifenex LA (slow release)

Guaifenex PPA (slow release)

Guaifenex PSE (slow release)

Guaimax-D (slow release)

Hydergine LC (sublingual)

Hytakerol (liquid filled)

Iberet (slow release)

ICAPS Plus (slow release)

ICAPS Time Release (slow release)

Ilotycin (enteric coated)

Imdur (slow release)

Inderal LA (slow release)

Indocin SR (slow release)

InnoPran XL (extended release)

Invegra (extended release)

Ionamin (slow release)

Isoptin SR (sustained release)

Isordil Sublingual (sublingual)

Isordil Tembids (slow release)

Isosorbide Dinitrate Sublingual (sublingual)

Kadian (extended release)

Kaletra (extended release)

Kaon-Cl (slow release)

K-Dur (slow release)

Klor-Con (slow release)

Klotrix (slow release)

K-Tab (slow release)

Letairis (protective coating)

Levbid (slow release)

Levsinex Timecaps (slow release)

Lithobid (slow release)

Macrobid (slow release)

Mestinon Timespans (slow release)

Metadate CD, ER (extended release)

Methylin ER (extended release)

Micro-K Extencaps (slow release)

Modane (enteric coated)

Motrin (taste)

MS Contin (slow release)

Mucinex (extended release)

Naprelan (slow release)

Nexium (sustained release)

Niaspan (extended release)

Nicotinic acid (slow release)

Nifedical XL (extended release)

Nitroglyn (slow release)

Nitrostat (sublingual)

Noctec (liquid within capsule)

Norflex (slow release)

Norpace CR (slow release)

Oramorph SR (slow release)

Orapred ODT (orally disintegrating)

Oruvail (extended release)

OxyContin (slow release)

Pancrease (enteric coated)

Pancrease MT (enteric coated)

Paxil CR (controlled release)

PCE (slow release)

Pentasa (controlled release)

Phazyme (slow release)

Phazyme 95 (slow release)

Phenytek (extended release)

Plendil (slow release)

Prelu-2 (slow release)

Prevacid, Prevacid SoluTab (delayed release)

Prilosec (slow release)

Prilosec OTC (delayed release)

Pro-Banthine (taste)

Procanbid (slow release)

Procardia XL (slow release)

Propecia (adverse effects when handled by pregnant women)

Proscar (adverse effects when handled by pregnant women)

Protonix (delayed release)

Proventil Repetabs (slow release)

Prozac Weekly (slow release)

Quibron-T/SR (slow release)

Quinaglute Duratabs (extended release)

Quinidex Extentabs (slow release)

Respaire SR (slow release)

Respbid (extended release)

Risperdal (orally disintegrating)

Risperdal M-Tab (delayed-release)

Ritalin-LA, -SR (slow release)

Rondec-TR (slow release)

Roxanol SR (sustained release)

Sinemet CR (slow release)

Slo-bid Gyrocaps (slow release)

Slo-Niacin (slow release)

Slo-Phyllin GG, Gyrocaps (slow release)

Slow FE (slow release)

Slow-K (slow release)

Slow-Mag (slow release)

Sorbitrate (sublingual)

Sotret (irritant)

Sudafed 12 Hour (slow release)

Sular (extended release)

Surfac Liquigels (liquid within capsule)

Taztia XT (extended release)

Tegretol-XR (extended release)

Ten-K (slow release)

Tenuate Dospan (slow release)

Tessalon Perles (slow release)

Theo-24 (slow release)

Theochron (slow release)

Theoclear LA (slow release)

TheoDur (extended release)

Thorazine Spansules (slow release)

Tiazac (sustained release)

Topamax (taste)

Toprol XL (extended release)

Trental (slow release)

Tylenol Extended Relief (slow release)

Uniphyl (slow release)

Uroxatral (extended release)

Vantin (taste)

Verelan, Verelan PM (slow release)

Volmax (slow release)

Voltaren (enteric coated)

Voltaren-XR (extended release)

Wellbutrin SR (sustained release)

Xanax XR (extended release)

Zerit XR (extended release)

Zomig-ZMT (delayed release)

ZORprin (slow release)

Zyban (slow release)

Zyrtec-D 12 hour (extended release)

Normal laboratory test values

Normal values may differ from laboratory to laboratory. Standard international units are abbreviated SI.

Hematology

Bleeding time
Template: 3–6 min (SI, 3–6 m)
Ivy: 3–6 min (SI, 3–6 m)
Duke: 1–3 min (SI, 1–3 m)

Fibrinogen, plasma
200–400 mg/dl (SI, 2–4 g/L)

Hematocrit
Men: 42%–52% (SI, 0.42–0.52)
Women: 36%–48% (SI, 0.36–0.48)

Hemoglobin, total
Men: 14–17.4 g/dl (SI, 140–174 g/L)
Women: 12–16 g/dl (SI, 120–160 g/L)

Partial thromboplastin time, activated
21–35 sec (SI, 21–35 sec)

Platelet aggregation
3–5 min (SI, 3–5 min)

Platelet count
140,000–400,000/mm^3 (SI, 140–400 $\times$ 10^9/L)

Prothrombin time
10–14 sec (SI, 10–14 sec); INR for patients not receiving warfarin, 1.12–1.46; INR for patients receiving warfarin, 2–3 (SI, 2–3) (those with prosthetic heart valve, 2.5–3.5 [SI, 2.5–3.5])

Red blood cell count
Men: 4.5–5.5 million/mm^3 (SI, 4.5–5.5 $\times$ 10^{12}/L) venous blood
Women: 4–5 million/mm^3 (SI, 4–5 $\times$ 10^{12}/L) venous blood

Red blood cell indices
Mean corpuscular volume: 82–98 femtoliters
Mean corpuscular hemoglobin: 26–34 picograms/cell
Mean corpuscular hemoglobin concentration: 31–37 g/dl

Reticulocyte count
0.5%–1.5% (SI, 0.005–0.025) of total RBC count

White blood cell count
4,500–10,500 cells/mm^3

White blood cell differential, blood
Neutrophils: 54%–75% (SI, 0.54–0.75)
Lymphocytes: 25%–40% (SI, 0.25–0.4)
Monocytes: 2%–8% (SI, 0.02–0.08)
Eosinophils: up to 4% (SI, up to 0.04)
Basophils: up to 1% (SI, up to 0.01)

Blood chemistry

Alanine aminotransferase
Adults: 10–35 units/L (SI, 0.17–0.6 µkat/L)
Newborns: 13–45 units/L (SI, 0.22–0.77 µkat/L)

Amylase, serum
Adults $\geq$ age 18: 30–175 units/L (SI, 0.5–2.83 µkat/L)

Arterial blood gases
pH: 7.35–7.45 (SI, 7.35–7.45)
Paco$_2$: 35–45 mm Hg (SI, 4.7–5.3 kPa)
Pao$_2$: 80–100 mm Hg (SI, 10.6–13.3 kPa)
HCO$_3^-$: 22–26 mEq/L (SI, 22–25 mmol/L)
Sao$_2$: 94%–100% (SI, 0.94–1.00)

Aspartate aminotransferase
Men: 14–20 units/L (SI, 0.23–0.33 µkat/L)
Women: 7–34 units/L (SI, 0.12–0.58 µkat/L)

Bilirubin, serum
Adults, total: 0.2–1 mg/dl (SI, 3.5–17 µmol/L)
Neonates, total: 1–10 mg/dl (SI, 17–170 µmol/L)
Neonates, unconjugated indirect: 0–10 mg/dl (SI, 0–170 µmol/L)

Blood urea nitrogen
8–20 mg/dl (SI, 2.9–7.5 mmol/L)

Calcium, serum
Adults: 8.2–10.2 mg/dl (SI, 2.05–2.54 mmol/L)
Children: 8.6–11.2 mg/dl (SI, 2.15–2.79 mmol/L)

Carbon dioxide, total blood
22–26 mEq/L (SI, 22–26 mmol/L)

Cholesterol, total serum
Men: < 205 mg/dl (SI, < 5.30 mmol/L) (desirable)
Women: < 190 mg/dl (SI, < 4.90 mmol/L) (desirable)

Creatine kinase, isoenzymes
CK–BB: none
CK–MB: 0–7%
CK–MM: 96–100%

Creatinine, serum
Adults: 0.6–1.3 mg/dl (SI, 53–115 µmol/L)

Glucose, plasma, fasting
70–110 mg/dl (SI, 3.9–6.1 mmol/L)

Glucose, plasma, 2-hour postprandial
< 145 mg/dl (SI, < 8 mmol/L)

Lactate dehydrogenase
Total: 71–207 units/L in adults (SI, 1.2–3.52 µkat/L)
LD1: 14%–26% (SI, 0.14–0.26)
LD2: 29%–39% (SI, 0.29–0.39)
LD3: 20%–26% (SI, 0.20–0.26)
LD4: 8%–16% (SI, 0.08–0.16)
LD5: 6%–16% (SI, 0.06–0.16)

Lipase
< 160 units/L (SI, < 2.72 µkat/L)

Magnesium, serum
1.8–2.6 mg/dl (SI, 0.74–1.07 mmol/L)

Phosphates, serum
2.7–4.5 mg/dl (SI, 0.87–1.45 mmol/L)

Potassium, serum
3.8–5 mEq/L (SI, 3.5–5 mmol/L)

Protein, serum
Total: 6.3–8.3 g/dl (SI, 64–83 g/L)
Albumin fraction: 3.5–5 g/dl (SI, 35–50 g/L)

Sodium, serum
135–145 mEq/L (SI, 135–145 mmol/L)

Triglycerides, serum
Men > age 20: 40–180 mg/dl (SI, 0.11–2.01 mmol/L)
Women > age 20: 10–190 mg/dl (SI, 0.11–2.21 mmol/L)

Uric acid, serum
Men: 3.4–7 mg/dl (SI, 202–416 µmol/L)
Women: 2.3–6 mg/dl (SI, 143–357 µmol/L)

English-to-Spanish drug phrase translator

Medication history

Do you take any medications?
– Prescription?
– Over-the-counter?
– Other?

¿Toma usted medicamentos?
– ¿Bajo receta?
– ¿De venta libre?
– ¿Otro?

Which prescription medications do you take routinely?

¿Qué medicamentos bajo receta toma como rutina?

Which over-the-counter medications do you take routinely?
– How often do you take them?
– Once daily?
– Twice daily?
– Three times daily?
– Four times daily?
– More often?

¿Qué medicamentos de venta libre toma como rutina?
– ¿Con qué frecuencia los toma?
– ¿Una vez al día?
– ¿Dos veces al día?
– ¿Tres veces al día?
– ¿Cuátro veces al día?
– ¿Con más frecuencia?

Why do you take these medications?

¿Por qué toma estos medicamentos?

What is the dosage for each medication?

¿Cuál es la dosis para cada medicamento?

Are you allergic to any medications?

¿Es usted alérgico(a) a algún medicamento?

Medication teaching

Purpose of the medication
This medication will:
– elevate your blood pressure.
– improve circulation to your _____.
– lower your blood pressure.
– lower your blood sugar.
– make your heart rhythm more even.
– raise your blood sugar.
– reduce or prevent the formation of blood clots.
– remove fluid from your body.
– remove fluid from your feet, ankles, or legs.

– remove fluid from your lungs so that they work better.
– remove fluid from your pancreas so that it works better.
– kill the bacteria in your _____.
– slow down your heart rate.
– soften your bowel movements.
– speed up your heart rate.
– help your body to use insulin more efficiently.

Este medicamento:
– elevará su presión sanguínea.
– mejorará la circulación a su _____.
– reducirá su presión sanguínea.
– reducirá el nivel de azúcar en su sangre.
– hará que su ritmo cardiaco sea más uniforme.
– elevará el nivel de azúcar en su sangre.
– reducirá o evitará la formación de coágulos.
– eliminará el liquido de su cuerpo.
– eliminará el liquido de sus pies, tobillos o piernas.
– eliminará el liquido de sus pulmones para que funcionen mejor.
– eliminará el liquido de su páncreas para que funcione mejor.
– matará las bacterias en su _____.
– hará más lento su ritmo cardiaco.
– ablandará sus evacuaciones intestinales.
– acelerará su ritmo cardiaco.
– ayudará a su cuerpo a usar la insulina de manera más eficaz.

This medication will help you to:
- breathe better.
- fight infections.
- relax.
- sleep.
- think more clearly.

This medication will relieve or reduce:
- the acid production in your stomach.
- anxiety.
- bladder spasms.
- burning in your stomach or chest.
- burning when you urinate.
- diarrhea.
- muscle cramps.
- nausea.
- pain in your _____.

Medication administration

I would like to give you:
- an injection.
- an I.V. medication.
- a liquid medication.
- a medicated cream or powder.
- a medication through your epidural catheter.

- a medication through your rectum.
- a medication through your _____ tube.
- a medication under your tongue.
- some pill(s).
- a suppository.

This is how you take this medication.

If you can't swallow this pill, I can get it in another form.

If you can't swallow a pill, you can crush it and mix it in soft food.

I need to mix this medication in juice or water.

I need to give you this injection in your:
- abdomen.
- buttocks.
- hip.
- outer arm.
- thigh.

Este medicamento le ayudará a:
- respirar mejor.
- combatir infecciones.
- relajarse.
- dormir.
- pensar con mayor claridad.

Este medicamento le aliviará o reducirá:
- la producción de ácido en su estómago.
- la ansiedad.
- los espasmos en la vejiga.
- el ardor en su estómago o pecho.
- el ardor al orinar.
- la diarrea.
- los calambres musculares.
- las nauseas.
- el dolor en su _____.

Quisiera darle:
- una inyección.
- un medicamento por vía intravenosa.
- un medicamento en forma líquida.
- un medicamento en pomada o polvo.
- un medicamento a través de su catéter epidural.
- un medicamento por vía rectal.
- un medicamento a través de su tubo de _____.
- un medicamento debajo de la lengua.
- algunas píldoras.
- un supositorio.

Así se toma este medicamento.

Si usted no logra tragar esta píldora, puede obtenerla en otra forma.

Si usted no logra tragar una píldora, puede molerla y mezclarla con alimentos blandos.

Necesito mezclar este medicamento en jugo o agua.

Necesito ponerle esta inyección en:
- el abdomen.
- las nalgas.
- la cadera.
- la parte externa el brazo.
- el muslo.

Some medications are coated with a special substance to protect your stomach from getting upset.

Do not chew:
– enteric-coated pills.
– long-acting pills.
– capsules.
– sublingual medication.

Ask your doctor or pharmacist whether you can:
– mix your medication with food or fluids.

– take your medication with or without food.

You need to take your medication:
– after meals.
– before meals.
– on an empty stomach.
– with meals or food.

Skipping doses
If you skip or miss a dose:
– Take it as soon as you remember it.
– Wait until the next dose.
– Call the doctor if you are not sure.
– Do not take an extra dose.

Adverse effects
Some common adverse effects of _____ are:

– constipation
– diarrhea
– difficulty sleeping
– dry mouth
– fatigue
– headache
– itching
– light-headedness
– nausea
– poor appetite
– rash
– upset stomach
– weight loss or gain
– frequent urination.

These adverse effects:
– will go away after your body gets used to the medication.
– may persist as long as you take the medication.

Algunos medicamentos están revestidos con una sustancia especial para protegerlo(a) contra malestar estomacal.

No masque:
– píldoras con recubrimiento entérico.
– píldoras de efecto prolongado.
– cápsulas.
– medicamentos sublinguales.

Pregunte a su médico o farmacéutico si usted puede:
– mezclar su medicamento con alimentos o líquidos.
– tomar su medicamento con o sin alimentos.

Usted debe tomar su medicamento:
– después de las comidas.
– antes de las comidas.
– con el estómago vacío.
– con comidas o alimentos.

Si usted se salta u omite una dosis:
– Tómela apenas se acuerde.
– Espere hasta la próxima dosis.
– Llame a su médico si no está seguro(a).
– No tome una dosis adicional.

Algunos afectos adversos comunes de _____ son:

– constipación
– diarrea
– dificultad para dormir
– boca seca
– fatiga
– dolor de cabeza
– picazón (comezón)
– mareos
– náuseas
– disminución del apetito
– erupción
– malestar estomacal
– aumento o pérdida de peso
– orinar con frecuencia.

Estos efectos adversos:
– desaparecerán cuanao su cuerpo se acostumbre al medicamento.
– podrán persistir mientras usted tome el medicamento.

If you have an adverse reaction to your medication, call your doctor right away.

Si usted tiene una reacción adversa a su medicamento, llame a su médico de inmediato.

Other concerns

Tell your doctor if you are pregnant or breast-feeding.

Dígale a su médico si usted está embarazada o amamantando.

While you are taking this medication, ask your doctor if:
– you can safely take other over-the-counter medications.
– you can drink alcoholic beverages.
– your medications interact with each other.

Mientras tome este medicamento, pregúntele a su médico si:
– usted puede tomar otros medicamentos de venta libre sin peligro.
– usted puede tomar bebidas alcohólicas.
– sus medicamentos tienen interacción entre si.

Storing medication

You should keep your medication:
– in a cool, dry place.
– in the refrigerator.
– at room temperature.
– out of direct sunlight.
– away from heat.
– away from children.

Usted debe guardar sus medicamentos:
– en un lugar fresco y seco.
– en el refrigerador.
– al temperatura ambiente.
– fuera de la luz directa del sol.
– lejos del calor.
– lejos del alcance de los niños.

Subcutaneous injection

To give yourself an injection, follow these steps:
– Draw up the medication.
– Replace the cap carefully.
– Decide where you are going to give the injection.
– Clean the skin area with alcohol.
– Gently pinch up a little skin over the area.

– Using a dartlike motion, stab the needle into your skin.
– Gently pull back on the plunger to see if there is any blood in the syringe.
– Steadily push the medication into your skin.

– Pull the needle out.
– Apply gentle pressure with the alcohol wipe.

– Dispose of the needle in a proper receptacle.

Para ponerse una inyección, haga lo siguiente:

– Extraiga el medicamento.
– Vuelva a colocar la tapa con cuidado.
– Decida dónde colocará la inyección.

– Limpie el área de la piel con alcohol.
– Suavemente, pellizque un poco de la piel sobre el área.
– Con un movimiento como si estuviera arrojando un dardo, penetre la piel con la aguja.
– Tire suavemente del émbolo para ver si hay sangre en la jeringa.
– Coloque el medicamento en la piel de manera uniforme.
– Retire la aguja.
– Aplique presión suave con un paño con alcohol.
– Deseche la aguja en un recipiente apropiado.

Insulin preparation and administration

The doctor has ordered insulin for you.

El médico le ha recetado insulina.

To draw up insulin, follow these steps:

Para extraer la insulina, siga los siguientes pasos:

– Wipe the rubber top of the insulin bottle with alcohol.

– Limpie la tapa de goma del frasco de insulina con alcohol.

– Remove the needle cap.
– Pull out the plunger until the end of the plunger in the barrel aligns with the number of units of insulin that you need.
– Push the needle through the rubber top of the insulin bottle.
– Inject the air into the bottle.
– Without removing the needle from the bottle, turn it upside down.
– Withdraw the plunger until the end of the plunger aligns with the number of units you need.
– Gently pull the needle out of the bottle.

To mix insulin, follow these steps:

– Wipe the rubber tops of the insulin bottles with alcohol.
– Gently roll the cloudy insulin between your palms.
– Remove the needle cap.
– Pull out the plunger until the end of the plunger in the barrel aligns with the number of units of NPH or Lente insulin that you need.
– Push the needle through the rubber top of the cloudy insulin bottle.
– Inject the air into the bottle.
– Remove the needle.
– Pull out the plunger until the end of the plunger in the barrel aligns with the number of units of clear regular insulin that you need.
– Push the needle through the rubber top of the clear insulin bottle.
– Inject the air into the bottle.
– Without removing the needle, turn the bottle upside down.
– Withdraw the plunger until it aligns with the number of units of clear regular insulin that you need.
– Gently pull the needle out of the bottle.
– Push the needle into the cloudy (NPH or Lente) insulin without injecting it into the bottle.
– Withdraw the plunger until you reach your total dosage of insulin in units (regular combined with NPH or Lente).
– We will practice again.

– Retire la tapa de la aguja.
– Tire del émbolo hasta que la extremidad del émbolo en la barril esté al nivel de la cantidad de unidades de insulina que usted necesita.
– Empuje la aguja a través de la tapa de goma del frasco de insulina.
– Inyecte el aire dentro del frasco.
– Sin retirar la aguja del frasco, gírelo boca abajo.
– Retire el émbolo hasta que la extremidad del émbolo esté al nivel de la cantidad de unidades que necesita.
– Suavemente, retire la aguja del frasco.

Para mezclar la insulina siga los siguientes pasos:

– Limpie las tapas de goma de los frascos de insulina con alcohol.
– Suavemente, gire el frasco de insulina turbia entre las palmas de la mano.
– Retire la tapa de la aguja.
– Tire del émbolo hasta que la extremidad del émbolo en el barril esté alineado con la cantidad de unidades de NPH o Lente que usted necesita.
– Empuje la aguja a través de la tapa de goma del frasco de insulina clara.
– Inyecte el aire en el frasco.
– Sin retirar la aguja, gire el frasco boca abajo.
– Tire del émbolo hasta que este al nivel de la cantidad de unidades de insulina común clara que usted necesita.
– Empuje la aguja a través de la tapa de goma del frasco de insulina clara.
– Inyecte el aire en el frasco.
– Sin retirar la aguja, gire el frasco boca abajo.

– Tire del émbolo hasta que al nive de la cantidad de unidades de insulina común clara que usted necesita.
– Suavemente, retire la aguja del frasco.
– Empuje la aguja hacia dentro de la insulina turbia (NPH o Lente) sin inyectarla en el frasco.

– Tire del émbolo hasta llegar ala dosis total de insulina en unidades (común combinada con NPH o Lente).
– Practicaremos nuevamente.

Home care phrases

Wash your hands before touching medications.	Lávese las manos antes de tocar medicamentos.
Check the medication bottle for name, dose, and frequency (how often it's supposed to be taken).	Verifique el nombre, dosis y frecuencia (cada cuanto lo debe tomar) en al frasco del medicamento.
Check the expiration date on all medications.	Verifique la fecha de vencimiento de todos los medicamentos.
Store medications according to pharmacy instructions.	Almacene los medicamentos de acuerdo con las instrucciones de la farmacia.
Under adequate lighting, read medication labels carefully before taking doses.	Con luz adecuada, lea las etiquetas de los medicamentos con mucho cuidado antes de tomar las dosis.
Don't crush medication without first asking the doctor or pharmacist.	No machaque el medicamento sin preguntar al médico o al farmacéutico.
Contact your doctor if a new or unexpected symptom or another problem appears.	Contacte a su médico si aparece u síntoma nuevo o imprevisto u otro problema.
Don't stop taking medication unless instructed by your doctor.	No deje de tomar el medicamento sin indicación médica.
Discard outdated medications.	Deseche los medicamentos vencidos.
Never take someone else's medications.	Nunca tome los medicamentos de otra persona.
Keep a record of your current medications.	Mantenga un registro de sus medicamentos actuales.

General drug therapy phrases

Drug classes

Analgesic	Analgésico
Anesthetic	Anestético
Antacid	Antiácido
Antianginal agent	Agente antianginal
Antianxiety agent	Agente ansiolítico
Antiarrhythmic agent	Agente antiarrítmico
Antibiotic	Antibiótico
Anticancer agent	Agente anticarcinógeno
Anticoagulant	Anticoagulante
Anticonvulsant	Anticonvulsivante
Antidepressant	Antidepresivo
Antidiarrheal	Antidiarreico
Antifungal agent	Agente antifúngico
Antigout agent	Agente antigota

Antihistamine	Antihistamínico
Antihyperlipemic agent	Agente hiperlipémico
Antihypertensive agent	Agente antihipertenso
Anti-inflammatory agent	Agente antiinflamatorio
Antimalarial agent	Agente antimalárico
Antiparkinsonian agent	Agente antiparkinsoniano
Antipsychotic agent	Agente antipsicótico
Antipyretic	Antipirético
Antiseptic	Antiséptico
Antispasmodic	Antiespasmódico
Antithyroid agent	Agente antitiroideo
Antituberculosis agent	Agente antituberculoso
Antitussive agent	Agente antitusígeno
Antiviral agent	Agente antiviral
Appetite stimulant	Estimulante para el apetito
Appetite suppressant	Supresor de apetito
Bronchodilator	Broncodilatador
Decongestant	Descongestivo
Digestant	Digestivo (agente que estimula la digestión)
Diuretic	Diurético
Emetic	Emético
Fertility agent	Agente para la fertilidad
Hypnotic	Hipnótico
Insulin	Insulina
Laxative	Laxante
Muscle relaxant	Relajante de músculos
Oral contraceptive	Anticonceptivo oral
Oral hypoglycemic agent	Agente hipoglucémico oral
Sedative	Sedante
Steroid	Esteroide
Thyroid hormone	Hormona de la glándula tiroides
Vaccine	Vacuna
Vasodilator	Vasodilatador
Vitamin	Vitamina

Preparations

Capsule	Cápsula
Cream	Pomada
Drops	Gotas
Elixir	Elixir
Inhaler	Inhalador

Injection	Inyección
Lotion	Loción
Lozenge	Pastilla
Powder	Polvo
Spray	Atomizador
Suppository	Supositorio
Suspension	Suspensión
Syrup	Jarabe
Tablet	Tableta

Frequency

Once daily	Una vez al día
Twice daily	Dos veces al día
Three times daily	Tres veces al día
Four times daily	Cuatro veces al día
In the morning	Por la mañana
With meals	Con las comidas
Before meals	Antes de las comidas
After meals	Después de las comidas
Before bedtime	Antes de acostarse
When you have_____	Cuando Ud. tome_____
Only when you need it	Sólo cuando lo necesite
Every four hours	Cada cuatro horas
Every six hours	Cada seis horas
Every eight hours	Cada ocho horas

Acknowledgments

We would like to thank the following companies for granting us permission to include their drugs in the full-color photoguide.

Abbott Laboratories
Depakote®
Hytrin®
Kaletra®

AstraZeneca LP
Arimidex®
Crestor®
Prilosec®
Tenormin®
Toprol-XL®

Aventis Pharmaceuticals
DiaBeta®
Lasix®

Bayer Pharmaceuticals Corporation
Cipro®
Levitra®
Nexavar®

Biovail Pharmaceuticals, Inc.
Cardizem®
Cardizem CD®
Cardizem LA®
Vasotec®

Bristol-Myers Squibb Company
Capoten®
Coumadin®
Monopril®
Pravachol®

CV Therapeutics
Ranexa®

Elan Pharmaceuticals, Inc.
Frova®

Forest Pharmaceuticals, Inc.
Campral®
Celexa®
Lexapro®

GlaxoSmithKline
Reproduced with permission of GlaxoSmithKline
Avandia®

Janssen Pharmaceutica, Inc.
Risperdal®
Risperdal® M-Tab™

King Pharmaceuticals, Inc.
Levoxyl®

Eli Lilly and Company
Copyright Eli Lilly and Company. Used with permission 2007.
Cymbalta®
Prozac®
Strattera®

Mallinckrodt, Inc.
Pamelor®

Merck & Co., Inc.
Used with permission of Merck & Co., Inc.
Cozaar®
Fosamax®
Januvia®
Mevacor®
Pepcid®
Prinivil®
Singulair®
Zocor®

Merck Santé
An associate of Merck KGaA, Darmstadt, Germany
Glucophage®
Glucophage XR®

Merck/Schering-Plough
Used with permission of Merck/Schering-Plough.
Zetia™

Novartis Pharmaceuticals, Inc.
Enablex®
Ritalin®

Ortho-McNeil Pharmaceutical
Levaquin®

Otsuka Pharmaceutical Company, Ltd.
Abilify®

Pfizer, Inc.
Used with permission from Pfizer Inc.
Accupril®
Celebrex®
Chantix®
Diflucan®
Dilantin® Kapseals®
Glucotrol®
Glucotrol XL®
Lipitor®
Neurontin®
Norvasc®
Procardia XL®
Sutent®
Viagra®
Zithromax®
Zoloft®

Pharmacia Corporation
Registered trademarks of
Pharmacia Corporation, a
Pfizer Inc. Corporation. All
rights reserved. Courtesy of
Pfizer Inc.
Calan®
Micronase®
Provera®
Xanax®

Proctor & Gamble Pharmaceuticals, Inc.
Actonel®

Purdue Pharma L.P.
OxyContin®

Roche Laboratories, Inc.
Valium®

Sanofi-Synthelabo, Inc.
Ambien®

Schering Corporation and Key Pharmaceuticals, Inc.
Clarinex ®
K-Dur®

Sepracor, Inc.
Lunesta®

Sucampo Pharmaceuticals, Inc.
Amitiza®

Tap Pharmaceuticals, Inc.
Prevacid®

Teva Neuroscience, Inc.
Azilect®

Warner Chilcott Laboratories, Inc.
Eryc®
Estrace®

Wyeth Pharmaceuticals
The capsules presented here
are trademarks of Wyeth
Pharmaceuticals, Philadelphia, Pa.
Effexor XR®

Index

Anxiety *(continued)*
  paroxetine for, 965–966
  prochlorperazine for, 1044
  sertraline for, 1129
  trifluoperazine for, 1266
  venlafaxine for, 1293
Anzemet, 434
Apacet, 100
APAP, **100–102**
Apidra, 687
Aplastic anemia, 1345
  lymphocyte immune glob-
    ulin for, 780
Apo-Alpraz ♦, 130
Apo-Amoxi, 148
Apo-Ampi ♦, 157
Apo-Atenol ♦, 180
Apo-Cephalex ♦, 291
Apo-Doxy ♦, 452
Apo-Erythro, 499
Apo-Erythro-ES ♦, 499
Apo-Erythro-S ♦, 499
Apo-Hydro ♦, 640
Apo-ISDN ♦, 707
Apo-Keto ♦, 717
Apo-Keto-E ♦, 717
Apo-Keto SR ♦, 717
Apokyn, 164
Apo-Metoclop ♦, 833
apomorphine hydrochloride,
    56, **164–166**
Apo-Napro-Na ♦, 885
Apo-Napro-Na DS ♦, 885
Apo-Nifed ♦, 904
Apo-Pen-VK ♦, 982
Apo-Sulfatrim ♦, 348
Apo-Sulfatrim DS ♦, 348
Apo-Sulin ♦, 1176
Apo-Tamox ♦, 1189
Apo-Tetra ♦, 1212
Apothecary measurement
    system, 4
Apo-Triazo ♦, 1265
Apo-Trihex ♦, 1268
Apo-Verap ♦, 1294
Appendicitis
  meropenem for, 810
  piperacillin and tazobac-
    tam for, 1010
aprepitant, **166–168**
Apresoline, 638
Apri, 528
Aptivus, 1238
Aquachloral Supprettes, 295
Aquasol A, 1302
Aquasol E Drops, 1307
Aquavit-E, 1307

Aquazide-H, 640
ara-C, **361–363**
Aralen Phosphate, 299
Aranesp, 373
Arava, 735
Aredia, 960
argatroban, 45, **168–170**
Aricept, 436
Aricept ODT, 436
Arimidex, 162, *C2*
aripiprazole, **170–173**, *C3*
Aristospan Intra-Articular,
    1260
Aristospan Intralesional,
    1260
Arixtra, 591
Arm and Hammer Pure
    Baking Soda, 1143
armodafinil, **173–174**
Aromasin, 543
Arrhythmias
  acebutolol for, 99
  adenosine for, 113
  amiodarone for, 140–141
  atenolol for, 180
  digoxin for, 412
  diltiazem for, 417
  disopyramide for, 423
  dofetilide for, 432
  edetate disodium for, 465
  esmolol for, 504
  flecainide for, 562
  heparin for, 633
  ibutilide for, 657
  isoproterenol for, 706
  lidocaine for, 757
  metoprolol for, 837
  mexiletine for, 842
  nadolol for, 877
  neostigmine for, 897
  phenylephrine for, 999
  phenytoin for, 1001
  procainamide for,
    1039–1040
  propafenone for, 1048
  propranolol for, 1051
  quinidine for, 1067
  sotalol for, 1158
  vasopressin for, 1289
  verapamil for, 1294
  warfarin for, 1311
Arterial blood gases, 1393t
Arterial occlusion
  alteplase for, 133–134
  streptokinase for, 1164
Arthralgia, 1345

Arthritis
  abatacept for, 92
  adalimumab for, 110
  anakinra for, 160
  aspirin for, 175
  azathioprine for, 192
  cefotaxime for, 274
  celecoxib for, 289
  chlorambucil for, 296
  chloroquine for, 300
  cyclophosphamide for,
    355
  cyclosporine for, 359
  diclofenac for, 405
  diflunisal for, 411
  epoetin alfa for anemia
    due to, 490
  etanercept for, 523
  etodolac for, 539
  high–molecular-weight
    hyaluronan for, 637
  hydroxychloroquine for,
    648
  ibuprofen for, 655
  indomethacin for, 674
  infliximab for, 677
  ketoprofen for, 717
  leflunomide for, 735
  meloxicam for, 800
  methotrexate for, 823
  nabumetone for, 876
  naproxen for, 885
  oxaprozin for, 940
  sulfasalazine for, 1173
  sulindac for, 1176
Artria S.R., 174
ASA, 174
Asacol, 811
ASA Enseals, 174
Asaphen ♦, 174
Ascites, mannitol for, 786
ascorbic acid, **1304–1306**
Ascor L500, 1304
Asmanex Twisthaler, 861
Asmol CFC-free, 115
Aspartate aminotransferase,
    1393t
Aspergillosis
  amphotericin B desoxy-
    cholate for, 150
  amphotericin B lipid com-
    plex for, 152
  amphotericin B liposomal
    for, 154
  caspofungin for, 263

Bacteremia *(continued)*
 ceftizoxime for, 283
 ceftriaxone for, 285
 daptomycin for, 372
 linezolid for, 759
 quinupristin and dalfo-
  pristin for, 1070
Bacterial infection
 amikacin for, 139
 amoxicillin and clavu-
  lanate potassium for,
  146
 amoxicillin for, 148–149
 ampicillin for, 157
 ampicillin sodium and sulbactam sodium for, 159
 azithromycin for, 194–195
 aztreonam for, 197
 cefadroxil for, 265
 cefazolin for, 267
 cefdinir for, 268
 cefditoren for, 270
 cefixime for, 272
 cefotaxime for, 273
 cefoxitin for, 275
 cefpodoxime for, 277
 cefprozil for, 278
 ceftazidime for, 280
 ceftibuten for, 282
 ceftizoxime for, 283
 ceftriaxone for, 285
 cefuroxime for, 287
 cephalexin for, 291
 ciprofloxacin for, 316
 clindamycin for, 325
 co-trimoxazole for,
  348–349
 daptomycin for, 372
 doripenem for, 439
 doxycycline for, 453
 ertapenem for, 496–497
 erythromycin for, 499–500
 gemifloxacin for, 615
 gentamicin for, 618–619
 imipenem and cilastatin
  sodium for, 665
 levofloxacin for, 751–753
 linezolid for, 759
 meropenem for, 810
 metronidazole for,
  839–840
 minocycline for, 850
 moxifloxacin for, 867–868
 nafcillin for, 879
 neomycin for, 895
 nitrofurantoin for, 906–907
 norfloxacin for, 917

Bacterial infection
 (continued)
 ofloxacin for, 924–925
 penicillin G benzathine for,
  974
 penicillin G potassium for,
  976
 penicillin G procaine for,
  978
 penicillin G sodium for,
  980
 penicillin V potassium for,
  982
 piperacillin and tazobactam for, 1010
 quinupristin and dalfo-
  pristin for, 1070
 retapamulin for, 1087
 streptomycin for, 1166
 telithromycin for, 1193
 tetracycline for, 1212
 ticarcillin and clavulanate
  potassium for, 1227
 ticarcillin for, 1225
 tigecycline for, 1230
 tobramycin for, 1240
 trimethoprim for,
  1270–1271
 vancomycin for,
  1284–1285
Bacterial vaginosis
 clindamycin for, 325
 metronidazole for, 840
 tinidazole for, 1232
Bactrim, 348
Bactrim DS, 348
Bactrim I.V., 348
balsalazide disodium,
  200–201
Balziva, 528
Banophen, 419
Banophen Caplets, 419
Baraclude, 480
Barbiturates, 57–59
 adverse reactions mis-
  interpreted as age-
  related changes,
  1388t–1389t
 drug interactions with,
  1368t–1369t
Baridium, 994
Bartter syndrome, in-
  domethacin for, 675
Basal cell carcinoma, fluorouracil for, 572
basiliximab, **202–203**
Basophils, 1393t

Bayer Aspirin, 174
BayHep B, 636
BayRho-D Full Dose, 1089
BayTet, 1211
BCNU, **259–261**
beclomethasone dipropi-
  onate, **203–205**
beclomethasone dipropi-
  onate monohydrate,
  205–206
Beconase AQ, 205
Bedoz ♦, 351
Behavior disorders, haloperi-
  dol for, 631
Behçet disease, colchicine
  for, 344
Bejel, penicillin G benzathine
  for, 974
Beldin, 419
Bell/ans, 1143
Benadryl, 419
Benadryl 25, 419
Benadryl Kapseals, 419
benazepril hydrochloride, 38,
  52, **206–208**
Benicar, 929
Benicar HCT, 1354
Benign prostatic hyperplasia
 alfuzosin for, 122
 doxazosin for, 443
 dutasteride for, 461
 finasteride for, 561
 prazosin for, 1029
 tamsulosin for, 1190
 terazosin for, 1202
Bentyl, 408
Bentylol ♦, 408
Benylin Cough, 419
Benzodiazepine reversal,
  flumazenil for, 570
Benzodiazepines, 59–60
 adverse reactions mis-
  interpreted as age-
  related changes,
  1388t–1389t
benztropine mesylate, 44,
  56, **208–209**
benzylpenicillin benzathine,
  974–976
benzylpenicillin potassium,
  976–978
benzylpenicillin sodium,
  980–981
Beriberi, thiamine for, 1217

Beta blockers, 40, 52, 60–61
  adverse reactions mis-
    interpreted as age-
    related changes,
    1388t–1389t
Betaloc♦, 837
Betaloc Durules♦, 837
betamethasone, 64
  drug interactions with,
    1366t–1367t
betamethasone sodium
    phosphate, 64
Betapace, 1158
Betapace AF, 1158
Betaseron, 695
betaxolol, 60
bevacizumab, **209–211**
Biaxin, 323
Biaxin XL, 323
Bicillin L-A, 974
BiCNU, 259
BiDil, 1354
Big Shot B-12, 351
bilberry, 1332
  drug interactions with,
    1377t
Biliary cirrhosis, colchicine
    for, 344
Biliary obstruction,
    cholestyramine for, 306
Biliary tract infection, cefa-
    zolin for, 267
Bilirubin, serum, 1393t
bimatoprost, **211–212**
Bipolar disorder
  aripiprazole for, 170–171
  carbamazepine for, 254
  fluoxetine for, 574
  lamotrigine for, 729
  lithium for, 765
  olanzapine for, 926–927
  quetiapine for, 1063–1064
  risperidone for, 1101
  ziprasidone for, 1320
Bisac-Evac, 213
bisacodyl, 74, **213–214**
Bisacodyl Uniserts, 213
Bisacolax♦, 213
Bisa-lax, 213
bismuth subgallate, 50,
    214–215
bismuth subsalicylate, 50,
    214–215
bisoprolol fumarate, 40, 52,
    60, **215–217**
bivalirudin, 45, **217–219**

Bladder atony, neostigmine
    for, 897
Bladder cancer
  cisplatin for, 319
  doxorubicin for, 448
  mitomycin for, 855
  thiotepa for, 1220
  vincristine for, 1298
Bladder overactivity
  darifenacin for, 376
  oxybutynin for, 945
  solifenacin for, 1153
  tolterodine for, 1243
  trospium for, 1273
Blastomycosis
  amphotericin B lipid com-
    plex for, 152
  itraconazole for, 711
Bleeding. See also Gastro-
    intestinal bleeding;
    Postpartum bleeding;
    Uterine bleeding;
    Variceal bleeding
  epinephrine for, 483
Bleeding time, 1393t
Blenoxane, 219
bleomycin sulfate, 43,
    219–220
Blood chemistry values, nor-
    mal, 1393t–1394t
Blood urea nitrogen, 1393t
Body surface area, to com-
    pute pediatric drug
    dose, 13
Bonamine♦, 794
Bone marrow transplant re-
    cipients
  amphotericin B desoxy-
    cholate for, 150
  filgrastim for, 559
  fluconazole for, 564
  immune globulin for, 669
  sargramostim for, 1121
Bone metastases, zoledronic
    acid for, 1322
Bone or joint infection
  aztreonam for, 197
  cefazolin for, 267
  cefotaxime for, 273
  cefoxitin for, 275
  ceftazidime for, 280
  ceftizoxime for, 283
  ceftriaxone for, 285
  cefuroxime for, 287
  cephalexin for, 291
  ciprofloxacin for, 316

Bone or joint infection
    (continued)
  imipenem and cilastatin
    sodium for, 665
  nafcillin for, 879
  ticarcillin and clavulanate
    potassium for, 1227
Bonine, 794
Boniva, 653
bortezomib, **221–222**
bosentan, **222–224**
Bowel evacuation after bari-
    um examination, lactu-
    lose for, 724
Bowel preparation
  bisacodyl for, 213
  magnesium citrate for,
    784
  polyethylene glycol and
    electrolyte solution for,
    1012
  sodium phosphate for,
    1148
  sodium phosphate mono-
    hydrate for, 1150
Bradycardia
  atropine for, 188
  isoproterenol for, 706
Brain tumor
  carmustine for, 259
  cisplatin for, 319
  lomustine for, 767
  procarbazine for, 1042
  vincristine for, 1298
Breast cancer
  anastrozole for, 162
  capecitabine for, 251
  carmustine for, 259
  cyclophosphamide for,
    355
  docetaxel for, 429
  doxorubicin for, 448
  epirubicin for, 486
  estradiol for, 509
  estrogens, conjugated,
    for, 515
  estrogens, esterified, for,
    517
  exemestane for, 543
  fluorouracil for, 572
  fulvestrant for, 605
  goserelin for, 627
  ifosfamide for, 660
  lapatinib for, 733
  megestrol for, 798
  paclitaxel for, 952

---

t refers to a table; **boldface** refers to the drug's monograph; **boldface italic** refers to a full-color photograph.

Breast cancer *(continued)*
  paclitaxel protein-bound
    particles for, 954
  pamidronate for, 960
  raloxifene to reduce risk
    of, 1074
  tamoxifen for, 1189
  testolactone for, 1206
  testosterone for, 1207
  thiotepa for, 1220
  trastuzumab for, 1253
  vinblastine for, 1296
  vincristine for, 1298
  vinorelbine for, 1300
Breast pain and engorge-
  ment, postpartum,
  testosterone for, 1208
Brethine, 1203
bretylium tosylate, 42
Brevibloc, 504
Brevicon, 528
Bricanyl, 1203
bromfenac ophthalmic solution, **224–225**
bromocriptine mesylate, 56,
  225–227
brompheniramine maleate,
  51
Bronchitis
  acetylcysteine for, 104
  cefdinir for, 268
  cefditoren for, 270
  cefixime for, 272
  cefpodoxime for, 277
  cefprozil for, 278
  ceftibuten for, 282
  cefuroxime for, 287
  clarithromycin for, 323
  co-trimoxazole for, 349
  fluticasone and salmeterol
    inhalation powder for,
    584
  formoterol fumarate in-
    halation powder for,
    593
  gemifloxacin for, 615
  levofloxacin for, 751
  moxifloxacin for, 867
  salmeterol for, 1117
  tiotropium for, 1236
Bronchoconstriction, for-
    moterol fumarate in-
    halation powder for,
    593
Bronchodilation, ephedrine
  for, 482

Bronchogenic cancer. *See
  also* Lung cancer
  mechlorethamine for, 792
Bronchospasm. *See also*
  Asthma
  albuterol for, 115
  epinephrine for, 483
  formoterol fumarate in-
    halation powder for,
    593
  ipratropium for, 698
  isoproterenol for, 706
  levalbuterol for, 740
  metaproterenol for, 814
  montelukast for, 863
  salmeterol for, 1117
  terbutaline for, 1203
  theophylline for, 1214
  tiotropium for, 1236
Brucellosis
  ofloxacin for, 924
  tetracycline for, 1212
Buccal drug administration,
  25
budesonide, **227–229**
budesonide (oral), **229–230**
Bulimia
  amitriptyline for, 143
  fluoxetine for, 574
bumetanide, 66, **231–232**
Bumex, 231
Buprenex, 232
buprenorphine hydrochlo-
  ride, **232–234**
buprenorphine hydrochloride
  and naloxone hydro-
  chloride dihydrate,
  232–234
bupropion hydrochloride,
  234–236
Burkitt lymphoma,
  methotrexate for, 823
Burn patients, vitamin C for,
  1304
Bursitis
  indomethacin for, 675
  naproxen for, 885
  sulindac for, 1176
Buscopan ◆, 1123
BuSpar, 236
buspirone hydrochloride,
  236–238
busulfan, 35, **238–240**
Busulfex, 238
butabarbital, drug interactions with, 1368t–1369t

butorphanol tartrate,
  240–241
Byclomine, 408
Bydramine Cough, 419
Byetta, 544

C
Cachexia
  megestrol for, 798–799
  somatropin for, 1155
Ca-DTPA, **987–989**
Caduet, 1355
Calan, 1294, *C16*
Calan SR, 1294
Cal-carb forte, 245
Cal-C-Caps, 245
Cal-CEE, 245
Calci-Chew, 245
Calciferol, 1306
Calcijex, 243
Calcimar, 241
Calcionate, 245
Calciquid, 245
calcitonin (salmon), **241–243**
calcitriol, **243–245**
Calcium, serum, 1394t
calcium acetate, **245–248**
calcium carbonate, 39,
  245–248
Calcium channel blockers,
  40, 53, 61–62
  adverse reactions mis-
    interpreted as age-
    related changes,
    1388t–1389t
calcium chloride, **245–248**
calcium citrate, **245–248**
Calcium Disodium Versen-
  ate, 463
calcium EDTA, **463–465**
calcium glubionate, **245–248**
calcium gluconate, **245–248**
calcium lactate, **245–248**
Calcium oxalate calculi, allopurinol for, 125
calcium phosphate, dibasic,
  245–248
calcium phosphate, tribasic,
  245–248
calcium polycarbophil, 50, 74
calfactant, **248–249**
Cal-Lac, 245
Calphron, 245
Camila, 915
Campath, 118
Campral, 96, *C2*

---

t refers to a table; **boldface** refers to the drug's monograph; *boldface italic* refers to a full-color photograph.

Edema *(continued)*
  hydrochlorothiazide for, 640
  indapamide for, 671
  mannitol for, 786
  metolazone for, 835
  spironolactone for, 1160
  triamterene for, 1263
edetate calcium disodium, **463–465**
edetate disodium, **465–466**
edrophonium, drug interactions with, 1370t–1371t
E.E.S., 499
E.E.S. Granules, 499
efalizumab, **466–468**
efavirenz, **468–470**
Effexor, 1292
Effexor XR, 1292, **C15**
Effusions, neoplastic
  bleomycin for, 219
  doxycycline for, 453
  thiotepa for, 1220
Efudex, 572
E-200 I.U. Softgels, 1307
E-400 I.U. Softgels, 1307
Eldepryl, 1126
Electroencephalography, chloral hydrate for, 295
Electrolyte replacement, sodium chloride for, 1145
eletriptan hydrobromide, **470–471**
Elidel, 1006
Eligard, 738
Elixophyllin, 1214
Ellence, 486
Eltor 120 ◆, 1056
Eltroxin ◆, 754
Embeline E, 327
Embolism. *See also* Pulmonary embolism
  alteplase for, 133
  dipyridamole for prevention of, 422
  heparin for prevention of, 633
  streptokinase for, 1164
Emend, 166
Emotional emergencies, hydroxyzine for, 651
Emphysema
  acetylcysteine for, 104
  formoterol fumarate inhalation powder for, 593

Emphysema *(continued)*
  salmeterol for, 1117
  tiotropium for, 1236
Empirin, 174
Empirin with Codeine No. 3, 1357
Empirin with Codeine No. 4, 1357
Emsam, 1126
emtricitabine, 76, **471–473**
Emtriva, 471
Enablex, 376, **C4**
enalaprilat, 38, 52, **473–475**
enalapril maleate, 38, 52, **473–475, C6**
Enbrel, 523
Encephalitis
  acyclovir for, 108
  levodopa and carbidopa for parkinsonism after, 747
  levodopa for parkinsonism after, 745
Encephalopathy
  bromocriptine for, 226
  lactulose for, 723
  thiamine for, 1217
Endocarditis
  amphotericin B desoxycholate for, 150
  cefazolin for, 267
  daptomycin for, 372
  flucytosine for, 566
  imipenem and cilastatin sodium for, 665
  nafcillin for, 879
  penicillin G sodium for, 980
  streptomycin for, 1166
Endocarditis prophylaxis
  amoxicillin for, 148
  ampicillin for, 157
  azithromycin for, 195
  clindamycin for, 325
  erythromycin for, 499
  gentamicin for, 619
  vancomycin for, 1285
Endocervical infection. *See also* Cervicitis
  ciprofloxacin for, 317
  doxycycline for, 453
  erythromycin for, 499
  levofloxacin for, 752
  minocycline for, 850
  tetracycline for, 1212
Endocet 5/325, 1357
Endocet 7.5/325, 1357

Endocet 7.5/500, 1357
Endocet 10/325, 1357
Endometrial ablation, goserelin for endometrial thinning before, 627
Endometrial cancer
  medroxyprogesterone for, 795
  megestrol for, 798
Endometrial hyperplasia, medroxyprogesterone for, 795
Endometriosis
  goserelin for, 627
  leuprolide for, 738
  norethindrone for, 916
Endometritis, piperacillin and tazobactam for, 1010
Endomyometritis, ertapenem for, 497
Endoscopic procedures
  diazepam for, 403
  midazolam for, 845
Endotracheal intubation
  atracurium for, 186
  dexmedetomidine for, 394
  midazolam for, 845
  pancuronium for, 962
  succinylcholine for, 1169
  vecuronium for, 1291
Endrate, 465
enfuvirtide, **475–476**
English-to-Spanish drug phrase translator, 1395–1402
Enjuvia, 515
enoxaparin sodium, 45, **476–478**
Enpresse, 528
entacapone, 56, **478–480**
entecavir, **480–481**
Enterococcus faecium infection, vancomycinresistant
  linezolid for, 759
  quinupristin and dalfopristin for, 1070
Enterocolitis, vancomycin for, 1285
Entocort EC, 229
Entrophen ◆, 174
Enulose, 723
Enuresis
  desmopressin for, 390
  imipramine for, 667
Eosinophilia, 1345

---

t refers to a table; **boldface** refers to the drug's monograph; ***boldface italic*** refers to a full-color photograph.

---

t refers to a table; **boldface** refers to the drug's monograph; ***boldface italic*** refers to a full-color photograph.

Gonococcal infection
(continued)
aztreonam for, 197
cefixime for, 272
cefotaxime for, 273–274
cefpodoxime for, 277
ceftriaxone for, 285
cefuroxime for, 287
ciprofloxacin for, 317
co-trimoxazole for, 349
doxycycline for, 453
erythromycin for, 499
levofloxacin for, 752
minocycline for, 850
norfloxacin for, 917
ofloxacin for, 924
probenecid for, 1038
tetracycline for, 1212
Gonococcal ophthalmia,
cefotaxime for, 274
goserelin acetate, **627–628**
Gout
allopurinol for, 125
colchicine for, 343
indomethacin for, 675
naproxen for, 885
probenecid for, 1038
sulfinpyrazone for, 1174
sulindac for, 1176
granisetron hydrochloride,
628–630
granulocyte colony-stimulating factor, **559–561**
granulocyte macrophage
colony-stimulating fac-
tor, **1121–1123**
Granuloma inguinale, erythromycin for, 500
grapeseed, 1338
drug interactions with,
1380t
Gray baby syndrome, 1345
green tea, drug interactions
with, 1380t
Growth failure
mecasermin for, 791
somatropin for, 1154,
1155
Growth hormone deficiency
mecasermin for, 791
somatropin for, 1154
Growth hormone release,
vasopressin provoca-
tive testing for, 1289
guaifenesin, **630–631**
guanfacine hydrochloride, 53
Guiatuss, 630

Gynecologic infection
ampicillin sodium and sulbactam sodium for, 159
aztreonam for, 197
cefotaxime for, 273
ceftazidime for, 280
ceftizoxime for, 283
ceftriaxone for, 285
ertapenem for, 497
imipenem and cilastatin
sodium for, 665
ticarcillin and clavulanate
potassium for, 1227
Gynodiol, 509
Gyromitra mushroom poi-
soning, pyridoxine for,
1060

H
Haemophilus ducreyi infec-
tion
azithromycin for, 195
co-trimoxazole for, 349
erythromycin for, 500
Haemophilus influenzae type
B infection, rifampin for
prevention of, 1094
Hair loss, finasteride for, 561
Hairy cell leukemia
fludarabine for, 567
interferon alfa-2b, recombinant, for, 692
Halcion, 1265
Haldol, 631
Haldol Decanoate, 631
Haldol LA ♦, 631
Half-life of drug, 1345
Halfprin, 174
Halofed, 1056
Halofed Adult Strength, 1056
haloperidol, **631–633**
haloperidol decanoate,
631–633
haloperidol lactate, **631–633**
Hartnup disease, niacin for,
902
hawthorn berry, drug interac-
tions with, 1380t–1381t
HBIG, 636
Headache. *See also* Cluster
headache; Migraine;
Vascular headache
paroxetine for, 966
Head and neck cancer
cetuximab or, 293
cisplatin for, 319

Head and neck cancer
(continued)
cyclophosphamide for,
355
docetaxel for, 429
hydroxyurea for, 650
isotretinoin for, 709
methotrexate for, 823
Health maintenance, folic
acid for, 590
Heart block, isoproterenol
for, 706
Heartburn
cimetidine for, 313
famotidine for, 548
magnesium hydroxide for,
784
nizatidine for, 913
omeprazole for, 934
pantoprazole for, 963
rabeprazole for, 1071
ranitidine for, 1080
Heart failure
acetazolamide for, 102
atorvastatin to reduce risk
for, 184
bisoprolol for, 216
bumetanide for, 231
candesartan for, 249
captopril for, 252
carvedilol for, 261
digoxin for, 412
dobutamine for, 427
enalapril for, 473
eplerenone for, 488
fosinopril for, 600
furosemide for, 606
heparin for, 633
hydralazine for, 639
isosorbide dinitrate for,
708
lisinopril for, 763
mannitol for, 786
metolazone for, 835
metoprolol for, 837
milrinone for, 848
nesiritide for, 899
nitroglycerin for, 908
nitroprusside for, 911
quinapril for, 1066
ramipril for, 1078
spironolactone for, 1160
torsemide for, 1248
trandolapril for, 1252
valsartan for, 1283

---

t refers to a table; **boldface** refers to the drug's monograph; ***boldface italic*** refers to a full-color photograph.

Insomnia *(continued)*
  temazepam for, 1196
  trazodone for, 1257
  triazolam for, 1265
  zaleplon for, 1314
  zolpidem for, 1326
Inspra, 488
Insta-Char Pediatric, 106
insulin aspart (rDNA origin)
  injection, **681–683**
insulin aspart (rDNA origin)
  protamine suspension
  and insulin aspart
  (rDNA origin) injection,
  681–683
insulin detemir, **683–685**
insulin glargine (rDNA),
  685–687
insulin glulisine (rDNA origin), **687–689**
Insulin growth factor-1 deficiency, mecasermin for,
  791
insulin (lispro), **689–692**
insulin lispro protamine and
  insulin lispro, **689–692**
insulin (regular), **689–692**
Insulin therapy replacement
  glipizide for, 622
  glyburide for, 625
Integrilin, 493
interferon alfa-2b, recombinant, **692–695**
interferon beta-1b, recombinant, **695–696**
interferon gamma-1b,
  697–698
Intermittent claudication
  cilostazol for, 311
  pentoxifylline for, 990
International units, 4
Intra-abdominal abscess,
  caspofungin for, 264
Intra-abdominal infection
  ampicillin sodium and sulbactam sodium for, 159
  anidulafungin for, 163
  aztreonam for, 197
  cefotaxime for, 273
  cefoxitin for, 275
  ceftazidime for, 280
  ceftizoxime for, 283
  ceftriaxone for, 285
  ciprofloxacin for, 316
  doripenem for, 439
  ertapenem for, 496

Intra-abdominal infection
  (continued)
  imipenem and cilastatin
  sodium for, 665
  moxifloxacin for, 868
  ticarcillin and clavulanate
  potassium for, 1227
  tigecycline for, 1230
Intracranial pressure elevation, mannitol for, 787
Intramuscular drug administration, 17–19
Intraocular pressure elevation
  acetazolamide for, 102
  bimatoprost for, 211
  dorzolamide for, 440
  mannitol for, 787
  travoprost for, 1255
Intravenous drug administration
  bolus, 15–16
  drip rates and flow rates
  for, 10
  through a secondary line,
  16–17
Intron-A, 692
Invanz, 496
Invega, 956
Invirase, 1119
Ionamin, 997
Ionsys, 553
Iosat, 1021
ipratropium bromide,
  698–699
irbesartan, 52, **699–701**
Ircon, 556
Iron deficiency
  ferrous fumarate for, 556
  iron dextran for, 701
  iron sucrose for, 702–703
  sodium ferric gluconate
  complex for, 1147
iron dextran, **701–702**
Iron overdose, polyethylene
  glycol and electrolyte
  solution for, 1012
iron sucrose, **702–704**
Irospan, 556
Irritability
  oxazepam for, 942
  risperidone for, 1102
Irritable bowel syndrome
  alosetron for, 128
  atropine for, 188
  dicyclomine for, 408
  octreotide for, 923

Isentress, 1075
ISMO, 707
isocarboxazid, drug interactions with, 1368t–1369t
Isochron, 707
isoniazid, **704–706**
Isoniazid poisoning, pyridoxine for, 1060
isonicotinic acid hydride,
  704–706
isophane insulin suspension,
  689–692
isophane insulin suspension
  and insulin injection
  combinations, **689–692**
isoproterenol hydrochloride,
  706–707
Isoptin SR, 1294
Isordil Titradose, 707
isosorbide dinitrate, 40,
  707–709
  drug interactions with,
  1370t–1371t
isosorbide mononitrate, 40,
  707–709
  drug interactions with,
  1370t–1371t
Isosporosis, pyrimethamine
  for, 1062
Isotamine ♦, 704
isotretinoin, **709–711**
Isuprel, 706
itraconazole, **711–714**
Iveegam EN, 669

J

Jantoven, 1311
Januvia, 1142, *C14*
Joint infection. *See* Bone or
  joint infection
Joint replacement surgery
  dalteparin for, 368
  enoxaparin for, 476
  fondaparinux for, 591
Jolivette, 915
Junel 1.5/30, 528
Junel 1/20, 528
Junel Fe 1/5/30, 528
Junel Fe 1/20, 528
Juvenile arthritis
  celecoxib for, 289
  etanercept for, 523
  meloxicam for, 800
  naproxen for, 885
  sulfasalazine for, 1173

---

t refers to a table; **boldface** refers to the drug's monograph; ***boldface italic*** refers to a full-color photograph.

K

K+ 8, 1017
K+ 10, 1017
Kadian, 865
Kaletra, 769, *C9*
kanamycin, drug interactions
 with, 1366t–1367t
Kaochlor, 1017
Kaodene Non-Narcotic, 714
kaolin and pectin mixtures,
 50, **714–715**
Kaolin w/Pectin, 714
Kaon, 1019
Kaon-Cl, 1017
Kaon-Cl-10, 1017
Kaon-Cl 20%, 1017
Kaopectate II Caplets, 768
Kaopectate (Regular), 214
Kao-Spen, 714
Kapectolin, 714
Kaposi sarcoma
 bleomycin for, 219
 daunorubicin citrate lipo-
  somal for, 381
 doxorubicin hydrochloride
  liposomal for, 450
 etoposide for, 541
 interferon alfa-2b, recom-
  binant, for, 692
 paclitaxel for, 952
 vinblastine for, 1296
 vincristine for, 1298
Kariva, 528
kava, 1339
 drug interactions with,
  1381t
Kawasaki syndrome
 aspirin for, 175
 immune globulin for, 670
Kay Ciel, 1017
Kayexalate, 1151
Kaylixir, 1019
K+ Care, 1017
K+ Care ET, 1016
K-Dur 10, 1017
K-Dur 20, 1017, *C12*
Keflex, 291
Kemstro, 198
Kenalog-10, 1260
Kenalog-40, 1260
Keppra, 742
Keratinization disorders,
 isotretinoin for, 709
Ketek, 1193
ketoconazole, **715–717**
ketoprofen, 75, **717–719**

ketorolac tromethamine, 75,
 719–721
ketotifen fumarate, **721–722**
K-G Elixir, 1019
Kidney dysfunction, mannitol
 test dose for, 786
Kidney transplant recipients
 azathioprine for, 191
 basiliximab for, 202
 cyclosporine for, 359
 cytomegalovirus immune
  globulin, intravenous,
  for, 363
 daclizumab for, 366
 lymphocyte immune glob-
  ulin for, 780
 muromonab-CD3 for, 871
 mycophenolate mofetil for,
  872
 sirolimus for, 1139
 tacrolimus for, 1183
 valganciclovir for, 1279
Kineret, 160
Kionex, 1151
Klonopin, 334
K-Lor, 1017
Klor-Con, 1017
Klor-Con 8, 1017
Klor-Con EF, 1017
Klor Con/EF, 1016
Klor-Con M10, 1017
Klor-Con M15, 1017
Klor-Con M25, 1017
Klorvess, 1017
Klotrix, 1017
K-Lyte, 1016
K-Lyte/Cl, 1017
Knee replacement surgery
 enoxaparin for, 476
 fondaparinux for, 591
Kraurosis vulvae, estradiol
 for, 509
Kristalose, 723
K-Tab, 1017
K-Vescent, 1017
Kytril, 628

L

LA-12, 351
Labels on drug containers,
 14
labetalol hydrochloride, 52,
 60, **722–723**
Labor, preterm
 magnesium chloride for,
  782
 terbutaline for, 1204

Laboratory test values, normal, 1393t–1394t
Labor induction, oxytocin,
 synthetic injection, for,
 950
Labor pain
 butorphanol for, 240
 meperidine for, 806
 pentazocine for, 986
Lactate dehydrogenase,
 1394t
lactulose, 74, **723–725**
Lamictal, 728
lamivudine, 76, **725–727**
lamivudine and zidovudine,
 727–728
lamotrigine, 46, **728–731**
Lanoxicaps, 412
Lanoxin, 412
lansoprazole, **731–733**, *C8*
Lantus, 685
lapatinib, **733–735**
Largactil ♦, 303
Lariam, 797
Larodopa, 745
Laryngitis, omeprazole for,
 934
Lasix, 606, *C7*
Lasix Special, 606
Laxatives, 74–75. *See also*
 Constipation
LCR, **1298–1300**
L-deprenyl hydrochloride,
 1126–1129
Lead encephalopathy, ede-
 tate calcium disodium
 for, 463
Lead poisoning
 edetate calcium disodium
  for, 463
 succimer for, 1168
leflunomide, **735–737**
Left ventricular dysfunction
 captopril for, 252
 carvedilol for, 261
 enalapril for, 473
 trandolapril for, 1252
 valsartan for, 1283
Left ventricular hypertrophy,
 losartan to reduce
 stroke risk in, 775
Left ventricular thrombi, heparin for, 633
Legionnaires' disease
 azithromycin for, 195
 erythromycin for, 499

---

t refers to a table; **boldface** refers to the drug's monograph; *boldface italic* refers to a full-color photograph.

---

t refers to a table; **boldface** refers to the drug's monograph; ***boldface italic*** refers to a full-color photograph.

Staff

Executive Publisher
Judith A. Schilling McCann, RN, MSN

Editorial Director
H. Nancy Holmes

Clinical Director
Joan M. Robinson, RN, MSN

Art Director
Elaine Kasmer

Clinical Manager
Janet Rader Clark, RN, BSN

Electronic Project Manager
John Macalino

Editorial Project Manager
Sean Webb

Editors
Christiane L. Brownell, ELS; Nancy Priff

Clinical Editors
Shari A. Regina-Cammon, RN, MSN, PCCN, TNCC;
Carol Romano, RN, MSN, CRNP

Copy Editors
Leslie Dworkin, Jenifer F. Walker

Digital Composition Services
Diane Paluba (manager), Joyce Rossi Biletz,
Donald G. Knauss

Associate Manufacturing Manager
Beth J. Welsh

Editorial Assistants
Karen J. Kirk, Jeri O'Shea, Linda K. Ruhf

Indexer
Deborah Tourtlotte

Visit our Web site at eDrugInfo.com

NSDH10010708
ISBN 13: 978-0-78178-883-0
ISBN 10: 0-78178-883-8
ISSN: 1941-739X

Tenth Edition

Nursing2009
STUDENT
DRUG
HANDBOOK™

Wolters Kluwer | Lippincott Williams & Wilkins
Health
Philadelphia · Baltimore · New York · London
Buenos Aires · Hong Kong · Sydney · Tokyo

IV Drug Compatibility Chart

	insulin (regular)	isoproterenol	lactated Ringer's	lidocaine	methylprednisolone sodium succinate	mezlocillin	midazolam	morphine sulfate	nafcillin	norepinephrine	normal saline solution	ondansetron	oxacillin	oxytocin	penicillin G potassium	phenylephrine	phenytoin	phytonadione	piperacillin	potassium chloride	procainamide	ranitidine	sodium bicarbonate	ticarcillin	tobramycin	vancomycin	verapamil
acyclovir		4		4			4	4					4		4				4	4		4	4	4	4		
albumin																											
amikacin		24				24		4		24	24	24	4		8		8		24			24	24			24	24
aminophylline		24	24	24	?			24			24		24						4			24	24				
amiodarone	24	24		24		24		24		24	24					4	24			24	24			4	4	24	
ampicillin	2							4			8							3	4			?	?			?	
calcium gluconate		24	24			24					24								4						1		48
cefazolin	2	24				24		4			24		4									?				?	24
cefoxitin	24	24						4			24		4									24		24	24		24
ceftazidime								4			24		4									?	6				
cimetidine	24	24			24	24		24					48		4		24		24							24	24
ciprofloxacin		48	24			24													24			24	24				24
clindamycin		24		24				4			24		4				24		48	24		?	24		48		24
dexamethasone sodium phosphate								4					4						4			24	4				
dextrose 5% in water (D5W)		24		24	?	24				24	24		48		6	6			24	24	24	48	24	24	24	24	
D5W in lactated Ringer's		24		24	?								24		24				24			24					24
D5W in normal saline solution		24		24	?						24		48		?				24	24		24		48			24
diazepam																						?					24
diphenhydramine					4		¼				4		4						4			1					
dobutamine		24	24	24				4		4	24		24						24	?		24	48				24
dopamine		48	24	18				4		4			48		24				24			48					24
epinephrine		24						4		4	24		24					3	4			24					24
erythromycin lactobionate		18									22											24	24		24	24	24
esmolol		24						24	8	24	24				24		24		24	24		24		24	24	24	
gentamicin	2	24						24		1			24	4			1					24					24
heparin sodium	2	24		24	?			24		1			4	4	4	?			4	6	24	4	24	6			24
hydrocortisone sodium succinate	4	4	24		?			24		4	4			4		4	24		4			4					24
insulin (regular)			24					24		1						2			4			24	3	2	2	2	48
isoproterenol			24								24								24			24					24
lactated Ringer's		24		24	?	72		24			24		24		24				24	24				24	24		24
lidocaine	24	24					4	48			24								24			24	24	24			48
methylprednisolone sodium succinate		?					24	4			?				24				?			48	2				24
mezlocillin		72									48																24
midazolam	24			24				24			24								24			24			24	24	
morphine sulfate	1			24			4				24		4	4	1				4	4		1	3	4	1	4	24
nafcillin		24	48					4			24											4					24
norepinephrine				24				4			24						4						4				24
normal saline solution		24		24	?	48		24					48	24		24			24	24	48	24	24	48	24		24
ondansetron		24						24			48								4	4		4		4			
oxacillin		24						4														4					24
oxytocin	2							1											4				24				24
penicillin G potassium		24		24				4															24				24
phenylephrine																			24				24				
phenytoin																											48
phytonadione		24																	4				24				
piperacillin		24		24			24	4			24											24					24
potassium chloride	4	24		?			24	4	24		24		4			4			24		4	48	24				24
procainamide		24									24											4	24				48
ranitidine	24	24		24	48			1			4		48			24			4	48	24		24	24	24		
sodium bicarbonate	3		24	2			3	24		24	24		24		24	24	24	24	24								
ticarcillin	2	24																				24					24
tobramycin	2	24					24	1			48											24					24
vancomycin	2	24					24	4			24											24					24
verapamil	48	24	24	48	24			24			24		24		24				24	24	48		24	24	24		